Complications in Small Animal Surgery

Dedication

À Emmanuel, pour ta presence et ta patience

To Maxime and Etienne, my amazing sons:

May this work inspire you to reach your full potential

—Dominique Griffon

To Bernard, for his infinite patience

To Sam and Zoé, who remind me every day the priorities of Life

—Annick Hamaide

Complications in Small Animal Surgery

Edited by

Dominique Griffon DMV, MS, PhD, DECVS, DACVS

Professor and Associate Dean for Research
College of Veterinary Medicine
Western University of Health Sciences
Pomona, CA, USA

Annick Hamaide DVM, PhD, Dipl ECVS

Associate Professor, Surgical Oncology
Department of Clinical Sciences (Companion Animals and Equids)
School of Veterinary Medicine
University of Liège
Liège, Belgium

WILEY Blackwell

This edition first published 2016 © 2016 by John Wiley & Sons, Inc.

Editorial offices: 1606 Golden Aspen Drive, Suites 103 and 104, Ames, Iowa 50010, USA
The Atrium, Southern Gate, Chichester, West Sussex, PO19 8SQ, UK
9600 Garsington Road, Oxford, OX4 2DQ, UK

For details of our global editorial offices, for customer services and for information about how to apply for permission to reuse the copyright material in this book please see our website at www.wiley.com/wiley-blackwell.

Library of Congress Cataloging-in-Publication Data

Complications in small animal surgery (2016)
  Complications in small animal surgery / edited by Dominique Griffon, Annick Hamaide.
     p. ; cm.
  Includes bibliographical references and index.
  ISBN 978-0-470-95962-6 (cloth)
  I. Griffon, Dominique., 1965– editor.   II. Hamaide, Annick., 1965– editor.   III. Title.
  [DNLM: 1. Animal Diseases—surgery.   2. Animals, Domestic—surgery.   3. Intraoperative Complications—veterinary.
4. Postoperative Complications—veterinary.   5. Surgical Procedures, Operative—veterinary.   SF 911]
  SF911
  636.0897—dc23
                                                                2015013294

A catalogue record for this book is available from the British Library.

Wiley also publishes its books in a variety of electronic formats. Some content that appears in print may not be available in electronic books.

Front cover images: Top left image: See figure 78.2's caption. Top middle image: See figure 2.1's caption. Top right image: See figure 113.9's caption. Main, central image: courtesy of Dominique Griffon.

Cover design by Matt Kuhns

Set in 9/11pt Minion Pro by Aptara Inc., New Delhi, India

Printed and bound in Singapore by Markono Print Media Pte Ltd

3 2018

Contents

List of Contributors

Davina Anderson, MA VetMB, PhD, DSAS(ST), DECVS, MRCVS
RCVS Recognized Specialist in Small Animal Surgery (Soft Tissue)
European Specialist in Small Animal Surgery
Anderson Moores Veterinary Specialists
Winchester UK
davina@andersonmoores.com

Maureen Anderson, DVM, DVSc, PhD, DAVCIM
Department of Pathobiology
University of Guelph
Guelph, Ontario, Canada
mander01@uoguelph.ca

Nicholas Bacon, MA, VetMB, CertVR, CertSAS, DECVS, DACVS, MRCVS
ACVS Founding Fellow, Surgical Oncology
Professor, Surgical Oncology
University of Surrey School of Veterinary Medicine
Clinical Director, Fitzpatrick Referrals Oncology and Soft Tissue
Guildford, Surrey, UK
baconn@ufl.edu

Stephen J. Baines, MA, VetMB, PhD, CertVR, CertSAS, DECVS, DipClinOnc, MRCVS
European Specialist in Small Animal Surgery
RCVS Specialist in Small Animal Surgery
RCVS Specialist in Veterinary Oncology
Willows Veterinary Centre and Referral Service
Solihull, West Midlands, UK
stephenbaines@gmail.com

Joseph W. Bartges, DVM, PhD, DACVIM (SA IM), DACVN
Professor of Medicine and Nutrition
The Acree Endowed Chair of Small Animal Research
Interim Department Head
Department of Small Animal Clinical Sciences
Veterinary Teaching Hospital
College of Veterinary Medicine
The University of Tennessee
Knoxville, TN, USA
jbartges@cuvs.org

Brian Beale, DVM, DACVS
Gulf Coast Veterinary Specialists
Houston, TX, USA
dogscopcr@aol.com

Jean-Philippe Billet, Doc Vét, Cert SAS, DECVS, MRCVS
Centre Hospitalier Veterinaire Atlantia
Nantes, France
jpbillet@hotmail.com

Christian Bolliger, Dr. med. vet. DACVS, DECVS
Surgical Referral Practice
Central Victoria Veterinary Hospital
Victoria, Canada
acbolliger@hotmail.com

Peter Böttcher, DECVS
Diplomate ECVS, European Veterinary Specialist in Surgery
Department of Small Animal Medicine
University of Leipzig
Leipzig, Germany
boettcher@kleintierklinik.uni-leipzig.de

Randy J. Boudrieau, DVM, DACVS, DECVS
Professor of Surgery
Cummings School of Veterinary Medicine at Tufts University
North Grafton, MA, USA
randy.boudrieau@tufts.edu

Jonathan Bray, MVSc, CertSAS, MSc(ClinOnc), MACVSc, DECVS
Associate Professor
Companion Animal Clinical Studies;
Head of Companion Animal Group
Institute of Veterinary, Animal and Biomedical Sciences
Massey University
Palmerston North, New Zealand
J.P.Bray@massey.ac.nz

Brigitte A. Brisson, DMV, DVSc, DACVS
Professor of Small Animal Surgery
Department of Clinical Studies
Ontario Veterinary College
University of Guelph
Guelph, Ontario, Canada
bbrisson@uoguelph.ca

Hervé Brissot, DEDV, MRCVS, DECVS
European Recognized Specialist in Small Animal Surgery
Honorary Associate Professor of Small Animal Surgery
University of Nottingham
Pride Veterinary Centre
Derby, UK
hbrissot@free.fr

Daniel J. Brockman, BVSc, DACVS, DECVS, FHEA, MRCVS
Professor of Small Animal Surgery
Head, Department of Clinical Science and Services
Royal Veterinary College
University of London
Hatfield, Hertfordshire, UK
djbrock@rvc.ac.uk

Paolo Buracco, DVM, DECVS
Full Professor of Veterinary Surgery
Department of Veterinary Science
University of Turin
Grugliasco, Turin, Italy
Paolo.buracco@unito.it

Rachel Burrow, BVetMed, MSc (Clin Onc), CertSAS, CertVR, DECVS, MRCVS
RCVS Recognized and European Specialist in Small Animal Surgery
Lecturer in Small Animal Soft Tissue Surgery
Small Animal Teaching Hospital
University of Liverpool
Leahurst, Neston, Wirral, UK
rburrow@liv.ac.uk

Carolyn A. Burton, BVetMed, PhD, MRCVS, CertVA, CertSAS, DECVS
RCVS Specialist in Small Animal Surgery (Soft Tissue)
European Veterinary Specialist in Small Animal Surgery
Davies Veterinary Specialists
Hertfordshire, UK
CBurton@vetspecialists.co.uk

Amanda Callens, BS, LVT
Veterinary Technician, Nephrology and Urology
Department of Small Animal Clinical Sciences
Veterinary Teaching Hospital
College of Veterinary Medicine
The University of Tennessee
Knoxville, TN, USA
acallens@utk.edu

Debra Canapp, DVM, CVA, CCRT, DACVSMR
Medical Director
Veterinary Orthopedic & Sports Medicine Group
Annapolis Junction, MD, USA
SCanapp@vosm.com

Sherman Canapp, Jr., DVM, MS, CCRT, DACVS, DACVSMR
Chief of Staff
Veterinary Orthopedic & Sports Medicine Group;
President & CEO
Orthobiologic Innovations, LLC
Annapolis Junction, MD, USA
DCanapp@vosm.com

Stéphanie Claeys, DVM, PhD, DECVS
Senior Lecturer
Department of Clinical Sciences (Companion Animals and Equids)
Faculty of Veterinary Medicine
University of Liège
Liège, Belgium
Stephanie.claeys@ulg.ac.be

Belinda Comito, DVM, DACVIM (Neurology)
Veterinary Specialty Center
Buffalo Grove, IL, USA
bindy_comito@yahoo.com

Jennifer Covey, DVM, DACVS-SA ACVS Founding Fellow
Surgical Oncology
Pittsburgh Veterinary Specialty and Emergency Center
Pittsburgh, PA, USA
jcovey10@gmail.com

Laura Cuddy, MVB, MS, DACVS-SA, DECVS
Lecturer
Small Animal Surgery
Department of Surgery
Section of Veterinary Clinical Studies
School of Agriculture, Food Science and Veterinary Medicine
University College Dublin
Dublin, Ireland
laura.cuddy@ucd.ie

Hilde de Rooster, DVM, MVM, PhD, DECVS
Department of Small Animal Medicine and Clinical Biology
Faculty of Veterinary Medicine
Ghent University
Ghent, Belgium
Hilde.DeRooster@Ugent.be

Jon Dee, DVM, MS, DACVS, ACVSMR
Hollywood Animal Hospital
Hollywood, FL, USA
jondee@bellsouth.net

Brigitte Degasperi, DVM, DECVS
Department for Companion Animals and Horses
University Clinic for Small Animals
Small Animal Surgery
University of Veterinary Medicine Vienna
Vienna, Austria
Brigitte.Degasperi@vetmeduni.ac.at

Jackie L. Demetriou, BVetMed, Cert SAS, DECVS, MRCVS
European Veterinary Specialist in Small Animal Surgery
Honorary Associate Professor of Small Animal Surgery
Dick White Referrals, Suffolk and University of Nottingham, Nottingham, UK
jd@dwr.co.uk / jd@dickwhitereferrals.com

Marjan Doom, DVM
Department of Morphology
Faculty of Veterinary Medicine
Ghent University
Ghent, Belgium
Marjan.Doom@UGent.be

Gilles Dupré, DECVS, Dipl. Pneumologie interventionnelle et thoracoscopie, Univ. Prof. Dr.med. Vet
Department for Companion Animals and Horses
University Clinic for Small Animals
Small Animal Surgery
University of Veterinary Medicine Vienna
Vienna, Austria
gilles.dupre@vetmeduni.ac.at

Jonathan Dyce, MA, VetMB, MRCVS, DSAO, DACVS
Associate Professor, Small Animal Surgery
Veterinary Medical Center
The Ohio State University
Columbus, Ohio
dyce.1@osu.edu

Maria Fahie, DVM, MS, DACVS
Western University of Health Sciences
College of Veterinary Medicine
Pomona, CA, USA
mfahie@westernu.edu

Lisa M. Fair, VT, CMT, CCRA
Orthopedic & Rehabilitation Technician
VCA Veterinary Referral Associates
Veterinary Orthopedic & Sports Medicine Group
Annapolis Junction, MD, USA
lisa.fair@handicappedpets.com

Valentina Fiorbianco, DVM, Dipl. Interpretation of Therapeutic Studies
Clinica Veterinaria CMV
Varese, Italy
allavale@libero.it

Noel Fitzpatrick, MVB, DUniv CVR, DSAS (Orth), ACVSMR, MRCVS
Director
Fitzpatrick Referrals Orthopedics and Neurology, Godalming, Surrey, UK
noelf@fitzpatrickreferrals.co.uk

Sonja Fonfara, DVM, Dr med vet, PhD, CertVC, DM-CA, PGCertTLHE, MRCVS
RCVS Recognized & European Specialist in Veterinary Cardiology
Senior Lecturer in Small Animal Cardiorespiratory Medicine
School of Veterinary Sciences
University of Bristol
Langford, Bristol, UK
sonjafonfara@googlemail.com

Kris Gommeren, DVM, DECVIM-CA
Emergency and Critical Care Unit
Department of Clinical Sciences (Companion Animals and Equids)
Faculty of Veterinary Medicine
University of Liège
Liège, Belgium
kris.gommeren@ulg.ac.be

Wanda Gordon-Evans, DVM, PhD, DACVS
Wisconsin Veterinary Referral Center
Waukesha, WI, USA
wgordonevans@gmail.com

Dominique Griffon, DMV, MS, PhD, DECVS, DACVS
Professor and Associate Dean for Research
College of Veterinary Medicine
Western University of Health Sciences
Pomona, CA, USA
dgriffon@westernu.edu

Tomas Guerrero, PD, Dr. med. vet., DECVS
Professor of Small Animal Surgery
St. George's University, School of Veterinary Medicine
True Blue, Grenada, West Indies
tguerrero@sgu.edu

Zoë Halfacree, MA, VetMB, CertVDI, CertSAS, FHEA, DECVS, MRCVS
Senior Lecturer in Small Animal Surgery
Department of Clinical Science and Services
The Royal Veterinary College
North Mymms, Hertfordshire, UK
zhalfacree@RVC.AC.UK

Annick Hamaide, DVM, PhD, DECVS
Associate Professor
Department of Clinical Sciences (Companion Animals and Equids)
School of Veterinary Medicine
University of Liège
Liège, Belgium
Annick.Hamaide@ulg.ac.be

Robert J. Hardie DVM, DACVS, DECVS
Clinical Associate Professor Small Animal General Surgery
The University of Wisconsin
School of Veterinary Medicine
Department of Surgical Sciences
Madison, WI, USA
hardier@svm.vetmed.wisc.edu

Galina Hayes, BVSc, PhD, DACVECC, DACVS
Cornell University
Ithaca, NY, USA
galinavet0@gmail.com

Cheryl Hedlund, DVM, MS, DACVS
Professor of Surgery
Department of Veterinary Clinical Sciences
Iowa State University
Ames, IA, USA
chedlund@iastate.edu

John Innes, BVSc, PhD, DSAS, MRCVS
CVS Vets
ChesterGates Veterinary Specialists
Chester, UK
Honorary Professor
University of Liverpool
Liverpool, Merseyside, UK
J.F.Innes@liverpool.ac.uk

Ann Johnson, MS, DVM, DACVS
Professor Emerita
College of Veterinary Medicine
University of Illinois
Champaign, IL, USA
aljohns@illinois.edu

Stanley Kim, BVSc, MS, DACVS
Department of Small Animal Clinical Sciences
University of Florida
Gainesville, FL, USA
stankim@ufl.edu

Barbara Kirby, BS, RN, DVM, MS, DACVS, DECVS
Associate Professor
Veterinary Surgery Discipline Leader
Section of Veterinary Clinical Studies
School of Veterinary Medicine
University College Dublin
Dublin, Ireland
barbara.kirby@ucd.ie

Anne Kummeling, DVM, PhD, DECVS
Assistant Professor in Soft Tissue Surgery
Division of Soft Tissue Surgery
Department of Clinical Sciences of Companion Animals
Faculty of Veterinary Medicine
Utrecht University
Utrecht, The Netherlands
A.Kummeling@uu.nl

Andrew Kyles, BVMS, PhD, DACVS
Blue Pearl Veterinary Partners
New York, NY
aekyles@gmail.com

Jane Ladlow, MA VetMB Cert VR, Cert SAS, DECVS, MRCVS
European and Royal College Specialist in Small Animal Surgery
Senior Lecturer in Small Animal Surgery
University of Cambridge
Cambridge, UK
jfl1001@cam.ac.uk

Outi Laitinen-Vapaavuori, DVM, PhD, DECVS
Professor, Small Animal Surgery
Department of Equine and Small Animal Medicine
Faculty of Veterinary Medicine
University of Helsinki
Helsinki, Finland
outi.vapaavuori@helsinki.fi

India Lane, DVM, MS, EdD (DACVIM-SAIM)
Professor of Medicine
Assistant Vice President for Academic Affairs and Student Success
Office of Academic Affairs and Student Success
The University of Tennessee
Knoxville, TN, USA
ilane@utk.edu

Lyon Lee, DVM, PhD, DACVAA
Professor, Anesthesiology
College of Veterinary Medicine
Western University of Health Sciences
Pomona, CA, USA
llyon@westernu.edu

Henry L'Eplattenier, Dr. med. vet., PhD, DECVS, MRCVS
VRCC Veterinary Referrals
Laindon, Essex, UK
h.leplattenier@googlemail.com

Julius Liptak, BVSc, MVetClinStud, FACVSc, DACVS, DECVS, ACVS Founding Fellow in Surgical Oncology
Staff Surgeon and Surgical Oncologist
Alta Vista Animal Hospital
Ottawa, Ontario, Canada
juliusliptak@mac.com

William Liska, DVM, DACVS
Global Veterinary Specialists
Sugar Land, TX, USA
billliska@aol.com

Federico Massari, DVM, DECVS
Soft Tissue and Oncologic Surgeon
Clinica Veterinaria Nerviano
Nerviano, Italy
fedemassari@hotmail.it

Joshua Milgram, DVM, BVSc (Hons), DECVS
Senior Lecturer
Veterinary Teaching Hospital
Koret School of Veterinary Medicine
Rehovot, Israel
josh.milgram@mail.huji.ac.il

Darryl Millis, MS, DVM, DACVS, CCRP, DACVSMR
Director, CARES Center for Veterinary Sports Medicine
Department of Small Animal Clinical Sciences
University of Tennessee College of Veterinary Medicine
Knoxville, TN, USA
dmillis@utk.edu

Eric Monnet, DVM, PhD, DACVS, DECVS
Professor
Small Animal Surgery
Colorado State University
Fort Collins, CO, USA
eric.monnet@colostate.edu

Alison Moores, BVSc(Hons), CertSAS, DECVS, MRCVS
European Specialist in Small Animal Surgery
Anderson Moores Veterinary Specialists
Winchester, Hampshire, UK
alisonmoores@googlemail.com

Abimbola Oshin, DVM, MS, MBA, MRCVS, DACVS, DECVS
North Georgia Veterinary Specialists
Buford, GA, USA
aoshin@ngvetspecialists.com

Laura J. Owen, BVSc, CertSAS, DECVS, MRCVS
European Specialist in Small Animal Surgery
Lecturer in Small Animal Surgery
University of Cambridge
Cambridge, UK
lo247@cam.ac.uk

Heidi Phillips, VMD, DACVS
Assistant Professor Small Animal Surgery
Department of Veterinary Clinical Medicine
University of Illinois College of Veterinary Medicine
Urbana, IL, USA
philli@illinois.edu

Alessandro Piras, DVM
Specialist in Veterinary Surgery
Sport Medicine Center & Surgical Referrals
Russi (RA), Italy
alexpvet@mac.com

G. Elizabeth Pluhar, DVM, PhD, DACVS
Department of Veterinary Clinical Sciences
College of Veterinary Medicine
University of Minnesota
St. Paul, MN, USA
pluha006@umn.edu

Cyril Poncet, DVM, Dip ECVS
C.H.V. Frégis
Arcueil, France
cponcet@fregis.com

Antonio Pozzi, DMV, MS, DACVS, DECVS, DACVSMR
Vetsuisse Faculty
University of Zurich
Zürich, Switzerland
antonio.pozzi@uzh.ch

Kathryn Pratschke, MVB, MVM, CertSAS, DECVS, MRCVS
Small Animal Surgical Specialist
Northeast Veterinary Referrals
Northumberland, UK
katnap@onetel.com

Lauren Pugliese, MS, DVM
The Ohio State University College of Veterinary
  Medicine
Columbus, OH, USA
lpugliesedvm@gmail.com

Guillaume Ragetly, DVM, PhD, DACVS, DECVS
Centre Hospitalier Vétérinaire Frégis
Paris, France
gragetly@yahoo.fr

Mark Rochat, DVM, MS, DACVS
College of Veterinary Medicine
Purdue University
West Lafayette, IN
mrochat@purdue.edu

Gian Luca Rovesti, drMedVet, DECVS
Clinica veterinaria M. E. Miller
Via della Costituzione 10 Cavriago
Italy
grovesti@clinicamiller.it

Jeffrey J. Runge, DVM, DACVS
Assistant Professor of Minimally Invasive Surgery
Head, Minimally Invasive Surgery
Department of Clinical Studies
School of Veterinary Medicine
University of Pennsylvania
Philadelphia, PA, USA
jeffreyjrunge@gmail.com

Chad Schmiedt, DVM, DACVS
Associate Professor
Small Animal Surgery
Department of Small Animal Medicine and Surgery
College of Veterinary Medicine
University of Georgia
Athens, GA, USA
cws@uga.edu

Reza Seddighi, DVM, MS, PhD, DACVAA
Associate Professor of Anesthesiology and Pain
  Management
College of Veterinary Medicine
The University of Tennessee
Knoxville, TN, USA
mseddigh@utk.edu

Ameet Singh, DVM, DVSc, DACVS
Assistant Professor of Small Animal Surgery
Department of Clinical Studies
University of Guelph
Guelph, Ontario, Canada
amsingh@uoguelph.ca

Lynne A. Snow, DVM, MS, DACVS (SA)
Southeast Veterinary Specialists
Metairie, LA, USA
lynne.snow@gmail.com

Gert ter Haar DVM, PhD, MRCVS, DECVS
Senior Lecturer
Soft Tissue Surgery
Head of the ENT, Brachycephaly and Audiology Clinic
Royal Veterinary College
North Mymms, Hatfield, Herts, UK
gterhaar@rvc.ac.uk

Anson J. Tsugawa, VMD, DAVDC
Dog and Cat Dentist, Inc.
Culver City, CA, USA
vetomfs@yahoo.com

Bart Van Goethem, DVM, DECVS
Small Animal Medicine and Clinical Biology
Faculty of Veterinary Medicine
Ghent University
Ghent, Belgium
bart.vangoethem@ugent.be

Aldo Vezzoni, Med. Vet., DECVS
Clinica Veterinaria Vezzoni srl
Via Angelo Massarotti 60/A
Cremona CR, Italy
aldo@vezzoni.it

Scott Weese, DVM, DVSc, DACVIM
Professor
Department of Pathobiology
University of Guelph
Guelph, Ontario, Canada
jsweese@uoguelph.ca

Angela Witzel, DVM, PhD, DACVN
Assistant Clinical Professor of Nutrition
University of Tennessee College of Veterinary Medicine
Knoxville, TN, USA
awitzel@utk.edu

Wing Tip Wong, DVM, MVS, MANZCVS
Referral Small Animal Orthopaedic Surgeon
WTW Veterinary Surgical Service
Gembrook, Australia
wtwong@bigpond.com

Andrew Worth, BVSc, PhD, FANZCVS
Associate Professor
Massey University Veterinary Teaching Hospital
Palmerston North, New Zealand
A.J.Worth@massey.ac.nz

Preface and Acknowledgements

Preface

Knowledge

"Through time comes wisdom, with wisdom comes knowledge,
The treasure we search through generations and civilizations;
This gem allows people to maintain an edge
Over others, in completing their work and missions.
This jewel allows us to create and evolve,
Allowing us to be the best and strongest.
To crush everything between our goal, to resolve
The obstacle before us and overcome the hardest
Problems. Books, the holders of knowledge, through scripts:
They tell the stories of people and mistakes
They made in search of different golden chips…"

Maxime Griffon

This book is designed to provide veterinary students and surgeons of all levels an up-to-date resource for diagnosing, managing, and preventing complications related to small animal surgery. Surgical complications are generally dreaded by owners and surgeons alike because of their morbidity for the patient, as well as the emotional and financial burdens caused on all parties involved. Managing surgical complications is often technically challenging, and revision surgeries tend to carry a less favorable prognosis than initial procedures. Yet, the literature related to that field consists largely of journal articles dealing with a specific procedure, short paragraphs in literature reviews, and book chapters dealing with other aspects of the surgical management of small animal diseases. Our objective was to provide a more detailed, and case-based approach to peri-operative complications.

This book is intended for the busy clinician in search of readily accessible and practical information to guide the management of a patient suspect of surgical complication. The format of this book was consequently selected to maximize ease of use and appealing presentation. The reader can easily locate information as definition, risk factors, diagnosis, treatment, outcome, and prevention of complications are consistently presented in each chapter. The use of bullet points and short sentences in these practical sections is intended to facilitate reading. Significant emphasis has been placed on illustrations, to allow case-based presentations and improve the clinical relevance of the content. Algorithms guide the reader through practical steps of diagnosis and management of complications. Tables provide quick references, summarizing facts or listing dosages.

For the scholars, each chapter ends with a scientific summary of recent and relevant literature. These reviews are intended to provide supporting evidence for the practical recommendations presented in the book and to outline current gaps in knowledge. Sections dealing with more advanced procedures will be especially relevant to specialists, as a source of recent references as well as practical information that may not yet be published.

This book could not have been completed without the invaluable input from world experts in small animal surgery. The authors of this textbook portray incredible clinical experience, combined with extensive studies of relevant sciences and literature. However, they also distinguish themselves by their willingness to share their expertise with the veterinary community and commitment toward this book. Words cannot express our gratitude for this generosity and dedication.

Dominique Griffon
Annick Hamaide

Acknowledgments

The authors would like to acknowledge John Greenwood for his efficient coordination and communication between authors, editors, and publishers.

About the companion website

This book is accompanied by a companion website:

www.wiley.com/go/griffon/complications

The website includes:

- Videos
- Figures from the book
- Linked references

The password for the companion website is the last word in the caption for Figure 5.1

SECTION 1

Surgical Infections

1 Surgical Wound Infections

Outi Laitinen-Vapaavuori

Department of Equine and Small Animal Medicine, Faculty of Veterinary Medicine, University of Helsinki, Helsinki, Finland

Surgical wound infections are the most common causes of postoperative morbidity and can cause serious complications after surgery despite constant improvements in surgical practice. In small animals, the overall postoperative wound infection rate ranges from 5.1% (Vasseur *et al.* 1988) to 5.8% (Eugster *et al.* 2004); however, the overall information available in the veterinary literature is still limited regarding the epidemiology of wound infections. The classification of surgical procedures has been based on the degree of bacterial contamination (Table 1.1). Infection rates have been reported as 2.5% to 4.9% in clean wounds, 4.5% to 5.9% in clean-contaminated wounds, 5.8% to 12.0% in contaminated wounds, and 10.1% to 18.1% in dirty wounds (Vasseur *et al.* 1988; Brown *et al.* 1997; Nicholson *et al.* 2002; Eugster *et al.* 2004). In addition to the degree of wound contamination, many other factors, both patient and operation related, are shown to influence the occurrence of surgical wound infection.

Definition

Surgical wound infection is not well defined in veterinary medicine. In humans, surgical wound infections are defined as those that occur within 30 days after a surgical operation or within 1 year if a surgical implant was left in place after the procedure. In most veterinary studies, surgical wounds are defined as infected if there is purulent discharge from the wound within 14 days after surgery. In

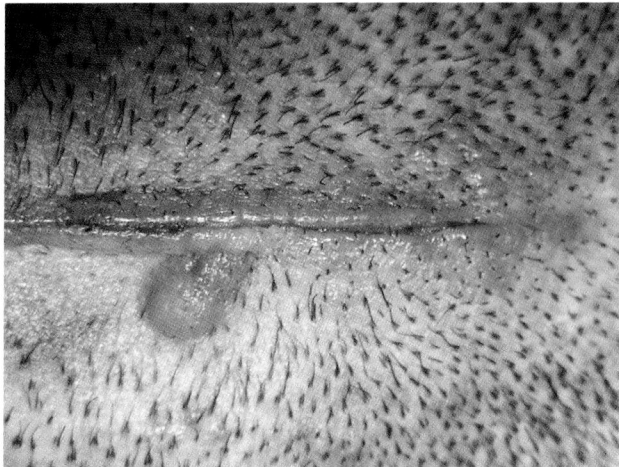

Figure 1.1 Surgical wound infection 6 days after surgery. Signs of redness, swelling, and purulent discharge are seen in the wound.

some studies, the definition also includes signs typical of infection such as redness, pain, swelling, and heat (Figure 1.1).

Risk factors

The factors that may influence the risk of veterinary surgical wound infection are adapted from human studies (Mangram *et al.* 1999; Owens and Stoessel 2008). In the following, the factors marked with asterisks have been shown to be associated with surgical wound infections in veterinary studies.

Patient-related factors include:
- Age*
- Nutritional status
- Diabetes
- Obesity*
- Colonization with microorganisms (particularly *Staphylococcus aureus*)
- Coexistent infections at a remote body site
- Altered immune status
- Length of preoperative stay

Table 1.1 Classification of operative wounds based on the degree of bacterial contamination

Clean	Nontraumatic, noninflamed operative wound
	No entry into the GI, urogenital, or respiratory tracts or oropharyngeal cavity
Clean contaminated	Entry into the GI, urogenital, or respiratory tracts or oropharyngeal cavity
	Clean procedure in which a drain is placed
	Minor break in aseptic technique
Contaminated	Spillage from the GI or urogenital tract
	Fresh traumatic wound (<4 hours old)
	Major break in aseptic technique
Dirty	Acute bacterial infection encountered
	Traumatic (>4 hours old) wound with devitalized tissues or foreign bodies or fecal contamination

GI, gastrointestinal.

Complications in Small Animal Surgery, First Edition. Edited by Dominique Griffon and Annick Hamaide.
© 2016 John Wiley & Sons, Inc. Published 2016 by John Wiley & Sons, Inc.
Companion website: www.wiley.com/go/griffon/complications

Operation-related factors include:
- Duration of surgical scrub
- Skin antisepsis*
- Preoperative hair clipping*
- Preoperative skin preparation*
- Duration of surgery and anesthesia*
- Antimicrobial prophylaxis*
- Operating room (OR) ventilation
- Inadequate sterilization of instruments
- Foreign material in the surgical site
- Surgical drains*
- Surgical technique

Diagnosis

The diagnosis is based on clinical signs and possible positive bacterial culture from the infection site. The identification of surgical wound infection is not always straightforward. If only redness, tenderness, swelling, or heat is present, one has to differentiate it from the normal inflammatory response that occurs in early wound healing. Normally, these signs subside within 24 to 48 hours after surgery.

   Local signs of wound infection include:
- Serosanguineous to purulent drainage from the wound or pus accumulation associated with
- Swelling, redness, heat, and pain or discomfort

Systemic signs and findings may include fever, tachypnea, and leukocytosis with a left shift. Fever and leukocytosis can also occur in the normal inflammatory response to the surgical wound.

If the infection involves deep tissues (bone or an organ), radiologic or ultrasonographic examinations may be warranted.

   Bacterial isolation and identification requires:
- Proper cleaning of the sampling site to avoid contamination of the sample with normal flora
- Taking samples aseptically by swabbing or aspiration depending on the infection site for aerobic and possibly anaerobic cultures and sensitivity testing
- Gram staining from the swab or aspirate in order to distinguish between gram-positive and gram-negative bacteria may aid in early selection of antimicrobials

Treatment

Treatment consists of surgical drainage or wound debridement (or both) depending on the extent of soft tissue or bone involvement and selection of appropriate antimicrobials, which should be based on bacterial culture results.

Drainage or debridement of the wound

- Adequate opening of the surgical incision and evacuation of purulent material are crucial (Figure 1.2). Systemic antimicrobials are not always necessary in patients lacking signs of deep infection or systemic signs.
- After drainage, the wound must be covered with a sterile dressing.
- Extensive soft tissue or bone involvement, the presence of implants, or systemic effects of the infection may warrant surgical exploration of the wound and debridement of all necrotic, devitalized tissue and foreign material.
- Lavage of the tissues can be done with sterile isotonic saline or local antiseptics, such as 0.05% chlorhexidine.
- If there are doubts as to the viability of the tissues, the wound should be treated as an open wound.

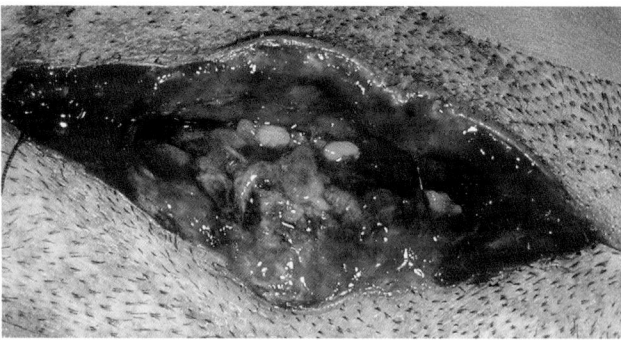

Figure 1.2 Surgical exploration of the infected surgical wound. This is the same wound as in Figure 1.1 after removal of the intradermal sutures.

Selection of antimicrobials

- If antimicrobials are indicated before the bacterial culture results are available, treatment should be started with an antimicrobial that is likely to have an effect against the most probable pathogens(s).
- When the results of the bacterial culture and sensitivity test are available, the antimicrobial should be changed if needed.

Other supportive treatment

- Pain control

Outcome

The prognosis depends on the location and extent of the wound infection and the causative agent. In any case, the wound infection prolongs recovery and causes discomfort to the patient along with increasing the costs of the treatment. The prognosis is good for superficial infections that involve the skin and subcutaneous tissues; however, if infection involves deep tissues or bone, it can seriously affect the outcome of the surgery.

Prevention

Preoperative

- Sterilization of surgical equipment
  ○ Routinely monitor the quality of sterilization process.
- Preparation of the patient
  ○ Identify and treat all infections remote to the surgical site before elective surgery.
  ○ Hair clipping should be done immediately before surgery.
  ○ Clean the clipped area with either a non-antiseptic or an antiseptic soap to remove gross contamination followed by drying the area. Wipe the area with suitable skin antiseptic (chlorhexidine–alcohol, povidone–iodine–alcohol, or 80% alcohol). Let the antiseptics have a proper influence time according to the manufacture's recommendations (usually 3 minutes).
- Preparation of the surgical team
  ○ Use surgical hand antisepsis with either a suitable antimicrobial soap or alcohol-based hand scrub. When using antimicrobial soap, scrub the hands and forearms for 2 to 5 minutes. When using alcohol-based surgical hand scrub, prewash hands and forearms with a non-antimicrobial soap and dry them completely. After application of alcohol-based product following the manufacturer's instructions for application

Table 1.2 Bacterial species colonizing different surgical sites and examples of the use of prophylactic antimicrobials*

Site	Species	Examples of Prophylactic Antimicrobials
Skin	Staphylococci, streptococci, corynebacteria	First-generation cephalosporins
Elective orthopedics	Skin flora as above	First-generation cephalosporins
Neurosurgery	Skin flora as above	First-generation cephalosporins
Oral cavity	Pasteurellae, streptococci, corynebacteria, actinomycetes fusobacteria, porphyromonas, *Prevotella,* bacteroides	Aminopenicillin (+/- clavulanate) or clindamycin
Upper GI tract	Staphylococci, streptococci, enterococci, clostridia, bacteroides, fusobacteria, other aerobic and anaerobic gram-positive cocci and rods, coliforms	Aminopenicillin (+/-clavulanate) or Aminopenicillin+ aminoglycoside
Lower GI tract	Clostridia, anaerobic positive cocci, bacteroides, fusobacteria, coliforms, enterococci, streptococci, gram-positive rods	Aminopenicillin (+/-clavulanate) or Aminopenicillin + aminoglycoside (+/-metronidazole)
Urinary tract	Coliforms, enterococci, staphylococci	Sulfonamides + trimethoprim Ampicillin if enterococci
Reproductive tract	Coliforms, streptococci, pasteurellae, staphylococci	Sulfonamides + trimethoprim

*A prophylactic antimicrobial should be targeted to the most likely organisms that cause wound infection. The selection is based on degree of contamination, operation type and degree of difficulty, knowledge of the local resistance situation, and possible regulatory issues such as local antimicrobial policy and legislation.

GI, gastrointestinal.

times, allow hands and forearms to dry completely before donning sterile gloves.
- Antimicrobial prophylaxis
  ◦ Use prophylactic antimicrobial agents in clean-contaminated and in clean surgeries lasting more than 90 minutes.
  ◦ Choose a narrow-spectrum antimicrobial that is effective on the bacteria likely to contaminate the surgery site (Table 1.2).
  ◦ Administer the antimicrobial by the intravenous route between 30 minutes and 1 hour before the incision to ensure that the bactericidal concentration of the drug is established in both serum and tissues.
  ◦ Maintain therapeutic levels of the drug in both serum and tissues throughout the operation. In clean and clean-contaminated surgeries, the antimicrobial rarely needs to be continued postoperatively. In contaminated and dirty surgeries, the antimicrobials are continued for treating the infection.

Intraoperative
- Surgical team
  ◦ Keep the amount of personnel to a minimum in the OR.
  ◦ Scrubbed surgical teams member should use facemasks, surgical caps, and sterile surgical gowns.
- Operative technique
  ◦ Gentle tissue handling
  ◦ Good hemostasis
  ◦ Obliteration of dead space
  ◦ Prevention of hypothermia during surgery
  ◦ Keep the operation and anesthesia time to a minimum.

Postoperative
- Wound care
  ◦ Protect the wound with a sterile dressing for 24 to 48 hours postoperatively if possible.
  ◦ Always follow strict hand hygiene when in contact with the wound.
- Adequate postoperative care
  ◦ Pain control
  ◦ Prevention of hypothermia and hypoperfusion

Surveillance
- Develop guidelines for controlling surgical wound infections and ensure that they are followed.
  ◦ Develop effective surveillance methods for surgical wound infections.
  ◦ For surveillance purposes, clear definitions of surgical wound infection are needed within an institution.

Relevant literature
The definition of *surgical wound infection* varies among veterinary reports. In human medicine, the term *surgical wound infection* was replaced in 1992 with the term *surgical site infection* (SSI), which was adapted to veterinary medicine by Frey *et al.* (2010) in a retrospective study on risk factors for SSI in anterior cruciate ligament (ACL) surgery. According to the Centers for Disease Control and Prevention, SSIs are divided into superficial (infection involves only subcutaneous tissue of the incision), deep (infection involves deep soft tissues such as fascial and muscle layers), and organ or space SSI (infection involves any part of the anatomy other than the incision) (Mangram *et al.* 1999). The identification of SSI involves interpretation of clinical as well as laboratory findings. There is also a need to standardize the definition of postoperative wound infections in veterinary medicine, too.

Several risk factors are identified in veterinary studies. When looking at **patient-related risk factors,** Nicholson *et al.* (2002) found that intact males and animals with endocrinopathy were at a higher risk for postoperative wound infections after clean-contaminated surgeries. Increasing weight of the dog was found to be a risk factor in a study in which the outcome was classified as infected or infected/inflamed (Eugster *et al.* 2004). In the same study, the authors also showed that an increasing American Society of Anesthesiologists score was associated with increasing wound infection rates. Further potential patient-related risk factors have been identified in human studies on different surgical procedures, including older age, preexisting infection, obesity, colonization with microorganisms, diabetes, preoperative anemia, use of corticosteroids, malnutrition, low serum albumin levels, and postoperative hyperglycemia (Mangram *et al.* 1999; Ata *et al.* 2010; Moucha *et al.* 2011). Some of the risk factors remain controversial, and more studies are needed to show their direct scientific evidence in various procedures.

Surgical site preparation is an important **operation-related risk factor.** Preoperative clipping immediately before surgery has been shown to decrease the risk of infection in small animals (Brown *et al.* 1997). Because the patient's skin is a major source of pathogens that cause wound infections, optimization of preoperative skin antisepsis is important. Nevertheless, study results are conflicting regarding the superiority of chlorhexidine–alcohol versus povidone–iodine (Darouiche *et al.* 2010) or chlorhexidine–alcohol versus povidone–iodine–alcohol for surgical site antisepsis in humans (Swenson *et al.* 2009). It was concluded, however, in a recent meta-analysis by Noorani *et al.* (2010) that preoperative cleansing with chlorhexidine is superior to povidone–iodine in reducing postoperative SSI after clean-contaminated surgery. In a recent canine study, it was shown that there was a reduction in bacterial counts from the skin with an increasing concentration of chlorhexidine gluconate from 1% to 4% (Evans *et al.* 2009).

The **duration of surgery** has been investigated in several studies, but drawing conclusions from these studies is challenging because variation is evident for the definition of surgical wound infection, the study design, antimicrobials regimen, and number of animals involved. However, it has been shown in one retrospective and two prospective studies that longer surgical procedures (>90 minutes) have a greater risk of infection (Vasseur *et al.* 1988; Brown *et al.* 1997; Eugster *et al.* 2004).

Increased **duration of anesthesia** has also shown to increase wound infection rates (Nicholson *et al.* 2002; Eugster *et al.* 2004; Owen *et al.* 2009). A 30% greater risk of postoperative wound infection in clean wounds for each additional hour of anesthesia has been reported (Beal *et al.* 2000). The proposed multifactorial causes resulting from anesthetic duration were impairment of function of phagocytic leukocytes (Mangram *et al.* 1999), prolonged use of anesthetic drugs (Beal *et al.* 2000), perioperative hypothermia (Dellinger 2006), and increased risk for wound contamination (Owen *et al.* 2009).

Wound infection rates increase with the **degree of bacterial contamination** (Vasseur *et al.* 1988; Brown *et al.* 1997; Eugster *et al.* 2004). The causative agent is most often endogenous, originating from the patient, and is site dependent (see Table 1.2). Surgical suction tips have been shown to become contaminated during surgery and could influence the risk of wound infection (Sturgeon *et al.* 2000). The use of adhesive incise drapes did not reduce wound contamination in clean surgeries in dogs (Owen *et al.* 2009), but it has also been reported that a sterile, impermeable barrier is needed in addition to sterile surgical drapes to prevent bacterial strikethrough when wrapping the distal limb in orthopedic surgeries (Vince *et al.* 2008).

In humans, there appears to be a clear consensus that **antimicrobial prophylaxis** is necessary and helpful in reducing the risk arising from bacterial contamination of the surgical wound in clean-contaminated procedures and in clean procedures that involve implantation of a graft or a device. In contaminated or dirty procedures, antimicrobials are administered with therapeutic intent (Mangram *et al.* 1999; Nichols 2004). Timing of the administration of prophylactic antimicrobials is crucial; 2 hours before surgery has shown to be effective in reducing surgical wound infections in humans (Classen *et al.* 1992). In veterinary medicine, only a few studies have been conducted on the effect of antimicrobial prophylaxis in clean and clean-contaminated procedures. In earlier reports, no difference

was found in infection rates between the group receiving antimicrobials or not (Vasseur *et al.* 1985; Brown *et al.* 1997; Nicholson *et al.* 2002). These contradictory findings compared with human studies are most probably attributable methodologic limitations. There is one prospective, randomized, controlled study by Whittem *et al.* (1999) in which there was a lower postoperative infection rate in dogs undergoing elective clean orthopedic surgery that received cefazolin or potassium penicillin within 30 minutes before the incision and received a second dose if surgery lasted longer than 90 minutes compared with placebo control animals. It is noticeable that antimicrobial prophylaxis was not continued after surgery.

When **selecting an antimicrobial** for prophylaxis, it should have activity against the pathogen most likely to contaminate the surgery site. Other factors that should be taken into consideration are pharmacokinetics, side effects, toxicity, and cost of the drug as well as the antibiotic resistance, which varies in different countries. Antimicrobials should be used in a targeted manner in which minimal use provides maximal effect with minimal adverse reaction. For most procedures, antimicrobials active against β-lactamase–producing staphylococci should be administered. These include β-lactamase–resistant penicillins and first-generation cephalosporins (Dunning 2003).

The duration of antimicrobial prophylaxis should encompass the entire procedure (Dohmen 2008); thus, redosing during surgery may be required depending on the half-life of the antimicrobial and the duration of the surgery. The majority of evidence in humans has demonstrated that antimicrobial prophylaxis after wound closure does not provide any additional protection against surgical wound infection (Evans and American Academy of Orthopaedic Surgeons Patient Safety Committee 2009b). Continuing antibiotic prophylaxis for longer than 24 hours after wound closure does not reduce rates of surgical infections, but it may contribute to the development of antimicrobial resistance (Dohmen 2008; Evans and American Academy of Orthopaedic Surgeons Patient Safety Committee 2009b). In veterinary studies, the postoperative use of antimicrobials has shown to increase the risk of wound infection in clean surgeries (Brown *et al.* 1997; Eugster *et al.* 2004), although contradictory findings have also been reported (Frey *et al.* 2010).

Despite the presence of strict protocols, discrepancies still exist between the protocols and practice. In one retrospective study in which the use of antimicrobials in ACL surgery was evaluated at a veterinary teaching hospital, it was noticed that whereas 85% of dogs received the first dose of antimicrobials within 60 minutes of the incision, 29% of dogs received antimicrobials after surgery (Weese and Halling 2006).

Minimizing the risk factors is the most effective way of **preventing** surgical wound infections. For instance, a **preoperative** issue that has been vigorously studied is hand cleansing before surgery. It has long been known that preoperative scrubbing with a brush has no advantage over nonscrubbing methods of hand preparation (Loeb *et al.* 1997). The current guidelines on hand hygiene are based on consensus recommendations that rely on the evidence of well-designed clinical and epidemiologic studies. According to the recommendations, surgical hand antisepsis should be done either by scrubbing with an antimicrobial soap or with non-antimicrobial soap followed by an alcohol-based hand rub (Boyce and Pittet 2002; Pittet *et al.* 2009; Verwilghen *et al.* 2010).

Intraoperatively, the number of persons in the OR during surgery should be kept to a minimum. For each additional person in the room, the risk for wound infection has shown to be 1.3 times higher (Eugster *et al.* 2004). Perioperative mild hypothermia has not shown to be a significant risk factor for wound infections in dogs and cats (Beal *et al.* 2000), but in human studies, there is evidence that systemic warming reduces wound infections and reduces blood loss and the need for transfusions (Leaper 2010). It has also been shown that supplemental administration of 80% oxygen in the recovery room could reduce SSIs (Qadan *et al.* 2009; Leaper 2010).

There are very few veterinary studies on **postoperative factors** associated with wound infections; however, the duration of the postoperative stay in the intensive care unit has been shown to be associated with SSI (Eugster *et al.* 2004).

The **surveillance** of surgical wound infections in humans has been effective in reducing SSIs (Owens and Stoessel 2008). Surveillance has an important information-gathering function that can be very helpful in the detection and prevention of nosocomial outbreaks.

References

Ata, A., Lee, J., Bestle, S.L., et al. (2010) Postoperative hyperglycemia and surgical site infection in general surgery patients. *Archives of Surgery* 145 (9), 858-864.

Beal, M.W., Brown, D.C., Shofer, F.S. (2000) The effects of perioperative hypothermia and the duration of anesthesia on postoperative wound infection rate in clean wounds: a retrospective study. *Veterinary Surgery* 29 (2), 123-127.

Boyce, J.M., Pittet, D. (2002) Guideline for hand hygiene in health-care settings: recommendations of the Healthcare Infection Control Practices Advisory Committee and the HICPAC/SHEA/APIC/IDSA hand hygiene task force. *American Journal of Infection Control* 30 (8), 1-46.

Brown, D.C., Conzemius, M.G., Shofer, F., et al. (1997) Epidemiologic evaluation of postoperative wound infections in dogs and cats. *Journal of the American Veterinary Medical Association* 210 (9), 1302-1306.

Classen, D.C., Evans, R.S, Pestotnik, S.L., et al. (1992) The timing of prophylactic administration of antibiotics and the risk of surgical wound infections. *The New England Journal of Medicine* 326 (5), 281-286.

Darouiche, R.O., Wall, M. J., Itani, K.M., et al. (2010) Chlorhexidine-alcohol versus povidone-iodine for surgical-site antisepsis. *The New England Journal of Medicine* 362 (2), 18-26.

Dellinger, E.P. (2006) Roles of temperature and oxygenation in prevention of surgical site infection. *Surgical Infection* 7 (Suppl. 3), 27-31.

Dohmen, P.M. (2008) Antibiotic resistance in common pathogens reinforces the need to minimise surgical site infections. *Journal of Hospital Infection* 70 (2), 15-20.

Dunning, D. (2003) Surgical wound infection and the use of antimicrobials. In: Slatter, D. (ed.) *Textbook of Small Animal Surgery*, vol. 1, 3rd edn. Saunders, Elsevier Science, Philadelphia, pp. 113-122.

Eugster, S., Schawalder, P., Gaschen, F., et al. (2004) A prospective study of postoperative surgical site infections in dogs and cats. *Veterinary Surgery* 33 (5), 542-550.

Evans R.P., American Academy of Orthopaedic Surgeons Patient Safety Committee (2009) Surgical site infection prevention and control: an emerging paradigm. *Journal of Bone and Joint Surgery* 91 (Suppl. 6), 2-9.

Evans, L.K., Knowles, T.G., Werrett, G., et al. (2009) The efficacy of chlorhexidine gluconate in canine skin preparation—practice survey and clinical trials. *Journal of Small Animal Practice* 50 (9), 458-465.

Frey, T.N., Hoelzler, M.G., Scavelli, T.D., et al. (2010) Risk factors for surgical site infection-inflammation in dogs undergoing surgery for rupture of the cranial cruciate ligament: 902 cases (2005-2006). *Journal of the American Veterinary Medical Association* 236 (1), 88-94.

Leaper, D.J. (2010) Risk factors for and epidemiology of surgical site infections. *Surgical Infection* 11 (3), 283-287.

Loeb, M.B., Wilcox, L., Smaill, F., et al. (1997) A randomized trial of surgical scrubbing with a brush compared to antiseptic soap alone. *American Journal of Infection Control* 25 (1), 11-15.

Mangram, A.J., Horan, T.C., Pearson, M.L., et al. (1999) Guideline for prevention of surgical site infection. *American Journal of Infection Control* 27 (2), 97-134.

Moucha, C.S., Clyburn, T., Evans, R.P. (2011) Modifiable risk factors for surgical site infection. *Journal of Bone and Joint Surgery* 93 (4), 398-404.

Nichols, R.L. (2004) Preventing surgical site infections. *Clinical Medicine & Research* 2 (2), 115-118.

Nicholson, M., Beal, M., Shofer, F. (2002) Epidemiologic evaluation of postoperative wound infection in clean-contaminated wounds: a retrospective study of 239 dogs and cats. *Veterinary Surgery* 31 (6), 577-581.

Noorani, A., Rabey, N., Walsh, S.R, et al. (2010) Systematic review and meta-analysis of preoperative antisepsis with chlorhexidine versus povidone-iodine in clean-contaminated surgery. *Bone and Joint Surgery* 97, 1614-1620.

Owen, L.J., Gines, J.A., Knowles, T.G. (2009) Efficacy of adhesive incise drapes in preventing bacterial contamination of clean canine surgical wounds. *Veterinary Surgery* 38 (6), 732-737.

Owens, C.D., Stoessel, K. (2008) Surgical site infections: epidemiology, microbiology and prevention. *Journal of Hospital Infection* 70 (Suppl. 2), 3-10.

Pittet, D., Allegranzi, B., Boyce, J. (2009) The World Health Organization guidelines on hand hygiene in health care and their consensus recommendations. *Infection Control and Hospital Epidemiology* 30 (7), 611-622.

Qadan, M., Akca, O., Mahid, S.S., et al. (2009) Perioperative supplemental oxygen therapy and surgical site infection. A meta-analysis of randomized controlled trials. *Archives of Surgery* 144 (4), 359-366.

Sturgeon, C., Lamport, A.I., Lloyd, D.H. (2000) Bacterial contamination of suction tips used during surgical procedures performed on dogs and cats. *American Journal of Veterinary Research* 61 (7), 779-783.

Swenson, B.R., Hedrick, T.L., Metzger, R., et al. (2009) Effects of preoperative skin preparation on postoperative wound infection rates: a prospective study of 3 skin preparation protocols. *Infection Control and Hospital Epidemiology* 30 (10), 964-971.

Vasseur, P.B., Levy, J., Dowd, E. (1988) Surgical wound infection rates in dogs and cats. Data from a teaching hospital. *Veterinary Surgery* 17 (2), 60-64.

Vasseur, P.B., Paul, H.A., Enos, L.R. (1985) Infection rates in clean surgical procedures: a comparison of ampicillin prophylaxis vs a placebo. *Journal of the American Veterinary Medical Association* 187 (8), 825-827.

Verwilghen, D., Mainil, J., Mastrocicco, E., et al. (2010) Surgical hand antisepsis in veterinary practice: evaluation of soap scrubs and alcohol based rub techniques. *The Veterinary Journal* 190 (3), 372-377.

Vince, K.J., Lascelles, B.D., Mathews, K.G. (2008) Evaluation of wraps covering the distal aspect of pelvic limbs for prevention of bacterial strike-through in an ex vivo canine model. *Veterinary Surgery* 37 (4), 406-411.

Weese, J.S., Halling, K.B. (2006) Perioperative administration of antimicrobials associated with elective surgery for cranial cruciate ligament rupture in dogs: 83 cases (2003-2005). *Journal of the American Veterinary Medical Association* 229 (1), 92-95.

Whittem, T.L., Johnson, A.L., Smith, C.W. (1999) Effect of perioperative prophylactic antimicrobial treatment in dogs undergoing elective orthopedic surgery. *Journal of the American Veterinary Medical Association* 215 (2), 212-216.

2 Sepsis

Galina Hayes[1] and Brigitte A. Brisson[2]

[1]Cornell University, Ithaca, NY, USA
[2]Department of Clinical Studies, Ontario Veterinary College, University of Guelph, Guelph, Ontario, Canada

Definition

The criteria for the diagnosis of sepsis consist of suspected or proven infection and concurrent systemic inflammatory response syndrome (SIRS). SIRS is classically diagnosed following identification of established criteria (Table 2.1) (Hauptman *et al.* 1997; Brady *et al.* 2000); however, any sick animal manifesting unexplained hemodynamic instability or thermoregulatory abnormality should be considered potentially septic.

Sepsis is a clinical diagnosis that does not require laboratory confirmation. Bacterial culture results are specific but not sensitive (Sands *et al.* 1997), and sepsis may be diagnosed on the basis of strong clinical suspicion, without microbiologic confirmation (Levy *et al.* 2003). Delaying intervention pending results of laboratory testing may result in missing the optimal intervention window and may worsen patient outcomes. Additional sepsis definitions are shown in Table 2.2 and are useful for further defining and prognosticating subsets of septic patients.

Risk factors

Severe sepsis and septic shock can develop as part of the primary disease process (e.g., perforating gastrointestinal [GI] foreign body) or secondary to treatment for another disorder (e.g., aspiration pneumonia after anesthesia). Hospital-acquired sepsis is typically diagnosed earlier in the clinical continuum, and the infective organism is more likely to be multidrug resistant, reflecting prior antibiotic exposure and a nosocomial origin. Amalgamating the results of several studies (*n* = 124 dogs), the source of the infective agent in septic dogs is most commonly the GI tract (37%) followed by the reproductive (21%), musculoskeletal (18%), pulmonary (17%), and urinary tracts (7%). Sepsis carries a mortality risk in dogs of 40% (Hauptman *et al.* 1997; de Laforcade *et al.* 2003, 2008; Gebhardt *et al.* 2009; Rogers and Rozanski 2010). Similar patterns have been reported in cats (*n* = 45) with species differences including increased pulmonary sources of infection (32%), increased incidence of viral or protozoal infective organisms compared with bacterial, and a tendency to manifest hypothermia as part of the sepsis syndrome (Brady *et al.* 2000; deClue *et al.* 2011).

Diabetic animals are at increased risk of postoperative sepsis and exhibit impaired hemodynamic and immunologic responses, likely resulting in higher mortality rates (Law *et al.* 1991; Greco and Harpold 1994). Immunologic compromise in diabetes is associated with altered lymphocyte populations with a lower CD4:8 ratio and depressed lymphocyte, neutrophil, and macrophage function (Mori *et al.* 2008).

Investigations of human patients in a critical care setting have found both parenteral nutrition or absence of nutrition to be risk factors for postoperative sepsis and have demonstrated enteral nutrition to be protective (Elke *et al.* 2008). Transfusion-associated immunomodulation, with decreased natural killer cell and macrophage function and a shift in T-cell phenotype, has also been associated with an increased incidence of postoperative sepsis (Prittie 2010). Finally, invasive devices, including urinary catheters, intravenous (IV) catheters, and drains, can act as conduits for microorganism invasion and colonization. The presence of these devices increases the risk of both nosocomial infection and sepsis in hospitalized animals (Ogeer-Gyles 2006; Szabo *et al.* 2011).

Risk factors for sepsis in dogs in some specific clinical contexts have been examined. The risk of intestinal leakage and septic peritonitis after GI surgery is higher in the face of **preoperative septic peritonitis**, **hypoalbuminemia**, and **hypotension** (Bentley *et al.* 2007; Grimes *et al.* 2011). The risk of sepsis in association with chemotherapy is higher with **doxorubicin or vincristine** or when the primary disease is **lymphoma** (Sorenmo *et al.* 2010).

Table 2.1 Criteria for diagnosis of the systemic inflammatory response syndrome (SIRS) in dogs and cats

Criteria	Limits for SIRS diagnosis in dogs (≥2/4 criteria needed)	Limits for SIRS diagnosis in cats (≥¾ criteria needed)
Rectal temperature (°C)	<38, >39	<37.8, >39.7
Heart rate (beats/min)	>120	<140, >225
Respiratory rate (breaths/min)	>20	>40
WBC count (×10³); % bands	<6, >16; >3%	<5, >19.5; >5%

WBC, white blood cell.
Source: Data from Hauptman *et al.* (1997) and Brady *et al.* (2000).

Table 2.2 Definitions of sepsis

Syndrome	Definition
Sepsis	Infection + systemic manifestations of infection
Severe sepsis	Sepsis + tissue hypoperfusion or sepsis-induced organ dysfunction
Septic shock	Sepsis-induced hypotension persisting despite adequate fluid resuscitation

Source: Levy *et al.*, 2003. Reproduced with permission from Wolters Kluwer Health.

Complications in Small Animal Surgery, First Edition. Edited by Dominique Griffon and Annick Hamaide.
© 2016 John Wiley & Sons, Inc. Published 2016 by John Wiley & Sons, Inc.
Companion website: www.wiley.com/go/griffon/complications

Table 2.3 Components and etiology of the shock state in sepsis

Type of shock	Etiology
Hypovolemic	• External losses: vomiting, polyuria • Third-space losses: peritonitis, pyothorax • Capillary leak: circulating intravascular volume → interstitial space secondary to endothelial damage + albumin extravasation

Vasodilatory	• Loss of autoregulation of vasomotor tone caused by
	   ○ Cytokine-mediated ↑ iNOS
	   ○ Activation of K_{ATP} channels secondary to ↑ intracellular H^+ + lactate
	   ○ ↓ Responsiveness to norepinephrine and angiotensin II potentiated by relative glucocorticoid deficiency
	   ○ Depletion of neurohypophyseal stores of vasopressin

Cardiogenic	• Cytokine- and NO-mediated ↓ systolic function + ↓ myocardial compliance secondary to:
	   ○ Downregulation of β-adrenergic receptors and postreceptor pathways
	   ○ Impaired calcium release from the sarcoplasmic reticulum
	   ○ Impaired electromechanical coupling

iNOS, inducible nitric oxide synthase; NO, nitric oxide.
Source: Data from Landry and Oliver (2001) and Rudiger and Singer (2007).

Mortality rates in animals with sepsis are high and have not changed significantly in the past 10 years (Bentley *et al.* 2007). Successful sepsis prevention strategies in postoperative patients may include careful consideration of morbidities associated with the process of care together with conservative use of indwelling devices, transfusion therapy, and glucocorticoids. Attention to the provision of early enteral nutrition and active monitoring for nosocomial infections may be of benefit.

Diagnosis

The classic shock state seen in sepsis has **vasodilatory, cardiogenic, and hypovolemic components**. Mechanisms are detailed in Table 2.3. SIRS is associated with an intense vasodilation that increases vascular capacitance and results in a decrease in arterial blood pressure. Reduced effective circulating volume caused by both fluid loss and translocation of fluid into the interstital space due to alterations in capillary permeability contributes to hypotension. This is further aggravated by reduced myocardial contractility. Sepsis syndrome in dogs is frequently manifested clinically as **hyperemic mucous membranes with rapid capillary refill**. Prominent peripheral pulses in the face of hypotension reflect low diastolic pressures and a widened pulse pressure. As the patient continues to decompensate, pulses become absent, and the extremities become cold to the touch. Tachycardia frequently becomes normocardia shortly before cardiac arrest and in the context of clinical hypoperfusion should signal imminent danger to the alert clinician.

Microbiologic sampling should not delay timely administration of antibiotics. However, obtaining appropriate cultures before antibiotic administration facilitates targeted administration and subsequent deescalation of antibiotic therapy. Cultures may be obtained from the suspected septic focus, or if this is not apparent, culture of blood and urine samples obtained with appropriate aseptic technique may yield the primary pathogen. Cultures obtained before antibiotic therapy or surgical intervention are typically the most predictive of the primary pathogen (Ogeer-Gyles 2006).

Timely **identification of a septic focus** facilitates surgical decision making and source control. In animals presenting with severe sepsis or septic shock, assessment of a suspected intracavitary focus with abdominal focused assessment with sonography for trauma (AFAST) or thoracic-focused assessment with sonography for trauma (TFAST) techniques (Lisciandro *et al.* 2008, 2009) and sampling of any free fluid identified should be performed concurrently with initial resuscitative efforts. In the absence of ultrasound, blind

needle or catheter abdominocentesis and thoracocentesis techniques are relatively safe, although they are less sensitive. **Cytology of the sample** can be performed expeditiously with basic equipment and definitive diagnosis obtained if infective organisms are identified. In the absence of infective organisms, the identification of suppurative inflammation with degenerate neutrophils may still be consistent with sepsis, particularly in the context of prior antibiotic administration or high GI perforation (Figure 2.1).

Assessment of glucose and lactate fluid:blood ratios on body cavity samples may also aid diagnosis in the acute context. Cut points of lactate 2 mmol/L higher in fluid compared with blood and glucose 20 mg/dL (1.1 mmol/L) lower in fluid compared with blood have been suggested (Bonczynski *et al.* 2003). However, for patients in the immediate post-operative period both blood:fluid ratios and the identification of degenerate neutrophils have been found to be unreliable (Szabo *et al.* 2011).

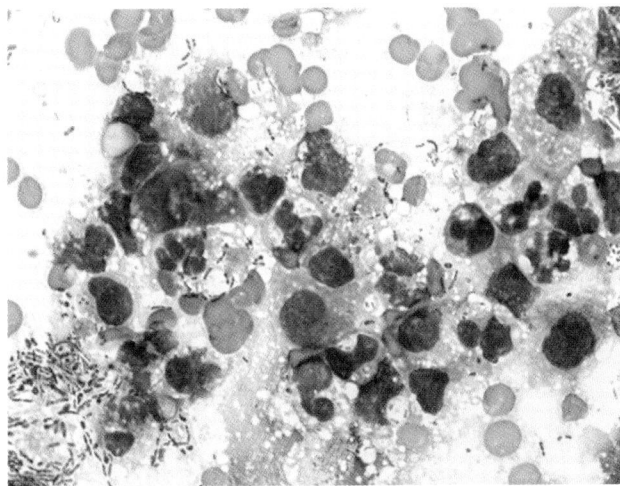

Figure 2.1 Cytology of abdominal fluid in a dog presenting with severe sepsis and gastrointestinal perforation. Free and intracellular bacteria are present. Circulating neutrophils exposed to bacterial toxins undergo altered cell membrane permeability with water influx and hydropic degeneration characterized by a loose, homogenous, eosinophilic nuclear chromatin pattern and are characterized as showing degenerate change. The nuclear:cytoplasmic ratio is increased. Neutrophils exhibiting toxic changes, characterized by Döhle bodies, toxic granulation, and foamy and basophilic cytoplasm, may also migrate into body cavity effusions; however, toxic changes occur in the bone marrow (Cowell *et al.* 1999). *Source:* D. Woods.

Imaging studies may be of assistance in confirming a potential source of infection and guiding surgical intervention. However, in the face of severe sepsis or septic shock, the potential benefits must be weighed against negatives, including additional delay, patient stress, and transfer to areas where resuscitative equipment and personnel may not be available.

Because of the morbidity associated with failure to identify a septic focus and achieve source control, a relatively low intervention trigger for timely surgical exploration should be maintained in animals with a suspicious clinical presentation.

Treatment

Monitoring

Successful titration of therapy in severe sepsis or septic shock requires end points to be assigned and monitored until the animal is stabilized. **Perfusion-associated physical examination findings**, including mentation, pulse quality, capillary refill time (CRT), and warmth of extremities, should be assessed every few minutes until stabilization is achieved. End points of resuscitation in septic shock include normalization of heart rate and CRT less than 2 seconds, normal pulses with mean arterial pressure (MAP) greater than 65 mm Hg, warm extremities, normal mental status, and urine output greater than 1 mL/kg/hr (Dellinger *et al.* 2008). Blood pressure should be monitored continuously in the resuscitation phase of therapy.

Direct blood pressure monitoring is recommended in the context of titration of pressors. However, obtaining an arterial catheter in a cat or small dog in decompensated septic shock may be unfeasible, in which case pressor therapy should be initiated and titrated to non-invasive blood pressure measurement methods or physical examination findings. Additional attempts to gain arterial access can be made after perfusion status is improved. **Continuous EKG** is helpful both for detection of acute arrhythmias and titration of cardiovascular resuscitative therapy. **Serial lactate assessments** reflect global perfusion dynamics, and lactate clearance is highly predictive of outcome (Arnold *et al.* 2009). **Central venous oxygen saturation** is a measure of the balance between tissue oxygen delivery and consumption; a therapeutic end point of 65% to 70% has been suggested in dogs (Hayes *et al.* 2011). There are recognized limitations to the use of **central venous pressure (CVP) targets** to direct fluid resuscitation (Magder 2005); however, an increase in CVP of greater than 5 mm Hg (7 cm H_2O) in response to fluid challenge without accompanying improvements in perfusion parameters may indicate that additional fluid challenge is likely to be unrewarding, and pressor therapy should be considered (Vincent and Weil 2006). Finally, possibly the most essential component of therapeutic success in a patient with severe sepsis or septic shock is the constant and undivided attention of a clinician able to integrate the monitored information and adjust therapy accordingly. Monitored information is of no benefit to the patient in the absence of intervention.

Initial resuscitation

A useful acronym to guide initial resuscitation therapy is VIP, which stands for ventilation, infusion, and pump (Weil and Shubin 1969). An algorithmic approach is outlined in Figure 2.2. In the following

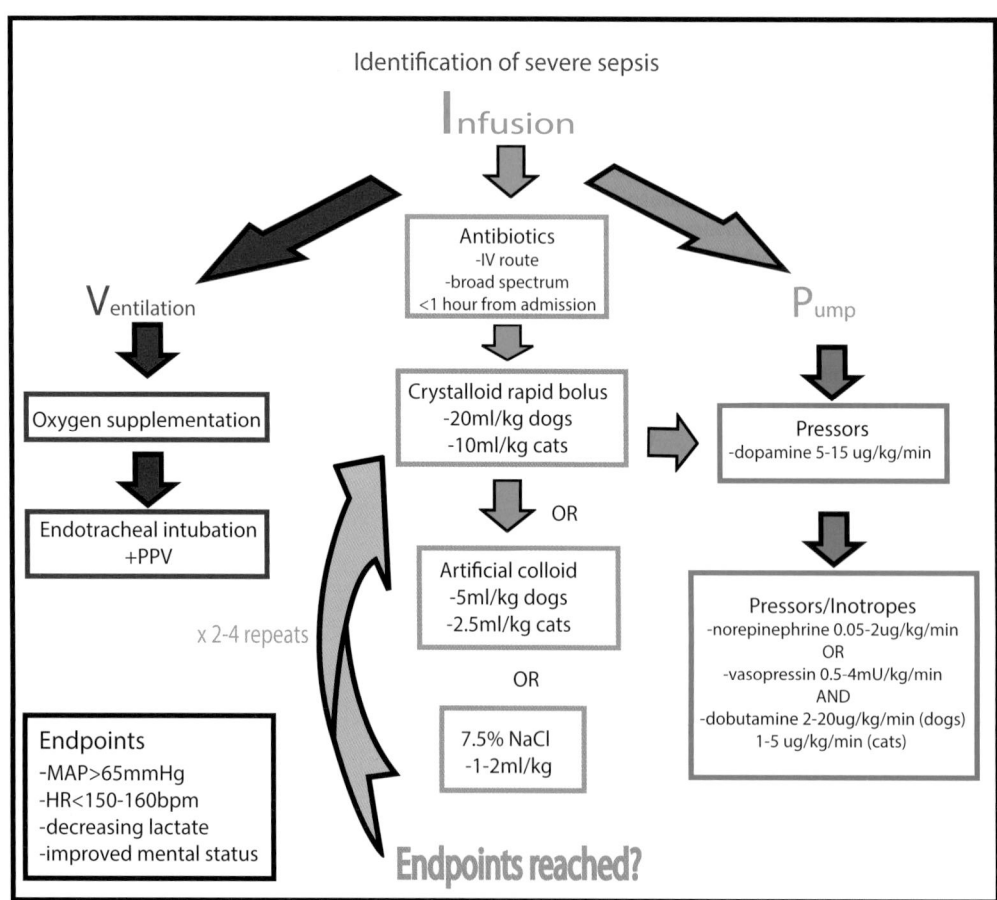

Figure 2.2 Algorithm for stabilization of severe sepsis and septic shock.

discussion, treatment recommendations are taken from the veterinary literature when good quality evidence is available and otherwise from the Surviving Sepsis Campaign Guidelines 2008, research using canine sepsis models, and the human critical care literature.

Antibiotic therapy

Intravenous antibiotic therapy should be started as soon as possible and **within 1 hour of recognition of severe sepsis or septic shock.** Each hour of delay in administration of effective antibiotics is associated with a measurable increase in mortality (Kumar *et al.* 2006). Empiric broad-spectrum antibiotic therapy should be targeted to likely pathogens and guided by local resistance patterns, with avoidance of antibiotics to which the patient has been recently exposed. **Deescalation** to the most appropriate single agent should be performed as soon as the susceptibility of the infective organism is known. Appropriate empiric broad-spectrum choices in the naïve context include cefoxitin, potentiated amoxicillin, or ampicillin with enrofloxacin. In the face of hospital-acquired severe sepsis or septic shock and likely antibiotic resistance, ticarcillin with clavulanate, meropenem, or imipenem should be considered.

Fluid therapy

Cardiovascular support is essential to maintain hemodynamic stability in severe sepsis or septic shock and bridge the delay until antibiotic therapy or surgical source control resolves the septic focus and allows the SIRS to abate (Natanson *et al.* 1990). Fluid therapy improves cardiac output by augmentation of preload and improves tissue microcirculation both through expansion of the intravascular blood volume and altered blood rheological characteristics (Piagnerelli *et al.* 2003; Bauer *et al.* 2009). Conversely, excessive fluid administration expands the interstitial space, adversely alters the capillary:cell oxygen diffusion gradient and Starling forces, increases the risk of respiratory failure, and is associated with increased morbidity. Fluid resuscitation should be performed using a fluid challenge technique in which sequential fluid boluses are administered under close monitoring to evaluate hemodynamic responses to fluid administration and avoid the development of pulmonary edema. One quarter of a shock volume (20 mL/kg in dogs; 10 mL/kg in cats) is administered every 10 to 15 minutes using a balanced electrolyte solution, and hemodynamic responses are assessed. Adjunctive bolus therapy using artificial colloids (2.5–5 mL/kg) or hypertonic saline (2 mL/kg) can also be considered. The intravascular volume deficit in septic animals is variable. However, if greater than 1 shock volume (80 mL/kg in dogs; 50 mL/kg in cat)s has been rapidly administered without hemodynamic improvement or if CVP increases by more than 5 mm Hg over the course of bolus therapy without hemodynamic improvement, then the addition of vasopressor therapy should be strongly considered. No definitive conclusions have been reached to date on the advantages of crystalloids vs colloids versus hypertonic saline in sepsis. However, several studies have reported an association between the use of hydroxyethyl starch and acute renal failure in the context of sepsis (Brunkhorst *et al.* 2008; Bayer *et al.* 2011), as well as a "rebound" effect on crystalloid requirements and increases in total body water suggesting rapid translocation of starches to the interstitial space caused by altered capillary micropermeability (Wills *et al.* 2005). Hypertonic saline modifies the inflammatory response as well has having fluid-sparing and antiedema effects (Bauer *et al.* 2009; Rahal *et al.* 2009). After stabilization, because of ongoing venodilation and capillary leak, continued fluid resuscitation with a positive fluid balance is typically required during the first few days of management. Input is typically much greater than output, and titration of fluids to input:output ratio has no role in this phase of management (Dellinger *et al.* 2008).

Vasopressor therapy

A key feature of sepsis pathophysiology is inappropriate vasodilation caused by the loss of autoregulation of vasomotor tone. Vasopressors are indicated when response to fluid therapy is inadequate or before full fluid resuscitation when emergency measures are required in a moribund patient. In this context, vasopressors can frequently be weaned with continued fluid resuscitation. Dopamine stimulates β_1 (inotrope), β_2 (vasodilator and bronchodilator), and α (vasoconstrictor) receptors, with β_1 and α effects dominant at the higher doses (5–15 µg/kg/min). Dopamine increases MAP and cardiac output by increasing stroke volume and heart rate. Norepinephrine has mainly α with some β_1 effects and increases MAP by vasoconstriction. Vasopressin is a pure vasoconstrictor acting via V1 receptors and counteracts septic vasodilation via closure of KATP channels (Schrier and Wang 2004). In a canine septic shock model, norepinephrine (0.2–2.0 µg/kg/min) and vasopressin (0.01–0.04 U/min) were found to be equivalent at improving survival, but epinephrine (0.2–2.0 µg/kg/min) worsened outcomes (Minnecl *et al.* 2004). Norepinephrine (0.01–0.2 µg/kg/min) and dopamine (5–20 µg/kg/min) were found to provide equivalent mortality outcomes for human patients with septic shock, with an increase in arrhythmias in the dopamine group (De Backer *et al.* 2010). Norepinephrine or dopamine is frequently used as a first-line agent, with the addition or substitution of vasopressin in refractory animals.

Inotropes

Canine sepsis is associated with ventricular dilation and a profound, although reversible, decrease in both systolic and diastolic cardiac function (Natanson *et al.* 1986). In the face of myocardial dysfunction, the use of vasoconstrictors may increase afterload and decrease cardiac output further. Dobutamine is recommended for animals with measured or suspected low cardiac output in the presence of adequate left ventricular filling pressure and MAP.

Source control

Surgical source control of a septic focus reduces patient exposure to microbiologic load. **Source control, hemodynamic stabilization, and timely antibiotic therapy** complete the triad of interventions that define successful sepsis management. Source control measures include abscess drainage, debridement of infected necrotic tissue, removal of an infected device or implant, and repair of a leaking viscus. Surgery should be performed on an emergency basis as soon as initial stabilization is complete. **Surgical intervention and the associated anesthesia impose an additional physiologic and inflammatory burden, and the lowest surgical dose necessary to achieve source control should be applied.** In the face of hemodynamic instability under anesthesia, a staged approach to surgical intervention should be considered. With this approach, the initial focus is on drainage and debridement of well-demarcated nonviable tissues, and definitive reconstruction or rerouting is delayed until all necrosis is declared, systemic instability addressed, and tissue perfusion restored.

Nutrition

Enteral nutrition via feeding tube should be initiated as soon as hemodynamic stability is achieved. Enteral feeding maintains the integrity of the gut mucosal barrier and normal gut flora, reducing bacterial invasion and portal vein bacteremia (Kudsk 2002).

Enteral feeding is immunomodulatory, promoting production of immunoglobulin A (IgA), interleukin-4 (IL-4) and IL-10, and Th2 CD4+ helper T-lymphocyte populations. Gut disuse, with or without parenteral nutrition, results in decreased IL-4 and IL-10 secretion while production of the proinflammatory cytokines is maintained. This unbalances the ratio of pro- to antiinflammatory responses. Decreased production of IL-4 and IL-10 results in increased expression of intercellular adhesion molecule 1 (ICAM-1) and E-selectin in both the pulmonary and intestinal microvasculature, promoting neutrophil migration and organ injury (Fukatsu 2000). Enteral nutrition has been consistently associated with a lower rate of infectious morbidity (McClave *et al.* 2009) compared with no or parenteral nutrition. Enteral nutrition should be targeted to provide at least 50% to 65% of resting energy requirements (RER) over the first week of hospitalization. Current human guidelines recommend the use of parenteral nutrition in the face of enteral intolerance only after 7 days of hospitalization for patients who were healthy before the critical illness or sooner in the face of preexisting protein calorie malnutrition (McClave *et al.* 2009).

Adjunctive therapies
Steroids
Corticosteroids have a permissive role in the control of vascular smooth muscle tone. Glucocorticoids enhance catecholamine-mediated pharmacomechanical coupling at multiple levels in vascular smooth muscle cells and suppress the production of endogenous vasodilators in endothelial cells (Yang and Shang 2004). Relative adrenal insufficiency has been documented in septic dogs and is associated with refractory hypotension (Burkitt *et al.* 2007). Current sepsis guidelines for human patients recommend the use of low-dose hydrocortisone only when blood pressure has been confirmed poorly responsive to aggressive fluid therapy and vasopressors. The role of adrenal stimulation testing to guide therapy in this context is controversial and is currently discouraged in the Surviving Sepsis Campaign guidelines. Recommended steroid doses are equivalent to 0.2 to 0.5 mg/kg IV every 6 to 12 hours of hydrocortisone or prednisone sodium succinate. Steroid use has been associated with an increased incidence of superinfections (Sprung *et al.* 2008).

Bicarbonate therapy
Current guidelines recommend that bicarbonate therapy only be considered with the goal of improving hemodynamics when pH is below 7.15 in association with lactic acidemia.

Complications
Septic shock and multiorgan dysfunction syndrome are the commonest causes of death in animals with sepsis. Comorbidities such as respiratory and renal dysfunction frequently develop after 2 to 3 days of management. Respiratory dysfunction is characterized by increased microvascular permeability, resulting in disruption of the endothelial–alveolar barrier and alveolar flooding with protein-rich edema fluid. The clinical presentation is progressive respiratory distress with an alveolar/interstitial lung pattern typically in dependent lung zones. Acute lung injury is diagnosed when the PaO_2-to-FiO_2 ratio is 300 or less and acute respiratory distress syndrome (ARDS) when the PaO_2-to-FiO_2 ratio is 200 or less (Ware and Matthay 2000). Treatment is supportive, with oxygen and mechanical ventilation if necessary (Figure 2.3). A conservative fluid strategy in the management of sepsis has been shown to decrease the requirement for ventilator support (ARDS Clinical Trials Network 2006).

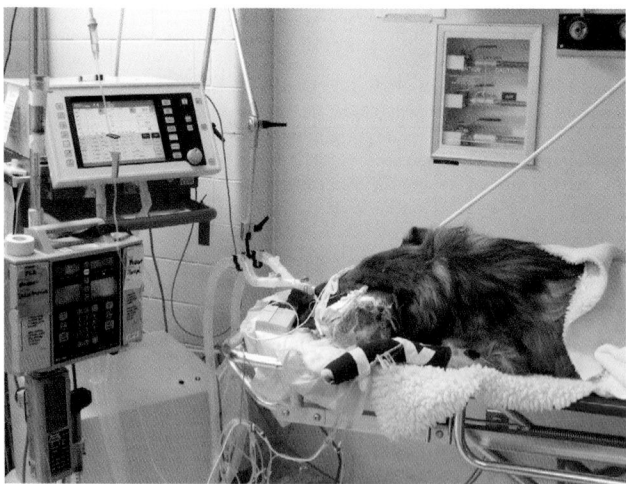
Figure 2.3 Dog with acute respiratory distress syndrome as a complication of septic peritonitis undergoing mechanical ventilator support.

Acute renal failure in sepsis is associated with hypotensive insult, failure of renal perfusion autoregulation mechanisms, microthrombosis, and exposure to endogenous and exogenous renal vasoconstrictors (e.g., norepinephrine or endothelin). Treatment is supportive.

Cellular pathophysiology of sepsis
The sepsis syndrome is the clinical result of multiple interactions between the host immune, inflammatory, and coagulation systems that culminate in disordered hemodynamics and a compromised microcirculation. Infective organisms have unique cell-wall molecules called pathogen-associated molecular patterns (PAMPs) that bind to pattern-recognition receptors (Toll-like receptors [TLRs]) on the surface of immune cells. PAMP binding initiates intracellular signal transduction pathways that activate cytosolic nuclear factor $\kappa\beta$ (NF-$\kappa\beta$). Activated NF-$\kappa\beta$ increases transcription of both pro- and antiinflammatory cytokines. Proinflammatory cytokines activate the adaptive immune response but also cause both direct and indirect host injury. Sepsis increases the activity of inducible nitric oxide synthase (iNOS), resulting in vasodilation. Endothelial cells exposed to cytokines increase the expression of adhesion receptors, binding neutrophils, macrophages, and platelets. In turn, these cells release proteases, oxidants, prostaglandins, and leukotrienes, injuring the endothelium and increasing permeability and vasodilation, as well as disrupting the anticoagulant surface (Figure 2.4).

Cytokine exposure activates the endothelial cells and circulating monocytes to express tissue factor. Tissue factor is the key in vivo initiator of coagulation. A series of events follow, resulting in activation of Va and VIIIa and the formation of the tenase and prothrombinase, culminating in the thrombin burst and the generation of microthrombi. Microvascular thrombi amplify injury through distal tissue ischemia and tissue hypoxia. Normally, natural anticoagulants protein C and S, antithrombin, and tissue factor pathway inhibitor (TFPI) dampen coagulation and enhance fibrinolysis. Thrombin binds thrombomodulin on endothelial cells, increasing the production of activated protein C. Activated protein C inactivates Va and VIIIa and decreases the synthesis of plasminogen activator inhibitor-1 (PAI-1). Sepsis decreases the levels of protein C, thrombomodulin, antithrombin, and TFPI as well and increases

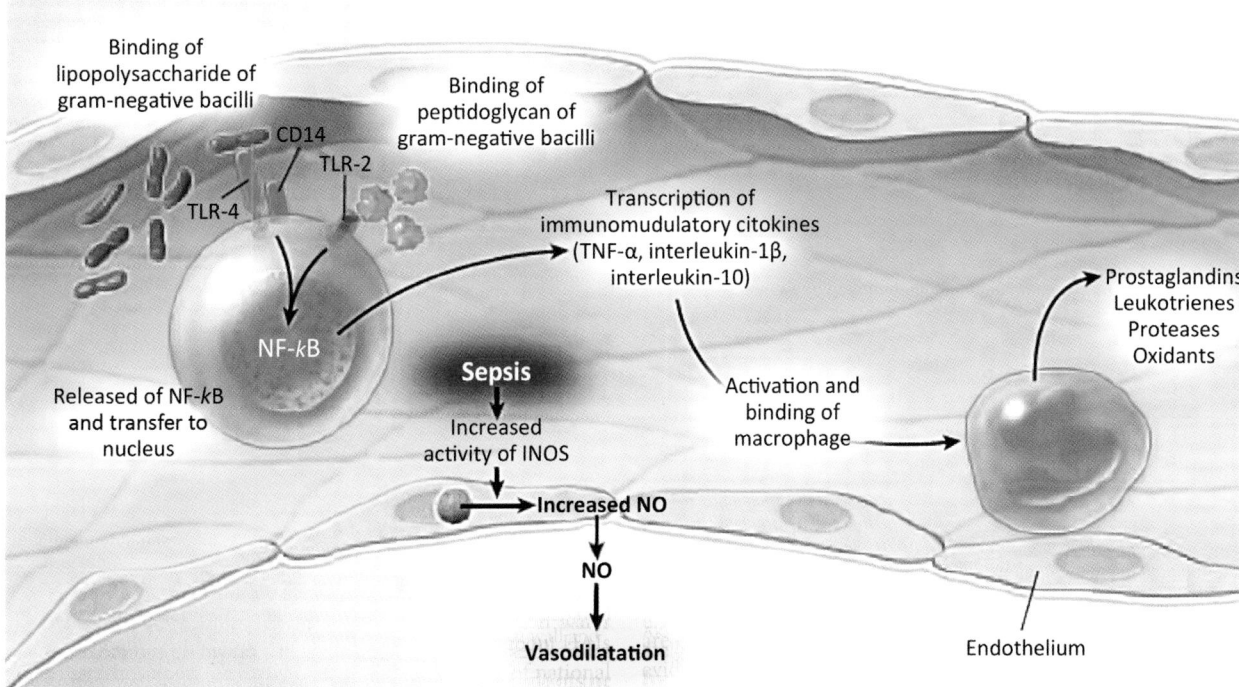

Figure 2.4 Inflammatory responses to sepsis. *Source:* Russell, 2006. Reproduced with permission from Massachusetts Medical Society.

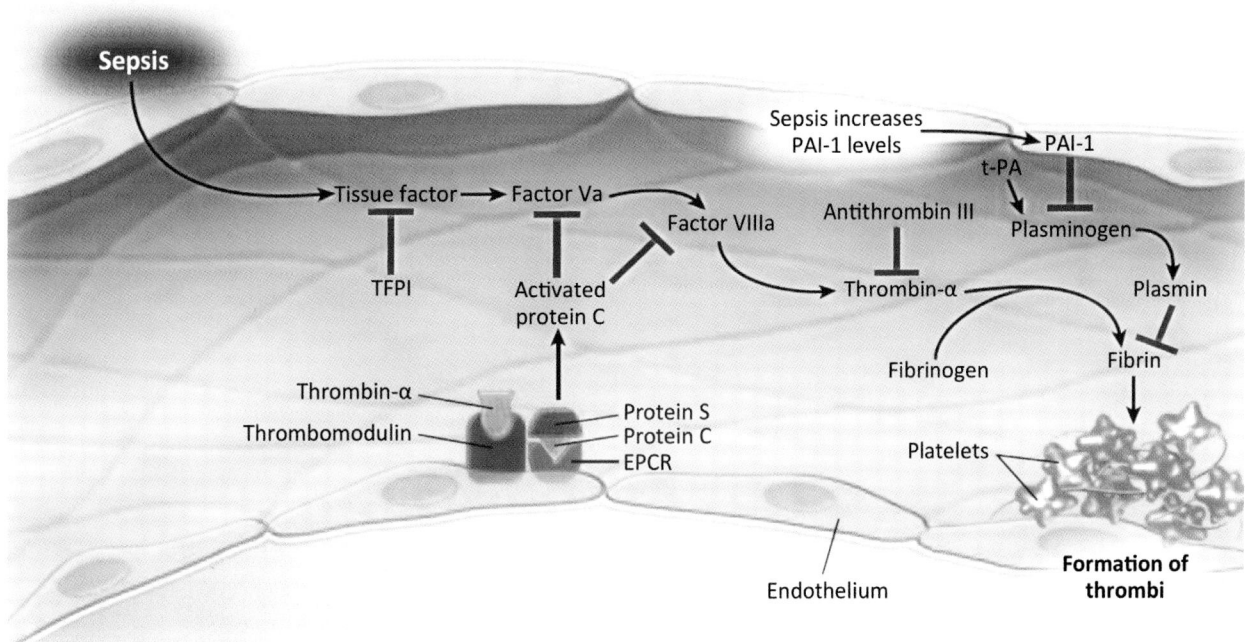

Figure 2.5 Procoagulant responses to sepsis. *Source:* Russell, 2006. Reproduced with permission from Massachusetts Medical Society.

PAI-1. This results in increases in the markers of disseminated intravascular coagulation and widespread organ dysfunction. As inflammation promotes coagulation, coagulation promotes inflammation in a positive feedback cycle. Thrombin, TF/VIIa, and Xa can activate pattern-recognition receptors on the surface of immune cells, further increasing neutrophil activation (Figure 2.5).

References

ARDS Clinical Trials Network (2006) Comparison of two fluid management strategies in acute lung injury. *The New England Journal of Medicine* 354, 2564-2575.

Arnold, R.C., Shapiro, N.I., Jones, A.E., et al. (2009) Multicenter study of early lactate clearance as a determinant of survival in patients with presumed sepsis. *Shock* 32 (1), 35-39.

Bauer, M., Kortgen, A., Hartog, C., et al. (2009) Isotonic and hypertonic crystalloid solutions in the critically ill. *Best Practice & Research Clinical Anaesthesiology* 23, 173-181.

Bayer, O., Reinhart, K., Saker, Y., et al. (2011) Renal effects of synthetic colloids and crystalloids in patients with severe sepsis: a prospective sequential comparison. *Critical Care Medicine* 39 (6), 1335-1342.

Bentley, A.M., Otto, C.M., Shofer, F.S. (2007) Comparison of dogs with septic peritonitis 1988-1993 versus 1999-2003. *Journal of Veterinary and Emergency Critical Care* 17 (4), 391-398.

Bonczynski, J.J., Ludwig, L.L., Barton, L., et al. (2003) Comparison of peritoneal fluid and peripheral blood pH, bicarbonate, glucose, and lactate concentration as a diagnostic tool for septic peritonitis in dogs and cats. *Veterinary Surgery* 31, 161-166.

Brady, C.A., Otto, C.M., Van Winkle, T., et al. (2000) Severe sepsis in cats: 29 cases (1986-1998). *Journal of the American Veterinary Medical Association* 217, 531:535.

Brunkhorst, F., Engel, C., Bloos, F. (2008) Intensive insulin therapy and pentastarch resuscitation in severe sepsis. *The New England Journal of Medicine* 358, 125-39.

Burkitt, J., Haskins, S., Nelson, R., et al. (2007) Relative adrenal insufficiency in dogs with sepsis. *Journal of Veterinary Internal Medicine* 21, 226-231.

Cowell, R.L., Tyler, R.D., Meinkoth, J.H. (1999) *Diagnostic Cytology and Hematology of the Dog and Cat*, 2nd edn. Mosby, St. Louis.

deClue, A.E., Delgado, C., Chang, C. (2011) Clinical and immunologic assessment of sepsis and the systemic inflammatory response in cats. *Journal of the American Veterinary Medical Association* 238, 890-897.

Dellinger, R.P., Levy, M.M., Carlet, J.M., et al. (2008) Surviving sepsis campaign: international guidelines for management of severe sepsis and septic shock. *Critical Care Medicine* 36, 296-327.

De Backer, D., Biston, P., Devriendt, J., et al. (2010) Comparison of dopamine and norepinephrine in the treatment of shock. *The New England Journal of Medicine* 362, 779-789.

De Laforcade, A.M., Freeman, L.M., Shaw, S.P., et al. (2003) Hemostatic changes in dogs with naturally occurring sepsis. *Journal of Veterinary Internal Medicine* 17, 674-679.

De Laforcade, A.M., Rozanski, E.A., Freeman, L.M., et al. (2008) Serial evaluation of protein C and antithrombin in dogs with sepsis. *Journal of Veterinary Internal Medicine* 22, 26-30.

Elke, G., Schadler, S., Engel, C., et al. (2008) Current practice in nutritional support and its association with mortality: a national, prospective, multicenter study. *Critical Care Medicine* 36 (6), 1762-1767.

Fukatsu, K., Lundberg, A.H., Hanna, M.K., et al. (2000) Increased expression of intestinal P-selectin and pulmonary E-selectin during intravenous total parenteral nutrition. *Archives of Surgery* 135, 1177-1182.

Gebhardt, C., Hirschberger, G., Rau, S., et al. (2009) Use of C-reactive protein to predict outcome in dogs with SIRS or sepsis. *Journal of Veterinary Emergency and Critical Care* 19 (5), 450-458.

Greco, D.S., Harpold, L.M. (1994) Immunity and the endocrine system. *Veterinary Clinics of North America: Small Animal Practice* 24 (4), 765-82.

Grimes, J.A., Schmiedt, C.W., Cornell, K.K., et al. (2011) Identification of risk factors for septic peritonitis and failure to survive following gastrointestinal surgery in dogs. *Journal of the American Veterinary Medical Association* 238, 486-494.

Hauptman, J.G., Walshaw, R., Olivier, N.B. (1997) Evaluation of sensitivity and specificity of diagnostic criteria for sepsis in dogs. *Veterinary Surgery* 26, 393-397.

Hayes, G., Mathews, K., Boston, S., et al. (2011) Low central venous oxygen saturation is associated with increased mortality risk in critically ill dogs. *Journal of Small Animal Practice* 52 (8), 433-440.

Kudsk, K.A. (2002) Current aspects of mucosal immunology and its influence by nutrition. *The American Journal of Surgery* 183, 390-398.

Kumar, A., Roberts, D., Woods, K.E., et al. (2006) Duration of hypotension prior to initiation of effective antimicrobial therapy is the critical determinant of survival in human septic shock. *Critical Care Medicine* 34, 1589-1596.

Landry, A.W., Oliver, J.A. (2001) The pathogenesis of vasodilatory shock. *The New England Journal of Medicine* 345 (8), 588-594.

Law, W.R., Moriarty, M.T., McLane, M.P. (1991) Cardiovascular sequelae of endotoxin shock in diabetic dogs. *Diabetologia* 34, 687-694.

Levy, M.M., Fink, M.P., Marshall, J.C., et al. (2003) 2001 SCCM/ESICM/ACCP/ATS/SIS International Sepsis Definitions Conference. *Critical Care Medicine* 31, 1250-1256.

Lisciandro, G.R., Lagutchik, M.S., Mann, K.A., et al. (2008) Evaluation of thoracic focused assessment with sonography for trauma (TFAST) protocol to detect pneumothorax and concurrent thoracic injury in 145 traumatized dogs. *Journal of Veterinary Emergency and Critical Care* 18 (3), 258-269.

Lisciandro, G.R., Lagutchik, M.S., Mann, K.A., et al. (2009) Evaluation of an abdominal fluid scoring system determined using abdominal focused assessment with sonography for trauma in 101 dogs with motor vehicle trauma. *Journal of Veterinary Emergency and Critical Care* 19 (5), 426-437.

Magder, S. (2005) How to use central venous pressure measurements? *Current Opinion in Critical Care* 11, 254-270.

McClave, S., Martindale, R., Vanek, V., et al. (2009) Guidelines for the provision and assessment of nutrition support therapy in the adult critically ill patient: Society of Critical Care Medicine (SCCM) and American Society for Parenteral and Enteral Nutrition (ASPEN). *Journal of Parenteral and Enteral Nutrition* 33, 277.

Minnecl, P., Deans, K., Banks, S., et al. (2004) Differing effects of norepinephrine, epinephrine, and vasopressin on survival in a canine septic shock model. *American Journal of Physiology* 287, H2545-2554.

Mori, A., Sagura, F., Shimizu, S., et al. (2008) Changes in peripheral lymphocyte subsets in type 1 diabetic dogs treated with insulin injections. *Journal of Veterinary Medical Science* 70 (2), 185-187.

Natanson, C., Fink, M., Ballantyne, H., et al. (1986) Gram negative bacteremia produces both severe systolic and diastolic cardiac dysfunction in a canine model that simulates human septic shock. *Journal of Clinical Investigation* 78, 259-270.

Natanson, C., Danner, R., Reilly, J., et al. (1990) Antibiotics versus cardiovascular support in a canine model of septic shock. *American Journal of Physiology* 259, 1440-1447.

Ogeer-Gyles, J.S., Mathews, K., Boerlin, P. (2006) Nosocomial infections and antimicrobial resistance in critical care medicine. *Journal of Veterinary Emergency and Critical Care* 16 (1), 1-18.

Piagnerelli, M., Boudjeltia, K.Z., Vanhaeverbeek, M., et al. (2003) Red blood cell rheology in sepsis. *Intensive Care Medicine* 29, 1052-1061.

Prittie, J.E. (2010) Controversies related to red blood cell transfusion in critically ill patients. *Journal of Veterinary Emergency and Critical Care* 20 (2), 167-176.

Rahal, L., Garrido, A.G., Cruz, R.J., et al. (2009) Fluid replacement with hypertonic or isotonic solutions guided by mixed venous oxygen saturation in experimental hypodynamic sepsis. *The Journal of Trauma* 67, 1205-1212.

Rogers, C.L., Rozanski, E.A. (2010) von Willebrand factor antigen concentration in dogs with sepsis. *Journal of Veterinary Internal Medicine* 24, 229-230.

Rudiger, A., Singer, M. (2007) Mechanisms of sepsis induced myocardial dysfunction. *Critical Care Medicine* 35, 1599-1608.

Russell, J. (2006) Management of sepsis. *The New England Journal of Medicine* 355, 1699-1713.

Sands, K.E., Bates, W.W., Lanken, P.N., et al. (1997) Epidemiology of sepsis syndrome in 8 academic medical centers. *Journal of the American Medical Association* 278 (3), 234-240.

Schrier, R., Wang, W. (2004) Acute renal failure in sepsis. *The New England Journal of Medicine* 351, 159-169.

Sorenmo, K.U., Harwood, L.P., King, L.G., et al. (2010) A case-control study to evaluate risk factors for the development of sepsis (neutropenia and fever) in dogs receiving chemotherapy. *Journal of the American Veterinary Medical Association* 236, 650-656.

Sprung, C., Annane, D., Keh, D., et al. (2008) Hydrocortisone therapy for patients with septic shock. *The New England Journal of Medicine* 358, 111-124.

Szabo, S.D., Jermyn, K., Neel, J., et al. (2011) Evaluation of postceliotomy peritoneal drain fluid volume, cytology, and blood-to-peritoneal fluid lactate and glucose differences in normal dogs. *Veterinary Surgery* 40 (4), 444-449.

Vincent, J.L., Weil, M.H. (2006) Fluid challenge revisited. *Critical Care Medicine* 34, 1333-1337.

Ware, L., Matthay, M. (2000) The acute respiratory distress syndrome. *The New England Journal of Medicine* 342 (18), 1334-1349.

Weil, M.H. & Shubin, H. (1969) The "VIP" approach to the bedside management of shock. *Journal of the American Medical Association* 207 (2), 337-340.

Wills, B.A., Nguyen, M.D., Ha, T.L., et al. (2005) Comparison of three fluid solutions for resuscitation in dengue shock syndrome. *The New England Journal of Medicine* 353, 877-889.

Yang, S., Shang, L. (2004) Glucocorticoids and vascular reactivity. *Current Vascular Pharmacology* 2, 1-12.

3

Pyothorax

Jackie L. Demetriou

Dick White Referrals, Suffolk and University of Nottingham, Nottingham, UK

Definition and pathophysiology

Pyothorax is the accumulation of exudate within the thoracic cavity. Under normal circumstances, a small amount of transudative fluid is present within the pleural space, allowing smooth movement of thoracic structures during the process of respiration. A pleural effusion develops when the production of pleural fluid exceeds absorption by alterations in hydrostatic and oncotic pressures, permeability in vascular membranes, and flow through the lymphatic system. This alteration in fluid dynamics can occur with a number of noninflammatory and inflammatory disease processes (MacPhail 2007). When infection affects the adjacent lung or vascular tissue, an immune response is activated, and pleural inflammation occurs, resulting in an increased vascular permeability and allowing migration of inflammatory cells (neutrophils, lymphocytes, and eosinophils) into the pleural space. Mediation of this inflammatory process occurs via a number of cytokines (e.g., interleukin-1, -6, and -8; tumor necrosis factor-α; and platelet activation factor), which are released by mesothelial cells lining the pleural space. This initial stage of pyothorax progresses to deposition of fibrin within the pleural space and eventually to the formation of scar tissue (Balfour-Lynn *et al.* 2005).

Etiology

The precise etiology of pyothorax in dogs and cats remains undefined in the majority of cases. In dogs, an underlying etiology has been definitively diagnosed in only 4% to 21%, with most studies suggesting an inhaled or penetrating foreign body being the likely source of infection (Demetriou *et al.* 2002; Rooney and Monnet 2002; MacPhail 2007; Boothe *et al.* 2010). Other reported causes in dogs include penetrating bite wounds, extension of bronchial or pulmonary infection, parasitic infection, pulmonary or thoracic wall trauma, hematogenous spread, or iatrogenic causes such as postoperative infection (MacPhail 2007). Grass awn foreign bodies are suspected to play an important role in the pathogenesis of pyothorax in dogs. Grass awns that are inhaled through the upper airway during exercise are thought to migrate down into bronchi and lungs and eventually penetrate through the pulmonary parenchyma into the thoracic cavity. A pulmonary abscess may or may not be found in association with a foreign body. However, one study that reported 182 cases of grass awn migration in dogs and cats found only three cases associated with thoracic migration, which casts some doubt on the purportedly close relationship between grass awns and pyothorax (Brennan and Ihrke 1983).

Possible routes of infection in cats are similar to those in dogs; however, evidence suggests that parapneumonic spread is the most common route of infection of the pleural space because bacterial isolates from the majority of cases of pyothorax in this species are polymicrobial and similar in composition to the normal feline oropharyngeal flora (Love *et al.* 1982; Barrs and Beatty 2009a). In earlier reports, it was thought that access of oropharyngeal flora to the thoracic space was via penetrating bite wounds, but more recent work suggests that aspiration of the flora is more significant (Barrs *et al.* 2005). Aspiration results in colonization of the lower respiratory tract with oropharyngeal bacteria and extension of infection into the pleural space from the bronchi or lungs. This is very similar to the pathophysiology of empyema in humans. Postmortem evaluation in cats with pyothorax has revealed an incidence of pneumonia or focal pulmonary abscessation in 7 of 15 (47%) cases (Hayward 1968; Davies and Forrester 1996). Furthermore, other reports have also consistently reported the presence of diffuse or focal pulmonary lesions in cats with pyothorax, which supports the link between pleural space infection and lower airway infection (Barrs and Beatty 2009a). One study reported that there was a higher likelihood of cats with pyothorax coming from multi-cat households (Waddell 2002), suggesting that increased aggression was the most likely reason, despite only 16% of cases having confirmed evidence of a thoracic bite wound on postmortem examination. The potential higher incidence of viral upper respiratory tract infections may be a viable alternative explanation for the increased incidence of pyothorax in this population.

Microbiology

Species of bacteria most commonly associated with pyothorax differ in cats versus dogs. In cats, *Pasteurella* spp. is by far the predominant species cultured; in dogs, a wider variety of bacteria have been associated with the condition, mainly obligate anaerobes or a mixture of obligate anaerobes with facultative aerobic bacteria. Table 3.1 illustrates bacterial species found in one study that looked at 50 cases of pyothorax, of which 36 were dogs and 14 were cats (Demetriou *et al.* 2002). In this study, cultures were positive in 33 cases with 8 of 33 (24%) cultures containing more than one organism. A further study examining the prevalence of aerobic bacteria in dogs and cats showed *Pasteurella* spp. to account for 70% of feline aerobic isolates compared with 37% of canine isolates (Walker *et al.* 2000). The most common anaerobic species isolated in dogs and cats were *Peptostreptococcus anaerobius* and *Bacteroides* spp., respectively, in this study.

Complications in Small Animal Surgery, First Edition. Edited by Dominique Griffon and Annick Hamaide.

© 2016 John Wiley & Sons, Inc. Published 2016 by John Wiley & Sons, Inc.

Companion website: www.wiley.com/go/griffon/complications

Table 3.1 Anaerobic and aerobic bacterial cultured from the pleural fluid of 33 cases of canine and feline pyothorax

Bacteria	Number of patients (%)	
	Dog	**Cat**
Anaerobic		
Bacteroides spp.	2	1
Peptostreptococcus anaerobius	4 (12.5)	0
Fusobacterium spp.	1	0
Clostridium spp.	1	0
Unidentified gram-negative rods	0	1
Aerobic		
Pasteurella spp.	7 (22)	5 (62.50)
Escherichia coli	3 (9)	0
Proteus spp.	1	0
Streptococcus spp.	2 (6)	0
Staphylococcus intermedius	1	0
Actinomyces spp.	3	0
Nocardia spp.	6 (19)	1
Unidentified filamentous organisms	1	

Source: Adapted from Demetriou *et al.* (2002).

Incidence

Four studies have examined the incidence of pyothorax from hospital records with varying conditions or procedures. A feline study evaluating severe sepsis in cats reported an incidence of pyothorax in 7 of 29 (24%), which was the most common diagnosis in this cohort of patients (Brady *et al.* 2000). In total, 24 of 29 (83%) of cats with severe sepsis had evidence of pulmonary or pleural disease, and the authors proposed that the lungs appear to be particularly susceptible to damage during shock or sepsis in cats. In a study that examined the etiology of canine pleural and mediastinal effusions (Mellanby *et al.* 2002), pyothorax was identified in 13 of 81 (16%) patients and was the most common cause of pleural or mediastinal effusion. In another retrospective study of 98 animals that underwent intrathoracic surgery (Tattersall and Welsh 2006), pyothorax was the diagnosis of 13/98 (13%) of cases undergoing thoracic surgery. Furthermore, a recent study evaluated the incidence of postoperative pyothorax in 232 dogs undergoing thoracic surgery (Meakin *et al.* 2010) identified 15 patients (6.5%) as having postoperative pyothorax.

Risk factors

Risk factors for pyothorax in cats and dogs can be broadly divided into factors relating to the development of preoperative or postoperative pyothorax.

Preoperative pyothorax

- Multi-cat household

Postoperative pyothorax

- Body weight
- Presence of preoperative pleural effusion
- Preoperative thoracocentesis
- Preoperative intrathoracic biopsy
- Diagnosis of chylothorax

- Duration of anaesthesia and surgery
- Number of postoperative thoracostomy tubes

Diagnosis

Signalment and clinical signs

The average age at presentation is between 4 and 5 years for cases of canine and feline pyothorax, although it may occur in all age groups. One report found that cats with pyothorax were significantly younger (mean, 3.83 ± 3.43 years) compared with a control population of cats (mean, 5.62 ± 5.27 years) (Waddell *et al.* 2002). A specific breed predisposition has not been identified, although Labrador retrievers, Springer spaniels, and Border collies appear to be the most common breeds affected. Males are more commonly affected, although this has not been demonstrated to be a significant finding. Clinical signs of pyothorax are well documented with the majority of dogs and cats presenting with dyspnea (69% and 79%, respectively). Other common clinical signs include tachycardia or bradycardia, pyrexia, depression or lethargy, weight loss, and hypersalivation (Demetriou *et al.* 2002; Waddell *et al.* 2002). The time to presentation from onset of clinical signs is usually several weeks. In one study, pyothorax was confirmed a medium of 7 days after surgery (range, 4–24 days) in patients developing the condition after thoracic surgery (Meakin *et al.* 2010).

Laboratory and diagnostic imaging findings

The most common **hematologic and biochemical findings** in canine and feline pyothorax are anemia, neutrophilic leucocytosis with a left shift, and hypoalbuminemia. Other findings may include elevations in ALT or ALP, hypoglycemia, hyperglobulinemia, elevated urea, elevated creatinine, electrolyte abnormalities (hyponatremia, hypochloremia) and increased bile acids. Information on the feline leukemia virus (FeLV) and feline immunodeficiency virus (FIV) status of cats with pyothorax is sparse, but in evidence collated from multiple studies, approximately 4% of cats with pyothorax tested positive for FeLV, and approximately 6% were positive for FIV. This compares with a prevalence of FIV of 1% to 14% in asymptomatic cats and 44% in symptomatic cats (Barrs and Beatty 2009).

Thoracocentesis typically reveals an opaque, flocculent fluid that may be hemorrhagic. A septic exudate is confirmed by **fluid analysis**, including cytology, with protein levels greater than 3.0 g/dL, specific gravity greater than 1.025, nucleated cell count greater than 3000 g/dL and the presence of degenerate neutrophils (the main cell type). Intracellular bacteria are commonly associated with an active infection but may not be present if antimicrobials have already been started. It is often the case that a mixed population of bacteria is present, so Gram staining can be helpful in determining the class of bacteria, which in turn can help guide antimicrobial drug choice.

Thoracic radiography will confirm the presence of a unilateral or bilateral pleural effusion, but this should be delayed if the patient is dyspneic and unstable. In addition to assessing the degree of pleural effusion and documenting whether it is unilateral or bilateral, thoracic radiography may also uncover a possible underlying cause or associated comorbidities such as a mediastinal or pulmonary mass, foreign body, pneumothorax, or pneumomediastinum.

Ultrasonography is also a central tool in the evaluation of pyothorax. It provides a dynamic assessment of the thorax and may estimate the size of the pleural collection, document the presence of septations or loculations, guide thoracostomy tube placement, and aid in aspiration of fluid.

Recently, the role of **computed tomography** (CT) has been examined in relation to surgical findings. A recent study evaluated and correlated CT and surgical findings in canine patients of pyothorax and reported how frequently CT accurately identified parameters that were later confirmed at surgery (Swinbourne *et al.* 2011). With many parameters, CT and surgical findings were similar (fluid, pleural thickening), but CT tended to identify focal disease more frequently than was identified at surgery. The significance of CT in the diagnosis of pyothorax is unclear, but its use may be helpful in guiding treatment decisions.

Treatment

Treatment of pyothorax in cats and dogs can be broadly divided into medical and surgical treatments.

Medical treatment may be conservative treatment (i.e., use of antimicrobials alone), but better treatment outcomes are achieved if this is combined with some form of drainage using thoracostomy tubes or large–bore catheters placed either unilaterally or bilaterally (Waddell *et al.* 2002; Boothe *et al.* 2010) as illustrated in Figure 3.1. Recently, there has been a trend to use small-bore thoracostomy tubes, which can be readily placed under sedation, tend to be less painful, and have been proven to be successful in cases of pyothorax (Frendin and Obel 1997; Valtolina and Adamantos 2009). One report (Johnson and Martin 2007) reported successful treatment of pyothorax in 15 cases that were managed with a single drainage technique under ultrasound guidance, so further consideration should be given to the use of imaging techniques to maximize drainage of the thoracic cavity or guide thoracostomy tube placement.

In addition to thoracic drainage, the pleural cavity can be lavaged, with the aim being to reduce the bacterial load and inflammatory mediators and prevent tube obstruction with exudate and breakdown of the fibrinous adhesions, which can separate the cavity and prevent adequate drainage. In dogs, thoracic lavage can be performed by instillation of warmed crystalloid solutions (typically 0.9% saline or lactated Ringer's solution) at a rate of 10 to 20 mL/kg into the thoracostomy tube in 1 to 3 aliquots. In cats, a total volume of 200 mL instilled in 50- to 100-mL aliquots was used in one study (Barrs and Beatty 2009b). The patient is then gently repositioned to encourage distribution of the fluid, and then the fluid is aspirated. One study suggested aspiration after a delay of 30 minutes; however,

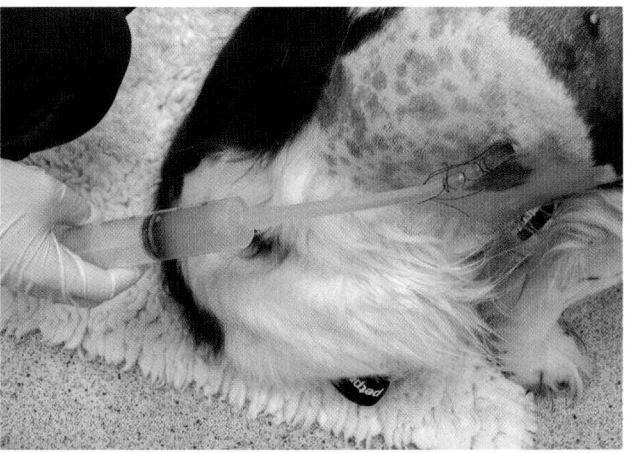

Figure 3.1 Drainage of a pyothorax using a wide-bore thoracostomy tube in a Springer spaniel.

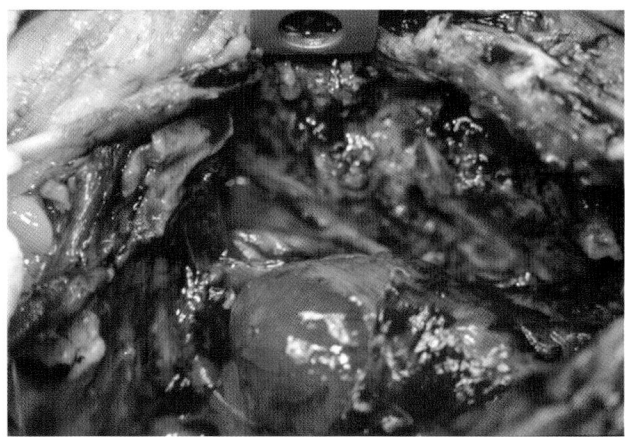

Figure 3.2 A median sternotomy to treat a pyothorax in a cat showing fibrinous material on the visceral surfaces and pericardium.

in this study, heparin was also used in the majority of patients, and this addition was found to provide a higher short-term survival rate (Boothe *et al.* 2010). Retrieval of a minimum of 75% of instilled lavage solution is expected. In most cases, lavage is performed more than once daily (usually between two and five times daily). Hypokalemia has been reported as a complication of thoracic lavage in cats. Antimicrobial choice should ideally be based on the culture and sensitivity result of the pleural fluid; however, empirically, it is prudent to select drugs that are effective against gram-positive and gram-negative aerobes and anaerobes. Treatment is usually administered for a minimum of 4 weeks, with recommendations of more than 6 weeks if *Actinomyces* spp. or *Nocardia* spp. are suspected or confirmed.

Surgical treatment involves exploratory thoracotomy (usually by median sternotomy) with debridement of the thoracic cavity and removal of any identifiable foreign bodies (Figure 3.2). From the limited number of surgical patients reported in the veterinary literature, open surgery, either by means of a median sternotomy or intercostal thoracotomy, results in good treatment outcomes, reported in the range of 70% to 100% (Demetriou *et al.* 2002; Rooney and Monnet 2002; Waddell *et al.* 2002; Boothe *et al.* 2010). The main aims of surgery are debridement of the thoracic cavity, removal of exudate, exploration of the thorax for any potential underlying cause, and lavage of the cavity to reduce the bacterial and inflammatory load. If both sides of the cavity are affected, a median sternotomy is likely to be the procedure of choice to allow a full and thorough inspection. Before closure, either unilateral or bilateral thoracostomy tubes are placed to continue drainage and possibly lavage. More recently, thoracoscopy has been described as a minimally invasive method of exploring pyothorax (Monnet 2009). Potential benefits of this procedure include guiding accurate thoracostomy tube placement and close assessment of the thorax with reduced morbidity compared with open procedures.

There is some debate regarding which treatment is better, but the majority of studies show that initial medical management in cases of spontaneous (i.e., nontraumatic) pyothorax, using thoracostomy tubes, with or without lavage, in combination with systemic antimicrobials is efficacious. Successful outcomes are achieved in 71% to 100% of cases managed by this method (Piek and Robben 2000; Demetriou *et al.* 2002; Barrs *et al.* 2005; Johnson and Martin 2007; Boothe *et al.* 2010). The main question that is as yet unanswered is at what point patients should undergo surgery (i.e., how is medical failure defined)? Most studies cite radiographic evidence

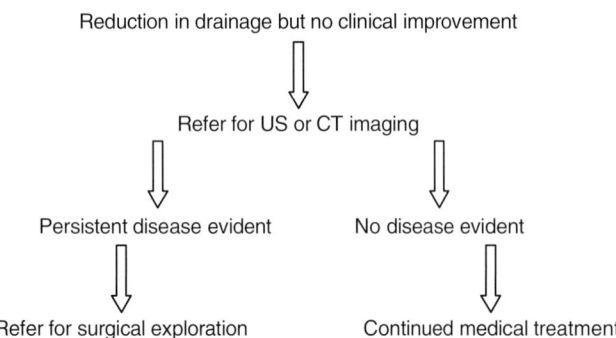

Figure 3.3 An algorithm that may be used to guide management of pyothorax in cats and dogs. CT, computed tomography; US, ultrasonography. *Source:* Adapted from St. Peter *et al.* (2009).

of pulmonary or mediastinal lesions or failure of medical management, although this appears to be highly subjective. The algorithm illustrated in Figure 3.3 can be used as a guide for treatment in cases in which initial medical management is appropriate. Certainly, in cases in which a foreign body is identified or there is a high index of suspicion of a foreign body, surgery should be considered as a first-line treatment. Cases that are medically managed with thoracostomy tubes should be monitored daily on the basis of clinical parameters, fluid production, and cytology results to assess the patient's progress, and the decision for surgical intervention should probably be based on deteriorating or nonimprovement of these three factors.

Outcomes and prognostic indicators

Both medical and surgical management of patients with pyothorax seem to be effective methods to treat the condition. Primary medical management using thoracostomy tubes and antimicrobials with or without lavage is still used in the majority of cases successfully. Various factors have been discussed in the veterinary literature in relation to outcomes and prognosis of pyothorax in either species.
- Surgery versus medical management
- Postoperative wound infection
- *Actinomyces* spp.
- Pleural lavage and heparin
- Low heart rates and hypersalivation
- Low white blood cell count

Relevant literature

Two studies have examined **risk factors** for the development of pyothorax in cats and dogs (Waddell *et al.* 2002; Meakin *et al.* 2010). One of the studies (Waddell *et al.* 2002) examined risk factors, prognostic indicators, and outcome of pyothorax in 80 cats. The authors found no specific gender, age, or breed predisposition. Cats with pyothorax were 3.8 times likely to come from **multi-cat households** and were 1.6 times as likely to have outdoor access compared with control animals, although the latter finding was not significant. Vaccination status was not significantly difference between cats with pyothorax and control animals.

The other study (Meakin *et al.* 2010) examining the risk factors for postoperative pyothorax in dogs found that **body weight** was significantly greater in dogs with postoperative pyothorax (37 ± 16 kg) compared with those without (22 ± 16 kg). Age, sex, National Research Council surgical site contamination classification, pericardial fluid, pneumothorax, primary diagnosis apart from idiopathic chylothorax, antibiotic use, and need for reoperation were not significantly associated with postoperative pyothorax.

Postoperative pyothorax was, however, significantly associated with **preoperative pleural fluid, preoperative thoracocentesis,** and **preoperative intrathoracic biopsy.** For the 15 dogs with postoperative pyothorax, 12 (80%) had preoperative pleural fluid; 13 (87%) underwent preoperative thoracocentesis, and 2 (13%) had a preoperative intrathoracic biopsy.

A diagnosis of **idiopathic chylothorax** was significantly associated with postoperative pyothorax, with 9 of 16 dogs with idiopathic chylothorax included in the study developing postoperative pyothorax.

Dogs diagnosed with pyothorax postoperatively also had significantly **longer mean duration of anesthesia and surgery** (306 ± 71 minutes and 197 ± 65 minutes) compared with those without (224 ± 93 minutes and 132 ± 64 minutes).

The **number of thoracostomy tubes placed postoperatively** was also significantly associated with the development of pyothorax. For the 217 dogs without postoperative pyothorax, 3 (1%), 208 (96%), and 6 (3%) had none, 1, and 2 postoperative thoracostomy tubes, respectively. In comparison, for the 15 dogs with pyothorax, 10 (67%) and 5 (33%) had 1 and 2 postoperative thoracostomy tubes, respectively.

In one study (Rooney and Monnet 2002), **surgical management** of pyothorax cases was reported to be associated with significantly better outcomes **compared with medical management**, with treatment more than five times more likely to fail in medically treated patients, although these results are not supported by a recent study that reported no difference between surgically and medically managed patients (Boothe *et al.* 2010).

A study that reported on factors that influenced the short-term outcomes of dogs undergoing thoracic surgery reported a higher incidence of **postoperative wound infections** in dogs having surgery to treat pyothorax (6 of 11; 11.5%), although the study also showed that any thoracic surgeries carried out by median sternotomy were associated with significantly more wound infections compared with surgeries approached by an intercostal thoracotomy (Tattersall and Welsh 2006). This study also reported a mean surgical time of 153.8 minutes, a mean thoracic drain placement time of 88.4 minutes, and short-term complications occurring in 7 of 13 (54%) pyothorax cases. Furthermore, 3 of 13 (27%) surgical case of pyothorax died within 2 weeks of surgery.

Actinomyces **spp.** has been reported to be associated with better outcomes if dogs positive for *Actinomyces* spp. are treated surgically rather than medically (Rooney and Monnet 2002). This is thought to be because *Actinomyces* spp. is most frequently associated with the presence of plant material.

Pleural lavage and heparin treatment may also increase the likelihood of short- and long-term survival (Boothe *et al.* 2010). The same study demonstrated that short-term survival rates were not related to bacterial species or volume of pleural fluid.

A feline study (Waddell *et al.* 2002) reported that nonsurvivors had significantly **lower heart rates** than survivors, and **hypersalivation** was significantly more common in nonsurvivors (11 of 39; 27%) than survivors (1 of 39; 3%). Furthermore, the **white blood**

cell count was significantly higher in survivors compared with those that died.

Several studies reported that patients with pyothorax were more likely to die within 48 hours of presentation, and if they survive beyond this time, then treatment is likely to be successful (Demetriou *et al.* 2002; Mellanby *et al.* 2002; Boothe *et al.* 2010).

The majority of human cases of empyema develop as a progression of a "simple" self-resolving parapneumonic pleural effusion into a "complicated" fibrinopurulent collection within the thoracic cavity. The development of empyema in conjunction with pneumonia is a progressive process and has been classified into three recognized stages as (1) a simple exudate, (2) a fibrinopurulent stage, and (3) a later organizing stage with scar tissue (pleural peel) formation. The vast majority of patients presenting at stage 1 are successfully managed by conservative (antimicrobial) treatment only. In cases of stage 2 and 3, further intervention is required, either with thoracostomy tubes or open or minimally invasive surgery. Evidence at present appears to indicate that primary medical management remains the first line of approach in treating patients with this condition (Balfour-Lynn *et al.* 2005). The use of fibrinolytic therapy in conjunction with thoracostomy tubes to aid breakdown of fibrin and pockets of fluid is common, although some debate still exists regarding their benefits. Video-assisted thoracoscopy is more widely used in the human field and appears to have at least equivalent, if not better, outcomes compared with open surgery in the treatment of patients with stage 2 disease.

References

Balfour-Lynn, I.M., Abrahamson, E., Cohen, G., et al. (2005) British Thoracic Society for the management of pleural infection in children. *Thorax* 60 (Suppl. I), i1-i21.

Barrs, V.R., Beatty, J.A. (2009a) Feline pyothorax: new insights into an old problem: part 1. Aetiopathogenesis and diagnostic investigation. *The Veterinary Journal* 179, 163-170.

Barrs, V.R., Beatty, J.A. (2009b) Feline pyothorax: new insights into an old problem: part 2. Treatment, recommendations and prophylaxis. *The Veterinary Journal* 179, 171-178.

Barrs, V.R., Martin, P., Allan, G.S., et al. (2005) Feline pyothorax: a retrospective study of 27 cases in Australia. *Journal of Feline Medicine and Surgery* 7, 211-222.

Boothe, H.W., Howe, L.M., Boothe, D.M. et al. (2010) Evaluation of outcomes in dogs treated for pyothorax: 46 cases (1983-2001). *Journal of the American Veterinary Medical Association* 236 (6), 657-663.

Brady, C.A., Otto, C.M., Van Winkle, T.J., et al. (2000) Severe sepsis in cats: 29 cases (1986-1998). *Journal of the American Veterinary Medical Association* 217 (4), 531-535.

Brennan, K.E., Ihrke, P.J. (1983) Grass awn migration in dogs and cats: a retrospective study of 182 cases. *Journal of the American Veterinary Medical Association* 182, 1201-1204.

Davies, C., Forrester, S.D. (1996) Pleural effusions in cats: 82 cases (1987-1995). *Journal of Small Animal Practice* 37, 217-224.

Demetriou, J.L., Foale, R.D., Ladlow, J., et al. (2002) Canine and feline pyothorax: a retrospective study of 50 cases in the UK and Ireland. *Journal of Small Animal Practice* 43, 388-394.

Frendin, J., Obel, N. (1997) Catheter drainage of pleural fluid collections and pneumothorax. *Journal of Small Animal Practice* 38, 237-242.

Hayward, A.H.S. (1968) Thoracic effusions in the cat. *Journal of Small Animal Practice* 9, 75-82.

Johnson, M.S., Martin, M.W.S. (2007) Successful medical treatment of 15 dogs with pyothorax. *Journal of Small Animal Practice* 48, 12-16.

Love, D.N., Jones, R.F., Bailey, M., et al. (1982) Isolation and characterisation of bacterial from pyothorax (empyaemia) in cats. *Veterinary Microbiology* 7, 455-461.

MacPhail, C.M. (2007) Medical and surgical management of pyothorax. *Veterinary Clinics of North America: Small Animal Practice* 37 (5), 975-988, vii.

Meakin, L., Salonen, L., Baines, S., et al. (2010) Post-operative pyothorax in dogs undergoing thoracic surgery: incidence and risk factors. In: Baines, S.J. (ed.) *Proceedings of the European College of Veterinary Surgeons*, Helsinki, p. 221.

Mellanby, R.J., Villiers, E., Herrtage, M.E. (2002) Canine pleural and mediastinal effusions: a retrospective study of 81 cases. *Journal of Small Animal Practice* 43, 447-451.

Monnet, E. (2009) Interventional thoracoscopy in small animals. *Veterinary Clinics of North America: Small Animal Practice* 39 (5), 965-975.

Piek, C.J., Robben, J.H. (2000) Pyothorax in nine dogs. *The Veterinary Quarterly* 22 (2), 107-111.

Rooney, M.B., Monnet, E. (2002) Medical and surgical treatment of pyothorax in dogs: 26 cases (1991-2001). *Journal of the American Veterinary Medical Association* 221 (1), 86-92.

St. Peter, S.D., Tsao, D., Harrison, C., et al. (2009) Thoracoscopic decortications vs tube thoracostomy with fibrinolysis for empyema in children: a prospective randomized trial. *Journal of Pediatric Surgery* 44, 106-111.

Swinbourne, F., Baines, E.A., Baines, S.J., et al. (2011) Computed tomographic findings in canine pyothorax and correlation with findings at exploratory thoracotomy. *Journal of Small Animal Practice* 52, 203-208.

Tattersall, J.A., Welsh, E. (2006) Factors influencing the short-term outcome following thoracic surgery in 98 dogs. *Journal of Small Animal Practice* 47, 715-720.

Valtolina, C., Adamantos, S. (2009) Evaluation of small-bore wire-guided chest drains for management of pleural space disease. *Journal of Small Animal Practice* 50, 290-297.

Waddell, L.S., Brady, C.A., Drobatz, K.J. (2002) Risk factors, prognostic indicators, and outcome of pyothorax in cats: 80 cases (1986-1999). *Journal of the American Veterinary Medical Association* 221 (6), 819-824.

Walker, A.L., Jang, S.S., Hirsh, D.C. (2000) Bacteria associated with pyothorax of dogs and cats: 98 cases (1989-1998). *Journal of the American Veterinary Medical Association* 216 (3), 359-363.

4 Peritonitis

Marjan Doom[1] and Hilde de Rooster[2]
[1]Department of Morphology, Faculty of Veterinary Medicine, Ghent University, Ghent, Belgium
[2]Department of Small Animal Medicine and Clinical Biology, Faculty of Veterinary Medicine, Ghent University, Ghent, Belgium

Peritonitis in dogs and cats is a potential postoperative complication but also a frequent indication for abdominal surgery. Moreover, peritonitis present before gastrointestinal (GI) surgery is a risk factor for postoperative leakage resulting in septic peritonitis. Consequently, a surgeon can be faced with the management of peritonitis under numerous circumstances. Whether the cause is iatrogenic or not, the condition is associated with high mortality rate.

Classification

Peritonitis can be classified as primary or secondary, aseptic or septic, and localized or generalized (Table 4.1).

Primary or spontaneous peritonitis is defined as an inflammation of the peritoneum in the absence of an apparent intraabdominal source of contamination or history of penetrating trauma. This condition is often associated with a compromised immunocompetence (Swann and Hughes 2000; Culp *et al.* 2009). It is very rare in dogs. In cats, primary peritonitis is occasionally encountered in the form of feline infectious peritonitis or as peritonitis without an identifiable underlying cause (Swann and Hughes 2000; Costello *et al.* 2004).

Secondary peritonitis is encountered by far more frequently in companion animals and is associated with a preexisting abdominal pathology (Swann and Hughes 2000; Culp and Holt 2010). It can be either aseptic (sterile) or septic.

Secondary aseptic peritonitis can be further categorized into mechanical and foreign body, granulomatous, chemical, or sclerosing encapsulating peritonitis. All abdominal surgeries result in aseptic peritonitis through the exposure of the mesothelial surface to air during celiotomy or laparoscopy. However, the evoked inflammation is usually mild and subclinical (Crowe and Bjorling 1993). Surgically induced peritonitis may be further enhanced by sterile foreign bodies such as suture material or a retained surgical sponge (Crowe and Bjorling 1993; Swann and Hughes 2000). Contamination with cornstarch surgical glove powder is associated with adhesion formation and granulomatous peritonitis (Edlich 2009). Sterile chemical substances induce inflammation and lead to chemical peritonitis. Sources of endogenous chemical contamination are gastric and pancreatic secretions, bile, and urine (Crowe and Bjorling 1993; McGrotty and Doust 2004). Exogenous chemical sources are usually iatrogenic such as intraperitoneal drug administration or sterile abdominal lavage solutions (Crowe and Bjorling 1993). Chemically induced aseptic peritonitis is prone to develop into septic peritonitis. Diffuse capillary damage by chemical burn facilitates migration of bacteria through the damaged intestinal wall (MacCoy 1981; Hosgood and Salisbury 1988). This is in particular the case for bile peritonitis (Ludwig *et al.* 1997). Sclerosing encapsulating peritonitis is a very rare chronic form of aseptic peritonitis in which the abdominal organs become encased in layers of connective tissue (Swann and Hughes 2000).

Secondary septic peritonitis is the most common form of peritonitis in small animal patients. In the majority of cases, the source of contamination is the GI tract. The urinary and reproductive tract, the hepatobiliary system, and the pancreas, as well as the external environment (through penetrating abdominal wounds) also represent potential infectious sources.

A recurrent or persistent intraabdominal infection after an apparently successful and adequate surgical source control of secondary peritonitis is called a **tertiary peritonitis** (Chromik *et al.* 2009). It has been reported in humans but not yet in companion animals.

Local host defense mechanisms attempt to contain and eliminate the insult, thus limiting the inflammation to a **localized peritonitis** (MacCoy 1981). Removal mechanisms (diaphragmatic lymphatic absorption) are used alongside the killing mechanisms (macrophages and polymorphonuclear leukocytes). Through the formation of fibrin, microorganisms are incorporated into a polymerizing matrix. Fibronectin in the peritoneal fluid acts as a nonspecific pathogen binding molecule (Dunn *et al.* 1985). Last but not least, the omentum plays a crucial role in the peritoneal host defense mechanism through formation of adhesions and its leukocyte aggregates, so-called the milky spots (Liebermann-Meffert 2000). If local defense mechanisms are unsuccessful, a local inflammatory process will evolve to **generalized peritonitis** (MacCoy 1981).

Complications in Small Animal Surgery, First Edition. Edited by Dominique Griffon and Annick Hamaide.
© 2016 John Wiley & Sons, Inc. Published 2016 by John Wiley & Sons, Inc.
Companion website: www.wiley.com/go/griffon/complications

Table 4.1 Classification of peritonitis

			Source of contamination	
Primary peritonitis			Absence of intraabdominal source	
Secondary peritonitis	Aseptic	Mechanical and foreign object	Iatrogenic	
		Granulomatous	Iatrogenic	
		Chemical	Endogenous or exogenous chemical source	
		Sclerosing encapsulating	Previous surgery or peritonitis; ingestion of glass fiber; idiopathic	
	Septic	Gastrointestinal tract	Leakage of content caused by trauma, infection or inflammation, neoplasia, obstruction, or foreign bodies. Changes in intestinal or uterine wall permeability	Iatrogenic
		Urinary tract		
		Reproductive tract		
		Hepatobiliary system		
		Exogenous environment	Penetrating trauma, ostium abdominale	
Tertiary peritonitis			Uncontrolled secondary peritonitis	

Pathophysiology

At the onset of peritonitis, mesothelial cellular damage results in a release of histamine, lysosomal enzymes, and kinins. This cascade leads to an increase in vascular permeability with a subsequent leakage of a protein-rich fluid as well as an influx of inflammatory cells into the peritoneal cavity (MacCoy 1981; Ludwig 2004). Given the large peritoneal surface, fluid and protein loss can be massive. Under normal circumstances, peritoneal fluid returns to the systemic circulation via the diaphragmatic lymphatics. However, in case of peritonitis, these lymphatics become blocked with fibrin, resulting in further fluid pooling (Holt and Brown 1999). The shift of the circulatory volume to the peritoneal cavity leads to a decrease in blood pressure countered by an increase in cardiac output and peripheral vasoconstriction. The subsequent fall in blood pressure deteriorates tissue perfusion, leading to a shift to anaerobic glycolysis and further damage to the capillary and intestinal walls. Intestinal bacteria and bacterial toxins may thereupon enter the bloodstream, resulting in bacteremia (MacCoy 1981).

Diagnosis

Clinical signs

Clinical signs of peritonitis are for the most part nonspecific. Depending on the severity of the disease and the extensiveness of the inflammatory process, clinical signs may vary greatly. Most animals are presented with a vague history of anorexia, vomiting, depression, or lethargy (Swann and Hughes 2000; Culp and Holt 2010). Nonetheless, some patients may present in acute collapse (Swann and Hughes 2000). The "praying position" is a clear sign of abdominal discomfort (Crowe and Bjorling 1993). Many animals have diffuse abdominal pain, although this pain is not always obvious on palpation. Cats in particular seem to be resistant to the expression of pain during abdominal palpation (Costello *et al.* 2004). A large effusion volume is rarely present. This may cause abdominal distention with a positive undulation and may secondarily lead to tachypnea and dyspnea (MacCoy 1981; Crowe and Bjorling 1993). The clinical manifestations of the circulatory changes mainly depend on the extensiveness of the fluid loss (MacCoy 1981; Swann and Hughes 2000).

Blood analysis

Blood gas analysis can reveal acidosis due to the shift to anaerobic glycolysis and the failure of compensatory mechanisms of acid–base balances (e.g., decreased renal blood flow with decreased secretion of acid metabolites). Other blood work findings are variable and nonspecific, although serum biochemistry might help to diagnose the type of peritonitis and the underlying cause. Anemia and leukocytosis are often encountered. However, the neutrophil count can be normal, elevated, or even low in patients with long-standing pathology, and a left shift may or may not be present (Crowe and Bjorling 1993; Swann and Hughes 2000; Culp and Holt 2010). Thrombocytopenia is a possible finding. A complete coagulation workup with platelet concentration, coagulation tests, and assessment of fibrinolysis via concentrations of fibrin degradation products is indicated when complications such as disseminated intravascular coagulation (DIC) are suspected (Crowe and Bjorling 1993; King 1994). Because of infection and the loss of large amounts of protein in the free peritoneal fluid, panhypoproteinemia may occur (McGrotty and Doust 2004). The loss of circulating volume may also lead to prerenal azotemia (Culp and Holt 2010).

Diagnostic imaging

Medical imaging is a useful tool in the diagnosis of peritonitis and the detection of the underlying cause. Abdominal effusion leads to increased diffuse and homogeneous intraabdominal radiopacity and loss of serosal detail, sometimes referred to as "ground glass" appearance (Figure 4.1). However, this sign is also present in young animals or patients in poor condition because of their lack of intraabdominal fat. Moreover, the effusion can be limited or absent in the early stages of peritonitis (Swann and Hughes 2000). Ultrasonography is a more sensitive technique to detect small or localized amounts of effusion, and it allows guided diagnostic abdominocentesis (Walters 2003).

Abdominocentesis and diagnostic abdominal lavage

The analysis of free abdominal fluid can be a rapid and accurate diagnostic tool in the work-up of peritonitis patients (Bonczynski *et al.* 2003; Connally 2003; Walters 2003). Clinical signs, blood

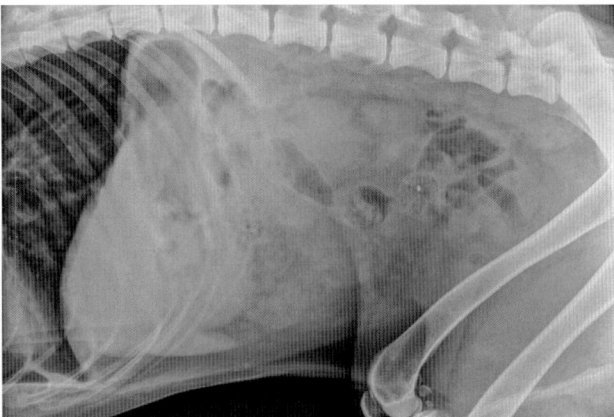

Figure 4.1 Lateral abdominal radiograph of a dog with septic peritonitis. Haziness and loss of abdominal detail are obvious in the mid-abdominal area.

analysis, and medical imaging are often too nonspecific to determine the therapeutic approach, particularly to decide whether or not to proceed surgically.

The sample can be obtained by abdominocentesis, four-quadrant paracentesis, or diagnostic abdominal lavage. Because obtaining a sample might introduce free air into the abdomen, which might interfere with the interpretation of abdominal radiographs or ultrasonography medical imaging should be performed beforehand.

For the four-quadrant paracentesis, four sites for needle placement are selected using the umbilicus as a center of reference. Multiple simultaneous needle placements provide an air vent that allows fluid to flow more fluently (Walters 2003). However, paramedian placement of the needle increases the risk of blood contamination of the sample. In abdominal lavage, warmed sterile saline is infused and then retrieved through a catheter (Walters 2003). Lavage is more sensitive but more invasive and is therefore performed only when abdominocentesis was unsuccessful. Indeed, in the presence of small amounts of fluid (<5–6 mL/kg body weight), false-negative results are likely (McGrotty and Doust 2004). Alternatively, ultrasound-guided aspiration can be performed (Walters 2003).

To perform abdominocentesis:

1   Place the animal in lateral recumbency.
2   Empty the bladder if interfering with sample collection.
3   Clip and surgically prepare an area around the umbilicus.
4   Introduce a needle or a catheter 1 to 3 cm caudal to the umbilicus in a caudodorsal direction.
5   Collect freely running fluid or apply gentle negative pressure with a syringe.
6   If no fluid collected, perform a four-quadrant paracentesis or a diagnostic abdominal lavage.
7   Perform cytologic evaluation (ethylenediaminetetraacetic acid [EDTA] tube).
8   Perform biochemical analysis (serum tube).
9   Submit fluid for bacterial culture and sensitivity testing (serum tube).

Sample analysis

A classification scheme for peritoneal effusions is proposed by Alleman (2003) and is based on pathophysiologic mechanisms (Table 4.2).

The appearance of the sample is evaluated grossly for color and turbidity. A clear, colorless sample excludes peritonitis caused by leakage of the GI tract unless the patient is sampled within 3 hours of visceral perforation (Connally 2003). A turbid tap is associated with a high cellularity. In case of uroabdomen, the odor of urine might be noticed; in bile peritonitis, bile-like fluid will be collected. Further cytologic and biochemical analysis of the sample provides a rapid, accurate tool to diagnose and classify peritonitis. Because of vasoactive and chemotactic products that cause an influx of protein-rich cellular fluid, the effusion in peritonitis is mostly categorized as an exudate. The protein content is up to 3 g/dL, and the total nuclear cell count (TNCC) is above 3000 cells/mL (Alleman 2003; Connally 2003). In addition to the presence of bacteria, the predominant cell type, the morphology of the neutrophils, and the glucose and lactate levels are considered helpful indicators to differentiate between nonseptic and septic exudates. These criteria are discussed later. The ratio of creatinine and potassium fluid to blood and the ratio of bilirubin fluid to blood can confirm the diagnosis of uroabdomen and bile peritonitis, respectively.

Table 4.2 Classification of effusions based on protein content, cell count, and cytology. Hematoxylin eosin–stained smears of noncentrifuged samples (scale bar, 20 µm).

	Total Protein(g/dL)	Cells/mL	Predominant cell types	Special features	
Pure transudate	<2.5	<1000	Mononuclear	Low cellularity	
Modified transudate	2.5–5	1000-8000	Mononuclear	Cell type varies with etiology	A
Septic exudate	>3	>3000	Neutrophils	Degenerate neutrophils	
Nonseptic exudate	>3	>3000	Neutrophils	Nondegenerate neutrophils	B
Hemorrhagic effusion	>3	Variable	Similar to blood	Erythrophagia or hemosiderin in macrophages	
Neoplastic effusion	>2.5	Variable	Tumor cells	Neoplastic cell population	C

A, Smear of a modified transudate caused by steroid-induced hepatopathy in a dog. Notice the low cell count and the presence of mononuclear cells and nondegenerate neutrophils.

B, Smear of a septic exudate of a dog. Notice the high cell count, the presence of degenerate neutrophils with an intracellular cocci-shaped bacterium (see box), and a macrophage with phagocytized cellular debris (upper right corner). Identification of intracellular bacteria is diagnostic for a septic effusion, but it may require adequate evaluation by an experienced cytologist.

C, Smear of a neoplastic effusion of a dog, most likely carcinomatosis. Notice the presence of various malignant cellular features such as nuclear crowding, the presence of multiple nuclei and nucleoli, and cytoplasmic vacuolization. A marked secondary inflammatory response is present.

Source: Data from Alleman (2003).

Secondary septic peritonitis

Definition
Secondary septic peritonitis can be defined as an infectious peritoneal effusion that occurs in conjunction with an intraabdominal pathology.

Risk factors
- Blunt or penetrating abdominal trauma
- Spontaneous or iatrogenic rupture of abdominal abscesses (e.g., pancreatic, prostatic)
- Pyometra
  ◦ Spontaneous or iatrogenic rupture (Figure 4.2)
  ◦ Leakage through the *ostium abdominale*
- Contamination of ovarian bursae
- Transmural migration of bacteria through the intestinal or uterine wall
- Surgically induced contamination
- Surgical wound dehiscence

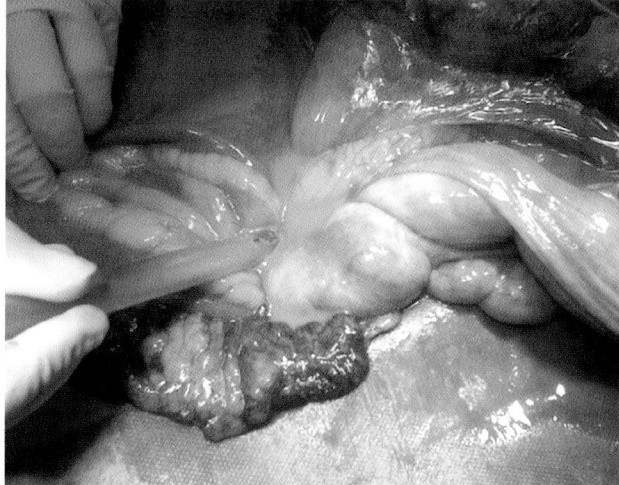

Figure 4.2 Spontaneous rupture of a pus-distended uterus in a bitch with pyometra.

Risk factors for leakage after GI surgery include the presence of pre-operative peritonitis (Allen *et al.* 1992; Ralph *et al.* 2003; Grimes *et al.* 2011), a left shift (Allen *et al.* 1992; Ralph *et al.* 2003), intraoperative hypotension (Grimes *et al.* 2011), low plasma protein and serum albumin concentrations (Ralph *et al.* 2003; Grimes *et al.* 2011), the extent of surgery (Wylie and Hosgood 1994), and the indication for abdominal surgery itself (Allen *et al.* 1992; Ralph *et al.* 2003). Cats appear to be less susceptible to intestinal dehiscence (Ralph *et al.* 2003).

Risk factors for contamination after ovari(ohyster)ectomy include pyometra cases in which excessive manipulation of the pus-filled uterus or rupture or spillage of uterine content occurs. Even in clinically normal bitches, opening of the ovarian bursa at the time of removal of the ovaries can lead to bacterial contamination of the abdominal cavity (de Rooster *et al.* 2010).

Urine-induced chemical peritonitis seldom progresses to septic peritonitis unless preexisting urinary tract infection was present (Crowe and Bjorling 1993).

Bile induces changes in the permeability of the intestinal wall, leading to bacterial translocation and infection of the peritoneal effusion. Moreover, the noxious effect of bile is enhanced by its impairing effect on local host defense mechanisms (Ludwig *et al.* 1997).

Diagnosis

Signs of the underlying pathology may be present. Fever is not a consistent sign. Moreover, patients with secondary septic peritonitis may be hypo-, normo- or hyperthermic. Cats with sepsis or septic peritonitis are on occasion presented with an inexplicable bradycardia (Costello *et al.* 2004).

Bacteriologic culture of the abdominal fluid remains the gold standard for diagnosing septic peritonitis but does not provide a fast diagnosis (Bonczynski *et al.* 2003). In contrast, **cytologic examination of the peritoneal fluid** is a rapid diagnostic test with a reported accuracy of identifying intracellular bacteria varying from 57% to 85% (King 1994; Lanz *et al.* 2001; Mueller *et al.* 2001). However, the presence of a localized process, previous antibiotic treatment, or limited experience of the cytologist reduces the accuracy of cytology (Ludwig 2004).

In septic effusions, the predominant cell type is the neutrophil (Alleman 2003). Based on their morphologic appearance, neutrophils can be classified as degenerate, nondegenerate, or toxic. Degenerate neutrophils demonstrate nuclear swelling, karyorrhexis, and karyolysis, manifestations of a quick cell death under the influence of bacterial toxins (Connally 2003). In contrast, pyknosis, characteristic of nondegenerate neutrophils, is an indication of slow cell death in a nonseptic environment (Alleman 2003; Connally 2003). Finally, toxic neutrophils may be observed in peripheral blood and abdominal effusions. The toxic changes occur during neutrophil maturation in the bone marrow in response to inflammatory or infectious processes. Their presence is associated with a poor prognosis (Aroch *et al.* 2005).

Ideally, the differentiation between septic and aseptic peritonitis should be based on a combination of diagnostic parameters in the peritoneal effusion.
- Degenerate neutrophils with intracellular bacteria
- More than 13,000 nucleated cells/μL
- A blood-to-fluid glucose difference greater than 20 mg/dL
- A blood-to-fluid lactate difference less than -2 mmol/L

The identification of intracellular bacteria is not always easy, and the interpretation of TNCC is hampered after an abdominal intervention because in those cases, the cell count in peritoneal fluid is always increased (Van Hoogmoed *et al.* 1999). A recent experimental study in healthy dogs undergoing an explorative celiotomy

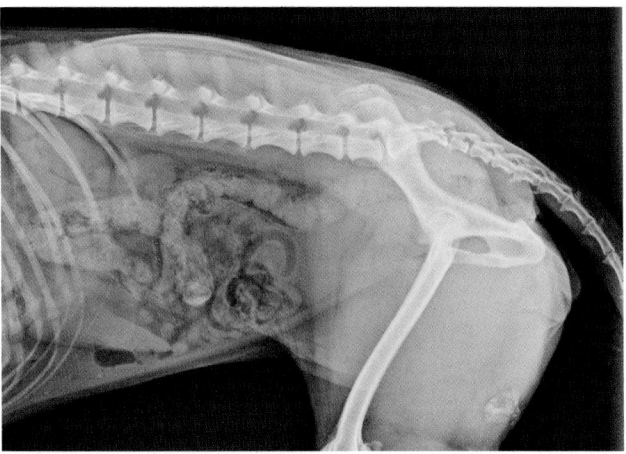

Figure 4.3 Lateral abdominal radiograph of a dog after a car accident. Free abdominal gas is present in the mid-abdomen ventral to the silhouette of the spleen.

suggests, however, that cytological and biochemical parameters in drain fluid should be interpreted with caution during the postoperative period to avoid overdiagnosing of septic conditions (Szabo *et al.* 2011).

The presence of **free abdominal gas on radiographs** is suggestive of GI perforation or penetrating trauma and is an indication for emergency surgical intervention (Figure 4.3). Recent abdominal surgery, however, can complicate the interpretation. **Ultrasonography** may prove useful to determine the region or the cause of the pathology. Focal changes in GI wall thickness, presence of a foreign body or mass, focal area of bright fat, and focal fluid collections aid in the diagnosis (Boysen *et al.* 2003).

Treatment

Medical management

The initial treatment goal is patient stabilization. Hypotension, hypoproteinemia, hypoglycemia, and electrolyte imbalances should be addressed before surgery (Swann and Hughes 2000; Ludwig 2004; McGrotty and Doust 2004).
- Administer crystalloids at shock infusion rates as described in Chapter 2.
- Use plasma (10–20 mL/kg) or synthetic colloids (maximum, 22 mL/kg/hr) if indicated.
- Monitor perfusion parameters.
- Monitor central venous and mean arterial blood pressures, electrolytes, and blood gases.

Hypoglycemia and electrolyte imbalances are corrected through intravenous supplementations. Metabolic acidosis is generally resolved by fluid therapy. If the response to fluid therapy is not adequate to stabilize the patient, vasopressor therapy is indicated. Pain management in patients with peritonitis should not be overlooked.

The use of heparin or other drugs to reduce fibrin formation and indirectly adhesion formation remains controversial.

Because the source of contamination is usually the intestinal tract, the most common isolates are *Escherichia coli*, *Enterococcus* spp., and *Clostridium* spp. (Swann and Hughes 2000; McGrotty and Doust 2004; Costello *et al.* 2004). An empirical treatment with broad-spectrum antimicrobials should be administered intravenously as soon as a peritoneal fluid sample has been obtained.

Table 4.3 Spectrum and posology of antimicrobial therapy for septic peritonitis in dogs and cats. In the perioperative period, antibiotics should be administered intravenously (IV). When the patient becomes clinically stable, the antibiotic treatment can be continued subcutaneously (SC) or orally (Ramsy 2007; Papich 2009). q, every.

	Main spectrum	Posology IV	Posology SC
Amoxycillin + clavulanic acid*	Gr+ Some Gr- (including Enterobacteriaceae) and various anaerobic	20 mg/kg q8h	12.5 mg/kg q24h
Enrofloxacin*	Gr-	5 mg/kg q24h Dilute and administer slowly	5 mg/kg q24h
Metronidazole†	Anaerobic	10 mg/kg q12h	15–25 mg/kg q12h
Cefazolin* (first-generation cephalosporin)	Gr+	20–35 mg/kg q8h	
Meropenem†	Gr-	24 mg/kg q24h	12 mg/kg q8h
		Only in case of multiresistant bacteria	
Amikacin†	Gr-	15–30 mg/kg q24h (dogs) 10–15 mg/kg q24h (cats)	15–30 mg/kg q24h (dogs) 10–15 mg/kg q24h (cats)
		Only in case of multiresistant bacteria Maintain adequate perfusion and monitor renal function and serum levels to minimize toxicity	

*Not registered for IV use in dogs or cats.

†Not registered for IV nor SC use in dogs or cats.

Antibiotics with a main activity against gram-positive, gram-negative, and anaerobic bacteria can be combined while awaiting the results of culture and sensitivity testing (Swann and Hughes 2000; Ludwig 2004) (Table 4.3). In the authors' experience, most bacteria isolated in peritonitis cases are sensitive to amoxicillin potentiated with clavulanic acid. In nonresponsive cases, the combination of amoxicillin–clavulanic acid, enrofloxacin, and metronidazole provides the broadest spectrum.

Surgical management

After patient stabilization, the elimination of the underlying cause is crucial, which in most cases involves surgical intervention. A complete abdominal exploration is required to eliminate the source of contamination and to identify possible other lesions, localized peritonitis, or abscesses (Crowe and Bjorling 1993; Swann and Hughes 2000; McGrotty and Doust 2004). Copious lavage is recommended to reduce the number of bacteria and the quantity of endotoxins, cytokines, and proteolytic enzymes and to remove material that promotes bacterial proliferation (Ludwig 2004). Factors required for fibrin formation such as fibrinogen, thromboplastin, and clotting factors are also diluted. As such, the risk of postoperative adhesion formation decreases (Crowe and Bjorling 1993). The inflammatory response evoked by lavage with isotonic saline can be considered

mild and transient in parallel to what has been described in ponies (Schneider 1988). The benefit of adding antibiotics or antiseptics to the lavage fluid remains controversial. Additives might increase the risk of chemical peritonitis without increasing the efficacy of the lavage (Crowe and Bjorling 1993). Lavage fluid left in the abdominal cavity impairs immune function by reducing chemotaxis of inflammatory cells, and it prevents antibiotics from reaching adequate concentrations (McGrotty and Doust 2004).

1 Perform a ventral midline laparotomy from the xyphoid process to the pubis.
2 Collect samples for aerobic and anaerobic cultures if not yet available.
3 Identify and eliminate the source of contamination.
4 Remove necrotic and fibrotic tissues.
5 Adjust surgical techniques and suture materials to the septic environment.
   ○ Simple interrupted sutures
   ○ Monofilament
6 Lavage with a minimum of 200 to 300 mL/kg warmed sterile 0.9% saline or until the returning fluid is clear (Figure 4.4).
7 Remove as much fluid as possible before closure.
8 Consider omental wrapping or serosal patching to support the suture lines.

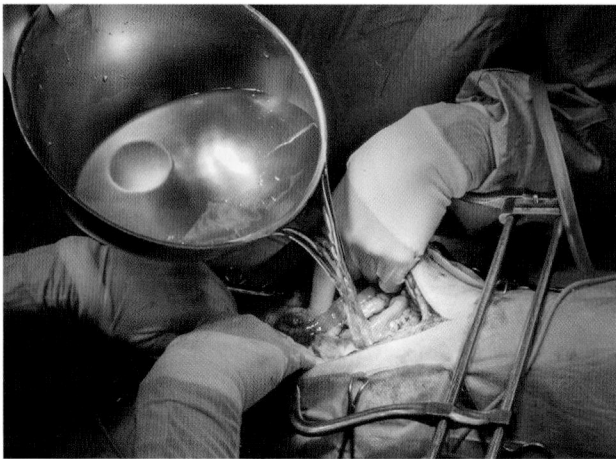

Figure 4.4 Septic peritonitis. At the end of the surgical intervention, copious lavage is performed.

The next dilemma in the surgeon's decision making is to whether or not close the abdomen at the end of the procedure.

In cases of generalized peritonitis in which intraoperative lavage seems insufficient to cleanse the peritoneal surface or when a continued septic inflammatory process is anticipated, postoperative abdominal drainage may be indicated (Woolfson and Dulish 1986). With this approach, exudates that may contain bacteria, toxins, fibrin, and foreign materials can be further evacuated during the postoperative period. Open abdominal drainage involves incomplete closure of the *linea alba* and skin (Figure 4.5). The ventral midline incision is covered with sterile dressings, which are changed on a regular basis.

Open drainage can only be considered when a 24-hour monitoring can be guaranteed (McGrotty and Doust 2004). Multiple complications have been reported with this approach. Fluid and protein loss through the abdominal wound can be massive. Other potential complications include electrolyte imbalances, enteric fistulas, evisceration, strangulation or adhesions of intestinal loops, anemia, or ascending nosocomial infections (Woolfson and Dulish 1986). Moreover, a second surgical procedure is necessary to close the abdomen. Cytologic examination of the discharge during bandage

changes will indicate if there is a need to reexplore or will define the ideal time to close the abdomen (Staatz *et al.* 2002). Whereas older reports showed a dramatic improvement on the survival of dogs treated with open drainage techniques, more recent studies failed to confirm these findings. In addition, the need for blood or plasma transfusion or the placement of a jejunostomy tube was significantly higher in these patients, and longer intensive care hospitalization was needed (Staatz *et al.* 2002). Most likely, improved surgical techniques, better intraoperative elimination of contamination, improved antibiotic options, and better postoperative management can explain the decrease in need for open abdominal drainage. If the inciting cause is adequately eliminated, if peritoneal lavage is performed, and if intensive postoperative medical support is installed, primary closure of the abdomen is a justifiable option (Lanz *et al.* 2001).

A potential alternative to the open abdominal drainage is the use of passive or active (closed-suction) drains. These can also allow intermittent postoperative abdominal lavage. Passive drains function by gravity, overflow, or capillarity. In active drains (e.g., Jackson-Pratt), the use of an external suction source with either a manual compressible or a rigid reservoir induces a negative pressure, which promotes peritoneal drainage (Figure 4.6). A variety of different materials and designs have been proposed. The functional characteristics of these drainage systems, such as initial suction generated and pressure–volume relationships during filling of the reservoir, vary greatly among systems (Mueller *et al.* 2001; Halfacree *et al.* 2009). The two most successful passive peritoneal drains in companion animals are the triple-lumen sump drain and the Parker peritoneal dialysis catheter (McGrotty and Doust 2004; Halfacree *et al.* 2009).

Complications associated with abdominal drains are nosocomial infections; adhesions; fluid production in response to the drain itself; and inefficient draining caused by fibrin, adhesions, or omental occlusion (Crowe and Bjorling 1993; Mueller *et al.* 2001; McGrotty *et al.* 2003). The use of active suction drains instead of passive drains reduces the risk of surgical site infection and occlusion of the drain by fibrin and adhesions.

For local foci of infection such as prostatic or pancreatic abscesses, omentalization represents an effective physiologic drain (White 2000; Johnson and Mann 2006).

There is current interest in the use of open abdomen techniques in combination with vacuum-assisted systems in canine peritonitis cases because this approach seems to work well in humans (Caro *et al.* 2011).

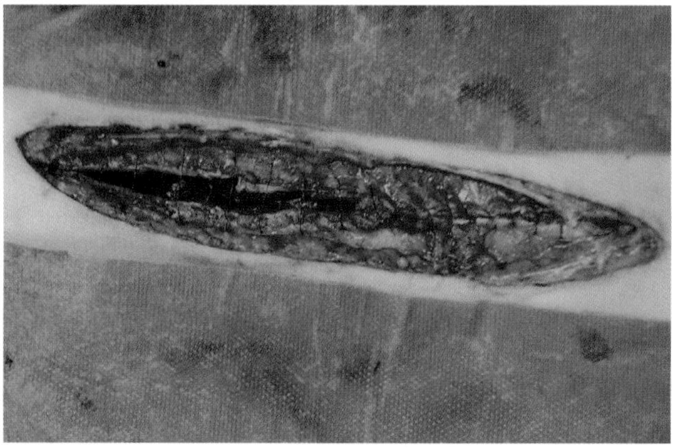

Figure 4.5 Open abdominal drainage. The linea alba and skin are incompletely closed to allow drainage of the abdomen into absorbent dressings.

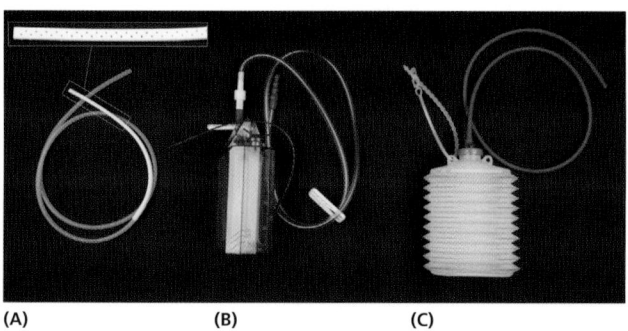

(A)   (B)   (C)

Figure 4.6 Active drains. **A,** Jackson-Pratt drain, here without reservoir. **B,** Active drain with rigid reservoir. **C,** Active drain with manual compressible reservoir

Outcome

Reported survival rates in canine and feline patients with septic peritonitis vary from 20% to 80% (Staatz *et al.* 2002). Refractory hypotension, acute collapse, and the development of respiratory distress or DIC are indicators of a poor prognosis (King 1994; Mueller *et al.* 2001).

Prevention

- Maintain blood pressure and restore protein levels in the perioperative period to optimize enteric perfusion and healing (Grimes *et al.* 2011).
- Limit surgical time. A prolonged length of surgery increases the risk of intestinal dehiscence (Allen *et al.* 1992).
- Preservation of a good blood supply and tissue apposition has been shown to affect healing of all intestinal segments (Wylie and Hosgood 1994).
- Keep the number of procedures during intestinal surgery to a minimum regardless of the segment involved. Animals undergoing more than one GI surgical procedure (e.g., enterotomy in addition to resection and anastomosis) have been reported as less likely to survive (Wylie and Hosgood 1994).
- Provide early postoperative feeding to supply nutrition and to support the health of the GI wall (Staatz *et al.* 2002; McGrotty and Doust 2004). Place a feeding tube if required.

References

Alleman, R. (2003) Abdominal, thoracic, and pericardial effusions. *Veterinary Clinics of North America: Small Animal Practice* 33, 89-118.

Allen, D.A., Smeak, D.D., Schertel, E.R. (1992) Prevalence of small intestinal dehiscence and associated clinical factors: a retrospective study of 121 dogs. *Journal of the American Animal Hospital Association* 28 (1), 70-76.

Aroch, I., Klement, E., Segev, G. (2005) Clinical, biochemical, and haematological characteristics, disease prevalence and prognosis of dogs presenting with neutrophil toxicity. *Journal of Veterinary Internal Medicine* 19, 64-73.

Bonczynski, J.J., Ludwig, L.L., Burton, L.J., et al. (2003) Comparison of peritoneal fluid and peripheral blood ph, bicarbonate, glucose, and lactate concentration as a diagnostic tool for septic peritonitis in cats and dogs. *Veterinary Surgery* 32, 161-166.

Boysen, S.R., Tidwell, A.S., Pennick, D.G. (2003) Ultrasonographic findings in dogs and cats with gastrointestinal perforation. *Veterinary Radiology and Ultrasound* 44 (5),556-564.

Caro, A., Olona, C., Jiménez, A., et al. (2011) Treatment of the open abdomen with topical negative pressure therapy: a retrospective study of 46 cases. *International Wound Journal* 8 (3), 274-279.

Chromik, A.M., Meiser, A., Hölling, J., et al. (2009) Identification of patients at risk for development of tertiary peritonitis on a surgical intensive care unit. *Journal of Gastrointestinal Surgery* 13 (7), 1358-1367.

Connally, H.E. (2003) Cytology and fluid analysis of the acute abdomen. *Clinical Techniques in Small Animal Practice* 18 (1), 39-44.

Costello, M.F., Drobatz, K.J., Aronson, L.R., et al. (2004) Underlying cause, pathophysiologic abnormalities and response to treatment in cats with septic peritonitis: 51 cases (1990-2001). *J Am Vet Med Assoc* 225 (6), 897-902.

Crowe, D.T., Bjorling, D.E. (1993) Peritoneum and peritoneal cavity. In: Slatter D.H. (ed.) *Textbook of Small Animal Surgery*, vol 1, 2nd edn. W.B. Saunders, London, pp. 407-445.

Culp, W., Holt, D. (2010) Septic peritonitis. *Compendium on Continuing Education for the Practicing Veterinarian* 32 (10), E1-E15.

Culp, W.T., Zeldis, T.E., Reese, M.S., et al. (2009) Primary bacterial peritonitis in dogs and cats: 24 cases (1990-2006). *Journal of the American Veterinarian Medical Association* 234 (7), 906-913.

de Rooster, H., Doom, M., Tas, O., et al. (2010) Bacterial contamination of the ovarian bursae in dogs with pyometra. In: *Proceedings of the European College of Veterinary Surgeons*. Helsinki, p. 216.

Dunn, D.L., Barke, R.A., Knight, N.B., et al. (1985) Role of resident macrophages, peripheral neutrophils, and translymphatic absorption in bacterial clearance from the peritoneal cavity. *Infection and Immunity* 49 (2), 257-264.

Edlich, R.F., Long, W.B., Gubler, D.K., et al. (2009) Dangers of cornstarch powder on medical gloves: seeking a solution. *Annals of Plastic Surgery* 63, 111-115.

Grimes, J.A., Schmiedt, C.W., Cornell, K.K., et al. (2011) Identification of risk factors for septic peritonitis and failure to survive following gastrointestinal surgery in dogs. *Journal of the American Veterinary Medical Association* 238 (4), 486-494.

Halfacree, Z.J., Wilson A.M., Baines S.J. (2009) Evaluation of in vitro performance of suction drains. *American Journal of Veterinary Research* 70 (2), 283-289.

Holt, D., Brown, D. (1999) Peritonitis. In: King, L. Hammond, R. (eds.) *Manual of Canine and Feline Emergency and Critical Care*. British Small Animal Veterinary Association, Cheltenham, UK, pp. 140-144.

Hosgood, G., Salisbury, S.K. (1988) Generalised peritonitis in dogs: 50 cases (1975-1986). *Journal of the American Veterinary Medical Association* 193 (11), 1448-1450.

Johnson, M.D., Mann, F.A. (2006) Treatment for pancreatic abscesses via omentalization with abdominal closure versus open peritoneal abdominal drainage in dogs: 15 cases (1994-2004). *Journal of the American Veterinary Medical Association* 228 (3), 397-402.

King, L.G. (1994) Postoperative complications and prognostic indicators in dogs and cats with septic peritonitis: 23 cases (1989-1992). *Journal of the American Veterinary Medical Association* 204 (3), 407-414.

Lanz, O.I., Ellison, G.W., Bellah, J.R., et al. (2001) Surgical treatment of septic peritonitis without abdominal drainage in 28 dogs. *Journal of the American Animal Hospital Association* 37, 87-92.

Liebermann-Meffert, D. (2000) The greater omentum. Anatomy, embryology, and surgical applications. *Surgical Clinics of North America* 80 (1), 275-293.

Ludwig, L.L. (2004) Improving survival in patients with septic peritonitis: what's new in diagnosis and treatment? In: *Scientific abstracts 2004 ACVS Veterinary Symposium*. ACVS, New York, pp. 424-428.

Ludwig, L.L., McLoughlin, M.A., Graves, T.K., et al. (1997) Surgical treatment of bile peritonitis in 24 dogs and 2 cats: a retrospective study (1987-1994). *Veterinary Surgery* 26, 90-98.

MacCoy, D. (1981) Peritonitis. In: Bojrab, M.J. (ed.) *Pathophysiology in Small Animal Surgery*, 1st edn. Lea & Febiger, Philadelphia, pp. 142-147.

McGrotty, Y.L., Doust, R.T. (2004) Management of peritonitis in cats and dogs. *In Practice*, 26, 385-367.

McGrotty, Y.L., Knottenbelt, C.M., Doust R.T., et al. (2003) Complications of open peritoneal drainage in nine dogs with gastrointestinal leakage. *Irish Veterinary Journal* 56 (7), 354-360.

Mueller, M.G., Ludwig, L.L., Burton, L.G. (2001) Use of closed-suction drains to treat generalised peritonitis in cats and dogs: 40 cases (1997-1999). *Journal of the American Veterinary Medical Association* 219 (6), 789-794.

Papich, M.G. (2009) Appendix I: Table of common drugs: approximate dosages. In: Bonagura, J.D. Twedt, D.C. (eds.) *Kirk's Current Veterinary Therapy*, 13th edn. Saunders Elsevier, St. Louis, pp. 1306-1334.

Ralph, S.C., Jessen, C.R., Lipowitz, A.J. (2003) Risk factors for leakage following intestinal anastomosis in dogs and cats: 115 cases (1991-2000). *Journal of the American Veterinary Medical Association* 223 (1), 73-77.

Ramsy, I. (2007) In: Ramsy, I. (ed.) *Small Animal Formulary*, 6th edn. British Small Animal Veterinary Medicine, Gloucester, UK.

Schneider, R.K., Meyer, D.J., Embertson, R.M., et al. (1988) Response of pony peritoneum to four peritoneal lavage solutions. *American Journal of Veterinary Research* 49 (6), 889-894.

Staatz, A.J., Monnet, E., Seim, B.S. (2002) Open peritoneal drainage versus primary closure for the treatment of septic peritonitis in dogs and cats: 42 cases (1993-1999). *Veterinary Surgery* 31, 174-180.

Swann, H., Hughes, D. (2000) Diagnosis and management of peritonitis. *Veterinary Clinics of North America: Small Animal Practice* 30 (3), 603-615.

Szabo, S.D., Jermyn, K., Neel, J., et al. (2011) Evaluation of postceliotomy peritoneal drain fluid volume, cytology, and blood to peritoneal fluid lactate and glucose differences in normal dogs. *Veterinary Surgery* 40 (4), 444-449.

Van Hoogmoed, L., Rodger, L.D., Spier, S.J., et al. (1999) Evaluation of peritoneal fluid pH, glucose concentration, and lactate dehydrogenase activity for detection of septic peritonitis in horses. *Journal of the American Veterinary Medical Association* 217 (7), 1032-1036.

Walters, J.M. (2003) Abdominal paracentesis and diagnostic peritoneal lavage. *Clinical Techniques in Small Animal Practice* 18 (1), 32-38.

White, R.A. (2000) Prostatic surgery in the dog. *Clinical Techniques in Small Animal Practice* 15 (1), 46-51.

Woolfson, J.M., Dulish, M.L. (1986) Open drainage in the treatment of generalised peritonitis in 25 dogs and cats. *Veterinary Surgery* 15 (1), 27-32.

Wylie, K.B., Hosgood, G. (1994) Mortality and morbidity of small and large intestinal surgery in dogs and cats: 74 cases (1980-1992). *Journal of the American Animal Hospital Association* 30 (5), 85-90.

5 Osteomyelitis

Dominique Griffon

College of Veterinary Medicine, Western University of Health Sciences, Pomona, CA, USA

Definition

Osteomyelitis is defined as an inflammation of the bone, typically due to an infectious process caused by bacteria or fungi. Osteomyelitis can be classified, based on its origin, as hematogenous or posttraumatic. Posttraumatic osteomyelitis is more common in small animals and results from direct inoculation of infectious agents during trauma or surgery.

Risk factors

Bone is naturally resistant to infection, and adjuvants play a crucial role in shifting surgical contamination toward bacterial proliferation (infection). Some of these factors are inherent to orthopedic procedures, such as the use of implants. However, surgeons must be especially cognizant of factors upon which they can have influence.

Factors affecting the host's ability to eradicate contamination include:
- Concurrent trauma or disease,
- Immunosuppression
- Preexisting infection
- Trauma to soft tissues adjacent to the surgery site, resulting from the initial injury, overzealous attempts at open fracture reduction, or manipulation of bone fragments
- Presence of dead space or necrotic tissue
- Instability at the fracture or osteotomy site

Factors influencing the bacterial load (number of bacteria or virulence) include:
- Duration of surgery
- Extent of the surgical approach
- Revision surgery
- Placement of implants (formation of a protective biofilm) (Figure 5.1)
- Placement of bone cement (polymethylmethacrylate [PMMA])
- Poor aseptic technique
- Use of skin staples in close proximity (<5 mm) to the bone, such as in tibial plateau leveling osteotomies (TPLOs)
- Patient is a carrier of methicillin-resistant bacteria

Diagnosis

In the acute phase, clinical signs of osteomyelitis are consistent with the presence of an inflammation at the surgical site and include localized swelling, pain, lameness, and fever. Osteomyelitis often

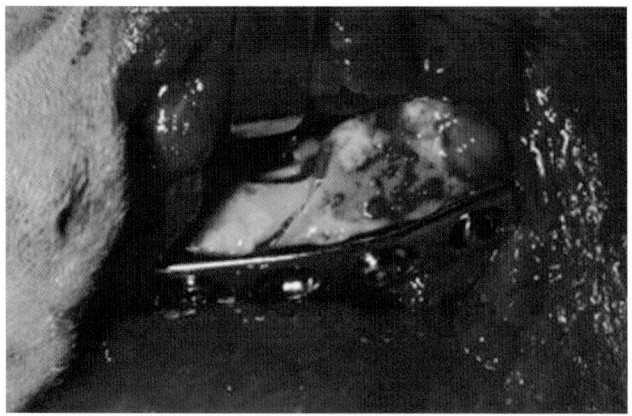

Figure 5.1 Role of orthopedic implant in osteomyelitis. After implantation, the biomaterial is covered with adsorbed macromolecules from local tissues (conditioning film), facilitating the adhesion of bacteria that produce exopolysaccharides (glycocalyx), thereby resulting in the formation of a protective biofilm.

results from an initial wound infection that gradually extends from the soft tissues into the bone. In the subacute (2 weeks) and chronic phase, clinical signs include lameness, drainage (Figure 5.2), and radiographic abnormalities.

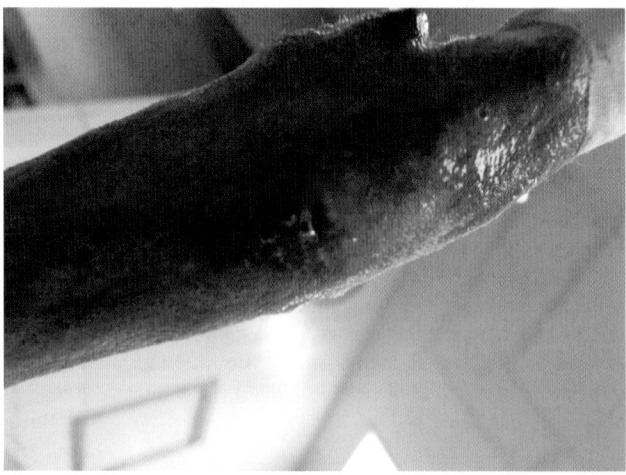

Figure 5.2 Wound dehiscence and drainage caused by osteomyelitis 12 weeks after fracture fixation in a dog.

Table 5.1 Specificity and sensitivity of diagnostic tests for osteomyelitis

Diagnostic technique	Sensitivity (%)	Specificity (%)
Plain radiography	62.5	57.1
Histopathology	33.3	86
Cultures	+ In ≤86%	Low*
Three-phase ^{99m}technetium scintigraphy	High (≥90%[†])	Low (70%[†])

*Smith *et al.* (1989): cultures were positive in 38% of healed uncomplicated fractures.
[†]Southwood *et al.* (2003): ^{99m}technetium ciprofloxacin in rabbits with experimental osteomyelitis.

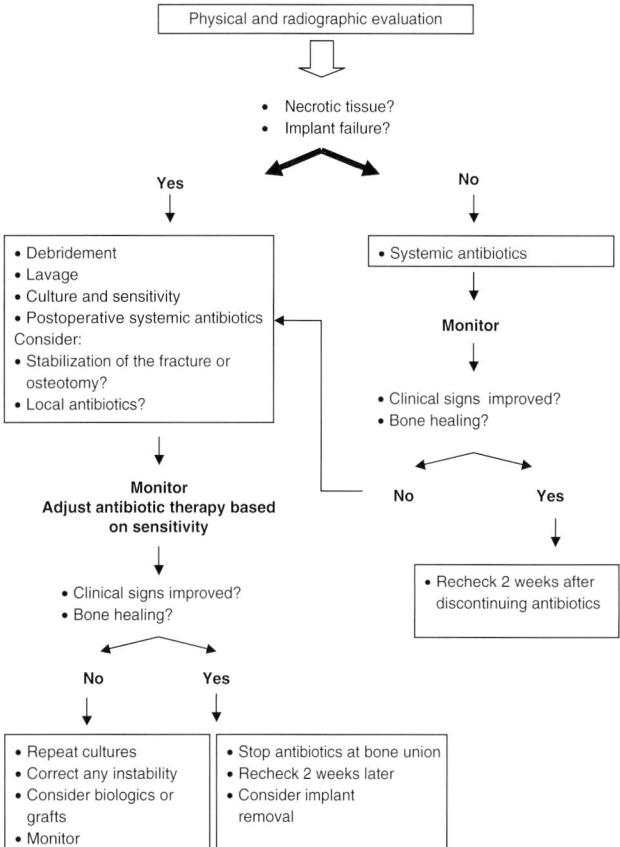
Figure 5.4 Proposed algorithm for the treatment of osteomyelitis.

Establishing a definitive diagnosis can be challenging, especially early in the disease process (Table 5.1). Osteomyelitis is most commonly diagnosed in small animals based on clinical signs combined with radiographic or microbiologic testing.

Radiographic signs (Figure 5.3) include:
- Presence of a well-defined segment of bone with increased radiopacity, consistent with a sequestrum. This segment may be surrounded by a radiolucent area with reactive tissues (involucrum) at the periphery.
- Evidence of bone resorption
- Implant failure: loosening or breakage

Microbiologic cultures:
- A swab should be obtained from deep tissues during surgical exploration, without skin contamination.
- Samples should be sent for aerobic and anaerobic cultures.
- The laboratory should be able to differentiate coagulase-positive staphylococci.
- Sensitivity results are crucial to guide antibiotic therapy.

Advanced imaging is rarely used in small animals. Nuclear scintigraphy is occasionally considered for early diagnosis; an increased uptake in the soft tissue phase is detected but is not specific for infection of the bone. An increased uptake during the delayed bone phase (24 hours after injection) is more consistent with osteomyelitis. Labeling nuclear agents (e.g., technetium) with antibiotics decreases the risk of false-positive diagnoses. Biopsy

and histopathology are indicated in cases with negative culture results, often resulting from fungal infections (e.g., *Blastomyces dermatitidis*).

Treatment

The treatment of patients with osteomyelitis varies with the stage of the disease, the severity of signs, and the underlying cause (Figure 5.4). Systemic antibiotic therapy remains the mainstay in the treatment of osteomyelitis in small animals. Selection is based on sensitivity, and systemic administration is continued for at least 6 weeks or until implant removal.

Amoxicillin–clavulanic acid is a good choice for empirical treatment of osteomyelitis, pending culture results. Special consideration should be given when antibiotics are selected to treat methicillin-resistant infections (see Chapter 7).

The initial approach to acute wound infection and osteomyelitis relies on systemic antibiotic therapy and protection of the surgical site (Elizabethan collar or bandage). Additional intervention should be considered to manage subacute and chronic osteomyelitis:

Debridement and lavage

Surgical debridement is indicated to remove nonviable tissues from the surgical site. Failed implants should be removed and cultures obtained from deep tissues. Infected joint prostheses require explantation in the vast majority of cases.

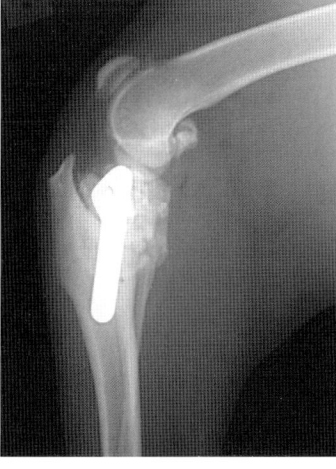
Figure 5.3 Radiographic signs of osteomyelitis 6 weeks after tibial plateau leveling osteotomy in a 4 year-old Labrador retriever. Lysis and sclerosis were present in the proximal tibia along with a loose proximal screw and collapse of the lateral proximal tibia.

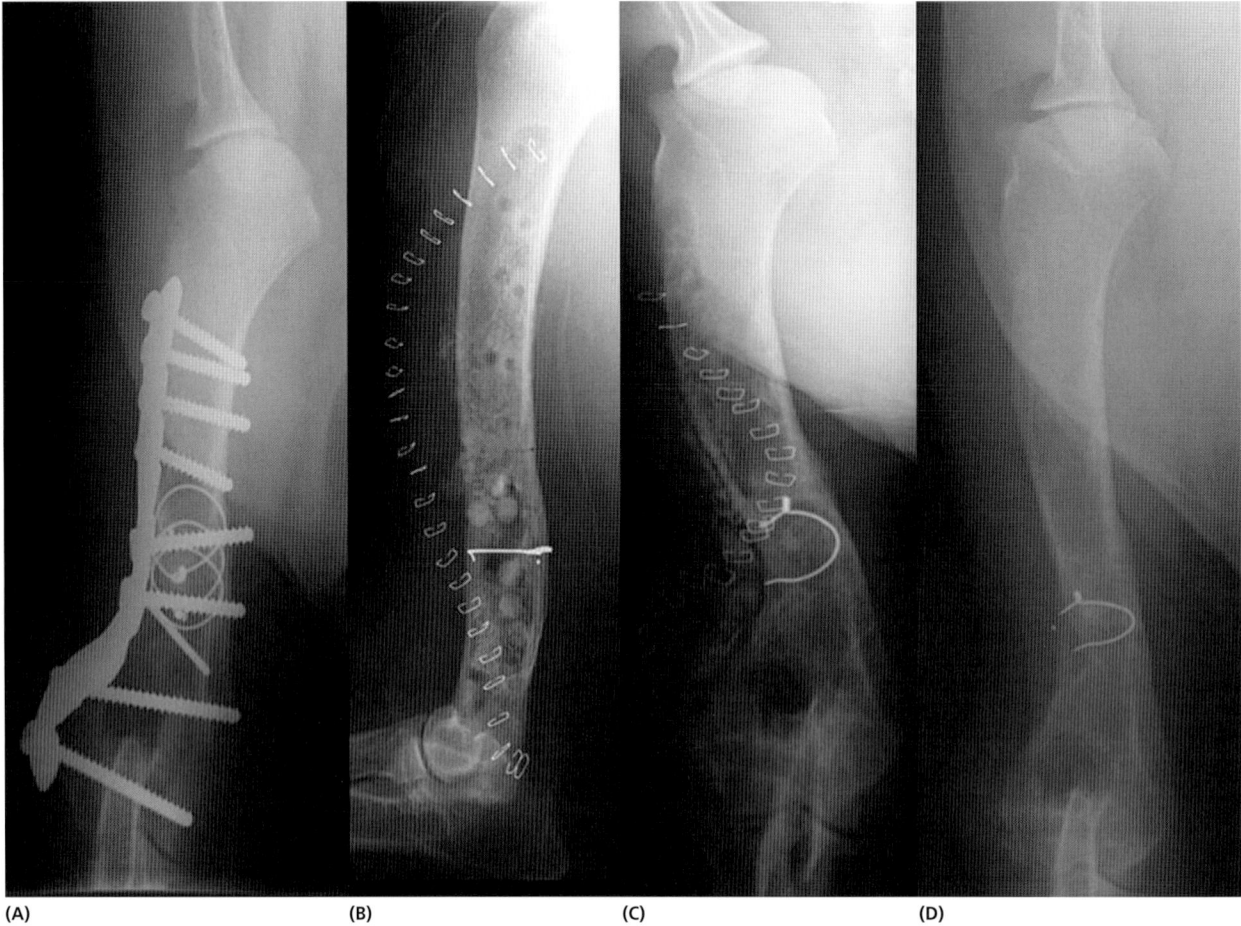

(A)   (B)   (C)   (D)

Figure 5.5 Local antibiotherapy as an adjunct treatment for osteomyelitis in a 7-year-old collie with a humeral fracture. **A,** Radiograph obtained 4 months after open fixation of the fracture with a plate and screws. The second most distal screw is loose and connected to a draining tract. **B** and **C,** Radiographs obtained after implant removal and lavage. A portion of cerclage wire embedded in bone could not be removed, prompting the placement of antibiotic-impregnated calcium sulfate beads. Antibiotics were prescribed for 6 weeks after surgery. **D,** Radiographs obtained 6 weeks later. Clinical signs have resolved.

Stabilization

Surgical stabilization of an infected site is indicated if instability is present at the fracture or osteotomy site. Revision may consist of the addition or replacement of implants. External fixation is generally preferred because of its versatility, placement away from the fracture site, and ease of postoperative adjustments and removal. Intramedullary fixation is typically avoided to preserve vascularization and limit intramedullary dissemination of bacteria from the fracture site.

Options after explantation of joint prostheses include excision arthroplasty, arthrodesis, amputation, or delayed revision (after eradication of infection).

Local antibiotherapy

This approach is designed to provide high local levels of antibiotics while limiting systemic distribution and toxicity. Local antibiotherapy is especially relevant in the treatment of:

- Infections caused by agents requiring administration of antibiotics with significant side effects (e.g., methicillin-resistant agents with sensitivity limited to aminoglycosides)
- Cases that fail to improve with systemic antibiotherapy
- Cases for which implants must be maintained within the fracture or osteotomy site (Figure 5.5)

The most common options for local antibiotherapy (Table 5.2) in small animals include:

- Preparation of PMMA beads impregnated with gentamicin. The release of antibiotic varies with types of PMMA, and the beads are not biodegradable, requiring removal.
- Preparation of calcium sulfate beads impregnated with vancomycin or tobramycin. These beads require the use of specific medical-grade calcium sulfate. They are biodegradable and disappear radiographically within 6 weeks of implantation

Biologic stimulation of bone healing

Strategies to stimulate bone healing in small animals include autogenous bone grafts, demineralized bone matrix, and osteoconductive agents. None of these agents has been proven to impact the outcome of osteomyelitis in small animals. Demineralized bone matrix impregnated with tobramycin and gentamicin has been investigated in vitro for potential application in nonunions in humans. This approach is appealing but warrants further evaluation. In the meantime, the addition of bone grafts or substitutes may be more advantageous after infection has been controlled and the environment is favorable as a strategy to accelerate bone healing.

Table 5.2 Examples of beads for local antibiotherapy

Bone cement	Quantity	Antibiotic	Bead diameter	Degradability	Reference
Polymethylmethacrylate*	10 g of powder and monomer	5 mL (500 mg) of gentamicin	5–7 mm by hand	No	Seddighi et al. 2007
Medical-grade calcium sulfate†	25 g of powder and 7.8 mL of diluent	1.2 g of tobramycin powder	7 mm in mold	6–8 weeks	Ham et al. 2008

*Simplex P, Howmedica ADS, Bloomington, IL.

†Fast Cure Osteoset, Wright Medical Technology, Arlington, TN.

Infection control program

The diagnosis of osteomyelitis should lead the clinician to question the need for preventing disease transmission and future hospital-associated infections (see Chapter 8).

Prognosis

The prognosis for osteomyelitis varies with the site of infection and consequences of the disease; the outcome is generally favorable with fractures and osteotomies and guarded to poor with osteomyelitis of a joint prosthesis. Early diagnosis and intervention improve the chances of recovery.

Prevention

Prevention of osteomyelitis starts with strict adherence to aseptic technique (see Chapter 8).

Patient preparation

- Surgical preparation of the surgical site is aimed at decreasing the presence of bacteria without damaging the skin. Aggressive clipping and scrubbing should be avoided.
- The distal extremities should be wrapped in layers, including a sterile impermeable barrier to prevent bacterial strike-through (Vince et al. 2008).

Preparation of the surgery team

- Hand preparation with hydroalcoholic solution is faster and more effective than traditional scrubbing techniques.
- Use of specially designed gloves or double gloving technique limits the risk of glove perforation during surgery.

Surgical technique

- Follow Halsted's principles of surgery.
- Minimally invasive approaches and procedures: use of arthroscopy and percutaneous fracture fixation (extrapolation from data in humans)
- Position skin incisions away from implants and close incisions overlying implants with suture rather than staples

Postoperative care

- Postoperative antibiotherapy has been found to decrease the risk of infections after tibial osteotomies (see relevant literature). Administration of amoxicillin–clavulanic acid for 48 to 72 hours after surgery may be a good compromise to limit the emergence of antibiotic resistance while controlling contamination until a fibrin seal has formed over the wound.
- Prevent licking of the surgical site with a dressing or Elizabethan collar, especially during the early postoperative phase.

Relevant literature

Osteomyelitis is well established as one of the most challenging complications after joint replacement, orthopedic reconstructive surgery, and fracture repair. Despite the refinement of powerful antibiotics, infection remains the most common complication associated with limb-sparing procedures in small animals, reported in up to 49% of patients. Surgeons have become increasingly aware of the risk of osteomyelitis after TPLO, which seems higher than after other elective orthopedic procedures. In fact, osteomyelitis has been reported as the single most common complication in a retrospective study of 253 TPLOs (Priddy et al. 2003). The majority of publications have since reported a percentage of infections after TPLOs approximating 7% to 8% and ranging from 3% to 10% (Frey et al. 2010; Bergh and Peirone 2012; Etter et al. 2013).

Although osteomyelitis may result from hematogenous spread, especially in immature patients, 90% of canine cases result from direct inoculation, such as bites, open fractures, foreign body penetration, gunshot injuries, or surgical procedures (Johnson 1994; Weese 2008). Under these circumstances, osteomyelitis results from an imbalance between the degree of contamination (bacterial load and virulence) and the host defense (systemic and local defense mechanisms). In dogs, the organisms most commonly isolated include gram-positive organisms, with *Staphylococcus intermedius* being the single most common bacteria. In a study of 21 TPLO plate removals because of postoperative infection, *Staphylococcus* spp. was isolated in 14 cases (Gallagher and Mertens 2012). *Staphylococcus pseudintermedius* was also reported in 13 of 15 (87%) of infected TPLOs, with four of those being methicillin resistant (Nazarali 2013). The increased awareness of surgeons for post-TPLO infections has been prompted by their unexpectedly high prevalence, as well as by the emergence of methicillin-resistant bacteria (see Chapter 7).

Substantial evidence emphasizes the role of adjuvant factors in transforming an initial contamination into an infection. In fact, the bacterial load required to induce osteomyelitis (10^8 colony-forming units of *Staphylococcus aureus*) is so high that it is often lethal in rodents. Experimental models therefore integrate adjuvant factors such as implants, PMMA, or sclerosing agents to reduce the bacterial inoculum. Surgeons greatly influence adjuvant factors such as soft tissue trauma, duration of surgery, and placement of implants. These factors aggravate any preexisting compromise of the host defense caused by systemic illness or local trauma and shift the balance from contamination to infection. The use of skin staples has recently been identified as a factor predisposing surgical wounds to infections. In humans, a meta-analysis of six studies including 683 wounds reported a fourfold increase in wound infections when the skin was closed with staples rather than sutures (Smith et al. 2010). Frey et al. (2010) reported a similar trend in dogs, in which the risk of wound infection or inflammation nearly doubled (factor 1.9) after staple closure in 902 cranial cruciate ligament repairs. The influence of simultaneous bilateral procedures has also been explored recently but with controversial results. Bilateral TPLOs were initially discouraged because of their high complication rate (40%) (Priddy et al. 2003). Diverging results were concurrently published by Barnhart (2003) in a study of 25 simultaneous TPLOs. The strongest evidence consisted of a study of 1000 dogs undergoing TPLOs, among which 65 were simultaneous and bilateral procedures (Fitzpatrick and

Solano 2010). This study found no difference in the rate of infection between unilateral and bilateral TPLOs, but the surgery time for bilateral procedures averaged 58 minutes, and wounds were covered with a dressing for 36 hours after surgery. Similar findings were later reported for tibial tuberosity advancement (TTA), although the sample size was limited to 33 bilateral procedures (of 68 TTAs) (Hirshenson *et al.* 2012). Overall, bilateral tibial osteotomies do not appear to increase the risk of infection as long as other adjuvant factors such as technique, duration, and prophylactic antibiotics are well controlled by the surgeon.

A tentative **diagnosis of osteomyelitis** is initially based on the history, clinical signs, and radiographic findings. A combination of clinical, laboratory, histopathology, microbiology, and imaging studies is typically needed to confirm the diagnosis because none of these modalities is accurate enough alone (see Table 5.1). Soft tissue swelling may appear radiographically within 24 to 48 hours, but bony changes are delayed by at least 10 to 14 days. Radiographs are therefore especially helpful to diagnose chronic osteomyelitis. In these cases, radiographic findings may include concurrent new bone formation and lysis, the presence of a sequestrum, and involucrum a few weeks after primary onset of the disease. Cultures derived from exudate in draining tracts are unreliable. Instead, a definitive diagnosis and antibiotherapy should be based on aerobic and anaerobic cultures obtained from deep aspiration or tissue biopsy. Much interest has focused on diagnostic tools to differentiate early osteomyelitis from inflammation to support early aggressive management of infection and decrease the morbidity associated with established osteomyelitis. Evaluation of the delayed bone phase of ^{99m}technetium-labeled monoclonal antibodies improves the otherwise low specificity of nuclear scintigraphy (Southwood *et al.* 2003). The use of computed tomography and magnetic resonance imaging in postoperative cases is limited by interference with metallic implants. In humans, a secondary increase of C-reactive protein after an initial postoperative decline is highly suggestive of infection (Trampuz and Zimmerli 2006).

The treatment of established osteomyelitis is usually based on surgical debridement and long-term systemic antibiotic therapy. The treatment should address the underlying environmental factors that caused the infection, such as the presence of necrotic tissue, impaired vascularization, loose metallic implants, and unstable fractures. Surgical management relies on extensive debridement and stabilization of unhealed fractures. External fixation is preferred because it eliminates the presence of implant at the surgical site and minimizes disruption of adjacent soft tissues. Intramedullary implants in fractures that are infected or predisposed to infection remain controversial. The management of surrounding soft tissues should prioritize blood supply, obliteration of dead space, and adequate drainage. Partial closure, delayed closure, or secondary healing is preferred to the placement of drains. The treatment of bone defects with autogenous cancellous graft is best delayed, especially in cases undergoing secondary closure. Traditional antibiotic treatment protocol for osteomyelitis includes long-term (minimum 6 weeks) systemic antibiotic therapy based on the results of antibiogram. Use of local depository systems for delivery of antibiotics has become common in the elimination of human infections and is gaining popularity in small animals as an adjunct to the traditional therapy of osteomyelitis. Local antibiotic implants and their applications in veterinary medicine have recently been reviewed (Hayes *et al.* 2013). These agents are designed to achieve high local concentrations of antibiotics and maintain prolonged activity without systemic toxicity (Weisman *et al.* 2000; Phillips *et al.* 2007, Seddighi *et al.* 2007;

Bridgens *et al.* 2008). As such, they defy the guidelines for selecting antibiotics based on antibiogram (minimum inhibitory concentration) and duration of treatment. Significant work is therefore warranted to refine the selection criteria for antibiotics and minimum duration of local release. In the meantime, the clinical application of tobramycin-impregnated calcium sulfate beads has been described in dogs (Ham *et al.* 2008). The safety of these beads has been confirmed in dogs that received the maximum dose prescribed in humans without adverse effects (Turner *et al.* 2005). In both studies, beads lost their radiopacity within 4 to 5 weeks after implantation. These beads compare favorably with gentamicin-impregnated PMMA beads because they are bioresorbable and osteoconductive. Demineralized bone matrix impregnated with gentamicin has been investigated in vitro for potential application in nonunions in humans (Lewis *et al.* 2012). The authors concluded that this carrier could release clinically relevant levels of antibiotics for 13 days, which is less than typically considered as appropriate for systemic antibiotherapy in small animals. Nonetheless, this approach is appealing because it would combine osteoinductive and osteoconductive properties in a cost-effective substitute. However, further studies are warranted to validate this approach in small animals.

Prevention of osteomyelitis via proper soft tissue and orthopedic surgical technique should be the goal of every surgeon. Prophylactic antibiotherapy is justified by placement of implants, duration of surgery, and preexisting compromise of trauma patients. A short course (3 days) of antibiotics has been recommended in humans after repair of open fractures (Holtom 2001). Interestingly, similar results have recently been published in 808 dogs treated with TPLOs; dogs that did not receive postoperative antibiotherapy were four times more likely to develop a surgical site infection than dogs treated with TPLO and postoperative antibiotics. They were also eight times more likely to develop surgical site infection than dogs treated with an extracapsular suture repair and postoperative antibiotics (Frey *et al.* 2010). These results were confirmed in another study of 1000 TPLOs in which the odds of postoperative infections were decreased by half in dogs that received postoperative antibiotics (Fitzpatrick and Solano 2010). The underlying cause of these findings may relate to early treatment of undiagnosed postoperative infection and control of postoperative contamination but remain undetermined at this point.

The role of intraoperative cultures during orthopedic procedures in the prevention of postoperative infections remains controversial. Several studies suggest that positive intraoperative cultures do not correlate with a higher risk of cultures (Stevenson *et al.* 1986; Lee and Kapatkin *et al.* 2002). However, animals with positive cultures are typically prescribed antibiotics, thereby potentially masking the impact of positive cultures. The author reviewed the records of 203 TPLOs in 178 dogs without routine postoperative antibiotherapy: 21 postoperative infections (equivalent to 10.3%) were reported, consisting of 9 incisional infections (4.4%) and 12 bone infections (5.9%). Cultures obtained at the time of initial TPLO were positive in 21 cases (10%) and were managed with antibiotherapy. Infections were subsequently diagnosed in 4 of these dogs (19%) compared with 12 of 172 TPLOs (10%) with negative cultures. Although not statistically significant, dogs with positive cultures were two times more likely to be diagnosed with infections.

Strategies currently explored to prevent implant-related osteomyelitis target the surface of fixation devices to inhibit bacterial attachment and biofilm formation (Harris and Richards 2006). For example, the surface of implants can be treated to modify its topography (polishing) and chemistry (nitrogen ion or titanium coating), thereby improving fibroblast attachment and growth while minimizing bacterial adhesion. Protein-resistant coatings such as albumin and hyaluronic acid are believed to interfere with the hydrophobic interactions occurring between the surface of the implant and the bacterial cell wall. These hydrophilic coatings would be especially relevant in locations where cell adhesion is undesirable, such as areas in contact with tendons. Antimicrobial coating is a concept derived from local antibiotic carriers, in which implant surfaces are coated with antibiotics, antiseptics, or ions (silver or nitrate) to control the local bacterial population. Although promising, none of these strategies fully prevents bacterial adhesion.

References

Barnhart, M.D. (2003) Results of single-session bilateral tibial plateau leveling osteotomies as a treatment for bilaterally ruptured cranial cruciate ligaments in dogs: (2000-2001). *Journal of the American Animal Hospital Association* 39 (6), 573-578.

Bergh, M.S., Peirone, B. (2012) Complications of tibial plateau leveling osteotomy in dogs. *Veterinary and Comparative Orthopaedics and Traumatology* 5 (5), 349-58.

Bridgens, J., Davies, S., Tilley, L., et al. (2008) Orthopaedic bone cement. Do we know what we are using? *The Journal of Bone and Joint Surgery* 90 (5), 643-647.

Etter, S.W., Ragetly, G.R., Bennett, R.A., et al. (2013) Effect of using triclosan-impregnated suture for incisional closure on surgical infection and inflammation following tibial plateau leveling osteotomy in dogs. *Journal of the American Veterinary Medical Association* 242 (3), 355-358.

Fitzpatrick, N., Solano, M.A. (2010) Predictive variables for complications after TPLO with stifle inspection by arthrotomy in 1000 consecutive dogs. *Veterinary Surgery* 39 (4), 460-474.

Frey, T.N., Hoelzler, M.G., Scavelli, T.D., et al. (2010) Risk factors for surgical site infection-inflammation in dogs undergoing surgery for rupture of the cranial cruciate ligament: 902 cases (2005-2006). *Journal of the American Veterinary Medical Association* 236 (1), 88-94.

Gallagher, A.D., Mertens, W.D. (2012) Implant removal rate from infection after tibial plateau leveling osteotomy in dogs. *Veterinary Surgery* 41 (4), 482-485.

Ham, K., Griffon, D., Sedighi, M.R., *et al.* (2008) Clinical application of tobramycin-impregnated calcium sulfate beads in dogs. *Journal of the American Animal Hospital Association* 44(6), 320-326.

Harris, L.G., Richards, R.G. (2006) Staphylococci and implant surfaces: a review. *Injury* 37 (Suppl.), S3-S14.

Hayes, G., Moens, N., Gibson, T. (2013) A review of local antibiotic implants and applications to veterinary orthopaedic surgery. *Veterinary and Comparative Orthopaedics and Traumatology* 26 (4), 251-259.

Hirshenson, M.S., Krotscheck, U., Thompson, M.S., et al. (2012) Evaluation of complications and short term outcome after unilateral or single-session bilateral tibial tuberosity advancement for cranial cruciate rupture in dogs. *Veterinary and Comparative Orthopaedics and Traumatology* 25, 402-409.

Holtom, P.D. (2001) Post-operative orthopedic infections. *Current Treatment Options in Infectious Diseases* 3, 309-314.

Johnson, K. (1994) Osteomyelitis in dogs and cats. *Journal of the American Veterinary Medical Association* 205, 1882-1887.

Lee, K.C., Kapatkin, A.S. (2002) Positive intraoperative cultures and canine total hip replacement: risk factors, periprosthetic infection and surgical success. *Journal of the American Animal Hospital Association* 38 (3), 271-278.

Lewis, C.S., Supronowicz, P.R., Zhukauskas, R.M., et al. (2012) Local antibiotic delivery with demineralized bone matrix. *Cell Tissue Bank* 13 (1), 119-127.

Nazarali, A. (2013) Peri-operative use of antibiotics in tibial plateau leveling osteotomy surgeries performed on dogs and its effect on surgical site infections: 224 cases (2008-2010). In *Proceedings of the ACVS Symposium*, San Antonio, October 23-26.

Phillips, H., Boothe, D.M., Shofer, F., et al. (2007) In vitro elution studies of amikacin and cefazolin from PMMA. *Veterinary Surgery* 36, 272-278.

Priddy II, N.H., Tomlinson, J.L., Dodam JR, et al. (2003) Complications with and owner assessment of the outcome of tibial plateau leveling osteotomy for treatment of cranial cruciate ligament rupture in dogs: 193 cases (1997-2001). *Journal of the American Veterinary Medical Association* 222 (12), 1726-1732.

Seddighi, M.R., Griffon, D.J., Constable, P., et al. (2007) Effects of porcine SIS on elution characteristics of gentamicin-impregnated POP. *American Journal of Veterinary* 69, 171-177.

Smith, T.O., Sexton, D., Mann, C., et al. (2010) Sutures versus staples for skin closure in orthopaedic surgery: meta-analysis. *British Medical Journal* 16, 340.

Southwood, L.L., Kawcak, C.E., McIlwraith, C.W., et al. (2003) Use of scintigraphy for assessment of fracture healing and early diagnosis of osteomyelitis following fracture repair in rabbits. *American Journal of Veterinary Research* 64, 736-745.

Stevenson, S., Olmstead, M.L., Kowalski, J. (1986) Bacterial culturing for prediction of postoperative complications following open fracture repair in small animals. *Veterinary Surgery* 15, 99-102.

Trampuz, A., Zimmerli, W. (2006) Diagnosis and treatment of infections associated with fracture-fixation devices. *Injury* 37 (Suppl.), S59-S66.

Turner, T.M., Urban, R.M., Hall, D.J., et al. (2005) Local and systemic levels of tobramycin delivered from calcium sulfate bone graft substitutes pellets. *Clinical Orthopaedics and Related Research* 437, 97-104.

Vince, K.J., Lascelles, B.D., Mathews, K.G., et al. (2008) Evaluation of wraps covering the distal aspect of pelvic limbs for prevention of bacterial strike-through in an ex vivo canine model. *Veterinary Surgery* 37 (4), 406-411.

Weese, J.S. (2008) A review of postoperative infections in veterinary orthopedic surgery. *Veterinary and Comparative Orthopaedics and Traumatology* 21, 99-105.

Weisman, D., Olmstead, M., Kowalski, J.J. (2000) In vitro evaluation of antibiotic elution from PPMA and mechanical assessment of antibiotic-PMMA composites. *Veterinary Surgery,* 29, 245-251.

6 Septic Arthritis

John Innes

CVS Vets, ChesterGates Veterinary Specialists, Chester, UK; University of Liverpool, Liverpool, Merseyside, UK

Definition

Septic (infective) arthritis is a microbial infection of the synovium and the synovial space. As a complication of orthopedic surgery, infective arthritis is generally bacterial in origin; this chapter is limited to this form of the condition. Bacterial invasion of joints in orthopedic surgery is most frequently caused by direct contamination during surgery but may also arise from postoperative hematogenous localization, or local spread from adjacent tissues. The most common bacteria isolated are representative of the most likely contaminants during surgery: *Staphylococcus intermedius, Staphylococcus aureus,* and β-hemolytic *Streptococcus* spp.

Risk factors

Postoperative infections after articular surgery probably represent the most frequent cause of infective arthritis in dogs and cats. Risk factors for bacterial infective arthritis can be divided in to those that are a product of the type of procedure performed and those that are patient-based risk factors. These are listed in Table 6.1.

Procedure-dependent factors

Placement of a biomaterial in the joint space

A biomaterial in the joint space, or in the synovium, appears to increase the risk of infection. Biomaterials can provide a surface

Table 6.1 Risk factors for postsurgical infective arthritis in dogs and cats

Procedure-based factors
• Placement of a biomaterial in the joint
• High risk: braided, permanent suture
○ High risk: humeral transcondylar screw
○ Moderate risk: intraarticular plate and screws
○ Low risk: absorbable suture
• Open arthrotomy (or arthroscopy)
• Prolonged surgery time
• Spread of infection from adjacent tissues

Patient-based factors
• Previous surgery in that anatomic region
• Reduced blood supply
• Immunosuppression
○ Cushing's syndrome or other immunosuppressive disorder
○ Systemic corticosteroids or other immunosuppressives
○ Local (depot) corticosteroids

for bacterial colonization with subsequent secretion of glycocalyx, which protects the bacteria from host immune cells and antibiotics. The risk of infection is low if absorbable biomaterials are used. However, permanent sutures, particularly braided materials, appear prone to infection, presumably because of the large surface area available for bacterial colonization. Bacterial infection rates after total joint arthroplasty in dogs appear relatively low, at approximately 1% (Dyce and Olmstead 2002; Schiffelers *et al.* 2005; Bergh *et al.* 2006). Late chronic infections can occur, and although these are thought to originate at the time of surgery, their presentation is delayed (6–24 months) because of a small inoculum or low bacterial virulence.

Type of surgery

Compared with open arthrotomy, arthroscopy seems associated with a very low infection rate, presumably because of the limited exposure of tissues and the constant lavage of the joint space during the procedure. Combined, these factors are expected to lower the intraoperative inoculation of bacteria. In line with general principles of surgery, duration of surgery correlates with risks of infection.

Spread of infection from adjacent tissues

Postoperative infective arthritis quite commonly results from an extension of an adjacent infection. One of the most common examples consists of the spread of infection from an infected lateral febellotibial suture into the stifle joint. However, spreading of osteomyelitis into an adjacent joint seems uncommon. In one retrospective series, only 2 of 58 cases resulted from an extension of osteomyelitis (Bennett and Taylor 1988).

Patient-dependent factors

Revision surgeries or the need for an additional surgery on a previously operated joint, appear to carry an approximately fivefold increase in the rate of infection (Olmstead *et al.* 1983).

Reduced blood supply to a particular joint will decrease the ability of the host immune system to respond to bacterial contamination or infection. Similarly, systemic or local immunosuppression through illness such as Cushing's syndrome, medication such as systemic immunosuppressive agents (corticosteroids or chemotherapeutic agents), or local injection of corticosteroids promotes bacterial colonization and increases the risk of postoperative infection.

Complications in Small Animal Surgery, First Edition. Edited by Dominique Griffon and Annick Hamaide.

© 2016 John Wiley & Sons, Inc. Published 2016 by John Wiley & Sons, Inc.

Companion website: www.wiley.com/go/griffon/complications

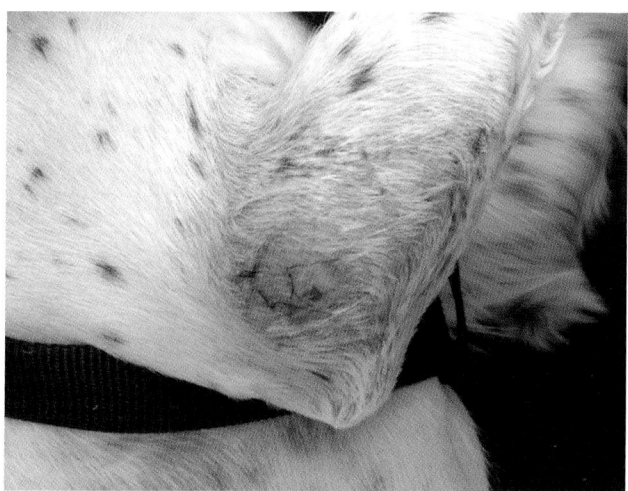

Figure 6.1 Draining sinus from the lateral aspect of the elbow joint of a Springer spaniel with incomplete ossification of the humeral condyle treated with a transcondylar lag screw.

Diagnosis of bacterial infective arthritis

Clinical signs of postoperative septic arthritis typically include loss of function, with a moderate to severe lameness, often with an acute onset. Additional signs may include:

- Joint swelling, redness, and palpable warmth
- Draining sinus (Figure 6.1)
- Pain on joint manipulation
- Local lymphadenopathy
- Pyrexia: detected in the minority of cases (Choi *et al.* 2009).
- Systemic depression or recumbency (uncommon)

Suspicion of infective arthritis should prompt immediate arthrocentesis. An algorithm for interpretation of synovial fluid analysis is presented in Figure 6.2. Typically, the synovial fluid is increased in volume and appears turbid (Figure 6.3A). Synovial fluid should be submitted for cytologic examination, including total and differential nucleated cell counts. Bacterial infective arthritis should be a working diagnosis ("probable" bacterial infective arthritis) if clinical signs and analysis of the affected synovial fluid suggest bacterial infective arthritis. Such synovial fluid has a high dominance of neutrophils. Degenerative and toxic changes such as pyknotic nuclei may be noted along with degranulation and cell rupture. Careful examination of the synovial fluid smear may allow identification of intracellular bacteria (Figure 6.3B); such a feature is pathognomonic for bacterial infection but is only seen in a minority of cases. An automated cell count of more than 5×10^9 cells/L with greater than 40% neutrophils should raise suspicion of postoperative bacterial infective arthritis. In acute cases, cell counts are usually very high, ranging between 100 and 250×10^9/L with 98% neutrophils (Table 6.2). However, in chronic cases, cell counts may be lower, approximating 40 to 100×10^9/L.

The result of bacteriologic culture of synovial fluid should *not* be used as a diagnostic criterion because of the risk of false-negative cultures in the presence of infection. Nonetheless, culture of synovial fluid should be attempted in all suspect cases of bacterial infective arthritis. The use of a blood culture medium is highly recommended to increase the likelihood of positive results when culturing synovial fluid. Initial incubation in this medium is also suggested to increase the sensitivity of the test.

Synovial biopsy for culture and histology may be justified in cases with negative synovial fluid cultures and persistent arthritis.

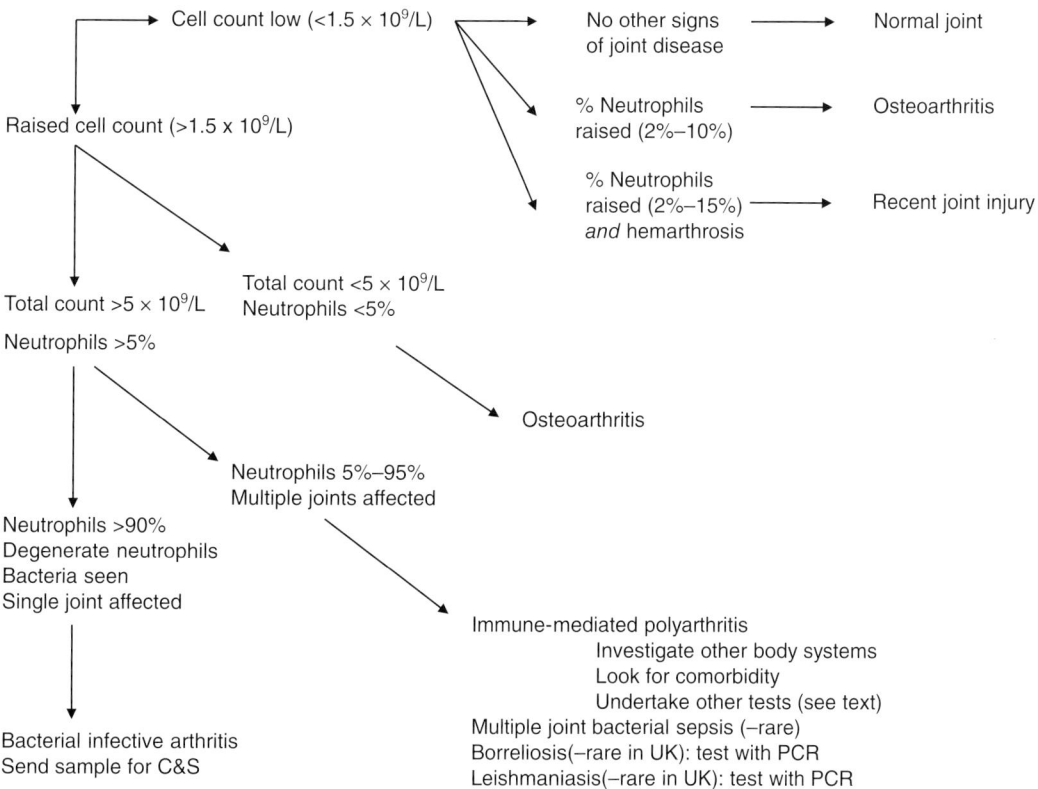

Figure 6.2 Algorithm for the interpretation of synovial fluid analysis. C&S, culture and sensitivity; PCR, polymerase chain reaction.

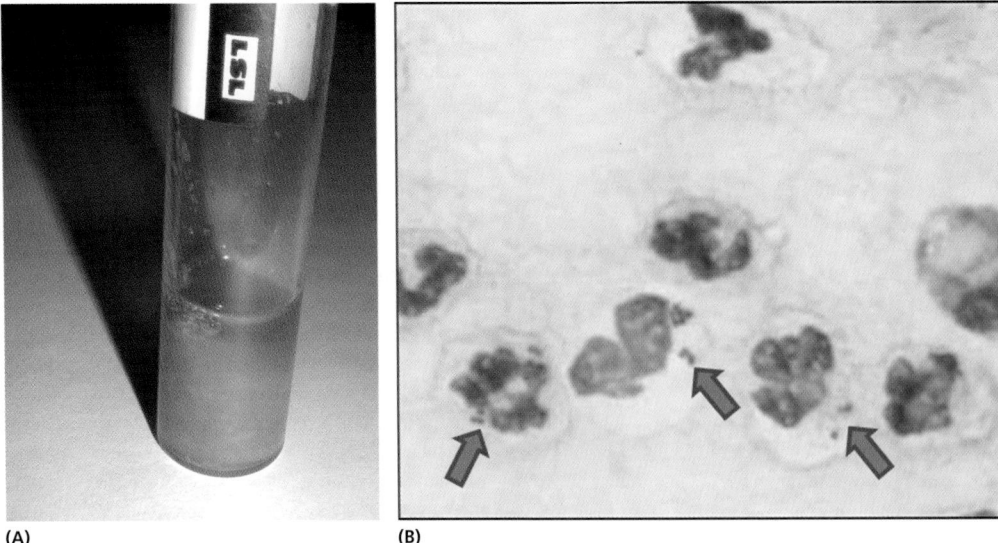

(A)   (B)

Figure 6.3 A, Gross appearance of synovial fluid from an infected stifle joint. **B,** Cytologic evaluation of synovial fluid showing intracellular bacteria.

Instances include failure of a case to respond to broad-spectrum antibiotic therapy or uncertain diagnosis, requiring synovial histology.

The author suggests that it is useful to use a criteria-based system for the diagnosis of bacterial infective arthritis. These criteria are listed in Table 6.2. A diagnosis of "definite" bacterial infective arthritis is based on the presence of all three criteria. A diagnosis of "probable" bacterial infective arthritis is based on the presence of criteria 1 and 2.

Although diagnostic imaging is not required for the diagnosis of bacterial infective arthritis, radiographs may help investigate the presence of contributing factors (e.g., loose intraarticular implants) and document any secondary changes. Nonspecific radiographic changes include soft tissue swelling centered on the joint line; joint effusion; and, with time, osteophytosis. Of course, in a postoperative situation, many of these features may already be present because of the original pathology or previous surgery. Joint effusion may be easily assessed in joints such as the stifle, where the infrapatellar fat pad allows delineation of the joint cavity. However, in other joints (e.g., shoulder or hip), the clinician may need to carefully compare the width of joint spaces between bilateral joints to evaluate synovial fluid volume. In some longer standing cases in which the bacteria initiate catabolic processes within tissues, erosive changes may appear in the subchondral bone. Such changes can appear within 10 to 14 days in uncontrolled infection, signaling significant damage to articular structures and a reduced prognosis for full recovery.

Table 6.2 Synovial fluid features in bacterial infective arthritis

Parameter	Typical result
Gross appearance	• Turbid • Yellow-orange-red-grey
Total cell count	• 100–250 × 10^9/L (acute cases) • 40–100 × 10^9/L (chronic cases)
Percentage neutrophils	• 97%–99% (acute cases) • 80%–99% (chronic cases)
Neutrophil morphology	• Degenerate • Intracellular bacteria may be seen

Treatment of postsurgical septic arthritis

The evidence base supporting treatment options for septic arthritis is currently small and consists of retrospective case series. Treatment can involve several approaches, which may be used in combination:

• Systemic antibiotics
• Joint aspiration (an inherent part of synovial fluid sampling)
• Joint irrigation
• Arthroscopic synovectomy
• Local antibiotic delivery systems

Systemic antibiotic therapy

Systemic antibiotics are a standard feature of all treatment regimens and are often initiated intravenously to rapidly gain effective tissue concentrations. Experimentally, antibiotic therapy commenced within 24 hours of infection decreases collagen loss from cartilage in septic arthritis but does not prevent glycosaminoglycan loss from the cartilage matrix (Ley *et al.* 2009).

Broad-spectrum antibiotics are administered while culture and sensitivity results are pending. Antibiotherapy is adjusted based on the results of bacterial culture and sensitivity testing. The author recommends a minimum of 28 days of therapy with repeat arthrocentesis and synovial fluid analysis at the end of that period. If the cell count has not returned to normal and the neutrophil percentage is still above 3%, antibiotic therapy is best continued until synovial fluid cytology is within the normal range (or one consistent with osteoarthrosis, if present).

Joint irrigation or surgical intervention at the time of initial presentation and in the absence of an infected surgical implant is controversial. The literature is based on retrospective studies and, as such, there may be bias as to whether clinicians opted for purely medical therapy or a combination of antimicrobials plus surgical intervention. Nevertheless, no convincing evidence support surgical intervention unless there is gross contamination of the joint or an infected implant, which will act as a nidus for ongoing bacterial colonization (Clements *et al.* 2005; Marquass *et al.* 2010). Surgical interventions can involve joint aspiration and irrigation, arthroscopic inspection and lavage of the joint, open exploratory arthrotomy, and local delivery of antibiotics.

Joint aspiration and irrigation

This procedure can be simply achieved with two needles placed in the joint at sites used for arthrocentesis. Copious quantities of sterile lactated Ringer's solution (or normal saline) are then injected to irrigate the joint.

Arthroscopic inspection and lavage of the joint

This approach is recommended if the joint must be explored to investigate other potential complications or to break down fibrin deposits in chronic infection. After inspection of the joint, synovial resection can be performed manually or with a powered shaver. However, no clinical evidence is available to support the benefit of synovial resection.

Open exploratory arthrotomy

Exploratory arthrotomy is generally best avoided, but it may be necessary in a minority of cases if arthroscopy is not available or if a surgical implant must be removed to eliminate the presence of nidus for infection.

Local delivery of antibiotics

Local antibiotics delivery systems may be used if the antibiotic of choice (based on culture and sensitivity results) has a toxicity profile precluding long-term systemic use. This approach requires local slow-release preparations, eluted over several weeks from carriers similar to those used to treat bone infections (see Chapter 5). Implantable carriers are used most frequently in the face of multiresistant organisms such as methicillin-resistant *S. aureus* (Horstman *et al.* 2004).

Drug delivery systems used for slow release may be divided into two groups: (1) nonbiodegradable and (2) biodegradable carriers. The nonbiodegradable carrier traditionally used for this purpose is polymethylmethacrylate (PMMA) (Figure 6.4). PMMA is commonly used as a bone cement in orthopaedic surgery because it becomes rigid after full polymerization. For the treatment of bacterial infective arthritis, preformed antibiotic-impregnated PMMA beads threaded on a wire are available commercially and are implanted into joint recesses.

The biodegradable carriers have the advantage of being degraded, mainly by hydrolysis, to nontoxic end products. Such carriers may

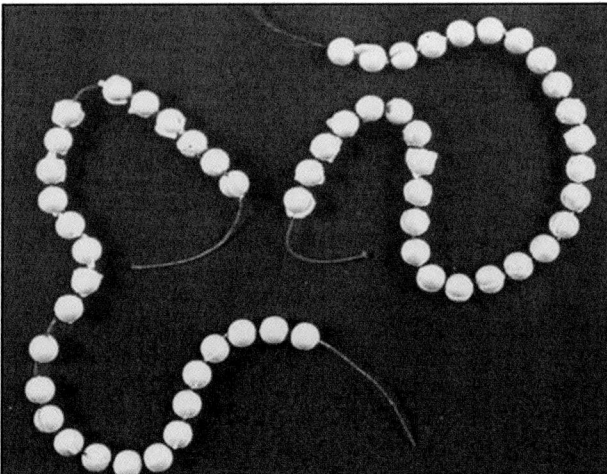

Figure 6.4 Polymethylmethacrylate beads impregnated with antibiotics, such as gentamicin, can be purchased in some territories or made at the tableside.

consist of inorganic salts (hydroxyapatite, tricalcium phosphate) or of polymeric biomaterials. Biodegradable polymeric carriers offer a broad range of characteristics, including degradability, permeability, and certain mechanical properties. Natural polymers consist of large proteins, such as processed fibers of bovine collagen, gelatin, and polysaccharides such as hyaluronan. Collagen antibiotic carriers are commercially available and have been used in dogs (Horstman *et al.*, 2004).

Outcome

Clinical response should be expected within 24 to 48 hours of treatment in acute cases. A reduction in pain and lameness along with resolution of pyrexia provide evidence that the treatment is effective. The author strongly recommends repeating synovial fluid analysis to monitor the efficacy of treatment and direct clinical decision making. Synovial fluid total and differential cell counts after 7 to 14 days of therapy should be compared with initial counts. The results of culture and sensitivity testing may justify a change in antibiotic therapy based on the resistance profile of the isolate. Treatment should be administered continuously for a minimum of 28 days or when clinical signs have resolved, whichever is longer. A repeat synovial fluid analysis should be performed before the withdrawal of antibiotic therapy; this is unlikely to be before 28 days. The author continues with antibiotic therapy until the cell count is within the normal or osteoarthritic range and the percentage of neutrophils is at or below 3%.

There is little information on the prognosis of dogs affected by bacterial infective arthritis. In one series, 17 of 32 joints recovered fully, 13 partially, and 2 failed to recover (Clements *et al.* 2005). Thus, in this series, infection was resolved in 94% of cases. Other reports document similar outcomes (Marquass *et al.* 2010). Despite these encouraging reports, clinicians should be aware that infected joints often have preexisting pathology (e.g., degenerative joint disease) that compromise expectations for full recovery.

Prevention

The role of antibiotics in preventing postoperative septic arthritis is somewhat controversial. A blinded, randomized, controlled trial of dogs undergoing elective orthopedic surgery at a U.S. veterinary teaching hospital found that the infection rate for control dogs (receiving saline injection only) was significantly higher than the rate for dogs treated with antimicrobials (penicillin or cefazolin) (Whittem *et al.* 1999). However, in a study of humans undergoing arthroscopic surgery, there appears to be no benefit from prophylactic antibiotic therapy in preventing postoperative joint sepsis (Nguyen *et al.* 2010). Of course, species and procedure differences are likely to be major factors for the opposing findings in these studies.

Relevant literature

The stifle, elbow, and carpus appear to be the joints most frequently affected by septic arthritis (Bennett and Taylor 1988; Marchevsky and Read 1999; Clements *et al.* 2005). Infection rates in dogs between 0% and 2.7% were reported for the major joints of the dog in one study with no significant differences among joints (Clements *et al.* 2005). In that study, the tarsus had the highest infection rate, although the stifle joint was the most frequently affected because of the large number of stifle surgeries performed.

Several routine surgeries appear associated with a higher frequency of septic arthritis. Lateral suture stabilization (LSS) of cranial cruciate ligament rupture involves the placement of a non-absorbable biomaterial close to the lateral aspect of the stifle joint. Although reported infection rates for LSS are within the expected infection rates for clean surgery in dogs (Casale and McCarthy 2009; Vasseur *et al.* 1988; Brown *et al.* 1997), the close proximity of the biomaterial to the stifle joint capsule increases the risk of implant-related infections. As a consequence, joint lavage is often necessary to manage these cases (Casale and McCarthy 2009). Treatment of incomplete ossification of the humeral condyle typically involves placement of a transcondylar screw. This procedure has been associated with unexpectedly high infection rates, approaching 30% (Hattersley *et al.* 2011). The risk of infection in dogs reportedly doubles with approximately every 70 minutes of surgery time (Brown *et al.* 1997).

Culture of synovium has been suggested to improve the sensitivity of bacterial cultures compared with synovial fluid aspirates. However, a study in horses suggested that culture from synovium was no more likely to yield a positive result than synovial fluid culture (Madison *et al.* 1991), and data in dogs support that finding (Montgomery *et al.* 1989).

Polymerase chain reaction (PCR) for bacterial DNA may be used to identify bacteria in synovial fluids. However, a study of humans with septic arthritis failed to demonstrate that bacterial PCR offered any advantage over standard culture methods (Jalava *et al.* 2001). In addition, PCR for canine bacterial DNA will likely lead to false-positive diagnoses for bacterial infective arthritis.

Initial systemic antibiotherapy in dogs suspect of septic arthritis relies on the following agents (Clements *et al.* 2005):
• Clavulanate-potentiated amoxicillin
• Cephalexin
• Clavulanate-potentiated amoxicillin combined with metronidazole
• Cephalexin combined with metronidazole

The degree of articular cartilage damage caused by bacterial infection is variable and depends on the number, type, and virulence of the organism present; the extent to which the organisms multiply; and the local and general immunity of the patient. Initially, infection causes inflammation of the synovium. This is reflected in the synovial fluid, which becomes hypercellular with high numbers of polymorphonuclear leukocytes. The hypercellular joint fluid is a potent source of lysosomal enzymes. Proteolytic enzymes such as matrix metalloproteinases are also released from the lysosomal granules of synovial cells, which may also result in synovial, cartilage, and bone catabolism. Macrophages in the synovium are activated by bacterial antigens such as lipopolysaccharide and release inflammatory cytokines such as tumor necrosis factor-α and interleukin-1. Such cytokines induce a catabolic response from synovium and cartilage, resulting in proteolysis.

As in other forms of cartilage catabolism, in experimental bacterial arthritis, glycosaminoglycans (GAGs) such as aggrecan are degraded in cartilage before collagen. The loss of GAGs allows degradation of the collagen network and irreversible change. Synovial fluid is usually free of all the factors of the blood clotting system, but in septic arthritis, fibrin deposits form. The deposition of fibrin on the cartilage surface limits the normal exchange of cartilage metabolites and nutrients with the synovial fluid, and this may a further contributor to cartilage damage. The extent of cartilage damage correlates with long-term outcome and justifies early diagnosis and treatment of this condition.

References

Bennett, D., Taylor, D.J. (1988) Bacterial infective arthritis in the dog. *Journal of Small Animal Practice* 29, 207-230.

Bergh, M.S., Gilley, R.S., Shofer, F.S., et al. (2006) Complications and radiographic findings following cemented total hip replacement—a retrospective evaluation of 97 dogs. *Veterinary and Comparative Orthopaedics and Traumatology* 19, 172-179.

Brown, D.C., Conzemius, M.G., Shofer, F., et al. (1997) Epidemiologic evaluation of postoperative wound infections in dogs and cats. *Journal of the American Veterinary Medical Association* 210, 1302-1306.

Casale, S.A., McCarthy, R.J. (2009) Complications associated with lateral fabellotibial suture surgery for cranial cruciate ligament injury in dogs: 363 cases (1997-2005). *Journal of the American Veterinary Medical Association* 234, 229-235.

Choi, H.J., Kwon, E., Lee, J.I., et al. (2009) Safety and efficacy assessment of mesenchymal stem cells from canine adipose tissue or umbilical cord blood in a canine osteochondral defect model. *Tissue Engineering and Regenerative Medicine* 6, 1381-1390.

Clements, D.N., Owen, M.R., Mosley, J.R., et al. (2005) Retrospective study of bacterial infective arthritis in 31 dogs. *Journal of Small Animal Practice* 46, 171-176.

Dyce, J., Olmstead, M.L. (2002) Removal of infected canine cemented total hip prostheses using a femoral window technique. *Veterinary Surgery* 31, 552-560.

Hattersley, R., Mckee, M., O'Neill, T., et al. (2011) Postoperative complications after surgical management of incomplete ossification of the humeral condyle in dogs. *Veterinary Surgery* 40, 728-733.

Horstman, C.L., Conzemius, M.G., Evans, R., et al. (2004) Assessing the efficacy of perioperative oral carprofen after cranial cruciate surgery using noninvasive, objective pressure platform gait analysis. *Veterinary Surgery* 33, 286-292.

Jalava, J., Skurnik, M., Toivanen, A., et al. (2001) Bacterial PCR in the diagnosis of joint infection. *Annals of the Rheumatic Diseases* 60, 287-289.

Ley, C., Ekman, S., Roneus, B., et al. (2009) Interleukin-6 and high mobility group box protein-1 in synovial membranes and osteochondral fragments in equine osteoarthritis. *Research in Veterinary Science* 86, 490-497.

Madison, J.B., Sommer, M., Spencer, P.A. (1991) Relations among synovial-membrane histopathologic findings, synovial-fluid cytologic findings, and bacterial culture results in horses with suspected infectious arthritis—64 cases (1979-1987). *Journal of the American Veterinary Medical Association* 198, 1655-1661.

Marchevsky, A.M., & Read, R.A. (1999) Bacterial septic arthritis in 19 dogs. *Australian Veterinary Journal* 77, 233-237.

Marquass, B., Somerson, J.S., Hepp, P., et al. (2010) A novel MSC-seeded triphasic construct for the repair of osteochondral defects. *Journal of Orthopaedic Research* 28, 1586-99.

Montgomery, R.D., Long, I.R., Milton, J.L., et al. (1989) Comparison of aerobic culturette, synovial-membrane biopsy, and blood culture-medium in detection of canine bacterial arthritis. *Veterinary Surgery* 18, 300-303.

Nguyen, T.G., Little, C.B., Yenson, V.M., et al. (2010) Anti-IgD antibody attenuates collagen-induced arthritis by selectively depleting mature B-cells and promoting immune tolerance. *Journal of Autoimmunity* 35, 86-97.

Olmstead, M.L., Hohn, R.B., Turner, T.M. (1983) A 5-year study of 221 total hip replacements in the dog. *Journal of the American Veterinary Medical Association* 183, 191-194.

Schiffelers, R.M., Xu, J., Storm, G., et al. (2005) Effects of treatment with small interfering RNA on joint inflammation in mice with collagen-induced arthritis. *Arthritis and Rheumatism* 52, 1314-1318.

Vasseur, P.B., Levy, J., Dowd, E., et al. (1988) Surgical Wound-infection rates in dogs and cats—data from a teaching hospital. *Veterinary Surgery* 17, 60-64.

Whittem, T.L., Johnson, A.L., Smith, C.W., et al. (1999) Effect of perioperative prophylactic antimicrobial treatment in dogs undergoing elective orthopedic surgery. *Journal of the American Veterinary Medical Association* 215, 212-216.

7 Methicillin-Resistant Staphylococcal Infections

Scott Weese

Department of Pathobiology, University of Guelph, Guelph, Ontario, Canada

Definition

Methicillin-resistant staphylococcal (MRS) infections are infections caused by staphylococci (Figure 7.1 and Table 7.1) that are resistant to methicillin and by extension to virtually all β-lactam antimicrobials. Postsurgical MRS infections in dogs are typically caused by *Staphylococcus pseudintermedius* (MRSP) or *Staphylococcus aureus* (MRSA), two varieties of bacteria that can reside in the nose, mouth, intestines, and skin of healthy dogs and humans.

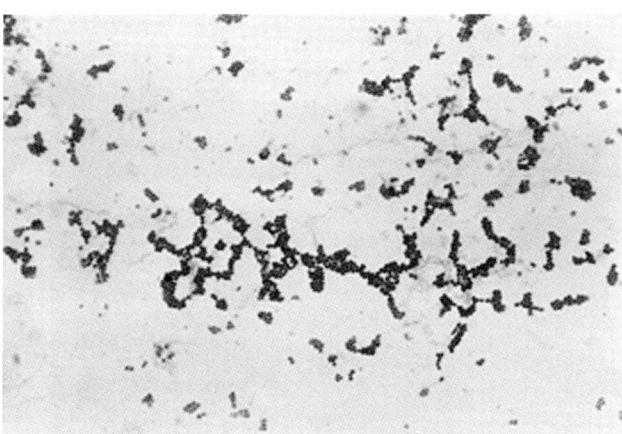

Figure 7.1 Gram stain appearance of *Staphylococcus aureus*. Note the gram-positive (purple) cocci that cluster together in clumps.

Table 7.1 Examples of coagulase-positive and coagulase-negative *Staphylococcus* species

Coagulase positive	Coagulase negative
S. aureus	S. epidermidis
S. pseudintermedius*	S. haemolyticus
S. schleiferi coagulans	S. schleiferi schleiferi
S. delphini*	S. hominis
S. hyicus†	S. warneri
S. intermedius*	S. felis
	S. cohnii
	S. auricularis

*S. intermedius group.

†Variable coagulase status.

Staphylococcus schleiferi subsp *coagulans* is another coagulase-positive *Staphylococcus* species that can cause infections in dogs and cats; however, it is predominantly a cause of pyoderma and otitis, not surgical site infections (SSIs).

Risk Factors

Risk factors predisposing patients to surgical infection in general include:

- Duration of surgery or anesthesia: This factor may explain the increased risk of infection associated with simultaneous bilateral orthopedic procedures.
- Placement of surgical implants: Surgical plates act as a nidus for infection and a site of biofilm formation, which can help the bacteria evade the immune system and antibiotics.
- Factors affecting the immune system: increasing age, immunosuppressive treatment, presence of comorbidity

Factors specifically predisposing dogs to MRSA or MRSP have not been extensively studied but may be extrapolated from studies in humans. These include:

- Previous exposure to antimicrobials
- Preoperative MRSA colonization

Diagnosis

Methicillin-resistant staphylococcal infections cannot be differentiated from infections caused by susceptible staphylococci or other opportunistic pathogens via clinical and radiographic examination (Figures 7.2 and 7.3). Culture and susceptibility testing are required for diagnosis. Culture is never contraindicated and should be undertaken in any suspected infection after placements of implants and in facilities with high incidences of methicillin-resistant surgical infections. The following measures should be considered to obtain a definitive diagnosis:

- Submit an appropriate sample from the surgical site, avoiding skin contamination because MRS can be skin commensals.
- Select a laboratory that will distinguish coagulase-positive from coagulase-negative strains and at a minimum differentiate *S. aureus* from other coagulase-positive staphylococci.
- Resistance to cefoxitin is indicative of methicillin resistance (MR) in *S. aureus*.
- Resistance to oxacillin is indicative of MR in infections caused by *S. pseudintermedius* and *S. schleiferi* subsp *coagulans*.

Complications in Small Animal Surgery, First Edition. Edited by Dominique Griffon and Annick Hamaide.

© 2016 John Wiley & Sons, Inc. Published 2016 by John Wiley & Sons, Inc.

Companion website: www.wiley.com/go/griffon/complications

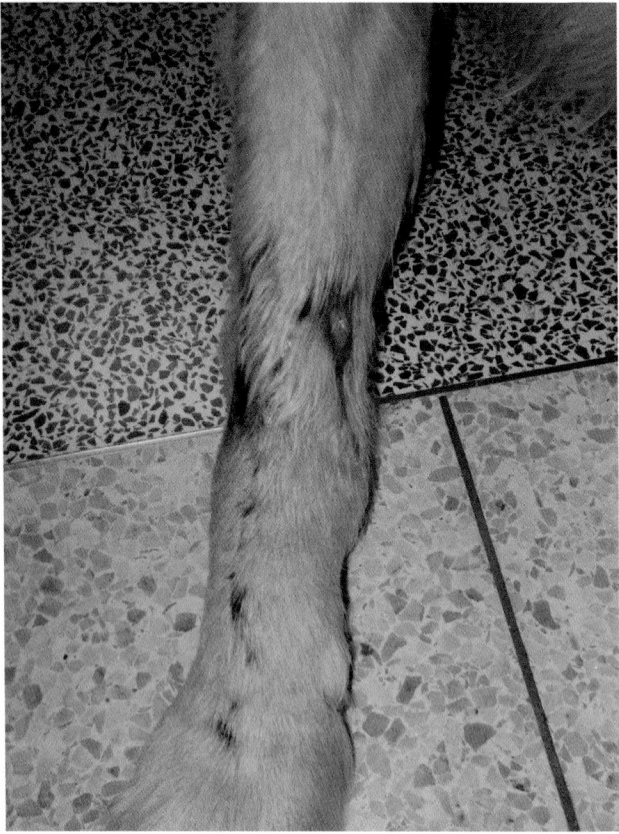

Figure 7.2 Draining tract in the forelimb of a dog with a surgical site infection caused by methicillin-resistant *Staphylococcus pseudintermedius*.

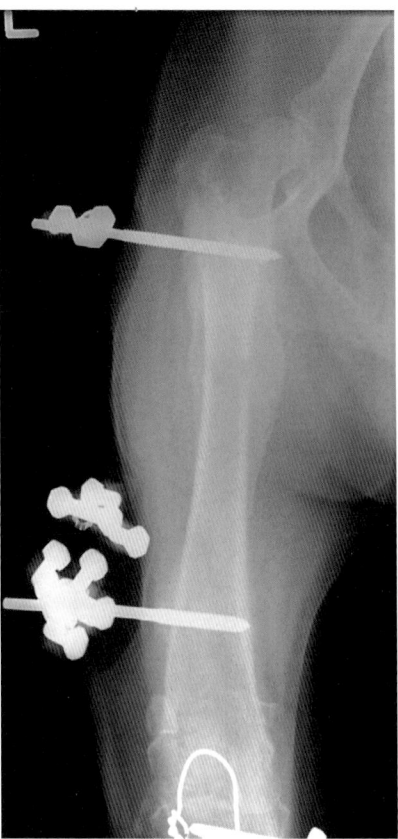

Figure 7.3 Implant-associated methicillin-resistant *Staphylococcus pseudintermedius* infection in a dog. Note the marked periosteal reaction around the proximal external fixator pin and extending distally on the femur. A draining tract was present surrounding the pin at its cutaneous insertion point.

Treatment

The principles relevant to the management of any opportunistic infections (Figure 7.4) (see Chapter 8) apply to the treatment of orthopedic infections caused by MRS. Antimicrobial therapy should be based on the susceptibility of the agent and warrants special considerations:

- All β-lactams, including carbapenems, are contraindicated, even if in vitro susceptibility to a particular β-lactam is reported.
- Fluoroquinolones are best avoided because of unpredictable response to treatment and the ease of emergence of resistance during treatment.
- Inducible clindamycin resistance is common in MRSA and occasionally found in MRSP. Clindamycin should be avoided in erythromycin-resistant staphylococci unless specific testing for inducible clindamycin resistance (e.g., D-test) has been performed.
- MRSA and MRSP are often susceptible to doxycycline, chloramphenicol, and amikacin, but resistance is increasingly common, particularly among MRSP.
- Implantation of antimicrobial-impregnated materials (e.g., polymethylmethacrylate [PMMA] beads, collagen sponges, gel matrices, calcium sulfate) can be useful along with other local or regional approaches such as regional limb perfusion.

Consideration must be given to measures that can be used to reduce the risk of transmission of MRS to owners, other patients, and clinic personnel. There is no standard approach to management of MRS in clinics, and factors such as clinic design, personnel availability, caseload, and risk aversion play roles in determining the type of infection control response. The bacterium that is involved

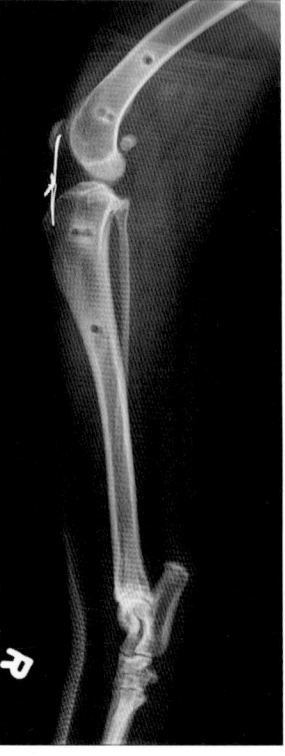

Figure 7.4 Surgical site infection shown in Figure 7.2 after removal of the pins and elimination of the infection.

Table 7.2 Examples of general infection control practices for management of animals with methicillin-resistant *Staphylococcus aureus* and methicillin-resistant *Staphylococcus pseudintermedius* infections.

Patient care	Personal hygiene	Facility measures
House in isolation or with barriers in main hospital.	Good attention to hand hygiene, including after glove removal	Good overall infection control program
Minimize of cross-use of items (e.g., bowls, leashes).	Do not wear clinic outerwear (e.g., lab coat, scrubs) home.	Written infection control protocols
Walk in separate area.		Surveillance for SSIs and recording of MRS infection rates
Use personal protective equipment (gloves, dedicated outerwear) when handling.		Good environmental cleaning and disinfection
Prevent contact of infected or colonized animals with other animals.		
Keep infected sites covered with an impermeable bandage whenever possible.		

MRS, methicillin-resistant staphylococcal; SSI, surgical site infection.

also plays a role because infection control measures are often more aggressive for MRSA because of the zoonotic infection concerns. The prevalence of MRS in the patient population also plays a role. For example, if a clinic has a busy dermatology service that is not physically or procedurally separated from the rest of the caseload (a common but undesirable situation) and if that dermatology population has a high prevalence of MRSP-infected patients that are not isolated, it is harder to justify strict isolation of a surgical patient with MRSP infection. Although there are no standard approaches, some general recommendations can be made (Table 7.2).

Given the low virulence and high prevalence of MR coagulase-negative staphylococci, measures beyond general infection control practices used for any patient are probably adequate. Owners should be notified about concerns regarding zoonotic transmission of MRS and counseled on basic infection control practices (Box 7.1). MRSA is the main concern, although the incidence of clinical MRSA infection from companion animals is probably very low. There is limited risk of zoonotic transmission of MRSP, but rare infections have been reported, so some degree of prudence is required. There is little to no evidence that MR coagulase-negative staphylococci are relevant zoonotic pathogens.

Box 7.1 Measures that can be recommended for home care of animals with methicillin-resistant *Staphylococcus aureus* and methicillin-resistant *Staphylococcus pseudintermedius* infections to reduce the risk of zoonotic transmission

---

Limit contact with high-risk sites on the animal (i.e. site of infection, mouth, nose, perineum).

Cover infected sites with an impermeable dressing whenever possible.

Wash hands after contact with the animal.

Wear gloves for any contact with an infected site and wash hands after glove removal.

Restrict contact of the infected animal with high-risk people (e.g., young children, elderly individuals, persons with compromised immune systems).

Restrict contact of the infected animal with animals outside of the household.

Regularly launder pet bedding in hot water and dry using a clothes dryer.

Ensure that people with skin lesions avoid contact with the animal or cover the lesions with an impermeable dressing before any contact with the animal.

Outcome

The outcome is highly dependent on the site and severity of infection, not the bacterium that is involved. MRS infections should not carry a poorer prognosis than infections caused by susceptible staphylococci (Faires *et al.* 2010) as long as the resistant infection is identified and appropriate treatment is started promptly. Rapid and accurate diagnosis may be the most important prognostic factor.

After successful treatment of MRS infection, nasal, pharyngeal, gastrointestinal, or skin colonization with the organism may persist. The goal of treatment is clinical cure, not microbiologic cure, so cultures are not indicated after successful treatment. It is important to be aware, however, of the potential (if not high likelihood) of at least transient colonization with MRS after elimination of infection. Accordingly, elimination of clinical infection does not necessarily mean that any infection control measures that have been implemented should be ceased.

Prevention

The prevention of MRSA and MRSP involves the general prevention of SSIs and the specific prevention of infections caused by MR agents, with the former component being the most important. General measures that can be undertaken to reduce the occurrence of *any* infection are the most important way to reduce the occurrence of MRS infections. This involves a wide range of measures that are used to reduce SSIs (see Chapter 8. Rarely, if ever, is screening of veterinary personnel for MRS colonization a useful infection prevention tool.

Relevant literature

Staphylococci are gram-positive cocci and a leading cause of opportunistic infections, including SSIs, in veterinary patients. Staphylococci are generally divided into two groups, coagulase positive and coagulase negative. Coagulase-positive staphylococci are the most virulent and most important causes of SSIs. Coagulase-negative staphylococci can cause infections but are of lesser virulence and are often found as contaminants.

One frustrating aspect of staphylococci is their tendency to become resistant to antimicrobials. Most notable is MR, mediated by the *mecA* gene, which confers resistance not just to methicillin but also to virtually all β-lactams (penicillins, cephalosporins, carbapenems). MRS often also acquire resistance to various other antimicrobials, and some can be highly drug resistant with few viable treatment options.

The two main MRS of concern in SSIs are *S. pseudintermedius* (MRSP) and *S. aureus* (MRSA). Both of these can be carried in the nose, mouth, or intestinal tract or on the skin of a small (but probably increasing) percentage of healthy dogs and cats. The incidence of MRS SSIs, particularly those caused by MRSP, appears to have dramatically increased over the past few years, and MRSP is the leading cause of SSIs in some facilities. *S. schleiferi* subsp *coagulans* is another coagulase-positive *Staphylococcus* species that can cause infections in dogs and cats; however, it is predominantly a cause of pyoderma and otitis, not SSIs. MR coagulase-negative staphylococci are commonly found in and on animals, yet when they are isolated from an SSI, it often represents contamination, not infection.

When overall infections are considered, prior antimicrobial exposure has been identified as a **risk factor** for both MRSA and MRSP versus their methicillin-susceptible counterparts in dogs (Faires *et al.* 2010; Soares Magalhães *et al.* 2010; Nienhoff *et al.* 2011). Previous hospitalization and the presence of a surgical implant have also been shown to be risk factors for MRSP colonization in dogs and for MRSA versus methicillin-susceptible *S. aureus* infection (Soares Magalhães *et al.* 2010). These studies have involved a combination of infection types, and although data specifically directed at SSIs are lacking, it is logical to assume that these factors are also important for MRSP and MRSA SSIs. However, prior antibiotic exposure is not an absolute requirement, and MRS infections can develop in any patient under any circumstances.

Because MRS are opportunistic pathogens, any factor associated with increased likelihood of SSI presumably increases the likelihood of MRS SSI, and the risk presumably increases further as MRS colonization rates increase in animals and veterinary personnel. Preoperative MRSA colonization is a risk factor for subsequent MRSA SSI in humans (Gupta *et al.* 2011; Murphy *et al.* 2011), and MRSA colonization at the time of hospital admission has been shown to be associated with increased risk of subsequent MRSA infection in horses (Weese *et al.* 2006a). The influence of preoperative MRS, particularly MRSP, colonization, in dogs has not been adequately investigated. Although is it reasonable to assume that preoperative colonization would increase the likelihood of infection, preliminary data suggest that this may not be a strong influence on MRSP SSI risk. A variety of other factors have been associated with increased MRSA SSI risk in humans, including increasing age, emergency procedures, presence of a comorbidity, immunosuppressive therapy, long surgical duration, and selected surgical procedures (e.g., undergoing joint replacement surgery, hip fracture repair) (Harbarth *et al.* 2008; Shukla *et al.* 2009; Murphy *et al.* 2011). It is reasonable to suspect that some of these might be a risk factor for MRSA or MRSP SSI in companion animals, but evidence is not yet available to substantiate this.

The diagnosis of MRS infections involves isolation of MRS from an infected site. MRS infections do not appear any different from infections caused by susceptible staphylococci or other opportunistic pathogens, so culture and susceptibility testing are required for diagnosis. The critical first step in diagnosis and management of MRS infection therefore is collection of an appropriate diagnostic sample. Culture and susceptibility testing should be considered for all SSIs, and is never contraindicated. Culture should be considered particularly important in areas where the prevalence of MR among staphylococci is high, in facilities where the incidence of MRS SSIs

is high, and whenever an outbreak is known or suspected. Culture should be considered mandatory in implant-associated infections and any other infections in which the implications of initial treatment failure may be profound.

Staphylococci are easy to grow in vitro, yet some factors must be considered when investigating SSIs. Because many staphylococci, including MRS, are common skin commensals, care should be taken to minimize the risk of contamination of samples with skin microflora. Culture results must always be interpreted with consideration of the type of sample, location the sample was from, degree of growth, whether there was mixed culture, and the staphylococcal species that was identified. Particular care must be taken when coagulase-negative staphylococci are isolated because they may be of limited pathogenicity, commonly present as skin commensals and often MR.

Isolation and testing of staphylococci are relatively straightforward; however, the ability of some diagnostic laboratories to identify MRS is still variable, largely because of the failure of some laboratories to use standard (e.g., Clinical and Laboratory Standards Institute) protocols. At a minimum, coagulase-positive and coagulase-negative staphylococci must be differentiated, and *S. aureus* must be differentiated from *S. pseudintermedius* (or *S. intermedius* group) because susceptibility breakpoints differ. Laboratories that report susceptibility data for undifferentiated "coagulase-positive *Staphylococcus* spp." are potentially providing erroneous data. Different methods can be used to identify MR. Methicillin is not usually tested because it is poorly stable in vitro. Oxacillin has traditionally been used as the marker of MR in MRSA, but it has been replaced by cefoxitin because cefoxitin is a better predictor of resistance in MRSA. However, cefoxitin is a poor indicator of MR in MRSP and MR-*S. schleiferi* (Bemis *et al.* 2006), so oxacillin is recommended for those species (Bemis *et al.* 2009). Some laboratories have offered *mecA* PCR tests from animal specimens as an MRSA diagnostic test, yet these are invalid because *mecA* can be found in a range of staphylococci. No rapid PCR tests for MRSA or MRSP are currently validated for animals.

The general therapeutic approach to MRS infections is no different than that for any other type of SSI. The presence of a multidrug resistant pathogen affects the choice of antimicrobial but not other aspects such as the need for systemic therapy or duration of therapy.

Superficial infections may respond to suture removal to facilitate drainage and local treatment with antiseptics (e.g., 4% chlorhexidine), antimicrobials (e.g., mupirocin, fusidic acid, silver sulfadiazine), or honey.

Systemic antimicrobial therapy is often required and should be based on culture and susceptibility data, with a few considerations. MRS are resistant to virtually all β-lactams, including carbapenems, so this class must not be used, even if in vitro susceptibility to a particular β-lactam is reported (something that a good diagnostic laboratory should not do). Fluoroquinolones are best avoided because of unpredictable response to treatment and the ease of emergence of resistance during treatment. Inducible clindamycin resistance is also a concern, particularly for MRSA (Faires *et al.* 2009; Rich *et al.* 2005). This phenomenon involves induction of resistance in isolates that appear to be susceptible in vitro. Clindamycin should be avoided in erythromycin-resistant MRSA isolates unless appropriate testing (D-test or equivalent) has indicated that inducible resistance is not present. The prevalence of inducible resistance appears to be low among MRSP (Faires *et al.* 2009); however, it should still be considered and appropriate testing sought, particularly for deep infections in which the implications of treatment failure are high.

MRSA and MRSP are often susceptible to doxycycline, chloramphenicol, and amikacin, but resistance is increasingly common, particularly among MRSP.

Adjunctive therapy is often required because of limited systemic antimicrobial options and difficulties treating certain types of infections. Implant-associated infections can be very difficult to treat, potentially because of the impact of bacterial biofilm on antimicrobial efficacy. Removal of the affected implant is recommended whenever possible. Systemic antimicrobial therapy may result in clinical improvement; however, signs of infection often return after cessation of therapy. Additional approaches such as implantation of antimicrobial-impregnated materials (e.g., PMMA beads, collagen sponges, gel matrices) can be useful, as can other local or regional approaches such as regional limb perfusion.

Because staphylococci are opportunists that are widely present on animals and humans and in the veterinary hospital environment, practices to **reduce the risk** of any opportunistic infection will reduce MRS infection rates. These strategies include a good general infection control program and proper peri-, intra-, and postoperative practices. In addition to these general principles of aseptic surgery, strategies may be designed to reduce the likelihood that, when a staphylococcal infection develops, the agent will be MR. This approach is hampered by limitations in knowledge of risk factors, although prudent use of antimicrobials would likely impact the risk of microbial resistance in a broad sense. Measures to reduce the overall use of antimicrobials and improve their selection when indicated may reduce selection pressure at the individual and population levels, thereby limiting the proportion of staphylococcal infections that are MR.

In humans, preoperative screening of high-risk patients (e.g., long-term care facility residents, patients transferred from other facilities, patients with prior MRSA infections) for MRSA colonization is used in some facilities as a means of reducing postoperative MRSA infections. With this approach, colonized patients undergo decolonization therapy before surgery or receive altered perioperative antimicrobial prophylaxis targeting MRSA. This approach may seem tempting for veterinary patients, particularly in terms of preoperative MRSP screening of orthopedic patients. However, several challenges need to be addressed before this preoperative screening may be implemented. These challenges stem from differences in the timing of surgical procedures and availability of specific assays between veterinary and human patients. In humans, surgical scheduling, routine preoperative testing in advance of surgery and the availability of rapid (real time PCR) screening facilitate preoperative screening for MRSA. These conditions do not necessarily apply to veterinary patients, in which preoperative assessment is more limited in cost and time. Furthermore, rapid MRSP screening tests have not yet been developed for animals, resulting in a delay of 2 to 5 days between sample collection and delivery of results. Additionally, no data are currently available to guide an appropriate response to a colonized animal, and there is no evidence that active decolonization measures (e.g., oral antimicrobials, intranasal antimicrobials, antiseptic baths) are effective in dogs and cats. However, preoperative screening could be useful for guiding the selection of antibiotics in procedures justifying prophylactic antimicrobial therapy. For example, cefazolin, an antimicrobial commonly administered before orthopedic procedures, could be complemented with amikacin in selected cases to expand the spectrum of activity in MRSP carriers. However, the efficacy of this approach has not been evaluated,

and care should be taken not to overuse the few treatment options for MRSP infections.

Transmission of MRSA and MRSP in veterinary hospitals, particularly surgical facilities, has become a major concern. It is beyond the scope of this chapter to provide a detailed description of proper practices for infection control, and objective data are lacking to support specific measures, but the key to prevention of hospital-associated transmission of MRS likely involves a good general infection control program, as described elsewhere (Anderson *et al.* 2008; British Small Animal Veterinary Association 2011).

Public health aspects must also be considered. MRSA is an important human pathogen, and transmission of this bacterium between humans and animals, in both directions, can occur (van Duijkeren *et al.* 2004; Strommenger *et al.* 2006; Weese *et al.* 2006b; Walther *et al.* 2012). The incidence of this is unknown, yet prudence dictates that good infection control measures be used in veterinary facilities and households to reduce the risk of human infection (Anderson *et al.* 2008). MRSP appears to be poorly adapted to infect humans, and reports of human MRSP infections are very rare, although transmission of MRSP between humans and animals can occur (van Duijkeren *et al.* 2011). There is limited concern about zoonotic transmission of other MRS.

References

Anderson, M.E.C., Montgomery, J., Weese, J.S., et al. (2008) **Infection Prevention and Control Best Practices for Small Animal Veterinary Clinics**. Canadian Committee on Antibiotic Resistance, Guelph, Ontario.

Bemis, D., Jones, R., Hiatt, L., et al. (2006) Comparison of tests to detect oxacillin resistance in *Staphylococcus intermedius*, *Staphylococcus schleiferi*, and *Staphylococcus aureus* isolates from canine hosts. *Journal of Clinical Microbiology* 44, 3374-3376.

Bemis, D.A., Jones, R.D., Frank, L.A., et al. (2009) Evaluation of susceptibility test breakpoints used to predict mecA-mediated resistance in *Staphylococcus pseudintermedius* isolated from dogs. *Journal of Veterinary Diagnostic Investigation* 21, 53-58.

British Small Animal Veterinary Association (2011) BSAVA practice guidelines—reducing the risk from MRSA and MRSP [Online]. Available: http://www.bsava.com/Advice/MRSA/tabid/171/Default.aspx [Accessed Sept 1 2011].

Faires, M., Gard, S., Aucoin, D., et al. (2009) Inducible clindamycin-resistance in methicillin-resistant *Staphylococcus aureus* and methicillin-resistant *Staphylococcus pseudintermedius* isolates from dogs and cats. *Veterinary Microbiology* 139 (3-4), 419-420.

Faires, M.C., Traverse, M., Tater, K.C., et al. (2010) Methicillin-resistant and -susceptible *Staphylococcus aureus* infections in dogs. *Emerging Infectious Diseases Journal* 16, 69-75.

Gupta, K., Strymish, J., Abi-Haidar, Y., et al. (2011) Preoperative nasal methicillin-resistant *Staphylococcus aureus* status, surgical prophylaxis, and risk-adjusted postoperative outcomes in veterans. *Infection Control and Hospital Epidemiology* 32, 791-796.

Harbarth, S., Huttner, B., Gervaz, P., et al. (2008) Risk factors for methicillin-resistant *Staphylococcus aureus* surgical site infection. *Infection Control and Hospital Epidemiology* 29, 890-893.

Murphy, E., Spencer, S.J., Young, D., et al. (2011) MRSA colonisation and subsequent risk of infection despite effective eradication in orthopaedic elective surgery. *The Journal of Bone & Joint Surgery* 93, 548-551.

Nienhoff, U., Kadlec, K., Chaberny, I.F., et al. (2011) Methicillin-resistant *Staphylococcus pseudintermedius* among dogs admitted to a small animal hospital. *Veterinary Microbiology* 150 (1-2), 191-197.

Rich, M., Deighton, L., Roberts, L. (2005) Clindamycin-resistance in methicillin-resistant Staphylococcus aureus isolated from animals. *Veterinary Microbiology* 111, 237-240.

Shukla, S., Nixon, M., Acharya, M., et al. (2009) Incidence of MRSA surgical-site infection in MRSA carriers in an orthopaedic trauma unit. *The Journal of Bone & Joint Surgery* 91, 225-228.

Soares Magalhães, R.J., Loeffler, A., Lindsay, J., et al. (2010) Risk factors for methicillin-resistant *Staphylococcus aureus* (MRSA) infection in dogs and cats: a case-control study. *Veterinary Research* 41, 55.

Strommenger, B., Kehrenberg, C., Kettlitz, C., et al. (2006) Molecular characterization of methicillin-resistant *Staphylococcus aureus* strains from pet animals and their relationship to human isolates. *Journal of Antimicrobial Chemotherapy* 57, 461-465.

Van Duijkeren, E., Wolfhagen, M.J., Box, A.T., et al. (2004) Human-to-dog transmission of methicillin-resistant *Staphylococcus aureus*. *Emerging Infectious Diseases Journal* 10, 2235-2237.

Van Duijkeren, E., Kamphuis, M., Van Der Mije, I.C., et al. (2011) Transmission of methicillin-resistant *Staphylococcus pseudintermedius* between infected dogs and cats and contact pets, humans and the environment in households and veterinary clinics. *Veterinary Microbiology* 150, 338-343.

Walther, B., Hermes, J., Cuny, C., et al. (2012) Sharing more than friendship—nasal colonization with coagulase-positive staphylococci (CPS) and co-habitation aspects of dogs and their owners. *PLoS ONE* 7, e35197.

Weese, J., Rousseau, J., Willey, B., et al. (2006a). Methicillin-resistant *Staphylococcus aureus* in horses at a veterinary teaching hospital: frequency, characterization, and association with clinical disease. *Journal of Veterinary* 20, 182-186.

Weese, J.S., Dick, H., Willey, B.M., et al. (2006b) Suspected transmission of methicillin-resistant *Staphylococcus aureus* between domestic pets and humans in veterinary clinics and in the household. *Veterinary Microbiology* 115, 148–155.

8 Hospital-Associated Infections

Maureen Anderson and Scott Weese
Department of Pathobiology, University of Guelph, Guelph, Ontario, Canada

Definition

Significant attention has recently focused on the increasing impact of nosocomial infections, more commonly and perhaps more accurately referred to as hospital-associated infections (HAIs). Although poorly quantified in veterinary medicine, the impact of HAIs in human medicine is profound, affecting tens of thousands of individuals, with an estimated economic impact in the United States alone of $28 to $49 billion per year (Scott 2009). Surgical site infections (SSIs) have been estimated to cost at least $10,000 to $25,000 per case annually (Anderson *et al.* 2007). Less is known about HAIs in veterinary hospitals, for many reasons, including lack of national surveillance programs, limited hospital-specific infection control surveillance and infection control efforts, and the limited involvement of veterinarians in this field of research. Although the scope of the problem remains poorly defined, the impact of HAIs in companion animal medicine is undeniable. SSIs are a readily apparent and relatively common type of HAI and can account for substantial morbidity, mortality, and treatment costs. Other HAIs such as diarrhea and upper respiratory infections can occur as sporadic cases or outbreaks in veterinary facilities. More insidious than any of these may be subclinical acquisition of opportunistic pathogens during hospitalization, particularly multidrug-resistant bacteria, with subsequent potential for infection after discharge from the hospital along with transmission to other animals or humans in the community.

A standard definition of what constitutes an HAI does not exist, nor is a single definition likely appropriate. An HAI may be broadly defined as any infection acquired by a patient during hospitalization. However, patients can develop infections during their hospitalization because of pathogens they were already carrying at the time of admission. In these cases, various stressors and hospital procedures such as surgery may contribute to decreased immune defenses (including broken skin), and disease develops in hospital even though the pathogen is not actually acquired in hospital. Conversely, patients can acquire pathogens during hospitalization but only develop clinical signs of infection after discharge. This scenario is of particular concern in veterinary medicine because of the typically short duration of patient hospitalization. Identifying infections that develop after discharge can be difficult, especially with mild disease (e.g., self-limiting diarrhea or respiratory disease) that owners may not report at all or with referral populations in which the primary care veterinarians may deal with minor complications.

Understanding the likely origin of the pathogen and the timing of disease development relative to hospitalization is crucial to developing effective strategies for surveillance, infection control, and outbreak response. Accordingly, HAIs can be divided into several subcategories following criteria similar to those widely used in human medicine (Table 8.1). However, these classifications are relatively empirical and should be considered general guidelines rather than absolute indicators of the source of infection. Their relevance may also vary among pathogens and syndromes. These limitations are especially relevant in veterinary medicine because the body of evidence related to the timing and origins of HAIs is even more limited in animals than in humans.

Risk factors

With the wide range of potential HAIs that may be encountered, the list of potential risk factors is equally broad. However, only a small portion of these factors has been objectively investigated with regard to their association with HAIs. In general, any factor that increases the likelihood of exposure to a pathogen (e.g., poor hand hygiene practices, direct or indirect contact with other animals, environmental contamination) or that increases susceptibility of the host (e.g., incisions, invasive devices, immunosuppression, antimicrobial administration, uncontrolled primary diseases, stress of hospitalization itself) can increase the likelihood of acquiring or developing infection in the hospital. Although some of these factors cannot be controlled, routine infection control protocols should be considered as the first line of defense to mitigate the risk of HAIs. Specific risk factors have been described for some HAIs such as SSIs, but overall, data are rather limited.

Table 8.1 Definitions of hospital- and community-associated infections

Category	Definition
Hospital-associated infections	Develop >48 hours after hospital admission
Hospital-associated, community-onset infections	Develop within 30 days of hospital discharge
Community-associated, hospital-onset infections	Develop <48 hours after hospital admission
Community-associated infections	Present at admission in patients with no history of hospitalization within 30 days

Complications in Small Animal Surgery, First Edition. Edited by Dominique Griffon and Annick Hamaide.
© 2016 John Wiley & Sons, Inc. Published 2016 by John Wiley & Sons, Inc.
Companion website: www.wiley.com/go/griffon/complications

Diagnosis

Hospital-associated infections encompass a wide range of syndromes and disease. The general diagnostic approach involves identification of a clinical abnormality followed by selection of specific tests to identify the cause. With HAIs, this process must be taken a step further to recognize the origin of the microbial agent relative to the hospital (Tables 8.1 and 8.2). An important component of infection control is making the connection between individual animal health and "hospital health." Although most HAIs are sporadic and not associated with outbreaks, recognition of HAIs remains important to understand disease trends, establish baseline infection rates, and facilitate early identification of outbreaks.

Treatment

The treatment of HAIs is twofold: treatment of the individual patient and "treatment" of the hospital. Both are important to optimize patient and facility health (Table 8.2).

Treatment of the patient depends on individual patient factors, the type of infection, and the severity. Many patients with HAIs can be treated at home, which is ideal because it decreases infection pressure within the hospital. Other cases require hospitalization, at which point the nature of the disease or pathogen, its mode of transmission, and measures to manage the infection safely must be carefully considered to reduce the risk of further transmission to patients and personnel. This should be done for

Table 8.2 Basic steps in identification and management of hospital-associated infections (HAIs), with emphasis on surgical site infections (SSIs).

Identification of suspected HAI	• Clinical signs in hospitalized patient or patient at recheck • Compatible clinical signs reported by owner and confirmed at recheck

Confirm infection	• Submit samples for testing
	  ◦ Culture and antimicrobial susceptibility testing
	  ◦ Other pathogens as indicated
	• For SSIs, differentiate wound infection vs. inflammation
	  ◦ See definitions of different types of SSIs (see Chapter 1)
	• Report occurrence of infection to clinic ICP
	  ◦ Facilitates detection of trends, especially in large clinics

Determine origin of infection (see Table 8.1)	• Hospital-associated vs. community associated • Hospital onset vs. community onset

Determine steps to treat patient	• Local therapy
	  ◦ Debridement and lavage
	  ◦ Topical antiseptics
	  ◦ Local antimicrobial therapy
	    – Intraarticular injection
	    – Regional limb perfusion
	    – Impregnated implants (beads, sponges)
	  ◦ Alternative therapy: honey, sugar
	• Systemic antimicrobial therapy
	  ◦ Empirical therapy should be revised based on C&S testing
	• Implant removal (if applicable)
	• Other supportive therapy as indicated (e.g., antiinflammatories, fluids, nutritional support)

Determine steps to treat hospital	• Take necessary precautions to reduce risk of spread to other patients
	  ◦ Emphasis on routine infection control precautions
	    – Hand hygiene
	• Avoid direct contact with infected wounds: bandaging
	  ◦ Contact precautions (e.g., gloves, designated or disposable gowns)
	  ◦ Isolation (particularly for multidrug-resistant pathogens)
	• Review patient record
	  ◦ Identify risk factors that were present for the patient
	    – Determine if these risk factors can be better addressed in future patients; amend protocols accordingly; educate and train staff
	  ◦ Identify any breaks in routine infection control practices
	    – Determine reason for break; amend protocols accordingly; educate and train staff
	• Review hospital records
	  ◦ Determine if infection rates have increased
	    – Overall HAI rate
	    – Overall SSI rate: procedure-specific rate (e.g., TPLOs)
	  ◦ Determine if other similar infections have occurred
	    – Identify potential common sources (e.g., equipment, environment, personnel), particularly if infections involve same pathogen
	• Address any common sources identified (e.g., enhanced cleaning and disinfection, amend protocols, educate and train staff)

Determine steps to protect public health	• Risk to humans (zoonotic risk)
	  ◦ In the clinic (i.e., staff)
	  ◦ At home (i.e., owners)
	  ◦ In the community
	• Risk to other animals
	  ◦ At home
	  ◦ In the community
	• Provide appropriate information and guidelines to owners and staff
	  ◦ Avoid high-risk contacts
	  ◦ Avoid contact with high-risk individuals
	• Encourage discussion with physician if zoonotic disease risk

C&S, culture and susceptibility; HAI, hospital-associated infection; ICP, infection control practitioner; SSI, surgical site infection; TPLO, tibial plateau leveling osteotomy.

any hospitalized patient with signs of infection, regardless of whether the original infection was hospital or community associated. A combination of routine infection control practices along with enhanced precautions (e.g., isolation) may be required, depending on the case. These measures are part of a complete clinic infection control program, which is further described later in the Prevention section.

Biocontainment of infectious cases

Preestablished protocols for infection control should be initiated as soon as an infectious or potentially infectious patient is identified (e.g., any animal with a potentially transmissible infection, whether it is hospital or community associated). Confirmatory testing is not required to initiate a response; a reasonable suspicion that the patient may be harboring a pathogen of concern should be enough to trigger an intervention. The handling of these cases varies with the pathogen (e.g., transmissibility, route of transmission), patient (e.g., severity of the disease or size of the patient might impact the housing of the animal within the hospital), and facility (e.g., availability of isolation wards, personnel constraints). Ideally, animals that are infectious or of uncertain risk should be housed in an isolation area using enhanced contact precautions (e.g., gloves, designated laboratory coat or gown). See Box 8.1 for a list of recommendations for isolation housing. Education of personnel regarding the reasons for isolation protocols and their importance

may help to increase compliance. When isolation is not possible, measures should be taken to provide as much **biocontainment** as possible, such as:

- Strategic placement of the animal or cage in the ward
- Temporary physical barriers to reduce exposure to neighboring animal
- Restricted access to common environmental areas (e.g., providing a separate area for a dog to urinate and defecate)
- Restricted handling
- Use of enhanced contact precautions when handling the animal
- Use of procedural methods to reduce the risk of cross-contamination (e.g., management by limited personnel, handling noninfectious patients first)

These measures can be adequate in many infectious cases, depending on the transmissibility of the pathogen, but in general, it is preferable to use physical and procedural measures, not just procedural measures, because the latter are more prone to breaches.

Enhanced contact precautions

Enhanced contact precautions and personal protective equipment (PPE), including but not limited to gloves, gowns, masks, face shields, and protective footwear, may be required when handling certain animals or specimens. Protocols should be in place to ensure that all clinic personnel are aware of when the use of such items is required, including how to put them on, take them off, and dispose of them without contaminating their skin, clothing, or the environment.

Treatment of contact areas

If a potentially infectious animal must be moved to another part of the clinic for procedures or diagnostic testing, if at all possible, this should be done at the end of the day or at a time when there is the least amount of animal and personnel movement in the clinic. Immediately after the patient leaves the area, all contact surfaces and equipment must be thoroughly cleaned and disinfected (Box 8.2). This also applies to the patient's housing area (isolation or elsewhere) after patient discharge. Allowing the room or area to stand empty after proper cleaning and disinfection does not decrease environmental contamination. Repeating cleaning and

Box 8.1 Checklist for isolation area for housing infectious and potentially infectious patients

- Clearly identified
- Restricted access (minimal number of personnel necessary)
- Located away from areas of normal personnel and animal flow
- Physically separated from rest of clinic (e.g., enclosed room with a door)
- Area is not used for temporary or long-term storage
- All surfaces are easy to clean and disinfect; surfaces must be kept in good repair (e.g., free of chips, cracks, scratches)
- There is dedicated equipment for each isolation patient (e.g., thermometer, stethoscope).
  ◦ All equipment remains in isolation until patient is discharged.
  ◦ All equipment is thoroughly cleaned and disinfected after patient discharge.
  ◦ Any consumable items left in the room are disposed after patient discharge.
- PPE (e.g., gloves, gown, or dedicated laboratory coat) is donned before entering the isolation area and removed at the threshold of the isolation area upon exiting.
  ◦ PPE is used in the isolation area regardless of whether there is direct contact with the patient.
  ◦ Gloves and disposable gowns are never reused (i.e., single-use only); dedicated laboratory coats (as well as other linens) are placed directly in a designated laundry bag after each use and laundered before being used again.
- Footbaths, footmats, or disposable shoe covers are used if there is a significant risk of contamination of the floor.
- Garbage and laundry from the isolation area are treated as potentially infectious.
- Dogs have a separate area to urinate and defecate that is not used by other patients; dogs are carried outside or transported on a designated gurney if possible.
- Air from isolation area is not circulated to other areas of the clinic.
  ◦ Vented directly to the outdoors
  ◦ HEPA filtration system in place if room cannot be vented to the outdoors

HEPA, PPE, personal protective equipment.

Box 8.2 General procedure for cleaning and disinfection of surfaces after direct or indirect contact with infectious and potentially infectious patients

- All surfaces are thoroughly cleaned to remove all organic debris.
  ◦ Surfaces are dampened before cleaning if there is risk of aerosolizing contaminated dust, hair, or dander.
  ◦ Use a general cleaner or detergent.
  ◦ Mechanical removal of debris through physical scrubbing (as necessary) is critical.
- Remove excess or standing water.
- An appropriate disinfectant is applied.
  ◦ Disinfectant selection is based on the pathogen(s) of concern.
  ◦ Manufacturer's instructions for contact time and concentration must be carefully followed.
  ◦ Disinfectant may be wiped or rinsed off surfaces after required contact time has elapsed (see manufacturer's recommendations).
- All surfaces are allowed to dry before admitting another patient.
  ◦ The area does not need to be left empty or unused for any particular amount of time after it is dry.
  ◦ Cleaning and disinfection may be repeated if desired (e.g., area was highly contaminated).

disinfection can be considered if concern about environmental contamination is very high (e.g., potential heavy contamination with a hardy pathogen such as clostridial spores), but careful cleaning and disinfection with an appropriate product once is more useful than repeated but less thorough attempts.

Outcome

The outcome of HAI cases varies widely according to the patient, the type of infection, and the disease severity. HAIs can range from unapparent to rapidly fatal. Similarly, from a hospital standpoint, HAIs can range from single sporadic cases to widespread outbreaks resulting in temporary facility closure. Some causes of HAIs are zoonotic, including many of the multidrug-resistant pathogens that may be involved in SSIs and bacterial enteropathogens that may cause diarrhea. This adds public health concerns for both owners and clinic personnel. As in animals, zoonotic infections in humans can range from unapparent to severe and rarely fatal disease and may occur as single cases to outbreaks involving numerous individuals with direct or indirect contact with the veterinary hospital. Veterinarians cannot provide medical advice to owners but should discuss the risk of zoonotic disease transmission and encourage owners to contact their physician regarding any personal medical concerns. Communication between physicians and veterinarians, with owner permission, particularly for those caring for humans and animals in the same household, should be promoted to help improve overall household healthcare.

Prevention and the components of an infection control plan

Hospital-associated infections are an inherent risk of exposure to the veterinary health care system. Regardless of the patient, there is always some risk of infection, albeit low in most situations. HAIs can be classified into two categories: preventable and nonpreventable. The "preventable fraction" is the percentage of infections that can be avoided through the use of reasonable, practical measures, such as good hygiene, proper antimicrobial use, and compliance with a sound overall infection control program. The "nonpreventable fraction" represents infections that develop despite best practices. Although it is often difficult to clearly differentiate preventable versus nonpreventable infections, it has been estimated that 30% to 70% of HAIs in human medicine are preventable. This relatively high proportion of preventable infections should prompt the veterinary community to endorse an active and dedicated approach to the prevention of HAIs. The impact of HAIs on patient morbidity, mortality, and financial costs fully justifies measures to address the preventable fraction of HAIs.

A complete description of measures to reduce the wide spectrum of potential HAIs is well beyond the scope of this chapter. Some control measures may apply only to specific pathogens or syndromes (e.g., control of fecal contamination for enteropathogens, precautions against aerosol transmission for respiratory pathogens); however, the core aspects of infection control are applicable to the majority of situations and facilities. Some of these key concepts are outlined below.

Every veterinary hospital, regardless of size or caseload, should have a formal infection control program. Such a program is designed to first of all prevent HAIs and to control HAIs when they do occur. A program may range from a basic manual of standard practices to a comprehensive program run by dedicated personnel,

including active surveillance activities. In most situations, implementing a basic infection control program is fairly straightforward and requires only a relatively small time and financial commitment. Some of the important components of a typical infection control program are described here, with particular mention of some that are pertinent to prevention of SSIs. Other components include policies and protocols regarding biocontainment of infectious patients (including isolation) and enhanced contact precautions discussed earlier under Treatment.

Infection control manual

A central written document outlining the required protocols for both routine (e.g., cleaning and disinfection) and uncommon (e.g., outbreak response, rabies exposure) events is a key component of the infection control program, serving as both a reference for and documentation of practices. Failure to adequately document protocols and practices can result in a loss of consistency as individuals modify practices, knowingly or otherwise, over time. Written documentation is also critical to demonstrate that an infection control program is in place if any issues regarding professional or legal liability arise. Finally, this central resource provides immediate guidance in case of HAIs, which can help to facilitate response of personnel and control of the infection. In its simplest form, creating an infection control manual may simply involve centralizing existing written protocols, with addition of other documents as needed. Broad guidelines are available that can be used as templates to help create tailored infection control manuals for individual clinics (Table 8.3).

Infection control personnel

Systems for proper program coordination will vary among clinics, but this is a key factor in maintaining an effective infection control program. Supervisors with expertise and experience in infection control are ideal but tend to be limited to large referral centers. However, coordination of a basic infection control program can be done by any veterinarian or technician, even if prior specific training is limited, as long as the individual has an interest in the field and good organizational skills. The program coordinator, regardless of experience, is designated as the clinic infection control practitioner (ICP). This individual ensures that appropriate and necessary protocols are developed and followed and that all staff (old and new) receive proper training. The ICP also acts as the central resource for questions related to infection control and directs any surveillance activities. This position is not necessarily cumbersome or time consuming because the day-to-day responsibilities are typically minimal.

Training and documentation

All personnel working in a clinic, from managers to temporary kennel staff and volunteers, must be trained with regards to infection control practices pertinent to their clinic duties. This training

Table 8.3 Resources related to infection control practices

Resource	Source
Infection Prevention and Control Best Practices for Small Animal Veterinary Clinics	Resources section of http://www.wormsandgermsblog.com
National Association of State Public Health Veterinarians Compendium of Veterinary Standard Precautions	http://www.nasphv.org/documentsCompendia.html
BSAVA practice guidelines—reducing the risk from MRSA and MRSP	http://www.bsava.com/Advice/MRSA/tabid/171/Default.aspx

BSAVA, British Small Animal Veterinary Association; MRSA, methicillin-resistant *Staphylococcus aureus*; MRSP, methicillin-resistant *Staphylococcus pseudintermedius*.

helps to maintain an appropriate standard of care for patients and is critical for protection of the clinic itself. Failure to perform and document training may expose the clinic to legal liability issues in the event of HAIs, outbreaks, or zoonotic infections of clinic personnel or owners. Relying solely on informal training, whereby new employees or volunteers simply imitate existing personnel, increases the likelihood of inadvertent modification of practices over time, and ultimately breaks in infection control procedures.

Surveillance

Identification of HAIs is critical for patient care and hospital infection control, and can be achieved through both formal and informal means. Routine clinical duties are at the forefront of disease surveillance, through identification of infections. Such a diagnosis must prompt consideration as to whether an infection may be hospital associated, and importantly, some form of reporting or recording of that fact. This constitutes the basis of infection control surveillance, a critical aspect of infection control. Although surveillance often sounds daunting, basic infection control surveillance is cost effective and easy to perform. Surveillance can be divided into three main categories: active surveillance, passive surveillance, and syndromic surveillance.

Active surveillance relies on the use of a formal and explicit approach to collecting data that goes beyond normal clinical activities. This involves specific time and effort directed to obtaining specific data. Examples of active surveillance include screening of patients for a certain pathogen (e.g., methicillin-resistant *Staphylococcus aureus*) or calling owners of discharged animals to identify potential infectious disease issues. Active surveillance can be time consuming and expensive and fortunately is rarely needed in most companion animal hospitals in the absence of an outbreak or particular disease concern. Perhaps the most common and useful form of routine active surveillance consists of calling owners of surgical patients to enquire about signs of SSI. This can be done a few days after discharge to detect early infections but is also important to do later on (e.g., 30 days for soft tissue procedures) to detect and record SSIs that were not identified at the time of suture removal and those that might have been treated at another veterinary facility.

Passive surveillance involves the use of data that are already available, such as SSI information obtained during routine rechecks or routine culture and susceptibility data obtained from patients for diagnostic purposes. Veterinary practices typically generate abundant passive surveillance data, but this information is rarely centrally recorded or readily accessible. Advances in electronic medical records systems facilitate access to large amounts of data that may be used to determine baseline infection rates (e.g., overall and procedure-specific SSI rates), culture results (e.g., typical pathogens and susceptibility patterns for infections such as SSIs and urinary tract infections), and similar basic but important data. However, this type of analysis requires proper data entry in a system allowing data search, retrieval, and summary. Passive surveillance data are inherently limited by incomplete or biased datasets (e.g., if cultures are only taken from serious or refractory infections). Nonetheless, properly collected and evaluated passive surveillance data can provide very useful information, especially in the early detection of rising infection rates. In this context, the ICP plays a critical role, assuming responsibility for the collation of disease reports that may not be directly available in the medical records system, and serving as "institutional memory." This facilitates prompt recognition of abnormal situations (e.g., a cluster of diarrhea cases in dogs that were recently hospitalized).

Syndromic surveillance relates to the collection of data about syndromes rather than specific diseases. Syndromes relevant to HAIs include fever, coughing, sneezing, diarrhea, and vomiting. These signs are readily identifiable by all personnel, thereby facilitating detection of potential HAIs. Prompt reporting of cases with these signs to the ICP can expedite the response to a developing problem and can help limit the risk of exposure for other patients and personnel to potentially infectious cases.

Environmental surveillance typically involves bacterial culture of environmental surfaces or objects. Although sometimes used by clinics, this form of surveillance is often overused and misused with a nontargeted approach, resulting in inefficient use of time, effort, and financial resources. The hospital environment is not meant to be sterile, and contamination of hospital environment by numerous opportunistic pathogens is fully expected, which hampers interpretation of random environmental cultures. Environmental surveillance should be initiated only in the following circumstances:

- Diagnosis of HAIs that are plausibly linked to the environment (e.g., affected animals were all kept in the same cage, clipped with the same set of clippers, treated with antiseptic from a particular container) *and* other potential sources of infection have been ruled out or are less likely
- A structured sampling program can be created, in terms of location and timing of sampling.
- An action plan has been predetermined for implementation based on environmental culture results (e.g., altering use of space or equipment, enhanced cleaning and disinfection procedures, follow-up surveillance of environment and patients to determine efficacy of intervention).

These factors are rarely present in veterinary hospitals, and environmental surveillance should be a rarely used infection control measure that is probably best performed in consultation with individuals with expertise in infection control.

Preventive measures involving the hospital environment
Clinic design and function

Animal and personnel flow within a clinic can influence the likelihood of pathogen transmission. General concepts in building design are aimed at limiting the incidence or risk of direct and indirect contact between animals. Sick animals should be kept away from healthy animals, especially from animals at increased risk of infection (e.g., immunosuppressed, very young, debilitated). The increasing prevalence of multidrug-resistant staphylococcal infection and colonization in some populations, particularly dermatology patients, should prompt strong consideration of hospital designs and other means of separating patients at high risk for infection (e.g., surgical patients) from patients at high risk for shedding important SSI pathogens (e.g., dogs with pyoderma). Traffic flow, both animal and human, should be evaluated as part of routine infection control reviews and carefully considered during clinic design or renovation.

Operating room design and function

Very few standards have been established to guide the design of veterinary surgical suites beyond the most basic requirements. Consideration should be given to the size of an operating room; it should allow necessary movement of personnel and equipment with limited risk of inadvertent contamination. Laminar airflow is

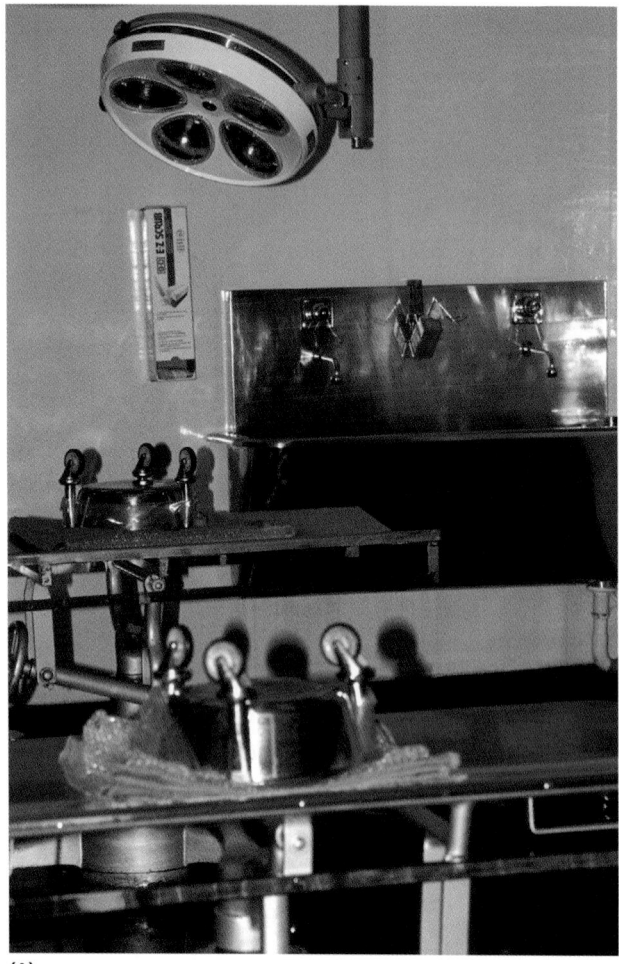
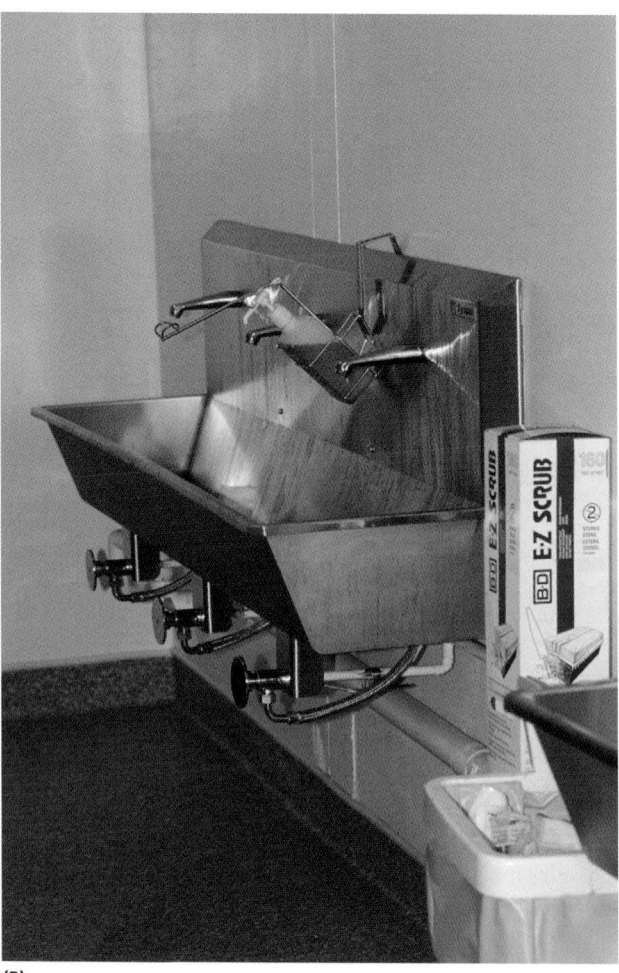

(A)
(B)

Figure 8.1 Hospital design and surgical site infections. **A,** Improper design of an operating room (OR): the scrubbing area is contained within the OR. **B,** This hospital was remodeled to move scrubbing area out of the OR. *Source:* D. Griffon, Western University of Health Sciences, Pomona, CA, 2014. Reproduced with permission from D. Griffon.

not essential, but due consideration of ventilation and assessment of airflow patterns is important to reduce airborne (and subsequently patient and equipment) contamination.

Operating rooms must only be used for surgical procedures. Ideally, clean procedures for which infection is of disastrous consequences (e.g., joint replacement and neurosurgery) should be carried out in rooms strictly dedicated to those procedures. In hospitals with the available facilities, a separate room is usually designated for contaminated orthopedic procedures and soft tissue surgery. Regardless of their primary use, surgery rooms should not be used as storage areas, they should be devoid of stand-alone cabinets and furniture, and they should not be allowed to become cluttered (Figure 8.1). The scrubbing area (e.g., scrub sink, if alcohol-based presurgical hand rubs are not used) should not be contained within the surgical suite, but if present, a sink should not be used when a patient or open surgical packs are present in the room.

Cleaning and disinfection

Cleaning and disinfection are key components of the infection control process, yet they are often performed incorrectly or inadequately. Some products facilitate removal of debris (cleaners, detergents, abrasives), and others are intended to kill microorganisms (disinfectants). Disinfectants vary in their spectrum of activity,

efficacy in the presence of organic debris, kill time, toxicity, and environmental impact, as well as compatibility with different cleaners (Table 8.4). This information should be provided by the manufacturer (ideally on the product label) and must be carefully considered when selecting a product for a given task, along with human safety issues, cost, and potential damage to surfaces. Cleaning and disinfection protocols should be reviewed to ensure that a relevant and acceptable level of disinfection is being achieved.

Ideally, a minimal number of cleaners and disinfectants should be available in a clinic to reduce the likelihood of misuse. During outbreaks, changes in disinfection protocols may be required to ensure that the relevant organisms are killed (see Box 8.1). Periodic cleaning with certain disinfectants that are not used on a daily basis may also be useful, particularly when the routinely used disinfectant has a limited spectrum of activity. For example, clostridial spores are resistant to most disinfectants and can therefore accumulate in the environment and cause outbreaks in veterinary clinics. Periodic cleaning with sporicidal disinfectants (e.g., accelerated hydrogen peroxide, bleach) may be useful as a routine measure or in response to specific concerns. Non-enveloped viruses such as parvovirus are also difficult to kill, and enhanced disinfection with parvocidal disinfectants (e.g., accelerated hydrogen peroxide, bleach, selected quaternary ammonium compounds) may be indicated after potential

Table 8.4 Antimicrobial spectrum of selected disinfectants

	Agent	Alcohols	Aldehydes	Alkalis: ammonia	Biguanides: chlorhexidine	Halogens: hypochlorite (bleach)	Oxidizing Agents	Phenols	Quaternary ammonium compounds
Most susceptible	Mycoplasmas	++	++	++	++	++	++	++	+
	Gram-positive bacteria	++	++	+	++	++	++	++	++
	Gram-negative bacteria	++	++	+	+	++	++	++	+
	Pseudomonads	++	++	+	±	++	++	++	±
	Enveloped viruses	+	++	+	++	++	++	++	+
	Chlamydiae	±	+	+	±	+	+	±	−
	Non-enveloped viruses	−	+	±	−	++	+	±*	−
	Fungal spores	±	+	+	±	+	±	+	±
	Acid-fast bacteria	+	++	+	−	+	±	++	−
	Bacterial spores	−	+	±	−	++	+	−	−
Most resistant	Coccidia	−	−	+	−	−	−	+	−

(left margin: Susceptibility of microorganisms to chemical disinfectants)

++ highly effective; + effective; ± limited activity; - no activity/

*In general, phenols are not effective against non-enveloped viruses, but they have been found to be effective against rotaviruses. They have been recommended for use on horse farms to help control equine rotaviral disease in foals. However, efficacy against small animal parvoviruses has not been demonstrated.

Examples of microorganisms from each category:

Mycoplasmas: *Mycoplasma canis* and *Mycoplasma felis*; **gram-positive bacteria:** *Staphylococcus* spp. and *Streptococcus* spp.; **gram-negative bacteria:** *Bordetella bronchiseptica* and *Salmonella* spp.; **pseudomonads:** *Pseudomonas aeruginosa*; **enveloped viruses:** influenza virus and herpesvirus; **chlamydiae:** *Chlamydophila psittaci*; **non-enveloped viruses:** feline panleukopenia virus and canine parvovirus; **fungal spores:** *Blastomyces dermatitidis* and *Sporothrix schenckii*; **acid-fast bacteria:** *Mycobacterium avium*; **bacterial spores:** *Clostridium difficile* and *Clostridium perfringens*; **coccidia:** *Cryptosporidium parvum*, *Isospora* spp., and *Toxoplasma gondii*.

Source: Adapted from Linton *et al.* (1987) and Block (2001).

environmental contamination if nonparvocidal agents are used for routine disinfection. Fortunately, typical SSI pathogens are relatively susceptible to most commonly used disinfectants.

Disinfection and sterilization of medical equipment

All medical equipment should be designated as requiring cleaning, low-level disinfection, high-level disinfection, or sterilization. Disinfection practices, including types of disinfectants, contact time, and general handling procedures, vary among these groups. Predetermination of the required disinfection level and written protocols for each level will facilitate proper disinfection practices.

Proper sterilization of surgical instruments and any items that might come in contact with the sterile surgical field is crucial. Poor sterilization or inappropriate handling of instruments after sterilization can result in contamination of sterile tissues during surgery. Steam sterilization (autoclaving) is most commonly used in veterinary clinics. Quality control testing of autoclaves should be performed regularly and documented. Sterility indicator strips should be placed in every surgical pack. External autoclave indicator tape is not a reliable indicator of the sterility of a pack's internal contents. Biological sterility indicators should be used periodically. These indicators contain bacterial spores, which are the most resistant form of bacteria, and can be processed in the clinic. In human health care facilities, it is recommended that these indicators are used daily or at least weekly. Weekly or biweekly use is likely adequate in most veterinary clinics, depending on how heavily the autoclave is used, as well as in the first cycle after the autoclave has been moved or repaired or when there has been any other indication of sterilization failure. Flash sterilization should not be used unless absolutely necessary in an emergency situation and should never be used for surgical implants.

"Cold-sterile" solutions are commonly used for high-level disinfection of selected items in veterinary clinics, yet they are often improperly used (e.g., inadequate contact time with instruments) and poorly maintained (e.g., improper dilution, failure to replace solution at recommended frequency). It is critical that the manufacturer's instructions for each specific product are carefully followed to ensure efficacy. Bacterial contamination of cold-sterile solutions is common (Murphy *et al.* 2010) and cold sterilization should not be used for any autoclavable items expected to have contact a sterile body site.

Preventive measures involving hospital personnel
Personal protective equipment

As a general preventive measure against HAIs, all personnel in a veterinary hospital should wear appropriate PPE to provide a barrier between patients (as well as specimens and the patient environment) and the person's body or clothing. Proper PPE are quickly and easily changed when contaminated and include laboratory coats, scrubs, and gowns. This apparel should be worn in all instances of contact between personnel and an animal or an animal's environment. Even if obvious contamination is not present, PPE should be changed regularly because contamination can occur in the absence of obvious soiling. Protective clothing should not be worn home because of the potential for transmission of pathogens to personal pets and family members. Clinic scrubs can be particularly problematic in this regard since they are more difficult to change and are more likely to be worn home. Surgical scrubs should never be directly exposed to the environment outside the surgical suite to reduce the risk of tracking contaminants into the surgical environment. When outside the surgical suite, such scrubs should always be covered with a clean laboratory coat.

Hand hygiene

Hand hygiene is widely considered as the single most important infection control measure in human health care, and there is no reason it should be considered as any less important in veterinary clinics. Hand washing has been shown to decrease the transmission of pathogens in human hospitals and in the community, yet compliance among veterinarians is typically poor (Wright *et al.* 2008; Shea and Shaw 2012). Measures to improve hand hygiene through education and improved access are essential. Alcohol-based hand sanitizers have become standard for routine hand hygiene in virtually all human hospitals and are gaining popularity in veterinary clinics. These agents have been shown to be more effective at eliminating bacterial contaminants on the hands of veterinary personnel compared with hand washing with antibacterial soap (Traub-Dargatz et al. 2006). These products are quick and easy to use, and because they contain emollients, they cause less skin irritation and damage than frequent hand washing. Alcohol-based hand sanitizers can easily be made available at any point of care in clinics and should be used between every animal contact. Gross soiling of hands or suspected contamination with an alcohol-resistant organism (i.e., non-enveloped viruses such as parvovirus, bacterial spores) warrants hand washing over the use of alcohol-based hand sanitizer. Non–alcohol-based hand sanitizers are also available, but their role in health care settings is currently unclear.

Surgeon preparation

The steps involved in the preparation of the surgery team for aseptic procedures have been well described, including surgical scrubbing and donning of surgical protective items (i.e., cap, mask, gown, gloves). Although a strict standard of care has not been established in this regard, observational data indicate that preparation practices vary greatly among veterinarians and may not meet the goals intended (Anderson and Weese 2011). Compliance of all members of the surgery team with regard to hand preparation (i.e., scrubbing) time is the most common challenge to proper preparation in human and veterinary surgery. Although the relative impact of poor practices has not been quantified, it is clear that there is significant room for improvement in compliance with typical recommendations among some veterinarians.

Although traditional surgical scrubbing with antiseptic soap and bristle sponges remains most commonly used in veterinary practices, the use of alcohol-based presurgical hand rubs is gaining popularity as an alternative. Although traditional scrubbing methods require timing or counting, the one-step alcohol-based presurgical hand preparation is simple and generally requires less time. These advantages are likely to improve the compliance of surgical personnel (Figure 8.2). This approach has been found to be more effective

than standard surgical scrub methods (Hobson et al. 1998; Verwilghen et al. 2011a) and is associated with less skin damage compared to repeated surgical scrubbing, yet veterinary surgeons have been slow to adopt this approach (Verwilghen et al. 2011b).

Preventive measures involving the surgical patient
Preoperative patient preparation

Patient preparation is an important aspect of SSI prevention, limiting contamination of sterile tissues by the patient's own endogenous flora at a time when these tissues are most vulnerable (i.e., during the surgical procedure itself). Surgical preparation of the patient is detailed elsewhere and traditionally involves at least a two-step scrubbing of the surgical site. One-step preparation kits used in human surgery were found equally effective as the traditional two-step method in healthy dogs undergoing elective surgery in one small study (Rochat et al. 1993), but they have not been objectively further evaluated. Overall, the relative impact of different patient preparation techniques has been inadequately investigated. Recent observational data have indicated marked variation in the time and quality of patient preparation in general small animal practices, with inadequately short or excessively long scrub times and inferior scrub methods identified in some cases (Anderson and Weese 2011). The goal of preoperative surgical site management is to eliminate potential pathogens without creating a physical environment that would be more conducive to bacterial colonization or infection postoperatively. Preoperative bathing of the patient is reasonable if there is significant contamination of the hair coat (Stick 2006). The patient's coat should be dried by the time of surgery because a wet coat promotes hypothermia and bacterial strike-through of sterile drapes. Minimizing skin damage during clipping and scrubbing is essential but often overlooked. Skin damage from excessive attempts at clipping every piece of hair or from forceful or prolonged scrubbing of the surgical site may predispose to infection rather than reduce the risk. Although objective data are lacking, anecdotal evidence supports the concept that excessive preparation may contribute to outbreaks of SSIs. Some indirect research data further support this concern. For example, Brown et al. reported that dogs clipped before anesthetic induction had higher SSI rates than those clipped after (Brown et al. 1997). Although the underlying cause of this finding could not be determined, it is certainly plausible that clipping a conscious animal could increase the risk of skin trauma and subsequent SSI. Surgical clipping is therefore always performed after induction of anesthesia. The only potential exception may be in dogs scheduled for joint replacement or other high risk (or high consequence) surgical procedures (e.g., tibial plateau leveling osteotomy) because some surgeons may choose to perform a rough clip of the surgical site before anesthetic induction to confirm the absence of skin lesions that would justify postponing the surgery. Clipping should always be done outside of the operating environment to reduce airborne contaminants such as hair and dander that may contact sterile sites or instruments.

Postoperative patient care

Postoperative care of the incision site may also be an important factor in preventing SSIs. The incision site is highly susceptible to opportunistic pathogens from the patient's own microflora, from the environment, or from hospital personnel. Contact with the surgical incision, particularly with bare hands, should be avoided. Covering or bandaging wounds for a minimum of 24 to 48 hours after surgery has been recommended in humans

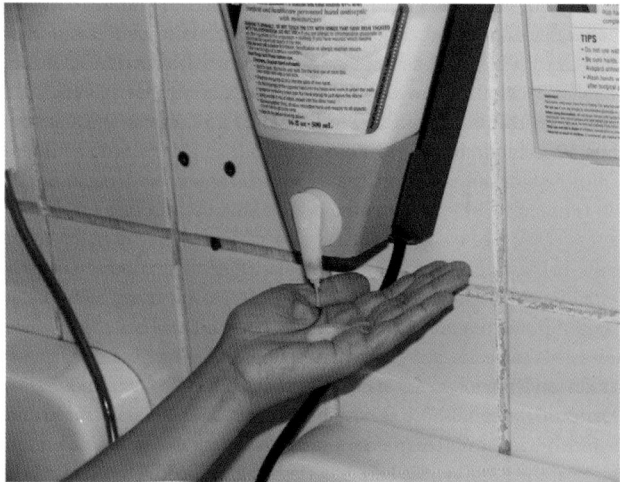

Figure 8.2 One-step preparation of the surgery team. This fast and simple technique is designed to improve compliance while maintaining efficacy. *Source:* D. Griffon, Western University of Health Sciences, Pomona, CA, 2014. Reproduced with permission from D. Griffon.

and horses (Mangram *et al.* 1999; Waguespack *et al.* 2006) and is a reasonable recommendation in small animals in most situations because a fibrin seal generally forms between the edges of a surgical wound within 24 hours. Bandage changes should be performed using aseptic technique (Mangram *et al.* 1999). Animal owners and handlers should be educated on proper incision management and signs of SSI. There is no objective information regarding the need to cover incisions beyond 48 hours in veterinary or human medicine, and arguments can be made either way. Prevention of surgical site trauma from licking or scratching by the patient is important because damage to the healing incision or associated skin can create a more hospitable site for bacterial growth, and such trauma can also result in the deposition of opportunistic pathogens. If surgical sites are bandaged, they should be inspected at least once daily to detect early signs of inflammation or infection, and the dressing must be kept as clean and dry as possible.

Conclusion

Infection control in veterinary medicine still lags behind that in human medicine. However, emergence of resistant agents, coupled with the risks of zoonoses and potential disastrous consequences of SSIs in patients, has raised the awareness of the veterinary community regarding the prevention and management of HAIs. Infection control targets multiple aspects of patient care, hospital protocols, and the clinical environment. Failure to meet standards in any of these areas will jeopardize the efficacy of the entire program. Veterinary facilities have an obligation to patients, clients, staff, and the public to take all reasonable precautions to reduce the risk of HAIs.

References

Anderson, D.J., Sexton, D.J., Kanafani, Z.A., et al. (2007) Severe surgical site infection in community hospitals: epidemiology, key procedures, and the changing prevalence of methicillin-resistant *Staphylococcus aureus. Infection Control and Hospital Epidemiology* 28, 1047-1053.

Anderson, M.E.C., Weese, J.S. (2011) Observation of patient and surgeon preparation in companion animal clinics. Annual Forum of the American College of Veterinary Internal Medicine, Denver, CO.

Block, S.S., ed. (2001) *Disinfection, Sterilization and Preservation*, 5th edn. 2001. Lippincott, Williams and Wilkins, Philadelphia.

Brown, D., Conzemius, M., Shofer, F., et al. (1997) Epidemiologic evaluation of postoperative wound infections in dogs and cats. *Journal of the American Veterinary Medical Association* 210, 1302-1306.

Hobson, D.W., Woller, W., Anderson, L., et al. (1998) Development and evaluation of a new alcohol-based surgical hand scrub formulation with persistent antimicrobial characteristics and brushless application. *American Journal of Infection Control* 26, 507-512.

Linton, A.H., Hugo, W.B., Russel, A.D. (1987) *Disinfection in Veterinary and Farm Practice.* Blackwell Scientific Publications, Oxford, England.

Mangram, A.J., Horan, T.C., Pearson, M.L., et al. (1999) Guidelines for prevention of surgical site infection, 1999. *Infection Control and Hospital Epidemiology* 20, 247-278.

Murphy, C.P., Weese, J.S., Reid-Smith, R.J., et al. (2010) The prevalence of bacterial contamination of surgical cold sterile solutions from community companion animal veterinary practices in southern Ontario. *The Canadian Veterinary Journal* 51, 634-636.

Rochat, M.C., Mann, F.A., Berg, J.N. (1993) Evaluation of a one-step surgical preparation technique in dogs. *Journal of the American Veterinary Medical Association* 203, 392-395.

Scott, R.D. (2009). The direct medical costs of healthcare-associated infection in U.S. hospitals and the benefits of prevention [Online]. Atlanta, GA: Division of Healthcare Quality Promotion, Centers for Disease Control and Prevention. Available: www.cdc.gov/ncidod/dhqp/pdf/scott_costpaper.pdf [Accessed Sept 5 2011].

Shea, A., Shaw, S. (2012) Evaluation of an educational campaign to increase hand hygiene at a small animal veterinary teaching hospital. *Journal of the American Veterinary Medical Association* 240, 61-64.

Stick, J.A. (2006) Preparation of the surgical patient, the surgery facility, and the operating team. In: Auer, J.A., Stick, J.A. (eds.). *Equine Surgery*, 3rd edn. Saunders Elsevier, Philadelphia.

Traub-Dargatz, J., Weese, J., Rousseau, J., et al. (2006) Pilot study to evaluate 3 hygiene protocols on the reduction of bacterial load on the hands of veterinary staff performing routine equine physical examinations. *The Canadian Veterinary Journal* 47, 671-676.

Verwilghen, D.R., Mainil, J., Mastrocicco, E., et al. (2011a) Surgical hand antisepsis in veterinary practice: Evaluation of soap scrubs and alcohol based rub techniques. *The Veterinary Journal* 190(3), 372-377.

Verwilghen, D., Grulke, S., Kampf, G. (2011b) Presurgical hand antisepsis: concepts and current habits of veterinary surgeons. *Vet Surgery* 40, 515-521.

Waguespack, R.W., Burba, D.J., Moore, R.M. (2006) Surgical site infection and the use of antimicrobials. In: Auer, J.A., Stick, J.A. (eds.). *Equine Surgery*, 3rd edn. Saunders Elsevier, Philadelphia.

Wright, J., Jung, S., Holman, R., et al. (2008) Infection control practices and zoonotic disease risks among veterinarians in the United States. *Journal of the American Veterinary Medical Association* 232, 1863-1872.

General Postoperative Complications

9 Dehiscence

Department of Clinical Sciences (Companion Animals and Equids), Faculty of Veterinary Medicine, University of Liège, Liège, Belgium

Disruption of apposed surfaces of a wound is a common complication. It may be caused by local or systemic factors. Several factors may be involved, either alone or in combination. Dehiscence involving skin, abdominal wall, and intestine is discussed in this chapter. Dehiscence involving other specific tissues is discussed in the related chapters.

Definition

Dehiscence can be defined as the disruption of wound edges. Any type of sutured wound may be concerned.

Risk factors

Inadequate technique

- Poor knot-tying technique
- Improper suture material selection (size, tensile strength, suture pattern, rate of resorption). Selection of suture material and size is dictated by the type of tissue to be sutured and the anticipated postoperative incisional forces. Multifilament material causes more tissue trauma and has increased capillarity, which may potentially increase bacterial contamination.
- Improper needle selection: Suture is more likely to cut through the tissue with cutting needles, especially if tension is present or if tissue is more fragile.
- Sutures may be placed too loosely because of anticipated edema. When edema subsides, the wound edges retract, leaving an incisional gap.
- Sutures may be placed too close to the wound margins. Collagenase activity is indeed high within 5 mm of the wound edges, making sutures placed in this zone more likely to cut through the tissue.
- Placement of sutures absorbing too quickly
- Moisture accumulation may contribute to tissue maceration, which in turn may induce dehiscence.
- Premature suture removal
- Suture placement in scar tissue, which has poor suture-holding ability
- Entrapment of fat between the wound edges may increase the risk of abdominal incisional hernia.

Excessive tension

Wound closure under a tension exceeding suture strength may lead to dehiscence by suture breakage. Excessive tension may also cause ischemic necrosis of the tissue, which results in suture cut-out (Figures 9.1 and 9.2). Excessive motion increases the risk of tension on the wound edges and dehiscence.

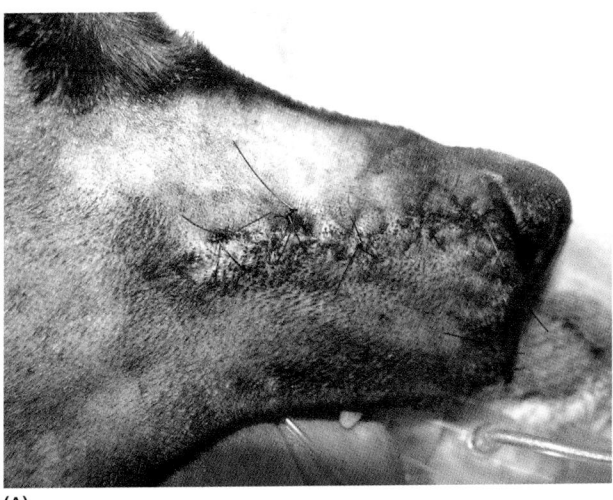

(A)

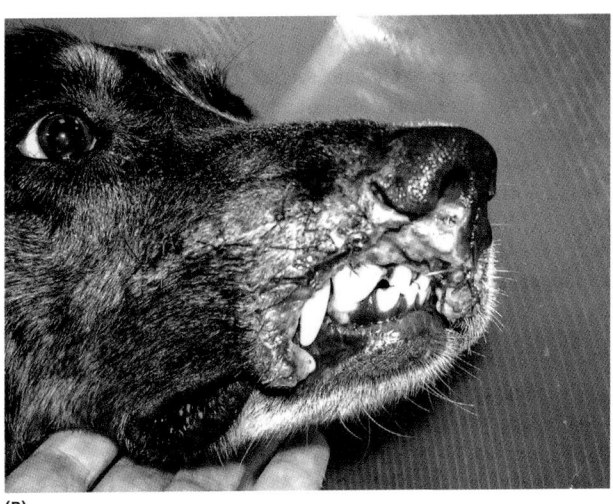

(B)

Figure 9.1 Lip advancement flap performed after tumor excision in a dog. **A,** Immediate postoperative view. **B,** Rostral dehiscence of the flap 11 days after surgery, most likely caused by a combination of excessive tension and self-trauma secondary to licking. *Source:* Julius Liptak, Alta Vista Animal Hospital, Ottawa, Ontario. Reproduced with permission from Julius Liptak.

Complications in Small Animal Surgery, First Edition. Edited by Dominique Griffon and Annick Hamaide.
© 2016 John Wiley & Sons, Inc. Published 2016 by John Wiley & Sons, Inc.
Companion website: www.wiley.com/go/griffon/complications

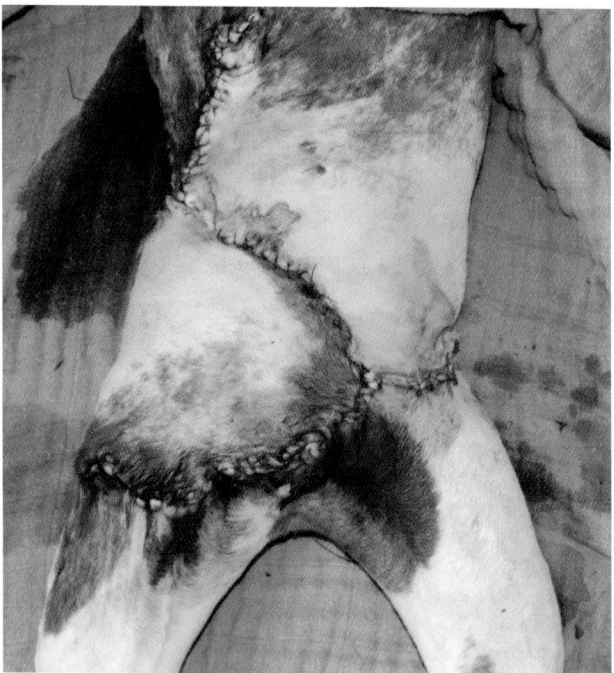

(A)

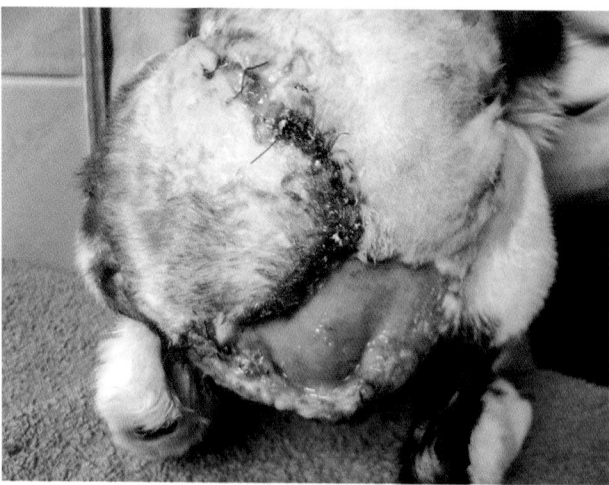

(B)

Figure 9.2 Bite wound covered by an inguinal fold flap in a cat.
A, Immediate postoperative view. **B,** Flap dehiscence secondary to
excessive tension. Note the presence of a purulent discharge, most likely
secondary to dehiscence. *Source:* Jean-Philippe Billet, Centre Hospitalier
Veterinaire Atlantia, Nantes, France. Reproduced with permission from
Jean-Philippe Billet.

Abdominal wall dehiscence may be secondary to excessive forces
placed on the incision, mainly caused by to excessive intraabdominal pressure or muscle tension. Uncontrolled activity, violent
coughing, or straining postoperatively predisposes to wound breakdown. Increased intraabdominal pressure may be observed in cases
of obesity, pregnancy, abdominal effusions, and organ distention
caused by ileus or obstruction (Smeak 2003).

Infection

Infection may be the primary reason for dehiscence or may be
secondary to it. Bacteria release proteolytic enzymes and other
substances that inhibit wound healing, therefore inducing wound
disruption. Other factors of dehiscence should, however, be ruled

out because some degree of infection is often associated with wound
disruption (see Figure 9.2B).

Underlying hematoma or seroma

Hematoma and seroma formation may provide a nutrient source
for bacteria, predisposing the wound to infection, which in turn
can result in wound dehiscence. Hematoma and seroma may also
increase the pressure underneath the suture line, increasing the risk
of disruption of the wound edges.

Suture of nonviable tissue

The viability of recently traumatized skin may be difficult to assess.
If a traumatic wound is closed too quickly, subsequent necrosis may
occur, resulting in dehiscence. In these cases, necrosis will usually
not be limited to the suture line but will concern larger areas.
Necrosis limited to the suture line may indicate ischemia secondary
to tight suture placement.

Underlying foreign body

The presence of an underlying foreign body may induce a persistent
wound drainage, which predisposes the wound to dehiscence.

Underlying neoplasia

Tumor infiltration after resection with incomplete surgical margins
may predispose the incision line to dehiscence. This is particularly
true with mast cell tumors (Figure 9.3).

Systemic factors

Endocrine imbalances (diabetes mellitus, Cushing's syndrome,
and hypothyroidism), nutritional deficiencies, hypoproteinemia,
hypovolemia, anemia, uremia, and obesity may delay wound healing and increase the risk of wound disruption (Figure 9.4). In
cats, feline leukemia virus, feline infectious peritonitis, and feline
immunodeficiency virus predispose to poor wound healing.

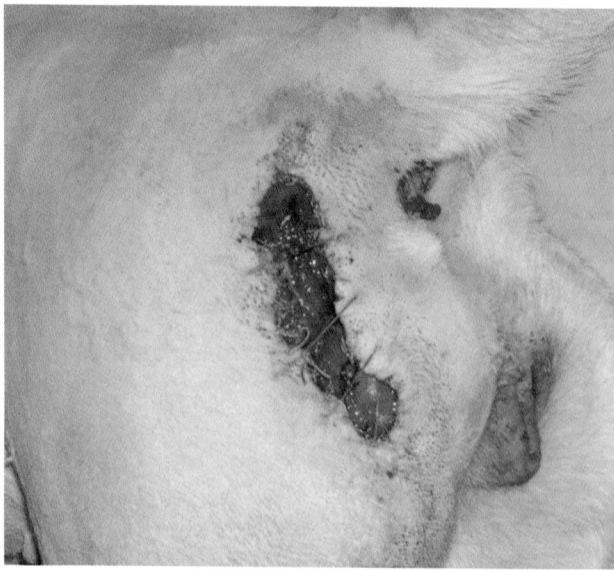

Figure 9.3 Wound dehiscence in a Labrador retriever after mast cell tumor
excision without clean margins in the caudal thigh region. Multiple closure
attempts had been made by the referring veterinarian. Wide en-bloc excision
of the wound was performed before closure of the defect using a rotation flap.
Clean margins were obtained, and the wound healed without complication.

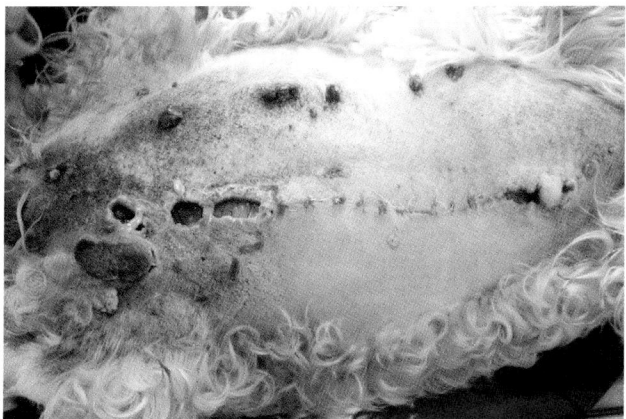

Figure 9.4 Wound dehiscence in a cocker spaniel after unilateral mastectomy. Excessive tension, severe obesity, chronic skin disease, and inadequate technique may all have contributed to dehiscence.

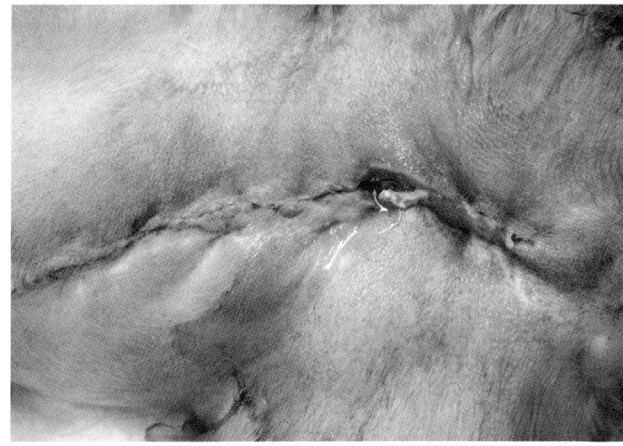

Figure 9.5 Wound dehiscence in a dog 4 days after mastectomy. Note the presence of serosanguineous discharge from the suture line, subcutaneous swelling and bruising, and necrosis of the skin edges.

Drugs such as corticosteroids and chemotherapeutic agents delay healing by decreasing fibroplasia and neovascularization.

Self-trauma
Molestation of the suture line may be an important cause of cutaneous dehiscence in animals (see Figure 9.1).

Radiation therapy
Radiation generates free radicals that damage DNA and associated proteins that affect all phases of wound healing. It mainly impairs wound healing by damaging fibroblasts and blood vessels. The damages caused by radiation are dose dependent and affect only exposed tissues. The maximum effect of radiation on wound healing usually occurs within 2 weeks of surgery.

Risk factors specific to intestinal dehiscence
Apart from the general risk factors listed earlier, reported risk factors for intestinal dehiscence after resection and anastomosis in dogs include intestinal obstruction by a foreign body, preexisting peritonitis, and serum albumin concentrations 2.5 g/dL or lower. Patients with two or more of those factors are predicted to be at high risk for developing anastomotic leakage (Ralphs *et al.* 2005).

Diagnosis

Cutaneous dehiscence
Cutaneous dehiscence may occur rapidly after surgery if caused by self-trauma or up to several weeks after surgery. It is usually observed 4 to 5 days after surgery. Clinical signs associated with cutaneous dehiscence are the presence of serosanguineous discharge from the suture line, subcutaneous swelling and bruising, and necrosis of the skin edges (Figure 9.5). Purulent discharge may be present if cutaneous disruption is associated with infection.

A deep sample should be taken for aerobic and anaerobic bacteriologic culture and sensitivity testing. Fungal culture may sometimes be recommended. Cytologic or histopathologic examination may be indicated to identify an underlying cause such as neoplasia.

If a systemic disease is suspected, the general health status of the animal should be assessed, and further work-up may be indicated.

Abdominal wall dehiscence
Abdominal wall dehiscence may occur acutely (within the first 7 days after surgery) or chronically (weeks to years after surgery). Clinical signs include wound edema and inflammation, serosanguineous drainage from the incision, and painless swelling. The overlying skin may remain intact, especially in chronic hernias, but the deeper layers have separated. Careful palpation may allow detection of the hernia. Abdominal radiographs, ultrasonography, or computed tomography may be needed to definitely identify disruption of the abdominal wall.

Evisceration is more common in acute hernias (often within 5 days of surgery). Exposure of abdominal organs is evident (Figure 9.6).

Intestinal dehiscence
Dehiscence after enteric suture leads to septic peritonitis. Clinical signs usually occur within 2 to 5 days after surgery and include depression, anorexia, vomiting, and abdominal pain. Some animals present with acute collapse. The diagnosis is based on blood analysis, abdominal radiography and ultrasonography, abdominal fluid

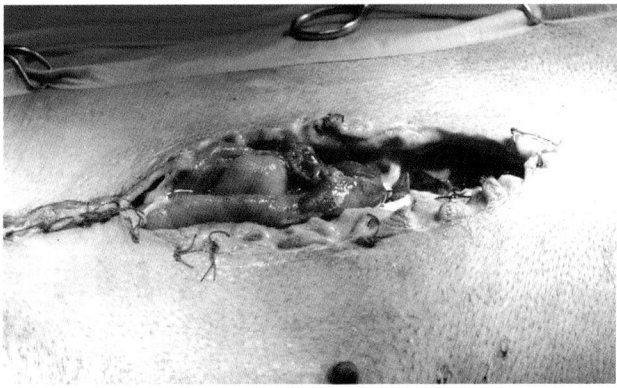

Figure 9.6 Evisceration 3 days after ovariohysterectomy in a dog. Exposure of abdominal organs is evident as well as necrosis of cutaneous wound edges.

analysis collected by abdominocentesis or peritoneal lavage (cytology and biochemical analysis), and bacteriologic culture of the fluid. Refer to Chapter 4 for more details.

Treatment

Cutaneous dehiscence
- Cutaneous dehiscence may be treated by wound lavage, debridement, and primary closure if infection has been ruled out.
- Penrose or closed-suction drains may be added to allow drainage and obliterate dead space, especially if seroma is suspected to have contributed to dehiscence.
- Delayed primary closure (before granulation tissue formation), secondary closure (after formation of a healthy granulation bed), or second intention healing are recommended in the presence of infection or if additional debridement is needed.
- Debridement may be performed surgically or conservatively with wet-to-dry dressings.
- Broad-spectrum antibiotics should be administered while waiting for sensitivity testing results. Antibiotic treatment may be changed accordingly.
- Systemic diseases that may interfere with healing should be treated concurrently.
- If excessive tension is suspected to have contributed to dehiscence, alternative closure techniques should be used. Walking sutures or tension-relieving suture patterns may be performed. If those are not sufficient to relieve enough tension, reconstructive flaps may be indicated. Free skin grafts may also be an option for distal extremity wounds covered with healthy granulation tissue.
- Bandaging may be indicated if excessive movement or self-trauma contributed to dehiscence.
- Animals should be confined and should wear an Elizabethan collar.

Abdominal wall dehiscence
- Acute abdominal wall dehiscence associated with exposure of abdominal organs (evisceration) or breakdown of the overlying skin should be treated immediately. These animals require early aggressive supportive care (fluids, antibiotic therapy, and so on). Herniated organs should be covered immediately with sterile dressings during stabilization of the patient. The approach is made over the original incision, and the entire abdominal cavity is explored. Damaged organs are repaired as needed, and the abdominal cavity is copiously lavaged. The abdomen is closed primarily or treated by open peritoneal drainage (see Chapter 4).
- In case of acute hernia without evisceration, the strongest holding layer of the abdominal wall is identified and used for closure. Only nonviable and necrotic tissues are debrided. Debridement of healthy tissue is not recommended in acute incisional hernias because it creates excessive unnecessary tissue trauma, spreads the contamination into sterile areas, and delays the onset of rapid strength gain of the wound (Smeak 2003).
- In cases of chronic incisional hernias, the skin overlying the hernia is usually intact, so these patients are usually not treated on an emergency basis.
- Some small asymptomatic chronic hernias may be treated conservatively if owners are attentive to any change of the hernia (color, pain, size) or any sign of deterioration of the condition of the animal.

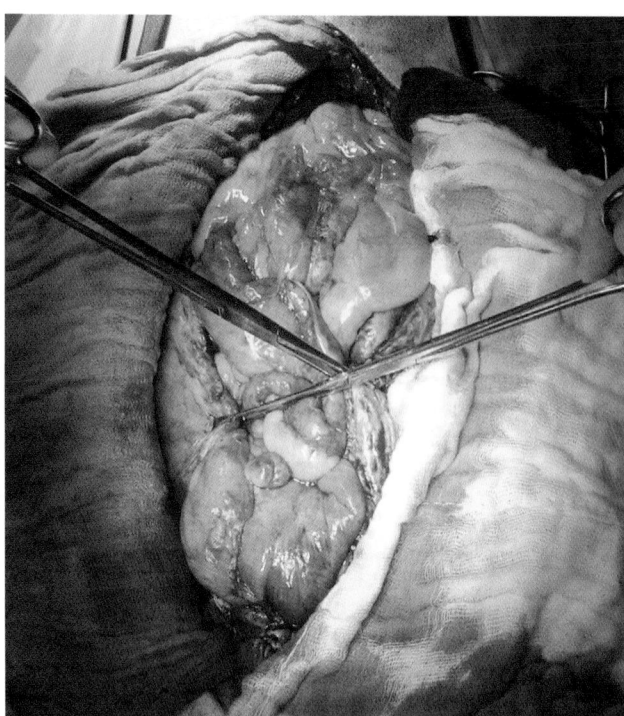

Figure 9.7 Chronic abdominal hernia with intact skin after laparotomy in a Labrador retriever. The referring veterinarian had debrided and closed the abdominal wall three times before referral, resulting in loss of domain. Abdominal wall could not be closed primarily, and a polypropylene mesh was used to allow closure without tension.

- Debridement of the scar tissue is recommended in chronic hernias to identify the holding layer. Excessive tension may be observed secondary to retraction of the wound edges and debridement.
- Large chronic defects may be impossible to close primarily because of loss of domain (Figure 9.7). In these cases, reduction of herniated organs back into the abdomen results in excessive tension on the incision and restriction of diaphragm movements. These defects require closure with prosthetic material (Smeak 2003).

Intestinal wound dehiscence
Patients with septic peritonitis require early intensive supportive care and should be returned to surgery to identify and correct the underlying problem (Figure 9.8). The dehiscence is corrected, and the abdominal cavity is copiously lavaged. The abdomen may be closed primarily, or open peritoneal drainage may be performed. Please refer to Chapter 4 for more details.

Outcome

Cutaneous dehiscence
The prognosis after repair of wound dehiscence is usually good as long as the causal factors are recognized and eliminated.

Abdominal wall dehiscence
Abdominal wall disruption with intact skin carries an excellent prognosis. Septic peritonitis associated with evisceration requires intense monitoring and treatment and dramatically changes prognosis. Early and aggressive medical and surgical intervention can however lead to a favorable outcome.

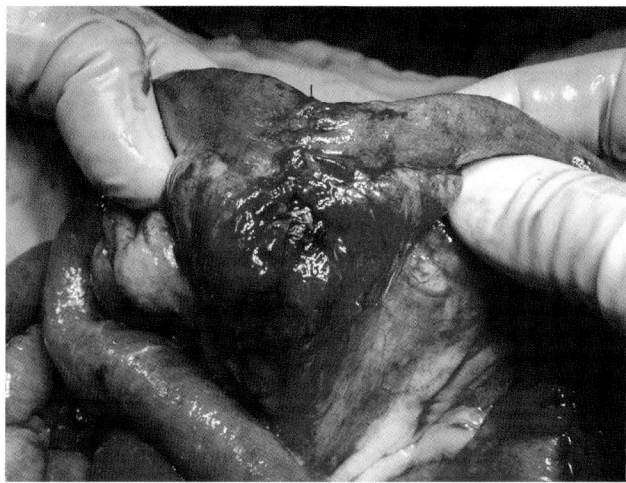

Figure 9.8 Intestinal dehiscence and secondary septic peritonitis 3 days after jejunal resection and anastomosis performed for obstruction by a foreign body in a dog. Anastomosis had been sutured by a simple continuous pattern using polydioxanone. Dehiscence of the suture line occurred at the level of the mesenteric border, which is often the case because of the presence of mesenteric fat obscuring the intestinal wall and making suturing more difficult at that location.

Intestinal wound dehiscence

Mortality rates of patients with septic peritonitis range from 29.0% to 73.7% (Woolfson and Dulisch 1986; Hosgood and Salisbury 1988; Allen *et al.* 1992; King 1994; Mueller *et al.* 2001; Lanz *et al.* 2001; Staatz *et al.* 2002). Reported indicators of a poor prognosis include refractory hypotension, cardiovascular collapse, and development of respiratory disease or disseminated intravascular coagulation (King 1994). Mortality rates between 73.7% and 85.0% are reported after intestinal dehiscence (Allen *et al.* 1992; Wylie and Hosgood 1994; Ralphs *et al.* 2003).

Prevention

Cutaneous dehiscence

- Adequate suturing technique (e.g., suture pattern, knot tying), suture material (e.g., type, size, tensile strength, resorption), and needle should be used.
- Excessive tension should be avoided. Tension-relieving techniques should be used if needed, as well as reconstructive flaps or free grafts when indicated.
- Hematoma and seroma formation should be prevented by adequate hemostasis, atraumatic surgical technique, and closure of dead space. Penrose or closed-suction drains may be placed at the time of surgery if seroma formation is anticipated.
- Severely traumatized skin should not be closed too quickly and should be monitored until viability is guaranteed.
- Proper bandaging should be used to immobilize areas of excessive motion. Circulatory compromise should, however, be avoided.
- An Elizabethan collar should be used to prevent self-trauma.
- Animals should be confined and exercise restricted for 2 weeks.
- Delaying chemotherapy until wound healing has begun (usually 7–10 days) has been recommended, although general recommendations are difficult to make based on the current literature given the influence of the type of agent, dose, and timing of administration.

- Postoperative radiation therapy should be delayed until 1 to 3 weeks after surgery.

Abdominal wall dehiscence

- Sutures must include the external rectus fascia.
- Preferred suture materials for celiotomy closure include polydioxanone, polyglyconate, polypropylene, and nylon. The tensile strength of fascia being only 20% of normal after 20 days, suture materials with a rapid loss of tensile strength should be avoided. Suture size should be adapted to the size of the animal.
- A continuous suture pattern, especially when using a monofilament suture, distributes the tension equally along the entire length of the incision and resists dehiscence as well as interrupted sutures do (Poole 1984).
- Sutures should be placed between 5 and 10 mm from the edges of the linea alba (Bellenger 2003).
- Suture interval in dogs and cats should be between 3 and 12 mm, depending on the size of the animal (Bellenger 2003).
- Activity should be restricted for 2 weeks.
- Conditions causing increased intraabdominal pressure (e.g., coughing, vomiting, straining) should be addressed pre- or postoperatively.

Intestinal wound dehiscence

- Adequate and atraumatic surgical technique should be used.
- Monofilament synthetic absorbable (polydioxanone or polyglyconate) or nonabsorbable (nylon or polypropylene) sutures are recommended for enteric closure. Staples are also a safe and quick alternative.
- A simple interrupted or simple continuous approximating suture pattern including the submucosa should be used.
- Omentum should be wrapped around the incision line.

Relevant literature

Cutaneous dehiscence

Cutaneous wound dehiscence is a common postoperative complication. Common causes and treatments are described in textbooks (Waldron and Zimmerman-Pope 2003; Friend 2009; Pavletic 2010).

Differences in wound healing have been reported in cats compared with dogs (Bohling *et al.* 2004). Sutured wounds in cats are indeed only half as strong as those in dogs 7 days after surgery. This may lead to dehiscence of cutaneous wounds when skin sutures are removed despite their healed appearance. Bohling *et al.* (2004) therefore recommend leaving skin sutures in place longer in cats than in dogs, especially in areas where excessive tension or motion is anticipated.

Cutaneous incisions performed with a carbon dioxide (CO_2) laser have been shown to heal more slowly and to have a lower tensile strength than incisions created by conventional surgical technique (Mison *et al.* 2003). Skin flaps created with a CO_2 laser may therefore be more susceptible to dehiscence.

Radiation therapy combined with surgery is becoming more common for management of veterinary cancer patients. Radiation has however detrimental effects on wound healing mainly by damaging fibroblasts and blood vessels. Irradiation decreases the ability of the fibroblasts to multiply and produce collagen (Denham and Hauer-Jensen 2002). When 18 Gy was delivered to guinea pigs before full-thickness wounding, wound bursting strength was decreased by 50% of normal 2 weeks after irradiation (Bernstein *et al.* 1993a).

Tolerance of cutaneous and mucosal flaps placed into a radiation therapy field has been evaluated clinically in 26 dogs (Séguin et al. 2005). Radiation therapy was performed either preoperatively (group 1) or postoperatively (group 2). In a third group, a flap was performed as a salvage procedure for management of complications or local tumor recurrence after radiation therapy. Complications (necrosis, local infection, dehiscence, or ulceration) were observed in 77% of the dogs, with dehiscence being the most common complication (62%). Some degree of dehiscence was noted in 6 of 8 dogs in group 1, 4 of 9 dogs in group 2, and 6 of 9 dogs in group 3. Flaps on previously irradiated surgical beds (groups 1 and 3) were at a higher risk for complication. The authors concluded that placing a cutaneous or mucosal flap into a radiation therapy field led to a successful outcome in 85% of the dogs but was associated with substantial morbidity. Whereas using a flap to correct a complication or failure of radiation therapy was more likely to result in a complication, planned preoperative irradiation increased the severity of the complications compared with postoperative irradiation. No recommendations regarding the time interval between the two treatment modalities were proposed by the authors. Postoperative radiotherapy was performed in this study a median of 33 days after surgery. Complications may have been worse if radiotherapy had been started earlier. Studies have, however, shown that wound healing was hardly affected if irradiation was delayed 7 days or more after wounding (Gorodetsky et al. 1988; Hidalgo and Carrasquillo 1992; Bernstein et al. 1993b; Panchal et al. 1993).

Abdominal wall dehiscence

In a study of 200 dogs and cats undergoing exploratory celiotomy, 8 (4%) incision-related complications were observed (Boothe et al. 1992). However, the rate of abdominal wall dehiscence was not specifically reported.

A continuous suture pattern using a monofilament suture resists dehiscence of the abdominal wall as well as simple interrupted sutures (Poole 1984; Kummeling and van Sluijs 1998). Moreover, closure of the rectus sheath with a continuous looped suture of polyglyconate and the skin with staples is equally safe and significantly faster than closure of the rectus sheath with simple interrupted sutures and the skin with a continuous subdermal suture (Kummeling and van Sluijs 1998).

A guarded prognosis is traditionally associated with abdominal evisceration because it is associated with septic peritonitis and requires intensive treatment and monitoring. Gower et al. (2009), however, reported a good outcome in eight dogs and four cats after major evisceration, eight of which were secondary to postsurgical dehiscence after ovariohysterectomy. All animals survived to discharge after a median hospitalization time of 4 days. This study shows that the prognosis after evisceration injuries may be favorable in cases of immediate and aggressive medical and surgical intervention.

Intestinal wound dehiscence

Intestinal wound dehiscence is reported to occur in 2.0% to 15.7% of patients (Allen et al. 1992; Wylie and Hosgood 1994; Weisman et al. 1999; Ralphs et al. 2003; Shales et al. 2005). Mortality rates between 73.7% and 85% have been reported after intestinal dehiscence (Allen et al. 1992; Wylie and Hosgood 1994; Ralphs et al. 2003). Reported risk factors for intestinal dehiscence after resection and anastomosis in dogs include intestinal obstruction by a foreign body, preexisting peritonitis, and serum albumin concentrations 2.5 g/dL or less (Allen et al. 1992; Ralphs et al. 2003). On the other hand, two studies did not identify hypoalbuminemia as a risk factor for leakage after full-thickness small intestinal biopsies (Harvey 1990; Shales et al. 2005).

No difference in the prevalence of dehiscence was identified between animals undergoing small versus large intestinal surgery (Wylie and Hosgood 1994). Smith et al. (2011) evaluated the complication rate after full-thickness gastrointestinal surgery in 70 cats with alimentary lymphosarcoma (LSA) and found no postoperative leakage from any biopsy or anastomosis site. Cats with alimentary LSA do not appear to be at high risk of postoperative dehiscence.

When comparing continuous with simple interrupted suture pattern for closure of enterotomy or anastomosis in 83 cases, one intestinal dehiscence was observed in each group (Weisman et al. 1999). A simple continuous closure pattern is therefore an acceptable alterative to simple interrupted sutures in intestinal closure. Stapling devices may also be a safe and quick alternative to traditional suturing techniques. Ullman et al. (1991) reported the use of gastrointestinal anastomosis (GIA) and thoracoabdominal (TA) stapling devices in 24 dogs and cats, with postoperative anastomotic leakage observed in 2 dogs and a localized abscess observed at the staple line in 1 cat. Similar results were obtained after stapled one-stage end-to-end resection and anastomosis in 30 dogs using GIA and TA stapling devices (Jardel et al. 2011). In that study, 1 dog had anastomotic leakage and died during the second surgery, and 1 dog presented a localized abscess at the transverse staple line. A modified technique using only a GIA stapling device was successfully used in 15 dogs to perform small intestinal anastomosis without postoperative dehiscence (White 2008).

References

Allen, D.A., Smeak, D.D, Schertel, E.R. (1992) Prevalence of small intestinal dehiscence and associated clinical factors: a retrospective study of 121 dogs. *Journal of the American Animal Hospital Association* 28, 70-76.

Bellenger, C.R. (2003) Abdominal wall. In: Slatter, D. (ed.) *Textbook of Small Animal Surgery*, vol. 1, 3rd edn. WB Saunders, Philadelphia, pp. 405-413.

Bernstein, E.F., Salomon, G.D., Harisiadis, L., et al. (1993a) Collagen gene expression and wound strength in normal and radiation-impaired wounds. *Journal of Dermatologic Surgery and Oncology* 19, 564-570.

Bernstein, E.F., Sullivan, F.J., Mitchell, J.B., et al. (1993b) Biology of chronic radiation effects on tissues and wound healing. *Clinics in Plastic Surgery* 20, 435-453.

Bohling, M.W., Henderson, R.A., Swaim, S.F., et al. (2004) Cutaneous wound healing in the cat: a macroscopic description and comparison with cutaneous wound healing in the dog. *Veterinary Surgery* 33, 579-587.

Boothe, H.W., Slater, M.R., Hobson, H.P., et al. (1992) Exploratory celiotomy in 200 nontraumatized dogs and cats. *Veterinary Surgery* 21, 452-457.

Denham, J.W., Hauer-Jensen, M. (2002) The radiotherapeutic injury—a complex wound. *Radiotherapy Oncology* 63, 129-145.

Friend, E. (2009) Complications of wound healing. In: Williams, J., Moores, A. (eds.) *BSAVA Manual of Canine and Feline Wound Management and Reconstruction*, 2nd edn. British Small Animal Veterinary Association, Gloucester, UK, pp. 254-270.

Gorodetsky, R., McBride, W.H., Withers, H.R. (1988) Assay of radiation effects in mouse skin as expressed in wound healing. *Radiation Research* 116, 135-144.

Gower, S.B., Weisse, C.W., Brown, D.C. (2009) Major abdominal evisceration injuries in dogs and cats: 12 cases (1998-2008). *Journal of the American Veterinary Medical Association* 234, 1566-1572.

Harvey, H.J. (1990) Complications of small intestinal biopsy in hypoalbuminemic dogs. *Veterinary Surgery* 19, 289-292.

Hidalgo, D.A., Carrasquillo, I.M. (1992) The treatment of lower extremity sarcomas with wide excision, radiotherapy, and free flap reconstruction. *Plastic and Reconstructive Surgery* 89, 96-101.

Hosgood, G., Salisbury, S.K. (1988) Generalized peritonitis in dogs: 50 cases (1975-1986). *Journal of the American Veterinary Medical Association* 193, 1448-1450.

Jardel, N., Hidalgo, N., Leperlier, D., et al. (2011) One stage functional end-to-end stapled intestinal anastomosis and resection performed by nonexpert surgeons for the treatment of small intestinal obstruction in 30 dogs. *Veterinary Surgery* 40, 216-222.

King, L.G. (1994) Postoperative complications and prognostic indicators in dogs and cats with septic peritonitis: 23 cases (1989-1992). *Journal of the American Veterinary Medical Association* 204, 407-414.

Kummeling, A., van Sluijs F.J. (1998) Closure of the rectus sheath with a continuous looped suture and the skin with staples in dogs: speed, safety, and costs compared to closure of the rectus sheath with interrupted sutures and the skin with a continuous subdermal suture. *Veterinary Quarterly* 20, 126-30.

Laing, E.J. (1990) Problems in wound healing associated with chemotherapy and radiation therapy. *Problems in Veterinary Medicine* 2, 433-441.

Lanz, O.I., Ellison, G.W., Bellah, J.R., et al. (2001) Surgical treatment of septic peritonitis without abdominal drainage in 28 dogs. *Journal of the American Animal Hospital Association* 37, 87-92.

Mison, M.B., Steficek, B., Lavagnino, M., et al. (2003) Comparison of the effects of the CO_2 surgical laser and conventional surgical techniques on healing and wound tensile strength of skin flaps in the dog. *Veterinary Surgery* 32, 153-160.

Mueller, M.G., Ludwig, L.L., Barton, L.J. (2001) Use of closed-suction drains to treat generalized peritonitis in dogs and cats: 40 cases (1997-1999). *Journal of the American Veterinary Medical Association* 219, 719-724.

Panchal, J.I., Agrawal, R.K., McLean, N.R., et al. (1993) Early postoperative brachytherapy following free flap reconstruction. *British Journal of Plastic Surgery* 46, 511-515.

Pavletic, M.M. (2010) *Atlas of Small Animal Wound Management and Reconstructive Surgery*, 3rd edn. Wiley-Blackwell, Ames, IA.

Poole, G.V., Meredith, J.W., Kon, N.D., et al. (1984) Suture technique and wound bursting strength. *American Journal of Surgery* 50, 569-572.

Ralphs, S.C., Jessen, C.R., Lipowitz, A.J. (2003) Risk factors for leakage following intestinal anastomosis in dogs and cats: 115 cases (1991-2000). *Journal of the American Veterinary Medical Association* 223, 73-77.

Séguin, B., McDonald, D.E., Kent, M.S., et al. (2005) Tolerance of cutaneous or mucosal flaps placed into a radiation therapy field in dogs. *Veterinary Surgery* 34, 214-222.

Shales, C.J., Warren, J., Anderson, D.M., et al. (2005) Complications following full-thickness small intestinal biopsy in 66 dogs: a retrospective study. *Journal of Small Animal Practice* 46, 317-321.

Smeak, D.D. (2003) Abdominal hernias. In: Slatter, D. (ed.) *Textbook of Small Animal Surgery*, vol. 1, 3rd edn. WB Saunders, Philadelphia, pp. 449-470.

Smith, A.L., Wilson, A.P., Hardie, R.J., et al. (2011) Perioperative complications after full-thickness gastrointestinal surgery in cats with alimentary lymphoma. *Veterinary Surgery* 40, 849-852.

Staatz, A.J, Monnet, E., Seim, H.B. (2002) Open peritoneal drainage versus primary closure for the treatment of septic peritonitis in dogs and cats: 42 cases (1993-1999). *Veterinary Surgery* 31, 174-180.

Ullman, S.L., Pavletic, M.M., Clark, G.N. (1991) Open intestinal anastomosis with surgical stapling equipments in 24 dogs and cats. *Veterinary Surgery* 20, 385-391.

Waldron, D.R., Zimmerman-Pope, N. (2003) Superficial skin wounds. In: Slatter, D. (ed.) *Textbook of Small Animal Surgery*, vol. 1, 3rd edn. WB Saunders, Philadelphia, pp. 259-273.

Weisman, D.L., Smeak, D.D., Birchard, S.J., et al. (1999) Comparison of a continuous suture pattern with a simple interrupted pattern for enteric closure in dogs and cats: 83 cases (1991-1997). *Journal of the American Veterinary Medical Association* 214, 1507-1510.

White, R.N. (2008) Modified functional end-to-end stapled intestinal anastomosis: technique and clinical results in 15 dogs. *Journal of Small Animal Practice* 49, 274-281.

Woolfson, J.M., Dulisch, M.L. (1986) Open abdominal drainage in the treatment of generalized peritonitis in 25 dogs and cats. *Veterinary Surgery* 15, 27-32.

Wylie, K.B., Hosgood, G. (1994) Mortality and morbidity of small and large intestinal surgery in dogs and cats: 74 cases (1980-1992). *Journal of the American Animal Hospital Association* 30, 469-474.

10 Suture Reactions

Outi Laitinen-Vapaavuori

Department of Equine and Small Animal Medicine, Faculty of Veterinary Medicine, University of Helsinki, Helsinki, Finland

Suture reactions are complications that are occasionally encountered in surgical patients. Suture materials influence patient morbidity through their interaction with the tissue. Many factors affect this interaction, including the composition and the amount of the suture material in the wound as well as the suturing technique (Boothe 1998).

Both the physical (monofilament vs. multifilament) and the chemical construction of the suture material affect the reactions that take place in the tissues. Monofilament suture material withstands contamination better than multifilament suture materials while minimizing tissue reactivity (Boothe 2003). Although bacteria can adhere to any suture material, multifilament suture surfaces bind larger numbers of bacteria than monofilament (Katz *et al.* 1981).

Surgical gut is a capillary multifilament suture that elicits a marked foreign body reaction when implanted in tissues because it is composed of collagen. In contrast, synthetic monofilament absorbable sutures such as polydioxanone, polyglyconate, and polyglecaprone 25, as well as synthetic multifilament absorbable sutures such as polyglycolic acid and polyglactin 610 cause a mild inflammatory response characterized by the presence of macrophages and fibroblasts at the wound site. Alternatively, synthetic nonabsorbable sutures such as nylon and polypropylene are biologically inert and cause minimal tissue reaction. Steel is biologically inert and incites no inflammatory reaction except for that caused by inflexible suture ends (Boothe 2003).

Inflammatory reactions to sutures are more pronounced near knots because they have highest amount of foreign material (van Rijssel *et al.* 1989). Knot size and volume depends on suture size and number of throws. Suture size is the principal influence on knot volume and tissue reactivity; an increase in suture size increases tissue reaction more than adding an extra throw to a knot (van Rijssel *et al.* 1989). Overly tight knot ties or closely placed sutures can promote ischemia and possible infection (see Chapter 1).

Definition

Suture reactions are inflammatory reactions induced by suture material.

Risk factors

- Inappropriate suture material
- Inappropriate suture technique

Diagnosis

The most common clinical signs include:
- Swelling around an individual suture or suture line (Figure 10.1)
- Isolated swelling filled with clear fluid around the knot placed in the subcutaneous tissue
- Draining track to the skin if the suture reaction is deeper in the tissues

Treatment

- Do nothing if the suture reaction is mild.
- Remove skin or subcutaneous suture(s) if the reaction is severe or does not resolve in 7 to 14 days.

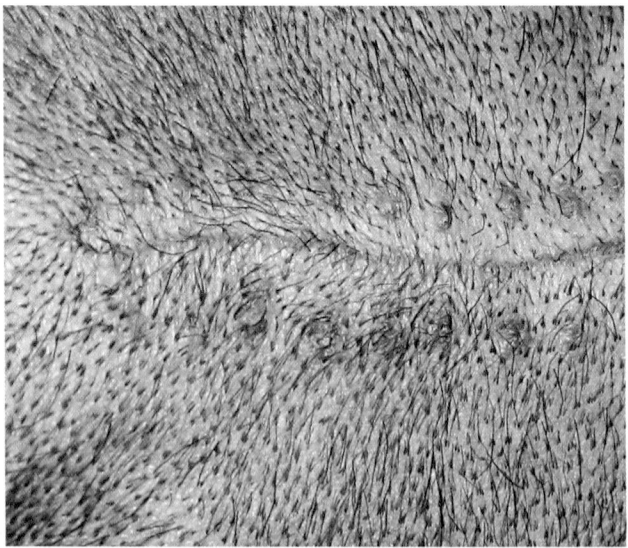

Figure 10.1 Suture reactions at suture removal 13 days after surgery.

Complications in Small Animal Surgery, First Edition. Edited by Dominique Griffon and Annick Hamaide.
© 2016 John Wiley & Sons, Inc. Published 2016 by John Wiley & Sons, Inc.
Companion website: www.wiley.com/go/griffon/complications

- Perform en-bloc resection of the suture(s) in severe cases. Samples of affected tissues are submitted for bacterial culture and histopathologic examination.
- After suture removal, close the wound with the most inert suture material available.

Outcome

Suture reactions can cause morbidity to the patient, prolong healing time, and increase the treatment costs; nonetheless, the prognosis is usually very good.

Prevention

Suture reactions are best prevented by:
- Using smallest suture size that is appropriate
- Minimizing the amount of suture material in the tissues
- Favoring monofilament suture material instead of multifilament
- Keeping the number of throws in a knot to a minimum without compromising the knot security
- Cutting the ends of the completed knot short, about 3 mm long for synthetic sutures
- Placing buried knots deep in the dermis when making intradermal closure of the skin

Relevant literature

When selecting an appropriate suture material, one must pay attention to the characteristics of the suture material, the condition of the wound environment in question, and its healing rate. In living tissues, any suture material acts as a foreign body and as such stimulates an inflammatory response. Choosing the smallest suture size and using the least amount of suture material with gentle tissue handling can decrease the risk of unnecessary suture reactions (Boothe 1998).

Uterine stump granulomas after ovariohysterectomy are complications occasionally encountered in dogs. Inflammation and granuloma formation can be caused by ligatures of nonabsorbable suture material, poor aseptic technique, or excessive residual tissue at the uterine body (van Goethem *et al.* 2006). Furthermore, fistulous tracts from the ligated ovarian pedicle can develop from inflammatory reaction to braided nonabsorbable suture material, which can even cause partial ureteral obstruction and hydronephrosis (Kanazono *et al.* 2010). Suture associated fistulous tracts can easily be prevented by using synthetic absorbable suture materials.

Suture remnants in the bladder can play an important role in the recurrence of cystoliths. In a study by Appel *et al.* (2008), suture-associated cystoliths were discovered to represent 9.4% of canine and 4% of feline recurrent cystoliths. Based on these findings, the authors recommended the avoidance of full-thickness bites, long-lasting suture materials, and nonabsorbable sutures in urinary tract surgery.

Although the use of nonabsorbable suture material, such as polypropylene, is a common and accepted practice in gastrointestinal surgery, it has been reported that when polypropylene is used in a continuous suture pattern in the small intestine, it can act as a site of attachment for a foreign body (Milovancev *et al.* 2004).

The use of multifilament suture material in extracapsular stabilization with lateral fabellar suture for cranial cruciate ligament injury has been shown to cause more suture complications than using monofilament nylon. Swelling associated with nylon has been reported to develop 6 to 44 weeks after surgery and to result in suture removal in 6 of 10 dogs (Casale and McCarthy 2009).

Species differences in the tissue response to the suture materials also appear to be evident. Cats seem to be more prone to experience incisional postoperative swelling than dogs (Runk *et al.* 1999; Papazoglou *et al.* 2010). The inflammatory reaction has been seen with different suture materials, usually subsiding within 7 to 14 days, and is typical in cats with thin skin and subcutaneous tissue (Muir *et al.* 1993; Runk *et al.* 1999). There are contradictory reports as to whether closing the subcutaneous tissue with sutures would help to prevent seroma formation in cats (Freeman *et al.* 1987; Muir *et al.* 1993). In dogs, when comparing buried continuous subcuticular pattern with polyglecaprone and a simple interrupted suture pattern with polypropylene in skin closure of ovariohysterectomy, it was noticed that the subcuticular closure demonstrated a higher rate of tissue reactivity 18 to 24 hours after surgery, but it was associated with significantly lower swelling or erythema scores 10 to 14 days after surgery (Sylvestre *et al.* 2002).

References

Appel, S.L., Lefebvre, S.L., Houston, D.M., et al. (2008) Evaluation of risk factors associated with suture-nidus cystoliths in dogs and cats: 176 cases (1999-2006). *Journal of the American Veterinary Medical Association* 233 (12), 1889-1895.

Boothe, H.W. (1998) Selecting suture materials for small animal surgery. *Compendium of Continuing Education* 20 (2), 155-163.

Boothe, H.W. (2003) Surgical materials, tissue adhesives, staplers, and ligating clips In: Slatter, D. (ed.) *Textbook of Small Animal Surgery*, vol. 1, 3rd edn. Saunders, Elsevier Science, Philadelphia, pp. 235-244.

Casale, S.A., McCarthy, R.J. (2009) Complications associated with lateral fabellotibial suture surgery for cranial cruciate ligament injury in dogs: 363 cases (1997-2005). *Journal of the American Veterinary Medical Association* 234 (2), 229-235.

Freeman, L.J., Pettit, G.D., Robinette, J.D. (1987) Tissue reaction to suture material in the feline alba. A retrospective, prospective, and histologic study. *Veterinary Surgery* 16 (6), 440-445.

Kanazono, S., Aikawa, T., Yoshigae, Y. (2009) Unilateral hydronephrosis and partial ureteral obstruction by entrapment in a granuloma in a spayed dog. *Journal of the American Animal Hospital Association* 45 (6), 301-304.

Katz, S., Izhar, M., Mirelman, D. (1981) Bacterial adherence to surgical sutures. A possible factor in suture induced infection. *Annals of Surgery* 194 (1), 35-41.

Milovancev, M., Weisman, D.L., Palmisano, M.P. (2004) Foreign body attachment to polypropylene suture material extruded into the small intestinal lumen after enteric closure in three dogs. *Journal of the American Veterinary Medical Association* 225 (11), 1713-1715.

Muir, P., Goldsmid, S.E., Simpson, D.J., et al. (1993) Incisional swelling following celiotomy in cats. *Veterinary Record* 132 (8), 189-190.

Papazoglou, L., G., Tsioli, V., Papaioannou, N., et al. (2010) Comparison of absorbable and nonabsorbable sutures for intradermal skin closure in cats. *The Canadian Veterinary Journal* 51 (7), 770-772.

Runk, A., Allen, S.W., Mahaffey, E.A. Tissue reactivity to poliglecaprone 25 in the feline linea alba. *Veterinary Surgery* 28 (6), 466-471.

Sylvestre, A., Wilson, J., Hare, J. (2002) A comparison of 2 different suture patterns for skin closure of canine ovariohysterectomy. *The Canadian Veterinary Journal* 43 (9), 699-702.

van Goethem, B., Schaefers-Okkens, A., Kirpensteijn, J. (2006) Making a rational choice between ovariectomy and ovariohysterectomy in the dog: a discussion of the benefits of either technique. *Veterinary Surgery* 35 (2), 136-143.

van Rijssel, E.J., Brand, R., Admiraal, C., et al. (1989) Tissue reaction and surgical knots: the effect of suture size, knot configuration, and knot volume. *Obstetrics and Gynecology* 74 (1),64-68.

11 Hyperthermia

Kris Gommeren

Emergency and Critical Care Unit, Department of Clinical Sciences (Companion Animals and Equids), Faculty of Veterinary Medicine, University of Liège, Liège, Belgium

In human literature, a general consensus exists that most cases of postoperative hyperthermia are of benign origin. In veterinary medicine, there is no uniform approach to deal with this complication to date.

Veterinarians often associate any elevation in temperature with fever, and normal temperature often gets associated with the absence of infectious disease (Miller 2010). However, human studies have shown that many patients get unnecessary treatment with antibiotics (Rybak *et al.* 2008). Furthermore, hyperthermia is only weakly associated with the presence of infection (Kennedy *et al.* 1997; Ward *et al.* 2010; Czaplicki *et al.* 2011) and hence has a low sensitivity and specificity as a diagnostic criterion for infection (Ghosh *et al.* 2006).

A complete infectious disease work-up and empirical coverage of all cases of postoperative hyperthermia with antibiotics are unnecessary, add unnecessary costs, and may have adverse medical consequences (Cunha 1999; Ward *et al.* 2010).

Despite all of this, the findings that human patients with postoperative hyperthermia are more likely to develop organ dysfunction and die and that peak temperature is a more powerful predictor of mortality than systemic inflammatory response syndrome (SIRS), emergency presentation, or APACHE (Acute Physiology and Chronic Health Evaluation) status (Barie *et al.* 2004) underline the importance of monitoring for this complication.

The incidence of postoperative hyperthermia has rarely been studied in veterinary medicine. In human studies, the prevalence of postoperative hyperthermia is 25% to 40%, but it can vary from 14% to 91% depending on the population and definition (de la Torre *et al.* 2003; Salom *et al.* 2003; Schey *et al.* 2005; Pile 2006; Rybak *et al.* 2008).

Definition

Hyperthermia is defined as an increase of the body temperature above a normal threshold. Unfortunately, there appears to be a lack of clear definition in veterinary medicine. Thresholds of 39.2°C, 39.3°C, or 40°C have been proposed for cats and dogs (Niedfeldt and Robertson 2006; Posner *et al.* 2007), or hyperthermia has been defined as an increase of body temperature compared with preoperative conditions (Posner *et al.* 2010).

True fever refers to a condition in which the set point of the thermoregulatory center, located in the anterior hypothalamus, is altered. In nonfebrile hyperthermic states, the set point is not altered, but because of (physio)pathological or pharmacologic conditions, heat gain exceeds heat loss (Miller 2010).

Risk factors

- Infectious causes
  - Wound infection
    - Iatrogenic infections
    - Surgical site infection
    - Catheter related causes
    - Urinary tract infection (UTI)
  - Pneumonia
- Noninfectious causes
  - Stress and agitation
  - Inflammatory hyperthermia
    - Phlebitis
    - Transfusion reactions
    - Acute pancreatitis
    - Malignancy and tumor lysis syndrome
  - Iatrogenic causes
    - Overheating
    - Pharmacologic agents
      - Feline opioid-induced hyperthermia
  - Neuromuscular disease
    - Seizures
    - Eclampsia
    - Hypothalamic lesions

Additionally, the incidence of postoperative hyperthermia in human medicine appears to be related to the length of operative time, lack of prophylactic antibiotics, estimated blood loss, patient's age, concurrent medical problems, obesity or cachexia, disease severity, and emergency presentation (Shackelford *et al.* 1999; Barie *et al.* 2004; Rybak *et al.* 2008).

Diagnosis

A careful history and physical examination should be performed if hyperthermia is detected to try to identify hyperthermic patients that would require immediate attention and further work-up (Pile 2006; Czaplicki *et al.* 2011).

Complications in Small Animal Surgery, First Edition. Edited by Dominique Griffon and Annick Hamaide.
© 2016 John Wiley & Sons, Inc. Published 2016 by John Wiley & Sons, Inc.
Companion website: www.wiley.com/go/griffon/complications

The work-up of hyperthermia should be tailored to the individual patient rather than in a "shotgun" fashion (Schey *et al.* 2005; Dionigi *et al.* 2006; Pile 2006; O'Grady *et al.* 2008).

History

- Previous anesthetic procedure (use of propofol or opioid drugs)
- Analgesia (use of opioid drugs)
- Blood products administration
- Vomiting, coughing, or diarrhea

Physical examination

- Vital signs
- Cardiac auscultation
- Respiratory auscultation
- Inspection of the surgical site
- Inspection of the catheter site
- Inspection of the urinary catheter
- Presence of skin rash
- Presence of joint inflammation

Treatment

- **True fever**
  - Nonsteroidal antiinflammatory drugs (NSAIDs)
    - Only in case of severe hyperthermia since NSAIDs
      - Prevent beneficiary effects of hyperthermia
      - Mask ongoing event
      - Can induce renal and gastro-intestinal complications
  - Antibiotics
  - Phenothiazines (hypotension!)
- **Nonfebrile hyperthermia**
  - Cool baths
  - Cool drinking water
  - Metal cage
  - Fans
  - Alcohol on footpads
    - Cool intravenous (IV) crystalloids: Avoid extreme cold because peripheral vasoconstriction will prevent heat loss.

Outcome

The prognosis largely depends on the underlying cause and to a lesser extent to the severity of the hyperthermia. Most causes of postoperative hyperthermia do not require any specific treatment. In case of severe hyperthermia, supportive care is indicated.

Prevention

- Prophylactic antibiotics
  - Important to follow a practice protocol
    - Time of injection before surgery
    - Repeat every 2 hours
    - Typical antibiotics for typical procedures
- Replace catheters as soon as the veins feel hard, the catheter site is dirty, or whenever they are present for longer than 3 to 5 days (depending on additional vascular access sites and the clinical situation). Label lines with the date of placement and when it was last checked and by whom.
- Hygiene of all indwelling tubes (endotracheal tubes transtracheal tubes, urinary catheters, oxygen probes, nutritional tubes)

INFECTIOUS HYPERTHERMIA

Wound infection

See Chapter 1

Surgical site infection

See Chapter 1

Catheter line infection

Definition

Catheter line infection is defined as bacterial infection of a peripheral or central catheter.

Risk factors

- Central venous catheters
- Infusion of dextrose-containing solutions
- Infusion of lipid-containing solutions

Diagnosis

- Culture of the catheter tip
- Blood culture

Treatment

- Removal of the catheter
- Antibiotherapy based on the antibiogram results

Outcome

- Good if there is early catheter removal and antibiotic treatment implementation

Prevention

- Good aseptic technique during catheter placement
- Regular check-up and cleansing of catheter sites
- Label lines (date, last check and by whom)
- Removal of catheters
  - After 3 to 5 days
  - When the veins feel hard
  - When the catheter site is dirty

Urinary tract infection

Definition

Urinary tract infection is defined as bacterial infection of the urinary tract, mostly the bladder.

Risk factors

- Residual bladder volume
- Nonambulatory patients
- Lack of voluntary urination
- Lack of perioperative antibiotic prophylaxis
- Perioperative hypothermia
- Longer duration of urethral catheterization
- Indwelling urethral catheters

Diagnosis

- A suspicion might be raised after the detection of smelly or cloudy urine with an active sediment and pyuria. The final diagnosis is based on urine culture and antibiogram results.

Treatment

- Treatment consists of urinary catheter removal and antibiotherapy.

Outcome

- The outcome is good after treatment with appropriate antibiotics and in case of normal bladder function with absence of a residual bladder volume.

Prevention

- Aseptic urinary catheter placement
- Vaginal or preputial flushing
- Minimal handling
- Good infection control
- Early removal of urinary catheters

Respiratory tract infection

Definition

- A respiratory tract infection is a bacterial infection of the respiratory tract, mostly the lungs.

Risk factors

- Vomiting
- Regurgitation
- Reflux
- Lateral recumbency
- Force feeding
- Swallowing disorders

Diagnosis

A suspicion might be raised on clinical examination because of the presence of abnormal lung sounds or in a coughing patient. Thoracic radiographs can provide a diagnosis and typically show an alveolar pattern in the right middle lung lobes. To identify the causative agent, culture of bronchoalveolar lavage (BAL) fluid can be performed.

Treatment

Treatment consists of the administration of antibiotics, which are usually empirically chosen, or adapted to the antibiogram of the BAL fluid. In severe cases of pneumonia, oxygen supplementation, clapping, and nebulization may be warranted.

Outcome

The outcome is guarded, depending on the severity of the respiratory signs.

Prevention

- Patient fasted before anesthesia
- Place an endotracheal tube with an inflated cuff
- Avoid dependent position of the head during anesthesia and recovery
- No force feeding of the hospitalized patient
- Antiemetic treatment
- Lift the head of patients with decreased consciousness

NONINFECTIOUS HYPERTHERMIA

Stress and agitation

Definition

Severely stressed and agitated animals may increase their heat production, resulting in hyperthermia.

Risk factors

- Overcrowded and noisy hospitalization
- Cats and dogs hospitalized together
- Uncomfortable, painful bedding
- Overexamination of the patient without sufficient time for the patient to rest

Diagnosis

Diagnosis is based on visual evaluation of the patient and exclusion of other causes for postoperative hyperthermia.

Treatment

Stress and agitation can be best treated by trying to calm the patient and decrease the amount of negative experiences for the patient while increasing the pleasant experiences.

Outcome

Good

Prevention

- Appropriate housing in a calm environment
- Application of the three to one rule: For every negative experience during hospitalization, the patient should experience three positive moments such as tender loving care, a walk, or food.

Inflammatory hyperthermia

Definition

A total of 50% to more than 90% of cases of postoperative hyperthermia occur secondary to noninfectious causes (Klimek *et al.* 1982; Fanning *et al.* 1998; Barie *et al.* 2004; Schey *et al.* 2005).

Benign postoperative hyperthermia is associated with increased levels of interleukin 6 (IL-6) and other proinflammatory mediators (e.g., interleukin 1 [IL-1], tumor necrosis factor α [TNF-α] and interferon-γ [INF-γ]). Peak temperatures have been correlated to IL-6 levels in patients after abdominal surgery (Wortel *et al.* 1993; McNally *et al.* 2000; Perlino 2001; Schey *et al.* 2005).

Risk factors

- Severe tissue trauma
- Ischemia
- Reperfusion
- Poor oxygenation
- Presence of necrotic tissue
- Malignancy and tumor lysis syndrome
- Transfusion therapy
- Phlebitis

Diagnosis

Inflammatory hyperthermia is often suspected when no obvious other cause is identified together with a positive response to treatment.

However, final diagnosis requires the analysis of proinflammatory mediators, which is only performed in research settings.

Treatment

Removal of any underlying cause is the first and paramount step. Local and systemic antiinflammatory treatment is made by cooling of inflamed tissue and administration of antipyretics.

Outcome

Good

Prevention

Minimize tissue trauma by applying a correct surgical technique. Use leukocyte-reducing filters to avoid hyperthermia caused by transfusions.

Overheating

Definition

Overheating is the result of extensive use of heating lamps, heating pads, warm water bottles, blankets, and bear huggers.

Risk factors

- Dark hair coat
- Heating pads without thermometers
- Placement of heating lamps too close to the patient
- Lack of ventilation of the patient cage

Diagnosis

The diagnosis is obtained by return to normal temperature after removal of the heating devices.

Treatment

The first treatment consists in the removal of all heating devices. In severe cases, the patient might need to be cooled down using the methods described earlier.

Outcome

The outcome is good if detected early and handled appropriately. Heating lamps can induce skin burns.

Prevention

Monitor the body temperature regularly while treating postoperative hypothermia. Provide sufficient ventilation and respect a minimal distance of 50 cm between heating lamps and the patient.

Pharmacologic agents

Definition

Malignant hyperthermia has been reported secondary to the administration of pharmacologic agents (e.g., halothane, succinylcholine) (Miller 2010). In humans, drug-related fever accounts for about 2% to 10% of postoperative hyperthermia, and most are hypersensitivity reactions, chemical phlebitis, and endogenous pyrogens (Cunha 1999; Dionigi et al. 2006).

In humans, malignant hyperthermia may occur up to 24 hours after surgery but tends to abate within 72 hours after discontinuation of the pharmacologic agent (Dionigi et al. 2006; Pile 2006).

Risk factors

- Genetic predisposition
- Inhalant anesthetics (halothane)

Diagnosis

Hyperthermia secondary to pharmacologic agents is suspected in case of short, severe bouts of hyperthermia after administration of a drug and is confirmed by the disappearance of hyperthermia after discontinuation of the drug.

Treatment

Treatment consists of discontinuation of the drug and unspecific methods to cool the patient.

Outcome

Good

Prevention

None

Opioid-induced hyperthermia

Definition

Postoperative hyperthermia can be observed in cats secondary to the administration of opioid medications. It has been reported with the use of hydromorphone, butorphanol, buprenorphine, morphine, and fentanyl. Hyperthermia appears to be dose dependent in cats at IV doses of morphine exceeding 1 mg/kg (Clark and Cumby 1978; Niedfeldt and Robertson 2006).

It is hypothesized that opioid derivatives (and μ-agonists in particular) reset the threshold point of the thermoregulatory center in the hypothalamus (Posner et al. 2010). In dogs, on the contrary, opioid therapy is associated with hypothermia (Niedfeldt and Robertson 2006; Posner et al. 2007, 2010).

Risk factors

- Severe postoperative hypothermia
- Coadministration of ketamine

Diagnosis

Hyperthermia secondary to opioid medications is suspected in cats with severe bouts of hyperthermia after administration of an opioid without any concurrent abnormalities on a physical examination. The diagnosis is confirmed by the disappearance of hyperthermia after discontinuation of the drug.

Treatment

Whereas naloxone reverses hyperthermia within 30 minutes, NSAIDs do not attenuate opioid-induced postoperative hyperthermia (Niedfeldt and Robertson 2006; Posner et al. 2010).

Outcome

Despite temperatures rising up to 42.5°C, opioid-associated hyperthermia does not appear to be associated with morbidity (Posner et al. 2007).

Prevention

None

Neuromuscular disease

Definition

Seizures and eclampsia caused by hypocalcemia result in extreme muscular activity, which can cause hyperthermia. Hypothalamic lesions and subsequent derangements in the thermoregulatory center can also cause hyperthermia (Miller 2010).

Risk factors

- Seizures
- Eclampsia
  - Hypothalamic lesions: Hypothermia during surgery can cause rebound hyperthermia.

Diagnosis

The diagnosis is based on the symptoms and physical examination for seizures; on the symptoms, history, and blood work for eclampsia; and on advanced diagnostic imaging for hypothalamic lesions.

Treatment

Treatment is nonspecific, and definitive treatment requires the underlying cause to be addressed.

Outcome

The outcome depends on the control of the underlying cause and the severity of the hyperthermia, with its possible complications.

Prevention

None

Relevant literature

Mild and moderate elevations in body temperature are rarely fatal and may even be beneficial by inhibition of viral replication, increased leukocyte function, and iron sequestration (Miller 2010). Temperatures under 41°C are rarely life threatening (except when prolonged), and a proper clinical evaluation should precede consideration of antipyretic usage (Miller 2010). Antipyretics block the hyperthermic defense mechanism and inhibit evaluation of hyperthermia afterward (Kennedy et al. 1997; Cunha 1999; Ghosh et al. 2006; Ward et al. 2010).

Additionally, humans with temperatures of 39.9° to 41.1°C have no prognostic difference (Cunha 1999), and clear scientific evidence of its benefit is lacking. Meanwhile, antipyretics may induce adverse effects on the gastric mucosa, renal blood flow, and coagulation (Barie et al. 2004). Hyperthermia above 41°C implies the risk of disseminated intravascular coagulation and organ damage and thus should be treated (Miller 2010).

Nonspecific therapy of severe true fever involves prostaglandin synthesis inhibition, usually by administration of NSAIDs. Glucocorticosteroid drugs are reserved for patients with noninfectious disease in which blocking of the acute-phase response is considered beneficial (e.g., immune-mediated hemolytic anemia) (Miller 2010). Phenothiazines may be valuable in stable hyperthermic patients because they depress thermoregulation and cause peripheral vasodilation, which increases heat dissipation. They are, however, sedatives and can cause hypotension, which makes them contraindicated in critical patients.

Severe hyperthermia can be managed with total body cooling by the use of cool (not cold) water and/or fans. One can also apply ice packs or alcohol on the footpads and IV crystalloid fluids

(Niedfeldt and Robinson 2006). This approach does not reset the thermoregulatory center in case of fever, with subsequent increased metabolism. Therefore, this approach is counterproductive in true fever. Conditions resulting in inadequate heat dissipation will not respond to antipyretics, but total-body cooling is indicated in these patients (Miller 2010).

Prophylactic and therapeutic antibiotics should be based on the expected flora, the infected tissue, known resistance patterns, pharmacokinetics, and culture and sensitivity test results (Howe and Boothe 2006).

Human studies in gynecology and orthopedic surgery have illustrated that an extensive work-up of postoperative hyperthermia has a low yield to determine the infectious cause, although it is performed in about half of patients (de la Torre et al. 2003; Schey et al. 2005; Ward et al. 2010).

The most commonly ordered laboratory tests are variable, with urinalysis and urine and blood cultures being the least or most often requested tests depending on the disease and the institution.

Neutrophil counts relate to the prevalence of hyperthermia (Lyon et al. 2000) but do not distinguish infectious from noninfectious causes of postoperative hyperthermia (Schey et al. 2005). All test results are rarely positive, with an overall yield of 10% to 30% (de la Torre et al. 2003; Rybak et al. 2008; Ward et al. 2010; Czaplicki et al. 2011). Blood cultures (5.6%–9.7%), urine culture (18.8%–22.4%), and thoracic radiographs (2%–14%) all had low yields (Schey et al. 2005). Furthermore, studies have shown that most patients with positive complementary test results had related signs on clinical examination and that positive examination results only rarely change the clinical management of these patients (Ward et al. 2010; Lesperance et al. 2011).

In asymptomatic, high-risk patients with low-grade fever, noninvasive routine examinations such as urine culture could be considered. In high-risk patients with high-grade fever (especially >72 hours after surgery), further evaluation remains preferable (Freischlag and Busuttil 1983; de la Torre et al. 2003).

Although these guidelines might seem to impose a risk to our veterinary hyperthermic patients, one should bear in mind that although human hospital records often reveal postoperative hyperthermia, a thorough evaluation is rarely performed. Furthermore, a prospective study in which additional testing was allowed only if abnormal findings besides fever were detected on clinical examination resulted in an important decrease of tests performed (in 11% of febrile patients), with a subsequent increase in their yield (80%–100%), but the procedure appeared to be safe for the patients (Schwandt et al. 2001).

Therefore, it appears that these guidelines are safe, and we should dare to implement them in veterinary medicine.

In human medicine, the most frequent risk factors for infectious hyperthermia are hyperthermia of longer duration and occurring later after surgery and more severe hyperthermia (Lyon et al. 2000; de la Torre et al. 2003; Barie et al. 2004; Schey et al. 2005; da Luz Moreira et al. 2008; Ward et al. 2010; Lesperance et al. 2011). On the first day after surgery, 80% of hyperthermic events were noninfectious in origin, and by the day after surgery, 60% were attributable to infectious hyperthermia (Schey et al. 2005).

Most cases of hyperthermia appearing within 48 hours after surgery are benign and self-limiting (Pile 2006). It has been mentioned that temperatures above 41.1°C are rarely of infectious origin but rather occur secondary to malignancy, hypothalamic disease, heat stroke, or are drug induced (Cunha 1999; Barie et al. 2004). Other human studies have indicated that patients fulfilling SIRS criteria and undergoing surgery for malignancy or bowel resection were more likely to have an infectious cause (de la Torre *et al.* 2003; da Luz Moreira *et al.* 2008).

Risk factors for urinary catheter-related infections are **patients that are nonambulatory, lack voluntary urination, lack periop-erative antibiotic prophylaxis, and have perioperative hypother-mia** (Stiffler *et al.* 2006).

Urinary catheterization has been associated with UTI in humans, dogs, and cats (Gregory *et al.* 1971; Biertuempfel *et al.* 1981; Bar-santi *et al.* 1985; Seguin *et al.* 2003; Bubenik and Hosgood 2008), and each additional day implies an increased risk (Barsanti *et al.* 1985; Smarick *et al.* 2004; Dionigi *et al.* 2006; Bubenik *et al.* 2007; Bubenik and Hosgood 2008). Risk for UTI in dogs appears to be most determined by duration rather than technique when compar-ing manual expression, indwelling catheters, and intermittent cath-eterization (Bubenik and Hosgood 2008).

Prevention of UTI consists mainly in good infection control and minimal handling (Dionigi *et al.* 2006).

In our veterinary patients, urinary catheters carry little risk if placed and maintained aseptically and for less than 3 days (Smarick *et al.* 2004). Vaginal or preputial flushing before placement might decrease risk, although a benefit has not been detected in humans (Smarick *et al.* 2004). Urinary catheters should be removed as soon as possible (Bubenik and Hosgood 2008). Prophylactic antibiotics are not recommended after urinary catheter placement because they increase the risk of antimicrobial-resistant bacteria (Barsanti *et al.* 1985; Saint and Lipsky 1999; Sedor and Mulholland 1999; Smarick *et al.* 2004).

References

Barie, P.S., Hydo, L.J., Eachempati, S.R. (2004) Causes and consequences of fever com-plicating critical surgical illness. *Surgical Infections* 5 (2), 145-159.

Barsanti, J.A., Blue, J., Edmunds, J. (1985) Urinary tract infection due to indwelling bladder catheters in dogs and cats. *Journal of the American Veterinary Medical Association* 187 (4), 384-388.

Biertuempfel, P.H., Ling, G.V., Ling, G.A. (1981) Urinary tract infection resulting from catheterization in healthy adult dogs. *Journal of the American Veterinary Medical Association* 178 (9), 989-991.

Bubenik, L.J., Hosgood, G.L., Waldron, D.R., et al. (2007) Frequency of urinary tract infection in catheterized dogs and comparison of bacterial culture and suscepti-bility testing results for catheterized and noncatheterized dogs with urinary tract infections. *Journal of the American Veterinary Medical Association* 231 (6), 893-899.

Bubenik, L., Hosgood, G. (2008) Urinary tract infection in dogs with thoracolumbar intervertebral disc herniation and urinary bladder dysfunction managed by man-ual expression, indwelling catheterization or intermittent catheterization. *Veteri-nary Surgery* 37 (8), 791-800.

Clark, W.G., Cumby, H.R. (1978) Hyperthermic responses to central and peripheral injections of morphine sulphate in the cat. *British Journal of Pharmacology* 63 (1), 65-71.

Cunha, B.A. (1999) Fever in the intensive care unit. Intensive Care Med 25 (7), 648-651.

Czaplicki, A.P., Borger, J.E., Politi, J.R., et al. (2011) Evaluation of postoperative fever and leukocytosis in patients after total hip and knee arthroplasty. *The Journal of Arthroplasty* 26 (8),1387-1389.

da Luz Moreira, A., Vogel, J.D., Kalady, M.F., et al. (2008) Fever evaluations after colo-rectal surgery: identification of risk factors that increase yield and decrease cost. *Diseases of the Colon and Rectum* 51 (5), 508-513.

de la Torre, S.H., Mandel, L., Goff, B.A. (2003) Evaluation of postoperative fever: use-fulness and cost-effectiveness of routine workup. *American Journal of Obstetrics and Gynecology* 188 (6), 1642-1647.

Dionigi, R., Dionigi, G., Rovera, F., et al. (2006) Postoperative fever. Surg Infect 7 (Suppl. 2), S17-S20.

Fanning, J., Neuhoff, R.A., Brewer, J.E., et al. (1998) Frequency and yield of postop-erative fever evaluation. *Infectious Diseases in Obstetrics and Gynecology* 6 (6), 252-255.

Freischlag, J., Busuttil, R.W. (1983) The value of postoperative fever evaluation. *Surgery* 94 (2), 358-363.

Ghosh, S., Charity, R.M., Haidar, S.G., et al. (2006) Pyrexia following total knee replace-ment. *The Knee* 13 (4), 324-327.

Gregory, J.G., Wein, A.J., Sansone, T.C., et al. (1971) Bladder resistance to infection. *The Journal of Urology* 105 (2), 220-222.

Howe, L.M., Boothe, H.W. Jr. (2006) Antimicrobial use in the surgical patient. *The Veterinary Clinics of North America: Small Animal Practice*, 36 (5), 1049-1060, vi.

Kennedy, J.G., Rodgers, W.B., Zurakowski, D., et al. (1997) Pyrexia after total knee replacement. A cause for concern? *The American Journal of Orthopedics* 26 (8), 549-552, 554.

Klimek, J.J., Ajemian, E.R., Gracewski, J., et al. (1982) Prospective analysis of hospital-acquired fever in obstetric and gynecologic patients. *The Journal of the American Medical Association* 247 (24), 3340-3343.

Lesperance, R., Lehman, R., Lesperance, K., et al. (2011) Early postoperative fever and the "routine" fever work-up: results of a prospective study. *The Journal of Surgical Research* 171 (1), 245-250.

Lyon, D.S., Jones, J.L., Sanchez, A. (2000) Postoperative febrile morbidity in the benign gynecologic patient. Identification and management. *The Journal of Reproductive Medicine* 45 (4), 305-309.

McNally, C.G., Krivak, T.C., Alagoz, T. (2000) Conservative management of isolated posthysterectomy fever. *The Journal of Reproductive Medicine* 45 (7), 572-576.

Miller, J.B. (2010) Hyperthermia and fever of unknown origin. In: Ettinger, S.J., Feld-mand, E.C. (eds.) *Textbook of Veterinary Internal Medicine*, vol. 7th edn. Saunders Elsevier, St. Louis, pp. 41-45.

Niedfeldt, R.L., Robertson, S.A. (2006) Postanesthetic hyperthermia in cats: a retro-spective comparison between hydromorphone and buprenorphine. *Veterinary Anaesthesia and Analgesia* 33 (6), 381-389.

O'Grady, N.P., Barie, P.S., Bartlett, J.G., et al. (2008) Guidelines for evaluation of new fever in critically ill adult patients: 2008 update from the American College of Crit-ical Care Medicine and the Infectious Diseases Society of America. *Critical Care Medicine* 36 (4), 1330-1349.

Perlino, C.A. (2001) Postoperative fever. *The Medical Clinics of North America* 85 (5), 1141-1149.

Pile, J.C. (2006) Evaluating postoperative fever: a focused approach. *Cleveland Clinic Journal of Medicine* 73 (Suppl. 1), S62-S66.

Posner, L.P., Gleed, R.D., Erb, H.N., et al. (2007) Post-anesthetic hyperthermia in cats. *Veterinary Anaesthesia and Analgesia* 34 (1), 40-47.

Posner, L.P., Pavuk, A.A., Rokshar, J.L., et al. (2010) Effects of opioids and anesthetic drugs on body temperature in cats. *Veterinary Anaesthesia and Analgesia*, 37 (1), 35-43.

Rybak, E.A., Polotsky, A.J., Woreta, T., et al. (2008) Explained compared with unex-plained fever in postoperative myomectomy and hysterectomy patients. *Obstetrics and Gynecology* 111 (5), 1137-1142.

Saint, S., Lipsky, B.A. (1999) Preventing catheter-related bacteriuria: should we? Can we? How? *Archives of Internal Medicine* 159 (8), 800-808.

Salom, E.M., Schey, D., Penalver, M., et al. (2003) The safety of incidental appendec-tomy at the time of abdominal hysterectomy. *American Journal of Obstetrics and Gynecology* 189 (6), 1563-1568.

Schey, D., Salom, E.M., Papadia, A., et al. (2005) Extensive fever workup produces low yield in determining infectious etiology. *American Journal of Obstetrics and Gyne-cology* 192 (5), 1729-1734.

Schwandt, A., Andrews, S.J., Fanning, J. (2001) Prospective analysis of a fever evalua-tion algorithm after major gynecologic surgery. *American Journal of Obstetrics and Gynecology* 184 (6), 1066-1067.

Sedor, J., Mulholland, S.G. (1999) Hospital-acquired urinary tract infections associated with the indwelling catheter. *The Urologic Clinics of North America* 26 (4), 821-828.

Seguin, M.A., Vaden, S.L., Altier, C., et al. (2003) Persistent urinary tract infections and reinfections in 100 dogs (1989-1999). *Journal of Veterinary Internal Medicine* 17 (5), 622-631.

Shackelford, D.P., Hoffman, M.K., Davies, M.F., et al. (1999) Predictive value for infec-tion of febrile morbidity after vaginal surgery. *Obstetrics and Gynecology* 93 (6), 928-931.

Smarick, S.D., Haskins, S.C., Aldrich, J., et al. (2004) Incidence of catheter-associated urinary tract infection among dogs in a small animal intensive care unit. *Journal of the American Veterinary Medical Association* 224 (12), 1936-1940.

Stiffler, K.S., Stevenson, M.A., Sanchez, S., et al. (2006) Prevalence and characteriza-tion of urinary tract infections in dogs with surgically treated type 1 thoracolumbar intervertebral disc extrusion. *Veterinary Surgery* 35 (4), 330-336.

Ward, D.T., Hansen, E.N., Takemoto, S.K., et al. (2010) Cost and effectiveness of post-operative fever diagnostic evaluation in total joint arthroplasty patients. *The Jour-nal of Arthroplasty* 25 (Suppl. 6), 43-48.

Wortel, C.H., van Deventer, S.J., Aarden, L.A., et al. (1993) Interleukin-6 mediates host defense responses induced by abdominal surgery. Surgery 114 (3), 564-570.

12 Hemorrhage

Jane Ladlow

University of Cambridge, Cambridge, UK

Definition

Postoperative hemorrhage can be primary or secondary depending on the time interval from surgery. **Primary hemorrhage** starts during surgery or after a postoperative increase in blood pressure (within 24 hours from surgery). This is usually a result of technical failure or failure to recognize small vessels during surgery, but in some patients, there may be an underlying coagulopathy. Primary hemorrhage may require reoperating or may result in hematomas with increased risk of infection or delayed wound healing.

Secondary hemorrhage occurs 1 to several days after the surgery and is usually a result of infection damaging vessels at the operative site or has been reported in the case of vaginal hemorrhage after ovariohysterectomy as a result of chromic gut ligatures pulling through and irritating the cervical lumen (Berzon 1979). Greyhounds and other sighthounds have an increased tendency to secondary bleeding linked to a problem with the fibrinolytic system and clot maintenance (Lara-Garcia *et al.* 2008).

Risk factors

A combination of patient and surgeon factors can contribute to a higher risk of postoperative hemorrhage.

Patient factors

- Coagulopathies
- Disease process
- Size or obesity
- Infection

Surgeon factors

- Drains
- Hemodilution
- Surgical experience
- Method of ligation

Diagnosis

- In human medicine, postoperative hemorrhage is defined as a decrease of 3 g/dL in hemoglobin concentration from baseline measures with a peripheral circulatory impairment requiring medical intervention. Although not all veterinary patients (particularly young animals undergoing elective procedures) have preoperative blood tests, the principle that a low hemoglobin concentration is considered alongside clinical assessment of perfusion (mucous membrane color and refill time, heart rate, temperature, pulse, and blood pressure) is useful for our patients. In practice, packed cell volume/total solids (PCV/TS) can be used if hemoglobin values are not readily available, but PCV does not initially decrease with hemorrhage until interstitial fluid is recruited into the intravascular system or crystalloid or colloid support is given. Also, because of splenic contraction, PCV depreciation may lag behind total solids; thus, these parameters should be considered in tandem and compared with a baseline value taken in the recovery stage. After surgery, PCV values should initially stabilize as intraoperative fluid supplementation is redistributed, and then start to increase. With postoperative hemorrhage, the PCV values continue decline. Thus, the trend in PCV/TS values is more important than single measurements.

"Practical tips": Clinical features of hemorrhage

- Pale mucous membranes
- Decreased capillary refill time
- Tachycardia
- Low blood pressure
- Thready pulse
- Decreased urine output
- Temperature: core–peripheral gap
- Tachypnea
- Clinical signs of hemorrhage at levels below 15% may be difficult to identify because the blood loss is compensated for by transcapillary refill. Changes in heart rate and blood pressure usually occur when there is between 15% and 30% loss of blood volume. This degree of bleeding will decrease the urine output (normally between 1 and 2 mL/kg/hr). More than 30% loss of blood volume marks the onset of decompensated hypovolemic shock when systemic vasoconstriction can no longer maintain organ perfusion.
- In patients at risk of postoperative hemorrhage, careful monitoring of peripheral perfusion is recommended at regular intervals (depending on the stability of the patient) for the initial 24 hours after surgery. Intervals between checks can then be adjusted depending on the stability of the patient. In critical patients and those in which hemorrhage is suspected, urine volume output, arterial blood pressure measurements, and central venous pressure aid in estimating the severity of the bleed and the response to fluid resuscitation, and blood gas analysis and venous lactate levels aid assessment of tissue perfusion.

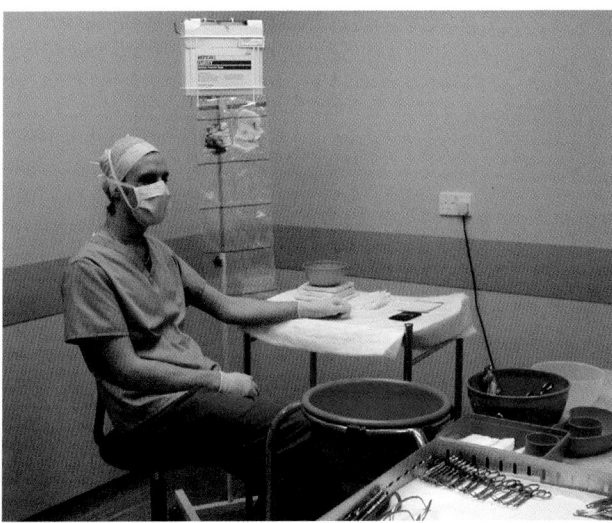

Figure 12.1 Quantitative blood loss assessment by weighing blood-soaked swabs. *Source:* J. Gasson, Animal Health Trust, Landwades Park, Suffolk. Reproduced with permission from J. Gasson.

- Blood loss estimation from a surface wound can be estimated by weighing the number of swabs used (1-g increase in weight = 1 mL of blood) or subjectively by visualization (Figure 12.1).
- The volume of blood lost into body cavities is far harder to estimate. With abdominal or thoracic bleeds, imaging in the form of ultrasonography, endoscopy, computed tomography, or radiography can give a rough approximation of volume lost and should be considered in conjunction with peripheral perfusion and PCV/TS of the cavitary fluid after thoracocentesis, paracentesis, or diagnostic peritoneal lavage. In patients at risk of postoperative cavitary hemorrhage (hepatic lobe resections, extensive tumor resection), the use of an active suction drain in the appropriate cavity for 24 hours after surgery allows earlier recognition of postoperative hemorrhage, although drains often underestimate blood loss (Gwozdziewicz et al. 2008).
- In patients in which an obvious source of bleeding cannot be identified and clotting abnormalities were noted at surgery (generalized oozing), investigations into abnormal coagulation should be performed in the postoperative period.
- Deciding on when to reoperate can be challenging, and the decision should be made by reviewing estimated blood loss, hemoglobin or hematocrit levels, and cardiovascular status. In human reviews, the time period to reoperation was often thought to be excessive (Karthik et al. 2004; Gwozdziewicz et al. 2008). Postoperative thromboelastography (TEG) is useful for differentiating surgical bleeding from coagulopathies (Essell et al. 1993; Johansson et al. 2010) and has resulted in a lower incidence of second surgeries in human cardiac, liver, and pediatric surgery. In patients with hemodynamic compromise and no evidence of coagulopathy, surgical exploration is warranted (Figure 12.2).

Treatment

Management of postoperative hemorrhage requires early recognition of bleeding, fluid support, and securing hemostasis when necessary.

Initial management involves fluid resuscitation, initially with crystalloids or colloids or more commonly a combination of both. Colloid administration is initially more effective than crystalloids or whole blood at maintaining cardiac output though in human medicine several studies have failed to establish an advantage of either type of fluid in decreased mortality rates (He et al. 2015, Guerci et al. 2014). Colloid use in humans has been associated with the induction of coagulopathies, impaired renal function and prolonged tissue storage with subsequent

pruritis (Mutter et al. 2013, Nepo et al. 2014). Similar results in elevated clotting times and decreased platelet counts have been found in dogs given low molecular weight hydroxyethyl starch, this was attributed to greater hemodulation effects with colloids compared to crystalloids (Gauthier et al. 2015). With either type of fluid, resuscitation needs to be monitored carefully because aggressive fluid resuscitation may increase blood pressure, dislodge clots, reverse vasoconstriction, and increase both blood loss and metabolic acidosis. Limited fluid resuscitation has been advocated in humans when the goal is a palpable radialis pulse.

Initial guidelines (Fischerova 2009) are resuscitation to:
- Systolic blood pressure of 80 to 100 mm/Hg, with
- Urine output of over 0.5 mL/kg/hr, with
- Arterial oxygen saturation of 93% or higher

When the patient is stable, fluid support is continued with a view to dropping lactate levels to normal and eliminating any metabolic acidosis. Estimation of the total resuscitation volume is given in Table 12.1.

After the fluid volume required has been calculated, the rate of fluid resuscitation can be determined by improvement in the patient's clinical signs of perfusion. If hemoglobin drops below 6 to 8 g/dL or hematocrit below 20%, volume replacement fluids require oxygen-carrying capacity in the form of red blood cells (RBCs) or hemoglobin/oxyglobin to prevent tissue hypoxia. A unit of packed RBCs (PRBCs) will increase hemoglobin by 1 to 1.2 g/dL and hematocrit by 3% to 4% more swiftly than whole blood (2 mL/kg to raise hematocrit by 1%). Whole blood, however, has the benefit of platelets, plasma proteins, and coagulation factors in animals that are hemodiluted or coagulopathic. Fresh whole blood is preferable to stored whole blood because there is a loss of platelet function and labile coagulation factor concentration (factor V and VIII) with storage longer than 8 hours. Whole blood or PRBCs should be given alongside crystalloids for volume resuscitation. Dogs should be blood typed and cross-matched before administration of blood products if possible to ensure donor and recipient compatibility. If blood typing is not possible, a donor that is negative for dog erythrocyte antigen 1.1 should be used. All cats require blood typing or cross-matching before blood products to avoid the risk of a potentially fatal transfusion reaction (Knottenbelt 2002). An alternative to blood products in dogs is a hemoglobin-based oxygen-carrying solution such as Oxyglobin or Biopure. Oxyglobin increases intravascular volume because of a colloidal oncotic pressure and is more efficient than RBCs at oxygen release (Muir and Wellman 2003). Oxyglobin can be given at a rate of up to 10 mL/kg/hr to a total recommended dose of 15 to 30 mL/kg.

Autotransfusion of blood involves returning the blood from a body cavity into the circulation. Prior to autotransfusion, the blood should be screened for bacteria, urine, or ingesta from an intestinal rupture. Autotransfused blood should be filtered with a micropore filter and given with an anticoagulant such as low-dose heparin or acid citrate dextrose. Autotransfused blood is usually very low in platelets and coagulation factors (Crowe 1980) (Figure 12.3).

If coagulopathies are identified by TEG or coagulation tests (prothrombin time [PT] or activated partial thromboplastin time [aPTT] >1.5 times the control value), fresh or fresh-frozen plasma should be given at 6 to 10 mL/kg/hr (Logan et al. 2001; Maegele 2009). If the platelet count has dropped below 50×10^9/L, platelet-rich plasma should be administered (Maegele 2009).

Any centrally hypothermic patients should be **gentled warmed** during resuscitation because hypothermia contributes to coagulopathy.

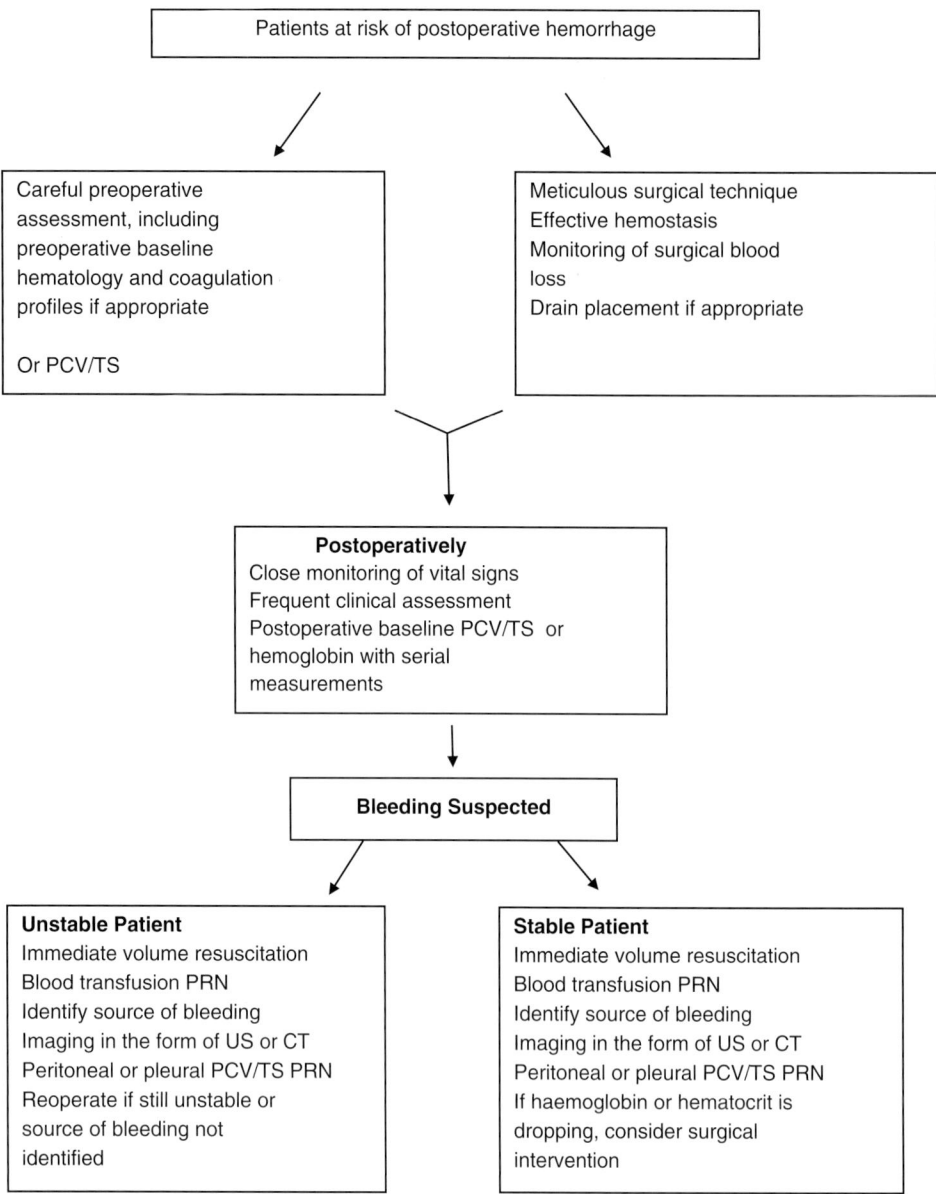

Figure 12.2 Algorithm to guide management of patients at risk of postoperative hemorrhage. CT, computed tomography; PCV, packed cell volume; PRN, as needed; TS, total solids; US, ultrasonography.

Table 12.1 Estimation of the total resuscitation volume

Estimation of the resuscitation volume	Method
Estimate normal blood volume	Dog weighing ~90 mL/kg Cat weighing ~60 mL/kg
Estimate % blood loss	Clinical signs develop >15% Hypovolemic shock >30% Increase in swab weight Subjective visual assessment
Calculate volume deficit (VD)	VD = BV × % loss BV
Resuscitation volume (RV)	RV = VD × 1.5 (colloids) RV = VD × 4 (crystalloids) RV = VD (whole blood)

Methods of controlling identified postoperative bleeding include dressing or applying direct pressure to a surface bleed; surgical reexploration and ligation of bleeding vessels using sutures, hemostatic clips, vessel-sealing devices, or laser application; and packing of hemorrhage sites with dressings or gauzes. Vessels larger than 2 mm in diameter usually require ligation to prevent bleeding.

Topical agents used to aid hemostasis include:

- Collagen sponges
- Microfibrillar collagen
- Gelatine sponges
- Oxidized regenerated cellulose
- Topical thrombin
- Fibrin sealants
- Microporous polysaccharide powder
- Chitosan and silica dressings.

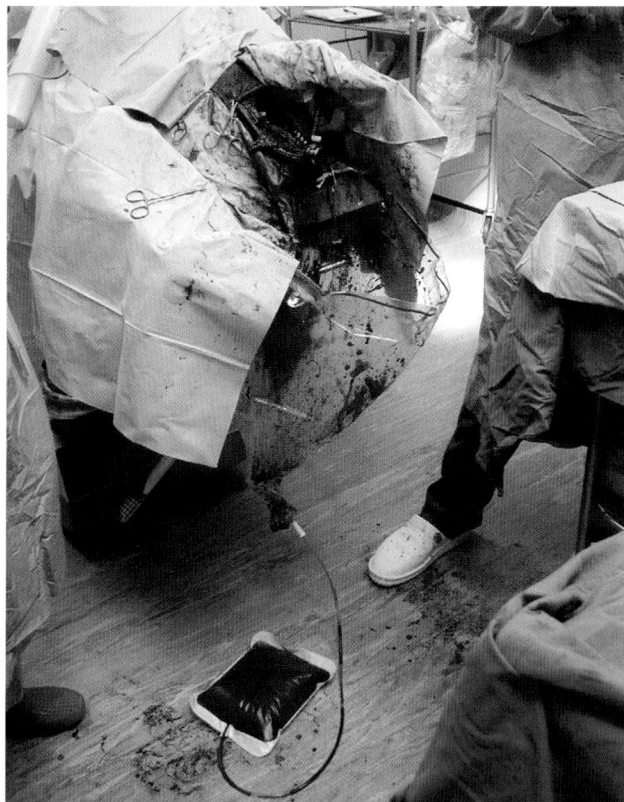

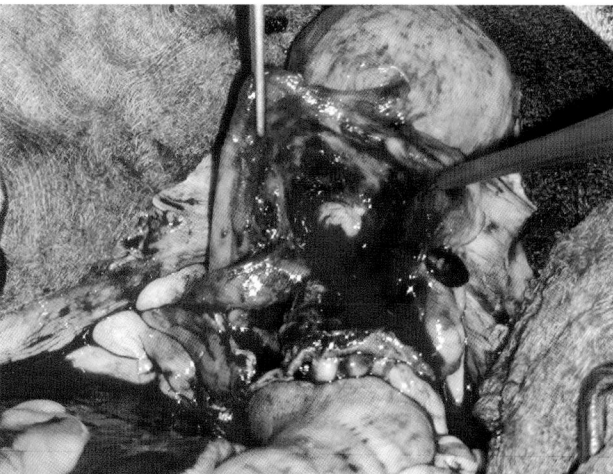

Figure 12.5 Reoperating on a cervical pedicle bleed after ovariohysterectomy.

Figure 12.3 Blood collection for autotransfusion following hemimaxillectomy for oral squamous cell carcinoma. *Source:* P. Neath, Oakwood Veterinary Referrals, Northwich, Cheshire, UK. Reproduced with permission from P. Neath.

In cases of hemoperitoneum, application of circumferential external counterpressure (body bandages) has shown efficacy in experimental studies (McAnulty and Smith 1986) (Figure 12.4). The body bandages consisted of a 0.45-kg roll of cotton wool formed into several layers that was applied from the pubis to the xiphoid and then covered by an elastic bandage. The central portion of the cotton roll was left intact to act as a stiff central spar, and the cranial part of

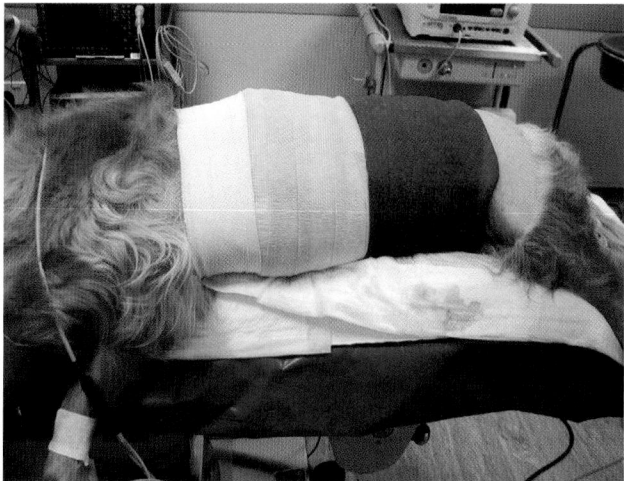

Figure 12.4 Use of a body bandage after postoperative hemorrhage after ovariohysterectomy.

the abdomen had extra padding to increase the compression under the rib cage. The body bandage increased intraabdominal pressure and reduced the decrease in mean arterial pressure, resulting in prolonged survival times in an experimental exsanguination study (McAnulty and Smith 1986). In human studies, antishock dressings are used primarily during transportation to surgical facilities, and in cases of massive abdominal hemorrhage, an abdominal wrap may aid preoperative stabilization.

In hemodynamically unstable patients, surgical procedures may need to be limited to damage control methods with a view to reoperating and performing definitive surgery when the patient is stable. The success of reoperation is facilitated by reasonable exposure and careful removal of blood clots that are obscuring the field of view (Figure 12.5).

Outcome

Postoperative hemorrhage is a significant cause of morbidity and increased mortality in human medicine, occurring in 1% to 9 % of surgical procedures (Berggvist and Kallero 1985; Gwozdziewicz *et al.* 2008; Heneghan *et al.* 2012). In human medicine, interventional radiography with angiographic embolization is the preferred method of stopping postoperative hemorrhage in certain procedures (Koukoutis *et al.* 2006; Sanjay *et al.* 2010).

In the human literature, reoperation for postoperative bleeding is associated with an increase in mortality, morbidity, and cost (Gwozdziewicz *et al.* 2008; Heneghan *et al.* 2012). Morbidity associated with postoperative hemorrhage (other than hypovolemic death if not successfully resuscitated) includes infected hematomas, respiratory complications, sepsis, or systemic inflammatory response syndrome–induced multiple organ failure, which can occur several days later.

There is little information in the veterinary literature on postoperative hemorrhage incidence and morbidity. The majority of the information available involves complications of elective neutering procedures at teaching hospitals (Berzon 1979; Burrow *et al.* 2005). These papers have intraoperative hemorrhage rates of 7% to 80% and postoperative hemorrhage rates of about 3%. The procedures were usually routine procedures performed by inexperienced surgeons (but supervised).

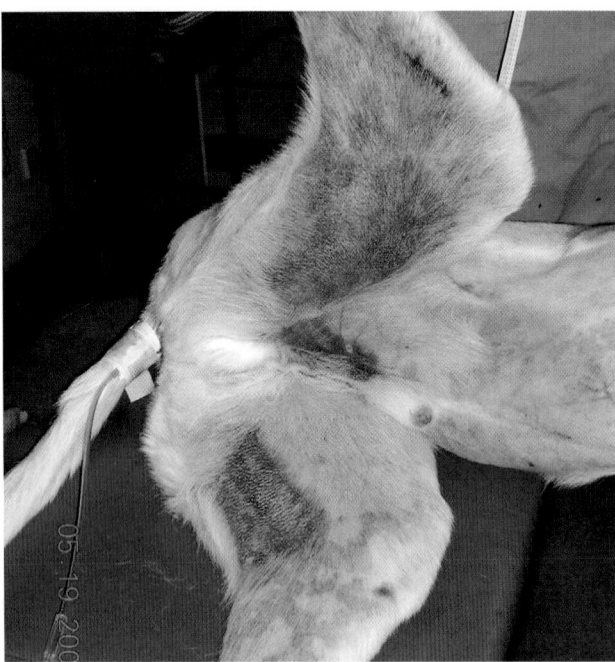

Figure 12.6 A greyhound with coagulopathy.

Prevention

Prevention of postoperative hemorrhage involves consideration of all the risk factors, meticulous surgical techniques, and having blood products available as necessary.

Before any surgery, a detailed history and clinical examination should be performed, including:

- Unexpected bruising
- Hematomas or bleeding episodes
- Problems with previous surgeries or injections
- Exposure to rodenticides
- Worming history in areas prevalent for *Angiostrongylus* infestation.
- Careful examination of mucous membranes
- Examination of the ventral abdominal skin to detect any petechia or ecchymosis indicative of thrombocytopathias or thrombocytopenias (Figure 12.6 and Table 12.2)

Primary hemostasis can be checked by a buccal mucosal bleeding time (BMBT) which is the time of hemorrhage from 1mm deep incisions of the oral mucosa to cessation of bleeding. Elevated times are those over 4.2 minutes in the dog and 2.4 minutes in the cat. BMBT will be elongated in disorders of primary hemostasis (von Willebrand's Disease), thrombopathia and thrombocytopenia. In certain breeds at risk of coagulopathies or in animals with suspicion of disseminated intravascular coagulation (DIC), those with liver disease and those with a focal splenic mass, a coagulation profile is taken before surgery, which includes:

- PT
- aPTT
- Platelet count
- Activated clotting time
- Fibrinogen concentration
- Fibrinogen degradation products

Alternatively, TEG (which gives information on clotting time, clot formation time, maximum clot firmness, and stability of the clot) can be used if available. Any detected preoperative anemia should be corrected if possible before surgery because anemia increases the risk of both postoperative mortality and infection (Brooks 1999; Dunne *et al.* 2002; Bischof *et al.* 2010). Animals with an underlying coagulopathy will ooze generally with surgical incision. Intravenous catheter placement before surgery may also be associated with excessive hemorrhage. Greyhound and other sighthounds have an increased tendency to delayed post-operative bleeding, with bleeding dogs having significantly lower activities of antiplasmin and antithrombin which has led to the theory that these dogs have a problem with the fibrinolytic system and clot maintenance (Lara-Garcia *et al.* 2008). In these breeds, fibrinolytic inhibitors such as epsilon aminocaproic acid or tranexamic acid have been shown to significantly decrease post-operative bleeding (Marin *et al.* 2012, Marin *et al.* 2012). The disease a patient presents with may increase the risk of hemorrhage. In some tumors such as hemangiosarcoma, half of patients have a coagulopathy that meets the criteria for DIC at presentation. Other diseases that predispose to DIC include pancreatitis, gastric dilatation and volvulus, major trauma, and sepsis. Animals with liver disease may present with various coagulopathies because of decreased coagulation factor production and reduced absorption of vitamin K.

Table 12.2 Common heritable bleeding disorders

Breed	Disorder or Deficiency	Appropriate test
Dobermans, others	von Willebrand's disease, type 1	BMBT
German shorthaired pointers	von Willebrand's disease, type 2	BMBT
Scottish and Manchester terriers, shelties, Chesapeake Bay retrievers, Dutch Kooikers	von Willebrand's disease, type 3	BMBT
Cocker spaniels, boxers	Factor II (prothrombin)	ACT, APTT, PT, TEG
Beagles, malamutes	Factor VII	PT, TEG
Many, cats	Factor VIII (hemophilia A)	ACT, aPTT, TEG
Many dog breeds	Factor IX (hemophilia B)	ACT, aPTT, TEG
Cocker spaniels, cats	Factor X	ACT, aPTT, PT, TEG
Kerry Blue, Great Pyrenees, English Springer spaniels	Factor XI	ACT, aPTT, TEG
Poodles, Sharpeis, cats	Factor XII	No bleeding ACT, aPTT
Devon Rexes	Vitamin K–dependent coagulopathy	ACT, aPTT, PT, TEG
American cocker spaniels, Smoke Persians, otterhounds, Great Pyrenees, Bassett hounds, boxers, Labrador retrievers, Spitzes	Platelet dysfunction: delta storage pool disease, Chédiak-Higashi syndrome, Glanzmann's thromboasthenia, thrombopathies	BMBT, TEG

ACT, activated clotting time; aPTT, activated partial thromboplastin time; BMBT, Buccal Mucosal Bleeding Time; PT, prothrombin time; TEG, thromboelastography.

Tumors are often problematic with regards to postoperative bleeding because of the new blood vessels that form around neoplasms that tend to be tortuous and friable. Postoperative bleeding is therefore common in cytoreductive surgery. Surgical planning in these cases should include methods to limit any postoperative bleeding. Thyroid adenomas or adenocarcinomas are notoriously hemorrhagic. Meticulous intraoperative hemostasis with early ligation of vessels is required for these tumors. Any thyroid tumors should be handled as gently as possible during surgery (avoiding direct manipulation of the tumor, even with stay sutures whenever possible). With large thyroid tumors and cytoreductive surgeries, it is sensible to have blood products available during the procedure.

Isovolemic hemodilution is a technique used to reduce transfusion requirements in the perioperative setting. This technique involves the preoperative removal of 1 unit of blood with volume replenishment with crystalloids. This unit of blood and viable platelets is then retransfused at the end of the surgical procedure. This technique reduces the number of RBCs lost per volume of blood. The hematocrit is usually dropped to greater than 28%, but hematocrits of 20% are tolerated (Hofland and Henny 2007).

Tourniquet use is a method to create a bloodless field when working on distal extremities. In human surgery, tourniquet use is associated with faster surgery times and less intraoperative bleeding but not a reduction in total blood loss (Tai et al. 2011). If used, tourniquets should be released completely after 1.5 hours or intermittently released for 10 minutes every hour to prevent postoperative ischemic muscle damage and pain (Heppenstall et al. 1979). Tourniquets are also associated with higher incidences of postoperative wound problems in the human literature (Tai et al. 2011). However, the use of a tourniquet in short duration distal limb surgeries can be of great benefit in regards to visibility and time. The limb should be dressed with a compression bandage before tourniquet release in anticipation of postoperative hemorrhage.

Relevant literature

Size and obesity affect postoperative hemorrhage, particularly in relation to elective neutering procedures. In one study on ovariohysterectomy, the intraabdominal hemorrhage rate for dogs weighing less than 22.7 kg was 2% compared with 79% for dogs weighing more than 22.7 kg (Berzon 1979).

In the human literature, **the presence of sepsis** is associated with late hemorrhage in pancreatectomy (Koukoutis et al. 2006), as is the presence of methicillin-resistant *Staphylococcus aureus* (MRSA) in abdominal drains (Sanjay et al. 2010). There is insufficient evidence in the veterinary literature as to whether MRSA or methicillin-resistant *Staphylococcus pseudintermedius* (MRSP) is increasing postoperative hemorrhage.

Early activation of **active closed-suction wound drains** can disrupt fibrin seals and potentially increase hemorrhage from a wound. One report in the veterinary literature describes two cases in which surgical drains were linked to postoperative hemorrhage resulting in hypovolemic shock, which required intervention (Lynch et al. 2011). In the human literature, there are reports of hemorrhage occurring with active suction drains, usually 2 to 5 days after surgery (Nomura et al. 1997; Tjalma 2006) in which delayed arterial hemorrhage was linked to pressure necrosis of the arterial wall. After major surgical resections, delaying drain activation for 4 to 6 hours after surgery and use of a low-pressure suction drainage such as the Jackson Pratt system are advisable. It is also good practice to avoid placing the drains close to major blood vessels. Fluid production from an active drain should be monitored, and if the appearance of the fluid changes to resemble frank blood, then a PCV/TS sample of the fluid should be performed and compared with a venous sample from the patient.

In the human literature, certain high-risk procedures (particularly coronary bypass) have higher postoperative hemorrhage rates recorded for patients who were on **nonsteroidal anti-inflammatory drugs** (NSAIDs; aspirin) before surgery (Karthik et al. 2004; Alghamdi et al. 2007). There is little information in the veterinary literature about NSAIDs, but with the majority of surgical procedures, they are unlikely to affect postoperative bleeding.

Initial circulatory support in intra- or postoperative hemorrhage is provided by intravenous crystalloid or colloid administration. **Hemodilution** with crystalloids results in a lower PCV and blood viscosity, which in turn increases blood flow velocity and decreases diffusional oxygen exit from the arterioles resulting in improved oxygen delivery to tissues. In experimental models of up to 60% dilution of blood volume, PT times are prolonged, but partial thromboplastin times are unaffected, indicating that the intrinsic clotting factors are relatively resistant to hemodilution (Schüriger et al. 2011). However, aggressive crystalloid administration can result in interstitial edema and the impairment of microcirculation (Knotzer et al. 2006). Colloid administration, particularly hydroxyethyl starch, influences coagulation more profoundly than crystalloids in experimental studies, causing the efflux of plasma proteins from blood to the interstitial space, a reduction in the plasma concentration of factor VIII and von Willebrand factor, the inhibition of platelet function, and reduced interaction of activated factor XIII with fibrin polymers. Low-weight hydroxyethyl starches (Hetastarch [HES] 130/0.4 and HES 200/0.5) have less effect on the coagulation process than higher weight hydroxethyl starch (HES 450/0.7) (Entholzner et al. 2000). However, in experimental dogs, low molecular weight hydroxylethyl starch (tetrastarch) still decreased aPPT in comparison to isotonic saline but did not alter ACT and PT (Gauthier et al. 2015). Colloids can also induce hypocalcemia, which further contributes to the coagulopathy. Gelatin-based colloids had less effect on coagulation time or clot firmness than hydroxyl starch when examined with TEG in a dilution study in humans (Fries et al. 2002). The effect of the colloids on coagulation profiles in clinical patients in vivo is less clear. Other colloid options include human serum albumin (HAS) which has been used in veterinary patients. Concerns over incomplete protein homology among species and reports of severe type III hypersensitivity reactions with HAS means other fluids types are more suitable for resuscitation (Martin et al. 2008, Powell et al. 2013).

If the studies on ovariohysterectomy and ovariectomy are compared with regard to **surgical experience**, intra- and postoperative hemorrhage complication rates for board-certified surgeons were minimal (Peeters and Kirpensteijn 2011) compared with rates of 6% to 20% and 3%, respectively, for final year veterinary students (Dorn and Swist 1977; Berzon 1979; Burrow et al. 2005).

The method of ligation can affect the rate of postoperative hemorrhage. Hemorrhage from vessels larger than 2 mm in diameter typically requires direct occlusion of the vessel to control the bleeding. Traditionally, ligatures were used, but recently, a variety of vessel-sealing systems have become available. Studies have demonstrated the vessel-sealing devices performed as well as a traditional surgeon's knot or metallic clip in vessels of 5 mm or smaller. The electrothermal bipolar vessel sealer system is suitable for vessels up to 7 mm in diameter, and the Harmonic (Ethicon, Johnson & Johnson, Somerville, NJ) scalpel is recommended for vessels up to 3 mm in diameter.

With regard to knot formulation, whereas the surgeon's knot has traditionally been thought to be the most secure for ligature formation, the square knot is preferable for tissue healing. However, the granny knot was shown to be as secure as a surgeon's knot when monofilament suture was used (Rajbabu *et al.* 2007). In an experimental model of a canine ovarian pedicle, the slip knot, modified transfixing ligature and the single-double other side knot had improved occlusion ability compare to the square knot or surgeon's knot (Leitch *et al.* 2012). Evaluation of postoperative hemorrhage after standard pulmonary resections in humans demonstrated that for larger bore arteries, the recommended transfixion suture was not absolutely safe to prevent slipping of ligatures from vessels, and a purse-string suture was advocated as a safer alternative (Péterffy and Henze 1983); alternatively, vascular clips could be used.

References

Alghamdi, A.A., Moussa, F., Fremes, S.E. (2007) Does the use of preoperative aspirin increase the risk of bleeding in patients undergoing coronary artery bypass grafting surgery? Systematic review and meta-analysis. *Journal of Cardiac Surgery* 22 (3), 247-256.

Berggvist, D., Kallero, S. (1985) Reoperation for postoperative haemorrhagic complications. Analysis of a 10-year series. *Acta Chirurgica Scandinavica* 151, 17-22.

Berzon, J.L. (1979) Complications of elective ovariohysterectomies in the dog and cat at a teaching institution: clinical review of 853 cases. *Veterinary Surgery* 8, 89-91.

Bischof, D., Dalbert, S., Zollinger, M., et al. (2010) Thromboelastography in the surgical patient. *Minerva Anestiologica* 76, 131-137.

Brooks, M. (1999) A review of canine inherited bleeding disorders. *The Journal of Heredity* 90, 112-118.

Burrow, R., Batchelor, D., Cripps, P. (2005) Complications observed during and after ovariohysterectomy of 142 bitches at a veterinary teaching hospital. *Veterinary Record* 157 (26), 829-833.

Crowe, D.T. (1980) Autotranfusions in the trauma patient. *Veterinary Clinics North America: Small Animal Practice* 10, 581-597.

Dorn, C.R., Swist R.A. 1977. Complications of canine ovariohysterectomy. *Journal of the American Animal Hospital Association* 13:720-724.

Dunne, J.R., Malone, D., Tracy, K.J., et al. (2002) Perioperative anaemia: an independent risk factor for infection, mortality, and resource utilisation in surgery. *Journal of Surgical Research* 102, 237-244.

Entholzner, E.K., Mielke, L.L., Calatzis, A.N., et al. (2000) Coagulation effects of a recently developed hydroxyethyl starch (HES 130/0.4) compared to hydroxyethyl starches with higher molecular weight. *Acta Anaesthesiologica Scandinavica* 44, 116-1121.

Essell, J.H., Martin, T.J., Salinas, J., et al. (1993) Comparison of thromboelastography to bleeding time and standard coagulation tests in patients after cardiopulmonary bypass. *Journal of Cardiothoracic and Vascular Anaesthesia* 7 (4), 410-415.

Fischerova, D. (2009) Urgent care in gynaecology: resuscitation and management of sepsis and acute blood loss. *Best Practice and Research clinical Obstetrics and Gynaecology* 23, 679-690.

Fries, D., Innerhofer, P., Klingler, A., et al. (2002) The effect of the combined administration of colloids and lactated ringer's solution on the coagulation system: an in vitro study using thromboelastograph coagulation analysis (ROTEG). *Anaesthesia and Analgesia* 94, 1280-1287.

Gauthier, V., Holowaychuk, M.K., Kerr, C.L., et al. (2015) Effect of Synthetic Colloid Administration on Coagulation in Healthy Dogs and Dogs with Systemic Inflammation. *Journal of Veterinary Internal Medicine* 29, 276-285.

Guerci, P., Tran, N., Menu, P., et al. (2014) Impact of fluid resuscitation with hypertonic-hydroxyethyl starch versus lactated ringer on hemorheology and microcirculation in hemorrhagic shock. *Clinics Hemorheology and Microcirculation* 56 (4), 301-317.

Gwozdziewicz, M., Olsak, P., Lonsky, V. (2008) Re-operations for bleeding in cardiac surgery: treatment strategy. *Biomedical Papers of the Medical Faculty of the University Palacky Olomouc Czech Republic* 152 (1), 159-162.

He, B., Xu, X., Li, L., et al Hydroxyethyl starch versus other fluids for non-septic patients in the intensive care unit: a meta-analysis of randomized controlled trials. *Critical Care* 2015, 19:92

Heneghan, H.M., Meron-Eldar, S., Yenumula, P., et al. (2012) Incidence and management of bleeding complications after gastric bypass surgery in the morbidly obese. *Surgery for Obesity and Related Disease* 8 (6), 729-735.

Heppenstall, R.B., Balderston, R., Goodwin, C. (1979) Pathophysiologic effects distal to a tourniquet in the dog. *Journal of Trauma* 19 (4), 234-238.

Hofland J., Henny, C.P. (2007) Bloodless (liver) surgery? The anesthetist's view. *Digestive Surgery* 24 (4), 265-273.

Johansson, P.I., Ostrowski, S.R., Secher, N.H. (2010) Management of major blood loss: an update. *Acta Anaesthesiologica Scandinavica* 54, 1039-1049.

Karthik, S., Grayson, A.D., McCarron, E.E., et al. (2004) Re-exploration for bleeding after coronary artery bypass surgery: risk factors, outcomes, and the effect of time delay. *The Annals of Thoracic Surgery* 78 (2), 527-534.

Knottenbelt, C.M. (2002) The feline AB blood group system and its importance in transfusion medicine. *Journal of Feline Medicine and Surgery* 4, 69-76.

Knotzer, H., Pajk, W., Maier, S., et al. (2006) Comparison of lactated Ringer's, gelatine and blood resuscitation on intestinal oxygen supply and mucosal tissue oxygen tension in haemorrhagic shock. *British Journal of Anaesthesia* 97 (4), 509-516.

Koukoutis, I., Bellagamba, R., Morris-Stiff, G., et al. (2006) Haemorrhage following pancreaticoduodenectomy: risk factors and the importance of sentinel bleed. *Digestive Surgery* 23 (4), 224-228.

Leitch, B.J., Bray, J.P., Kim, N.J., et al. (2012) Pedicle ligation in ovariohysterectomy: an in vitro study of ligation techniques. *J Small Anim Pract*. 53(10), 592-8.

Logan, J.C., Callan, M.B., Drew, K., et al. (2001) Clinical indications for use of fresh frozen plasma in dogs. *Journal of the American Veterinary Medical Association* 218, 1449-1455.

Lynch, A.M., Bound, N.J., Halfacree Z.J., et al. (2011) Postoperative haemorrhage associated with active suction drains in two dogs. *Journal of Small Animal Practice* 52, 172-174.

Maegele, M. (2009) Frequency, risk stratification and therapeutic management of acute post-traumatic coagulopathy. *Vox Sanguinis* 97, 39-49.

Marin, L.M., Iazbik, M. C., Zaldivar-Lopez, S., et al. (2012) Retrospective evaluation of the effectiveness of epsilon aminocaproic acid for the prevention of postamputation bleeding in retired racing Greyhounds with appendicular bone tumours: 46 cases (2003-2008). *Journal of Veterinary Emergency Critical Care* 22(3), 332-340.

Marin, L.M., Iazbik, M. C., Zaldivar-Lopez, S., et al. (2012) Epsilon aminocaproic acid for the prevention of delayed postoperative bleeding in retired racing greyhounds undergoing gonadectomy. *Veterinary Surgery* 41, 594-603.

Martin, L.G, Luther, T.Y., Alperin, D. C., et al. (2008) Serum antibodies against human albumin in critically ill and healthy dogs. *Journal of the American Veterinary Medical Association* 232(7), 1004–1009.

McAnulty, J.F., Smith, G.K. (1986) Circumferential external counterpressure by abdominal wrapping and its effect on simulated intra-abdominal hemorrhage. *Veterinary Surgery* 3, 270-274.

Muir, W.M., Wellman, M.L. (2003) Hemoglobin solutions and tissue oxygenation. *Journal of Veterinary Internal Medicine* 17, 127-135.

Mutter, T.C., Ruth, D.A., Dart, A.B. (2013) Hydroxyethyl starch (HES) versus other fluid therapies: effects on kidney function. *Cochrane Database Systemic Reviews* 23;7 CD007594

Neto, A.S, Veelo, D.P., Peireira, V.G.M., (2014) Fluid resuscitation with hydroxyethyl starches in patients with sepsis is associated with an increased incidence of acute kidney injury and use of renal replacement therapy: A systematic review and meta-analysis of the literature. *Journal of Critical Care* 29 185.e1-185.e7.

Nomura, T., Shitia, Y., Okamoto, H., et al. (1997) Massive postmastectomy hemorrhage caused by a suction drain. *Surgery* 121, 477.

Peeters, M.E., Kirpensteijn, J. (2011) Comparison of surgical variables and short-term postoperative complications in healthy dogs undergoing ovariohysterectomy or ovariectomy. *Journal of the American Veterinary Medical Association* 238, 189-194.

Péterffy, A., Henze, A. (1983) Haemorrhagic complications during pulmonary resection. A retrospective review of 1428 resections with 113 haemorrhagic episodes. *Scandinavian Journal of Thoracic and Cardiovascular Surgery* 17 (3), 283-287.

Powell, C., Thompson, L., Murtaugh, R.J. (2013) Type III hypersensitivity reaction with immune complex deposition in 2 critically ill dogs administered human serum albumin. *Journal of Veterinary Emergency Critical Care* 23(6), 598–604.

Rajbabu, K., Barber, N.J., Choi, W., et al. (2007) To knot or not to knot? Sutureless hemostasis compared to the surgeon's knot. *Annals of the Royal College of Surgeons England* 89 (4), 359-362.

Sanjay, P., Fawzi, A., Fulke, J.L., et al. (2010) Late post pancreatectomy haemorrhage. Risk factors and modern management. *Journal of the Pancreas* 11 (3), 220-225.

Schüriger, B., Inaba, K., Barmparas, G., et al. (2009) A new survivable damage control model including hypothermia, hemodilution, and liver injury. *Journal of Surgical Research* 169, 99-105.

Tai, T.W., Lin C.J., Jou, I.M., et al. (2011) Tourniquet use in total knee arthroplasty: a meta-analysis. *Knee Surgery, Sports Traumatology, Arthroscopy* 19 (7), 1121-1130.

Tjalma, W.A.A. (2006) Suction drain-induced haemorrhage after nerve-and vessel-sparing axillary lymph node dissection for breast cancer. *The Breast* 15, 442-444.

13 Anorexia

Angela Witzel

University of Tennessee College of Veterinary Medicine, Knoxville, TN, USA

An old Chinese proverb states: "He that takes medicine and neglects diet wastes the skills of the physician." Good nutrition is essential for repairing the wounds of surgery. Unfortunately, anorexia is one of the most common and most neglected postoperative complications. Starvation in the intensive care setting is an insidious process. Poor nutrition rarely causes death directly, but it can contribute to numerous other complications, including weakened immune function, wound dehiscence, bacterial translocation in the gastrointestinal (GI) tract, and longer hospital stays. The goals of this chapter are to discuss the causes, consequences, and management of anorectic patients in the postsurgical setting.

Definition

Anorexia can be defined as a lack or loss of appetite for food. Anorexia may be **complete**, meaning the patient will eat no food, or **partial**, meaning the patient consumes less food than needed to maintain a neutral energy balance. **Starvation** is a term used to describe prolonged anorexia. There are two categories of starvation, which are described next.

Simple starvation

The body's response to starvation varies with the circumstances surrounding anorexia. **Simple starvation** is a term used to describe metabolic changes occurring when an animal is free of disease but does not eat for several days. For example, a cat that becomes locked in a neighbor's garage without food for 1 week would be in a state of simple starvation. Several hours after a meal, glycogen (storage form of glucose) is released from the liver to maintain blood glucose levels. After about 12 to 24 hours, the glycogen reserves in the liver are depleted, and the body must rely on synthesis of new glucose molecules (gluconeogenesis) from endogenous protein and amino acids. Because of their carnivorous nature, cats have lower liver glycogen stores and are constantly gluconeogenic (Zoran 2002). During simple starvation, the body slows down its metabolic rate, and the liver produces ketone bodies from adipose stores as a way to decrease the need for glucose and limit muscle catabolism (Saker and Remillard 2010). In humans, more than 90% of caloric needs are met through fat metabolism in simple starvation (Demling 2009). In summary, after several days of simple starvation, the body becomes primed to use fat stores for energy and decreases its overall energy consumption to minimize protein and muscle wasting.

Stress starvation

Stress starvation describes a condition in which a patient is anorectic secondary to a disease process. The metabolic changes associated with stress starvation are quite different from a simply starved patient. Activation of the sympathetic nervous system and the release of hormones such as cortisol, adrenocorticoids, catecholamines, and glucagon lead to insulin resistance and increased gluconeogenesis, proteolysis and lipolysis, and basal metabolic rate. Elevated glucose production combined with increased energy demands cause rapid protein and muscle breakdown. Therefore, malnutrition occurs more quickly in a stress-starved patient. It should also be noted that protein catabolism is prominent in obese patients undergoing stress starvation, and despite ample fat stores, these patients are also at risk for malnutrition after surgery.

Refeeding syndrome

Refeeding syndrome is a response to nourishment, particularly carbohydrates, after long periods of anorexia (~5 days) or malnourishment. When a patient is malnourished, the intracellular concentrations of certain electrolytes are diminished because of a lack of intake. When a carbohydrate-containing meal is given, insulin is released, and glucose enters the cells. This stimulates adenosine triphosphate (ATP) production. Potassium, phosphorus, and magnesium follow insulin into the cells to support glucose metabolism. As a result, blood concentrations of these electrolytes can fall dramatically. Hypophosphatemia is the most common manifestation of refeeding syndrome, and levels below 1.5 mg/dL are associated with muscle weakness, respiratory distress, heart failure, hemolysis, and death. Hypokalemia is also associated with muscle weakness, cardiac arrhythmias, and death. Hypomagnesemia can also lead to muscle cramps, tetany, and seizure and can exacerbate cardiac arrhythmias. Magnesium is essential for potassium uptake into cells, and magnesium depletion should be suspected in cases of refractory hypokalemia (Adkins 2009).

Patients at risk for refeeding syndrome should have electrolytes measured before providing nutrition. If phosphorus, potassium, or magnesium is below the reference range, patients should be supplemented before giving food. After a meal is given, a chemistry and electrolyte panel should be repeated within 12 to 24 hours. One should also check a packed cell volume to look for red blood cell hemolysis and monitor for hyperglycemia. Refeeding syndrome

Complications in Small Animal Surgery, First Edition. Edited by Dominique Griffon and Annick Hamaide.

© 2016 John Wiley & Sons, Inc. Published 2016 by John Wiley & Sons, Inc.

Companion website: www.wiley.com/go/griffon/complications

typically occurs within the first 24 to 48 hours but may take up to 4 days to manifest.

Risk factors

Loss of appetite is one of the most common and vague maladies affecting our patients. The potential risk factors for anorexia after surgery are numerous and include:

- Pain
- Nausea
- Psychological stress
- GI stasis or ileus
- Release of inflammatory mediators
- Pain medications and antibiotics
- Organ dysfunction

Many causes of anorexia after surgery cannot be eliminated, but one should attempt to minimize stress, provide antiemetics, manage pain appropriately, and assess the need for GI protectants or prokinetics.

Treatment

Patient selection

When determining if a patient should receive assisted feeding after surgery, one should consider several factors. The first consideration should be the patient's nutritional history. Is the patient currently underweight or overweight? Was the patient anorectic or hyporexic before surgery? In general, aggressive nutritional support in the form of a feeding tube or parenteral nutrition should be considered after 3 days of complete anorexia or about 5 days of partial anorexia (consuming <50% of resting energy requirements [RERs]). The next factor to consider is weight loss. After a patient is rehydrated, a loss of more than 5% of its previous body weight is a sign of malnourishment. Some laboratory parameters can also be used to assess nutritional status, such as low albumin and elevated creatinine kinase, but these are often altered by surgery and may not change significantly with acute anorexia. However, patients with low protein concentrations are in greater need of nutritional support to prevent further muscle wasting and protein catabolism. Another consideration when assessing the need for nutritional support is a patient's anticipated length of anorexia. For example, if a patient has been anorectic for 3 days after surgery but has a sudden positive change in attitude and alertness, one may decide to wait 1 more day before placing a feeding tube. In contrast, a surgeon may preemptively place a feeding tube in a historically nonanorectic patient during surgery if it is expected to be anorectic after a procedure.

After surgery, most patients are cage confined with little activity. Although stress starvation increases the basal metabolic rate of animals compared with simple starvation, limited activity and the potential complications of hyperglycemia, diarrhea, and refeeding syndrome cause most nutritionists to recommend feeding at or below RER for the first few days after surgery.

resting energy requirements can be calculated using the following formula:

$$\text{Body weight}_{kg}^{0.75} \times 70 - \text{kcal/day}.$$

If an animal is overweight or obese, its ideal body weight should be used in the formula because adipose tissue contributes little to overall energy needs. After the need for nutritional support is established, the route of nutrition must be chosen (Figure 13.1).

Enteral feeding

If a patient will not consume enough calories voluntarily to meet its RER, a feeding tube should be considered. Enteral feeding using the GI tract is always preferred to parenteral (intravenous [IV]) nutrition. Enterocytes in the intestine rely on nutrients within the GI lumen for energy. Therefore, enteral feeding prevents villous atrophy and may reduce the risk of bacterial translocation through the intestines. Enteral feeding also promotes peristalsis and often improves the patient's appetite. The type of feeding tube chosen is based on expected duration of anorexia, a patient's ability to undergo anesthesia, and the need to bypass certain regions of the GI tract.

Nasoesophageal and nasogastric feeding tubes

Feeding tubes placed through the nasal cavity can either extend to the caudal esophagus (nasoesophageal tube) or into the stomach (nasogastric tube). The small diameter of the tube (5–8 Fr) usually does not elicit gastric reflux; however, nasoesophageal tubes are preferred to minimize this potential side effect. The main advantage to use nasal feeding tubes is they can be placed with little or no sedation. They are appropriate for patients needing 3 to 7 days of assisted feeding but often become irritating to the nasal cavity if used beyond 7 days. The small diameter of nasal feeding tubes limits their use to liquid formulations.

To place a nasoesophageal tube:

- Begin by numbing the nose with 0.5% proparacaine hydrochloride (0.5–1 cc for cats and small dogs; 1–2 cc for large dogs). Cats and small dogs can typically accept a 5-Fr tube, and larger dogs can tolerate an 8-Fr tube.
- Measure the desired tube length by running your tube along the side of the animal from the caudal margin of the last rib to the nasal planum. This places the end of your tube in the stomach. If you pull the end of the tube 1 to 5 cm proximal to the caudal rib (or make the total length about 75% of the original length), the tube will end in the caudal esophagus.
- Place a butterfly tape at the proximal end of the tube where it will exit the nose.
- Begin passing the lubricated tube in a caudoventral and medial direction. When you are 1 to 2 mm inside the nostril, push the external nares dorsally to open the ventral meatus. After inserting the tube another 3 to 5 cm, flex the animal's head ventrally to help the tube pass into the esophagus.
- Continue inserting the tube until the butterfly tape is reached; then suture or glue the tape to the skin.
- To determine if the feeding tube is correctly placed in the gastrointestinal tract instead of the respiratory tract, two-view chest radiographs should be performed. One can also attach a syringe to the end of the tube and pull back. If there is negative pressure, the tube is probably in the GI tract. You can also place the end of the tube in a cup of water and look for bubbles of air. If a capnometer is available, high levels of carbon dioxide coming from the feeding tube would be indicative of respiratory tract placement. One could also inject 1 to 2 cc of sterile saline into the tube and watch for coughing (Bosworth *et al.* 2004; Saker and Remillard 2010).

Esophagostomy tubes

Esophagostomy tubes are simple to place and can be used for several months of assisted feeding. They require heavy sedation or anesthesia for placement, and the most common complication is tube site infection. Esophagostomy tubes are larger in diameter

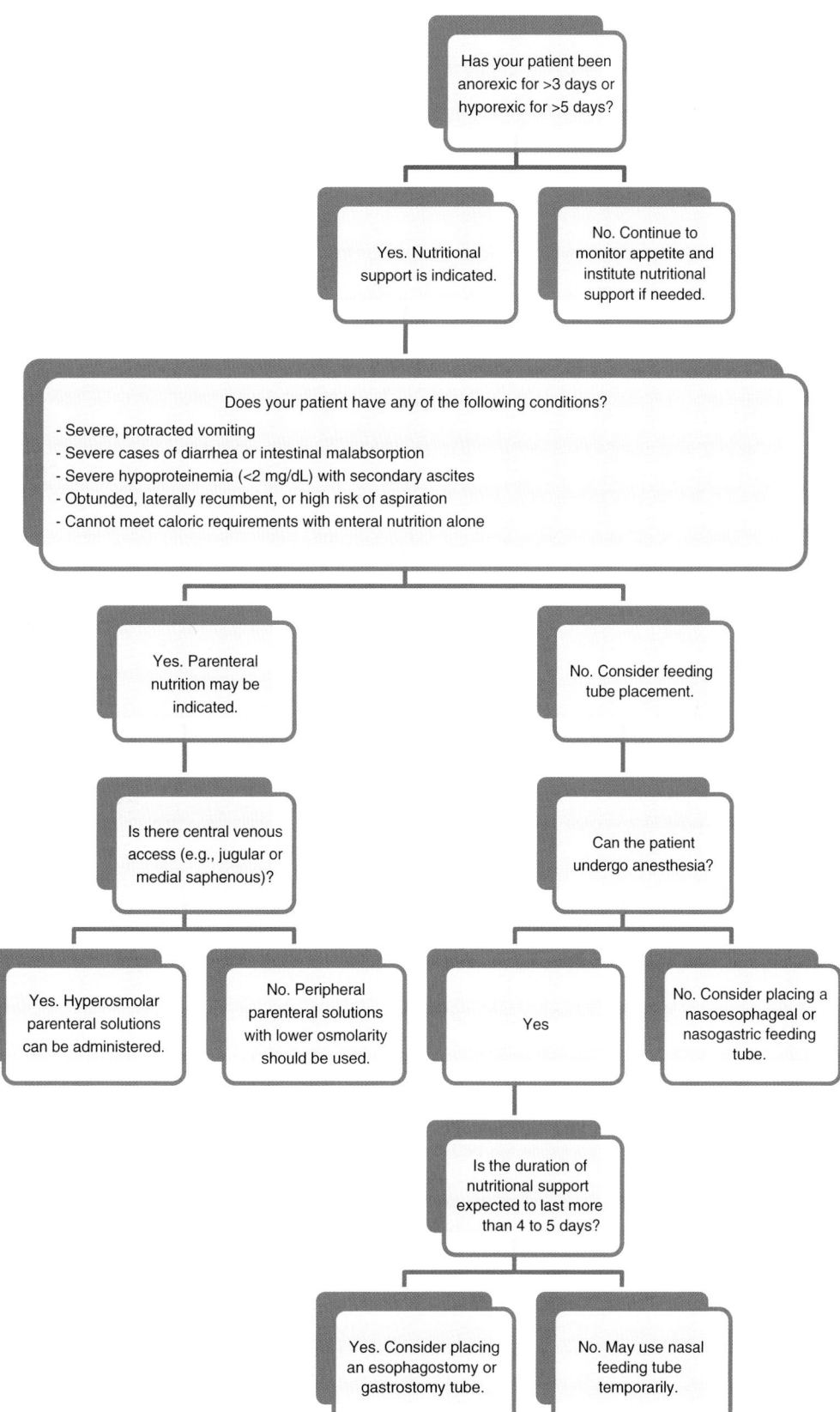

Figure 13.1 Decision-making algorithm for an anorectic patient.

(usually 12–19 Fr) than nasal feeding tubes, so most canned foods can be blenderized with water and used for feeding. Placement of esophagostomy tubes is described in the main surgical textbooks.

Gastrostomy tubes

Gastrostomy tubes (G-tubes) are useful for patients that require long-term assisted feeding or need to bypass the esophagus. Gastrostomy tubes can be placed surgically or percutaneously using an endoscope. The most significant complication of G-tubes is peritonitis if the tube displaces and food is placed into the abdomen. G-tubes must also be left in place for 1 week to 10 days before being removed so that a stoma can be formed. The larger diameter of the gastrostomy tubes allows for a great variety of foods, including dry kibble soaked in water. Placement of gastrostomy tubes is described in the main surgical textbooks.

Managing feeding tubes

After placing a feeding tube and allowing the patient to recover from anesthesia, one should begin with a few milliliters of room temperature water. If no vomiting occurs, food can be initiated. Most patients with feeding tubes have been anorectic for several days and are prone to diarrhea, ileus, and refeeding syndrome. Therefore, feeding should begin with only one third of the patient's RER on the first day, divided into four to six small meals. Before each feeding, one should attach a syringe and attempt to aspirate fluid from the stomach. If less than 5 cc is aspirated, continue with feeding. If more than 5 cc is collected, skip the feeding and consider a prokinetic agent like metoclopramide. Next, inject 3 to 5 cc of warm water to assure tube patency. Food injected into the syringe should be at room temperature or warm and given slowly over 5 to 10 minutes. If using a nasal feeding tube, constant-rate infusions using a syringe pump can also be used. After feeding, flush the tube with 3 to 5 cc of warm water to prevent clogging. If no vomiting or diarrhea occurs in the first day of feeding, then increase to 2/3 of RER on day 2, and achieve full RER on day 3. After a patient is able to tolerate feeding its RER, the frequency of meals can decrease and the volume increase. Avoid giving more than 20 mL/kg per feeding in cats and 60 mL/kg per feeding in dogs.

Parenteral feeding

Although enteral feeding is preferred to parenteral feeding for most patients, some animals are unable to obtain sufficient nutrients from enteral routes and require IV nutrition. Parenteral nutrition provides macronutrients in the form of proteins, carbohydrates, and lipids intravenously. Parenteral nutrition can be classified as total parenteral nutrition (TPN) or partial/peripheral parenteral nutrition (PPN). The term TPN implies a solution containing all of the nutrients needed for long-term health. In veterinary medicine, patients are rarely on TPN more than a couple of weeks, and we often do not formulate TPN to be a complete and balanced diet. TPN solutions have very high osmolarity and must be given through a central line jugular or medial saphenous catheter. PPN solutions may contain one, two, or all macronutrient components but have lower osmolarity (usually 450–600 mOsm) and can be given through peripheral catheters. It is recommended to consult with a veterinary nutritionist when formulating and initially using parenteral nutrition (see the list of recommended veterinary nutrition consultants below).

Indications for parenteral nutrition:
- Severe, protracted vomiting
- Severe cases of diarrhea or intestinal malabsorption

- Severe hypoproteinemia (<2 mg/dL) as low oncotic pressure can inhibit nutrient absorption in the GI tract
- Obtunded, laterally recumbent patient, or at risk for aspiration
- Any case in which you cannot meet caloric requirements with enteral nutrition alone

Outcome

As described earlier, stress starvation is associated with increased basal energy requirements and rapid protein catabolism. As a result, human surgical patients who do not receive adequate nutritional support have delayed wound healing, GI villus atrophy, decreased immune function, and longer hospital stays compared with well-nourished patients (Lidder and Lewis 2004; Demling 2009). Data comparing the use of nutritional support postoperatively in veterinary patients is sparse, but adequate caloric intake is associated with higher hospital discharge rates (Brunetto et al. 2010). Enteral nutrition also improves gut mucosal integrity and improves outcomes in dogs with pancreatitis and parvovirus (Qin et al. 2002; Mohr et al. 2003).

Prevention

Preventing anorexia in surgical patients is a challenging task, and management with feeding tubes and parenteral nutrition is often required. However, some strategies to minimize anorexia include:
- Try to mimic a normal feeding environment.
  - Take patients outside or to a quiet room.
  - Kitchen or laundry rooms may resemble home.
- Minimize stress as much as possible.
- Avoid the food server being the person who performs procedures or restrains.
- Normalize feeding times.
  - What is the typical feeding schedule at home?
  - Maintain light–dark cycles in the intensive care unit.
- Feed cats with wide, shallow bowls so that whiskers are not in the way.
- Remove physical constraints such as e-collars while feeding.
- Increase palatability.
  - Canned food is sometimes preferred; it is typically higher in fat and protein.
  - Remove uneaten canned food after 30 to 45 minutes to avoid food aversions.
  - Try foods that are rare but not foreign. If a cat only eats dry food at home, canned food may be too foreign. Try a small variety of both canned and dry foods.
  - Increase freshness and aroma by heating foods.
- Use antiemetics if nausea suspected. Many patients receiving pain medications often feel nauseous even if no vomiting is present.

Relevant literature

Good nutrition is essential to the repair and recovery of patients after surgery. The metabolic consequences of malnourishment in the immediate postoperative period can result in decreased wound healing, immunosuppression, and longer hospital stays. In a recent study, hospitalized dogs and cats that received no nutritional support had a much lower discharge rate (38.4%) than anorectic dogs and cats receiving some form of nutrition (~70% discharge rate) (Brunetto et al. 2010). Clinicians should evaluate patient needs carefully and then institute aggressive nutritional intervention in anorectic patients.

Recommended veterinary nutrition consultants include:

- University of Tennessee Veterinary Medical Center: phone: 865-974-8387, email: UTVNS@utk.edu, https://vetmed.tennessee.edu/vmc/SmallAnimalHospital/Nutrition
- University of California, Davis Veterinary Medical Teaching Hospital: phone: 530-752-1393, http://www.vetmed.ucdavis.edu/vmth/small_animal/nutrition/index.cfm
- Dr. Rebecca Remillard: phone: 508-429-4845, email: petdiets@att.net, http://www.petdiets.com
- Contact the American College of Veterinary Nutritionists for additional suggestions: phone: 508-429-4845; fax: 800-649-2043; email: petdiets@att.net, http://acvn.org

References

Adkins, S. (2009) Recognizing and preventing refeeding syndrome. *Dimensions of Critical Care Nursing* 28, 53-58.

Bosworth, C., Bartges, J., Snow, P. (2004) Nasoesophageal and nasogastric feeding tubes. *Veterinary Medicine* July, 590-594.

Brunetto, M., Gomes, M., Andre, M., et al. (2010) Effects of nutritional support on hospital outcome in dogs and cats. *Journal of Veterinary Emergency and Critical Care* 20, 224-231.

Demling, R. (2009) Nutrition, anabolism, and the wound healing process: an overview. *Eplasty* 9, 65-94.

Lidder, P., Lewis, S. (2004) Perioperative and postoperative nutrition. *Journal of Hospital Medicine* 65, 717-720.

Mohr, A. J., Leisewitz, A. L., Jacobson, L. S., et al. (2003) Effect of early enteral nutrition on intestinal permeability, intestinal protein loss, and outcome in dogs with severe parvoviral enteritis. *Journal of Veterinary Internal Medicine* 17, 791-798.

Qin H.L., Su Z.D., Gao Q., Lin Q.T. (2002) Early intrajejunal nutrition: bacterial translocation and gut barrier function of severe acute pancreatitis in dogs. *Hepatobiliary & Pancreatic Diseases International* 1, 150-154.

Saker, K., Remillard, R. (2010) Critical care nutrition and enteral-assisted feeding. In: Hand, M., Thatcher, C., Remillard, R., et al. (eds.) *Small Animal Clinical Nutrition*, 5th edn. Topeka, KS, Mark Morris Institute.

Zoran, D. L. (2002) The carnivore connection to nutrition in cats. *Journal of the American Veterinary Medical Association* 221, 1559-1567.

14 Management of Surgical Pain

Lyon Lee[1] and Reza Seddighi[2]
[1]Western University of Health Sciences, Pomona, CA, USA
[2]College of Veterinary Medicine, The University of Tennessee, Knoxville, TN, USA

Definition

Surgical pain is associated with surgery performed in many areas of the body, including the muscles, bones, tendons, ligaments, nerves, and abdominal organs. Although general anesthesia allows the patient to undergo surgery without pain, modern inhalation anesthetics such as isoflurane and sevoflurane carry minimal residual analgesia, justifying adjunct interventions after the animal recovers from unconsciousness to provide adequate postoperative analgesia. The most commonly prescribed analgesics for perioperative periods are opioids and nonsteroidal antiinflammatory drugs (NSAIDs) because of their proven efficacy. Therefore, an overview of these analgesic agents is provided below to begin with followed by a synopsis of other atypical analgesics such as anticonvulsants and psychotropic drugs, which have gained popularity in animals in recent years. In addition, knowledge of the pathophysiology of pain and the pharmacology of analgesics is critical for successful therapeutic outcomes in animals, so a quick description of these topics is also provided in this chapter.

Risk factors for inadequate pain control

Surgery inherently leads to tissue damage and nociceptive pain. The degree or intensity of postoperative pain seems closely related to the type of surgical procedures. Table 14.1 describes the level of pain associated with common surgical procedures. Inadequate analgesic dosing and frequency, improper selection of analgesics, and poor techniques will result in failure to control perioperative pain. The stress response triggered by surgery and anesthesia further contributes to postoperative pain. Poor management of the pain and stress response may not only delay healing but also result in adverse effects such as cardiac arrhythmias, disuse atrophy of muscles, and metabolic disorders.

Diagnosis

Assessment of pain

Assessment of pain for a given animal is typically inferred because no machine can measure pain. Animals are generally less expressive of pain than humans because it offers survival advantages against potential predators. The obvious lack of communication dictates that pain assessment in veterinary patients rely extensively on observation of behavior (Figure 14.1). Altered behavior to human contact routinely serves as an indicator discomfort. The ability to relate such signs with pain management is a prerequisite to effective pain control.

Signs of acute postoperative pain include:
- Guarding and aversion to manipulation of the surgical site
- Vocalization may indicate discomfort, but lack of vocalization should not be interpreted as a lack of pain.
- Self-mutilation: Moderate discomfort often leads to attempts to bite or scratch the site.
- Activity: Whereas animals in visceral pain tend to exhibit restlessness and agitation, those in somatic pain typically are reluctant to move.

Cats and dogs share some signs of pain but also differ markedly in their behavioral responses. Cats tend to demonstrate fewer signs of pain compared with dogs in response to surgical procedures that may inflict similar tissue damage such as an ovariohysterectomy. However, this does not necessarily indicate that the cat feels less pain than the dog but rather an inter-species difference in expressing pain, requiring species specific methods of assessment. Table 14.2 describes some examples of differences in painful behavior between dogs and cats.

Table 14.1 Severity of pain based on invasiveness of surgical procedures

Grade	Invasiveness	Examples	Level of pain
1	Mild	Skin excision, microchip implant, toenail clipping	Minor
2	Intermediate	Tooth extraction, Unilateral cricoarytenoid lateralization, PEG tube placement	Mild
3	Major	Cruciate repair, bone plate, bowel resection, Mammary gland resection	Moderate
4	Very major	PSS, PDA, THR, limb amputation	Severe

PEG, percutaneous endoscopic gastrostomy; PSS, portosystemic shunt; PDA, patent ductus arteriosis; THR, total hip replacement

Complications in Small Animal Surgery, First Edition. Edited by Dominique Griffon and Annick Hamaide.
© 2016 John Wiley & Sons, Inc. Published 2016 by John Wiley & Sons, Inc.

Companion website: www.wiley.com/go/griffon/complications

Dog's name_____ Hospital number_____ Date_____

Time_____ Procedure_____

A. Look at dog in kennel
Is the dog?
(i)

		(ii)		(iii)	
Quiet	☐	Ignoring any wound, painful area	☐	Normal	☐
Crying or whimpering	☐	Licking, looking or rubbing it	☐	Hunched/tense	☐
Groaning	☐	Chewing it	☐	Rigid	☐
Screaming	☐				

For clinical reasons it may not be possible to carry out question B

Please tick if this is the case ☐ and then proceed to C

B. Put lead on dog and lead out of kennel

When the dog rises/walks is it?
(iv)

Normal	☐
Lame	☐
Slow/reluctant	☐
Stiff	☐
It refuses to move	☐

C. If it has a wound/painful area apply gentle pressure 2 inches round the site
Does it?
(v)

Do nothing	☐
Flinch	☐
Growl/guard area	☐
Snap	☐
Cry	☐

D. Overall
Is the dog?
(vi)

Happy and content/happy and bouncy	☐
Quiet or indifferent	☐
Aggressive	☐
Nervous/anxious/fearful	☐
Depressed/uninterested	☐

Is the dog?
(vii)

Comfortable	☐
Uncomfortable	☐

Figure 14.1 Modified form of the Glasgow pain scale. *Source:* Murrell *et al.*, 2008. Reproduced with permission from BMJ.

Table 14.2 Clinical signs attributed to pain in cats and dogs

Behavior	Dogs	Cats
Vocalization	Groan, whine, whimper, growl	Groan, purr, hiss
Facial expression	Fixed stare, glazed appearance, dilated pupil	Furrowed brow, squinted eyes, dilated pupil
Body posture	Hunched, laterally recumbent, prayer position	Generally sternal, laterally recumbent
Self-awareness (guarding and self mutilating)	Protective of wounds; licking, chewing, and rubbing wounds and surgical sites; limping; loss of weight bearing	Protective of wounds; licking, chewing, and rubbing wounds and surgical sites; limping; loss of weight bearing
Activity	Restless or restricted movement, trembling (shivering)	Restricted movement, stereotypies (meaningless encircling movement)
Attitude: Socialization and comfort or attention seeking	Increased aggressiveness or timidity (fearfulness)	Comfort seeking or hiding; aggressiveness
Appetite	Decreased	Decreased
Urinary and bowel habits	Increased urination, urinary retention, noncompliance to house training	Failure to use litter box
Grooming	Loss of sheen in hair coat, particularly in chronically painful dogs	Failure to groom, particularly in chronically painful cats
Response to palpation	Protecting, biting, vocalizing, withdrawing, orienting, escape	Protecting, biting, scratching, vocalizing, withdrawing, orienting, escape

Source: Adapted from Carrol (1998).

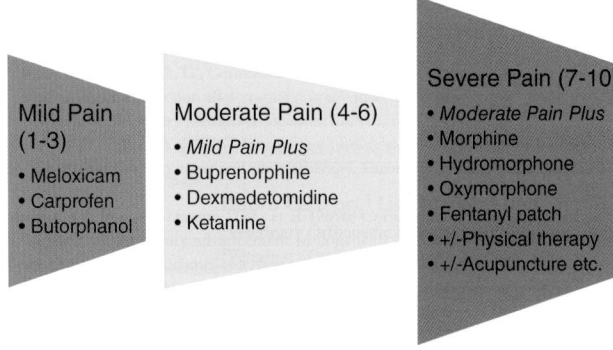

Figure 14.2 Option to achieve analgesia based on severity of surgical pain.

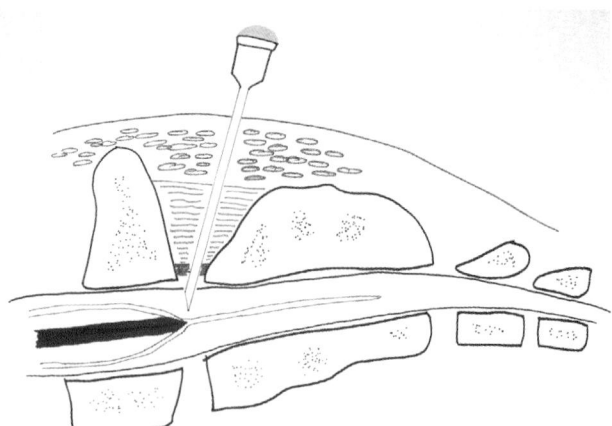

Figure 14.4 Lateral view of the lumbosacral epidural area with a spinal needle placed in the epidural space, illustrating the "hanging drop" epidural anesthetic technique.

Treatment of pain

Several classes of analgesics are available, but the most effective agents belong to the class of opioids (see additional information under relevant literature). However, mild surgical pain such as a cutaneous wound closure can be successfully managed with non-opioid analgesics such as NSAIDs (see Chapter 15). More invasive surgical procedures, such as fracture repairs, justify administration of opioids, and patients frequently require increased dosing or frequency of analgesic administration. Figure 14.2 lists examples of analgesic choices in relation to severity of pain.

Previous studies indicate that veterinarians and technicians tend to underestimate the level of pain in patients and are overly anxious about potential side effects of the drugs. In addition, the use of opioids is subject to strict government regulations, which complicate their access and administration. Practitioners may also be concerned about potential drug abuse by owners or hospital staff with access to these medications. Alternative options that are not subject to these concerns include NSAIDs, corticosteroids, α_2 agonists, and sodium channel blockers (local and systemic).

Although perioperative pain management commonly involved a multimodal approach (Figure 14.3), with adjunct strategies such as local anesthesia (Figure 14.4) and physical therapies including massage, ultrasound therapy, acupuncture, transcutaneous electrical nerve stimulation (TENS), laser irradiation, and magnetic field therapy, this chapter focuses on pharmacologic management of

surgical pain. Table 14.3 and Table 14.4 list analgesic agents commonly administered in dogs and cats along with modalities for administration (Figure 14.5).

Prevention

To reduce or prevent surgical pain, several factors need to be taken into account.

- Select minimally invasive surgical techniques (e.g., laparoscopic cholecystectomy vs. open abdominal cholecystectomy) whenever feasible.
- Strict adherence to Halsted's principles of surgery is a prerequisite to minimize tissue injury and functional impairment, including inflammation.
- Clinicians should be familiar with the clinical pharmacology of key analgesics used in veterinary medicine to effectively treat pain.
- Preemptive analgesia with proper selection of analgesic drug and dosage should be given.
- Aim for a multimodal analgesic approach to pain management (see Figure 14.3); different classes of analgesics are used simultaneously to benefit from the resulting synergism.

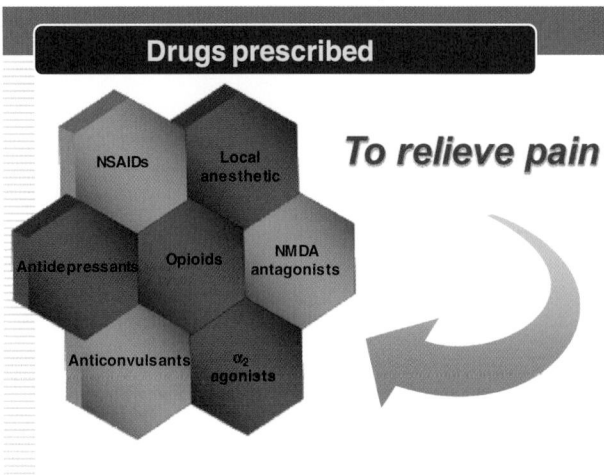

Figure 14.3 Options for pharmacologic management of pain.

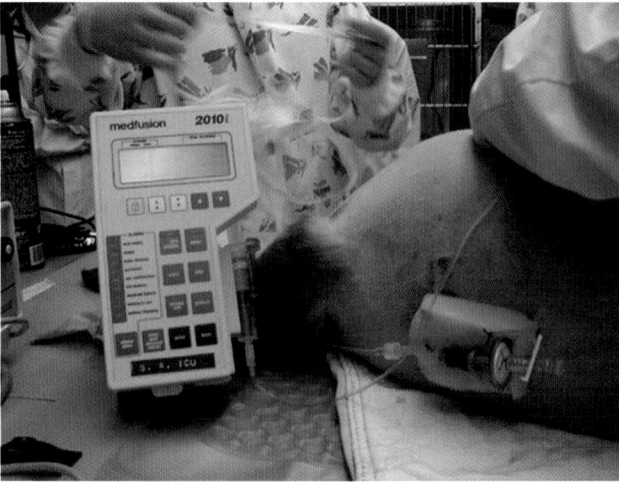

Figure 14.5 Application of a constant-rate infusion of morphine using an indwelling epidural catheter and a syringe pump.

Table 14.3 Analgesic agents commonly used for perioperative management of pain in small animals

Drug	Dose in Dogs (mg/kg)	Dose in Cats (mg/kg)	Comments
Morphine	0.25–0.5 IV, IM, or SC	0.05–0.1 IV, IM, or SC	Gold standard narcotic analgesic; inexpensive; vomiting frequent; histamine release when given IV (hypotension); 1–3 hours of duration; q8h
Hydromorphone	0.05–0.2 IV, IM, or SC	0.05–0.1 IV, IM, or SC	Occasional vomiting; mild to moderate sedation; panting; 1–3 hours of duration; q8h
Oxymorphone	0.05–0.2 IV, IM, or SC	0.05–0.1 IV, IM, or SC	Minimal vomiting; mild to moderate sedation; panting; 1–3 hours of duration; q8h; interrupted supplies
Butorphanol	0.2–0.4 IV, IM, or SC	0.2–0.4 IV, IM, or SC	Minimal vomiting; less panting; mild sedation; 1–2 hours of duration; less respiratory depression than pure agonists but less reliable analgesia
Fentanyl	0.002–0.01 IV, IM, or SC		Minimal vomiting; mild to moderate sedation; panting; 0.3–2.0 hours of duration; CRI, available as a transdermal patch or solution for extended analgesia (≤3–4 days)
Buprenorphine	0.005–0.02 IV, IM, or SC	0.005–0.02 IV, IM, or SC	Slow onset of analgesia but extended 4 or 6 hours' analgesic duration with less respiratory depression than pure agonists; q12h; also available in sustained-release polymer preparation designed to release buprenorphine over a 72-hour period
Dexmedetomidine	0.001–0.01 IV, IM, or SC	0.002–0.02 IV, IM, or SC	Replaced medetomidine as active enantiomer; potent sedation with profound cardiovascular effect (bradycardia and depressed myocardial contractility); 1–3 hours of duration
Carprofen	2–4 PO, IV, IM, or SC	1–4 PO, IV, IM, or SC	Use with opioids or other analgesics has been proven to provide a superior analgesic through synergism; q24h
Ketoprofen	0.25–2 PO, IV, IM, or SC	0.25–2 PO, IV, IM, or SC	Similar to carprofen; commonly used as part of multimodal analgesic therapy; q24h
Meloxicam	0.025–0.2 PO, IV, or SC	0.025–0.2 PO, IV, or SC	Similar to carprofen and ketoprofen; commonly used as part of multimodal analgesic therapy; q24h
Local anesthetics; lidocaine, bupivacaine	L: 2–4 B: 1–2	L: 1–2 B: 0.5–1	For local anesthesia or adjunct to general anesthesia; specific or regional nerve blocks require much less than infiltration local anesthesia over the surgical site; recently, lidocaine has proved be a useful analgesic in CRI at much lower doses as part of multimodal anesthetic therapy (see Table 14.3)

CRI, constant-rate infusion; IM, intramuscular; IV, intravenous; PO, oral; q, every; SC, subcutaneous.

Table 14.4 Analgesia via constant-rate of infusion of various analgesic agents*

Analgesic drugs	Comments
Fentanyl	Infuse with a syringe or infusion pump at a rate of 5–20 µg/kg/hr
Morphine	0.05–0.25 mg/kg/hr; may use an infusion pump or gravity flow with IV drip set prepared in one of the following diluents: 5% dextrose, saline, or isotonic crystalloids
Ketamine	0.06–0.6 mg/kg/hr or 1–10 µg/kg/min (60 mg into a 1000-mL diluent solution infused at 1–10 mL/kg/hr) with a loading dose of 0.1–0.5 mg/kg
Dexmedetomidine	0.5–2 µg/kg/hr with close monitoring of heart rate and blood pressure
Morphine–ketamine (cats) or morphine–ketamine–lidocaine mixture (dogs)	Infuse at a rate of 4–8 mL/kg/hr from a preparation of the mixture; 60 mg of morphine, 60 mg of ketamine, and 500 mg of lidocaine into a single 500-mL diluent bag (*Note:* Because of increased toxicity to lidocaine, only the morphine–ketamine mixture is used in cats.)

*This modality allows immediate titration to effect.

IV, intravenous.

- Caretakers should be familiar with the pain behavior of the animal to provide timely intervention with analgesics for breakthrough pain.
- Recovery in a stress-free environment under vigilant observation should be provided.
- Proper postoperative care of the surgical site should be provided to promote healing.

Relevant literature

Physiology of pain

Studies of analgesics are based on experimental "analgesiometry." However, the results of many of these investigations may bear little relation to the apparent efficacy of analgesics in the clinical setting, where multiple pathophysiologic conditions coexist and influence the types and intensities of pain. Therefore, a good understanding of the pathophysiology of pain is critical to the clinician's ability to control postoperative pain. This section includes a brief review of the extensive literature covering this topic (Levine and Alessandri-Haber 2007; Maddison *et al.* 2008; Riviere and Papich 2009; Stone and Molliver 2009; Bredersona *et al.* 2013).

The receptors that mediate the noxious signal that is ultimately converted to the pain sensation are called nociceptors. Pain pathways can be subdivided into transduction, transmission, modulation, and perception, and understanding of these pathways is beneficial when treating pain in animals (Figure 14.6). Noxious stimuli activate nociceptors that are at the termination of free nerve

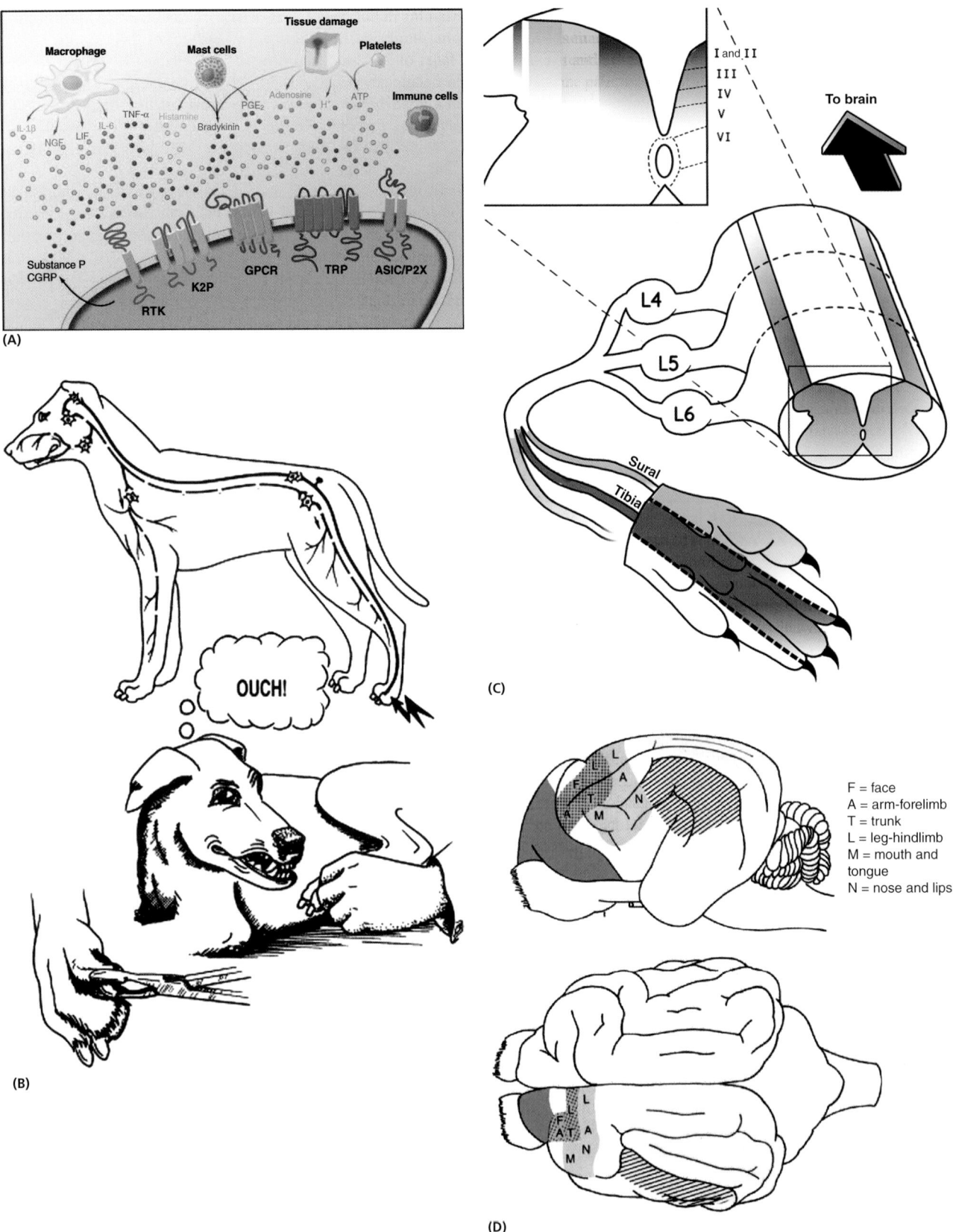

Figure 14.6 Four main pathways of pain: transduction of the noxious signals in the periphery (**A**), transmission of the signals via peripheral nerves (**B**), modulation at the dorsal horn of the spinal cord (**C**), and perception of the pain in the cerebrum (**D**). ATP, adenosine triphosphate; ASIC, Acid-Sensing Channel; CGRP, calcitonin gene-related peptide; IL, interleukin; K2P, two-pore domain potassium channels; LIF, leukemia inhibitory factor; NGF, nerve growth factor; P2X, P2 purinoreceptors; PG, prostaglandin; RTK, receptor tyrosine kinase; TNF, tumor necrosis factor; TRP, transient receptor potential channel. *Sources:* Basbaum *et al.*, 2009. Reproduced with permission from Elsevier (**A**); van Nes *et al.*, 2009. Reproduced with permission from Elsevier (**B**); Corder *et al.*, 2010. Reproduced with permission from Elsevier (**C**); Miller, 2008. Reproduced with permission from Elsevier (**D**).

endings of A-δ and C afferent fibers. The pain sensory fibers (nociceptors) have cell bodies in dorsal root ganglia and project to the dorsal horn of the spinal cord where they synapse in Rexed laminae I, II, V, VII, and X. After synapses at this level, the information is transmitted further via several spinal tracts, most notably the spinothalamic tract, to the supraspinal level. The synapses at the level of the thalamus then transmit the information diffusely to the cerebral cortex (thalamocortical projection). Pain perception takes place when the cerebral cortex processes the information as noxious.

Different neurotransmitters are involved in these pathways, including γ-aminobutyric acid (GABA), glutamate, endogenous opioids, substance P, norepinephrine, and many other neuropeptides. The effects of these neurotransmitters can be modulated at each step in the pathway (providing basis for the multimodal, or balanced, analgesic approach). Pain can be characterized as acute or chronic based on the duration, and somatic, visceral, or neuropathic based on the origin and the involvement of the damaged tissues. Tissue injury such as surgery initiates release of cytokines that transduce the thermomechanoceptive signal to electrical signals. Damage to nerves and tissues in the periphery increases afferent signals and induces central wind-up, contributing to the development of neuropathic pain. Full details of the pathophysiology, including pain mechanisms and definitions of analgesic terms, have been described (Stoelting and Hillier 2005; Gaynor and Muir 2008; Maddison et al. 2008; Riviere and Papich 2009; Clarke et al. 2013).

Methods for assessment of pain
To improve the effectiveness of pain management, various methods have been developed to assess pain, but all carry several limitations:
- Simple descriptive scales (SDS) use word scales presenting a patient in pain with predetermined words such as "no," "moderate," "severe," or "very severe." This method requires minimal training and is simpler than NRS or VAS (see below) to apply but has wide interobserver variability with low sensitivity. Because there are only four or five categories, small changes in pain response may not get reflected appropriately, thus limiting effective pain management.
- **Numeric rating scales (NRS):** The intensity of pain is scored from 0 to 10, where 0 represents no pain and 10 the worst possible pain. Interpretation of pain intensity may be widely variable, thereby increasing interobserver variability, and differences of pain intensity among categories are undefined and inconsistent. NRS requires training and experience.
- **Visual analog scales (VAS)** are variations of NRS in which a line is displayed on a page without numbers. The left end is marked as no pain, and the right end represents the worst possible pain. The observer places a mark along the line representing the intensity of pain the animal seems to be experiencing. This assessment is also limited by interobserver variability. It requires more training and experience to use than NRS because interpretation of pain intensity may be widely variable.
- **Composite scoring system (CSS):** Two or more different pain assessment scales are combined to improve the accuracy of the pain measurement. This approach may require more time and effort but has been found to improve pain assessment, limiting errors and enhancing clinicians' ability to manage pain in animals (Murrell et al. 2008; van Loon et al. 2014). The form in Figure 14.1 is an example of CSS and can be downloaded from the publisher's website (veterinaryrecord.bmj.com) and used in assessing the pain in animals in clinical practice.

Analgesics
These medications (Figure 14.3) target the sources of pain by acting on pain transduction, transmission, modulation, projection, and perception in both the peripheral and the central nervous systems. Itravenous (IV), intramuscular (IM), and subcutaneous (SC) routes of administration are favored during the perioperative period because of their quick onset and control of pharmacologic effect, but analgesics may also be administered via transdermal, oral, and rectal routes.

Multimodal approach allows for synergism, and analgesics of different classes such as opioids, NSAIDs, α₂ agonists, and NMDA (N-methyl-D-aspartate) antagonists may be co-administered in the same patient. An analgesic drug may also be combined with an anxiolytic or sedative to enhance analgesia, suggesting that pain is a complex phenomenon influenced by behavior modification.

Opioids
All opioids (including endogenous and exogenous substances that possess morphine-like properties) are chemically related and subject to regulatory controls that are governed by the Controlled Substance Act 1970. In humans and dogs, these are the mainstay of perioperative analgesia, before, during, and after surgery. The potential excitement caused by opioids in cats limited the use of these drugs in the past, but newer opioids and the availability of sedatives have expanded the use of opioids in this species. Selection of a specific opioid is based on several considerations, including time of administration.

For use at premedication, a long-acting opioid should be selected to have an effect before, during, and after surgery. Hypnosis and sedation are acceptable side effects and are often desired to facilitate catheterization, anesthetic induction, and preparation of the surgical site. An opioid may induce respiratory depression, warranting monitoring of ventilation. Opioid-induced vomiting may be an acceptable side effect, but ideally, one should select the dose, route, and drug that will minimize the incidence.

During the intraoperative period, a very short-acting and very potent drug with a rapid onset of action is generally prescribed. Respiratory depression is acceptable as long as artificial ventilation can be initiated if needed. In dogs, fentanyl is suitable, but intermittent positive-pressure ventilation (IPPV) is essential.

During the postoperative period, drugs are selected to cause minimal respiratory depression. A long-acting agent (e.g., buprenorphine) is required, but initial dosing should take into consideration potential residual effects of drugs administered during surgery, which may be synergistic. For this reason, a short-acting analgesic such as fentanyl or remifentanil may be preferred initially followed later by a longer acting drug.

Clinical pharmacology of opioid analgesics
Opioids commonly used in small animals cause varying degrees of depression or stimulation depending on factors such as dose, receptor type, and species. "Depression" causes analgesia (desired effect), hypnosis (possibly useful), respiratory depression and bradycardia (side effects), and depression of the cough reflex (care needed during recovery). "Stimulation" causes the generalized excitement seen in horses and cats (often accompanied by tachycardia), euphoria (resulting in a tendency toward physical dependence in humans), dysphoria (side effects), and vomiting and defecation (side effects). Opioids do not cause myocardial depression and are therefore commonly used for induction of anesthesia in human patients with cardiac disease. They can cause very severe bradycardia, which can

be counteracted with anticholinergics. In dogs, some opioids may cause hypotension, and in cats, excitement is accompanied by tachycardia and hypertension.

Mechanism of action

All opioids have a similar mode of action, but their activity varies depending on degree of affinity toward the specific receptor subtypes. They all stimulate opioid receptors, modulating inhibitory and excitatory effects in the central nervous system (CNS). Their action causes analgesia and sedation to a lesser extent. Clinically important subtypes of opioid receptors are $\mu 1$, $\mu 2$, κ, and δ subtypes. Stimulation of these receptor subtypes induces the following activities:

μ_1: supraspinal analgesia, euphoria, and sedation
μ_2: respiratory depression, bradycardia, increased gastrointestinal transmit time, hypothermia, and physical dependence
κ: spinal analgesia, sedation, and dysphoria
δ: spinal analgesia and respiratory depression

Classification

Opioids are generally classified as pure agonists, antagonists, partial agonists, and mixed agonists–antagonists. Pure agonists (morphine, hydromorphone, fentanyl, meperidine) produce a "maximal" biologic response through binding of opioid receptors. In general, a pure μ agonist provides the best analgesia, with a dose-related effect. Unfortunately, this analgesia currently remains accompanied by respiratory depression and liability associated with addiction and abuse. Antagonists (naloxone, nalmefene, naltrexone) are drugs that competitively reverse (antagonize) the effects of agonists by preventing their access to a receptor. They have low (or no) intrinsic activity at the receptors themselves. Partial agonists are drugs that produce a partial response at a particular receptor type, even at high doses. The slope of their dose-response curve is not as steep as that of pure (full) agonists. The dose-response curve also exhibits a "ceiling" effect, explaining the partial response. Concomitant administration of a partial with a pure agonist can reduce (antagonize) the pure agonist's clinical effects. The analgesic properties of partial agonists are quite reduced (except for buprenorphine) but induce less respiratory depression and are often less subject to regulations. Partial agonists often have a bell-shaped dose-response curve; after maximal analgesia is achieved, further doses only reverse the effect. Therefore, if these partial agonists prove ineffective, repeat administrations are not recommended. Partial agonists also have a tendency to cause dysphoria, with unpleasant hallucinatory effects, and are therefore less likely to cause abuse. Mixed agonists–antagonists have divergent activities on different receptors, acting simultaneously as an agonist at one receptor (e.g., κ or δ receptors) while acting as an antagonist at another (e.g., μ receptors). Examples include butorphanol and nalbuphine.

Being familiar with the classification of opioid analgesics is important when several agents are administered in order to understand the potential for antagonism. For example, naloxone antagonizes morphine very well but is less efficient in its antagonism of the partial agonist buprenorphine. Administering butorphanol to a dog previously treated with morphine will result in partial antagonism, reducing the total analgesia even despite the analgesic properties of each drug. Ideally, agonist and partial agonist drugs should not be combined to obtain analgesia in an animal. However, if a partial agonist fails to be effective, a pure agonist at higher than normal doses may be effective. The term "sequential analgesia" has been used to describe the use of the partial agonists such as buprenorphine or nalbuphine to reverse a pure agonist while maintaining some analgesia.

Opioid agonists

Morphine

Morphine is the gold standard against which other opioids are compared, and it is classed as the prototype opioid agonist. It functions primarily as a μ agonist, with a lesser degree of κ and δ agonism. It provides excellent analgesia with some sedation in most species, including dogs, but must be used with care in some species such as cats and horses, generally at a maximum dose of 0.2 mg/kg, preferably with sedation. It can be used at all perioperative stages and is relatively inexpensive. The time of onset after IV injection is 5 to 10 minutes, but it is longer after IM administration. Rapid IV injection causes more predictable histamine release, which induces significant hypotension. Slow administration is therefore recommended for IV administration. Doses of 0.25 to 2.0 mg/kg provide 4 hours of analgesia in dogs. Adverse side effects include vomiting and defecation, as well as urinary retention and constipation with prolonged use.

Hydromorphone

Hydromorphone is a μ agonist, approximately five times more potent than morphine when administered at 0.05 to 0.2 mg/kg. The incidence of vomiting is not as common as with morphine, but is more common than seen with oxymorphone. Sedation is superior than that induced by morphine or oxymorphone. Panting should be expected but is of little clinical significance as overall minute ventilation is not impaired. Unlike morphine, IV injection is not associated with histamine release, and the duration of action is slightly shorter than morphine. It is more expensive than morphine, but more cost effective than oxymorphone and is therefore frequently used as a substitute for oxymorphone.

Oxymorphone

Oxymorphone is a μ agonist and is very similar to morphine but has approximately 10 times greater potency when administered at 0.05 to 0.1 mg/kg. This agent rarely induces vomiting and does produce mild sedation. Unlike morphine, IV injection of oxymorphone is not associated with histamine release. Its duration of action is similar or marginally shorter than that of morphine. Panting should be expected but is of little clinical significance. The cost is greater than that of hydromorphone or morphine, and the current supply in the United States is very limited because of a reduction in manufacturing.

Meperidine (pethidine)

Meperidine is a semisynthetic μ and κ agonist and is one fifth as potent as morphine. Doses of 1 to 3 mg/kg are required in dogs, and doses of 1 to 2 mg/kg may be administered in cats to induce a short-lasting analgesia (2 hours). This agent provides less sedation than morphine and does not induce vomiting. IV administration occasionally causes a severe anaphylactic reaction and is therefore not recommended. Meperidine depresses myocardial function and tends to increase heart rate because of the similarity of its molecular structure with atropine. The main advantage of meperidine consists of smooth muscle relaxation, justifying its use in horses with spasmodic colic and in biliary and renal colic in all species.

Methadone

Methadone is a synthetic pure μ agonist that is equipotent to morphine but prolongs analgesia, with less sedation and vomiting. Doses up to 1 mg/kg may be administered in dogs and cats. IV administration does not cause histamine release and may therefore be used for a faster onset of drug action. Its NMDA antagonistic activity may provide an additional mode of analgesia and prevent opioid tolerance.

Fentanyl

Fentanyl is a short-acting μ agonist with strong potency and a quick onset of analgesic properties. It does not cause histamine release and is popular for intraoperative and postoperative constant-rate infusion (CRI). Analgesia is dose related but accompanied by respiratory depression, and at high doses (≥20 μg/kg), it may only be used with O_2 and IPPV. In dogs, an infusion can start with a 3 to 5 μg/kg bolus followed by an infusion of 3 to 6 μg/kg/hr. In cats, half of these doses can be used. Cardiovascular effects are minimal, but bradycardia may be seen. Other congeners (e.g., sufentanil, remifentanil, alfentanil) are costly, limiting their current veterinary use. The transdermal fentanyl patch offers the advantage of a prolonged duration of effect for postoperative management of patients with severe pain. The patches come in several doses based on patient sizes. The patch must be applied for at least 12 hours before reaching effective plasma levels in dogs. However, after the plasma level is established, analgesia lasts for a few days. Transdermal fentanyl solution (Recuvyra) has recently become available to provides up to 4 days of analgesia with a single dose, applied 2 to 4 hours before surgery.

Opioid antagonists

The principles for application of antagonists are similar to those for sedative antagonists. Clinicians must match the duration of action of agonists and antagonists and remember that opioid antagonists will reverse analgesia.

Naloxone, naltrexone, and nalmefene

These drugs have pure antagonist effects, binding to opioid receptors but without any other intrinsic effect. The most common indications are to reverse opioid-induced sedation, respiratory depression, and excitement. Naloxone is recommended for treating opioid overdose in animals and humans, with doses ranging from 5 to 40 μg/kg. Naltrexone and nalmefene are longer acting pure antagonists but have been used less frequently than naloxone. If the duration of action of the antagonist is shorter than that of the agonist, the animal may return to sleep or experience respiratory depression. Close observation must be continued until the negative agonist effect fully wanes. Administration of an opioid antagonist will reverse analgesia and will complicate further postoperative analgesia with opioids.

Opioid partial agonists and mixed agonist–antagonists
Buprenorphine

Buprenorphine is a μ partial agonist and κ antagonist that is widely used in dogs and cats at doses ranging from 5 to 20 μg/kg. It is an effective analgesic, with the advantage of a prolonged duration of action (6–8 hours). It takes up to 45 minutes for full action even after being given through IV injection and delays recovery from anesthesia. Its disadvantages include the prolonged induction time and a "bell-shaped" dose-response curve,

in which increasing doses antagonize the analgesia that is already present. Therefore, if analgesia is inadequate after its use, further doses must not be given. Instead, any μ agonist, such as morphine or hydromorphone, is preferable. Its high affinity to μ receptors implies that reversal will be difficult because of a very slow dissociation from those receptors. If naloxone does not reverse respiratory depression, doxapram can be used for temporary reversal. Buprenorphine causes severe hallucinations in ambulatory human patients (as opposed to postoperatively), prompting its reclassification from a class V drug to a class III drug as awareness for abuse potential emerged.

Nalbuphine

Nalbuphine is a κ partial agonist and μ antagonist. This relatively new agent has been found to provide effective analgesia and is widely used in laboratory animals. Effects last 1 to 2 hours, and the drug is not classified as a controlled substance.

Butorphanol

Butorphanol is a κ partial agonist and μ antagonist, similar to nalbuphine, initially used as a cough suppressant in animals. It is 5 to 10 times more potent than morphine, with much lower analgesic efficacy. Potency should not be confused with efficacy, and both can be differentiated by understanding the use of dose-response curves to compare drugs. Most investigations failed to prove effective surgical pain management with butorphanol, warranting adjunct therapy when butorphanol is chosen as the main opioid used for pain management. Butorphanol provides mild sedation with minimal cardiopulmonary effects, and increasing doses lead to a ceiling effect on respiratory depression (i.e., further increases do not increase respiratory depression). The recommended dose is 0.1 to 0.5 mg/kg in dogs and 0.1 to 0.4 mg/kg in cats, with a duration of action approximating 2 hours. Intramuscular injection is painful, and it is recommended to take precautions not to be bitten when it is administered this way.

Development of new opioids

The research for new opioids is to identify alternatives to morphine that limit respiratory depression. However, thus far, no suitable alternatives have been found because a reduction in respiratory depression appears to result in a decrease in analgesia as well. The ideal opioid should also reduce the potential for abuse. Most partial agonists cause dysphoria, which is an unpleasant side effect and limits the potential for drug abuse. A specific and potent opioid with a reduction in side effects such as vomiting, excitement, euphoria, dysphoria, and vagal stimulation is also desirable. The more specific a drug is for opioid receptors, the less likely are the side effects, other than those related to stimulation of that receptor. A variety of pharmacokinetic ranges is desirable so that the length of action (longer or shorter) or the speed of onset of action can be adjusted to the needs. Currently, a good selection of options is available to alter the duration of drug action.

Use of opioids with sedatives

Sedative and opioid drugs have been combined for synergistic (i.e., the total effects are greater than the sum of the effects of the two drugs used individually) effects as early as 1932. In addition to the synergism of the sedative effect, the sedative was expected to counteract the undesirable effects of opioids (in particular, excitement and muscle rigidity) without increasing the opioid induced respiratory depression. Opioids were initially combined with "neuroleptic" agents such as the phenothiazines, hence the terms *neuroleptanalgesia* and *neuroleptanesthesia*. Neuroleptanalgesia was first used to produce sedation with higher doses of a potent opioid to produce a level of analgesia conducive to surgery. The concept has since been extended to include the use of any sedative type drug (i.e., benzodiazepines and α_2 adrenoceptor agonists) in combination with the opioids, and thus the term *neuroleptanalgesia* has been replaced by *sedative/opioid combinations*.

Nonsteroidal antiinflammatory drugs

Chapter 15 provides extensive information on these drugs. This section focuses specifically on the application of these agents for pain management in surgical patients. With the advent of potent NSAIDs such as carprofen and meloxicam, NSAIDs have become the analgesics of choice to manage acute perioperative pain in veterinary patients. However, the impact of carprofen on intraoperative surgical anesthesia remains controversial, ranging from little to no effect on the minimum alveolar concentration (MAC) of volatile anesthetics (Alibhai and Clarke 1996) to significant reduction of MAC by 15% (Yamashita *et al.* 2008). The discrepancy between these studies may reflect differences in administration because carprofen was administered subcutaneously 1 hour before anesthetic induction in the second study, but it was administered intravenously just before MAC determination in the first one. Compared with opioids, NSAIDs have the advantage of not decreasing consciousness or causing respiratory depression. Their antiinflammatory action contributes to healing and decreases pain. However, prolonged administration can result in drug accumulation and associated toxicity. Doses and new information cannot be transposed between species because of species differences in elimination times and toxicity. Cardiovascular support must precede IV administration of these drugs during anesthesia because the delay in elimination resulting from anesthetic-induced cardiovascular depression increases their toxicity.

NSAIDs exert analgesia by preventing formation of inflammatory mediators such as prostaglandins via inhibition of cyclooxygenase (COX) enzyme. Tissue injury induces the release of inflammatory mediators that stimulate pain sensation via nociceptor-mediated neuronal signaling. NSAIDs prevent this peripheral sensitization by blocking the synthesis of prostaglandins and other inflammatory mediators. Efforts have focused on the production of NSAIDs that inhibit the inducible COX-2 while sparing the physiological benefits of native COX-1 (see Chapter 15). As a result, newer NSAIDs have successfully reduced the incidence of side effects compared with earlier nonspecific COX inhibitors. Many small animal patients are now prescribed COX-2 selective NSAIDs for treatment of chronic pain such as osteoarthritis, thereby reducing the incidence of adverse effects. Selective COX-2 inhibitors also have a reduced influence on platelet activities, decreasing the risk of postoperative bleeding.

Carprofen (Rimadyl) has been widely used as an analgesic in dogs and appears very effective at doses of 4 mg/kg IV or SC given at premedication or induction. It is very long acting and has a much greater safety margin than flunixin. Other NSAIDs relevant to perioperative management of pain include meloxicam, ketoprofen, firocoxib, etodolac, and tepoxalin. Many NSAIDs, including carprofen, may be given by the oral route, facilitating their application in later stages of postoperative analgesia.

α_2 Adrenoceptor agonists

The α_2 agonists most commonly used in small animals include dexmedetomidine, medetomidine, romifidine, and xylazine. These drugs reduce the dose of anesthetics required to maintain anesthesia and provide some analgesia, especially against visceral rather than somatic pain. However, this analgesia is accompanied by sedation, as well as undesirable effects such as profound bradycardia, limiting their postoperative use. Although no premixed combination is commercially available, α_2 agonist and opioid combinations show marked synergism, generating various degrees of sedation and, in some cases, anesthesia. α_2 Agonists can provide effective analgesia with minimal side effects when used by the epidural route. If antagonists such as atipamezole, yohimbine, or tolazoline have been used, analgesia is reversed alongside sedation and other adverse side effects.

Other nonopioid, non-NSAID analgesics

Tramadol

Tramadol acts as a μ opioid agonist and as a monoamine reuptake inhibitor. This agent may be used as an alternative analgesic to NSAIDs in animals. However, possible side effects include stomachache, agitation, salivation, excitement, constipation, miosis, and bradycardia. Severe overdose potentiates seizures.

Tramadol comes in tablets, capsules, or ampules, but in some countries (e.g., the United States), the injectable form is not yet available. It has a bitter taste and therefore is usually mixed with syrups to increase acceptance by the animal. Recommended doses range between 4 and 8 mg/kg every 6 to 8 hours in dogs and 1 to 2 mg/kg every 12 hours in cats. Tramadol can be co-administered for a synergistic effect with gabapentin, NSAIDs, opioids, and amantadine but must not be used with tricyclic antidepressants (TCAs), selective serotonin reuptake inhibitors, or monoamine oxidase inhibitors.

Tapentadol

Tapentadol is structurally and functionally similar to tramadol, with a central analgesic property and a dual mode of action as an agonist at the μ opioid receptor and as a norepinephrine reuptake inhibitor (Tzschentke *et al.* 2007). Its analgesic efficacy is considered similar to that of tramadol with a potency intermediate between tramadol and morphine. However, unlike tramadol, it does not require metabolic activation and does not have isomer-dependent pharmacodynamics (Power 2011). Tramadol is approved by the U.S. Food and Drug Administration for treating moderate to severe acute pain in humans. However, its dual mode of action has resulted in off-label use for treating chronic pain. Use of serotonin and norepinephrine reuptake inhibitors has been proven effective in chronic pain management by increasing the effectiveness of opioids, NSAIDs, NMDA antagonists, and α_2 agonists against neuropathic pain such as human fibromyalgia and diabetic neuropathy. It is probable that some neuropathic pain in small animals could be effectively treated using this medication, but currently, few data are available regarding its dosing and frequency in small animals.

Gabapentin

Gabapentin is a GABA analog originally developed to treat epilepsy and later found useful in treating chronic neuropathic pain in humans. The mechanism of action for this analgesia is not well understood but may involve GABA synthesizing enzymatic activities and calcium channel blockade. Gabapentin has also been proposed to exert its pharmacologic effect by modulating synthesis of GABA and glutamate via the action of the GABA synthetic enzyme, glutamic acid decarboxylase (GAD), and the glutamate synthesizing enzyme and branched-chain amino acid transaminase (Taylor 1997). Gabapentin binds to the α2δ subunit of voltage-dependent calcium channels in the CNS to reduce calcium influx and inhibits the release of neurotransmitters, including norepinephrine and glutamate, resulting in subsequent analgesia or an antiepileptic effect (Powers *et al.* 1994; Davies *et al.* 2007).

Gabapentin has been successfully used in humans as an adjunct treatment for neuropathic pain when opioids and other analgesic classes do not provide adequate pain relief. However, in veterinary medicine, it has been more commonly used as an anticonvulsant rather than an analgesic. Nevertheless, this agent has the potential to provide similar benefits for veterinary patients as it does for humans, particularly in animals with neuropathic pain or pain associated with orthopedic procedures. The most common side effect in small animals consists of a mild sedation and ataxia. Gabapentin is typically administered orally in dogs, with an onset of effect within 1 to 2 hours. The recommended dose rate is 10 mg/kg twice daily for treating pain; higher doses and increased frequency are required for treating seizures. Although the drug dose and frequency is not well established in cats for analgesic use, a lower dose is suggested.

Pregabalin

Similar to gabapentin, pregabalin binds to the α2δ subunit of the voltage-dependent calcium channels in the CNS and inhibits the release of neurotransmitters, including norepinephrine and glutamate. Pregabalin increases neuronal GABA levels by producing a dose-dependent increase in glutamic acid carboxylase activity, which converts the excitatory neurotransmitter glutamate into the inhibitory GABA in a single step. This explains the increased efficacy of co-administered barbiturates and benzodiazepines in the presence of pregabalin. The main advantages of this agent over gabapentin include an accelerated onset of drug action and predictable duration of effect because of its linear pharmacokinetic profiles. Currently, the only evidence available regarding the use of pregabalin in small animals is limited to a few, anecdotal, positive reports in Internet-based discussion boards. Clinical trials are warranted to establish data on safe use of the drug in small animals.

Ketamine

Ketamine is classified as a dissociate anesthetic, frequently administered at induction to facilitate endotracheal intubation, or as a maintenance agent for short surgical or diagnostic procedures. Its analgesia is primarily mediated through NMDA antagonism. Tiletamine belongs to the same class but is only available in combination with zolazepam as telazol, limiting its practical use as an analgesic. Ketamine and other NMDA antagonists tend to offer a better somatic analgesia over a visceral one. Recently, using very low doses of ketamine (Table 14.4) given by CRI has gained popularity, frequently mixed with other classes of analgesics, including morphine and lidocaine, to manage perioperative pain and neuropathic pain refractory to opioids. Extended administration of ketamine may lead to accumulation, with associated hallucination, delirium, or excessive salivation.

Amantadine

Amantadine was originally developed as an antiviral agent to treat influenza infection but was subsequently found effective against Parkinson's syndrome and neuropathic pain. These effects may be mediated via dopaminergic agonism and NMDA receptor antagonism, respectively. Amantadine may be considered in animals with cancer, osteoarthritis, hyperalgesia, allodynia, and other types of neuropathic pain at dosages ranging from 2 to 4 mg/kg twice daily in dogs. Side effects in humans include hallucination, seizure, hyperactivity, dizziness, arrhythmia, diarrhea and flatulence.

Tricyclic antidepressants (amitriptyline, clomipramine)

The TCAs act primarily as serotonin-norepinephrine reuptake inhibitors, elevating extracellular concentrations of serotonin or norepinephrine and enhancing the availability of these neurotransmitters responsible for mood elevation. Additionally, they may also interact with NMDA receptors and transmembraneous sodium channels, which may account for their analgesic effect. These agents are mainly applied for treating depression, but amitriptyline is the most commonly prescribed TCA to treat neuropathic pain in dogs and humans. Many side effects may be related to the antimuscarinic properties of the TCAs, including dry mouth, mydriasis, constipation, drowsiness, agitation, sweating, muscle twitches, tachycardia, and rarely, irregular heart rhythms. The TCAs must not be co-administered with tramadol because of potential serotonergic storm. The recommended dosage ranges from 1 to 6 mg/kg twice daily in dogs for behavior modification or cataplexy, but few data are available regarding doses for analgesia.

Physical therapy, including acupuncture and transcutaneous electrical nerve stimulation

Alternative methods are gaining popularity as adjunct therapy for acute or chronic pain. Modalities include acupuncture, TENS, therapeutic ultrasound application, laser irradiation, and magnetic field therapy. The mechanism of action of acupuncture is not fully understood, but the gate control theory proposed by Melzack and Wall (1965) seems to offer a partial explanation for the analgesic properties of acupuncture or TENS. Briefly, the gate control theory postulates that both thin (sensory) and large-diameter (motor) nerve fibers carry information from the periphery into the dorsal horn of the spinal cord, where signal transmission synapses at different speeds. These differences explain why rubbing of a hand that has been hit by a hammer relieves the pain sensation and that analgesia achieved by acupuncture or TENS is achieved primarily through stimulation of large-diameter fiber transmission. An alternative theory proposes that TENS and acupuncture provide pain relief by stimulating the endogenous pain suppression system (e.g., release of endogenous opioid peptides).

Although many advocate strongly for the efficacy of TENS and recognize its unique place in pain management, this modality has not gained wide acceptance. TENS can be applied at high frequency (>50 Hz) with an intensity below motor contraction (sensory intensity) or low frequency (<10 Hz) with an intensity that produces motor contraction (Robinson and Snyder-Mackler 2007). Studies have demonstrated marked increases in β-endorphin and met-enkephalin in response to low-frequency TENS, with these antinociceptive effects being reversible by naloxone (Clement-Jones *et al.* 1980). However, high-frequency TENS analgesia was not reversed by naloxone, implicating a naloxone-resistant, dynorphin-binding receptor effect. Dynorphin levels were increased in the cerebrospinal fluid of these subjects. Application of TENS in animals poses a greater challenge because of their inability to tolerate noxious stimulation of electrical frequency, pulse duration, and amplitude necessary for optimal results. Consideration should be given to gradual acclimatization to TENS for animals with chronic pain and limited pharmacologic options.

Local and regional anesthesia

Several features of local anesthesia render it particularly useful in veterinary practice. Although many surgical procedures can be carried out satisfactorily under local anesthesia alone, sedation or general anesthesia may become necessary depending on the species, temperament, and health of the animal and on the type of procedure. Preemptive local anesthesia in animals undergoing general anesthesia reduces the amount of general anesthetic that is required, thus minimizing cardiopulmonary depression and accelerating recovery. In addition, local anesthesia provides pain relief extending past full recovery from general anesthesia. Local anesthesia can be largely subdivided into surface (or topical) anesthesia, infiltration anesthesia, intrasynovial anesthesia, and epidural anesthesia.

Local anesthesia has been most commonly carried out with sodium channel blockers such as lidocaine and bupivacaine. However, more recently, other classes of analgesics, including opioids, α2 agonists, NMDA antagonists, and NSAIDs, have gained popularity in small animals, particularly for epidural anesthesia in cranial laparotomies or hindlimb orthopedic procedures. These nonconventional local analgesics provide equal or superior analgesia for extended periods along with a reduction of side effects either when used alone or with a sodium channel blocker. This section focuses on various analgesics currently used for epidural anesthesia in small animals.

Anatomy and techniques for epidural anesthesia in dogs and cats

The epidural injection site in dogs and cats is located at the lumbosacral junction between the seventh lumbar (L7) and the first sacral vertebra (S1), with the animal in lateral or sternal recumbency (personal preference; see Figure 14.4). Because the canine spinal cord terminates around L6 to L7, anterior epidural anesthesia may be safely and easily induced at the lumbosacral junction. To locate the site, the iliac prominences on either side are identified, and an imaginary line is drawn between them, crossing the dorsal spinous process of the last lumbar segment. A spinal needle should be inserted on the midline, immediately caudal to this point. The epidural space is located immediately below the ligamentum flavum, separating the dura mater from the vertebral periosteum. The epidural space is identified by advancing the needle from an area of high resistance (ligamentum flavum) to an area of low resistance (epidural space). This is usually accomplished using the "hanging drop" or the "lack of resistance" technique during injection. Dangers of spinal and epidural block include hypotension, hindlimb motor paralysis, infection, and irritation.

Epidural injection should be differentiated from spinal (or intrathecal) injection, in which the anesthetic is injected into the subarachnoid space between the arachnoid membrane and the pia mater (space for injection of contrast media in myelograms). Anesthetic agents injected into the subarachnoid space (spinal injection) produce true spinal anesthesia because of the lack of protection provided by the dura mater and arachnoid meninges. Consequently, the volume of the anesthetic solution must be reduced by one third. These injections are prone to induce hypotension and should not be carried out without prior placement of an IV catheter for urgent fluid therapy.

A multimodal approach to epidural anesthesia offers several advantages, including reduced adverse effects, prolonged duration, and superior analgesia. CRI of analgesics has now become more frequent because of a prolonged duration of effect and ease of analgesic administration (see Figure 14.5). **Further studies are warranted to optimize agent selection and dosing in multimodal epidural anesthesia.**

Pharmacologic choices for epidural anesthesia
Sodium channel blockers

Sodium channel blockers interfere with nerve conduction by inhibiting the influx of sodium ions through ion-selective sodium channels in the nerve membrane, impairing the generation of an action potential. This effect blocks both sensory input and motor activity of the innervated area, thereby providing local anesthesia.

Lidocaine and bupivacaine are the two most commonly used sodium channel blockers in veterinary medicine. Lidocaine possesses a reasonably rapid onset of action, with good dispersal properties, and remains effective for 1 to 2 hours. Bupivacaine has a prolonged duration of action, lasting up to 8 hours, and is therefore preferred over lidocaine for epidural anesthesia, particularly for prolonged surgery and for postoperative analgesia.

Several precautions must be taken when using sodium channel blocker. Accidental IV injection is the most common cause of adverse reaction; excessive plasma concentrations may block cardiac sodium channels, depressing conduction and automaticity, potentially leading to cardiac arrest. It is therefore imperative to draw back on the syringe to check that the needle is not in a vein before injecting a sodium channel blocker local anesthetic. The toxic dose of lidocaine can be approximated to 8 mg/kg (much lower in cats, 3 mg/kg) and 4 mg/kg of bupivacaine (Chadwick 1985; Feldman et al. 1991; Lemo et al. 2007; Clarke et al. 2013). This amount can easily be reached with solutions at standard concentrations in very small animals such as domestic cats, small dogs, goat kids, birds, and small mammals. Solutions should therefore be diluted before administration.

The dose of sodium channel blocker indicated for epidural use is well below the toxic level, ranging between 2 and 4 mg/kg for lidocaine or 0.5 to 1 mg/kg of bupivacaine in dogs. Undesirable signs of overdose include initial sedation, which can be followed by twitching, convulsions, coma, and death with increasing doses. A common acceptable side effect consists of temporary hindlimb paralysis after recovery. Clinical research and observations support the combination of analgesics of different classes, such as opioids and α2 agonists, to extend the duration of epidural analgesia and improve motor function compared with animals treated with sodium channel blockers alone.

Opioids

Since the potential of opioids for epidural analgesia was recognized in the 1980s, they have gained a wider acceptance in human and veterinary medicine, and indeed the authors prefer opioids over sodium channel blockers in epidural anesthesia in small animals. Opioids have become the second most popular pharmacologic agents behind sodium channel blockers for epidural anesthesia. Among those, morphine and, to a lesser extent, hydromorphone are the most commonly used. The drugs bind to opioid receptors in the CNS to produce spinal analgesia. The major advantages of opioids include prolonged analgesia either alone or in combination with a sodium channel blocker and a motor-sparing effect that maintains the patient ambulatory. In a study by Kona-Boun et al. (2006), epidural administration of morphine (0.2 mg/kg) combined with bupivacaine (1 mg/kg) provided superior and prolonged analgesia compared with morphine (0.2 mg/kg) alone in dogs. The main concern after opioid epidural analgesia consists

Table **14.5** Examples of local and regional analgesic techniques in dogs and cats

Type	Nerves and coverage	Local anesthetic	Comments
Brachial plexus block	C5–C8 and T1; covers the midhumerus and down the digits	Lidocaine up to 4 mg/kg, bupivacaine up to 2 mg/kg; may mix with lidocaine and bupivacaine 1:1 for faster onset and extended duration	The needle must not enter the thorax or a major artery
RUMM nerve block	RUMM covers the distal thoracic limb	Lidocaine 2% or bupivacaine 0.5%, 0.1–0.15 mL/kg	Potential hematoma from arterial puncture and IV injection
Dental nerve block)	Maxillary, mandibular, mental, infraorbital	Lidocaine 2% or bupivacaine 0.5%, 0.3 to 1.5 mL per nerve	Same as above

IV, intravenous; RUMM, radial, ulna, median, and musculocutaneous.

Source: Campoy and Read, 2013. Reproduced with permission from John Wiley & Sons.

of urinary retention: urinary output should be closely monitored for 24 to 48 hours, occasionally requiring urinary catheterization, particularly in patients with a CRI epidural infusion, to avoid inadvertent bladder rupture.

α_2 Agonists

The mechanism of action of α_2 agonists is mainly mediated through their agonist activity at presynaptic α_2 adrenergic receptors, decreasing the release of norepinephrine from adrenergic nerve terminals in the CNS and periphery. This effect causes sedation, decreased sympathetic activity, analgesia, and hypotension. α_2 Agonists are mainly indicated to decrease anxiety, provide chemical restraint with relatively dependable sedation, potentiate effects of other drugs, and provide analgesia. The duration of action after systemic administration is dose dependent and typically results in 10 to 30 minutes of sedation and restraint for xylazine and 60 to 90 minutes for medetomidine. The ability to pharmacologically reverse them with α_2 adrenergic antagonists (atipamezole, yohimbine, and tolazoline) makes them very attractive.

α_2 Agonists, such as xylazine and detomidine, have been popular for epidural analgesia in large animals, including horses, because they induce less ataxia and have an extended duration of effect than lidocaine. In dogs, epidurally administered xylazine (0.25 mg/kg) provides analgesia and more than 4 hours of analgesia (Rector *et al.* 1998). Combining α_2 agonists with lidocaine or bupivacaine is believed to allow synergy, with superior and longer lasting analgesia than when a sodium channel blocker is used alone.

NMDA antagonists

The NMDA antagonists used in veterinary medicine include ketamine and tiletamine. Their mechanism of action is mediated through antagonistic effects on NMDA glutamate receptors, inhibiting neurotransmission and causing a variety of pharmacological effects, including analgesia. Because tiletamine is only available as a combined agent with zolazepam, ketamine is more practical for epidural administration. Epidural administration of ketamine at 0.4 to 1 mg/kg resulted in 90 to 240 minutes of analgesia in dogs (Rao *et al.* 1999; Acosta *et al.* 2005). Currently, better alternatives are available to provide epidural analgesia in small animals.

Summary

The selection of agents or methods (systemic or locoregional) to control pain control should be tailored to meet the individual needs of each patient, taking into consideration the nature of the surgical procedure, severity of pain, presence of risk factors for complications, and cost. Our understanding of pain in regards to its manifestation, mechanisms, assessment, and alleviation in animals is still evolving. Further work is needed to optimize safe and appropriate use of analgesics in animals. Finally, pharmacologic intervention should always be combined with comprehensive supportive care to effectively control pain in animals during healing and recovery from a surgery.

References

Acosta, A.D., Gomar, C., Correa-Natalini, C., et al. (2005) Analgesic effects of epidurally administered levogyral ketamine alone or in combination with morphine on intraoperative and postoperative pain in dogs undergoing ovariohysterectomy. *American Journal Veterinary Research* 66 (1), 54-61.

Alibhai, H.I.K., Clarke, K.W. (1996) Influence of carprofen on minimum alveolar concentration of halothane in dogs. *Journal of Veterinary Pharmacology and Therapeutics* 19 (4), 320-321.

Basbaum, A.I., Bautista, D.M., Scherrer, G. (2009) Cellular and molecular mechanisms of pain. *Cell* 139 (2), 267-284.

Bredersona, J., Kyma, P.R., Szallasi, A. (2013) Targeting TRP channels for pain relief. *European Journal of Pharmacology* 716 (1–3), 61-76.

Carrol, G.L. (1998) *Small Animal Pain Management.* American Animal Hospital Association Press, Lakewood, CO.

Chadwick, H.S. (1985) Toxicity and resuscitation in lidocaine- or bupivacaine-infused cats. *Anesthesiology* 63 (4), 385-390.

Clarke, K.W., Trim, C.M., Hall, L.W. (2013) *Veterinary Anaesthesia*, 11th edn. Saunders Elsevier, London.

Clement-Jones, V., McLoughlin, L., Tomlin, S., et al. (1980) Increased beta-endorphin but not met-enkephalin levels in human cerebrospinal fluid after acupuncture for recurrent pain. *Lancet* 2 (8201), 946-949.

Corder, G., Siegel, A., Intondi, A.B. (2010) A novel method to quantify histochemical changes throughout the mediolateral axis of the substantia gelatinosa after spared nerve injury: characterization with TRPV1 and substance. *The Journal of Pain* 11 (4), 388-398.

Davies, A., Hendrich, J., Van Minh, A.T., et al. (2007) Functional biology of the alpha(2)delta subunits of voltage-gated calcium channels. *Trends in Pharmacological Science* 5, 220-228.

Feldman, H.S., Arthur, G.R., Pitkanen, M., et al. (1991) Treatment of acute systemic toxicity after the rapid intravenous injection of ropivacaine and bupivacaine in the conscious dog. *Anesthesia & Analgesia* 73 (4), 373-384.

Gaynor, J.S., Muir, W.W. (2008) *Handbook of Pain Management*, 2nd edn. Mosby-Elsevier, Missouri.

Kona-Boun, J.J., Cuvelliez, S., Troncy, E. (2006) Evaluation of epidural administration of morphine or morphine and bupivacaine for postoperative analgesia after premedication with an opioid analgesic and orthopedic surgery in dogs. *Journal of the American Veterinary Medical Association* 229, 1103-1112.

Lemo, N., Vnuk, D., Radisic, B., et al. (2007) Determination of the toxic dose of lidocaine in dogs and its corresponding serum concentration. *Veterinary Record* 160 (11), 374-375.

Levine, J.D., Alessandri-Haber, N. (2007) TRP channels: targets for the relief of pain. *Biochimica et Biophysica Acta* 1772 (8), 989-1003.

Maddison, J.E., Page, S.W., Church, D.B. (2008) *Small Animal Clinical Pharmacology*, 2nd edn. Saunders, Philadelphia.

Melzack, R., Wall, P.D. (1965) Pain mechanisms: a new theory. *Science* 150 (699), 971-979.

Miller, P.E. (2008) Structure and function of the eye. In: Maggs, D., Miller, P., Ofri, R. (eds.) *Slatter's Fundamentals of Veterinary Ophthalmology,* 4th edn. Saunders Elsevier, St. Louis, pp. 1-19.

Murrell, J.C., Psatha, E.P., Scott, E.M., et al. (2008) Application of a modified form of the Glasgow pain scale in a veterinary teaching centre in the Netherlands. *Veterinary Record* 162, 403-408.

Pablo, E., Campoy, L., Read, M. (2013) Epidural and spinal anesthesia. In: Campoy, L., Read, M. (eds.) *Small Animal Regional Anesthesia and Analgesia,* 1st edn. Wiley-Blackwell, Ames, IA, pp. 227-259.

Power, I. (2011) An update on analgesics. *British Journal of Anaesthesia* 107 (1), 19-24.

Powers, P.A., Scherer, S.W., Tsui, L.C., et al. (1994) Localization of the gene encoding the alpha 2/delta subunit (CACNL2A) of the human skeletal muscle voltage-dependent Ca2+ channel to chromosome 7q21-q22 by somatic cell hybrid analysis. *Genomics* 1, 192-193.

Rao, K.N.M., Rao, K.V., Makkera, S., et al. (1999) Ketamine as epidural anaesthetic in dogs. *Indian Veterinary Journal* 76, 61-62.

Rector, E., Kramer, S., Kietzmann, M., Hart, S., et al. (1998) Evaluation of the antinociceptive effect of systemic and epidurally applied xylazine in general anesthesia with isoflurane in dogs and the effect of atipamezole injection on postoperative analgesia. *Berl Munch Tierarztl Wochenschr* 111 (11-12), 438-451.

Riviere, J.E., Papich, M.G. (2009) *Veterinary Pharmacology and Therapeutics,* 9th edn. Wiley-Blackwell, IA.

Robinson, A.J., Snyder-Mackler, L. (2007) *Clinical Electrophysiology: Electrotherapy and Electrophysiologic Testing,* 3rd edn. Lippincott Williams & Wilkins, Baltimore.

Stoelting, R.K., Hillier, S.C. (2005) *Pharmacology and Physiology in Anesthetic Practice,* 4th edn. Lippincott Williams & Wilkins, Baltimore.

Stone, L.S., Molliver, D.C. (2009) In search of analgesia: emerging roles of GPCRs in pain. *Molecular Interventions* 9 (5), 234-251.

Taylor, C.P. (1997) Mechanisms of action of gabapentin. *Revista de Neurologia (Paris)* 153 (Suppl. 1), S39-S45.

Tzschentke, T.M., Christoph, T., Kögel, B., et al. (2007) (1R,2R)-3-(3-dimethylamino-1-ethyl-2-methyl-propyl)-phenol hydrochloride (tapentadol HCl): a novel μ-opioid receptor agonist/norepinephrine reuptake inhibitor with broad-spectrum analgesic properties. *Journal of Pharmacology and Experimental Therapeutics* 323 (1), 265-276.

van Loon, J.P., Jonckheer-Sheehy, V.S., Back, W., et al. (2014) Monitoring equine visceral pain with a composite pain scale score and correlation with survival after emergency gastrointestinal surgery. *Veterinary Journal* 200 (1), 109-115.

van Nes, J.J., Meij, B.P., van Ham, L. (2009) Nervous system. In: Rijnberk, A., van Sluijs, F. (eds.) *Medical History and Physical Examination in Companion Animals,* 2nd edn. Saunders Elsevier, St. Louis, pp. 160-174.

Yamashita, K., Okano, Y., Yamashita, M. (2008) Effects of carprofen and meloxicam with or without butorphanol on the minimum alveolar concentration of sevoflurane in dogs. *The Journal of Veterinary Medical Science* 70 (1), 29-35.

15 Complications Associated with Nonsteroidal Antiinflammatory Drugs

Reza Seddighi[1] and Lyon Lee[2]

[1]College of Veterinary Medicine, The University of Tennessee, Knoxville, TN, USA
[2]Western University of Health Sciences, Pomona, CA, USA

Nonsteroidal antiinflammatory drugs (NSAIDs) are the oldest and, undoubtedly, one of the most successful drug classes used in modern medicine. NSAIDs are used to treat mild to moderate pain, fever, and inflammation. NSAIDs mediate their effects via inhibition of the synthesis of prostaglandins (PGs). PGs are products of the metabolism of arachidonic acid, a component of membrane glycerophospholipids of mammalian cells. Arachidonic acid subsequently interacts with two enzymes, lipoxygenase (LOX), and cyclooxygenase (COX), and produces leukotrienes and PGs, respectively (Vane 2000) (Figure 15.1). PGs act locally in different tissues (Table 15.1) and are involved in a number of processes such

Table 15.1 Main prostaglandins and their target tissues

	TxA_2	PGD_2	PGE_2	PGI_2	$PGF_{2\alpha}$
Tissues	Platelets	Mast cells	Brain	Endothelium	Uterus
	Vascular smooth muscle	Brain	Kidney	Vascular smooth muscles	Airways
	Macrophages	Airways	Vascular smooth muscle	Platelets	Vascular smooth muscles
	Kidney		Platelets	Kidney	Eyes
				Brain	

PG, prostaglandin; Tx, thromboxane.

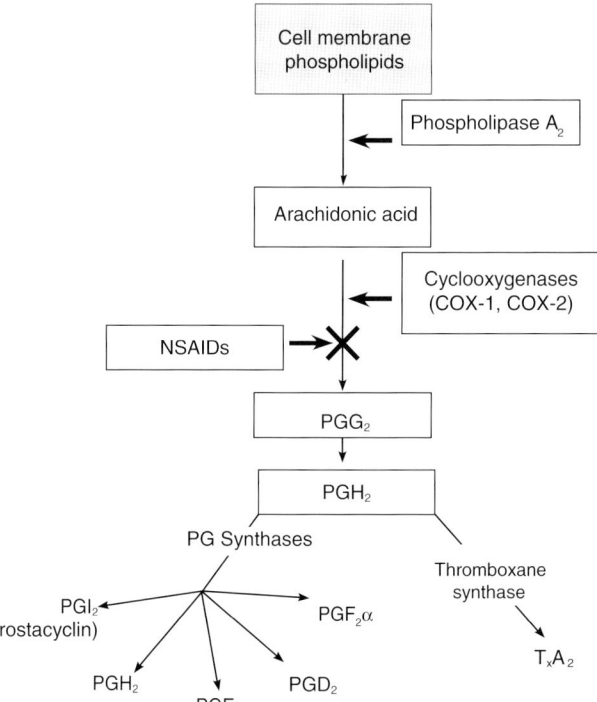

Figure 15.1 Mechanisms of action of nonsteroidal antiinflammatory drugs (NSAIDs) relative to synthesis pathway for prostaglandins. COX, cyclooxygenase; PG, prostaglandin; Tx, thromboxane.

as inflammation and blood clotting. The primary PGs and their target tissues are listed in Table 15.1.

The adverse effects of NSAIDs are also essentially related to their inhibition of COX isoenzymes and their resulting interference with PG formation (Figure 15.2). COX-1 is referred to as the constitutive or "housekeeping" isoform, and COX-2 is the inducible isoform. The genes coding for COX-1 and COX-2 are quite different in size, as are their respective mRNAs (Smith *et al.* 2000). COX-2 is induced, particularly in endothelial cells and monocytes, in response to proinflammatory cytokines. A third isoform, COX-3, a splice variant of COX-1, was cited as a target for acetaminophen and dipyrone (Chandrasekharan *et al.* 2002); however, this speculation does not appear to be of real significance (Kis *et al.* 2005).

Although COX-1 and COX-2 share similar structures, minor differences carry significant consequences in terms of drug development. An example is the exchange of isoleucine in COX-1 for valine in COX-2 at positions 434 and 523 (Flower 2003). These differences allow for a larger and more flexible channel for arachidonic acid binding to COX-2. This structural difference served as a basis in the development of NSAIDs that are selective for COX-2, the so-called "coxib" drugs. The term "coxib" is loosely used to define newer drugs that are designed to selectively inhibit COX-2; however, the term is vague because it neither denotes a chemical or pharmacologic class (Mitchell and Warner 2006).

Complications in Small Animal Surgery, First Edition. Edited by Dominique Griffon and Annick Hamaide.
© 2016 John Wiley & Sons, Inc. Published 2016 by John Wiley & Sons, Inc.
Companion website: www.wiley.com/go/griffon/complications

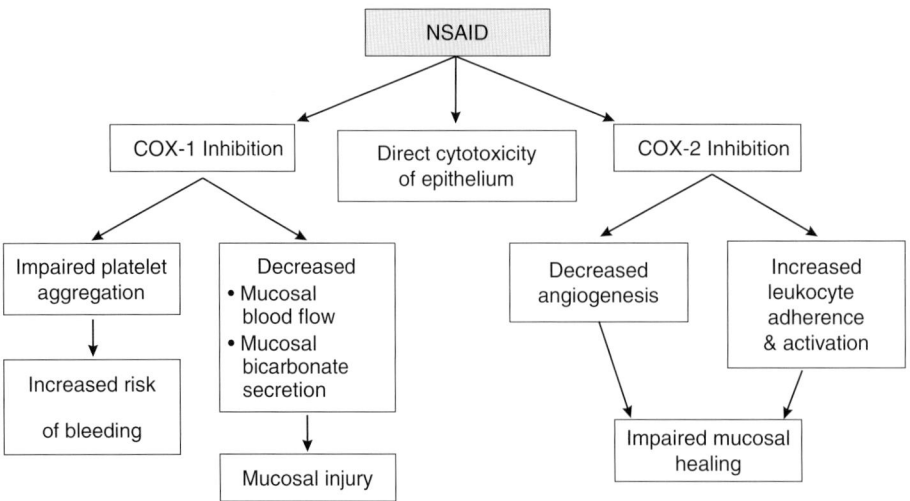

Figure 15.2 Pathophysiology of nonsteroidal antiinflammatory drug–induced gastric mucosal damage. COX, cyclooxygenase; NSAID, nonsteroidal antiinflammatory drug.

Gastrointestinal damage

Definition

The gastrointestinal (GI) toxicity of NSAIDs is considered to be their most common adverse effect (Table 15.2) and may range from mild gastritis, to gastroduodenal erosion and stricture, ulceration, perforation, bleeding, and even death (Jones *et al.* 1992; Bergh and Budsberg 2005).

Risk factors

Risk factors have not been extensively evaluated in animals; however, based on the literature on this topic in humans (Laine *et al.* 2002; Silverstein *et al.* 2000) and on data available for animals (Dow *et al.* 1990; Bergh and Budsberg 2005; Curry *et al.* 2005; KuKanich *et al.* 2012), the following may increase the risk of adverse effects of NSAIDs:

- Age: pediatric or geriatric patients
- Previous history of gastric ulceration
- Concurrent administration of NSAIDs, glucocorticoids, or corticosteroids
- Anticoagulant therapy
- Spinal disease (risk of colonic ulceration)
- Conditions affecting the perfusion of the gastric mucosa: dehydration, anesthesia, or critical illness (Vonderhaar and Salisbury 1993).

Diagnosis and clinical signs

The clinical signs of NSAID-induced GI toxicity range from vomiting, anorexia, and diarrhea to hematochezia or melena and death (KuKanich *et al.* 2012).

Gastrointestinal perforation was reported in 29 dogs that were administered celecoxib (Lascelles *et al.* 2005a). In most of those dogs, the first clinical sign associated with ulceration was vomiting, which was followed by anorexia and lethargy. It should be considered that animals with vomiting, diarrhea and anorexia may not always have GI erosions or ulcers because clinical signs may correlate poorly with GI tract injury (Dow *et al.* 1990). On the other hand, clinical effects may not always be present when erosions and ulcerations are present (Stanton and Bright 1989; Wooten *et al.* 2010).

Gastrointestinal injury may occur in different regions of the GI tract. In the aforementioned study, perforation was predominantly located in the pylorus or pyloroduodenal junction followed by the body of the stomach and duodenum and the jejunum (Lascelles *et al.* 2005a).

The onset of development of GI lesions depend on multiple factors such as the dose of NSAID administered, preexistent GI lesions, duration of the treatment, and co-administration of other NSAIDs or glucocorticoids. Twenty-six (90%) of the latter dogs were given deracoxib at a greater than the Food and Drug Administration–(FDA) approved dosage or at least one other NSAID or a corticosteroid in close temporal association with deracoxib administration (Lascelles *et al.* 2005a). The mean duration of NSAID administration before identification of GI perforation in the latter study was approximately 20 days.

Endoscopy of the GI tract is a common technique for determining the presence of NSAID-induced GI lesions (Dowers *et al.* 2006). Other techniques, such as contrast radiography, are also used. Some lesions, such as perforations, may be diagnosed (or treated) via exploratory laparotomy or may be diagnosed during necropsy (Lascelles *et al.* 2005a).

Prevention and treatment

Prevention of GI toxicity is based on identifying patients at risk, avoiding NSAIDs in the at-risk population, selecting NSAIDs with a greater safety profile (i.e., COX- I- sparing NSAIDs), and using NSAIDs in a dosing regimen that results in the lowest exposure necessary for efficacy. NSAIDs that undergo enterohepatic circulation (e.g., naproxen, carprofen, etodolac) may be associated with a greater incidence of GI adverse effects and should be used cautiously in at-risk animals (Boothe 2012). Decreasing the need for NSAID use, by co-administration of other analgesics and supportive disease-modifying agents should also be considered in susceptible populations. Enteric coatings and alternative routes of administration of NSAIDs (e.g., ketoprofen as a topical preparation) may also be considered (Mason *et al.* 2004; Boothe 2012). Additionally, because of their effects on healing, NSAIDs should be avoided or used cautiously in animals that have preexisting GI damage such as ulceration, are undergoing surgical intervention, or are

Chapter 15 Complications Associated with Nonsteroidal Antiinflammatory Drugs **99**

Table 15.2 Recommended dosages for use of nonsteroidal antiinflammatory drugs in small animals

NSAID	COX selectivity	Canine IC50 ratio	Dose (mg/kg) Dogs	Cats	Primary adverse effects	Comments
Aspirin	Preferential COX-1 inhibitor	—	10–25 PO q12h	10–20 PO q48–72h	Risk of subclinical GI bleeding (even after a single dose) Altered hemostasis Hypersensitivity in dogs Teratogenicity	Enteric-coated tablets are not recommended for dogs because of incomplete absorption. Buffering hastens gastric emptying of aspirin, thus decreasing the contact time of aspirin with the gastric mucosa and decreasing gastric absorption. Should be given with food to reduce GI irritation.
Carprofen	Preferential COX-2 inhibitor	6.5–15	2.0–4.4 IV, SC, IM, or PO q12–24h	2.0–4.0 (single dose) IV, SC, or IM	Typical NSAID toxicity Idiosyncratic hepatotoxicity Duodenal perforation in cats (when used for 7 days)	Repeated administration is not recommended in cats.
Deracoxib	Preferential COX-2 inhibitor	12–36.5	1–4 PO q24h	—	Typical NSAID toxicity	
Dipyrone	COX-3 (and some COX-1) inhibitor	—	25 IV or PO q8–12h	Same as dogs	Bone marrow toxicosis and teratogenicity Hypersensitivity in cats	Very limited use in veterinary medicine Irritation after IM or SC administration
Etodolac	Preferential COX-2 inhibitor	4.2	10–15 PO q24h	—	GI toxicity (when used at three times the dose) Transient decrease in serum proteins in chronic use Excessive hemorrhage during surgery	GI lesions similar to carprofen and less significant than buffered aspirin
Firocoxib	Highly selective COX-2 inhibitor	380	5 PO q24h	—	Typical NSAID toxicity	Not approved for use in cats
Ketoprofen	Nonselective COX inhibitor	0.2	0.25-1 IV, SC, IM, or PO q24h	1 SC or PO q24h for 3–5 days	Vomiting GI ulceration (risk greater than with carprofen but less than with aspirin)	Mainly used for short duration
Meloxicam	Preferential COX-2 inhibitor Equipotent COX-1 and COX-2 inhibitor (based on some studies)	2.1–10	0.2 (initial dose) SC or PO followed by 0.1 PO q24h	0.1–0.2 IM or SC (single dose) 0.025–0.05 PO q24h for ≤4 days	Typical NSAID toxicity	
Paracetamol (acetaminophen)	Inhibitor of the splice variant of COX-1 (COX-3) 5-HT3 inhibition?	—	10–15 PO q8h		Dogs: Hepatic dysfunction and secondary GI and CNS signs Methemoglobinemia and respiratory distress Keratoconjunctivitis sicca Acute renal failure GI toxicity

Cats: Edema of the face, cyanosis and methemoglobinemia, anemia, hemoglobinuria, icterus, and acute renal failure | Highly toxic in cats |
| Tepoxalin | COX/LOX inhibitor (dual inhibitor) | — | 10–20 PO followed by 10 mg/kg PO q24h | 5.0 PO q12h | Typical NSAID toxicity | |

CNS, central nervous system; COX, cyclooxygenase; GI, gastrointestinal; IM, intramuscular; IV, intravenous; LOX, lipoxygenase; NSAID, nonsteroidal antiinflammatory drug; PO, oral; q, every; SC, subcutaneous; IC50 ratio, COX-1/COX-2 inhibitory ratio, the ratio of 50% inhibition of COX-1 and COX-2.

Source: Data from Hanson and Maddison (2008), Boothe (2012), and Alwood (2009a,b).

concurrently being treated with glucocorticoids (Dow *et al.* 1990; Lascelles *et al.* 2005a; Narita *et al.* 2007).

Because of the failure of selective COX-2 inhibitors to eliminate the GI toxicity of NSAIDs, investigators have considered alternative strategies to improve the therapeutic index. Strategies include co-administration of pharmaceutical agents that decrease gastric acid secretion, replace PGs, or protect the damaged mucosa (Giannoukas *et al.* 1996; Dickman and Ellershaw 2004). Among the antisecretory drugs, proton pump inhibitors (PPIs), such as omeprazole, may be a safe, cost-effective method of reducing NSAID-induced gastropathy (Hawkey *et al.* 1998; Abraham *et al.* 2008; Scheiman *et al.* 2011). Although routine use of PPIs in apparently healthy animals may not be indicated, strong consideration should be given to their use in animals at risk of NSAID toxicity. PPIs generally have proved to be more effective than H_2 receptor blockers for this purpose (Boothe 2012).

Misoprostol, a synthetic PGE1 analog, is effective in treating and preventing NSAID-induced GI lesions in humans (Silverstein et al. 1995). In a study of six dogs treated with aspirin, concurrent administration of misoprostol effectively decreased the severity of endoscopically detectable gastroduodenal lesions (Johnston et al. 1995). Misoprostol has potentiated the antiinflammatory effect of a variety of compounds in animals and appears to have analgesic effects at high concentrations, acting synergistically with NSAIDs (Shield 1998). Misoprostol may be more effective in the presence of agents that decrease gastric acid secretion (Giannoukas et al. 1996). More recently, DA-9601, an antioxidant with antiinflammatory and cytoprotective effects, was shown to be more effective than misoprostol in decreasing the GI effects of NSAID therapy in human patients (Lee et al. 2011).

Although the efficacy of antisecretory drugs and PG substitutes is shown in human medicine, their clinical benefits in dogs remain unclear, and the results of different studies are somewhat controversial (Boulay et al. 1986; Jenkins et al. 1991). For instance, omeprazole (0.7 mg/kg orally [PO] every 24 hours), misoprostol (2 mcg/kg PO every 8 hours), or placebo administered to dogs treated with glucocorticoids for intervertebral disc disease did not create any significant difference in decreasing endoscopic gastric mucosal scores (Neiger et al. 2000). However, omeprazole (1.0–2.5 mg/kg PO every 24 hours) increased gastric pH significantly more than famotidine (1.0–1.3 mg/kg PO every 24 hours) and placebo in laboratory dogs (Tolbert et al. 2011). Also, omeprazole (1.0 mg/kg PO every 24 hours) significantly decreased exercise-induced gastritis in sled dogs compared with famotidine (2 mg/kg PO every 24 hours) or placebo (Williamson et al. 2010).

Gastroprotectants are the other group of pharmaceuticals that are used to protect from GI adverse effects of NSAIDs and include sucralfate and potentially glucosamine and chondroitin products. The benefits of sucralfate in the treatment of NSAID-induced adverse GI events include binding to and protecting damaged mucosa, increasing PG synthesis, angiogenesis, and sulfhydryl production at the site of damage. The advantage of the combined use of glucosamine and NSAIDs is the potential for gastroprotection caused by enhanced mucopolysaccharide production (Boothe 2012).

Despite these strategies to limit the GI adverse effects of NSAIDs, research continues to focus on the development of **novel NSAIDs** to improve their safety, such as p**hosphatidylcholine- (PC-) conjugated NSAIDs**. Surface-active phospholipids contribute to the GI mucosal barrier, thereby playing a protective role against cellular damage. Pre-association of NSAIDs with phospholipids preserves the protective effects of the surface-active phospholipid layer and prevents gastric damage. The use of aspirin pre-associated with PC in humans and rats (Kurinets and Lichtenberger 1998; Anand et al. 1999) and ibuprofen–PC in rats (Lichtenberger et al. 2001) have yielded encouraging results.

Another category of novel NSAIDs are **gaseous mediator-releasing NSAIDs.** Nitric oxide (NO) and hydrogen sulfide (H$_2$S) are endogenous gaseous mediators that produce many of the same physiological effects as PGs in the GI tract (Wallace and Miller 2000; Fiorucci et al. 2006). Administration of NO or H$_2$S donors increases the resistance of the gastric mucosa to the NSAID-induced damage (Fiorucci et al. 2005; MacNaughton et al. 1989; Whittle et al. 1990) and accelerates the healing of ulcers in rodents (Konturek et al. 1993; Elliott et al. 1995). NO also stimulates the release of vascular endothelial growth factor (Ma et al. 2002), which can promote angiogenesis and ulcer healing (Wallace 2008). In animal studies (Wallace et al. 1994b; Wallace et al. 1994a) and human clinical trials (Fiorucci et al. 2003; Hawkey et al. 2003), NO-releasing NSAIDs, described as COX-inhibiting nitric oxide donors (CINODs) produce significantly less GI injury than the parent NSAIDs. NO- and H$_2$S-releasing NSAIDs also protect the heart from ischemia/reperfusion injury in animal models (Rossoni et al. 2004; Rossoni et al. 2008).

Outcome

The prognosis for GI lesions depends on the extent of the damage and early diagnosis. In a retrospective study on 29 dogs that developed GI perforation, primarily caused by NSAID overdosage, 20 dogs died or were euthanatized because of the extent of the lesions, and only 9 survived (Lascelles et al. 2005a). Therefore, considering the wide range of clinical presentations and the weak correlation between GI damage and the clinical signs, it is imperative that animals with a history of NSAID therapy that exhibit clinical signs of GI irritation (e.g., vomiting), lethargy, or anorexia be further evaluated and treated.

Renal disease

Definition

The most common adverse renal effects of NSAIDs are interference with fluid and electrolyte homeostasis. Less frequently, adverse effects include acute renal failure, interstitial nephritis, nephritic syndrome, atrophy of subcapsular cortex in dogs, and renal papillary necrosis. Rats and dogs usually exhibit greater susceptibility than humans to renal papillary necrosis (Khan and Alden 2002).

Risk factors

Based on studies of human patients, the following can be listed as potential risk factors for veterinary patients in development of renal toxicity (Mathews et al. 1990; Mathews 1996; Curry et al. 2005; Narita et al. 2007):

- Preexisting renal disease
- Chronic use of NSAIDs
- Geriatric or very young animals
- Anesthesia, dehydration, shock
- Hepatic insufficiency
- Concurrent use of nephrotoxic drugs (e.g., aminoglycosides)
- Concurrent use of corticosteroids
- Co-administration of angiotensin-converting enzyme inhibitors
- Concurrent diseases (e.g., hypertension, diabetes, cardiac failure)

Diagnosis

The diagnosis of NSAID-induced acute renal failure is based on the history of NSAID use and clinical signs such as sudden onset of depression, lethargy, anorexia, vomiting, diarrhea, oliguria, or polyuria (Senior 1999). Laboratory findings in these animals are usually nonspecific and may include azotemia, changes in fractional clearance, and an increase in urine-specific gravity (Lobetti and Joubert 2000). In dogs with renal toxicity induced by NSAIDS, renal blood flow (RBF) may decrease without any alteration in the glomerular filtration rate (GFR) (Feigen et al. 1976; Rodriguez et al. 2000), suggesting that GFR is not an appropriate indicator of acute NSAID-induced renal toxicity.

Prevention

In contrast to NSAID-associated GI adverse events, the risk of renal adverse effects may not necessarily be reduced with the use of newer COX-2–selective drugs. Currently, preventive measures, including therapy with sodium-containing fluids, minimizing drug interactions, and avoidance of NSAIDS in patients at risk, appear to be the best methods for avoiding nephrotoxicity (KuKanich et al. 2012). Anesthesia and hypotension may contribute to NSAID renal toxicity because inhalational anesthetics cause a dose-dependent decrease in RBF in dogs (Hartman et al. 1992; Takeda et al. 2002). Therefore, during anesthesia, careful monitoring of the cardiovascular status and concurrent administration of intravenous (IV) fluids to ensure adequate perfusion of vital organs, including the kidneys, is imperative and helps to minimize the risk for renal toxicity. Animals with decreased serum sodium concentrations or decreased renal perfusion (e.g., shock, dehydration, hemorrhage) should only be given NSAIDs after their cardiovascular status has been stabilized.

Treatment

Several studies have attempted to identify methods to prevent or treat NSAID-induced nephropathies. Misoprostol does not have a recognized role in the prevention or treatment of NSAID-induced nephrotoxicity (Boothe 2012). N-acetylcysteine has been studied experimentally, and its protective mechanism is thought to be due to vasodilation (D'Angio 1987; Aitio 2006). Although animal models support the efficacy of this approach, clinical trials, including meta-analyses, have failed to provide conclusive evidence of efficacy (Levin et al. 2007). Nonetheless, in the absence of effective therapies, N-acetylcysteine is generally recommended (~10 mg/kg or more PO twice daily) preventively for drug-induced toxicity (Boothe 2012).

Outcome

Favorable prognosis can be expected in animals that are diagnosed early in the course of the disease and when NSAID treatment is discontinued before significant renal damages are sustained.

Hepatic disease

Definition

The clinical presentation of NSAID-induced hepatic injury ranges from mild cholestasis to severe hepatocellular injury. Hepatotoxicity caused by NSAIDs has been proposed to be either idiosyncratic (unpredictable, not dose-related) or intrinsic (predictable and dose-related), due to a direct action on cells or tissue (Bjorkman 1998; Tolman 1998). The toxicity of acetaminophen, aspirin, and phenylbutazone is considered intrinsic (Papich 2008; Bjorkman 1998). The hepatotoxic effects of aspirin are predominantly dose dependent, anicteric (not associated with jaundice), rarely fatal, and usually reversible upon cessation of treatment (Bjorkman 1998). A breed predisposition for carprofen-induced idiosyncratic hepatotoxicosis is reported in Labrador retriever dogs (MacPhail et al. 1998).

Risk factors

- Animals with underlying hepatic disease (slower elimination of NSAIDs, greater risk for GI adverse effects)
- Large doses of NSAIDs (?)

Diagnosis

Nonspecific clinical signs such as vomiting, diarrhea, anorexia, lethargy, depression, and icterus may suggest hepatic toxicity. Early intensive monitoring of hepatic function is recommended because

hepatic toxicity is more likely to occur during the first few weeks of treatment (MacPhail et al. 1998; Lascelles et al. 2005b). Cholestatic injury results from impairment of bile secretion, resulting in an increase in alkaline phosphatase activity and bilirubin but with little change in aminotransferases activity (Zimmerman and Lewis 1987). Hepatocellular injury from metabolic inhibition, oxygen radical toxicity, immunologically mediated damage, or some other mechanism results predominantly in increases in aminotransferase activity, with smaller increases in alkaline phosphatase activity or bilirubin (Boelsterli et al. 1995; Manoukian and Carson 1996). The intervals for laboratory retesting can be extended depending on the dog's response. It seems prudent to determine baseline renal and hepatic panels before initiating chronic NSAID therapy and to repeat testing within the first 2 weeks and periodically thereafter (KuKanich et al. 2012).

Prevention

Preexisting hepatic disease is not necessarily a contraindication to administration of an NSAID (Papich 2008); however, it is not clear whether NSAIDs can be safely administered to patients with hepatic disease (Laffi et al. 1997). The consumption of NSAIDs by humans with chronic liver disease can provoke hepatorenal syndrome, diuretic-resistant ascites, and gastroesophageal ulceration, which are likely the result of COX inhibition in the kidney and GI tract. There is no evidence that prior hepatic disease predisposes an animal to NSAID-induced liver injury, and drug enzyme systems are remarkably preserved in hepatic disease (Papich 2008).

Nevertheless, because of the risk of decreased elimination, administration of NSAIDs to animals with hepatic diseases may warrant extra caution. Additionally, because animals with liver disease may be more prone to GI ulceration (Stanton and Bright 1989), independent of NSAID administration, it is possible that the administration of NSAIDs to these patients may increase the risk of this complication (KuKanich et al. 2012). Therefore, when an animal is receiving an NSAID, any unexplained increase in hepatic enzyme activity or bilirubin concentration, 7 to 90 days after initiating NSAID administration, should be investigated (Papich 2008).

Acetaminophen, an atypical NSAID, is the second most common cause of NSAID toxicity in small animals (see Table 15.2). These toxicities occur after an accidental exposure or deliberate administration in dogs and cats. Toxicity from acetaminophen results when the metabolic pathways for glucuronidation and sulfation are absent or depleted and the toxic metabolite N-acetyl-p-benzoquinone-imine (NAPQI) accumulates, causing oxidative injury (Alwood 2009).

Cats are genetically sensitive to acetaminophen because they lack the glucuronyl transferase enzyme required to detoxify the reactive biotransformation metabolites (Wilcke 1984; Robertson 2008) and acetaminophen-induced hepatotoxicity and icterus are cats is well known (Robertson and Taylor 2004; Taylor and Robertson 2004; Robertson 2008). Acetaminophen toxicity may result from doses exceeding 75 mg/kg in dogs, but doses as low as 10 mg/kg have been associated with toxicity in cats. Therefore, use of acetaminophen in cats, at any dose, is contraindicated (Jones et al. 1992; Alwood 2009). In addition, acetaminophen is known to cause Heinz body formation, methemoglobinemia, anemia, and hemoglobinuria in cats (Finco et al. 1975; Allen 2003).

Outcome

The clinical course of the hepatic toxicity induced by NSAIDs is variable; however, in most animals, resolution of the clinical signs and improvement or resolution of biochemical abnormalities occurs soon after discontinuation of the NSAID and administration of supportive care.

Interference with coagulation and hematopoiesis

Definition
Prolongation of bleeding times and the tendency for bleeding, especially in at-risk populations, is reported in animals that have received NSAIDs. Thromboxane A2 (TxA2) is primarily associated with platelets, stimulating their aggregation along with vasoconstriction, thereby enhancing coagulation and blood clot formation. Inhibition of COX-1 produces an anticoagulant effect (KuKanich et al. 2012).

Risk factors
- von Willebrand's disease (Dobermans and Scottish terriers)
- Chronic administration of NSAIDs
- Administration of high doses of NSAIDs

Diagnosis
Coagulation tests (e.g., bleeding time) should be performed in animals that have the tendency to bleed or have been receiving NSAIDs.

Prevention
The baseline coagulation status of at-risk animals should be determined before NSAID therapy. Although the use of aspirin as an antithrombotic agent is not common in animals, administration at inappropriate dose or in at-risk animals may result in bleeding caused by irreversible effects on platelets (Sakai et al. 2003). In suspected cases of coagulopathy, discontinuation of NSAID administration at least 1 week before major surgeries, especially in the case of aspirin, may be necessary.

Outcome
Myelotoxicity (agranulocytosis) occurs relatively commonly in humans but is rare in dogs. Blood dyscrasias have been reported occasionally in association with the use of phenylbutazone in dogs (Hanson and Maddison 2008). COX-2 activity results in vasodilation and inhibition of platelet aggregation, producing an antagonistic effect to TxA_2 (Simmons et al. 2004). Therefore, exclusive inhibition of COX-2 produces a procoagulant effect. However, there is no evidence for increased cardiovascular events with COX-2 selective NSAIDs in dogs (Hanson and Maddison 2008). The platelet dysfunction induced by NSAIDs is unlikely to result in spontaneous bleeding in normal animals but may aggravate a bleeding tendency in animals with inherited disorders of hemostasis or in animals undergoing surgery (Littlewood 1999).

Interference with bone and cartilage metabolism

Definition
Although controversial, NSAIDs are reported to cause some adverse effects on bone healing. A greater risk for nonunion and decrease in the biochemical properties of the callus are reported, especially when NSAIDS are used for longer period of time or at greater doses (Bergenstock et al. 2005; Bergmann et al. 2005; Goodman et al. 2005). In laboratory animals, inhibition of angiogenesis resulted in nonunion or delayed union, even in the case of COX-2 inhibitors (Murnaghan et al. 2006). Chronic NSAID therapy may also worsen cartilage degeneration in animals with osteoarthritis through impaired proteoglycan synthesis, although its clinical importance is unclear (Abernathy et al. 1992).

Risk factors
- Compromised fracture healing
- Very young or old animals

Diagnosis
The diagnosis is based on serial radiographs and clinical orthopedic examinations in suspected animals with a history of NSAID treatment.

Prevention
Avoid long-term or high doses of NSAIDs after fracture repair, especially in at-risk animals (with infected, complicated fractures).

Outcome
No firm evidence-based recommendation can be made regarding the use of NSAIDs in fracture treatment. The risk of delayed bone healing with long-term administration or greater doses of these drugs, especially in patients with compromised fracture healing, may further delay the repair. However, the benefits of short-term administration of NSAIDs, within recommended doses (see Table 15.2), outweigh the risk of compromised bone healing (Griffon 2010).

Relevant literature

Epidemiology
The incidence of NSAID-induced toxicity on each body system in veterinary patients is unclear; however, based on the human data, NSAIDs induce gastric ulceration occurs in up to 4% of human patients after chronic administration, and the incidences of adverse gastric events in at-risk human patients taking traditional NSAIDs and COX-2 selective NSAIDs are 17.1% and 16.5%, respectively (Silverstein et al. 2000). **GI toxicity** is the most predictable and serious adverse effect associated with NSAIDs use in human beings and companion animals (Collins and Tyler 1985; Jones et al. 1992; Meddings et al. 1995; Hunt and Yuan 2011) (see Table 15.2).

Renal toxicity is considered the second most likely adverse effect of NSAIDs, especially in at-risk animals, and is primarily attributable to reduced RBF and GFR secondary to inhibition of renal PG synthesis. Most clinically used NSAIDs have been implicated in renal damage. In contrast to humans and horses, there are no comprehensive data on the prevalence of NSAID-associated renal toxicity in dogs and cats (Hanson and Maddison 2008). Nevertheless, it is reported that 50% of the surveyed cases of acute renal failure in cats were associated with NSAID therapy (Steagall et al. 2009; Boothe 2012), which underlines the need for monitoring of renal function in cats being treated with NSAIDs long term, particularly if other risk factors for renal disease are present.

Although the risk of **NSAID-associated hepatotoxicity** is considerably less than that of upper GI complications, NSAIDs have been associated with hepatotoxicity in humans and animals (Bjorkman 1998; Lee 2003; Nakagawa et al. 2005). All NSAIDs, regardless of their COX selectivity, have the potential for causing hepatic injury (Lee 2003). Acute idiosyncratic hepatotoxicosis was reported in a group of dogs treated with carprofen for an average of 19 days (MacPhail *et al.* 1998). In the latter study, Labrador retrievers were the most common breed affected (MacPhail *et al.* 1998). Labrador retrievers are the most popular breed in the United States and are often affected by musculoskeletal disorders such as osteoarthritis, hip dysplasia, and rupture of the cranial cruciate ligament; therefore, the increased incidence of toxicity in Labrador retrievers is probably a reflection of breed popularity and frequency of NSAID administration in that breed (KuKanich *et al.* 2012).

The potential **interference of NSAIDs with bone healing** has been questioned because of the role PGs play during fracture repair (Raisz 1990; Kawaguchi *et al.* 1995). However, the incidence of these adverse effects is much less than GI complications. Experimental data have also been published on the **deleterious effects of NSAIDs on cartilage metabolism**, especially with chronic administration. In a canine cartilage explant model, carprofen directly decreased proteoglycan synthesis by chondrocytes (Benton *et al.* 1997). Aspirin seems to have the most consistent adverse effect on matrix production (Johnston and Budsberg 1997). However, large doses of NSAIDs are needed to produce these lesions (Palmoski and Brandt 1983), and it is not known if NSAIDs administered at the recommended doses to clinical patients would contribute to cartilage degradation (Papich 1997).

Overall, experimental data support the notion that long-term administration of NSAIDs may interfere with fracture healing and cartilage metabolism, but no clinical evidence of these adverse effects have been reported in small animals. Aspirin, indomethacin, ibuprofen, and naproxen caused increased cartilage degeneration in arthritic and unstable joints in experimental murine and canine models, but ketoprofen and diclofenac did not (Palmoski and Brandt 1982, 1983). Meloxicam does not appear to adversely affect synthesis of cartilage proteoglycans in vitro. Carprofen may adversely affect chondrocyte metabolism but only if present in synovial fluid at large concentrations that do not appear to be reached in vivo (Hanson and Maddison 2008). Therefore, the benefits of short-term administration of therapeutic doses of NSAIDs seem to overweigh the potential risk of interference with bone or cartilage metabolism.

Interference with PGs by NSAIDs can be expected to result in **adverse effects on platelet function, hematopoiesis, and thrombosis**. Inhibition of platelet aggregation and a predisposition to bleeding are potential concerns with all NSAIDs (Weiss 2000). Chronic administration of aspirin should be discontinued at least 1 week before surgery to reduce the likelihood of intraoperative bleeding (Curry *et al.* 2005). Aplastic anemia may occur with phenylbutazone administration because of its selective toxicity on hematopoietic stem cells of the bone marrow. This toxicity occurs sporadically, generally after long-term treatment; is not dose dependent; and may or may not resolve after discontinuation of the drug (Boudreaux 2000). From a clinical standpoint, commonly used doses of ketoprofen and diclofenac (Naclerio-Homem *et al.* 2009), meloxicam (Rinder *et al.* 2002), and nimesulide (Marbet *et al.* 1998) did not alter the coagulation profile of healthy human patients. Similarly, administration of NSAIDs to healthy animals at clinically relevant doses has not been associated with significant changes in coagulation. Meloxicam did not adversely affect the coagulation profile in dogs undergoing orthopedic surgery when administered either as a single subcutaneous dose (0.2 mg/kg) at premedication or daily oral dosing (0.1 mg/kg)

for 5 days followed by a single subcutaneous administration (0.2 mg/kg) preoperatively (Kazakos *et al.* 2005). In another study in dogs, meloxicam (0.2 mg/kg IV immediately before induction of anesthesia) or ketoprofen (2 mg/kg IV 30 minutes before the end of surgery) had no significant effects on buccal mucosal bleeding and whole blood clotting times (Deneuche *et al.* 2004). Overall, it appears that the clinical significance of the bleeding predisposition (i.e., platelet inhibition) primarily depends on the type of NSAID, dosage, and underlying disease that may predispose the animal to development of adverse effects. For instance, a decrease in the production of TxA_2 subsequent to COX-1 inhibition may predispose thrombocytopenic animals or those with coagulopathies (e.g., von Willebrand's disease, hemophilia, liver failure, rodenticide intoxication) to bleeding (Weiss 2000).

Roles of cyclooxygenase isoenzymes and cyclooxygenase selectivity

Various measures such as the **IC50 ratio** (**COX-1/COX-2 inhibitory ratio**; the ratio of 50% inhibition of COX-1 and COX-2) are used to present the safety of NSAIDs, although the clinical applicability of these is limited. For instance, the IC50 ratio is determined in vitro conditions may not correspond to effective doses or minimize adverse effects (KuKanich *et al.* 2012). Additionally, species-specific differences in the COX inhibitory concentrations have been documented for some NSAIDs (Lees *et al.* 2004). For example, the reported IC50 COX-1/COX-2 ratio for carprofen is 0.020 (COX-1 preferential) in humans to 16.8 (COX-2 preferential) in dogs (Warner *et al.* 1999; Streppa *et al.* 2002). Therefore, extrapolations of COX inhibitory ratios between species may not be accurate and should be avoided (KuKanich *et al.* 2012). Nevertheless, the same ratio has been used as a measure to primarily compare the safety of different NSAIDs (see Table 15.2).

Gastrointestinal complications result essentially from the **suppressive effects of NSAIDs on the synthesis of PGs**. PGs protect the mucosa through several mechanisms, including inhibiting acid secretion, dilating the vessels in the gastric mucosa, and stimulating the secretion of mucus and duodenal bicarbonate. COX-1 and COX-2 seem to contribute to gastric mucosal defense, COX-1 predominating in healthy mucosa, and COX-2 expression occurring after events such as mucosal irritation (Gretzer *et al.* 2001) or when COX-1 is suppressed (Davies *et al.* 1997). Selective COX-2 inhibitors (coxibs) were developed with the hope of decreasing the prevalence of GI adverse effects by specifically targeting the COX-2 pathway. It is now evident that NSAID-induced gastropathy necessitates that COX-1 and COX-2 be inhibited because when COX-1–sparing NSAIDs are used in humans the incidence of adverse effects was decreased by half but not eliminated (Scheiman 1996; Kawai 1998; Silverstein *et al.* 2000). Similar results are reported from animal studies (Wright 2002; Bergh and Budsberg 2005). The fact that the COX-2 enzyme may also have a protective effect on GI mucosal border and is important in maintaining mucosal health (Gretzer *et al.* 2001) and GI healing (Mizuno *et al.* 1997) explains the unexpected incidence of adverse effects with selective COX-2 inhibitors. Administration of a selective COX-1 inhibitor does not cause mucosal injury, and COX-1–deficient mice do not spontaneously develop gastric ulceration and are actually less susceptible to NSAID toxicity than normal mice (Sigthorsson *et al.* 2002). COX-2–deficient mice develop more severe ulceration after NSAID treatment than do normal mice (Langenbach *et al.* 1995), and co-administration of a selective COX-1 and a selective COX-2 inhibitor causes hemorrhagic ulceration (Wallace *et al.* 2000).

Both COX isoforms are present in the kidney, and in animals, COX-1 and COX-2 co-localize in the macula densa (Smith and Bell 1978). COX selectivity does not seem to translate into renal-sparing effects, presumably because the constitutive expression of COX-2 influences salt and water regulation and hemodynamics in the kidney, thereby maintaining normal RBF, GFR, and electrolyte excretion (Harris et al. 1994; Rossat et al. 1999; DeMaria and Weir 2003). Glomeruli and arterioles synthesize the vasodilatory PGs, PGE_2 and PGI_2, and the vasoconstrictor TxA_2. The primary renal cortical actions of these PGs (PGE_2 and PGI_2) are renal vasodilation and maintenance of GFR or renal vasoconstriction and reduction of GFR (TxA_2) (Dunn et al. 1984). Although RBF is normally not dependent on PGs, formation of renal eicosanoids becomes crucial to the maintenance of renal homeostatic mechanisms under conditions that may be relevant to surgical patients (Knights et al. 2005). For instance, during volume depletion, the renin–angiotensin system is activated to increase vascular resistance and maintain systemic blood pressure; renal PGs are released to offset the effect of vasoconstriction and maintain perfusion of the kidneys (Dunn et al. 1984). These patients become more vulnerable to the renal adverse effects of NSAIDs.

Regarding hepatic toxicity with NSAIDs, at least in the case of intrinsic (dose-dependent) toxicity, COX selectivity does not have a significant effect in dogs, and all NSAIDs have the potential for causing hepatic injury (Lee 2003; KuKanich et al. 2012).

Pathogenesis of complications associated with nonsteroidal antiinflammatory drugs

Local and systemic mechanisms have been implicated in the **pathogenesis of NSAIDs-induced GI damage** (Box 15.1). GI-induced NSAID toxicity may result indirectly through the inhibition of PGE2 and directly by irritating the GI mucosa. NSAID-associated GI ulcers are most commonly reported in the proximal duodenum and pylorus of dogs (Stanton and Bright 1989; Dow et al. 1990; Lascelles et al. 2005a). There is a suggestion that long-term usage of NSAIDs, including COX-2–selective NSAIDs, increases the incidence of duodenal ulcers (Hanson and Maddison 2008).

Box 15.1 Pathogenesis of NSAIDs-induced gastric damage

NSAIDs can damage the gastric epithelium by a number of mechanisms, which may be topical or systemic:
- Some NSAIDs can directly kill epithelial cells (Tarnawski et al. 1988; Allen et al. 1993), which may be attributable to a number of mechanisms, including uncoupling of oxidative phosphorylation (Somasundaram et al. 1995) and trapping of charged NSAIDs within the cell (Schoen and Vender 1989).
- By decreasing mucus and bicarbonate secretion, NSAIDs decrease the effectiveness of the juxtamucosal pH gradient in protecting epithelial cells (Palileo and Kaunitz 2011).
- NSAIDs can disrupt surface-active phospholipids, rendering the mucosa susceptible to acid damage (Darling et al. 2004). Certain NSAIDs undergo enterohepatic circulation, thus leading to repeated exposure of the upper intestinal tract epithelial cells to these drugs (Reuter et al. 1997).
- Under certain conditions, NSAIDs can increase gastric acid secretion (Feldman and Colturi 1984).
- An import mechanism in the NSAID-induced decrease in mucosal blood flow is the triggering of neutrophil adhesion to vascular endothelium. Activated neutrophils are a source of free radicals and have been implicated in the pathogenesis of NSAID-induced gastric ulceration (Wallace et al. 1990).

NSAID, nonsteroidal antiinflammatory drug.

COX-1 and COX-2 are constitutively expressed in the canine GI tract, and their inhibition can lead to GI adverse effects, including gastritis, enteritis, ulceration, and perforation. The lesser frequency of GI adverse effects is reported when only one isoform of COX is inhibited and is thought to be due to upregulation of the other isoform because both isoforms produce PGE_2 (Wooten et al. 2008). The decreased incidence of adverse effects with some recently licensed veterinary NSAIDs may be attributable to less than complete inhibition of COX-1, resulting in continued PGE_2 production in the GI tract by COX-1 (Reimer et al. 1999; Nishihara et al. 2001; Luna et al. 2007). PGE_2 and PGI_2, have important gastroprotective effects, including increased mucosal blood flow, increased mucus production, increased bicarbonate production, decreased acid secretion, and increased turnover of GI epithelial cells (Wolfe et al. 1999; Simmons et al. 2004; Whittle 2004). In a study evaluating the adverse effects of long-term (90 days) administration of carprofen, etodolac, flunixin, ketoprofen, or meloxicam to dogs, carprofen was associated with the least frequency and severity of GI adverse effects (Luna et al. 2007); however, no study has comprehensively compared all of the FDA-approved veterinary NSAIDs (KuKanich et al. 2012). Nevertheless, the safety of COX-1–sparing NSAIDs may be lost at high doses (Wolfe et al. 1999). Meloxicam has also been associated with GI toxicity (including GI perforation) at higher doses (Reed 2002). Therefore, dose and treatment recommendations should be closely followed to minimize the potential for toxicity of NSAIDs, including COX-1–sparing drugs.

Gastric bleeding after NSAID administration is, in part, caused by inhibition of TxA_2 in platelets, which is synthesized via the COX-1 pathway (Wallace 2008). Hence, the relative decrease in gastric toxicity with COX-2 selective inhibitors is probably caused by their lack of effect on TxA_2 synthesis. The delayed ulcer healing with NSAIDs is also caused, in part, by their effect on platelets. The beneficial effect of platelets on ulcer healing is perhaps attributable to their effects on vascular endothelial growth factor (VEGF) because VEGF is a potent stimulus for angiogenesis (Ma et al. 2001). By decreasing mucus and bicarbonate secretion, NSAIDs decrease the effectiveness of the juxtamucosal pH gradient in protecting epithelial cells (Palileo and Kaunitz 2011). NSAIDs can disrupt surface-active phospholipids, rendering the mucosa susceptible to acid damage (Darling et al. 2004). The decrease in mucosal blood flow caused by NSAIDs triggers the adhesion of neutrophils to the vascular endothelium. Activated neutrophils are a source of free radicals and have been implicated in the pathogenesis of NSAID-induced gastric ulceration (Wallace et al. 1990). COX-2 is thought to promote ulcer healing (Jones et al. 1999, Hirose et al. 2002) by increasing angiogenesis at the edge of gastric ulcers by inhibiting cellular kinase activity and increasing production of PGE_2 and VEGF (KuKanich et al. 2012). Therefore, inhibition of COX-2 in an animal with preexisting GI damage, regardless of COX-1 inhibition, can result in delayed or inhibited healing of the GI tissues which in turn can lead to severe adverse effects, including perforation and death (Goodman et al. 2009).

Other mechanisms involved in GI toxicity of NSAIDs may include increased production of leukotrienes, alteration of ion channel conductance, inhibition of PGI_2, and inhibition of aspirin triggered lipoxin (Wallace et al. 2000; Simmons et al. 2004; Wooten et al. 2008). Additionally, NSAIDs can occasionally stimulate the secretion of gastric acid (Feldman and Colturi 1984). Toxicity may be more severe with NSAIDs that undergo enterohepatic circulation (e.g., naproxen and tolfenamic acid) because of repeated exposure of the upper intestinal tract epithelial cells to these drugs (Reuter et al. 1997).

Although the **decrease in renal function** resulting from NSAIDs is primarily caused by inhibition of COX-1 (Vane 1971), nonselective COX inhibitors and COX-2 selective inhibitors cause a transitory decrease in urinary sodium excretion (Catella-Lawson et al. 1999) and therefore COX-selective NSAIDs may not be any safer. The consequences of COX-2 inhibition may include decreased RBF and GFR, combined with an imbalance in electrolyte excretion (Harris et al. 1994; Rossat et al. 1999; DeMaria and Weir 2003). Based on experimental data in rats, NSAIDs are also suspected to interfere with oxidative phosphorylation, potentially generating free radicals that contribute to renal toxicity (Okada et al. 1998).

The **pathophysiology of hepatic damage** caused by NSAIDs is difficult to define but does not appear linked to PG biosynthesis or to the ability of an NSAID to inhibit COX enzymes (Bjorkman 1998). Idiosyncratic reaction is the most common cause of hepatotoxicity resulting from administration of NSAIDs. The FDA adverse drug event reports for veterinary-approved NSAIDs suggest that hepatic toxicity can occur with any veterinary NSAID, and there is no reports identifying a particular NSAID as having an increased risk of idiosyncratic hepatic toxicity in dogs (KuKanich et al. 2012). This reaction is associated with an immunologic response occurring after metabolic transformation of the NSAID to reactive acyl glucuronate derivatives (Manoukian and Carson 1996). These derivatives form an immunogenic adduct with either intracellular or plasma membrane proteins (Boelsterli et al. 1995; Manoukian and Carson 1996).

When hepatic toxicity becomes clinically significant, signs usually appear within the first 3 weeks of administration of the NSAID (Lascelles et al. 2005b). An increase in aminotransferase activity can be expected after administering any NSAIDs; however, this increase is generally not clinically relevant, and enzyme activity returns to normal upon cessation of treatment (Manoukian and Carson 1996; Zimmerman 1990; Chitturi and George 2002).

Acetaminophen, an agent with many similarities to NSAIDs, deserves discussion because its use in some animals, particularly cats, may cause serious hepatic complications. It is rapidly absorbed from the GI tract and is conjugated, in most species, by sulfation or glucuronidation. Cats are considered more susceptible to NSAID toxicity, particularly acetaminophen-induced hepatotoxicity (Robertson and Taylor 2004; Taylor and Robertson 2004; Robertson 2008). Acetaminophen reactive metabolites bind to cellular macromolecules and cause hepatic necrosis (Jones et al. 1992). In addition, acetaminophen is known to cause Heinz body formation, methemoglobinemia, anemia, hemoglobinuria, and icterus in cats (Finco et al. 1975; Allen 2003). Therefore, acetaminophen is strictly contraindicated, at any dose, in cats (Jones et al. 1992).

The COX-2 isoenzyme has been implicated in the signaling and coordination of **ossification** and inflammation after bone fracture (Simon et al. 2002). This isoenzyme regulates the genes required for bone formation (Zhang et al. 2002), and COX-2–generated PGs may alter bone metabolism by regulating osteoblasts (Bergh and Budsberg 2005). Thus, COX-2 inhibitors may delay the early stages of bone healing and potentially contribute to nonunions (Gerstenfeld et al. 2003; Aspenberg 2004). Experimental studies in rodents and dogs support this theory, and this evidence has been recently reviewed (Griffon 2010). For example, rats and mice treated with celecoxib or rofecoxib had delayed fracture healing compared with those taking placebo (Simon et al. 2002). In dogs, long-term (120 days) administration of carprofen inhibited normal bone healing after tibial osteotomy (Ochi et al. 2011). However, these adverse effects appear to be reversible if NSAIDs are only administered for a short period (Zhang et al. 2002).

Interspecies differences in nonsteroidal antiinflammatory drug toxicity

There appears to be significant interspecies differences in the ratio of COX-1 and COX-2 expression and susceptibility to the adverse effects of COX inhibition. For example, susceptibility of cats, dogs, and horses to the adverse effects of nonselective NSAIDs is greater than that of humans (Mahmud et al. 1996). Dogs are less tolerant of nonselective NSAIDs than humans and more at risk of nonselective NSAID-induced gastropathy (Elliott et al. 1988; Forsyth et al. 1998) (see Table 15.2). Naproxen is well tolerated by mice, rabbits, monkeys, and pigs; less well tolerated by rats; and poorly tolerated by dogs (Hallesy et al. 1973).

Cats are generally more susceptible to the toxic effects of NSAIDs because of decreased clearance and dose-dependent elimination. The toxic effects of salicylates in cats are well documented. Affected cats may develop hyperthermia, respiratory alkalosis, metabolic acidosis, methemoglobinemia, hemorrhagic gastritis, and kidney and liver injury (Davis 1980). As was mentioned earlier, cats lack the glucuronyl transferase enzyme, which further predisposes them to the adverse effects of drugs (e.g., acetaminophen) that require glucuronidation before elimination (Court and Greenblatt 1997). Until recently, the long-term administration of the oral suspension of meloxicam, a COX-2 preferential NSAID, to cats at a dose of 0.05 mg/kg was recommended for control of inflammation and pain in chronic musculoskeletal conditions (Gunn-Moore 2010). However, per FDA request, Boehringer Ingleheim Vetmedica, the manufacturer for meloxicam, has recently added a "Boxed Warning Label for Use of Meloxicam in Cats" to inform veterinarians of the serious risks associated with extralabel use of meloxicam in cats. Veterinarians are encouraged to periodically refer to the updated information regarding meloxicam use in cats to the guidelines of the American Association of Feline Practitioners (http://www.aafponline.org). The administration of carprofen to cats has also been discouraged because of reports of gastroduodenal toxicosis when it was administered according to canine dose rates (Papich 2008).

Gastric adaptation is an interesting mechanism described in dogs, humans, and rats by which the inherent susceptibility of those species to the adverse effects of NSAIDs is reduced by chronic administration. Mechanisms involved in gastric adaptation include an increase in gastric blood flow, a decrease in inflammatory cell infiltration, and an increase in mucosal cell regeneration and mucosal content of epidermal growth factor (Konturek et al. 1994). Gastric adaptation occurs by about day 14 of continuous aspirin therapy in dogs (Hurley and Crandall 1964). Whether such adaptation also applies to the small intestine is still debated (Hanson and Maddison 2008).

Conclusions

Nowadays, NSAIDs are one of the first-line drugs for treatment of fever and inflammation and for the relief of mild to moderate pain. NSAIDs have stood the test of time and are efficacious; nevertheless, their use has been associated with adverse effects on several organ systems, especially in susceptible animals. GI, renal, and hepatic toxicities are the most frequently reported complications of NSAID use, but adverse effects on bone, cartilage growth, and coagulation are also reported. Although management of pain and discomfort in animals is foremost, judicious use of NSAIDs is warranted to minimize their toxicity. Further studies are necessary to develop new generations of NSAIDs with a greater therapeutic index, and progress is being made toward this end.

References

Abernathy, C.O., Zimmerman, H.J., Ishak, K.G., et al. (1992) Drug-induced cholestasis in the perfused rat liver and its reversal by tauroursodeoxycholate: an ultrastructural study. *Proceedings of the Society for Experimental Biology and Medicine* 199, 54-58.

Abraham, N.S., Hartman, C., Castillo, D., et al. (2008) Effectiveness of national provider prescription of PPI gastroprotection among elderly NSAID users. *American Journal of Gastroenterology* 103, 323-332.

Aitio, M.L. (2006) N-acetylcysteine—passe-partout or much ado about nothing? *British Journal of Clinical Pharmacology* 61, 5-15.

Allen, A., Flemstrom, G., Garner, A., et al. (1993) Gastroduodenal mucosal protection. *Physiological Reviews* 73, 823-857.

Allen, A.L. (2003) The diagnosis of acetaminophen toxicosis in a cat. *Canadian Veterinary Journal* 44, 509-510.

Alwood, A.J. (2009). Acetaminophen. In: Silverstein, D.C., Hopper, K. (eds.) *Small Animal Critical Care Medicine*. Elsevier Saunders, Philadelphia, pp. 334-337.

Anand, B.S., Romero, J.J., Sanduja, S.K., et al. (1999) Phospholipid association reduces the gastric mucosal toxicity of aspirin in human subjects. *American Journal of Gastroenterology* 94, 1818-1822.

Aspenberg, P. (2004) Differential inhibition of fracture healing by non-selective and cyclooxygenase-2 selective non-steroidal anti-inflammatory drugs. *Journal of Orthopedic Research* 22, 684, author reply 685.

Benton, H.P., Vasseur, P.B., Broderick-Villa, G.A., et al. (1997) Effect of carprofen on sulfated glycosaminoglycan metabolism, protein synthesis, and prostaglandin release by cultured osteoarthritic canine chondrocytes. *American Journal of Veterinary Research* 58, 286-292.

Bergenstock, M., Min, W., Simon, A.M., et al. (2005) A comparison between the effects of acetaminophen and celecoxib on bone fracture healing in rats. *Journal of Orthopedic Trauma* 19, 717-723.

Bergh, M.S., Budsberg, S.C. (2005) The coxib NSAIDs: potential clinical and pharmacologic importance in veterinary medicine. *Journal of Veterinary Internal Medicine* 19, 633-643.

Bergmann, H.M., Nolte, I.J., Kramer, S. (2005) Effects of preoperative administration of carprofen on renal function and hemostasis in dogs undergoing surgery for fracture repair. *American Journal of Veterinary Research* 66, 1356-1363.

Bjorkman, D. (1998) Nonsteroidal anti-inflammatory drug-associated toxicity of the liver, lower gastrointestinal tract, and esophagus. *American Journal of Medicine* 105, 17S-21S.

Boelsterli, U.A., Zimmerman, H.J., Kretz-Rommel, A. (1995) Idiosyncratic liver toxicity of nonsteroidal antiinflammatory drugs: molecular mechanisms and pathology. *Critical Reviews in Toxicology* 25, 207-235.

Boothe, D.M. (2012). Antiinflammatory drugs. In: Boothe, D.M. (ed.) *Small Animal Clinical Pharmacology & Therapeutics*, 2nd edn. Elsevier, St. Louis, pp. 1045-1094.

Boudreaux, M.K. (2000). Aquired platelet dysfunction. In: Feldman, B., Zinkl, J. Jain, N. (eds.) *Schalm's Veterinary Hematology.* Lippincott Williams and Wilkins, Philadelphia, pp. 496-500.

Boulay, J.P., Lipowitz, A.J., Klausner, J.S. (1986) Effect of cimetidine on aspirin-induced gastric hemorrhage in dogs. *American Journal of Veterinary Research* 47, 1744-1746.

Catella-Lawson, F., McAdam, B., Morrison, B.W., et al. (1999) Effects of specific inhibition of cyclooxygenase-2 on sodium balance, hemodynamics, and vasoactive eicosanoids. *Journal of Pharmacology and Experimental Therapeutics* 289, 735-741.

Chandrasekharan, N.V., Dai, H., Roos, K.L., et al. (2002) COX-3, a cyclooxygenase-1 variant inhibited by acetaminophen and other analgesic/antipyretic drugs: cloning, structure, and expression. *Proceeding of the National Academy of Sciences* 99, 13926-13931.

Chitturi, S., George, J. (2002) Hepatotoxicity of commonly used drugs: nonsteroidal anti-inflammatory drugs, antihypertensives, antidiabetic agents, anticonvulsants, lipid-lowering agents, psychotropic drugs. *Seminars in Liver Disease* 22, 169-183.

Collins, L.G., Tyler, D.E. (1985) Experimentally induced phenylbutazone toxicosis in ponies: description of the syndrome and its prevention with synthetic prostaglandin E2. *American Journal of Veterinary Research* 46, 1605-1615.

Court, M.H., Greenblatt, D.J. (1997) Molecular basis for deficient acetaminophen glucuronidation in cats. An interspecies comparison of enzyme kinetics in liver microsomes. *Biochemical Pharmacology* 53, 1041-1047.

Curry, S.L., Cogar, S.M., Cook, J.L. (2005) Nonsteroidal antiinflammatory drugs: a review. *Journal of American Animal Hospital Association* 41, 298-309.

D'Angio, R.G. (1987) Nonsteroidal antiinflammatory drug-induced renal dysfunction related to inhibition of renal prostaglandins. *Drug Intelligence & Clinical Pharmacology* 21, 954-960.

Darling, R.L., Romero, J.J., Dial, E.J., et al. (2004) The effects of aspirin on gastric mucosal integrity, surface hydrophobicity, and prostaglandin metabolism in cyclooxygenase knockout mice. *Gastroenterology* 127, 94-104.

Davies, N.M., Sharkey, K.A., Asfaha, S., et al. (1997) Aspirin causes rapid up-regulation of cyclo-oxygenase-2 expression in the stomach of rats. *Alimentary Pharmacology & Therapeutics* 11, 1101-1108.

Davis, L.E. (1980) Clinical pharmacology of salicylates. *Journal of Amrican Veterinary Medical Association* 176, 65-66.

DeMaria, A.N., Weir, M.R. (2003) Coxibs—beyond the GI tract: renal and cardiovascular issues. *Journal of Pain and Symptom Management* 25 (Suppl.), S41-S49.

Deneuche, A.J., Dufayet, C., Goby, L., et al. (2004) Analgesic comparison of meloxicam or ketoprofen for orthopedic surgery in dogs. *Veterinary Surgery* 33, 650-660.

Dickman, A., Ellershaw, J. (2004) NSAIDs: gastroprotection or selective COX-2 inhibitor? *Palliative Medicine* 18, 275-286.

Dow, S.W., Rosychuk, R.A., McChesney, A.E., et al. (1990) Effects of flunixin and flunixin plus prednisone on the gastrointestinal tract of dogs. *American Journal of Veterinary Research* 51, 1131-1138.

Dowers, K.L., Uhrig, S.R., Mama, K.R., et al. (2006) Effect of short-term sequential administration of nonsteroidal anti-inflammatory drugs on the stomach and proximal portion of the duodenum in healthy dogs. *American Journal of Veterinary Research* 67, 1794-1801.

Dunn, M.J., Scharschmidt, L., Zambraski, E. (1984) Mechanisms of the nephrotoxicity of non-steroidal anti-inflammatory drugs. *Archives of Toxicology Supplement* 7, 328-337.

Elliott, G.A., Purmalis, A., VanderMeer, D.A., et al. (1988) The propionic acids. Gastrointestinal toxicity in various species. *Toxicologic Pathology* 16, 245-250.

Elliott, S.N., McKnight, W., Cirino, G., et al. (1995) A nitric oxide-releasing nonsteroidal anti-inflammatory drug accelerates gastric ulcer healing in rats. *Gastroenterology* 109, 524-530.

Feigen, L.P., Klainer, E., Chapnick, B.M., et al. (1976) The effect of indomethacin on renal function in pentobarbital-anesthetized dogs. *Journal of Pharmacology and Experimental Therapeutics* 198, 457-463.

Feldman, M., Colturi, T.J. (1984) Effect of indomethacin on gastric acid and bicarbonate secretion in humans. *Gastroenterology* 87, 1339-1343.

Finco, D.C., Duncan, J.R., Schall, W.D., et al. (1975) Acetaminophen toxicosis in the cat. *Journal of the American Veterinary Medical Association* 166, 469-472.

Fiorucci, S., Santucci, L., Gresele, P., et al. (2003) Gastrointestinal safety of NO-aspirin (NCX-4016) in healthy human volunteers: a proof of concept endoscopic study. *Gastroenterology* 124, 600-607.

Fiorucci, S., Antonelli, E., Distrutti, E., et al. (2005) Inhibition of hydrogen sulfide generation contributes to gastric injury caused by anti-inflammatory nonsteroidal drugs. *Gastroenterology* 129, 1210-1224.

Fiorucci, S., Distrutti, E., Cirino, G., et al. (2006) The emerging roles of hydrogen sulfide in the gastrointestinal tract and liver. *Gastroenterology* 131, 259-271.

Flower, R.J. (2003) The development of COX2 inhibitors. *Nature Reviews Drug Discovery* 2, 179-191.

Forsyth, S.F., Guilford, W.G., Haslett, S.J., et al. (1998) Endoscopy of the gastroduodenal mucosa after carprofen, meloxicam and ketoprofen administration in dogs. 39, 421-424.

Gerstenfeld, L.C., Thiede, M., Seibert, K., et al. (2003) Differential inhibition of fracture healing by non-selective and cyclooxygenase-2 selective non-steroidal anti-inflammatory drugs. *Journal of Orthopedic Research* 21, 670-675.

Giannoukas, A.D., Baltoyiannis, G., Milonakis, M., et al. (1996) Protection of the gastroduodenal mucosa from the effects of diclofenac sodium: role of highly selective vagotomy and misoprostol. *World Journal of Surgery* 20, 501-5 discussion 505-6.

Goodman, L., Torres, B., Punke, J., et al. (2009) Effects of firocoxib and tepoxalin on healing in a canine gastric mucosal injury model. *Journal of Veterinary Internal Medicine* 23, 56-62.

Goodman, S.B., Ma, T., Mitsunaga, L., et al. (2005) Temporal effects of a COX-2-selective NSAID on bone ingrowth. *Journal of Biomedical Materail Research Part A* 72, 279-287.

Gretzer, B., Maricic, N., Respondek, M., et al. (2001) Effects of specific inhibition of cyclo-oxygenase-1 and cyclo-oxygenase-2 in the rat stomach with normal mucosa and after acid challenge. *British Journal of Pharmacology* 132, 1565-1573.

Griffon, D.J. (2010) Secondary (indirect) bone healing. In: Bojrab, M.J., Monnet, E. (eds.) *Mechanisms of Disease in Small Animal Surgery*, 3rd edn. Teton New Media, Jackson, WY, pp. 513-516.

Gunn-Moore, D. (2010) NSAIDs and cats—it's been a long journey. *Journal of Feline Medicine & Surgery* 12, 519.

Hallesy, D.W., Shott, L.D., Hill, R. (1973) Comparative toxicology of naproxen. *Scandinavian Journal of Rheumatology - Supplement*, 2, 20-28.

Hanson, P.D., Maddison, J.E. (2008) Nonsteroidal anti-inflammatory drugs and chondroprotective agents. In: Maddison, J.E., Page, S.W. (eds.) *Small Animal Clinical Pharmacology*, 2nd edn. Saunders/Elsevier, Edinburgh, pp. 287-306.

Harris, R.C., McKanna, J.A., Akai, Y., et al. (1994) Cyclooxygenase-2 is associated with the macula densa of rat kidney and increases with salt restriction. *Journal of Clinical Investigation* 94, 2504-2510.

Hartman, J.C., Page, P.S., Proctor, L.T., et al. (1992) Influence of desflurane, isoflurane and halothane on regional tissue perfusion in dogs. *Canadian Journal of Anaesthesia* 39, 877-887.

Hawkey, C.J., Karrasch, J.A., Szczepanski, L., et al. (1998) Omeprazole compared with misoprostol for ulcers associated with nonsteroidal antiinflammatory drugs. Omeprazole versus Misoprostol for NSAID-induced Ulcer Management (OMNIUM) Study Group. *New England Journal of Medicine* 338, 727-734.

Hawkey, C.J., Jones, J.I., Atherton, C.T., et al. (2003) Gastrointestinal safety of AZD3582, a cyclooxygenase inhibiting nitric oxide donor: proof of concept study in humans. *Gut* 52, 1537-1542.

Hirose, M., Miwa, H., Kobayashi, O., et al. (2002) Inhibition of proliferation of gastric epithelial cells by a cyclooxygenase 2 inhibitor, JTE522, is also mediated by a PGE2-independent pathway. *Alimentary Pharmacology & Therapeutics* 16 (2), 83-89.

Hunt, R.H., Yuan, Y. (2011) Acid-NSAID/aspirin interaction in peptic ulcer disease. *Digestive Diseases* 29, 465-468.

Hurley, J.W., Crandall, L.A. Jr. (1964) The effect of salicylates upon the stomachs of dogs. *Gastroenterology* 46, 36-43.

Jenkins, C.C., DeNovo, R.C., Patton, C.S., et al. (1991) Comparison of effects of cimetidine and omeprazole on mechanically created gastric ulceration and on aspirin-induced gastritis in dogs. *American Journal of Veterinary Research* 52, 658-661.

Johnston, S.A., Budsberg, S.C. (1997) Nonsteroidal anti-inflammatory drugs and corticosteroids for the management of canine osteoarthritis. *Veterinary Clinics of North America: Small Animal Practice* 27, 841-862.

Johnston, S.A., Leib, M.S., Forrester, S.D., et al. (1995) The effect of misoprostol on aspirin-induced gastroduodenal lesions in dogs. *Journal of Veterinary Internal Medicine* 9, 32-38.

Jones, M.K., Wang, H., Peskar, B.M., et al. (1999) Inhibition of angiogenesis by nonsteroidal anti-inflammatory drugs: insight into mechanisms and implications for cancer growth and ulcer healing. *Nature Medicine* 5, 1418-1423.

Jones, R.D., Baynes, R.E., Nimitz, C.T. (1992) Nonsteroidal anti-inflammatory drug toxicosis in dogs and cats: 240 cases (1989-1990). *Journal of the American Veterinary Medical Association* 201, 475-477.

Kawaguchi, H., Pilbeam, C.C., Harrison, J.R., et al. (1995) The role of prostaglandins in the regulation of bone metabolism. *Clinical Orthopaedics and Related Research* 313, 36-46.

Kawai, S. (1998) Cyclooxygenase selectivity and the risk of gastro-intestinal complications of various non-steroidal anti-inflammatory drugs: a clinical consideration. *Inflammation Research* 47 (Suppl. 2), S102-106.

Kazakos, G.M., Papazoglou, L.G., Rallis, T., et al. (2005) Effects of meloxicam on the haemostatic profile of dogs undergoing orthopaedic surgery. *Veterinary Record* 157, 444-446.

Khan, N., Alden, C. (2002) Kidney. In: Haschek, W., Rousseux, C., Walling, M. (eds.) *Handbook of Toxicologic Pathology*, vol. 2, Academic Press, San Diego, pp. 272-274.

Kis, B., Snipes, J.A., Busija, D.W. (2005) Acetaminophen and the cyclooxygenase-3 puzzle: sorting out facts, fictions, and uncertainties. *Journal of Pharmacology and Experimental Therapeutics* 315, 1-7.

Knights, K.M., Tsoutsikos, P., Miners, J.O. (2005) Novel mechanisms of nonsteroidal anti-inflammatory drug-induced renal toxicity. *Expert Opinion on Drug Metabolism & Toxicology* 1, 399-408.

Konturek, S.J., Brzozowski, T., Majka, J., et al. (1993) Inhibition of nitric oxide synthase delays healing of chronic gastric ulcers. *European Journal of Pharmacology* 239, 215-217.

Konturek, S. J., Brzozowski, T., Stachura, J., et al. (1994) Role of gastric blood flow, neutrophil infiltration, and mucosal cell proliferation in gastric adaptation to aspirin in the rat. *Gut* 35, 1189-1196.

KuKanich, B., Bidgood, T., Knesl, O. (2012) Clinical pharmacology of nonsteroidal anti-inflammatory drugs in dogs. *Veterinary Anaesthesia and Analgesia* 39, 69-90.

Kurinets, A., Lichtenberger, L.M. (1998) Phosphatidylcholine-associated aspirin accelerates healing of gastric ulcers in rats. *Digestive Diseases and Sciences* 43, 786-790.

Laffi, G., La Villa, G., Pinzani, M., et al. (1997) Arachidonic acid derivatives and renal function in liver cirrhosis. *Seminars in Nephrology* 17, 530-548.

Laine, L., Bombardier, C., Hawkey, C.J., et al. (2002) Stratifying the risk of NSAID-related upper gastrointestinal clinical events: results of a double-blind outcomes study in patients with rheumatoid arthritis. *Gastroenterology* 123, 1006-1012.

Langenbach, R., Morham, S.G., Tiano, H.F., et al. (1995) Prostaglandin synthase 1 gene disruption in mice reduces arachidonic acid-induced inflammation and indomethacin-induced gastric ulceration. *Cell* 83, 483-492.

Lascelles, B.D., Blikslager, A.T., Fox, S.M., et al. (2005a) Gastrointestinal tract perforation in dogs treated with a selective cyclooxygenase-2 inhibitor: 29 cases (2002-2003). *Journal of the American Veterinary Medical Association* 227, 1112-1117.

Lascelles, B.D., McFarland, J.M., Swann, H. (2005b) Guidelines for safe and effective use of NSAIDs in dogs. *Veterinary Therapeutics* 6, 237-251.

Lee, K.N., Lee, O.Y., Choi, M.G., et al. (2011) Prevention of NSAID-associated gastroduodenal injury in healthy volunteers-a randomized, double-blind, multicenter study comparing DA-9601 with misoprostol. *Journal of Korean Medical Science*, 26, 1074-1080.

Lee, W.M. (2003) Drug-induced hepatotoxicity. *The New rEngland Journal of Medicine* 349, 474-485.

Lees, P., Landoni, M.F., Giraudel, J., et al. (2004) Pharmacodynamics and pharmacokinetics of nonsteroidal anti-inflammatory drugs in species of veterinary interest. *Journal of Veterinary Pharmacology and Therapeutics* 27, 479-490.

Levin, A., Pate, G.E., Shalansky, S., et al. (2007) N-acetylcysteine reduces urinary albumin excretion following contrast administration: evidence of biological effect. *Nephrology Dialysis Transplantation* 22, 2520-2524.

Lichtenberger, L.M., Romero, J.J., de Ruijter, W.M., et al. (2001) Phosphatidylcholine association increases the anti-inflammatory and analgesic activity of ibuprofen in acute and chronic rodent models of joint inflammation: relationship to alterations in bioavailability and cyclooxygenase-inhibitory potency. *Journal of Pharmacology and Experimental Therapeutics* 298, 279-287.

Littlewood, J.D. (1999) Diseases of blood and blood-forming organs. In: Dunn, J.K. (ed.) *TEXTBOOK of Small Animal Medicine*. W.B. Saunders, London, p. 800.

Lobetti, R.G., Joubert, K.E. (2000) Effect of administration of nonsteroidal anti-inflammatory drugs before surgery on renal function in clinically normal dogs. *American Journal of Veterinary Research* 61, 1501-1507.

Luna, S.P., Basilio, A.C., Steagall, P.V., et al. (2007) Evaluation of adverse effects of long-term oral administration of carprofen, etodolac, flunixin meglumine, ketoprofen, and meloxicam in dogs. *American Journal of Veterinary Research* 68, 258-264.

Ma, L., Elliott, S.N., Cirino, G., et al. (2001) Platelets modulate gastric ulcer healing: role of endostatin and vascular endothelial growth factor release. *Proceedings of the National Academy of Sciences* 98, 6470-6475.

Ma, L., del Soldato, P., Wallace, J.L. (2002) Divergent effects of new cyclooxygenase inhibitors on gastric ulcer healing: shifting the angiogenic balance. *Proceedings of the National Academy of Sciences* 99, 13243-13247.

MacNaughton, W.K., Cirino, G., Wallace, J.L. (1989) Endothelium-derived relaxing factor (nitric oxide) has protective actions in the stomach. *Life Sciences* 45, 1869-1876.

MacPhail, C.M., Lappin, M.R., Meyer, D.J., et al. (1998) Hepatocellular toxicosis associated with administration of carprofen in 21 dogs. *Journal of the American Veterinary Medical Association* 212, 1895-1901.

Mahmud, T., Rafi, S.S., Scott, D.L., et al. (1996) Nonsteroidal antiinflammatory drugs and uncoupling of mitochondrial oxidative phosphorylation. *Arthritis & Rheumatism* 39, 1998-2003.

Manoukian, A.V., Carson, J.L. (1996) Nonsteroidal anti-inflammatory drug-induced hepatic disorders. Incidence and prevention. *Drug Safety* 15, 64-71.

Marbet, G.A., Yasikoff Strub, M.L., Macciocchi, A., et al. (1998) The effect of nimesulide versus placebo on hemostasis in healthy volunteers. *European Journal of Clinical Pharmacology* 54, 383-387.

Mason, L., Moore, R.A., Edwards, J.E., et al. (2004) Topical NSAIDs for acute pain: a meta-analysis. *BMC Family Practice* 5, 10.

Mathews, K.A. (1996) Nonsteroidal anti-inflammatory analgesics in pain management in dogs and cats. *Canadian Veteterinary Journal* 37, 539-545.

Mathews, K.A., Doherty, T., Dyson, D.H., et al. (1990) Nephrotoxicity in dogs associated with methoxyflurane anesthesia and flunixin meglumine analgesia. *Canadian Veterinary Journal* 31, 766-771.

Meddings, J.B., Kirk, D., Olson, M.E. (1995) Noninvasive detection of nonsteroidal anti-inflammatory drug-induced gastropathy in dogs. *American Joyurnal of Veterinary Research* 56, 977-981.

Mitchell, J.A., Warner, T.D. (2006) COX isoforms in the cardiovascular system: understanding the activities of non-steroidal anti-inflammatory drugs. *Natural Reviews Drug Discovery* 5, 75-86.

Mizuno, H., Sakamoto, C., Matsuda, K., et al. (1997) Induction of cyclooxygenase 2 in gastric mucosal lesions and its inhibition by the specific antagonist delays healing in mice. *Gastroenterology* 112, 387-397.

Murnaghan, M., Li, G., Marsh, D.R. (2006) Nonsteroidal anti-inflammatory drug-induced fracture nonunion: an inhibition of angiogenesis? *The Journal of Bone & Joint Surgery* 88 (3), 140-147.

Naclerio-Homem, M.G., Deboni, M.C., Rapoport, A., et al. (2009) Effects of ketoprofen and diclofenac potassium on blood coagulation tests after removal of third molars. *Quintessence International* 40, 321-325.

Nakagawa, K., Yamagami, T., Takemura, N. (2005) Hepatocellular toxicosis associated with the alternate administration of carprofen and meloxicam in a siberian husky. *Journal of Veterinary Medical Sciences* 67, 1051-1053.

Narita, T., Sato, R., Motoishi, K., et al. (2007) The interaction between orally administered non-steroidal anti-inflammatory drugs and prednisolone in healthy dogs. *Journal of Veterinary Medical Sciences* 69, 353-363.

Neiger, R., Gaschen, F., Jaggy, A. (2000) Gastric mucosal lesions in dogs with acute intervertebral disc disease: characterization and effects of omeprazole or misoprostol. *Journal of Veterinary Internal Medicine* 14, 33-36.

Nishihara, K., Kikuchi, H., Kanno, T., et al. (2001) Comparison of the upper gastrointestinal effects of etodolac and aspirin in healthy dogs. *Journal of Veterinary Medical Sciences* 63, 1131-1133.

Ochi, H., Hara, Y., Asou, Y., et al. (2011) Effects of long-term administration of carprofen on healing of a tibial osteotomy in dogs. *American Journal of Veterinary Research* 72, 634-641.

Okada, A., Kinoshita, Y., Waki, S., et al. (1998) Rat gastric mucosal cells express ICAM-1 and proinflammatory cytokines during indomethacin-induced mucosal injury. *Journal of Laboratory and Clinical Medicine* 131, 538-547.

Palileo, C., Kaunitz, J.D. (2011) Gastrointestinal defense mechanisms. *Current Opinion in Gastroenterology* 27, 543-548.

Palmoski, M.J., Brandt, K.D. (1982) Aspirin aggravates the degeneration of canine joint cartilage caused by immobilization. *Arthritis & Rheumatism* 25, 1333-1342.

Palmoski, M.J., Brandt, K.D. (1983) In vivo effect of aspirin on canine osteoarthritic cartilage. *Arthritis & Rheumatism* 26, 994-1001.

Papich, M.G. (1997) Principles of analgesic drug therapy. *Seminars in Veterinary Medical Surgery (Small Animal)* 12, 80-93.

Papich, M.G. (2008) An update on nonsteroidal anti-inflammatory drugs (NSAIDs) in small animals. *Veterinary Clinics of North America: Small Animal Practice* 38, 1243-1266.

Raisz, L.G. (1990) The role of prostaglandins in the local regulation of bone metabolism. *Progress in Clinical Biological Research,* 332, 195-203.

Reed, S. (2002) Nonsteroidal anti-inflammatory drug-induced duodenal ulceration and perforation in a mature rottweiler. *Canadian Veterinary Journal* 43, 971-972.

Reimer, M.E., Johnston, S.A., Leib, M.S., et al. (1999) The gastroduodenal effects of buffered aspirin, carprofen, and etodolac in healthy dogs. *Journal of Veterinary Internal Medicine* 13, 472-477.

Reuter, B.K., Davies, N.M., Wallace, J.L. (1997) Nonsteroidal anti-inflammatory drug enteropathy in rats: role of permeability, bacteria, and enterohepatic circulation. *Gastroenterology* 112, 109-117.

Rinder, H.M., Tracey, J.B., Souhrada, M., et al. (2002) Effects of meloxicam on platelet function in healthy adults: a randomized, double-blind, placebo-controlled trial. *Journal of Clinical Pharmacology* 42, 881-886.

Robertson, S.A. (2008) Managing pain in feline patients. *Veterinary Clinics of North America: Small Animal Practice* 38, 1267-1290.

Robertson, S.A., Taylor, P.M. (2004) Pain management in cats—past, present and future. Part 2. Treatment of pain—clinical pharmacology. *Journal of Feline Medicine & Surgery* 6, 321-333.

Rodriguez, F., Llinas, M.T., Gonzalez, J.D., et al. (2000) Renal changes induced by a cyclooxygenase-2 inhibitor during normal and low sodium intake. *Hypertension* 36, 276-281.

Rossat, J., Maillard, M., Nussberger, J., et al. (1999) Renal effects of selective cyclooxygenase-2 inhibition in normotensive salt-depleted subjects. *Clinical Pharmacology & Therapeutics* 66, 76-84.

Rossoni, G., Manfredi, B., Del Soldato, P., et al. (2004) The nitric oxide-releasing naproxen derivative displays cardioprotection in perfused rabbit heart submitted to ischemia-reperfusion. *Journal of Pharmacology and Experimental Therapeutics* 310, 555-562.

Rossoni, G., Sparatore, A., Tazzari, V., et al. (2008) The hydrogen sulphide-releasing derivative of diclofenac protects against ischaemia-reperfusion injury in the isolated rabbit heart. *British Journal of Pharmacology* 153, 100-109.

Sakai, M., Watari, T., Miura, T., et al. (2003) Effects of DDAVP administered subcutaneously in dogs with aspirin-induced platelet dysfunction and hemostatic impairment due to chronic liver diseases. *The Journal of Veterinary Medical Science* 65, 83-86.

Scheiman, J.M. (1996) NSAIDs, gastrointestinal injury, and cytoprotection. *Gastroenterology Clinics of North America* 25, 279-298.

Scheiman, J.M., Devereaux, P.J., Herlitz, J., et al. (2011) Prevention of peptic ulcers with esomeprazole in patients at risk of ulcer development treated with low-dose acetylsalicylic acid: a randomised, controlled trial (OBERON). *Heart* 97, 797-802.

Schoen, R.T. and Vender, R.J. (1989) Mechanisms of nonsteroidal anti-inflammatory drug-induced gastric damage. *American Journal of Medicine* 86, 449-458.

Senior, D.F. (1999). Diseases of the urinary system. In: Dunn, J.K. (ed.) *TEXTBOOK of Small Animal Medicine.* W.B. Saunders, London, pp. 612-623.

Shield, M.J. (1998) Diclofenac/misoprostol: novel findings and their clinical potential. *The Journal of Rheumatology Supplement* 51, 31-41.

Sigthorsson, G., Simpson, R.J., Walley, M., et al. (2002) COX-1 and 2, intestinal integrity, and pathogenesis of nonsteroidal anti-inflammatory drug enteropathy in mice. *Gastroenterology* 122, 1913-1923.

Silverstein, F.E., Graham, D.Y., Senior, J.R., et al. (1995) Misoprostol reduces serious gastrointestinal complications in patients with rheumatoid arthritis receiving nonsteroidal anti-inflammatory drugs. A randomized, double-blind, placebo-controlled trial. *Annals of Internal Medicine* 123, 241-249.

Silverstein, F.E., Faich, G., Goldstein, J.L., et al. (2000) Gastrointestinal toxicity with celecoxib vs nonsteroidal anti-inflammatory drugs for osteoarthritis and rheumatoid arthritis: the CLASS study: a randomized controlled trial. Celecoxib Long-term Arthritis Safety Study. *Journal of the American Medical Association* 284, 1247-1255.

Simmons, D.L., Botting, R.M., Hla, T. (2004) Cyclooxygenase isozymes: the biology of prostaglandin synthesis and inhibition. *Pharmacological Reviews* 56, 387-437.

Simon, A.M., Manigrasso, M.B., O'Connor, J.P. (2002) Cyclo-oxygenase 2 function is essential for bone fracture healing. *Journal of Bone and Mineral Research* 17, 963-976.

Smith, W.L., Bell, T.G. (1978) Immunohistochemical localization of the prostaglandin-forming cyclooxygenase in renal cortex. *American Journal of Physiology* 235, F451-F457.

Smith, W.L., DeWitt, D.L., Garavito, R.M. (2000) Cyclooxygenases: structural, cellular, and molecular biology. *Annual Review of Biochemistry* 69, 145-182.

Somasundaram, S., Hayllar, H., Rafi, S. et al. (1995) The biochemical basis of nonsteroidal anti-inflammatory drug-induced damage to the gastrointestinal tract: a review and a hypothesis. *Scandinavian Journal of Gastroenterology* 30, 289-299.

Stanton, M.E., Bright, R.M. (1989) Gastroduodenal ulceration in dogs. Retrospective study of 43 cases and literature review. *Journal of Veterinary Internal Medicine* 3, 238-244.

Steagall, P.V., Moutinho, F.Q., Mantovani, F.B., et al. (2009) Evaluation of the adverse effects of subcutaneous carprofen over six days in healthy cats. *Research in Veterinary Science* 86, 115-120.

Streppa, H.K., Jones, C.J., Budsberg, S.C. (2002) Cyclooxygenase selectivity of nonsteroidal anti-inflammatory drugs in canine blood. *American Journal of Veterinary Research* 63, 91-94.

Takeda, S., Sato, N., Tomaru, T. (2002) Haemodynamic and splanchnic organ blood flow responses during sevoflurane-induced hypotension in dogs. *European Journal of Anaesthesiology* 19, 442-446.

Tarnawski, A. Brzozowski, T., Sarfeh I.J., et al. (1988) Prostaglandin protection of human isolated gastric glands against indomethacin and ethanol injury. Evidence for direct cellular action of prostaglandin. *Journal of Clinical Investigation* 81, 1081-1089.

Taylor, P.M., Robertson, S.A. (2004) Pain management in cats—past, present and future. Part 1. The cat is unique. *Journal of Feline Medicine & Surgery* 6, 313-320.

Tolbert, K., Bissett, S., King, A., et al. (2011) Efficacy of oral famotidine and 2 omeprazole formulations for the control of intragastric pH in dogs. *Journal of Veterinary Internal Medicine* 25, 47-54.

Tolman, K.G. (1998) Hepatotoxicity of non-narcotic analgesics. 105, 13S-19S.

Vane, J.R. (1971) Inhibition of prostaglandin synthesis as a mechanism of action for aspirin-like drugs. *Nat New Biol* 231, 232-235.

Vane, S.J. (2000) Aspirin and other anti-inflammatory drugs. *Thorax* 55 (Suppl. 2), S3-S9.

Vonderhaar, M.A., Salisbury, S.K. (1993) Gastroduodenal ulceration associated with flunixin meglumine administration in three dogs. *JAMA* 203, 92-95.

Wallace, J.L. (2008) Prostaglandins, NSAIDs, and gastric mucosal protection: why doesn't the stomach digest itself? *Physiological Reviews* 88, 1547-1565.

Wallace, J.L., Miller, M.J. (2000) Nitric oxide in mucosal defense: a little goes a long way. *Gastroenterology* 119, 512-520.

Wallace, J.L., Keenan, C.M., Granger, D.N. (1990) Gastric ulceration induced by nonsteroidal anti-inflammatory drugs is a neutrophil-dependent process. *American Journal of Physiology* 259, G462-G467.

Wallace, J.L., Reuter, B., Cicala, C., et al. (1994a) A diclofenac derivative without ulcerogenic properties. *European Journal of Pharmacology* 257, 249-255.

Wallace, J.L., Reuter, B., Cicala, C., et al. (1994b) Novel nonsteroidal anti-inflammatory drug derivatives with markedly reduced ulcerogenic properties in the rat. *Gastroenterology* 107, 173-179.

Wallace, J.L., McKnight, W., Reuter, B.K., et al. (2000) NSAID-induced gastric damage in rats: requirement for inhibition of both cyclooxygenase 1 and 2. *Gastroenterology* 119, 706-714.

Warner, T.D., Giuliano, F., Vojnovic, I., et al. (1999) Nonsteroid drug selectivities for cyclo-oxygenase-1 rather than cyclo-oxygenase-2 are associated with human gastrointestinal toxicity: a full in vitro analysis. *Proceedings of the National Academy of Science* 96, 7563-7568.

Weiss, D.J. (2000). Aplastic anemia. In: Feldman, B., Zinkl, J., Jain, N. (eds.) *Schalm's Veterinary Hematology.* Lippincott Williams and Wilkins, Philadelphia, pp. 213-215.

Whittle, B.J. (2004) Mechanisms underlying intestinal injury induced by anti-inflammatory COX inhibitors. *Eur J Pharmacol* 500, 427-39.

Whittle, B.J., Lopez-Belmonte, J., Moncada, S. (1990) Regulation of gastric mucosal integrity by endogenous nitric oxide: interactions with prostanoids and sensory neuropeptides in the rat. *British Journal of Pharmacology,* 99, 607-11.

Wilcke, J.R. (1984) Idiosyncrasies of drug metabolism in cats. Effects on pharmacotherapeutics in feline practice. *Veterinary Clinics of North America: Small Animal Practice* 14, 1345-1354.

Williamson, K.K., Willard, M.D., Payton, M.E., et al. (2010) Efficacy of omeprazole versus high-dose famotidine for prevention of exercise-induced gastritis in racing Alaskan sled dogs. *Journal of Veteterinary Internal Medicine* 24, 285-8.

Wolfe, M.M., Lichtenstein, D.R., Singh, G. (1999) Gastrointestinal toxicity of nonsteroidal antiinflammatory drugs. The New England *Journal of Medicine* 340, 1888-99.

Wooten, J.G., Blikslager, A.T., Ryan, K.A., et al. (2008) Cyclooxygenase expression and prostanoid production in pyloric and duodenal mucosae in dogs after administration of nonsteroidal anti-inflammatory drugs. *American Journal of Veterinary Research* 69, 457-464.

Wooten, J.G., Lascelles, B.D., Cook, V.L., et al. (2010) Evaluation of the relationship between lesions in the gastroduodenal region and cyclooxygenase expression in clinically normal dogs. *American Journal of Veterinary Research* 71, 630-635.

Wright, J.M. (2002) The double-edged sword of COX-2 selective NSAIDs. *Canadian Medical Association Journal* 167, 1131-1137.

Zhang, X., Schwarz, E.M., Young, D.A., et al. (2002) Cyclooxygenase-2 regulates mesenchymal cell differentiation into the osteoblast lineage and is critically involved in bone repair. *Journal of Clinical Investigation* 109, 1405-1415.

Zimmerman, H.J. (1990) Update of hepatotoxicity due to classes of drugs in common clinical use: non-steroidal drugs, anti-inflammatory drugs, antibiotics, antihypertensives, and cardiac and psychotropic agents. *Seminars in Liver Disease* 10, 322-38.

Zimmerman, H.J., Lewis, J.H. (1987) Drug-induced cholestasis. *Medical Toxicology* 2, 112-160.

16 Complications Associated With External Coaptation

Dominique Griffon

College of Veterinary Medicine, Western University of Health Sciences, Pomona, CA, USA

External coaptation includes the use of casts, splints, bandages, slings, or hobbles to help stabilize fractures or luxations, reduce postoperative swelling, or help to protect wounds (Weinstein and Ralphs 2004).

Degenerative Joint Disease
See Chapter 18.

Bone Resorption
See Chapter 97.

Malunion
See Chapter 100.

Nonunion
See Chapter 99.

Premature Physeal Closure
See Chapter 95.

Quadriceps Contracture
See Chapter 103.

Carpal Contracture
See Chapter 102.

Neurapraxia
See Chapter 82.

Edema

Definition
Edema is accumulation of fluid in the intercellular space. Edema secondary to external coaptation most commonly involves the

STAGE	SKIN	LESIONS
I	Intact	Edema, erythema that does not blanch with pressure
II	Partial thickness lesion	Superficial lesion limited to the epidermis and dermis. Subcutaneous tissues are not visible.
III	Full thickness lesion	Extension into the subcutaneous tissue, intact fascia. No bone exposed
IV	Full thickness lesion	Lesion extends into muscle. Bone is exposed. Eschar may be present

Figure 16.1 Classification of wounds based on increasing severity.

digits or distal limbs. Edema may be considered as the milder and earlier stage of soft tissue disease caused by external coaptation (Figure 16.1)

Risk factors
- Placement of circumferential tape around the limb (Figure 16.2)
- Excessive tension applied on the bandage
- Insufficient padding in the secondary layer
- Bandage placed on a limb without extending distally to the toes
- Movement of the bandage slipping along the limb

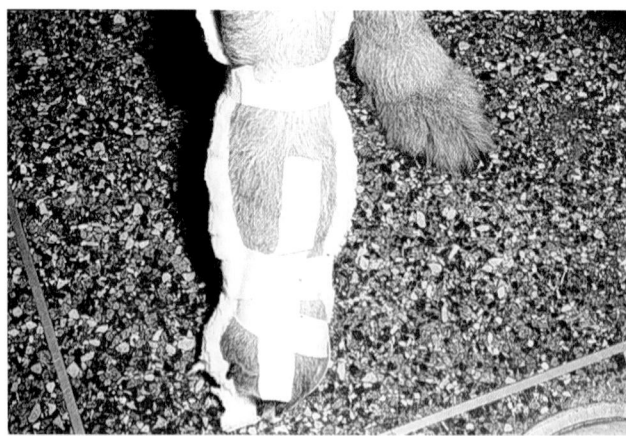

Figure 16.2 Edema secondary to placement of a bandage on the limb. Tape had been applied circumferentially around the limb to prevent migration of stir-ups and maintain the bandage in position. The tape acted as tourniquet, inducing edema of the distal limb.

Complications in Small Animal Surgery, First Edition. Edited by Dominique Griffon and Annick Hamaide.

© 2016 John Wiley & Sons, Inc. Published 2016 by John Wiley & Sons, Inc.

Companion website: www.wiley.com/go/griffon/complications

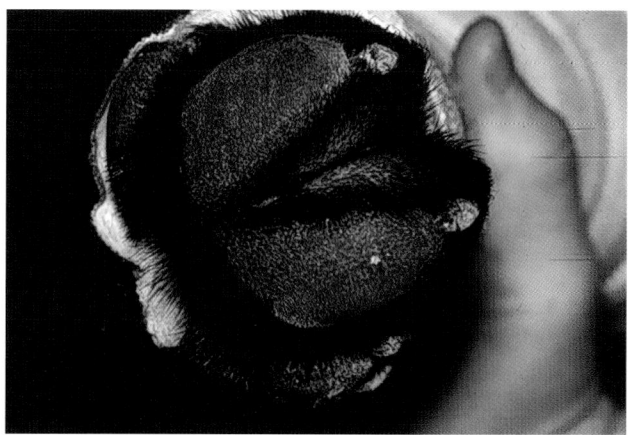

Figure 16.3 Edema of the toes secondary to bandaging of the limb. Notice the divergent appearance of the two central digits along with the impossibility of placing a finger between the two toes.

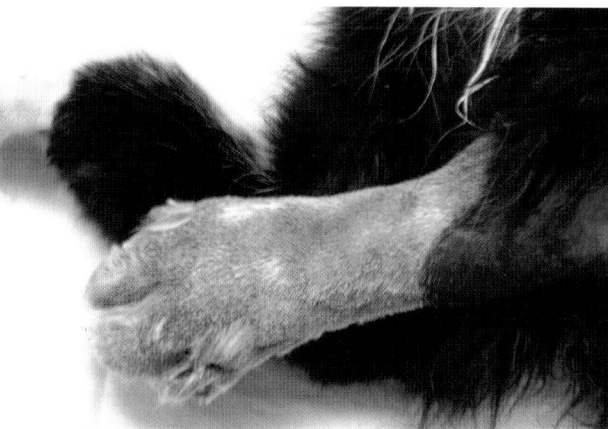

Figure 16.4 Erythema and swelling of the foot after application of a cast in a cat.

- Preexisting inflammation, swelling, or soft tissue disease
- Concurrent disease predisposing to edema (e.g., hypoproteinemia, cardiac disease)

Diagnosis
- Swollen toes (Figure 16.3)
- Toes will feel cooler than the proximal limbs
- Pain: licking or chewing, decreased use of the limb, vocalization, change in behavior
- Erythema and swelling of the foot (Figure 16.4)

Treatment
- Remove the device.
- Hydrotherapy with warm water
- Massage the limb in a distal to proximal direction to stimulate drainage.
- Pain management
- If indicated, replace the bandage with extra padding (e.g., Robert Jones bandage) and change every 12 hours for physical therapy until resolution.
- Consider alternatives to external coaptation (Table 16.1).

Outcome
Edema secondary to external coaptation carries an excellent prognosis if recognized and treated early. Delayed diagnosis allows progression to more serious lesions, such as pressure sores, compartment syndrome, or ischemia of the skin (see later).

Prevention
The most effective prevention consists of using alternatives to external coaptation when indicated (see Table 16.1).

If a bandage must be applied, preventive measures include:
- Incorporate "stir-ups," two long pieces of tape on the skin, on each side of the limb and parallel to the long axis of the limb, folded over the secondary layer to maintain the bandage in place (Figure 16.5).

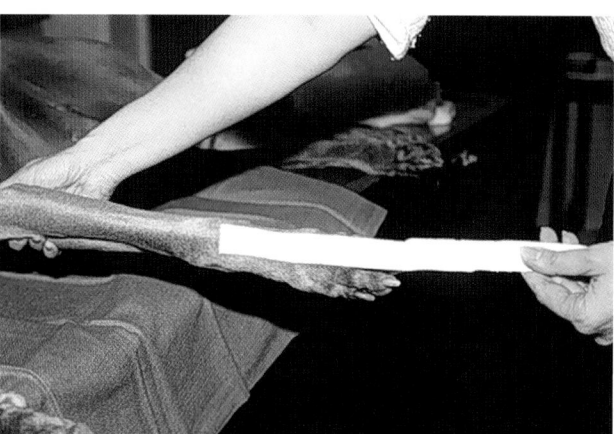

Figure 16.5 Proper application of tape to prevent bandage migration. Tape is applied parallel to the long axis of the bone on each side of the limb to avoid interference with the blood supply.

Table 16.1 Alternatives to external coaptation

External coaptation	Indication	Alternative
Bandage	Protect surgical wound (primary closure) and control postoperative swelling	Limit to the first 48 hours and combine with compresses, massage, and passive range of motion
Splint or cast	Fracture treatment	Select fixation techniques and implant that will allow early return to function without adjunct support
Splint	Arthrodesis	Alternative plate selection and location (see Chapter 108)
Splint	Elbow luxation	Flexible external fixation (Schwartz and Griffon 2008)
Splint	Achilles tendon or tarsal collateral ligament injuries	External fixation rigid or flexible (Schwartz and Griffon 2008)
Ehmer sling	Coxofemoral luxation	Open reduction and fixation or flexible external fixation (Schwartz and Griffon 2008)

- Include generous amount of padding into the secondary layer of the bandage to prevent it from acting as a tourniquet when tension is applied.
- Always place bandage material distal to proximal, alternating the direction of rotation while applying the secondary layer, to distribute tension evenly.
- Splint material should not be placed in direct contact with the skin.
- A bandage applied on a limb should always extend to the digits.
- Unless the entire foot must be incorporated in the bandage or splint, digits 3 and 4 should be allowed to protrude to allow monitoring.
- There should be enough room to slide a finger between the toes and between the limb and the external coaptation device.
- Provide detailed instructions to the primary caregiver regarding the monitoring and management of the external coaptation device.

Pyodermatitis

Definition

Pyodermatitis is a suppurative inflammation of the skin. Pyodermatitis secondary to external coaptation is usually associated with the presence of moisture around the skin and is especially common between the toes and pads of a bandaged foot. This complication is more common with devices that cover large areas of skin, such as bandages, splints, or casts, compared with slings or hobbles. Local lesions are commonly referred to as "hot spots" or moist dermatitis.

Risk factors

Patient-related risk factors include:
- Preexisting dermatitis affecting an area of skin covered by the external coaptation device
- Inclusion of the entire foot in a bandage, splint, or cast (management of phalangeal, metacarpal, or metatarsal injuries)
- Presence of open wounds
- Immunocompromised patient or skin (Figure 16.6)

Risk factors related to the management of the external coaptation device include:
- Inadequate wound management
- Insufficient frequency of bandage changes (see Figure 16.6)
- Postoperative soiling of the device by fluids (urine)
- Lack of protection of the device during outdoor walks

Diagnosis

- Foul odor
- Interdigital dermatitis can be diagnosed with the device in place if the toes are exposed.
- Moist or mutilated bandage
- Strikethrough of wound exudate
- Upon bandage removal, the skin is softened and appears white or grey. Exudate is usually present over open wounds.

Treatment

Open wounds covered by the device should be treated with lavage and wet-to-dry bandages and changed at least once a day until healthy granulation tissue covers the area. At this point, secondary healing or delayed primary closure is considered (see Figure 16.5).

Interdigital dermatitis can be treated with topical antibiotics, such as neomycin (Neo-Predef with tetracaine powder, Zoetis, Florham Park, NJ). If external coaptation is removed, an Elizabethan collar should be placed to prevent licking until lesions have resolved. If external coaptation must be maintained, daily changes are required initially along with preventive measures (see later discussion).

Outcome

Pyodermatitis responds to treatment and usually resolves after external coaptation can be discontinued. Early diagnosis and treatment are important to prevent spreading of the infection into deeper tissues, including osteomyelitis.

Prevention

General preventive measures include:
- Appropriate selection of the dressing in contact with the skin, especially if an open wound is covered by the device

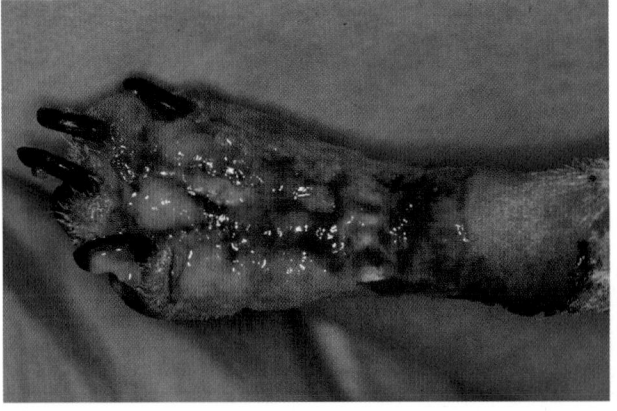 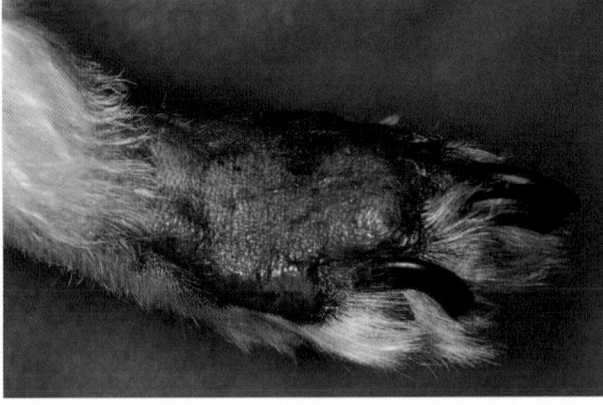

(A) (B)

Figure 16.6 Pyodermatitis secondary to external coaptation. **A,** Appearance of the surgical wound after removal of a hemangiopericytoma in a 12-year-old miniature Schnauzer. After surgical excision of the tumor, the wound was bandaged with a hydrogel dressing and treated via brachytherapy for 5 days, preventing bandage change. Open wound management with wet-to-dry bandages was applied until coverage by granulation tissue. **B,** Appearance of the wound 6 weeks after application of a full-thickness mesh graft.

- Appropriate frequency of bandage change:
  - At least once a day initially if an open wound is covered by the device
  - Every time the external coaptation device is soiled
  - At least once weekly if the device is placed over intact skin
- External coaptation should be kept dry and clean at all times.
  - Instruct the caregiver to monitor the device and cover it with a waterproof layer if the patient is taken outside.
  - The waterproof layer should be removed soon as the patient returns in the house to prevent moisture built-up.

In addition to the strategies above, preventive measures specific to interdigital dermatitis include:

- Unless the entire foot must be covered by the external coaptation device (e.g., lesions of the digits), the two central digits should be left out of the bandage to allow monitoring.
- Place absorbent material (cotton) between the toes and pads before placing any external coaptation device over a limb.
- Check the toes once daily for moisture (sliding a finger between the toes) and erythema.

Abrasions, pressure sores, and ulcers

Definition

Abrasions are partial-thickness cutaneous lesions caused by blunt trauma or a shearing force (Hosgood 2012). Pressure sores result from excessive pressure localized to an area of skin. Pressure sores are more common over bony prominences and vary in severity based on the intensity and duration of the pressure applied. Initial erythema progresses into open wounds, increasing in size and depth (Figure 16.7). Ulcers are full-thickness skin defects combined with tissue necrosis, which compromising their healing potential (Figure 16.8). Ischemia is a serious complication because compression compromises blood supply and lead to ischemia, potentially extending over large areas of the limb (Figure 16.9).

Risk factors

Abrasions, pressure sores, ulcers, and ischemia of the limb are all related to friction, excessive compression, either generalized or localized over a specific area.

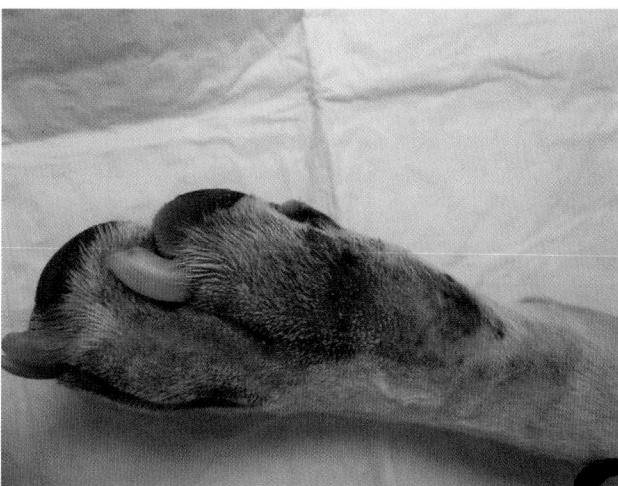

Figure 16.7 Cast sores after application of a splint in a mixed breed dog. In addition to general erythema, note the presence of small open wounds over areas of localized pressure.

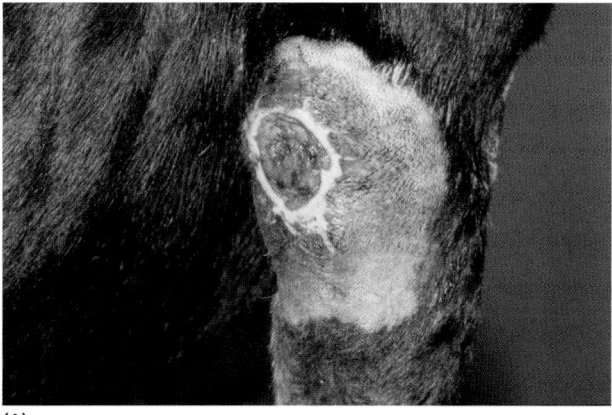

(A)

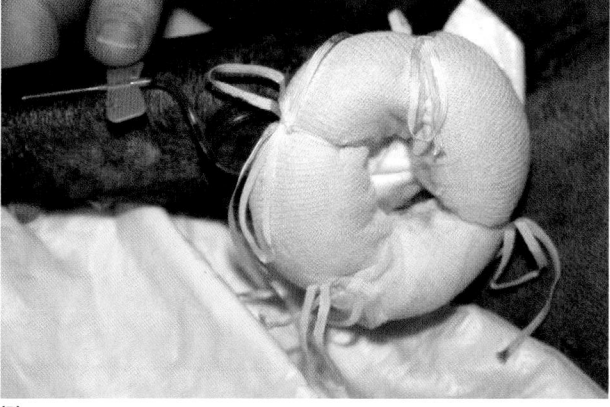

(B)

Figure 16.8 Ulcer over the elbow of a 1-year-old Rottweiler. The dog was referred after the limb had been bandaged for several weeks to manage in a hygroma. **A,** Appearance of the open wound after bandage removal. The ulcer extends beyond the subcutaneous layer, exposing bone. **B,** Postoperative bandage. After excision of nonviable tissues, a closed-suction drain (modified butterfly catheter) was placed in the defect, and a random flap, rotated over the wound, was sutured lateral to the olecranon. Stay sutures were placed around the elbow to secure a "doughnut" made of a stockinette and eliminate pressure over the bony prominence. The limb was placed in a bandage changed once daily until removal of the drain.

Specific risks factors include:
- Presence of sharp edges along the coaptation device (e.g., fiberglass edges in a splint)
- Insufficient padding between the edges of rigid material and underlying skin (abrasions and pressure sores)
- Insufficient padding over bony prominences (pressure sores and ulcers)
- Tight coaptation devices extending near areas of high motion such as the elbow or stifle (Figure 16.10)
- Insufficient padding or excessive tension (ischemia)
- Duration of immobilization
- Infrequent changes
- Constant motion between the edges of the coaptation device and skin (sores and open wounds along the proximal and distal edges of splints, bandages, casts, or slings (see Figure 16.10)
- -Young or active patient (increases the risk of motion and friction)
- -Patients with compromised health

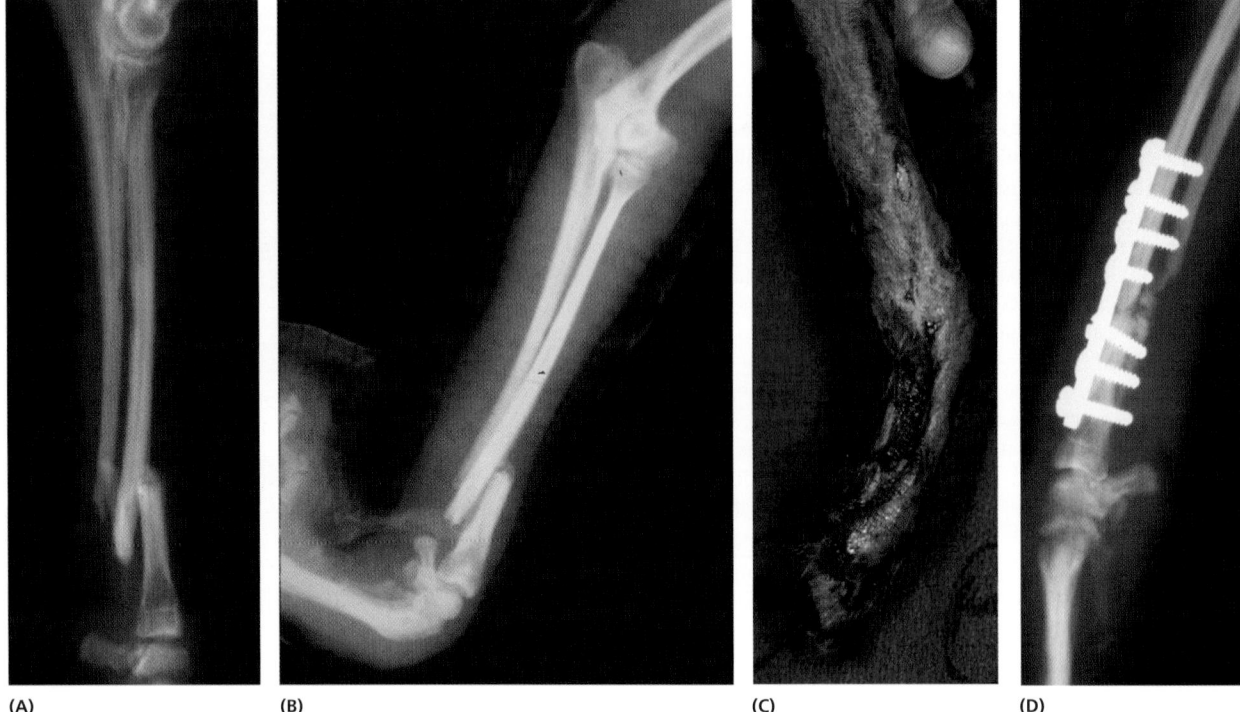

(A) (B) (C) (D)

Figure 16.9 Ischemic lesions after application of a cast in a young toy breed dog. **A,** Radiograph obtained after initial trauma showing displaced closed short oblique fractures of the distal radius and ulna. **B,** Radiograph obtained at the time of referral. The limb had been kept in a cast, with the carpus in a flexed position, for 6 weeks. Note the absence of contact between the proximal and distal fracture segments along with resorption of the ulna. **C,** Appearance of the limb after cast removal. Wounds ranging from abrasions to deep ulcers filled with necrotic tissues and exposed bone are present along the distal limb. **D,** The dog regained use of the limb after plate fixation of the fracture, open wound management, and rehabilitation.

Diagnosis

Patients with cutaneous wounds secondary to external coaptation may show signs of discomfort, decreased use of the limb, or attempting at mutilating the coaptation device. However, these signs may be initially difficult to differentiate from postoperative morbidity associated with the condition being treated. A definitive diagnosis is established by direct visualization of the skin covered by the device.

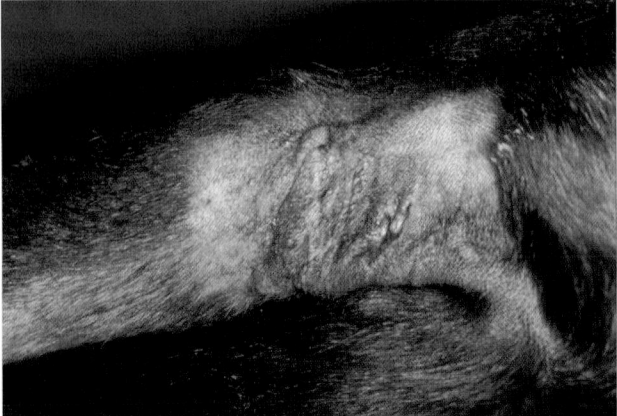

Figure 16.10 Open wound over the cranial surface of the elbow in a dog. A splint had been applied over the forelimb, extending from the foot to the elbow.

Treatment

The goal of treatment is to reach the best compromise between:
- Severity of the soft tissue lesions
- Importance of external coaptation to manage the primary (orthopedic) condition

The primary layer of the external coaptation device needs to be altered to match the needs of the cutaneous lesions. Abrasions may be treated with a hydrogel bandage, but open wounds (e.g., sores, ulcers, or ischemic lesions) require frequent lavages and wet-to-dry bandages. Surgical debridement may first be required to remove necrotic tissues in ulcers and ischemic lesions (see Figures 16.8 and 16.9).

Minor lesions respond well if the external coaptation can be removed. If support is required, alternatives to external coaptation should be considered (see Table 16.1). If these are not an option, the device may be replaced after preventive measures (see later discussion).

Outcome

Abrasions and small wounds (sores) respond well to treatment. The prognosis for ulcers and ischemic lesions is more guarded because the healing potential of these wounds is affected by compromised biological factors. Depending on the extent and duration of vascular compromise, lesions will respond to aggressive treatment after blood supply is restored, or they may warrant amputation. Ulcers deep enough to expose the bone generally require long-term treatment and have a high risk of dehiscence or recurrence.

Prevention

- Adjust positioning of the device around areas of high motion (joints) and localized pressure (bony prominence).
- Trim any sharp edges (especially on the distal end) along the splint material and ensure placement of padding material between the edges of the splint and the skin.
- To avoid folds in synthetic casting tape, the material can be rotated horizontally to change direction over flexed joints (Keller and Montavon 2006b).
- If folds are created in synthetic casting tape, the tape should be cut through the folds and smoothed over (Keller and Montavon 2006b).
- Add padding in the secondary layer.
- Modify the bandage to protect areas of localized pressure (see Figure 16.8).
- Frequent bandage change until resolution of skin lesions
- Daily monitoring of the device by the caregiver

Abnormal range of motion

Definition

These are changes in range of motion (ROM) of the affected joints secondary to external coaptation. These changes result directly from immobilization and generally consist in a loss of ROM of the joints included in the device. They may be beneficial in some patients and justify the application of external coaptation in the management of joint instability caused by ligament or capsular tears. In other patients, loss of motion caused by immobilization represents a side effect inherent to prolonged external coaptation.

On the other end of the spectrum, joint laxity is an uncommon complication of external coaptation, most commonly affecting the carpal joint in immature dogs.

Risk factors

Changes in ROM are most common after:
- Prolonged immobilization
- Complete immobilization of joints (hobbles are unlikely to induce undesirable changes)

Carpal laxity is more common after immobilization of the forelimb of immature dogs in a splint or cast, especially if the limb is maintained in extension.

Stiffness is more common in older patients with preexisting joint disease.

Diagnosis

The diagnosis is based on orthopedic examination of the limb after removal of the external coaptation. Based on goniometry, the ROM of the immobilized joint is decreased compared with the contralateral limb, pretreatment ROM of the same joint, or normal values published in dogs (Table 16.2). Loss of ROM may be accompanied by a stiff gait or lameness.

Young dogs with iatrogenic carpal laxity stand with a palmigrade stance. The degree of extension of the affected joint is greater than that of the contralateral limb and normal values.

Treatment

Loss of ROM after immobilization can be managed with:
- Pain management
- Passive ROM
- Rehabilitation therapy
- Treatment of any underlying joint disease (e.g., degenerative joint disease)

Table 16.2 Range of motion of various appendicular joins measured by goniometry in 16 healthy Labrador retrievers

Joint	Position	Mean (degrees)	95% CI of the mean (degrees)
Carpus	Flexion	32	31–34
	Extension	196	194–197
	Valgus	12	11–13
	Varus	7	6–8
Elbow	Flexion	36	34–38
	Extension	165	164–167
Shoulder	Flexion	57	54–59
	Extension	165	164–167
Tarsus	Flexion	39	37–40
	Extension	164	162–166
Stifle	Flexion	42	40–43
	Extension	162	160–164
Hip	Flexion	50	48–52
	Extension	162	160–164

CI, confidence interval.

Source: Data from Jaegger *et al.* (2002).

Carpal laxity secondary to immobilization is generally managed with gradual loading of the limb:
- Casts may be replaced by splints or Robert Jones bandages.
- After removal of the external coaptation device, exercise is limited to walks on surfaces that provide good muscle traction such as carpets, grass, or rubber mats for 1 to 3 weeks.
- Nutrition should consist of a balanced diet for immature dogs.

Outcome

Range of motion generally improves after removal of external coaptation and physical therapy.

Prevention

General prevention against changes in ROM secondary to immobilization focuses on:
- Avoiding external coaptation and considering alternative options (see Table 16.1)
- Aiming for early return to function and joint mobilization
- Limiting the duration of immobilization
- Rehabilitation therapy in conjunction with external coaptation

External coaptation of the forelimb should maintain the carpus in 10 to 15 degrees of flexion and varus position to minimize the risk of carpal laxity (Keller and Montavon 2006b).

Osteofascial compartment syndrome

Definition

This is neuromuscular ischemia caused by increased pressure in a compartment anatomically confined by bone and fascia.

Risk factors

- Fracture repair of the tibia, femur, or radius with severe soft tissue trauma
- Acute trauma within a known compartment:
  - Craniolateral crus
  - Caudal crus
  - Caudal antebrachium
  - Quadriceps

- Surgical closure of the fascia within a compartment after severe soft tissue trauma (high-energy fractures)
- Injection or leaking of large amount of fluids (e.g., blood) within a compartment
- Patients with coagulation disorders
- Tight bandages or splints

Diagnosis

Clinical signs are not specific but should trigger a tentative diagnosis:

- Pain levels exceeding expectations based on injury and patient
- Neurologic impairment, including paresis or sensory deficits

The diagnosis is confirmed by measuring compartmental pressure with a pressure catheter or an 18-gauge needle connected to a three-way stopcock and saline-filled central venous pressure manometer. Normal intrafascial pressure should range between –2.7 and 11 cm of water (equivalent to –2 and +8 mm Hg). Pressures exceeding 40 cm of water (30 mm Hg) are clinically significant.

Treatment

The goal of the treatment for compartment syndrome is to relieve tissue pressure as soon as possible. Surgical fasciotomy is recommended if compartmental pressure exceeds 40 cm of water (30 mm Hg). Incision of the fascia is combined with debridement of necrotic tissues. The cutaneous incision is generally closed to prevent contamination of the tissues, especially if a fracture has been fixed internally. Placement of drains should be considered to prevent fluid accumulation after surgery.

Outcome

Compartment syndrome is much less commonly recognized in dogs than in humans and may be underdiagnosed. Based on evidence limited to case reports, dogs diagnosed with compartment syndrome respond favorably to surgical treatment and regain function of the affected limb. However, compartment syndrome has been proposed as a cause of muscle contracture (Taylor and Tangner 2007).

Prevention

Compartment syndrome is a rare complication in small animals, and no specific preventive measure has been established. It may be reasonable to leave the fascia at least partially open in tibial, radial, and femoral fractures with significant swelling of the soft tissues. This strategy seems especially relevant if significant tension is generated while attempting to close the fascia over known compartments in dogs.

Relevant literature

Although prolonged immobilization was common practice after orthopedic procedures 20 years ago, the standard of care has evolved toward early return to function combined with physical therapy, thereby decreasing external coaptation in small animals. This evolution has been facilitated by a deeper understanding of the morbidity associated with immobilization combined with development of new implants, surgical techniques, and postoperative physical therapy. Today, bandages are still routinely placed over the limbs to control postoperative swelling but are generally limited to the first 48 hours before discharge from the hospital. The primary layer (in contact with the wound) generally consists of nonadhesive, semiocclusive dressing. The amount of padding placed in the secondary layer of the bandage should be proportional to the amount of compression expected from the bandage. Finally, a tertiary layer is applied without tension to protect the bandage from external contamination. Prolonged application of bandages is indicated in the treatment of soft tissue lesions, such as open wounds, that may be associated with orthopedic diseases. In these instances, the primary layer is selected to address the objectives of wound management and match the phase of wound healing. The secondary layer assists with absorption of fluids from the wound. Splints are designed to provide some biomechanical support to the affected limb by incorporation of a hard material, such as low-temperature thermoplastics, plastic, or aluminum (Johnson *et al.* 2003). Splints may be used for preoperative stabilization of fractures, for conservative management of selective fractures or soft tissue injuries (tendons or ligaments), or as an adjunct to fixation of an arthrodesis or ligament repair. Casts include a rigid material on the outer surface and circumferentially around the limb (Keller and Montavon 2006a). Slings are indicated to restrict motion of a joint (Velpeau and Ehmer slings) or prevent weight bearing (carpal flexion sling). They may be applied after closed reduction of a luxation or as an adjunct to internal reduction and immobilization of a luxated joint. Hobbles allow weight bearing but prevent abduction via placement of tape encircling contralateral fore- or hindlimbs.

The most common complications associated with external coaptation consist of **soft tissue damage**. Although most are minor complications, these affect the patient's comfort and can lead to severe consequences. A retrospective study of 60 small animals described soft tissue injuries associated with cast application for distal limb orthopedic conditions (Meeson *et al.* 2011). Soft tissue injuries were recorded in 63% cases, with 60% of those considered as mild, 20% as moderate, and 20% as severe. Mild lesions consisted of swelling, erythema, and partial thickness sores that did not require specific treatment. Moderate lesions extended deeper, were combined with infection, and required specific treatment. Severe lesions included full-thickness wounds and necrosis, all associated with loss of function or systemic signs of disease. The mean time from casting to diagnosis of injuries was 23 days ± 17. Sighthounds were predisposed to these complications, but cross-breeds were less likely to be affected. These breed differences could be attributable to differences in limb conformation and soft tissue coverage over bony prominences. The most common indications for casting were tarsal arthrodesis and common calcanean tendon injuries. All dogs with Achilles tendon reconstruction in this series ($n = 6$) had soft tissue complications. This finding is consistent with a retrospective study of 28 cases of Achilles tendon repair in dogs in which complications were generally attributable to external coaptation rather than to the primary tendon repair (Nielsen and Pluhar 2006). Complications caused by external coaptation are also well recognized after carpal and tarsal arthrodeses. In fact, the relatively high incidence of splint- or cast-related complications has prompted the search for castless alternatives. In a recent clinical comparison of plate fixation techniques for pancarpal arthrodesis, external coaptation related complications occurred in 32% of cases with hybrid dynamic compression plates and 18% of cases with CastLess Plate (Bristow *et al.* 2015). In the same study, limbs immobilized for more than 14 days were more likely to have a related complication if a cast was placed (44.4%) compared with other forms of external coaptation (20.7%).

Although most soft tissue related lesions caused by external coaptation generally carry a good prognosis, **ischemic bandage injuries** can have devastating consequences, requiring extensive treatment, potentially including amputation. In a case series of 11 small animals with such injuries, 5 required full-thickness skin grafts, 3 digit amputations, and 2 limb amputations (Anderson and White 2000). Nine of these patients survived, but only 4 regained full function of the affected limb. Loss of digital flexor tendons was associated with a worse prognosis for return to function because of hyperextension and pressure necrosis on weight-bearing areas. Interestingly, the duration of application varied from 1 to 14 days before the lesion was first diagnosed, suggesting that ischemia can develop fairly quickly. The authors concluded that ischemic injuries were sustained within the first 24 to 48 hours after bandage application and therefore recommended evaluation of the bandage during that time.

Compartment syndrome is a well-established condition in humans and was first described in 1881 by Volkmann, who accurately recognized the etiology of muscle contracture secondary to application of a constrictive bandage over the distal limb and ischemic destruction of the muscle. The condition is much less documented in small animals, and the literature consists essentially of case reports and review articles (de Haan and Beale 1993; Fitch *et al.* 1997). Most of our understanding of the pathogenesis of compartment syndrome in dogs is derived from that described in humans, in whom the condition is believed to arise from (1) increased compartment volume (bleeding, fluid accumulation, or injection), (2) postischemic tissue swelling (after vascular surgery), or (3) excessive external pressure (tight external coaptation). In humans, compartment syndrome exists in an acute (especially after tibial fractures) and chronic (associated with exercise in young male runners), but in dogs, only the acute form has been reported. Because tissue perfusion correlates inversely with compartment pressure, the higher the pressure, the shorter the time required to produce irreversible damage. In the acute form, compartment pressure results from soft tissue damage, bleeding, or constriction secondary to external coaptation. These factors may be combined with the high-energy fractures associated with this syndrome in dogs. The few case reports published in dogs involved (1) the antebrachium (laceration of the median artery secondary to a gunshot wound and radial fracture; Olivieri 1978), (2) the femoral compartment (secondary to closure of the fascia under tension after fracture repair; Basinger *et al.* 1987), (3) the femoral compartment (after repair of a comminuted femoral fracture; de Haan and Beale 1993), and (4) caudal crus (secondary to a bite wound; Williams *et al.* 1993). Although the true incidence of compartment syndrome is unknown, their apparent lower predisposition compared with humans has been attributed to two main factors: (1) underdiagnosis because intracompartment pressure is not routinely measured in dogs and (2) a superior collateral circulation in dogs (de Haan and Beale 1993). Based on the limited evidence available in the veterinary literature, dogs diagnosed with compartment syndrome and treated by emergency fasciotomy respond well to treatment.

Prevention of complications associated with external coaptation relies on three main strategies: (1) case selection, (2) proper selection and application of external coaptation, and (3) proper management and monitoring until removal of the device. The first line of management should focus on alternatives to external coaptation; ligament injuries may be better treated with hinged or flexible external fixators that limit the ROM of the affected joint within safe limits. Implants and fixation technique for fracture repair should generally strive to provide a suitable biomechanical environment without adjunct support. Alternatives are becoming available to eliminate the need for or reduce the duration of external coaptation after joint arthrodesis (see Chapter 108). If external coaptation is necessary, the device should be properly placed to avoid localized pressure areas, remain

in place and provide the support required without compromising the vascular supply to the area (Oakley 1999; Keller and Montavon 2006a). In a review of complications of fractures repaired with casts and splints, the authors concluded that most complications resulted from improper application of the device or poor management of the patient (Tomlinson 1991). Indeed, the patient's temperament and the owner's ability for compliance must be evaluated when selecting treatment modalities. Detailed instructions should be provided to the caretaker to ensure proper maintenance and monitoring of the device. However, in a study of soft tissue injuries caused by casts, 80% of the lesions were diagnosed by the attending clinician during scheduled follow-up examinations, although owners had been instructed to monitor the casts (Meeson *et al.* 2011). The authors concluded that the only reliable method to identify complications was inspection of the limb by a veterinarian. Combined with the report of ischemic lesions early after application of external coaptation (Anderson and White 2000), these publications emphasize the importance of close veterinary monitoring.

References

Anderson, D.A., White, R.A.S., (2000) Ischemic bandage injuries: a case series and review of the literature. *Veterinary Surgery* 29 (6), 488-498.

Basinger, R.R., Aron, D.N., Crowe, D.T., et al. (1987) Osteofascial compartment syndrome in the dog. *Veterinary Surgery* 16 (6), 427-434.

Bristow, P.C., Meeson, R.L., Thorne, R.M., et al. (2015) Clinical comparison of the hybrid dynamic compression plate and the castless plate for pancarpal arthrodesis in 219 dogs. *Veterinary Surgery* 44 (1), 70-77.

De Haan, J.J., Beale, B.S. (1993) Compartment syndrome in the dog: case report and literature review. *Journal of the American Animal Hospital Association* 29, 134-140.

Fitch, R., Montgomery, R., Jaffe, M. (1997) Muscle injuries in dogs. *Compendium on Continuing Education for the Practicing Veterinarian* 19 (8) 947-957.

Hosgood, G. (2012) Open Wounds. In: Tobias, K.M., Johnston, S.A. (eds.) *Veterinary Surgery: Small Animal.* Elsevier Saunders, St. Louis.

Jaegger, G., Marcellin-Little, D.J., Levine, D. (2002) Reliability of goniometry in Labrador Retrievers. American Journal of Veterinary Researc 63 (7), 979-986

Johnson, R.P., Steiss, J.E., Sorjonen, D.C. (2003) Thermoplastic materials for orthotic design. *Compendium on Continuing Education for the Practicing Veterinarian* 25 (1) 20-28.

Keller, M.A., Montavon, P.M. (2006a) Conservative fracture treatment using casts: indications, principles of closed fracture reduction and stabilization, and cast materials. *Compendium on Continuing Education for the Practicing Veterinarian* 29 (9), 631-641.

Keller, M.A., Montavon, P.M. (2006b) Conservative Fracture treatment using casts: application of a full-leg cast. *Compendium on Continuing Education for the Practicing Veterinarian* 29 (9), 642-651.

Meeson, R.L., Davidson, C., Arthurs, G.I. (2011) Soft-tissue injuries associated with cast application for distal limb orthopaedic conditions. A retrospective study of sixty dogs and cats. *Veterinary and Comparative Orthopaedics and Traumatology* 24 (2), 126-131.

Nielsen, C., Pluhar, G.E. (2006) Outcome following surgical repair of Achilles tendon rupture and comparison between postoperative tibiotarsal immobilization methods in dogs: 28 cases (1997-2004). *Veterinary and Comparative Orthopaedics and Traumatology* 19 (4), 246-249.

Oakley, R.E. (1999) External coaptation. *Veterinary Clinics of North America: Small Animal Practice* 29 (5), 1083-1095.

Olivieri, M. (1978) Compartment syndrome of the front leg of a dog due to rupture of the median artery. *Journal of the American Animal Hospital Association* 14, 210-248.

Schwartz, Z., Griffon, D. (2008) Nonrigid external fixation of the elbow, coxofemoral, and tarsal joints in dogs. *Compendium on Continuing Education for the Practicing Veterinarian* 30 (12), 648-653.

Taylor, J., Tangner, C.H. (2007) Acquired muscle contractures in the dog and cat. A review of the literature and case report. *Veterinary and Comparative Orthopaedics and Traumatology* 20(2), 79-85.

Tomlinson, J. (1991) Complications of fractures repaired with casts and splints. *Veterinary Clinics of North America: Small Animal Practice* 21 (4), 735-44.

Weinstein, J., Ralphs, S.C. (2004) External coaptation. *Clinical Techniques in Small Animal Practice* 19 (3), 98-104.

Williams, J., Bailey, M.Q., Schertel, E.R., et al. (1993) Compartment syndrome in a Labrador retriever. *Veterinary Radiology & Ultrasound* 34, 244-248.

17 Complications Associated with Rehabilitation Modalities

Debra Canapp,[1] Lisa M. Fair,[1] and Sherman Canapp[2]
[1]Veterinary Orthopedic & Sports Medicine Group, Annapolis Junction, MD, USA
[2]Veterinary Orthopedic & Sports Medicine Group; Orthobiologic Innovations, LLC, Annapolis Junction, MD, USA

Pain and inflammation

Definition

Pain is an unpleasant sensation occurring in varying degrees of severity as a consequence of injury, disease, or emotional disorder.

Inflammation is defined as a localized, protective reaction of tissue to irritation, injury, or infection characterized by pain, redness, swelling, and sometimes loss of function.

Risk factors

Pain associated with rehabilitation is more common with:
- Therapeutic ultrasonography
- Cryotherapy
- Therapeutic heat
- Cold laser
- Electrical stimulation
- Therapeutic exercise

Diagnosis

Clinical signs of pain and methods used to assess pain in small animals are described in Chapter 14. Patients undergoing rehabilitation should be monitored closely during applications of therapy. The first signs of pain (Figure 17.1) include change in behavior, agitation, discomfort, unrest or evidence of cutaneous erythema during treatment (Figure 17.2).

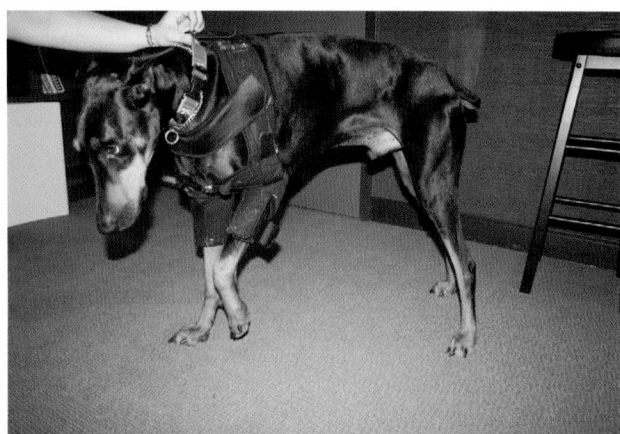

Figure 17.1 Evidence of pain in a dog undergoing rehabilitation. Signs of pain include offweighting of a limb and changes in expression.

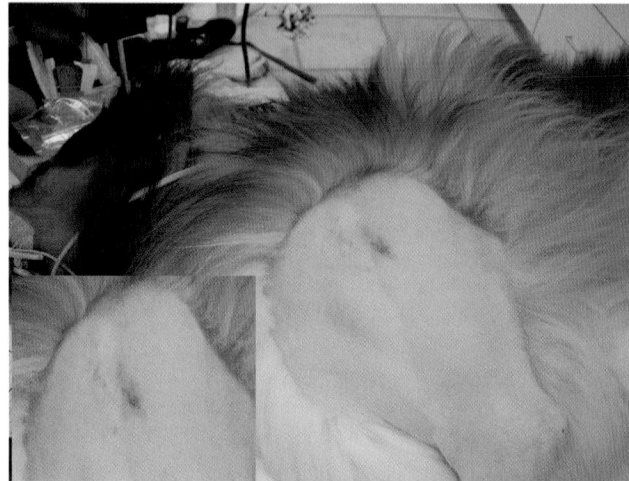

Figure 17.2 Cutaneous inflammation after therapeutic ultrasonography. Continuous application at excessive intensity caused inflammation across the spinous process of the scapula.

Treatment

- Immediate removal of the modality
- Medical management of pain (see Chapter 14) and inflammation (see Chapter 15) via oral or topical routes

Prevention

Preventive measures vary with the modality considered.
Therapeutic ultrasonography:
- Use appropriate settings for the size of the patient and the anatomic area treated.
- Apply generous amounts of coupling gel before application.
- Avoid application over boney prominences.
- Maintain the ultrasound probe in continuous movement during treatment.

Cryotherapy:
- Avoid in areas of decreased sensation or on anesthetized patients.

Therapeutic heat:
- Avoid on sedated or immobile patients.
- Monitor the temperature of the treated site.
- Place a fabric buffer between the heat source and patient.

Complications in Small Animal Surgery, First Edition. Edited by Dominique Griffon and Annick Hamaide.
© 2016 John Wiley & Sons, Inc. Published 2016 by John Wiley & Sons, Inc.
Companion website: www.wiley.com/go/griffon/complications

Cold laser:
- Avoid high dosage use of class IV lasers.
- Keep class IV laser probes in continuous movement during application.

Electrical stimulation:
- Avoid application of direct currents.
- Use pulsed setting and fresh patches with sufficient amounts of evenly distributed coupling gel.

Therapeutic exercise:
- Tailor therapeutic exercises to the phase of healing and individual needs of the patient.
- Alter the number of repetitions and duration based on patient's athletic ability and overall pain tolerance.
- Consider preemptive analgesia.

Primary or latent infection

Definition
This kind of infection is a primary or lingering invasion by and multiplication of pathogenic microorganisms in a bodily cavity or within tissues. Latent infections may lead to tissue injury and progress to overt disease through a variety of cellular and toxic mechanisms. Latent infections may remain dormant in the body for a period of time and become active under conditions depressing the immune response, such as surgical stress.

Risk factors
- Therapeutic ultrasonography
- Electrical stimulation
- Hydrotherapy

Diagnosis
A presumptive diagnosis can be made based on signs of infection subsequent to therapeutic ultrasonography, electrical stimulation, or hydrotherapy. These signs may consist of:
- Surgical wound infection
- Pyodermatitis (Figure 17.3)
- Systemic signs of infection

A definitive diagnosis may be made based on similarities of culture and sensitivity between samples obtained from the patient compared with those obtained from the therapeutic unit.

Treatment
- Discontinuation of modality
- Antibiotherapy based on culture and sensitivity results
- Open wound management of the surgical wound is indicated in case of dehiscence.
- Treatment should be pursued until complete resolution of infection, confirmed by negative culture results.
- Take actions to control a hospital-associated infection (see Chapter 8).

Prevention
- Avoid therapeutic ultrasonography, electrical stimulation, and hydrotherapy in patients with confirmed or suspected infections, such as dermatitis, abscesses, or osteomyelitis in the area to be treated.
- Covering small localized skin wounds on patients requiring hydrotherapy is a strategy to prevent cross-contamination while allowing them to benefit from this treatment modality.
- Delay hydrotherapy in patients with more generalized infections such as those affecting the urinary tract, skin, open wounds, or gastrointestinal tract until they have been successfully treated. Patient triage is essential to prevent hydrotherapy from becoming a source of infectious agents.
- Proper equipment cleaning, sanitation, and management (Figures 17.4 to 17.6) are crucial to control contamination from unidentified infected cases.

Cutaneous burns

Definition
A cutaneous burn is an injury to the skin caused by exposure to heat or an electrical, chemical, or radioactive agent.

Risk factors
- Therapeutic ultrasonography
- Cryotherapy
- Therapeutic heat
- Cold laser
- Electrical stimulation

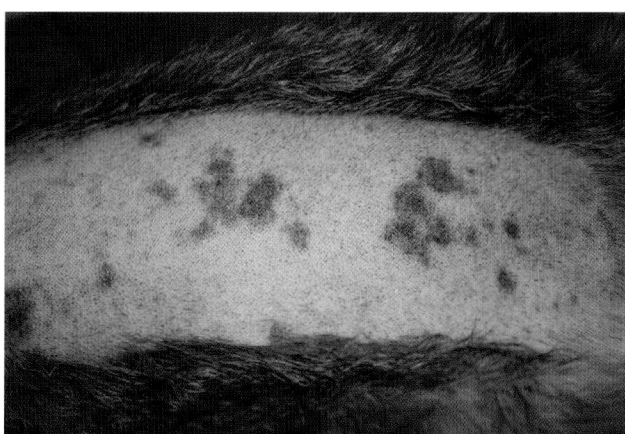

Figure 17.3 Staphylococcus pyodermatitis. This patient should not be allowed in hydrotherapy. Modalities such as electrical stimulation and therapeutic ultrasonography should be avoided on the affected skin until this infection is resolved.

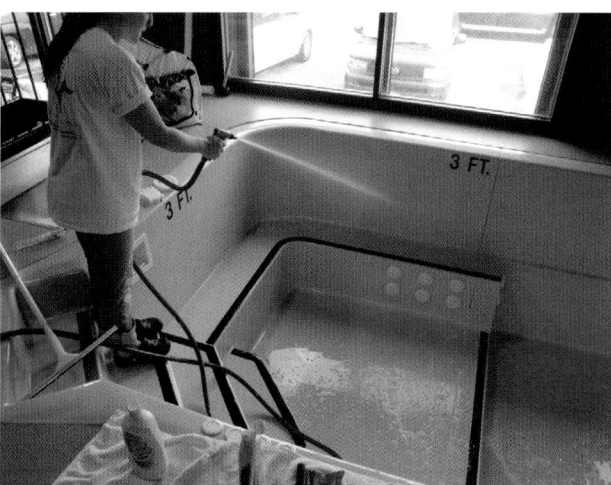

Figure 17.4 Cleaning of the swimming pool. Proper disinfection on a routine basis decreases cross-contamination and prevents this modality from acting as a source of infection for patients.

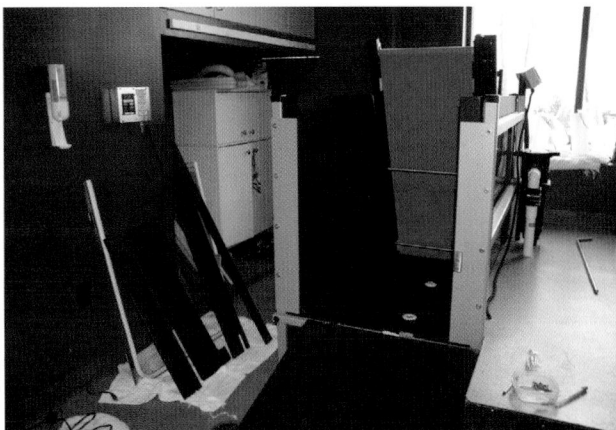

Figure 17.5 Cleaning of an underwater treadmill. Weekly, thorough cleaning should include bleaching and steaming down to the tread to reduce bacterial load and risk of infections in regular patients.

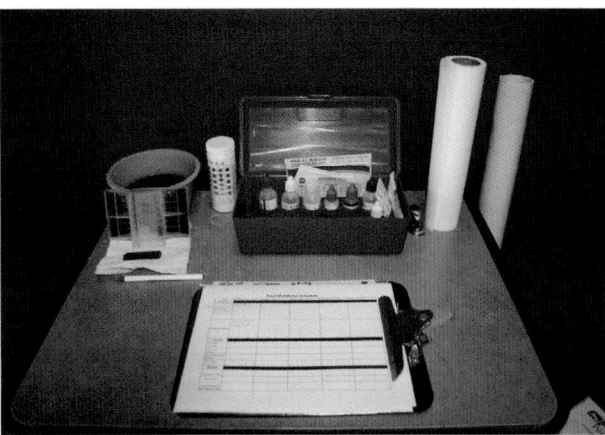

Figure 17.6 Water maintenance. Daily water chemical and chlorine maintenance is key in keeping the water safe for exercise and minimize the risk of cross-contamination between patients.

Diagnosis

Diagnosis is made by monitoring patients closely during modality applications and acknowledging the first signs of change in behavior, agitation, pain, or unrest. Cutaneous burns are diagnosed by direct observation of skin lesions, including severe erythema, blisters, or open wounds (Figure 17.7) during treatment.

Treatment

- Immediately discontinue application of the treatment modality.
- Systemic antibiotherapy
- Pain management
- Local treatment of the burns with topical agents or open wound management depending on the severity of the wound (see Figure 17.7).
- Protect the wound (bandage) from mutilation and contamination.

Prevention

Therapeutic ultrasonography:
- Use appropriate settings based on patient size and anatomic area treated.
- Apply generous amounts of coupling gel.
- Use the continuous mode only when medically indicated.
- Move the ultrasound probe continuously during application.

Cryotherapy:
- Avoid in areas of decreased sensation or on anesthetized patients; monitor temperature of skin to avoid frostbite.

Therapeutic heat:
- Avoid on sedated or immobile patients; monitor temperature of site being treated and use fabric buffer between the heat source and the patient.

Cold laser:
- Avoid high dosage use of class IV lasers; keep the head of class IV laser probes moving.

Electrical stimulation:
- Avoid direct currents.
- Use pulsed setting.
- Use fresh, moist patches with sufficient amounts of evenly distributed coupling gel. Discard old and dried out patches (Figure 17.8).

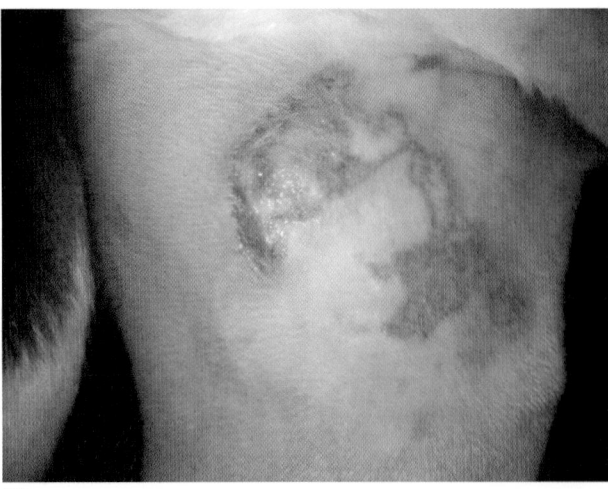
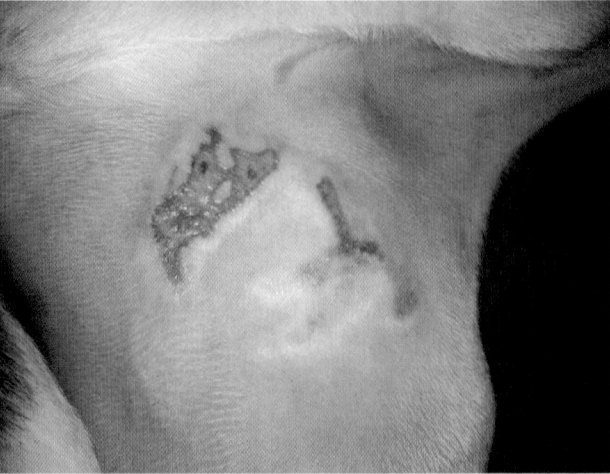

(A)   (B)

Figure 17.7 Cutaneous burn caused by application of an old electrical stimulation patch. **A,** Initial appearance of the lesions. **B,** Lesions responded to open wound management. Prevention focuses on the use of electric stimulation patches that are new and well hydrated. Patches should be placed in good contact with the patient, with sufficient and evenly distributed coupling gel to avoid superficial skin burns during neuromuscular stimulation.

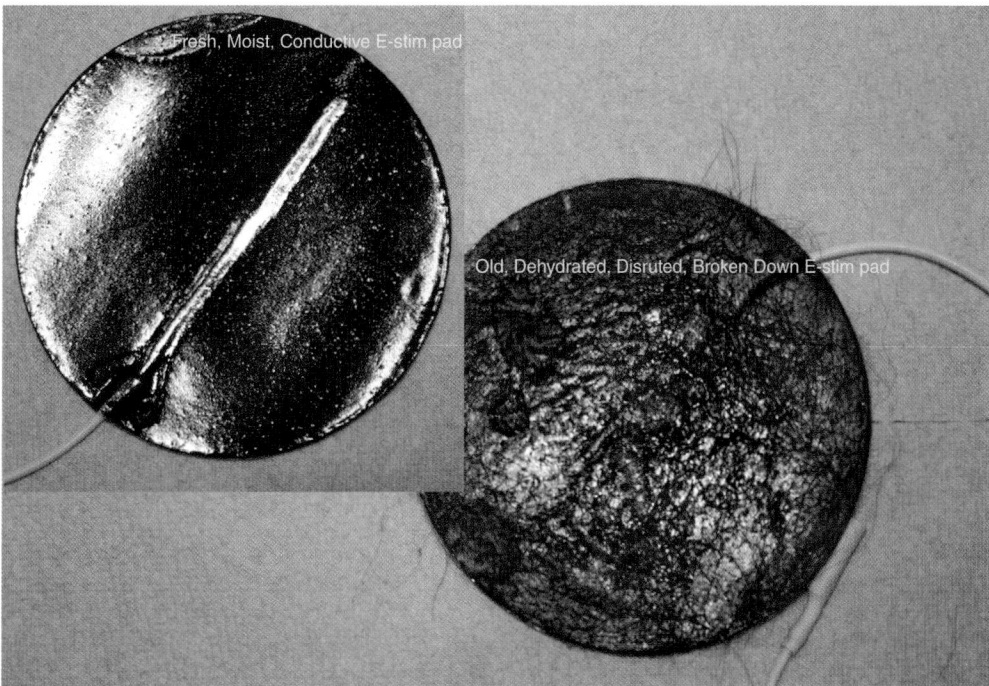

Figure 17.8 Appearance of patches used for electrical stimulation. Old and worn electrical stimulation patches (bottom right) should be discarded and replaced with new and well-hydrated patches (top left) to avoid burns and skin injury.

Retinal burns

Definition
A retinal burn is a retinal lesion induced by prolonged exposure to high-powered laser energy. Most retinal burns create permanent damage.

Risk factors
Retinal burns occur as a result of cold laser therapy under the following conditions:
- Prolonged exposure to lower power (5–250 MW)
- Shorter exposure times to power lasers in excess of 500 MW

Diagnosis
The diagnosis is based on recognizing direct, prolonged exposure of a patient's eye to laser energy. Retinal lesions are confirmed during ophthalmic examination.

Treatment
There is no treatment for a true retinal burn. Steroids have been successfully used to treat retinal inflammation. The authors are not aware of any publication reporting cold laser retinal burns in the veterinary literature.

Prevention
- Eye protection is available for patients (Laser Safety Doggles; Laservision, Saint Paul, MN) and is especially indicated when using class IV higher powered lasers.
- Attentive application of cold laser therapy to patient is needed to avoid inadvertent eye exposure.

Traumatic injuries to the digits and tail

Definition
This is a bodily wound caused by sudden physical damage or harm.

Risk factors
- Underwater treadmill exercise
- Decreased proprioception
- Exhaustion

Diagnosis
Diagnosis is done through direct observation of the patient during underwater treadmill exercise; a body part becomes entrapped in the revolving tread, creating significant injury of varying depth and severity.

Treatment
- Turn the treadmill off as quickly as possible, using the emergency shut-off button, if available.
- Begin draining the water while an assistant calms and restrains the patient.
- Safely enter the treadmill and dislodge the appendage. This can be done by reversing the tread, prying downward on the belt, or levering upward or removing the ledge.
- Take the patient out of the water, apply pressure if bleeding, assess injuries, and begin appropriate treatment.
- Open wound management is generally indicated to treat the injuries.
- The patient should be fully healed before hydrotherapy is reintroduced.

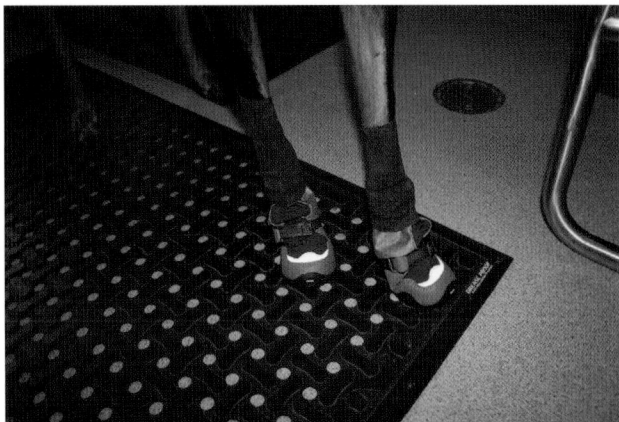

Figure 17.9 Prevention of treadmill-induced injuries to the toes. Using booties on the paws of patients can protect the toes from getting caught in the tread.

Prevention

- Monitor the patient's position in the underwater treadmill; do not allow the patient to drop too far back, risking entrapment.
- Apply booties (Figure 17.9) or wrap the tail to prevent entrapment under the tread.
- Placing bumpers behind the patient (Figure 17.10) helps maintain the position of the patient away from the rear of the treadmill, where entrapment is most likely to occur.

Muscle and tendon fatigue

Definition

This is loss of muscle or tendon function caused by excessive stimulation or prolonged exertion.

Risk factors

- Hydrotherapy
- Therapeutic exercise
- Electrical stimulation

Diagnosis

The diagnosis is based on visual inspection of the patient (Figure 17.11), recognizing the inability or diminishing capacity of the patient or the muscle being treated to complete the exercise at hand.

Treatment

Depending on the patient's needs and medical state, nonsteroidal pain medication can be used to reduce any inflammation or pain caused by excessive exercise. When the patient is back in a comfortable state, the exercise regimen or protocol for electrical neuromuscular stimulation should be readjusted to match the ability of the patient or muscle to perform the movement and avoid aggravation of the initial injury.

Prevention

- Monitor the patient and muscle during the exercise; form, strength, and ability should be maintained during the session particularly towards the end.

- Develop a rehabilitation program that is individually adapted to each patient's injuries, abilities, and goals.
- Move progressively through the program at a pace that is challenging but not to the point of affecting healing and strength recovery to avoid delays in return to function.

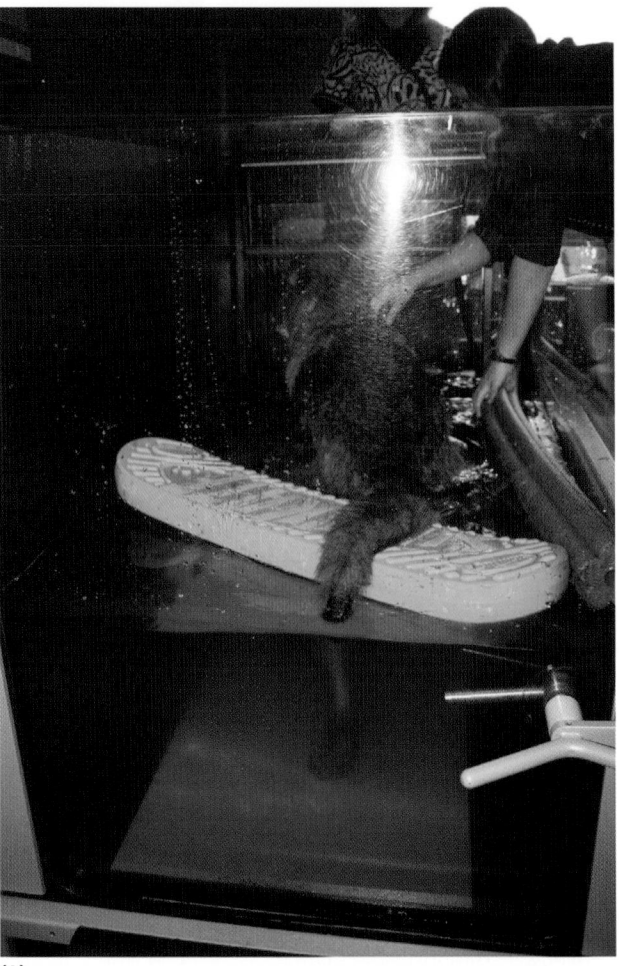

(A)

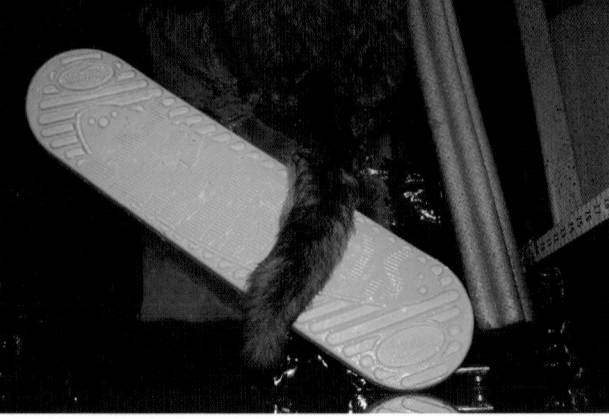

(B)

Figure 17.10 Prevention of treadmill-induced lesions to the tail. Placing bumpers behind the patient (**A**) and under the tail (**B**) of patients with neurologic conditions with decreased tail tone can help prevent entrapment in the tread.

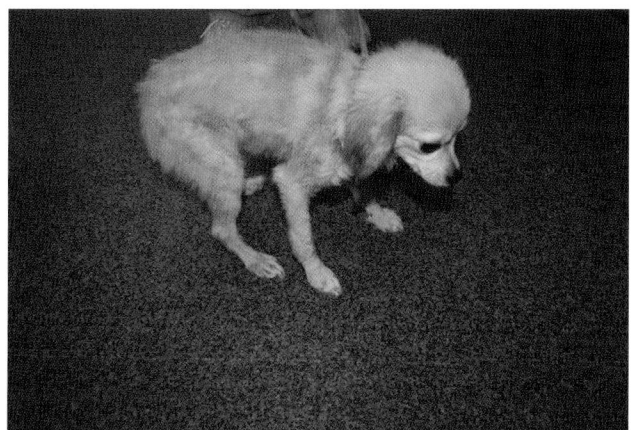

Figure 17.11 Muscle fatigue secondary to strenuous exercise. Clinical signs may include a wide-based stance and a roached back. This posture is often seen in patients with neurologic conditions after prolonged exertion or excessive stimulation of weak or compromised muscles.

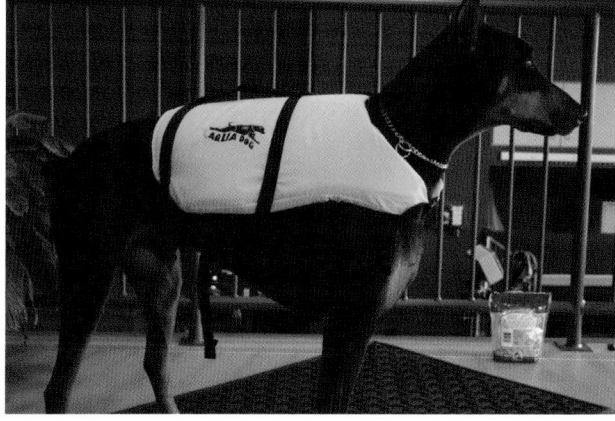

Figure 17.12 Placement of a life vest before hydrotherapy. Proper fitting is important to aid in flotation and prevent drowning while limiting interference with swimming.

Peripheral nerve injury

Definition
Peripheral nerve injury is iatrogenic damage inflicted on a peripheral nerve.

Risk factors
- Cryotherapy

Diagnosis
The diagnosis is based on neurologic examination of a patient before and after treatment.
- Neuropraxia of a peripheral nerve incorporated into the area treated with cryotherapy, inducing loss of superficial sensation or motor function.

Treatment
- Discontinue the use of cryotherapy and gradually warm the area to normal body temperature.
- If neuropraxia persists, the affected area may need to be protected with a bandage or e-collar until function has returned.

Prevention
- Avoid placement of the cold therapy device close to superficial peripheral nerves.
- Regulate the time and temperature of application.
- Monitor the patient for signs of discomfort during cold therapy because this may precede neuropraxia.
- Check skin temperature if the patient becomes agitated or exhibits signs of pain.

Drowning

Definition
Drowning is death secondary to immersion in water, depriving the patient of oxygen and ending in suffocation.

Risk factors
- Hydrotherapy
- Inadequate patient monitoring
- Inadequate patient support

Diagnosis
- Suffocation by immersion in water followed by cessation of the heartbeat and death

Treatment
- Initiate cardiopulmonary resuscitation (CPR)

Prevention
- Patients should wear properly fitted life vests (Figure 17.12) during hydrotherapy.
- Accompany patients during deep-water therapy.
- Supplement floatation (Figure 17.13) with neck or midbody rolls in older, debilitated patients or those with neurologic conditions; these rolls may be needed to increase buoyancy and to keep patients properly placed with the head above the water surface.

Relevant literature
Therapeutic modalities are gaining popularity in small animal rehabilitation, paralleling the expansion of therapy centers and the growing number of trained individuals dedicated to the field.

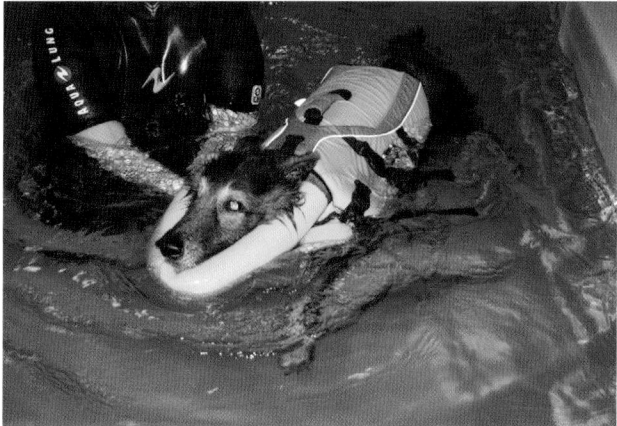

Figure 17.13 Head support during hydrotherapy. Some patients with neurologic conditions need additional head support or flotation to prevent aspiration of water or drowning.

Although rare when administered by a trained and highly educated individual, complications associated with all forms of rehabilitation may occur at any time. In a national survey published in 2003, 26% of 903 human athletic trainers reported complications, and a total of 362 complications were documented (Nadler *et al.* 2003). Cryotherapy was involved in 42% of complications, with allergic reactions, burns, and intolerance or pain most commonly listed. Electric stimulation accounted for 29% of complications, with skin irritation, burns, and intolerance or pain most commonly listed. Therapeutic heat accounted for 22% of complications; therapeutic exercise accounted for 7% of complications. Unfortunately, limited information has been published on this topic in small animals because of the relative infancy of veterinary rehabilitation. A thorough understanding of the physics behind modalities is a prerequisite to ensure safe application and positive outcomes. Nonetheless, even when the utmost care is taken, complications may happen because of an individual patient reaction. This section discusses complications associated with modalities used in rehabilitation along with their prevention.

Cryotherapy is one of the most commonly used modalities both after surgery and after injury in both humans and animals. Peripheral nerve injury can occur with cryotherapy, temporarily affecting the patient's function. Pain and frostbite are also frequently encountered. These complications are easy to avoid by avoiding placement of the cold therapy device on superficial peripheral nerves and regulating the time and temperature of application (Bassett *et al.* 1992). Direct observation of the skin also helps early detection of complications. Thorough monitoring and careful application of cryotherapy are especially relevant when treating patients with decreased sensation or anesthesia because they may not show signs of discomfort or adverse reaction.

Therapeutic heat is another common and simple rehabilitation modality designed to stimulate drainage in chronic inflammation. Misuse of thermal applications can result in severe burns, leading to tissue death and infection. Heating pads are one of the most common causes of **thermal burns** both in human and veterinary medicine. Burns, dermatitis, and pain can all occur during use of any thermal modality, including hot water bottles, warm moist heat, hot packs, electric heating pads, and thermal therapeutic ultrasonography (Nadler *et al.* 2003). Avoiding electric heating pads, especially on sedated or immobile patients, is highly recommended. Monitoring temperature and placing a fabric buffer between the patient and heat source will help avoid these injuries. Water bottles exceeding 45°C will induce thermal burns when placed in direct contact with the skin of a dog (Dunlop *et al.* 1989). Extreme caution is therefore warranted when applying heat to an anesthetized or sedated patient because the normal pain response will be absent. Forced-air warming blankets are preferred for that purpose. If those are not available, a thin blanket or cloth should be placed between a heating pad and the underlying skin.

Complications associated with **therapeutic ultrasonography** can generally be avoided by avoiding obvious contraindications such as application over growth plates, infected sites, and major vessels. The most significant contraindication to ultrasound therapy consists of application in the presence of infection. Failure to comply will invariably lead to an aggravation or spread of the infection. Thorough screening of patients before application is therefore crucial to avoid application over an undiagnosed infected site. Most other complications occur when therapeutic ultrasonography are set in the continuous setting. These adverse reactions can affect both soft tissues and bone. **Inflammation** may be observed over

the site undergoing treatment, in which case a pulsed mode may be appropriate. Patients may feel pain or irritation over the site treated with ultrasonography if an insufficient amount of coupling gel is applied to protect the skin. The same deficiency can lead to superficial **cutaneous burns** (Singer *et al.* 1998). Periosteal reaction may occur if the depth and intensity are too high or if the area being treated includes superficial boney prominences. Bone marrow lesions have also been reported and can be avoided with proper probe movement during treatment and using correct unit settings. Patients may also experience redness or irritation to the specific agents used in the gel during phonophoresis. Most of these complications are preceded by **pain** and can therefore be prevented by monitoring the patient's reactions closely. As soon as adverse signs are observed, the clinician should terminate the session and reevaluate the treatment regimen, including settings. Prevention of complications relies so heavily on patient's response that therapeutic ultrasonography should be avoided in anesthetized patients.

Moderate- and high-power **laser therapy** is potentially hazardous because of the associated risks of **retinal and cutaneous burns**. Wearing safety goggles eliminates the risk of retinal damage. There is relatively little risk or complications noted when cold laser therapy is delivered to tissues with a class 3b machine. Patients have been found to tolerate 360 J/cm^2 equally well as those treated with 36 J/cm^2 (Sasaki *et al.* 1992; Sasaki and Oshiro 1997). These results, along with others, support the concept of cold laser as a safe therapy that does not cause tissue damage on normal treated tissue even at high doses (Yoshida *et al.* 1991; Calderhead and Inomata 1992). Extrapolation of these results to clinical patients warrants caution because they were generated on normal, healthy tissues, and injured or diseased tissue may react differently. Doses should therefore be carefully selected and adjusted to the injury or tissue type being treated. Concerns have also been expressed regarding new "high-powered" class IV lasers that emit more than 1000 MW into a single site. With these units, the potential for tissue damage and skin burns is highly increased, although no current research is noted.

The most common complications associated with **electrical stimulation**, including iontophoresis, include **cutaneous irritation, burns, and pain** (Nadler *et al.* 2003). Skin irritation can result from the product used with iontophoresis or even consist of an individual reaction to the adhesive comprising the patches. Burns can occur when old, dried out patches are used, even without direct contact with the skin. Burns also occur if a coupling agent has not been distributed in sufficient quantity and evenly throughout the hair or skin. In these situations, the electrical current is not uniformly distributed; instead, the electrical energy becomes delivered over small areas, creating superficial burns. Cutaneous burns are usually preceded by discomfort and can be avoided via patient monitoring. Patients with neurologic deficits lack this sensory response and therefore warrant extra precautions during gel application. Most of the complications observed with electrical stimulation occur as a result of uninterrupted direct current technique and can be avoided by eliminating this modality. Most protocols in veterinary medicine rely on pulsed settings and therefore lessen the probability for complications. Electrical stimulation at the motor level can cause undesirable tension of the muscle fibers, tendons, or bony insertion. This side effect can aggravate preexisting weakness or injury. **Muscle fatigue** can also develop if the duty cycle, or repetition of contraction, is too high, thus depleting the energy and reducing muscle function. Intense or prolonged stimulation may result in muscle spasm or muscle soreness, which contradicts the purpose of rehabilitation via electrical stimulation. Indeed, these side effects can affect limb function, therefore promoting loss of muscle tone and mass. Similar to other modalities, patients should be carefully screened for infection before therapeutic ultrasonography is initiated to avoid extension of infection.

Complications associated with **underwater treadmill** usage can be classified as mechanical or physiological. Mechanical complications essentially involve **impingement** of appendages into the back of the belt treadmill interface if the patient is not kept moving forward. This situation can result in a minor complication or significant tissue loss over the digits. Control of the tail is often impaired in patients with neurologic deficits. If the tail is long enough, this deficit increases the risk of impingement and degloving injury. Physiological complications include benign **dermatitis** caused by exposure to sanitation chemicals. Proper monitoring is necessary and can often be helpful in avoiding this simple problem. A more serious complication involves water aspiration leading to tracheitis. This complication is caused by an irritation produced by the chlorine and can lead to pneumonia. These incidents are more frequent during jet or whirlpool therapy (Aksamit 2003). Proper head support and avoiding feeding during the session help to circumvent these issues. **Bacterial infection**, usually dermatitis, can occur if water sanitation and regulation of the chemicals are defective. Patients with open wounds or with a history of urinary tract infections or dermatitis can contaminate the water with potential pathogens. Daily monitoring and intermittent culturing of the treadmill should be part of the routine maintenance of the equipment. Among bacterial infections, *Pseudomonas* infection has been reported in human pools and has been found problematic in veterinary aquatic therapy (Schlech *et al.* 1986). Parasitic infections can also be spread to other patients, thereby emphasizing the importance of screening patients before their introduction to the water.

The most common complications reported in human patients attending **therapeutic exercises** include **swelling, pain, and aggravation of the injury** (Aksamit 2003). Some patients may experience muscle soreness or fatigue when flexibility or strengthening exercises are initiated. Symptoms usually subside with or without modifications to the treatment plan. However, persistence of signs should prompt a reevaluation of the exercise regimen and the ability of the patient to perform them. Adjusting the exercises to the individual ability of the patient is crucial to avoid aggravation of the initial injury. In general, when performed correctly, therapeutic exercise

and manual therapy (unless referring to cross-frictional massage or fiber breakdown) should not induce significant discomfort or soreness. Nonsteroidal agents may be prescribed to reduce the inflammation during initiation of the therapy, but in the long term, irritation should not subsist if the therapeutic exercise and manual therapy program match the stage of healing and the individual surgery or injury.

Conclusion

The body of evidence regarding complications secondary to modalities used in physical therapy is limited in the human peer-reviewed literature and is virtually nonexistent in the literature relevant to small animals. Complications secondary to rehabilitation may therefore be more common and different than reported here. The expansion of small animal rehabilitation justifies a survey aimed at documenting the relative frequency of adverse effects of modalities.

References

Aksamit, T.R. (2003) Hot tub lung: infection, inflammation, or both? *Seminars in Respiratory Infections* 18 (1), 33-39.

Bassett, F., Kirkpatrick, J.S., Englehardt, J.L., et al. (1992) Cryotherapy-induced nerve injury. *The American Journal of Sports Medicine* 20, 516-518.

Calderhead, R.G., Inomata, K. (1992) A study of the possible haemorrhagic effects of extended infrared diode laser irradiation on encapsulated and exposed synovial membrane articular tissue of the rat. *Laser Therapy* 4, 65-69.

Dunlop, C.I., Daunt, D.A., Haskins, S.C. (1989) Thermal burns in four dogs during anesthesia. *Veterinary Surgery* 18 (3), 242-246.

Nadler, S.F., Prybicien, M., Malanga, G.A., et al. (2003) Complications from therapeutic modalities: results of a national survey of athletic trainers. *Archives of Physical Medicine and Rehabilitation* 84, 849-853.

Sasaki, K., Ohshiro, T. (1997) Assessment in the rat model of the effects of 830 nm diode laser irradiation in a diachronic wound healing study. *Laser Therapy* 9, 25-32.

Sasaki, K., Calderhead, R.G., Chin, I., et al. (1992) To examine the adverse photothermal effects of extended dosage laser therapy in vivo on the skin and subcutaneous tissue in the rat model. *Laser Therapy*, 4, 69-74.

Schlech, E.F., Simonsen, N., Sumarah, R., et al. (1986) Nosocomial outbreak of pseudomonas aeruginosa folliculitis associated with physiotherapy pool. *Canadian Medical Association Journal* 134 (8), 909-913.

Singer, A.J., Homan, C.S., Church, A.L., et al. (1998) Low-frequency sonophoresis: pathologic and thermal effects in dogs. *Academic Emergency Medicine* 5, 35-40.

Yoshida, K., et al. (1991) *The effect of low power semiconductor laser to stellate ganglion.* Presented at the IX Congress International Society for Laser Surgery and Medicine, Anaheim, CA.

18 Degenerative Joint Disease

Guillaume Ragetly[1] and Dominique Griffon[2]

[1]Centre Hospitalier Vétérinaire Frégis, Paris, France
[2]College of Veterinary Medicine, Western University of Health Sciences, Pomona, CA, USA

Degenerative joint disease (DJD) results from both mechanical and biologic events that destabilize the normal coupling of degradation and synthesis of articular cartilage and subchondral bone. These events ultimately lead to morphologic, biochemical, molecular, and biomechanical changes affecting the chondrocytes and surrounding matrix. The clinical impact of DJD includes pain, decreased range of motion (ROM), crepitus, and variable degree of inflammation.

Degenerative joint disease is a common disease in small animals, affecting approximately 20% of dogs older than 1 year of age (Johnston 1997). The prevalence increases with age, and radiographic evidence of DJD was recently detected in 90% of cats older than 12 years of age (Hardie 2002; Lascelles 2010). Factors involved in the pathogenesis of DJD include metabolic disorders, supraphysiologic overload, or progression of an isolated lesion caused by macrostructural failure (Cole and Malek 2004). This failure appears to be traumatic in origin and accounts for about 25% of degenerative joint lesions in cats (Clarke *et al.* 2005). The incidence of trauma as a cause of DJD is unknown in dogs. In both species, cartilage trauma can be a direct consequence of surgery.

Although articular cartilage resurfacing procedures have reached clinical applications, DJD remains a common postoperative complication. This outcome was first described more than 30 years ago, but further studies are indicated to establish the prevalence of postoperative DJD and clearly define the role of causative factors.

Infection: septic arthritis (see Chapter 1)

Iatrogenic damage
Definition
Iatrogenic articular damage is an injury to the cartilage caused by a diagnostic or therapeutic procedure. Iatrogenic articular damage, although largely unreported, is likely the most common surgical complication leading to DJD. Damage can result from direct trauma to the articular surface, leading to tracklike fissures or patchlike defects, potentially extending into superficial layers of subchondral bone. Cartilage lesions can also develop secondary to penetration of an implant in the subchondral bone or in the deeper layer of the cartilage, affecting the tissue biomechanics and leading to DJD.

Risk factors
- Technical errors leading to intraarticular placement of surgical implants (Figure 18.1)
- Implant migration: may result from improper technique, poor implant selection, or postoperative loosening

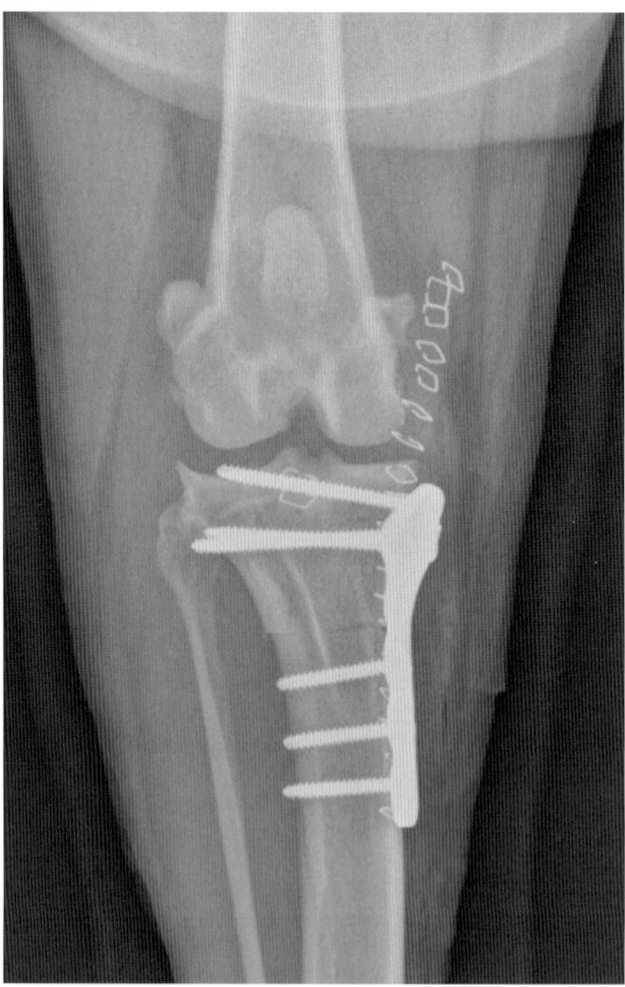

Figure 18.1 Postoperative radiograph after a tibial plateau leveling osteotomy. The most proximal screw enters the joint, leading to iatrogenic cartilage damage. *Source:* Reproduced with permission from G. Ragetly.

Complications in Small Animal Surgery, First Edition. Edited by Dominique Griffon and Annick Hamaide.
© 2016 John Wiley & Sons, Inc. Published 2016 by John Wiley & Sons, Inc.
Companion website: www.wiley.com/go/griffon/complications

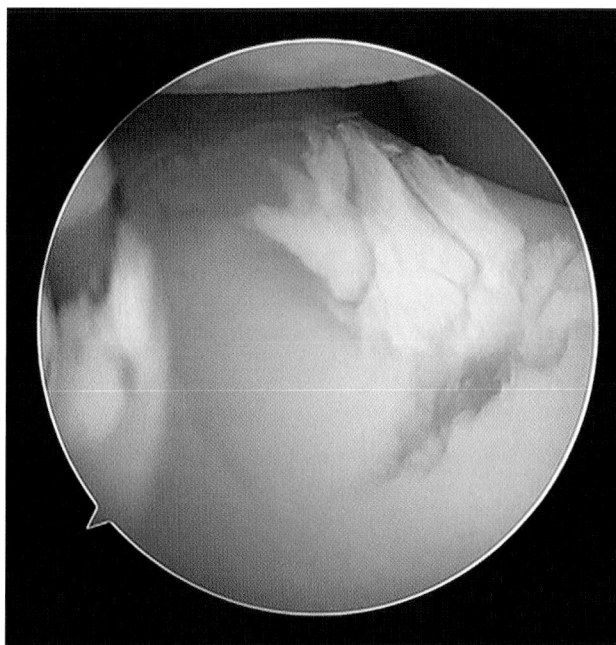

Figure 18.2 Arthroscopic appearance of an elbow with acute, iatrogenic cartilage damage. A tracklike fissure is present secondary to the placement of the arthroscopic portal. *Source:* Reproduced with permission from G. Ragetly.

- Improper instrumentation: direct trauma to the cartilage during intraarticular surgery (arthroscopy or arthrotomy)
- Surgical procedures that alter load distribution throughout the joint, such as meniscectomy and meniscal release
- Radioablation: thermal damage occurs if the tip of the radioablator contacts or comes close to cartilage, especially in small joints, or if lavage or perfusion is insufficient.

Diagnosis
Intraoperatively
Diagnosis can be made by direct visualization of fissures or exposure of subchondral bone: the edges of the lesions are fresh without evidence of remodeling, supporting the diagnosis of acute damage. Lesions created during placement of an arthroscope are visible after placement of the arthroscope (Figure 18.2) (see chapter 116). Inadvertent incision of the cartilage may occur during open or arthroscopic exploration of a joint or intraarticular placement of a pin or screw.

Postoperatively
- Postoperative pain, limb function, and ROM that do not match expectations for normal postoperative recovery; auscultation facilitates the detection of crepitus when the affected joint is mobilized
- Radiographs: poor implant placement (postoperatively) or signs of DJD (long term)
- Computed tomography (CT) is occasionally indicated if intraarticular placement of an implant is suspected but cannot be confirmed on radiographs.

Treatment
Immediate removal of the intraarticular implant is indicated to prevent postoperative pain and limit the progression of degenerative changes. Conservative treatment is considered when the long-term function is expected to be worse with implant revision

(e.g., fracture that cannot be revised safely, transarticular pining for complex joint luxation).

Full-thickness cartilage damage should be treated intraoperatively with micropicking. Long-term medical management for DJD should be instituted in all cases (weight loss, rehabilitation, nutraceuticals with or without antiinflammatory therapy). Figure 18.3 summarizes the multimodal approach to managing postoperative DJD. Administration of nonsteroidal antiinflammatory drugs (NSAIDs) remains the mainstay for managing DJD (Table 18.1). This approach is indicated in dogs when nutritional and exercise management fail to produce satisfactory results. Revision surgery or salvage procedures (joint replacement, excision arthroplasty, arthrodesis) are considered in most severe cases. Alternative and regenerative medicine provides new options in dogs failing to respond to NSAIDs, especially if surgical treatment is contraindicated or not possible.

Prevention
Proper use of instrumentation
- Placement of implants under fluoroscopic guidance if technique (minimally invasive osteosynthesis) or fracture location affects visualization
- Use of intraoperative radiographs as an alternative to intraoperative fluoroscopy to confirm proper placement of implants
- Use of cannulated guides to direct the placement of implants (e.g., a C-clamp has been designed to guide screw fixation of humeral condylar fractures)
- Use of guidewires: After appropriate placement of a fine wire has been confirmed, a cannulated drill bit is placed over the wire to ensure proper positioning of the screw or pin. Alternatively, guidewires may serve as landmarks for placement of pins or screws. In addition, wires immobilize the fracture during implant placement and can therefore prevent inadvertent loss of reduction during fracture repair.
- Use of cannulated instrumentation and proper selection of instrument size during arthroscopy (Table 18.2).

Proper surgical technique
Fracture fixation via intramedullary pins
- Humerus: The pin should be advanced in a craniolateral direction during retrograde placement.
- Tibia: The pin should be directed in a craniomedial direction during retrograde placement.

Arthroscopic trauma (see also Chapter 116)
- Distension of the joint before insertion of a cannula
- Injection of saline before creating a camera portal
- Closure of the egress before insertion of subsequent cannulas.
- Application of traction on the joint to increase the intraarticular space (Figure 18.4)

Use of anatomic landmarks Arthroscopy:
- Placement of camera and instrument portals warrants caution, especially for arthroscopy of the carpus, tarsus, elbow, and hip.
- A needle can be used to locate the position of the joint and serve as a guide.
- Arthroscopy of the hip: The arthroscope portal is placed 0 to 10 mm cranial and 12 to 18 mm proximal to the greater trochanter.
- Arthroscopy of the elbow: The arthroscope portal should be placed distal (~1–2 cm) and caudal (~5 mm) to the medial humeral

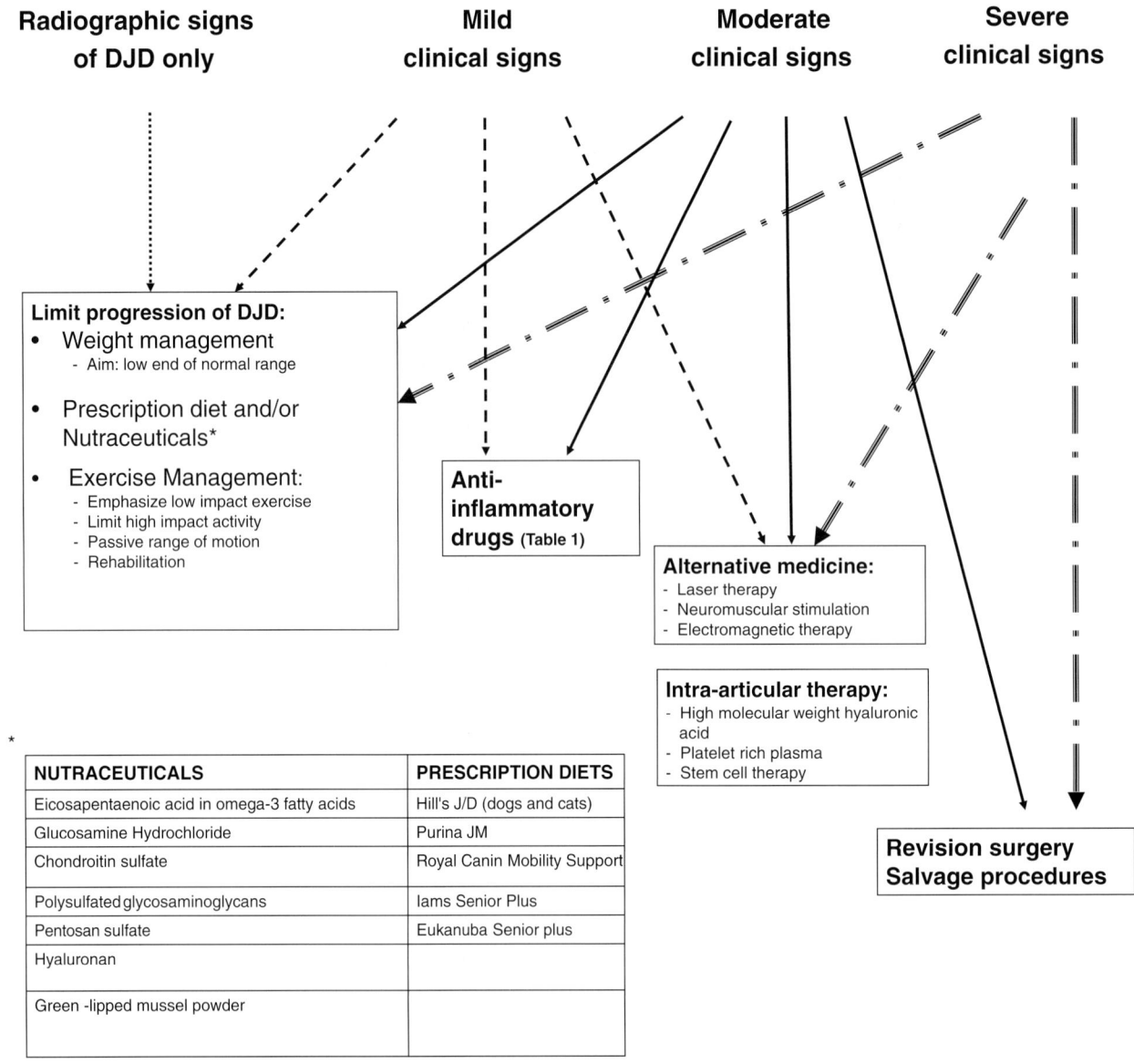

Figure 18.3 Algorithm for managing postoperative degenerative joint disease (DJD).

Table 18.1 Common nonsteroidal antiinflammatory drugs used for medical management of degenerative joint disease in small animals

	Agent	Dose	Frequency	Specific side effects
Dogs				
Metacam	Meloxicam	0.2 mg/kg once; then 0.1 mg/kg PO	Once daily	
Rimadyl	Carprofen	4.4 mg/kg PO	Once daily	Hepatopathy in <0.05% of dogs
Previcox	Firocoxib	5 mg/kg PO	Once daily	
Deramaxx	Derocoxib	1–2 mg/kg PO	Once daily	
Etogesic	Etodolac	10–15 mg/kg PO	Once daily	Keratoconjunctivitis sicca
Cat				
Ketofen	Ketoprofen	1 mg/kg PO	Once daily for ≤5 days	
Metacam	Meloxicam	0.1 mg/kg PO initially followed by 0.05 mg/kg for 3 days and then 0.025 mg/kg every other day		

PO, orally.

Table 18.2 Recommended diameters of arthroscopes based on patient size and joints*

	Medium to large dogs	Small dogs	Cats
Shoulder (mm)	2.7 (4.0 in giant breed)	1.9–2.4	1.9
Elbow (mm)	1.9–2.4	1.9	1.9
Carpus (mm)	1.9 (2.4 in giant breed)	1.9	1.9
Hip (mm)	2.7	1.9–2.4	1.9
Stifle (mm)	2.7	2.4	2.4
Tarsus (mm)	1.9 (2.4 in giant breed)	1.9	1.9

*Smaller arthroscopes minimize the risk of iatrogenic damage but limit the field of visualization.

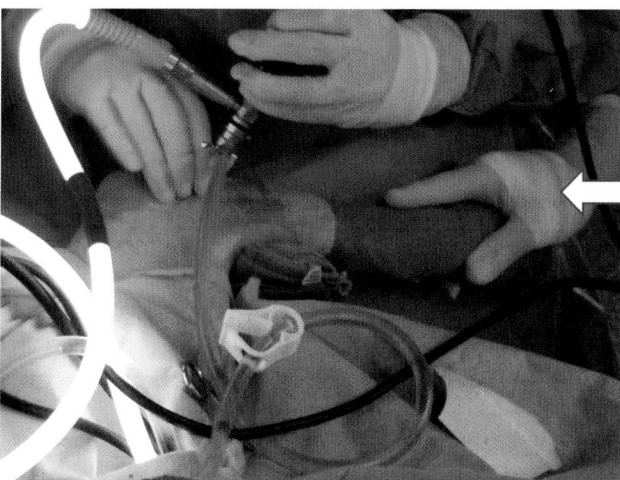

Figure 18.4 Distal distraction and abduction of the joint minimize the risk of iatrogenic trauma during introduction of instruments. The assistant is applying pressure (arrow) on the distal limb to distract the elbow joint. *Source:* Reproduced with permission from G. Ragetly.

epicondyle. The distance between the epicondyle and the joint can be measured on preoperative craniocaudal radiographs or via CT.
- Instrument portals, if needed, are placed under direct visualization.
Fracture repairs and osteotomies:
- During tibial plateau leveling osteotomy (TPLO), the safe zone for probing the stifle joint with a needle is located on the medial aspect of the joint at one third of the distance between the cranial border of the collateral ligament and the medial edge of the patellar ligament.
- During fixation of epiphyseal femoral fractures, pins may be placed to a distance equal to 80% (or 65% if the placement is eccentric) of the contralateral intact proximal femoral epiphysis depth or pubic bone as measured from a ventrodorsal radiograph with minimal risk of penetration though the cartilage.
- During repair of fractures involving the lateral portion of the humeral condyle, a compression screw should be located slightly craniodistal to the lateral epicondyle. It can be safer for inexperienced veterinarians to drill the initial gliding hole from the fracture surface laterally to exit to this point.

Malreduction

Definition
Malreduction is failure to restore the anatomic apposition of fracture fragments. Malreduction of articular fractures alter contact

areas and biomechanical loads distribution across the affected joint, initiating cartilage breakdown.

Risk factors
- Articular fractures affecting weight-bearing areas of the joint
- Presence of a step between articular surfaces relative to the patient. A gap greater than 1 mm will result in fibrocartilage formation. Anatomic reduction and compression of articular fractures are therefore recommended.
- Complex fractures are generally more challenging to reduce than simple fractures. In some cases, the degree of comminution or the size of fragments may preclude anatomic reduction.
- Lack of surgical access may affect the ability to manipulate fragments and visualize articular surfaces.

Diagnosis
Intraoperative diagnosis
Fracture reduction is generally assessed by direct visualization of articular surfaces or adjacent landmarks. When this is not possible, fluoroscopy and arthroscopy should be considered.

Postoperative diagnosis
Fracture reduction is assessed via radiography immediately after surgery. The presence of a gap or step between articular surfaces on postoperative radiographs establishes the diagnosis (Figure 18.5). However, superimposition with adjacent structures or implants may affect the detection of minor articular gaps. In these cases, oblique projections and CT should be considered to confirm anatomic fracture reduction. Failure to detect malreduction immediately after surgery will lead to the presence of callus and degenerative joint changes on long-term radiographic evaluations.

Treatment
- Long-term medical management (see Iatrogenic damage earlier) for DJD should be instituted in all cases.
- Surgical revision of the fracture repair is recommended when the articular surfaces are misaligned by more than 1.5 mm.
- Total joint replacement, arthrodesis, or excision arthroplasty may be considered if the diagnosis of malreduction has been delayed.

Prevention
Proper technique and intraoperative visualization of the articular surface limit the risk of malreduction.

Malunion (see Chapter 100)

Fracture disease

Definition
Fracture disease encompasses all pronounced manifestations of the immobilization associated with fracture management. Quadriceps contracture (see Chapter 103) and disuse osteoporosis are examples of fracture disease. However, this chapter focuses on the role of immobilization on DJD. Disuse associated with pain, postoperative external coaptation, or iatrogenic neurologic complications can lead to cartilage disuse atrophy and increase the vulnerability of cartilage to injury.

Risk factors
- The duration of immobilization has a direct effect on cartilage matrix, synovial production, and cellular components. Articular

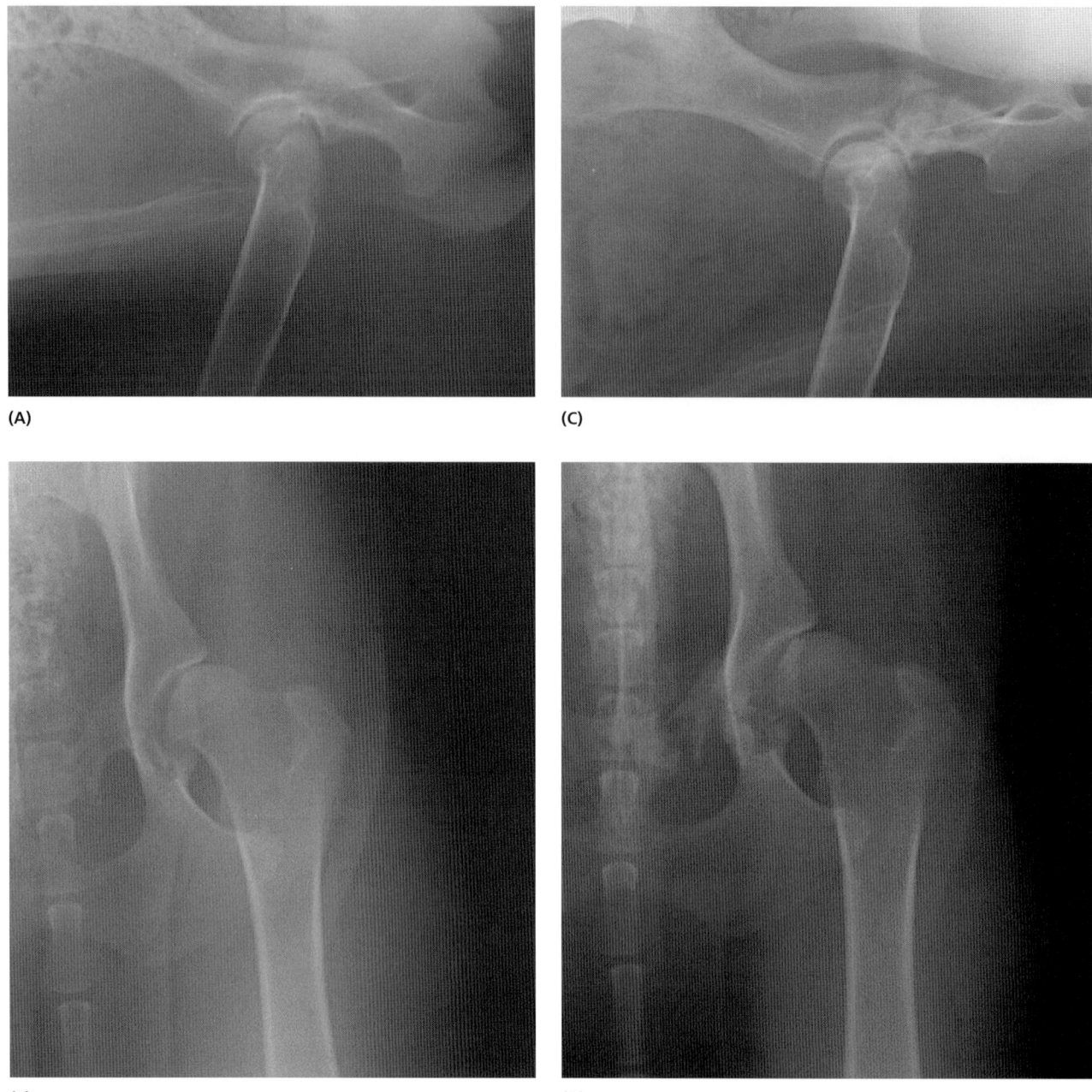

(A)

(C)

(B)

(D)

Figure 18.5 Progression of degenerative joint disease caused by misalignment of an intraarticular fracture. **A** and **B,** Initial close-up radiographic appearance of a caudal acetabular fracture in a 2-year-old German pointer with hip dysplasia. **C** and **D,** Radiographs obtained 4 weeks after conservative management. Notice the remodeling and widening of the fracture site along with progression of degenerative joint disease. *Source:* D. Griffon, Western University of Health Sciences, Pomona, CA, 2014. Reproduced with permission from D. Griffon.

and periarticular changes occur with as little as 2 weeks of immobilization. Irreversible damage to the cartilage can happen if immobilization is prolonged, starting after 11 weeks.
* Severe contracture caused by periarticular adhesions can lead to permanent immobilization of the joint. Young patients are at risk of severe contracture. The most frequent contracture is the quadriceps contracture caused by femoral fracture.

Diagnosis
The diagnosis is based on the presence of DJD in a patient with a history of postoperative disuse of the limb because of pain or external coaptation. Early signs consist of lameness or loss of ROM. Radiographic signs of DJD are present in chronic cases.

Treatment
* Control of inflammation and pain, combined with early physical rehabilitation and active motion, can counteract many of the changes caused by postsurgical disuse, improving limb use and accelerating return to function.
* Rehabilitation help restore limb function in dogs with contractures that have not yet matured.

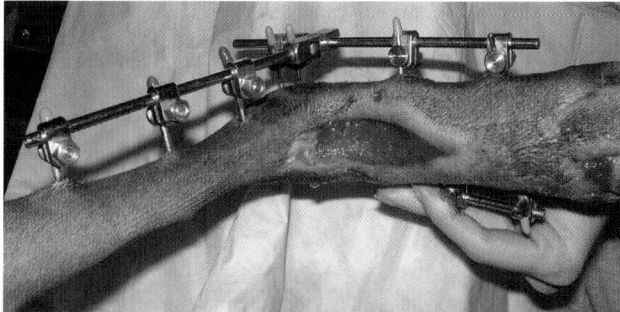

Figure 18.6 Postoperative flexible external fixation of the tarsus. A hinged external fixator is centered over the tibiotarsal joint after surgical repair of collateral ligament injuries. *Source:* D. Griffon, Western University of Health Sciences, Pomona, CA, 2014. Reproduced with permission from D. Griffon.

- Surgical intervention is warranted when a severe and chronic contracture is present (see Chapter 103).

Prevention
Alternatives to postoperative immobilization of joints
- Appropriate use of implants for fracture fixation
- Nonrigid or flexible external fixation after surgical treatment of luxations and ligamentous injuries (Figure 18.6 and **Video 18.1**)
- Promote early ROM and return to function via rehabilitation. Postoperative rehabilitation generally includes three stages:
  - The initial 2 weeks are aimed at decreasing pain and inflammation, improving ROM, weight bearing, and limiting muscle atrophy. Sessions are recommended twice daily and include passive ROM, massage, and weight-bearing exercises.
  - The second stage is initiated when the level of pain decreases (at 2–3 weeks). The goals are to normalize motion, improve muscular strength, and establish neuromuscular control. Exercises include stretching, longer walks, hydrotherapy, and proprioceptive exercises. An advanced strengthening stage starts 6 weeks after the surgery after pain free ROM has returned to normal. At this point, the program is designed to increase muscle strength and neuromuscular control in preparation for a return to sport activities. Strategies focus on increasing the frequency, duration, and the distance of walks.
  - The last stage, usually initiated after 12 weeks, corresponds to a return to a normal activity level.

Progression of presurgical degenerative joint disease

Definition
Progression of DJD is a common complication after surgical treatment of joint diseases, probably because treatment is not initiated before secondary changes occur in the affected joint. In most cases, this progression occurs despite an acceptable clinical outcome.

The surgery corrects the predisposing cause but cannot correct secondary degenerative changes, thereby allowing the breakdown cycle of articular cartilage.

Risk factors
- Preoperative cartilage lesions
- Meniscal lesions present at the time of stifle surgery (Figure 18.7)
- Duration of intraarticular disease

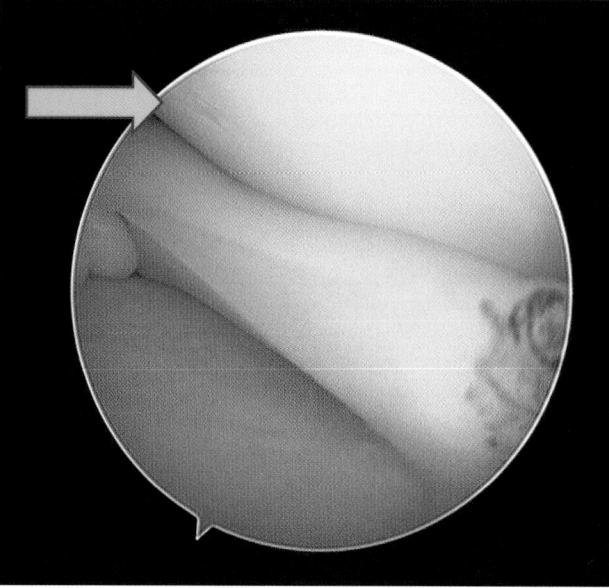

Figure 18.7 Arthroscopic appearance of a meniscal tear. Note the focal cartilage damage already present on the femoral condyle (arrow) *Source:* D. Griffon, Western University of Health Sciences, Pomona, CA, 2014. Reproduced with permission from D. Griffon.

- Preoperative joint instability, such as cranial cruciate ligament deficiency or collateral ligament damage
- Postoperative joint instability such as persistent cranial drawer or recurrent joint luxation
- More invasive joint approaches such as arthrotomies compared with arthroscopic approaches
- Surgeries improving, but not fully restoring contact between articular surfaces (triple pelvic osteotomy, fragment removal in osteochondritis dissecans)

Diagnosis
The diagnosis is determined through progression of degenerative changes on serial postoperative radiographs.

Treatment
- Long-term medical management for DJD should be instituted in all cases (see earlier section "Iatrogenic damage").
- Revision may be corrected if initial surgical treatment failed to correct the primary disease:
  - Consider subtotal coronoidectomy or humeral/ulnar osteotomy in cases that fail to respond to removal of a fragmented medial coronoid process.
  - Consider tibial osteotomies in cases with early postoperative instability after lateral fabellar repair of cranial cruciate ligament instability.

Prevention
Evidence is lacking regarding the efficacy of postoperative interventions in preventing the progression of preexisting osteoarthrosis. However, the following strategies may be considered:
- Early diagnosis and treatment of joint diseases
- Rehabilitation and low-impact exercise
- Nutritional management of patients with DJD (see Figure 18.3)
- Arthroscopy may be considered to assess the cartilage covering the weight-bearing portion of the acetabulum before triple pelvic osteotomy. This preoperative evaluation may improve the

selection of candidates for triple pelvic osteotomy and carry a prognostic value.
- A minimally invasive approach to the joint should be preferred whenever possible.
- Owners should be well informed regarding postoperative function, especially if a pet has severe DJD before surgery.

Relevant literature

Iatrogenic damage is probably one of the most common surgical complications leading to DJD, yet it is likely underreported in the veterinary literature (Klein and Kurze 1986; Byrd 2000). This may result from a reporting bias or a lack of awareness from the surgeon. For example, articular trauma was not reported as a potential disadvantage of transarticular pining (Keeley 2007). Similarly, intraarticular radiofrequency was applied for years until its detrimental effects on cartilage were documented in experimental studies (Lu 2007; Horstman 2009). Occasional damage is unavoidable with arthroscopy but is rarely reported in clinical studies (Byrd 2000). However, experimental studies have been performed to improve portal placement for arthroscopy of the elbow and hip joints (Saunders et al. 2004; Jardel et al. 2010). Jardel et al. confirmed the safety of elbow medial arthroscopic portals but found that the camera portal was close to the ulnar nerve. Saunders et al. suggested that the ideal limb position for canine coxofemoral arthroscopy required holding the limb in slight adduction, 30 degrees of hip flexion, with the stifle in a neutral position. With this position, the arthroscope portal could safely be placed 5 mm cranial and 15 mm proximal to the greater trochanter. The instrument portal should be located 10.2 mm cranial and 14 mm proximal to the greater trochanter. Joint distraction and distension also help reducing iatrogenic trauma during arthroscopy. Stifle probing for TPLO has also been improved with the description of a safe zone for needle insertion (O'Brien and Martinez 2009). This safe zone was defined as the third of the distance from the cranial border of the medial collateral ligament to the medial edge of the patellar ligament.

Intraarticular placement of implants can occur during osteotomies or fracture repair. In several initial studies on TPLO, 1% or fewer of the cases had intraarticular placement of screws or jig pins (Pacchiana et al. 2003; Priddy et al. 2003). Juxtaarticular fractures are likely at risk for implant misplacement. CT may develop as a valuable approach to better evaluate implant position in specific cases such as vertebral and pelvic fractures (Hettlich et al. 2010).

Intramedually pinning can also lead to severe osteoarthritis caused by placement or migration of the implant (Bardet et al. 1983; Lesser 1984). Most postoperative complications associated with pin fixation develop because of technical errors. Those complications can be traced to problems encountered during surgery (Schrader 1991). Both humeral and tibial pinning techniques have been improved; the risk of complication decreases with retrograde placement in a craniolateral direction during humeral pinning and with retrograde placement in a craniomedial direction during tibial pinning (Dixon et al. 1994; Sissener et al. 2005). Similarly, Lorinson et al. (1998) determined the depth of the femoral epiphysis on radiographs and provided landmarks to prevent cartilage penetration with the pins during epiphyseal femoral fracture repairs. Based on their results, pins should be placed to a distance equal to 80% of the contralateral intact epiphysis or pubic bone width as measured on ventrodorsal radiographs.

Lack of evidence may also lead to the use of techniques that are deleterious to the joints. For example, meniscal release has been performed for many years without strong evidence for its benefit. This procedure has since been shown to increase DJD and dysfunction (Luther et al. 2009).

Malreduction is considered as a major cause for DJD after repair of articular fractures, aggravating the direct impact of the initial trauma. This concern justifies the recommendation for anatomic reduction and interfragmentary compression as principles for managing articular fractures. However, the relationship between the magnitude of the postoperative misalignment of articular surfaces (or step) and the progression of DJD has not been clearly established. In fact, no correlation was found between the fracture reduction and osteoarthritis scores in an experimental study (Gordon et al. 2003). These results may reflect the presence of confounding factors such as joint trauma at the time of fracture, iatrogenic trauma during the repair, and postoperative activity. The incidence of postoperative DJD is especially high after repair of distal humeral articular repair. In fact, osteoarthrosis progressed radiographically in all 15 elbows with condylar fractures repaired surgically and followed for 43 months (Vannini et al. 1988; Gordon et al. 2003). The high incidence of DJD has been attributed to the difficulty visualizing articular surfaces via arthrotomy, thereby increasing the risk of malreduction. However, the same study reported that the vertical impulses of operated limbs were similar to those of sound contralateral limbs (Gordon et al. 2003). These results, combined with the good to excellent function reported in 80% of dogs with distal humeral articular fractures, raise questions as to the clinical relevance of mild malreduction. In a study in which reduction of humeral condylar fractures was assessed via fluoroscopy, 91% of cases had a malreduction of less than 1 mm, leading to an excellent outcome (Cook et al. 1999). The difficulty in determining the clinical significance of malreduction stems from the lack of correlation between radiographic evidence and clinical signs of DJD along with the short-term follow-up period reported in most studies. A case report recently described severe DJD and loss of ROM in a dog with incomplete ossification of the humeral condyle evaluated over 10 years (von Pfeil et al. 2010).

The causes of articular cartilage degeneration caused by **fracture disease** are complex and involve interrelated biologic, mechanical, and structural pathways. Prolonged immobilization leads to DJD, loss of muscle mass, and loss of bone mineral content (Namba et al. 1991; Bruce et al. 2002; Jaeger et al. 2005; Moores and Sutton 2009). The lack of cyclic weight bearing and movement affect the flow of synovial fluid and the diffusion of nutrients within articular structures. Postoperative immobilization decreases synovial fluid production, cartilage stiffness, and thickness. These changes eventually lead to ulcerative lesions over opposing surfaces of articular cartilage. The glycosaminoglycans and collagen concentrations were reduced by 20% and 14%, respectively, in articular cartilage of beagles after 11 weeks of immobilization (Haapala et al. 1999). These concentrations failed to return to normal after 50 weeks of remobilization. The negative impacts of postoperative immobilization prompted the development of implants for fracture fixation in the early 20th century, and this trend was more recently expanded to the surgical management of joint diseases (Marsolais et al. 2002; Johnson et al. 2005). External coaptation is typically limited to the first 24 hours after surgery as a mean to control postoperative swelling. Early postoperative rehabilitation is becoming standard of care after joint surgery (Marsolais et al. 2002). Hinged fixators offer alternatives to external fixation after collateral ligament repair, preserving ROM in the axis of the joint (Schwartz and

Griffon 2008). Flexible fixation of the coxofemoral and elbow joints has been described to control ROM after reduction of a traumatic luxation (Schwartz and Griffon 2008).

Surgical treatment of joint diseases typically occurs after the onset of secondary changes. **Postoperative progression of DJD** is an outcome expected after most intraarticular surgeries and is especially well documented in common procedures. Progression of DJD occurs in 40% to 76% of dogs after TPLO (Lineberger *et al.* 2005; Boyd *et al.* 2007; Hurley *et al.* 2007), 55% of stifles treated via tibial tuberosity advancement (Morgan *et al.* 2010), and in 100% of cases treated with intracapsular techniques (Boyd *et al.* 2007). The progression of DJD was not different between dogs treated with TPLO and the Tightrope® CCL technique (Arthrex, Naples, FL; Cook *et al.* 2010). Second-look arthroscopic findings 2 to 69 months after TPLO include cartilage lesions, meniscal damage, and caudal cruciate ligament fraying (Hulse *et al.* 2010). The changes are consistent with a progression of DJD and correlate with the initial severity of cranial cruciate ligament disease. Another study documented a correlation between the progression of DJD and the severity of cartilage lesions at surgery (Morgan *et al.* 2010). Minimally invasive joint surgery has been proposed to limit the progression of DJD postoperatively (Lineberger *et al.* 2005). However, this recommendation must be weighed against the risk of iatrogenic trauma and warrants further studies. Similarly, the influence of ligamentous remnants in cases of partially ruptured cranial cruciate ligament remains controversial (Breshears *et al.* 2010). Ligamentous remnants have been proposed to act as a source of postoperative inflammation and osteoarthritis, thereby justifying their removal. However, some evidence in human patients with partial anterior cruciate tears suggests that remnants may serve as a source of vascular supply and improve proprioception, thereby enhancing healing (Sonnery-Cottet *et al.* 2014). In dogs with medial patellar luxation, DJD has been found to progress significantly and similarly in stifles treated conservatively or surgically, prompting authors to recommend against surgery in grade I patellar luxations (Roy *et al.* 1992). Trochlear wedge and en-bloc recessions effectively consist in intraarticular fractures that result in a misalignment of articular surfaces and potential motion at the fracture site. An individual approach to the management of patellar luxation, precluding systematic trochleoplasty, may decrease the progression of DJD (Linney *et al.* 2011). However, in a recent study of 124 dogs with congenital medial patellar luxation, trochlear wedge recession resulted in a 5.1-fold reduction in postoperative reluxation when combined with tibial tuberosity transposition (Cashmore *et al.* 2014).

All videos cited in this chapter can be found on the book companion website at www.wiley.com/go/griffon/complications.

References

Bardet, J.F., Hohn, R.B., Rudy, R.L., et al. (1983) Fractures of the humerus in dogs and cats: a retrospective study of 130 cases. *Veterinary Surgery* 12, 73-77.

Boyd, D.J., Miller, C.W., Etue, S.M., et al. (2007) Radiographic and functional evaluation of dogs at least 1 year after tibial plateau leveling osteotomy. *Canadian Veterinary Journal* 48, 392-396.

Breshears, L.A., Cook, J.L., Stoker, A.M., et al. (2010) Detection and evaluation of matrix metalloproteinases involved in cruciate ligament disease in dogs using multiplex bead technology. *Veterinary Surgery* 39 (3), 306-314.

Bruce, W.J., Frame, K., Burbridge, H.M., et al. (2002) A comparison of the effects of joint immobilization, twice-daily passive motion, and voluntary motion on articular cartilage healing in sheep. *Veterinary and Comparative Orthopaedics and Traumatology* 15, 23-29.

Byrd, J.W. (2000) Avoiding the labrum in hip arthroscopy. *The Journal of Arthroscopic and Related Surgery* 16 (7), 770-773.

Cashmore, R.G., Havlicek, M., Perkins, N.R., et al. (2014) Major complications and risk factors associated with surgical correction of congenital medial patellar luxation in 124 dogs. *Veterinary and Comparative Orthopaedics and Traumatology* 27, 263-270.

Clarke, S.P., Mellor, D., Clements, D.N., et al. (2005) Prevalence of radiographic signs of degenerative joint disease in a hospital population of cats. *Veterinary Record* 157, 793-799.

Cole, B.J., Malek, M.M. (2004) *Articular Cartilage Lesions: A Practical Guide to Assessment and Treatment.* New York, Springer.

Cook, J.L., Tomlinson, J.L., Reed, A.L. (1999) Fluoroscopically guided closed reduction and internal fixation of fractures of the lateral portion of the humeral condyle: prospective clinical study of the technique and results in ten dogs. *Veterinary Surgery* 28 (5), 315-321.

Cook, J.L., Luther, J.K., Beetem, J. (2010) Clinical comparison of a novel extracapsular stabilization procedure and tibial plateau leveling osteotomy for treatment of cranial cruciate ligament deficiency in dogs. *Veterinary Surgery* 39, 315-323.

Dixon, B.C., Tomlinson, J.L., Wagner, C.C. (1994) Effects of three intramedullary pinning techniques on proximal pin location and articular damage in the canine tibia. *Veterinary Surgery* 23, 448-455.

Gordon, W.J., Besancon, M.F., Conzemius, M.G., et al. (2003) Frequency of posttraumatic osteoarthritis in dogs after repair of a humeral condylar fracture. *Veterinary and Comparative Orthopaedics and Traumatology* 16, 1-5.

Haapala, J., Arokoski, J.P., Hyttinen, M.M., et al. (1999) Remobilization does not fully restore immobilization induced articular cartilage atrophy. *Clinical Orthopedic and Related Research* 362, 218-229.

Hardie, E.M., Roe, S.C., Martin, F.R. (2002) Radiographic evidence of degenerative joint disease in geriatric cats: 100 cases (1994-1997). *Journal of the American Veterinary Medical Association* 220(5), 628-632.

Hettlich, B.F., Fosgate, G.T., Levine, J.M., et al. (2010) Accuracy of conventional radiography and computed tomography in predicting implant position in relation to the vertebral canal in dogs. *Veterinary Surgery* 39 (6), 680-687.

Horstman, C.L., McLaughlin, R.M., Elder, S.H., et al. (2009) Changes to articular cartilage following remote application of radiofrequency energy and with or without Cosequin therapy. *Veterinary and Comparative Orthopaedics and Traumatology* 22, 103-112.

Hulse, D., Beale, B., Kerwin, S. (2010) Second look arthroscopic findings after tibial plateau leveling osteotomy. *Veterinary Surgery* 39, 350-354.

Hurley, C.R., Hammer, D.L., Shott, S. (2007) Progression of radiographic evidence of osteoarthritis following tibial plateau leveling osteotomy in dogs with cranial cruciate ligament rupture: 295 cases (2001-2005). *Journal of the American Veterinary Medical Association* 230, 1674-1679.

Jaeger, G.H., Wosar, M.A., Marcellin-Little, D.J., et al. (2005) Use of hinged transarticular external fixation for adjunctive joint stabilization in dogs and cats: 14 cases (1999-2003). *Journal of the American Veterinary Medical Association* 227 (4), 586-591.

Jardel, N., Crevier-Denoix, N., Moissonnier, P., et al. (2010) Anatomical and safety considerations in establishing portals used for canine elbow arthroscopy. *Veterinary and Comparative Orthopaedics and Traumatology* 23, 75-80.

Johnson, A.L., Houlton, J.E.F., Vannini R. (2005) *AO Principles of Fracture Management in the Dog and Cat.* AO Publishing, Switzerland.

Johnston, S.A. (1997) Osteoarthritis: joint anatomy, physiology and pathobiology. *Veterinary Clinics of North America Small Animal Practice* 27, 699-723.

Klein, W., Kurze, V. (1986) Arthroscopic arthropathy: iatrogenic arthroscopic joint lesions in animals *Arthroscopy: The Journal of Arthroscopic & Related Surgery* 2 (3), 163-168.

Keeley, B., Glyde, M., Guerin, S., *et al.* (2007) Stifle joint luxation in the dog and cat: the use of temporary intraoperative transarticular pinning to facilitate joint reconstruction. *Veterinary and Comparative Orthopaedics and Traumatology* 20, 198-203.

Lascelles, B.D. (2010) Prevalence of radiographic signs of degenerative joint disease in a hospital population of cats. *Veterinary Surgery* 39, 2-13.

Linney, W.R., Hammer, D.L., Shott, S. (2011) Surgical treatment of medial patellar luxation without femoral trochlear groove deepening procedures in dogs: 91 cases (1998-2009). *Journal of the American Veterinary Medical Association* 238, 1168-1172.

Lesser, A.S. (1984) Complications from improper intramedullary pin placement in tibial fractures. *Modern Veterinary Practice* 65, 940-944.

Lineberger, J.A., Allen, D.A., Wilson, E.R., et al. (2005) Comparison of radiographic arthritic changes associated with two variations of tibial plateau leveling. *Veterinary and Comparative Orthopaedics and Traumatology* 18, 13-17.

Lu, Y., Meyer, M.L., Bogdanske, J.J., et al. (2007) The effects of radiofrequency energy probe speed and application force on chondrocyte viability. *Veterinary and Comparative Orthopaedics and Traumatology* 20, 34-37.

Luther, J.K., Cook, C.R., Cook, J.L. (2009) Meniscal release in cruciate ligament intact stifles causes lameness and medial compartment cartilage pathology in dogs 12 weeks postoperatively. *Veterinary Surgery* 38, 520-529.

Marsolais, G.S., Dvorak, G., Conzemius, M.G. (2002) Effects of postoperative rehabilitation on limb function after cranial cruciate ligament repair in dogs. *Journal of the American Veterinary Medical Association* 220 (9), 1325-1330.

Moores, A.P., Sutton, A. (2009) Management of quadriceps contracture in a dog using a static flexion apparatus and physiotherapy. *Journal of Small Animal Practice* 50, 251-254.

Morgan, J.P., Voss, K., Damur, D.M., et al. (2010) Correlation of radiographic changes after tibial tuberosity advancement in dogs with cranial cruciate-deficient stifles with functional outcome. *Veterinary Surgery* 39, 425-432.

Namba, R.S., Kabo, J.M., Dorey, F.J., et al. (1991) Continuous passive motion versus immobilization. The effect on post-traumatic joint stiffness. *Clinical Orthopedic and Related Research* 267, 218-223.

O'Brien, C.S., Martinez, S.A. (2009) Potential iatrogenic medial meniscal damage during tibial plateau leveling osteotomy. *Veterinary Surgery* 38, 868-873.

Pacchiana, P.D., Morris, E., Gillings, S.L., et al. (2003) Surgical and postoperative complications associated with tibial plateau leveling osteotomy in dogs with cranial cruciate ligament rupture: 397 cases (1998-2001). *Journal of the American Veterinary Medical Association* 222, 184-193.

Priddy, N.H., Tomlinson, J.L., Dodam, J.R., et al. (2003) Complications with and owner assessment of the outcome of tibial plateau leveling osteotomy for treatment of cranial cruciate ligament rupture in dogs: 193 cases (1997-2001). *Journal of the American Veterinary Medical association* 222, 1726-1732.

Roy, R.G., Wallace, L.J., Johnston, G.R., et al. (1992) A retrospective evaluation of stifle osteoarthritis in dogs with bilateral medial patellar luxation and unilateral surgical repair. *Veterinary Surgery* 21, 475-479.

Saunders, W.B., Hulse, D.A., Schulz, K.S. (2004) Evaluation of portal locations and periarticular structures in canine coxofemoral arthroscopy: a cadaver study. *Veterinary and Comparative Orthopaedics and Traumatology* 17, 184-188.

Schrader, S.C. (1991) Complications associated with the use of Steinmann intramedullary pins and cerclage wires for fixation of long-bone fractures. *Veterinary Clinics North America Small Animal Practice* 21, 686-703.

Schwartz, Z., Griffon, D.J. (2008) Nonrigid external fixation of the elbow, coxofemoral, and tarsal joints in dogs. *Compendium: Continuing Education for Veterinarians* 30 (12), 648-660.

Sissener, T.R., Jones, E., Langley-Hobbs, S.J. (2005) Effects of three intramedullary pinning techniques on pin location and articular damage in the canine humerus. *Veterinary and Comparative Orthopaedics and Traumatology* 18, 153-156.

Sonnery-Cottet, B, Bazille, C, Hulet, C, et al. (2014): Histological features of the ACL remnant in partial tears. *Knee* 21 (6), 1009-1013.

Vannini, R., Smeak, D.D., Olmstead, M.L. (1988) Evaluation of surgical repair of 135 distal humeral fractures in dogs and cats. *Journal of American Animal Hospital Association* 24, 537-545.

von Pfeil, D.J., DeCamp, C.E., Agnello, C., et al. (2010) Deformity secondary to bilateral incomplete ossification of the humeral condyle in a German Shorthaired Pointer dog: a case report with ten-year follow-up. *Veterinary and Comparative Orthopaedics and Traumatology* 23, 468-471.

Surgery of the Head and Neck

19 Dorsal Rhinotomy

Gert ter Haar

ENT, Brachycephaly and Audiology Clinic, Royal Veterinary College, North Mymms, Hatfield, Herts, UK

Rhinotomy is indicated for removal of nasal foreign bodies that cannot be removed using endoscopy, as part of a combination therapy (radiotherapy before or after surgery) for intranasal neoplasia, and for the treatment of chronic infectious rhinitis associated with nasal obstruction (especially in cats). Most surgeons prefer a dorsal approach to the nasal cavity and paranasal sinuses because of enhanced accessibility to the cribriform plate and frontal sinuses, but ventral rhinotomy may be indicated in selected patients with focal abnormalities in the ventral meatus or nasopharynx. Even with proper patient selection and thorough diagnostic work-up and preoperative evaluation of rhinologic patients, dorsal rhinotomy with unilateral or bilateral turbinectomy is a major surgical procedure. Complications associated with dorsal rhinotomy include entrance into the cranial vault and hemorrhage during and after surgery (epistaxis). In addition, early postoperative complications include pneumocephalus and septic meningoencephalitis, subcutaneous emphysema, failure to mouth breathe, aspiration pneumonia, persistent anorexia, and pain. Persistent nasal discharge or respiratory noise and recurrence of disease are considered late postoperative complications. Oronasal fistula formation has been reported after ventral rhinotomy only, but chronic fistulization after wound dehiscence and osteomyelitis or osteonecrosis is possible after dorsal rhinotomy in patients that have received radiation therapy before surgery.

Hemorrhage

See also Chapter 12.

Etiopathogenesis

The nasal bones, nasal cavity, nasal turbinates, and overlying mucosa receive an abundant blood supply from branches of the maxillary artery, including the sphenopalatine, ethmoid, greater palatine, dorsal, and lateral nasal and maxillary labial arteries. Standard dorsal midline rhinotomy causes mild hemorrhage of the incised periosteum and nasal bone. Disruption of the extensive arterial network within the nasal cavity during turbinectomy causes considerable hemorrhage.

Diagnosis

Blood loss is inevitable and obvious during or after surgery (Figure 19.1). Whether or not blood loss is clinically relevant depends on:
• The amount of blood loss, which can be quantified by measuring aspired contents in suction bottles (taking the contribution of aspired lavage fluid into consideration) and counting surgical sponges
• Patient evaluation (pale mucous membranes, prolonged capillary refill time, hypotension, hypothermia)
• Serial monitoring of packed cell volume (PCV) or hematocrit and total protein. Hemorrhage should be considered to be clinically significant when blood loss approaches 25% of total blood volume, PCV is less than 20%, total protein is less than 3.5 g/dL, or there is any deterioration in clinical status related to the hemorrhage. Despite significant blood loss, most patients do not require a blood transfusion after rhinotomy.

Treatment

Intraoperative uncontrolled nasal hemorrhage can be managed by:
• Quickly but carefully completing the turbinectomy. Hemorrhage is much easier controlled when all turbinates are removed.
• Packing the nasal cavity temporarily with sterile gauzes under pressure for 5 minutes.

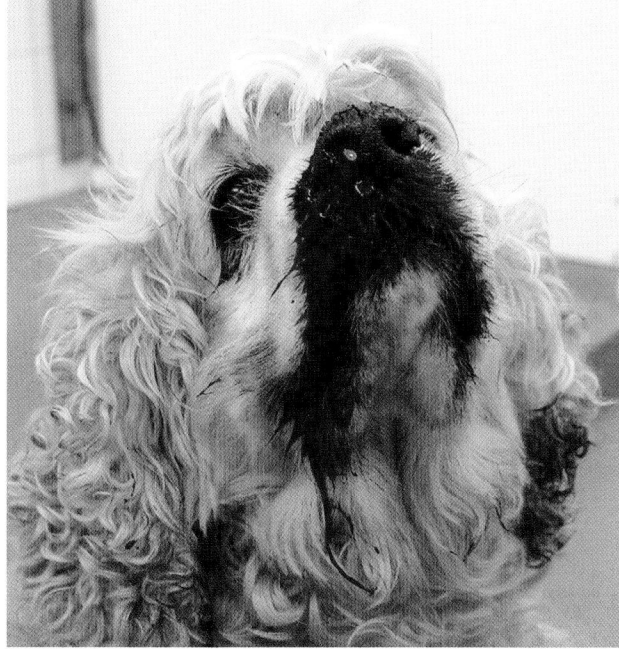

Figure 19.1 Patient with epistaxis.

Complications in Small Animal Surgery, First Edition. Edited by Dominique Griffon and Annick Hamaide.

© 2016 John Wiley & Sons, Inc. Published 2016 by John Wiley & Sons, Inc.

Companion website: www.wiley.com/go/griffon/complications

After removal of the gauzes, active bleeding can usually be controlled with direct electrocautery, using metal Frazier or Adson suction cannulae as conductor while "fixating" the end of the vessel with the tip of the suction tube and clearing the surgical area of blood at the same time.

- Packing the nasal cavity with sterile gauze strip placed in accordion fashion and exiting through the nostril, in case of persistent hemorrhage. The strip is subsequently removed in stages during the first several days after surgery. This is painful, and sedation is usually necessary.
- Alternatively, packing the nasal cavity with absorbable gelatine sponges at the end of surgery. These sponges do not need to be removed and are usually sneezed out or swallowed in the week after surgery. However, this is not an option for bilateral turbinectomy because it leads to obstructed breathing after surgery.
- Providing additional medical treatment in case of clinically significant ongoing hemorrhage, which involves intravenous (IV) administration of a balanced electrolyte solution or hypertonic saline in severe cases. Whole blood should be administered when blood loss approaches 25% of total blood volume, if the PCV drops below 20%, or if the patient is clinically affected by the amount of blood loss.

Prevention

Excessive blood loss during dorsal rhinotomy can be prevented by:

- Having the procedure performed with speed, accuracy, and efficiency by a rhinologic surgeon with thorough knowledge of the regional anatomy and experience with the technique
- Ligation of the paired sphenopalatine arteries on the lateral floor of the nasal cavity and using electrocautery to seal other vessels during surgery
- Application of iced saline lavage or application of topical 0.5% cocaine to provide hemostasis
- Assessing the patient coagulation function before surgery because massive hemorrhage may occur if a coagulopathy is present
- Temporary unilateral or bilateral occlusion of the common carotid artery, which has been reported to minimize hemorrhage (Hedlund *et al.* 1983). This does not eliminate hemorrhage but reduces expected blood loss. Extensive extracranial vascular anastomoses provide sufficient blood supply to the brain during occlusion in dogs. Carotid artery occlusion is not recommended in cats because their collateral blood supply is inadequate to maintain cerebral perfusion and occlusion can lead to postoperative death (Holmberg *et al.* 1989, 1996). In one large study, no difference in the need for a blood transfusion was noted when comparing animals with or without carotid artery occlusion (Holmberg 1996).

Entrance into the cranial vault

Etiopathogenesis

Inadvertent penetration into the cranial vault is possible during turbinectomy of the ethmoturbinates, especially when resecting tumors that have invaded the cribriform plate.

Diagnosis

Entrance into the cranial vault and penetration of the cribriform plate will allow brain tissue to herniate and become visible in the surgical field. Clinical signs will be present after surgery and can range from minimal to severe depending on the severity of central nervous system trauma and associated brain edema.

Treatment

Brain edema should be treated with:
- Rapid-acting IV corticosteroids
- Osmotic agents such as mannitol (not when active hemorrhage is present because it may permit increased bleeding and worsen clinical signs)
- Hyperventilation
- Hyperbaric oxygen
- Calcium channel blockers
- Antioxidants

Prevention

Entrance into the cranial vault is prevented by:
- Having thorough knowledge of the regional anatomy
- Preoperative computed tomography to assess tumor invasion into and erosion of the cribriform plate
- Exercising extreme care when performing turbinectomy of the ethmoturbinates

Pneumocephalus and septic meningoencephalitis

Recently, pneumocephalus and septic meningoencephalitis was reported secondary to dorsal rhinotomy for removal of nasal polyps in a dog (Fletcher *et al.* 2006). The authors proposed that the pneumocephalus resulted from damage to the cribriform plate at the time of rhinotomy or from a congenital nasoencephalocele that was present concurrently with the nasal disease and that the olfactory bulb had been inadvertently damaged at the time of surgery. Clinical signs consisted of lethargy, anorexia, and pyrexia after the initial surgery. In addition, neurologic signs such as ataxia, loss of proprioception, and seizures developed. CT revealed a defect in the cribriform plate and pneumocephalus. Conservative and medical treatment with broad-spectrum antibiotics and corticosteroids was attempted first followed by reconstruction and closure of the defect in the cribriform plate. However, the dog subsequently developed septic meningoencephalitis and was euthanized.

Subcutaneous emphysema

Etiopathogenesis

Subcutaneous emphysema is caused by the flow of air from the nasal cavity into the subcutaneous tissue around the rhinotomy site. It may be precipitated by:
- Violent episodes of sneezing
- Rostral obstruction to nasal airflow (nasal packing, blood clots, or inadequate removal of rostral nasal turbinates)
- Inadequate closure of nasal bone periosteum over the defect.

Diagnosis

Subcutaneous emphysema is diagnosed hours to days after surgery by physical and visual examination. Crepitation and swelling initially involve the area immediately adjacent to the rhinotomy site but may extend to involve the entire head, face, and neck.

Treatment

Subcutaneous emphysema is usually self-limiting and resolves without treatment in 10 to 14 days. If desired, a small stab incision can

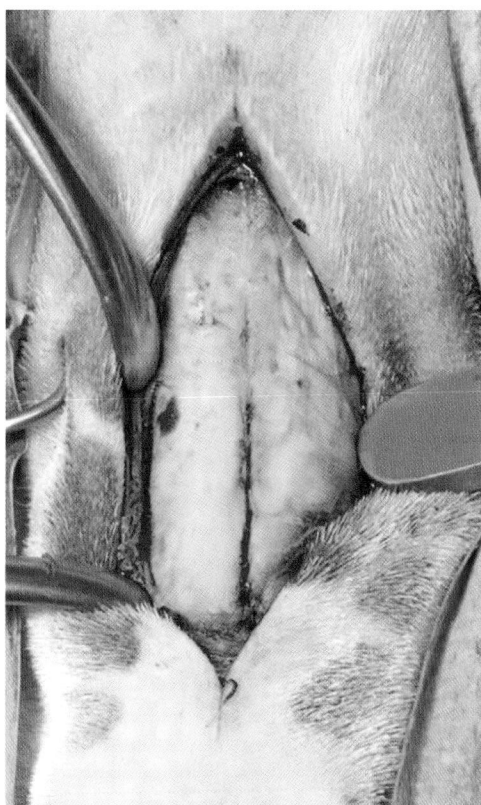

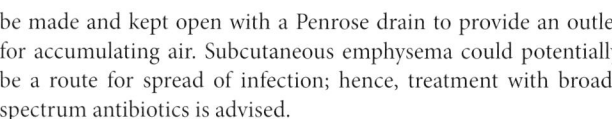

Figure 19.2. Dorsal rhinotomy. Undermining of the periosteum over the nasal bone with periosteal elevators is necessary to preserve it for closure.

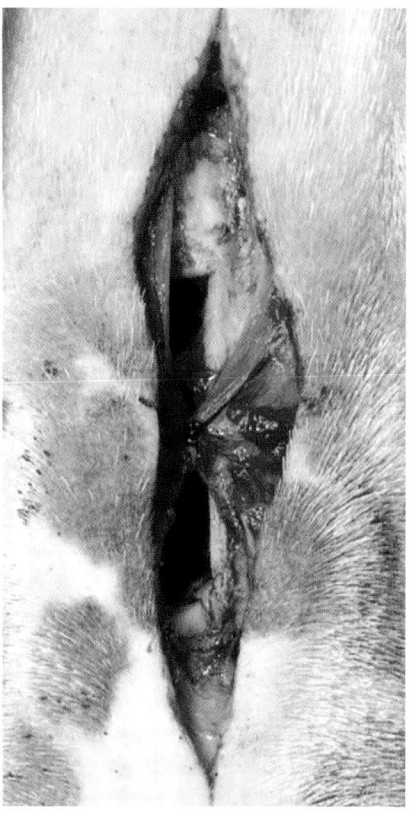

Figure 19.3. Dorsal rhinotomy. Airtight closure of the periosteum using interrupted sutures of a monofilament absorbable material is critical in preventing postoperative subcutaneous emphysema.

be made and kept open with a Penrose drain to provide an outlet for accumulating air. Subcutaneous emphysema could potentially be a route for spread of infection; hence, treatment with broad-spectrum antibiotics is advised.

Prevention
Subcutaneous emphysema is prevented by:
- Maintaining normal nasal airflow (remove all turbinates, including the rostral maxilloturbinates; remove all large blood clots; avoid excessive packing with gauze strips or gelatin sponges; and remove dried blood that is crusted on the external nares after surgery)
- Eliminating sites of possible air leakage: Replacement of the bone flap after dorsal rhinotomy has little effect on the incidence of subcutaneous emphysema, but airtight closure of the periosteum is critical. Undermining the periosteum over the nasal bone and preserving it carefully while creating and removing the nasal bone flap can accomplish this (Figures 19.2 and 19.3). A tie-over bandage can be used to apply pressure over small areas of potential leakage.
- Providing an alternate pathway for air to escape: The use of rhinostomy tubing after surgery has been recommended to allow air to escape, or a temporary rhinotomy can be performed by modifying the standard rectangular dorsal rhinotomy bone flap into a keyhole shape and leaving the caudal circular area open to heal by second intention.
- Using a ventral rather than dorsal rhinotomy technique

Failure to mouth breathe

Etiopathogenesis
Complete bilateral obstruction of nasal airflow by blood clots or nasal packing necessitates open mouth breathing. This complication is rare, but in animals that fail to mouth breathe, it can lead to acute respiratory distress. This is of particular concern in brachycephalic breeds with pharyngeal and laryngeal hypoplasia and secondary collapse.

Diagnosis
All animals, but specifically brachycephalic breeds, should be closely monitored after dorsal rhinotomy for respiratory compromise caused by failure to mouth breathe. Signs indicative of (pre)hypoxemia are anxiousness, excitation or agitation, obstructive breathing pattern with pharyngeal and laryngeal stridor, gagging, retching, and syncope. Arterial blood gas analysis measuring PO_2 and PCO_2 can quantitate blood oxygenation.

Treatment
Animals that are reluctant to or unable to mouth breathe should be:
- Positioned in sternal recumbency with the chin supported without causing pressure on the pharynx and larynx and tongue pulled out as far as possible
- Provided with supplemental oxygen by nasal tube or placed in an oxygen cage
- Kept in a cool, quiet environment with normal humidity

- Given antiinflammatory doses of corticosteroids to decrease turbinate and pharyngeal or laryngeal edema
- Handled with care and minimal stress so that acute respiratory decompensation is avoided
- Given tranquilizers and narcotic analgesics because anxiety and pain are major exacerbating factors in reluctance to mouth breathe. However, these should be used with extreme caution in brachycephalic dogs!

In severe cases, placement of an endotracheal tube or emergency tracheostomy can be lifesaving.

Prevention

Animals that are expected to be reluctant to or unable to mouth breathe after rhinotomy should:

- Always be observed during recovery and recover in a quiet, clean, oxygen rich environment.
- Be kept intubated until near complete recovery and only be extubated, with a slightly inflated cuff, when they have become aware of the endotracheal tube.
- Have all airways checked for blood clots, saliva, and lavage fluids before extubation.
- Receive antiinflammatory doses of corticosteroids upon anesthetic induction.
- Receive local (infraorbital foramen block) and systemic analgesic drugs.

Aspiration pneumonia

Etiopathogenesis

Aspiration pneumonia after dorsal rhinotomy is uncommon but may be caused by aspiration of blood, saliva, or lavage fluids that have accumulated in the nasopharynx during recovery from surgery.

Diagnosis

Aspiration pneumonia is suspected when animals present with tachypnea, dyspnea or coughing, pyrexia, and inappetence after surgery. Auscultation of the chest is both an insensitive and nonspecific indicator of pneumonia in dogs and cats. The diagnosis should be based on a complete blood count, thoracic radiography (radiographic signs of aspiration pneumonia may be minimal in acute stages), and transtracheal or bronchoscopy-assisted aspiration of airway contents for cytology and culture and sensitivity testing.

Treatment

Aspiration pneumonia is treated with broad-spectrum antibiotics, aggressive supportive therapy, coupage, and nebulization. The antibiotic sensitivity of bacteria associated with pneumonia is varied, so sensitivity testing is indicated in all cases. Pending culture and sensitivity results, amoxicillin with clavulanic acid or first-generation cephalosporins are recommended because they have excellent efficacy against both gram-positive and gram-negative aerobes and most anaerobic bacteria. Antibiotics should be continued for a minimum of 3 to 4 weeks or at least 10 days after resolution of pneumonia, as confirmed by thoracic radiographs.

Prevention

Aspiration pneumonia is prevented by:

- Maintaining a properly inflated endotracheal tube cuff at all times during the procedure

- Packing several gauze sponges around the endotracheal tube at the glottis before surgery (count them and make note!)
- Suctioning all debris, blood, saliva, and lavage fluid from the oropharynx and nasopharynx at the end of surgery
- Placing animals in a head-down position during recovery
- Delaying endotracheal tube removal until well-developed swallowing and cough reflexes are present and with the cuff kept partially inflated

Anorexia and pain

Also see Chapter 13.

Etiopathogenesis

Partial or complete anorexia is expected after dorsal rhinotomy, especially in cats. Cats depend heavily on their extensive ethmoturbinates for olfaction and appetite stimulation. In both dogs and cats, dorsal rhinotomy produces acute postoperative pain, which will contribute to postoperative anorexia.

Diagnosis

Some degree of decreased appetite is expected after dorsal rhinotomy, but continued anorexia beyond 1 to 2 weeks postoperatively is unusual in dogs. The contribution of pain to the anorexia is difficult to assess because even animals with severe postoperative pain may show no overt clinical signs. Responses that indicate pain after dorsal rhinotomy include face rubbing, vocalization, aggression, trembling, and attempts to escape.

Treatment

- Treatment of anorexia and pain is usually only required in cats.
- Animals should be encouraged to eat tempting foods or hand fed as needed.
- Appetite stimulants such as diazepam or oxazepam can be provided and are helpful in some cases.
- Supportive alimentation is required for animals that are unable to maintain nutritional needs with oral feeding.
- Placement of an oesophageal or gastric feeding tube allows long-term feeding with a blended slurry and can be easily managed at home.
- Patients with postoperative pain should be treated with narcotic analgesics such as methadone, buprenorphine, fentanyl (patch), butorphanol, or oxymorphone in combination with nonsteroidal antiinflammatory drugs (unless long-term corticosteroid use is indicated at the same time). Tramadol in combination with narcotic analgesics can be given to patients that are concurrently treated with corticosteroids.

Prevention

Some degree of decreased appetite and postoperative pain can not be prevented, but ensuring unobstructed nasal airflow and an intraoperative start with a proper analgesic protocol, including topical and systemic administration of analgesic agents, aid in preventing excessive postoperative anorexia and pain.

Persistent nasal discharge or respiratory noise and recurrence of disease

Etiopathogenesis

Nasal airflow should improve after dorsal rhinotomy and nasal stridor should be minimal, but some degree of serosanguineous nasal discharge is expected to persist in all patients.

- Persistence of (excessive) discharge or recurrence of discharge, stridor, and nasal obstruction can be caused by turbinate damage, inflammation, turbulent airflow, and loss of normal defense mechanisms. Although dorsal rhinotomy and turbinectomy may be curative for chronic nasal infections associated with granulomatous or polypous lesions, these can still lead to persistent nasal discharge. In addition, if the primary cause of the rhinitis (viral infection, allergy, hypersensitivity, fungal infection, chronic nonspecific inflammation) is not addressed, some clinical signs are likely to persist or recur after surgery.
- Dorsal rhinotomy alone for nasal neoplasia will neither cure the disease nor increase life expectancy. However, nasal airflow should improve temporarily after surgery. Some degree of nasal stridor and serosanguineous nasal discharge is expected to persist because of residual inflammation or remaining tumor growth or because of tumor recurrence.
- Wound dehiscence, wound infection, and fistula formation as a result of radiation induced delayed wound healing or (nasal) bone necrosis can occur when dorsal rhinotomy for cytoreductive surgery is performed after radiation therapy (Figures 19.4 to 19.7).

Diagnosis
- The underlying primary cause of the rhinitis should be identified on preoperative evaluation of the patient or histopathologic examination of the removed turbinates.
- Persistent nasal stridor or progressive nasal discharge is abnormal, and chronic infection must be differentiated from tumor recurrence in these animals. CT with rhinoscopy and collection of rhinoscopy-assisted biopsies and material for culture and sensitivity testing is indicated for differentiation of the causes of persistent discharge.
- Wound dehiscence, wound infection, and fistula formation are usually evident by 7 to 10 days after surgery (see Figure 19.4), but late osteomyelitis or osteonecrosis can lead to fistulization weeks to months after surgery.

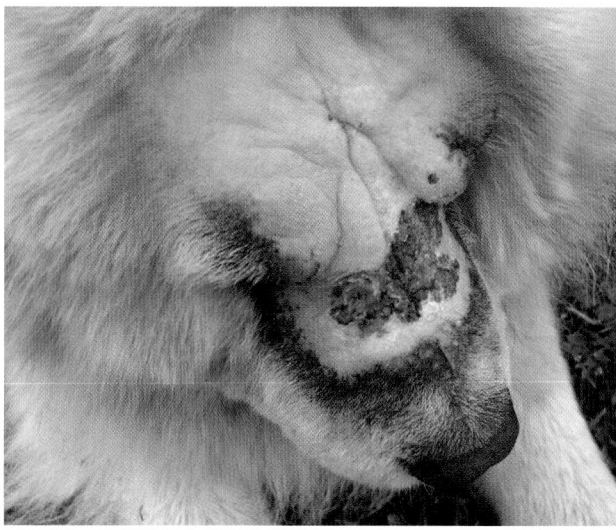

Figure 19.5. Postirradiation wound complications. Six weeks after dorsal rhinotomy and 11 weeks after irradiation, healing of a large part of the wound can be seen. Midnasally, crust formation and dermatitis are still present.

Treatment
- Chronic nasal infections caused by turbinate removal and loss of normal defense mechanisms are usually controlled but not cured by long-term antibiotic therapy. Choice of antibiotic should be based on results of culture and sensitivity tests. In addition, in most animals, corticosteroids are indicated to suppress turbinate mucosal swelling and inflammation, especially in cases with allergy, hypersensitivity–based, or chronic nonspecific rhinitis.
- In case of recurrence of malignant nasal neoplasia after combined cytoreductive surgery and radiation therapy, a second course of radiation therapy may be attempted. Alternatively, the secondary inflammation is treated with corticosteroids and broad-spectrum antibiotics.

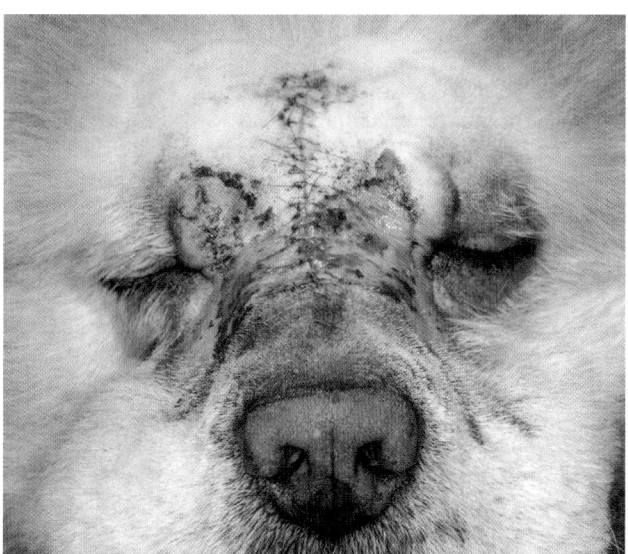

Figure 19.4. Postirradiation dermatitis. Dorsal rhinotomy with turbinectomy was performed in this patient 5 weeks after radiotherapy demonstrating irradiation induced dermatitis.

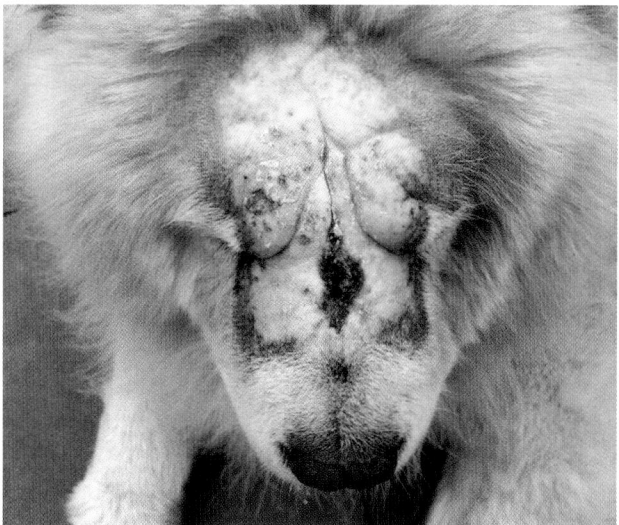

Figure 19.6. Postirradiation wound complications. Nine weeks after surgery, partial wound dehiscence, wound infection, and fistula formation are present.

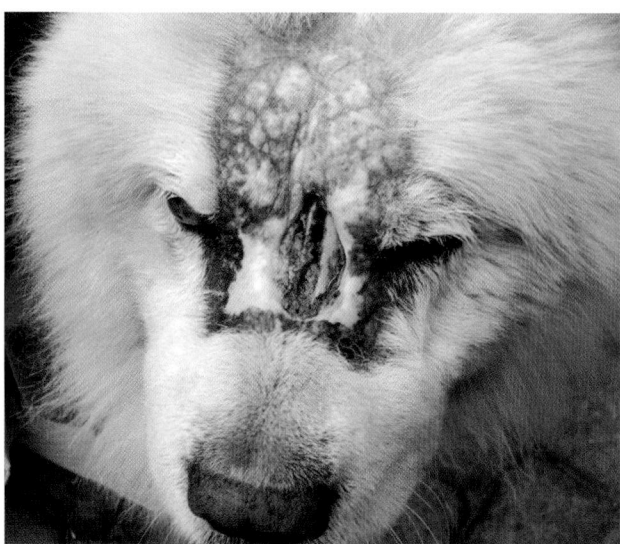

Figure 19.7. Postirradiation wound complications. Fourteen weeks after surgery, a nonhealing wound and osteomyelitis are present, and a chronic fistula has formed.

• Wound dehiscence and infection are treated with proper wound management and systemic antibiotics until viability of tissues can be properly assessed and a healthy recipient bed has formed. Reconstruction and closure of the defect with local or axial pattern flaps can subsequently be performed.

Prevention

The nasal cavity will never be anatomically or functionally normal after turbinectomy, and some degree of nasal discharge is inevitable after dorsal rhinotomy. Therefore, proper client education is essential. In most cases of persistent rhinitis:

• Clinical signs can be controlled with medical treatment directed at the primary cause of the rhinitis.
• Most tumors of the nasal cavity recur after surgery, but time to recurrence and survival are significantly prolonged with ancillary radiation therapy.
• Dorsal rhinotomy after radiotherapy is probably best performed after complete recovery of the patient and after radiation-induced dermatitis and osteomyelitis have subsided.

Relevant literature

Dorsal rhinotomy for removal of nasal foreign bodies is becoming a rare occurrence because advanced diagnostic imaging (CT or magnetic resonance imaging) can pinpoint the exact location of a focal abnormality, and modern rhinoscopy equipment and experience with it is readily available. Dorsal rhinotomy with turbinectomy (Spreull 1963, 1971) is also rarely indicated for treatment of chronic infectious rhinitis in dogs and cats. In dogs with fungal infections, surgery is best avoided (White 2006), with rare exceptions (Claeys et al. 2006), and most patients are best treated with intranasal application of antimycotic agents via either clotrimazole soaks (with or without intrasinusal clotrimazole or bifonazole cream) or tube placement and daily enilconazole flushing (Sissener et al. 2006; White 2006; Schuller and Clercx 2007; Billen et al. 2010). In cats with viral or nonspecific rhinitis, surgery is only indicated if associated with polyp formation, impaction of the

frontal sinus with mucus, or nasal obstruction caused by granulomatous turbinate expansion (Demko and Cohn 2007). However, the use of rhinotomy in combination with radiotherapy is gaining momentum for treatment of intranasal neoplasia. Canine nasal tumors are difficult to control with surgery alone, and survival times are similar with or without surgical treatment (Beck and Withrow 1985, Greenfield 2003). Radiotherapy is currently recognized as the most effective sole treatment modality, but local recurrence rates reportedly exceed 60%, and median survival time is approximately only 12 to 14 months (Beck and Withrow 1985; Straw et al. 1986; Theon et al. 1993; Adams et al. 1998; LaDue et al. 1999; Northrup et al. 2001; Mellanby et al. 2002; Lana et al. 2004; Adams et al. 2005, Gieger et al. 2008; Adams et al. 2009; Elliot and Mayer 2009). Some strategies, such as chemoradiotherapy (median survival, 19.3 months) (Lana et al. 2004), accelerated radiation therapy (median survival, 19.7 months), or preoperative accelerated radiation therapy (median survival, 47.7 months) may lead to improved survival times (Adams et al. 2005et al, 2009). A combination of surgery followed by orthovoltage radiation was reported to result in a median survival time of 23 months (Thrall and Harvey 1983); however, more recent studies (Evans et al. 1989; Northrup et al. 2001) have not substantiated these results. Megavoltage radiotherapy given soon after nasal turbinectomy does not appear to improve survival times compared with megavoltage radiotherapy alone (LaDue et al. 1999; Adams et al. 2005). The use of chemotherapy in combination with radiotherapy has met with limited success (Hahn et al. 1992; Lana et al. 2004; Nadeau et al. 2004).

Previous results of combining radiotherapy and surgery for the treatment of intranasal neoplasia have involved administration of external-beam fractionated radiotherapy beginning 14 to 21 days after nasal turbinectomy (Thrall and Harvey 1983; Adams et al. 1987; Evans et al. 1989; Northrup et al. 2001). Studies on the effect of resection of residual tumor after radiotherapy have demonstrated much better and significantly increased survival time rates (median survival, 47.7 months)(Adams et al. 2005). However, dogs that underwent dorsal rhinotomy with turbinectomy after radiotherapy had a substantial risk of developing postoperative complications (Adams et al. 2005).

Complications reported after dorsal rhinotomy with turbinectomy include **entrance into the cranial vault, hemorrhage, pneumocephalus and septic meningoencephalitis, subcutaneous emphysema, failure to mouth breathe, aspiration pneumonia, persistent anorexia and pain**, and **recurrence of disease** (Spreull 1963; Cook 1964; Spreull 1971; Baker 1972; Hoerlein 1975; Hedlund et al. 1983; Legendre et al. 1983; Beck and Withrow 1985; Birchard 1988; Holmberg et al., Holmberg 1996; McCarthy 1996; Hedlund 1998; Adams et al. 2005). Dogs with nasal neoplasia that are operated upon after radiotherapy in particular have an significantly higher risk of developing **chronic or recurrent rhinitis and osteomyelitis** with subsequent late **wound dehiscence and fistula formation** than dogs that underwent radiotherapy alone (Adams et al. 2005). Although these complications did not appear to affect outcome, **chronic bacterial or fungal rhinitis** resulted in long-term management responsibilities for the owners (Adams et al. 2005). A **chronic nasal discharge** is common in dogs that undergo turbinectomy (without radiotherapy) but commonly resolves within a few months after surgery, although a serous or purulent discharge may persist (Greenfield 2003, Adams et al. 2005). It is hypothesized that in dogs that undergo radiotherapy before nasal turbinectomy, the compromised blood supply in the underlying bone could impair healing of the exposed bone surfaces, resulting in poorly vascularized granulation tissue that is susceptible to opportunistic infection (Adams *et al.* 2005). One approach that might help to reduce this problem would be to resect turbinates only in the area of any persistent or recurrent tumor. The incidence of postsurgical rhinitis and osteomyelitis may also be reduced by preserving the periosteal lining of the nasal cavity to minimize compromise to the blood supply to the bone surfaces (Adams *et al.* 2005). Currently, long-term treatment with broad-spectrum antibiotics is recommended to reduce the incidence and severity of secondary bacterial rhinitis for these patients. The time between radiotherapy and nasal turbinectomy may influence the occurrence of these late complications; however, insufficient data are currently available to determine the optimum time frame.

The current treatment of nasal neoplasia in small animals has not developed to its full potential. Radiotherapeutic success can potentially be improved by changing treatment protocols or increasing dose or reirradiation after tumor recurrence (Bommarito *et al.* 2011). Increasing the doses used for radiotherapy will lead to a higher incidence of **severe acute mucositis**, **ocular inflammation**, **skin necrosis**, and **dental problems** (Gieger *et al.* 2008; Elliot and Mayer 2009; Belshaw *et al.* 2011; Bommarito *et al.* 2011).

References

Adams, W.M., Withrow, S.J., Walshaw, R., et al. (1987) Radiotherapy of malignant nasal tumors in 67 dogs. *Journal of the American Veterinary Medical Association* 191 (3), 311-315.

Adams, W.M., Miller, P.E., Vail, D.M., et al. (1998) An accelerated technique for irradiation of malignant canine nasal and paranasal sinus tumors. *Veterinary Radiology & Ultrasound* 39 (5), 475-481.

Adams, W.M., Bjorling, D.E., McAnulty, J.E., et al. (2005) Outcome of accelerated radiotherapy alone or accelerated radiotherapy followed by exenteration of the nasal cavity in dogs with intranasal neoplasia: 53 cases (1990-2002). *Journal of the American Veterinary Medical Association* 227 (6), 936-941.

Adams, W.M., Kleiter, M.M., Thrall, D.E., et al. (2009) Prognostic significance of tumor histology and computed tomographic staging for radiation treatment response of canine nasal tumors. *Veterinary Radiology & Ultrasound* 50 (3), 330-335.

Baker, G.J. (1972) Treatment of malignant neoplasia. Surgical management. *The Journal of Small Animal Practice* 13 (7), 373-379.

Beck, E.R., Withrow, S.J. (1985) Tumors of the canine nasal cavity. *The Veterinary clinics of North America. Small Animal Practice* 15 (3), 521-533.

Belshaw, Z., Constantino-Casas, F., Brearley, M.J., et al. (2011) COX-2 expression and outcome in canine nasal carcinomas treated with hypofractionated radiotherapy. *Veterinary and Comparative Oncology* 9 (2), 141-148.

Billen, F., Guieu, L.V., Bernaerts, F., et al. (2010) Efficacy of intrasinusal administration of bifonazole cream alone or in combination with enilconazole irrigation in canine sino-nasal aspergillosis: 17 cases. *The Canadian Veterinary Journal* 51 (2), 164-168.

Birchard, S.J. (1988) A simplified method for rhinotomy and temporary rhinostomy in dogs and cats. *Journal of the American Animal Hospital Association* 24, 69-72.

Bommarito, D.A., Kent, M.S., Selting, K.A., et al. (2011) Reirradiation of recurrent canine nasal tumors. *Veterinary Radiology & Ultrasound,* 52 (2), 207-212.

Claeys, S., Lefebvre, J.B., Schuller, S., et al. (2006) Surgical treatment of canine nasal aspergillosis by rhinotomy combined with enilconazole infusion and oral itraconazole. *The Journal of Small Animal Practice* 47 (6), 320-324.

Cook, W.R. (1964) Observations on the upper respiratory tract of the dog and cat. *Journal of Small Animal Practice* 5, 309-329.

Demko, J.L., Cohn, L.A. (2007) Chronic nasal discharge in cats: 75 cases (1993-2004). *Journal of the American Veterinary Medical Association* 230 (7), 1032-1037.

Elliot, K.M., Mayer, M.N. (2009) Radiation therapy for tumors of the nasal cavity and paranasal sinuses in dogs. *The Canadian Veterinary Journal* 50 (3), 309-312.

Evans, S.M., Goldschmidt, M., McKee, L.J., et al. (1989) Prognostic factors and survival after radiotherapy for intranasal neoplasms in dogs: 70 cases (1974-1985). *Journal of the American Veterinary Medical Association* 194 (10), 1460-1463.

Fletcher, D.J., Snyder, J.M., Messinger, J.S., et al. (2006) Ventricular pneumocephalus and septic meningoencephalitis secondary to dorsal rhinotomy and nasal polypectomy in a dog. *Journal of the American Veterinary Medical Association* 229 (2), 240-245.

Gieger, T., Rassnick, K., Siegel, S., et al. (2008) Palliation of clinical signs in 48 dogs with nasal carcinomas treated with coarse-fraction radiation therapy. *Journal of the American Animal Hospital Association* 44 (3), 116-123.

Greenfield, C.L. (2003) Respiratory tract neoplasia. In: *Slatter Textbook of Small Animal Surgery*, 3rd edn. W.B. Saunders, Philadelphia, pp. 2474-2487.

Hahn, K.A., Knapp, D.W., Richardson, R.C., et al. (1992) Clinical response of nasal adenocarcinoma to cisplatin chemotherapy in 11 dogs. *Journal of the American Veterinary Medical Association* 200 (3), 355-357.

Hedlund, C.S., Tangner, C.H., Elkins, A.D., et al. (1983) Temporary bilateral carotid artery occlusion during surgical exploration of the nasal cavity of the dog. *Veterinary Surgery* 12 (2), 83-85.

Hedlund, C.S. (1998) Rhinotomy techniques. In: Bojrab, M.J. (ed.) *Current Techniques in Small Animal Surgery*, 4th edn. Williams & Wilkins, Baltimore, pp. 346-354.

Hoerlein, B.F. (1975) The nasal cavity. In: Bojrab, M.J. (ed.) *Current Techniques in Small Animal Surgery*. Lea & Febiger, Philadelphia, pp. 174-182.

Holmberg, D.L., Fries, C., Cockshutt, J., et al. (1989) Ventral rhinotomy in the dog and cat. *Vet Surg* 18 (6), 446-449.

Holmberg, D.L. (1996) Sequelae of ventral rhinotomy in dogs and cats with inflammatory and neoplastic nasal pathology: a retrospective study. *The Canadian veterinary journal,Can Vet J* 37 (8), 483-485.

LaDue, T.A., Dodge, R., Page, R.L., et al. (1999) Factors influencing survival after radiotherapy of nasal tumors in 130 dogs. *Veterinary Radiology & Ultrasound* 40 (3), 312-317.

Lana, S.E., Dernell, W.S., Lafferty, M.H., et al. (2004) Use of radiation and a slow-release cisplatin formulation for treatment of canine nasal tumors. *Veterinary Radiology & Ultrasound* 45 (6), 577-581.

Legendre, A.M., Spaulding, K., Krahwinkel, D.J. (1983) Canine nasal and paranasal sinus tumors. *Journal of the American Animal Hospital Association* 19, 115-123.

McCarthy, R.J. (1996) Surgery of the head & neck; dorsal rhinotomy. In: Lipowitz, A.J., Caywood, D.D., Cann, C.C., et al. (eds.) *Complications in Small Animals Surgery*. Lippincott, Williams & Wilkins, Philadelphia, pp. 99-107.

Mellanby, R.J., Stevenson, R.K., Herrtage, M.E., et al. (2002) Long-term outcome of 56 dogs with nasal tumours treated with four doses of radiation at intervals of seven days. *The Veterinary Record* 151 (9), 253-257.

Nadeau, M.E., Kitchell, B.E., Rooks, R.L., et al. (2004) Cobalt radiation with or without low-dose cisplatin for treatment of canine naso-sinus carcinomas. *Veterinary Radiology & Ultrasound,* 45 (4), 362-367.

Northrup, N.C., Etue, S.M., Ruslander, D.M., et al. (2001) Retrospective study of orthovoltage radiation therapy for nasal tumors in 42 dogs. *Journal of Veterinary Internal Medicine* 15 (3), 183-189.

Schuller, S., Clercx, C. (2007) Long-term outcomes in dogs with sinonasal aspergillosis treated with intranasal infusions of enilconazole. *Journal of the American Animal Hospital Association* 43 (1), 33-38.

Sissener, T.R., Bacon, N.J., Friend, E., et al. (2006) Combined clotrimazole irrigation and depot therapy for canine nasal aspergillosis. *The Journal of Small Animal Practice* 47 (6), 312-315.

Spreull, J.S.A. (1963) Surgery of the Nasal cavity of the dog and cat. *The Veterinary Record* 75 (5), 105-113.

Spreull, J.S.A. (1971) Surgery of the nasal cavity of the dog. In: Kirk, R.W. IV (ed.) *Current Veterinary Therapy*. W.B. Saunders, Philadelphia, pp. 125-128.

Straw, R.C., Withrow, S.J., Gillette, E.L., et al. (1986) Use of radiotherapy for the treatment of intranasal tumors in cats: six cases (1980-1985). *Journal of the American Veterinary Medical Association* 189 (8), 927-929.

Theon, A.P., Madewell, B.R., Harb, M.F., et al. (1993) Megavoltage irradiation of neoplasms of the nasal and paranasal cavities in 77 dogs. *Journal of the American Veterinary Medical Association* 202 (9), 1469-1475.

Thrall, D.E., Harvey, C.E. (1983) Radiotherapy of malignant nasal tumors in 21 dogs. *Journal of the American Veterinary Medical Association* 183 (6), 663-666.

White, D. (2006) Canine nasal mycosis—light at the end of a long diagnostic and therapeutic tunnel. *The Journal of small animal practice* 47 (6), 307.

20 Sublingual and Mandibular Sialadenectomy

Cheryl Hedlund

Department of Veterinary Clinical Sciences, Iowa State University, Ames, IA, USA

Resection of the sublingual and mandibular salivary glands is most often performed to treat salivary mucoceles (sialoceles) or neoplasia (Hedlund 2007). Cervical (Figure 20.1), sublingual (ranula) (Figure 20.2), and pharyngeal mucoceles (Figure 20.3) are caused by leakage of saliva into the surrounding tissues. Trauma, foreign bodies, sialoliths (calcium phosphate or carbonate), neoplasia, or inflammation can lead to leakage of saliva (Griffiths *et al.* 2000; Ryan *et al.* 2008). Saliva irritates surrounding tissues, causing inflammation and formation of granulation tissue, which encapsulates the saliva.

Leakage of saliva is most often associated with the polystomatic portion of the sublingual gland, but both the mandibular and sublingual glands are removed because the sublingual gland is intimate with the mandibular salivary gland duct (Figure 20.4).

Sialadenectomy is also indicated to remove salivary tumors. Adenocarcinoma is the most common tumor of the mandibular salivary gland in cats (Figure 20.5) and the parotid gland in dogs. Another indication for removing the salivary glands may be trauma caused by bites or puncture wounds, which may result in chronic inflammation, infection, or fistula formation.

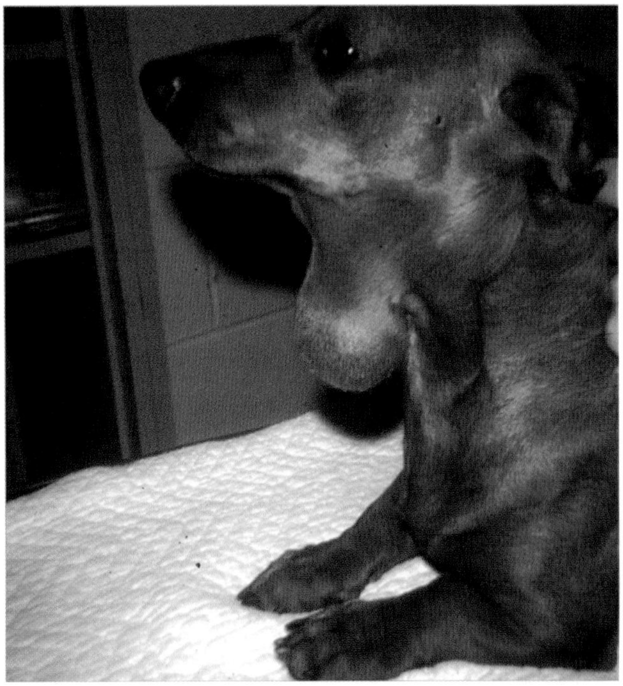

Mucocele recurrence

Definition
A salivary mucocele is a collection of saliva that has leaked from a damaged salivary duct or gland and is surrounded by granulation tissue. Mucoceles recur when there is failure to remove the damaged duct–gland tissue at the origin of the mucocele.

Risk factors
- Prior drainage of a mucocele by paracentesis alone
- Failure to dissect the sublingual gland beyond the origin of the mucocele
- Tearing of the duct–gland complex caudal to the duct–gland defect and failure to remove the orad gland
- Failure to identify the correct side of the damaged salivary gland or duct (right vs. left)

Figure 20.1 Identifying which salivary glands should be excised is easier if the cervical mucocele is lateralized rather than being pendulous and more midline in locations such as in this dog. *Source:* A. Hamaide, University of Liège, Liège, Belgium, 2014. Reproduced with permission from A. Hamaide.

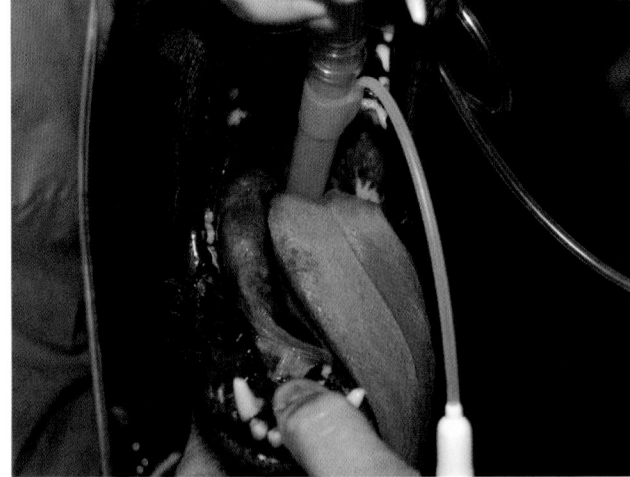

Figure 20.2 Ranula or sublingual mucoceles are located ventral to the tongue and lateral to the frenulum, indicating the side of glandular or duct leakage. *Source:* A. Hamaide, University of Liège, Liège, Belgium, 2014. Reproduced with permission from A. Hamaide.

Complications in Small Animal Surgery, First Edition. Edited by Dominique Griffon and Annick Hamaide.
© 2016 John Wiley & Sons, Inc. Published 2016 by John Wiley & Sons, Inc.
Companion website: www.wiley.com/go/griffon/complications

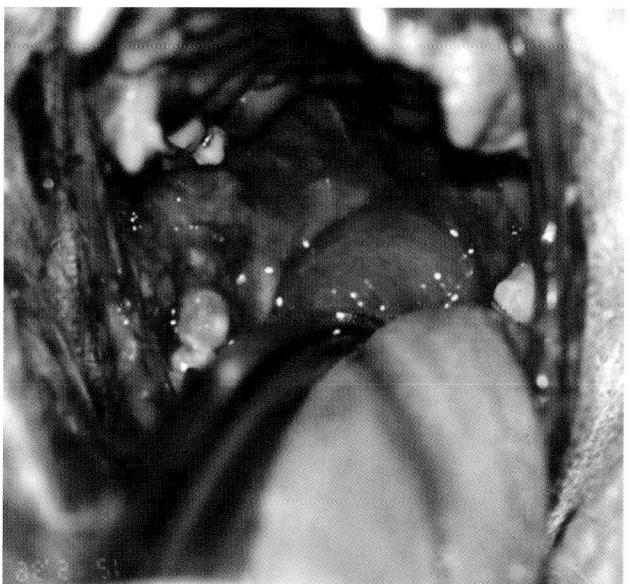

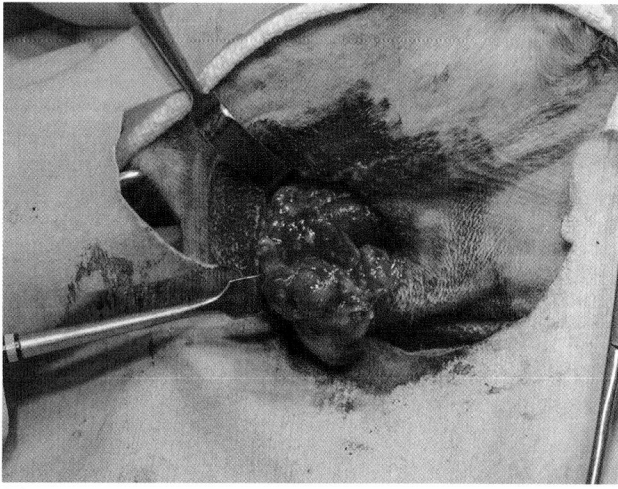

(A)

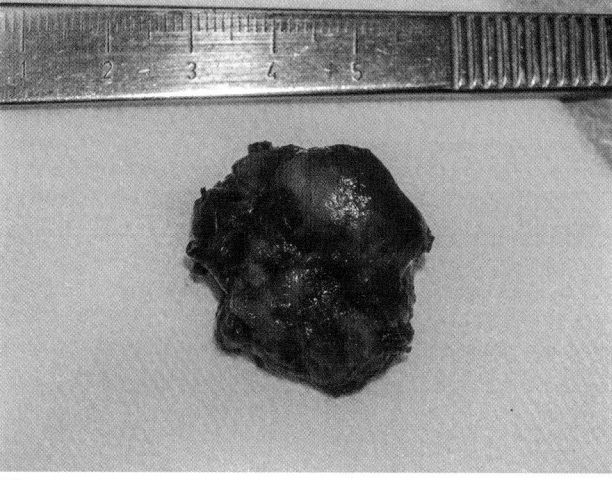

(B)

Figure 20.5 This cat presented with a firm, circular mass between the maxillary and linguofacial veins, which was diagnosed as a mandibular salivary gland adenocarcinoma.

Figure 20.3 Pharyngeal mucocele obstructing the airway. These are often seen in conjunction with cervical mucoceles.

- Misidentification and removal of lymph node rather than salivary gland(s)
- Mistaking a cyst (lymph node, tonsil, thyroglossal, Rathke's pouch, branchial cleft, or choristoma; Bentley 2006) for a salivary mucocele. The cyst will recur if the salivary glands are removed because the lining is of epithelial origin and will continue to secrete.

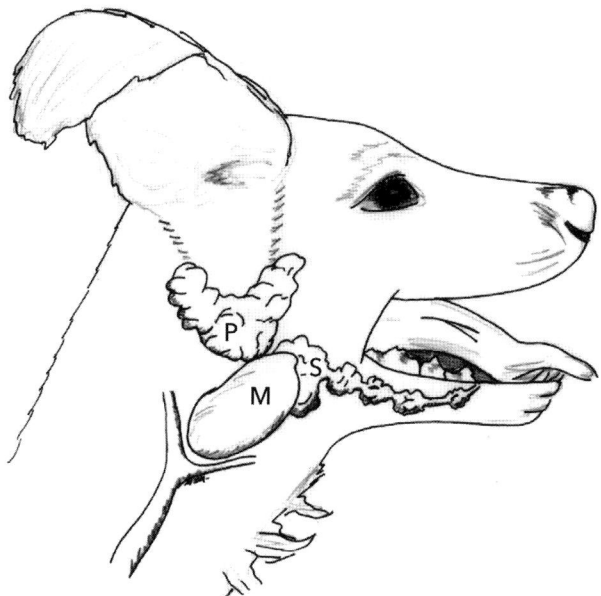

Figure 20.4 The mandibular salivary gland (M) is found ventral to the parotid salivary gland (P) at the base of the horizontal ear canal and between the maxillary and linguofacial veins near their junction. The monostomatic portion of the sublingual gland (S) cups the rostral aspect of the mandibular gland. The polystomatic portion of the sublingual gland travels with the mandibular duct toward the oral cavity.

Diagnosis

Mucocele recurrence must be differentiated from a postoperative seroma, which may occur with inadequate drainage after surgery, or the development of a second mucocele from the gland on the opposite side of the head. The diagnosis is most often made based on history, clinical signs, and cytology findings (Figure 20.6). Determination of the correct side is sometimes difficult for cervical mucoceles, which may appear to be on the midline. It is sometimes helpful to examine the animal in dorsal recumbency because the swelling may fall to the affected side. Sometimes diagnostic imaging and histopathology are necessary (Figure 20.7).

A diagnostic tree for evaluation of a soft tissue swelling in the cervical region is shown in Figure 20.8.

Treatment

The treatment consists of exploration, identification, and removal of the remaining salivary tissue on the involved side to resolve the mucocele. Dissection rostral to the lingual nerve may be necessary

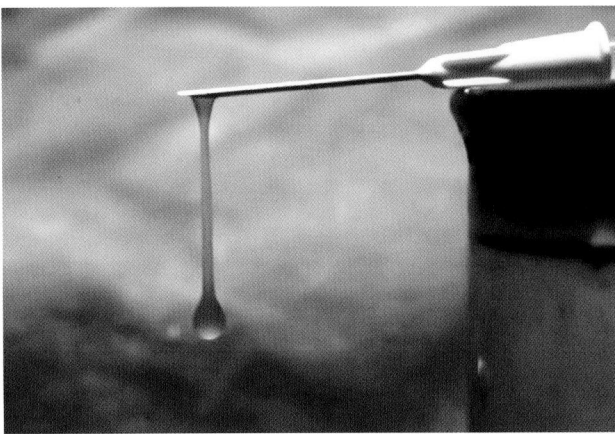

Figure 20.6 Mucocele fluid is usually yellowish and viscid. Fluid within a seroma is less tenacious and serosanguineous than that of a mucocele.

to remove the entire sublingual gland. This may be accomplished from a ventral (intermandibular), lateral, or possibly an oral approach.

- Ventral approach: Incise from the level of the linguofacial vein to the rostral intermandibular area. Locate the digastricus muscle and isolate remnants of the sublingual gland and mandibular duct. Undermine the digastricus muscle and pull any remaining glandular tissue rostrally. Identify the lingual nerve and then incise the mylohyoideus muscle to allow rostral dissection of the remaining sublingual gland to where it terminates near the sublingual caruncle.
- Lateral approach: Divide or retract the digastricus muscle to access the intermandibular area. Visualization and dissection of the polystomatic sublingual tissue is more challenging using this approach (Figure 20.9).
- Oral approach: Identify the sublingual caruncle and incise the mucosa to gain access to the intermandibular area. Contamination and subsequent infection are greater risks with this approach.

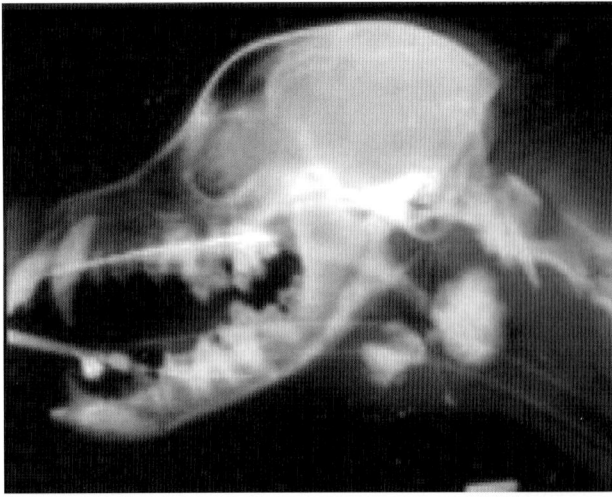

Figure 20.7 Sialograms may help identify the origin of the mucocele and help differentiate a mucocele from a cyst. Duct catheterization is challenging, especially in small dogs and cats.

Outcome

Mucocele resolution occurs when the damaged gland or duct has been removed. Animals moisten food adequately even after mandibular and sublingual glands have been removed bilaterally.

Prevention

Mucocele recurrence is prevented by correctly identifying the side of origin and by meticulous dissection beyond the damaged gland or duct. The dissection should be continued along the mandibular duct and polystomatic portion of the sublingual gland until the lingual nerve is identified. Then, rather than ligating and transecting the duct at this site, continue rostral dissection until no more glandular tissue is identifiable. Accomplish this by passing the mandibular duct with attached sublingual glands dorsal to the digastricus muscle and then incising the mylohyoideus muscle to expose the most rostral lobules of salivary tissue. A ventral approach facilitates more rostral dissection.

Respiratory and swallowing problems

Definition

Dyspnea may be caused by nasopharyngeal or oropharyngeal obstruction of the airway. This may be caused by a pharyngeal mucocele or tumor bulging into the pharynx (Figures 20.3 and 20.10).

Dysphagia may be caused by sublingual or oropharyngeal obstruction of food passage or difficulty with food prehension and movement into the esophagus secondary to pain or nerve damage. Damage to the hypoglossal or lingual nerves may cause loss of sensation and motor control to the tongue, lower jaw, lip, cheek, and mucosa.

Risk factors

- Animals with pharyngeal mucoceles
- Animals with tumors protruding into the pharynx (see Figure 20.10).
- Animals with ranulas may bite or traumatize the mucocele, causing oral pain and reluctance to pick up and chew food.
- Failure to identify and protect nerves during dissection leading to operative trauma to branches of the trigeminal or hypoglossal nerves (Figure 20.11)

Diagnosis

Clinical signs and visual examination of the mouth and oropharynx are often diagnostic.

- Presence of a soft, fluctuant, nonpainful mass → pharyngeal mucocele
- Presence of a firm and fixed mass → tumor
- Abnormal tongue movements, difficulty in picking up or moving food into esophagus → nerve damage

The diagnosis may be confirmed by cytology or histopathology which can differentiate among a mucocele, tumor, or cyst. Ultrasonography, computed tomography, or sialography may help localize the lesion. A neurologic examination to assess cranial nerve function and a contrast swallowing study may help explain abnormal swallowing.

Treatment

Respiratory problems are alleviated by draining the mucocele, resecting redundant oropharyngeal tissues, and removing damaged glandular tissue and ducts.

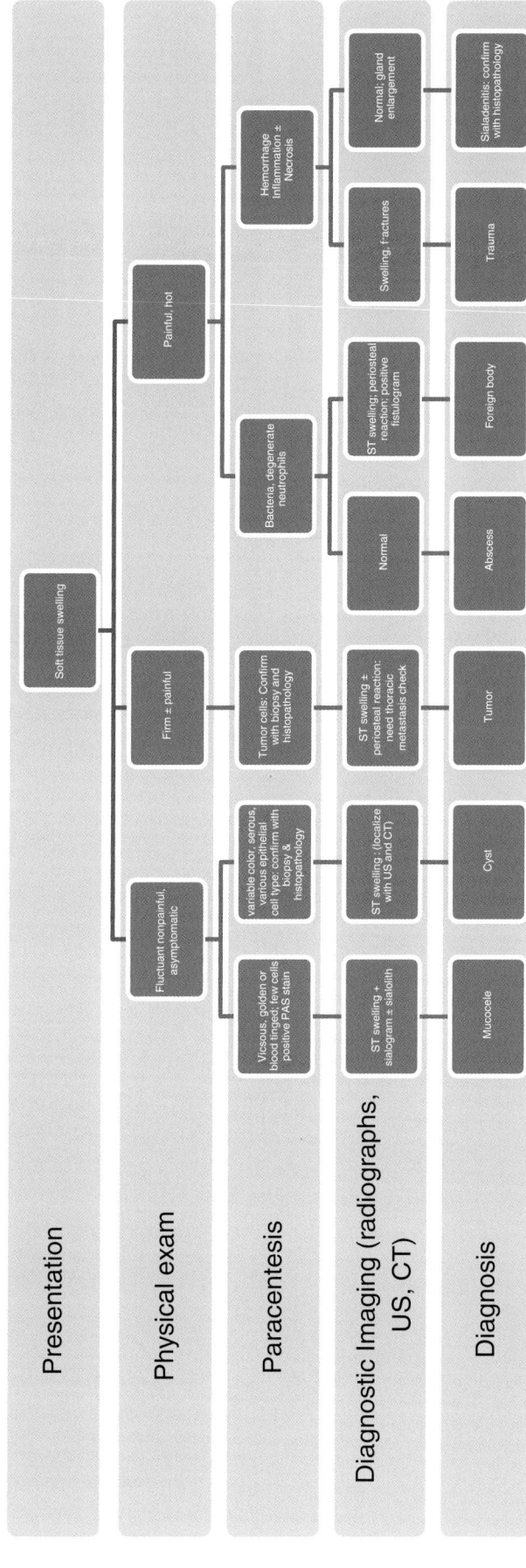

Figure 20.8 Diagnostic tree for evaluation of a soft tissue (ST) swelling in the cervical region. CT, computed tomography; US, ultrasonography. PAS, period acid-Schiff.

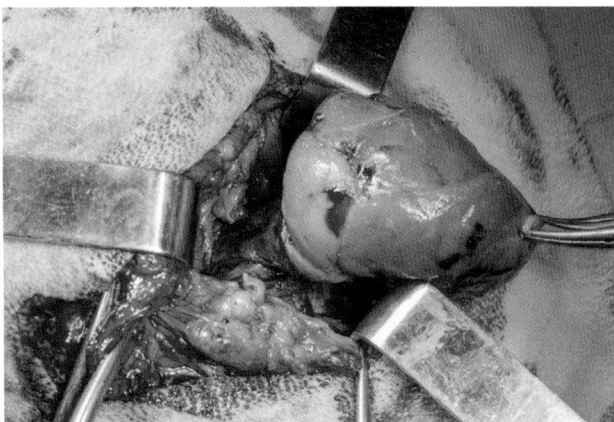

Figure 20.9 The mandibular and sublingual glands exposed using a lateral approach and freed from the capsule.

- Treat acute, severe dyspnea by aspirating fluid from the mucocele and if necessary placing a tracheostomy tube.
- Marsupialize the mucocele to prolong drainage. Incise and remove an ellipse of mucosa overlying the mucocele; then suture the granulation tissue lining to the oral (ranula) or oropharyngeal (pharyngeal mucocele) mucosa.
- Resect residual salivary tissue as described for recurrent mucoceles.
- Treatment of salivary gland tumors includes resection of the involved glands, radiation therapy, and/or chemotherapy.

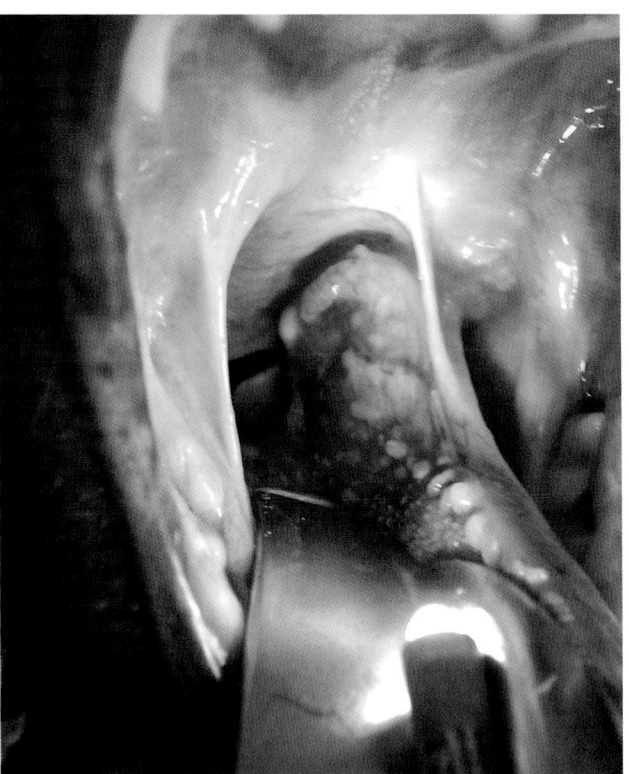

Figure 20.10 Partial obstruction of the airway and pharynx as a result of inward bulging of a mandibular salivary gland adenocarcinoma in a cat.

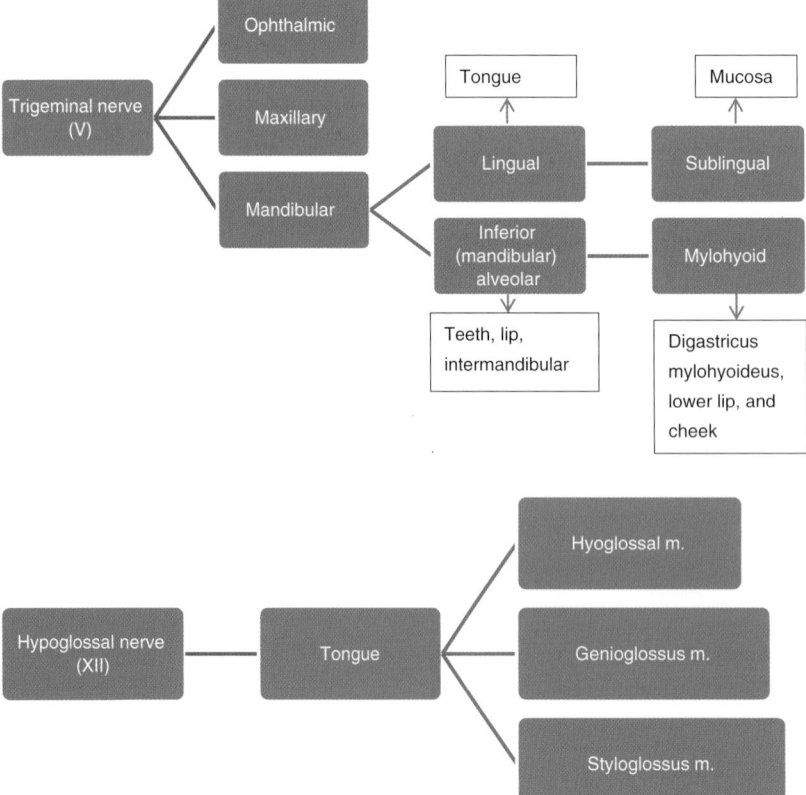

Figure 20.11 Trauma to branches of cranial nerves V and XII may result in problems with prehension of food and pushing the food bolus into the pharynx.

- Swallowing abnormalities caused by nerve trauma may gradually improve with time. Antiinflammatory drugs may be beneficial if nerves are inflamed.

Outcome

Evacuation of the mucocele alleviates associated respiratory problems. Mucoceles will not recur after complete removal of the involved mandibular and sublingual glands. New mucoceles, however, can develop from salivary glands not previously involved (opposite side).

The prognosis for long-term survival after salivary gland tumor resection is guarded because most tumors are malignant. The reported median survival times when treated by resection with and without adjunctive radiation therapy are 550 days in dogs and 516 days in cats (Hammer *et al.* 2001).

Abnormal nerve function may improve over time.

Prevention

Mucocele drainage and meticulous dissection to completely remove the glandular tissue and prevent damage to the hypoglossal or lingual nerves avoid these complications.

Relevant literature

The reported incidence of salivary gland disease in dogs is less than 0.3% (Carberry *et al.* 1988; Spangler and Culbertson 1991; Hammer *et al.* 2001). The most common surgical disease affecting the salivary glands is mucocele (Bellenger and Simpson 1992). Other conditions affecting the salivary glands include tumors (Carberry *et al.* 1988; Spangler and Culbertson 1991; Hammer *et al.* 2001), trauma (Griffiths *et al.* 2000), and sialadenitis (McGill *et al.* 2009).

Treatment of mucoceles by aspiration alone results in recurrence in 42% of affected animals within 48 hours (Bellenger and Simpson 1992). Recurrence after complete salivary gland resection of the involved gland(s) is not expected (Ritter *et al.* 2006; McGurk *et al.* 2008).

References

Bellenger, C.R., Simpson, D.J. (1992) Canine sialocoeles—60 clinical cases. *Journal of Small Animal Practice* 33, 376-380.

Bentley, A.M., Goldschmidt, M.H., Bennett, R.A. (2006) Intestinal choristoma in the midcervical region of a dog. *Journal of the American Animal Hospital Association* 42, 223-225.

Carberry, C.A., Flanders, J.A., Harvey, H.J., et al. (1988) Salivary gland tumors in dogs and cats: A literature and case review. *Journal of the American Animal Hospital Association* 24, 561-67.

Griffiths, L.G., Tiruneh, R., Sullivan, M., et al. (2000) Oropharyngeal penetrating injuries in 50 dogs: a retrospective study. *Veterinary Surgery* 29, 383-388.

Hammer, A., Getzy, D. Ogilvie, G., et al. (2001) Salivary gland neoplasia in the dog and cat: survival times and prognostic factors. *Journal of the American Animal Hospital Association* 37, 478-482.

Hedlund, C.S. (2007) Surgery of the Digestive System. In: Fossum, T.W. (ed.) *Small Animal Surgery*. Mosby Elsevier, St. Louis, pp. 367-372.

McGurk, M., Eyeson, J., Thomas, B., et al. (2008) Conservative treatment of oral ranula by excision with minimal excision of the sublingual gland: Histological support for a traumatic etiology. *Journal of Oral and Maxillofacial Surgery* 66, 2050-2057.

McGill, S., Lester, N., McLachlan, A., et al. (2009) Concurrent sialocoele and necrotizing sialadenitis in a dog. *Journal of Small Animal Practice* 50, 151-156.

Ritter, M.J., von Pfeil, D.J.F., Hauptman, J.B., et al. (2006) Mandibular and sublingual sialocoeles in the dog: A retrospective evaluation of 41 cases, using the ventral approach for treatment. *New Zealand Veterinary Journal* 54 (6),333-337.

Ryan, T., Welsh, E., McGorum I., (2008) Sublingual salivary gland sialolithiasis in a dog. *Journal of Small Animal Practice* 49, 254-256.

Spangler, W.L., Culbertson, M.R. (1991) Salivary gland disease in dogs and cats: 245 cases (1985-1988). *Journal of the American Veterinary Medical Association* 198 (3), 465-469.

21 Incisional Drainage of Aural Hematomas

Cheryl Hedlund
Department of Veterinary Clinical Sciences, Iowa State University, Ames, IA, USA

Aural hematomas are fluctuant to firm, fluid-filled swellings on the concave surface of the pinna. The pinna's entire concave surface or just a portion may be involved. Aural hematoma is one of the most common diseases of the external ear. Seen most commonly in dogs with pendulous ears, they also occur in dogs with erect ears and cats. The auricular cartilage is pierced by many foramina through which numerous branches of the caudal auricular artery pass. Traumatic shearing forces may tear these vessels, resulting in a hematoma. Bleeding and accumulation of blood force apart the cartilage layers. Bleeding continues until the pressure created by the pooling blood equalizes with that of the bleeding arteries. Evacuation and drainage of blood and clots is necessary to avoid disfiguring scar formation caused by the auricular cartilages' potential for chondrogenesis (Kagan 1983).

Incisional drainage and suturing is probably the most successful method of resolving the hematoma but has the greatest risk of cosmetic alterations. Other treatment methods include placement of a teat cannula (Wilson 1983), tube (Kagan 1983), or suction drain (Swaim and Bradley 1996) (Figure 21.1).

Drainage of the hematoma reduces pain, self-mutilation, and healing by fibrous contraction (Figure 21.2). Careful surgical technique and attention to postoperative management prevent most complications. Cosmetic alterations to the pinna and recurrence of the hematoma are the most common complications associated with drainage. Contributing causes such as otitis externa, otitis media, external parasites, and atopy or systemic disease (i.e., Cushing's disease, immune mediated) must be concurrently treated to diminish hematoma recurrence.

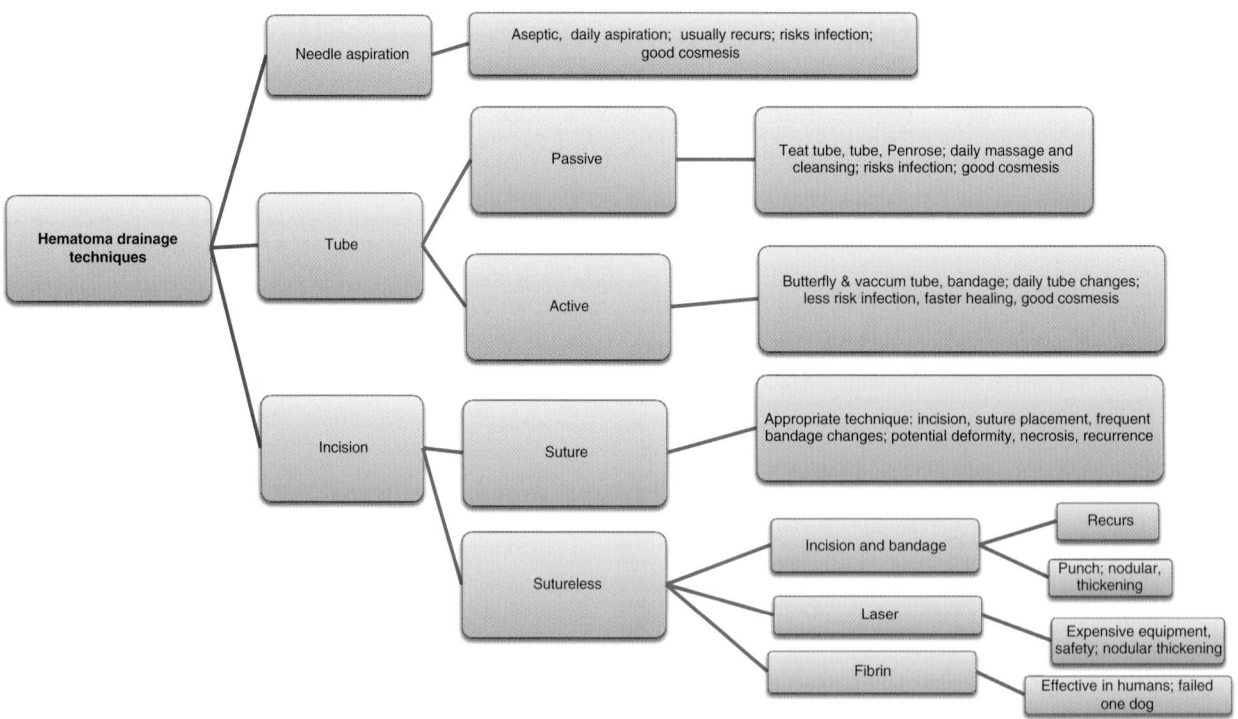

Figure 21.1 Aural hematoma: drainage techniques and expectations.

Complications in Small Animal Surgery, First Edition. Edited by Dominique Griffon and Annick Hamaide.
© 2016 John Wiley & Sons, Inc. Published 2016 by John Wiley & Sons, Inc.
Companion website: www.wiley.com/go/griffon/complications

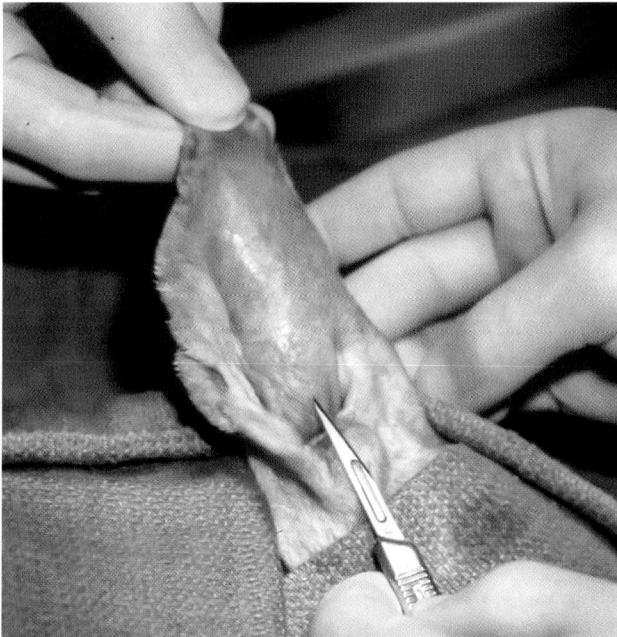

Figure 21.2 Aural hematomas are fluctuant to firm, fluid-filled swellings on the concave surface of the pinna. Drainage of the hematoma reduces pain, self-mutilation, and healing by fibrous contraction.

Cosmetic alterations

Definition
Cosmetic alterations are mild to severe thickening and wrinkling of the pinna. They are caused by healing with secondary contracture and are usually related to excessive suture tension or delayed treatment. All ears with hematomas are at risk for cosmetic alterations. Chronicity and severe cartilage damage cause the pinna to shrink and resemble a cauliflower (Figure 21.3).

Risk factors
- Delayed hematoma treatment and resolution
- Severely damaged auricular cartilage
- Improper technique: bad incision orientation, placing sutures too tight
- Self-mutilation
- Failure to maintain bandage and Elizabethan collar

Diagnosis
The diagnosis is made on visual inspection and palpation. The pinna is thickened and wrinkled to various degrees. Identification of predisposing causes may require otoscopic examination, specimen cytology, culture, and histopathology, and skull imaging. Additionally, allergy testing and other testing may be indicated to identify systemic diseases.

Treatment
The best treatment is prevention. Cosmetic alterations caused by pinna contracture are irreparable. Some acute thickening of the pinna may resolve over 2 to 3 months as inflammation resolves and fibrous tissue matures.

Outcome
Little to no improvement is expected.

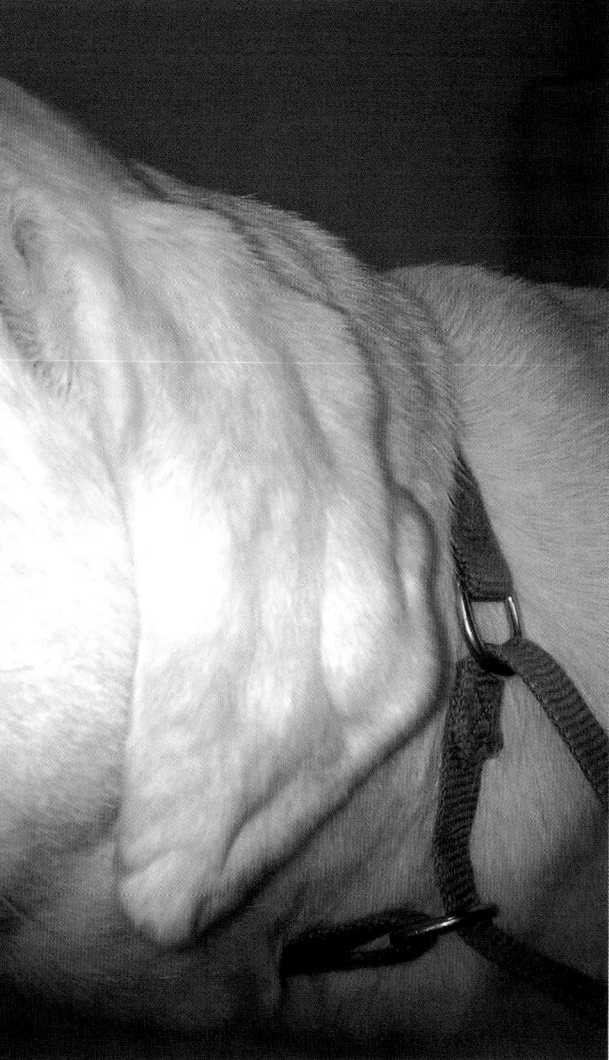

Figure 21.3 This pinna has irregular thickening after resolution of an aural hematoma and is often described as a "cauliflower ear."

Prevention
If owners are unwilling to risk cosmetic alterations, alternative drainage techniques can be attempted such as using the sutureless technique (Bojrab and Constantinescu 1998; Dye *et al.* 2002; Blättler *et al.* 2007), placing a teat cannula (Wilson 1983), or inserting closed-suction drains (Swaim and Bradley 1996) (see Figure 21.1).
- Treat hematomas soon after they form, preferably within the first few days. Bleeding within the cartilage continues until the pressure in the cavity equals the pressure in the bleeding arteries. Additional trauma causes resumption of bleeding and further separation of cartilage. Additionally, auricular chondrogenesis associated with trauma leads to thickening and irregularity.
- Create an S-shaped incision so longitudinal contraction is less likely to occur.
- Place sutures that appose the cartilage with both skin surfaces but are loose enough to allow passage of a needle holder tip to the boxlock (Henderson and Horne 2003). Tightly tied sutures cause discomfort, pain, irritation, edema, and necrosis.
- Leave a gap between incised skin and cartilage edges.

- Some suggest suturing through sheets of plastic, foam, or similar object to help distribute suture tension over a larger area and compress tissue planes. This is not necessary if enough sutures are placed.
- Place a bandage and Elizabethan collar immediately postoperatively to prevent self-mutilation.
- Treat the underlying cause: otitis, parasites, atopy, neoplasm, or systemic disease.
- Administer analgesics and sedation as necessary until pain and the underlying disease is controlled.

Recurrence of hematoma

Definition
Hematoma recurrence is the collection of blood within the cartilage plate of the pinna after drainage. It may occur at the original site, but it often affects an adjacent area.

Risk factors
- Associated with improper surgical technique: too few sutures, improper location
- Associated with failure to correct the underlying cause of the condition or predisposing factors: unresolved otitis, atopy, parasites, neoplasm, and so on.
- Animals with coagulopathies

Diagnosis
The diagnosis is made on visual inspection and palpation. There is a fluctuant to firm swelling of the concave surface of the pinna. Pain and various degrees of cartilage thickening may be present. Identification of predisposing causes may require otoscopic examination, specimen cytology, culture and histopathology, and skull imaging. Additionally, allergy testing and other testing may be indicated to identify systemic diseases.

Treatment
The cause of recurrence must be identified and corrected. The hematoma should be managed surgically with attention to detail.
- Create an S-shaped incision over the entire hematoma on the concave surface of the ear (Figure 21.4).
- Evacuate blood and fibrin clots; then flush the cavity.
- Hold the cartilage in apposition with suture until scar tissue forms. Depending on the size of the cavity, place two to five rows of sutures (see Figure 21.4).
- Place sutures parallel to the major branches of the caudal auricular artery with bites approximately 0.5 to 1 cm long penetrating the skin on the concave surface and the cartilage and then engaging the dermis on the convex surface but not necessarily penetrating it (see Figure 21.4 insert).
- Place enough sutures to prevent pockets for fluid accumulation by staggering rows. Space each suture approximately 0.5 to 1 cm apart and each row is approximately 0.5 to 1 cm away from the previous row.
- Leave a gap between incised skin edges.
- Protect and immobilize the ear postoperatively with a bandage and Elizabethan collar to prevent head shaking, scratching, and rubbing. Change the bandage at least weekly and maintain the bandage for an additional week after suture removal at 14 to 21 days.

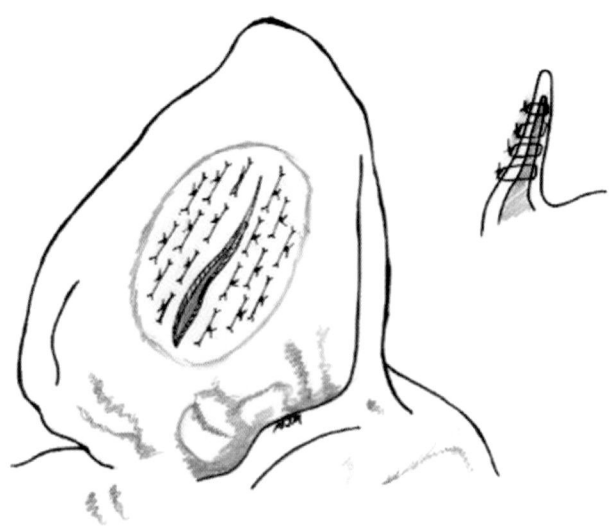

Figure 21.4 Incisional drainage and suture of the hematoma cavity with sutures placed parallel to vasculature in staggered rows to hold tissue planes in apposition. Sutures are placed full thickness through the pinna or engaging only the dermis on the convex surface (insert).

Outcome
Repeat occurrences increase the risk of cosmetic alterations; however, resolution of the hematoma is expected.

Prevention
- Use careful surgical technique and attention to postoperative management.
- Incise the entire length of the hematoma.
- Appose tissue layers beginning at the edges of the hematoma cavity.
- Prevent violent head shaking and self-inflicted trauma from scratching and rubbing.
- Effectively treat predisposing conditions.

Pinna necrosis

Definition
Pinna necrosis is ischemic degeneration of a portion or the entire pinna.

Risk factors
- Incorrect suture placement

Diagnosis
The diagnosis is made on visual inspection and palpation. A portion of the pinna is greenish black, insensitive, and cold and fails to bleed when cut.

Treatment
Resect the necrotic portion of the pinna, contouring the edges so the cosmetic result is more acceptable. Suture the haired skin edge to the thinner, relatively hairless skin on the concave surface of the pinna. Avoid penetrating the cartilage edge with the needle. Prevent trauma from scratching, rubbing, and shaking by bandaging the ear and placing an Elizabethan collar.

Outcome

The symmetrical appearance of the ears is lost and the cosmetic appearance of the involved ear disappointing (smaller, shorter, notched, and so on).

Prevention

Careful surgical technique and attention to postoperative management.

- Visualize the three main branches of the caudal auricular artery (lateral, intermediate, medial) on the convex (haired, external) aspect of the pinna.
- Avoid placing sutures around the ascending branches of the caudal auricular artery.
- Tie sutures so tissues are just apposed but not strangulated. Sutures tied too tightly can cause discomfort, pain, irritation, edema, and necrosis.

Relevant literature

Incisional drainage of aural hematomas may be the best treatment for chronic hematomas, but its risks for cosmetic alterations are greater than some alternative techniques. Alternative techniques are often preferred for acute aural hematomas because there is less risk of ear thickening, wrinkling, and contraction (Kagan 1983; Wilson 1983; Swaim and Bradley 1996). Teat tube placement is a simple and inexpensive method effective in 85% of animals with aural hematomas, and cosmetic alterations are minimal (Wilson 1983) (Figure 21.5 and Box 21.1).

Disadvantages of the teat tube technique include owner compliance to massage and cleanse the site daily and the risk of ascending infections associated with an unbandaged drain. Similar advantages and disadvantages are associated with tube drainage as described by Kagan (1983). The suction-drain technique described by Swaim and Bradley (1996) is another simple technique that

Box 21.1 Technique for teat tube management of aural hematomas

Teat Tube Technique

Collared, tapered, fenestrated teat tube with "fingers"

Remove half of collar and discard cap.

Technique

Puncture the distal aspect (tip) with a 12- or 14-gauge needle or #11 blade.

Evacuate and flush the hematoma cavity.

Insert the teat tube, engaging "fingers"; place the flat side of the collar to the pinna.

Optional: Secure with a suture through the collar.

Daily: Massage gently to "milk" accumulated fluid and cleanse area.

Maintain for 3 to 4 weeks.

Remove tube.

Continue daily massage and cleansing until the tract is healed.

uses a closed-suction drain easily made from a butterfly catheter and an evacuated blood collection tube (Figure 21.6 and Box 21.2). The advantages of this technique include faster healing, less risk of ascending infection, few complications, and measureable fluid accumulation. Disadvantages might include bandage maintenance, needle breakage, and owner compliance with changing tubes as recommended.

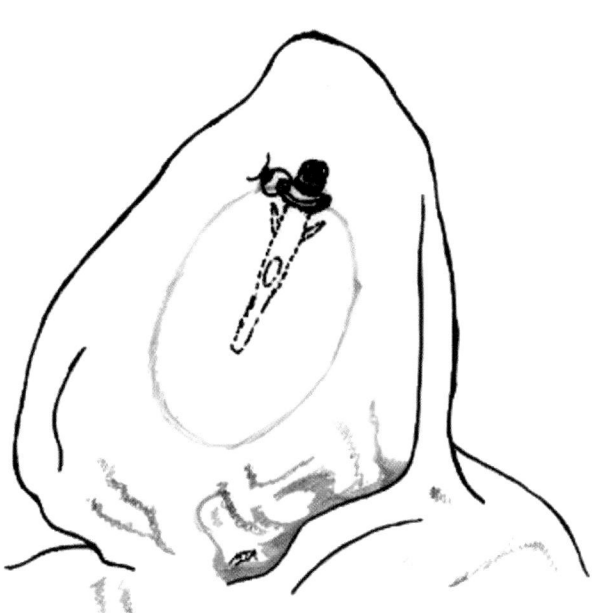

Figure 21.5 Teat tube placement is a simple and inexpensive method effective method of aural hematomas drainage.

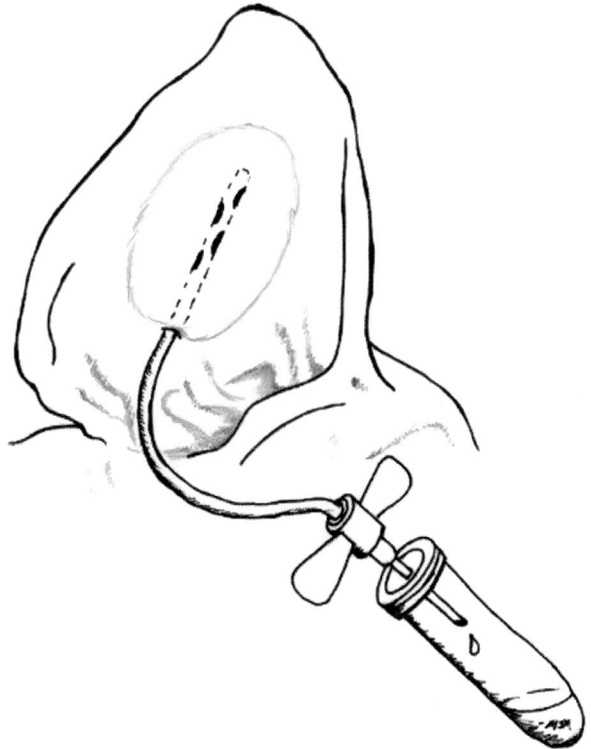

Figure 21.6 The suction-drain technique is a simple technique that uses a closed-suction drain easily made from a butterfly catheter and an evacuated blood collection tube.

Box 21.2 Technique for management of aural hematomas using the closed-suction drainage technique

Closed-Suction Drainage

Butterfly catheter: fenestrate; remove syringe adaptor

5 to 10 mL evacuated blood collection tube

Technique

Evacuate and flush the hematoma with an 18-gauge needle and syringe.

Enlarge the puncture with a #11 blade.

Insert a catheter and secure.
- Interrupted suture distally through catheter
- Purse-string at puncture

Attach to suction tube.

Bandage ear overhead; change bandage weekly or as needed.

Change tube.
- Two to three times daily the first 2 or 3 days
- Modify the frequency with declining fluid collection

Expect tube removal at ~7 to 10 days.

Replace bandage for an additional 7 days.

Sutureless, drainless techniques have also been suggested (Cowley 1976; Bojrab and Constantinescu 1998; Dye *et al.* 2002; Blättler *et al.* 2007). Recurrence was high after creation of a long incision spanning the length of the hematoma cavity and bandaging without the placement of sutures as described by Bojrab and Constantinescu (1998). The use of a punch to create a series of small holes thru the cartilage and concave surface of the pinna followed by bandaging

for 10 days was reported to be effective (Cowley 1976). Similarly, smaller, full-thickness holes were created with a carbon dioxide laser to stimulate adhesion between tissue layers (Dye *et al.* 2002). Laser treatment of the hematoma cavity and an adjacent margin of tissue followed by bandaging resulted in resolution in all ten ears. However, 2 of 10 recurred and required additional treatment. Laser treated pinnas were inflamed and thickened for several weeks, this gradually resolved leaving a slightly too moderately thickened, nodular pinna. A case report suggested coating the hematoma cavity with fibrin sealant to promote adhesion because this is described as an effective treatment in humans with similar problems (Blättler *et al.* 2007). The initial success in this case was followed by recurrence, possibly caused by premature removal of a protective collar.

References

Blättler, U., Harlin, O., Mattison, R.G., et al. (2007) Fibrin sealant as a treatment for canine aural haematoma: a case history. *The Veterinary Journal* 173, 697-700.

Bojrab, M.J., Constantinescu, G.M. (1998) Sutureless technique for repair of aural hematoma. In Bojrab, M.J., Ellison, G.W., Slocum, B. (eds.) *Current Techniques in Small Animal Surgery*, 4th edn. Williams & Wilkins, Baltimore, pp. 97-98.

Cowley, F. (1976) Treatment of hematoma of the canine ear. *Veterinary Medicine and Small Animal Clinician,* 71, 283.

Dye, T.L., Teque, H.D., Ostwald, D.A., et al. (2002) Evaluation of a technique using the carbon dioxide laser for the treatment of aural hematomas. *Journal of the American Animal Hospital Association* 38, 385-390.

Henderson, R.A., Horne, R. (2003) Pinna. In: Slatter, D. (ed.) *Textbook of Small Animal Surgery*, 3rd edn.. Saunders, Philadelphia, pp 1737-1741.

Kagan, K.G. (1983) Treatment of aural hematoma with an indwelling drain. *Journal of the American Veterinary Medical Association* 183 (9), 972-974.

Swaim, S.F., Bradley, D.M. (1996) Evaluation of closed-suction drainage for treating auricular hematomas. *Journal of the American Animal Hospital Association* 32, 36-43.

Wilson, J.W. (1983) Treatment of aural hematomas using a teat tube. *Journal of the American Veterinary Medical Association* 182, 1081-1083.

22 Ear Canal Surgery

Gert ter Haar

ENT, Brachycephaly and Audiology Clinic, Royal Veterinary College, North Mymms, Hatfield, Herts, UK

An otologic surgeon must face the particular challenges inherent to performing surgery in an area with complex anatomy and close proximity to major vascular and neurologic structures where small errors can lead to serious complications. The variation in anatomy of the ear within dog and cat breeds and the high number of bacteria inhabiting the ear canal of patients that require surgery create additional elements of unpredictability that, despite every effort, can lead to undesirable results and outcomes. It is therefore important to master the complex anatomy and physiology of the outer, middle, and inner ear and to master techniques to avoid surgical pitfalls and methods to manage complications before performing even "routine" procedures on the external ear canal. Avoidance of complications is commonly achieved with the use of proper patient selection, precise technique, proper instrument and tissue handling, sound judgment, and a realistic goal of what can be achieved in a particular situation. Ear canal surgery is reserved for cases in which proper medical treatment for otitis externa has failed and for ear canal neoplasia. Surgical techniques that have been described for the external auditory canal include lateral ear canal resection (LECR; Zepp and Lacroix modification), vertical ear canal resection or ablation (VECA), and total ear canal ablation (TECA) with lateral bulla osteotomy (LBO). Specific indications and complications are associated with each of these procedures. Prevention of complications requires proper patient selection. Intraoperative management of complications requires experience with all techniques described below and judgment on the part of the surgeon. During the postoperative period, it also requires the cooperation and involvement of the patient and animal owner.

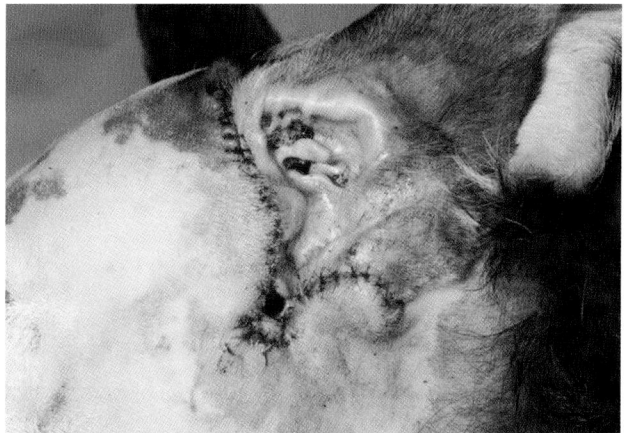

Figure 22.1 End-result after ear canal resection according to Lacroix. En-bloc resection of a mastocytoma in the skin overlying the lateral wall of the vertical ear canal.

processes (tumors, polyps, or wounds) truly limited to the vertical ear canal.

Complications associated with both lateral and vertical ear canal resections include infection, incisional dehiscence, stenosis of the remaining horizontal ear canal, and failure to alleviate clinical signs when performed for otitis externa. Complications only seen after VECA include facial nerve palsy and failure of erect ears to stand (cosmetic complication).

Lateral and vertical ear canal resection

Traditionally, LECR and VECA were performed as part of the treatment of medically nonresponsive chronic otitis externa. However, in the author's opinion, LECR should be reserved for the removal of small neoplasms restricted to the lateral wall of the vertical ear canal or for en-bloc resection of skin or subcutaneous neoplasms overlying the lateral ear canal. In these cases, LECR according to Lacroix is indicated because the lateral ear canal wall is removed during surgery, and no ventral drain board is created (Figure 22.1).

LECR according to Zepp, in which the lateral wall of the vertical ear canal is reflected to form a ventral drain board, theoretically can be used when dealing with small tumors limited to the very distal part of the lateral ear canal wall. VECA is indicated for disease

Infection
See Chapter 1.

Incisional dehiscence

Etiopathogenesis
Incisional dehiscence is common after both LECR and VECA and is caused by:
- Inappropriate tissue handling or traumatic surgical technique
- Closure of the incision under tension
- Automutilation
- Infection

Complications in Small Animal Surgery, First Edition. Edited by Dominique Griffon and Annick Hamaide.
© 2016 John Wiley & Sons, Inc. Published 2016 by John Wiley & Sons, Inc.
Companion website: www.wiley.com/go/griffon/complications

Diagnosis

Incisional dehiscence is usually noticed within the first 7 days after surgery. Clinical signs of infection are usually present as well. The most common sites of dehiscence are the medial ear canal wall just above the horizontal canal for LECR and the horizontal aspect of the suture line when T-shaped closure was used for VECA or at the ventral aspect of the auricular suture line when a cosmetic closure technique has been used (see cosmetic complications of total ear canal resection with lateral bulla osteotomy [TECALBO]).

Treatment

Small areas of dehiscence and localized infection usually resolve with appropriate systemic antibiotic therapy and second-intention healing. Larger areas should be debrided and resutured or secondary fibrous contracture and stenosis of the horizontal ear canal are likely.

Prevention

- Atraumatic surgical technique with the use of Adson-Brown or Debakey forceps is advised for tissue handling. Swaged reverse-cutting or tapered cutting needles facilitate atraumatic needle passage through both the aural epithelium and skin. Absorbable monofilament suture material of an appropriate size should be used for the subcutaneous tissues, and nonabsorbable monofilament material should be used for apposition of the skin. Full-thickness sutures should be placed through both cartilage and aural epithelium if the epithelium is too weak or damaged to hold sutures alone.
- Decrease tension on the suture lines by placing sutures in the subcutaneous tissues and perichondrium before apposing the skin to the aural epithelium. In addition, take larger than normal tissue bites on the skin side of the closure to spread any tension over a larger area.
- Attention to postoperative care is important; trauma to the surgical site caused by self-mutilation can be prevented by bandaging the ear over the head or by application of an Elizabethan collar. Judicious use of the combination of nonsteroidal and opioid analgesics should be part of postoperative care in all animals.
- Bacterial contamination of the surgical field is inevitable from the infected external ear canal, so prophylactic antibiotics are indicated to help prevent infection. Cefazolin or amoxicillin with clavulanic acid is effective against the most commonly encountered bacterial species in the ear canal (staphylococcal species, anaerobes, and gram-negative bacteria). In addition, copious lavage of the surgical site and elimination of dead space further help to reduce the risk of infection.
- Postoperative inflammation of aural tissues can be prevented by elimination of technical errors and appropriate selection of patients. Adequate ventral drain board reflection in LECR needs to be assured by continuing the cuts deep enough into the proximal aspect of the horizontal ear canal. If otitis media is present and left untreated, failure is inevitable after either of these procedures. Persistent inflammation of the skin lining the horizontal ear canal is likely after either LECR or VECA when performed for management of otitis externa, and continued medical management is required.

Stenosis of the horizontal ear canal

Etiopathogenesis

Stenosis of the horizontal ear canal is reported more frequently after LECR than VECA. Complete obstruction will lead to para-aural abscessation and fistulation (see TECA). Stenosis is caused by:

- Incisional dehiscence; healing of the wound by second intention healing may lead to fibrous contracture and stenosis of the horizontal ear canal.
- Persistent ear canal inflammation and ulceration may cause granulation tissue and scar tissue formation.

Diagnosis

- Stenosis of the horizontal ear canal is usually clinically noticeable within the first several months after surgery when the newly created stoma progressively retracts and narrows or after incisional dehiscence and second intention healing.
- Failure to address and control inflammation of the remaining parts of the ear canal is usually evident in the immediate postoperative period. Concurrent otitis media may explain treatment failure and is reportedly the most common cause of persistent inflammation of the ear canal. The diagnosis of otitis media is based on a thorough history and physical, neurologic, otoscopic examinations and diagnostic imaging of the middle ear cavities.

Treatment

- Revision of the original surgery if inadequate ventral drain board reflection after LECR is inhibiting drainage from the horizontal canal
- Animals with persistent ear canal inflammation after either LECR or VECA are treated according to the cause of surgical failure. Otitis media can initially be treated by myringotomy, middle ear lavage, and systemic antibiotics, but ventral bulla osteotomy (VBO) or LBO is usually required to completely eliminate middle ear disease. Persistent inflammation in the residual medial wall of the vertical ear canal after LECR is alleviated by conversion of the LECR into a VECA.
- If severe disease is present in the horizontal canal after either LECR or VECA, TECALBO is indicated.

Prevention

- Atraumatic surgical technique
- Attention to postoperative care (see prevention of incisional dehiscence)
- Persistent ear canal inflammation should be addressed appropriately.

Facial nerve palsy

Facial nerve palsy is rare after VECA and has not been reported after LECR. It occurs only when dissections are continued deep along the horizontal canal (see discussion of TECALBO).

Cosmetic complications

Erect ears may fail to stand after VECA because of loss of support to the base of the pinna when currently described surgical techniques are used. A technique to prevent this cosmetic complication is described in the discussion of TECALBO.

Relevant literature

The purpose of LECR is to provide an alteration in the ear canal microenvironment by increasing ventilation so moisture, humidity, and temperature are decreased. LECR also provides drainage for exudates and moisture in the ear canal (Coffey 1975; Getty 1979; Harvey 1980; Gregory and Vasseur 1983; Bradley 1988; Hobson 1988; Elkins 1991; McCarthy and Caywood 1992; Layton 1993; McCarthy and McCarthy 1994; McCarthy 1996; Bojrab and Constantinescu 1998; White 1998; Lanz and Wood 2004).

LECR has primarily been used to aid management of chronic otitis externa. It is reportedly contraindicated if there is stenosis or obstruction of the horizontal ear canal; concurrent otitis media; or severe, proliferative epithelial ear canal disease with calcification of the auricular cartilage (Layton 1993). However, previous studies have indicated that the failure rate of this procedure is high (between 35% and 62%) despite what seemed to be an appropriate selection of cases (Tufvesson 1955; Gregory and Vasseur 1983; Lane and Little 1986; Sylvestre 1998; Doyle *et al.* 2004). Most animals do not show an improvement of clinical signs after surgery and still need topical medication. Breed has been correlated with the outcome though. The procedure failed in 86.5% of the cocker spaniels, but Sharpeis had a tendency to have better outcomes, even though they were found to have an ear canal of small diameter compared with that of other breeds (Sylvestre 1998). The procedure is seldom necessary and in the author's opinion is best reserved for oncologic surgery. VECA can be used for more severe cases of otitis externa, including cases with irreversible disease of the medial wall of the vertical ear canal. However, a patent healthy horizontal ear canal and absence of otitis media are required. If hearing has already been significantly affected before surgery, TECA is preferred over VECA. Results after VECA are reported to be excellent in 72%, improved in 24%, and poor in 4% of animals, and complications of the procedure are fewer than those reported for LECR (Siemering 1980; Tirgari and Pinniger 1986; Tirgari 1988; McCarthy and Caywood 1992; McCarthy 1996). Dehiscence and stenosis may be less likely after VECA when the "pull-through" modification is used because the vertical aspect of the incision is eliminated (Tirgari and Pinniger 1986; Tirgari 1988). This technique does not appear to offer major advantages over the traditional technique and has not gained popularity.

Total ear canal resection with lateral bulla osteotomy

Total ear canal ablation is indicated for management of end-stage otitis externa, ear canal neoplasia, and aural cholesteatoma. The procedure must be combined with bulla osteotomy when concurrent otitis media is present. The combination of TECA with LBO is most commonly performed and is associated with complications in about 50% of dogs. Complications can be divided into intraoperative bleeding as a result of damage to vascular structures, peripheral nerve and inner ear injury, cosmetic alterations, infection and recurrence of aural inflammation manifested as para-aural cellulitis, abscessation, and fistulation. Cholesterol granulomas and cholesteatomas have recently been reported as late sequelae to this procedure as well.

Hemorrhage
Also see Chapter 12.

Etiopathogenesis
Severe hemorrhage during surgery is rare but may be caused by:
- Damage to the retroarticular vein; the retroarticular vein exits the retroarticular foramen just caudodorsal to the retroarticular process and rostral to the external auditory meatus (Figure 22.2).

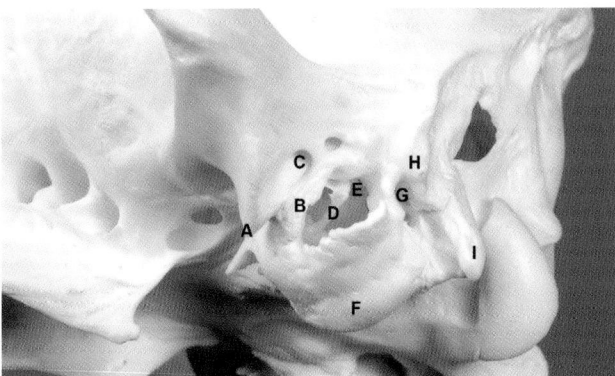

Figure 22.2 Left lateral view of the canine skull. **A**, Retroarticular process. **B**, External bony acoustic meatus. **C**, Retroarticular foramen. **D**, Handle of the malleus. **E**, Round window. **F**, Tympanic bulla. **G**, Stylomastoid foramen. **H**, Mastoid process. **I**, Jugular process.

It is most often damaged during detachment of the horizontal ear canal epithelium from the bone, excessive curettage in this area, or when removing bone with rongeurs for bulla osteotomy.
- Damage to the external carotid artery and maxillary vein that lie immediately ventral to the tympanic bulla. Damage occurs only when dissections are continued deep along the ventral aspect of the tympanic bulla when performing a wide LBO.
- Damage to the internal carotid artery. The carotid canal that houses the internal carotid artery runs longitudinally through the medial wall of the osseous bulla. The internal carotid can be damaged if the thin bone between the carotid canal and tympanic cavity is disrupted by curettage in a medial direction or when the medial wall of the bulla has been eroded by the disease process and is damaged during epithelial stripping.

Treatment
- Hemorrhage from the retroarticular vein can usually be controlled with digital pressure for several minutes or placement of bone wax into the retroarticular foramen.
- Damage to the external carotid artery or maxillary vein is difficult to control because of low visibility and poor accessibility of the area. Digital pressure and temporary tight placement of gauzes while stopping further dissection usually controls the bleeding. Sometimes vascular clips can be applied when the vessel can be visualized.
- Hemorrhage from the internal carotid artery was treated successfully by ligation of the left common carotid artery with blood transfusion in one report. However, tight placement of absorbable gelatin sponges into the tympanic bulla followed by digital pressure for several minutes usually controls the bleeding.

Prevention
- Damage to the retroarticular vein can be prevented by keeping deep dissections as close as possible to the perichondrium of the horizontal canal and periosteum of the tympanic bulla and by using delicate curved Kelly or Toennis-Adson dissecting scissors (Figure 22.3). In addition, the rostroventral area of the bony meatus should be spared when performing LBO.
- Damage to the external carotid artery and maxillary vein is best avoided by careful elevation of the periosteum from the lateroventral bulla before LBO and ensuring that only bone is included within the jaws of rongeurs during osteotomy.

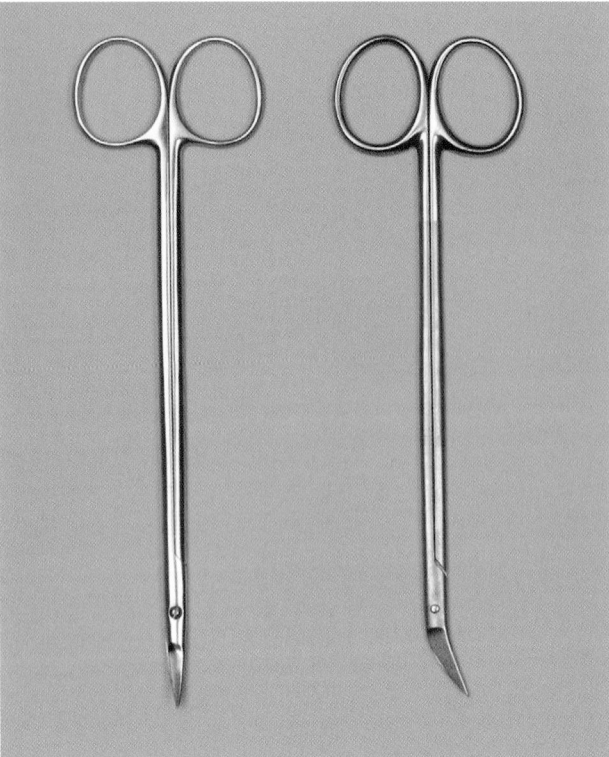

Figure 22.3 Two types of Toennis-Adson dissecting scissors.

- Damage to the internal carotid artery can be avoided by careful curettage of the medial part of the bulla guided by preoperative computed tomography (CT) information on the petrosal bone involvement.

Facial nerve palsy

Etiopathogenesis
Facial nerve palsy is the most common neurologic complication after TECALBO in dogs and occurs in 13% to 36% of the procedures (Figure 22.4). It is usually temporary with full resolution of clinical signs within several weeks; fewer than half are permanent in dogs. In cats, the frequency of facial nerve palsy can be as high as 74% after TECALBO with a reported 20% to 47% being permanent. Temporary deficits are probably the result of excessive facial nerve retraction to expose the bulla during deep dissection or dissecting to close to the stylomastoid foramen where the nerve exits (see Figure 22.2).

Diagnosis
Facial nerve palsy is usually evident directly upon full recovery of the patient after surgery and is manifested by absence of a blink reflex and a pendulous lower lip on the ipsilateral side.

Treatment
All patients with facial nerve deficits should be treated with corneal protectants for at least the first 3 days after surgery and thereafter if tear production is decreased until full recovery of the facial nerve function.

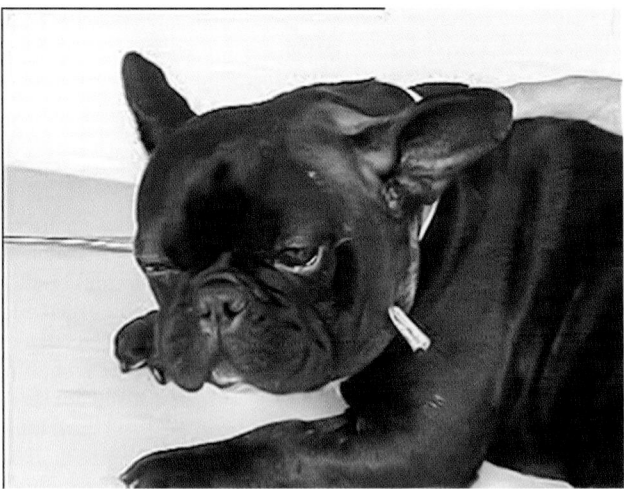

Figure 22.4 French bulldog showing left-sided facial nerve palsy after total ear canal resection with lateral bulla osteotomy.

Prevention
- Limiting wound retractor placement directly around the facial nerve and avoiding excessive traction on tissues lateral or more superficial to the course of the nerve
- Early isolation and protection of the facial nerve during deep dissection and removal of the horizontal ear canal
- Keeping deep dissections near the caudoventral bony acoustic meatus and bulla as close as possible to the perichondrium and periosteum by using delicate curved Kelly or Toennis-Adson dissecting scissors (see Figure 22.3)

Horner's syndrome

Etiopathogenesis
Horner's syndrome is rarely, if ever, encountered in dogs after TECALBO. In cats, it may appear in up to 53% of patients, possibly because of the greater fragility of the feline tympanic plexus compared with dogs. Although many affected cats have temporary nerve damage, 7% to 27% develop permanent Horner's syndrome.

Diagnosis
Horner's syndrome can be present upon recovery after anaesthesia or develop within the first 6 to 12 hours after surgery. Ptosis, miosis, enophthalmus, and protrusion of the third eyelid can be seen on the ipsilateral eye (Figure 22.5).

Treatment
This complication is usually short lived (3–21 days) and reversible. Treatment is not required.

Prevention
Excessive curettage of the promontory should be avoided. However, it is more important to remove all abnormal middle ear mucosa than to try to attempt avoiding damage to the sympathetic nerves.

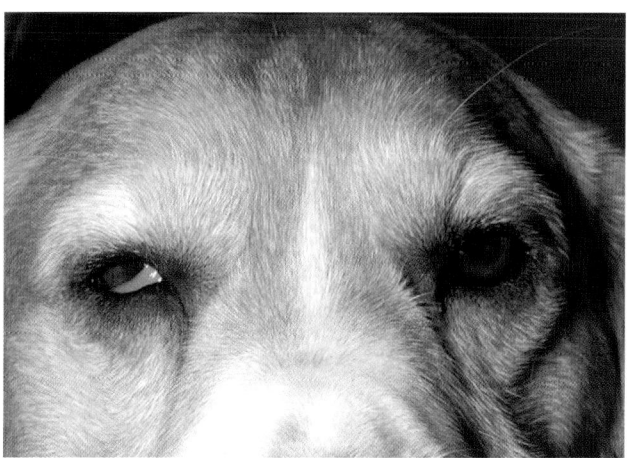

Figure 22.5 Beagle showing right-sided Horner's syndrome as a result of chronic otitis media.

Other neurologic complications

Etiopathogenesis
- Hypoglossal nerve dysfunction occurs rarely in the early postoperative period and has only been documented in dogs. The hypoglossal nerve lies superficial to the hypopharyngeal muscle, which overlies the ventral and lateral aspects of the bulla. Overzealous ventral retraction and inappropriate sharp dissection may damage it.
- Inner ear damage (peripheral vestibular ataxia and hearing loss) occurs after TECALBO surgery in 3% to 8% of dogs but has not been documented in cats. It is thought to be the result of damage to the round or oval window during removal of tissue or debris from the epitympanic recess and promontory areas.

Diagnosis
- Damage to the hypoglossal nerve can be clinically diagnosed when tongue paralysis, excessive drooling, and dysphagia are seen after surgery. When the tongue is protruded, it deviates toward the side of the injury because of the normally functioning genioglossus muscle and intrinsic muscles of the tongue.
- Whereas nystagmus, ataxia, circling, and head tilt suggest trauma to the vestibulum, hearing loss indicates trauma to the cochlea. Definitive diagnosis of hearing impairment caused by TECALBO requires hearing assessment using brainstem evoked response audiometry (bone conduction).

Treatment
- Damage to the hypoglossal nerve usually does not require treatment, although dietary alterations may improve prehension and swallowing function.
- Initial treatment of vestibular injury should include antiinflammatory doses of corticosteroids and antibiotics based on the results of culture and sensitivity testing from the middle ear. Occasionally, vomiting is severe, and H1 histaminergic receptor antagonists, M1 cholinergic receptor antagonists, or vestibulosedative drugs can be administered for 2 to 3 days to alleviate the emesis associated with motion sickness.

- Hearing impairment after TECA-LBO usually does not require treatment because dogs have adjusted to the deficits before surgery. Sensorineural hearing loss as a result of cochlear damage cannot be treated. Middle ear implants could potentially restore auditory function after TECALBO if sensory transduction of the cochlea is not impaired.

Prevention
- Meticulous dissection and avoidance of aggressive retraction in tissues deep to the tympanic bulla should help avoid glossopharyngeal nerve dysfunction.
- Adequate exposure and avoidance of curettage in the dorsal aspect of the tympanic cavity (epitympanic recess) are important technical steps to avoid inner ear damage during TECALBO.

Cosmetic complications

Etiopathogenesis
Cosmetic alterations after TECALBO are minimal in floppy-eared dogs, such as cocker spaniels, but erect ears may fail to stand because of loss of support to the base of the pinna, especially if ear canal excision is extended well up into the base of the pinna, including the anthelix.

Prevention
Loss of support to the base of the pinna can be prevented by:
- Using a subtotal ear canal ablation that preserves part of the dorsal vertical ear canal when the disease process is limited to the horizontal ear canal
- Using a ventrally based advancement skin flap as has been proposed to maintain ear carriage after TECA in cats.

However, because removal of all diseased tissue and control or elimination of signs of ear disease are the goals of surgery, preserving ear carriage is best achieved by using a technique originally described by Venker-van Haagen (1983).
- TECA is started with a V-shaped incision in the skin from the intertragic incisure to the palpable ventral limit of the vertical ear canal and from the tragohelicine incisure to the same ventral point. The triangular skin flap is lifted at this point with Adson forceps and is dissected free toward the tragus at the level of the dermis and retracted dorsally with Allis forceps. The cranial, lateral, and caudal aspects of the distal vertical ear canal are exposed by blunt and sharp dissection of the subcutaneous tissue and muscles with scissors. This dissection is continued until strong Mayo-Noble dissecting scissors can be advanced from the cranial and caudal side of the vertical ear canal under the cartilage of the auricle on the medial side. The cartilage and the skin of the medial wall of the ear canal are then freed from the remaining auricular cartilage in an inverted U-V shape (Figure 22.6). Dissection of the ear canal is continued in a routine fashion, and LBO is performed when indicated. Closure after TECA starts with remodelling of the auricle. The caudal part of the pinna is folded forward toward the cranial part using the most natural folding point at the base of the pinna as the point of rotation. These parts are then sutured together, starting at this folding point with monofilament absorbable suture material (2-0), leaving the ends of the sutures long to facilitate removal later on (Figures 22.7 and 22.8). The remainder of the wound is closed routinely.

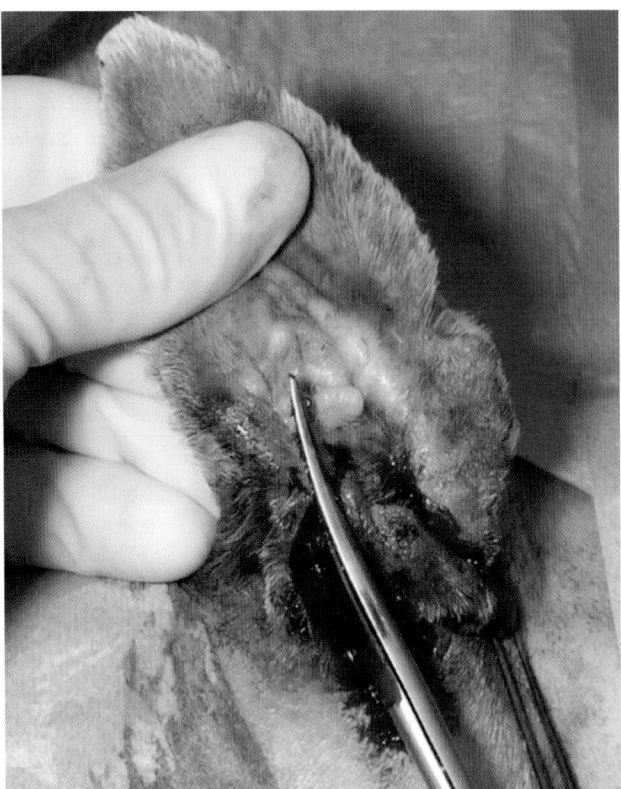

Figure 22.6 Cosmetic remodeling of the auricle for total ear canal ablation. The cartilage and the skin of the medial wall of the ear canal are freed from the remaining auricular cartilage in an inverted U-V shape.

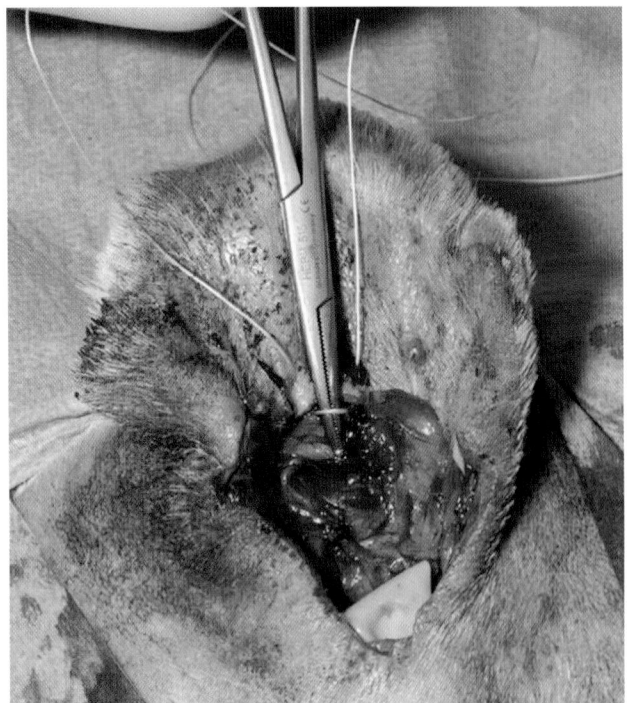

Figure 22.7 Cosmetic remodeling of the auricle for total ear canal ablation. The caudal part of the pinna is folded forward toward the cranial part using the most natural folding point at the base of the pinna as the point of rotation. These parts are then sutured together, starting at this folding point.

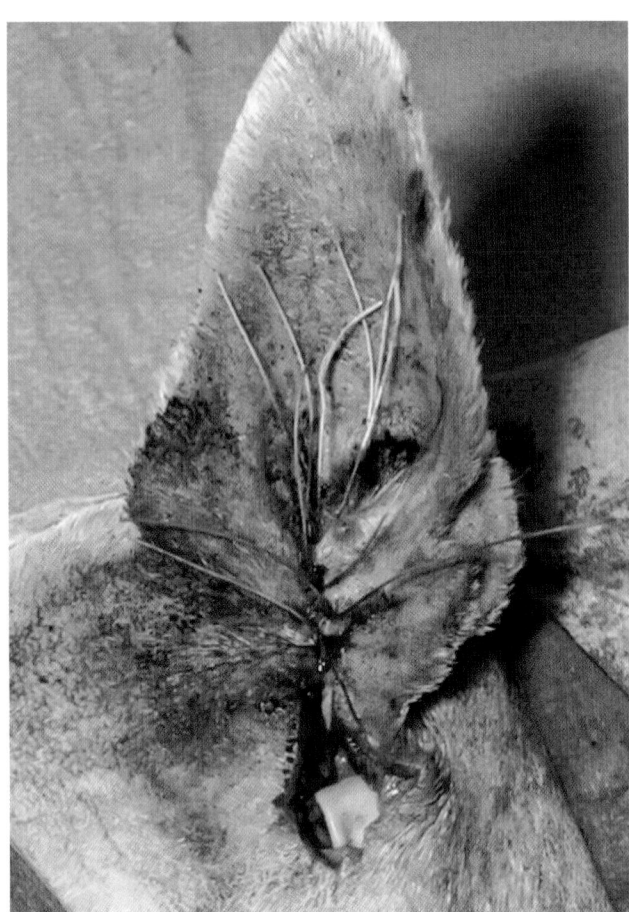

Figure 22.8 Cosmetic remodeling of the auricle for total ear canal ablation. Suturing of the auricle is completed, the ends of the sutures are left long to facilitate removal later on.

Infection, cellulitis, abscessation, and fistulation

Etiopathogenesis

Extensive contamination by spillage of debris and exudate during horizontal ear canal removal is inevitable despite proper wound preparation. Acute wound complications are therefore common (8%–31%) and include acute cellulitis, incisional dehiscence, extended wound drainage, abscessation, and fistulation. Abscessation and fistulation can occur weeks, months, and even years after surgery and are caused by incomplete removal of all infected tissue (epithelial lining of the horizontal ear canal or middle ear mucosa).

Diagnosis

Wound infection after surgery usually is clinically evident 3 to 5 days after surgery and is diagnosed on the classical signs of infection, including pain, redness, swelling, purulent discharge, fever, and wound dehiscence. Culture with susceptibility testing will reveal the microorganisms involved in the infection. *Staphylococcus aureus*, *Streptococcus* spp., *Escherichia coli*, *Proteus* spp., and *Pseudomonas* spp. are the organisms most likely to be isolated.

Treatment

- Most wound complications are treated successfully with appropriate antibiotic therapy and local wound care until second intention healing occurs.
- When drainage and signs of infection persist beyond several weeks, deeper sources of infection, such as otitis media or retained secretory epithelium, should be investigated.
- Delayed abscess and fistula formation occasionally responds to simple antibiotic therapy. Most animals, however, require reoperation to identify and remove retained secretory epithelium and infected foci. Either a ventral approach or a repeated lateral approach can be performed. VBO is performed in healthy tissue but removal of secretory epithelium (usually from a retained portion of the horizontal canal) is difficult. This is easier from the original lateral approach, but scar tissue resulting from the previous surgery and subsequent cellulitis or abscessation make dissection difficult, and facial nerve damage is likely. About 85% of animals that undergo reoperation for persistent infection are cured.

Prevention

- Appropriate perioperative antibiotic administration
- Meticulous wound dissection to avoid tissue devitalization
- Copious lavage during surgery to help remove contamination and debris from the wound
- Complete removal of the lateral and ventral walls of the tympanic bulla is required to provide good ventral drainage, but more important, to aid in removing all infected tissue remnants that are otherwise potentially missed at the entrance to the bony horizontal ear canal and within the bony canal itself. In some animals with long-standing chronic otitis externa, a greenish-brown soft tissue extrusion can be seen ventral to the bony meatus as a result of widening of the ear canal and stretching of the ligament anchoring the horizontal ear canal to the external acoustic bony meatus. This extrusion must be gently dissected free or delayed abscess and fistula formation are inevitable.
- Careful apposition of the wound edges
- No difference was found in wound complication rates when TECALBO procedures were closed primarily with or without drainage in a large retrospective study. Whether or not to use drains (active or passive) therefore depends on the surgeon's preference.

Relevant literature

The management of complications of TECALBO starts preoperatively with choosing the proper diagnostic work-up and selecting the appropriate treatment for the patient. Advanced imaging with CT or magnetic resonance imaging is necessary for evaluation of the middle ear (and inner ear to some extent) and is advised for all patients needing ear canal surgery (Ter Haar 2006). TECA must be reserved for cases in which proper medical treatment has failed (usually end-stage proliferative otitis externa or chronic ulcerative otitis externa with a *Pseudomonas* spp. superinfection) and ear canal neoplasia (Ter Haar 2006). Otitis externa is a multifactorial, often systemic disease of dogs and cats, and surgery should be considered to be only a part of the overall treatment plan. Careful consideration should be given to the presence of generalized skin disorders, endocrine dysfunction, allergic diseases, and concurrent otitis media. Appropriate treatment of underlying disorders increases the success rate of the surgical procedure. **Persistent dermatitis of the**

auricle is seen in up to 21% of dogs after TECA but has not been documented in cats (Smeak and Kerpsack 1993; Matousek 2004; Saridomichelakis *et al.* 2007). This complication results from progression of an underlying dermatologic problem or incomplete removal of affected skin at the base of the pinna. Ceruminal glands can be found in the skin of the cavum conchae up to the level of the anthelix, which should be included in the resection.

Overall complication rates of TECA ran as high as 82% with chronic deep wound infection, abscessation, and debilitating fistula formation developing in 10% of the cases in early studies (Smeak and Dehoff 1986; Mason *et al.* 1988; Matthieson and Scavelli 1990; Sharp 1990). Since then, it has been shown that retained epithelium within the bony ear canal or tympanic bulla was the underlying cause for most persistent infections (Smeak and Dehoff 1986; Smeak and Kerpsack 1993; McAnulty *et al.* 1995; Smeak *et al.* 1996; Smeak and Inpanbutr 2005; Doust *et al.* 2007; Hardie *et al.* 2008). Therefore, TECA with adequate tympanic cavity exposure is currently considered the gold standard treatment for end-stage ear canal disease (McAnulty *et al.* 1995; Smeak and Inpanbutr 2005). The procedure is considered to be very **painful**; hence, pre-, intra-, and post-operative administration of analgesic agents (opioids, nonsteroidal antiinflammatory drugs, local blocks) is necessary to assure postoperative patient comfort and assist an uneventful recovery (Buback *et al.* 1996; Wolfe *et al.* 2006). Recent studies on the complications after TECALBO show an overall trend toward a decrease in the rate of most complications over time, particularly in early wound related problems (Beckman *et al.* 1990; White and Pomeroy 1990; Williams and White 1992; Marino *et al.* 1994; Devitt *et al.* 1997; Doyle *et al.* 2004; Mathews *et al.* 2006).

Severe **hemorrhage** during surgery is rare but has been reported and may result in death of the patient (Smeak 2011). In most cases, bleeding can be prevented by using a meticulous surgical technique and controlled with judicious use of electrocautery, ligation, bone wax, or digital pressure (White and Pomeroy 1990; Smeak and Inpanbutr 2005). Rarely is ligation of the carotid artery or blood transfusion necessary (Matthieson and Scavelli 1990). Partial necrosis of the auricle from damage to the vasculature during medial dissection of the vertical ear canal is rare and is most often found along the caudal pinna margin (Smeak and Dehoff 1986). Complete necrosis of the auricle has been reported in one dog (Matthieson and Scavelli 1990). Therapy for partial or complete necrosis of the auricle consists of (partial) pinnal amputation.

The incidence of **facial nerve palsy** after TECALBO has decreased over time with fewer than 4% to 6% of the procedures resulting in accidental transection of the nerve and permanent facial nerve paralysis in dogs (Beckman *et al.* 1990; Devitt *et al.* 1997; Doyle *et al.* 2004). This is possibly the result of increased experience with the technique and improved tissue and instrument handling or might reflect a patient selection bias toward performing surgery earlier in the disease process before severe proliferative calcifying otitis externa has developed. Cats with ear canal neoplasia are twice as likely to have facial nerve paralysis postoperatively compared with cats with other aural diseases (Marino *et al.* 1994; Bacon *et al.* 2003).

Acute cellulitis or abscessation, wound dehiscence, infection, and extended wound drainage are wound complications associated with TECALBO still reported commonly in the literature, ranging from 8% to 31% (Smeak and Dehoff 1986; Matthieson and Scavelli 1990; Devitt *et al.* 1997; Doyle *et al.* 2004). Although wound drainage after TECALBO with active or passive drains has always been recommended to combat incisional complications in early reports, no difference in wound complication rates was seen when TECALBO procedures were closed primarily with or without drainage (Devitt *et al.* 1997). Appropriate perioperative antibiotic administration, aseptical surgical technique, atraumatic tissue handling to avoid tissue devitalization, and copious lavage during surgery remain the advocated methods to help prevent serious early wound-related complications (Smeak and Kerpsack 1993; Devitt *et al.* 1997).

The most serious long-term complication encountered after TECALBO in dogs involves **para-aural infection** (otitis media), **abscessation,** and **fistula** formation (Smeak and Kerpsack 1993; Smeak 2011). Even with wide LBO, recurrent deep infection rates are still as high as 2% to 10% (Smeak and Dehoff 1986; Beckman *et al.* 1990; Matthieson and Scavelli 1990). When performed for aural cholesteatoma, recurrent deep infection rate approaches 50% (Hardie *et al.* 2008). Deep wound infections are less common in cats (Williams and White 1992; Marino *et al.* 1994). Clinical signs of pain upon opening the mouth, para-aural swelling, and the development of draining tracts can appear from 1 month to years after TECALBO (Holt *et al.* 1996; Smeak *et al.* 1996; Hardie *et al.* 2008; Smeak 2011). Incomplete removal of secretory epithelium lining the tympanic bulla or osseous canal, retained infected ear canal cartilage, osteomyelitis of the ossicles, inadequate drainage of the middle ear through the Eustachian tube, and parotid salivary gland damage are factors implicated in the etiopathogenesis (Holt *et al.* 1996; Smeak *et al.* 1996; Hardie *et al.* 2008; Smeak 2011). Performing TECA with VBO instead of LBO does not reduce the risk of deep infection (Sharp 1990). A surgical treatment is recommended for recurrent deep infection and can include a lateral approach to the middle ear and VBO (Holt *et al.* 1996; Smeak *et al.* 1996; Hardie *et al.* 2008). If diagnostic imaging demonstrates signs of remnant tissue of the horizontal ear canal or tissue suggestive of retained epithelium within the external bony meatus, a lateral approach is preferred. In all other cases, it depends on the surgeon's preference (Holt *et al.* 1996; Smeak 2011) .

A **cholesterol granuloma** was reported recently as a long-term complication of TECA 3 years after the original procedure, in a 13-year-old Cocker spaniel (Riedinger *et al.* 2011). The dog presented with signs of pain upon opening the mouth. MRI revealed a large mass arising from the tympanic bulla. Cytology of aspirates revealed a chronic suppurative inflammatory reaction and numerous cholesterol crystals. Intraoperative hemorrhage and surgical trauma in this case during the primary procedure were proposed to have been responsible for erythrocyte accumulation at the surgical site, subsequent cholesterol deposition, and a significant inflammatory reaction. **Cholesteatoma** formation after TECA has been reported recently in three dogs, including two brachycephalic dogs (Hardie *et al.* 2008; Schuenemann and Oechtering 2012). This epidermoid cyst containing keratotic material is surrounded by keratinizing squamous epithelium, which is continuously shedding keratin debris within the middle ear cavity, leading to expansion of the cyst and tympanic cavity with eventual destruction of the adjacent tissue by increasing pressure and osteoclastic bone resorption. Most cholesteatomas in dogs are thought to arise secondary to otitis media (Little *et al.* 1991), but a recent publication mentioned auditory tube dysfunction as a potential cause for otitis media with effusion, specifically in brachycephalic dogs (Hayes *et al.* 2010), which can lead to subsequent cholesteatoma formation. Cholesteatoma formation after TECA may occur because stratified squamous epithelium has not been completely removed during surgery (Hardie *et al.* 2008). Complete removal of epithelium can be especially challenging in brachycephalic animals, making them potentially more

prone to cholesteatoma development (Schuenemann and Oechtering 2012).

Most dogs with chronic external and middle ear infection have **diminished hearing ability** as a result of conduction problems (obstruction of the ear canal, fluid in middle ear cavity) or sensorineural loss (otitis interna, ototoxicity) before surgery (Smeak and Kerpsack 1993). After experimental TECALBO in normal dogs, all were found to be deaf as determined by air-conducted brainstem evoked response audiometry (McAnulty *et al.* 1995). If the tympanic membrane and ossicles are not removed during surgery, some air-conducted hearing remains (Payne *et al.* 1989; Krahwinkel *et al.* 1993). Bone-conducted hearing is not lost if the sensorineural pathways have not been damaged (McAnulty *et al.* 1995). Bone-conducted hearing is clinically not very relevant, though. To reduce the chance of late deep infection after TECA, removal of the tympanic membrane despite the risk of decreasing hearing ability is recommended (McAnulty *et al.* 1995; Smeak and Inpanbutr 2005). In the near future, middle ear implants could potentially restore conductive hearing loss in dogs after TECA (Ter Haar *et al.* 2010, 2011).

Some owners of erect-eared dogs complain about **poor ear carriage** after TECALBO. A subtotal ear canal ablation that preserves part of the dorsal vertical ear canal may be indicated when the disease process is limited to the horizontal ear canal and when any systemic skin disease is expected to be controlled (Mathews *et al.* 2006). A ventrally based advancement skin flap has been proposed to maintain ear carriage after TECA in cats (McNabb and Flanders 2004). The Venker-van Haagen technique described in this chapter for remodeling of the auricle yields excellent cosmetic results while not making concessions to the amount of tissue removed and is therefore the technique of choice for maintaining ear carriage (Venker-van Haagen 1983).

References

Bacon, N.J., Gilbert, R.L., Bostock, D.E., et al. (2003) Total ear canal ablation in the cat: indications, morbidity and long-term survival. *Journal of Small Animal Practice* 44 (10), 430-434.

Beckman, S.L., Henry, W.B. Jr., Cechner, P. (1990) Total ear canal ablation combining bulla osteotomy and curettage in dogs with chronic otitis externa and media. *Journal of the American Veterinary Medical Association* 196 (1), 84-90.

Bojrab, M.J., Constantinescu, G.M. (1998) Treatment of otitis externa. In Bojrab, M.J. (ed.) *Current Techniques in Small Animal Surgery*, 4th edn. Williams & Wilkins, Baltimore, pp. 98-101.

Bradley, R.L. (1988) Surgical management of otitis externa. *The Veterinary Clinics of North America. Small Animal Practice* 18 (4), 813-819.

Buback, J.L., Boothe, H.W., Carroll, G.L., et al. (1996) Comparison of three methods for relief of pain after ear canal ablation in dogs. *Veterinary Surgery* 25 (5), 380-385.

Coffey, D.J. (1975) Lateral Ear drainage for otitis externa. In Bojrab, M.J. (ed.) *Current Techniques in Small Animal Surgery*. Lea & Febiger, Philadelphia, pp. 64-67.

Devitt, C.M., Seim, H.B.,3rd, Willer, R., et al. (1997) Passive drainage versus primary closure after total ear canal ablation-lateral bulla osteotomy in dogs: 59 dogs (1985-1995). *Veterinary Surgery* 26 (3), 210-216.

Doust, R., King, A., Hammond, G., et al. (2007) Assessment of middle ear disease in the dog: a comparison of diagnostic imaging modalities. *Journal of Small Animal Practice* 48 (4), 188-192.

Doyle, R.S., Skelly, C., Bellenger, C.R. (2004) Surgical management of 43 cases of chronic otitis externa in the dog. *Irish Veterinary Journal* 57 (1), 22-30.

Elkins, A.D. (1991) Surgery of the external ear canal. *Problems in Veterinary Medicine* 3 (2), 239-253.

Getty, R. (1979) The ear. In Evans, H.E., Christensen, G.C. (eds.) *Miller's Anatomy of the Dog*, 2nd edn. W.B. Saunders, Philadelphia, pp. 1059-1072.

Gregory, C.R., Vasseur, P.B. (1983) Clinical results of lateral ear resection in dogs. *Journal of the American Veterinary Medical Association* 182 (10), 1087-1090.

Hardie, E.M., Linder, K.E., Pease, A.P. (2008) Aural cholesteatoma in twenty dogs. *Veterinary Surgery* 37 (8), 763-770.

Harvey, C.E. (1980) Ear canal disease in the dog: medical and surgical management. *Journal of the American Veterinary Medical Association* 177 (2), 136-139.

Hayes, G.M., Friend, E.J., Jeffery, N.D. (2010) Relationship between pharyngeal conformation and otitis media with effusion in Cavalier King Charles spaniels. *The Veterinary Record* 167 (2), 55-58.

Hobson, H.P. (1988) Surgical management of advanced ear disease. *The Veterinary Clinics of North America. Small Animal Practice,* 18 (4), 821-844.

Holt, D., Brockman, D.J., Sylvestre, A.M., et al. (1996) Lateral exploration of fistulas developing after total ear canal ablations: 10 cases (1989-1993). *Journal of the American Animal Hospital Association* 32 (6), 527-530.

Krahwinkel, D.J., Pardo, A.D., Sims, M.H., et al. (1993) Effect of total ablation of the external acoustic meatus and bulla osteotomy on auditory function in dogs. *Journal of the American Veterinary Medical Association* 202 (6), 949-952.

Lane, J.G., Little, C.J.L. (1986) Surgery of the canine external auditory meatus: a review of failures. *Journal of Small Animal Practice* 27, 247-254.

Lanz, O.I., Wood, B.C. (2004) Surgery of the ear and pinna. *The Veterinary Clinics of North America. Small Animal Practice* 34 (2), 567-599, viii.

Layton, C.E. (1993) The role of lateral ear resection in managing chronic otitis externa. *Seminars in Veterinary Medicine and Surgery (Small Animal)* 8 (1), 24-29.

Little, C.J., Lane, J.G., Gibbs, C., et al. (1991) Inflammatory middle ear disease of the dog: the clinical and pathological features of cholesteatoma, a complication of otitis media. *Veterinary Record* 128 (14), 319-322.

Marino, D.J., MacDonald, J.M., Matthieson, D.T., et al. (1994) Results of surgery in cats with ceruminous gland adenocarcinoma. *Journal of the American Animal Hospital Association* 30, 54-58.

Mason, L.K., Harvey, C.E., Orsher, R.J. (1988) Total ear canal ablation combined with lateral bulla osteotomy for end-stage otitis in dogs. Results in thirty dogs. *Veterinary Surgery* 17 (5), 263-268.

Mathews, K.G., Hardie, E.M., Murphy, K.M. (2006) Subtotal ear canal ablation in 18 dogs and one cat with minimal distal ear canal pathology. *Journal of the American Animal Hospital Association* 42 (5), 371-380.

Matousek, J.L. (2004) Diseases of the ear pinna. *The Veterinary clinics of North America. Small animal practice* 34 (2), 511-540.

Matthieson, D.T., Scavelli, T. (1990) Total ear canal ablation and lateral bulla osteotomy in 38 dogs. *Journal of the American Animal Hospital Association, J Am Anim Hosp Assoc* 26, 257-267.

McAnulty, J.F., Hattel, A., Harvey, C.E. (1995) Wound healing and brain stem auditory evoked potentials after experimental total ear canal ablation with lateral tympanic bulla osteotomy in dogs. *Veterinary Surgery* 24 (1), 1-8.

McCarthy, P.E., McCarthy, R.J. (1994) Surgery of the ear. *The Veterinary Clinics of North America. Small Animal Practice,* 24 (5), 953-969.

McCarthy, R.J., Caywood, D.D. (1992) Vertical ear canal resection for end-stage otitis externa in dogs. *Journal of the American Animal Hospital Association* 28, 545-549.

McCarthy, R.J. (1996) Surgery of the head & neck; lateral and vertical ear canal resection. In Lipowitz, A.J., Caywood, D.D., Cann, C.C., et al. (eds.) *Complications in Small Animals Surgery*. Lippincott, Williams & Wilkins, Philadelphia, pp. 114-118.

McNabb, A.H., Flanders, J.A. (2004) Cosmetic results of a ventrally based advancement flap for closure of total ear canal ablations in 6 cats: 2002-2003. *Veterinary Surgery* 33 (5), 435-439.

Payne, J.T., Shell, L.G., Flora, R.M., et al. (1989) Hearing loss in dogs subjected to total ear canal ablation. *Veterinary Surgery* 18, 60.

Riedinger, B., Albaric, O., Gauthier, O. (2011) Cholesterol granuloma as long-term complication of total ear canal ablation in a dog. *Journal of Small Animal Practice* 53, 188-191.

Saridomichelakis, M.N., Farmaki, R., Leontides, L.S., et al. (2007) Aetiology of canine otitis externa: a retrospective study of 100 cases. *Veterinary Dermatology* 18 (5), 341-347.

Schuenemann, R.M., Oechtering, G. (2012) Cholesteatoma after lateral bulla osteotomy in two brachycephalic dogs. *Journal of the American Animal Hospital Association* 48, 261-268.

Sharp, N.J. (1990) Chronic otitis externa and otitis media treated by total ear canal ablation and ventral bulla osteotomy in thirteen dogs. *Veterinary Surgery* 19 (2), 162-166.

Siemering, G.H. (1980) Resection of the vertical ear canal for treatment of chronic otitis externa. *Journal of the American Animal Hospital Association* 16, 753.

Smeak, D.D. (2011) Management of complications associated with total ear canal ablation and bulla osteotomy in dogs and cats. *Veterinary Clinics of North America Small Animal Practice* 41, 981-994.

Smeak, D.D., Dehoff, W.D. (1986) Total ear canal ablation: clinical results in the dog and cat. *Veterinary Surgery* 15, 161-170.

Smeak, D.D., Kerpsack, S.J. (1993) Total ear canal ablation and lateral bulla osteotomy for management of end-stage otitis *Seminars in Veterinary Medicine and Surgery (Small Animal)* 8 (1), 30-41.

Smeak, D.D., Inpanbutr, N. (2005) Lateral approach to subtotal bulla osteotomy in dogs. *Compendium on Continuing Education for the Practicing Veterinarian* 27, 377-384.

Smeak, D.D., Crocker, C.B., Birchard, S.J. (1996) Treatment of recurrent otitis media that developed after total ear canal ablation and lateral bulla osteotomy in dogs: nine cases (1986-1994). *Journal of the American Veterinary Medical Association* 209 (5), 937-942.

Sylvestre, A.M. (1998) Potential factors affecting the outcome of dogs with a resection of the lateral wall of the vertical ear canal. *The Canadian Vreterinary Journal* 39 (3), 157-160.

Ter Haar, G. (2006) Basic principles of surgery of the external ear (pinna and ear canal). In Kirpensteijn, J. Klein, W.R. (eds.) *The Cutting Edge: Basic Operating Skills for the Veterinary Surgeon*, 1st edn. Roman House Publishers, London, UK, pp. 272-283.

Ter Haar, G., Mulder, J.J., Venker-van Haagen, A.J., et al. (2010) Treatment of Age-related hearing loss in dogs with the vibrant soundbridge middle ear implant: short-term results in 3 dogs. *Journal of Veterinary Internal Medicine* 24 (3), 557-564.

Ter Haar, G., Mulder, J.J., Venker-van Haagen, A.J., et al. (2011) A surgical technique for implantation of the vibrant soundbridge middle ear implant in dogs. *Veterinary Surgery* 40 (3), 340-346.

Tirgari, M. (1988) Long-term evaluation of the pull-through technique for vertical canal ablation for the treatment of otitis externa in dogs and cats. *Journal of Small Animal Practice* 29, 165-175.

Tirgari, M., Pinniger, R.S. (1986) Pull-through technique for vertical canal ablation for the treatment of otitis externa in dogs and cats. *Journal of Small Animal Practice* 27 (3), 123-131.

Tufvesson, G. (1955) Operation for otitis externa in dogs according to Zepp's method; a statistical analysis of follow-up examinations and a study of possible age, breed, or sex disposition to the disease. *American Journal of Veterinary Research* 16, (61), 565-570.

Venker-van Haagen, A.J. (1983) *Managing Diseases of the Ear.* W.B. Saunders, Philadelphia, pp. 47-52.

White, R.A. (1998) The ear: surgery for chronic otitis. *Veterinary Quarterly* 20 (Suppl 1), S7-S9.

White, R.A.S., Pomeroy, C.J. (1990) Total ear canal ablation and lateral bulla osteotomy in the dog. *Journal of Small Animal Practice* 31, 547-553.

Williams, J.M., White, R.A.S. (1992) Total ear canal ablation combined with lateral bulla osteotomy in the cat. *Journal of Small Animal Practice* 33, 225-227.

Wolfe, T.M., Bateman, S.W., Cole, L.K., et al. (2006) Evaluation of a local anesthetic delivery system for the postoperative analgesic management of canine total ear canal ablation—a randomized, controlled, double-blinded study. *Veterinary Anaesthesia and Analgesia* 33 (5), 328-339.

23 Ventral Bulla Osteotomy

Cheryl Hedlund

Department of Veterinary Clinical Sciences, Iowa State University, Ames, IA, USA

Ventral bulla osteotomy (VBO) is most commonly indicated to remove tumors or polyps from the middle ear and to treat chronic or recurring otitis media refractory to other treatments (Box 23.1). It allows exploration of the bulla and provides a temporary path for continuous drainage from the bulla. VBO provides the best exposure of the tympanic cavity or bulla and allows better drainage than does lateral bulla osteotomy (LBO). Excellent long-term results are expected, but complications can occur.

Infection

Definition

A definitive diagnosis of infection is made when greater than 10^5 microorganisms are identified per gram of tissue collected from the middle ear. After VBO, infection may be manifested as incisional swelling, inflammation, drainage, abscessation, fistulous tracts, or vestibular signs (extension into the brain).

Risk factors

- Preoperative infection that is undiagnosed or ineffectively treated before surgery

Box 23.1 Potential indications for ventral bulla osteotomy

- Infection (bacterial, yeast, fungus)
  - Most common
  - Concurrent otitis externa
- Neoplasia
  - Primary uncommon
  - Most extend from external ear
  - Benign > malignant
    - Papillary adenoma
    - Fibroma
    - Squamous cell carcinoma (cats)
- Polyps
  - Cats primarily (Pratschke 2003)
    - Ascending infection
    - Congenital
- Cholesteatomas (epidermal cysts)
- Otoliths (mineral opacities, concretions) (Ziemer et al. 2003)
- Trauma
- Foreign bodies
- Congenital palatine defects (Gregory 2000)

- Selection of antimicrobials based on external ear cultures and susceptibility results rather than those obtained from the middle ear
- Microorganisms that are resistant to administered or available antimicrobials
- Inadequate closure of dead space
- Inadequate irrigation or drainage

Diagnosis

Heat, pain, and **swelling** at the surgical site may indicate infection. **Reluctance to or pain on opening the mouth** and draining tracts are other clinical signs of infection. An **acute worsening of signs of middle or inner ear disease** may indicate abscess formation within the bulla or extension into the brain (Sturges *et al.* 2006).

Skull radiographs and **cross-sectional imaging** are helpful in identifying otitis media. The most valuable radiographic view of the bulla is the frontal open-mouth (rostrocaudal open-mouth) view (Figure 23.1). Abnormal findings with otitis media include opacification of the air-filled bulla and thickening and sclerosis of the bulla walls. Lysis or periosteal reaction of the bulla and petrous temporal bone suggests a neoplastic process. Nearly 25% to 33% of animals with middle ear disease will have normal-appearing bulla on radiographs (Remedios *et al.* 1991; Love *et al.* 1994). Cross-sectional imaging is preferred because of the lack of superimposition and increased sensitivity in detecting abnormalities. Animals with otitis media have thickening and irregularity of the bulla walls; they may also have lysis, luminal soft tissue and signs of otitis externa. Contrast computed tomography (CT) shows increased uptake in regions of infections (abscesses, fistulous tracts). CT is most beneficial for delineating destructive lesions of bone; however, abnormal changes in extracranial soft tissues, meninges, and brain parenchyma may exist on normal CT images. Therefore, if it is suspected that otitis media or interna has extended into the brainstem, magnetic resonance imaging (MRI) will yield a more accurate assessment (Sturges *et al.* 2006). After intravascular contrast is given, MRI is superior for visualizing changes in extracranial and intracranial soft tissue structures (Sturges *et al.* 2006).

Specimen collection and identification of microorganisms at greater than 10^5/g tissue provides a definitive diagnosis of ear infection. Organisms isolated from the external ear canal may be different than the organisms present in the bulla (Cole *et al.* 1998; Hettlich *et al.* 2005). Analysis of a cerebrospinal fluid specimen with culturing (aerobic, anaerobic, fungal) is recommended when extension of infection into the brain is suspected (Sturges *et al.* 2006).

Complications in Small Animal Surgery, First Edition. Edited by Dominique Griffon and Annick Hamaide.
© 2016 John Wiley & Sons, Inc. Published 2016 by John Wiley & Sons, Inc.
Companion website: www.wiley.com/go/griffon/complications

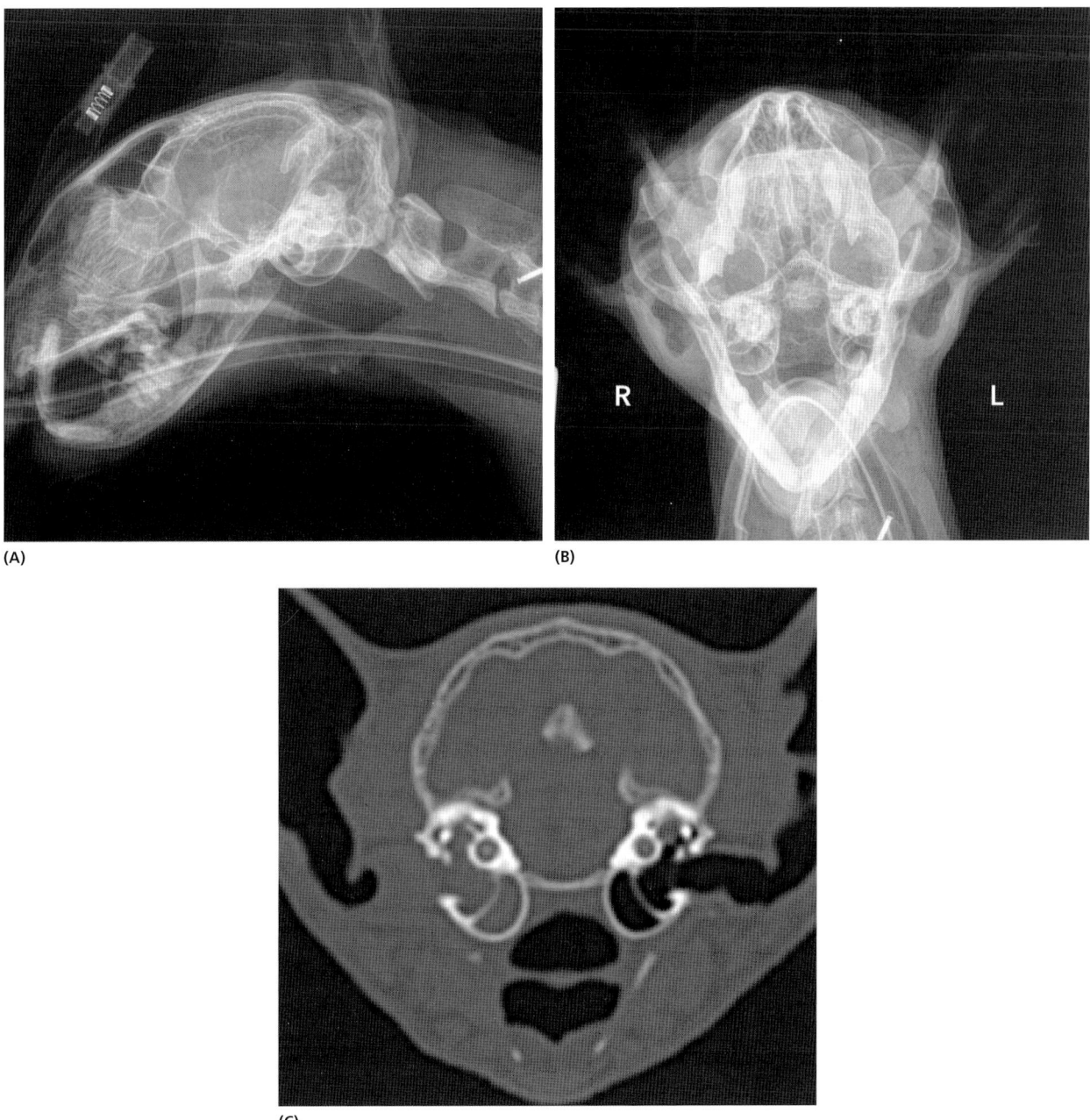

(A)

(B)

(C)

Figure 23.1 Lateral (**A**) and frontal open-mouth (**B**) views of a cat skull compared with a computed tomography scan (**C**) showing a soft tissue opacity in the right bulla.

Treatment

- Administer antimicrobials based on bacterial susceptibility and continue for a minimum of 4 weeks when the disease is confined to the ear and for a minimum of 3 to 4 months when infection extends into the brain.
- Allow incisions that have dehisced to heal by second intention.
- Lance abscesses, allowing them to drain.
- Reexpose the bulla and curette the remaining epithelium when abscesses recur or chronic fistulas develop.

Outcome

Ventral bulla osteotomy is effective in resolving infections of the middle ear if epithelium and debris are completely removed.

Infections resolve with drainage and prolonged administration of effective antibiotics.

Prevention

- Completely remove the epithelial lining and debris from the bulla. When VBO is performed for recurrent infection after a total ear canal ablation with lateral bulla osteotomy (TECALBO), remnants of epithelium are commonly found just dorsal to and inside the osseous portion of the external ear canal or just caudal to the external acoustic meatus within the tympanic cavity (Smeak *et al.* 1996) (Figure 23.2).
- Irrigate the bulla and surgical site profusely before closure (300–500 mL of sterile saline).

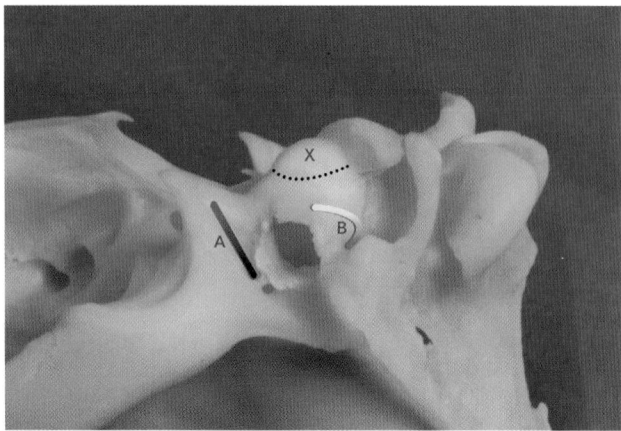

Figure 23.2 The skull is positioned in dorsal recumbency to illustrate the anatomic structures surrounding the tympanic bulla. The external acoustic meatus is shaded. B identifies the facial nerve caudal to the bulla, A identifies the retroarticular vein rostral to the external acoustic meatus, x approximates the site for entrance into the bulla, and the dashed line suggests the lateral extent of ventral bulla osteotomy.

- Administer antimicrobials effective against the organisms cultured from the bulla taken during surgery. Systemic antibiotics are indicated because highly vascular mucous membrane lining the cavity of an inflamed middle ear promotes diffusion of drugs from the blood into the bulla.
- Place a closed-suction drain in the bulla after osteotomy to evacuate blood and fluid accumulation (Figure 23.3).
- In cats, open, curette, and evacuate both the large ventromedial compartment and the smaller dorsolateral (craniolateral) compartment of the bulla (Figures 23.4 and 23.5)

Hemorrhage

Definition
Hemorrhage related to VBO can be defined as the escape of blood from vascular structures surrounding the bulla or external ear canal.

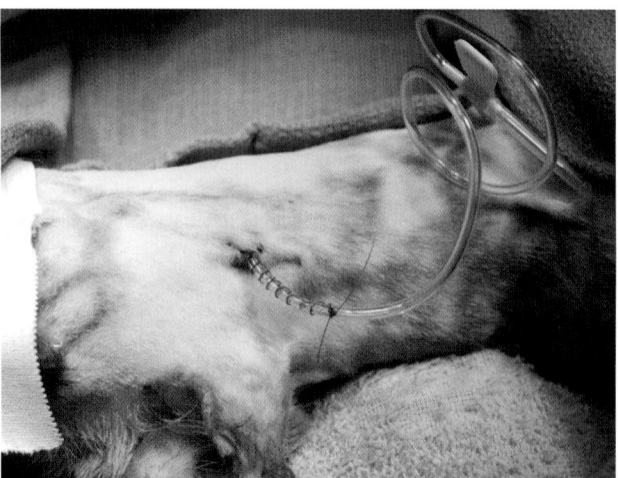

Figure 23.3 A modified butterfly catheter is placed into the tympanic bulla after ventral bulla osteotomy and secured with a figure-trap suture. The needle will be inserted into an evacuated tube to provide closed suction drainage.

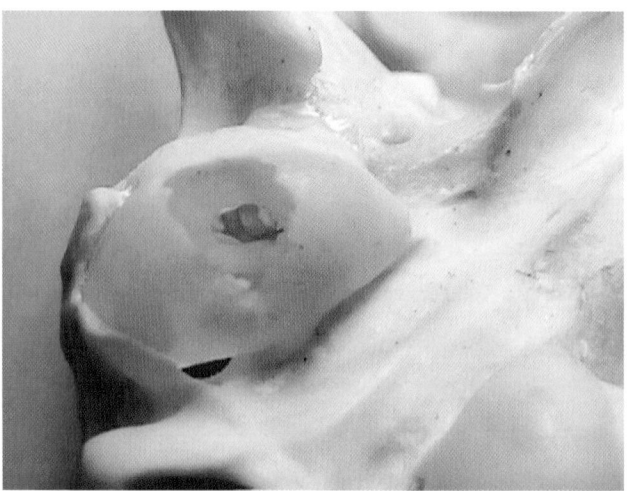

Figure 23.4 A cat skull showing entry into the large ventromedial compartment and with a smaller osteotomy through the wall of the smaller dorsolateral compartment.

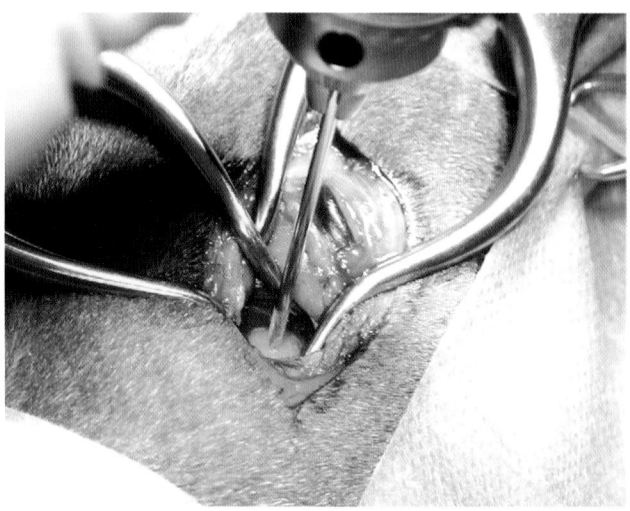

(A)

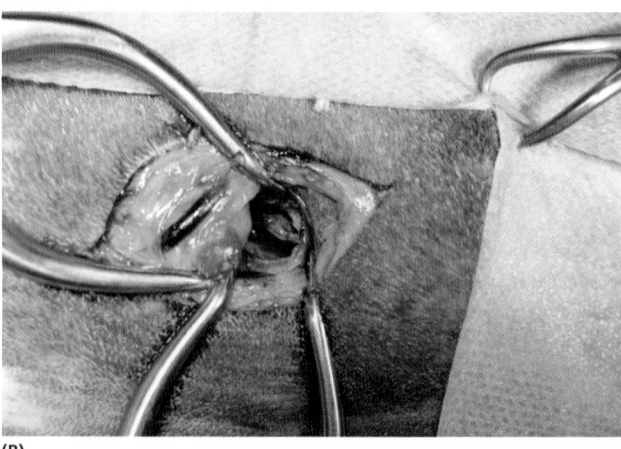

(B)

Figure 23.5 Ventral bulla osteotomy in a cat. **A,** Entry into the tympanic bulla with an intramedullary pin. **B,** View of the osteotomy site after bulla curettage. Both compartments are visible. *Source:* A. Hamaide, University of Liège, Liège, Belgium, 2014. Reproduced with permission from A. Hamaide.

Vessels most at risk for hemorrhage during VBO are the lingual artery, linguofacial vein, external carotid artery, internal carotid artery, external maxillary vein, and retroarticular vein (Figures 23.2 and 23.6).

Risk factors
- Lack of anatomic familiarity
- Excessive dissection and disruption of vasculature in the region of the bulla
- Proliferative reaction of the bulla, which may incorporate the vascular structures
- Coagulopathy

Diagnosis
- Blood is observed during surgery and may be difficult to control and obscures visualization.
- Postoperatively, hemorrhage may be recognized in the collection receptacle connected to the drain or soaking through the incision and bandage material. Excessive hemorrhage may cause signs upper respiratory obstruction.
- Aspiration of cervical swelling may confirm hemorrhage.

Treatment
- Identify the bleeding vessel and occlude with ligatures, electrocoagulation, or vascular sealing during surgery. Sustained pressure for 3 to 5 minutes may be necessary to control hemorrhage when the vessel cannot be identified or accessed.

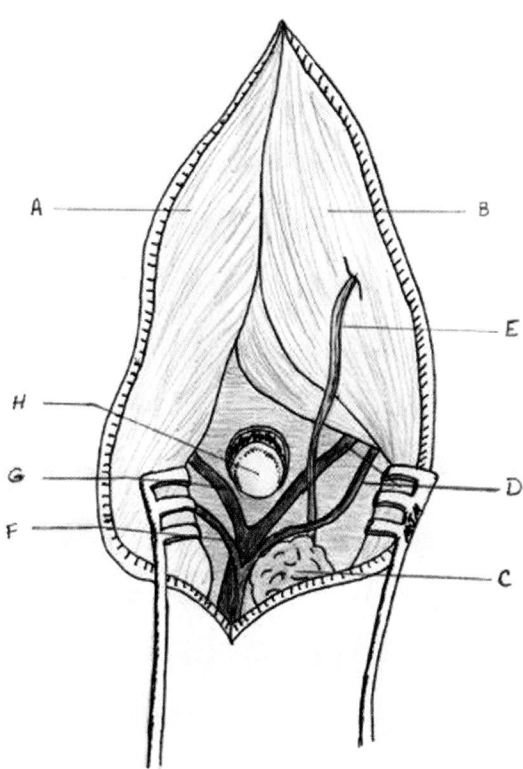

Figure 23.6 Exposure of the tympanic bulla (H) with a ventral approach requires separation of the digastric muscle (A) from the styloglossus and hyoglossus (B) muscles. Other anatomic structures that should be protected during the procedure include the mandibular salivary gland (C), lingual artery and vein (D), hypoglossal nerve (E), external carotid artery (F), and maxillary artery (G).

- Loosen head bandages if respiratory distress becomes moderate to severe postoperatively.
- Severe postoperative hemorrhage that does not subside may require exploration of the surgical site to achieve control. Carotid artery ligation may be performed for arterial bleeding.

Outcome
- Hemorrhage is usually successfully controlled. Excessive use of suction rather than pressure and patience to control hemorrhage and improve visualization can result in exsanguination if branches of the carotid artery are hemorrhaging.

Prevention
- Be meticulous.
- Dissect with care and be familiar with the vessels and nerves adjacent to the bulla (see Figures 23.2 and 23.6). The lingual artery lies medial to the digastric muscle and courses in a caudoventral direction with the hypoglossal nerve. The external carotid artery can overlie the bulla or lie medial to the bulla. The external maxillary vein lies beneath the mylohyoid muscle. The retroarticular vein lies a few millimeters rostral to external acoustic meatus (see Figure 23.2). Avoid excessive medial pressure during curettage of the medial bulla wall to prevent disruption of the internal carotid artery.

Incisional swelling

Definition
Incisional swelling is an abnormal enlargement or increase in volume of the tissues surrounding the operative site.

Risk factors
- Uncontrolled hemorrhage
- Seroma formation
- Contamination of soft tissues with bacteria
- Traumatic surgical technique
- Failure to close dead space

Diagnosis
Visualization of facial and neck asymmetry and palpation of an enlargement at or adjacent to the incision are sufficient for diagnosing incisional swelling. Although usually unnecessary, diagnostic imaging (ultrasonography, CT scan, and radiographs) may be useful in localizing the extent of involvement.

Swelling together with a restrictive bandage can impair respiration.

Treatment
- Apply cold compresses several times a day for 24 to 48 hours after surgery and then warm compresses for 48 to 72 hours.
- Loosen restrictive bandages.
- Drain excessive fluid accumulation.
- Monitor closely for respiratory distress and, if necessary, place a tracheostomy tube.
- Administer antimicrobials indicated by susceptibility results from bulla specimens to control soft tissue infection and abscessation.

Outcome
Incisional swellings resolve with appropriate treatment.

Prevention

- Be meticulous.
- Dissect with care and be familiar with the vessels and nerves adjacent to the bulla. Elevate soft tissue from the bulla before enlarging the osteotomy. Lavage the bulla and soft tissue thoroughly during and after surgery. Place a closed-suction drain before wound closure and appose dead space and tissue planes with nonreactive monofilament suture material.

Horner's syndrome

Definition

Horner's syndrome can be defined as the neurologic signs occurring secondary to traumatizing the sympathetic trunk (probably the oculosympathetic trunk), including ptosis, miosis, enophthalmos, and protrusion of the third eyelid (Figure 23.7 and Box 23.2).

Risk factors

- Cats requiring VBO, especially with inflammatory polyps
- Careless penetration of the bulla causing damage to the sympathetic fibers associated with the promontory, oval or round windows
- Poor knowledge of the anatomy and careless surgical technique

Diagnosis

Diagnosis is made when the clinical signs of ptosis, miosis, enophthalmos, and protrusion of the third eyelid are observed.

Treatment

There is no specific treatment for these signs after VBO. Signs gradually resolve with time.

Outcome

Signs of Horner's syndrome usually resolve in 2 to 4 weeks (Faulkner and Budsberg 1990; Kapatkin and Matthiesen 1990; Anders *et al.* 2008). It is reported to persist long term in fewer than 25% of the cases (Faulkner and Budsberg 1990). Those with Horner's syndrome persisting beyond 6 weeks are unlikely to fully recover.

Box 23.2 Clinical signs of Horner's syndrome

Ptosis

Miosis

Enophthalmos

Protrusion of third eyelid

Prevention

- Careful surgical technique and knowledge of regional anatomy
- In cats, avoid traumatizing the plexus of postganglionic sympathetic nerves on the promontory that is near the fissure between the ventromedial and dorsolateral compartments of the bulla
- Visualization of the postganglionic sympathetic nerves is difficult, so magnification may aid identification.

Facial nerve palsy

Definition

Facial nerve palsy is a condition identified by deficiencies in facial nerve function recognized by poor or no palpebral reflex, lip droop, facial spasms, and loss of parasympathetic innervation to the lacrimal glands (Figure 23.8 and Box 23.3). It is an uncommon complication of VBO unless total ear canal ablation is concurrently performed. Preoperative facial nerve paralysis suggests that the facial nerve is embedded in the inflammatory or proliferative reaction of the horizontal canal or that serious concurrent middle ear disease is present.

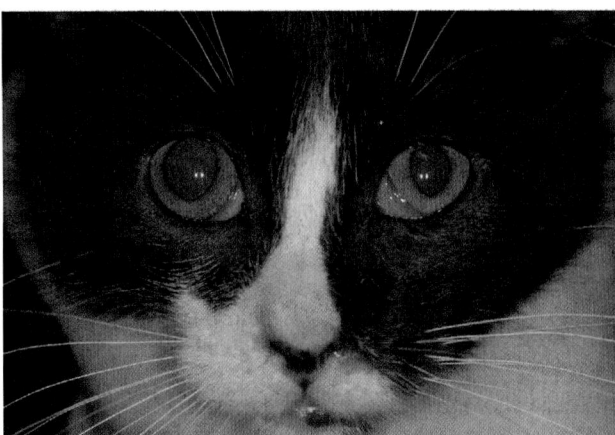

Figure 23.7 A cat with postoperative Horner's syndrome after left side ventral bulla osteotomy for inflammatory polyp removal. *Source:* Dr. S. Monclin. Reproduced with permission from Dr. S. Monclin.

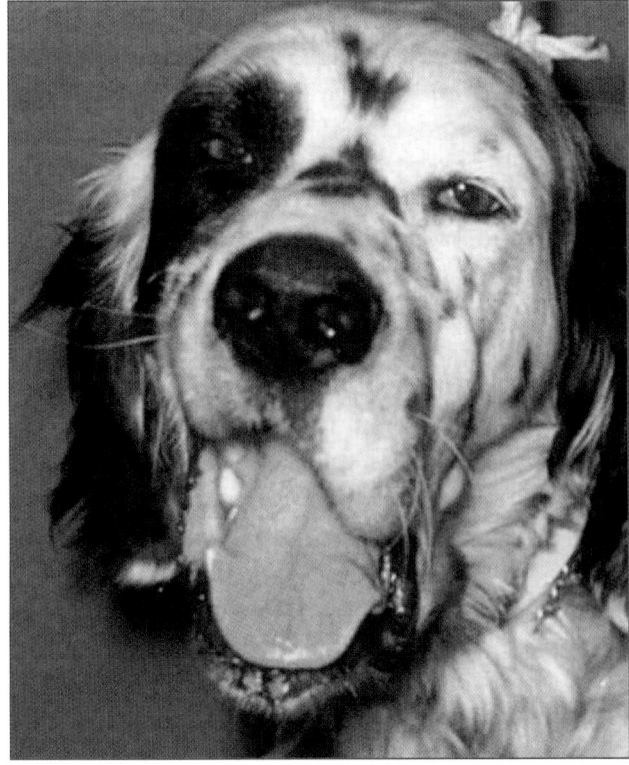

Figure 23.8 Lip droop associated with facial nerve palsy. *Source:* Dr. J. P. Toombs, Iowa State University, Ames, IA. Reproduced with permission from Dr. J. P. Toombs.

Box 23.3 Clinical signs of facial nerve palsy

> Reduced palpebral reflex
>
> Widened palpebral fissure
>
> Blepharospasm
>
> Drooping of lip and ear
>
> Excessive drooling
>
> Elevation and wrinkling of lip
>
> Caudal displacement of lip commissures
>
> Elevation of ear on affected side
>
> Reduced lacrimal secretions

Risk factors

- Poor knowledge of the anatomy and careless surgical technique
- Concurrent otitis externa with entrapment of the facial nerve in the inflammatory reaction
- Concurrent lateral or vertical ear canal resection or total ear canal ablation with manipulation of the facial nerve. In one study (Sharp 1990), 31% of patients developed facial nerve paralysis when VBO was performed in conjunction with total ear canal ablation.
- Stretching of the facial nerve during soft tissue retraction
- Fracture of the bulla wall into the stylomastoid foramen while enlarging the osteotomy site

Diagnosis

Facial nerve paralysis is diagnosed initially when the patient is noted to have a slow or nonexistent palpebral reflex. Other signs include a wide palpebral fissure, lip droop, and lack of lacrimal secretion on the ipsilateral side. Facial nerve tests include the menace response (mediated by the optic and facial nerves) and the palpebral reflexes (mediated by trigeminal and facial nerves).

Treatment

- Lubricate the eye with artificial tears or ophthalmic lubricant until lacrimal gland function returns.
- Function generally returns within 4 to 6 weeks.
- Eliminate swelling and inflammation to reduce nerve irritation by applying cold compresses for 48 to 72 hours followed by warm compresses for 48 to 72 hours and administer nonsteroidal antiinflammatory drugs.

Outcome

Facial nerve paralysis caused by stretching or retraction of the nerve usually resolves within a few days to weeks of surgery. If the nerve is severely stretched or severed, damage is permanent.

Prevention

- Identification and protection of the facial nerve as it travels from the stylomastoid foramen on the medial and caudal aspect of the horizontal canal and then courses ventral to the horizontal canal close to the middle ear (see Figure 23.2)
- Atraumatic dissection and gentle retraction
- Avoid taking large bites of bone with the rongeur when enlarging the osteotomy site to avoid fracture into the stylomastoid foramen.

Vestibular syndrome

Definition

Vestibular syndrome is one or more of a group of neurologic signs, including circling, nystagmus, loss of balance, and head tilt (Box 23.4).

Both central and peripheral vestibular syndrome can occur with otitis media or interna; peripheral vestibular syndrome is more common unless infection or neoplasia extends into the brainstem.

Risk factors

- Otitis interna or severe otitis media
- Poor knowledge of the anatomy and careless surgical technique
- Curettage of the dorsomedial region of the bulla
- Polyps or mucous material within the bulla that puts pressure on the labyrinthine structures

Diagnosis

Diagnosis is usually based on clinical recognition of neurologic abnormalities, including ataxia, head tilt, circling, and nystagmus. Vestibular nerve tests can also be evaluated, including righting reflex and the doll's head reflex (rapid head movement in horizontal and vertical planes normally induces a physiologic nystagmus in each plane). In vestibular disorders, the slow component is abnormal, and the fast phase is compensatory with its direction opposite the side of the lesion.

Treatment

Nonsteroidal antiinflammatory drugs may reduce swelling and irritation of the nerves, but evidence is lacking as to their efficacy. Meclizine, an antiemetic antihistamine (12.5 mg orally each day), is sometimes recommended to minimize vestibular signs.

Outcome

Neurologic signs may persist, especially those that were present before surgery. Animals with head tilt before surgery may improve, but most retain some degree of head tilt. Most cats adjust well to persistent head tilt and maintain a near normal level of activity. Neurologic signs caused by surgery are usually temporary.

Prevention

- Avoid curettage and manipulation in the dorsomedial aspect of the bulla to preserve the auditory ossicles and bony labyrinth of the inner ear containing the semicircular canals and cochlea.
- Obtain specimens from the middle ear and treat infections with antimicrobials based on susceptibility results for a minimum of 4 months (Palmeiro *et al.* 2004).

Box 23.4 Clinical signs of vestibular dysfunction

> - Toward affected side:
>   - Head tilt
>   - Circling
>   - Falling
>   - Rolling
> - Away from affected side:
>   - Fast component of nystagmus (rotary or horizontal)
> - Asymmetric ataxia with persistent strength
> - Positional or vestibular strabismus
>   - Eye ipsilateral to affected side deviated ventrally
> - Postural reactions

Relevant literature

Recognition of otitis media can be challenging because some animals show no signs of middle or inner ear disease. Typical signs are head shaking, pain, head tilt, and otitis externa. Less common preoperative signs may include Horner's syndrome, vestibular syndrome, and facial nerve palsy (Little *et al.* 1991; Remedios *et al.* 1991; Trevor & Martin 1993). A review of a large number of necropsied cats (*n* = 3442), which excluded those with neoplastic ear disease and polyps, found an incidence of 1.7% for non-neoplastic diseases of the middle ear (Schlicksup *et al.* 2009). Only 10% of cats with these abnormal bullae had clinical signs (Schlicksup *et al.* 2009).

Diagnosis involves otoscopic examinations, cultures, cytology, and imaging in addition to the history and clinical signs. Otoscopic examination may reveal tympanic membrane rupture (95%; Palmeiro *et al.* 2004) or an intact membrane that is bulging, opaque, and thickened or relatively normal (71%; Little *et al.* 1991; Cole *et al.* 1998). Sometimes the tympanic membrane cannot be visualized because of hyperplasia and stenosis of the external ear canal. Cultures must be taken to determine susceptibility. Different organisms will be cultured with different susceptibilities in the external ear canal and the middle ear (89.5%; Cole *et al.* 1998) and from the middle ear before and after lavage (91% for gram-positive and 65% for gram-negative organisms; Hettlich *et al.* 2005). Other imaging might include radiographs, CT, or MRI to better visualize and localize the involvement of the middle ear. When comparing surgical confirmation of otitis media with imaging, it appeared that radiographs identified 66% of abnormal bullae, and CT scan identified 83% of abnormal bullae (Love *et al.* 1994). MRI is effective in identifying intracranial extension of otitis media or interna and in characterizing the location and extent of the pathologic changes intracranially as well as within the middle or inner ear (Sturges *et al.* 2006).

Rigorous medical treatment of otitis media (lavage and prolonged, appropriate antibiotic therapy) results in resolution of the condition within 4 months in the majority (82%) of dogs (Palmeiro *et al.* 2004). Cases that are refractory to medical therapy because of resistant microorganisms or the presence of a mass may require surgery for resolution. TECALBO is recommended for cases with otitis externa and media. Even though exposure of the bulla is better with a VBO, it has been demonstrated that complications are similar when performing a VBO in conjunction with total ear canal ablation (Sharp 1990). Dogs and cats with primary otitis media caused by infection or masses and those with recurrent otitis after a total ear canal resection are candidates for VBO. Successful resolution of otitis media requires that all the epithelial lining of the bulla be removed except that which lines the dorsomedial recess to avoid the auditory ossicles and bony labyrinth (contains semicircular canals and cochlea) of the inner ear (Kapatkin and Matthiesen 1990; Sharp 1990). Epithelial remnants that remain cause recurrence of otitis media, possible extension into the inner ear and brain, abscesses, and draining tracts. Residual epithelium after TECALBO is frequently found just dorsal to the external ear canal or just caudal to the external acoustic meatus (Smeak *et al.* 1996). After VBO, the bulla rapidly reforms with no deleterious effect on hearing in most dogs (McAnulty *et al.* 1995). Resolution of otitis media is expected to occur after VBO, but preoperative neurologic abnormalities and hearing deficits are unlikely to improve (Remedios *et al.* 1991; Trevor and Martin 1993; McAnulty *et al.* 1995; Anders *et al.* 2008).

Complications of otitis media or VBO include hemorrhage, infection, swelling, Horner's syndrome, facial nerve palsy, and vestibular syndrome. Postoperative Horner's syndrome occurs in most cats and is expected to resolve within the first week, but it can be permanent in up to 25% (Faulkner and Budsberg 1990; Kapatkin and Matthiesen 1990; Trevor and Martin 1993; Anders *et al.* 2008). Postoperative facial nerve palsy is expected to improve over days to months (Kapatkin and Matthiesen 1990; Trevor and Martin 1993). Postoperative vestibular signs occurring in 4% (Kapatkin and Matthiesen 1990) to 42% (Faulkner and Budsberg 1990) of the cases are usually transient and mild but may persist for the long term in up to 17% (Faulkner and Budsberg 1990).

References

Anders, B.B., Hoelzler, M.G., Scavelli, T.D., et al. (2008) Analysis of auditory and neurologic effects associated with ventral bulla osteotomy for removal of inflammatory polyps or nasopharyngeal masses in cats. *Journal of the American Veterinary Medical Association* 233, 580-585.

Cole, L.K., Kwochka, K.W., Hillier A.(1998) Microbial flora and antimicrobial susceptibility patterns of isolated pathogens from the horizontal ear canal and middle ear in dogs with otitis media. *Journal of the American Veterinary Medical Association* 212, 534-538.

Faulkner, J.E., Budsberg, S.C.(1990) Results of ventral bulla osteotomy for treatment of middle ear polyps in cats. *Journal of the American Animal Hospital Association* 26, 496-499.

Gregory, S.P. (2000) Middle ear disease associated with congenital palatine defects in seven dogs and one cat. *Journal of Small Animal Practice* 41, 398-401.

Hettlich, B.F., Boothe, H.W., Simpson, R.B., et al. (2005) Effects of tympanic cavity evacuation and flushing on microbial isolates during total ear canal ablation with lateral bulla osteotomy in dogs. *Journal of the American Veterinary Medical Association* 227, 748-755.

Kapatkin, A.S., Matthiesen, D.T. (1990) Results of surgery and long-term follow-up in 31 cats with nasopharyngeal polyps. *Journal of the American Animal Hospital Association* 26, 387-392.

Little, C.J.L., Lane, J.G., Pearson, G.R. (1991) Inflammatory middle ear disease of the dog: the pathology of otitis media. *Veterinary Record* 128, 293-296.

Love, N.E., Kramer, R.W., Spodnick, G.J., et al. (1995) Radiographic and computed tomographic evaluation of otitis media in the dog. *Veterinary Radiology & Ultrasound* 36 (5), 375-379.

McAnulty, J.F., Hattel, A., Harvey, C.E. (1995) Wound healing and brain stem auditory evoked potentials after experimental ventral tympanic bulla osteotomy. *Veterinary Surgery* 24, 9-14.

Palmeiro, B.S., Morris, D.J., Wiemelt, S.P., et al. (2004) Evaluation of outcome of otitis media after lavage of the tympanic bulla and long-term antimicrobial drug treatment in dogs: 44 cases (1998-2002). *Journal of the American Veterinary Medical Association* 225 (4), 548-553.

Pratschke, K.M. (2003) Inflammatory polyp in the middle ear in 5 dogs. *Veterinary Surgery* 32, 292-296.

Remedios, A.M., Fowler, J.D., Pharr, J.W. (1991) A comparison of radiographic versus surgical diagnosis of otitis media. *Journal of the American Animal Hospital Association* 27, 183-188.

Schlicksup, M.D. Van Winkle, T.J., Holt, D.E. (2009) Prevalence of clinical abnormalities in cats found to have non-neoplastic middle ear disease at necropsy: 59 cases (1991-2007). *Journal of the Ameraicn Veterinary Medical Association* 235 (7), 841-843.

Sharp, N.J.H. (1990) Chronic otitis externa and media treated by total ear canal ablation and ventral bulla osteotomy in thirteen dogs. *Veterinary Surgery* 19 (2), 162-166.

Smeak, D.D., Crocker, C.B., Birchard, S.J. (1996) Treatment of recurrent otitis media that developed after total ear canal ablation and lateral bulla osteotomy in dogs: nine cases (1986-1994). *Journal of the American Veterinary Medical Association* 209 (5), 937-942.

Sturges, B.K., Dickinson, P.J., Kortz, G.D., et al. (2006) Clinical signs, magnetic resonance imaging features, and outcome after surgical and medical treatment of otogenic intracranial infection in 11 cats and 4 dogs. *Journal of Veterinary Internal Medicine* 20, 648-656.

Trevor, P.B., Martin, R.A. (1993) Tympanic bulla osteotomy for treatment of middle ear disease in cats: 19 cases (1984-1991). *Journal of the American Veterinary Medical Associationr* 202 (1), 123-128.

Ziemer, L.S., Schwarx, T. Sullivan, M. (2003) Otolithiasis in three dogs. *Veterinary Radiology & Ultrasound* 44 (1), 28-31.

24 Surgical Management of Brachycephalic Airway Obstructive Syndrome

Cyril Poncet
C.H.V. Frégis, Arcueil, France

Brachycephalic airway obstructive syndrome (BAOS) is a complex entity characteristic of brachycephalic breeds. This syndrome is not limited to stenotic nares and elongated soft palate; these primary malformations can be associated with numerous other anomalies of the respiratory, cardiovascular, or even gastrointestinal (GI) systems. The complexity of this syndrome leads to increased perianesthetic mortality rates in brachycephalic breeds and a high risk of complications after the surgical management of BAOS.

Anesthetic complications

Definition
There is a known increase in anesthetic risk in brachycephalic breeds, irrespective of the type of general anesthesia or surgical procedure.

The anesthetic risk is linked to various particularities of these breeds:
- Primary anatomic malformations of the respiratory system (elongated soft palate, stenotic nares, macroglossia, tracheal hypoplasia)

and secondary (everted laryngeal saccules, laryngeal collapse, oropharyngeal inflammation), leading to disturbed spontaneous ventilation during the induction and recovery phases
- Cardiovascular and pulmonary diseases secondary to the chronic upper airway obstruction (Figure 24.1)
- Increased vagal tone, leading to bradycardia
- Anomalies of the GI system, which may lead to ptyalism, regurgitation, vomiting, and gastroesophageal reflux during the perianesthetic period
- Defective thermoregulation at the nasal cavities, leading to hyperthermia

Risk factors
- Absence of endotracheal intubation with oxygenation during anesthesia
- Severity of respiratory disorders and advanced age of the animal
- Animals with known cardiac and pulmonary disorders
- State of stress of the animal or emergency surgery
- Associated GI disorders

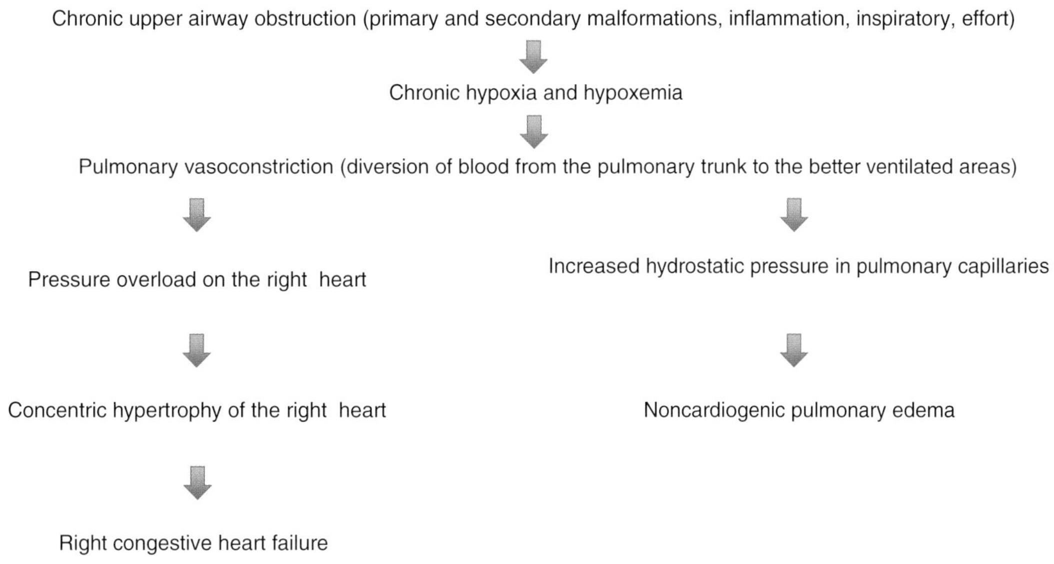

Chronic upper airway obstruction (primary and secondary malformations, inflammation, inspiratory, effort)

⇩

Chronic hypoxia and hypoxemia

⇩

Pulmonary vasoconstriction (diversion of blood from the pulmonary trunk to the better ventilated areas)

⇩   ⇩

Pressure overload on the right heart   Increased hydrostatic pressure in pulmonary capillaries

⇩   ⇩

Concentric hypertrophy of the right heart   Noncardiogenic pulmonary edema

⇩

Right congestive heart failure

Figure 24.1 Pathophysiology of cardiovascular diseases associated with brachycephalic airway obstructive syndrome.

Complications in Small Animal Surgery, First Edition. Edited by Dominique Griffon and Annick Hamaide.
© 2016 John Wiley & Sons, Inc. Published 2016 by John Wiley & Sons, Inc.
Companion website: www.wiley.com/go/griffon/complications

Diagnosis

All phases of general anesthesia are delicate in brachycephalic dogs. The induction phase may be hindered by great difficulty in intubating these animals or finding an endotracheal tube of the right size. General anesthesia may be punctuated by phases of apnea or cardiac rhythm disorders (bradycardia, other arrhythmias). The recovery phase is also critical with animals presenting with airway obstruction leading to severe dyspnea.

Treatment

- Use of medication (acepromazine, glycopyrrolate) to control stress and the increased vagal tone
- Endotracheal intubation with an appropriately sized endotracheal tube, often small in these animals, which have a tendency toward tracheal hypoplasia (English and French bulldogs in particular) or tracheomalacia (Pug). Thoracic radiography can be used to evaluate the size of the tracheal lumen.
- Oxygenation during the recovery phase (nasotracheal tube) and prepare for temporary tracheostomy placement if necessary

Outcome

The anesthetic mortality rate is linked to the severity of preoperative respiratory disorders and preexisting pulmonary or cardiac sequelae.

Prevention

- Preoxygenation of the animal before induction
- Premedication with a vagolytic (glycopyrrolate)
- Sedation (phenothiazines) to reduce stress and potentiate the effect of the anesthetic agents, thus ensuring a more rapid recovery
- Preoperative detection of cardiovascular and pulmonary disorders
- Preoperative management of GI disorders: ensure prolonged preoperative fasting, investigate and treat any GI disorders (cf. GI complications)
- Systematic intubation with an appropriately sized endotracheal tube
- Minimal oropharyngeal inflammation during the surgical procedure by any means possible
- Increased and prolonged monitoring during the recovery period

Postoperative upper airway obstruction

Definition

Dyspnea during the hours after the recovery phase from surgery for BAOS is the main postoperative complication. It is usually caused by upper airway obstruction; the causes vary as a function of the individual and the type of surgery:
- Inflammatory edema at the surgical site after palatoplasty or ventriculectomy
- Wound dehiscence or necrosis of the surgical site after palatoplasty
- Persistence of upper airway obstruction in case of insufficient palatoplasty or untreated laryngeal collapse
- Upper airway obstruction by excessive mucus production that the animal cannot expectorate.

Risk factors

- An insufficient or excessively traumatic surgical procedure combined with perioperative inflammation of the tissues may cause severe dyspnea. Recent studies emphasize the advantages

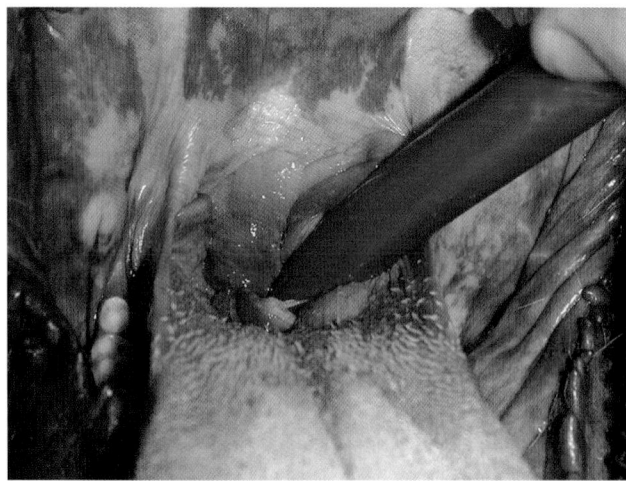

Figure 24.2 Severe laryngeal inflammation after ventriculectomy. An emergency temporary tracheostomy was required.

of surgically thinning the soft palate to relieve nasopharyngeal obstruction.
- The surgical wound is highly solicited during the recovery phase. Poor suture placement may promote dehiscence and oropharyngeal inflammation.
- Ventriculectomy may promote perioperative oropharyngeal inflammation (Figure 24.2).
- The presence of severe laryngeal collapse (common in pugs) at the time of intervention promotes airway obstruction.

Diagnosis

Immediately after recovery, inflammatory edema, the presence of mucus, and the persistence of an obstruction are the most common causes. The animal may be anesthetized again to determine the cause of the complication and implement appropriate measures.

After the animal has been through a satisfactory recovery phase, the two most common complications are then dehiscence of the palatoplasty site or inflammatory edema. This may also necessitate endoscopy to reevaluate the surgical site (Figure 24.3).

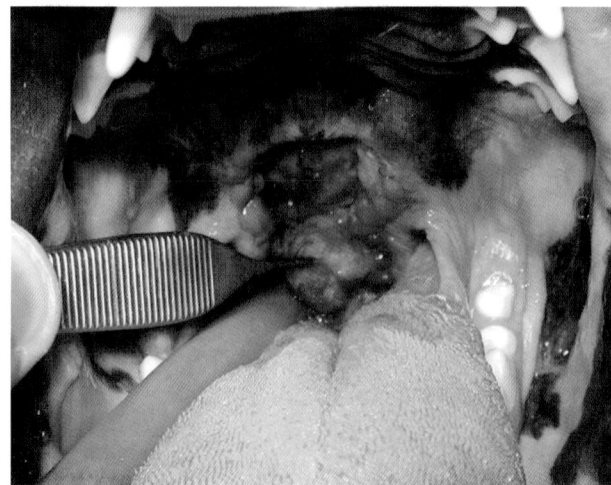

Figure 24.3 Wound dehiscence after palatoplasty (modified palatoplasty technique). The animal presented with sudden onset of dyspnea 72 hours after the surgical procedure.

Treatment

- Clapping can be performed to limit tracheal and pharyngeal congestion by provoking expectoration; this is an effective technique in the hours after the surgical procedure to facilitate the expectoration of mucus.
- In the presence of inflammatory edema associated with moderate inspiratory dyspnea, the use of steroidal antiinflammatory drugs, continued oxygen therapy via a nasotracheal tube, and a quiet recovery of the animal may be sufficient as an initial approach.
- In cases of severe dyspnea, the decision to perform a temporary tracheostomy should be rapidly envisaged to ensure sufficient patency of the airways. The tube is then left in place for 3 to 5 days until the inflammation has subsided.
- Further surgery may be needed in case of persistence of oropharyngeal obstruction caused by insufficient palatoplasty, wound dehiscence, or severe laryngeal collapse. The various surgical solutions include the placement of a permanent tracheostomy.

Outcome

Oropharyngeal obstruction during the immediate postoperative period may be rapidly fatal if the airways are not cleared.

Prevention

- Delayed extubation until a good laryngeal reflex is present
- Postoperative oxygen therapy
- Surgical reduction of excessive thickness of the soft palate in addition to reducing its length
- Minimal postoperative inflammation by gentle handling of the soft tissues, use of a laser, use of steroidal antiinflammatory drugs, control of polypnea and hyperthermia
- Secure sutures by use of polyfilament suture, which generally provides more secure knots (although the use of monofilament material may reduce the local inflammatory reaction).

Nasal wound healing complications

Definition

Rhinoplasty may be associated with immediate (bleeding, inflammation, wound dehiscence, alar necrosis) or delayed complications (discoloration of the nose, weakening of the nasal alae, asymmetry of the nostrils, persistence of stenotic nares, strident breathing sounds).

Risk factors

- Electrocautery and laser techniques can cause inflammation and necrosis of the nostrils.
- Overly tight or poorly tied sutures create discomfort, promoting scratching and dehiscence.
- If the alar cartilages (internal part of the nostril) are not excised at the same time as the cuneiform resection of the nares, nasal obstruction will usually persist.

Diagnosis

Inspection of the nostrils while the animal is awake is sufficient to assess unfavorable scarring or persistent stenotic nares (generally restricted to the nasal vestibule).

Treatment

- An Elizabethan collar is advisable to prevent scratching, and antiinflammatory drugs are prescribed if the wound is inflamed.

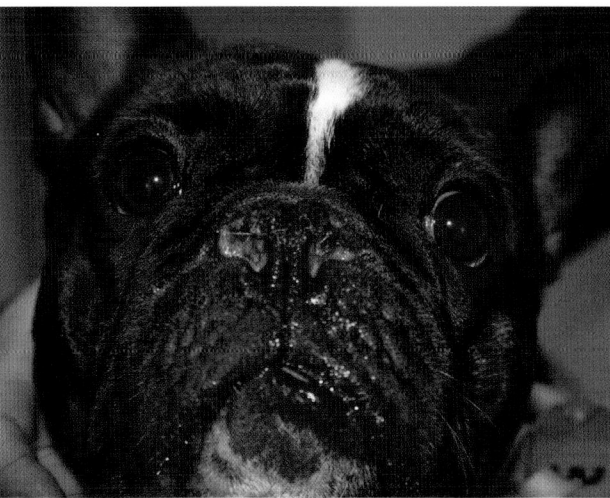

Figure 24.4 Necrosis of the nares secondary to rhinoplasty performed with a diode laser. Second intention healing and repigmentation are to be expected.

- The application of Vaseline on the wound promotes healing.
- If the stenosis persists, another rhinoplasty can be performed, and surgical treatment of other malformations leading to upper airway obstruction is indicated.
- Discoloration of the nose around the wound site is temporary; repigmentation occurs after a few weeks (Figure 24.4).

Outcome

The complications of nostril surgery are uncommon and often easy to treat.

Prevention

- Surgery with a cold scalpel blade and good hemostasis should limit inflammation and postoperative bleeding.
- Symmetrical excision at the level of the nares and the alar cartilage is essential for a satisfactory esthetic result.
- The rhinoplasty should include resection of the alar cartilages located in the internal part of the nostril, this zone being largely responsible for nasal obstruction (rhinoplasty by cuneiform resection of part of the epithelium and of the medial fold of the alar cartilage).
- The use of rapidly resorbable monofilament suture material limits inflammation at the wound site and eliminates the need for manual suture removal. The knots should be securely tied to prevent dehiscence.
- An alapexy technique can be used for nostrils with a very flaccid alar cartilage.

Aspiration pneumonia

Definition

This is infection of the lungs caused by aspiration of food particles or fluids into the lungs.

Risk factors

- Presence of GI disorders
- Clinical signs of lower respiratory tract disorders (coughing, expiratory noise)

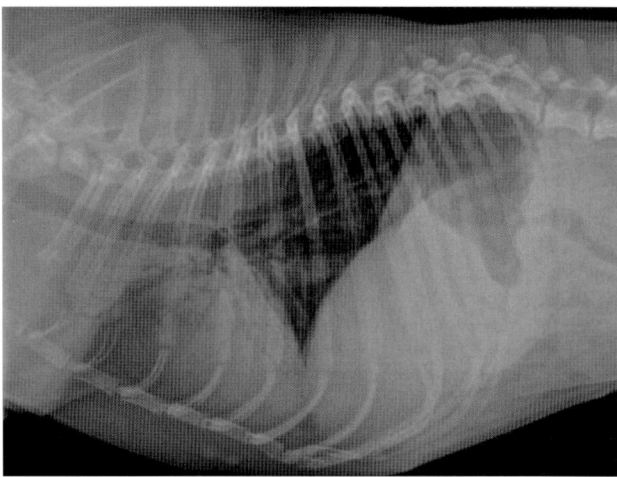

Figure 24.5 Lateral thoracic radiograph of a French bulldog with severe postoperative aspiration pneumonia. Note the cranial and ventral alveolar pattern with air bronchograms.

- Presence of an abnormal thoracic radiographic pattern before the intervention

Diagnosis
- Per-acute respiratory distress within hours of aspiration. There may be a sudden onset of coughing before the development of respiratory distress.
- Cardiovascular shock may occur.
- Signs of vomiting and regurgitation with phases of coughing may be reported.
- Depression and pyrexia develop rapidly.
- Pulmonary auscultation reveals crackles and sometimes wheezing, especially in the dependent (usually cranioventral) lung fields.
- Thoracic radiographs show a bronchoalveolar pattern involving primarily the dependant lung lobes. Consolidation may be present (Figure 24.5).

Treatment
- Immediate oxygen supplementation
- Intravenous fluid therapy is indicated. High volumes may be needed initially to treat shock. Overhydration may contribute to the formation of pulmonary edema.
- Tracheal aspiration
- Clapping
- Bronchodilators and corticosteroids are justified in the first 24 to 48 hours.
- Use of first-line, broad-spectrum antibiotics; amoxicillin–clavulanate is a good initial choice

Outcome
The prognosis depends on the amount and character of the material aspirated, the condition of the animal before aspiration, and the cause of the aspiration.

Prevention
- Systematic preoperative thoracic radiographs to detect current or chronic pulmonary lesions and to detect tracheal hypoplasia that could alter the function of the mucociliary apparatus
- Fasting of the animal for at least 24 hours before surgery
- Detection and preventive treatment of any GI disorders
- Recent advances in palatoplasty techniques and the multimodal management of these animals both at a respiratory and GI level could reduce the incidence of aspiration bronchopneumonia.
- Increased and prolonged monitoring during the recovery period

Perioperative gastrointestinal signs

Definition
Perioperative GI disorders include vomiting, regurgitation, gastroesophageal reflux, and ptyalism that could exacerbate the respiratory status. The concomitance of anatomic malformations of the upper respiratory and GI tracts and the close interactions between respiratory and GI disorders indicate a common pathophysiological etiology to explain the correlation in the severity of GI and respiratory disorders (Figure 24.6).

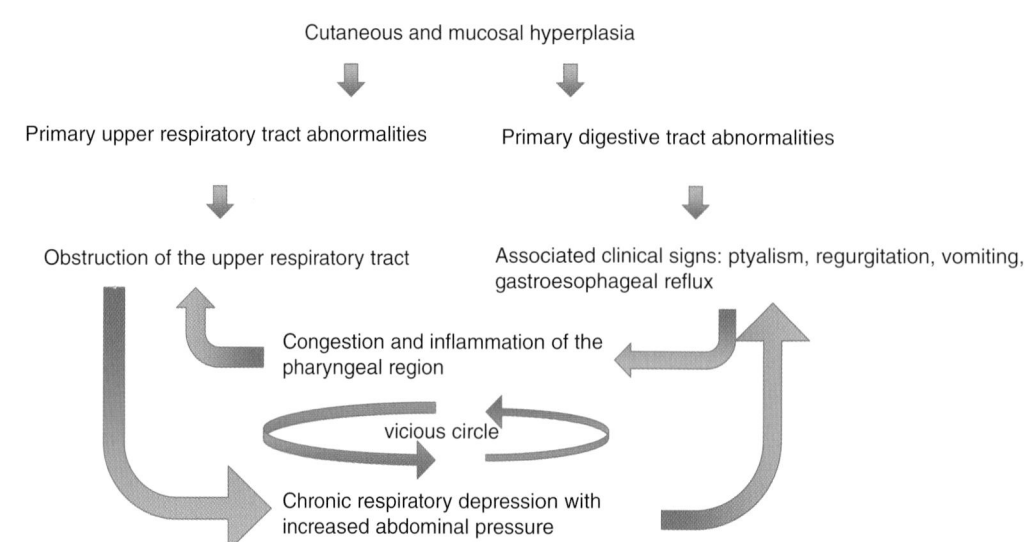

Figure 24.6 Common pathophysiology pathway of digestive and respiratory diseases in brachycephalic airway obstructive syndrome.

Risk factors

- Presence of GI signs before surgery (chewing, hypersalivation, vomiting, regurgitation, spitting jets of foam when excited)
- Reduced fasting period
- Difficult recovery with inspiratory dyspnea

Diagnosis

- Vomiting (with gastric juices or food, indicating gastric retention)
- Regurgitation (may or may not be exercise induced but very frequent when the animal gets excited)
- Eructation
- Ptyalism
- Repeated swallowing
- Ingestion of grass or pica

Treatment

Treatment is mainly medical; the most commonly used agents are antacids (omeprazole), GI protectants (sucralfate, aluminium phosphate), and prokinetics (metoclopramide) associated with corticosteroids (prednisolone) when gastroduodenal inflammation is marked.

Surgical treatment, when necessary, of GI anomalies detected on gastroscopy (hiatal hernia or true pyloric stenosis) is not performed at the same time as the correction of respiratory anomalies. It should be differed by a few weeks, and interim medical treatment should be implemented.

Prevention

- It is important to provide a water-only diet for 24 hours before surgery in animals with gastric retention.
- Upper GI endoscopy provides a view of the GI lesions to enable implementation of medical management combined with surgical

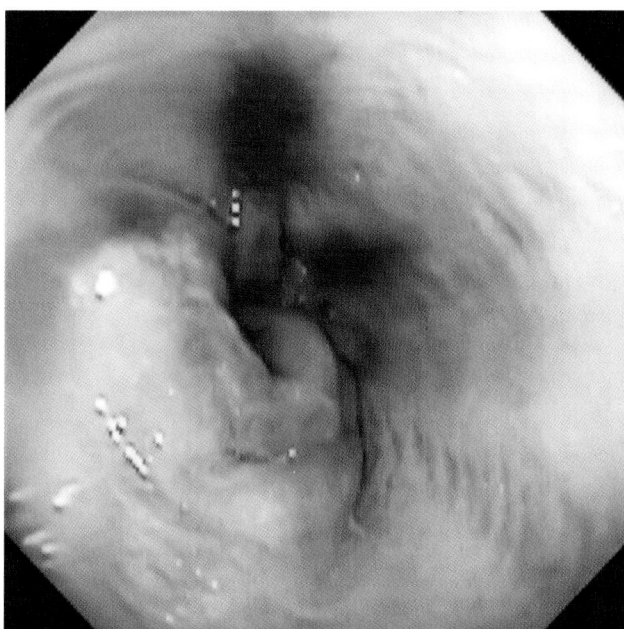

Figure 24.7 Endoscopy of the upper gastrointestinal (GI) tract in an English bulldog before surgery on the upper airways. There is severe reflux esophagitis. Specific treatment should be instigated to control postoperative GI disorders.

correction of upper airway obstruction. There are three types of anomaly for each segment of the GI tract:
- **Anatomic anomalies,** which may be congenital malformations or acquired lesions of the upper GI tract (e.g., esophageal deviation, pyloric stenosis, hiatal hernia)
- **Functional anomalies,** including gastric atony, duodenogastric reflux, and so on
- **Inflammatory lesions,** generally secondary to the first two anomalies described (esophagitis, gastritis) (Figure 24.7)

Gastrointestinal endoscopy also enables the practitioner to take gastroduodenal biopsy samples to assess the intensity of the inflammatory infiltrate via histology because the correlation between the macroscopic appearance of the lesions and histology results is not good.

Outcome

The surgical correction of airway obstruction improves GI symptoms. Similarly, medical treatment of GI disorders should improve the prognosis of operated animals. Thus, the systematic detection of GI lesions and the implementation of medical treatment for gastric disorders could help to reduce respiratory disorders and improve the prognosis of animals undergoing surgery for airway obstruction syndrome.

Persistent signs of upper airway obstruction

Definition

Clinical signs of upper airway obstruction may persist or recur several months or years after the surgical procedure. They can be identified by persistent upper airway stertor or stridor, recurrence of less extreme upper airway signs, and voice changes. The causes are multiple:
- Onset or worsening of secondary lesions such as everted laryngeal saccules or laryngeal collapse
- Presence of obstructive lesions that were not treated initially (excessive ethmoidal turbinates, laryngeal collapse, macroglossia)
- Recurrent obstruction caused by wound failure on the soft palate or persistence of excess thickness in the soft palate
- Stenotic nares
- Persistence of pharyngeal inflammation after GI disorders

Risk factors

- Severe cases or elderly animals
- Inadequate surgical treatment for the primary or secondary anatomic respiratory anomalies (Figure 24.8)
- Failure to treat GI disorders

Diagnosis

Exploration of the upper airways should be envisaged under general anesthesia. Respiratory endoscopy is indicated in first intention combined with cross-sectional imaging techniques (magnetic resonance imaging, computed tomography [CT]).

Outcome and treatment

The treatment and prognosis are variable and depend on the cause. Laryngeal collapse is the hardest complication to deal with as the flaccidity of the arytenoid cartilages often renders techniques for lateralizing the arytenoid cartilages ineffective. Stiffening or partial

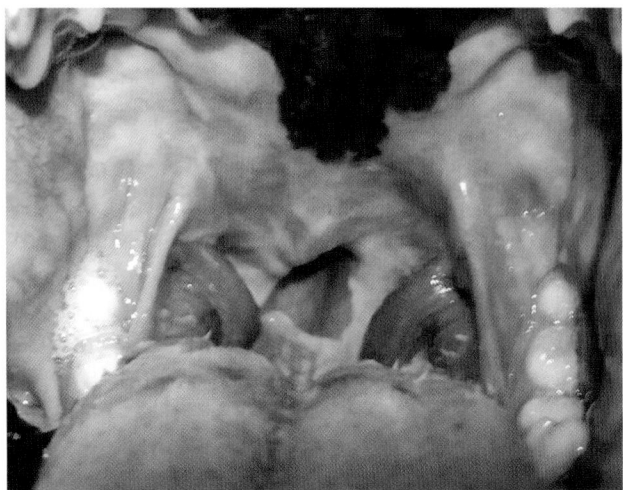

Figure 24.8 Wound failure after palatoplasty. Fibrous tissue scarring is visible, leading to narrowing of the nasopharynx.

excision of the arytenoid cartilages with a laser can be considered. As a last resort, a permanent tracheostomy can be proposed.

Prevention

Exhaustive investigation, including any GI anomalies, is essential for the correct surgical treatment of BAOS. The treatment, whether surgical or medical, is multimodal and highly variable as a function of the brachycephalic breed, and the nature and severity of the anomalies observed.

Relevant literature

The most common complications are undoubtedly **postoperative upper airway obstructions**, which can jeopardize the recovery phase of the animal.

Surgical lasers are particularly interesting for palate surgery by reducing surgical time, bleeding, tissue inflammation, and postoperative pain. A recent retrospective study (Dunie-Merigot *et al.* 2010) demonstrated the significant advantages of a carbon dioxide laser compared with other techniques (diode laser and electrocautery). This technique is particularly interesting for thinning the soft palate, which requires incision through the muscular and highly vascularized part of the soft palate. Another study (Brdecka *et al.* 2008) demonstrated the possibility of using a bipolar sealing device for the resection of the elongated part of the soft palate. The use of such techniques reduces inflammatory edema during the postoperative phase.

It is likely that the everted laryngeal saccules play a role in the obstruction of the upper airways. However, resection of the saccules causes edema and laryngeal hemorrhage, which is likely to increase the anesthetic risk on recovery and may necessitate the placement of a temporary tracheostomy. A study of 25 cases of BAOS treated surgically reported significantly inferior results after resection of the saccules (60% good results compared with 83.3% in the absence of ventriculectomy) (Ducarouge 2002). Based on these observations, systematic ventriculectomy has become increasingly controversial (Poncet *et al.* 2006; Riecks *et al.* 2007; Dunie-Merigot *et al.* 2010) especially because one can postulate that these lesions may be reversible after satisfactory resolution of the upper airway

obstruction. The author currently only advise its use in cases of significant eversion, ulceration, or formation of an inflammatory granuloma over these saccules.

The onset of severe dyspnea during the postoperative period with the suspicion of pharyngeal edema or severe laryngeal collapse may necessitate the placement of a temporary tracheostomy tube (Torrez and Hunt 2006; Riecks *et al.* 2007; Dunie-Merigot *et al.* 2010). In addition to providing an alternate airway, it also allows oxygen therapy and the provision of ventilatory support if necessary (Hoareau *et al.* 2011). No recent study advises systematic tracheostomy placement. However, one study demonstrated the advantages of placing a nasotracheal tube for oxygen supplementation during the recovery phase (Senn *et al.* 2011).

The high prevalence of **GI problems** has been identified clinically, endoscopically, and histologically in these animals with upper respiratory problems, and there is a proven correlation between the severity of the GI and respiratory signs (Poncet *et al.* 2005).

The onset of GI disorders in the postoperative period has been widely demonstrated in several recent studies with signs of regurgitation and vomiting present in nearly 20% of the cases operated (Torrez and Hunt 2006; Fasanella *et al.* 2010). These GI disorders may promote the onset of **aspiration bronchopneumonia** during the postoperative period. Fasting the animal for at least 24 hours before surgery, premedication, and early medical treatment of GI disorders helps to limit complications related to aspiration during the recovery phase (rhinitis, bronchopneumonia). In a retrospective study on 51 animals operated on for BAOS, endoscopic exploration and systematic histologic examination of the upper GI tract and combination of medical treatment of GI disorders with upper airway surgery were shown to possibly reduce the risks of complications and improve the prognosis of these animals (Poncet *et al.* 2006). This study did not report any cases of aspiration bronchopneumonia in the 6 months after their medical and surgical treatment.

The persistence of inspiratory noise is commonly described, with some animals remaining dyspneic or with delayed onset of relapsing dyspnea. One study reported that 73.9% of dogs always present with snoring in the postoperative phase and that 21.7% remain dyspneic (Torrez and Hunt 2006).

One explanation is the persistence of pharyngeal obstruction by the **residual soft palate**. Indeed, a recent study on the conformation of the soft palate using CT confirmed the presence of excessive thickness of the soft palate in these animals (Grand and Bureau 2011). A histologic study in brachycephalic dogs confirmed this study by demonstrating features such as thickened superficial epithelium, extensive edema of the connective tissue, mucous gland hyperplasia, and several muscular alterations (Pichetto *et al.* 2011). This excessive thickness in the soft palate had already been highlighted (Poncet *et al.* 2006), and techniques to thin the soft palate have been proposed (Dupre *et al.* 2005; Findji and Dupre 2008; Dunie-Merigot *et al.* 2010). No oropharyngeal disorders were reported in either of these studies. Other authors advised sectioning a larger portion of the soft palate than previously described (Brdecka *et al.* 2008). In the author's opinion, shortening the soft palate so that its free border lies at the tip of the epiglottis, as is recommended as the "conventional" palatoplasty, may be insufficient and could lead to potential residual signs.

The protrusion of the ethmoidal turbinates in the nasopharyngeal duct and the presence of distorted ethmoidal turbinates within the nasal cavities may have a role to play in the persistence of respiratory signs (nasal snoring). Pugs appear to be particularly predisposed to this type of anomaly (Ginn *et al.* 2008). Laser-assisted turbinectomy is the only technique described to date with the objective of reducing resistance to airflow through the nasal cavities (Oechtering *et al.* 2007).

The diagnosis of **laryngeal collapse** complicates the prognosis in these animals. The collapse seems to appear progressively over time after chronic respiratory obstruction even though puppies can also show this type of anomaly (Pink *et al.* 2006). In the more severe cases, the corniculate processes collapse, and laryngomalacia becomes apparent (often in pugs). If palatoplasty and rhinoplasty do not produce sufficient clinical improvement, surgical alternatives are limited. Partial laryngoplasty could be associated with high mortality rates and significant risks of aspiration pneumonia. Permanent tracheostomy can be proposed as a last resort in these animals.

References

Brdecka, D.J., Rawlings, C.A., Perry, A.C., et al. (2008) Use of an electrothermal, feedback-controlled, bipolar sealing device for resection of the elongated portion of the soft palate in dogs with obstructive upper airway disease. *Journal of the American Veterinary Medical Association* 233, 1265-1269.

Ducarouge, B. (2002) Le syndrome obstructif des voies respiratoires supérieures chez les chiens brachycéphales. Etudes clinique à propos de 27 cas. Doctoral thesis. Lyon, France; p. 142.

Dunie-Merigot, A., Bouvy, B., Poncet, C. (2010) Comparative use of CO laser, diode laser and monopolar electrocautery for resection of the soft palate in dogs with brachycephalic airway obstructive syndrome. *Veterinary Record* 167, 700-704.

Dupre, G., Findji, L., Poncet, C. (2005) The folded flap palatoplasty: a new technique for treatment of elongated soft palate in dogs. 14th Annual Scientific Meeting of European College of Veterinary Surgeons. Marcy L'Etoile, France, p. 3.

Fasanella, F.J., Shivley, J.M., Wardlaw, J.L., et al. (2010) Brachycephalic airway obstructive syndrome in dogs: 90 cases (1991-2008). *Journal of the American Veterinary Medical Association* 237, 1048-1051.

Findji, L., Dupre, G. (2008) Folded flap palatoplasty for treatment of elongated soft palates in 55 dogs. *Wien Tierärztl Mschr* 95, 56-63.

Ginn, J.A., Kumar, M.S., McKiernan, B.C., et al. (2008) Nasopharyngeal turbinates in brachycephalic dogs and cats. *Journal of the American Animal Hospital Association* 44, 243-249.

Grand, J.G., Bureau, S. (2011) Structural characteristics of the soft palate and meatus nasopharyngeus in brachycephalic and non-brachycephalic dogs analysed by CT. *Journal of Small Animal Practice* 52, 232-239.

Hoareau, G.L., Mellema, M.S., Silverstein, D.C. (2011) Indication, management, and outcome of brachycephalic dogs requiring mechanical ventilation. *Journal of Veterinary Emergency and Critical Care* 21,226-235.

Oechtering, G., Hueber, J., Kiefer, I. (2007) Laser-assisted turbinectomy (LATE)—A novel approach to brachycephalic airway syndrome. *Veterinary Surgery* 36, E11.

Pichetto, M., Arrighi, S., Roccabianca, P., et al. (2011) The anatomy of the dog soft palate. ii. histological evaluation of the caudal soft palate in brachycephalic breeds with grade i brachycephalic airway obstructive syndrome. *Anatomical Record* 294, 1267-1272.

Pink, J.J., Doyle, R.S., Hughes, J.M., et al. (2006) Laryngeal collapse in seven brachycephalic puppies. *Journal of Small Animal Practice* 47, 131-135.

Poncet, C.M., Dupre, G.P., Freiche, V.G., et al. (2005) Prevalence of gastrointestinal tract lesions in 73 brachycephalic dogs with upper respiratory syndrome. *Journal of Small Animal Practice* 46, 273-279.

Poncet, C.M., Dupre, G.P., Freiche, V.G., et al. (2006) Long-term results of upper respiratory syndrome surgery and gastrointestinal tract medical treatment in 51 brachycephalic dogs. *Journal of Small Animal Practice* 47, 137-142.

Riecks, T.W., Birchard, S.J., Stephens, J.A. (2007) Surgical correction of brachycephalic syndrome in dogs: 62 cases (1991-2004). *Journal of the American Veterinary Medical Association* 230, 1324-1328.

Senn, D., Sigrist, N., Forterre, F., et al. (2011) Retrospective evaluation of postoperative nasotracheal tubes for oxygen supplementation in dogs following surgery for brachycephalic syndrome: 36 cases (2003-2007). *Journal of Veterinary Emergency and Critical Care* 21, 261-267.

Torrez, C.V., Hunt, G.B. (2006) Results of surgical correction of abnormalities associated with brachycephalic airway obstruction syndrome in dogs in Australia. *Journal of Small Animal Practice* 47, 150-154.

25 Surgical Management of Laryngeal Paralysis

Gert ter Haar

ENT, Brachycephaly and Audiology Clinic, Royal Veterinary College, North Mymms, Hatfield, Herts, UK

The larynx is a complex cartilaginous organ that serves many functions but is primarily used to separate the respiratory tract from the digestive tract. The intrinsic and extrinsic muscles of the cricoid, thyroid, and paired arytenoid cartilages and the epiglottis interact under the control of the neuromuscular system of the larynx to move the larynx in swallowing, protect the lower airways (coughing), facilitate and regulate the respiratory airflow, and vocalize.

Therefore, surgeons must be thoroughly aware of the potential effects on all of these functions when performing surgery on the larynx. A perturbation of any of these important tasks may have a marked impact on a patient. Some laryngeal procedures have an expected set of sequelae, but unexpected complications related to a surgical intervention are not uncommon either, especially when treating laryngeal trauma or neoplasia. However, laryngeal surgery in dogs is most commonly performed for acquired and sometimes for congenital laryngeal paralysis (Harvey and Venker-van Haagen 1975; Venker-van Haagen et al. 1978; Amis et al. 1986; Venker-van Haagen 1992; Nelson 1993; Holt and Harvey 1994; Monnet 2003; Mercurio 2011).

Various surgical treatment methods for laryngeal paralysis have been described, including bilateral arytenoid lateralization, unilateral arytenoid lateralization (UAL), partial arytenoidectomy, unilateral and bilateral ventriculocordectomy, and castellated laryngofissure (Harvey and O'Brien 1982; Rosin and Greenwood 1982; Gourley et al. 1983; Harvey 1983; White 1989; Burbridge et al. 1991; Ross et al. 1991; Lozier and Pope 1992; Nelson 1993; Trout et al. 1994; McCarthy 1996; Alsup et al. 1997; Gilson 1998; Holt 1998; LaHue 1998; Smith 1998; Griffiths et al. 2001; Demetriou and Kirby 2003; Snelling and Edwards 2003; Schofield et al. 2007). Neuromuscular pedicle grafts have been investigated in an attempt to restore the normal arytenoid abduction mechanism, but the technique is not useful in clinical practice (Greenfield et al. 1988; Payne et al. 1990; Monnet 2003; Mercurio 2011). UAL is currently the standard and recommended treatment for canine laryngeal paralysis (MacPhail and Monnet 2001; Bureau and Monnet 2002; Snelling and Edwards 2003; Hammel et al. 2006; Greenberg et al. 2007a; White 2009; Mercurio 2011). It involves fixation of the arytenoid cartilage to either the thyroid (TAL) or cricoid (CAL) cartilage using one or two strands of nonabsorbable suture material. Modifications with and without cricothyroid disarticulation and interarytenoid band transection are described, but all techniques lead to the same degree of clinical success and have comparable complication rates. The reported complication rate with UAL is high, ranging from 10% to 58% (White 1989; McCarthy 1996; Alsup et al. 1997; Gilson 1998;

LaHue 1998; Griffiths et al. 2001; MacPhail and Monnet 2001; Monnet 2003; Snelling and Edwards 2003; Hammel et al. 2006). Potential perioperative complications associated with surgery for laryngeal paralysis include hemorrhage, penetration into the laryngeal lumen, esophageal laceration, and cartilage laceration and fracture. Postoperative complications include postoperative edema, aspiration pneumonia and coughing and gagging when eating and drinking, seroma formation, and persistent upper airway obstruction (continued dyspnea and stridor). Voice change is reported in all cases after surgery and should be considered to be a normal sequela to the surgical treatment of laryngeal paralysis. Arytenoidectomy, ventriculocordectomy, and castellated laryngofissure are all associated with an unacceptable high complication rate, including all complications mentioned earlier, transverse laryngeal webbing and stenosis and are not recommended. UAL is a technically challenging procedure and should only be performed by an experienced surgeon with thorough knowledge of the regional anatomy and physiology who performs the procedure on a regular basis.

Hemorrhage

See also Chapter 12.

Hemorrhage during UAL is usually mild and easily controlled with pressure and judicious use of electrocoagulation. However, meticulous hemostasis is important to prevent submucosal bleeding and subsequent airway diameter compromise (Monnet 2003; Mercurio 2011). It is also important with respect to maintenance of proper visualization of the surgical field and dissection of the arytenoid. Avoiding arterial hypertension by choosing a fitting anaesthesia protocol is helpful in minimizing diffuse bleeding after cutting the thyropharyngeus and dorsal cricoarytenoid muscles. Venous bleeding may be minimized with proper patient positioning, ensuring avoidance of compression on the jugular veins. Continued hemorrhage after surgery can lead to aspiration of blood into the lower airways, causing pneumonia.

Penetration into the laryngeal lumen

Etiopathogenesis

Penetration into the laryngeal lumen is most likely during disarticulation and dissection of the cricoarytenoid joint and disarticulation of the interarytenoid band.

Complications in Small Animal Surgery, First Edition. Edited by Dominique Griffon and Annick Hamaide.
© 2016 John Wiley & Sons, Inc. Published 2016 by John Wiley & Sons, Inc.
Companion website: www.wiley.com/go/griffon/complications

178

Diagnosis

Inadvertent penetration into the laryngeal lumen may be visible during surgery or cause intraluminal hemorrhage and edema after surgery and clinical signs of upper airway obstruction. Fresh blood visible during throat inspection during or after surgery is indicative of penetration of the mucosa. Large perforations with severe damage to laryngeal mucosa may lead to granulomatous tissue formation, stenosis, and webbing.

Treatment

- Small lacerations can be left to heal by second intention healing.
- Large lacerations should be carefully sutured.

If inadvertent penetration into the laryngeal lumen causes laryngeal hemorrhage and edema:

- Closely monitor animals for clinical signs of upper airway obstruction.
- Avoid unnecessary manipulations and stress.
- Provide supplemental oxygen.
- Use tranquilizers and anxiolytic drugs when indicated.
- Administer corticosteroids.

Prevention

Inadvertent penetration into the laryngeal lumen is prevented by thorough knowledge of local anatomy, careful surgical technique, and the use of delicate instruments.

Esophageal laceration

Esophageal laceration has been reported in one dog that underwent a modified cricoidarytenoid lateralization procedure in which no cricoarytenoid disarticulation was performed (Payne *et al.* 1990). The laceration occurred during dissection of the cricopharyngeal and thyropharyngeal muscles, which are just dorsal to the esophagus. The laceration was diagnosed during surgery and closed with sutures after copious lavage. Despite antibiotic treatment, the dog died 8 days after surgery from aspiration pneumonia. Although an extremely rare complication, identification of the esophagus and avoidance of it during dissection are recommended.

Cartilage laceration and fracture

Etiopathogenesis

Laryngeal cartilage laceration and fracture can occur:

- Upon passage of or tying of the CA or TA sutures when the arytenoid cartilages are appreciably mineralized
- Upon improper handling of the thyroid cartilage and manipulation of it using grasping forceps during exposition of the larynx
- In small animals, brachycephalic breeds and cats with weak laryngeal cartilages

Diagnosis

Fragmentation of the cartilage can be noticed during tying of the sutures or manipulation of the cartilages during surgery. Breaking or pull-out of the suture after surgery will lead to recurrence of the initial signs of laryngeal paralysis.

Treatment

- In case of fragmentation of the arytenoid or suture pull-out, perform arytenoid lateralization on the contralateral side (Monnet 2003).

- Small lacerations of the thyroid do not need any repair; large fragments or devitalized tissue need to be removed.

Prevention

- Fragmentation of the arytenoid is less likely to occur if the arytenoid is pulled into position toward the caudal thyroid or cricoid after dissection and preplacement of the sutures using an Allis forceps on the remnants of the cricoarytenoid dorsal muscle rather than pulling on the sutures themselves.
- Use delicate forceps and gentle tissue handling when manipulating the laryngeal cartilages.
- Use noncutting needles and small sized suture material in weak cartilages.

Postoperative edema

Etiopathogenesis

Tissues of the larynx are extremely sensitive to handling, and even minimal manipulation can cause considerable edema. Swelling causes increased airway resistance and increased negative pressure during inspiration, thereby contributing to further edema and airway obstruction. Postoperative edema may be related to:

- Airway swelling from surgical trauma to the laryngeal tissues
- Airway swelling related to the anesthesia technique, intubation, and inflation of the cuff
- Postoperative panting, tachypnea, or dyspnea as a result of inadequate opening of the rima glottidis

Diagnosis

Clinical signs of laryngeal inflammation and swelling vary with severity of the swelling:

- Up to 50% of the airway can be compromised without causing obvious clinical signs (Lozier and Pope 1992).
- Mild swelling may cause gagging, retching, and intermittent coughing, especially when the animal drinks water. In some animals, an obstructive breathing pattern, characterized by slow inspiratory phase followed by a rapid expiratory phase and laryngeal stridor, can be detected (Lozier and Pope 1992).
- More severe swelling may cause anxiousness or agitation and pronounced inspiratory dyspnea, stridor, increased respiratory rate, and open mouth breathing. The forelimbs may be abducted during breathing, and animals may become hyperthermic (Gourley *et al.* 1983; McCarthy 1996).
- Pulmonary edema can develop in animals with upper airway obstruction because of abnormal reduction in intrathoracic negative pressure during inspiration and may be detected on thoracic radiographs (Smith *et al.* 1986; McCarthy 1996).

Hypoxemia is difficult to diagnose on mucous membrane color because cyanosis is not clinically detectable until arterial pO2 is less than 60 mm Hg. Determination of arterial blood gases quantitates blood oxygenation and true hypoxemia. In stressed patients, noninvasive monitoring of saturated oxygen level by pulse oxymetry is helpful as well.

Treatment

- Use tranquilizers and anxiolytic drugs when indicated,
- Administer corticosteroids,
- In severe cases of laryngeal edema, a temporary tracheostomy should be performed. Silastic tracheal cannulas or stainless steel cannulas with an inner cannula that can be removed and

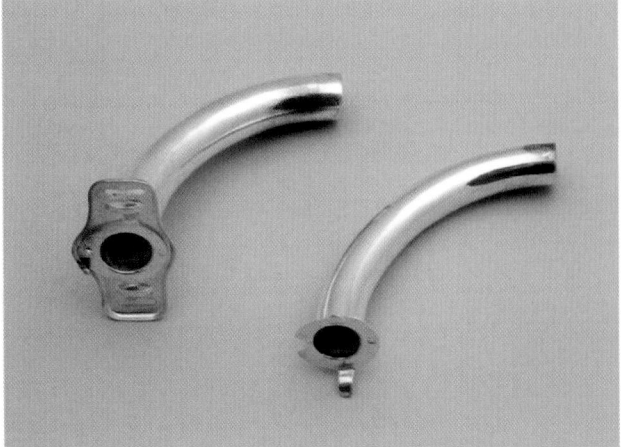

Figure 25.1 Stainless steel tracheal cannulas. A stainless steel outer and inner tracheal cannula is shown. Several sizes are available.

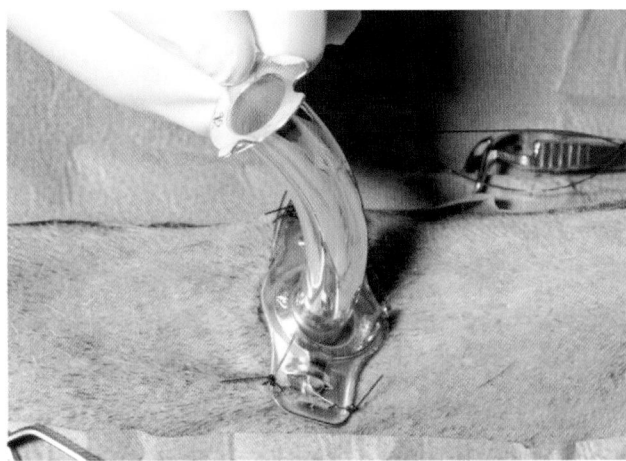

Figure 25.3 Temporary tracheostomy. The outer cannula is sutured to the skin with four sutures, after which the inner cannula can be inserted.

cleaned are preferred (Figure 25.1). A transverse skin incision of approximately 2 cm is made over the trachea at the midpoint between the larynx and the thoracic inlet. The subcutaneous fat and the left and right sternothyroid and sternohyoid muscles are divided in the midline by blunt dissection (Figure 25.2). The ligament between two adjacent rings is incised, and small forceps are placed on one of the tracheal rings beside the incision. A round piece of tracheal cartilage and intercartilage ligament is removed to produce an opening of the same size and shape as the tracheal tube or cannula. The oropharyngeal endotracheal tube is removed and replaced by the endotracheal cannula that is inserted through the tracheal window. The cannula is sutured to the skin with four sutures (Figure 25.3). In addition, two cotton ribbons are attached to the wings of the tracheal cannula and tied around the neck (Figure 25.4). Silastic cannulas have an inner cannula that should be cleaned every 2 hours. After the cannula is removed, the tracheostomy wound is not sutured but left open to heal spontaneously.

- Supplemental oxygen should be provided for all animals with clinically significant laryngeal edema by means of:
  - Nasal tube: Advantages are easy access to the patient without interrupting oxygen flow, low costs, and ready availability for all patient sizes,
  - Enrichment of inspired air with oxygen by partly closing an Elizabethan collar with transparent film, leaving the back of the collar open for administration of oxygen and air circulation
  - Oxygen cage: humidification of inspired oxygen is important to prevent drying of the mucous membranes of the respiratory tract.

Prevention
- Having detailed knowledge of the regional anatomy and experience with the procedure
- Meticulous surgical technique: Gentle tissue handling is important, and stay sutures should be used rather than forceps for tissue retraction whenever possible. Excessive use of electrocoagulation should be avoided as well as inadvertent penetration into the laryngeal lumen.

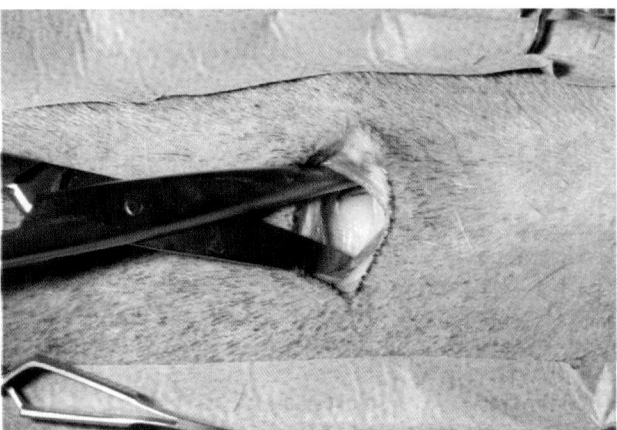

Figure 25.2 Temporary tracheostomy. A transverse skin incision midway between the larynx and the thoracic inlet has been made followed by blunt dissection toward the trachea.

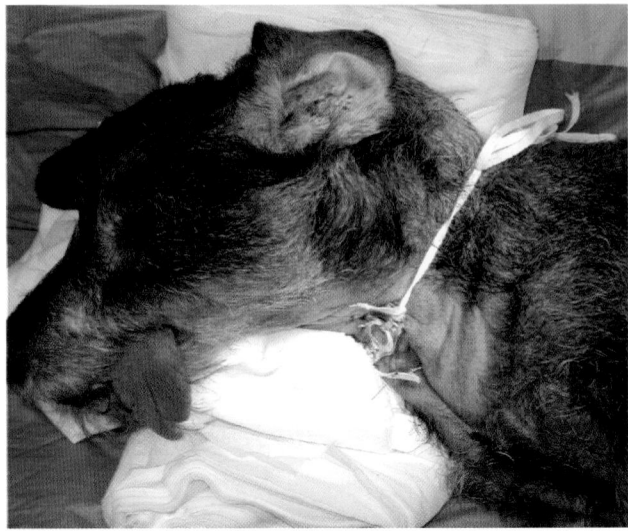

Figure 25.4 Temporary tracheostomy. Two cotton ribbons are attached to the wings of the tracheal cannula and tied around the neck.

- Administration of corticosteroids at induction of surgery (e.g., dexamethasone sodium phosphate, 0.1–1.0 mg/kg intravenously) has been advocated to help reduce inflammation (Mercurio 2011). There is no evidence that corticosteroids need to be continued for more than 24 to 48 hours after surgery.

Aspiration pneumonia and coughing and gagging with eating and drinking

Etiopathogenesis
The most common complication after UAL is aspiration pneumonia, occurring in 18% to 28% of dogs after surgery (Gaber *et al.* 1985; Burbridge 1995; Alsup *et al.* 1997; Gilson 1998; MacPhail and Monnet 2001; Hammel *et al.* 2006; Kogan *et al.* 2008; Mercurio 2011). Coughing and gagging, especially after eating or drinking, are common sequelae of arytenoid lateralization and are probably associated with chronic laryngitis or minor incidents of aspiration. Aspiration pneumonia results from inhalation of oropharyngeal or gastrointestinal contents into the respiratory tract, causing chemical, bacteriologic, and immunologic damage to the airways. Damage to the cranial laryngeal nerve, responsible for sensory innervation of the laryngeal mucosa during incision of the thyropharyngeal muscle, may predispose animals to aspiration pneumonia.

Diagnosis
- Clinical signs of fever, depression, tachypnea or dyspnea, and moist cough
- High body temperature, tachypnea, increased pulmonary sounds on auscultation of the chest, and coughing upon palpation of the trachea or percussion of the lungs
- On thoracic radiographs, depending on the position of the animal when aspiration occurs (usually in lateral or dorsal recumbency), alveolar infiltrates can be seen in the dependent lung lobes.
- Cytology and culture and sensitivity testing of transtracheal aspirates or preferably bronchoalveolar lavage (McCarthy 1996; Jeffery *et al.* 2006; Kogan *et al.* 2008).

Treatment
- First-generation cephalosporins can be used pending culture and sensitivity results because they have excellent efficacy against both gram-positive and gram-negative aerobes in addition to anaerobic bacteria. Alternatively, amoxicillin with clavulanic acid in combination with metronidazole can be used. Antibiotics should be continued for a minimum of 4 weeks or at least 10 days after thoracic radiographic findings indicate resolution of the pneumonia (McCarthy 1996; Kogan *et al.* 2008).
- Fluid therapy
- Oxygen supplementation
- Coupage
- Nebulization

Prevention
- Control intraoperative and postoperative hemorrhage.
- Maintain a properly inflated endotracheal tube cuff at all times during the procedure.
- Avoid damage to the cranial laryngeal nerve during dissection (Figure 25.5).
- Suction all fluids and debris from both the oropharynx and nasopharynx at the completion of surgery.
- Place the animal in a head-down position during recovery.

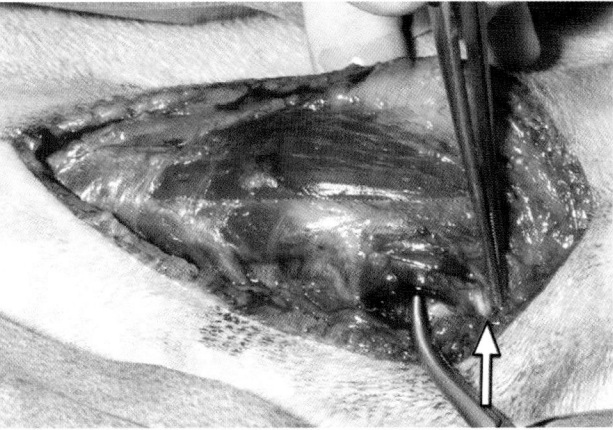

Figure 25.5 Thyroid arytenoid lateralization (TAL). Left lateral view of a patient in dorsal recumbency during TAL. The head is on the right side of the photograph. When incising the thyropharyngeal muscle, care should be taken not to damage the cranial laryngeal nerve (arrow).

- Delay removal of the endotracheal tube until well-developed swallowing and cough reflexes are present. When the endotracheal tube is removed, the cuff should be kept partially inflated.
- Avoid excessive abduction of the arytenoids.
- Observe per os the size of the laryngeal opening during surgery (Weinstein and Weisman 2010). Unfortunately, intraoperative visualization of the larynx requires removal of the endotracheal tube, causing a temporary loss of airway control.

Seroma formation
Seroma formation after arytenoid lateralization is common and is caused by dead space formation as a result of blunt dissection in approaching the thyroid cartilage in a highly mobile area. The diagnosis is made on palpation of a soft tissue swelling at the surgical site in absence of clinical signs of infection and upon fine-needle aspiration of the fluid. Small accumulations of fluid usually resolve without treatment, but large seromas require drainage. Seromas can be prevented by the use of atraumatic technique, meticulous attention to hemostasis, and careful tissue apposition with the obliteration of dead space. Closing the subcutaneous space in two layers might help preventing seroma formation.

Persistent upper airway obstruction

Etiopathogenesis
Unilateral arytenoid lateralization procedures involve placement of extraluminal sutures between the muscular process of the arytenoid cartilage and the caudodorsal edge of either the thyroid cartilage or cricoid cartilage (White 1989; Lozier and Pope 1992; Venker-van Haagen 1992; LaHue 1998; Griffiths *et al.* 2001; Bureau and Monnet 2002; Demetriou and Kirby 2003). The need for cricothyroid, cricoarytenoid, and interarytenoid disarticulations is still open for debate, but they are advised by this author. Unilateral CAL or TAL restores normal pattern of breathing in dogs having experimental laryngeal paralysis, significantly improves arterial oxygen tension, and results in an excellent clinical outcome in more than 90% of reported cases (Harvey and Venker-van Haagen 1975; Love *et al.* 1987; White 1989; McCarthy 1996; LaHue 1998; Smith 1998;

Snelling and Edwards 2003; Hammel *et al.* 2006; Mercurio 2011). However, little or no improvement is reported in about 10% of dogs, and most dogs have at least some degree of persistent respiratory stridor (White 1989). Failure to alleviate clinical signs may be caused by:
- Loss of arytenoid abduction because of suture pull-out
- Inadequate arytenoid abduction because of insufficient suture tension
- Limitations of the surgical procedure itself.

Diagnosis
Careful laryngoscopic examination should be performed on dogs having continued clinical signs after arytenoid lateralization to determine the cause. The diagnosis of adequate degree of arytenoid abduction is somewhat subjective, but arytenoid position should be similar to that recorded at surgery. Loss of arytenoid abduction suggests that the sutures have pulled out.

Treatment
Treatment of persistent clinical signs after arytenoid lateralization depends on the cause of the problem.
- Inadequate arytenoid abduction caused by cartilage fracture or suture pull-out requires arytenoid lateralization surgery on the opposite side.
- If insufficient suture tension is the cause of inadequate arytenoid abduction, the suture can be replaced and tightened further.
- If suture tension is sufficient but the glottic diameter remains inadequate, a bilateral procedure can be performed, but owners should be warned of the potential risk of aspiration pneumonia.
- Some animals with generalized neuromuscular disorders respond poorly despite apparently appropriate surgery. These animals can be treated with exercise restriction, environmental control, tranquilizers, and corticosteroids, but the prognosis is poor.

Prevention
Correct suture placement and tension are required to produce adequate arytenoid abduction and eliminate clinical signs. Good suture purchase must be obtained in the muscular process of the arytenoid cartilage, and excessive suture tension should be avoided (McCarthy 1996). Metallic suture material tends to cut through tissue, so monofilament nonabsorbable suture such as polypropylene is preferred (White 1989). CAL procedures that place sutures between the muscular process of the arytenoid cartilage and the caudodorsal edge of the cricoid cartilage more closely mimic the normal pull of the cricoarytenoideus dorsalis muscle and increase rima glottis diameter by approximately 200% (Payne *et al.* 1990; LaHue 1998; Demetriou and Kirby 2003; Greenberg *et al.* 2007a). TAL procedures require less dissection and can be performed more rapidly and still provide efficient caudolateralization while increasing the rima glottis diameter by approximately 140%. When sutures are placed through the muscular process of the arytenoid and the cuneiform process, a larger increase in rima glottis diameter can be achieved during TAL (Figure 25.6). Care has to be taken as not to overlateralize the arytenoid because this might predispose the animal to the development of aspiration pneumonia. With all UAL techniques, it is important to temporarily extubate the animal during surgery to confirm adequate arytenoid abduction by oral examination. It has been suggested that animals with severe cartilage calcification may not be appropriate candidates for UAL because it may not be possible to abduct the cartilages with sutures (McCarthy 1996).

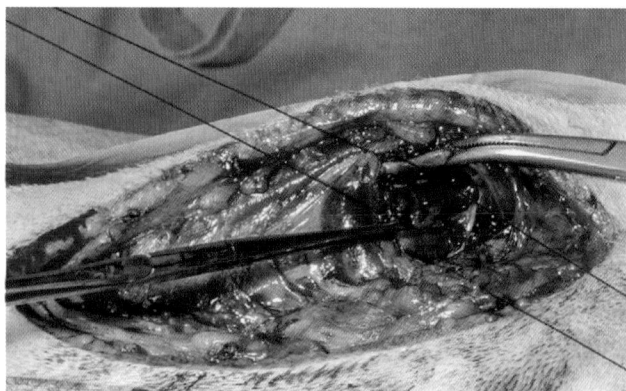

Figure 25.6 Thyroid arytenoid lateralization. Same view as in Figure 25.5. Two Prolene sutures have been placed—one through the caudal thyroid and the muscular process and one through the caudal thyroid (cranial to the other suture) and the cuneiform process of the arytenoid to maximize caudolateralization.

Relevant literature
The cause of laryngeal paralysis, the complexity of laryngeal and pharyngeal anatomy and physiology, and the effects of surgical techniques and perioperative care are all factors influencing the prognosis. Factors that were significantly associated with a higher risk of dying or of developing complications in one large study included age, temporary tracheostomy placement, concurrent respiratory tract abnormalities, concurrent esophageal disease, postoperative megaesophagus, concurrent neoplastic disease, and concurrent neurologic disease (MacPhail and Monnet 2001). Another study demonstrated that increasing familiarity with the technique favorably influenced the incidence of complications and the success rate (White 1989).

The most common and serious complication after UAL is aspiration pneumonia (McCarthy 1996; MacPhail and Monnet 2001; Hammel *et al.* 2006; Mercurio 2011). Aspiration is prevented in normal animals by closure of the rima glottis by the arytenoid cartilage and vocal fold adductors and by coverage of the rima glottis by the epiglottis during swallowing (Venker-van Haagen *et al.* 1978; Venker-van Haagen *et al.* 1986). Thus, the risk of aspiration pneumonia is high when the rima glottis diameter is mechanically increased beyond closure of epiglottis coverage by lateralization surgery, or because normal glottic closure during swallowing is dysfunctional as a result of laryngeal paralysis or surgery to correct it (damage to cranial laryngeal nerve) or underlying generalized neuromuscular disease.

Whereas CAL procedures increase the rima glottis diameter to a greater degree than TAL procedures do (200% versus 140% respectively), there is no difference reported between these two techniques with regards to development of aspiration pneumonia. In addition, there are no clinical studies available evaluating or demonstrating increased risk of aspiration pneumonia after cricothyroid, cricoarytenoid, and interarytenoid disarticulations during CAL or TAL. Dogs that underwent bilateral arytenoid lateralization however were significantly more likely to develop complications and significantly less likely to survive than were dogs that underwent UAL in one large study (MacPhail and Monnet 2001).

Recent studies show accumulative evidence that an underlying neuromuscular disease process is involved in the etiology of acquired laryngeal paralysis (Gabriel *et al.* 2006; Jeffery *et al.* 2006;

Shelton 2010; Thieman *et al.* 2010) Generalized neuromuscular disease that affects normal swallowing and airway protective mechanisms may significantly increase the risk of aspiration pneumonia (Mercurio 2011). A recent study prospectively evaluated esophageal dysfunction in dogs with idiopathic laryngeal paralysis using esophagrams evaluating oropharyngeal and esophageal function under fluoroscopic guidance (Stanley *et al.* 2010). Approximately 70% of dogs with idiopathic laryngeal paralysis were found to have some degree of esophageal dysfunction, with the cervical and cranial thoracic esophagus most notably affected. The degree of preoperative esophageal dysfunction was significantly higher in dogs that developed aspiration pneumonia after UAL (Stanley *et al.* 2010). It is therefore recommended that all dogs evaluated for suspected acquired laryngeal paralysis have a thorough clinical history taken regarding clinical signs consistent with esophageal dysfunction and undergo a complete neurologic examination prior to surgery (Mercurio 2011).

The surgical approach itself for either CAL or TAL lateralization should be considered as well, especially with respect to identification and protection of the cranial laryngeal nerve and the anatomy and physiology of the upper esophageal sphincter. The cranial laryngeal nerve courses over the cranial aspect of the thyropharyngeal muscle and innervates sensory receptors on the epiglottis and the luminal mucosa of the larynx. These receptors initiate the closure reflex of the glottis during swallowing and initiate the cough reflex in case of threatening aspiration (Venker-van Haagen *et al.* 1978, 1986). When the cranial sensory laryngeal nerve is traumatized during surgery, as a result of potential failure to elicit a proper cough reflex, these animals may be predisposed to aspiration pneumonia.

The upper esophageal sphincter is anatomically composed primarily of the cricopharyngeus and thyropharyngeus muscles and relaxes/opens during swallowing, vomiting, and eructation (Venker-van Haagen *et al.* 1986; Sivarao and Goyal 2000). After gastroesophageal reflux, this sphincter is the only remaining physical barrier against entry of the refluxate into the pharynx and potentially the larynx and airway (Sivarao and Goyal 2000; Shaker and Hogan 2000). As part of the surgical approach for UAL however, the thyropharyngeus muscle is routinely transected. The consequence of transecting this muscle on upper esophageal sphincter function has not been evaluated. Transection may impair its function as a sphincter and increase the risk of aspiration after surgery (Mercurio 2011). Another factor to consider with regards to impairment of upper esophageal sphincter function, is general anesthesia. The reported incidence of gastroesophageal reflux under general anesthesia varies from 17% to greater than 50% (Galatos and Raptopoulos 1995a, 1995b; Wilson *et al.* 2005; Wilson *et al.* 2006). In approximately 25% of patients under general anesthesia that develop gastroesophageal reflux, the refluxed contents reach the pharynx in sufficient quantity to place the patient at risk for aspiration (Wilson *et al.* 2006). In a prospective clinical trial, the use of high-dose metoclopramide resulted in a 54% reduction in the relative risk of developing gastroesophageal reflux (Wilson *et al.* 2006). Dogs undergoing surgical treatment for laryngeal paralysis and receiving metoclopramide perioperatively had a lower prevalence of aspiration pneumonia than did dogs that did not receive metoclopramide in a retrospective study (Greenberg *et al.* 2007b). Additional studies are needed to determine optimal dosing and long-term efficacy of perioperative metoclopramide use to reduce the prevalence of aspiration pneumonia after UAL (Greenberg *et al.* 2007b).

References

Alsup, J.C., Greenfield, C.L., Hungerford, L.L., et al. (1997) Comparison of unilateral arytenoid lateralization and ventral ventriculocordectomy for the treatment of experimentally induced laryngeal paralysis in dogs. *The Canadian Veterinary Journal* 38 (5), 287-293.

Amis, T.C., Smith, M.M., Gaber, C.E., et al. (1986) Upper airway obstruction in canine laryngeal paralysis. *American Journal of Veterinary Research* 47 (5), 1007-1010.

Burbridge, H.M. (1995) A review of laryngeal paralysis in dogs. *British Veterinary Journal* 151 (1), 71-82.

Burbridge, H.M., Goulden, B.E., Jones, B.R. (1991) An experimental evaluation of castellated laryngofissure and bilateral arytenoid lateralisation for the relief of laryngeal paralysis in dogs. *Australian Veterinary Journal* 68, 268.

Bureau, S., Monnet, E. (2002) Effects of suture tension and surgical approach during unilateral arytenoid lateralization on the rima glottidis in the canine larynx. *Veterinary Surgery* 31 (6), 589-595.

Demetriou, J.L., Kirby, B.M. (2003) The effect of two modifications of unilateral arytenoid lateralization on rima glottidis area in dogs. *Veterinary Surgery* 32 (1), 62-68.

Gaber, C.E., Amis, T.C., LeCouteur, R.A. (1985) Laryngeal paralysis in dogs: a review of 23 cases. *Journal of the American Veterinary Medical Association* 186 (4), 377-380.

Gabriel, A., Poncelet, L., Van Ham, L., et al. (2006) Laryngeal paralysis-polyneuropathy complex in young related Pyrenean mountain dogs. *Journal of Small Animal Practice* 47 (3), 144-149.

Galatos, A.D., Raptopoulos, D. (1995a) Gastro-oesophageal reflux during anaesthesia in the dog: the effect of age, positioning and type of surgical procedure. *The Veterinary Record* 137 (20), 513-516.

Galatos, A.D., Raptopoulos, D. (1995b) Gastro-oesophageal reflux during anaesthesia in the dog: the effect of preoperative fasting and premedication. *The Veterinary Record* 137 (19), 479-483.

Gilson, S.D. (1998) Treatment of Laryngeal paralysis with arythenothyroid lateralization. In Bojrab, M.J. (ed.) *Current Techniques in Small Animal Surgery*, 4th edn. Williams & Wilkins, Baltimore, pp. 365-370.

Gourley, I.M., Paul, H., Gregory, C. (1983) Castellated laryngofissure and vocal fold resection for the treatment of laryngeal paralysis in the dog. *Journal of the American Veterinary Medical Association* 182 (10), 1084-1086.

Greenberg, M.J., Bureau, S., Monnet, E. (2007a) Effects of suture tension during unilateral cricoarytenoid lateralization on canine laryngeal resistance in vitro. *Veterinary Surgery* 36 (6), 526-532.

Greenberg, M.J., Reems, M.R., Monnet, E. (2007b) Use of perioperative metoclopramide in dogs undergoing surgical treatment of laryngeal paralysis: 43 cases (1999-2006). *Veterinary Surgery* 36, pp. E11.

Greenfield, C.L., Walshaw, R., Kumar, K., et al. (1988) Neuromuscular pedicle graft for restoration of arytenoid abductor function in dogs with experimentally induced laryngeal hemiplegia. *American Journal of Veterinary Research* 49 (8), 1360-1366.

Griffiths, L.G., Sullivan, M., Reid, S.W. (2001) A comparison of the effects of unilateral thyroarytenoid lateralization versus cricoarytenoid laryngoplasty on the area of the rima glottidis and clinical outcome in dogs with laryngeal paralysis. *Veterinary surgery* 30 (4), 359-365.

Hammel, S.P., Hottinger, H.A., Novo, R.E. (2006) Postoperative results of unilateral arytenoid lateralization for treatment of idiopathic laryngeal paralysis in dogs: 39 cases (1996-2002). *Journal of the American Veterinary Medical Association* 228 (8), 1215-1220.

Harvey, C.E. (1983) Partial laryngectomy in the dog. II. Immediate increase in glottis area obtained compared with other laryngeal procedures. *Veterinary Surgery* 12, 197.

Harvey, C.E., Venker-van Haagen, A.J. (1975) Surgical management of pharyngeal and laryngeal airway obstruction in the dog. *The Veterinary Clinics of North America: Small Animal Practice* 5 (3), 515-535.

Harvey, C.E., O'Brien, J.A. (1982) Treatment of laryngeal paralysis in dogs by partial laryngectomy. *J Am Anim Hosp Assoc* 18, 551.

Holt, D.E. (1998) Treatment of Laryngeal paralysis by bilateral ventriculocordectomy. In Bojrab, M.J. (ed.) *Current Techniques in Small Animal Surgery*, 4th edn. Williams & Wilkins, Baltimore, pp. 362-365.

Holt, D.E., Harvey, C.E. (1994) Idiopathic laryngeal paralysis: results of treatment by bilateral vocal fold resection in 40 dogs. *Journal of the American Animal Hospital Association* 30, 389-395.

Jeffery, N.D., Talbot, C.E., Smith, P.M., et al. (2006) Acquired idiopathic laryngeal paralysis as a prominent feature of generalised neuromuscular disease in 39 dogs. *Veterinary Record* 158 (1), 17.

Kogan, D.A., Johnson, L.R., Sturges, B.K., et al. (2008) Etiology and clinical outcome in dogs with aspiration pneumonia: 88 cases (2004-2006). *Journal of the American Veterinary Medical Association* 233 (11), 1748-1755.

LaHue, T.R. (1998) Treatment of laryngeal paralysis with unilateral cricoarythenoid laryngoplasty. In Bojrab, M.J. (ed.) *Current Techniques in Small Animal Surgery*, 4th edn. Williams & Wilkins, Baltimore, pp. 370-374.

Love, S., Waterman, A.E., Lane, J.G. (1987) The assessment of corrective surgery for canine laryngeal paralysis by blood gas analysis: a review of thirty-five cases. *Journal of Small Animal Practice* 28, 597.

Lozier, S., Pope, E. (1992) Effects of arytenoid abduction and modified castellated laryngofissure on the rima glottidis in canine cadavers. *Veterinary Surgery* 21 (3), 195-200.

MacPhail, C.M., Monnet, E. (2001) Outcome of and postoperative complications in dogs undergoing surgical treatment of laryngeal paralysis: 140 cases (1985-1998). *Journal of the American Veterinary Medical Association* 218 (12), 1949-1956.

McCarthy, R.J. (1996) Surgery of the head & neck; surgical management of laryngeal paralysis. In Lipowitz, A.J., Caywood, D.D., Cann, C.C., et al. (eds.) *Complications in Small Animals Surgery*. Lippincott, Williams & Wilkins, Philadelphia, pp. 176-182.

Mercurio, A. (2011) Complications of upper airway surgery in companion animals. *The Veterinary Clinics of North America: Small Animal Practice* 41 (5), 969-980.

Monnet, E. (2003) Laryngeal paralysis and devocalization. In Slatter, D. (ed.) *Textbook of Small Animal Surgery*, 3rd edn. Saunders, Philadelphia, pp. 837-845.

Nelson, W.A. (1993) Upper respiratory system. In Slatter, D. (ed.) *Textbook of Small Animal Surgery*, 2nd edn. Saunders, Philadelphia, pp. 733-776.

Payne, J.T., Martin, R.A., Rigg, D.L. (1990) Abductor muscle prosthesis for correction of laryngeal paralysis in 10 dogs and one cat. *Journal of the American Animal Hospital Association* 26, 599.

Rosin, E., Greenwood, K. (1982) Bilateral arytenoid cartilage lateralization for laryngeal paralysis in the dog. *Journal of the American Veterinary Medical Association* 180 (5), 515-518.

Ross, J.T., Matthiesen, D.T., Noone, K.E., et al. (1991) Complications and long-term results after partial laryngectomy for the treatment of idiopathic laryngeal paralysis in 45 dogs. *Veterinary Surgery* 20 (3), 169-173.

Schofield, D.M., Norris, J., Sadanaga, K.K. (2007) Bilateral thyroarytenoid cartilage lateralization and vocal fold excision with mucosoplasty for treatment of idiopathic laryngeal paralysis: 67 dogs (1998-2005). *Veterinary Surgery* 36 (6), 519-525.

Shaker, R., Hogan, W.J. (2000) Reflex-mediated enhancement of airway protective mechanisms. *The American Journal of Medicine* 108 (Suppl. 4a), 8S-14S.

Shelton, G.D. (2010) Acquired laryngeal paralysis in dogs: evidence accumulating for a generalized neuromuscular disease. *Veterinary Surgery* 39 (2), 137-138.

Sivarao, D.V., Goyal, R.K. (2000) Functional anatomy and physiology of the upper esophageal sphincter. *The American Journal of Medicine* 108 (Suppl. 4a), 27S-37S.

Smith, M.M. (1998) Treatment of laryngeal paralysis with modified castellated laryngofissure. In Bojrab, M. (ed.) *Current Techniques in Small Animal Surgery*, 4th edn. Williams & Wilkins, Baltimore, pp. 375-376.

Smith, M.M., Gourley, I.M., Kurpershoek, C.J., et al. (1986) Evaluation of a modified castellated laryngofissure for alleviation of upper airway obstruction in dogs with laryngeal paralysis. *Journal of the American Veterinary Medical Association* 188 (11), 1279-1283.

Snelling, S.R., Edwards, G.A. (2003) A retrospective study of unilateral arytenoid lateralisation in the treatment of laryngeal paralysis in 100 dogs (1992-2000). *Australian Veterinary Journal* 81 (8), 464-468.

Stanley, B.J., Hauptman, J.G., Fritz, M.C., et al. (2010) Esophageal dysfunction in dogs with idiopathic laryngeal paralysis: a controlled cohort study. *Veterinary Surgery* 39 (2), 139-149.

Thieman, K.M., Krahwinkel, D.J., Sims, M.H., et al. (2010) Histopathological confirmation of polyneuropathy in 11 dogs with laryngeal paralysis. *Journal of the American Animal Hospital Association* 46 (3), 161-167.

Trout, N.J., Harpster, N.K., Berg, J. (1994) Long-term results of unilateral ventriculocordectomy and partial arytenoidectomy for the treatment of laryngeal paralysis in 60 dogs. *Journal of the American Animal Hospital Association* 30, 401-407.

Venker-van Haagen, A.J. (1992) Diseases of the larynx. *Veterinary Clinics North America: Small Animal Practice* 22, 1155.

Venker-van Haagen, A.J., Hartman, W., Goedegebuure, S.A. (1978) Spontaneous laryngeal paralysis in young Bouviers. *Journal of the American Animal Hospital Association* 14, 714-720.

Venker-van Haagen, A.J., Hartman, W., Wolvekamp, W.T. (1986) Contributions of the glossopharyngeal nerve and the pharyngeal branch of the vagus nerve to the swallowing process in dogs. *American Journal of Veterinary Research* 47 (6), 1300-1307.

Weinstein, J., Weisman, D. (2010) Intraoperative evaluation of the larynx following unilateral arytenoid lateralization for acquired idiopathic laryngeal paralysis in dogs. *Journal of the American Animal Hospital Association* 46 (4), 241-248.

White, R.A. (2009) Canine laryngeal surgery: time to rethink? *Veterinary Surgery* 38 (4), 432-433.

White, R.A.S. (1989) Unilateral arytenoid lateralisation: an assessment of technique and long term results in 62 dogs with laryngeal paralysis. *Journal of Small Animal Practice* 30, 543-549.

Wilson, D.V., Evans, A.T., Miller, R. (2005) Effects of preanesthetic administration of morphine on gastroesophageal reflux and regurgitation during anesthesia in dogs. *American Journal of Veterinary Research* 66 (3), 386-390.

Wilson, D.V., Evans, A.T., Mauer, W.A. (2006) Influence of metoclopramide on gastroesophageal reflux in anesthetized dogs. *American Journal of Veterinary Research* 67 (1), 26-31.

26 Thyroidectomy

Chad Schmiedt

Small Animal Surgery, Department of Small Animal Medicine and Surgery, College of Veterinary Medicine, University of Georgia, Athens, GA, USA

In dogs, thyroidectomy is most frequently indicated for removal of nonfunctional thyroid carcinoma. In cats, thyroidectomy is indicated for removal of functional thyroid adenomas, although other treatment modalities have largely replaced thyroidectomy in the treatment of feline hyperthyroidism.

Anesthetic risks of thyrotoxicosis

Definition

Thyrotoxicosis is defined as having systemic pathologies secondary to elevated thyroid hormone concentrations. The major systemic consequences of thyrotoxicosis are increased basal metabolic rate, positive chronotropic and ionotropic cardiac effects, reduction in systemic vascular resistance by vasodilation of the resistance arterioles, increase in cardiac output because of renin–angiotensin activation and increased cardiac preload, cardiomyopathy, and increased glomerular filtration rate. The possibility of a thyroid storm, or an acute thyrotoxic crisis, should also be considered. This can occur before, during, or after anesthesia and is characterized by increased heart rate and blood pressure, cardiac dysrhythmias, elevated body temperature, and shock.

Hyperthyroidism may increase the metabolic rate, so hyperthyroid patients may metabolize anesthetic or analgesic drugs more rapidly and have a higher oxygen and glucose demands.

Risk factors
General thyrotoxicosis
- Presence of a functional thyroid tumor
- Inadequate treatment before anesthesia

Thyroid storm
- Catecholamine release from stress
- Rapid change in thyroid hormone concentration
- Thyroid surgery
- Administration of iodinated contrast dyes or free iodine
- Radioactive iodine therapy
- Vigorous thyroid palpation
- Ingestion of excessive thyroid hormone supplementation

Diagnosis

Hyperthyroidism can be easily diagnosed before surgery by evaluation of thyroid hormone concentrations. Clinical signs of hyperthyroidism include, but are not limited to, a palpable thyroid mass, thin body condition, polyphagia, vomiting, tachypnea, dyspnea, hypertension, a gallop heart rhythm, or a heart murmur. Clinical signs of thyroid storm are listed in Box 26.1. Under anesthesia, thyroid storm may resemble malignant hyperthermia because patients become hyperthermic, hypertensive, tachycardic, or develop cardiac arrhythmias.

Treatment

Treatment of thyrotoxicosis is best done before anesthesia (see later under Prevention).

Treatment of thyroid storm should focus on reducing the production of more thyroid hormone, reducing the systemic effects of thyroid hormone, symptomatically supporting the animal, and removing the inciting cause. Methimazole (in cats, 5 mg twice a day, orally [PO], rectally, or transdermally) will prevent synthesis of new thyroid hormone. Potassium iodate (in cats, 25 mg every 8 hours) will also help reduce the formation of additional thyroid hormone. β-Blockers such as propranolol (in cats, 5 mg PO every 8 hours or 0.2 mg/kg intravenously [IV] over 1 minute) or atenolol (1 mg/kg every 24 hours) will reduce the systemic effects of excessive thyroid hormone. Esmolol (0.5 mg/kg IV loading dose followed by infusion of 10–200 μg/kg/min) is a short acting β-blocker and may be useful as treatment for an acute thyrotoxic crisis during anesthesia.

Box 26.1 Clinical signs of thyroid storm (Ward, 2007)

Tachycardia
Tachypnea
Hyperthermia
Respiratory distress
Cardiac arrhythmia or murmur
Sudden blindness
Auscultatory crackles
Severe muscle weakness
Ventroflexion of the neck
Neurologic abnormalities
Absent motor limb function
Neurologic abnormalities
Sudden death

Complications in Small Animal Surgery, First Edition. Edited by Dominique Griffon and Annick Hamaide.
© 2016 John Wiley & Sons, Inc. Published 2016 by John Wiley & Sons, Inc.
Companion website: www.wiley.com/go/griffon/complications

Additionally, providing appropriate systemic support (IV fluids, fans, ice, dextrose supplementation, and so on) is also important, as are identification and correction of the potential inciting event.

Outcome
Most patients with hyperthyroidism have minimal anesthetic effects, especially if preanesthetic preventative treatment is used.

Prevention
- Delay elective surgeries until hyperthyroidism is controlled with methimazole or radioactive iodine treatment.
- Pretreatment with β-blockers will reduce the systemic consequences of hyperthyroidism.
- Use anesthetic agents which decrease the catecholamine response to minimize the risk of a catecholamine-induced thyroid storm. Acepromazine and opioids work well for this purpose.
- Avoid mask inductions because they are associated with high levels of stress.
- Consider supplementing glucose (2.5% or 5%) during anesthesia to support the increased glucose demands in hyperthyroid patients.
- Avoid dissociative and anticholinergic drugs because a rapid heart rate might cause a reduction in diastolic filling.

Hypothyroidism

Definition
Surgical removal of both lobes of the thyroid gland may result in hypothyroidism (Figure 26.1). Hypothyroidism occurs when the concentration of thyroid hormone is less than normal.

Risk factors
- Bilateral thyroidectomy

Diagnosis
Hypothyroid dogs and cats have decreased metabolic rates, resulting in lethargy, obesity, or weakness. Dermatologic problems (alopecia, scaly skin, seborrhea, pyoderma) are common in hypothyroid animals. Less commonly, hypothyroid animals may have

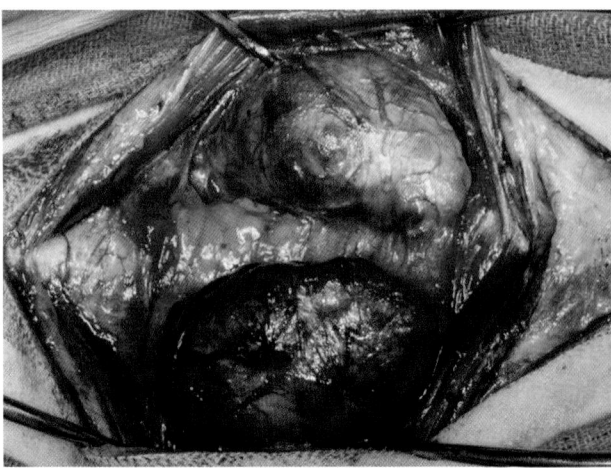

Figure 26.1 Bilateral thyroid carcinoma in a dog. Bilateral thyroidectomy increases the risk of postoperative hypocalcemia.

abnormalities of the neurologic, cardiovascular, or other endocrine systems (Scott-Moncrieff 2007). Diagnosis of hypothyroidism is more difficult than diagnosis of hyperthyroidism and is commonly performed by measuring the concentration of total thyroxine, free thyroxine, and thyroid-stimulating hormone. Interpretation of these tests should be made in light of clinical signs. Diagnosis of hypothyroidism is difficult because concomitant disease, recent anesthesia and surgery, or drug administration (steroids, non-steroidal antiinflammatory drugs, clomipramine, sulfonamides, and phenobarbital) may reduce thyroid function test results, creating false–positive test results (euthyroid sick, and so on). Resolution of clinical signs during a levothyroxine trial and recurrence of clinical signs after discontinuation of levothyroxine will confirm the diagnosis.

Treatment
Treatment of hypothyroidism involves administration of levothyroxine (0.02 mg/kg PO every 12 hours to start and then every 24 hours to maintain). The efficacy of treatment is determined by resolution of clinical signs. Monitoring total thyroxine levels 4 to 6 weeks after beginning therapy will prevent oversupplementation.

Outcome
Generally, dogs and cats have adequate ectopic thyroid tissue to prevent clinically significant hypothyroidism after bilaterally thyroidectomy (Scott-Moncrieff 2007). However, if clinical signs exist, and supplementation is required, clinical signs should resolve.

Prevention
- Prophylactic supplementation of levothyroxine after bilateral thyroidectomy

Hemorrhage
See also Chapter 12.

Definition
Acute severe hemorrhage secondary to arterial invasion has been reported in a dog with thyroid carcinoma (Slensky *et al.* 2003). More commonly, hemorrhage is encountered during surgery because of the abundant blood supply to the thyroid gland (Figure 26.2). Bleeding is especially common in dogs during removal or debulking of invasive thyroid carcinomas (Figure 26.3).

Risk factors
- Invasive (nonmoveable) thyroid tumor
- Thyroid carcinoma
- Coagulopathy
- Inadequate intraoperative hemostasis
- Inadequate surgical exposure

Diagnosis
Intraoperative hemorrhage is an obvious diagnosis made by the surgeon. Postoperatively, hemorrhage may result in a hemorrhagic discharge from the surgical incision, swelling of the neck, dyspnea, or subcutaneous bruising. Evaluation of serial packed cell volume measurements and total protein concentrations may support the diagnosis of hemorrhage. Cervical ultrasonography can be used to identify free fluid or a blood clot around the surgical site.

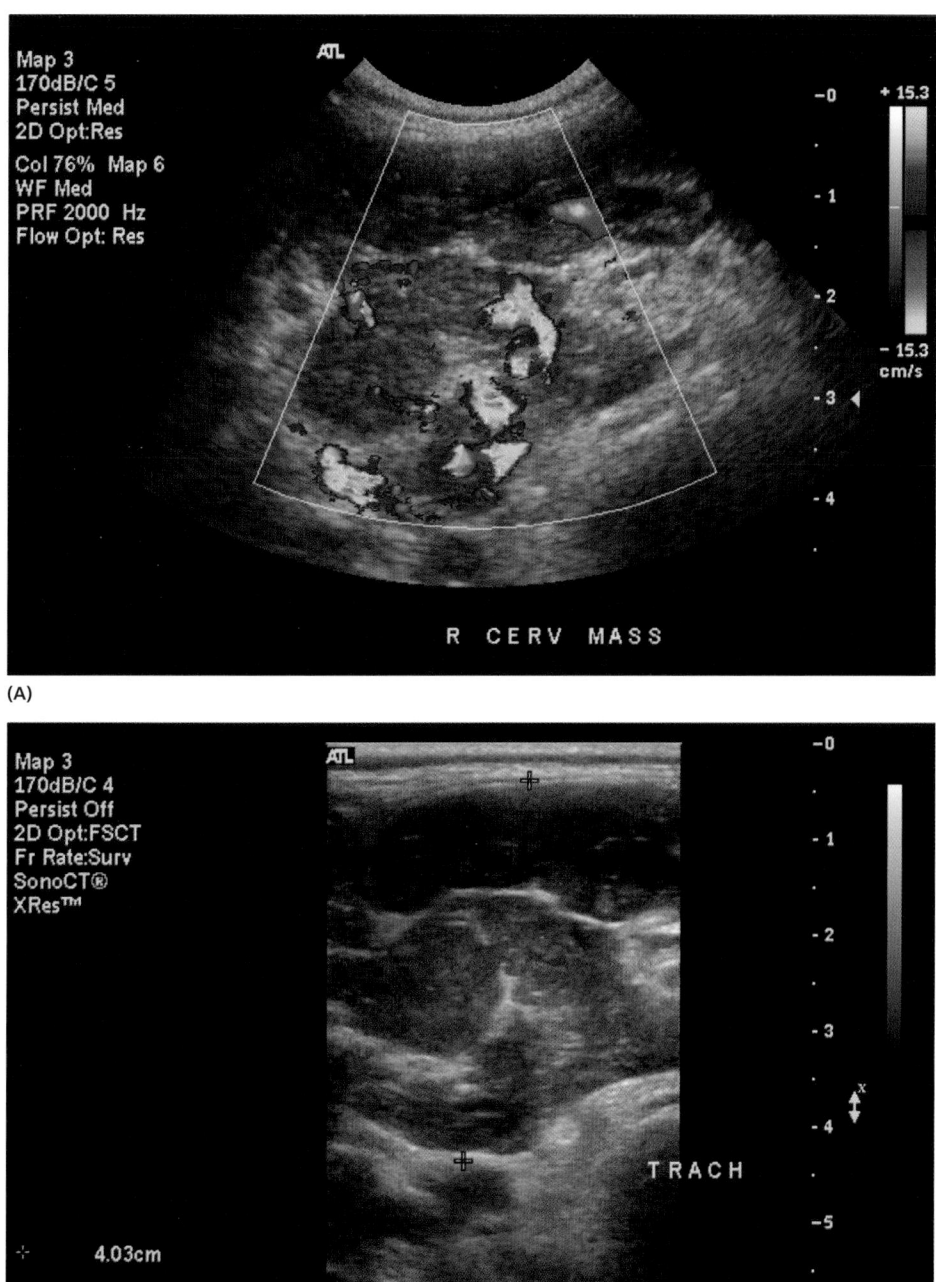

Figure 26.2 Transverse ultrasound image of a thyroid carcinoma in a dog (**A**) with and (**B**) without power Doppler. Thyroid carcinomas have significant blood flow. Hemorrhage before, during, and after surgery is a potential complication.

Treatment

Intraoperatively, accurate and thorough hemostasis is necessary to prevent hemorrhage and optimize the accuracy of surgical dissection. Improving surgical exposure will assist the surgeon in identifying and controlling hemorrhage. Postoperatively, if significant hemorrhage is present, reoperation may be necessary to identify and ligate bleeding vessels. Alternatively, if hemorrhage is mild, a soft padded bandage may provide adequate compression for coagulation. Systemic support with blood products may be necessary if hemorrhage is severe.

Outcome

After hemorrhage is controlled and, if needed, blood products are administered, the patient has a good prognosis.

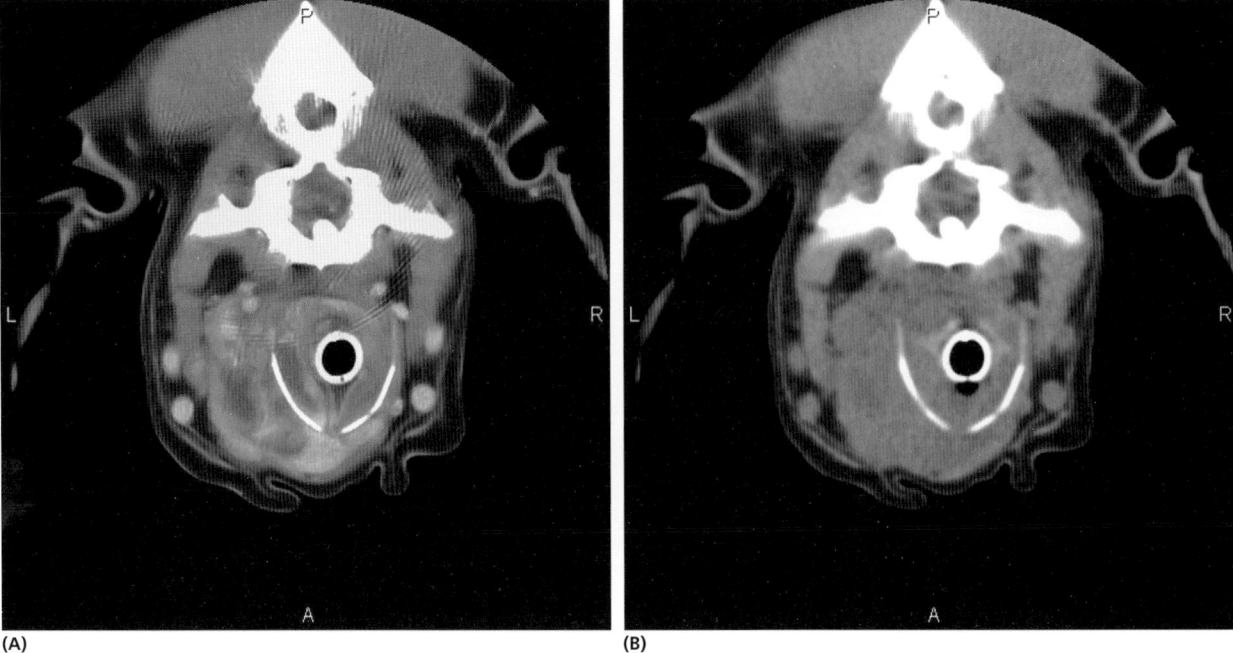

(A)   (B)

Figure 26.3 Transverse computed tomography images with (**A**) and without (**B**) contrast administration of an invasive thyroid carcinoma in a dog. The mass is moderately heterogenous with irregular contrast enhancement. The tumor surrounds the esophagus and trachea. Resection of this tumor is not possible, and treatment with radiation therapy should be considered. (Courtesy of Shannon Holmes, DVM, MSc, DACVR.)

Prevention
- Accurate and thorough intraoperative hemostasis
- Adequate surgical exposure
- Preoperative surgical planning for invasive (nonmoveable) masses
- Assessment of coagulation function before surgery
- Ensuring blood products are available if they are required

Hypocalcemia

Definition
Hypocalcemia is the presence of blood total or ionized calcium concentrations less than the normal range. Hypocalcemia after thyroidectomy occurs because of concurrent parathyroidectomy or iatrogenic damage to the parathyroid glands or the blood supply to those glands (Figure 26.4). Clinical signs of hypocalcemia can occur 1 to 4 days after surgery. Hypocalcemia is only a potential complication if bilateral thyroidectomy is performed because normal blood calcium concentrations can be maintained with one parathyroid gland.

Risk factors
- Bilateral thyroidectomy
- Extracapsular dissection technique

Diagnosis
Clinical signs of hypocalcemia include facial pruritus; ataxia; a tense, "sardonic" grin with the ears folded caudally; muscle weakness; tremors; convulsions; or cardiac arrhythmias. The diagnosis is confirmed by documenting total or ionized blood calcium concentrations.

Treatment
Animals with mild hypocalcemia may not require treatment. In cats, hypocalcemia secondary to complete thyroparathyroidectomy should gradually resolve over 12 weeks despite persistently low parathyroid hormone levels (Flanders *et al.* 1991).

Animals with moderate hypocalcemia should be started on oral calcitriol therapy. Animals symptomatic for hypocalcemia or with severe hypocalcemia are treated initially with IV calcium gluconate. (For acute signs: 0.5–1.5 mL/kg of 10% calcium gluconate IV over 20 minutes, monitor for bradycardia, cardiac arrhythmias,

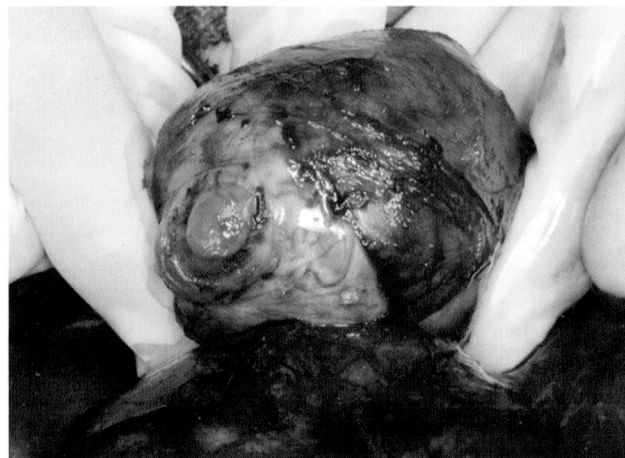

Figure 26.4 The external parathyroid gland on the surface of the thyroid tumor. The blood supply to this parathyroid has been disturbed by the thyroid tumor and the surgical dissection. This parathyroid gland was removed with the associated thyroid tumor.

or ST segment elevation. For chronic supplementation: 10–15 mL of 10% solution/kg/day IV or subcutaneously [SC].) Patients are transitioned to oral calcitriol (2.5–10 ng/kg/day divided) with or without oral calcium supplementation. Dogs fed an appropriate diet should not require additional calcium supplementation. Occasionally, dogs with concomitant gastrointestinal disease do not absorb oral calcitriol and respond more favorably to SC calcitriol administration.

Outcome

In cats that become hypocalcemic after thyroidectomy, hypocalcemia is often transient and should normalize within 1 to 12 weeks (Flanders *et al.* 1991; Naan *et al.* 2006). One might expect a similar course in dogs, but little information is available in dogs with hypocalcemia after bilateral thyroidectomy. In animals with hypocalcemia, calcium concentrations should be monitored regularly and supplementation reduced slowly.

Prevention

- Staged thyroidectomy
- Parathyroid autotransplantation
- Staged thyroidectomy with parathyroid autotransplantation during the first surgery
- Preservation of at least one parathyroid gland during thyroidectomy
- Preservation of the cranial thyroid artery and the vasculature to the parathyroid during dissection
- Supplementation in calcitriol several days before surgery

Recurrence of signs

Definition

After thyroidectomy in cats with hyperthyroidism, recurrence of signs associated with hyperthyroidism may be caused by contralateral occurrence, local (ipsilateral) recurrence, or the presence of ectopic adenomatous thyroid tissue. In dogs with thyroid adenocarcinomas, local recurrence or distant metastasis may be responsible for the recurrence of hyperthyroidism (if the tumor is functional) or the presence of a cervical mass or pulmonary metastasis. Animals with intravascular invasion are more likely to develop metastasis (Figure 26.5) (Liptak 2007).

Risk factors

- Ectopic thyroid tissue
- Unilateral thyroidectomy in cats with hyperthyroidism
- Intracapsular technique
- Malignant thyroid tumor

Diagnosis

After surgical thyroidectomy in cats, thyroxin concentrations should be evaluated regularly or if signs of hyperthyroidism recur (typically, weight loss, strong appetite, hyperactivity). An elevated total and free thyroxin concentration will be present in most cats, although normal results may not rule out hyperthyroidism. Thyroid scintigraphy is effective for documentation of hyperfunctioning adenomatous tissue, especially when ectopic adenomatous tissue is suspected (Figure 26.6). In dogs, routine monitoring for recurrence should include cervical palpation, thoracic radiography, and ultrasound imaging.

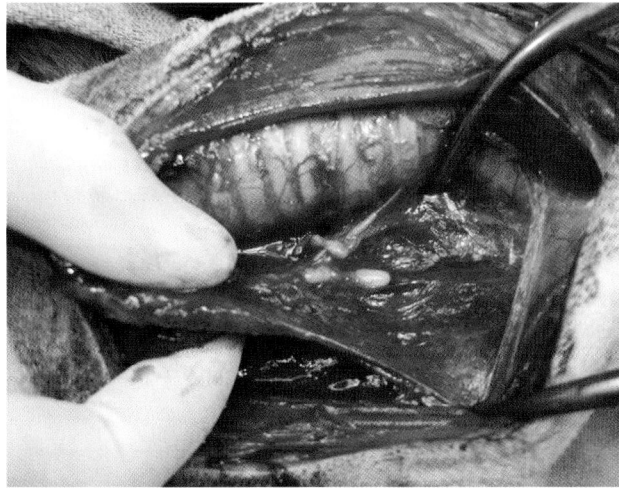

Figure 26.5 The thyroid tumor has an intravascular component within the caudal thyroid vein, which can be seen as a pale structure extending caudally. The patient's head is to the left.

Treatment

Cats with recurrent clinical signs should have definitive treatment after restaging with imaging studies. Because ectopic adenomatous tissue may be responsible for clinical signs, complete staging is required before a second surgery. Alternatively, recurrence may be treated with radioactive iodine therapy, which will destroy adenomatous thyroid tissue, no matter its location.

Dogs with recurrent signs secondary to local recurrence or distant metastasis of thyroid carcinoma should be completely staged before therapy and may benefit from chemotherapy or radiation therapy.

Outcome

In animals with recurrence of signs, the outcome will depend on the reason for recurrence and the specific pathologic diagnosis of the tumor. Whereas local recurrence of benign disease has a good prognosis, distant metastasis of malignant disease has a poor prognosis.

Prevention

- Completely stage patients before surgery.
- Perform a bilateral (staged or simultaneous) modified extracapsular thyroidectomy technique in cats.
- Avoid intracapsular dissection or perform a modified intracapsular technique.
- Avoid surgery in cases with ectopic adenomatous thyroid tissue.
- Consider postoperative chemotherapy or radiation therapy in animals with malignant thyroid disease.

Neurologic complications

Definition

Neurologic complications after thyroidectomy result from nerve injury during thyroid dissection. Specifically, the vagosympathetic trunk and the recurrent laryngeal nerve are in close proximity to the thyroid. This complication is more of a concern when invasive thyroid adenocarcinomas are removed. Damage to the nerves may be permanent or transient depending on the degree of injury.

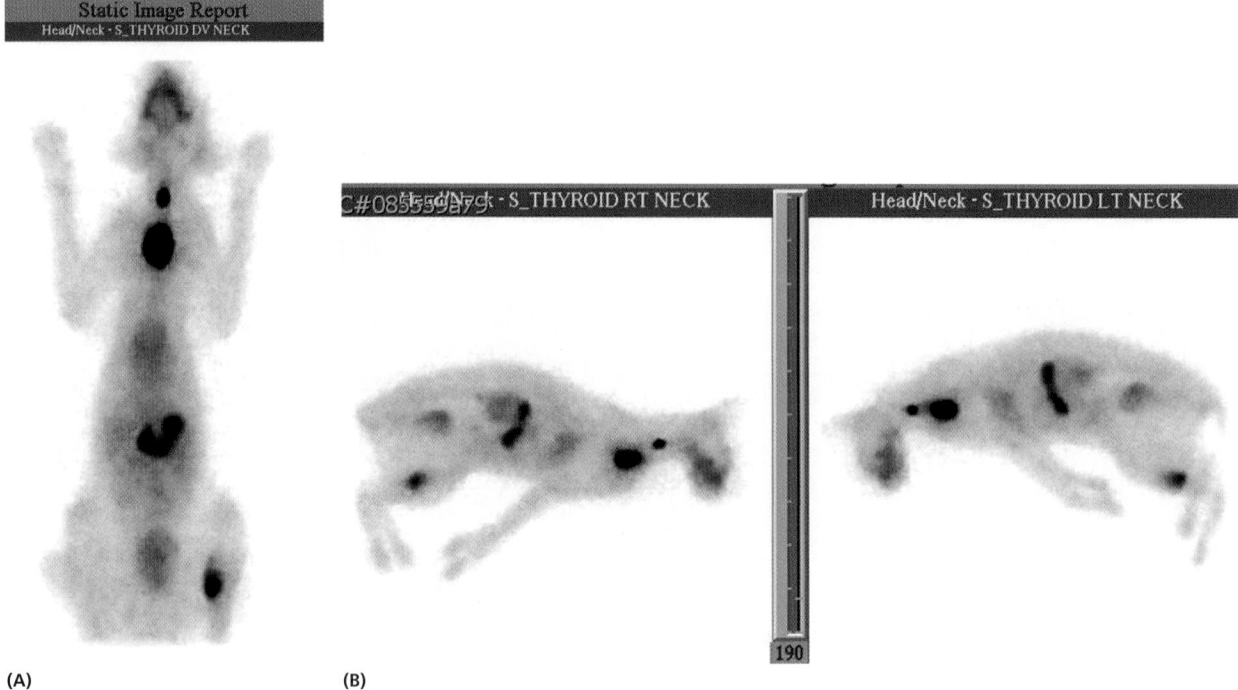

Figure 26.6 Ventral (**A**) right- and left-sided (**B**) images of thyroid scintigraphy in a cat 20 minutes after intravenous administration of technetium pertechnetate ($^{99m}TcO_4$). Radiopharmaceutical uptake is present in the thorax, consistent with ectopic thyroid tissue. Additional areas of uptake are present in the thyroid glands and stomach. Thyroid uptake is substantially greater than that of the zygomatic/molar salivary glands because of adenomatous hyperplasia. Focal uptake at the injection site is present in the left pelvic limb. (Courtesy of David Jiménez DVM, DACVR.)

Neurologic complications should be minimal after removal of thyroid adenomas.

Risk factors
- Invasive thyroid tumor
- Aggressive surgical dissection
- Inadequate knowledge of local anatomy
- Previous cervical surgery

Diagnosis
Diagnosis of neurologic complications after thyroidectomy is based on observation of characteristic clinical signs. Animals with injury to the vagosympathetic trunk will have Horner's syndrome on the affected side. Animals with unilateral injury to the recurrent laryngeal nerve may develop a change in voice, have mild inspiratory stridor, or be asymptomatic. Unilateral lack of arytenoid abduction will be observed during laryngeal examination. If bilateral injury occurs to the recurrent laryngeal nerve, clinical significant inspiratory dyspnea will occur.

Treatment
Treatment of neurologic complications is generally not necessary. However, if an animal is symptomatic for an upper airway obstruction secondary to recurrent laryngeal nerve damage, a unilateral arytenoid lateralization surgery should be performed.

Outcome
Unless bilateral injury is present, the consequences to neurologic injury during thyroid dissection are minimal. If bilateral injury occurs to the vagosympathetic trunk or recurrent laryngeal nerve, significant morbidity should be expected.

Prevention
In cases of invasive disease, accurate surgical planning and execution are necessary to minimize collateral iatrogenic injury to nerves surrounding the thyroid gland.

Relevant literature

Feline
Thyroidectomy in cats is almost always performed for treatment of hyperthyroidism secondary to benign adenomatous thyroid tissue, although thyroid carcinoma has been reported in cats (Naan *et al.* 2006; Hibbert *et al.* 2009). Although medical and radiotherapeutic treatment strategies are commonly used to treat benign thyroid adenomas, multiple surgical techniques are also described (Flanders 1999). Given the widespread availability of radioactive iodine therapy and the lack of associated complications, thyroidectomy in cats is not commonly performed. However, if surgery is elected as the treatment of choice, a thyroid scan is indicated to document the presence of ectopic thyroid tissue. Approximately 20% of cats are reported to have ectopic thyroid tissue, which would cause a surgical failure or recurrence if thyroidectomy alone was used to treat hyperthyroidism (Naan *et al.* 2006; Harvey *et al.* 2009). Cats with ectopic thyroid tissue are best treated with radioactive iodine therapy or maintained on daily medical management.

The extracapsular thyroidectomy technique was the first and most basic technique and involves ligation of the cranial and caudal thyroid vessels and complete removal of the thyroid and parathyroid glands (Holzworth *et al.* 1980). Although ectopic parathyroid tissue may eventually cause normocalcemia (Flanders *et al.* 1991), 82% of the cats became hypocalcemic after extracapsular thyroidectomy (Flanders *et al.* 1987). Because of the high incidence of hypocalcemia, surgeons tended toward intracapsular dissection. The disadvantage of intracapsular dissection is that abnormal adenomatous thyroid tissue may remain attached to the capsule resulting in a high rate of local recurrence. In one study of 23 cats with recurrence of hyperthyroidism after thyroidectomy, 11 cats had an intracapsular dissection, and 1 cat had an extracapsular dissection (Welches *et al.* 1989).

Modifications of the extracapsular and intracapsular techniques have been reported to minimize the occurrence of hypocalcemia and recurrence, respectively. The modified extracapsular technique involves removal of the internal or cranial parathyroid gland with no disruption of the cranial thyroid artery and its branches to the external parathyroid gland. This strategy requires intracapsular dissection only around the external parathyroid, essentially leaving a cuff of thyroid capsule just subjacent to the external parathyroid gland and its associated vasculature. This approach has a reported postoperative hypocalcemia rate of 23% and a recurrence rate of 4% (Welches *et al.* 1989).

In the modified intracapsular technique, the surgeon performs an intracapsular dissection and then resects the capsule that is not associated with the external parathyroid gland. This technique also has a low reported rate of recurrence, ranging from 0% to 4.9% (Welches *et al.* 1989; Naan *et al.* 2006).

Another described variation of thyroidectomy technique is performing a staged thyroidectomy compared with a bilateral simultaneous thyroidectomy. A staged thyroidectomy is advocated by some because of the reduced risk of postoperative hypocalcemia (Flanders *et al.* 1987). Using a staged technique, the rate of postoperative hypocalcemia was reduced to 11% compared with 82% for simultaneous extracapsular dissections and 36% for simultaneous intracapsular dissections (Flanders *et al.* 1987).

A final modification is autotransplantation of the parathyroid glands in a strap muscle at the time of thyroidectomy (Padgett *et al.* 1998). This technique resulted in cats becoming normocalcemic after a median of 14 days after thyroparathyroidectomy (Padgett *et al.* 1998).

The largest study of outcomes after bilateral thyroidectomy evaluated 101 cats that underwent a modified intracapsular technique (Naan *et al.* 2006). In that study, 9 cats had ectopic thyroid tissue, which was associated with a significantly higher recurrence rate. Two cats died perioperatively, 5 developed transient hypocalcemia, and 5 had recurrence.

Canine

Ninety percent of dogs with thyroid neoplasia have thyroid carcinomas, and most are nonfunctional (Wucherer and Wilke 2010). Thyroid follicular adenocarcinomas and thyroid medullary carcinomas are reported, and their clinical behavior has been compared in dogs. Medullary thyroid carcinomas may have less malignant behavior compared with thyroid adenocarcinomas (Carver *et al.* 1995). Functional thyroid carcinomas and adenomas have also been reported in dogs (Melian *et al.* 1996; Itoh *et al.* 2007; Malik 2007; Simpson and McCown 2009; Wuchener and Wilke 2010).

Dogs with thyroid tumors often present for cervical masses, dyspnea, or coughing (Harari *et al.* 1986). Tumors can be unilateral or bilateral, but unilateral tumors occur more commonly (Liptak 2007). Ectopic thyroid tumors may occur anywhere from the tongue to the base of the heart. Thyroid tumors have variable degrees of invasiveness to surrounding tissues; this characteristic is most easily determined during the physical examination by palpation of the mass. Whereas thyroid tumors that are easily moveable during palpation are generally resectable, tumors that are fixed and not moveable may not be resectable.

Staging of thyroid tumors consists of aspiration cytology and imaging. Although cytology is frequently performed, the results are commonly unrewarding because of blood contamination and a nondiagnostic sample (Harari *et al.* 1986). Surgical biopsy is not commonly performed because of the risk of hemorrhage and a high degree of clinical suspicion in most cases. Three-view thoracic radiographs, cervical and abdominal ultrasound examination, and cervical computed tomography or magnetic resonance imaging define the local and systemic extent of the disease.

Results of surgical therapy have been reported in several limited studies (Harari *et al.* 1986; Carver *et al.* 1995; Klein *et al.* 1995). If thyroid tumors are freely moveable, the reported median survival time is about 3 years; however, if the tumor is fixed and not moveable, the survival time falls to about 6 to 12 months (Harari *et al.* 1986; Carver *et al.* 1995; Klein *et al.* 1995). Nonresectable tumors may be treated with radiation therapy with good success; in one study, 80% of dogs had progression-free survival at 1 year and 72% had progression-free survival at 3 years (Theon *et al.* 2000). Another study reports a median survival time of 24.5 months after radiation therapy for invasive thyroid tumors in dogs (Pack *et al.* 2001). Radioactive iodine therapy has also been reported as the sole treatment or as a adjunct to surgical therapy in invasive thyroid tumors (Worth *et al.* 2005). Chemotherapy may also be indicated in dogs with incompletely resected, nonresectable, or metastatic disease (Liptak 2007).

References

Carver, J.R., Kapatkin, A., Patnaik, A.K. (1995) A comparison of medullary thyroid carcinoma and thyroid adenocarcinoma in dogs: a retrospective study of 38 cases. *Veterinary Surgery* 24, 315-319.

Flanders, J.A. (1999) Surgical options for the treatment of hyperthyroidism in the cat. *Journal of Feline Medicine and Surgery* 1, 127-134.

Flanders, J.A., Harvey, H.J., Erb, H.N. (1987) Feline thyroidectomy. A comparison of postoperative hypocalcemia associated with three different surgical techniques. *Veterinary Surgery* 16, 362-366.

Flanders, J. A., Neth, S., Erb, H.N., et al. (1991) Functional analysis of ectopic parathyroid activity in cats. *American Journal of Veterinary Research* 52, 1336-1340.

Harari, J., Patterson, J.S., Rosenthal, R.C. (1986) Clinical and pathologic features of thyroid tumors in 26 dogs. *Journal of the American Veterinary Medical Association* 188, 1160-1164.

Harvey, A.M., Hibbert, A., Barrett, E.L., et al. (2009) Scintigraphic findings in 120 hyperthyroid cats. *Journal of Feline Medicine and Surgery* 11, 96-106.

Hibbert, A., Gruffydd-Jones, T., Barrett, E.L., et al. (2009) Feline thyroid carcinoma: diagnosis and response to high-dose radioactive iodine treatment. *Journal of Feline Medicine and Surgery* 11, 116-124.

Holzworth, J., Theran, P., Carpenter, J.L., et al. (1980) Hyperthyroidism in the cat: ten cases. *Journal of the American Veterinary Medical Association* 176, 345-353.

Itoh, T., Kojimoto, A., Nibe, K., et al. (2007) Functional thyroid gland adenoma in a dog treated with surgical excision alone. *Journal of Veterinary Medical Science* 69, 61-63.

Klein, M.K., Powers, B,E., Withrow, S.J., et al. (1995) Treatment of thyroid carcinoma in dogs by surgical resection alone: 20 cases (1981-1989). *Journal of the American Veterinary Medical Association* 206, 1007-1009.

Liptak, J. M. (2007) Canine thyroid carcinoma. *Clinical Techniques in Small Animal Practice* 22, 75-81.

Malik, R. (2007) Dog with a functional intra-thoracic thyroid tumour. *Journal of Small Animal Practice* 48, 474; author reply 474.

Melian, C., Morales, M., Espinosa De Los Monteros, A., et al. (1996) Horner's syndrome associated with a functional thyroid carcinoma in a dog. *Journal of Small Animal Practice* 37, 591-3.

Naan, E.C., Kirpensteijn, J., Kooistra, H.S., et al. (2006) Results of thyroidectomy in 101 cats with hyperthyroidism. *Veterinary Surgery* 35, 287-293.

Pack, L., Roberts, R.E., Dawson, S.D., et al. (2001) Definitive radiation therapy for infiltrative thyroid carcinoma in dogs. *Veterinary Radiology and Ultrasound* 42, 471-474.

Padgett, S. L., Tobias, K. M., Leathers, C. W., et al. (1998) Efficacy of parathyroid gland autotransplantation in maintaining serum calcium concentrations after bilateral thyroparathyroidectomy in cats. *Journal of the American Animal Hospital Association* 34, 219-224.

Scott-Moncrieff, J. C. (2007) Clinical signs and concurrent diseases of hypothyroidism in dogs and cats. *Veterinary Clinics of North America: Small Animal Practice* 37, 709-22, vi.

Simpson, A.C., McCown, J.L. (2009) Systemic hypertension in a dog with a functional thyroid gland adenocarcinoma. *Journal of the American Veterinary Medical Association* 235, 1474-1479.

Slensky, K.A., Volk, S.W., Schwarz, T., et al. (2003) Acute severe hemorrhage secondary to arterial invasion in a dog with thyroid carcinoma. *Journal of the American Veterinary Medical Association* 223, 649-653.

Theon, A.P., Marks, S.L., Feldman, E.S., et al. (2000) Prognostic factors and patterns of treatment failure in dogs with unresectable differentiated thyroid carcinomas treated with megavoltage irradiation. *Journal of the American Veterinary Medical Association* 216, 1775-1779.

Ward, C.R. (2007) Feline thyroid storm. *Veterinary Clinics of North America: Small Animal Practice* 37, 745-754, vii.

Welches, C.D., Scavelli, T.D., Matthiesen, D.T., et al. (1989) Occurrence of problems after three techniques of bilateral thyroidectomy in cats. *Veterinary Surgery* 18, 392-396.

Worth, A.J., Zuber, R.M., Hocking, M. (2005) Radioiodide (131I) therapy for the treatment of canine thyroid carcinoma. *Australian Veterinary Journal* 83, 208-214.

Wucherer, K.L., Wilke, V. (2010) Thyroid cancer in dogs: an update based on 638 cases (1995-2005). *Journal of the American Animal Hospital Association* 46, 249-254.

27 Parathyroidectomy

Chad Schmiedt

Small Animal Surgery, Department of Small Animal Medicine and Surgery, College of Veterinary Medicine, University of Georgia, Athens, GA, USA

Parathyroidectomy is most commonly indicated in dogs with functional parathyroid adenomatous tissue resulting in hypercalcemia. Parathyroidectomy is also occasionally performed with thyroidectomy.

Hypercalcemia

Definition

Most commonly, parathyroidectomy is performed to remove a functional parathyroid adenoma (Figure 27.1), although occasionally multiple parathyroid adenomas, parathyroid hyperplasia, or a parathyroid adenocarcinoma may be present. Successful surgical treatment of any of those results in an immediate decline in total or ionized blood calcium concentration (Figure 27.2). In a patient without exogenous calcium supplementation, ionized and total calcium concentrations should not be elevated within 24 to 36 hours after surgery. Hypercalcemia after parathyroidectomy occurs when postoperative blood calcium concentrations remain greater than normal limits. Alternatively, an initial normalization of calcium may be followed by a chronic increase in calcium concentration in the months after surgery.

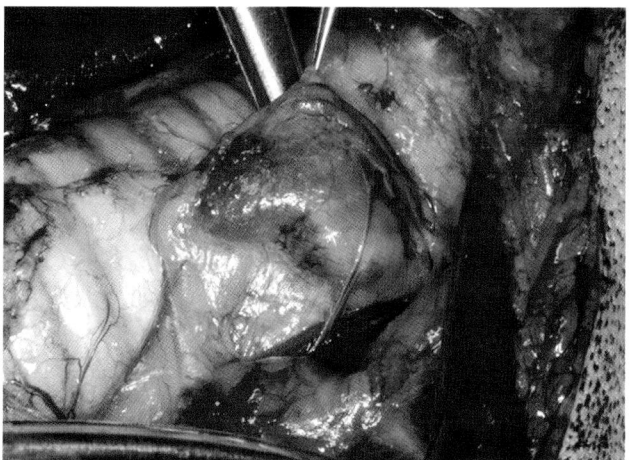

Figure 27.1 Intraoperative photograph of a functional parathyroid adenoma in a dog. The adenoma is arising from the internal parathyroid gland, which is just medial to the thyroid gland. Resection of the parathyroid adenoma is possible without removing the associated thyroid gland.

Risk factors

- Incomplete excision of functional autonomous parathyroid tissue
- Metastasis of parathyroid tumor
- Recurrence of parathyroid tumor
- Alternate cause of hypercalcemia (e.g., renal disease, other neoplasia, nutritional)
- Excessive prophylactic calcium supplementation

Diagnosis

Clinically, hypercalcemic animals may be weak, may have polyuria or polydipsia, have a reduced appetite and activity level, or may be prone to develop cystoliths and present for signs of cystitis or urethral obstruction. Hypercalcemic animals may be asymptomatic. A serum biochemical profile will rule out some of the other systemic causes of hypercalcemia. Evaluation of parathyroid hormone (PTH), parathyroid hormone–related protein (PTH-rP), and ionized blood calcium concentrations helps identify the cause of postoperative hypercalcemia (Table 27.1). With persistently elevated PTH, imaging studies (cervical ultrasonography, computed tomography, or magnetic resonance imaging) of the entire neck and cranial thorax may identify ectopic or metastatic, autonomous PTH-producing tissue.

If the PTH concentration is appropriately low, especially if the PTH-rP is elevated, consider repeating the physical examination, paying special attention to skeletal abnormalities, anal sacs, mammary glands, and lymph nodes, and perform abdominal and thoracic imaging, bone marrow and lymph node aspirates, and an adrenocorticotropic hormone stimulation test.

Treatment

Treatment options depend on the cause of the persistent hypercalcemia. If the surgeon is suspicious of incomplete excision, imaging studies should be performed to direct a second surgery.

One challenging clinical scenario is the diagnosis of multiple hyperplastic parathyroid glands. Hyperplastic glands are not neoplastic, but they are enlarged and secrete excessive PTH, causing hypercalcemia. Removal of multiple (two to four) glands may be required to resolve hypercalcemia. If complete parathyroidectomy is performed, animals need to be chronically managed for hypocalcemia (see later discussion). Depending on the animal's degree of hypercalcemia and the owner's physical and financial ability to chronically medicate the animal, this may be a reasonable solution; however, chronic calcitriol therapy is expensive.

Complications in Small Animal Surgery, First Edition. Edited by Dominique Griffon and Annick Hamaide.

© 2016 John Wiley & Sons, Inc. Published 2016 by John Wiley & Sons, Inc.

Companion website: www.wiley.com/go/griffon/complications

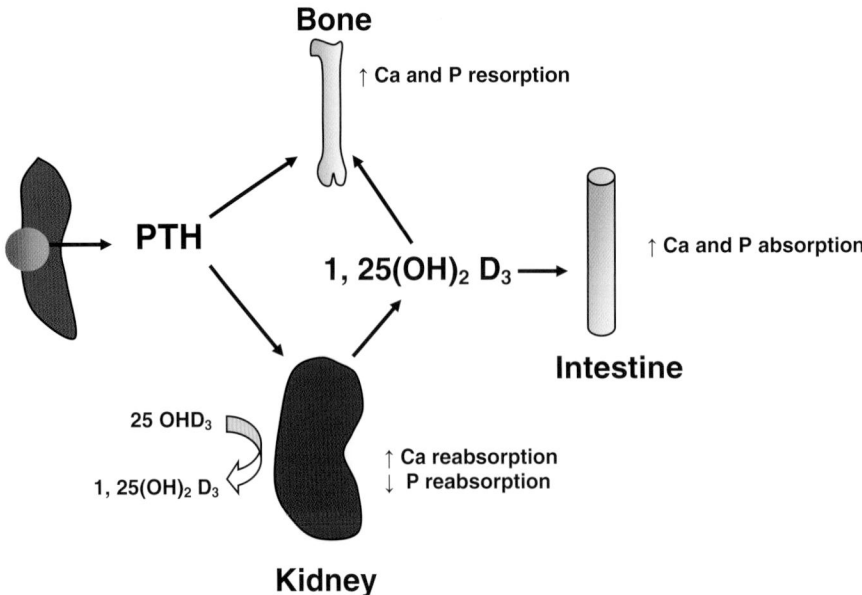

Figure 27.2 Physiology of parathyroid hormone (PTH). PTH regulates systemic calcium concentrations through its actions on the bone, kidney, and intestine. In the kidney, PTH increases the formation of 1,25-dihydroxycholecalciferol (1,25-$(OH)_2D_3$), which acts both on bone and intestine. Furthermore, PTH causes the kidney to excrete phosphorus and reabsorb more calcium. In the bone, PTH initially causes osteocytes to resorb calcium and phosphorus from the bone and chronically causes osteoclastic-mediated reabsorption of bone. 1,25-$(OH)_2D_3$ is believed to enhance movement of calcium across the cellular membranes. In the intestine, 1,25-$(OH)_2D_3$ dramatically increases absorption of calcium and phosphate.

Autotransplantation of parathyroid tissue has been described; parathyroid tissue is removed, sliced into thin sections, and implanted into the strap musculature of the ventral neck (Padgett *et al.* 1998). Its location is marked with a nonabsorbable suture. The goal is for revascularization of the transplanted parathyroid glands within the muscle. If hypercalcemia persists after surgery, then the autotransplanted parathyroid tissue may be partially or completely removed with a relatively more simple surgery. Parathyroid autotransplantation is also used to avoid hypoparathyroidism after thyroidectomy.

If a second surgery is not an option or if no surgical lesion can be identified, generic medical therapy for hypercalcemia may be instituted, including fluid therapy (0.9% NaCl at 90–180 mL/kg/day), furosemide (2–4 mg/kg twice or thrice a day, only in well-hydrated patients), prednisone (2 mg/kg orally twice a day), or bisphosphonates (Hostutler *et al.* 2005).

Outcome

The outcome varies with the reason for the persistent hypercalcemia. If additional functional parathyroid tissue is identified and removed, the prognosis is good.

Table 27.1 Parathyroid hormone, parathyroid hormone–related protein, and ionized serum calcium for common causes of hypercalcemia

	PTH	PTH-related protein	Ionized calcium concentration
Parathyroid adenoma	↑ or normal	↓↓	↑↑
Chronic kidney disease	↑	↑	↑ or normal
Vitamin D intoxication	↓↓	↓↓	↑↑
Malignant lymphoma or other neoplasia	↓	↑↑	↑↑

PTH, parathyroid hormone.

Prevention

- Complete and accurate staging before surgery
- Delicate tissue handling and meticulous hemostasis to optimize exposure and identification of abnormal tissue during surgery
- Complete intraoperative exploration of all parathyroid glands

Hypocalcemia

Definition

Hypocalcemia is the presence of blood total or ionized calcium concentrations less than the normal range. Hypocalcemia may occur after parathyroidectomy because PTH production from autonomous adenomas results in negative feedback to the normal parathyroid glands and downregulation of PTH production in normal glands (Figure 27.3). After removal of the autonomously producing tissue, calcium homeostasis requires several days to 1 week to be reestablished through upregulation of PTH production by the remaining normal parathyroid glands. Hypocalcemia usually occurs 24 to 48 hours after parathyroidectomy. Clinical signs of hypocalcemia include facial pruritus; ataxia; a tense, "sardonic" grin with the ears folded caudally; muscle weakness; tremors; convulsions; or cardiac arrhythmias (Figure 27.4).

Risk factors

Risk factors have not been identified definitively, although these anecdotal characteristics are routinely cited:

- Chronicity of hypercalcemia
- Degree of hypercalcemia (higher calcium concentrations lead to more negative feedback and more potential for hypocalcemia)
- Osteopenia
- Concurrent renal disease
- Complete parathyroidectomy

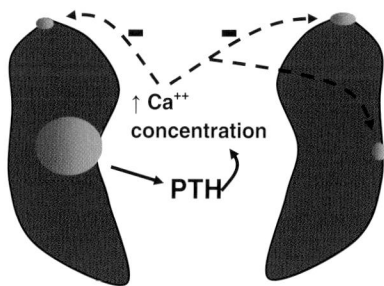

Figure 27.3 Excessive parathyroid hormone (PTH) secretion results in hypercalcemia through the mechanisms discussed in Figure 27.2. Increased serum ionized calcium concentrations have a negative feedback to the remaining parathyroid glands, causing them to shrink and halt production of PTH. Clinically, this means it may be several days after excision of the parathyroid adenoma before the remaining parathyroid tissue become active.

Diagnosis

Total or ionized calcium concentrations should be monitored postoperatively. Because ionized calcium represents the metabolically active form of calcium, this test may more accurately predict the occurrence of clinical signs. Calcium concentrations are monitored every 6 to 12 hours after surgery depending how quickly the calcium concentration is falling and if clinical signs have been noted. The diagnosis of hypocalcemia is made when ionized or total calcium concentrations fall below the low normal reference range. Animals with mild hypocalcemia frequently do not have clinical signs.

Treatment

Animals with mild hypocalcemia may not require treatment. Animals with moderate hypocalcemia should be started on oral calcitriol therapy. Animals symptomatic for hypocalcemia or with severe hypocalcemia are treated initially with intravenous (IV) calcium gluconate (for acute signs, 0.5–1.5 mL/kg of 10% calcium gluconate IV over 20 minutes with monitoring for bradycardia,

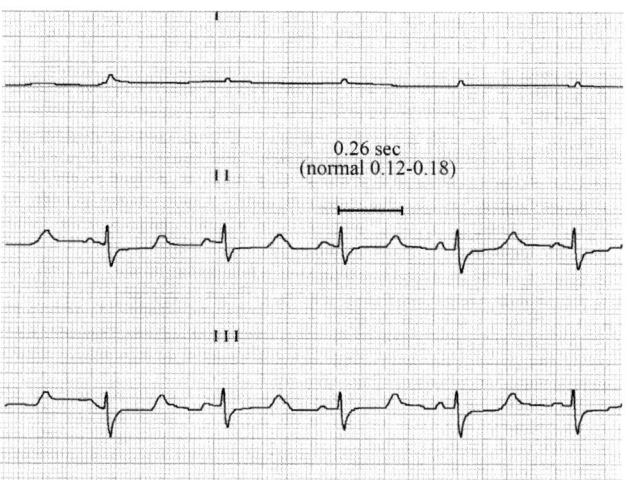

Figure 27.4 Hypocalcemia can result in cardiac arrhythmias. This is an electrocardiogram from a cat that developed hypocalcemia after thyroidectomy. Notice the prolongation of the QT interval. This resolved after calcium supplementation.

cardiac arrhythmias, and ST segment elevation; for chronic supplementation, 10–15 mL of 10% solution/kg/day IV or subcutaneous [SC]). Patients are transitioned to oral calcitriol (2.5–10 ng/kg/day divided) with or without oral calcium supplementation. Dogs fed an appropriate diet should not require additional calcium supplementation. Occasionally, dogs with concomitant gastrointestinal disease do not absorb oral calcitriol and respond more favorably to SC calcitriol administration.

Outcome

Most dogs that become hypocalcemic normalize within 1 week. If oral calcitriol supplementation has been started, calcium is rechecked 1 to 2 weeks after discharge, and the patient is gradually weaned off the drug over a 4- to 6-week period. Calcium is monitored during the weaning process. After complete parathyroidectomy, animals may require oral calcitriol supplementation for life.

Prevention

The following are used routinely to prevent hypocalcemia, although their efficacy has not been critically evaluated:
• Preoperative calcitriol administration
• Preoperative calcium-lowering therapy (e.g., fluid diuresis, steroids)

Neurologic complications

Definition

Neurologic complications after parathyroidectomy are the result of alterations in calcium homeostasis as described earlier. Clinically, animals with hypocalcemia may be depressed, weak, or ataxic or have tremors or convulsions. Animals with hypercalcemia may have muscle weakness or lethargy.

Rarely, aggressive dissection around the thyroid or parathyroid gland will result in damage to the caudal laryngeal nerve, which is the continuation of the recurrent laryngeal nerve (Figure 27.5). Bilateral damage to these nerves will result in clinical signs consistent with laryngeal paralysis (inspiratory dyspnea).

Risk factors
• Moderate to severe abnormal calcium concentrations
• Aggressive surgical dissection
• Inadequate knowledge of local anatomy
• Previous cervical surgery

Diagnosis

The diagnosis of neurologic complications is made by observation of neurologic clinical signs in a patient with concomitant abnormal calcium concentrations and that resolves when the blood calcium concentration is normalized. A laryngeal examination under sedation is necessary to determine laryngeal function.

Treatment

Correction of calcium concentrations rapidly resolves neurologic signs. Clinical signs resulting from recurrent laryngeal nerve damage may improve with conservative management depending on the amount of nerve damage. A unilateral arytenoid lateralization surgery or tracheostomy is indicated in dogs with severe inspiratory dyspnea secondary to nerve damage.

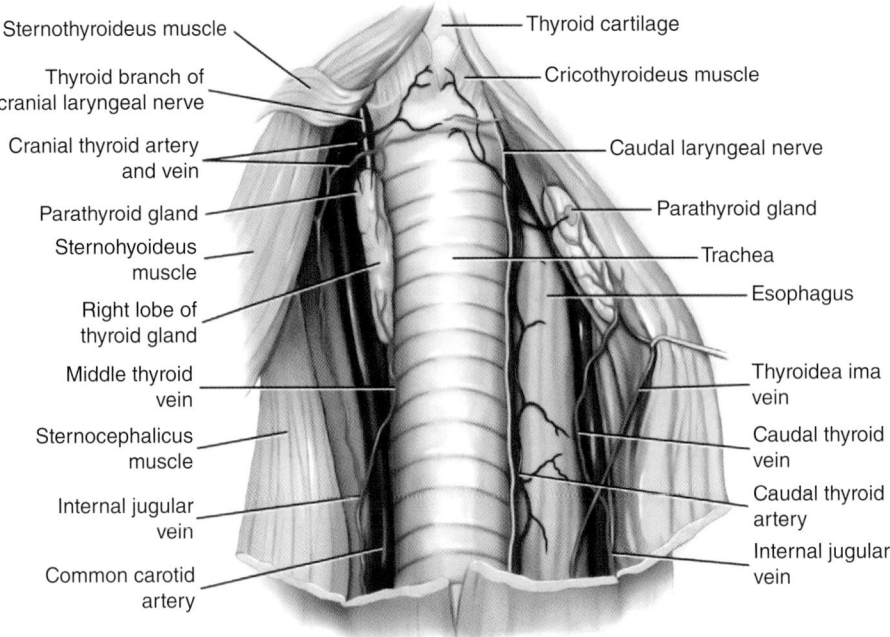

Sternothyroideus muscle

Thyroid branch of
cranial laryngeal nerve

Cranial thyroid artery
and vein

Parathyroid gland

Sternohyoideus
muscle

Right lobe of
thyroid gland

Middle thyroid
vein

Sternocephalicus
muscle

Internal jugular
vein

Common carotid
artery

Thyroid cartilage

Cricothyroideus muscle

Caudal laryngeal nerve

Parathyroid gland

Trachea

Esophagus

Thyroidea ima
vein

Caudal thyroid
vein

Caudal thyroid
artery

Internal jugular
vein

Figure 27.5 The thyroid and parathyroid glands sit immediately adjacent to the caudal laryngeal nerve, which is the cranial continuation of the recurrent laryngeal and innervates the muscles of laryngeal abduction. This nerve can be damaged during surgery, especially if the patient had surgery before, there is poor exposure, or the surgeon is not familiar with the local anatomy. *Source:* Evans, 2013. Reproduced with permission from Elsevier.

Outcome

The prognosis for resolution of calcium-associated neurologic signs is good. The prognosis for return to function after nerve damage depends on the degree of nerve damage.

Prevention

- Accurate tissue dissection
- Diligent assessment of calcium concentration
- Rapid identification of subtle changes in clinical signs

Relevant literature

Primary hyperparathyroidism has been reported in a variety of breeds and has been documented as an autosomal dominant, genetically transmitted condition in Keeshonden (Feldman *et al.* 2005; Goldstein *et al.* 2007). Dogs tend to be older (mean age, ~11 years) and most commonly present for signs associated with the urinary tract (urolithiasis, urinary tract infection, polyuria and polydipsia) (Feldman *et al.* 2005; Gear *et al.* 2005). The degree to which renal disease accompanies primary hyperparathyroidism varies (Feldman *et al.* 2005; Gear *et al.* 2005).

Most parathyroid tumors are functional adenoma, although parathyroid carcinomas have also been reported (Sawyer *et al.* 2012). In that study, dogs with parathyroid carcinomas had very similar clinical signs, and outcomes compared to what is reported in dogs with parathyroid adenomas. None had metastatic disease.

The diagnosis of primary hyperparathyroidism is based on characteristic laboratory results, including an elevated calcium concentration with a normal or elevated PTH concentration and a low PTH-rP concentration. A rapid PTH assay has been validated in

dogs and can be used intraoperatively to measure local PTH concentrations and confirm resection of a PTH-secreting tumor (Ham *et al.* 2009). In dogs that are hypercalcemic secondary to a malignancy, the PTH-rP can be a useful diagnostic tool and was found elevated in 12 of 14 dogs with hypercalcemia secondary to malignancy (Mellanby *et al.* 2006).

Identification of a parathyroid nodule with ultrasonography or other advanced imaging helps to confirm the diagnosis and plan surgery. Ultrasound evaluation was shown to identify a nodule in 26 of 27 dogs with a parathyroid nodule and identified the correct side in 13 of 14 studies when a side was recorded (Gear *et al.* 2005).

Several different strategies have been investigated to remove or ablate parathyroid adenomas. Traditionally, surgical exploration of the ventral cervical area and resection of the nodule (parathyroidectomy) has been the standard of care. Ultrasound-guided radiofrequency or 96% ethanol injection has also been described (Long *et al.* 1999; Pollard *et al.* 2001). The three techniques were compared, and it was reported that parathyroidectomy, radiofrequency ablation, and ethanol ablation resulted in 94%, 90%, and 72% control for 561, 540, and 581 days, respectively (Rasor *et al.* 2007). Significantly more dogs undergoing surgery had resolution of hypercalcemia compared with dogs undergoing ethanol ablation (Rasor *et al.* 2007).

Most surgeons view very elevated preoperative calcium levels (total calcium >14 mg/dL) as a risk factor for development of hypocalcemia postoperatively. Although it has been demonstrated that dogs that become hypocalcemic after parathyroidectomy have a greater preoperative total calcium concentration (Gear *et al.* 2005), this arbitrary cut-off has not been confirmed.

References

Feldman, E.C., Hoar, B., Pollard, R., et al. (2005) Pretreatment clinical and laboratory findings in dogs with primary hyperparathyroidism: 210 cases (1987-2004). *Journal of the American Veterinary Medical Association* 227, 756-761.

Gear, R.N., Neiger, R., Skelly, B.J., et al. (2005) Primary hyperparathyroidism in 29 dogs: diagnosis, treatment, outcome and associated renal failure. *Journal of Small Animal Practice* 46, 10-16.

Goldstein, R.E., Atwater, D.Z., Cazolli, D.M., et al. (2007) Inheritance, mode of inheritance, and candidate genes for primary hyperparathyroidism in Keeshonden. *Journal of Veterinary Internal Medicine* 21, 199-203.

Ham, K., Greenfield, C.L., Barger, A., et al. (2009) Validation of a rapid parathyroid hormone assay and intraoperative measurement of parathyroid hormone in dogs with benign naturally occurring primary hyperparathyroidism. *Veterinary Surgery* 38, 122-132.

Hostutler, R.A., Chew, D.J., Jaeger, J.Q., et al. (2005) Use and effectiveness of pamidronate disodium for treatment of dogs and cats with hypercalcemia. *Journal of Veterinary Internal Medicine* 19, 29-33.

Long, C.D., Goldstein, R.E., Hornof, W.J., et al. (1999) Percutaneous ultrasound-guided chemical parathyroid ablation for treatment of primary hyperparathyroidism in dogs. *Journal of the American Veterinary Medical Association* 215, 217-221.

Mellanby, R.J., Craig, R., Evans, H., et al. (2006) Plasma concentrations of parathyroid hormone-related protein in dogs with potential disorders of calcium metabolism. *Veterinary Record* 159, 833-838.

Padgett, S.L., Tobias, K.M., Leathers, C.W., et al. (1998) Efficacy of parathyroid autotransplantation in maintaining serum calcium concentrations after bilateral thyroparathyroidectomy in cats. *Journal of the American Animal Hospital Association* 34, 219-234.

Pollard, R.E., Long, C.D., Nelson, R.W., et al. (2001) Percutaneous ultrasonographically guided radiofrequency heat ablation for treatment of primary hyperparathyroidism in dogs. *Journal of the American Veterinary Medical Association* 218, 1106-1110.

Rasor, L., Pollard, R., Feldman, E.C. (2007) Retrospective evaluation of three treatment methods for primary hyperparathyroidism in dogs. *Journal of the American Animal Hospital Association* 43, 70-77.

Sawyer, E.S., Northrup, N.C., Schmiedt, C.W., et al. (2012) Outcome in 19 dogs with parathyroid carcinoma after surgical excision. *Veterinary and Comparative Oncology* 10, 57-64.

28 Tracheal Surgery

Barbara Kirby

Section of Veterinary Clinical Studies, School of Veterinary Medicine, University College Dublin, Dublin, Ireland

Surgery of the trachea in dogs and cats is indicated in a variety of emergent and elective clinical situations. The three most common open surgeries involving the trachea in small animals are temporary tracheostomy, permanent tracheostomy, and tracheal resection and anastomosis. Primary repair of tracheal lacerations associated with bite wounds, projectile injuries, or impalements and primary repair of iatrogenic tracheal lacerations or ruptures associated with endotracheal intubation are occasionally required. In addition, both open and endoscopically assisted minimally invasive techniques are available for support of tracheal collapse.

The trachea is composed of variable numbers of C-shaped hyaline cartilage rings, 35 to 46 rings in dogs (Sura and Durant 2012) and 38 to 43 rings in cats (Hardie 2014). There is a gap between the ends of each cartilage ring dorsally. This gap is filled by the dorsal longitudinal ligament composed of four tissue layers: tracheal mucosa, transverse tracheal muscle, annular ligament composed of fibrous and elastic tissue, and adventitia (Evans and de Lahunta 2013). Adjacent rings are attached cranially and caudally by the annular ligament, with a gap of variable width between adjacent cartilage rings. The tracheal lumen is lined throughout its length with ciliated columnar epithelium containing goblet cells. The tracheal lumen is widest at the level of the cricothyroid junction and progressively tapers to its narrowest point at the thoracic inlet. Brachycephalic dogs have a significantly smaller trachea than nonbrachycephalic dogs, with English bulldogs having a significantly smaller trachea than other brachycephalic breeds (Sura and Durant 2012). Tracheal size in dogs as a proportion of tracheal diameter:thoracic inlet diameter measured from lateral thoracic radiographs is reported as 0.20 ± 0.03 in nonbrachycephalic breeds, 0.16 ± 0.03 in brachycephalic breeds except English bulldogs, and 0.13 ± 0.38 in English bulldogs (Sura and Durant 2012). Tracheal diameter in normal domestic short-haired (DSH) cats is reported as 18% of the diameter of the thoracic inlet In Persian cats, it is reported as 20% of the diameter of the thoracic inlet. In cats, tracheal lumen diameter measurements are similar between brachycephalic and nonbrachycephalic breeds at 5.4 and 5.6 mm, respectively (Hammond *et al.* 2011). The difference for tracheal diameter:thoracic inlet diameter between DSH and Persian cats is attributed to a proportional dorsoventral compression of the thoracic inlet itself in Persian cats (Hammond *et al.* 2011).

Temporary tracheostomy

Temporary tube tracheostomy is most commonly indicated in emergency situations to bypass the proximal part of the upper airway. Emergency temporary tracheostomy may be indicated in upper airway obstruction secondary to functional abnormalities of the larynx such as laryngeal paralysis, laryngeal or upper airway edema after upper airway surgery such as brachycephalic obstructive airway syndrome, and after trauma to the head or neck such as from dog bites, among other reasons. Elective temporary tracheostomy may be indicated for long-term mechanical ventilation and for anesthetic and perioperative management of selected oral, pharyngeal, and laryngeal surgical procedures.

Temporary tube tracheostomy is ideally performed by tracheotomy incision at the level of the third, fourth, or fifth tracheal ring. Transverse tracheotomy between the third and fourth or fourth and fifth tracheal rings is most commonly recommended. Placement of stay sutures around cartilage rings cranial and caudal to the tracheotomy incision is recommended to facilitate replacement of the tube in the event of occlusion or dislodgement. Other tracheotomy incisions that have been described include vertical and inverted U-flap tracheotomy. In vertical tracheotomy, a ventral midline incision across tracheal rings 3 through 5 is recommended (Smith *et al.* 1995). Most authors conclude that the type of tracheotomy incision plays only a minor role in tracheal stenosis after temporary tube tracheostomy (Hedlund 1994); however, in a study of 25 dogs cannulated for 14 days, there was more tracheal distortion with a vertical incision than with an inverted U-flap (Smith *et al.* 1995).

Excisional tracheotomy by removal of a small ellipse of cartilage ring on each side of a horizontal tracheotomy has been recommended for cases when insertion of the tracheostomy tube proves difficult (Hedlund 1994). Excisional tracheotomy by removal of a rectangle of ventral tracheal wall has also been described but is considered a suboptimal technique (Smith *et al.* 1995). The author of this chapter does not recommend either of these excisional tracheotomy techniques for temporary tracheostomy and prefers the transverse tracheotomy incision technique.

In transverse tracheotomy, the length of tracheotomy incision should be limited to no more than one third the circumference of the trachea. Large tracheal wounds (>50% of the tracheal diameter) may heal with excess granulation tissue, resulting in

Complications in Small Animal Surgery, First Edition. Edited by Dominique Griffon and Annick Hamaide.
© 2016 John Wiley & Sons, Inc. Published 2016 by John Wiley & Sons, Inc.
Companion website: www.wiley.com/go/griffon/complications

concentric contracture (Smith *et al.* 1995). Clinical signs of upper airway obstruction associated with tracheal stenosis are usually inapparent until more than 50% of the tracheal lumen is compromised (Smith *et al.* 1995). Differences in healing of various tracheotomy incisions in temporary tracheostomy are generally clinically insignificant.

Complication rates for temporary tracheostomies are high in small animals, with a 43% complication rate in one retrospective study including both dogs and cats (Harvey and O'Brien 1982), 86% reported retrospectively in 42 dogs (Nicholson and Baines 2012), and 87% reported retrospectively in 23 cats (Guenther-Yenke and Rozanski 2007). Cats are generally considered less tolerant of temporary tracheostomy than dogs because of their small tracheal diameters, limiting the choice of available tracheostomy tubes and their propensity to produce large quantities of viscous mucus.

A variety of tubes can be used as temporary tracheostomy tubes, both commercially available and home-made. Tracheostomy tubes made of plastic, silicone, and metal are commercially available. There are no studies comparing complication rates related to these tube types in clinical settings. Double-cannula tubes and tubes with obturators are generally considered easier to clinically manage to prevent obstruction of the tube with clotted blood or secretions, although these tubes are generally not available in sizes small enough to be suitable for use in cats. A variety of other tube types can be modified for use as temporary tracheostomy tubes; standard orotracheal tubes can be shortened, but their straight tube configuration makes them less than ideal. Commercial tracheostomy tubes or shortened orotracheal tubes with cuffs should be used only in situations requiring manual or mechanical ventilation. Temporary tracheostomy tubes should fill no more than 50% of the lumen of the trachea and should not be excessively long, extending no more than a few centimeters into the tracheal lumen distal to the tracheotomy incision.

Tracheostomy-associated stenosis is considered primarily the result of tube selection (Hedlund 1994). Stenosis may occur at the site of insertion, at the level of the cuff, or at the level of the tip of the tube. Movement of the tube at any of these sites may result in irritation to the tracheal mucosa or necrosis of the tracheal cartilage, resulting in healing with excessive granulation tissue and stenosis. Excessively long tubes erode the tracheal wall at contact points. Tubes that are too small or mobile allow excess movement of the tube within the tracheal lumen, also resulting in tracheal injury and stenosis.

Definition

Major short-term complications of temporary tracheostomy include dislodgement of the tracheostomy tube or any event causing total occlusion of the airway requiring immediate intervention (Guenther-Yenke and Rozanski 2007). **Other serious complications** include stricture formation or stenosis, respiratory infections, tracheal rupture, and pneumothorax (Hoareau *et al.* 2011).

Minor complications are defined as non–life-threatening events. Minor complications reported **in cats** with temporary tracheostomies include (Guenther-Yenke and Rozanski 2007):

- Increased respiratory rate and effort associated with partial obstruction of the tube (Figure 28.1)
- Hyperthermia
- Pneumomediastinum
- Subcutaneous emphysema
- Edema at the tracheostomy site
- Horner's syndrome
- Iatrogenic laryngeal paralysis
- Cough
- Vomiting associated with tube suctioning
- Dislodgement of tracheal stay sutures

Complications and percentage of cases with each complication reported **in 42 dogs** with temporary tracheostomies are listed below (Nicholson and Baines 2012). Survival rate was 60% with euthanasia caused by the underlying disease reported in 21% of cases.

- Pneumomediastinum (50%)
- Obstruction of the tube or airway (26%)
- Dislodgement of the tube (21%)
- Pneumothorax (17%)
- Subcutaneous emphysema (12%) (Figure 28.2)
- Hemorrhage (12%)
- Regurgitation (10%)
- Sinus bradycardia during manipulation of the tube or during airway suctioning (10%)
- Vomiting (6%)
- Cough (6%)

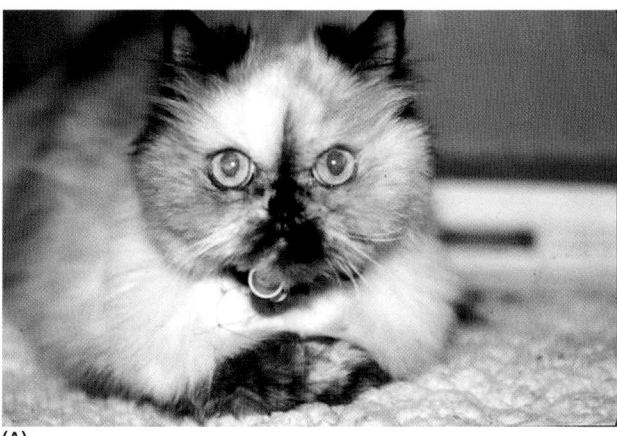

(A)

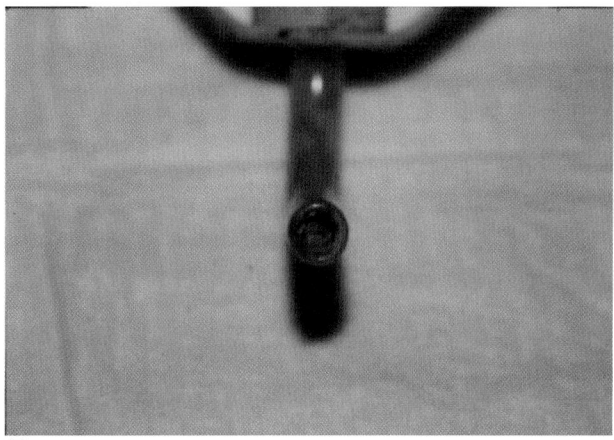

(B)

Figure 28.1 A, Cat with temporary tracheostomy tube placed after per os biopsy of laryngeal mass. **B,** Complete occlusion of the tracheostomy tube lumen by a blood and mucus plug at the time of tube change.

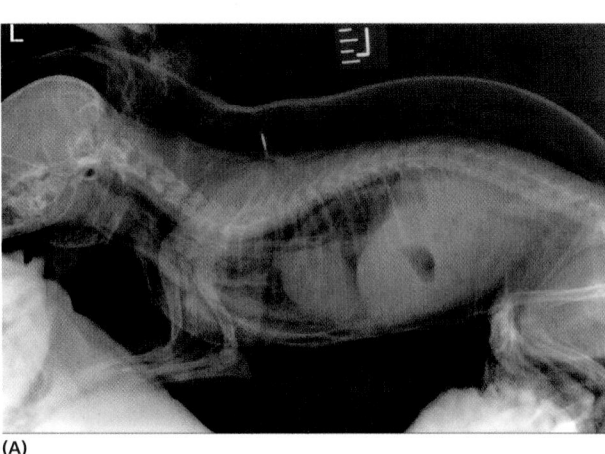

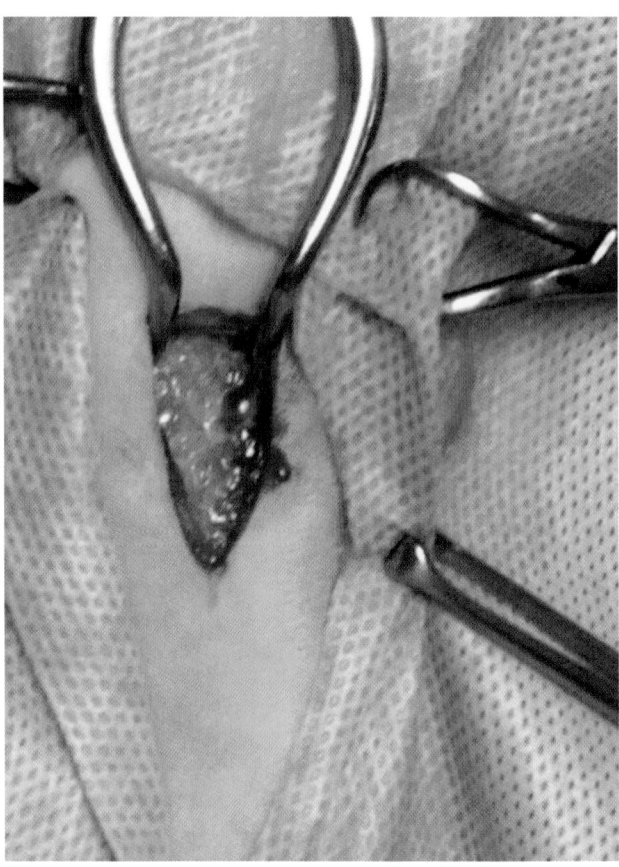

(A)   (B)

Figure 28.2 A, Lateral cervicothoracic radiograph of a 6-month-old, 1.4-kg Chihuahua puppy with severe subcutaneous emphysema and severe, progressive upper airway obstruction secondary to iatrogenic tracheal intubation injury 6 days previously. This puppy and its littermate were intubated with cuffed endotracheal tubes of unknown type for ovariohysterectomy. Both puppies developed subcutaneous emphysema immediately after surgery, and the littermate died a few days after surgery. **B,** Cervical subcutaneous emphysema at the surgical site at the time of temporary tracheostomy tube placement. The subcutaneous emphysema and upper airway obstruction resolved without further surgical intervention, allowing tracheostomy tube removal 5 days after its placement.

- Excessive serosanguineous discharge from stoma (5%)
- Head tremor, seizures, pyothorax (2% each)

Other reported complications in dogs and cats (Harvey and O'Brien 1982):

- Gagging, vomiting, coughing (73%)
- Complete or partial obstruction (18%)
- Tube dislodgement (12.5%)
- Tracheal stenosis
- Aspiration pneumonia
- Pneumothorax, subcutaneous emphysema, pneumomediastinum
- Tracheocutaneous or tracheoesophageal fistulae
- Tracheomalacia

Risk factors

In dogs (Nicholson and Baines 2012):

- Brachycephalic dogs, particularly French and English bulldogs, pugs, and Boston terriers
- Dogs with large amount of ventral neck tissue, such as bulldogs, were prone to dislodge their tubes likely because of the tube being relatively too short for the depth of tissue between the skin and tracheal stoma.
- Brachycephalic breeds requiring mechanical ventilation

- Animals with severe peristomal swelling
- Younger dogs
- Dogs with bradycardia requiring treatment

In cats (Guenther-Yenke and Rozanski 2007):

- Cats with a laryngeal mass were more likely to have tube occlusion than those without a laryngeal mass.

Diagnosis

Diagnosis of **short-term** serious **complications** of temporary tracheostomy are usually made by direct observation of the patient in the intensive care unit. Animals with temporary tracheostomy tubes require continuous direct observation. Monitoring of respiratory rate and effort, oxygen saturation, and body temperature may assist in early detection of partial or complete tube obstruction.

Diagnosis of **long-term complication**, such as stenosis, is most often made by tracheoscopy in animals presenting with signs of respiratory obstruction. Survey lateral cervical or thoracic radiographs are recommended by some clinicians 2 to 3 months after surgery to screen for tracheal stenosis. In the author's opinion, the risk of sedation for imaging outweighs the potential benefit in clinically asymptomatic animals, particularly in brachycephalic breeds.

Treatment

Specific treatment of complications of temporary tracheostomy depends on the specific complication(s) encountered. Items that should be readily available at the cage side include sterile saline for loosening secretions within the tube and sterile suction catheters for suctioning partially obstructed tubes. Regularly scheduled hydration and suctioning of temporary tracheostomy tubes is recommended, with high frequency of tube suction in the early hours after placement as required and then progressively decreasing. Scissors to release the tube ties and replacement tube of the same and smaller diameter should be immediately available in the event of complete obstruction or dislodgement of the tube. In cats, the tube should probably be replaced once daily because of the high risk of complete obstruction of these small-diameter tubes with mucus plugs and the difficulty of clearing the tube lumen in the small, single cannula pediatric tubes that are sufficiently small for the cat trachea. However, the potential benefits of tube replacement must be weighed against the potential risk of acute respiratory decompensation in stressed or fractious cats. The author does not recommend routine daily replacement of tubes in dogs.

Perioperative prophylactic antibiosis is recommended for temporary tube tracheostomy placement because of entry into the contaminated tracheal lumen. Continued postoperative antibiotic therapy is only rarely indicated and may induce colonization or infection with multidrug-resistant bacteria. In most cases, topical treatment of the tracheostomy site is sufficient.

Outcome

The outcome in dogs and cats with temporary tracheostomies largely depends on the underlying reason for tube placement. In a retrospective study of 15 brachycephalic dogs, most commonly with aspiration pneumonia as the underlying disease, the rate of discharge from the hospital was only 27% (Hoareau *et al.* 2011). In the Nicholson and Baines (2012) study of complications associated with temporary tracheostomy tubes in 42 dogs, the survival rate was 60%; 21% were euthanized because of their underlying disease, 10% were euthanized with complications associated with the tube influencing the decision for euthanasia, and 10% died. Management of the tracheostomy tube was considered a failure in 19% of the cases in this study. In the 23 cats with temporary tracheostomies reported by Guenther-Yenke and Rozanski (2007), 7 required permanent tracheostomy, and 6 died or were euthanized in the hospital. Seven of the 10 cats that were discharged had permanent tracheostomies, with only 1 long-term survivor. The outcome in cats with temporary tracheostomy appears worse than for dogs. The complication rates and outcomes in both dogs and cats are worse than those reported in humans, with a 66% complication rate reported for operative tube tracheostomy and an 11% complication rate reported for percutaneous tube tracheostomy in humans (Hedlund 1994).

Prevention

Prevention of complications in temporary tracheostomy requires careful and meticulous anesthetic and surgical techniques, including:

- Control of the airway by orotracheal intubation in most cases allows appropriate positioning, preparation for aseptic surgery, and controlled dissection for exposure of the trachea. The "slash" technique can generally be avoided.
- Proper surgical technique, including:
  - Transverse tracheotomy incision between the third and fourth or fourth and fifth tracheal rings (Figure 28.3)

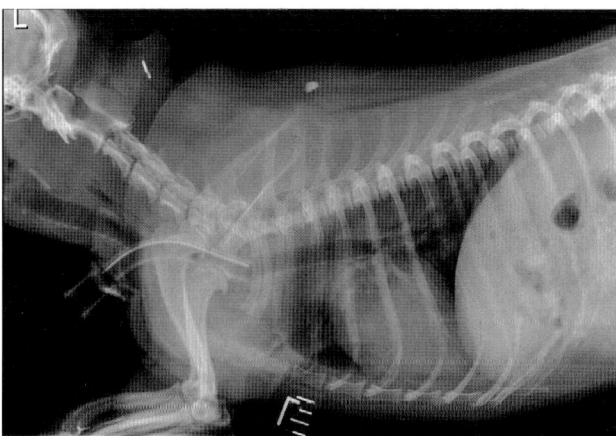

Figure 28.3 Lateral cervicothoracic radiograph of an adult Parson Russell terrier with cervical bite wounds and an emergency temporary tube tracheostomy placed at the local emergency clinic. Technical errors included oversized tube filling 100% of the tracheal lumen and incorrect site of tracheotomy incision at the thoracic inlet. This dog required a permanent tracheostomy because of multiple hyoid apparatus fracture or luxation and laryngeal paralysis. A tracheal resection and anastomosis was required at the temporary tracheostomy site. If the tracheotomy for temporary tracheostomy had been correctly sited in the proximal trachea, the resection and anastomosis would not have been required.

  - Tracheotomy incision of approximately one third the tracheal circumference
  - Placement of stay sutures cranial and caudal to the tracheotomy incision
  - Tube selection, including tube type, diameter, and length most appropriate for the individual patient
    - Double-cannula or obturator tubes preferred
    - Avoid cuffed tubes unless ventilation required
    - Tube occupying no more that 50% of tracheal lumen
    - Proportionately long tube for English and French bulldogs
  - Secure the tube with ties (e.g., umbilical tape) around the neck to prevent dislodgement of the tube and movement of the tube within the tracheal lumen.
  - Avoid suturing the tube directly to the skin because this delays tube replacement in the event the tube becomes dislodged.
  - Avoid excessive bandaging around the neck, which may obstruct or dislodge the tube.

Critical care and nursing care of the patient and tube in the postoperative period, including:

- Continuous patient monitoring
- Rapid intervention for dyspnea, tube dislodgement, or tube obstruction
- Regular "tracheal toilette," including
  - Aseptic technique for all tube manipulations
  - Preoxygenation for tube suctioning, cleaning, or replacement
  - Regular cleaning of the peristomal skin and application of petrolatum to prevent adherence of mucus and exudates to the skin
  - Monitoring for vagally mediated bradycardia associated with manipulation or suctioning of the tube, particularly in brachycephalic dogs
    - Pretreatment with atropine or glycopyrrolate in animals after a single incident of bradycardia
  - Daily tube replacement in cats

- Supportive care. including
  - Maintenance of hydration
  - Appropriate analgesic and antiinflammatory management
  - Nutritional support
  - TLC (tender loving care)

Permanent tracheostomy

Permanent tracheostomy is most commonly considered a salvage or palliative procedure. Permanent tracheostomy is always an elective procedure and should not be the chosen technique for emergency tracheostomy.

Permanent tracheostomy may be indicated for advanced laryngeal collapse, laryngeal masses, or laryngeal trauma. Permanent tracheostomy may also be indicated after temporary tube tracheostomy for any reason when extubation is not tolerated. Permanent tracheostomy is a necessary component of complete laryngectomy.

Permanent tracheostomy involves creation of a permanent opening between the tracheal lumen and the skin. Precise planning and construction of the tracheostomy is required for optimal outcome (see Prevention later). Appropriate patient selection and committed owner(s) are also required for successful outcome.

Definition

The most common long-term complications of permanent tracheostomy are stenosis of the tracheostoma and skin-fold occlusion of the tracheostoma. Transient intermittent occlusion of the stoma may be related to posture in some animals. Obstruction or collapse at the tracheostomy site may be caused by concurrent tracheal collapse, tracheomalacia, or creation of an excessively large stoma (Hedlund 1994). Sixty percent of dogs and cats with permanent tracheostomy (without laryngectomy) lose their ability to vocalize normally. In cats, occlusion of the stoma by mucus plugs is a potentially life-threatening complication both in the short and long terms. Additional minor complications include subcutaneous emphysema, peristomal hematoma or seroma, peristomal dermatitis, and peristomal skin trauma associated with scratching.

Additional long-term complications in some animals include risk of death by drowning and tracheal irritation from environmental factors such as smoke and dust inhalation. Inhalation of foreign bodies through the stoma is a potential risk but has not been described to date.

Risk factors and outcome

Permanent tracheostomy is associated with particularly high complication and mortality rates in cats compared with dogs. Permanent tracheostomy is rare in both cats and dogs, perhaps even more rare in cats than dogs. In a retrospective study involving six veterinary medical teaching hospitals over a period of 18 years, only 21 cats undergoing permanent tracheostomy were identified (Stepnik *et al.* 2009). All 21 survived the surgical procedure, but 11 died (6 while hospitalized and 5 after discharge), 7 were euthanized for progression of neoplastic disease, and only 2 were still alive at the time of the study. Mean survival time in 20 cats with follow-up data was only 20.5 days. Mucus plugs at the stoma or elsewhere in the respiratory tract, including 3 cats with mucus plugs in the bronchi at necropsy, appeared to be the primary cause of both morbidity and mortality.

In Gunther-Yenke and Rozanski's (2007) study of 23 cats with tracheostomies cited earlier, 7 cats required permanent tracheostomies and were discharged from the hospital, but only one cat was alive long term. Six cats died between 2 and 281 days, 2 with confirmed occlusion of the tracheostomy site.

In a study of long-term outcome of permanent tracheostomies in 21 dogs, 50% had major complications, including 20% that required revision surgery (Occhipinti and Hauptman 2014). The most common complications were aspiration pneumonia and occlusion of the stoma by skin folds or stenosis. Preoperative diagnoses in these cases included laryngeal collapse associated with brachycephalic airway obstructive syndrome (BAOS) ($n = 5$), bilateral laryngeal paralysis ($n = 5$), laryngeal neoplasia ($n = 2$), severe laryngospasm ($n = 2$), traumatic laryngeal collapse caused by cervical bite wounds ($n = 2$), and laryngeal malformation ($n = 3$). Seventeen of 21 dogs had received airway surgery before permanent tracheostomy. The median survival time was 328 days with acute death caused by respiratory obstruction in 26%, euthanasia caused by respiratory disease in 21%, and death or euthanasia caused by nonrespiratory disease in 53%. Long-term survival (1–9 years) was achieved in 50% of cases, with 25% surviving 1321 days or longer. Diagnosis was the only factor that approached significance when evaluating survival times.

Diagnosis

- Diagnosis of aspiration pneumonia is made on the basis of clinical signs, thoracic radiographs, and bronchoalveolar lavage sampling for cytology and bacterial culture.
- Collapse or folding of the tracheostoma caused by tracheal collapse, tracheomalacia, or excessively large tracheostomy can be diagnosed by cervical radiographs or tracheoscopy. In some cases, fluoroscopic imaging may be useful to diagnose dynamic, intermittent, or postural collapse.
- Diagnosis of skin-fold occlusion, stomal stenosis, peristomal dermatitis, and other local problems such as hair ingrowth are made by direct observation. Bacterial fungal culture of severe peristomal dermatitis is useful in directing treatment.

In cats, detection of mucus plugs at the tracheostoma can usually be made by direct observation. Mucus plugs in the bronchi in three cats reported by Stepnik (2009) were detected only at necropsy.

Treatment

- Nebulization of cats with permanent tracheostomies every 2 to 8 hours after surgery has been recommended in an attempt to decrease the incidence of mucus plug formation, although the efficacy of this treatment is unknown (Stepnik *et al.* 2009). The efficacy of treatment with mucolytics and other agents is also unknown. Overly aggressive or frequent airway suctioning may promote mucus secretion. Suction using sterile catheters should be limited to superficial airways at negative pressures no greater than 120 mm Hg. Limited suctioning of the airway on an as-needed only basis is recommended in humans and may limit complications in other species as well (Stepnik *et al.* 2009).
- Occlusion of the tracheostoma by skin folds is an indication for revision surgery. Revision may also be considered in stomal stenosis, although stenosis of 10% to 35% of the original stomal area is expected and not usually associated with clinical signs.
- Aspiration pneumonia is treated with appropriate antibiosis based on culture and sensitivity testing. Nebulization and chest coupage may assist mobilization and expectoration of purulent secretions. Supportive care, including maintenance of hydration and nutrition, is important.
- Peristomal dermatitis is usually treated topically. Overly aggressive cleaning of peristomal skin may contribute to the occurrence

of peristomal dermatitis. Appropriate technique for hair clipping and skin care should be demonstrated to the owners.

Prevention

Prevention of complications of permanent tracheostomy require meticulous surgical planning and surgical technique including:

- Excision of a rectangular segment of tracheal wall centered ventrally of three to fourth cartilage widths in length and one third the circumference of the tracheal circumference. Preservation of the lateral aspects of the tracheal walls is important to prevent collapse or bending of the trachea at the tracheostomy site (Hedlund 1994).
- Ventral deviation of the trachea reduces tension on the mucocutaneous junction during healing. This is accomplished by creation of a sternohyoid muscle sling by adequate dissection of the sternohyoid muscles bilaterally and apposition of their medial edges dorsal to the trachea.
- Placement of a series of interrupted intradermal sutures between the skin and peritracheal tissues lateral to the proposed tracheostoma and between the skin and annular ligaments proximal and distal to the proposed tracheostoma promotes adhesion between the trachea and skin, reducing skin-fold problems.
- Careful handling of the tracheal mucosa to create a circumferential rim of mucosa around the incised cartilage edges minimizes tracheal stenosis.
- Excision of a large amount of skin and subcutaneous fat in animals with loose neck skin or excessive fat reduce postoperative skin-fold occlusion of the stoma (Figure 28.4).
- Polypropylene tracheal ring prostheses may be beneficial at the time of initial tracheostomy construction to support the stoma in patients with concurrent tracheal collapse or tracheomalacia.
- Gentle cleaning of the stoma and surrounding skin in the postoperative period prevents irritation or disruption of the tracheal mucosa at the mucocutaneous junction.

Tracheal resection and anastomosis

Tracheal resection and anastomosis may be required for a variety of conditions in dogs and cats, including tracheal stenosis (Figure 28.5), tracheal rupture, tracheal avulsion, tracheal or peritracheal masses

(e.g., benign or malignant neoplasia, granulomas, intramural hematomas), and iatrogenic injuries to the tracheal wall associated with improper temporary tracheostomy technique (Figure 28.6).

Definition

Complications of tracheal resection and anastomosis have only rarely been reported. Iatrogenic laryngeal paralysis may result from damage to one or both recurrent laryngeal nerves. Tracheal devascularization and necrosis may result from overly aggressive peritracheal dissection (Kirby *et al.* 1991). Excessive tension at the anastomosis site may lead to partial or complete disruption of the anastomosis. Partial dehiscence of the anastomosis may lead to partial tracheal wall necrosis with resultant healing by granulation tissue formation, scarring, and stenosis.

Intrathoracic tracheal avulsion is reported in cats, most often associated with blunt traumatic incident (White and Burton 2000). Most cats are presented 1 to 3 weeks after the traumatic incident with progressively worsening dyspnea. Rupture of the trachea occurs 1 to 4 cm cranial to its bifurcation with maintenance of the tracheal lumen by development of a pseudotrachea or pseudoairway of mediastinal tissue. Clinical signs result from obstruction or stenosis of the lumen of the trachea at both transected ends. Resection of four to eight tracheal rings and anastomosis resulted in long-term resolution in all cats reported (White and Burton 2000).

Tracheal rupture has also been reported in 16 cats, most commonly associated with cats anaesthetized for dental procedures (Hardie *et al.* 1999). In a cadaver study in cats in this same report, tracheal rupture was induced in 7 of 10 cats with endotracheal tube cuff inflation with more than 6 mL of air. Rupture of the trachealis muscle from its attachment to the tracheal cartilages on the left side occurred consistently, with the mediastinal coverage remaining intact and expanding. This phenomenon likely explains the pseudotrachea formation observed in the traumatic tracheal avulsion cats reported by White and Burton. Hardie *et al.* further reported a study of 20 clinically normal cats undergoing anaesthesia, where the volume of air needed for endotracheal tube cuff inflation to obtain an airtight seal was only 1.6 ± 0.7 mL (range, 0–3 mL) ,concluding that the tracheal rupture in the 16 reported clinically affected cats was most likely iatrogenic in origin and associated with overly zealous cuff inflation (Hardie *et al.* 1999).

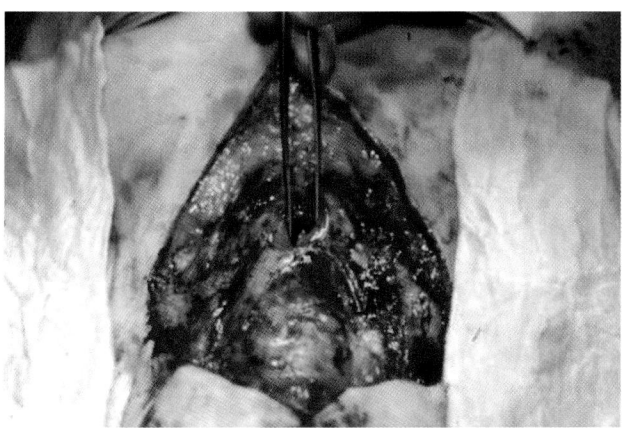

(A)

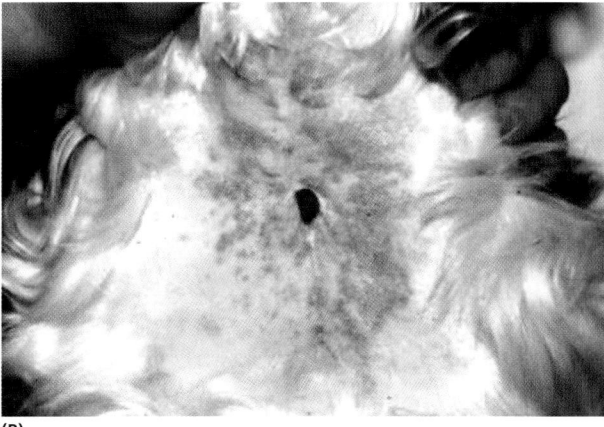

(B)

Figure 28.4 A, Intraoperative photograph of large skin and subcutaneous tissue excision at the time of construction of a permanent tracheostomy to reduce the risk of postoperative skin fold occlusion of the stoma in an adult Cavalier King Charles spaniel with grade 3 laryngeal collapse. **B,** Clinically insignificant stenosis of the stoma and mild peristomal dermatitis at the 6-month postoperative follow-up.

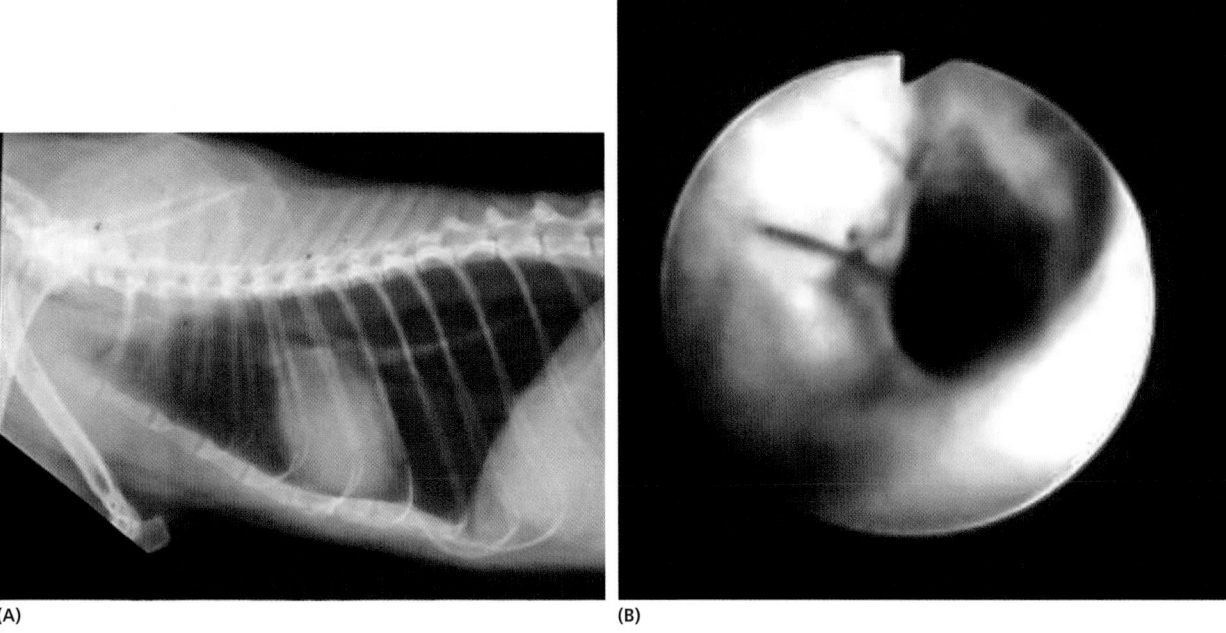

(A)   (B)

Figure 28.5 A, Tracheal stenosis in an adult cat caused by iatrogenic tracheal injury. Tracheal resection and anastomosis were required. **B,** Endoscopic appearance of the site of anastomosis 3 months after surgery. Note the polypropylene sutures covered with respiratory mucosa visible at the anastomosis site and absence of tracheal stenosis.

Risk factors
- Tracheal devascularization
- Excessive tension at anastomotic site

Diagnosis
- Clinical signs may be absent despite extensive tracheal necrosis (Kirby *et al*. 1991).
- Dyspnea, tachypnea, or subcutaneous emphysema may be observed.
- Radiographic or tracheoscopic diagnosis of tracheal stenosis

Treatment
- Varies with the cause of anastomotic failure
- Revision surgery with resection of additional tracheal rings and repeat tracheal anastomosis may be indicated.
- Placement of vertical mattress sutures around tracheal rings distant from the site of anastomosis helps reduce tension at the anastomosis site.
- Omentalization of potentially devitalized trachea or anastomosis site with compromised blood supply

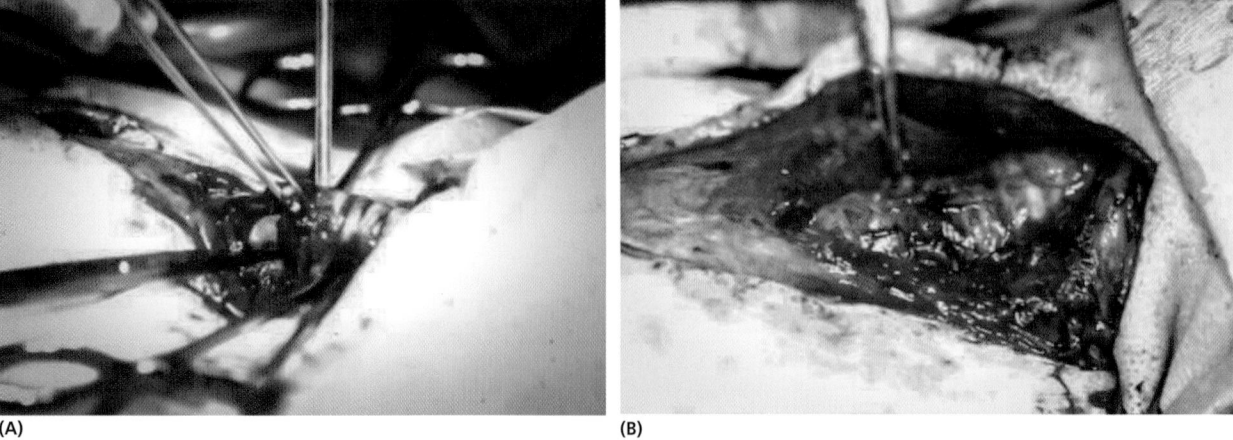

(A)   (B)

Figure 28.6 A, Intraoperative photograph of an adult Chow with inappropriate temporary tracheostomy technique via excision of a large ventrolateral tracheal window necessitating tracheal reconstruction by resection of five tracheal rings and end-to-end anastomosis. **B,** Note the polypropylene vertical mattress tension-relieving sutures supporting the primary suture line.

Outcome

- There are no large prospective or retrospective case series reporting outcomes in tracheal resection and anastomosis in dogs or cats.
- Good outcome reported in 16 cats with tracheal rupture (Hardie *et al.* 1999) and 9 cats with tracheal avulsion (White and Burton 2000) treated with tracheal resection and anastomosis.

Prevention

- The laryngeal and vagus nerves must be protected from iatrogenic injury during peritracheal dissection.
- Identification and preservation of the main tracheal blood supply (cranial and caudal thyroid arteries) and segmental tracheal blood supply are important for successful surgery. The segmental vessels supplying the area of trachea to be resected should be carefully isolated and individually ligated.
- Blood supply to the site of anastomosis can be augmented in cases of trauma with suspected major vascular disruption and cases with suspected iatrogenic devascularization by omentalization of the anastomosis (Fujiwara *et al.* 1994).
- A martingale head restraint maintaining flexion of the neck may prevent excessive tension at the anastomosis site in animals with large cervical tracheal resections, although there are no specific reports of use of this technique in small animals.

References

Evans, H.E., de Lahunta, A. (2013) The respiratory system. In Evans, H.E., de Lahunta, A. (eds.) *Miller's Anatomy of the Dog*, 4th edn, Elsevier, St. Louis, pp. 349-350.

Fujiwara, K., Nakahara, K., Fujii, Y., et al. (1994) Effect of omentopexy on wound healing of the extensively detached and anastomosed canine trachea. *Surgery* 115, 227-232.

Guenther-Yenke, C. L., Rozanski, E.A. (2007) Tracheostomy in cats: 23 cases (1998-2006). *Journal of Feline Medicine and Surgery* 9, 451-457.

Hammond, G., Geary, M., Coleman, E., et al. (2011) Radiographic measurements of the trachea in domestic shorthair and Persian cats. *Journal of Feline Medicine and Surgery* 13, 881-884.

Hardie, E.M. (2014) In Langley-Hobbs, S.J., Demetriou, J.L., Ladlow, J. F. (eds.) *Feline Soft Tissue and General Surgery*. Saunders Elsevier, Edinburgh, pp. 531-540.

Hardie, E.M., Spodnick, G. J., Gilson, S.D., et al. (1999) Tracheal rupture in cats: 16 cases (1983-1998). *Journal of the American Veterinary Medical Association* 214, 508-512.

Harvey, C.E., O'Brien, J.A. (1982) Tracheotomy in the dog and cat: analysis of 89 episodes in 79 animals. *Journal of the American Animal Hospital Association* 18, 563-566.

Hedlund, C.S. (1994) Tracheostomies in the management of canine and feline upper respiratory disease. *Veterinary Clinics of North America: Small Animal Practice* 24, 873-886.

Hoareau, G.L., Mellema, M.S., Silverstein, D.C. (2011) Indication, management, and outcome of brachycephalic dogs requiring mechanical ventilation. *Journal of Veterinary Emergency and Critical Care* 21, 226-35.

Kirby, B.M., Bjorling, D.E., Rankin, H.G., et al. (1991) The effect of surgical isolation and application of polypropylene spiral prostheses on tracheal blood flow. *Veterinary Surgery* 20, 49-54.

Nicholson, I., Baines, S. (2012) Complications associated with temporary tracheostomy tubes in 42 dogs (1998 to 2007). *Journal of Small Animal Practice* 53, 108-114.

Occhipinti, L. L., Hauptman, J. G. (2014) Long-term outcome of permanent tracheostomies in dogs: 21 cases (2000-2012). *The Canadian Veterinary Journal* 55, 357-360.

Smith, M.M., Saunders, G.K., Leib, M.S., et al. (1995) Evaluation of horizontal and vertical tracheotomy healing after short-duration tracheostomy in dogs. *Journal of Oral Maxillofacial Surgery* 53, 289-294.

Stepnik, M.W., Hehl, M.L, Hardie, E.M., et al. (2009) Outcome of permanent tracheostomy for treatment of upper airway obstruction in cats: 21 cases (1990-2007). *Journal of the American Veterinary Medical Association* 234, 638-643.

Sura, P.A., Durant, A.M. (2012) Trachea and bronchi. In Tobias, K.M., Johnston, S.A. (eds.) *Veterinary Surgery Small Animal*. Elsevier, St. Louis, pp. 1734-1751.

White, R.N., Burton, C.A. (2000) Surgical management of intrathoracic tracheal avulsion in cats: long-term results in 9 consecutive cases. *Veterinary Surgery* 29, 430-435.

Laura Cuddy

Small Animal Surgery, Department of Surgery, Section of Veterinary Clinical Studies, School of Agriculture, Food Science and Veterinary Medicine, University College Dublin, Dublin, Ireland

Intraluminal tracheal stenting was initially developed for treatment of intrathoracic tracheal collapse in dogs and is now routinely used for treatment of both intra- and extrathoracic tracheal collapse (Barras and Myers 2000; Gellasch *et al.* 2002). Although earlier versions were fabricated from stainless steel, the tracheal stents currently used most widely are composed of nitinol, a biocompatible alloy of nickel and titanium, with the properties of thermal shape memory, superelasticity, and force hysteresis (Barras and Myers 2000; Sura and Krahwinkel 2008; Durant *et al.* 2012). These self-expanding metallic stents exert a continuous outward radial force against the tracheal wall to resist collapse of the chondromalacic cartilage during changes in airway pressure to maintain tracheal patency.

There are two broad categories of tracheal stents: (1) woven, knitted, or mesh or (2) laser cut. The tracheal stent used most widely is the mesh, nitinol Vet Stent-Trachea (Infiniti Medical, Menlo Park, CA). These stents are reconstrainable and undergo a degree of foreshortening after release from the outer sheath, meaning they may shorten over time, with the degree of shortening depending on tracheal diameter. Newer iterations include variable lumen stents to accommodate those patients with significant disparity in intraluminal diameter between the cervical and thoracic trachea.

Tracheal stents may be deployed under either endoscopic or fluoroscopic guidance (Sura and Krahwinkel 2008; Durant *et al.* 2012). Because of the frequency of complications associated with intraluminal stenting, this procedure is still widely considered as a salvage procedure for patients who are refractory to conservative management or have extensive intrathoracic tracheal collapse and as a less invasive alternative to extraluminal tracheal ring prostheses. The advantages of intraluminal tracheal stents include the relatively noninvasive and rapid nature of the procedure.

Complications associated with deployment

Definition

Suboptimal positioning of a tracheal stent, typically resulting from a technical error, may result in the absence of bridging of collapsed areas of the trachea or impingement of the stent on the larynx cranially or on the carina caudally. Malpositioning of a tracheal stent has been documented postoperatively in up to 50% of cases when using a cord mechanism for deployment (Sura and Krahwinkel 2008).

Risk factors

- Inaccurate measurement and selection of appropriate stent diameter or length on preprocedural cervical and thoracic radiographs, resulting in stent over- or under-sizing
- Inappropriate selection of the starting point for stent deployment caudally
- Inadvertent retraction of the stent during or after deployment

Diagnosis

- If the stent is deployed under fluoroscopic guidance, identification of malpositioning is readily achieved on lateral cervical and thoracic fluoroscopic images (Figure 29.1).
- If the stent is deployed under endoscopic guidance, malpositioning may be identified during endoscopic visualization or on postprocedural radiographs (Figure 29.2).

Treatment

- If feasible, the stent may be reconstrained and repositioned before redeployment.
- If the stent has been completely deployed and cannot be reconstrained, it may be withdrawn from the trachea in its entirety by

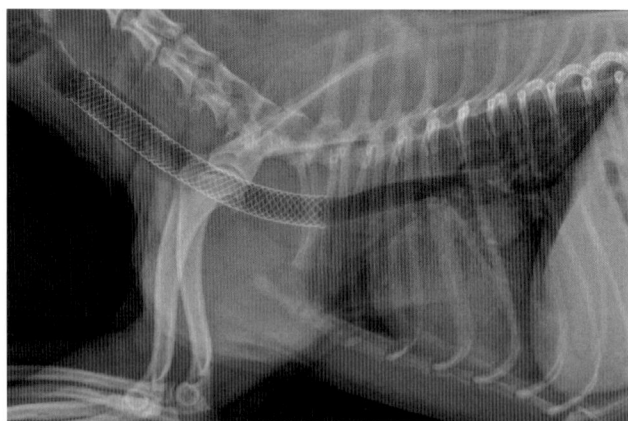

Figure 29.1 Lateral radiograph obtained immediately after stent deployment. There is impingement of the cranial aspect of the stent on the cricoid cartilage caused by inaccurate selection of the caudal point for initiation of stent deployment. This translated clinically as a persistent cough.

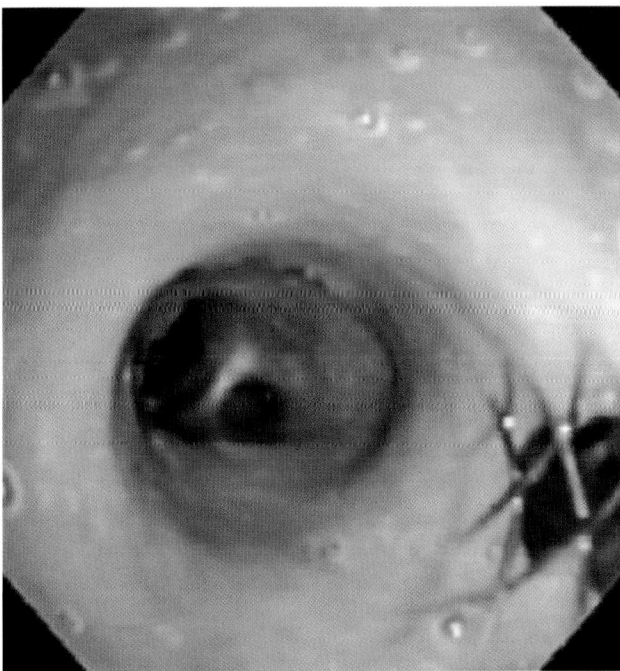

Figure 29.2 Endoscopic image of a tracheal stent extending caudally into a mainstem bronchus. *Source:* C. Weisse, 2014. Reproduced with permission from C. Weisse.

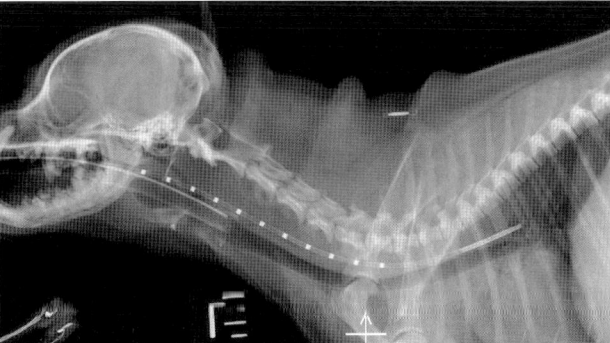

Figure 29.3 Lateral radiograph of the cervical and thoracic regions with the endotracheal tube withdrawn to the level of the larynx under a breath-hold of 20 cm H$_2$O. A measuring catheter with radiopaque markers is present in the esophagus.

grasping the cranial end with an alligator forceps and sliding an endotracheal tube down over the stent (Gary Ellison, personal communication). A new stent can subsequently be deployed.
• If the stent cannot be reconstrained or withdrawn and is not bridging the collapsed areas sufficiently, a second stent may be deployed within the lumen of the first stent.

Outcome
• This complication can be overcome if a stent is successfully redeployed to bridge the collapsed areas of the trachea.
• If an excessively long or malpositioned stent is impinging on the carina or the cricoid cartilage, persistent coughing may be expected.
• A stent that is too short or malpositioned, and therefore incompletely bridging areas of collapse, typically results in persistence of clinical signs.

Prevention
• The length of collapsed trachea should be estimated on an unsedated fluoroscopic examination, ideally during induced coughing if this does not place the patient at undue risk. The stent should extend at least 1 to 2 cm cranial and caudal to the collapsed area or from 1 cm caudal to the cricoid cartilage to 1 cm cranial to the carina if planning to stent the trachea in its entirety. A repeatable landmark, such as an adjacent rib or intercostal space, should be identified at the optimal location of the caudal aspect of the stent to facilitate accurate positioning during fluoroscopic-assisted deployment.
• A measuring catheter with radiopaque marks, typically at 10-mm intervals, should be placed into the esophagus to account for radiographic magnification (Figure 29.3).
• Accurate measurements of the maximal tracheal diameter should be obtained from preprocedural lateral radiographs of the thorax

and cervical region. These should be obtained under general anesthesia with the endotracheal tube withdrawn to the level of the larynx and using positive-pressure ventilation to facilitate a breath-hold at 20 cm H$_2$O (see Figure 29.3).
• A stent 10% to 20% times the maximal diameter of the trachea is selected to minimize the risk of stent migration (Sura and Krahwinkel 2008). The length should at least encompass the area of collapse, as well as 1 to 2 cm on either side. Consideration may be given to stenting the entire length of the intra- and extrathoracic trachea to prevent subsequent collapse of the trachea adjacent to the stent.
• A shortening chart should be consulted so that the expected length of the deployed stent can be estimated based on tracheal diameter.
• It is ideal to maintain a selection of stents in 2-mm-diameter increments in stock because stent deployment ideally immediately follows acquisition of measurements.
• All manipulations of the deployment system should be performed under direct fluoroscopic or endoscopic guidance. Care should be taken to gently advance the deploying hand while simultaneously withdrawing the outer sleeve to prevent a shift in the site of deployment. The stent should not be advanced while the sheath is stationary.

Anesthetic complications

Definition
Lack of coordination between surgeon and anesthesiologist during stent placement may result in temporary inadequate delivery of oxygen and inhaled anesthetic agent, which may compromise homeostatic processes and complicate control of the depth of anesthesia. Entrapment of the deployed stent in the endotracheal tube may result in inadvertent stent removal during extubation.

Risk factors
• Inadequate endotracheal tube size
• Lack of a radiopaque marker at the distal extent of the endotracheal tube
• Unavailability of a right-angled bronchoscope adapter for the endotracheal tube (Figure 29.4)
• Lack of additional or total intravenous anesthesia (TIVA)
• Inexperience of the anesthesiologist or surgeon
• Poor communication between the anesthesiologist and surgeon

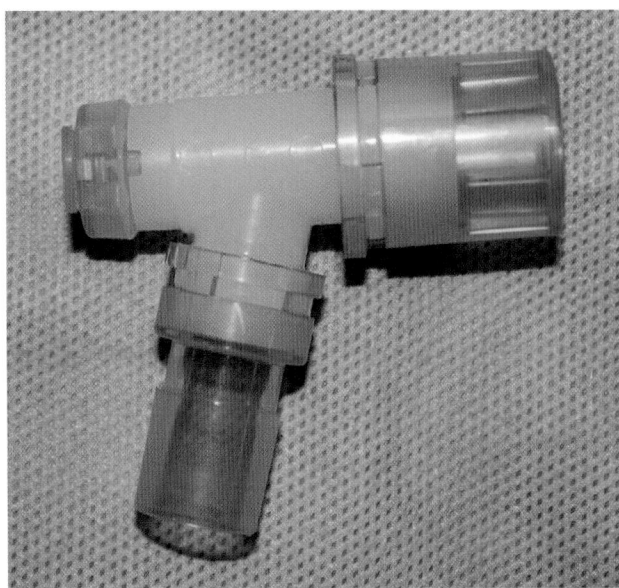

Figure 29.4 A right-angled bronchoscope adapter permits administration of oxygen through a side channel during stent placement.

Diagnosis
- Hypoxemia may be recognized on arterial blood gas analysis or via pulse oximetry.
- Inadequate depth of anesthesia may result in coughing and other movements, which may complicate stent deployment.
- Entrapment of the endotracheal tube by the stent may be identified during fluoroscopy if a radiopaque marker is incorporated in the distal aspect of the tube.

Treatment
- Communication between the anesthesiologist and surgeon is key to limit the duration of limited airway access and facilitate simultaneous endotracheal tube withdrawal to the level of the larynx during stent deployment.

Outcome
- Anesthetic complications and compromised airway access may lead to periprocedural death.
- If preventive measures are instituted, the duration of hypoxia and exposure of staff to inhalant anesthetics can be limited.

Prevention
- Intubation should be achieved with the largest endotracheal tube possible to facilitate the stent delivery system while simultaneously permitting adequate oxygen delivery.
- A right-angled bronchoscope adapter allows the anesthesiologist to administer oxygen during stent deployment (see Figure 29.4).
- TIVA with oxygen supplementation is preferable to reduce unnecessary exposure of staff to inhalant anesthetics.
- A radiopaque marker should be incorporated into the distal aspect of the endotracheal tube to prevent inadvertent deployment of the stent within the tube. The endotracheal tube should be withdrawn to the larynx as the stent is deployed to minimize the risk of entrapment.

Stent obstruction caused by granuloma formation

Definition
This is obstruction of the internal lumen of the endotracheal stent and trachea by granulation tissue forming secondary to a foreign body reaction or persistent tracheitis. This was recorded in 2 of 12 dogs in a case series (Sura and Krahwinkel 2008).

Risk factors
- Stainless steel stents may be less biologically inert than their nitinol counterparts.
- Persistent sterile or bacterial tracheitis may stimulate the production of exuberant granulation tissue.

Diagnosis
- Granulation tissue can be identified at the cranial or caudal aspect of the stent–trachea interface as a radiopaque thickening of the tracheal wall on lateral radiographic projections (Figure 29.5).
- Obstruction of the tracheal lumen can be further characterized by endoscopic visualization (Figure 29.6).

Treatment
- Medical therapy with antiinflammatory doses of corticosteroids (prednisone 0.25 mg/kg orally [PO] every 24 hours) is initially recommended.
- Additional treatment with colchicine (0.03 mg/kg PO every 24 hours) has been reported to resolve granulation tissue associated with endotracheal stenting (Moritz *et al.* 2004; Brown *et al.* 2008; Sura and Krahwinkel 2008). Colchicine is an alkaloid derivative that inhibits microtubule formation, stimulates tissue collagenase production, and has antiinflammatory effects, thereby inhibiting collagen synthesis and subsequent deposition of fibrous tissue.
- Doxycycline is a tetracycline antibiotic that also has an immunomodulatory function as a matrix metalloproteinase inhibitor. The dual function of this drug may resolve the underlying infection and dampen the inflammatory response of the tracheal mucosa.
- Targeted antibiotic therapy for bacterial tracheitis may be warranted.
- Endoscopic laser ablation of granulation tissue may be performed (Figure 29.7).

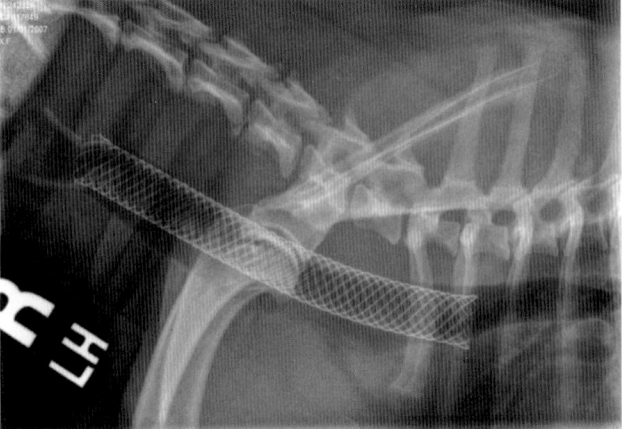

Figure 29.5 Right lateral radiograph of the cervical and cranial thoracic region demonstrating thickening of the tracheal lumen at the caudal aspect of the stent consistent with granuloma formation. *Source:* A. Gallagher, 2014. Reproduced with permission from A. Gallagher.

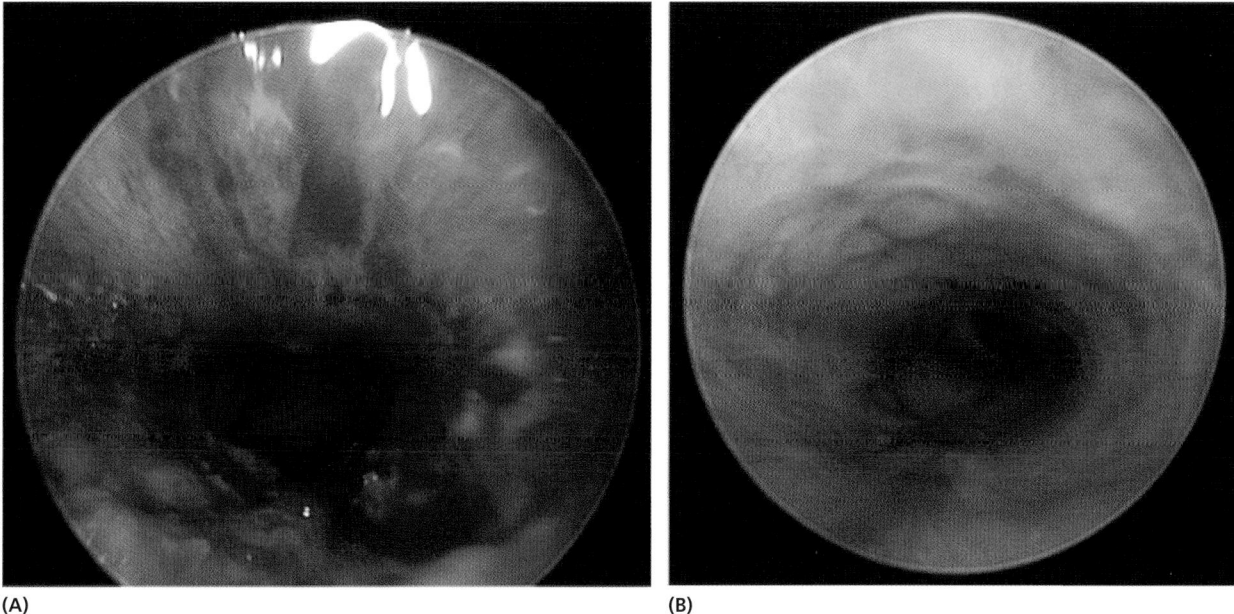

(A)   (B)

Figure 29.6 Endoscopic visualization of granuloma formation at the cranial (**A**) and caudal (**B**) aspects of a tracheal stent in the dog in Figure 29.5. *Source:* A. Gallagher, 2014. Reproduced with permission from A. Gallagher.

Outcome

A single case has been reported describing the resolution of granulation stenosis after treatment with corticosteroids, colchicine, and doxycycline in a Yorkshire terrier (Brown *et al.* 2008). Anecdotally, although the initial response to treatment may be positive, the outlook for long-term management or resolution of granulation tissue appears guarded, with many patients succumbing to worsening of their clinical signs because of progressive obstruction of the tracheal lumen.

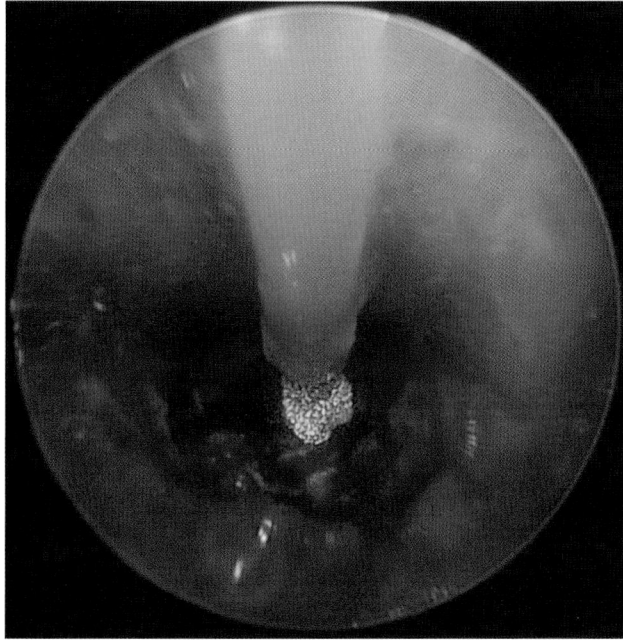

Figure 29.7 Laser ablation of the granulation tissue within the endotracheal stent and tracheal lumen of the dog in Figure 29.5. *Source:* A. Gallagher, 2014. Reproduced with permission from A. Gallagher.

Prevention

• Minimizing bouts of tracheitis and recurrent tracheal infection is warranted, with administration of intermittent antiinflammatory doses of corticosteroids and empirical broad-spectrum antibiotic therapy.
• The use of nitinol stents may reduce the risk of granuloma formation because of their relatively inert nature compared with stainless steel (Moritz *et al.* 2004; Sura and Krahwinkel 2008). Newer generations of Vet Stent-Trachea (Infiniti Medical, LLC, Menlo Park, CA) have a proprietary PurLux high-definition stent surface to enhance biocompatibility.

Stent migration

Definition

Stent migration is dislodgement and movement of an endotracheal stent from its initial position at the time of deployment, typically occurring in a cranial direction. In extreme circumstances, expectoration of the stent may occur.

Risk factors

• Persistent coughing caused by tracheal or laryngeal irritation, interference with the mucociliary apparatus, or mainstem bronchial collapse results in cranial propulsive forces.
• Iatrogenic endotracheal stent dislodgement can occur with traumatic endotracheal intubation at subsequent general anesthetic procedures.

Diagnosis

Orthogonal radiographs of the cervical and thoracic regions can be used to document stent location relative to adjacent ribs or absence of the stent in cases of expectoration.

Treatment

• In the absence of significant worsening of clinical signs, treatment may not be necessary.

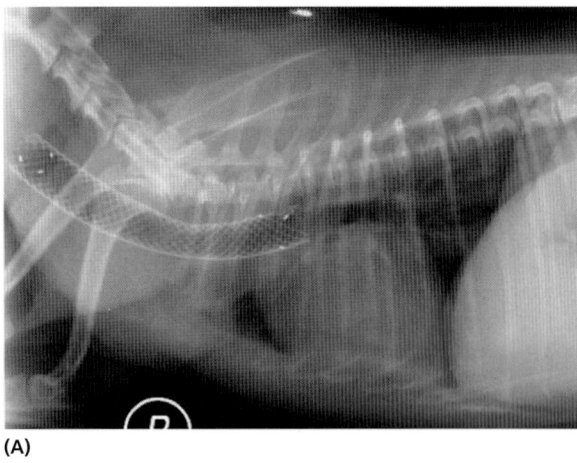
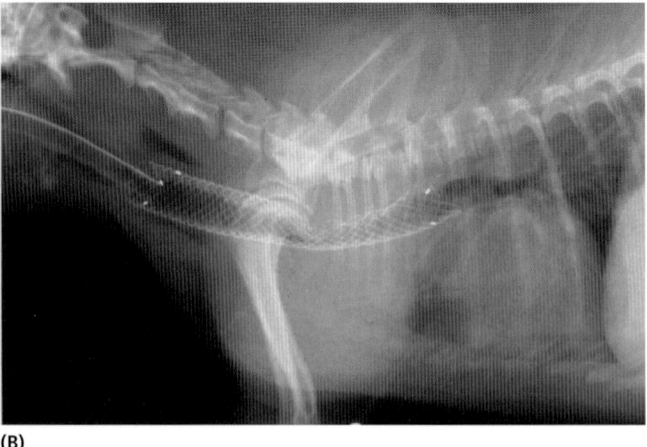

(A)   **(B)**

Figure 29.8 Right lateral thoracic radiographs demonstrating fraying (**A**) and subsequent fracture (**B**) of a tracheal stent. *Source:* G. W. Ellison, University of Florida, Gainesville, FL, 2014. Reproduced with permission from G. W. Ellison.

- If clinical signs result from collapse of areas from which the stent has migrated, deployment of a second stent to bridge the affected areas may be warranted.

Outcome
- The outcome may be favorable if stent migration is an incidental radiographic finding, although close monitoring for recurrence of clinical signs is warranted.
- Fatal laryngeal spasm secondary to stent migration has been reported (Moritz *et al.* 2004; Sura and Krahwinkel 2008).

Prevention
- The tracheal stent selected should be 10% to 20% greater than the maximum tracheal diameter at a breath-hold of 20 cm H_2O to minimize the risk of undersizing and subsequent migration.
- Early and aggressive treatment of persistent coughing with combinations of antitussive medications, including butorphanol (0.5–1 mg/kg PO every 6–12 hours), diphenoxylate hydrochloride with atropine (0.2–0.5 mg/kg PO every 12 hours), or hydrocodone (0.22 mg/kg PO every 6–12 hours), should be instituted to minimize stent migration. Sedation with acepromazine (0.5–2 mg/kg PO as needed) may be required to minimize excitement or stress. Bronchodilators such as theophylline (10–20 mg/kg PO every 12 hours) may also be warranted.
- Continued medical management, including reduction of environmental stressors, weight loss, and the use of a harness in place of a neck leash, is advised. Management of comorbidities, including cardiac disease or pulmonary disease, may reduce the frequency of coughing.
- A note should be made on the medical record to ensure careful intubation with a smaller diameter endotracheal tube during subsequent general anesthesia to minimize the risk of iatrogenic dislodgement.

Stent fracture

Definition
Stent fracture is disruption or fraying of the fibers of the tracheal stent caused by cyclic loading and fatigue. This typically occurs at or cranial to the thoracic inlet or at the caudal aspect of the stent and may result in narrowing of the tracheal lumen. This was reported as

the second most common complication, after bacterial tracheitis, in one case series, occurring in 42% of dogs (Ouellet *et al.* 2006; Sura and Krahwinkel 2008).

Risk factors
Continued coughing caused by tracheal or laryngeal irritation or mainstem bronchial collapse results in repeated cyclic forces and eventual fatigue fracture of the nitinol stent in the areas of highest motion

Diagnosis
- Stent fracture or fraying of the caudal end of the stent at the stent–trachea interface is usually associated with an acute worsening of clinical signs, although it can be an incidental finding on routine recheck radiographs.
- Orthogonal cervical and thoracic radiographs are usually sufficient to make the diagnosis (Figure 29.8), although tracheoscopy may be used as an adjunct diagnostic modality. Stent fracture should not be confused with the normal radiographic appearance of the free wire ends at the caudal aspect of certain brands of stent (Figure 29.9).

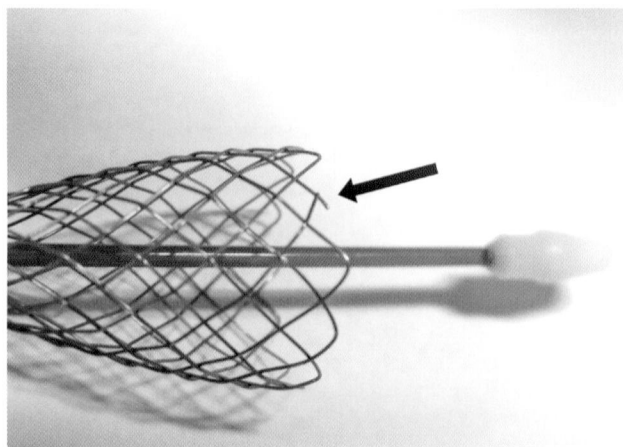

Figure 29.9 The normal appearance of the distal end of the Vet Stent-Trachea (Infiniti Medical, Menlo Park, CA). The free wire ends (arrow) do not represent a manufacturing defect. *Source:* Dr. F. Billen. Reproduced with permission of Dr. F. Billen.

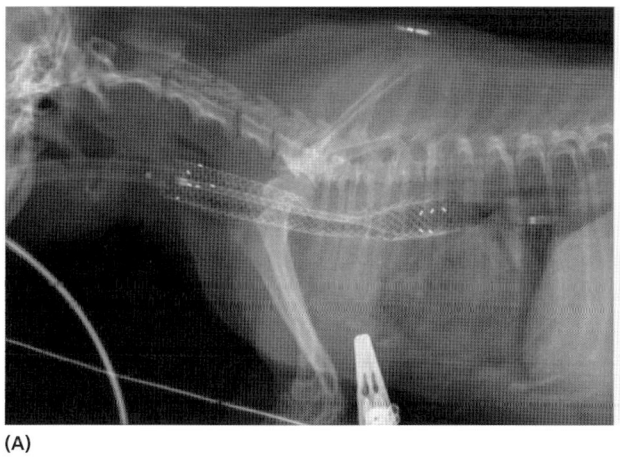
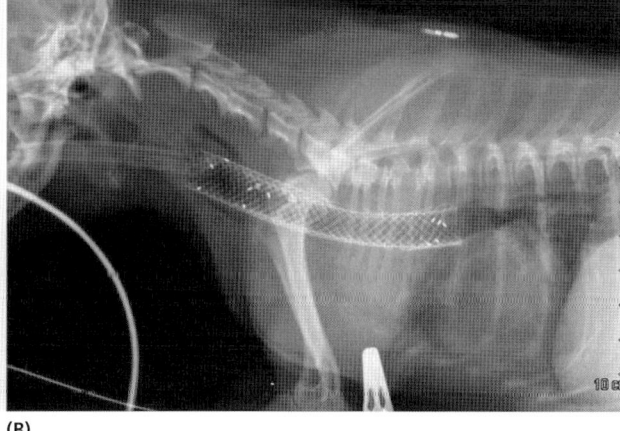

(A)   **(B)**

Figure 29.10 Intra- (**A**) and postprocedural (**B**) lateral radiographs obtained during deployment of a second endotracheal stent within the lumen of the fractured stent in the dog in Figure 29.8. *Source:* G. W. Ellison, University of Florida, Gainesville, FL, 2014. Reproduced with permission from G. W. Ellison.

Treatment

- An incidental finding of stent fracture or fraying may be managed conservatively. Corticosteroids may be prescribed to reduce periprosthetic inflammation. Any underlying reason for persistent coughing should be treated aggressively.
- Acute failure of the stent may warrant deployment of a second stent within the lumen of the fractured stent (Figure 29.10) (Mittleman *et al.* 2004; Ouellet *et al.* 2006; Woo *et al.* 2007; Sura and Krahwinkel 2008). Tracheal resection and anastomosis or partial or complete surgical stent removal with extraluminal ring prosthesis has also been described (Mittleman *et al.* 2004; Woo *et al.* 2007; Sura and Krahwinkel 2008).

Outcome

The outcome is variable depending on the severity of the associated clinical signs and if restenting is feasible.

Prevention

- Underlying comorbidities precipitating coughing should be addressed while strict environmental control is concurrently instituted.
- Early and aggressive treatment of persistent coughing with combinations of antitussive medications, including butorphanol, diphenoxylate, or hydrocodone, should be instituted to minimize coughing and stent fatigue.

Tracheitis

Definition

Tracheitis is inflammation of the tracheal mucosa, either secondary to a foreign body reaction to the stent or inhaled irritants or a superficial bacterial or viral infection. Bacterial tracheitis was the most common complication reported in one case series, occurring in 58% of dogs (Sura and Krahwinkel 2008). The interval from stent placement to tracheitis ranges from 1 to 3 months.

Risk factors

- Continued exposure to inhaled irritants may predispose to secondary bacterial tracheitis

- Undersized stents that do not become embedded in the tracheal epithelium interrupt the normal mucociliary apparatus and may permit biofilm formation, permitting reinfection (Figure 29.11).

Diagnosis

- Thoracic radiographs may not demonstrate significant abnormalities.
- Tracheoscopy may reveal inflammation or superficial erosion of the tracheal mucosa, with associated increased fluid production (see Figure 29.11).
- A tracheal wash may be performed to obtain fluid for cytological analysis and routine culture, as well as special culture for *Mycoplasma* spp. In the case of bacterial tracheitis, degenerative neutrophils containing intracellular bacteria may be present on cytologic evaluation (Figure 29.12). The most common bacterial isolates reported include *Pasteurella multocida*, α-hemolytic *Streptococcus* spp., and gram-negative rods (Sura and Krahwinkel 2008; Adamama-Moraitou *et al.* 2011).

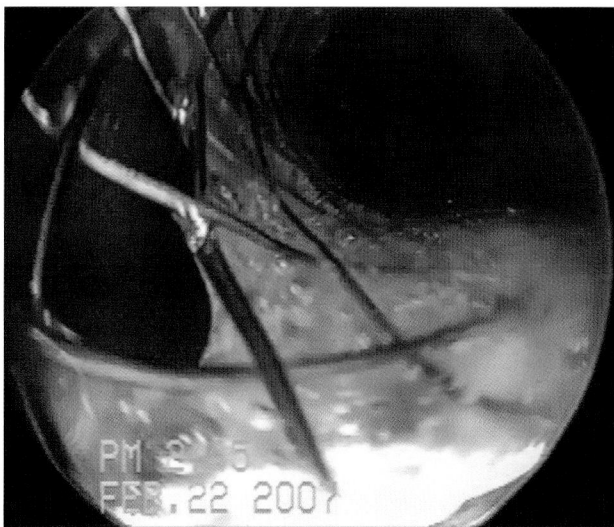

Figure 29.11 Endoscopic image of an undersized tracheal stent. *Source:* C. Weisse, 2014. Reproduced with permission from C. Weisse.

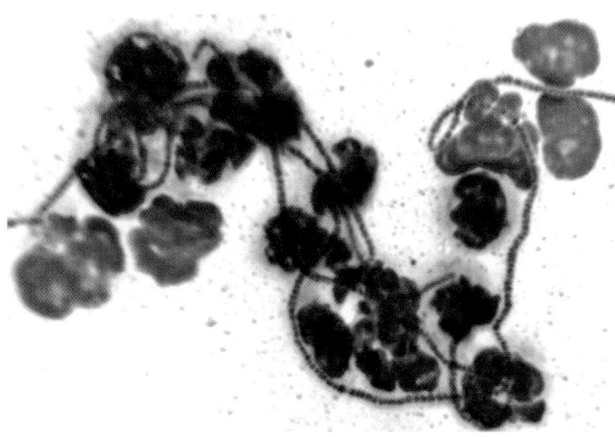

Figure 29.12 Cytology of a tracheal wash consistent with bacterial tracheitis. Multiple lysed, degenerate neutrophils are present along with a long chain of cocci. *Source:* H. Wamsley, 2014. Reproduced with permission from H. Wamsley.

Treatment

A course of antibiotic therapy should be prescribed for a minimum of 14 days based on the results of culture and sensitivity. Prolonged courses of antibiotics may be required for deep-seated infections. Doxycycline is typically prescribed for confirmed infection associate with *Mycoplasma* spp.

Outcome

With appropriate diagnostic and therapeutic intervention, the clinical signs typically resolve during antibiotic therapy; however, recurrence is common.

Prevention

- Reduction of environmental stressors is warranted to reduce inhaled irritants that may lead to tracheitis and secondary bacterial infection.
- Undersizing of the stent at deployment may prevent appropriate integration into the tracheal mucosa and permit trapping of mucus and inhaled irritants, predisposing to tracheitis.
- Pulse antibiotic therapy may be required for recurrent infections.

Bacterial pneumonia

Definition

Bacterial pneumonia is an inflammatory condition of the lower airways and pulmonary parenchyma associated with bacterial colonization.

Risk factors

Primary bacterial pneumonia may occur because of impaired clearance of respiratory secretions caused by disruption of the mucociliary apparatus. Dogs undergoing tracheal stenting may be predisposed to aspiration pneumonia, particularly if undergoing general anesthesia on multiple occasions.

Diagnosis

- Bacterial pneumonia may be suspected based on a sudden increase in respiratory rate and effort, accompanied by lethargy and pyrexia.
- Thoracic radiographs typically confirm the diagnosis.

Treatment

Bacterial pneumonia is treated supportively with supplemental oxygen if necessary, nebulization and coupage, and antibiotic therapy prescribed either empirically or on the basis of culture and sensitivity from bronchoalveolar lavage.

Outcome

The prognosis depends on the cause and severity of clinical signs. Dogs with few clinical signs and limited radiographic changes are more likely to have a favorable outcome.

Prevention

- If possible, avoid placement of stents in dogs with active respiratory infections.
- The number of general anesthetics should be limited when possible. This relies on maintaining a stock of standard sizes of tracheal stents.

Progressive tracheal collapse or mainstem bronchus collapse

Definition

This is progressive collapse of the trachea in the region cranial or caudal to the tracheal stent or of the mainstem bronchi, which may result in worsening of clinical signs.

Risk factors

- Tracheal collapse occurs secondary to progressive degeneration of the tracheal rings caused by hypocellularity and decreased glycosaminoglycan content. Stenting of the trachea is merely a palliative procedure that does not mitigate this degenerative process.
- Foreshortening, or gradual shortening of the stent over time, may occur in woven or knitted stents, resulting in collapse of segments previously supported by the stent.

Diagnosis

- Inspiratory and expiratory lateral radiographs of the cervical and thoracic regions permit evaluation of the entire length of the trachea (Figure 29.13).
- Fluoroscopy is typically the modality of choice to evaluate for dynamic collapse, particularly of the mainstem bronchi, which is typically identified on expiration.

Treatment

- A second stent may be deployed within the lumen of the first stent to support the area of collapsed trachea (see Figure 29.13).
- Mainstem bronchial collapse often involves the secondary and tertiary bronchi concurrently. Therefore, placement of stents within the mainstem bronchi themselves is considered futile.

Prevention

- There has been no documented correlation between stent length and complication rate, with some veterinarians routinely stenting the entire length of the trachea from 1 cm caudal to the cricoid cartilage to 1 cm cranial to the carina in anticipation of progressive tracheal degeneration.
- Endotracheal stenting in the face of concurrent mainstem bronchial collapse is controversial. Endotracheal stenting may be

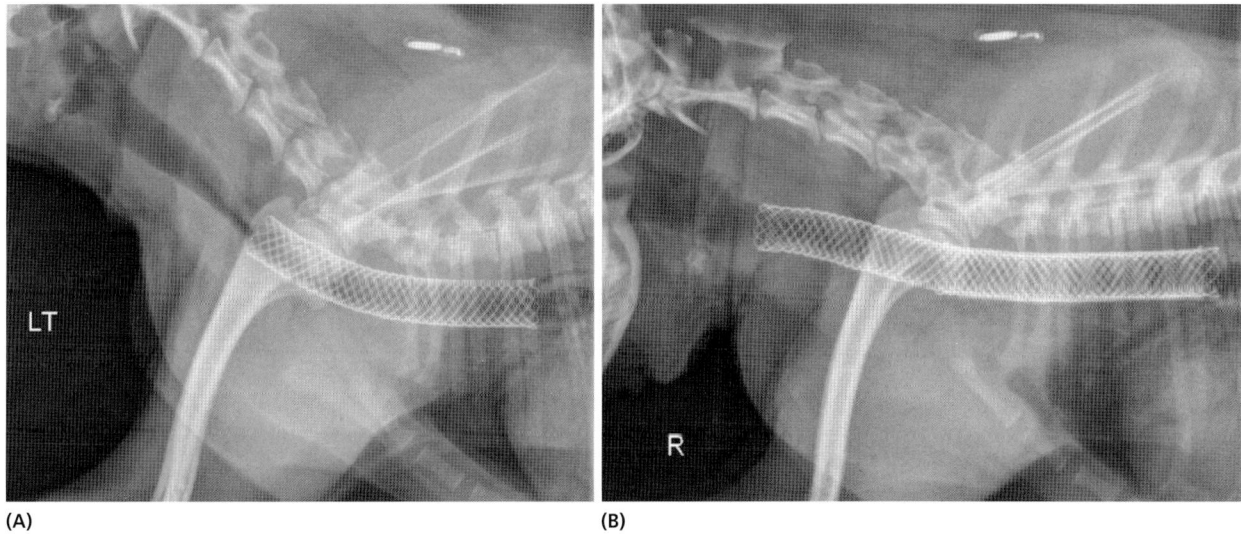

Figure 29.13 Lateral thoracic and cervical radiographs demonstrating progressive tracheal collapse cranial to the stent (**A**) and placement of a second stent spanning the collapsed area (**B**).

necessary as a lifesaving measure or to permit a reasonable quality of life. Owners, however, should be warned that the prognosis for resolution of clinical signs, in particular coughing, and subsequently the longevity of the stent is more guarded because of the cyclic fatigue of the stent.

- Recent prospective controlled clinical studies documented efficacy of the anabolic steroid, stanozolol (0.15 mg/kg PO twice a day for 60 days and tapered over 15 days), in the strengthening of the chondromalacic tracheal cartilages (Adamama-Moraitou *et al.* 2011; Durant *et al.* 2012). This treatment may provide benefit for patients with adjacent tracheal collapse or mainstem bronchial collapse after tracheal stenting.

Persistent clinical signs with extratracheal complications

Definition
Comorbidities have been reported associated with the spasmodic increase in intraabdominal pressure caused by persistent coughing. These include perineal hernia with bladder entrapment and rectal prolapse (Durant *et al.* 2012).

Risk factors
Persistent coughing caused by sterile or bacterial tracheitis, mainstem bronchial collapse, subsequent tracheal collapse, or granuloma formation may result in periodic increases in intraabdominal pressure. Concomitant cortico steroid therapy may weaken the pelvic diaphragm, predisposing to perineal hernia.

Diagnosis
- Clinical signs typically reflect those related to perineal hernia or rectal prolapse, and a diagnosis can typically be made on clinical examination.
- Thoracic radiographs, fluoroscopy, tracheoscopy, and tracheal wash may be warranted to determine underlying causes for persistent coughing.

Treatment
The underlying cause of coughing should be investigated and treated aggressively. The secondary extratracheal abnormalities may need to be addressed surgically.

Outcome
The outcome depends on the cause and severity of clinical signs associated with the extratracheal complication.

Prevention
Investigation and aggressive treatment for persistent coughing and judicious use of corticosteroids are warranted.

Relevant literature
Two retrospective case series have documented the use of nitinol stents for tracheal collapse (Sura and Krahwinkel 2008; Durant *et al.* 2012). Sura and Krahwinkel (2008) reported a series of 12 dogs in which nitinol tracheal stents were used. Overall, 83% had long-term improvement of their clinical condition. However, 25% of dogs had died within 6 months, with just over 50% surviving more than 2 years. Tracheal disease was directly associated with death in 56% of dogs. The main reported complication was stent fracture, which occurred in 5 of 12 cases (42%). Other complications reported include granuloma formation, tracheitis, and pneumonia. A more recent review by the same group (Durant *et al.* 2012) reviewed 18 dogs, with a comparable 11.1% mortality rate within 60 days, with 50% of cases experiencing postoperative complications. An unpublished study has revealed fewer short-term complications in patients undergoing intraluminal stenting compared with extraluminal ring prosthesis. This study reported an immediate mortality rate of 9% in 75 dogs in which extraluminal rings were placed compared with 3% in 32 dogs receiving tracheal stents; however, a comparison of long-term outcome has not yet been undertaken (Kelley M. Thieman-Mankin, personal communication). On the basis of these studies, owners should be informed that although tracheal stenting is typically rewarding in the short term, long-term complications often necessitating intervention are not unexpected.

References

Adamama-Moraitou, K.K., Pardali, D., Athanasiou, L.V., et al. (2011) Conservative management of canine tracheal collapse with stanozolol: a double blinded, placebo control clinical trial. *International Journal of Immunopathology and Pharmacology* 24 (1), 111-118.

Barras, C.D.J., Myers, K.A. (2000) Nitinol—its use in vascular surgery and other applications. *European Journal of Vascular and Endovascular Surgery* 19 (6), 564-569.

Brown, S.A., Williams, J.E., Saylor, D.K. (2008) Endotracheal stent granulation stenosis resolution after colchicine therapy in a dog. *Journal of Veterinary Internal Medicine* 22 (4), 1052-1055.

Durant, A.M., Sura, P., Rohrbach, B., et al. (2012) Use of nitinol stents for end-stage tracheal collapse in dogs. *Veterinary Surgery* 41 (7), 807-817.

Gellasch, K.L., Da Costa Gomez, T., McAnulty, J.F., et al. (2002) Use of intraluminal nitinol stents in the treatment of tracheal collapse in a dog. *Journal of the American Veterinary Medical Association* 221 (12), 1719-1723.

Mittleman, E., Weisse, C., Mehler, S.J., et al. (2004) Fracture of an endoluminal nitinol stent used in the treatment of tracheal collapse in a dog. *Journal of the American Veterinary Medical Association* 225 (8), 1217-1221.

Moritz, A., Schneider, M., Bauer, N. (2004) Management of advanced tracheal collapse in dogs using intraluminal self expanding biliary wallstents. *Journal of Veterinary Internal Medicine* 18 (1), 31-42.

Ouellet, M., Dunn, M.E., Lussier, B., et al. (2006) Noninvasive correction of a fractured endoluminal nitinol tracheal stent in a dog. *Journal of the American Animal Hospital Association* 42 (6), 467-471.

Sura, P.A., Krahwinkel, D.J. (2008) Self-expanding nitinol stents for the treatment of tracheal collapse in dogs: 12 cases (2001-2004). *Journal of the American Veterinary Medical Association* 232 (2), 228-236.

Woo, H.-M., Kim, M.-J., Lee, S.-G., et al. (2007) Intraluminal tracheal stent fracture in a Yorkshire terrier. *The Canadian Veterinary Journal* 48 (10), 1063-1066.

Dental and Oral Surgery

30 Repair of Mandibular and Maxillary Fractures

Christian Bolliger

Surgical Referral Practice, Central Victoria Veterinary Hospital, Victoria, Canada

Fractures of the jaw in dogs and cats are common after road accidents, bite wounds, violent kicks, and gunshots or part of the highrise syndrome, particularly in cats (Umphlet and Johnson 1988, 1990; Lopes *et al.* 2005). Pathologic fractures occur during dental extractions as a consequence of infection, neoplasia, or metabolic diseases. In cats, traumatic separation of the mandibular symphysis is most common, but dogs present more frequently with mandibular body fractures (Table 30.1) (Umphlet and Johnson 1988, 1990; Zetner 1992; Lopes *et al.* 2005). In case of orofacial trauma, additional trauma may occur to the teeth, gingiva, tongue, or lips as well as the nasal passages, eyes, or brain.

Postoperative complications are more common with mandibular than with maxillary fractures. Overall complications reported after mandibular fracture treatment account for 15% and 34% in dogs and cats, respectively. Preoperative complications include airway obstruction and brain injury, and malocclusion is the main intraoperative complication. Nonunion is a possible postoperative complication, as well as temporomandibular joint (TMJ) disease (luxation, ankylosis), which can develop later on.

Airway obstruction

Definition
Upper airway obstruction can be caused by displaced bone fragments, damaged turbinates, blood clots, swelling of the nasopharyngeal mucosa, or rarely foreign bodies. Thoracic trauma with lower airway disease can also be present.

Risk factors
- Narrow upper airways in brachycephalic dogs and cats
- Profuse nasal bleeding

Table 30.1 Distribution of mandibular fractures

Localization of mandibular fractures	Cats (*n* = 190)	Dogs (*n* = 257)
Symphysis and parasymphysis	114	57
Body	73	155
Coronoid process	13	9
Condylar process	25	8

Data from Umphlet and Johnson 1988 and 1990; Lopes et al. 2005; and Zetner 1992.

- Compression or unstable fracture of maxilla
- Caudal mandibular fractures
- Preexisting tracheal collapse or lower airway disease
- Thoracic trauma

Diagnosis
The **most common clinical sign is** an obstructive breathing pattern with an open mouth. In case of pharyngeal or laryngeal obstruction, life-threatening dyspnea can develop, possibly leading to ventilatory failure.

Additional clinical signs include:
- Epistaxis
- Stridor, stertor, blocked nose, or cyanosis
- Pharyngeal soft tissue swelling
- Deviation of the maxillary bones
- Signs of lower airway disease

Diagnostic imaging can be helpful; computed tomography (CT) is the modality of choice to evaluate the airways, brain tissue, skull, neck, and thorax (Figures 30.1 and 30.2); however, radiography can help diagnosing skull fractures, cervical instability, and thoracic trauma.

Treatment
- Oxygen administered by mask. Avoid nasal catheters after trauma to nasal cavity.
- Intubation or tracheostomy if severe dyspnea is present, especially in brachycephalic breeds and unconscious animals
- Cardiovascular stabilization with crystalloids, hypertonic saline, colloids, or blood products
- Hemostasis
- Sedation and analgesia to reduce stress and oxygen consumption and improve ventilation if pain is present (benzodiazepines combined with microdoses of a short-acting opioid is a good choice because both can be reversed if needed).
- Dexamethasone sodium phosphate (0.2–0.4 mg/kg intravenously [IV], intramuscularly, or subcutaneously) to reduce mucosal inflammation and swelling.

Outcome
Upper airway obstruction is common with orofacial trauma.

In combination with lower airway disease or brain trauma, rapid decompensation has to be anticipated. The obstructive breathing

Complications in Small Animal Surgery, First Edition. Edited by Dominique Griffon and Annick Hamaide.
© 2016 John Wiley & Sons, Inc. Published 2016 by John Wiley & Sons, Inc.
Companion website: www.wiley.com/go/griffon/complications

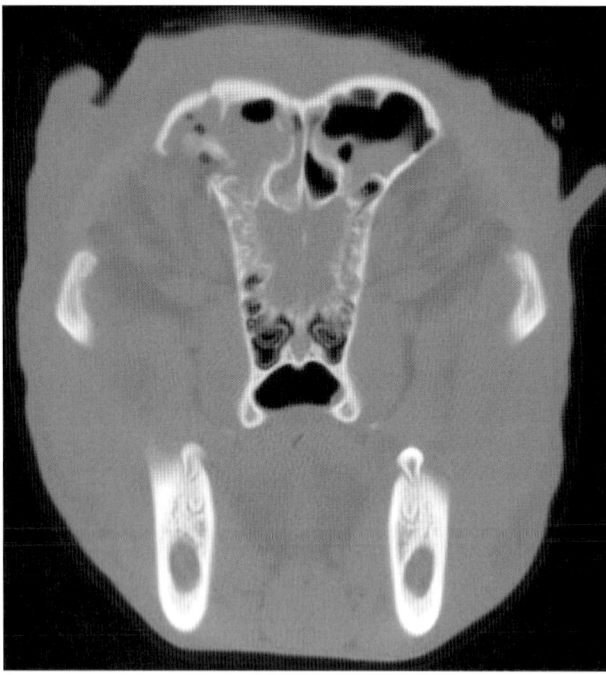

Figure 30.1 Partial airway obstruction. Transverse computed tomography image of a penetrating trauma into the right nasal cavity and sinus. *Source:* Dr. E. Carmel, University of Montréal, Montréal, QC. Reproduced with permission from Dr. E. Carmel.

pattern will further increase mucosal swelling and place the animal at risk for aspiration pneumonia or noncardiogenic pulmonary edema.

Prevention
- Calm and careful handling of the animal to reduce stress and oxygen consumption

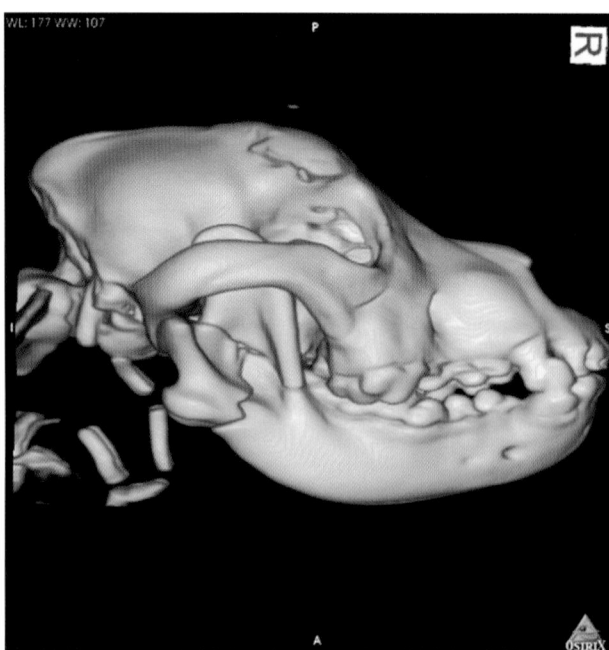

Figure 30.2 Right caudal mandibular fracture, sinus and nasal fracture. Three-dimensional reconstruction of Figure 30.1. *Source:* Dr. E. Carmel, University of Montréal, Montréal, QC. Reproduced with permission from Dr. E. Carmel.

- Oxygen administration
- Tracheostomy when marked upper airway obstruction is present, especially in brachycephalic breeds

Brain injury

Definition
Initial brain injury is defined as primary blunt or penetrating trauma causing direct damage to the neurovascular tissues of the brain through compressive and shearing forces.

Secondary brain injury is initiated by biochemical changes such as ischemia; intracellular accumulation of sodium and calcium; elevation of extracellular excitatory neurotransmitter glutamate; and release of free radicals, which peak hours to days after the primary trauma (Figure 30.3) (Wilkinson 1999; Leach 2009; Syring 2011).

Risk factors
- Orofacial fractures
- Depressed or deteriorating mental status
- Abnormal neurologic examination findings
- Arterial hypotension
- Hypoxia
- Infection
- Hematoma
- Edema
- Seizure

Diagnosis
- Stabilize the animal before evaluation of consciousness because altered mentation is common in shock.

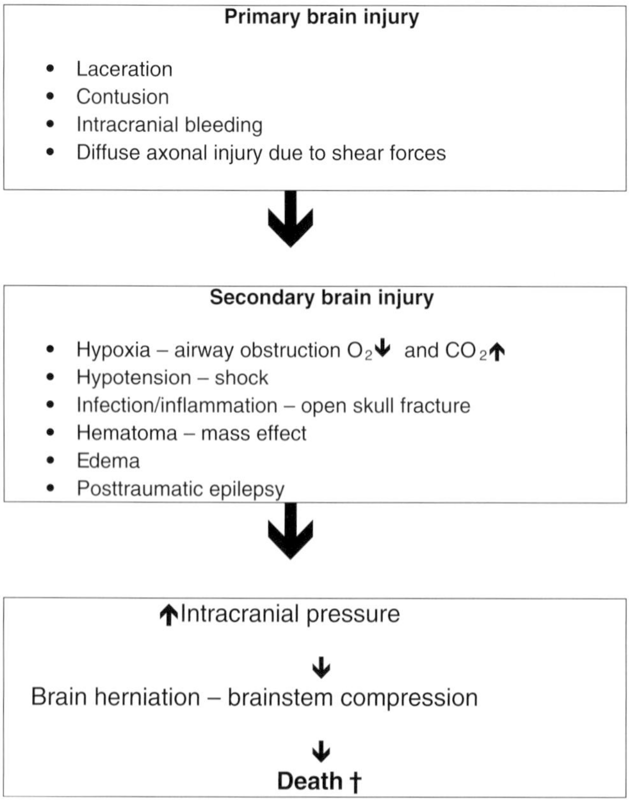

Primary brain injury
- Laceration
- Contusion
- Intracranial bleeding
- Diffuse axonal injury due to shear forces

Secondary brain injury
- Hypoxia – airway obstruction $O_2\downarrow$ and $CO_2\uparrow$
- Hypotension – shock
- Infection/inflammation – open skull fracture
- Hematoma – mass effect
- Edema
- Posttraumatic epilepsy

$\uparrow$Intracranial pressure

Brain herniation – brainstem compression

Death †

Figure 30.3 Progressive traumatic brain injury.

- Proceed carefully because cervical instability and loose skull fragments may be present.
- Examine cortical and brainstem function.
  ∘ Level of consciousness
  ∘ Pupil size, symmetry, and light response
  ∘ Motor activity: normal, hemi- or tetraparesis, extensor rigidity
    ▪ Decerebrate rigidity: stupor or coma and opisthotonus with hyperextension of all limbs (after herniation under tentorium cerebelli and brainstem compression).
    ▪ Decerebellate rigidity: normal awareness and consciousness and opisthotonus with hyperextension of front legs and flexion of hind legs (after herniation through foramen magnum)
- Pulse rate and blood pressure (a decreased pulse rate associated to an increased blood pressure indicate cerebral-ischemic response reflex or Cushing's reflex, indicating elevated intracranial pressure [ICP])
- Modified Glasgow Coma Scale (GCS) score aids in formulating prognosis by evaluating function of the cerebrum, midbrain, pons, and medulla.
- Direct measurement of ICP is used in human medicine but is rarely performed in veterinary medicine because of cost and high technical complexity.
- Magnetic resonance (MRI) or CT imaging: brain edema, hemorrhage, and brain shifts are indirect indicators of raised ICP (Figure 30.4).

Treatment
- Correction of life-threatening abnormalities according to the ABC principles (airway, breathing, cardiovascular support). This will also reduce secondary brain damage.
- Maintenance of adequate **ventilation and oxygenation** to keep SaO_2 above 95% and PaO_2 above 90 mm Hg. Oxygen is given by mask, hood, or nasal tubes when nasal passages are not traumatized. Consider intubation or tracheostomy.
  ∘ Hyperventilating to a PCO_2 below 30 mm Hg is an emergency procedure only because brain ischemia will worsen.
  ∘ Keep a low normal PCO_2 between 35 and 40 mm Hg.

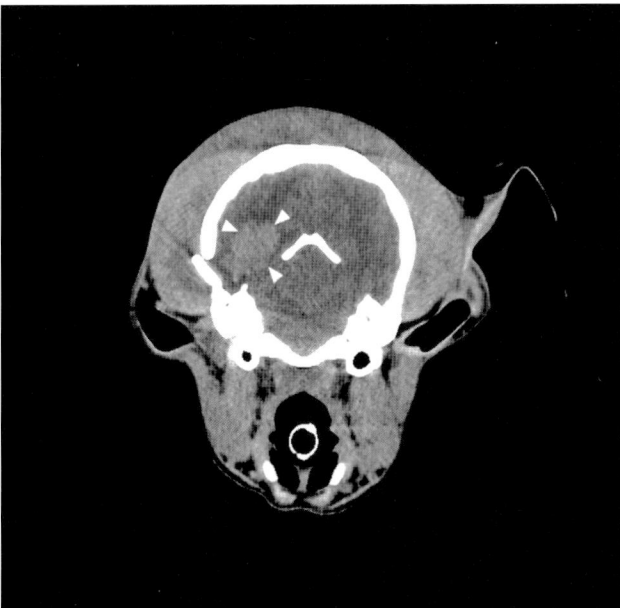

Figure 30.4 Skull fracture causing intraparenchymal hematoma (arrows). *Source:* Dr. E. Carmel, University of Montréal, Montréal, QC. Reproduced with permission from Dr. E. Carmel.

- **Shock** treatment with isotonic crystalloids, hypertonic saline, colloids, or blood products. Hypertonic saline also decreases ICP and is advantageous in brain trauma. Avoid hypernatremia.
- **Hemostasis**
- **Mannitol** 1 g/kg given slowly IV over 15 to 20 minutes
- **Furosemide** 2 mg/kg has a synergistic effect on lowering ICP, especially when given before mannitol.
- Establish baseline **neurologic examination**.
- **Benzodiazepines** with a short-acting μ-opioid sedate agitated or hysteric animals and reduce brain activity (and so oxygen consumption) and can be reversed. The neurologic examination findings will be altered.
- **Surgical decompression** of the brain is indicated in case of:
  ∘ Worsening of neurologic signs despite medical therapy
  ∘ Open skull fractures
  ∘ Severe displacement of bone fragments
  ∘ Subdural hematoma: in rare situations the drainage of an enlarging hematoma may be indicated. There is a risk that further bleeding is precipitated. Advanced imaging is mandatory for this procedure.
- **Position** the patient in sternal recumbency with the head raised to a 30-degree angle to improve venous return. Do not compress the jugular vein or use for blood sampling.
- Start basic nursing care to avoid pressure ulcers and aspiration pneumonia.

Outcome
The nursing care of patients with neurologic conditions is demanding and often prolonged. Cortical lesions carry a better prognosis, but posttraumatic seizures may develop. Comatose animals rarely recover to a functional state when decerebrate rigidity and apnea caused by brainstem hemorrhage are present or progressive tentorial herniation develops.

The modified GCS takes into account motor activity, brainstem reflexes, and level of consciousness with a maximum possible score of 18. In a retrospective study of 38 dogs, those with a score of 8 at admission had a 50% probability of survival at 48 hours (Platt *et al.* 2001). No studies are available in veterinary medicine to evaluate the functional recovery after moderate to severe brain trauma.

Prevention
- Stabilization of blood pressure
- Treatment of hypoxia
- Prevention of infection
- Reduction of cerebral edema
- Decompression of enlarging hematoma
- Frequent neurologic examination
- Advanced imaging

Malocclusion

Definition
Malocclusion is defined as the inability to properly close the mouth because of abnormal interdigitation of teeth in the mandible and maxilla. Malocclusion can be present intraoperatively or develop postoperatively and originates most of the time in the mandible (Figures 30.5 to 30.7). Breed-related malocclusion or deformities already present before the trauma caused by a short or long mandible should be considered.

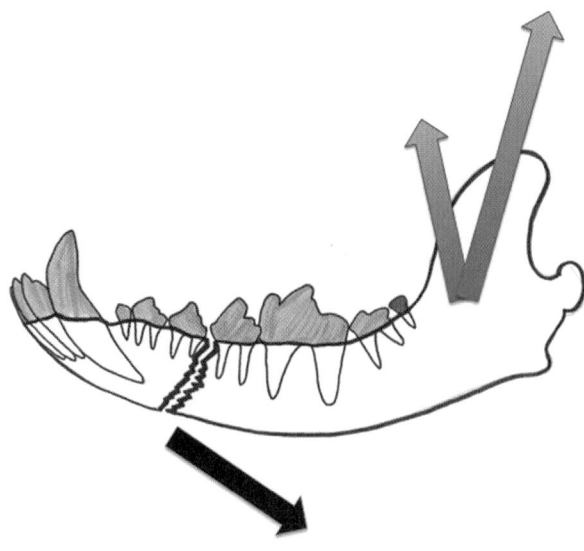

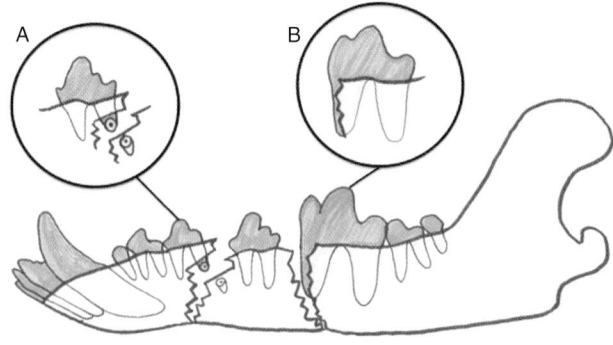

A: Tooth root fracture
B: Tooth root exposure

Figure 30.7 Mandibular fractures with fracture of tooth root (**A**) rostrally (vascularization impaired) and exposure of tooth root caudally (**B**) (vascularization preserved). *Source:* Tutt, 2006. Reproduced with permission from John Wiley & Sons.

Figure 30.5 Favorable fracture line (dorsal to rostroventral). The action of the masticatory muscles will compress the fracture line. *Source:* Tutt, 2006. Reproduced with permission from John Wiley & Sons.

Risk factors
- Bilateral fractures
- Comminuted fracture
- Bone loss, resulting in gap formation or reduced jaw length
- Tooth loss
- Inadequate implant position or choice
- Overtightened interfragmentary or circumferential wire
- Implant failure
- Growing animal
- TMJ luxation
- Severe soft tissue swelling preventing assessment of occlusion
- Oral intubation

- Nonunion or malunion of jaw fracture
- Mandibular resection

Diagnosis
Signs of malocclusion include:
- Mandibular shift
- Mandibular or maxillary instability
- Dropped jaw
- Inability to close the mouth
- Crepitation
- Soft tissue damage
- Grinding teeth
- Enamel damage of the opposing teeth

Intraoral radiographs are mandatory to evaluate the presence of tooth and bone pathology. CT imaging is the best modality to evaluate the TMJ.

Treatment
- Endotracheal intubation via pharyngostomy to allow intraoperative assessment of occlusion
- Debridement of soft tissue, suture of gingiva
- Extraction of damaged or loose teeth
- Anatomic reduction and stabilization of fracture fragments; corrective osteotomy if postoperative malocclusion, orthodontics, endodontics, or tooth extraction
- Bone graft or substitute if fracture gap present
- Various techniques of resection of the mandible as a salvage procedure

Multiple techniques for stabilization have been described and can be used in oral surgery. Interdental wire and composite bar offer a very versatile and biomechanically sound fixation for most fractures and nonunions (Figures 30.8 and 30.9). External fixators, bone plates, or maxillary–mandibular composite fixations (MMFs) are indicated for highly unstable or comminuted fractures, fractures caudal to first molar (M1), and fractures with tooth or bone loss. MMF should be delayed if nasal obstruction is present.

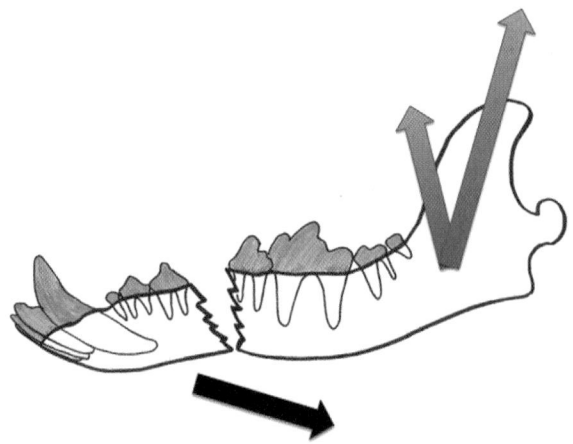

Figure 30.6 Unfavorable fracture line (dorsal to caudoventral). The action of the masticatory muscles will open the fracture line, and fixation has to more solid. *Source:* Tutt, 2006. Reproduced with permission from John Wiley & Sons.

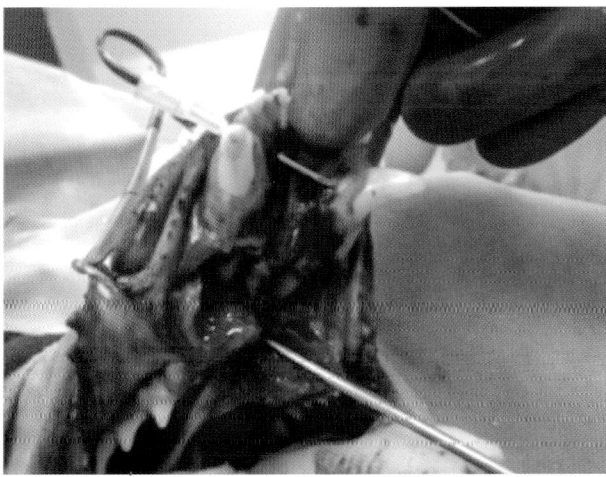

Figure 30.8 Highly unstable bilateral fracture of the rostral mandible. Fixation with interdental and interfragmentary wire. Although vascular supply to the canine was interrupted, the two teeth provided important strength for the fracture fixation. Endodontic treatment or extraction after bone fusion should be considered.

Outcome

In several studies, malocclusion was the most common complication, occurring in 23 of 122 dogs and 12 of 129 cats (Umphlet and Johnson 1988, 1990; Zetner 1992; Owen *et al.* 2004). The healing time for jaw fractures depends on the location and age of the animal but is usually between 6 and 12 weeks (Boudrieau and Kudisch 1996; Owen *et al.* 2004).

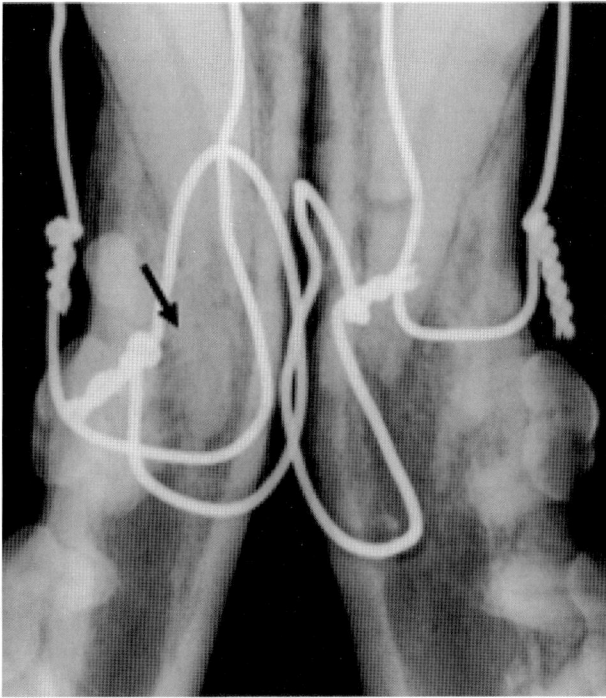

Figure 30.9 Intraoral radiography 7 weeks after fracture repair. Tooth root fracture of right canine visible (arrow).

Prevention
- Identification of TMJ luxation or second fracture
- Anatomic fracture reduction and stable fixation
- Preservation of dental occlusion intraoperatively
- Avoid exaggerated fragment compression
- Restoration of jaw length by using bone grafts

Nonunion

Definition
Nonunion is a fracture that has failed to heal. Nonunions with variable callus formation, which fail to bridge the fracture gap, are called biologically active nonunions, and those without callus formation are called nonviable or avascular nonunions. Nonunions affect mostly the mandibular bone and are rather rare in the maxillary bone (Boudrieau 2005).

Risk factors
- Fracture instability
- Loss of soft tissue and vascularization
- Bone loss
- Comminuted bone fracture
- Bone gap
- Osteomyelitis
- Tooth fracture
- Avascular tooth
- Endodontic disease
- Implant failure or inadequate implant position

Diagnosis
- Difficulties in prehension and mastication
- Malocclusion
- Instability
- Pain
- Swelling
- Draining tract
- Foul odor
- Gingival ulceration, necrosis, or discoloration

Intraoral radiographs are invaluable to evaluate bone pathology and teeth at the fracture site and are more sensitive than CT scan, which may suffer from artifacts due to the presence of implants.

Radiographs should be evaluated for:
- Callus formation
- Avascular nonunion
- Favorable versus nonfavorable fracture configuration
- Bone resorption at the fracture site
- Bone resorption around the tooth root
- Fractured tooth in the fracture line
- Osteomyelitis
- Sequestrum formation
- Presence of implants
- Implant loosening or broken implants
- Fibrous nonunion without clinical signs may be discovered incidentally during the acquisition of dental radiographs.

Treatment
- Mobilization of gingival flaps to gain access to the fracture site
- Extraction of loose, infected, or avascular teeth; tooth cleaning; or endodontic treatment if needed

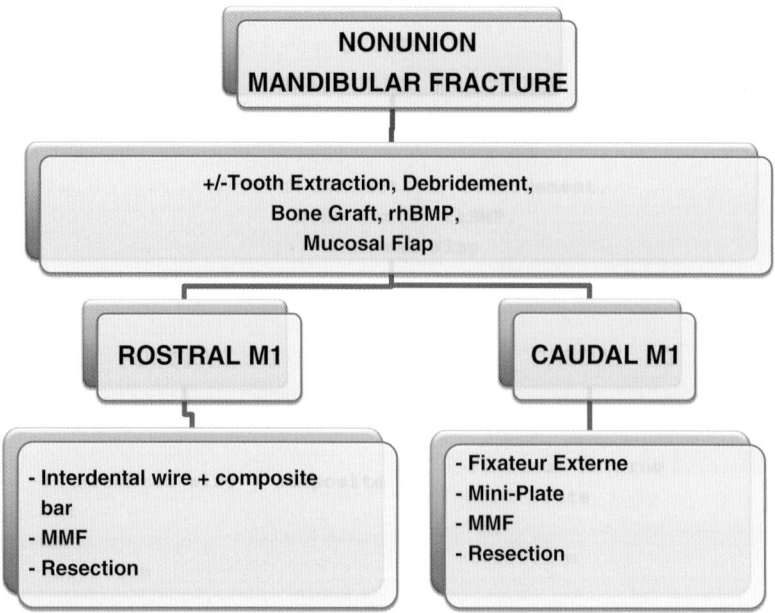

Figure 30.10 Treatment options for nonunion mandibular fractures. rhBMP, recombinant human bone morphogenetic protein; M1, first molar; MMF, maxillary-mandibular composite fixation.

- Removal of loose implants
- Debridement of fibrous, infected, or necrotic soft and hard tissue followed by copious lavage
- Bone grafting or bone substitute
- Restoration of dental occlusion
- Stable fixation (Figure 30.10)
- Soft tissue closure
- Antibiotherapy according to results of sensitivity test. In specific cases, antibiotic-impregnated sponges or polymethylmetacrylate beads may be indicated.
- Hemi-, segmental-, or rostral mandibulectomies are salvage procedures for patients with extensive osteomyelitis or severe bone loss.
- Commissurorrhaphy can support the jaw in case of extensive periodontal disease and replacement by fibrous tissue.

Outcome
Extensive osteomyelitis and large bone gaps are negative prognostic factors and often require mandibular resection as a salvage procedure. Nonunions without large gaps heal in the same time frame as fresh fractures when treated appropriately (Boudrieau and Kudisch 1996; Owen *et al.* 2004).

Prevention
- Application of basic principles of osteosynthesis
- Preservation of vascularization
- Bone graft or bone substitutes to fill gaps
- Prophylactic antibiotherapy
- Injection of recombinant human bone morphogenetic protein (rhBMP-2) into the fracture site
- Shockwave therapy

Temporomandibular joint luxation, dysplasia, fracture, or locked coronoid process
The TMJ is formed by the transversely elongated mandibular condyle, intraarticular disc, mandibular fossa, and joint capsule, which is laterally thickened. The TMJ moves in flexion and extension and to a lesser degree in translation (rostral and lateral movement). Several pathologies in the TMJ or the surrounding tissues (bulla, caudal mandibular ramus, zygomatic arch, orbit) can interfere with range of motion.

Definition
- TMJ luxation occurs as a result of trauma, with or without dysplasia of the condyle or fossa, and is frequently in a rostrodorsal direction, causing malocclusion with the mouth open. The retroarticular process prevents caudal luxation of the mandibular condyle unless it is fractured (Figure 30.11).
- Condylar dysplasia (congenital or acquired) with or without dysplasia of the mandibular fossa has primarily been reported in Basset hounds, Irish setters, bullmastiffs, Cavalier King Charles spaniels, golden and Labrador retrievers, Bernese mountain dogs, and Dobermans, as well as Siamese and Persian cats.
- Fracture of the condylar process, mandibular fossa or retroarticular process can occur isolated or in combination with luxation of the TMJ.
- Hypermobility of the TMJ with or without dysplasia can lead to lateral movement of the coronoid process, which may become locked at the zygomatic arch (Figure 30.12).

Risk factors
- Trauma
- Growing animal with large callus formation
- Dysplasia of the mandibular condyle with or without dysplasia of the mandibular fossa
- Symphyseal laxity
- Neoplasia

Diagnosis
- TMJ luxation: mandible deviates to the contralateral side
- Locked TMJ: bulge can be palpated lateral to the zygomatic arch and occurs with the mouth open

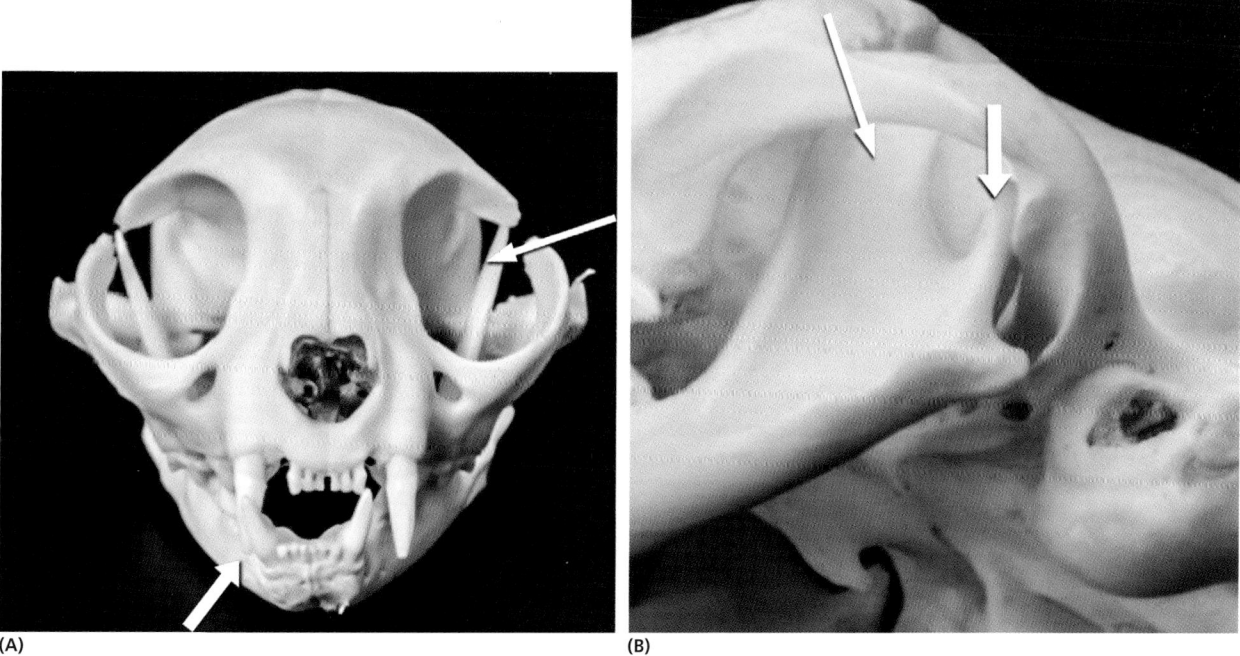

(A)   (B)

Figure 30.11 Temporomandibular joint luxation in a cat. **A,** Cranial aspect. The small arrow shows the coronoid process, and the large arrow show the mandibular drift to the right. **B,** Lateral aspect. The small arrow shows the coronoid process, and the large arrow shows the condyle luxated dorsorostrally.

- TMJ fracture: mandible may deviate to the ipsilateral side
- Palpation: range of motion, crepitus, pain, swelling
- Radiography: four radiographic views are required to evaluate properly the TMJ joint (i.e., dorsoventral or ventrodorsal, right and lateral oblique, and intraoral open-mouth radiographs)

- CT is the gold standard for examination of the TMJ and surrounding tissues (Figure 30.13).

Treatment

Treatment of TMJ luxation, TMJ fracture, and locked coronoid is detailed in Figure 30.14.

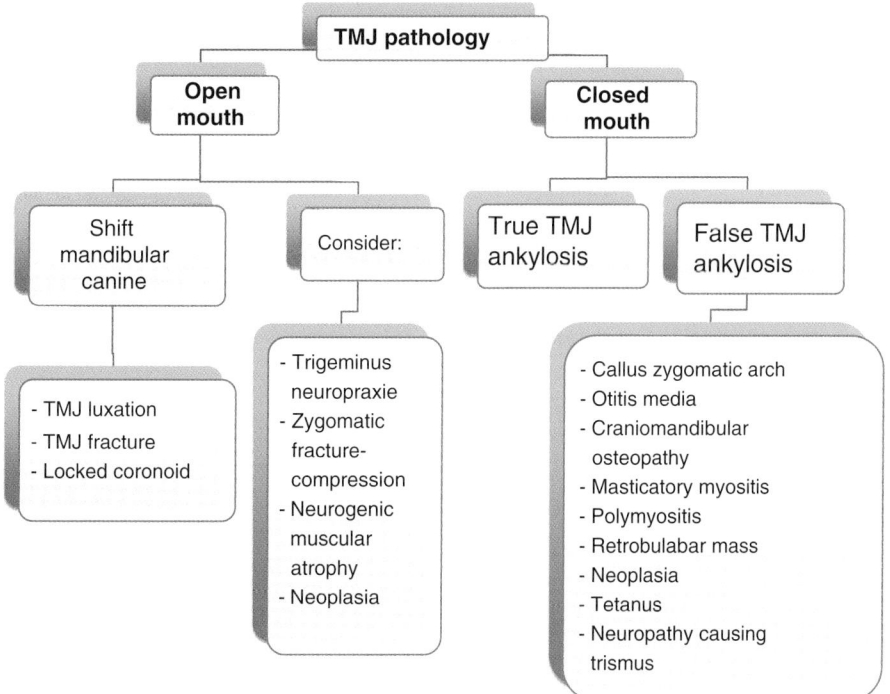

Figure 30.12 Temporomandibular joint (TMJ) pathologies. *Source:* Adapted from Rawlinson, J. (2008), with permission.

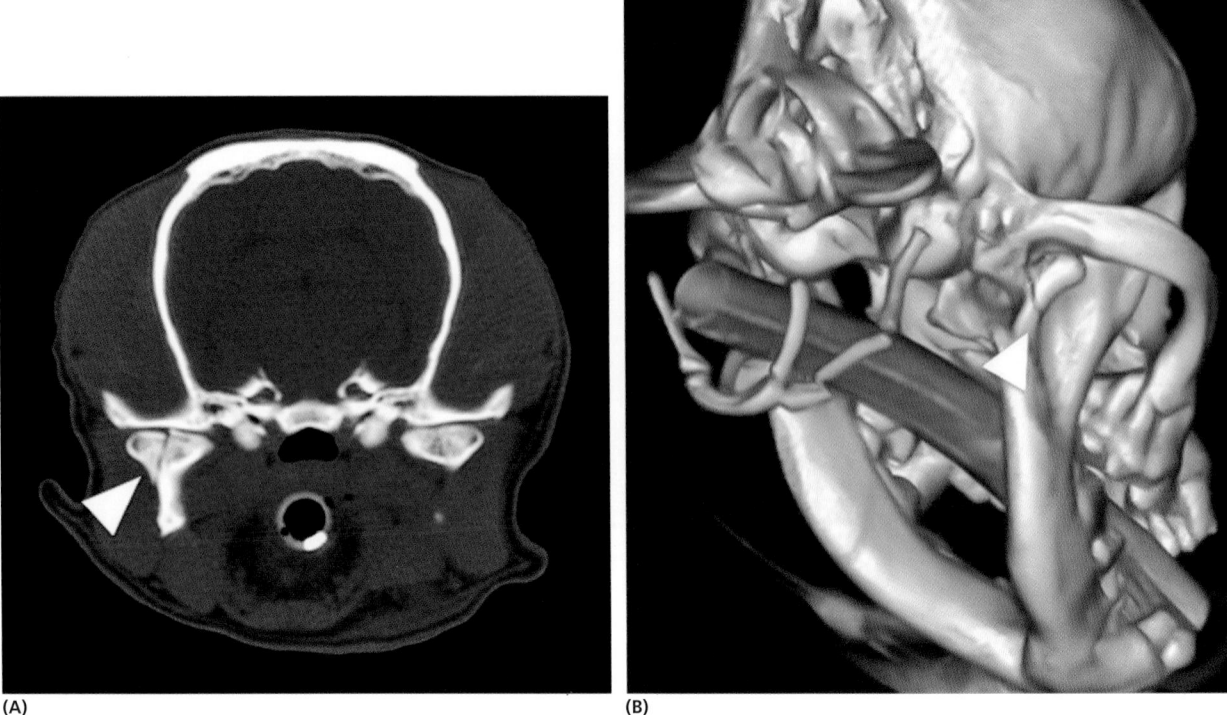

(A) (B)

Figure 30.13 A, Transverse computed tomography image of a condylar fracture on the right side (arrowhead). **B,** Three-dimensional reconstruction of the same condylar fracture (arrowhead). *Source:* Dr. E. Carmel, University of Montréal, Montréal, QC. Reproduced with permission from Dr. E. Carmel.

Outcome

Animals with a traumatic TMJ luxation without fractures show an excellent prognosis after closed reposition.

Fractures of the TMJ can heal by bony union or as a pain-free functional non-union although osteoarthritis or ankylosis may develop, necessitating a condylectomy (Lobprise 2007; Rawlinson 2008).

Prevention

• Immobilize the TMJ after closed reposition for 1 to 2 weeks with a muzzle or MMF.

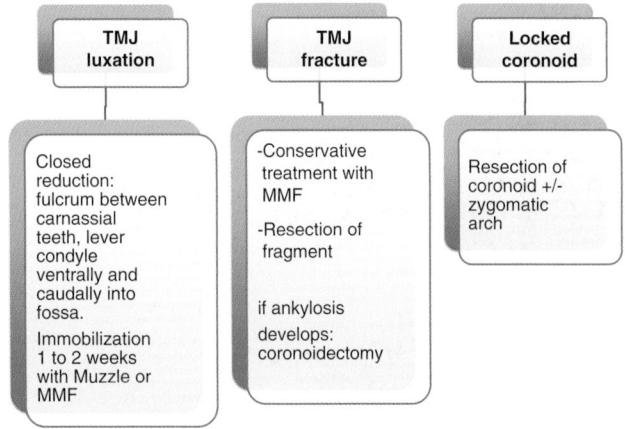

Figure 30.14 Treatment of temporomandibular joint (TMJ) luxation and fracture and locked coronoid. MMF, maxillary–mandibular composite fixation.

Temporomandibular joint ankylosis

Definition

Ankylosis is a stiffness of the TMJ caused by abnormal adhesions and rigidity of the joint, which is most often the result of injury. The rigidity may be partial or complete and results in progressive inability to open the mouth. Whereas true ankylosis results from intraarticular pathology, false ankylosis describes extraarticular pathology.

Risk factors

• Trauma to the TMJ or zygomatic arch, especially in growing animals
• Prolonged MMF
• Otitis media
• Craniomandibular osteopathy
• Neoplasia

Diagnosis

• Progressive inability to open the mouth. This may result in malnutrition and dehydration.
• Radiographs show loss of regular joint space and mandibular contour and osteophyte formation.
• Irregular new bone formation in close proximity of the TMJ. Signs of otitis.
• Orbital mass
• CT and three-dimensional reconstruction of the TMJ and orbit is the preferred imaging modality.

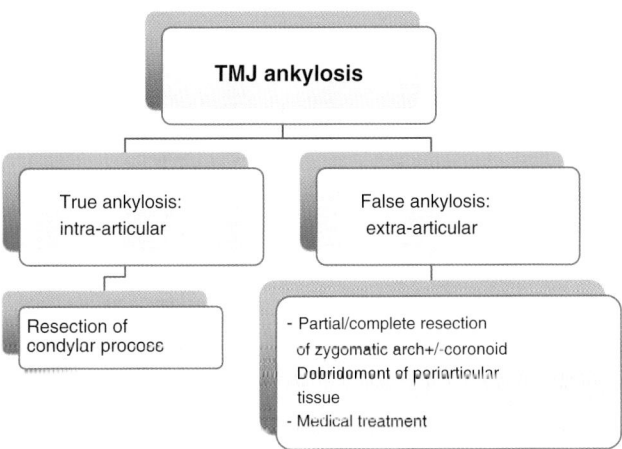

Figure 30.15 Treatment of temporomandibular joint (TMJ) ankylosis.

Treatment

Treatment of TMJ ankylosis is described in Figure 30.15.

Outcome

The resection of ankylosing tissue in false ankylosis or gap arthroplasty in true ankylosis was successful in all of the trauma-induced cases (Maas and Theyse 2007). Animals tolerate reasonably well a resection of the condylar or coronoid process.

Prevention

- Coronoidectomy if large fracture fragments are present
- Limited immobilization in case of intraarticular fractures
- Physical therapy

Relevant literature

Animals presenting with orofacial trauma are often in shock and may have **brain injury**. Arterial hypotension or hypoxia, infection, and intracranial hematoma may cause further mechanical compression of the brain, potentially leading to increased ICP, brain herniation, brainstem compression, and death (Wilkinson 1999).

These secondary brain injuries can be minimized by an efficient emergency medical treatment with the objective of improving perfusion and oxygen delivery and reducing brain swelling. Hyperventilation to a PCO_2 below 30 mm Hg is only an emergency procedure. Low PCO_2 causes a strong cerebral vasoconstriction in noninjured regions, which reduces cerebral blood flow and ICP and reduces brain volume while redirecting blood flow to the injured parts of the brain. However, long-term vasoconstriction will add to the global ischemia and should be avoided. Current recommendations are to keep a low normal PCO_2 between 35 and 40 mm Hg to avoid vasoconstriction or vasodilation (Mishra et al. 2006; Armitage-Chen et al. 2007; Leach 2009; Syring 2011).

The cerebral blood flow (CBF) depends on the cerebral perfusion pressure (CPP), mean arterial blood pressure (MABP), and ICP according to the following equation: CPP = MABP – ICP. Between the MABP extremes of 50 and 150 mmHg, ICP remains constant between 5 and 12 mm Hg in dogs and cats (Syring 2011). This autoregulation of the brain to stabilize CPP and ICP is overwhelmed when cerebral edema or hemorrhage is present (Leach 2009). Therefore, the traumatized animal should rapidly be stabilized to return MABP in the normal range. Hypertonic saline may

be superior to isotonic saline in head-injured patients. A smaller volume increases rapidly cardiac output, MABP, and tissue perfusion (Mishra et al. 2006; Syring 2011).

Mannitol is a potent diuretic. It should not be used before the patient is hemodynamically stabilized. The osmotic effect depends on an intact blood–brain barrier. Intracranial hemorrhage may theoretically worsen interstitial edema through extravasation of mannitol, but this has not been proven clinically in human head trauma patients (Berger et al. 1995, Rosner et al. 1995).

Mannitol has also rheologic properties with some radical scavenging properties. An immediate plasma-expanding effect improves blood flow. The hyperosmotic effect is evident within 15 to 20 minutes of administration by drawing fluid into the intravascular space, which reduces cerebral edema.

In veterinary medicine, there is a lack of studies to evaluate the outcome **of cranial decompression** caused by intractable elevation of ICP after closed head trauma. One case report describes the successful surgical treatment of a traumatic intracranial epidural hematoma in a dog (Cabassu et al. 2008).

The majority of jaw fractures (~70%) are open and contaminated (Umphlet and Johnson 1988, 1990). Small fracture gaps can heal as long as vascularity is preserved and infection prevented (Marretta et al. 1990; Smith and Kern 1995). Antibiotic therapy is indicated in the majority of jaw fractures and reduces the occurrence of osteomyelitis (Umphlet and Johnson 1990; Legendre 2005). The treatment of **bone infection** requires long-term antibiotic treatment, debridement, and stable fracture fixation. Antibiotic-impregnated beads have been successfully used in orthopedic surgery to deliver antibiotics locally at a high concentration over weeks to months. Currently, research is focused around antibiotic-impregnated bioabsorbable bone substitutes to improve the consistency of elution and to avoid a second surgery (Kanellakopoulou and Giamarellos-Bourboulis 2000; Garvin and Feschuk 2005; McKee et al. 2010; Lewis et al. 2011). Another product uses denatured bovine collagen sponges impregnated with gentamicin for its hemostatic properties in addition to the antibacterial effect (Kanellakopoulou and Giamarellos-Bourboulis 2000; Pico et al. 2008; McKee et al. 2010).

Malocclusion followed by **nonunion** and osteomyelitis are the most frequent complications reported after fracture repair of the jaw (Umphlet and Johnson 1988, 1990; Zetner 1992; Owen et al. 2004).

Malocclusion interferes with eating, is a source of pain, and may promote nonunion of the fracture because of abnormal stress. It cannot be overemphasized that occlusion has to be achieved and must be evaluated during surgery. The endotracheal tube has to be outside of the mouth, introduced through pharyngostomy or tracheostomy. To promote rapid healing, proper soft tissue debridement and closure over the fracture site is mandatory (Boudrieau and Kudisch 1996).

A major factor in the successful repair of jaw fractures is the **choice of implants**. Interfragmentary wire is commonly used for its versatility in thin, flat bones and in all size animals (Umphlet and Johnson 1988). Jaw bones are not loaded with weight-bearing forces and can heal with less rigid fixations than long bones. With multiple fractures, wires should be sequentially tightened with the jaw kept closed. Overtightened wire may reduce bone length or tilt the mandibular canines during symphyseal fracture repair, resulting in malocclusion. Occlusion is always prioritized over fragment compression in oral surgery. Bone and teeth loss may prevent fragment compression by the wire, resulting in instability and diminished neovascularization (Davidson and Bauer 1992; Smith 2004;

Legendre 2005). If bone healing results in malocclusion, corrective osteotomy, orthodontics, endodontics, or tooth extraction may be required (Boudrieau et al. 1994, 2004; Lobprise 2007; Bar-Am and Verstraete 2010).

Bending forces are the primary forces acting on the mandible. The tension side of the mandible and maxilla is at the alveolar border, which is biomechanically the optimal position for implants (Boudrieau et al. 1992, 2005; Smith and Kern 1995). Interdental wire and composite bar are a very versatile and solid fixation technique for the majority of fractures and many nonunions when teeth are present on both sides (Kern et al. 1995). No foreign material is placed inside the fracture, which preserves the vascularity and eliminates the risk of damaging delicate bone, neurovascular structures, or tooth roots. Wires can progressively be tensioned to achieve the desired fracture reduction and dental occlusion. In the same fashion, the composite is applied and shaped to promote normal occlusion. Interdental wire stabilizes the fragments, and the composite adds rigidity. Maxillary teeth occlude to the outside of the mandibular teeth; therefore, wire twists and interdental composite splints are positioned lingually in mandibular fractures and buccally in maxillary fractures (Kern et al. 1993; Smith and Kern 1995, 2004; Eickhoff 2005; Legendre 2005; Lobprise 2007).

Caudally located fractures, TMJ luxations or fractures, and multiple fractures, as well as comminuted fractures with some loss of length can be anatomically stabilized with MMF by composite as a two- or four-point fixation. Intact canine teeth or extension tubes placed over broken teeth are required to apply the composite (Zetner 1992; Bennett et al. 1994; Eickhoff 2005; Legendre 2005; Beckman and Smith 2009; Hoffer et al. 2011). MMF with a circular external skeletal fixator (ESF) has also been described in a dog for the successful treatment of bilateral caudal mandibular fractures (Marshall et al. 2010).

Many animals can eat liquid food with a MMF, but an esophagostomy tube is a convenient and easy way to meet the caloric requirement (Ireland et al. 2003).

If a more rigid fixation is required, particularly after large bone loss, ESF or bone plates are indicated (Kern et al. 1995). Large tooth roots and alveolar canal occupy the majority of the mandibular bone and limit available bone stack for implant position. The ESF is very versatile in application if silicon tubing filled with composite is used to connect the pins. The composite is hardened with the jaw in closed position. The use of threaded pins, at least two pins per fragment, reduces the risk for premature implant loosening, which is common in the thin bones of mandible and maxilla (Davidson and Bauer 1992; Clary and Roe 1995; Owen et al. 2004). Mandibular fractures in the rostral and very caudal aspect of the mandible are less suited for ESF fixation.

In a study with clinical patients, mandibular fractures stabilized with ESF healed within 4 to 16 weeks in dogs and 4 to 10 weeks in cats (Owen et al. 2004).

Bone plates offer the most rigid fixation in both mandibular and maxillary fractures when prolonged healing time is anticipated. They are placed in a buttress or neutralization fashion with or without bone grafts. Mini-reconstruction plates with locking screws are preferred in thin bones because the thread pitch of the smallest screws allows bone purchase in any thickness greater than 1 mm, and three-dimensional contouring is possible (Boudrieau et al. 1994; Boudrieau and Kudisch 1996, 2005; Vérez-Fraguela and Vives Vallés 2000; Bilgili and Kurum 2003).

In an experimental study with 15 dogs undergoing a mandibular osteotomy with plate and screw fixation, 10 dogs showed ulceration of the overlying mucosa postoperatively, which exposed the plate to the oral milieu. Dental pathology was histologically seen in around 61% of the screws (Verstraete and Ligthelm 1992). Clinically, periapical inflammatory bone resorption after trauma may not be evident at the time of fracture healing and therefore missed. This can lead to painful conditions weeks to months later. If tooth viability is doubtful, radiographs should be repeated, and if pathologic changes develop, endodontic treatment or extraction should be performed.

Another concern with bone plates and ESF pins is their ventral position toward the compression side of the bone to avoid tooth roots, which is biomechanically less solid (Boudrieau and Kudisch 1996; Boudrieau 2005, Sverzut et al. 2008).

Small fracture gaps should be filled with cancellous bone graft or synthetic bioactive ceramics or glass. These synthetic bone grafts proved to be valuable in fracture healing by their osteoconductive and osteoinductive properties (Boudrieau et al. 1994, 2004; Kaufmann et al. 2000; Au et al. 2007; Lewis et al. 2008; Chim and Gosain 2009, Gorustovich et al. 2010). Bone morphogenetic protein is a growth factor that is widely used in orofacial and orthopedic surgery to enhance bone healing (Zimmermann et al. 2006; Milovancev et al. 2007; Spector et al. 2007; Elsalanty et al. 2008; Lewis et al. 2008; Boyce et al. 2009; Giannoudis et al. 2009).

Large fracture gaps are grafted with various bone autografts or allografts stabilized with screws and plates. Successful incorporation in the mandible has been reported with rib segments, cortical diaphyseal ulnar segments, free vascularized coccygeal vertebra, and vascularized medial tibial bone (Yeh and Hou 1994; Boudrieau et al. 1994, 2004; Bebchuck et al. 2000; Lewis et al. 2008; Nolff et al. 2009).

Maxillary fractures present much fewer complications than mandibular fractures. The maxilla is formed by thin bone lamellae, has a broad base, is immobile, and is less exposed than the mandible. Many maxillary fractures heal after apposition of soft tissue or with interfragmentary wire or pin fixation. In highly unstable fractures, mini-plate fixation can be applied (Boudrieau and Kudisch 1996; Vérez-Fraguela and Vives Vallés 2000).

The **TMJ** should always be examined when dental occlusion is affected or problems exist to open or close the mouth. Multiple radiographic views have been recommended because superimposition with other bones of the skull limits visualization of the TMJ. CT imaging is the modality of choice to examine the TMJ and periarticular tissue, including bulla, mandibular ramus, zygomatic arch, and orbit (Schwarz et al. 2002; Gatineau et al. 2008; Soukup et al. 2009). Most **TMJ luxations** are reduced in closed fashion followed by 1 or 2 weeks of immobilization (Eickhoff 2005; Klima 2007; Lobprise 2007). Open reduction may be successful in chronic luxations.

Intraarticular fractures of the TMJ are more frequently treated by immobilization, fragment excision, or condylectomy when ankylosis develops (Legendre 2005; Klima 2007; Scott and McLaughlin 2007). Prolonged complete immobilization by MMF will reduce range of motion of the TMJ (Jermyn et al. 2007). Internal fixation of the fractured condyle is rarely performed because of the limited exposure possible.

Locked jaw syndrome can occur with the mouth open or closed. **Open-mouth jaw locking** secondary to displacement of the mandibular coronoid process ventrolateral to the zygomatic arch is caused by TMJ dysplasia, flattening of the zygomatic arch, excessive mandibular symphyseal laxity, previous maxillofacial trauma, and breed-specific skull conformation (Soukup et al. 2009). Under sedation, the displaced coronoid process is repositioned medially. Frequently, locking will reoccur, and a resection of the coronoid process, zygomatic arch, or both has to be performed (Maas and Theyse 2007; Gatineau *et al.* 2008; Soukup *et al.* 2009).

Closed-mouth locking jaw is most commonly caused by TMJ ankylosis. Orofacial trauma, TMJ fracture, retrobulbar abscess, foreign body, neoplasia, trigeminal neuropathy causing trismus, masticatory muscle myositis or fibrosis and polymyositis, tetanus, otitis media, and craniomandibular osteopathy are reported to cause true or false ankylosis. Idiopathic cases are also possible (Maas and Theyse 2007; Gatineau *et al.* 2008). Proper diagnosis of the pathology is mandatory to choose the appropriate treatment.

A major problem is encountered when the animal is anesthetized. Vomiting during induction has to be avoided by selecting appropriate drugs. If the mouth is locked closed, intubation is performed with endoscopic assistance, symphysiotomy, and transoral intubation or tracheostomy (Nanai *et al.* 2009; Maas and Theyse 2007).

References

Armitage-Chan, E.A., Wetmore, L.A., Chan, D.L. (2006) Anesthetic management of the head trauma patient. *Journal of Emergency and Critical Care* 17 (1), 5-14.

Au, A.Y., Au, R.Y., Al-Talib, T.K., et al. (2008) Consil bioactive glass particles enhance osteoblast proliferation and maintain extracellular matrix production in vitro. *Journal of Biomedical Materials Research Part A*. 86 (3), 678-684.

Bar-Am, Y., Verstraete, F.J.M. (2010) Elastic training for the prevention of mandibular drift following mandibulectomy in dogs: 18 cases (2005-2008). *Veterinary Surgery* 39 (5), 574-580.

Bebchuck, T.N., Degner, D.A., Walshaw, R., et al. (2000) Evaluation of a free vascularised medial tibial bone graft in dogs. *Veterinary Surgery* 29 (2), 128-144.

Beckman, B., Smith, M.H. (2009) Interarcade bonding for non-invasive mandibular fracture repair. *Journal of Veterinary Dentistry* 26 (1), 62-66.

Bennett, J.W., Kapatkin, A.S., Maretta, S.M. (1994). Dental composite for the fixation of mandibular fractures and luxations in 11 cats and 6 dogs. *Veterinary Surgeryr* 23, 190-194.

Berger, S., Schürer, L., Härtl, R., et al. (1995) Reduction of post-traumatic intracranial hypertension by hypertonic/ hypertonic/hyperoncotic saline/dextran and hypertonic mannitol. *Neurosurgery* 37 (1), 98-107.

Bilgili, H., Kurum, B. (2003) Treatment of fractures of the mandible and maxilla by mini titanium plate fixation systems in dogs and cats. *Australian Veterinary Journal* 81 (11), 671-673.

Boudrieau, R.J. (2005) Fractures of the maxilla. In Johnson, A.L., Houlton, J.E.F., Vannini R. (eds.) *AO Principles of Fracture Management in the Dog and Cat*. Thieme, Stuttgart, pp. 99-129.

Boudrieau, R.J., Kudisch, M. (1996) Miniplate fixation for repair of mandibular and maxillary fractures in 15 dogs and 3 cats. *Veterinary Surgery* 25, 277-291.

Boudrieau, R.J., Tidwell, A.S. Ullman, S.L., et al. (1994) Correction of mandibular nonunion and malocclusion by plate fixation and autogenous cortical bone grafts in two dogs. *Journal of the American Veterinary Medical Association* 204 (5), 744-750.

Boudrieau, R.J., Mitchell, S.L., Seeherman, H. (2004) Mandibular reconstruction of a partial hemimandibulectomy in a dog with severe malocclusion. *Veterinary Surgery* 33 (2), 119-130.

Boyce, A.S., Reveal, G., Scheid, D.K., et al. (2009) Canine investigation of rhBMP-2, autogenous bone graft for the healing of a large segmental tibial defect. *Journal of Orthopaedic Trauma* 23 (10), 685-692.

Cabassu, J.B., Cabassu, J.P., Brochier, L., et al. (2008) Surgical treatment of a traumatic intracranial epidural haematoma in a dog. *Veterinary and Comparative Orthopaedics and Traumatology* 5, 457-461.

Chim, H., Gosain, A.K. (2009) Biomaterials in craniofacial surgery. *The Journal of Craniofacial Surgery* 20 (1), 29-32.

Clary, E.M., Roe, S.C. (1995) Enhancing external skeletal fixation pin performance: consideration of the pin-bone interface. *Veterinary and Comparative Orthopaedics and Traumatology* 8, 8-12.

Davidson, J.R., Bauer, M.S. (1992) Fractures of the mandible and maxilla. *Veterinary Clinics Of North America: Small Animal Practice. Feline Dentistry* 22 (1), 109-119.

Eickhoff, M. (2005) *Zahn-, Mund- und Kieferheilkunde bei Klein- und Heimtieren*. Enke Verlag, Stuttgart, 158-167.

Elsalanty, M.E., Genecov, D.G., Salyer, K.E., et al. (2008) Recombinant human BMP-2 enhances the effects of materials used for reconstruction of large cranial defects. *Journal Oral Maxillofacial Surgery* 66 (2), 277-285.

Garvin, K., Feschuk, C. (2005) Polylactide-polyglycolide antibiotic implants. *Clinical Orthopaedics and Related Research* 437, 105-110.

Gatineau, M., El-Warrak, A.O., Maretta, S.M., et al. (2008) Locked jaw syndrome in dogs and cats: 37 cases (1998-2005). *Journal of Veterinary Dentistry* 25 (1), 16-22.

Giannoudis, P.V., Kanakaris, N.K., Dimitriou, R. (2009) The synergistic effect of autograft and BMP-7 in the treatment of atrophic non-unions. *Clinical Orthopaedics and Related Research* 467 (12), 3239-3248.

Gorustovich, A.A., Roether, J.A., Boccaccini, A.R. (2010) Effect of bioactive glasses on angiogenesis: a review of in vitro and in vivo evidences. *Tissue Engineering Part B Reviews* 16 (2), 199-207.

Hoffer, M., Maretta, S.M., Kurath, P., et al. (2011) Evaluation of composite resin materials for maxillomandibular fixation in cats for treatment of jaw fractures and temporomandibular joint luxations. *Veterinary Surgery* 40 (3), 357-368.

Ireland, L.M., Hohenhaus, A.E., Broussard, J.D., et al. (2003) A comparison of owner management and complications in 67 cats with esophagostomy and percutaneous endoscopic gastrostomy feeding tubes. *Journal of the American Animal Hospital Association* 39, 241-246.

Jermyn, K., Farrell, M., Bennett, D. (2007) Maxillomandibular external skeletal fixation as an alternative technique for treatment of caudal mandibular fractures or instability in 2 dogs and 3 cats. Proceedings of the British Small Animal Veterinary Congress, Birmingham UK.

Kanellakopoulou, K., Giamarellos-Bourboulis, E.J. (2000) Carrier systems for the local delivery of antibiotics in bone infections. *Drugs* 59 (6), 1223-1232.

Kaufmann, E.A., Ducheyne, P., Shapiro, I.M. (2000) Effect of varying physical properties of porous, surface modified bioactive glass 45S5 on osteoblast proliferation and maturation. *Journal of Biomedical Materials Research* 52 (4), 783-796.

Kern, D.A., Smith, M.M., Grant, J.W., et al. (1993) Evaluation of bending strength of five interdental fixation apparatuses applied to canine mandibles. *American Journal of Veterinary Research* 54 (7), 1177-1182.

Kern, D.A., Smith, M.M., Stevenson, S., et al. (1995) Evaluation of three fixation techniques for repair of mandibular fractures in dogs. *Journal of the American Veterinary Medical Association* 12, 1883-1890.

Klima, L.J. (2007) Temporomandibular joint luxation in the cat. *Journal of Veterinary Dentistry* 24 (3), 198-201.

Leach, R. (2009) Head injury. Leach, R (ed.) *Acute and Critical Care Medicine at a Glance*, 2nd edn. Wiley-Blackwell, Oxford, UK, pp. 112-113.

Legendre, L. (2005) Maxillofacial fracture repairs. *Veterinary Clinics of North America: Small Animal Practice. Dentistry* 35 (4), 985-1008.

Lewis, C.S., Supronowicz, P.R., Zhukauskas, R.M., et al. (2011) Local antibiotic delivery with demineralised bone matrix. *Cell and Tissue Banking* 13 (1), 119-127.

Lewis, J.R., Boudrieau, R.J., Reiter, A.M., et al. (2008) Mandibular reconstruction after gunshot trauma in a dog by use of recombinant human bone morphogenetic protein-2. *Journal of the American Veterinary Medical Association* 233 (10), 1598-1604.

Lobprise, H.B. (2007) Maxillary and mandibular fractures. Temporomandibular joint disorders. In Lobprise, H.B. (ed.) *Small Animal Dentistry*. Blackwell Publishing, Ames, IA, pp. 289-302.

Lopes, F.M., Gioso, M.A., Ferro, D.G., et al. (2005) Oral fractures in dogs of Brazil—a retrospective study. *Journal of Veterinary Dentistry* 22 (2), 86-90.

Maas, C.P.H.J., Theyse, L.F.H. (2007) Temporomandibular joint ankylosis in cats and dogs. *Veterinary and Comparative Orthopaedics and Traumatology* 3, 192-197.

Marretta, M.S., Schrader, S.C., Matthiesen, D.T. (1990) Problems associated with the management and treatment of jaw fractures. *Problems in Veterinary Medicine* 2, 220-247.

Marshall, W.G., Farrell, M., Chase, D., et al. (2010) Maxillomandibular circular external skeletal fixation for repair of bilateral fractures of the caudal aspect of the mandible in a dog. *Veterinary Surgery* 39 (6), 765-770.

McKee, M.D., Li-Bland, E.A., Wild, L.M., et al. (2010) A prospective, randomized clinical trial comparing an antibiotic-impregnated bioabsorbable bone substitute with standard antibiotic-impregnated cement beads in the treatment of chronic osteomyelitis and infected non-union. *Journal of Orthopedic Trauma* 24 (8), 483-490.

Milovancev, M., Muir, P., Manley, P.A., et al. (2007) Clinical application of recombinant human bone morphogenetic protein-2 in 4 dogs. *Veterinary Surgery* 36 (2), 132-140.

Mishra, L.D., Rajkumar, N., Hancock, S.M. (2006) Current controversies in neuroanesthesia, head injury management and neuro critical care. *Continuing Education in Anesthesia & Critical Care and Pain* 6 (2), 79-82.

Nanai, B., Phillips, L., Christiansen, J., et al. (2009) Life threatening complication associated with anesthesia in a dog with masticatory muscle myositis. *Veterinary Surgery* 38 (5), 645-649.

Nolff, M.C., Gellrich, N.C., Hauschild, G., et al. (2009) Comparison of two beta-tricalcium phosphate composite grafts used for reconstruction of mandibular critical size bone defects. *Veterinary and Comparative Orthopaedics and Traumatology* 2, 96-102.

Owen, M.R., Langley Hobbs, S.J., Moores, A.P., et al. (2004) Mandibular fracture repair in dogs and cats using epoxy resin and acrylic external skeletal fixation. *Veterinary and Comparative Orthopaedics and Traumatology* 4, 189-197.

Pico, R.B., Jimenez, L.A., Sanchez, M.C., et al. (2008) Prospective study comparing the incidence of wound infection following appendectomy for acute appendicitis in children: conventional treatment versus using reabsorbable antibacterial suture or gentamycin-impregnated collagen fleeces. *Cirugia Pediatrica* 21 (4), 199-202.

Platt, S.R., Radaelli, S.T., McDonnell J.J., et al. (2001) The prognostic value of the modified Glasgow Coma Scale in head trauma in dogs. *Journal of Veterinary Internal Medicine* 15, 581-584.

Rawlinson, J. (2008) Unraveling the mysteries of the TMJ. *Proceedings of the American College of Veterinary Internal Medicine*. San Antonio, TX.

Rosner, M.J., Rosner, S.D., Johnson, A.H. (1995) Cerebral perfusion pressure: management protocol and clinical results. *Journal of Neurosurgery* 83 (6), 949-962.

Schwarz, T., Weller, R., Dickie, A.M., et al. (2002) Imaging of the canine and feline temporomandibular joint: a review. *Veterinary Radiology & Ultrasound* 43 (2), 85-97.

Scott, H.W., McLaughlin, R. (2007) Temporomandibular joint injury. In Scott, H.W., McLaughlin, R. (eds.) *Feline Orthopedics*. Manson Publishing, London, p. 273.

Smith, M.M. (2004) Oral fracture repair using interdental wire and acrylic. Proceedings of the World Small Animal Veterinary Association World Congress, Dentistry.

Smith, M.M., Kern, D.A. (1995) Skull trauma and mandibular fractures. *Veterinary Clinics of North America: Small Animal Practice. Management of Orthopedic Emergencies* 25 (5), 1127-1147.

Spector, D.I., Keating, J.H., Boudrieau, R.J. (2007) Immediate mandibular reconstruction of a 5cm defect using rhBMP-2 after partial mandibulectomy in a dog. *Veterinary Surgery* 36 (8), 752-759.

Soukup, J.W., Snyder, C.J., Gengler, W.R. (2009) Computed tomography and partial coronoidectomy for open-mouth jaw locking in two cats. *Journal of Veterinary Dentistry* 6 (4), 226-233.

Sverzut, C.E., Lucas, M.A., Sverzut, A.T., et al. (2008) Bone repair in mandibular body osteotomy after using 2.0 miniplate system—histological and histometric analysis in dogs. *International Journal of Experimental Pathology,* 89 (2), 91-97.

Syring, R.S. (2011) Traumatic brain injury. Drobatz, K.J., Beal, M.W., Syring, R.S. (eds.) *Manual of Trauma Management in the Dog and Cat.* Wiley-Blackwell, Oxford UK, pp. 136-156.

Tutt, C. (2006) Jaw fracture repair. In Tutt, C. (ed.) *Small Animal Dentistry.* Blackwell Publishing, Oxford, UK, pp. 174-195.

Umphlet, R.C., Johnson, A.L. (1988) Mandibular fractures in the cat. *Veterinary Surgery* 17 (6), 333-337.

Umphlet, R.C., Johnson, A.L. (1990) Mandibular fractures in the dog. *Veterinary Surgery* 19 (4), 272-275.

Vérez-Fraguela, J.L., Vives Vallés, M.A. (2000) Maxillofacial surgery: maxillary osteosynthesis craniomaxillofacial CMS-titanium plates. *Veterinary and Comparative Orthopaedics and Traumatology* 13, 119-122.

Verstraete, M., Ligthelm, A.J. (1992) Dental trauma caused by screws in internal fixation of mandibular osteotomies in the dog. *Veterinary and Comparative Orthopaedics and Traumatology* 5, 104-108.

Wilkinson, I.M.S. (1999) Head injury. In Wilkinson, I.M.S. (ed.) *Essential Neurology.* Blackwell Science, Oxford, UK, pp. 53-63.

Yeh, L.S., Hou, S.M. (1994) Repair of a mandibular defect with a free vascularised coccygeal vertebra transfer in a dog. *Veterinary Surgery* 23 (4), 281-285.

Zetner, K. (1992) Treatment of jaw fractures in small animals with parapulpar pin composite bridges. *Veterinary Clinics Of North America: Small Animal Practice. Feline Dentistry* 22 (6), 1461-1467.

Zimmermann, G., Moghaddam, A., Wagner, C., et al. (2006) Clinical experience with bone morphogenetic protein 7 in nonunions of long bones. *Unfallchirurgie* 109 (7), 528-537.

31 Partial Mandibulectomy

Julius Liptak

Alta Vista Animal Hospital, Ottawa, Ontario, Canada

Mandibulectomy procedures are most commonly performed for the treatment of benign and malignant oral tumors. Other indications for mandibulectomy include treatment of mandibular fractures and osteomyelitis and palliation of diseases involving the temporomandibular joint (TMJ). Mandibulectomy procedures include unilateral and bilateral rostral mandibulectomy, segmental mandibulectomy, caudal mandibulectomy, and subtotal and total hemimandibulectomy.

The complication rate after all types of mandibulectomy procedures is 22% in dogs (Schwarz *et al.* 1991). In a retrospective study of 42 cats treated with various mandibulectomy procedures, short- and long-term complications were reported in 98% and 76% of cats, respectively (Northrup *et al.* 2006). Local tumor recurrence and distant metastasis will not be considered as complications of mandibulectomy for the purposes of this chapter; however, it should be noted that complete histologic excision of malignant oral tumors is important to decrease local tumor recurrence rates and improve survival times.

Hemorrhage

Definition
Intraoperative hemorrhage is defined as blood loss, usually from the inferior alveolar artery, resulting in poor visualization of the surgical field, hypotension, and anemia.

Risk factors
• Subtotal and total hemimandibulectomy

Diagnosis
• Intraoperative observation of brisk or profuse bleeding

Treatment
• Ligation of the inferior alveolar artery and vein
• Bleeding from the inferior alveolar artery is rarely severe enough to warrant a blood transfusion, but a cross-matched compatible blood transfusion should be considered if hematocrit acutely decreases below 15% to 30%, particularly if this occurs in combination with hypotension (mean blood pressure <80 mm Hg or systolic blood pressure <100 mg Hg); hypoxia;

or clinical, biochemical, or echocardiographic evidence of anaerobic metabolism.

Outcome
Blood loss from the inferior alveolar artery is rarely severe enough to warrant a blood transfusion; hence, the outcome is usually not affected by blood loss if treated appropriately.

Prevention
• Ligation of the inferior alveolar artery before transection as it courses over the caudomedial aspect of the mandible, TMJ, and pterygoid muscles before entering the mandibular foramen

Incisional swelling

Definition
Incisional swelling is defined as swelling of the surgical incision.

Risk factors
Swelling of the surgical site is more common after nonrostral mandibulectomies (i.e., segmental and caudal mandibulectomy and subtotal and total hemimandibulectomy) because of more extensive tissue manipulation and dissection.

Diagnosis
A cosmetic defect characterized by swelling at and adjacent to the incision site is usually the only clinical sign associated with incisional swelling. The incision may be painful on palpation.

Treatment
Ice packing every 4 hours and the administration of nonsteroidal antiinflammatory drugs (NSAIDs) may assist in decreasing the severity of postoperative swelling.

Outcome
Swelling resolves spontaneously in 5 to 7 days.

Prevention
• Gentle intraoperative tissue handling and prophylactic ice packing and administration of NSAIDs

---

Complications in Small Animal Surgery, First Edition. Edited by Dominique Griffon and Annick Hamaide.
© 2016 John Wiley & Sons, Inc. Published 2016 by John Wiley & Sons, Inc.
Companion website: www.wiley.com/go/griffon/complications

Ranula-like lesions

Definition
Ranula-like lesions are uncommon and appear as soft, fluctuant, nonpainful swellings in the frenulum of the tongue ipsilateral to the mandibulectomy procedure (Figure 31.1). Ranula-like lesions may be caused by trauma to the mandibular and sublingual salivary ducts, but hematoma or seroma formation is more likely.

Risk factors
Ranula-like lesions are more common after subtotal or total hemimandibulectomy. These mandibulectomy procedures involve more extensive dissection of the intermandibular tissues.

Diagnosis
Ranula-like lesions are often asymptomatic, and the diagnosis is made by intraoral examination. Rarely, ranula-like lesions are large enough to interfere with lingual function and cause prehension difficulties.

Treatment
None

Outcome
Ranula-like lesions usually resolve spontaneously within 5 to 7 days.

Prevention
Preventive factors are not known, but gentle tissue handle, careful dissection, meticulous hemostasis, and preservation of the salivary ducts (if they can be identified and are not involved in the neoplastic process) may decrease the risk of this complication.

Wound dehiscence

Definition
Wound dehiscence is the breakdown of the surgical wound with separation of the wound edges. The two most common sites for incisional dehiscence are the occlusal margin after rostral and segmental mandibulectomies and the rostral aspect of a cheiloplasty

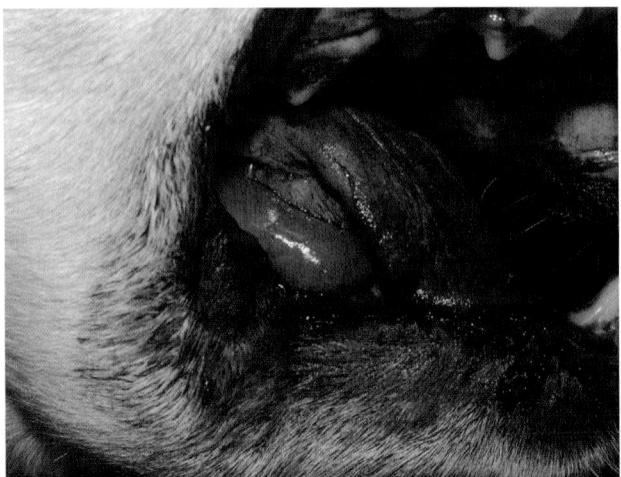

Figure 31.1 A ranula-like lesion in a dog 1 day after subtotal hemimandibulectomy for a mandibular osteosarcoma.

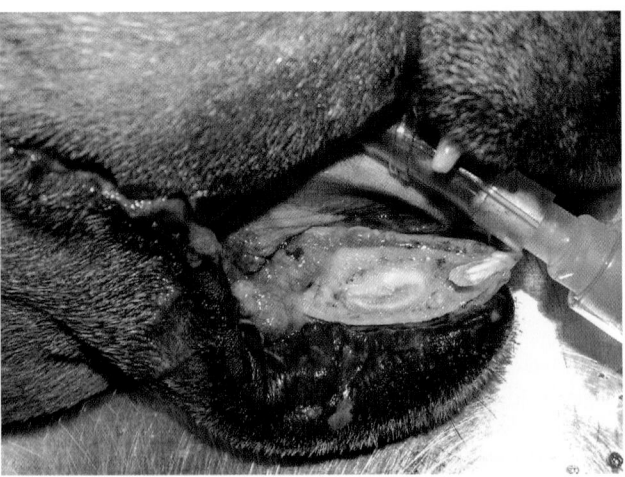

Figure 31.2 Dehiscence of both the intraoral surgical wound and cheiloplasty after total hemimandibulectomy for a mandibular osteosarcoma. Although many intraoral dehiscences can be managed with second intention healing, larger lesions such as this require debridement; occasionally, extraction of teeth on the occlusal margin of the osteotomy; and resuturing.

(which is performed after a total hemimandibulectomy to prevent protrusion of the tongue) (Figure 31.2).

Risk factors
- Wound tension
- Self-induced trauma, especially the tongue
- Chewing of hard foods, sticks, and so on
- Use of cautery to incise oral mucosa
- Use of rapidly absorbable suture material (i.e., catgut or polyglecaprone 25)
- Closure of surgical wounds with a single layer of suture material
- Poor wound healing because of radiation therapy, chemotherapy, or debilitation

Diagnosis
Wound dehiscence typically occurs 3 to 7 days after surgery and is often asymptomatic. Clinical signs of intraoral wound dehiscence are rare but may include inappetence and halitosis; cosmetic disruption of the incision is the most obvious clinical sign associated with dehiscence of cheiloplasty wounds.

Treatment
Treatment of intraoral surgical wound dehiscence depends on the size of the defect. Wound dehiscence can be managed with either second intention healing if the dehisced area is small and granulating or debridement and resuturing if the defect is large or rostral. If dehiscence is detected early in the postoperative period, then serial debridement and delayed closure are recommended. Dehiscence of cheiloplasty wounds usually requires surgical revision with the use of tension-relieving sutures. If the tongue is the cause of tension and dehiscence, then tube feeding may be required for 1 to 2 weeks.

Outcome
Conservative management with second intention healing and surgical treatment of dehisced wounds usually results in an uncomplicated recovery with no functional consequences or cosmetic defects.

Prevention

The risk of wound dehiscence can be minimized by tension-free closure of the mucosal suture line. This can be achieved with sufficient undermining of the labial mucosal–submucosal flap and angling the dorsal (occlusal) bone margin away from the lesion during rostral and horizontal mandibulectomies (which may require additional extraction of teeth) and then suturing the mucosa over the tapered bone. Two-layer closures with long-lasting absorbable suture material (i.e., polydioxanone) are recommended. Cautery should only be used for hemostasis purposes during mandibulectomy procedures. Chewing on hard foods and materials should be avoided until the surgical wound has healed, typically 2 to 3 weeks. If the tongue is the cause of tension and dehiscence, then tube feeding may be required for 1 to 2 weeks.

Ptyalism

Definition

Ptyalism is an excessive drooling of saliva.

Risk factors

- Bilateral rostral mandibulectomy in cats and dogs
- Resection of more than 50% of the mandible in cats

Diagnosis

Ptyalism is typically diagnosed by observation of excessive drooling and salivation. Cheilitis and facial dermatitis are common in chronic cases.

Treatment

- Daily washing with an antiseptic solution
- Cheiloplasty

Outcome

Ptyalism will either resolve spontaneously or significantly reduce in volume after several weeks in the majority of animals. However, for cats and dogs with persistent drooling, cheilitis and facial dermatitis are common sequelae.

Prevention

Cheiloplasty should be performed in cats after resection of more than 50% of the mandible. Other preventive factors are not known.

Mandibular drift and malocclusion

Definition

Mandibular drift is characterized by the medialization of the mandible toward the side of the resection (Figure 31.3).

Risk factors

Mandibular drift is common after segmental mandibulectomy and subtotal and total hemimandibulectomy. Mandibular drift is caused by a loss of mandibular support at either the mandibular symphysis or TMJ.

Diagnosis

Mandibular drift is common, but it rarely causes a clinical problem. For this reason, mandibular drift is often diagnosed by

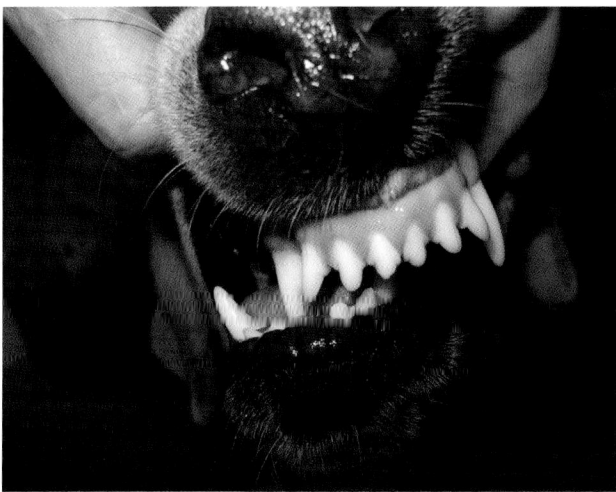

Figure 31.3 Mandibular drift in a dog after a large segmental mandibulectomy for a mandibular fibrosarcoma. Mandibular drift results in medialization of the mandible toward the midline and malocclusion, but clinical problems are rare as a result of this complication.

visual inspection of the oral cavity. Mandibular drift will cause malocclusion, which may result in audible clicking of teeth, prehension difficulties, ulceration of the hard palate secondary to trauma from the mandibular canine tooth, and halitosis secondary to periodontal disease.

Treatment

Mandibular drift does not require treatment unless it results in complications. Extraction or shortening of the mandibular canine tooth is required for cases in which malocclusion results in trauma to the hard palate. Reconstruction of the mandible with either an ulnar or rib autograft and promotion of osseous ingrowth with bone morphogenetic protein-2 (BMP-2) has been described to treat mandibular drift.

Outcome

- Mandibular drift often remains asymptomatic.
- Malocclusion may predispose to periodontal disease.
- Histologic, but not clinical or radiographic, evidence of TMJ osteoarthritis has been reported.

Prevention

- Rim resection for benign oral tumors with a biradial oscillating saw to preserve the ventral mandibular cortex and hemimandible integrity (Figure 31.4)
- Reconstruction of the mandible with either an ulnar or rib autograft and promotion of osseous ingrowth with BMP-2 has been described to prevent mandibular drift but is rarely required and is associated with increased expense and risk of complications.
- Elastic training, consisting of an orthodontic elastic rubber chain between an orthodontic button on the lingual aspect of the intact mandible canine tooth and buccal aspect of the maxillary fourth premolar tooth has been described to maintain occlusion and prevent mandibular drift after mandibulectomy in dogs.

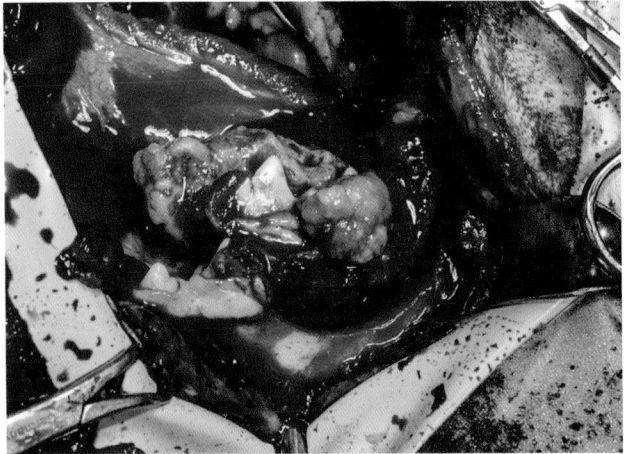

Figure 31.4 A rim resection has been performed for removal of an acanthomatous ameloblastoma with 1-cm margins. Note that the ventral cortex of the mandible has been preserved. Preservation of the ventral cortex prevents the development of mandibular drift and malocclusion.

Eating difficulties

Definition
Eating difficulties are defined as difficulty prehending food, dysphagia, or inappetence.

Risk factors
- Cats: Dysphagia and inappetence are very common regardless of the mandibulectomy procedure
- Bilateral rostral mandibulectomy with resection of both canine teeth, particularly the more aggressive bilateral procedures extending caudally to the second premolar teeth, results in prehension difficulties in dogs.
- Rarely, hypoglossal nerve damage, mandibular drift, and ranula-like lesions may be responsible for prehension difficulties and dysphagia.

Diagnosis
Eating difficulties are best diagnosed through observation in the hospital and by the owners. In cases that have not resolved within 2 weeks, a cranial nerve examination may be required to assess hypoglossal nerve function.

Treatment
A feeding tube should be inserted at the time of mandibulectomy in all cats because of their high risk of inappetence and dysphagia. An esophageal or gastric feeding tube is preferred because of the ability to maintain and use these feeding tubes for a prolonged period (Figure 31.5). The feeding tube should be removed when the cat begins to eat voluntarily and consistently.

Prehension difficulties are more common in dogs, and most adapt within 2 weeks. Supplemental feeding may be required during this period, such as force feeding, tube feeding, or feeding soft foods made into a ball. Hand feeding and trying foods with different consistencies may be necessary. Oral feeding should be encouraged to allow the animal to adapt and develop a new prehensile function of the tongue.

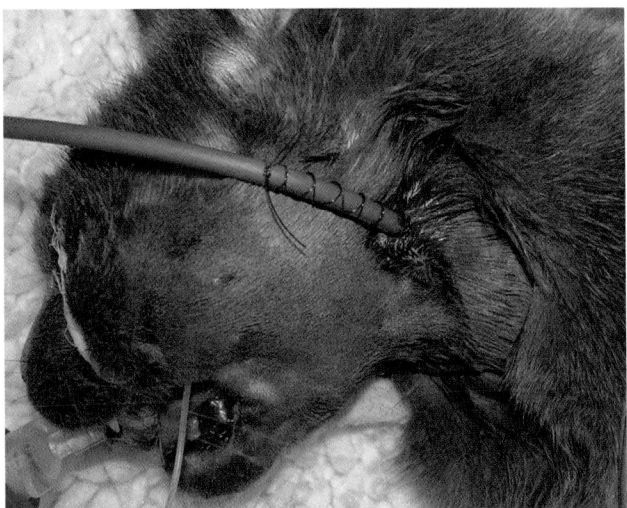

Figure 31.5 A feeding tube, in this case an esophagostomy tube, should be inserted in all cats after any type of mandibulectomy.

Outcome
Most cats return to the ability to eat, but this can take weeks to months. Some cats will never eat voluntarily again and will require lifelong tube feeding.

Prehension difficulties will often resolve within 2 weeks in dogs.

Prevention
Prehension difficulties, dysphagia, and inappetence are difficult to prevent because they are either inherent with the species (i.e., cat) or the procedure (i.e., bilateral rostral mandibulectomy caudal to the canine teeth in dogs). Owner education is imperative, particularly in cats, to prepare them for the postoperative management and care.

Grooming difficulties

Definition
Difficult with grooming is a specific complication in cats after mandibulectomy whereby cats are either unable or unwilling to groom.

Risk factors
The risk factors are unknown, but possible causes for grooming difficulties after mandibulectomy in cats include
- Ptyalism
- Tongue protrusion
- Mandibular drift
- Pain

Diagnosis
- Unkempt physical appearance with a matted hair coat

Treatment
If cats do not resume grooming behavior, then owners must groom cats with brushing once to twice daily, depending on the length of the hair coat.

Outcome
- Unkempt physical appearance with a matted hair coat

Prevention

Preventive factors are not known.

Tongue protrusion

Definition

Tongue protrusion is defined as the tongue protruding either rostrally or laterally from the oral cavity.

Risk factors

- Bilateral rostral mandibulectomy caudal to the second premolar teeth for rostral tongue protrusion in dogs
- Hemimandibulectomy for lateral tongue protrusion in dogs
- Any mandibulectomy procedure in cats

Diagnosis

Diagnosis made through observation of the tongue protruding either rostrally (Figure 31.6) or laterally (Figure 31.7). Prehension is rarely affected, although eating difficulties may be observed for 1 to 2 weeks after aggressive bilateral rostral mandibulectomy procedures.

Treatment

- No treatment is necessary for rostral tongue protrusion.
- No treatment is usually necessary for lateral tongue protrusion, but cheiloplasty can be performed if tongue protrusion is causing clinical problems.

Outcome

Rostral tongue protrusion after aggressive bilateral rostral mandibulectomy can cause initial eating difficulties; however, dogs typically adjust and eat without difficulty within 1 to 2 weeks. Otherwise, the only outcome is a different cosmetic appearance.

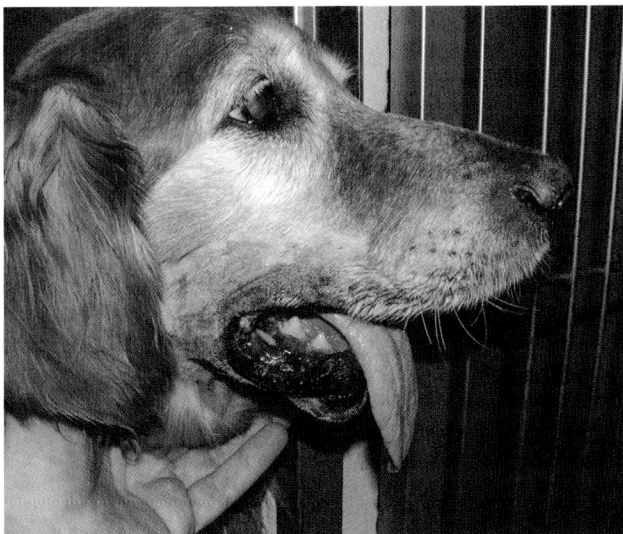

Figure 31.6 The tongue protruding rostrally after bilateral rostral mandibulectomy caudal to the second premolar teeth for resection of a malignant melanoma. Eating difficulties can be observed for 1 to 2 weeks after surgery, but this is uncommon, and most dogs can eat unassisted without difficulty.

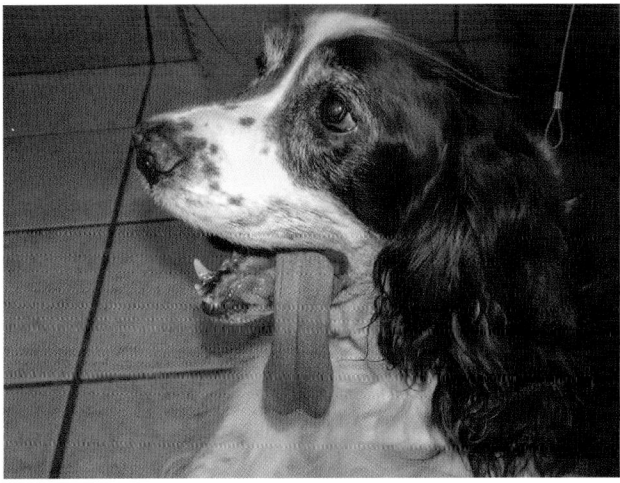

Figure 31.7 The tongue protruding laterally after total hemimandibulectomy for resection of a mandibular osteosarcoma. This is typically a cosmetic defect, and functional consequences, such as difficulty eating, are very rare.

Prevention

Cheiloplasty after hemimandibulectomy may decrease the incidence or severity of lateral tongue protrusion after hemimandibulectomy. There is no known prevention of rostral tongue protrusion after bilateral rostral mandibulectomy caudal to the second premolar teeth.

Relevant literature

The majority of mandibulectomy complications in dogs are minor and can be treated conservatively. Complications are more common with total hemimandibulectomies, accounting for 56% of all mandibulectomy complications with 38% (10 of 26) of dogs treated with total hemimandibulectomy experiencing one or more complications (Schwarz *et al.* 1991). In comparison, complications were reported in 33% (2 of 6) of dogs treated with segmental hemimandibulectomy, 19% (3 of 16) of dogs treated with bilateral rostral hemimandibulectomy, and 12% (3 of 25) of dogs treated with unilateral rostral hemimandibulectomy (Schwarz *et al.* 1991).

In contrast to dogs, complications are common after mandibulectomy in cats, and these complications can have a significant impact on the quality of life and management of cats postoperatively (Hutson *et al.* 1992; Northrup *et al.* 2006). In one study of 42 cats, 98% of cats had complications in the short term (≤4 weeks), and 76% had complications in the long term (Northrup *et al.* 2006). Complications were common regardless of the mandibulectomy technique. Short- and long-term complications were reported in 92% (11 of 12) and 50% (5 of 10) of cats after bilateral rostral mandibulectomy, 67% (2 of 3) and 67% (2 of 3) of cats after segmental mandibulectomy, 100% (19 of 19) and 84% (16 of 19) of cats after hemimandibulectomy, and 100% and 100% of six cats after resection of more than 50% of the mandible, respectively (Northrup *et al.* 2006). The most common complication was inappetence or dysphagia, which was reported in 76% of cats (and 12% never regained the ability to eat voluntarily). Despite the high morbidity rate, 83% of owners were satisfied with the outcome.

Swelling of the surgical site was a common finding in 12 dogs treated with total hemimandibulectomy in one study, but these all resolved without further treatment within 3 to 5 days (Salisbury and Lantz 1988). Incisional swelling was a common complication after total hemimandibulectomy in two other studies, but the number of dogs affected was not reported (Withrow and Holmberg 1983; Bradley *et al*. 1984). In another study, incisional swelling and drainage were reported in both dogs treated with a caudal mandibulectomy (White *et al*. 1985). Incisional swelling is rare after rostral mandibulectomies because tissue dissection is not as aggressive (Withrow and Holmberg 1983; Bradley *et al*. 1984; Salisbury and Lantz 1988).

Ranula-like lesions are uncommon in dogs and rare in cats and appear as soft, fluctuant, nonpainful swellings in the frenulum of the tongue ipsilateral to the mandibulectomy procedure (Withrow and Holmberg 1983; Bradley *et al*. 1984; Salisbury and Lantz 1988; Kosovsky *et al*. 1991; White 1991; White *et al*. 1995; Dernell *et al*. 1998; Northrup *et al*. 2006). They are most frequently observed after either subtotal or total hemimandibulectomy and have been reported in 8% of 12 dogs after total hemimandibulectomy and 14% (1 of 7) of dogs after bilateral rostral mandibulectomy (Salisbury and Lantz 1988). Ranula-like lesions may be caused by trauma to the mandibular and sublingual salivary ducts, but hematoma or seroma formation is more likely. Removal of the mandibular and sublingual salivary glands is not necessary (Withrow and Holmberg 1983; Dernell *et al*. 1998). If this is a true ranula, then ligation or inflammation of the salivary ducts will lead to atrophy of these salivary glands (Withrow and Holmberg 1983; Dernell *et al*. 1998). Ranula-like lesions usually resolve spontaneously, and treatment is rarely required.

Wound dehiscence is reported in 13% of cats and 8% to 33% of dogs after mandibulectomy (Withrow and Holmberg 1983; Bradley *et al*. 1984; Lantz and Salisbury 1987; Salisbury and Lantz 1988; Kosovsky *et al*. 1991; White 1991; Dernell *et al*. 1998; Northrup *et al*. 2006). The incidence of wound dehiscence in dogs depends on the mandibulectomy procedure and has been reported in 8% (5 of 65) and 19% (5 of 26) of dogs after total hemimandibulectomy, 17% (1 of 6) of dogs after segmental mandibulectomy, and 2% (1 of 41) and 8% (6 of 78) of dogs after rostral mandibulectomy (Kosovsky *et al*. 1991; Schwarz *et al*. 1991). In another report of 30 dogs treated with various mandibulectomy procedures, 75% (6 of 8) of dogs had dehiscence of their surgical wound over the rostral end of either a rostral or horizontal osteotomy (Salisbury and Lantz 1988). Tension is the most likely cause of dehiscence, although the use of cautery, rapidly absorbing suture material, or single-layer closures and poor wound healing capabilities as a result of radiation therapy, chemotherapy, or debilitation may also contribute to wound dehiscence (Withrow and Holmberg 1983; Bradley *et al*. 1984; Salisbury and Lantz 1988; Kosovsky *et al*. 1991; White 1991; Dernell *et al*. 1998; Northrup *et al*. 2006). Tapering the rostral end of the mandible before suturing has been recommended to reduce the risk of this complication (Lantz and Salisbury 1987). Closure of rostral dehiscences has been recommended for functional and cosmetic purposes (Kosovsky *et al*. 1991), but this is rarely necessary. Dehiscence of the commissure of the lip usually requires surgical revision to improve the cosmetic appearance and the use of tension-relieving sutures, such as a vertical mattress pattern (Dernell *et al*. 1998).

Excessive drooling is common, particularly after bilateral rostral mandibulectomy in cats and dogs and resection of more than 50% of the mandible in cats (Withrow and Holmberg 1983; Bradley *et al*. 1984; Salisbury and Lantz 1988; Kosovsky *et al*. 1991; White 1991; Hutson *et al*. 1992; Dernell *et al*. 1998; Northrup *et al*. 2006).

Ptyalism was reported in 50% of cats after bilateral rostral mandibulectomy, 37% of cats after hemimandibulectomy, and 83% of cats after resection of more than 50% of the mandible (Northrup *et al*. 2006). Ptyalism either resolves spontaneously or significantly reduces in volume after several weeks in the majority of dogs and cats. Persistent ptyalism was reported in 30% of cats after bilateral rostral mandibulectomy, 21% of cats after hemimandibulectomy, and 33% of cats after resection of more than 50% of the mandible (Northrup *et al*. 2006). For cats and dogs with persistent drooling, cheilitis and facial dermatitis are common sequelae.

Mandibular drift is common after segmental, subtotal, and total hemimandibulectomies because of loss of mandibular support at either the mandibular symphysis or TMJ. Despite its commonality, mandibular drift rarely causes clinical problems in dogs. Mandibular drift results in malocclusion. Drift of the mandibular canine tooth toward the midline can cause ulceration and trauma to the overlying hard palate. This is rarely a problem in dogs, reported in 2% (2 of 81) and 5% (3 of 65) of dogs (Kosovsky *et al*. 1991; Schwarz *et al*. 1991), but has been reported in up to 18% of cats, especially after segmental mandibulectomy (67%), hemimandibulectomy (16%), and resection of more than 50% of the mandible (33%) (Hutson *et al*. 1992; Northrup *et al*. 2006). Mandibular drift does not require treatment unless the drift results in complications. For animals with secondary hard palate trauma, the lower canine tooth should either be extracted or shortened with vital pulpotomy (Dernell *et al*. 1998).

Reconstruction of the mandible with either ulnar or rib autografts and promotion of osseous ingrowth with BMP-2 have been described to prevent or treat mandibular drift (Boudrieau *et al*. 1994; Bracker and Trout 2000; Boudrieau *et al*. 2004; Spector *et al*. 2007), but this is rarely required and is associated with increased expense and risk of complications.

Mandibular drift can be prevented in dogs with benign oral tumors by preserving the ventral mandibular cortex in a procedure called rim resection. Rim resection involves using a biradial oscillating saw of appropriate diameter to excise an oral tumor with a minimum of 10-mm margins around the tumor while preserving the ventral cortex of the mandible. Mandibular drift is prevented by minimizing soft tissue dissection and preserving the integrity of the hemimandible. Rim resection has been described in 11 dogs with good results (Reynolds *et al*. 2009; Arzi and Verstraete 2010).

The prevention of mandibular drift after segmental mandibulectomy or hemimandibulectomy was reported in 18 dogs using elastic training (Bar-Am and Verstraete 2010). This technique involves the placement of an orthodontic elastic rubber chain between an orthodontic button on the lingual aspect of the intact mandible canine tooth and buccal aspect of the maxillary fourth premolar tooth. The orthodontic elastic rubber chain was adjusted weekly to maintain occlusion and prevent mandibular drift. With the orthodontic elastic rubber chain in situ, all dogs maintained normal occlusion and jaw function. However, normal occlusion and TMJ stability was maintained in 50% (8 of 16) of dogs at up to 6 months after removal of the orthodontic elastic rubber chain, but mandibular drift recurred in the remaining 50% of dogs (Bar-Am and Verstraete 2010).

Eating difficulties are reported in 44% dogs and 72% cats after mandibulectomy (Withrow and Holmberg 1983; Bradley *et al*. 1984; Salisbury and Lantz 1988; Kosovsky *et al*. 1991; White 1991; Dernell *et al*. 1998; Northrup *et al*. 2006). In one study, voluntary eating returned by day 1 in 30%, day 2 in 70%, day 3 in 90%, and day 4 in 97% of dogs regardless of the mandibulectomy procedure

(Salisbury and Lantz 1988). In another study, all dogs were eating voluntarily within 3 days of their mandibulectomy procedure (White *et al.* 1985). Dogs tend to start eating later after total hemimandibulectomy (median, 2.5 days) compared with unilateral (median, 1 day) and bilateral (median, 2 days) rostral mandibulectomies (White *et al.* 1985; Salisbury and Lantz 1988). In another study, prehension difficulties were more common after bilateral rostral mandibulectomies with resection of both canine teeth, particularly the more aggressive bilateral procedures extending caudally to the second premolar teeth because of the loss of bone and soft tissue support of the tongue (Schwarz *et al.* 1991). The majority of dogs with prehension difficulties adapt within 2 weeks. Supplemental feeding may be required during this period, such as force feeding, tube feeding, or feeding soft foods made into a ball. If prehension difficulties continue beyond 2 weeks, then other causes should be investigated. Injury to the hypoglossal nerve and mandibular drift can also occasionally result in difficulties in prehending and eating food (Withrow and Holmberg 1983; Bradley *et al.* 1984; Salisbury and Lantz 1988; Kosovsky *et al.* 1991; White 1991; Dernell *et al.* 1998; Northrup *et al.* 2006).

In cats, eating difficulties are common regardless of the mandibulectomy procedure. In the short term (≤4 weeks), inappetence or dysphagia was reported in 84% (10 of 12) of cats after bilateral rostral mandibulectomy, 74% (14 of 19) of cats after hemimandibulectomy, 83% (5 of 6) of cats after resection of more than 50% of the mandible, and 73% of all cats (Northrup *et al.* 2006). Inappetence and dysphagia were also common in the long term with 10% (1 of 10) of cats with bilateral rostral mandibulectomy, 53% (9 of 19) of cats with hemimandibulectomy, 83% (5 of 6) of cats with resection of more than 50% of the mandible, and 42% of all cats experiencing eating difficulties (Northrup *et al.* 2006). Furthermore, 12% (5 of 42) of cats never regained the ability to eat voluntarily after mandibulectomy, with half of these cats treated with resection of more than 50% of the mandible (Northrup *et al.* 2006). A feeding tube should be inserted at the time of mandibulectomy in cats because of this high risk of inappetence and dysphagia. The feeding tube should be removed if and when the cat begins to eat voluntarily and consistently.

Grooming difficulties are a specific complication in cats and have been reported in 17% (2 of 12) of cats after bilateral rostral mandibulectomy, 26% (5 of 19) of cats after hemimandibulectomy, 17% (1 of 6) of cats after resection of more than 50% of the mandible, and in 20% of cats overall (Northrup *et al.* 2006). The cause of these grooming difficulties may be related to ptyalism, tongue protrusion, mandibular drift, and possibly pain. They are difficult to manage, and in these cases, owners must groom their cats. In one retrospective review of mandibulectomy in cats, grooming difficulties were infrequent (18%) but had a major impact on the perceived quality of life for affected cats (Northrup *et al.* 2006).

Tongue protrusion is relatively common in dogs after bilateral rostral mandibulectomies extending caudal to the second premolar teeth and total hemimandibulectomy, especially when a cheiloplasty is not performed. Protrusion of the tongue is also common in cats, but it occurs regardless of the mandibulectomy procedure. Tongue protrusion is reported in up to 33% of cats after bilateral rostral mandibulectomy, up to 42% of cats after hemimandibulectomy, up to 50% of cats after resection of more than 50% of the mandible, and up to 38% of cats overall (Hutson *et al.* 1992; Northrup *et al.* 2006). Prehensile function is rarely affected with tongue protrusion after total hemimandibulectomy, but it can take up to 2 weeks for dogs to adapt to loss of tongue support after

bilateral rostral mandibulectomies caudal to the second premolar teeth (Dernell *et al.* 1998).

The **cosmetic appearance** of cats and dogs after mandibulectomy is usually good to excellent. Owner acceptance of postoperative appearance and function is improved with a thorough discussion, including the use of pre- and postoperative images of the appropriate procedure before surgery. Owner satisfaction with the cosmetic appearance and functional outcome after mandibulectomy is high with 83% and 85% to 100% of owners satisfied after mandibulectomy in cats and dogs, respectively (Salisbury and Lantz 1988; Fox *et al.* 1997; Northrup *et al.* 2006).

The cosmetic appearance of dogs is not altered after unilateral rostral, segmental, and caudal mandibulectomy. However, ipsilateral temporal muscle atrophy was reported as a common sequela to nonrostral mandibulectomies in one study (White *et al.* 1985). Bilateral rostral mandibulectomy results in the most cosmetically challenging of the mandibulectomy procedures in both cats and dogs because of mandibular shortening; excessive drooling and cheilitis; and the tongue hanging out, especially when panting or excited (Salisbury and Lantz 1988). Subtotal and total hemimandibulectomy results in a mild concavity on the resected side, which is rarely appreciable; mandibular drift; and the tongue hanging out on the resected side (Withrow and Holmberg 1983; Bradley *et al.* 1984; Salisbury and Lantz 1988; Kosovsky *et al.* 1991; Schwarz *et al.* 1991; White 1991; Dernell *et al.* 1998; Northrup *et al.* 2006).

Infection is very rare after mandibulectomy because of the rich vascular supply to the oral cavity (Dernell *et al.* 1998). Infection has been reported in one dog in which bone screws were used to stabilize the mandibular rami (White *et al.* 1985).

Osteoarthritis of the TMJ has been investigated in 10 dogs after hemimandibulectomy and resultant mandibular drift. The TMJ was radiographically normal at 6 months, but joint asymmetry was noted in 3 dogs at 3 months and 4 dogs at 6 months. The TMJs were grossly normal at necropsy at 6 months, but there were degenerative changes in the articular cartilage and subchondral bone consistent with osteoarthritis in all joints (Umphlet *et al.* 1988). Although osteoarthritis of the TMJ may be a common histologic feature in dogs with mandibular drift, it rarely manifests as a clinical problem (Dernell *et al.* 1998). Crepitus of the TMJ was reported in 5% of cats after various mandibulectomy procedures, and, although unlikely, this may have contributed to the high incidence of inappetence and dysphagia in cats (Northrup *et al.* 2006). If degenerative joint disease of the TMJ causes pain on opening of the jaw or eating difficulties, then an NSAID and a chondroprotective agent should be administered.

References

Arzi, B., Verstraete, F.J. (2010) Mandibular rim excision in seven dogs. *Veterinary Surgery* 39, 226-231.

Bar-Am, Y., Verstraete, F.J.M. (2010) Elastic training for the prevention of mandibular drift following mandibulectomy in dogs: 18 cases (2005-2008). *Veterinary Surgery* 39, 574-580.

Boudrieau, R.J., Tidwell, A.S., Ullman, S.L., et al. (1994) Correction of mandibular nonunion and malocclusion by plate fixation and autogenous cortical bone grafts in two dogs. *Journal of the American Veterinary Medical Association* 204, 744-750.

Boudrieau, R.J., Mitchell, S.L., Seeherman, H. (2004) Mandibular reconstruction of a partial hemimandibulectomy in a dog with severe malocclusion. *Veterinary Surgery* 33, 119-130.

Bracker, K.E., Trout, N.J. (2000) Use of a free cortical ulnar autograft following en bloc resection of a mandibular tumor. *Journal of the American Animal Hospital Association* 36, 76-79.

Bradley, R.L., MacEwen, E.G., Loar, A.S. (1984) Mandibular resection for removal of oral tumors in 30 dogs and 6 cats. *Journal of the American Veterinary Medical Association* 184, 460-463.

Dernell, W.S., Schwarz, P.D., Withrow, S.J. (1998) Mandibulectomy. In Bojrab, M.J., Ellison, G.W., Slocum, B. (eds.) *Current Techniques in Small Animal Surgery.* Baltimore: Williams & Wilkins, pp. 132-142.

Fox, L.E., Geoghegan, S.L., Davis, L.H., et al. (1997) Owner satisfaction with partial mandibulectomy or maxillectomy for treatment of oral tumors in 27 dogs. *Journal of the American Animal Hospital Association* 33, 25-31.

Hutson, C.A., Willauer, C.C., Walder, E.J., et al. (1992) Treatment of mandibular squamous cell carcinoma in cats by use of mandibulectomy and radiotherapy: seven cases (1987-1989). *Journal of the American Veterinary Medical Association* 201, 777-781.

Kosovsky, J.K., Matthiesen, D.T., Marretta, S.M., et al. (1991) Results of partial mandibulectomy for the treatment of oral tumors in 142 dogs. *Veterinary Surgery* 20, 397-401.

Lantz, G.C., Salisbury, S.K. (1987) Partial mandibulectomy for treatment of mandibular fractures in dogs. Eight cases (1981-1984). *Journal of the American Veterinary Medical Association* 191, 243-245.

Northrup, N.C., Selting, K.A., Rassnick, K.M., et al. (2006) Outcomes of cats with oral tumors treated with mandibulectomy: 42 cases. *Journal of the American Animal Hospital Association* 42, 350-360.

Reynolds, D., Fransson, B., Preston, C (2009) Cresentic osteotomy for resection of oral tumours in four dogs. *Veterinary Comparative Orthopedics and Traumatology* 22, 412-416.

Schwarz, P.D., Withrow, S.J., Curtis, C.R., et al. (1991) Mandibular resection as a treatment for oral cancer in 81 dogs. *Journal of the American Animal Hospital Association* 27, 601-610.

Salisbury, S.K. (1991) Problems and complications associated with maxillectomy, mandibulectomy, and oronasal fistula repair. *Problems in Veterinary Medicine* 3, 153-169.

Salisbury, S.K., Lantz, G.C. (1988) Long-term results of partial mandibulectomy for treatment of oral tumors in 30 dogs. *Journal of the American Animal Hospital Association* 24, 285-294.

Spector, D.I., Keating, J.H., Boudrieau, R.J. (2007) Immediate mandibular reconstruction of a 5 cm defect using rhBMP-2 after partial mandibulectomy in a dog. *Veterinary Surgery* 36, 752-759.

Umphlet, R.C., Johnson, A.L., Eurell, J.C., et al. (1988) The effect of partial rostral hemimandibulectomy on mandibular mobility and temporomandibular joint morphology in the dog. *Veterinary Surgery* 17, 186-193.

White, R.A.S. (1991) Mandibulectomy and maxillectomy in the dog: Long-term survival in 100 cases. *Journal of Small Animal Practice* 32, 69-74.

White, R.A.S., Gorman, N.T., Watkins, S.B., et al. (1985) The surgical management of bone-involved oral tumours in the dog. *Journal of Small Animal Practice* 26, 693-708.

Withrow, S.J., Holmberg, D.L. (1983) Mandibulectomy in the treatment of oral cancer. *Journal of the American Animal Hospital Association* 19, 273-286.

32 Partial Maxillectomy

Julius Liptak
Alta Vista Animal Hospital, Ottawa, Ontario, Canada

Maxillectomy procedures are most commonly performed for the treatment of benign and malignant oral tumors. Maxillectomy procedures include unilateral and bilateral rostral maxillectomy, radical bilateral rostral maxillectomy, hemimaxillectomy, and caudal maxillectomy.

The complication rate after all types of maxillectomy procedures is less than 33% in dogs (Salisbury *et al.* 1986; Schwarz *et al.* 1991; Wallace *et al.* 1992; Kirpensteijn *et al.* 1994; Lascelles *et al.* 2003, 2004) but has not been reported in cats. Cats likely have a similar risk of complications as dogs. Local tumor recurrence and distant metastasis will not be considered as complications of maxillectomy for the purposes of this chapter; however, it should be noted that complete histologic excision of malignant oral tumors is important to decrease local tumor recurrence rates and improve survival times.

Intraoperative hemorrhage

Definition
Intraoperative hemorrhage is defined as blood loss, usually from either the maxillary or major palatine arteries, resulting in poor visualization of the surgical field, hypotension, and anemia.

Risk factors
- Maxillectomy procedures involving the caudal maxilla and inferior orbit

Diagnosis
- Intraoperative observation of brisk or profuse bleeding

Treatment
- Ligation of the maxillary and major palatine arteries
- A cross-matched compatible blood transfusion should be considered if hematocrit acutely decreases below 15% to 30%, particularly if this occurs in combination with hypotension (mean blood pressure <80 mm Hg or systolic blood pressure <100 mg); hypoxia; or clinical, biochemical, or echocardiographic evidence of anaerobic metabolism.

Outcome
Blood loss from the maxillary and major palatine arteries is rarely life threatening, and the outcome is usually not affected by blood loss if treated appropriately.

Prevention
- Ligation of the maxillary artery before transection as it courses over the ventral aspect of the inferior orbit
- Temporary occlusion of the carotid arteries may be effective in reducing bleeding from the major palatine artery, but it should only be performed in dogs because carotid artery occlusion can be fatal in cats.

Incisional swelling

Definition
Incisional swelling is swelling of a surgical incision (Figure 32.1).

Risk factors
- Caudal maxillectomy through the combined intraoral–dorsolateral approach
- Radical bilateral rostral maxillectomy

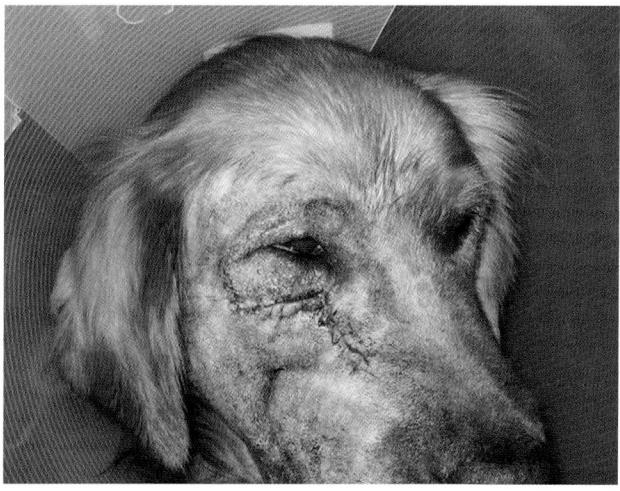

Figure 32.1 Incisional swelling after a caudal maxillectomy via a combined intraoral–dorsolateral approach for resection of a histologically low-grade and biologically high-grade fibrosarcoma. *Source:* Dr. L. Selmic, Colorado State University, Fort Williams, CO. Reproduced with permission of Dr. L. Selmic.

Complications in Small Animal Surgery, First Edition. Edited by Dominique Griffon and Annick Hamaide.
© 2016 John Wiley & Sons, Inc. Published 2016 by John Wiley & Sons, Inc.
Companion website: www.wiley.com/go/griffon/complications

Diagnosis

A cosmetic defect characterized by swelling at and adjacent to the incision site is usually the only clinical sign associated with incisional swelling. The incision may be painful on palpation.

Treatment

Ice packing every 4 hours and the administration of nonsteroidal antiinflammatory drugs (NSAIDs) may assist in decreasing the severity of postoperative swelling.

Outcome

Swelling resolves spontaneously in 5 to 7 days.

Prevention

• Gentle intraoperative tissue handling and prophylactic ice packing and administration of NSAIDs

Wound dehiscence and oronasal fistula

Definition

Wound dehiscence is breakdown of a surgical wound with separation of the wound edges. Wound dehiscence after maxillectomy often results in an oronasal fistula, which is defined as a communication between the oral and nasal cavities (Figure 32.2).

Risk factors

• Wound tension, especially tumors that cross the midline of the hard palate
• Movement and tension of the submucosal–mucosal labial flap with swallowing and tongue movement, especially after rostral maxillectomies
• Closure of surgical wounds with a single layer of suture material
• Self-induced trauma, especially from the tongue
• Chewing of hard foods, sticks, and so on
• Use of cautery to incise the oral mucosa
• Suturing the mucosa adjacent to a tooth on the occlusal margin of the ostectomy

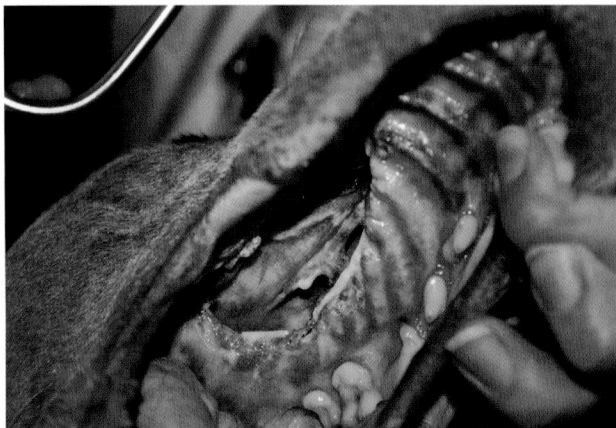

Figure 32.2 Wound dehiscence and with resultant oronasal fistula after maxillectomy of an irradiated oral tumor. Although there are many potential causes of wound dehiscence, pre- or postoperative radiation therapy is a common cause of poor wound healing and wound dehiscence. The management of these cases can be difficult because the most common flaps used to reconstruct these defects have also often been irradiated. *Source:* N. Bacon, University of Florida, Gainesville, FL. Reproduced with permission from N. Bacon.

• Use of rapidly absorbable suture material (i.e., catgut or poliglecaprone 25)
• Ischemic necrosis of the mucosal–submucosal labial flap
• Poor wound healing because of radiation therapy, chemotherapy, or debilitation
• Local tumor recurrence

Diagnosis

Wound dehiscence typically occurs 3 to 7 days after surgery. If there is no communication with the nasal cavity or the oronasal fistula is small, then wound dehiscence may not be associated with any clinical signs. However, if the oronasal fistula is large, then clinical signs can include unilateral nasal discharge and coughing and respiratory signs with secondary aspiration pneumonia.

Treatment

• The full extent of dehiscence should be assessed.
• A biopsy of the dehisced wound is recommended to evaluate for local tumor recurrence.
• If dehiscence is associated with the mucosa being sutured adjacent to a tooth on the occlusal margin of the ostectomy, it should be treated by extracting the tooth, elevating the palatal and labial gingiva, and suturing the mucosal flaps over the alveolar bone.
• Dehiscence without an oronasal fistula can be managed with either second intention healing if small or debridement and resuturing if large.
• If dehiscence is associated with an oronasal fistula, then surgical debridement and reconstruction of the defect should be performed. A number of surgical techniques have been described for the management of oronasal fistulae such as the mucoperiosteal flap and bilateral overlapping mucosal flaps. However, these may not be possible after maxillectomy because much of the available buccal mucosal or mucoperiosteal tissue typically used for these reconstructions has either been excised or used for reconstruction of the original maxillectomy defect. In these cases, angularis oris axial pattern buccal flaps, advancement of skin flaps into the oral cavity, or free microvascular grafts of the rectus abdominus muscle may be useful.

Outcome

• Conservative or surgical management of dehisced wounds without oronasal fistula usually results in an uncomplicated recovery with no functional consequences or cosmetic defects.
• Surgical management of wound dehiscence with oronasal fistula can be complicated by the lack of available tissue; however, healing is usually uncomplicated in a nonirradiated field. Recurrent dehiscence and poor wound healing are common after radiation therapy, even with advancement of healthy nonirradiated tissue into the defect.

Prevention

The risk of wound dehiscence can be minimized by tension-free closure of the suture line. This can be achieved with a two-layer closure, preferably using bone tunnels for the first layer; sufficient undermining of the labial mucosal–submucosal flap; use of long-lasting absorbable suture material (i.e., polydioxanone); and minimizing the use of cautery for hemostasis purposes. Chewing on hard foods and materials should be avoided until the surgical wound has healed, typically 2 to 3 weeks. If the tongue is the cause of tension and dehiscence, then tube feeding may be required for 1 to 2 weeks.

Ulcer formation secondary to trauma by teeth

Definition
This is ulcer formation on the upper lip caused by trauma by the teeth, usually the mandibular canine tooth. The lip is drawn medially into the occlusal plane of the teeth after rostral maxillectomy procedures (Figure 32.3).

Risk factors
- Unilateral (± bilateral) rostral maxillectomy
- Loss of sensation to the upper lip after transection of the infraorbital nerve

Diagnosis
- Ulcer formation on the mucosal or cutaneous surface of the upper lip adjacent to teeth from the ipsilateral mandible

Treatment
The tooth causing ulceration of the upper lip can either be extracted or shortened with vital pulpotomy (Figure 32.4).

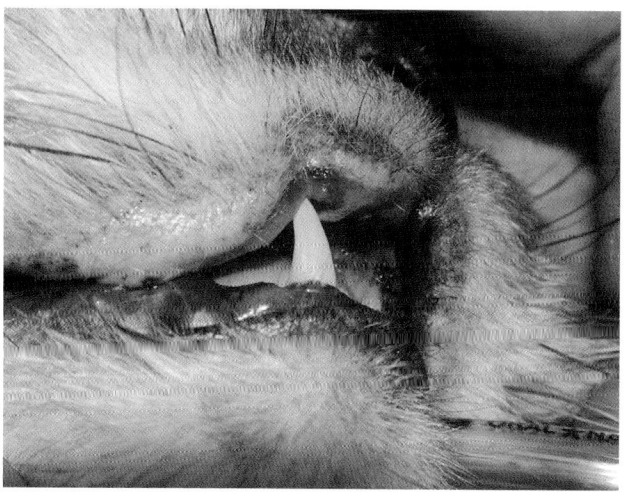

Figure 32.3 Ulcer formation on the upper lip after unilateral rostral maxillectomy in a cat for resection of an odontoma.

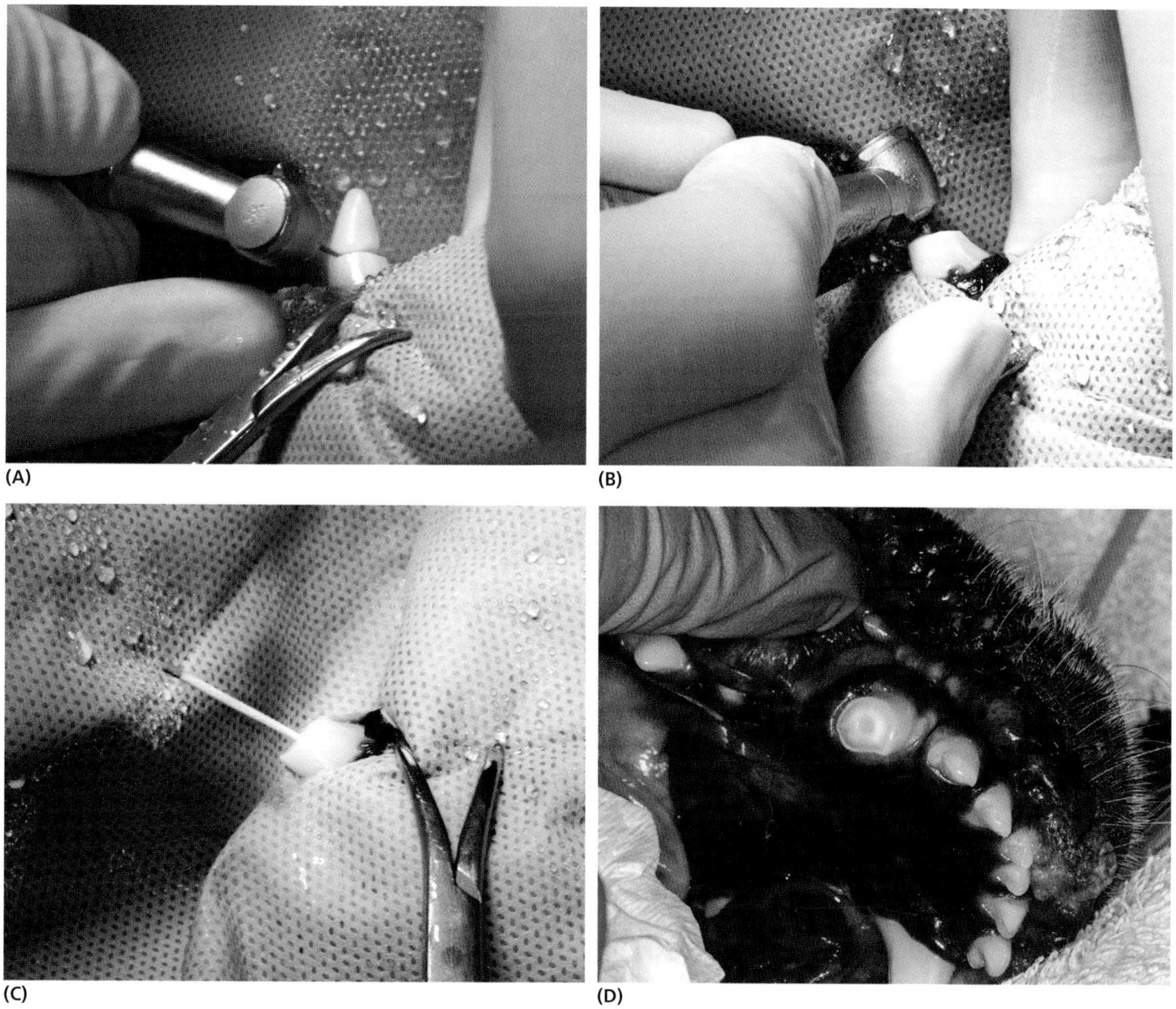

(A)

(B)

(C)

(D)

Figure 32.4 A vital pulpotomy is being performed in a dog to prevent further lip ulceration after a hemimaxillectomy for treatment of a histologically low-grade and biologically high-grade fibrosarcoma. **A**, The coronal portion of the mandibular canine tooth is being removed with a high-speed burr; **B**, The pulp tissue is removed with a high-speed burr; **C**, Bleeding is controlled with sterile paper points in the canal; **D**, After inserting calcium hydroxide into the canal, the coronal surface is covered with an intermediate layer and restorative. *Source:* Dr. R. Cavanaugh, VCA Alameda East Veterinary Hospital, Fort Myers, FL. Reproduced with permission from Dr. R. Cavanagh.

Outcome
Ulceration resolves after appropriate treatment.

Prevention
Ulceration of the lip is difficult to prevent, but sufficient undermining of the labial mucosal–submucosal flap and preservation of the infraorbital nerve (and hence lateral facial sensation) may decrease the incidence of lip ulceration.

Eating difficulties
Eating difficulties are uncommon after the majority of maxillectomy procedures in cats and dogs. Dogs treated with radical maxillectomy may have difficulty eating dry food and may also require initial assistance in feeding. This includes manual feeding or feeding from an inclined bowl. However, the majority of dogs adapt to unassisted eating within 2 to 3 weeks.

Supplemental feeding may be required for up to 1 week in cats after bilateral rostral maxillectomy, with or without nasal planum resection, or radical maxillectomy.

Definition
Eating difficulties are defined as difficulty prehending food, dysphagia, or inappetence.

Risk factors
• Radical bilateral rostral maxillectomy

Diagnosis
Eating difficulties are best diagnosed through observation in the hospital and by the owners.

Treatment
Treatment consists of assisted feeding, either by hand or feeding from an inclined or flexible dish (Figure 32.5), until the resumption of unassisted feeding.

Outcome
Dogs and cats can eat unassisted within 2 to 3 weeks.

Prevention
Preventive factors are not known.

Cosmetic appearance

Definition
The cosmetic appearance of cats and dogs after various maxillectomy procedures is usually good to excellent. Poor cosmesis is defined as dissimilar pre- and postoperative cosmetic appearances.

Risk factors
• Unilateral rostral maxillectomy
• Bilateral rostral maxillectomy
• Bilateral rostral maxillectomy combined with nasal planum resection
• Radical bilateral rostral maxillectomy

Diagnosis
Poor cosmetic results are best diagnosed through observation in hospital and by the owners.
• Unilateral rostral maxillectomy: medialization of the upper lip with possible exposure of the ipsilateral mandibular canine tooth lateral to the upper lip (Figure 32.6)
• Bilateral rostral maxillectomy: drooping of the rostral nose because of loss of bony support (Figure 32.7)
• Bilateral rostral maxillectomy combined with nasal planum resection: mild to moderate prognathism (Figure 32.8)
• Radical bilateral rostral maxillectomy: marked prognathism (Figure 32.9)

Treatment
• Cantilever suture technique to lift the muzzle after bilateral rostral maxillectomy

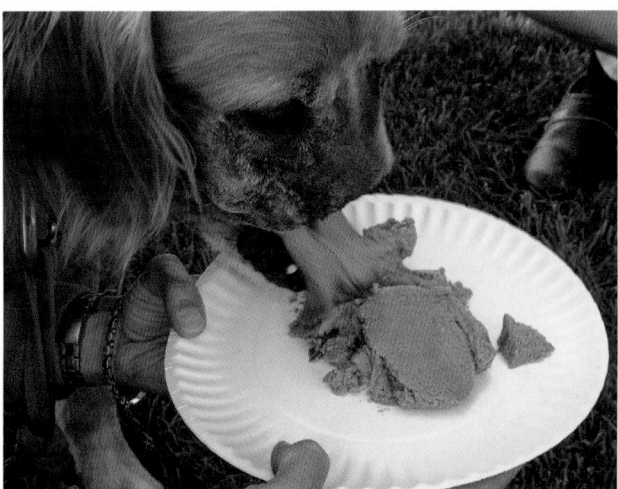

Figure 32.5 A dog 1 day after radical bilateral rostral maxillectomy for resection of a histologically low-grade and biologically high-grade fibrosarcoma. This is the only maxillectomy procedure that may result in eating difficulties. Assisted feeding, either manually or using an inclined bowl or flexible dish (pictured), may be required for up to 2 to 3 weeks until the resumption of voluntary eating.

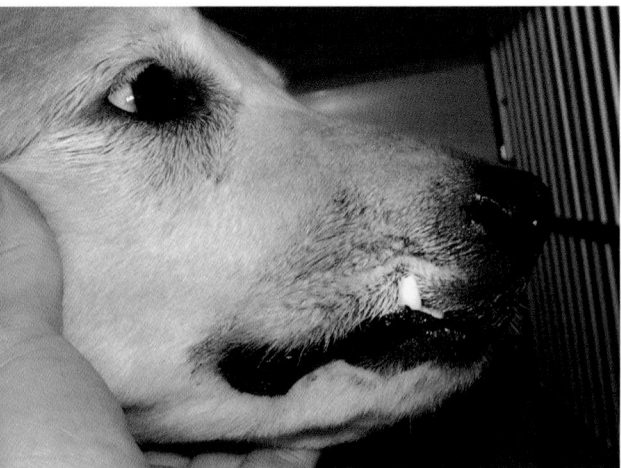

Figure 32.6 Medialization of the upper lip with exposure of the ipsilateral mandibular canine tooth lateral to the upper lip after unilateral rostral maxillectomy for resection of a fibrosarcoma. This can result in ulceration of the upper lip. There is no treatment for this defect. Vital pulpotomy (see Figure 32.4) or tooth extraction may be required if the tooth causes ulceration of the upper lip.

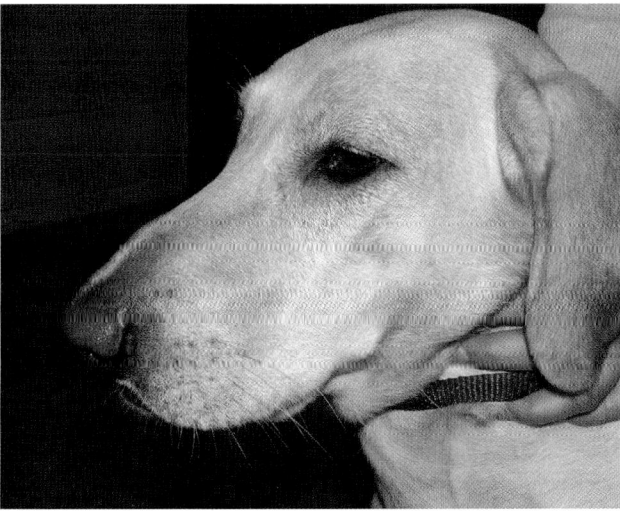

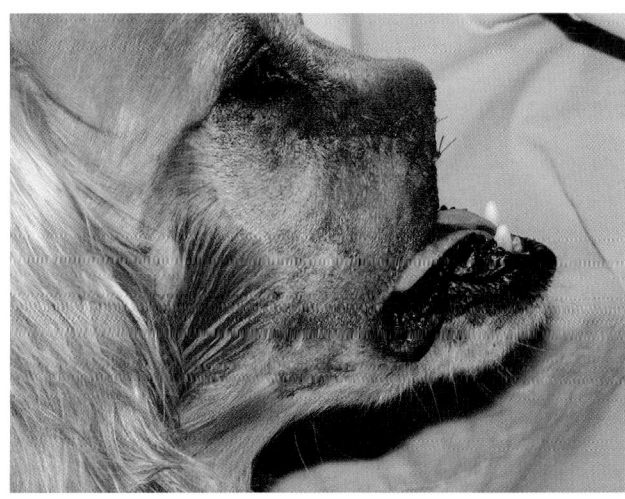

Figure 32.9 Radical bilateral rostral maxillectomy is the most cosmetically challenging of the maxillectomy procedures. Despite the cosmetic appearance, dogs and cats eat well, function normally, and have excellent tumor control.

Figure 32.7 Drooping of the nose after bilateral rostral maxillectomy for resection of an acanthomatous ameloblastoma. This cosmetic defect does not cause any functional problems. A cantilever suture technique can be used to prevent or correct this defect.

- No treatment for unilateral rostral maxillectomy and radical bilateral rostral maxillectomy

Outcome

- Cosmetic appearance is an aesthetic consideration for owners, but the vast majority of owners are satisfied with the cosmetic appearance after rostral maxillectomy procedures. Acceptance of cosmetic appearance is improved when owners are specifically informed and educated about what appearance to expect after

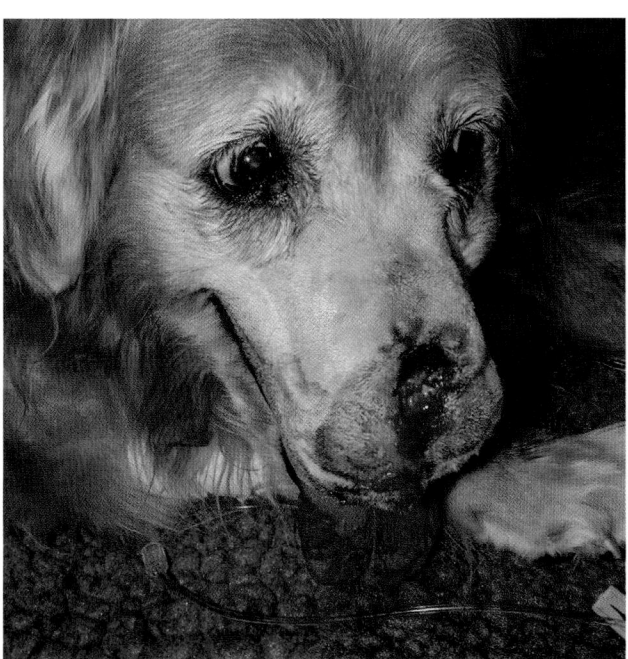

Figure 32.8 Bilateral rostral maxillectomy combined with resection of the nasal planum for treatment of a dog with squamous cell carcinoma of the nasal planum. This technique results in mild prognathism but no functional problems.

surgery. Despite poor cosmesis for some procedures, especially radical bilateral rostral maxillectomy, it is important to note that the patient's behavior is not altered, and function remains good to excellent.

- The most significant functional effects after radical bilateral rostral maxillectomy include difficulty or inability in retrieving or picking up items, difficulty in eating dry food, and messy eating and drinking. Functional sequelae to other maxillectomy procedures in cats and dogs are rare.
- Ulceration of the upper lip secondary to trauma from the ipsilateral mandibular teeth can occur after unilateral rostral maxillectomy.

Prevention

Although the cosmetic appearance often cannot be altered, especially with radical bilateral rostral maxillectomy, owner acceptance of postoperative appearance and function is improved with a thorough discussion, including the use of pre- and postoperative images of the appropriate procedure, before surgery.

Relevant literature

The majority of maxillectomy complications in both cats and dogs are relatively minor and can be treated either conservatively or with minor surgical revisions. The incidence of complications with various maxillectomy procedures has not been compared. However, some complications are more commonly associated with particular maxillectomy procedures, such as intraoperative blood loss with caudal maxillectomies (Lascelles *et al.* 2003), incisional swelling with radical bilateral rostral maxillectomy and caudal maxillectomy via a combined intraoral–dorsolateral approach (Lascelles *et al.* 2003, 2004), eating difficulties with radical bilateral rostral maxillectomy (Lascelles *et al.* 2004), and cosmetic appearance with rostral maxillectomy procedures (Lascelles *et al.* 2004).

   Intraoperative blood loss is more common during caudal maxillectomy procedures, either through an intraoral or combined intraoral–dorsolateral approach, because of transection of the maxillary artery as it courses over the ventral aspect of the inferior orbit. Ligation of the maxillary artery before transection is preferred, but exposure is limited, and hence identification and ligation of the maxillary artery is not always possible. For this reason, the caudal osteotomy is performed last so that the maxillary bone segment can be quickly removed from the surgical field to allow rapid identification and ligation of the maxillary artery (Lascelles et al. 2003). Blood loss from the major palatine artery can also be brisk but is usually easier to control.

Hemorrhage from either the maxillary or major palatine artery can be severe enough to warrant a whole-blood transfusion. In one study, one dog died because of intraoperative blood loss and hypovolemic shock, and a further 9% of dogs (6 of 69) had blood loss that did not require a blood transfusion (Wallace et al. 1992). Significant blood loss requiring transfusion was reported in 12% dogs (2 of 17) and 0% cats (0 of 3) (Salisbury et al. 1986) in another study. These studies did not detail which procedures were more commonly associated with blood loss. However, Lascelles et al. (2003) documented significant blood loss in 75% (15 of 20) dogs treated with a caudal maxillectomy via a combined intraoral–dorsolateral approach with a mean decrease in packed cell volume of 15.4%. Thirty percent (6 of 20) of these dogs required a whole-blood transfusion. Trauma to the maxillary artery and its infraorbital branch during the caudal osteotomy were considered the most likely cause for intraoperative hemorrhage (Lascelles et al. 2003).

Ligation of the maxillary or major palatine arteries does not affect healing of the labial mucosal–submucosal flap. The labial mucosal blood supply is derived from the lateral nasal artery, a branch of the maxillary artery, and the angular artery of the mouth and superior labial artery, branches of the facial artery. Adequate circulation is maintained to the labial mucosa after ligation of the maxillary artery via the branches of the facial artery and contralateral maxillary artery (Salisbury et al. 1986; Dernell et al. 1998).

Temporary occlusion of the carotid arteries may be effective in reducing bleeding from the maxillary and major palatine arteries, particularly when a blood transfusion is not available, but this should only be performed in dogs as carotid artery occlusion can be fatal in cats (Holmes and Wolstencroft 1959; Gillian 1976; Hedlund et al. 1983; Holmberg 1996; Holmberg and Pettifer 1997).

Swelling of the surgical site is common after caudal maxillectomy, particularly via the combined intraoral–dorsolateral approach, and radical maxillectomy (Salisbury et al. 1986; Lascelles et al. 2003, 2004). Swelling usually resolves spontaneously within 3 weeks. Ice packing every 4 hours and the administration of NSAIDs may assist in decreasing the severity of postoperative swelling.

Wound dehiscence is the most common complication after maxillectomy (White et al. 1985; Withrow et al. 1985; Harvey 1986; Salisbury et al. 1986; Schwarz et al. 1991; White 1991; Wallace et al. 1992; Fox et al. 1997; Dernell et al. 1998; Lascelles et al. 2003). The incidence of partial wound dehiscence after various maxillectomy procedures has been reported in 7% (5 of 69) of dogs (Wallace et al. 1992), 15% (3 of 20) of cats and dogs (Salisbury et al. 1986), and 33% (21 of 60) of dogs (Schwarz et al. 1991). A 5% (1 of 20) dehiscence rate was reported in a case series of caudal maxillectomy via a combined intraoral–dorsolateral approach (Lascelles et al. 2003). For rostral maxillectomies, partial dehiscence was reported in 29% (2 of 7) dogs after radical bilateral rostral maxillectomy (Lascelles et al. 2004) and 67% (2 of 3) dogs after combined bilateral rostral maxillectomy and nasal planum resection (Kirpensteijn et al. 1994). The cause was not always identified in these studies, but local tumor recurrence was noted in 33% (1 of 3) of dogs with partial dehiscence in one study (Salisbury et al. 1986) and 55% (11 of 20) of dogs in another study (Schwarz et al. 1991). Schwarz et al. (1991) also investigated adjunctive therapies and found that 55% (11 of 20) of dogs with dehiscence were also treated with either pre- or postoperative radiation therapy, and 100% (3 of 3) of dogs treated with both radiation therapy and chemotherapy developed partial wound dehiscence. For dogs treated with rostral maxillectomies, surgical debridement and resuturing were effective in all cases (Kirpensteijn et al. 1994; Lascelles et al. 2004). Although success rates were not reported, 30% (6 of 20) of dogs with dehiscence in one study were treated conservatively with second intention healing, and the remaining 70% (14 of 20) of dogs were treated with debridement and resuturing (Schwarz et al. 1991). In another study, all dogs (3 of 3) with dehiscence were treated successfully with debridement and resuturing (Salisbury et al. 1986).

Ulcer formation caused by trauma from the ipsilateral mandibular teeth, particularly the canine tooth, is a potential complication after unilateral rostral maxillectomies and hemimaxillectomies (White et al. 1985; Withrow et al. 1985; Harvey 1986; Salisbury et al. 1986; White 1991; Fox et al. 1997; Dernell et al. 1998; Lascelles et al. 2003). In one study of dogs treated with caudal maxillectomy via an intraoral–dorsolateral approach, lip ulceration because of interference from the ipsilateral mandibular canine tooth was reported in 10% (2 of 20) dogs (Lascelles et al. 2003). However, lip ulceration was not reported in two large studies totaling 130 dogs (Schwarz et al. 1991; Wallace et al. 1992).

The ulcerated region is usually caused by the ipsilateral mandibular canine tooth and results from the lip being drawn medially into the occlusal plane of the teeth. Ulcer formation is potentiated by the loss of sensation to the upper lip after severance of the infraorbital nerve. After the source of the ulceration has been identified, the tooth or teeth are removed or capped. In one study, however, the mandibular teeth caused mild ulceration of the mucosal–submucosal labial flap, but this did not cause a clinical problem and resolved without treatment within 2 to 3 weeks (Salisbury et al. 1986).

Eating difficulties are uncommon after the majority of maxillectomy procedures in cats and dogs, with all animals eating within 1 to 3 days (White et al. 1985; Withrow et al. 1985; Salisbury et al. 1986; Schwarz et al. 1991 White 1991; Wallace et al. 1992; Fox et al. 1997; Dernell et al. 1998; Lascelles et al. 2003). Eating difficulties were more common after radical bilateral rostral maxillectomy in one cat and six dogs (Lascelles et al. 2004). Inappetence was reported in one dog, and this dog required supplemental feeding via a pharyngostomy tube for 6 days. Although not inappetent, two dogs required hand feeding for 3 weeks before resuming normal eating. One of these dogs required lip revision because the rostral lips interfered with eating. Eating was considered normal at follow-up examinations ranging from 11 to 66 months in one cat and five dogs. One dog would not eat dry food; otherwise, all other animals would eat both canned and dry food without difficulty. However, eating and drinking were messy. An angled or flexible bowl aided eating in some dogs (Lascelles et al. 2004).

The **cosmetic appearance** of cats and dogs after various maxillectomy procedures is usually good to excellent. The major exceptions are bilateral rostral maxillectomy combined with nasal planum resection and radical bilateral radical maxillectomy. Owner acceptance of postoperative appearance and function is improved with a thorough discussion, including the use of pre- and postoperative images of the appropriate procedure, before surgery. Owner satisfaction with the cosmetic appearance and functional outcome after maxillectomy is high with 85% of dog owners satisfied after partial maxillectomy (Fox *et al.* 1997), 100% of owners (20 of 20) after caudal maxillectomy via a combined intraoral–dorsolateral approach (Lascelles *et al.* 2003), and 100% of owners (7 of 7) after radical bilateral rostral maxillectomy (Lascelles *et al.* 2004.).

Postoperative swelling can be significant, particularly if venous drainage has been compromised during tumor excision, but this usually subsides within 3 weeks, resulting in an improved cosmetic appearance. The lateral aspect of the lip overlying the maxillectomy site often moves with respiration for the first 24 to 48 hours postoperatively (Salisbury *et al.* 1986; Lascelles *et al.* 2003).

After unilateral rostral and caudal maxillectomies, the skin and lip are often drawn medially toward the midline, and the extent of this will depend on the medial extent of the resection and the degree of undermining of the mucosal–submucosal labial flap, resulting in a dished in appearance (Salisbury *et al.* 1986; Fox *et al.* 1997; Dernell *et al.* 1998). Depending on the extent of this medialization of the lip, the ipsilateral mandibular canine tooth may protrude lateral to the upper lip after maxillectomy procedures involving the rostral maxilla (Salisbury *et al.* 1986).

The most common cosmetic defect after bilateral rostral maxillectomy is drooping of the nose because of loss of ventral support (White *et al.* 1985; Withrow *et al.* 1985; Salisbury *et al.* 1986; Schwarz *et al.* 1991; White 1991; Wallace *et al.* 1992; Lascelles *et al.* 2003). Pavletic (1999) described the cantilever suture technique to correct drooping of the nose after bilateral rostral maxillectomy. Another common cosmetic defect is protrusion of the mandibular canine teeth rostral to the resected maxilla after bilateral rostral maxillectomy combined with nasal planum resection and radical bilateral rostral maxillectomy (Kirpensteijn *et al.* 1994; Dernell *et al.* 1998; Lascelles *et al.* 2004).

The cosmetic appearance of dogs after radical bilateral rostral maxillectomy is the most challenging of all maxillofacial resections (Lascelles *et al.* 2004). Owners should be thoroughly counseled before surgery of the expected appearance of their dog, and the use of postoperative images of dogs treated with radical bilateral rostral maxillectomy can facilitates this discussion. Despite the change in cosmetic appearance, it is important to note that their behavior is not altered, and their function remains good to excellent. The most significant functional effects include difficulty or inability in retrieving or picking up items, difficulty in eating dry food, and messy eating and drinking.

Other complications reported after maxillectomy include pain, infection, subcutaneous emphysema, epistaxis, nasal discharge, epiphora, and nasal stenosis.

Pain has specifically been mentioned as being minimal and well controlled with standard analgesic drugs in earlier reports of maxillectomies in cats and dogs (Salisbury *et al.* 1986; Wallace *et al.* 1992). Lascelles *et al.* (2004) noted pain or irritation for 3 to 4 weeks after surgery in 29% (2 of 7) of animals treated with radical bilateral rostral maxillectomy, and all responded well to multimodal analgesic protocols. Pawing and rubbing the mouth have also been described, but this could also result from irritation caused by the suture ears on adjacent mucosa (Dernell *et al.* 1998).

Infection is very rare after maxillectomy because of the rich vascular supply to the oral cavity (Dernell *et al.* 1998). Infection was reported in 2% (1 of 61) dogs in one study (Schwarz *et al.* 1991) but has not been reported in any other study of maxillectomy in cats and dogs.

The lateral aspect of the lip overlying the maxillectomy site often moves with respiration for the first 24 to 48 hours postoperatively (Salisbury *et al.* 1986; Lascelles *et al.* 2003). However, **subcutaneous**

emphysema is rare despite exposure of the surgical site to the nasal cavity (Dernell *et al.* 1998). If present, the subcutaneous emphysema is usually mild and nonprogressive and resolves spontaneously within 7 days.

Dyspnea can occur secondary to subcutaneous emphysema, but this has been reported in numerous series of maxillectomies in cats and dogs. In one study of 17 dogs and three cats treated with various maxillectomy procedures, one dog developed dyspnea and cyanosis after bilateral premaxillectomy because of occlusion of the nasal passages with blood clots and reluctance to acutely mouth breathe (Salisbury *et al.* 1986). This dog responded well to sedation. Based on this case, animals should be observed for hypoxia after bilateral maxillectomy procedures because nasal packing causes arterial hypoxia and hypercarbia in conscious normal dogs (Cavo *et al.* 1975).

Ipsilateral **epistaxis** is common after caudal maxillectomy (Figure 32.10) and hemimaxillectomy but typically resolves within 1 to 3 days.

A mild but persistent **nasal discharge** can be observed after maxillectomy procedures in which the nasal turbinates have been exposed (White *et al.* 1985; Withrow *et al.* 1985; Harvey 1986; Salisbury *et al.* 1986; Schwarz *et al.* 1991; White 1991; Wallace *et al.* 1992; Fox *et al.* 1997; Dernell *et al.* 1998; Lascelles *et al.* 2003). This is usually rare for most maxillectomy procedures but is very common after radical bilateral rostral maxillectomy (Lascelles *et al.* 2004). This discharge is usually clear but can occasionally be mucoid to mucopurulent. This did not cause a concern to any animal and did not result in moisture dermatitis (Lascelles *et al.* 2004). Treatment is rarely required, but culture-directed antibiotics may be necessary if an infected rhinitis is suspected.

Epiphora can occur secondary to nasolacrimal duct damage during caudal maxillectomies (Salisbury *et al.* 1986; Lascelles *et al.* 2003) (Figure 32.11). This was not considered significant by the author or owners in one study of 20 dogs treated with caudal maxillectomy via a combined intraoral–dorsolateral approach (Lascelles *et al.* 2003). However, Salisbury *et al.* (1991) recommended stenting the nasolacrimal duct if damaged for 1 month to allow epithelialization of a new duct.

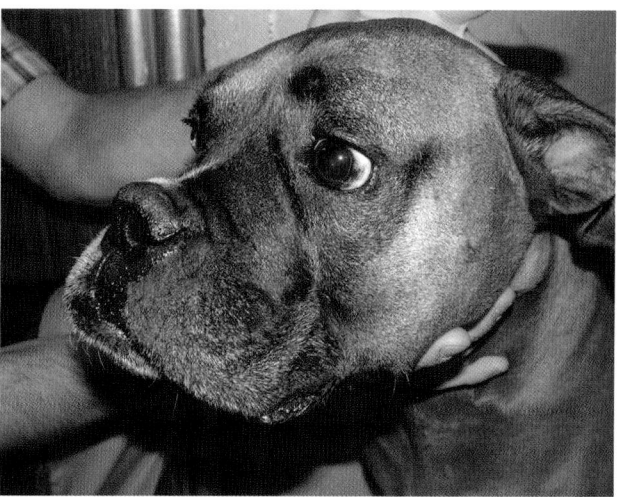

Figure 32.10 Epistaxis after intraoral caudal maxillectomy for resection of a fibrosarcoma. The epistaxis is usually mild and resolves spontaneously within 1 to 3 days.

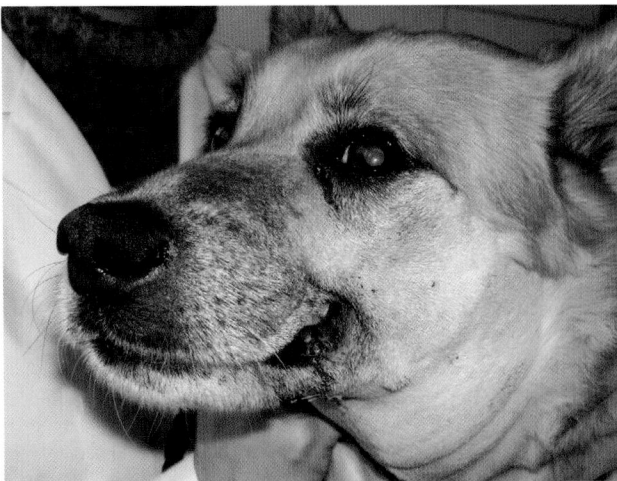

Figure 32.11 Mild epiphora in a dog after maxillectomy for the treatment of an oral tumor. Epiphora typically occurs secondary to damage to the nasolacrimal duct during caudal maxillectomies. *Source:* Dr. B. van Goethem, Ghent University, Gent, Belgium.

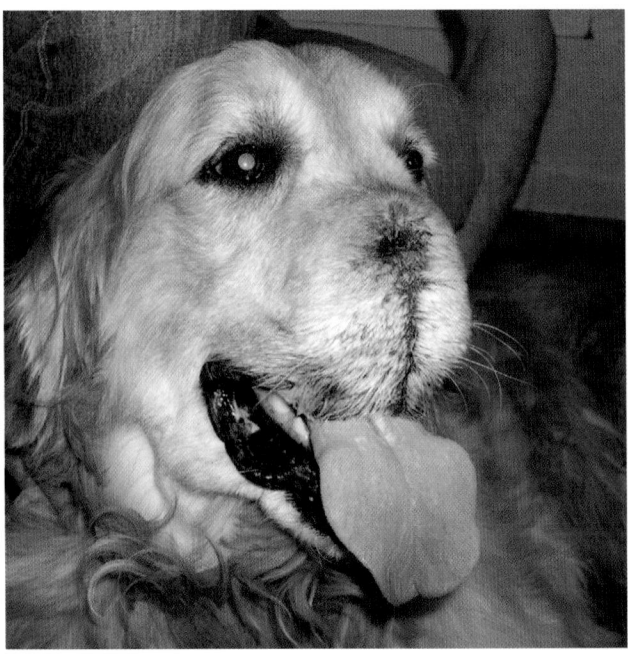

Figure 32.12 Stenosis of the nasal aperture after purse-string closure after combined bilateral rostral maxillectomy and nasal planum resection for treatment of a nasal planum squamous cell carcinoma. Attempts at correcting nasal stenosis are often unsuccessful, but dogs seem to adapt well with no respiratory difficulties. Simple interrupted closure is preferred to purse-string closure to minimize the risk of nasal stenosis. *Source:* A. Hamaide, University of Liège, Liège, Belgium, 2014. Reproduced with permission from A. Hamaide.

Stenosis of the nasal apertures has been described in 14% (1 of 7) of animals after radical bilateral rostral maxillectomy and 33% (1 of 3) of dogs after bilateral rostral maxillectomy combined with nasal planum resection (Kirpensteijn *et al.* 1994) (Figure 32.12). In both cases, attempts at surgical reconstruction failed, and stenosis recurred. However, both dogs were able to breathe without difficulty, and hence further reconstruction or stenting was not attempted or deemed necessary. The risk of nasal stenosis can be minimized by closing the wound in a simple interrupted suture pattern rather than a purse-string suture pattern.

References

Cavo, J.W., Kawamoto, S., Berlin, B.P., et al. (1975) Arterial blood gas changes following nasal packing in dogs. *Laryngoscope* 85, 2055-2068.

Dernell, W.S., Schwarz, P.D., Withrow, S.J. (1998) Maxillectomy and premaxillectomy. In Bojrab, M.J., Ellison, G.W., Slocum, B. (eds.) *Current Techniques in Small Animal Surgery*. Williams & Wilkins, Baltimore, pp. 124-132.

Fox, L.E., Geoghegan, S.L., Davis, L.H., et al. (1997) Owner satisfaction with partial mandibulectomy or maxillectomy for treatment of oral tumors in 27 dogs. *Journal of the American Animal Hospital Association* 33, 25-31.

Gillian, L.A. (1976) Extra- and intra-cranial blood supply to brains of dog and cat. *American Journal of Anatomy* 146, 237-253.

Harvey, C.E. (1986) Oral surgery: radical resection of maxillary and mandibular lesions. *Veterinary Clinics of North America: Small Animal Practice* 16, 983-993.

Hedlund, C.S., Tangner, C.H., Elkins, H.D., et al. (1983) Temporary bilateral carotid artery occlusion during surgical exploration of the nasal cavity of the dog. *Veterinary Surgery* 12, 83-85.

Holmberg, D.L. (1996) Sequelae of ventral rhinotomy in dogs and cats with inflammatory and neoplastic nasal pathology: a retrospective study. *Canadian Veterinary Journal* 37, 483-485.

Holmberg, D.L., Pettifer, G.R. (1997) The effect of carotid artery occlusion on lingual arterial blood pressure in dogs. *Canadian Veterinary Journal* 38, 629-631.

Holmes, R.L., Wolstencroft, J.H. (1959) Accessory sources of blood supply to the brain of the cat. *Journal of Physiology* 148, 93-107.

Kirpensteijn, J., Withrow, S.J., Straw, R.C. (1994) Combined resection of the nasal planum and premaxilla in three dogs. *Veterinary Surgery* 23, 341-346.

Lascelles, B.D., Thomson, M.J., Dernell, W.S., et al. (2003) Combined dorsolateral and intraoral approach for the resection of tumors of the maxilla in the dog. *Journal of the American Animal Hospital Association* 39, 294-305.

Lascelles, B.D., Henderson, R.A., Seguin, B., et al. (2004) Bilateral rostral maxillectomy and nasal planectomy for large rostral maxillofacial neoplasms in six dogs and one cat. *Journal of the American Animal Hospital Association* 40, 137-146.

Pavletic, M.M. (1999) Cantilever suture technique. In Pavletic, M.M. (ed.) *Atlas of Small Animal Reconstructive Surgery*. Saunders, Philadelphia, pp. 408-411.

Salisbury, S.K., Richardson, D.C., Lantz, G.C. (1986) Partial maxillectomy and premaxillectomy in the treatment of oral neoplasia in the dog and cat. *Veterinary Surgery* 15, 16-26.

Schwarz, P.D., Withrow, S.J., Curtis, C.R., et al. (1991) Partial maxillary resection as a treatment for oral cancer in 61 dogs. *Journal of the American Animal Hospital Association* 27, 617-624.

Wallace, J., Matthiesen, D.T., Patnaik, A.K. (1992) Hemimaxillectomy for the treatment of oral tumors in 69 dogs. *Veterinary Surgery* 21, 337-341.

White, R.A.S. (1991) Mandibulectomy and maxillectomy in the dog: Long-term survival in 100 cases. *Journal of Small Animal Practice* 32, 69-74.

White, R.A.S., Gorman, N.T., Watkins, S.B., et al. (1985) The surgical management of bone-involved oral tumours in the dog. *Journal of Small Animal Practice* 26, 693-708.

Withrow, S.J., Nelson, A.W., Manley, P.A., et al. (1985) Premaxillectomy in the dog. *Journal of the American Animal Hospital Association* 21, 49-55.

33 Lingual Surgery

Julius Liptak
Alta Vista Animal Hospital, Ottawa, Ontario, Canada

Tongue surgery is most commonly performed for the treatment of benign and malignant tumors, but ischemic necrosis and trauma have also been reported as causes for partial resection. Tongue resection has been classified according to the amount of tongue removed as partial glossectomy, subtotal glossectomy, near-total glossectomy, and total glossectomy (Dvorak *et al.* 2004). Partial glossectomy involves excision of part or all of the body of the tongue rostral to the frenulum. Subtotal glossectomy involves the entire free portion of the tongue and a portion of the genioglossus or geniohyoid muscles (or both muscles) caudal to the frenulum. Near-total glossectomy is defined as resection of 75% or more of the tongue. Total glossectomy is amputation of the entire tongue (Dvorak *et al.* 2004).

The complication rate depends on the type of glossectomy. For partial and subtotal glossectomies, short-term complications (<2 weeks) are reported in 54% (7 of 13) of dogs and long-term complications in 23% (3 of 13) of dogs (Syrcle *et al.* 2008). All dogs with near-total and total glossectomy developed changed eating habits, but otherwise these procedures were well tolerated in the long term (Dvorak *et al.* 2004). Local tumor recurrence and distant metastasis will not be considered as complications of glossectomy procedures for the purposes of this chapter; however, it should be noted that complete histologic excision of malignant oral tumors is important to decrease local tumor recurrence rates and improve survival times.

Intraoperative hemorrhage

Definition
Intraoperative hemorrhage is defined as blood loss during surgical resection of portions of the tongue.

Risk factors
- Any glossectomy procedure because of the rich vasculature of the tongue

Diagnosis
- Intraoperative observation of brisk or profuse bleeding

Treatment
- Ligation or cautery of bleeding vessels

Outcome
Blood loss from the tongue is very rarely severe enough to warrant a blood transfusion; hence, the outcome is usually not affected by blood loss if treated appropriately.

Prevention
Temporary occlusion of the carotid arteries may be effective in reducing intraoperative bleeding, but this is rarely necessary and should only be performed in dogs because carotid artery occlusion can be fatal in cats.

Wound dehiscence

Definition
Wound dehiscence is the breakdown of the surgical wound with separation of the wound edges (Figure 33.1).

Risk factors
- Wound tension
- Chewing of hard foods, sticks, and so on
- Use of cautery or laser to incise oral mucosa
- Use of rapidly absorbable suture material (i.e., catgut or poliglecaprone 25)
- Poor wound healing because of radiation therapy, chemotherapy, or debilitation

Diagnosis
Wound dehiscence typically occurs 3 to 7 days after surgery and is often asymptomatic. Clinical signs of intraoral wound dehiscence are rare but may include inappetence and halitosis.

Treatment
Treatment of wound dehiscence depends on the size of the defect. Wound dehiscence can be managed with either second intention healing if the dehisced area is small and granulating or debridement and resuturing if the defect is large.

Outcome
Conservative management with second intention healing and surgical treatment of dehisced wounds usually results in an uncomplicated recovery with no functional consequences.

Complications in Small Animal Surgery, First Edition. Edited by Dominique Griffon and Annick Hamaide.
© 2016 John Wiley & Sons, Inc. Published 2016 by John Wiley & Sons, Inc.
Companion website: www.wiley.com/go/griffon/complications

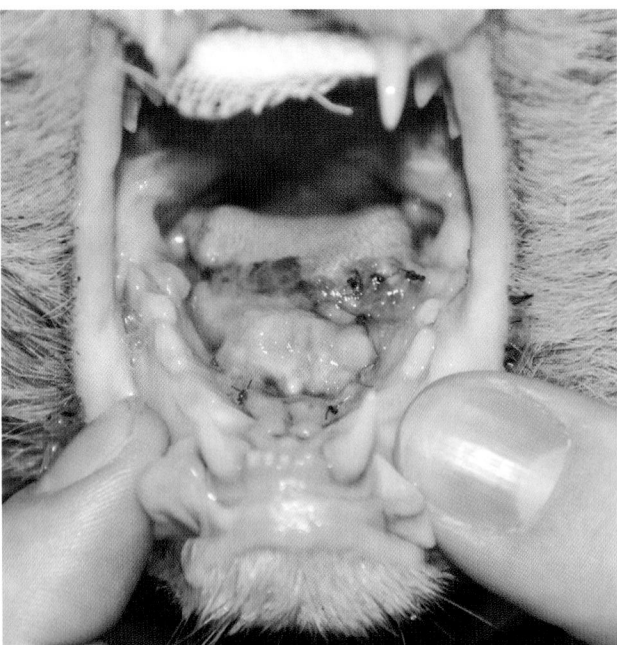

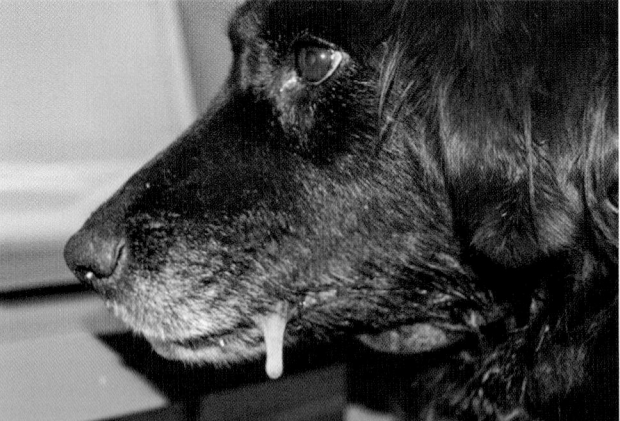

Figure 33.2 Ptyalism in a dog with a tongue tumor. Ptyalism can occur postoperatively after various glossectomy procedures. Cheilitis and facial dermatitis are common in chronic cases of ptyalism. Medical management is usually unsuccessful, although sialadenectomy has reduced the volume of saliva in one dog. *Source:* A. Hamaide, University of Liège, Liège, Belgium, 2014. Reproduced with permission from A. Hamaide.

Figure 33.1 Dehiscence of mucosal flaps used to reconstruct the tongue after traumatic avulsion of the tongue. Depending on the size of the dehiscence, the defect can be allowed to heal by second intention if small or debridement and resuturing if large. *Source:* Dr. B. van Goethem, Ghent University, Gent, Belgium.

Prevention

The risk of wound dehiscence can be minimized by avoiding the predisposing factors to dehiscence, in particular restricting the use of cautery or laser for hemostasis only, using long-lasting absorbable monofilament suture material, closing the glossectomy defect in two layers, and avoiding chewing on hard food and toys until the surgical wound has healed.

Ptyalism

Definition

Ptyalism is an excessive drooling of saliva or inability to retain saliva in the oral cavity (Figure 33.2).

Risk factors

- Partial glossectomy
- Subtotal glossectomy
- Near-total glossectomy
- Total glossectomy

Diagnosis

Ptyalism is typically diagnosed by observation of excessive drooling and salivation. Cheilitis and facial dermatitis are common in chronic cases.

Treatment

- Daily washing with an antiseptic solution
- Cheiloplasty
- Sialadenectomy

Outcome

Ptyalism will either resolve spontaneously or significantly reduce in volume after several weeks in the majority of animals. However, for cats and dogs with persistent drooling, cheilitis and facial dermatitis are common sequelae.

Prevention

Preventive factors are not known.

Eating difficulties

Definition

Eating difficulties are defined as difficulty prehending food, dysphagia, or inappetence.

Risk factors

- Near-total glossectomy
- Total glossectomy

Diagnosis

- Difficulty eating food or drinking unassisted with inability to maintain food boluses in the oral cavity, difficulty in propelling food boluses into the pharynx, and dribbling of water from the oral cavity.

Treatment

- All dogs should initially be offered meat balls of canned food, either offered by hand or placed on a flat dish rather than a bowl.
- Transition from meat balls to a diet consisting of free choice canned food when voluntary eating resumes.
- Food requiring extensive chewing or lapping should be avoided because they are not well tolerated.
- Water should be provided in a bucket or deep pan so that dogs could compensate for their inability to lap fluids by learning to immerse their muzzles into the water and suck.

Outcome

- After an initial learning period of 2 to 3 weeks, dogs are able to compensate for the near or total loss of their tongues and eat voluntarily and unassisted.
- Major glossectomy should not be performed in cats because of a poor ability to eat, drink, and groom.

Prevention

Preventive factors are not known.

Relevant literature

Major functions of the tongue during the oral and pharyngeal phases of swallowing include formation of a food bolus, keeping the bolus positioned between the teeth during mastication, and moving the bolus into the pharyngeal area immediately before swallowing (Lobprise and Wiggs 1993). The tongue is also important for grooming and thermoregulation (Lobprise and Wiggs 1993).

Complications of glossectomy include intraoperative hemorrhage and postoperative dehiscence; prehension difficulties; ptyalism; tongue necrosis; heat stress; and, particularly in cats, grooming difficulties (Beck *et al.* 1986; Carpenter *et al.* 1993; Dvorak *et al.* 2004; Syrcle *et al.* 2008). Although some of these complications are common, especially short-term eating difficulties, most are self-limiting and mild, particularly for partial and subtotal glossectomies (Syrcle *et al.* 2008).

Intraoperative hemorrhage is common because of the rich vasculature of the tongue. However, bleeding during glossectomy is usually easily controlled with cautery and ligatures. Temporary occlusion of the carotid arteries may decrease the risk of hemorrhage and blood loss in dogs but is rarely required (Hedlund *et al.* 1983; Holmberg and Pettifer 1997). Carotid artery occlusion should not be performed in cats (Holmes and Wolstencroft 1959; Gillian 1976; Holmberg 1996).

Dehiscence has been reported but is usually minor and heals rapidly by second intention because of the vascularity of the tongue (Dvorak *et al.* 2004; Syrcle *et al.* 2008). Dehiscence has been reported in 23% (3 of 13) and 25% (2 of 8) of dogs after partial or subtotal glossectomy for the management of tongue tumors (Carpenter *et al.* 1993; Syrcle *et al.* 2008). In one study, both dogs with dehiscence were treated with a transverse partial glossectomy, and disruption to the rostral vascular blood supply was proposed as the most likely cause of these dehiscences (Carpenter *et al.* 1993). In Syrcle *et al.* (2008), laser was used for resection of the tongue in two dogs (six dogs in total). Of the three dogs with dehiscence in this latter study, two dogs were managed conservatively with second intention healing, and one dog was managed with surgical debridement and resuturing. All dogs healed uneventfully (Syrcle *et al.* 2008).

Necrosis of the free portion of the tongue has been reported after minor glossectomy, presumably because of compromise to both of the paired lingual arteries (Carpenter *et al.* 1993; Dvorak *et al.* 2004). For this reason, one of these paired arteries should be preserved during partial or subtotal lateral glossectomy procedures (Carpenter *et al.* 1993).

Ptyalism was reported in 38% (5 of 13) dogs after partial and subtotal glossectomy (Syrcle *et al.* 2008) and 20% (1 of 5) dogs after major glossectomy (Dvorak *et al.* 2004). Ptyalism tends to either resolve spontaneously or significantly reduce in volume after several weeks in the majority of animals treated with partial or subtotal glossectomy (Syrcle *et al.* 2008). However, ptyalism did not resolve in one dog after major glossectomy. This dog did not respond to oral glycopyrrolate but showed a partial response to sialadenectomy of the ipsilateral mandibular and sublingual salivary glands and duct (Dvorak *et al.* 2004). Other proposed treatments include salivary duct ligation and salivary duct diversion (Dvorak *et al.* 2004).

Heat stress is a possible complication after major glossectomy (Dvorak *et al.* 2004). The dorsal surface of the canine tongue contains numerous arteriovenous anastomoses, which are necessary for thermoregulation (Chibuzo 1979). The tongue is also important for heat dissipation through panting. Major glossectomy removes these arteriovenous anastomoses and reduces the effectiveness of panting. The risk of heat stress can be minimized by avoiding hot environments, minimizing activity during warmer periods of the day, and immediate cooling if the dog becomes hot through excessive activity or excitation.

The tongue plays an important role in the prehension of food and swallowing. **Eating is rarely affected** after minor glossectomies (partial and subtotal glossectomies), even in cats, but major glossectomy (near-total and total glossectomies) in both cats and dogs can prevent normal eating because the tongue is integral during the oral phase and initiates the pharyngeal phase of swallowing. This effect is usually temporary in dogs but permanent in cats.

In one study of eight dogs treated with partial or subtotal glossectomies for management of tongue tumors, it was noted that most dogs ate better when hand fed or when food was placed on a flat dish rather than in a bowl (Carpenter *et al.* 1993). Food requiring extensive chewing or lapping was not well tolerated. Water was better in a bucket or deep pan so that dogs could compensate for their inability to lap fluids by learning to immerse their muzzles into the water and suck (Carpenter *et al.* 1993). These findings were supported by a later study in which 100% (6 of 6) of dogs ate without difficulty within 2 weeks of partial or subtotal glossectomy (Syrcle *et al.* 2008).

In one study of major glossectomy in five dogs, dogs were able to eat and drink unassisted by 24 hours (*n* = 1), 3 weeks (*n* = 2), and 4 weeks (*n* = 2) (Dvorak *et al.* 2004). Supplemental nutrition via a feeding tube was used in all dogs until they were able to be trained to eat and drink unassisted. Dogs were trained to eat and drink unassisted by throwing chilled meat balls into the air, and after dogs were able to pick up the chilled meat balls, they were encouraged to drink by placing the meatballs in bowls of water (Dvorak *et al.* 2004). Eating habits changed in one dog that ate dry food by throwing her head back to assist in swallowing the kibble, and soft food tended to lodge in the intermandibular space and cause problems (Dvorak *et al.* 2004). In another study, 15% (2 of 13) of dogs had long-term complications with eating such as dropping food and dribbling water (Syrcle *et al.* 2008). In the study by Dvorak *et al.* (2004), four dogs sucked water from a bucket, but one dog did not learn how to do this but received his water requirements from soaked dry food (Dvorak *et al.* 2004). Major glossectomy is not recommended in cats because of a poor ability to eat, drink, and groom.

Other complications are rarely reported but include mild to moderate postoperative dehydration in dogs with more than 50% of the tongue resected (Carpenter *et al.* 1993) and salivary mucocele in one dog after a major glossectomy (Dvorak *et al.* 2004).

References

Beck, E.R., Withrow, S.J., McChesney, A.E., et al. (1986) Canine tongue tumors: a retrospective review of 57 cases. *Journal of the American Animal Hospital Association* 22, 525-532.

Carpenter, L.G., Withrow, S.J., Power, B.E., et al. (1993) Squamous cell carcinoma of the tongue in 10 dogs. *Journal of the American Animal Hospital Association* 29, 17-24.

Chibuzo, G.A. (1979) The tongue. In Evans, H.E., Christensen, G.C. (eds.) *Miller's Anatomy of the Dog*. Saunders, Philadelphia, pp. 423-445.

Dvorak, L.D., Beaver, D.P., Ellison, G.W., et al. (2004) Major glossectomy in dogs: a case series and proposed classification system. *Journal of the American Animal Hospital Association* 40, 331-337.

Gillian, L.A. (1976) Extra- and intra-cranial blood supply to brains of dog and cat. *American Journal of Anatomy* 146, 237-253.

Hedlund, C.S., Tangner, C.H., Elkins, H.D., et al. (1983) Temporary bilateral carotid artery occlusion during surgical exploration of the nasal cavity of the dog. *Veterinary Surgery* 12, 83-85.

Holmberg, D.L. (1996) Sequelae of ventral rhinotomy in dogs and cats with inflammatory and neoplastic nasal pathology: a retrospective study. *Canadian Veterinary Journal* 37, 483-485.

Holmberg, D.L., Pettifer, G.R. (1997) The effect of carotid artery occlusion on lingual arterial blood pressure in dogs. *Canadian Veterinary Journal* 38, 629-631.

Holmes, R.L., Wolstencroft, J.H. (1959) Accessory sources of blood supply to the brain of the cat. *Journal of Physiology* 148, 93-107.

Lobprise, H.B., Wiggs, R.B. (1993) Anatomy, diagnosis and management of disorders of the tongue. *Journal of Veterinary Dentistry* 10, 16-23.

Syrcle, J.A., Bonczynski, J.J., Monnette, S., et al. (2008) Retrospective evaluation of lingual tumors in 42 dogs: 1999-2005. *Journal of the American Animal Hospital Association* 44, 308-319.

34 Tooth Extractions

Anson J. Tsugawa

Dog and Cat Dentist, Inc., Culver City, CA, USA

Extraction procedures are the most commonly performed oral surgery in dogs and cats (Wiggs and Lobprise 1997). Permanent teeth are most commonly extracted for the treatment of severe periodontal disease, tooth resorption, or when traumatized (e.g., fractured teeth with pulp exposure; irreversible pulpitis or nonvital teeth; subluxated, luxated, or intruded teeth). Tooth extraction may also be indicated for oncologic and orthodontic purposes or when performing maxillofacial fracture repair. Extraction of the deciduous dentition is performed in the case of delayed tooth exfoliation (persistent deciduous teeth) or traumatized deciduous teeth with pulp exposure or in the treatment of deciduous dental or skeletal malocclusions (i.e., interceptive orthodontics).

Complications arising from tooth extractions are common and can vary from the routine, fracturing of a root during an extraction to the more difficult to treat and potentially very severe mandibular fracture, oronasal fistula formation, or even orbital penetration. Alveolar osteitis "dry socket," in which there is lysis of the mature blood clot before its being replaced by granulation tissue, a well-known complication in humans, does not appear to be common in dogs and cats (Van Cauwelaert de Wyels 1998). Dysanesthesias, or nerve injuries, secondary to extraction may also occur but are more than likely underdiagnosed in dogs and cats. Proper extraction technique can minimize complications, but perhaps more important is the accurate assessment and handling of these complications when they occur. Tooth extractions, the concept of loss of teeth, and how the dog or cat will function or eat after extractions are very sensitive issues with clients and should not be overlooked in their importance.

Retention of broken tooth roots

Definition
This is the fracture or separation of the tooth root from its crown that occurs during an extraction and the portion of the root or root tip remains within the socket. In cats, the intentional retention of resorbing tooth roots with dentoalveolar ankylosis secondary to tooth resorption may be acceptable (DuPont 1995).

Risk factors
- Tooth resorption with dentoalveolar ankylosis, previous endodontic therapy, or other intrinsic root pathologies influencing the integrity of the root

- Root morphology (root curvature or dilaceration)
- Incomplete assessment or failure to obtain preoperative radiographs of the tooth to be extracted
- Poor extraction technique or exposure

Diagnosis
Retained tooth roots may be diagnosed by clinical appearance, in which visually, the smooth apical portion of the root tip is absent; a portion of the root is visible emerging from the oral soft tissues; by the audible sound of the fracturing of a root during the extraction; or more reliably, through the use of dental radiography. Although the standard dental radiography views may be applied for this purpose, obtaining an orthogonal view (Figure 34.1), in which the tooth sockets are visualized end on, is often the easiest method for determining whether tooth material remains in the socket. The identification of root tips that have migrated from the immediate tooth socket may require use of radiographic markers or application of dental radiographic principles to facilitate their localization (Figure 34.2). Diagnostic radiographs should show the associated structures (mental foramen) that may be affected by the surgery to retrieve the root fragment (Dennis 2009).

Treatment
Because tooth extractions in dogs and cats are usually performed to treat infected teeth, removal of any fractured portions of the root is indicated. Radiographically confirmed root tips are best addressed by improving the exposure and access to the root tip, either by elevation of a periodontal flap, if one has not already been raised, or by apical extension of the vertical releasing incision of an existing flap followed by the necessary buccal alveolectomy or periradicular bone removal with dental bur to improve visibility of the root tip, allowing an elevator, luxator, or root tip pick to access the periodontal ligament space around to root tip. Typically, the diameter of the alveolus will need to be enlarged approximately 30% wider than the diameter of the root fragment (Woodward 2006). For less accessible root tips, use of a root canal file, threaded into the canal of the root tip, may prove helpful. Specialized tips that are available for use with piezoelectric ultrasonic units can be used for root tip retrieval as well. Proper patient positioning, magnification (loupes), local hemorrhage control, and lighting (preferably headlight illumination) will aid tremendously in the successful removal of retained root tips.

Complications in Small Animal Surgery, First Edition. Edited by Dominique Griffon and Annick Hamaide.
© 2016 John Wiley & Sons, Inc. Published 2016 by John Wiley & Sons, Inc.
Companion website: www.wiley.com/go/griffon/complications

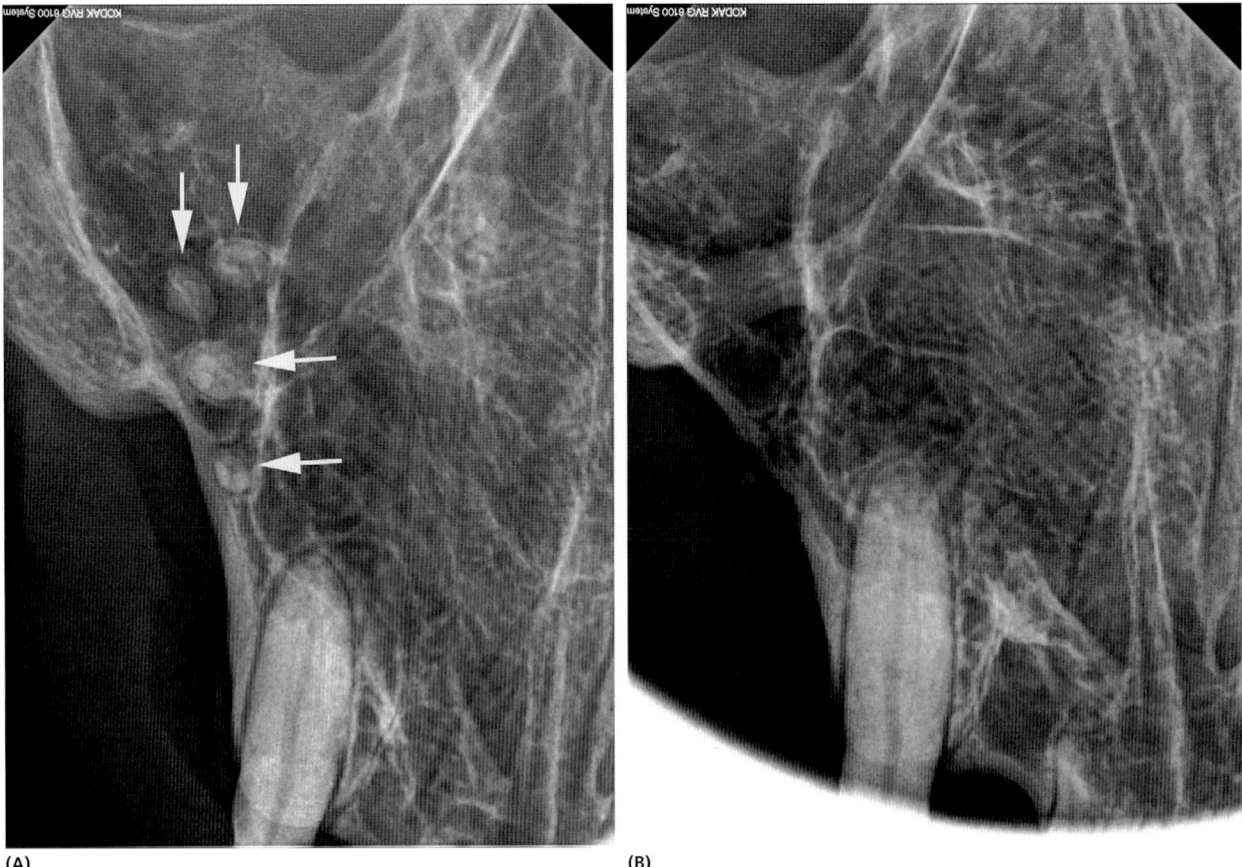

(A)   **(B)**

Figure 34.1 Intraoral radiographs of a cat with gingivostomatitis undergoing retrieval of root fragments from a previous extraction procedure. **A,** Intraoral dorsoventral radiographic view of the right maxilla. Notice the root tips (arrows) of the right maxillary second premolar, distal root of the right maxillary third premolar, and mesial roots of the right maxillary fourth premolar. **B,** Postoperative radiograph revealed vacated tooth sockets.

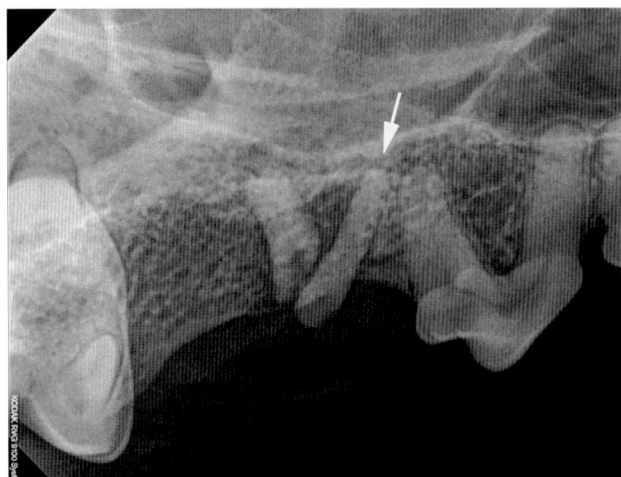

Figure 34.2 Radiograph demonstrating the use of a dental radiographic principle (same lingual opposite buccal [SLOB] rule) for proper orientation and localization of the retained mesial root tips of the right maxillary fourth premolar. To obtain this bisecting-angle technique view, the x-ray tube head was angled from the front of the patient, creating radiographic separation of the mesial root tips of the right maxillary fourth premolar; the palatal root is identified as the root closest to the incoming x-ray beam (arrow).

Outcome

The prognosis and outcome after the retrieval of root tips is good and this retrieval is medically necessary unless the collateral damage to the adjacent anatomy that is likely to be incurred during the process of retrieving the root tip is too great and not in the best interest of the patient. In the case of the latter, the client must be informed regarding the retained root(s) and given the opportunity for referral of the patient to a veterinary dental specialist, or the retained root should be monitored clinically and radiographically.

Prevention

- Proper patient positioning and lighting to perform extractions
- Use of proper extraction technique and instruments; avoidance of uncontrolled force with extraction forceps
- Preoperative intraoral dental radiographic assessment: dentoalveolar ankylosis, hypercementosis, periapical pathology or root resorption, previous endodontic treatment, root morphology (root divergence, dilaceration, concrescence, fused roots, supernumerary roots)
- Conservative but deliberate and adequate alveolar bone removal to expedite and provide proper visualization of the root, which will simultaneously facilitate the extraction and minimize collateral damage to the oral hard and soft tissues.

Oronasal communication and fistula

Definition

The extraction of the maxillary canine and less commonly the incisor teeth may result in a communication between the oral and nasal cavities when a section of bone from the palatal wall of socket is removed along with a tooth root or when a deep periodontal pocket that communicates or nearly communicates with the nasal cavity is revealed after extraction of the tooth. If this complication is not addressed, a fistula (i.e., an epithelium-lined communication between the oral and nasal cavities) may develop.

Risk factors

- Narrow-nosed small dogs (Rossman *et al.* 1985)
- Presence of severe periodontitis with deep periodontal pockets along the palatal surface of a maxillary tooth.
- Extractions performed in a previously irradiated region of the mouth
- Oronasal communication that is iatrogenically induced during extraction or after maxillectomy
- Failure to close the socket(s) of severely diseased maxillary teeth
- After oncologic surgery, for example, partial rostral maxillectomy or mandibulectomy with associated mandibular drift, in which there is the potential for traumatic occlusion of the mandibular canine tooth into the opposing oral soft tissues and subsequent traumatic oronasal fistula formation

Diagnosis

Oronasal communication at an extraction site, which is a risk factor for fistula formation, is often noted at the time of extraction when a portion of the palatal wall of the alveolus bone is found adhered to the extracted root tip; epistaxis from the ipsilateral nostril is identified; or a fenestration through the alveolus into the nasal cavity is directly visualized as a black hole, which may be accompanied by additional hemorrhage from the local area secondary to turbinate trauma (Figure 34.3). In patients with severe periodontitis, especially smaller breed dogs, the epistaxis may be bilateral, attributable to the extensiveness of the secondary bone destruction in the area even if the oronasal communication is unilateral in nature.

The presence of oronasal communication may also be identified at postoperative follow-up as a dehiscence of the surgical flap, fenestration in a compromised portion of the flap (i.e., a thin portion of the flap, or region of the flap overlying an undercontoured ridge of alveolar bone), or at an extraction site that was never closed as a black hole. The client may also report that the patient has been sneezing or that there has been nasal discharge immediately after consumption of food or water. In the case of oronasal communication at a dehisced or fenestrated surgical flap, additional healing time may be warranted before a diagnosis of a fistula is made.

Treatment

Although small communications may heal spontaneously, the majority of oronasal communications require closure to prevent food, water, and air from the mouth from traveling into the nasal cavity. For cases of oronasal communication identified at the time of the extraction, the communication should be addressed by careful closure of the site using an appropriate flap, usually a buccal flap, which, if successful, will avoid development of a fistula. When oronasal communication is identified during a subsequent tooth extraction follow-up visit as a dehiscence of a periodontal flap, early in the course of healing (i.e., within 2 weeks of the extraction), additional healing time is warranted before intervening surgically

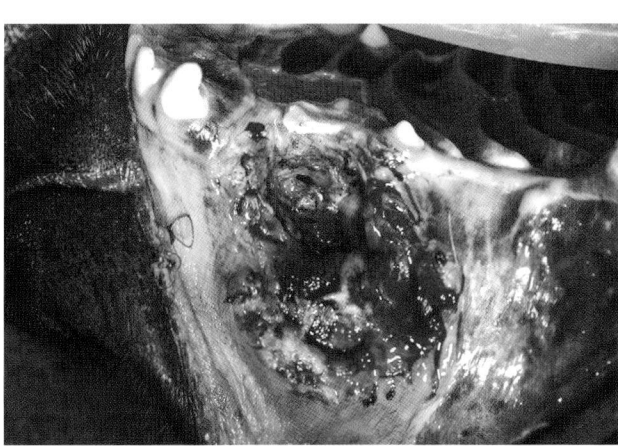
(A)

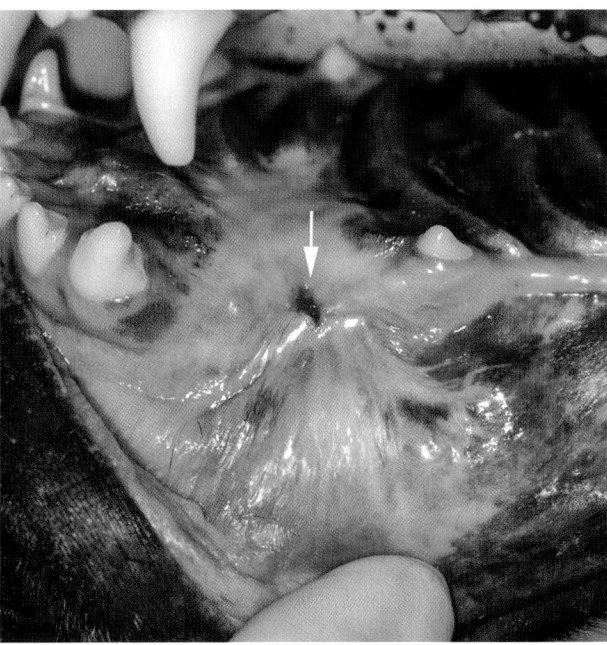
(B)

Figure 34.3 Dog after dehiscence of a right maxillary canine tooth extraction site. **A,** Notice the significant inflammation of the adjacent tissues. Surgical closure, if attempted immediately, would be at high risk for repeat dehiscence; tissue handling would be challenging because of the degree of inflammation and require significant tissue debridement, compromising the width of the vestibule and pulling the lip in a palatal direction. **B,** The same extraction site, without surgical intervention, 1 month later. Notice that the area of oronasal communication (arrow) is limited to a much smaller area.

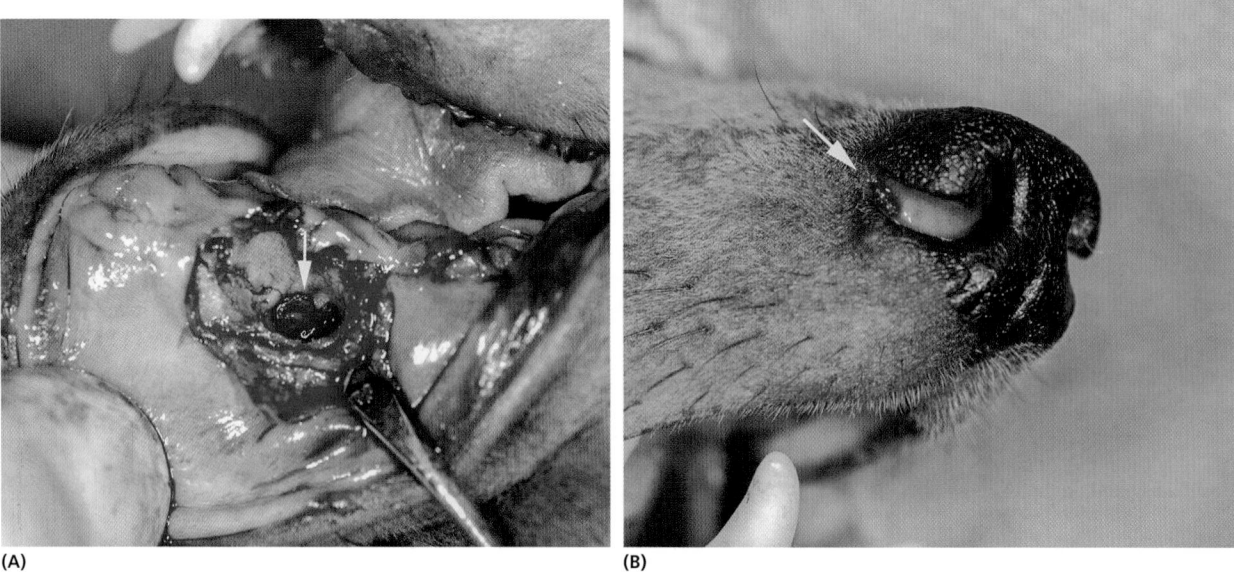

(A)   **(B)**

Figure 34.4 Oronasal communication at a maxillary canine extraction socket. **A,** Oronasal communication (arrow) is identified at the extraction socket of the right maxillary canine tooth in a dog. **B,** Epistaxis (arrow) from the right nostril, confirming the presence of oronasal communication at the right maxillary canine tooth socket.

and assuming that the area of communication will become a fistula, from the standpoint that the area may contract and close; heal further, making it a smaller defect to repair (Figure 34.4); and improve overall tissue handling when the closure is attempted after the initial inflammation has resolved. In the case of a preexisting area of communication at an extraction site that went undiagnosed and was never closed at the time of the extraction, a fistula is more than likely present and will not close without surgical intervention (Figure 34.5).

Outcome

The outcome after identification and immediate surgical repair of iatrogenic oronasal communication is good, and a resultant fistula will be averted. The treatment success of oronasal fistulas, especially fistulas that are recurrent and when adjacent oral soft tissues are in limited supply, can be challenging, and success is directly related to appropriate surgical flap selection and technique. Treatment success can be improved by performing surgical closure on healed, noninflamed soft tissue and avoiding the temptation to approach surgery prematurely when tissues are still severely inflamed and sutures are more likely to pull through.

Prevention

- Avoid excess apical or lateral luxation forces on the root.
- Closure of extraction sites along the rostral maxillary arch (incisors and canines) when there is radiographic (Figure 34.6) or intraoperative identification of pathologic or iatrogenic oronasal communication or when teeth, especially the maxillary canines, are extracted by simple technique or simply fall out with minimal force. The latter is an indication of severe attachment loss and alveolar bone loss, with a high risk of oronasal communication.
- Do not probe sockets to determine if communication is present; communication could be created that was not present or damage an intact membrane (Dennis 2009).

- Development of full-thickness tension-free flaps for closure and positioning of wound edges over sound bone
- Accurate flap adaptation and suturing technique

Fractured mandible

Definition

This is an incomplete or complete fracture of the mandibular bone that occurs during tooth extraction, most commonly in small or toy breed dogs at the level of the mandibular first molar roots, or through the lingual wall of the alveolus of the mandibular canine (Figure 34.7), adjacent to the mandibular symphysis, in the presence of compromised bone quality, periodontitis, or poor extraction technique. In cats, iatrogenic mandibular fractures most frequently occur at the level of the mandibular canines; however, because of their small skull size, poor extraction technique can lead to fracture at any level of the mandibular body. As a rule, all mandibular fractures that occur in this fashion are considered open fractures because they occur through the periodontal ligament space of the tooth.

Risk factors

- Compromised mandibular bone quality secondary to severe periodontitis, periapical disease, other infection (osteomyelitis), neoplasia, trauma, developmental, or metabolic disease
- Unfavorable root morphology (dilaceration of the mandibular first molar roots) or dentoalveolar ankylosis (Figure 34.8)
- Use of extraction instruments with excessive force; performing a mandibular extraction with forceps only or using a one-handed technique, without use of the operator's other hand to stabilize the mandible, when tooth sectioning and a surgical (open) extraction technique is indicated

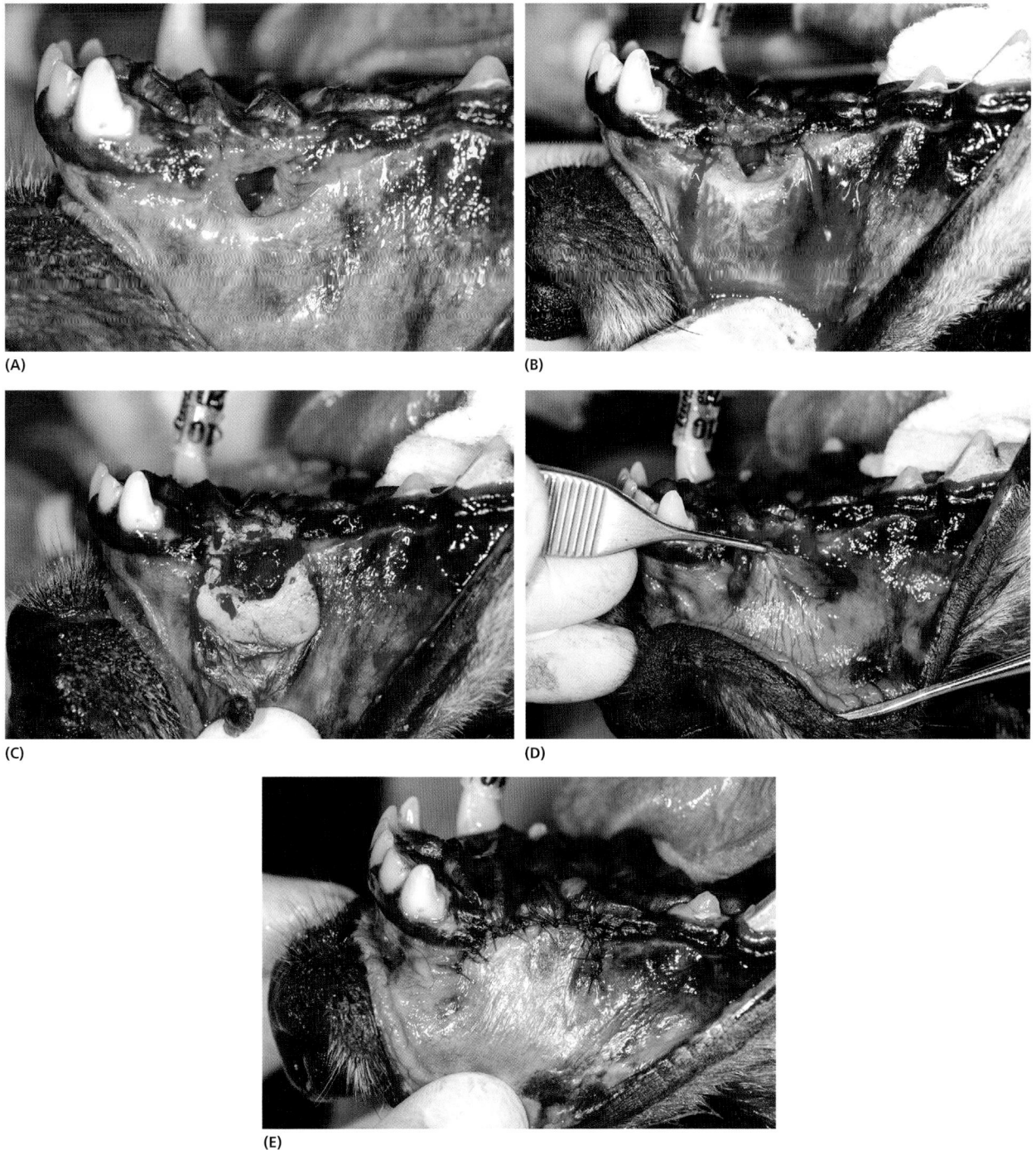

Figure 34.5 Closure of an oronasal fistula using a single full-thickness buccal alveolar mucosa pedicle flap. **A,** Oronasal fistula at the socket of a previously extracted right maxillary canine tooth. **B,** Development of a full-thickness buccal alveolar mucosa pedicle flap. **C,** Sharp debridement of the lining of the fistula. **D,** Tension-free flap. **E,** Simple interrupted closure of the flap using absorbable monofilament suture.

Diagnosis

Mandibular fractures that occur during the course of tooth extraction are almost always immediately clinically diagnosed, an audible fracturing or splintering sound of the mandibular bone is often heard, or there is palpable instability of the mandible. Radiographs, either extraoral skull views or intraoral dental views, are indicated for confirmation and treatment planning (Figure 34.9).

Treatment (Figure 34.10)

Mandibular fractures at the level of the mandibular canine: interdental wire and splinting or external skeletal fixation

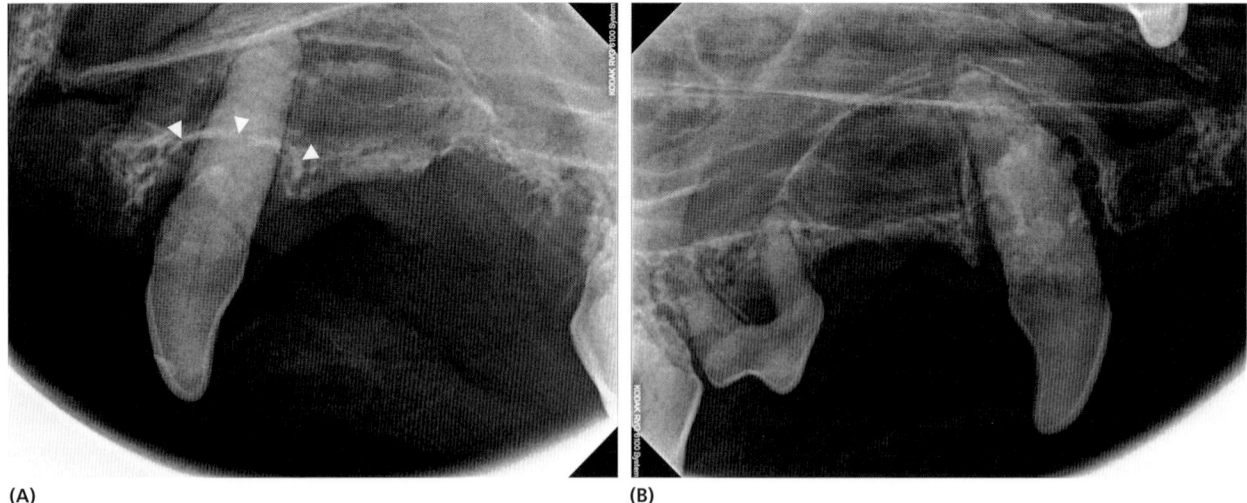

(A)   **(B)**

Figure 34.6 Intraoral lateral radiographic views of the maxillary canine teeth in a dog with oronasal communication at the right maxillary canine tooth. **A,** The left maxillary canine tooth in a dog. Notice the radiodense line (arrowheads), which is the radiographic appearance of the nasal surface of the alveolar process of the maxilla, the radiographic separation of the oral and nasal cavities. **B,** In the same patient, the radiographic view of the contralateral right maxillary canine reveals the absence of the radiodense line that is the nasal surface of the alveolar process of the maxilla, which correlates clinically with oronasal communication along the palatal aspect of the right maxillary canine tooth.

(Modified-Gunning splint with circum-mandibular wire or interdental full-pin technique) (Cook *et al.* 2001) (Figure 34.11)

- Mandibular body fractures: interdental wire and splinting in combination with intraosseous wire or intraosseous wire alone and plate (miniplate or extraoral bicortical plate) fixation with graft if needed (Boudrieau and Kudisch 1996; Chiodo and Milles 2009; Gorzelnik and Kozlovsky 2009)
- Mandibular body fractures with associated severe concomitant infectious pathology (pathologic fracture secondary to severe periodontal disease): delayed fixation, after infection is resolved, or leave as a nonunion fracture and perform occlusal adjustment or commissuroplasty on the affected side to achieve additional mandibular support without primary osteosynthesis

Outcome

The prognosis for mandibular fracture secondary to tooth extraction varies depending on whether the fracture was caused by poor technique or compromised bone quality. In the case of poor

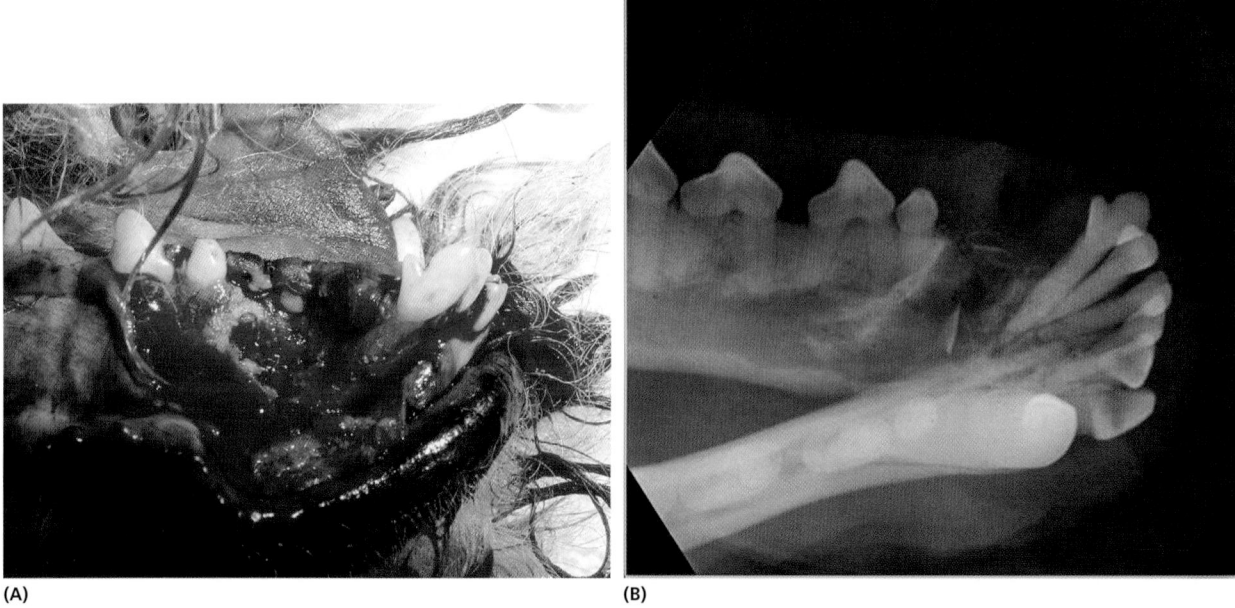

(A)   **(B)**

Figure 34.7 Mandibular fracture at the level of the right mandibular canine tooth extraction socket. **A,** Fracture through the lingual wall of the alveolus of the right mandibular canine tooth. **B,** Intraoral lateral radiographic view of the rostral right mandible of the fracture through the right mandibular canine tooth socket.

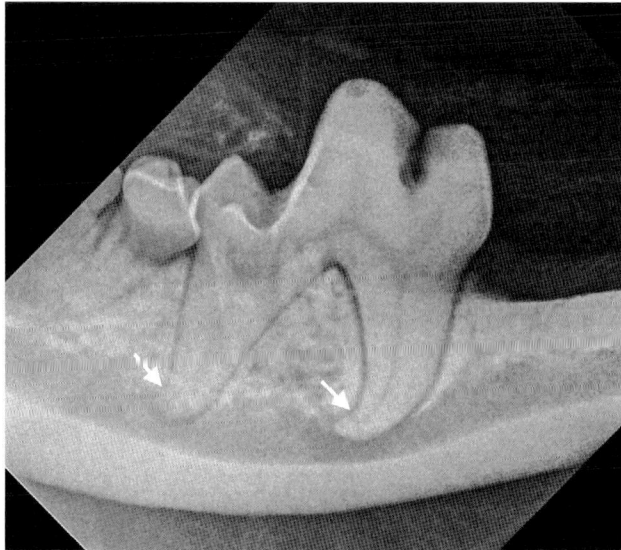

Figure 34.8 Intraoral paralleling technique radiographic view of the right mandibular first molar. Notice the severe dilaceration (arrows) of both roots of the mandibular first molar.

technique, with appropriately timed intervention and use of appropriate osteosynthesis techniques, without additional damage to adjacent teeth, a complete restoration of function can be expected. When there is preexisting poor bone quality, the combination of the missing tooth and bone in the area, bone that is often carried away with the extracted tooth roots, may result in a critical defect in the bone, which will necessitate repair with a graft, which engenders a guarded prognosis, or left as a nonunion fracture, a poor prognosis.

Prevention
- Use proper extraction technique and tooth sectioning and minimize buccal alveolar bone removal

- Preoperative identification of areas of potential concern for fracture using appropriate imaging (intraoral dental radiography and computed tomography [CT]) when applicable
- Inform clients regarding the risk of possible fracture.

Persistent hemorrhage
See Chapter 13.

Migration of roots

Definition
This is the displacement of tooth roots into unfavorable anatomic spaces such as the nasal cavity, mandibular canal, periorbital tissues, submandibular space, gastrointestinal tract, or airway during extraction (Figure 34.12). Although veterinary patients are under general anesthesia and intubated for tooth extractions, any tooth debris or pharyngeal (gauze) packing material that remains in the mouth after extubation can compromise the patient's airway and less commonly, the gastrointestinal tract, requiring airway support, bronchoscopy, or even endoscopy for retrieval (Pacchiana *et al.* 2001).

Risk factors
- Radiographic documentation when root tips are in close proximity to the mandibular canal or nasal cavity
- Caudal maxillary tooth extractions (fourth premolar and molars) when there is existing bone destruction associated with periodontal or endodontic disease
- Use of a simple or closed surgical extraction technique when an open surgical extraction is warranted
- Excessive application of apical extraction force
- Species or breed predisposition (cats and small or toy breed dogs)

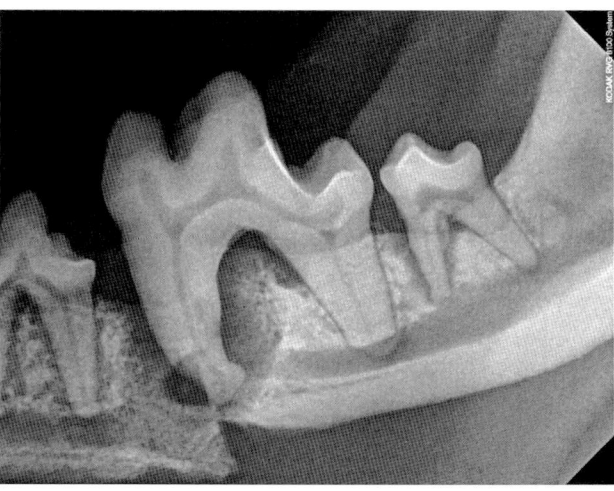

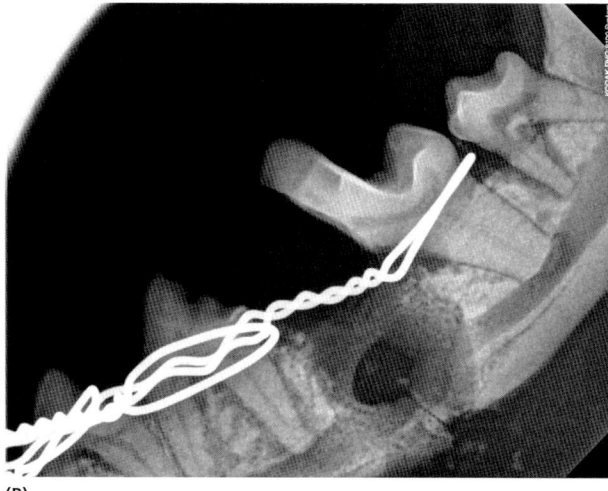

(A)   (B)

Figure 34.9 Mandibular body fracture at the level of the left mandibular first molar. **A,** Fracture at the level of the mesial root of the left mandibular first molar with preexisting endodontic and periodontic disease. **B,** Extraction of the diseased left mandibular first molar followed by immediate stabilization of the fracture segments using interdental wire.

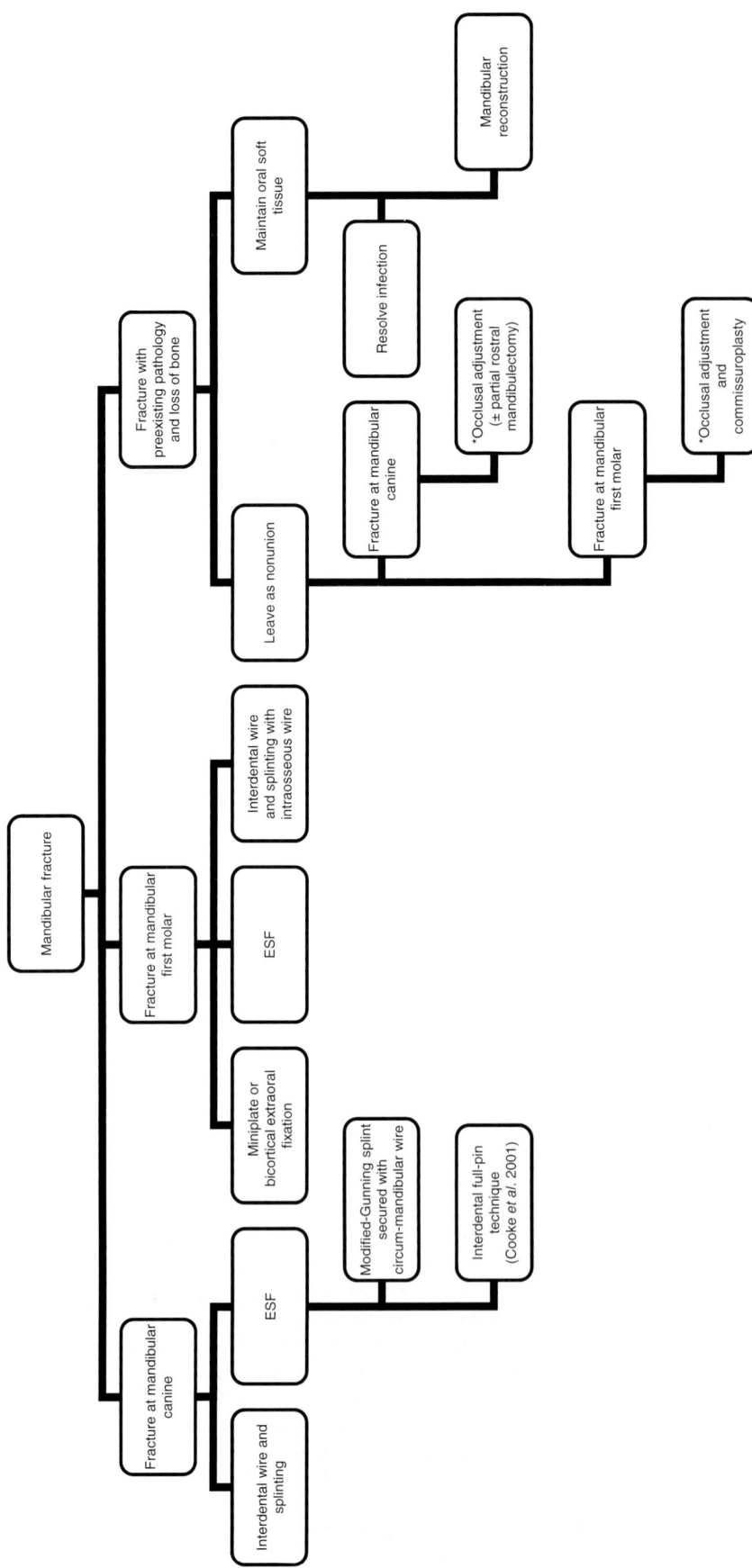

Figure 34.10 Decision tree in case of mandibular fracture. Asterisk indicates that occlusal adjustment is the modification of the patient's occlusion to address the traumatic occlusion of mandibular teeth into the opposing oral soft tissues associated with the instability or drift of the mandible as a result of leaving the mandibular fracture as a nonunion.

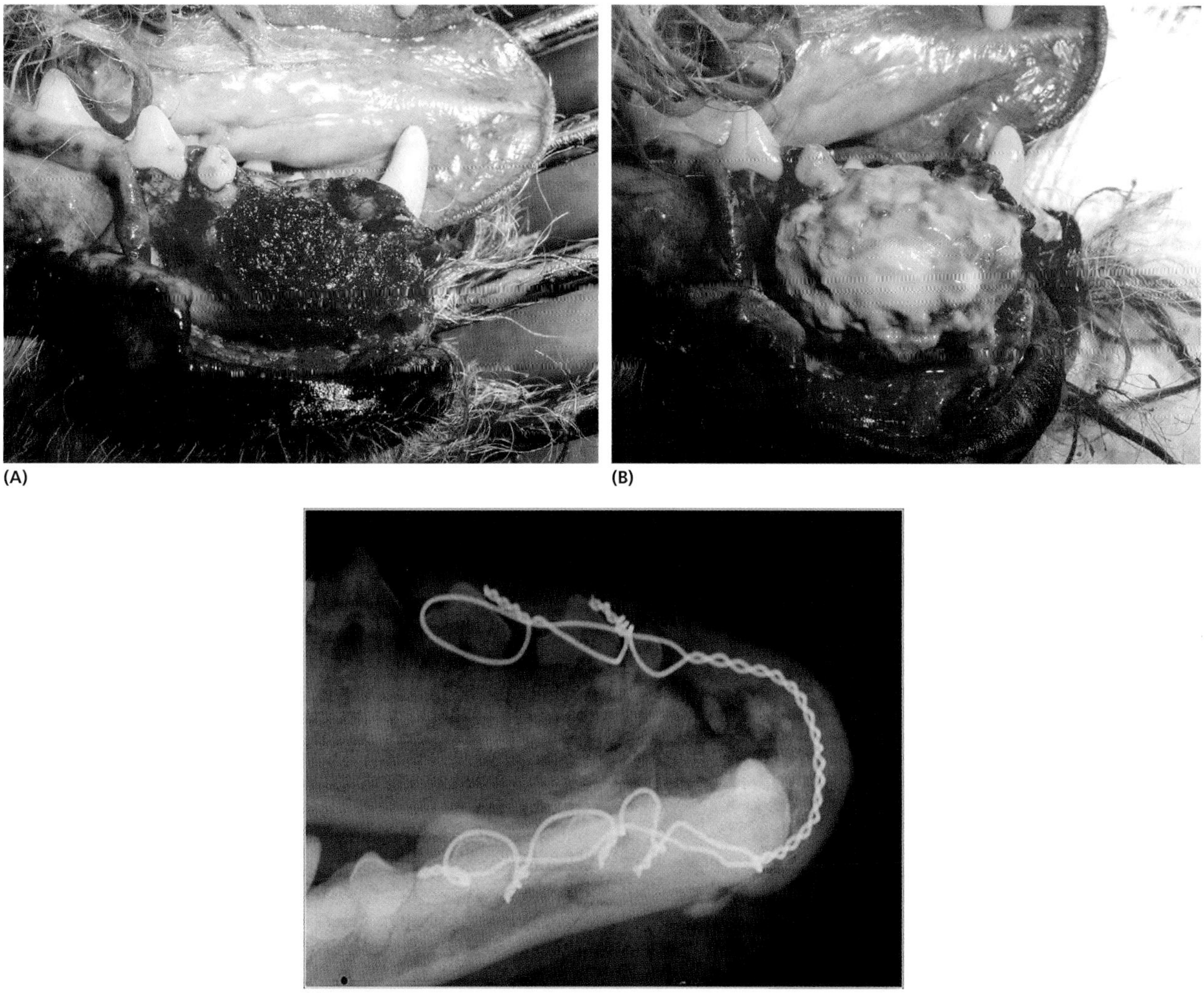

Figure 34.11 Interdental wire and splint repair of a mandibular fracture at the level of the right mandibular canine tooth. **A,** Xenograft incorporated with autogenous platelet-rich plasma placed into right mandibular canine socket and fracture site. **B,** Calcium sulfate bone graft barrier applied over graft to prevent epithelial disturbance and repopulation of the graft. **C,** Immediate postoperative intraoral lateral radiographic view of the completed interdental wire and splint stabilization of the mandibular fracture.

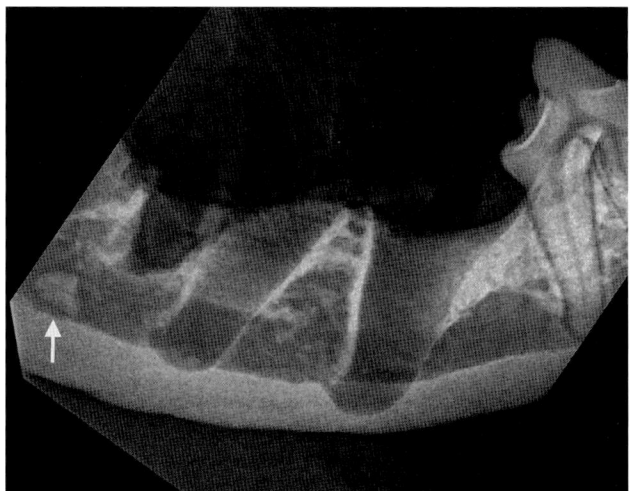

Figure 34.12 Intraoral paralleling technique radiographic view of the caudal right mandible. Notice the displaced root fragment (arrow) in the mandibular canal.

Diagnosis

The position and size of the tooth or tooth fragment (entire root or root tip) should be documented radiographically. Use of radiographic markers placed at the level of the root tip may aid in localization. Other imaging modalities may be indicated, such as skull radiographs, CT, or more recently, cone-beam computed tomography (CBCT), depending on the anatomic location of the displaced tooth fragment. CT and CBCT have the advantage of elimination superimposition of anatomic structures (Chrcanovic *et al.* 2010).

Treatment

A displaced tooth, tooth roots or large root fragments that were being extracted for the treatment of infection (e.g., periodontitis or periapical pathosis) should be removed to avoid potential infection related sequelae as long as the surgical procedure for retrieval itself does not have an unfavorable complication rate (Figure 34.13). In the case of the latter, careful monitoring and follow-up are advised. Very small fragments may be better off left in place. The careful use of suction and an appropriately sized suction tip directed at the socket can sometimes aid in recovery of the tooth (Ness and Peterson 2004).

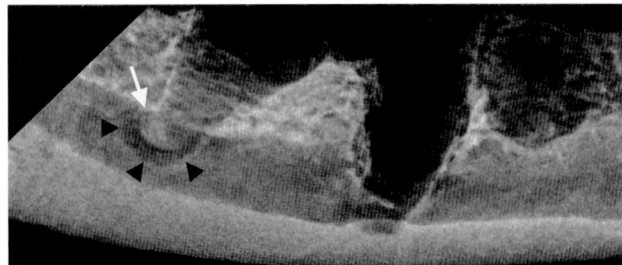

Figure 34.13 Intraoral paralleling technique radiographic view of the caudal right mandible. Notice the periapical radiolucency (arrowheads) surrounding the root tip fragment (arrow) of the distal root of the right mandibular first molar and proximity of the fragment to the mandibular canal.

Outcome

The outcome of migrated tooth roots is directly related to any potential infection-related sequelae if the roots are not retrieved, and if retrieved, the extensiveness of the tissue dissection, collateral damage that is incurred to gain access to the tooth fragment. When retrieving root tips that have been displaced into the mandibular canal, atraumatic bone removal (alveolectomy) and extraction technique are necessary to avoid traumatizing the inferior alveolar neurovascular bundle. Exploration within the nasal cavity can result in excessive damage to the turbinates, local hemorrhage that will impair visualization, postoperative epistaxis, and subcutaneous emphysema. The resultant oronasal communication will also necessitate careful flap closure to prevent development of a chronic oronasal fistula. Exploration for tooth fragments in the caudal maxilla and the soft tissue floor of the orbit may result in orbital cellulitis, or worse, penetrating trauma to the globe.

Prevention

- Awareness of the regional anatomy, preparation, and having an action plan available in the event of root displacement
- Avoid the application of uncontrolled apical force with extraction instruments
- Proper grasp of sharp instruments near the working end may limit potentially dangerous slippage of the instrument
- Where visualization is lacking, create the necessary access, and utilize an open surgical extraction technique

Infection and osteomyelitis

See Chapter 5.

Bacteremia and septicemia

See Chapter 2.

Traumatic occlusion

Definition

Traumatic occlusion after tooth extraction is a complication limited, for the most part, to cats; when there is an injurious occlusion of an opposing tooth into the oral soft tissues where a tooth has been extracted, usually after extraction of the mandibular first molar; or

in the case of the extracted maxillary canine tooth, when the opposing mandibular canine tooth becomes entrapped extraoral to the maxillary lip, resulting in ulceration or even puncture injury of the lip (Figure 34.14). Injury to the intraoral soft tissues, particularly of the vestibular mucogingival tissues of the mandibular first molar teeth, ranges from ulceration (indentation of the cusp tip in the mucosa) to development of mucosal polyp formation or pyogenic granuloma; which may be easily mistaken in clinical appearance for neoplasia (i.e., squamous cell carcinoma) (Figure 34.15).

Risk factors

- Brachycephalic cat breeds and cat breeds such as Siamese cats, which have a triangular or wedge-shaped face, are at risk for the development of traumatic occlusion of the mandibular canine into the maxillary lip when the maxillary canine is extracted.

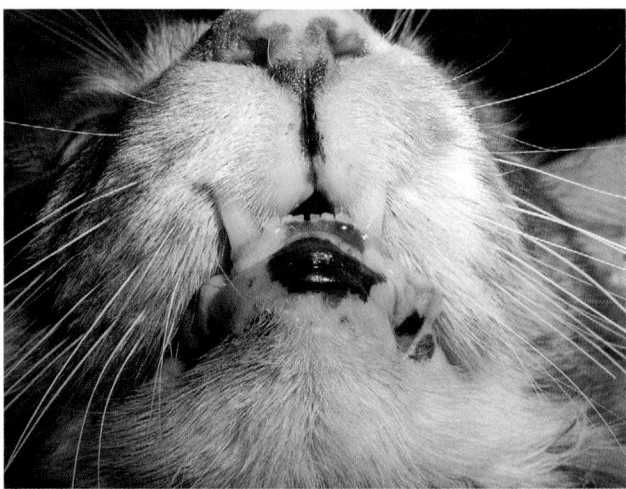

Figure 34.14 Bilateral maxillary lip entrapment in a cat after extraction of both maxillary canine teeth.

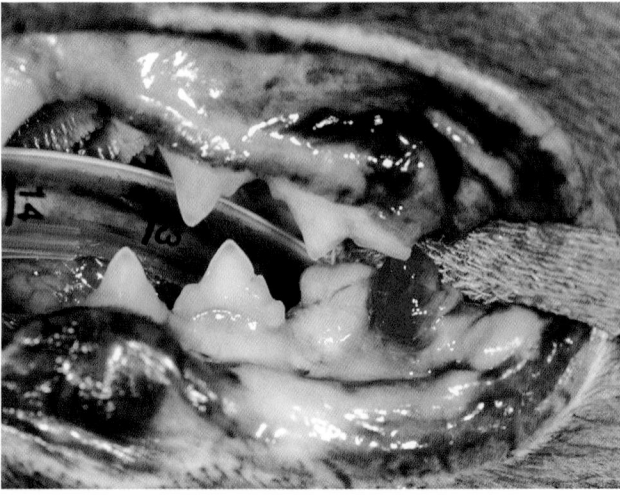

Figure 34.15 Traumatic occlusion of the left maxillary fourth premolar in a cat after extraction of the left mandibular first molar. Notice the proliferative inflammatory tissue in the buccal alveolar mucosa at the level of the previously extracted left mandibular first molar.

- After rostral or partial rostral maxillectomy
- Aggressive buccal alveolectomy during surgical extraction of the maxillary canine tooth

Diagnosis

Clinical signs of maxillary lip entrapment range from an indentation in the oral soft tissues, ulceration to puncture of the infolding maxillary lip that occurs after the extraction of the maxillary canine or oral mucosal polyp, and pyogenic granuloma of the vestibular mucogingival tissues of the extracted mandibular first molar where the cusp tip of the maxillary fourth premolar is occluding

Treatment (Figure 34.16)

- If the patient shows the ability to self-correct the lip entrapment and there is no resultant soft tissue trauma, treatment is not indicated.
- If the maxillary lip is swollen secondary to the extraction procedure, antiinflammatory medications may be successful at reducing the swelling, and the entrapment may resolve uneventfully after the swelling subsides.
- Conservative odontoplasty, without entry into the pulp chamber, blunting of the cusp tip of the offending tooth using a dental finishing bur
- Crown-height reduction of the mandibular canine followed by vital pulp therapy or standard root canal treatment (Figure 34.17)
- Extraction of the offending tooth: maxillary fourth premolar or mandibular canine

Outcome

The outcome after appropriate management of a patient's traumatic occlusion is good and will result in resolution of the associated soft tissue lesions and a rapid return to comfort.

Prevention

- Client communication regarding the potential for the occurrence of traumatic occlusion after the extraction of the maxillary canine or mandibular first molar teeth in cats; offer options to treat for such an outcome concurrently with the extraction or outline an appropriate action plan in the event of its occurrence
- Be conservative with buccal bone plate removal (alveolectomy) when extracting the maxillary canine tooth.
- Offer alternatives to extraction, such as root canal therapy for a fractured tooth.
- Treat for the potential traumatic occlusion at the same time as the extraction of the maxillary canine or mandibular first molar.

Relevant literature

In humans, one of the most frequent complications associated with tooth extractions is fracture of a portion of the root (Ness and Peterson 2004). Although the frequency of **root fracture** associated with tooth extractions in dogs and cats is unknown, it is routine (Harvey and Emily 1993). Every attempt should be made to extract infected roots. Infected tooth roots with radiolucencies around the root apex should not be left behind (Peterson 2003). In humans, uninfected roots left within the alveolar bone may become incorporated into the bone and remain in place without complications (Knutsson *et al.* 1989).

The probability that **oronasal fistula** will occur is said to be related to both the size and management of the communication (Peterson 2003). In dogs and cats, the etiology of chronic oronasal fistula is usually associated with canine tooth extraction or extraction of canine teeth with severe periodontitis (Smith 2000). Specific defect size guidelines for repair of oronasal communications incurred at the time of extraction in dogs and cats, aside from the obvious, do not exist. However, in humans, oronasal communications larger than 6 mm typically require more advanced repair, with a buccal flap, but those between 2 to 6 mm may be managed more conservatively with a collagen sponge pledget and figure of eight suture (Dennis 2009). The marked inflammatory response of the adjacent nasal structures and osteitis of the maxillary bone should be allowed to subside, usually for 2 months, before attempting closure of a fistula (Ross and Goldstein 1986).

The most severe complication associated with exodontia is **mandibular fracture**, which may occur during the extraction or as a later occurrence, usually within the first 4 weeks of the extraction (Bodner *et al.* 2011). The frequency of iatrogenic mandibular fracture in veterinary species is unknown, but in humans, this complication is rare, reported between 0.0034% and 0.0075% (Bodner *et al.* 2011). Predisposing factors for surgical-related mandibular fracture in humans include deep impaction, age, gender (male), dentoalveolar ankylosis, cyst formation, and other pathologic lesions (Pippi *et al.* 2010). The volume of mandible or the ratio of tooth to jaw bone has been reported to an important predisposing factor for mandibular fracture in humans and can be assessed before extraction by CT with buccolingual reconstruction (Wagner *et al.* 2005). Similarly, dogs, particularly smaller dogs, that have proportionally larger mandibular first molar teeth relative to mandibular height compared with larger dogs, may be prone to pathologic or extraction-induced fracture (Gioso *et al.* 2001). When the pathologic process has destroyed the lingual alveolar bone and the buccal alveolar bone is removed for the extraction, the risk of mandibular fracture during surgery is increased (Pippi *et al.* 2010). The buccal alveolar bone plate of the mandible is also approximately twice as thick as that of the maxilla; which creates significant resistance to extraction forces and a tendency to use heavier force (Scheels and Howard 1993). In the human literature, the mandibular third molar is the most common tooth involved in extraction-related mandibular fractures, but in dogs, the mandibular first molar and canine teeth appear to be the most commonly involved (Pippi *et al.* 2010). The symphysis and parasymphysis and mandibular body are locations of mandibular fracture predisposition in dogs and cats (Umphlet and Johnson 1988, 1990; Lopes *et al.* 2005). Iatrogenic mandibular fractures can be minimized through conservative bone removal and tooth sectioning (Iizuka *et al.* 1997). In dogs and cats, the use of a lingual approach may minimize the risk of mandibular fracture with mandibular canine extraction (Smith 1996). A technique involving application of a miniplate near or alongside the alveolar margin on the buccal side of the mandible to avoid rotational movements and postoperative mandibular fracture has been described (Pippi *et al.* 2010).

Tooth or root displacement into the nasal cavity or sinus is a complication associated with extraction of teeth (Kapatkin *et al.* 1990). Severe periodontal disease and tooth mobility may decrease the intrusive force necessary to induce orbital and nasal penetration of tooth roots (Ramsey *et al.* 1996; Taylor *et al.* 2004). The relative proximity of the caudal maxillary tooth roots to the orbit floor warrants great care when performing extractions in this area (Smith

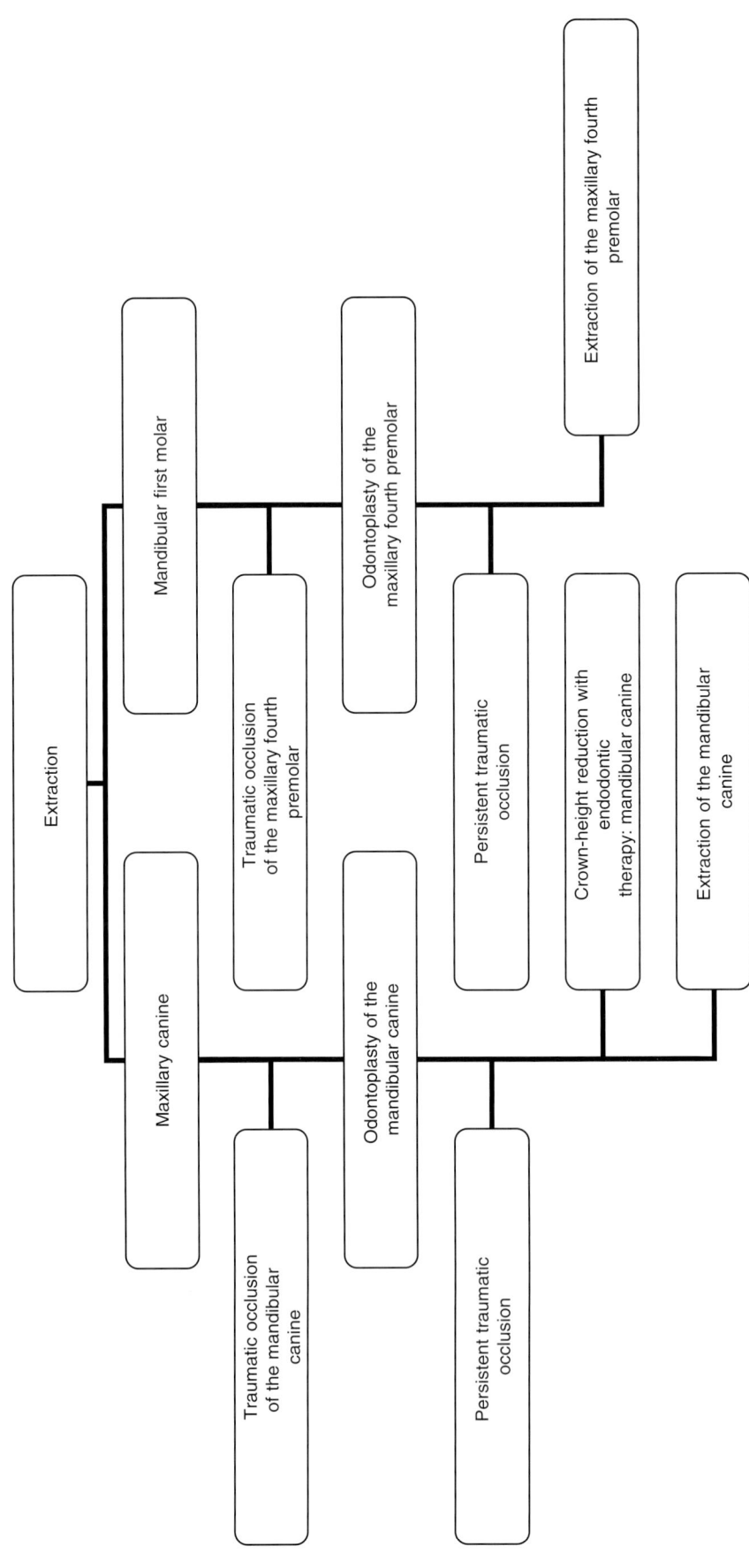

Figure 34.16 Decision tree for the management of traumatic occlusion.

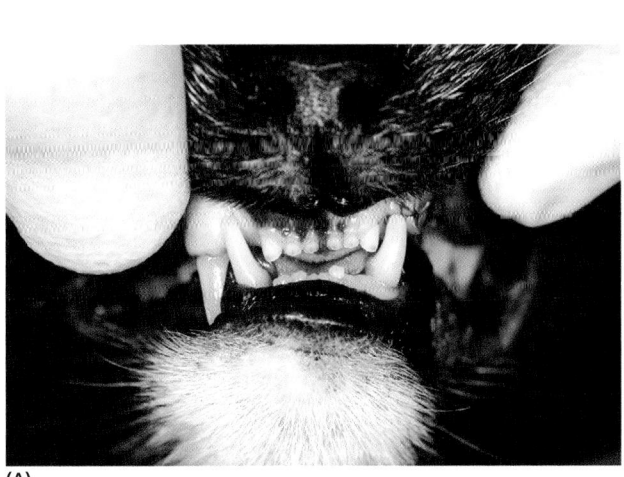
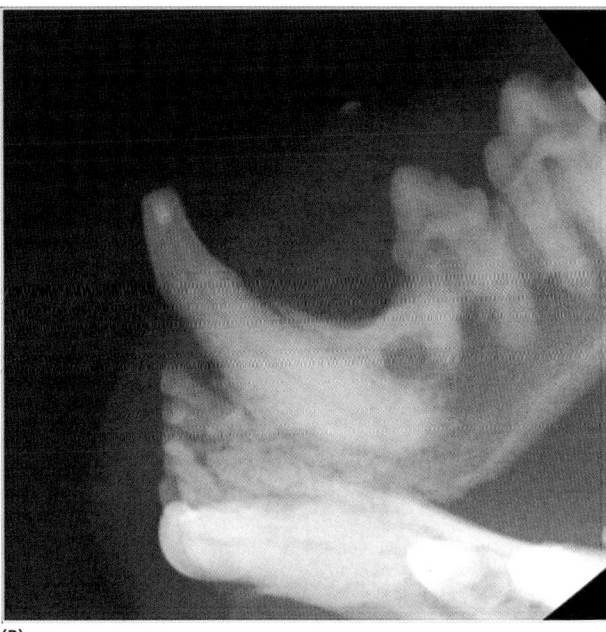

(A)   (B)

Figure 34.17 Crown-height reduction with vital pulpotomy of the left mandibular canine tooth performed immediately after extraction of the left maxillary canine tooth. **A,** Immediate postoperative clinical appearance of the extracted left maxillary canine and completed crown-height reduction and vital pulp therapy procedure on the left mandibular canine tooth. **B,** Intraoral lateral radiographic view of the left mandibular canine tooth after crown-height reduction and vital pulp therapy.

et al. 2003). Teeth displaced into the nasal cavity are foreign bodies and should be removed (Taylor *et al.* 2004).

Functional abnormalities after tooth extraction in dogs and cats are rare, even if all the teeth have been removed (Rossman *et al.* 1985). Glossoptosis, or ventral deviation of the tongue, is perhaps the most frequently mentioned of these abnormalities in dogs and lesser so in cats after extraction of the mandibular canine teeth (Wiggs and Lobprise 1997). In clinical practice, traumatic occlusions after exodontia are not uncommon, accompany extraction of the maxillary canine and mandibular first molar in cats, and should be a consideration before the extraction of these teeth. In a recent veterinary proceedings, chronic inflammation and local tissue irritation caused by bruxism was reviewed as a cause for the development of oral mucosal polyps adjacent to the mandibular first molar in cats (Lyon and Okuda 2009). Similar lesions in a case series of eight cats were reported as pyogenic granulomas; traumatic contact of the maxillary carnassial with the opposing mandibular oral soft tissues was suggested as the etiopathogenic mechanism (Riehl *et al.* 2014). Interestingly, however, missing mandibular first molar teeth were reported in only one cat, and traumatic contact of the ipsilateral maxillary carnassial with the lesions was identified in only 50% of the cases (Riehl *et al.* 2014). The relative omission in the literature of this clinically common complication is perhaps related to its subliminal inclusion in discussions regarding the rationale for endodontic therapy as an alternative to extraction of these strategic teeth.

References

Bodner, L., Brennan, P.A., McLeod, N.M. (2011) Characteristics of iatrogenic mandibular fractures associated with tooth removal: review and analysis of 189 cases. *British Journal of Oral and Maxillofacial Surgery* 49, 567-572.

Boudrieau, R.J.. Kudisch, M. (1996) Miniplate fixation for repair of mandibular and maxillary fractures in 15 dogs and 3 cats. *Veterinary Surgery* 25, 277-291.

Chiodo, T.A., Milles, M. (2009) Use of monocortical miniplates for the intraoral treatment of mandibular fractures. *Atlas of the Oral and Maxillofacial Surgery Clinics of North America* 17, 19-25.

Chrcanovic, B.R., Bueno, S.C., Da Silveira, D.T., et al. (2010) Traumatic displacement of maxillary permanent incisor into the nasal cavity. *Oral and Maxillofacial Surgery* 14, 175-182.

Cook, W. T., Smith, M. M., Markel, M. D., et al. (2001) Influence of an interdental full pin on stability of an acrylic external fixator for rostral mandibular fractures in dogs. *American Journal of Veterinary Research* 62, 576-580.

Dennis, M. J. (2009) Exodontia for the general dentist: complications. *Today's FDA* 21, 14-19.

Dupont, G. (1995) Crown amputation with intentional root retention for advanced feline resorptive lesions—a clinical study. *Journal of Veterinary Dentistry* 12, 9-13.

Gioso, M. A., Shofer, F., Barros, P. S., et al. (2001) Mandible and mandibular first molar tooth measurements in dogs: relationship of radiographic height to body weight. *Journal of Veterinary Dentistry* 18, 65-68.

Gorzelnik, L., Kozlovsky, E. (2009) Bicortical extraoral plating of mandibular fractures. *Atlas of Oral and Maxillofacial Surgery Clinics of North America* 17, 35-43.

Harvey, C.E., Emily, P.P. (1993) Oral surgery. In *Small Animal Dentistry.* Mosby-Year Book, St. Louis, pp. 312-377.

Iizuka, T., Tanner, S., Berthold, H. (1997) Mandibular fractures following third molar extraction. A retrospective clinical and radiological study. *International Journal of Oral and Maxillofacial Surgery* 26, 338-343.

Kapatkin, A.S., Manfra Marretta, S., Schloss, A. J. (1990) Problems associated with basic oral surgical techniques. *Problems in Veterinary Medicine* 2, 85-109.

Knutsson, K., Lysell, L., Rohlin, M. (1989) Postoperative status after partial removal of the mandibular third molar. *Swedish Dental Journal* 13, 15-22.

Lopes, F.M., Gioso, M.A., Ferro, D.G., et al. (2005) Oral fractures in dogs of Brazil—a retrospective study. *Journal of Veterinary Dentistry* 22, 86-90.

Lyon, K.F., Okuda, A. (2009) Feline oral mucosal inflammatory polyps. *Proceedings of the 23rd Annual Veterinary Dental Forum*, Scottsdale, AZ.

Ness, G.M., Peterson, L.J. (2004) Impacted teeth. In Miloro, M., Ghali, G.E., Larsen, P.E., Waite, P.D. (eds.) *Peterson's Principles of Oral and Maxillofacial Surgery,* 2nd edn. BC Decker, Hamilton, Ontario pp. 139-156.

Pacchiana, P.D., Burnside, P.K., Wilkens, B.E., et al. (2001) Primary bronchotomy for removal of an intrabronchial foreign body in a dog. *Journal of the American Animal Hospital Association* 37, 582-585.

Peterson, L.J. (2003) Prevention and management of surgical complications. In Peterson, L.J., Ellis, E. III, Hupp, J.R. Tucker, M.R. (eds.) *Contemporary Oral and Maxillofacial Surgery*, 4th edn. Mosby, St. Louis, pp. 221-237.

Pippi, R., Solidani, M., Broglia, S., et al. (2010) Prevention of mandibular fractures caused by difficult surgical extractions: report of a borderline case. *Journal of Oral and Maxillofacial Surgery* 68, 1162-1165.

Ramsey, D.T., Marretta, S.M., Hamor, R.E., et al. (1996) Ophthalmic manifestations and complications of dental disease in dogs and cats. *Journal of the American Animal Hospital Association* 32, 215-224.

Riehl, J., Bell C.M., Constantaras M., et al. (2014) Clinicopathologic characterization of oral pyogenic granuloma: a previously unnamed mucogingival lesion in cats—8 cases. *Journal of Veterinary Dentistry* 31 (2), 80-86.

Ross, D.L., Goldstein, G. S. (1986) Oral surgery. Basic techniques. *Veterinary Clinics of North America: Small Animal Practice* 16, 967-981.

Rossman, L.E., Garber, D.A., Harvey, C.E. (1985) Disorders of teeth. In Harvey, C.E. (ed.) *Veterinary Dentistry*. WB Saunders, Philadelphia, pp. 79-105.

Scheels, J.L., Howard, P. E. (1993) Principles of dental extraction. *Veterinary Medicine and Surgery (Small Animal)* 8, 146-154.

Smith, M.M. (1996) Lingual approach for surgical extraction of the mandibular canine tooth in dogs and cats. *Journal of the American Animal Hospital Association* 32, 359-364.

Smith, M.M. (2000) Oronasal fistula repair. *Clinical Techniques in Small Animal Practice* 15, 243-250.

Smith, M.M., Smith, E.M., La Croix, N., et al. (2003) Orbital penetration associated with tooth extraction. *Journal of Veterinary Dentistry* 20, 8-17.

Taylor, T.N., Smith, M.M., Snyder, L. (2004) Nasal displacement of a tooth root in a dog. *Journal of Veterinary Dentistry* 21, 222-225.

Umphlet, R.C., Johnson, A.L. (1988) Mandibular fractures in the cat. A retrospective study. *Veterinary Surgery* 17, 333-337.

Umphlet, R.C., Johnson, A.L. (1990) Mandibular fractures in the dog. A retrospective study of 157 cases. *Veterinary Surgery* 19, 272-275.

Van Cauwelaert De Wyels, S. (1998) Alveolar osteitis (dry socket) in a dog: a case report. *Journal of Veterinary Dentistry* 15, 85-87.

Wagner, K.W., Otten, J.E., Schoen, R., et al. (2005) Pathological mandibular fractures following third molar removal. *International Journal of Oral and Maxillofacial Surgery* 34, 722-726.

Wiggs, R.B., Lobprise, H.B. (1997) Oral surgery. In Wiggs, R.B., Lobprise, H.B. (eds.) *Veterinary Dentistry: Principles and Practice*. Lippincott-Raven, Philadelphia, pp. 232-258.

Woodward, T.M. (2006) Extraction of fractured tooth roots. *Journal of Veterinary Dentistry* 23, 126-129.

35 Tonsillectomy

Jonathan Bray

Institute of Veterinary, Animal and Biomedical Sciences, Massey University, Palmerston North, New Zealand

Surgical removal of the palatine tonsils is performed for three reasons: (1) cases of persistent tonsillitis that are unresponsive to antibiotic therapy, (2) to remove neoplastic growths that may develop on the tonsil, and (3) as part of management of brachycephalic airway syndrome (Dean 1991; Montague *et al.* 2002; Fasanella *et al.* 2010; Mathews 2012).

Specific complication rates after tonsillectomy are not reported but are generally considered to be very low (Dean 1991; Mathews 2012). For malignant neoplasia, persistence of clinical signs and tumor recurrence are the main postoperative concerns (Todoroff and Brodey 1979; Mathews 2012).

Hemorrhage
See Chapter 13.

Pharyngeal edema
See Chapter 25.

Aspiration pneumonia
See Chapter 25.

Recurrence of disease

Definition
Clinical signs of tonsillar disease include dysphagia, odynophagia (pain on swallowing), or obstruction of the pharynx caused by a physical mass. Persistence or recurrence of these clinical signs may occur in cases of neoplasia.

Risk factors
- Neoplastic disease affecting the tonsil is the most common reason for clinical signs to persist or recur after tonsillectomy.
- Regrowth of hyperplastic tissue may occur in inflammatory or infectious disease if incomplete removal of all tonsillar tissue was performed during the initial surgery.

Diagnosis
- Neoplastic disease may recur locally or arise from regional lymph nodes. Diagnosis is usually confirmed by fine-needle aspiration or biopsy of affected tissues.
- Thoracic radiographs or abdominal ultrasonography may be required to diagnose the development of distant metastatic disease affecting the lungs, liver, or other sites.

Treatment
- Treatment options for recurrent neoplastic disease are very limited, with most animals being euthanized as a consequence of poor quality of life (Todoroff and Brodey 1979; Mas *et al.* 2011; Mathews 2012).
- Repeated surgical resection of regrown tonsillar tissue may be considered for infectious or inflammatory disease.

Outcome
The prognosis for tonsillar carcinoma is very poor, and no single treatment or combination of treatments has been shown to be highly effective.

Prevention
The use of adjuvant treatments such as radiotherapy or chemotherapy may improve disease-free intervals after surgical excision of tonsillar tumors.

Relevant literature
Complications after routine tonsillectomy for infectious or benign inflammatory or neoplastic are infrequent, and precise incidences are not published. The absence of published data would suggest that with appropriate care, tonsillectomy can be accomplished with few consequences.

In human surgery, a variety of techniques are used for adenotonsillectomy, a technique that is considered to be one of the most commonly performed in the world (O-Lee and Rowe 2004; Johnson *et al.* 2008). Techniques include the use of scalpel and scissors; tonsillar snare; electrocautery; and a combination of more advanced technologies, including harmonic scalpel. Electrocautery ablation techniques have been shown to be associated with decreased bleeding and shortened surgery time, with consequent cost savings through improved operative efficiency (O-Lee and Rowe 2004; Johnson *et al.* 2008). Similar comparative studies are not available in the veterinary literature (Mathews 2012).

Tonsillar carcinomas have usually infiltrated local tissues and metastasized by the time of diagnosis, so surgery alone is often ineffective at providing prolonged disease control. Tumor development has also been reported to occur in the contralateral tonsil, even if gross enlargement is not present at the time of surgery. Bilateral tonsillectomy is therefore recommended in all cases (Mathews 2012).

The prognosis after surgery for tonsillar carcinoma is very poor, with median survival times reported between 110 and 270 days (Todoroff and Brodey 1979; MacMillan *et al.* 1982; Brooks *et al.* 1988; Schmidt *et al.* 2001; de Vos *et al.* 2005; Murphy *et al.* 2006; Mas *et al.* 2011). Published case series are typically small and retrospective in nature.

There is some evidence to suggest that the use of piroxicam may increase disease-free interval and overall survival times for patients with tonsillar carcinoma, but results of larger prospective trials are required (Schmidt *et al.* 2001; de Vos *et al.* 2005).

The use of treatments such as radiotherapy or chemotherapy may improve disease-free intervals without surgical excision of tonsillar tumors (MacMillan *et al.* 1982; Brooks *et al.* 1988).

Although some individual animals can enjoy prolonged survival times of 2 years or more after diagnosis, predicting long-term survivors is difficult. In one study, patients with anorexia or lethargy at the time of diagnosis had a poorer prognosis (Mas *et al.* 2011).

References

Brooks, M.B., Matus, R.E., Leifer, C.E., et al. (1988) Chemotherapy versus chemotherapy plus radiotherapy in the treatment of tonsillar squamous cell carcinoma in the dog. *Journal of Veterinary Internal Medicine* 2, 206-211.

de Vos, J.P., Burm, A.G., Focker, A.P., et al. (2005) Piroxicam and carboplatin as a combination treatment of canine oral non-tonsillar squamous cell carcinoma: a pilot study and a literature review of a canine model of human head and neck squamous cell carcinoma. *Veterinary Comparative Oncology* 3, 16-24.

Dean, P.W. (1991) Surgery of the tonsils. *Problems in Veterinary Medicine* 3, 298-303.

Fasanella, F.J., Shivley, J.M., Wardlaw, J.L., et al. (2010) Brachycephalic airway obstructive syndrome in dogs: 90 cases (1991-2008). *Journal of the American Veterinary Medical Association* 237, 1048-1051.

Johnson, K., Vaughan, A., Derkay, C., et al. (2008) Microdebrider vs electrocautery: a comparison of tonsillar wound healing histopathology in a canine model. *Otolaryngology Head and Neck Surgery* 138, 486-491.

MacMillan, R., Withrow, S.J., and Gillette, E.L. (1982) Surgery and regional irradiation for treatment of canine tonsillar squamous cell carcinoma: retrospective review of eight cases. *Journal of the American Animal Hospital Association* 18, 311-314.

Mas, A., Blackwood, L., Cripps, P., et al. (2011) Canine tonsillar squamous cell carcinoma—a multi-centre retrospective review of 44 clinical cases. *Journal of Small Animal Practice* 52, 359-364.

Mathews, K.G. (2012) Tonsillectomy. In Verstraete, F.J.M., Lommer, M.J. (eds.) *Oral and Maxillofacial Surgery in Dogs and Cats.* Elsevier, St. Louis, pp. 343-350.

Montague, A.L., Markey, B.K., Bassett, H.F., et al. (2002) A study of greyhounds with tonsillar enlargement and a history of poor racing performance. *Veterinary Journal* 164, 106-115.

Murphy, S., Hayes, A., Adams, V., et al. (2006) Role of carboplatin in multi-modality treatment of canine tonsillar squamous cell carcinoma—a case series of five dogs. *Journal of Small Animal Practice* 47, 216-220.

O-Lee, T.J., and Rowe, M. (2004) Electrocautery versus cold knife technique adenotonsillectomy: a cost analysis. *Otolaryngology Head and Neck Surgery* 131, 723-726.

Schmidt, B.R., Glickman, N.W., DeNicola, D.B., et al. (2001) Evaluation of piroxicam for the treatment of oral squamous cell carcinoma in dogs. *Journal of the American Veterinary Medical Association* 218, 1783-1786.

Todoroff, R.J., Brodey, R.S. (1979) Oral and pharyngeal neoplasia in the dog: a retrospective survey of 361 cases. *Journal of the American Veterinary Medical Association* 175, 567-571.

36 Repair of Congenital Defects of the Hard and Soft Palates

Jonathan Bray

Institute of Veterinary, Animal and Biomedical Sciences, Massey University, Palmerston North, New Zealand

Congenital defects of the hard or soft palate can arise because of failure of embryonic structures to fuse on the midline, with subsequent disruption of normal tissue differentiation at these sites (Kelly and Bardach 2012). Fusion of the central palate structures should occur at crucial times in the embryo, and a range of genetic and environmental factors have been implicated that could disrupt this process (Richtsmeier *et al.* 1994; Elwood and Colquhoun 1997; Kemp *et al.* 2009; Davies 2011; Kelly and Bardach 2012). Affected animals can often have other developmental defects, including polydactyly, middle ear disease, hydrocephalus, microphthalmia, atresia ani, kyphosis, and limb deformities (Gregory 2000; White *et al.* 2009; Kelly and Bardach 2012; Woodbridge *et al.* 2012).

Surgical repair of the defect is usually essential to enable the animal to achieve a normal degree of independence for eating and drinking. In most cases, repair is delayed until the patient is 3 to 4 months of age; at this age, the patient is larger, so there is more tissue available for the closure, and the impact of growth retardation on maxillary growth will be less (Waldron and Martin 1991; Kelly and Bardach 2012; Marretta 2012). Because successful resolution relies on a client who is able to make a significant commitment to supporting the patient's dietary needs until closure is achieved, an early assessment on the viability of a repair is essential. Some defects are too large to close, and others may require multiple procedures to achieve complete resolution.

Hemorrhage
See Chapter 13.

Pharyngeal edema
See Chapter 25.

Aspiration pneumonia
See Chapter 25.

Dehiscence and oronasal fistula formation

Definition
This is separation or breakdown of the original repair. Dehiscence can develop anywhere along the repair, but the most frequent site is in the area of the incisive foramen (Waldron and Martin 1991; Marretta 2012) (Figure 36.1).

When dehiscence occurs, communication between the oral and nasal cavities is reestablished with creation of an oronasal fistula. Food, liquid, or other material can be forced into the fistula during swallowing, causing irritation of the nasal tissues.

Risk factors
Wound dehiscence is the most common complication after attempted cleft palate repair. Successful healing of the initial repair depends on creation of a tension-free closure and maintenance of a secure blood supply (Waldron and Martin 1991; Marretta 2012).

- Recommended techniques for closure of large hard palate defects usually rely on mucoperiosteal flaps (i.e. either the von Langenbeck or overlapping flap techniques). These flaps are completely reliant on the palatine artery for their survival (Fernandes *et al.* 2002; Kelly and Bardach, 2012). Care is therefore essential during elevation of the flap to avoid lacerating, attenuating or disrupting the palatine arteries as they exit the major palatine foramen (Figure 36.2).

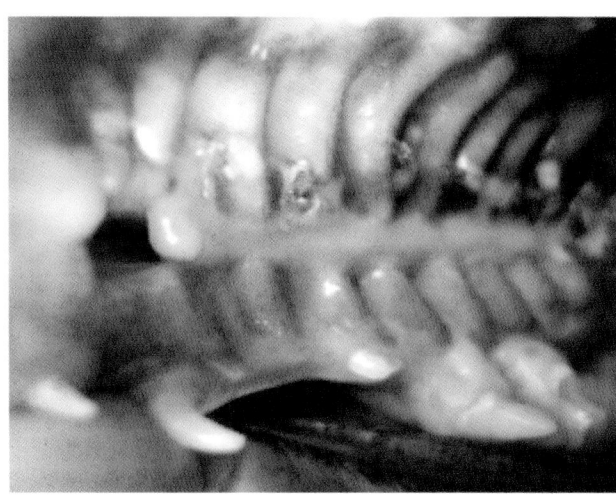

Figure 36.1 A common site for failure of a congenital hard palate repair is around the incisive foramen.

Complications in Small Animal Surgery, First Edition. Edited by Dominique Griffon and Annick Hamaide.
© 2016 John Wiley & Sons, Inc. Published 2016 by John Wiley & Sons, Inc.
Companion website: www.wiley.com/go/griffon/complications

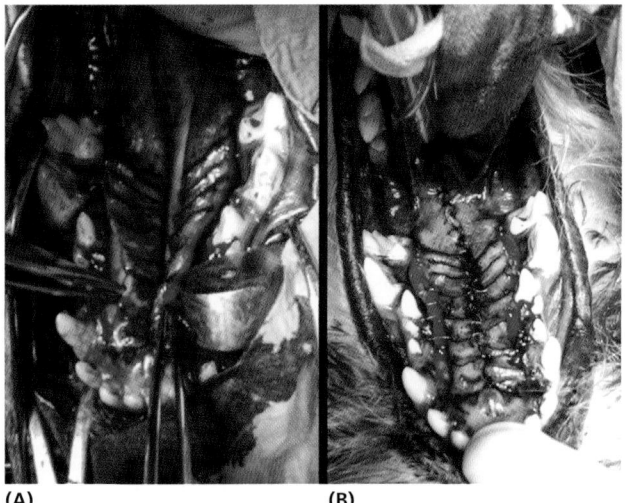

(A)   **(B)**

Figure 36.2 Optimal repair of a congenital hard palate defect is achieved by adherence to good surgical principles. This includes maintenance of a secure blood supply to the raised mucoperiosteal flaps (**A**) and a tension-free closure (**B**).

- Repair of cleft soft palate defects is usually more successful because tissue at this site is more flexible, and a two-layer closure is often achievable (Waldron and Martin 1991; Griffiths and Sullivan 2001; Warzee *et al.* 2001; Headrick and McAnulty 2004; Marretta 2012). However, some animals with a hypoplastic soft palate may continue to have signs of oronasal reflux even if an effective tissue barrier has been created. This is because the reconstructed mucosal shelf cannot replicate the contribution a normal palatine muscle would make to the coordinated swallowing activities of the tongue, pharynx, and larynx; as a consequence, food particles may become refluxed during deglutition.
- Some authors recommend the use of feeding tubes to reduce contamination and continual abrasion to the primary repair, but this is probably not required in every case (Marretta 2012).

Diagnosis

Dehiscence is usually diagnosed by visual evaluation of the oral cavity defect in the postoperative period or because of signs associated with the oronasal fistula, which may include sneezing, gagging, nasal discharge, and halitosis (Marretta 2012).

Small defects can often be associated with more clinical signs than larger defects because objects become trapped in the nasal tissues and cannot be expelled.

Treatment

- Treatment of a dehiscence is usually only necessary if clinical signs are present.
- Any attempted repair is best delayed for 4 to 6 weeks. The patient may need to be supported during this period with the use of feeding tubes (Marretta 2012).
- Options for treatment of a dehisced wound depend on the reason for the dehiscence and the location of the dehiscence.
- Repair solutions using autogenous tissue may include simple resuturing (with or without reelevation of the mucoperiosteal flap), single-layer vestibular flaps, flaps raised from the skin, or the angularis oris axial pattern buccal flap.
- A variety of prosthetic appliances made from silicone, stainless steel, titanium, or soft polymethyl methacrylate have been described, with mixed success.

Outcome

Although successful repair after dehiscence can often be achieved in time, owners need to be willing to persist with patient care and financial commitments in the meantime.

Prevention

Management of dehiscence from a cleft palate repair can be very difficult, and every effort should be taken for the first repair to be successful by adhering to sound surgical technique. If wound repair has failed because of poor owner or patient compliance, these issues need to be addressed before progressing with subsequent attempts at repair.

Success with closure of a wound dehiscence for a cleft palate and associated oronasal fistula will decline with each subsequent repair attempt. Optimal results are achieved during the first surgery.

Growth abnormalities

Definition

Elevation of mucoperiosteal flaps disrupts growth centers on the palate. Therefore, if these flaps are elevated too early in life, various maxillofacial deformities may arise.

Risk factors

Elevation of mucoperiosteal flaps before full rostral growth of the maxilla may cause shortening of the maxillofacial region.

Diagnosis

Potential problems include dental malocclusion and alterations in maxillary height, width, and length. However, clinical problems associated with growth abnormalities have not been reported in dogs or cats.

Treatment

No treatment is generally required.

Prevention

Although clinical problems have not been reported, it is still recommended that attempted repair of congenital oronasal fistula be delayed until the animal is at least 3 to 4 months of age, particularly if mucoperiosteal flaps are going to be used in the repair.

Relevant literature

Dogs have acted as surrogate models for investigation of congenital palatine defect repair in humans since the 1950s (Kelly and Bardach 2012). Consequently, an extensive amount of experimental research is available. Perhaps because a significant component of cleft palate repair success in humans is focused around maintenance of speech (Kelly and Bardach 2012), some nuances of repair in humans are less relevant for veterinary patients. For example, the ability to create intelligible speech depends on a functional velopharyngeal valve. This can become incompetent when the soft palate and the lateral or posterior pharyngeal walls fail to separate the oral cavity from the nasal cavity during speech (Havstam *et al.* 2010). The hypothesis that early elevation of mucoperiosteal flaps could interfere with normal maxillofacial development was first proposed in the 1940s (Kelly and Bardach 2012). Accumulated experimental evidence since then has tended to support this hypothesis, although the precise mechanism remains unclear (Alkhairy 1993; Bardach *et al.* 1993, 1994; Leenstra *et al.* 1995a, 1999; Ascherman *et al.* 2000). Clinical consequences of maxillofacial deformities have not been reported in dogs or cats, but it is still recommended to delay repair until maxillary longitudinal growth is largely completed at 4 to 5 months of age. In veterinary patients, the rationale for waiting to this time period is more influenced by the observation that there is more palatal tissue to work with by this age, and the tissues are more robust and tolerant of surgical manipulation (Waldron and Martin 1991; Wijdeveld *et al.* 1991; Marretta 2012).

Wound dehiscence is the most common complication after attempted cleft palate repair (Waldron and Martin 1991; Marretta 2012). The surgical wound is subject to constant contamination from food, bacteria, saliva, nasal secretions, and other liquids. Constant abrasion of the wound surface by the tongue also occurs. Successful healing depends on creation of a tension-free closure and maintenance of a secure blood supply.

Some authors recommend the use of feeding tubes (e.g., naso-esophageal, esophageal, or percutaneous endoscopic gastrostomy tubes) in the postoperative period to reduce contamination and continual abrasion to the primary repair. There is insufficient evidence to suggest that the use of a feeding tube would eliminate the risk of dehiscence in all cases. However, the use of a feeding tube may be a useful consideration for a repair that is believed to be at more risk of dehiscence because of increased tension or other local factors (Marretta, 2012).

Treatment of a dehiscence may only be necessary if clinical signs of oronasal fistulation are present. Many small defects (<3 mm in size) will ultimately contract or may persist with no detrimental impact on the patient. In most cases, any attempted repair is best delayed for 4 to 6 weeks. This allows inflammation and neutrophilic activity at the dehisced edges to resolve, provides an opportunity for the microcirculation to recover from the previous surgical insult, and ensures the remaining sections of the wounded tissue have gained more strength. The patient may need to be supported during this period with the use of feeding tubes to ensure daily calorie requirements are maintained, and localized irritation by the continued presence of foreign material (food particles etc) within the fistulous tract can be negated.

Options for treatment of a dehisced wound depend on the reason for the dehiscence and the location of the dehiscence. The principles of repair remain as for the initial repair: tension-free closure with robust, well-vascularized tissue. Although a two-layer closure is optimal, this may not be achievable in all cases. When this is not possible, choosing a technique that avoids the primary suture line being located over the primary defect is desirable.

Repair solutions using autogenous tissue may include simple resuturing (with or without elevation of the mucoperiosteal flap), single-layer vestibular flaps, flaps raised from the skin, or the angularis oris axial pattern buccal flap (Luskin 2000; Bryant *et al.* 2003; Dundas *et al.* 2005; Sivacolundhu 2007; Yates *et al.* 2007; Marretta 2012). These techniques are more typically described for the management of traumatically created defects in the palate, so they are often better suited to small, localized lesions. However, their ability to reach lesions in the middle of the palate may restrict their use. There are no specific reports that details precise management of complications of dehiscence after repair of a congenial cleft palate, so the clinician will need to evaluate the suitability of these options for the specific defect they are attending to.

Transplanted free grafts of auricular cartilage have also been reported for the management of small persistent oronasal fistulae in the dog and cat (Cox *et al.* 2007; Soukup *et al.* 2009). The edges of the cartilaginous graft are placed into a mucosal pocket created about the circumference of the fistula and sutured in place. The exposed surface of the cartilaginous graft covers the fistula and provides a shelf for granulation and mucosal epithelialization on the oral and nasal sides of the graft. In one study, auricular cartilage grafts proved successful in achieving closure of chronic small oronasal fistulae in five cats (Cox *et al.* 2007).

If adequate autogenous tissue is no longer available for creation of a suitable flap, a variety of prosthetic appliances made from silicone, stainless steel, titanium, or soft polymethyl methacrylate have been described for chronic oronasal fistulae, with mixed success (Smith and Rockhill 1996; Smith 2000; Kuipers von Lande *et al.* 2012; Marretta 2012). In one report, a nasal septal button (designed for human use) was trimmed to successfully close an oronasal fistula in a cat (Smith and Rockhill, 1996). Rapid prototype modeling of a titanium plate has also been reported for closure of persistent oronasal fistula in a dog (Kuipers von Lande *et al.* 2012). In both cases, the prosthodontic provided an effective barrier against food and liquid passing though the oronasal fistula and allowed clinical signs relating to the fistula to be well controlled. However, food particles and other material (e.g., grass, fur) can become entrapped around the edge of the device; regular cleaning by rinsing the area with saline was required to control halitosis.

References

Alkhairy, F. (1993) Effect on craniofacial growth of simultaneous cleft lip and palate repair. *Plastic and Reconstructive Surgery* 92, 379-380.

Ascherman, J.A., Marin, V.P., Rogers, L., et al. (2000) Palatal distraction in a canine cleft palate model. *Plastic and Reconstructive Surgery* 105, 1687-1694.

Bardach, J., Kelly, K.M., Salyer, K.E. (1993) A comparative study of facial growth following lip and palate repair performed in sequence and simultaneously: an experimental study in beagles. *Plastic and Reconstructive Surgery* 91, 1008-1016.

Bardach, J., Kelly, K.M., Salyer, K.E. (1994) Relationship between the sequence of lip and palate repair and maxillary growth: an experimental study in beagles. *Plastic and Reconstructive Surgery* 93, 269-278.

Bryant, K.J., Moore, K., McAnulty, J.F. (2003) Angularis oris axial pattern buccal flap for reconstruction of recurrent fistulae of the palate. *Veterinary Surgery* 32, 113-119.

Cox, C.L., Hunt, G.B., Cadier, M.M. (2007) Repair of oronasal fistulae using auricular cartilage grafts in five cats. *Veterinary Surgery* 36, 164-169.

Davies, M. (2011) Excess vitamin A intake during pregnancy as a possible cause of congenital cleft palate in puppies and kittens. *Veterinary Record* 169, 107.

Dundas, J.M., Fowler, J.D., Shmon, C.L., et al. (2005) Modification of the superficial cervical axial pattern skin flap for oral reconstruction. *Veterinary Surgery* 34, 206-213.

Elwood, J.M., Colquhoun, T.A. (1997) Observations on the prevention of cleft palate in dogs by folic acid and potential relevance to humans. *New Zealand Veterinary Journal* 45, 254-256.

Fernandes, A., Wafae, N., Yamashita, H.K. (2002) Angiographic study of the arterial supply to the palatine mucoperiosteum. *Annals of Anatomy* 184, 41-44.

Gregory, S.P. (2000) Middle ear disease associated with congenital palatine defects in seven dogs and one cat. *Journal of Small Animal Practice* 41, 398-401.

Griffiths, L.G., Sullivan, M. (2001) Bilateral overlapping mucosal single-pedicle flaps for correction of soft palate defects. *Journal of the American Animal Hospital Association* 37, 183-186.

Havstam, C., Sandberg, A.D., Lohmander, A. (2011) Communication attitude and speech in 10-year-old children with cleft (lip and) palate: An ICF perspective. *International Journal of Speech-Language Pathology* 13, 156-164.

Headrick, J.F., McAnulty, J.F. (2004) Reconstruction of a bilateral hypoplastic soft palate in a cat. *Journal of the American Animal Hospital Association* 40, 86-90.

Kelly, K.M., Bardach, J. (2012) Biologic basis of cleft palate and palatal surgery. In Verstraete, F.J.M., Lommer, M.J. (eds.) *Oral and Maxillofacial Surgery in Dogs and Cats*. Elsevier, St. Louis, pp. 343-350.

Kemp, C., Thiele, H., Dankof, A., et al. (2009) Cleft lip and/or palate with monogenic autosomal recessive transmission in Pyrenees shepherd dogs. *The Cleft Palate-Craniofacial Journal* 46, 81-88.

Kuipers von Lande, R.G., Worth, A.J., Peckitt, N.S., et al. (2012) Rapid prototype modeling and customized titanium plate fabrication for correction of a persistent hard palate defect in a dog. *Journal of the American Veterinary Medical Association* 240, 1316-1322.

Leenstra, T.S., Kuijpers-Jagtman, A.M., Maltha, J.C., et al. (1995a) Palatal surgery without denudation of bone favours dentoalveolar development in dogs. *International Journal of Oral and Maxillofacial Surgery* 24, 440-444.

Leenstra, T.S., Maltha, J.C., Kuijpers-Jagtman, A.M., et al. (1995b) Wound healing in beagle dogs after palatal repair without denudation of bone. *The Cleft Palate- Craniofacial Journal* 32, 363-369; discussion 369-370.

Leenstra, T.S., Kuijpers-Jagtman, A.M., Maltha, J.C. (1999) The healing process of palatal tissues after operations with and without denudation of bone: an experimental study in dogs. *Scandinavian Journal of Plastic and Reconstructive Surgery and Hand Surgery* 33, 169-176.

Luskin, I.R. (2000) Reconstruction of oral defects using mucogingival pedicle flaps. *Clinical Techniques in Small Animal Practice* 15, 251-259.

Maretta, S.M. (2012) Repair of acquired palatal defects. In Verstraete, F.J.M., Lommer, M.J. (eds.) *Oral and Maxillofacial Surgery in Dogs and Cats*. Elsevier, St. Louis, pp. 343-350.

Marretta, S.M. (2012) Cleft palate repair techniques. In Verstraete, F.J.M., Lommer, M.J. (eds.) *Oral and Maxillofacial Surgery in Dogs and Cats*. Elsevier, St. Louis, pp. 351-361.

Richtsmeier, J.T., Sack, G.H. Jr., Grausz, H.M., et al. (1994) Cleft palate with autosomal recessive transmission in Brittany spaniels. *The Cleft Palate-Craniofacial Journal* 31, 364-371.

Sivacolundhu, R.K. (2007) Use of local and axial pattern flaps for reconstruction of the hard and soft palate. *Clinical Techniques in Small Animal Practice* 22, 61-69.

Smith, M.M. (2000) Oronasal fistula repair. *Clinical Techniques in Small Animal Practice* 15, 243-250.

Smith, M.M., Rockhill, A.D. (1996) Prosthodontic appliance for repair of an oronasal fistula in a cat. *Journal of the American Veterinary Medical Association* 208, 1410-1412.

Soukup, J.W., Snyder, C.J., Gengler, W.R. (2009) Free auricular cartilage autograft for repair of an oronasal fistula in a dog. *Journal of Veterinary Dentistry* 26, 86-95.

Waldron, D.R., Martin, R.A. (1991) Cleft palate repair. *Problems in Veterinary Medicine* 3, 142-152.

Warzee, C.C., Bellah, J.R., Richards, D. (2001) Congenital unilateral cleft of the soft palate in six dogs. *Journal of Small Animal Practice* 42, 338-340.

White, R.N., Hawkins, H.L., Alemi, V.P., et al. (2009) Soft palate hypoplasia and concurrent middle ear pathology in six dogs. *Journal of Small Animal Practice* 50, 364-372.

Wijdeveld, M.G., Maltha, J.C., Grupping, E.M., et al. (1991). A histological study of tissue response to simulated cleft palate surgery at different ages in beagle dogs. *Archives of Oral Biology* 36, 837-843.

Woodbridge, N.T., Baines, E.A., Baines, S.J. (2012) Otitis media in five cats associated with soft palate abnormalities. *Veterinary Record* 171, 124.

Yates, G., Landon, B., and Edwards, G. (2007) Investigation and clinical application of a novel axial pattern flap for nasal and facial reconstruction in the dog. *Australian Veterinary Journal* 85, 113-118.

SECTION 5

Thoracic Surgery

37 General Complications

Hervé Brissot

University of Nottingham, Pride Veterinary Centre, Derby, UK

Postoperative complications after thoracic surgery are mainly associated with surgical wound complications, pleural effusion, pulmonary complications, hypothermia, cardiac arrhythmias, postoperative pain, and inadequate ventilation. Wound complication appears to be the most common complication of thoracic surgery and is reported in 20% to 40% of the cases (Tattersall and Welsh 2006; Moores *et al.* 2007). Seroma, wound inflammation, infection, and postoperative lameness are the most reported complications.

Early signs of postoperative complication include alteration of the respiratory function and development of dyspnea, which should be closely monitored during the first postoperative hours and days (Sigrist *et al.* 2011)(Figure 37.1).

Hemothorax

Definition

Hemothorax is the accumulation in the pleural space of a hemorrhagic effusion with a packed cell volume (PCV) equal to or greater than PCV of circulating blood (or superior to 20%).

Risk factors

- Clotting disorder, platelet dysfunction
- "En-bloc" lobectomy (mechanical but more often hand made)
- Inflamed and neovascularized serosa (pleura or pericardium)
- Lung metastases, atrial tumor

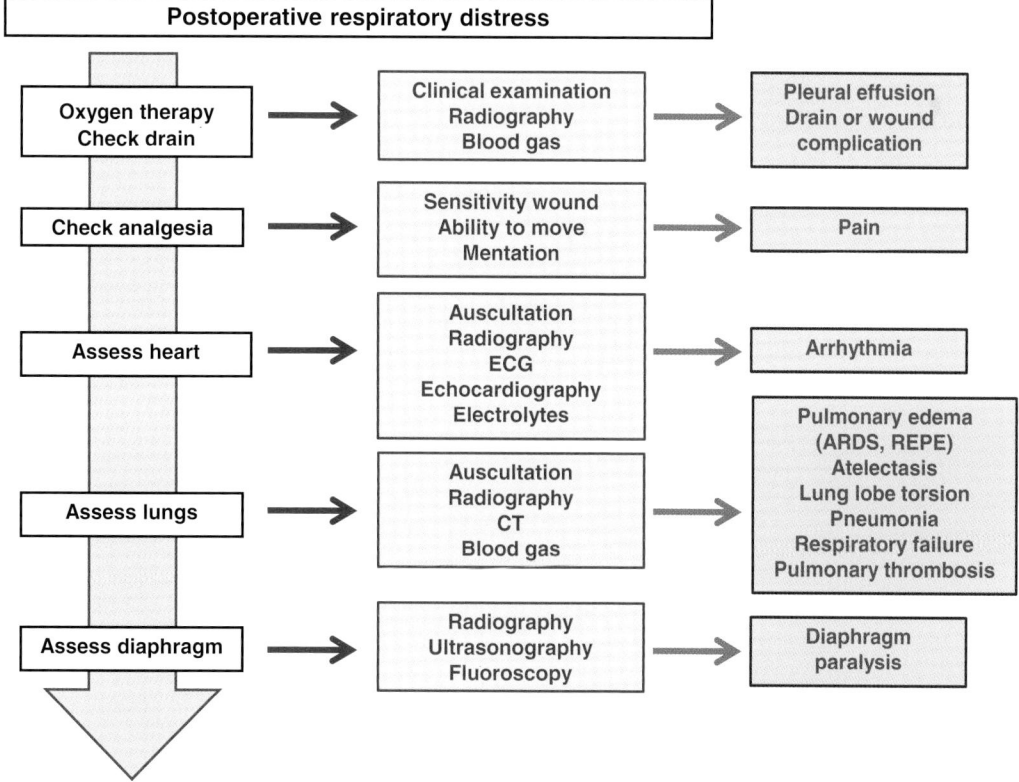

Figure 37.1 Differential diagnosis of postoperative dyspnea after thoracic surgery. ARDS, acute respiratory distress syndrome; CT, computed tomography; ECG, electrocardiography; REPE, reexpansion pulmonary edema.

Complications in Small Animal Surgery, First Edition. Edited by Dominique Griffon and Annick Hamaide.
© 2016 John Wiley & Sons, Inc. Published 2016 by John Wiley & Sons, Inc.
Companion website: www.wiley.com/go/griffon/complications

Diagnosis

- Clinical signs of pleural effusion
  - Dyspnea
  - Muffled cardiopulmonary noises during auscultation
- Clinical signs of acute blood loss
  - Depression
  - Tachycardia
  - Hypothermia
  - Hypotension
  - Discolored mucosa
  - Prolonged capillary refill time
- Radiographic signs of pleural effusion
- Definitive diagnosis is achieved by direct sampling of the pleural space through the chest drain or via thoracocentesis (Figure 37.2).

Treatment (Figure 37.3)

- Initial assessment requires quantifying the amount of blood loss and, if necessary, to replace it and to monitor the severity and progression of the bleeding.
- A clotting profile and full blood count should be performed to rule out coagulopathy or platelet disorder.
- If a large effusion is present and ventilation has been objectively assessed as adequate, full drainage of the chest may not be necessary because blood is expected to be reabsorbed through the pleura.
- Initially, the blood lost is replaced with intravenous (IV) fluid therapy using crystalloid or colloid solutions (or both).
- Treatment is based on the evolution of the circulating blood PCV (PCVb) and PCV of the effusion (PCVe). This comparison should be repeated every 10 to 15 minutes to assess the progression of the hemorrhage. With time, PCVb should drop because of the blood loss (independently of it being controlled or not) and con-

comitant fluid therapy. If hemorrhage is active in the chest, PCVe should drop similar to PCVb. If hemorrhage has stopped, PCVe should remain stable or even increase with transpleural red blood cell (RBC) reabsorption.

- In compromised animals, appropriate blood products or hemoglobin-based oxygen-carrying solutions should be administered. Autotransfusion could be considered.
- Reoperation is required in cases of
  - Rapid blood loss via the chest drain
  - Significant pleural effusion on thoracic radiographs
  - Persistent hypovolemia despite transfusion
  - Hypoxemia caused by a large-volume effusion
  - Uncontrolled hemorrhage and PCVb less than 20%

Outcome

Given the high vascular supply of the intrathoracic structures, hemorrhage can be severe and in some cases associated with acute exsanguination and death. Because of the high blood flow in the pulmonary arteries and veins, hemorrhage directly from these structures is often too severe to be successfully rescued in surgery.

Prevention

- Most of the time, postoperative hemothorax is secondary to trauma to the intercostal vessels or internal thoracic arteries during opening or closure of the thorax. Careful closure of the chest wall and identification of these structures should prevent the complication.
- Sutures placed in highly perfused vessels, especially pulmonary or lobar arteries, can loosen or get dislodged after completion of the procedure because of the ventilatory motion or the pulsatile motion of the vessels. Double ligation and transfixing sutures should ensure safe vessel occlusion.

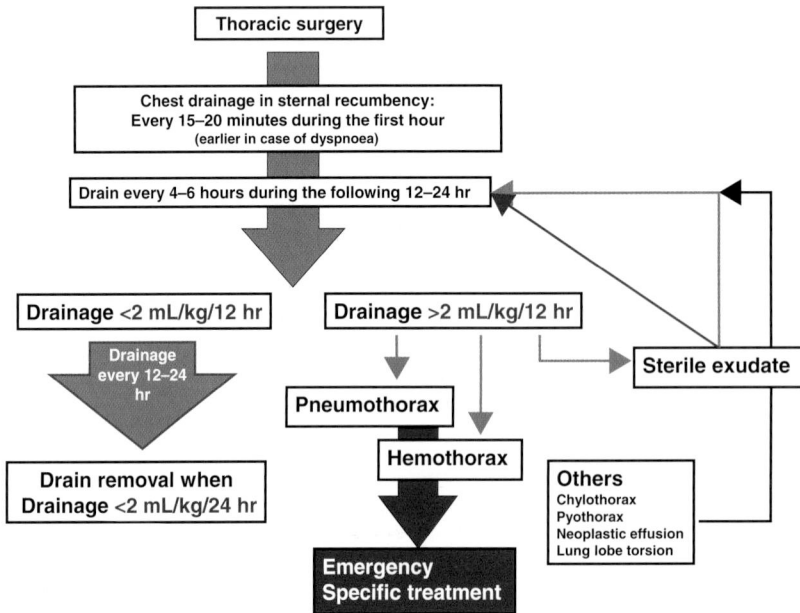

Figure 37.2 General recommendations for chest drainage after thoracic surgery.

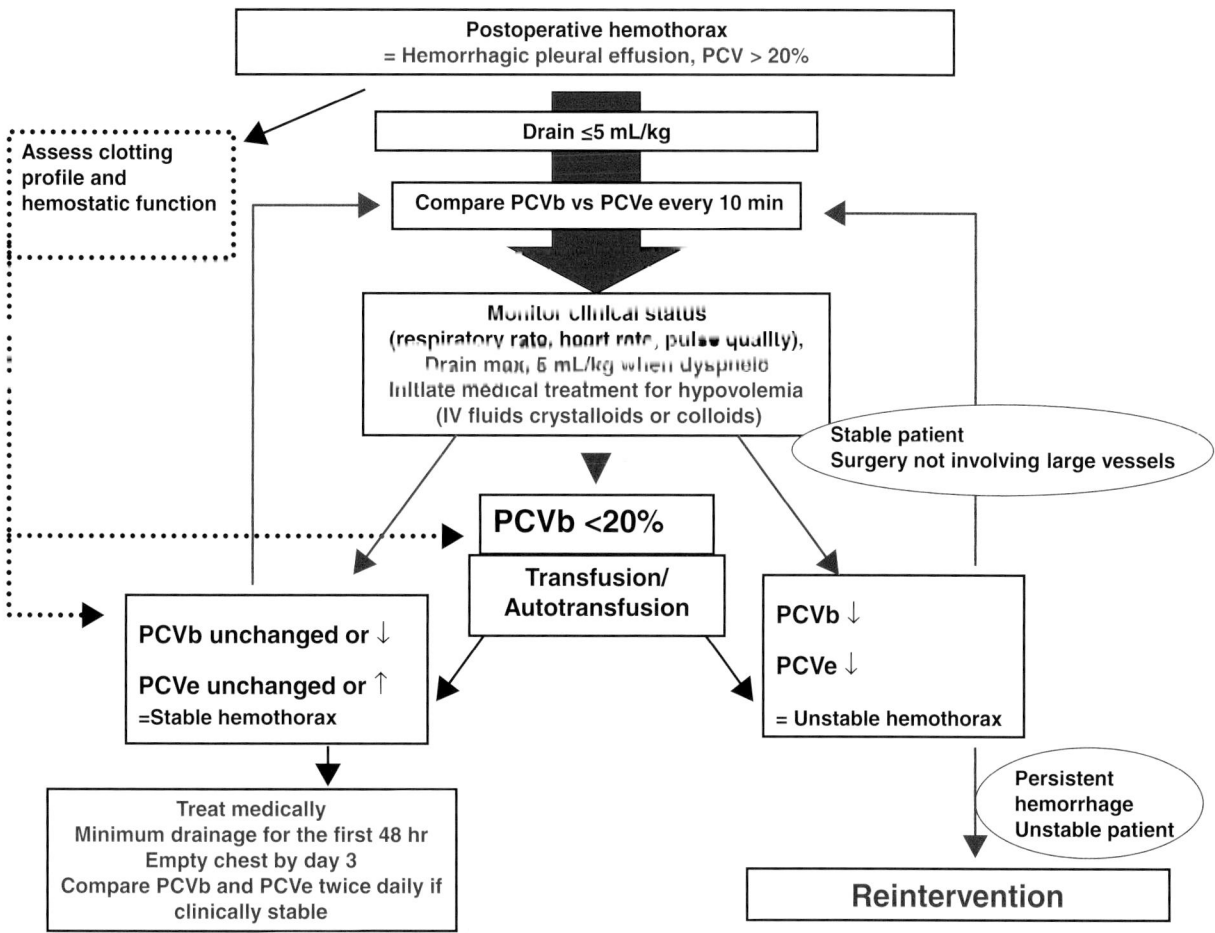

Figure 37.3 Algorithm for treatment of postsurgical hemothorax. IV, intravenous; PCV, packed cell volume; PCVb, packed cell volume of circulating blood; PCVe, packed cell volume of pleural effusion.

Pneumothorax

Definition
Pneumothorax is the accumulation of air in the pleural space.

Risk factors
- Inadequate closure of the surgical wound
- Chest drain or thoracocentesis (Tattersall and Welsh 2006; Moores et al. 2007)
- Tracheal, bronchial, or pulmonary complications
- Esophageal laceration
- Surgery for spontaneous pneumothorax
- Lung emphysema; pulmonary bullae or blebs

Diagnosis
- Clinical signs of pleural effusion:
  - Dyspnea
  - Muffled cardiopulmonary noises during auscultation
- Radiographic signs: increased radiolucency from the presence of air in the pleural cavity secondary to lung atelectasis and free gaseous space (Figure 37.4)

- Definitive diagnosis is achieved by removing free gas from the pleural space via the chest drain or by thoracocentesis.

Treatment (Figure 37.5)
- Chest drainage: Emergency thoracocentesis is possible if drain has not been placed during the surgery. In this case, a chest drain should be promptly place after the emergency treatment.
- Oxygen therapy
- Analgesia
- Restoration of the pleural subatmospheric pressure via direct intermittent aspiration or continuous suction (onsite designed "three-bottle suction system" or Pleurovac)
- Record the amount and rate of effusion.
- Transient air-thigh seal can be achieved in dressing non air-thigh seal wounds with swabs covered with a thick layer of petrolatum jelly or any antiseptic ointment.
- Pneumothorax caused by drain complication can be difficult to rule out, especially in dogs with poor subcutaneous tissue. In these cases, it is sometimes difficult to achieve seal during drainage as manual aspiration suctioned air around the drain from the outside. Removing the drain after a drainage attempt and monitoring the possible recurrence of the effusion can allow to

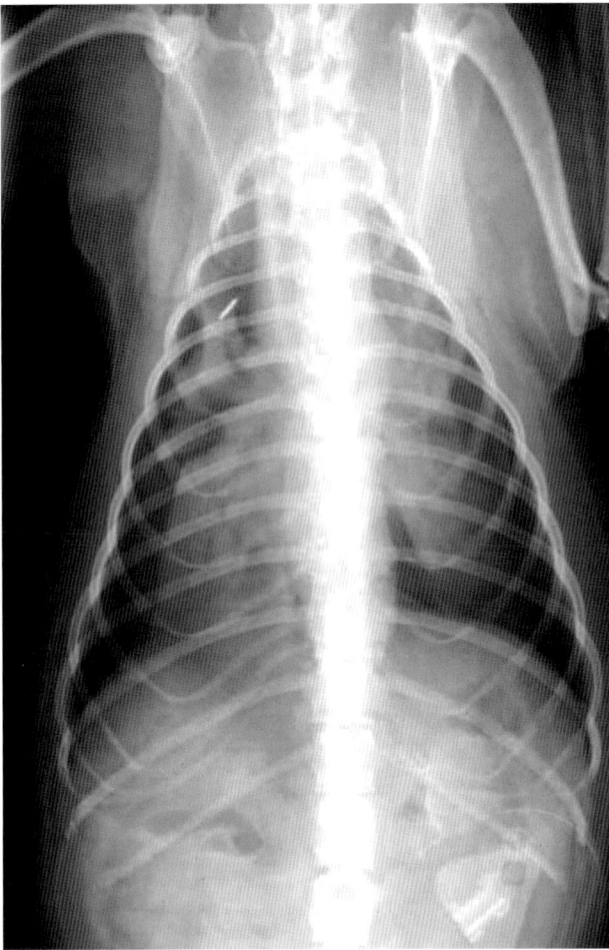

Figure 37.4 Bilateral postoperative pneumothorax a few hours after the endoscopic removal of an intrathoracic esophageal foreign body. A 2-year-old female Springer spaniel was presented with dysphagia, and examination showed a large piece of bone (chop bone) wedged in her caudal thoracic esophagus. This initially was treated with chest drainage and eventually with exploratory thoracotomy and closure of the esophageal laceration.

definitively diagnose recurring pneumothorax that deserves surgical attention.
- Reintervention is indicated when:
  ○ Air seal can not be achieved by drainage,
  ○ Pleural effusion is greater than 2 mL/kg/hr or lasts longer than 7 days
- If reintervention is necessary, careful examination of each potential source of air leak (surgical access, chest drain, trachea, esophagus, pulmonary tissue and bronchus) should be checked. For all intrathoracic structures, the "immersion test" should be used.

Outcome

Minor pulmonary leaks tend to seal spontaneously when pleural subatmospheric pressure is restored because it allows serosal contact and fibrin clots formations. After removal of large mass or extensive pneumonectomy, low-rate but long-duration effusion (up to 5 to 7 days) could be expected.

Postoperative pneumothorax in dogs with primary spontaneous pneumothorax might carry a less favorable prognosis because the origin of the air leak might be associated with diffuse parenchymal disease or remaining pulmonary bullae missed during surgery.

Prevention
- Pneumothorax associated with patient interference can be prevented with careful monitoring, use of an Elizabethan collar, and prompt removal of the chest drain when drainage is no longer necessary.
- Keep the latissimus dorsi muscle intact during surgical approach to improve air seal after thoracotomy closure (Figure 37.6).
- Check for any air leak when performing any lung or bronchial surgery.

Pyothorax

Definition

Pyothorax is the accumulation of a septic pleural exudate in the pleural cavity.

Risk factors
- Break of sterility during surgery
- Leakage through esophageal sutures
- Ascending infection from the chest drain
- Persistence of contaminated foreign material within the thoracic cavity
- Long-lasting surgery (>2 hours)
- Secondary infection of a preexisting sterile effusion (blood, transudate)
- Preexisting pyothorax

Diagnosis
- Clinical signs of pleural effusion
- Clinical signs of sepsis
  ○ Depression
  ○ Tachycardia
  ○ Hyperthermia and, when severe, hypothermia
  ○ Hypotension
  ○ Leukocytosis
- Radiographic signs of pleural effusion with possible lung consolidation or intrathoracic mass
- Definitive diagnosis is achieved by direct sampling of the pleural space (Figure 37.7). Examination of the fluid typically shows a high protein level and nucleated cell count with predominance of degenerate neutrophils and presence of bacteria. A sample should be submitted for culture and sensitivity. Despite the septic origin, culture and sensitivity testing results are not always significant (Demetriou *et al.* 2002).

Treatment
- Chest drainage via thoracocentesis as an emergency procedure in case of acute dyspnea. Then a chest drain has to be placed systematically.
- Chest lavage with 10 to 20 mL/kg of sterile isotonic solution at body temperature twice daily. Up to 10% of saline reabsorption is to be expected when lavaging the chest. The usual guidelines are to leave the lavage solution within the chest for 10 to 20 minutes before drainage. However, the author prefers to drain straight after injecting the saline (5–10 mL/kg) and to repeat the lavage

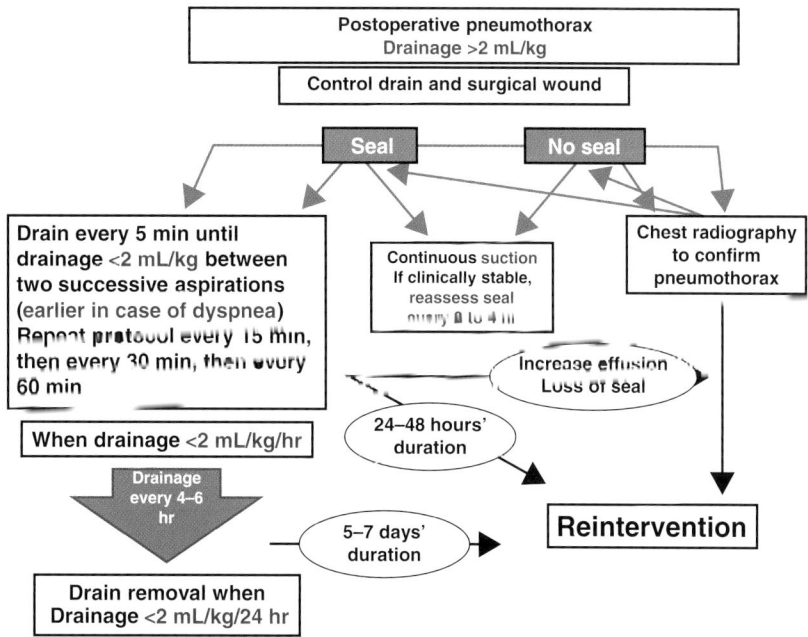

Figure 37.5 Algorithm for treatment of postsurgical pneumothorax.

several times until the macroscopic aspect of the drained solution appears grossly clear. Chest drainage and lavage is stopped when daily effusion is less than 2 mL/kg.

- Antibiotic therapy according to culture and sensitivity testing.
- Reintervention has to be considered:
  ○ In the absence of improvement in the effusion after 7 days of treatment
  ○ If there is an inability to achieve adequate drainage (consider thoracoscopic exploration (Figure 37.8)

○ Suspicion of pulmonary, mediastinal mass, or abscess
○ Suspicion of esophageal leakage (consider contrast study or endoscopy)
- In case of reintervention, lavage and drainage should be initially performed to achieve full exploration of the pleural cavity. All necrotic and infected tissues should be removed. The aim of the procedure is to establish a large cavity suitable for postoperative lavage and drainage.
- In case of abscesses that could not been fully excised, transdiaphragmatic omentalization can be performed (Franklin *et al.* 2011).
- In case of large infected cavity after lobectomy or pneumonectomy, thoracoplasty with a latissimus dorsi pedicle flap or with a large omental flap is indicated.

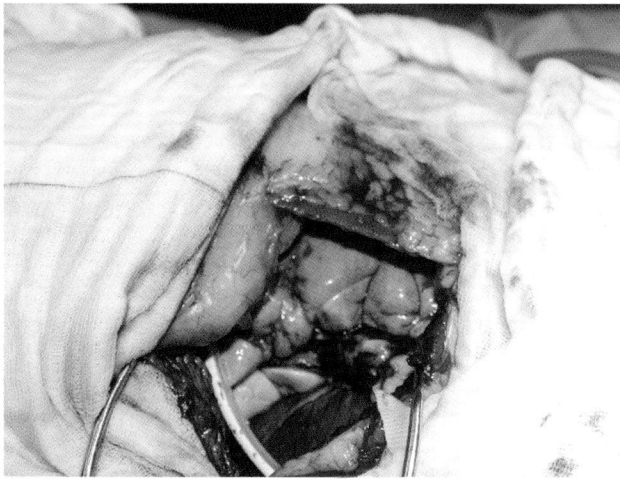

Figure 37.6 Preservation of the latissimus dorsi muscle during lateral thoracotomy (fifth intercostal space). The intact latissimus dorsi would be used to cover the intercostal wound. This would improve the postoperative seal above the wound and limit the risks of postoperative pneumothorax or subcutaneous emphysema.

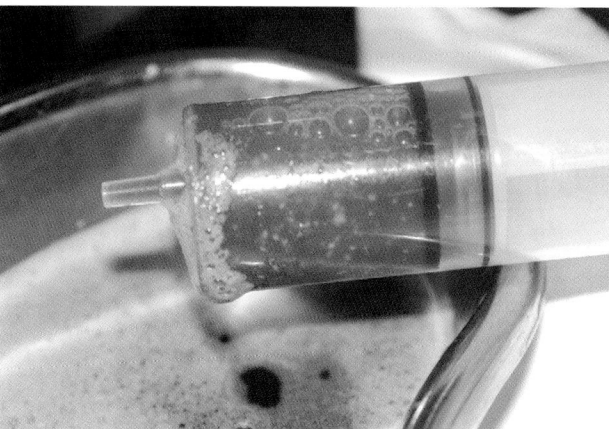

Figure 37.7 Drainage of a pyothorax. Note the small floating particles of fibrin.

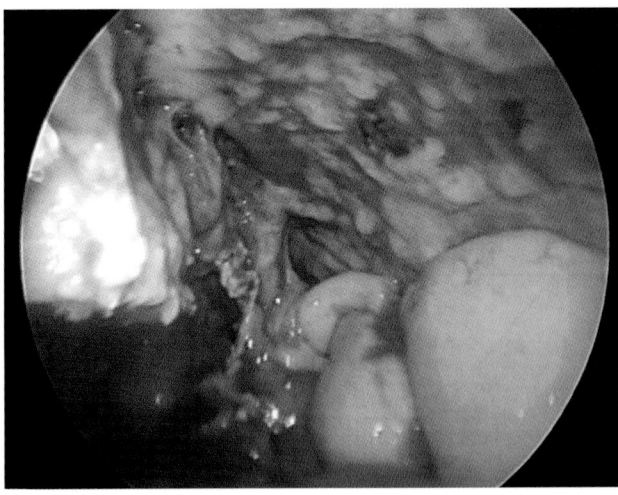

Figure 37.8 Thoracoscopy could be used to investigate postoperative pyothorax. In this view, the lungs are partially inflated in the lower right part of the picture along the very inflamed parietal pleura patched with fibrin plaques. This approach is suitable for the removal of devitalized tissues to establish large draining cavities and optimum chest drain placement.

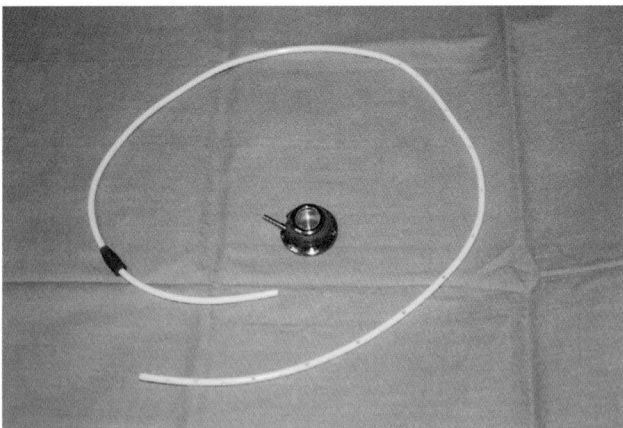

Figure 37.9 View of a pleural port. The multifenestrated silicone drain (white tube) is introduced in the pleural space and runs subcutaneously before being connected to a chamber designed for multiple puncture (middle). The chamber metallic case is fixed over the epiaxial muscles fascia in a small subcutaneous pocket. The middle of the metallic case is covered by a thick sheet of silicone (septum). This will seal itself after being punctured by Hubert point needles and allowed percutaneous repeated drainage.

Outcome

Postoperative pyothorax is a serious complication, especially when esophageal rupture is suspected. Complications associated with retained swabs are subjectively associated with a better prognosis after the removal of the material, providing that this could be done with minimal morbidity.

Prevention

A strict record of the number of swabs used during the surgery should prevent swab retention. The use of swabs knitted with radiodense markers allows postoperative radiographic control.

Neoplastic effusion

Definition

Neoplastic effusion often starts a few days (sometimes weeks or months) after surgery.

Risk factors
- Mediastinal lymphoma
- Diffuse lung tumor with hilus invasion
- Lung tumor with preoperative pleural effusion or signs of pleural infiltration

Diagnosis

Clinical signs of pleural effusion
- Radiographic signs of pleural effusion with possible lung mass or metastases or mediastinal lymph nodes enlargements
- Definitive diagnosis requires cytological examination of the effusion. Thoracoscopic exploration could be considered to collect samples for histopathology.

Treatment

Chest drainage via a chest drain
- Metastasectomy
- Intracavitary chemotherapy

- Systemic chemotherapy
- Subcutaneous pleural port for iterative drainage (Figures 37.9 and 37.10)
- Pleurodesis

Outcome

The prognosis appears poor, but long-term palliation can be achieved with pleural port. In humans, pleurodesis appears to be the method of choice for neoplastic effusion. In normal dogs, however, mechanical or talc-induced pleurodesis attempts were not successful (Jerram *et al.* 1999).

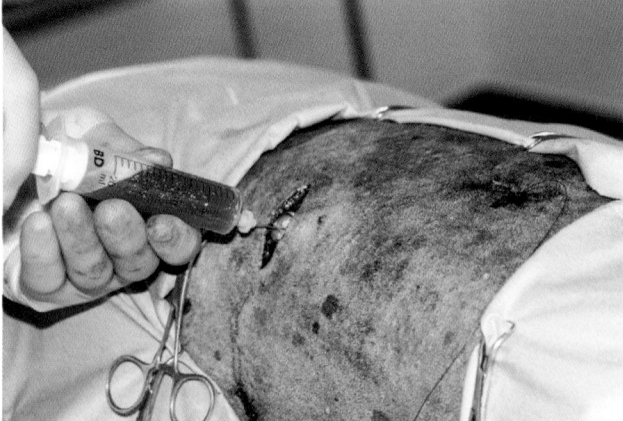

Figure 37.10 View of a pleural port. The system has been placed. The position and the connection of the port and drain are checked before closure of the surgical wounds. Note the aspect of the pleural effusion collected in the syringe and the small surgical access wound performed over the intercostal space to introduce the drain in the pleural space. When in place, the skin is sutured over the chamber, and further drainage will be performed percutaneously.

Prevention

The complication is associated with the nature of the disease rather than with technical mistake. However, because pulmonary tumor could spread by contact, prevention of pleural contamination and further implantation of tumoral cells should be done during surgery.

Chylothorax

Definition

Chylothorax is postoperative accumulation of chyle in the pleural cavity.

Risk factors

- Preexisting chylothorax
- Lung lobe torsion
- Mediastinal tumor
- Extensive dissection of the caudal mediastinum

Diagnosis

- Clinical signs of pleural effusion
- Radiographic signs of pleural effusion possibly associated with lung lobe torsion
- Chylothorax is suspected (but not confirmed) after collection of a milklike pleural effusion (Figure 37.11).
- Definitive diagnosis is made after comparison of the cholesterol and triglyceride concentrations between the effusion and the circulating blood. Chylothorax is diagnosed when the triglyceride concentration in the effusion is 10 to 100 times superior to the serum concentration and when cholesterol concentration remains similar in both. Additional diagnostic tests for chylous effusion include a cholesterol-to-triglyceride ratio in the fluid less than 1, the presence of chylomicrons seen microscopically on a wet mount preparation, fluid that clears with the addition of ether, and fluid that is positive for the presence of lipid droplets with Sudan III stain (Monnet 2003).

Treatment

The usual treatment of the postoperative chylous effusion is medical with chest drainage and institution of a low-fat diet. If the effusion fails to resolve after 5 to 10 days of conservative treatment, then surgical management should be considered (Hodges *et al.* 1993).

Outcome

Iatrogenic chylothorax consecutive to traumatic laceration of normal thoracic duct should resolve with medical treatment, and patients should not need surgery. However, it appears to be a frequent complication after or in conjunction with lung lobe torsion (Neath *et al.* 2000). In these cases, the general prognosis is guarded.

Pulmonary atelectasis

Definition

Atelectasis is defined as airway closure (permanent or intermittent) and subsequently alveolar collapse. The nonventilated alveoli are still perfused, so atelectasis contributes to the development of "shunt" and hypoxemia.

Risk factors

- General anesthesia
- 100% O_2 ventilation
- Dorsal or lateral recumbency
- Pulmonary compression (high interpleural pressure, large mass, diaphragmatic hernia)

Treatment

- Intraoperative reexpansion of atelectatic lungs via high pressure lung inflation has to be avoided. Atelectatic lungs should be reexpanded postoperatively with gentle restoration of pleural subatmospheric pressure.
- Postoperatively, gentle physiotherapy has to be performed. Early mobilization of the patient with frequent position changes, favoring early walks, gentle chest percussion (clapping) (Figure 37.12), and even encouraging barking (Dunning *et al.* 2005). These exercises inspired by human medicine improve clearance of the airways and ventilation (Duggan and Kavanagh 2005; Cavenaghi *et al.* 2009).
- In the case of very productive airways, suction is indicated, but practically, this can only be performed in patients with a tracheostomy.

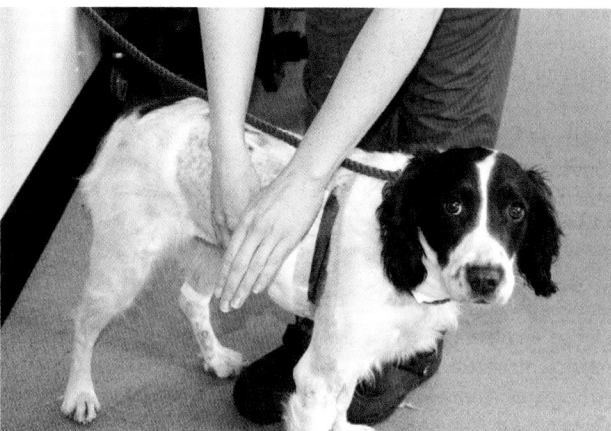

Figure 37.12 Postoperative physiotherapy after thoracic surgery. This young Springer spaniel had an intercostal thoracotomy to remove a large lung abscess. Twenty-four hours after the surgery, she is encouraged to walk and sustained gentle clapping of her chest. Note the "cuplike" shape of the hands during gentle percussion of the thoracic wall.

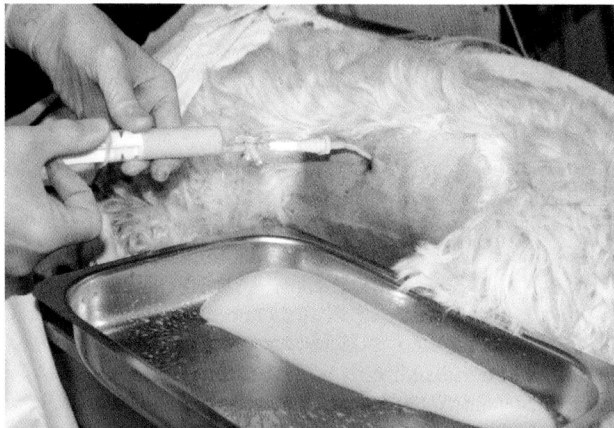

Figure 37.11 Chylothorax. Note the "milklike" aspect of the pleural effusion.

• In case of severe dyspnea, oxygen therapy and, as a last resort, mechanical ventilation are indicated.

Outcome

When the origin of the atelectasis is relieved providing that the animal achieved correct oxygenation and ventilation, recovery should be achieved with gentle reopening of the atelectatic area (Van der Kloot *et al.* 2000). One should be careful during this period because overzealous therapy might create life-threatening pulmonary reexpansion edema.

Prevention

Per-anesthetic prevention of atelectasis **on healthy lungs** can be achieved with "recruitments maneuvers":

• Long-duration and high-pressure inspirations can reopen collapsed lungs and reduce atelectasis (maximum inflation pressure of 20 cm H_2O).
• Minimize gas resorption in avoiding 100% oxygen as the only ventilating gas.
• Systematic application of positive end-expiratory pressure (PEEP) (Duggan and Kavanagh 2005)
• Tracheal and bronchial secretions should be aspirated intraoperatively to prevent subsequent airways obstruction.

Reexpansion pulmonary edema

Definition

Reexpansion pulmonary edema (REPE) is a noncardiogenic acute and diffuse pulmonary edema that develops on previously atelectatic lungs after acute decompression or reexpansion (Jordan *et al.* 2000).

Risks factors

• Long-lasting atelectasis (>12 hours)
• Acute relieve of long-lasting atelectasis
• Fluid overload
• Cats
• Diaphragmatic hernia (Worth and Machon 2005)
• Pectus excavatum (Soderstrom *et al.* 1995)
• Pulmonary decortication (Fossum *et al.* 1992).

Diagnosis

Reexpansion pulmonary edema can develop immediately and up to 3 days after lung reexpansion. Diagnosis is based on clinical examination (increased respiratory frequency, pulmonary auscultation with crackles, absence of pleural effusion), demonstration of increased pulmonary edema (intraoperative obstruction of the endotracheal tube can be observed), and imaging studies (showing lung consolidation and air bronchograms).

Treatment

• Oxygen therapy
• Discontinuation of IV crystalloids
• Diuretics +/− colloid infusion
• Mechanical ventilation

Outcome

The condition in cats appears particularly severe and, when observed, is often fatal (Fossum *et al.* 1992; Soderstrom *et al.* 1995; Worth and Machon 2008).

Prevention

• Positive-pressure ventilation in surgery should be carefully performed to prevent barotrauma to the lungs. The usual guidelines are to inflate to a maximum inspiratory pressure of 15 to 20 cm H_2O (Worth and Machon 2008), but much lower pressures (6–8 cm H_2O) are preferable in cats and smaller dogs.
• Chronically collapsed lungs should not been forced to reexpand with forced inspiratory pressure. The collapse should resolve postoperatively after restoration of normal pulmonary mechanics.
• Gentle reinstallment of the pleural subatmospheric pressure via the chest drain over several hours is recommended. If atelectasis is severe, acute restoration of a large negative pressure can stretch the lungs and induce REPE. The clinician could be guided by the use of pleural manometry to directly measure the pleural depression and prevent further lung damage induced by intrapleural depression (Doelken *et al.* 2004; Echevarria *et al.* 2008; Worth and Machon 2008). In dogs, the pleural depression at the end of inspiration should be between −5 cm H_2O and −8 cm H_2O (Tucker 2003). Some authors recommend gentle repeated aspirations every hour to achieve full reexpansion 12 to 24 hours after surgery (Echevarria *et al.* 2008; White 2008; Worth and Machon 2008).

Secretion retention (sputum)

Definition

Failure to clear bronchial secretions can result in bronchial obstruction, atelectasis, lobar collapse, and secondary pulmonary infection (Figures 37.13 and 37.14).

Risk factors

• Pulmonary infection or lung abscess
• Tracheitis
• Tracheostomy
• Atelectasis
• Hypoventilation

Diagnosis

• Dyspnea or increased lung noises during auscultation
• Hypoxemia
• Radiographic changes of lung consolidation

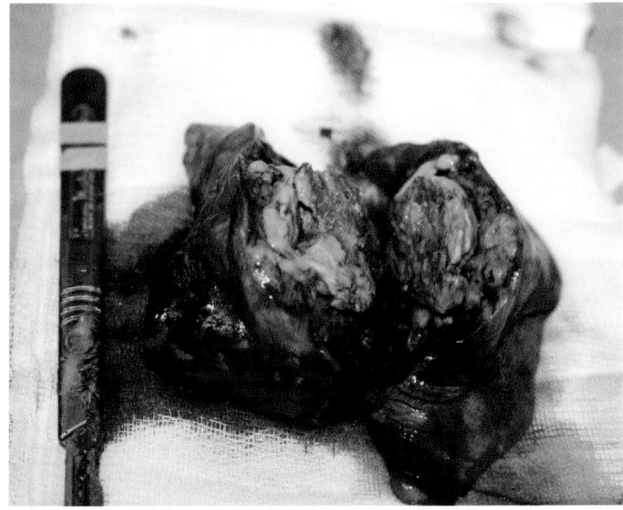

Figure 37.13 Postsurgical view of a lung abscess.

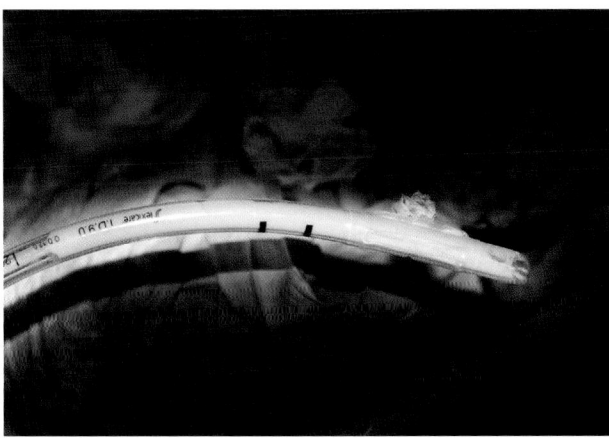

Figure 37.14 View of the endotracheal tube of the same dog as in Figures 37.12 and 37.13. Note the accumulation of secretion that spilled within the airways during the surgery. Early physiotherapy is indicated to help clearance of the secretions and prevent further pneumonia or atelectasis.

Treatment
- Prevention of airway obstruction during surgery
- Intraoperative suction of the airways
- Nebulization and airway physiotherapy

Outcome
Sputum without associated pneumonia should carry a good prognosis after release. When not diagnosed, it could be source of lung infection and, pending its location, could create major airway obstruction and possible fatal asphyxia.

Prevention
- Adequate postoperative pain relief to favor deep inspiration and expiration
- Chest physiotherapy

Humidification of inspired oxygen and bronchodilator therapy when oxygen therapy is performed

Pneumonia

Definition
Pneumonia is a pulmonary infection.

Risk factors
- Sputum
- Atelectasis
- Aspiration pneumonia (megaesophagus, gastritis)
- Hypoventilation
- Preexisting infection
- Mechanical ventilation
- Tracheostomy

Diagnosis
Nosocomial pneumonia must be suspected in all patients that develop pyrexia, increased respiratory frequency, and tachycardia.

When clinical examination and chest auscultation raise suspicion of early pneumonia, the diagnosis should be confirmed radiographically (lung lobe consolidation or diffuse interstitial pattern).

Treatment
- Oxygen therapy
- Bronchoalveolar lavage (BAL) and further submission of samples for culture and sensitivity. If the clinical status of the patient excludes performing a BAL, transtracheal aspiration could be performed. Otherwise, empirical treatment with broad-spectrum antibiotics should be prescribed.
- Postoperative physiotherapy

Outcome
The prognosis for postoperative pneumonia remains guarded pending the general status of the patient before the infection, the extent of the disease, and how quickly the condition has been diagnosed and treated.

Prevention
- Favor physiological ventilation (analgesia)
- Early physiotherapy

Lung lobe torsion

Definition
Lung lobe torsion consists in the torsion of a lung lobe along its long axis associated with the torsion of its vascular pedicle.

Risk factors
- Deep-chested dog
- Afghan and pugs
- Concomitant pleural effusion (mainly chylothorax)
- Previous removal of a large intrathoracic mass or released of caudal lung lobe mediastinal ligament

Diagnosis
- Clinical presentation
  - Predisposed breed with acute dyspnea
  - Pleural effusion
  - Tachycardia and pyrexia
- Imaging (radiography, computed tomography, ultrasonography) will show signs of pleural effusion and lung lobe consolidation, as well as an abnormal direction of the main bronchus of the consolidated lobe.
- Bronchoscopy can document torsion of the bronchus.
- Analysis of the pleural effusion can be consistent with mere transudate, septic exudate, neoplastic exudate or chylothorax (Neath *et al.* 2000).

Treatment
- Oxygen therapy
- Chest drainage
- Lung lobe resection (Figure 37.15)

Outcome
The prognosis is guarded, especially in large breed dogs in which studies show high postoperative morbidity and mortality. The most frequent postoperative complications observed with lung torsion were chylothorax, pneumothorax, and thoracic neoplasia. Postoperative fatal acute respiratory distress syndrome was also reported (Parent *et al.* 1996, Syrja *et al.* 2009).

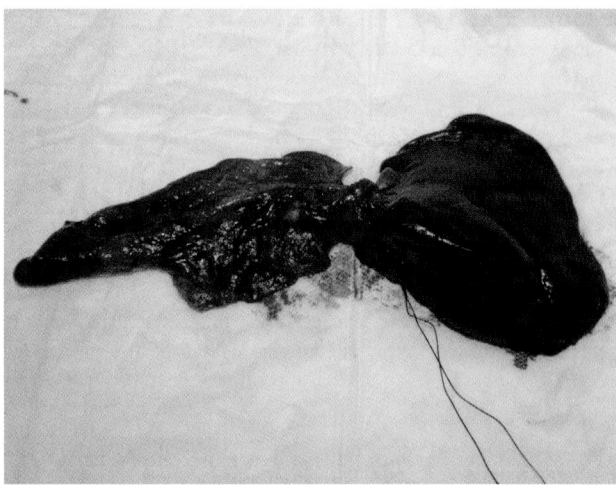

Figure 37.15 View of the left cranial lung lobe of an adult Afghan diagnosed with lung lobe torsion. In this case, the caudal part of the left cranial lung lobe twisted around her basis with minimum change in the cranial part of the lobe. This was possible because of a very deep fissure between both units. Note the congestion and the difference in size and density of both segments.

Prevention

The exact physiopathology of the torsion remains unknown. Fixation of mobile lung lobe after thoracic exploration might prevent the complication.

Hypoxemia

Definition

Hypoxemia can be defined as a PaO_2 of less than 60 mm Hg when the patient is breathing room air.

Risk factors

- Atelectasis
- Anemia
- Pulmonary edema
- Pulmonary embolism
- Pleural effusion
- Aspiration pneumonia
- Bronchospasm
- Upper airway obstruction
- Hypoventilation (breathing room air)

Diagnosis

- Hypoxemia can be difficult to detect but may manifest as an increase in respiratory rate. Cardiovascular effects may include arrhythmias and hypertension. Central nervous system effects, including changes in mentation, are late signs that are only apparent with severe hypoxemia.
- Arterial blood gas (ABG) analysis is the gold standard for the assessment of hypoxemia. The presence of an arterial catheter is invaluable in allowing repeated ABG evaluation. Pulse oximeters provide a safe, reliable, and noninvasive method of continuous arterial oxygen saturation monitoring. In general, an SpO2 below 95% warrants intervention.

Treatment

- Oxygen therapy
- Correction of the underlying cause
- Mechanical ventilation

Outcome

When the origin of disorder is transient, quick improvement should be observed after correction (e.g., pleural effusion). For more severe causes (e.g., severe pneumonia, too large lung resection), the prognosis appears much more guarded.

Prevention

- Prevention of atelectasis
- Preemptive analgesia to ensure correct ventilation
- Removal of less than 55% of the lung parenchyma
- Postoperative oxygen therapy

Hypoventilation

Definition

Hypoventilation is defined by a lack of alveoli ventilation. There is an inability to remove an adequate volume of CO_2, and thus hypercapnia occurs. Hypercapnia can generally be defined as a $PaCO_2$ greater than 45 mm Hg when the patient is breathing spontaneously. When severe hypoventilation occurs in an animal breathing room air, hypoxemia may result.

Risk factors

- Residual effects of volatile agents
- Associated underlying neuromuscular disease (e.g., thymoma, myasthenia gravis)
- Drugs, including opioids and neuromuscular blocking agents
- Decreased inspiratory effort resulting from:
  - Pain
  - Dressings restricting thoracic movement
  - Flail chest
- Airway obstruction
- Pleural effusion

Diagnosis

- Clinical signs may not be obvious but may manifest as increases in respiratory rate or effort. Severe hypoventilation can lead to CO_2-induced narcosis. Moderate hypercapnia will cause blood pH changes, which may compound preexisting blood gas abnormalities. Hypercapnia can also result in cardiovascular effects caused by sympathetic stimulation.
- ABG analysis is the gold standard for the assessment of adequacy of ventilation. A $PaCO_2$ of greater than 60 mm Hg usually warrants intervention to support ventilation.
- Capnography may be used as a noninvasive and continuous monitor of the adequacy of ventilation. The gradient between the end-tidal CO_2 (obtained by capnography) and the $PaCO_2$ (obtained by ABG analysis) is normally small (<5 mm Hg). When there is increased dead space ventilation (i.e., ventilation of areas that are not perfused), the difference between arterial and end-tidal CO_2 may become much greater (low cardiac output, pulmonary thromboembolism, or ventilation with very high PEEP).

Treatment
- Analgesia (consider local blockade) + physiotherapy
- Stable chest wall reconstruction
- Look for underlying neuromuscular disorder
- Pleural drainage
- Mechanical ventilation
- Consider sedation in stressed patients without pleural or parietal dysfunction

Outcome
The origin of the hypoventilation and its prompt resolution will predict the outcome of the hypercapnia. Because CO_2 exchanges are fast, quick improvement should be observed when adequate ventilation is restored.

Prevention
- Analgesia
- Stable reconstruction of the chest wall
- Prevention of accumulation of any pleural effusion

Phrenic nerve injury

Anatomy
The phrenic nerve arises from the fifth, sixth, and seventh cervical nerves. Its branches run along the external jugular vein and fuse at the level of the thoracic inlet to form the phrenic nerve. Within the thorax, each nerve runs along the lateral surface of the mediastinum ventral to the large vessels and to the pulmonary hilus. It crosses the upper third of the pericardium and runs caudally medial to the ligament of the caudal pulmonary lungs. It then divides over the surface of its respective half of the diaphragm. The phrenic nerve is essentially a motor nerve for the diaphragm. Damage to the nerve is associated with paralysis of its associated hemidiaphragm (Kitchell and Evans 1993, De Troyer *et al.* 2009).

Risk factors
- Cranial mediastinal surgery
- Cardiac or pericardial surgery
- Caudal lung lobectomy or pneumonectomy (Burns and Dunning 2011)

Diagnosis
- Increased inspiratory effort and paradoxical abdominal motion caused by paralysis of the hemidiaphragm
- Radiographic examination, fluoroscopy, and ultrasonography have all proved useful to confirm the suspicion (Vignoli *et al.* 2002). Asymmetry of the diaphragm crus during inspiration has been reported on radiographs. Decreased contractility of the paralyzed hemidiaphragm has been observed on fluoroscopy and during ultrasound examination.

Treatment
- Oxygen therapy
- Surgery could be considered in dogs with clinically significant dyspnea. Diaphragmatic plicature has been widely used in human surgery (Burns and Dunning 2011) and has been described in experimental settings in unilaterally paralyzed dogs (Takeda *et al.* 1995).

Outcome
- Unilateral damages are often clinically nonrelevant.
- Diaphragm plicature has improved ventilation during experimental studies.

Prevention
- Anatomic dissection and identification and retraction of the nerve in the areas where traumas are possible (lateral aspect of the mediastinum, pericardium, at the level of the heart base)

Postoperative pain
The use of multimodal analgesic techniques may minimize postoperative pain, therefore improving pain-free ventilation despite surgical trauma. In veterinary practice, several local anesthetic techniques may be used to improve analgesic efficacy and reduce the reliance on systemic drug administration with their associated side effects:
- Intercostal nerve blocks (e.g., bupivacaine 1.5 mg/kg) during lateral thoracotomies
- Interpleural analgesia (e.g., bupivacaine 1.5 mg/kg every 6–8 hours) via a pleural catheter or chest drain
- Local infiltration (e.g., bupivacaine 1 mg/kg) along the sternotomy incision (Figure 37.16)
- Wound catheter through which local anesthetics can be administered (e.g., bupivacaine 1.5 mg/kg every 6–8 hours)

Relevant literature
In case of postoperative hemothorax, autotransfusion could be considered when no other options are available and in the absence of possible bacterial or neoplastic effusion or contamination. Actual recommendations advise using a blood giving set with filter to readminister blood. The value of systematic mixing of the autotransfused blood with anticoagulant is unclear because blood collected from pleural effusion is unlikely to clot (Crow 2010; Devey 2010).

Concurrent fresh-frozen plasma administration may be advised at the time of autotransfusion because the blood from the pleural effusion can trigger disseminated intravascular coagulation (Devey 2010).

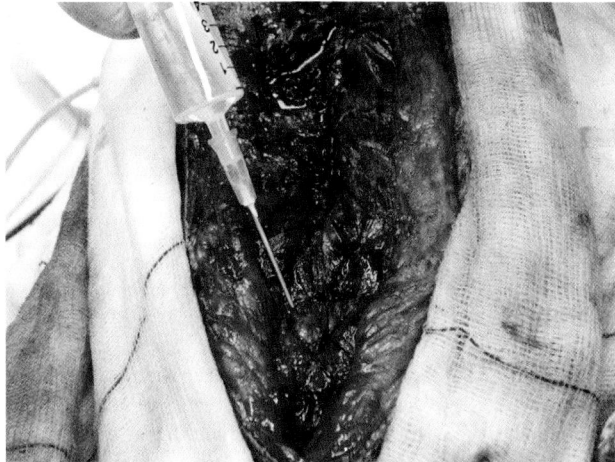

Figure 37.16 Operative view of a sternotomy closure. Local infiltration is performed along the sternotomy incision.

Using a "cell-salvage procedure" has also been described as a safer but more expensive alternative compared with simple autotransfusion. Namely, the pleural effusion is collected and then "washed" to only keep viable RBCs that are subsequently mixed with sterile saline solution to be readministered as a globular concentrate (PCV 60%). This procedure is technically challenging and expensive. Therapeutically, as the plasma is discarded during the procedure, the benefits of injecting a colloid solution in association with oxygen carrier are lost. On the other hand, the process appears to increase the range of applications to effusion potentially contaminated with bacteria or neoplastic cells (Chan 2009).

Pneumothorax associated with patient interference (mutilation of the surgical wound or the chest drain) has been observed and can be fatal (Salci *et al.* 2005; Tattersall and Welsh 2006; Moores *et al.* 2007). Protection of the wounds and chest drains should be done systematically. If necessary, a muzzle or a long Elizabethan collar should be used. For the same reason, it is advisable to remove the chest drain as soon as possible (Tattersall and Welsh 2006; Moores *et al.* 2007).

Reexpansion pulmonary edema is a well-known condition in human surgery. When the lung has been collapsed for more than 3 days, severe parenchymal edema can be observed as it rapidly expands (Jordan *et al.* 2000, Echevarria *et al.* 2008; Sohara 2008). Typically, REPE is observed in humans after acute drainage of a very large effusion. Consequently, to prevent REPE, human medicines guidelines recommend that complete emptying of the pleural space should not be attempted at once and that a maximum volume of 1.5 L should be removed by drainage. There are no such evidence-based guidelines in veterinary surgery.

Different pathogeneses have been reported for REPE. The condition results from the association of histologic and mechanical factors (Jordan *et al.* 2000, Sohara 2008). Lung collapse is associated with rapidly occurring fibrotic changes of the endothelium of the pulmonary vessels, resulting in diminished "flexibility." When stretched during lung reexpansion, the permeability of these vessels increases and allows fluids leak in the interstitium.

It is suspected that the release of free radicals in the reexpanded lung, the sequestration of neutrophils and the modification of the surfactant within the collapsed lung are part of the process and aggravate the process induced by the histologic lesions (Sohara 2008, Worth and Machon 2008). The use of small-caliber drains has been associated with slower aspiration of the intrapleural air and has been reported to reduce the risks of REPE in human patients. Because manometry has never been described in small animal surgery, the therapeutic pleural pressure to achieve during drainage is unknown, and no recommendation can yet be issued.

The etiology of **lung lobe torsion** is unknown, but it is suspected that mechanisms increasing lung mobility (pleural effusion, lung atelectasis, and surgical manipulations) could increase the risks of subsequent torsion. Deep-chested dogs are predisposed, but surprisingly, pugs appear as susceptible to develop the condition as Afghans (Neath 2000). Despite being commonly reported as a potential complication of thoracic surgery, lung lobe torsion is more likely to present as a primary condition often secondarily complicated by or associated with other thoracic conditions (e.g., chylothorax) (Neath 2000). In human medicine, however, intraoperative fixation of mobile lung lobe in prevention of possible postoperative torsion has been recommended (Ferretti *et al.* 2009). In a population of 21 dogs that underwent surgery for diagnosed lung lobe torsion, only 11 were discharged alive from the hospital. Three

of them died of respiratory disorder in the 6 years after the surgery (Neath 2000).

Reports of **iatrogenic phrenic section** and subsequent diaphragm paralysis are rare in veterinary surgery. Phrenic nerve paralysis has been described as an iatrogenic complication during video-assisted pericardiectomy in dogs (Jackson *et al.* 1999) and as a self-resolving condition after blunt chest traumas in cats (Vignoli *et al.* 2002).

References

Burns, J., Dunning, J. (2011) Is the preservation of the phrenic nerve important after pneumonectomy? *Interactive Cardiovascular and Thoracic Surgery*, 12, 47-50.

Cavenaghi, S., Garcia de Moura, S.C., Da Silva, T.H., et al. (2009) Importance of pre- and postoperative physiotherapy in pediatric cardiac surgery. *Revista Brasileira de Cirurgia Cardiovascular*, 24 (3), 397-400.

Chan, D.L. (2009) Autotransfusion using cell-saver devices. *Proceedings of the International Emergency and Critical Care Symposium*, Chicago, September.

Crow, T. (2010) Cases that should not have recovered but did: lessons learned. *Proceedings Atlantic Coast Veterinary Conference*, Atlantic City, October.

Demetriou, J.,L., Foale, R.,D., Ladlow, J., et al. (2002) Canine and feline pyothorax: a retrospective study of 50 cases in the UK and Ireland. *Journal of Small Animal Practice* 43, 388-394.

De Troyer, A., Leduc, D., Cappello, M. (2009) Bilateral impact on the lung of hemidiaphragmatic paralysis in dog. *Respiratory Physiology & Neurobiology*, 166, 68-72.

Devey, J.J. (2010) Crystalloid and colloid fluid therapy. In Ettinger, S.J., Feldman, E.C. (eds.) *Textbook of Small Internal Medicine*, 7th edn. WB Saunders, Philadelphia, 487-495.

Doelken, P., Huggins, J.T., Pastis, N.J., et al. (2004) Pleural manometry: technique and clinical implications. *Chest* 126, 1764-1769.

Duggan, M., Kavanagh, B.P. (2005) Pulmonary atelectasis. *Anesthesiology* 102, 838-854.

Dunning, D., Halling, K.B., Ehrhart, N. (2005) Rehabilitation of medical and acute care patients. *Veterinary Clinics of North America: Small Animal Practice*, 35 (6), 1411-1426.

Echevarria, C., Twomley D., Dunning, J., et al. (2008) Does reexpansion pulmonary oedema exist? *Interactive Cardiovascular & Thoracic Surgery*, 7, 485-489.

Ferretti, G., Brichon, P.Y., Jankowski A., et al. (2009) Postoperative complications after thoracic surgery. *Journal of Radiology*, 90, 1001-1012.

Fossum, T.W., Evering, W.N., Miller, M.W., et al. (1992) Severe fibrosing pleuritis with chronic chylothorax in five cats and two dogs. *Journal of the American Veterinary Medical Association*, 201 (2), 317-324.

Franklin, A.D., Fearnside, S.M., Brain, P.H. (2011) Omentalisation of a caudal mediastinal abscess in a dog. *Australian Veterinary Journal*, 89, 217-220.

Hodges, C.C., Fossum, T.W., Evering, W. (1993) Evaluation of thoracic duct healing after experimental laceration and transaction. *Veterinary Surgery*, 22 (6), 431-435.

Jackson, J., Richter, K.P., Launer, D.P. (1999) Thoracoscopic partial pericardiectomy in 13 dogs. *Journal of Veterinary Internal Medicine*, 13, 529-533.

Jerram, R.M., Fossum, T.W., Berridge, B.R., et al. (1999) The efficacy of mechanical abrasion and talc slurry as methods of pleurodesis in normal dogs. *Veterinary Surgery*, 28, 322-332.

Jordan, S., Mitchell, J.A., Quinlan, G.J., et al. (2000) The pathogenesis of lung injury following pulmonary resection. *European Respiratory Journal*, 15, 790-799.

Kitchell, R.E., Evans, H.E. (1993) The spinal nerves: nerves to the diaphragm. In Ed Evans, H.E. (ed.) *Anatomy of the Dog*, 3rd edn. WB. Saunders, Philadelphia, pp. 840-841.

Monnet, E. (2003) Pleura and pleural space. In Slatter, D. (ed.) *Textbook of Small Animal Surgery*, 3rd edn. WB Saunders, Philadelphia, pp. 387-405.

Moores, A.L., Halfacree, Z.J., Baines, S.J., et al. (2007) Indications, outcomes and complications following lateral thoracotomy in dogs and cats. *Journal of Small Animal Practice*, 48, 695-698.

Neath, P.J., Brockman, D.J., King, L.C. (2000) Lung lobe torsion in dogs: 22 cases (1981-1999). *Journal of the American Veterinary Medical Association*, 217, 1041-1044.

Parent, C., King, L.G., Van Winkle, T.J., et al. (1996) Respiratory function and treatment in dogs with acute respiratory distress syndrome: 19 cases (1985-1993). *Journal of the American Veterinary Medical Association*, 208 (9), 1428-1433.

Salci, H., Sami Bayram, A., Ozyigit, O., et al. (2007) Comparison of different bronchial closure techniques following pneumonectomy in dogs. *Journal of Veterinary Science*, 8 (4), 393-399.

Sigrist, N.E., Adamik, K.N., Doherr, M.G., et al. (2011) Evaluation of respiratory parameter at presentation as clinical indicators of the respiratory localization in dogs and cats withy respiratory distress. *Journal of Veterinary Emergency and Critical Care* 21 (1), 13-23.

Soderstrom, M.J., Gilson, S.D., Gulbas, N., et al. (1995) Fatal reexpansion pulmonary edema in a kitten following surgical correction of pectus excavatum. *Journal of the American Animal Hospital Association,* 31 (2), 133-436.

Sohara, Y. (2008) Reexpansion pulmonary edema . *Annals of Thoracic & Cardiovascular Surgery,* 14 (4), 205-209.

Syrja, P., Saari, S., Rajamaki, M., et al. (2009) Pulmonary histopathology in dalmatians with familial acute respiratory distress syndrome (ARDS). *Journal of Comparative Pathology,* 141, 254-259.

Takeda, S., Nakahara, K., Fuji, Y., et al. (1995) Effects of diaphragmatic plication on respiratory mechanics in dogs with unilateral and bilateral phrenic nerve paralysis. *Chest* 107 (3), 798-804.

Tattersall, J.A., Welsh, E. (2006) Factors influencing the short-term outcome following thoracic surgery in 98 dogs. *Journal of Small Animal Practice,* 47, 715-720.

Tucker, A. (2003) Respiratory pathophysiologie. In Slatter, D. (ed.) *Textbook of Small Animal Surgery,* 3rd edn. WB Saunders, Philadelphia, pp. 781-797.

Van der Kloot, T.E., Blanch, L., Youngblood, A.M., et al. (2000) recruitment maneuvers in three experimental models of acute lung injury. *American Journal of Respiratory and Critical Care Medicine,* 161, 1485-1494.

Vignoli, M., Toniato, M., Rossi, F., et al. (2002) Transient post-traumatic hemidiaphragmatic paralysis in two cats *Journal of Small Animal Practice,* 43, 312-316.

White, R.N. (2008) Updates in diaphragmatic hernia. *Proceedings European College of Veterinary Surgery Symposium,* Basel.

Worth, A.J., Machon, R.G. (2005) Traumatic diaphragmatic herniation: pathophysiology and management. *Compendium of Continuing Education for the Practicing Veterinarian* 27 (3), 178-191.

Worth, A.J., Machon, R.G. (2008) Prevention of reexpansion pulmonary edema and ischemia-reperfusion injury in the management of diaphragmatic herniation *Compendium of Continuing Education for the Practicing Veterinarian,* 28 (7), 178-191

38 Thoracostomy and Thoracocentesis

Alison Moores

Anderson Moores Veterinary Specialists, Winchester, Hampshire, UK

Thoracic drainage, via thoracocentesis or thoracostomy tube placement, is used for the diagnosis and treatment of pleural space disease, including pneumothorax, pyothorax, malignant pleural effusions, chylothorax, and hemothorax. Both techniques can be used for the removal of air or fluid after thoracic surgery, with thoracostomy tubes being preferred if ongoing fluid or air production is expected. Tubes can be used to instill pharmaceutical agents into the interpleural space (e.g., local anesthetic for analgesia after thoracotomy or chemotherapeutic agent for treating pleural mesothelioma).

Thoracocentesis may be performed using a butterfly needle or vascular catheter, usually attached to a syringe via extension tubing and a three-way tap. Although described in many papers, there is little information on complications associated with the technique. Thoracocentesis has also been described using the temporary placement of a small-bore wire-guided thoracostomy tube.

Until recently, most thoracostomy tubes were wide-bore tubes requiring a trocar to place them. In humans, these techniques are no longer recommended because of high complication rates. Similarly, in animals, complication rates up to 58% have been described with large-bore tubes. The use of small-bore (14-gauge) wire-guided thoracostomy tubes has been described (Valtolina and Adamantos 2009). Placement can be performed in conscious or lightly sedated animals, and the rate of complications is lower than with large-bore tubes.

Inability to place a tube

Definition
Occasionally, technical difficulties are encountered, and it is difficult to get the tube into the pleural space.

Risk factors
- Trocar tubes: Some animals, especially small dogs and cats, have high thoracic wall compliance. The ribs tend to flatten, and the thoracic wall moves toward the table when pressure is placed down on the trocar. A larger degree of force is required for the trocar to enter the pleural space, so there may be an increased risk of iatrogenic damage.

- Non trocar tube placement may be technically harder to perform than trocar tube placement in nonsurgical patients. Reasons for failure may include large patient size, failure to tunnel under the latissimus dorsi muscle, not using a large enough forceps to penetrate the intercostal muscles, or failure to find the hole in the intercostal muscles when placing the tube.

Treatment
- Dogs with high chest wall compliance may benefit from nontrocar tube placement or a small-bore wire-guided chest tube.
- Consider whether thoracocentesis can be performed instead.

Outcome
Treatment is usually successful when technical issues are resolved.

Prevention
- Difficult to avoid but have other options for tube placement available

Improper tube placement

Definition
This is failure to place the tube within the pleural space or placement of the tube in an abnormal location within the pleural space.

Risk factors
- Failure for the tube to penetrate the full extent of the thoracic wall (i.e., subcutaneous location)
- Tubes placed through a caudal intercostal space or placed in a caudal direction may enter the abdominal cavity directly or after penetrating the diaphragm (Figure 38.1)
- Tube not correctly advanced into the cranial thorax (Figure 38.2)
- Tube embedded in pleural folds or mediastinum

Diagnosis
- Orthogonal radiographs should be taken after tube placement to document its position and allow many irregularities to be noted (e.g., subcutaneous or abdominal placement).
- Failure to achieve thoracic drainage.

Complications in Small Animal Surgery, First Edition. Edited by Dominique Griffon and Annick Hamaide.

© 2016 John Wiley & Sons, Inc. Published 2016 by John Wiley & Sons, Inc.

Companion website: www.wiley.com/go/griffon/complications

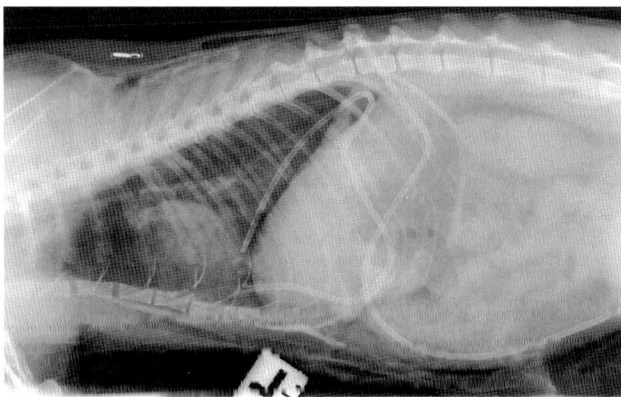

Figure 38.1 Radiograph showing a small-gauge chest tube entering the abdominal cavity rather than the pleural cavity. In this patient, tube placement had been attempted in the caudal thoracic cavity caudal to bite wounds causing trauma to the thoracic wall at the normal site of tube insertion. A second drain has been correctly placed within the thoracic cavity.

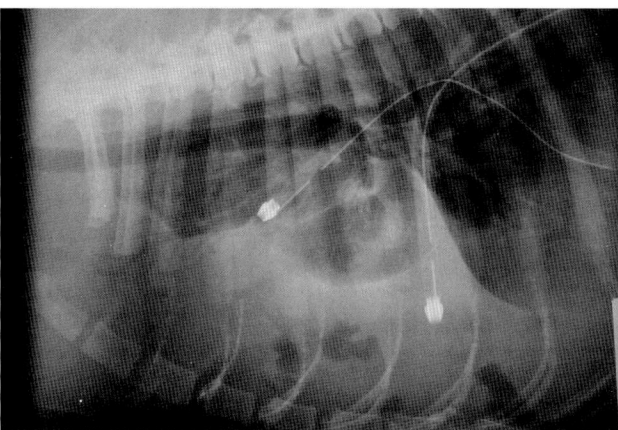

Figure 38.2 Placement of bilateral trocar chest drains into the pleural cavity for the treatment of chylothorax in a dog. The short length of the tubes means that they do not reach the suggested correct location at the second intercostal space.

Treatment

Figure 38.3 as an algorithm on treatment after improper tube placement.

Outcome

During tube placement, it is usually easier to replace the tube than to try to manipulate it into the correct position. After tube placement, malpositioning is very difficult to rectify unless it can be done by slightly withdrawing the tube. Most cases require new tube placement.

Prevention

- Place the tube at the correct intercostal space.
- Tunnel the tube under the skin in a cranioventral direction.
- Penetrate the thoracic wall aiming cranioventrally.
- Trocar tubes: after penetrating the intercostal muscles, advance the tube 1 to 2 cm further before removing the stylet. Care must be taken not to advance the trocar too far because it may cause iatrogenic damage.
- Check that thoracic drainage can be achieved before ending the procedure.
- Obtain radiographs (two views) to confirm correct positioning.

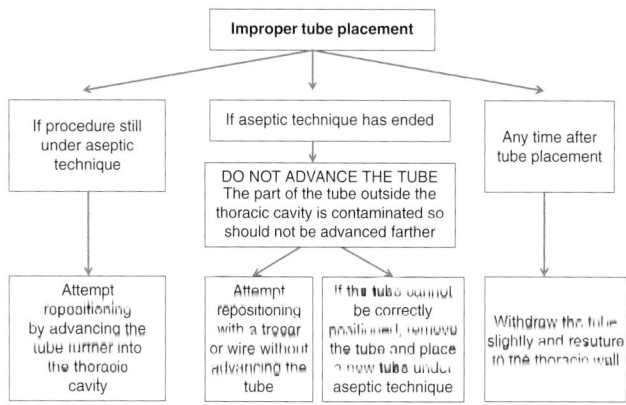

Figure 38.3 Algorithm on improper tube placement.

Problems with tube maintenance

Definition

- Inadvertent slippage or removal (e.g., caught in kennel door, stood on by patient)
- Patient interference (e.g., chewing holes in tube, chewing through tube, pulling tube out)
- Seroma or fluid leakage around tube
- Subcutaneous emphysema
- Leakage around tube, causing pneumothorax

Risk factors

- Tube not secured properly to skin
- Tube not appropriately covered
- Patient not prevented from interfering with tube
- Incision in skin too large
- Subcutaneous tunnel not made (large-bore tubes)
- Seroma or fluid leakage around the tube may be caused by a high volume of pleural fluid rather than a problem with the tube itself

Diagnosis

Diagnosis is obtained through clinical examination.

Treatment

Figure 38.4 is an algorithm on problems with tube maintenance.

- Consider whether a tube is still necessary if there are complications with its use. It is often better to remove a tube than to try to manage one that is not functioning properly. A new tube can be placed at the same time if it is needed or subsequently be placed if clinical evidence suggests it is necessary. The paper by Marques *et al.* (2009) suggests that tubes can be removed even in the presence of ongoing pleural fluid production and that the presence of the tube itself may incite some of the fluid production.

Outcome

- Rapid and potentially fatal tension pneumothorax is a risk when the tube is accidently removed or displaced.
- Tubes can easily be removed and replaced with a new tube in most individuals. If an animal's clinical condition precludes anesthesia, a small-bore wire-guided catheter can be placed in most conscious or sedated animals.
- Seroma, fluid leakage around the tube, and subcutaneous emphysema are likely to continue for as long as the tube remains in place but should resolve rapidly after tube removal.

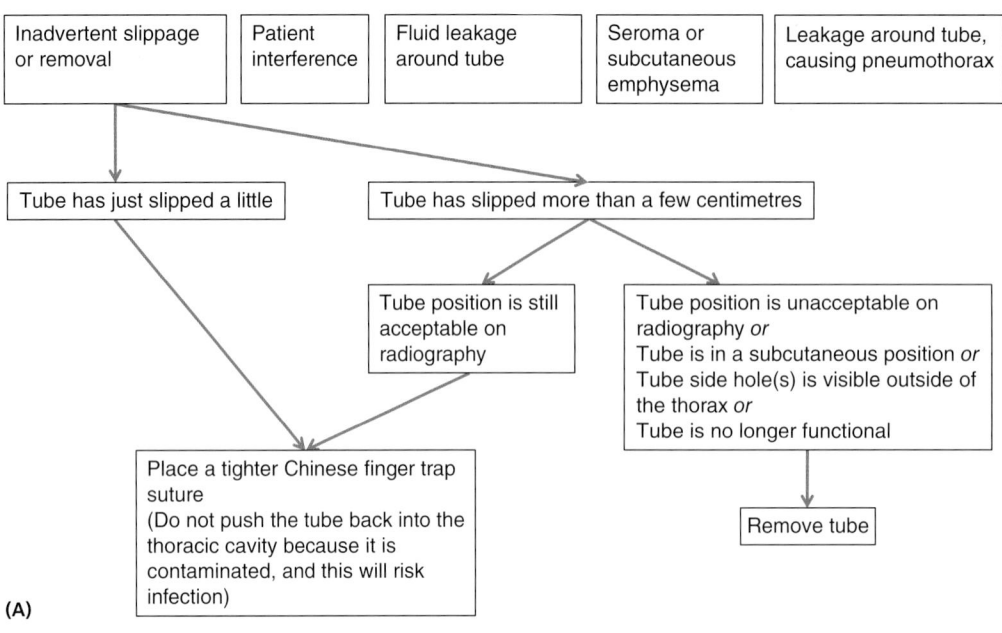

Figure 38.4 Algorithm on problems with tube maintenance. **A,** Inadvertent slippage or removal. **B,** Patient interference. **C,** Fluid leakage around the tube. **D,** Seroma and subcutaneous emphysema. **E,** Leakage around the tube, causing pneumothorax.

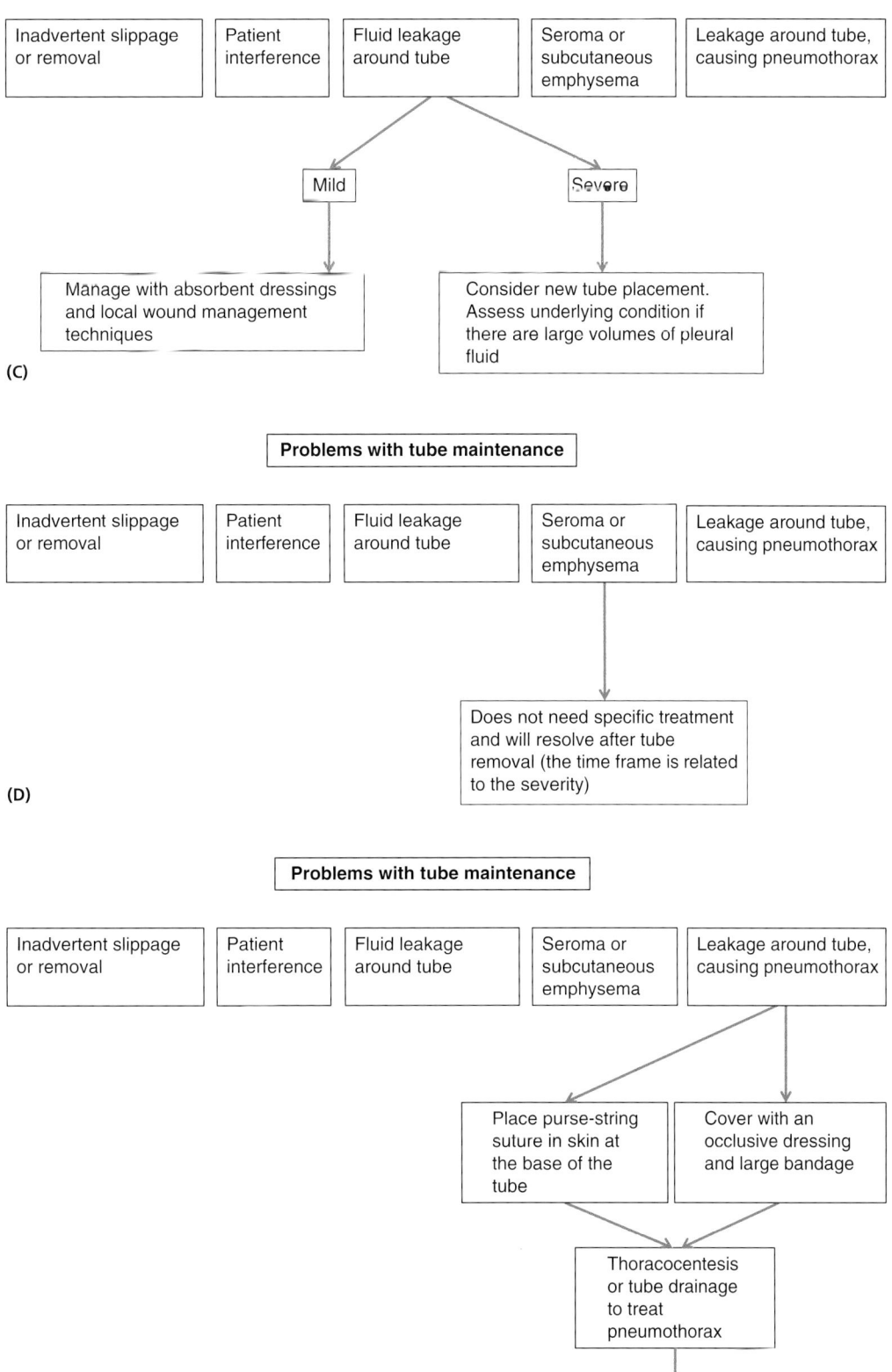

Figure 38.4 *Continued*

Prevention

- Make a skin incision no larger than the tube. If the skin incision is too large, place a purse-string suture in the skin around the tube.
- Create a subcutaneous tunnel when placing large-bore tubes. Small-bore tubes placed by the Seldinger technique are less likely to leak and can be placed without a tunnel.
- Place a secure Chinese finger trap suture from the skin to the tube. Large gauge suture material (e.g., 3 metric nylon) allows the suture to be pulled tighter than smaller gauge suture because it is less likely to break. The sutures should be pulled tightly enough to make a small indentation in the tube.
- Prevent patient interference and inadvertent removal in cage doors:
  - 24-hour monitoring
  - Buster collar
  - Cover drain with dressings

Iatrogenic intrathoracic or abdominal damage

Definition

The effects of needles scratching the lungs are commonly seen at thoracotomy in animals that have had thoracocentesis, especially multiple times. Major damage to intrathoracic structures by needles or catheters during thoracocentesis or thoracic tubes during tube placement is extremely rare and mostly unreported in the literature. Anecdotal reports suggest that penetration and damage to the heart, lungs, stomach, liver, and biliary tract can occur. The effects of iatrogenic damage may include:

- Intercostal vessel puncture or laceration
  - Hematoma
  - Hemorrhage around the tube or (more rarely) from a thoracocentesis site
  - Interpleural hemorrhage
  - Hypovolemic shock
- Lungs
  - Superficial damage (scratching) of lungs during needle thoracocentesis
  - Lung penetration (chest tubes) (Figure 38.5)
    - Pneumothorax
    - Hemorrhage

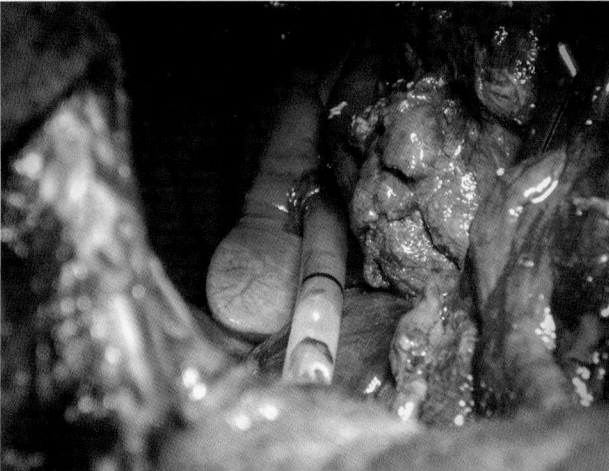

Figure 38.5 A chest tube has inadvertently penetrated a lung lobe. © Davina Anderson

- Heart or great vessels
  - Superficial damage
    - Arrhythmia
    - Muscle damage
    - Coronary vessel laceration
  - Full-thickness cardiac wall or vessel penetration with significant hemorrhage (especially when the tube is withdrawn)
  - Pericardial effusion
- Abdominal cavity
  - Stomach: misdiagnosis of pyothorax if fluid examined cytologically. The presence of bacteria in the absence of neutrophils should alert the clinician that the fluid is gastric in origin.
  - Liver, gallbladder
- Sympathetic nerve (preganglionic): Horner's syndrome (Boydell *et al.* 1997).

Risk factors

- Damage to intercostal neurovascular bundle: entering the intercostal space along the caudal aspect of a rib
- Using the wrong intercostal space. Damage to the heart may occur if a cranial position is used, and damage to the abdominal organs may occur if a caudal space is used. Lung damage can occur even if the correct position is used.
- Aiming thoracic tubes in the wrong direction (e.g., caudally)
- Placing the tube too far cranially (i.e., cranial to second intercostal space): damage to ocular sympathetic nerve pathway in cranial thorax
- Animal moving or inappropriately restrained. However, it should be noted that some conscious animals prefer a "hands-off approach" and struggle more with restraint.
- It has been suggested that the risk of lung damage is higher when draining pleural fluid than air because the lungs are likely to be closer to the thoracic wall.
- Thoracocentesis
  - Needle too long or wide gauge
  - Failure to hold the needle still
  - Holding needle perpendicular to thoracic cavity rather than at an angle
- Small-gauge wire-guided catheter
  - Iatrogenic damage is rare because the needles and catheters are small.
- Trocar catheter
  - Placement through a highly compliant thoracic wall because more force must be applied
  - Applying too much pressure during tube application where it is not required
  - Failure to hold the tube tightly adjacent to the thoracic wall thus allowing the tube to enter the thorax with too much force and for too great a distance
- Nontrocar catheter (closed thorax)
  - Iatrogenic damage is rare because the incision for the tube is made under more controlled conditions than a trocar tube. However, it is more difficult to place a tube by this method than a trocar tube in most cases.
- Trocar or nontrocar catheter (open thorax)
  - Failure to visualize and protect thoracic organs. However, iatrogenic damage is extremely rare because the tube can be seen entering the pleural space, and the thoracic wall can be supported making tube placement easier.

Diagnosis

- Pneumothorax (see Chapter 37)
- Hemorrhage: Clinical signs, including hypovolemic shock and marked dyspnea, may develop rapidly if there is significant hemorrhage (see Chapters 12 and 37), although this is rare. More minor bleeding is unlikely to have a significant effect on blood volume. Hemorrhage from intercostal vessels may be obvious if the blood runs along the tube or if a swelling develops. Aspiration will yield blood (packed cell volume [PCV] initially the same as peripheral blood). Pleural hemorrhage will be noted at subsequent tube drainage or can be diagnosed by thoracocentesis for animals without a tube in place. PCV should be obtained on any pleural fluid that looks bloody because it may be hard to differentiate blood from sanguinous fluid on visual inspection, although fresh blood will clot.
- Sympathetic nerve damage: presence of Horner's syndrome, mydriasis 20 to 45 minutes after ocular phenylephrine 10% administration

Treatment

- Damage to intercostal blood vessels
  - Treatment for blood loss and hypovolemic shock as necessary (see Chapter 12)
  - Specific treatment is rarely required if occurs after thoracocentesis.
  - Removal of the tube and placement at an adjacent intercostal space.
  - Very rarely, a surgical approach to the bleeding vessel for ligation is required.
- Superficial damage (scratching) of lungs is unlikely to have any clinical effect and should not require treatment. Penetration of a lung lobe by a trocar or tube will require partial or complete lung lobectomy (depending on the site of damage) only if hemorrhage or pneumothorax does not resolve spontaneously. Mild cases can be given time to resolve without surgical treatment. If there is significant or uncontrollable hemorrhage or pneumothorax, thoracotomy may need to be performed as an emergency procedure.
- Penetration of the heart or great vessels may not be instantly apparent if the tube remains in the heart or vessel but should be obvious when the trocar is removed because frank blood will be withdrawn from the tube. Treatment would require rapid thoracotomy. Removal of the tube before thoracotomy will be associated with significant hemorrhage and is likely to be rapidly fatal, so the tube is left in position until thoracotomy has been performed and it can be removed under direct visualization. Penetration of great vessels would require cross- or side-clamping of the vessel, tube removal, and vessel repair. Cardiac repair is often possible. Effects of superficial damage rarely require treatment, although some arrhythmias may be clinically significant and require antiarrhythmic medication.
- In extreme cases of intrathoracic bleeding (heart, great vessels, intercostal vessels), the blood can be collected by thoracocentesis and autotransfused, assuming that appropriate equipment is available, it can be performed under aseptic conditions, and the animal does not have an underlying disease that would preclude autotransfusion (e.g., neoplasia, chylothorax, pyothorax).
- Abdominal cavity or organ penetration after thoracocentesis should not require treatment unless there is leakage of fluid from a hollow viscus or significant hemorrhage from a solid organ.

Tubes may cause more significant damage and necessitate repair of these tissues.
- Sympathetic nerve damage: Remove the tube when no longer needed.

Outcome

- Damage to intercostal blood vessels: Significant blood loss and hypovolemic shock are rare, and it is unlikely that the vessel will need to be ligated. A hematoma will resolve with time and is unlikely to require intervention. There is a small risk of infection in a hematoma, and its presence may make subsequent intercostal thoracotomy more awkward to perform.
- Superficial damage of lungs after thoracocentesis is unlikely to be clinically significant. Lung damage by tubes can be cured by lobectomy if necessary, but there is the potential for death if hemorrhage or pneumothorax is severe.
- Full-thickness cardiac wall or vessel penetration with significant hemorrhage is likely to be fatal. Successful surgical treatment will occasionally be possible if the tube seals the defect and the appropriate facilities and expertise for cardiovascular surgery are available. More superficial cardiac damage is unlikely to be fatal unless there is significant arrhythmia or coronary vessel damage, and most cases are self-limiting.
- Clinically significant complications after penetration of abdominal organs during thoracocentesis are rare. More significant damage may occur with trocar tubes, including leakage from hollow organs and bleeding from solid organs.
- Sympathetic nerve damage is consistent with neuropraxia and should resolve after tube removal.

Prevention

- Enter the intercostal space midway between the ribs or toward the cranial edge of a rib to avoid the intercostal vessels on the caudal edge of the rib.
- Choose the correct intercostal space to avoid the heart, sympathetic nerve, and abdominal cavity.
- Thoracocentesis
  - Consider placement of a small-gauge wire-guided catheter instead of thoracocentesis for the following instances:
    - Thick thoracic wall (require long needles)
    - Agitated animal: A small-gauge wire-guided catheter can be placed after brief sedation, and thoracic drainage can be performed in a more controlled manner.
    - Large volume of pleural fluid or air that will take a long time to drain and may need repeated passes of a needle with an inherent risk of lung damage at each needle entry point
    - Likely need for repeated thoracocentesis
  - Choose an appropriate sized needle or catheter.
  - When the needle is in thoracic cavity, angle it cranioventrally to avoid the lungs.
  - Hold the needle still during drainage.
  - Stop thoracocentesis if the needle is felt to scratch the expanding lung.
- Small-gauge wire-guided catheter: Carefully follow instructions on catheter placement.
- Trocar catheter
  - Consider a different tube type in animals with highly compliant thoracic walls.
  - Avoid applying too much pressure to a tube where it is not required.

- The hand that is holding the tube should grip it firmly so that the closed fist will abut the thoracic wall and stop the tube from advancing any further after it has penetrated the intercostal muscles. The position of this hand should be such that only the tip of the tube will initially penetrate the muscles. The rest of the tube can then be advanced in a more controlled manner.
- Nontrocar catheter (closed thorax)
  - Careful placement technique
  - Use of blunt, right-angled forceps for controlled penetration of the intercostal muscles
- Trocar or nontrocar catheter (open thorax)
  - Visualize tube placement from within the thoracic cavity.
  - Protect the intrathoracic organs with laparotomy swabs during tube placement.

Insufficient pleural drainage

Definition
This is an inability of thoracocentesis or a chest tube to remove part or all of the pleural fluid or air.

Risk factors
- Thoracocentesis
  - Catheter or needle not long enough (i.e., in subcutaneous position)
  - Catheter kinked during placement or as chest wall moves with breathing
  - Catheter or needle in wrong position (e.g., in dorsal thorax it will be difficult to drain fluid)
  - Fluid in pockets or one hemithorax
- Chest tube
  - Tube malposition (see earlier)
  - Tube obstruction: blood clots, purulent material
  - Connectors not open (e.g., gate clamp, three-way tap)
  - Heimlich valve getting wet

Diagnosis
- Failure of drainage even after tube flushing
- Radiographic signs of the presence of pleural effusion or pneumothorax

Treatment
- Reposition the needle or tube.
- Change the animal's position and try to drain again.
- Check that connectors are all open.
- Repeat flushing the tube.
- Remove the nonfunctioning Heimlich valve and use an alternative method of drainage.
- Remove the tube and replace it with a new tube if it is still needed.

Outcome
A blocked tube can usually be flushed successfully.

Prevention
- Use large-bore tubes for hemothorax or pyothorax or regularly flush smaller tubes.
- Place extra holes in large-bore trocar or nontrocar tubes.
- Avoid Heimlich valves in the presence of pleural fluid and in animals weighing less than 15 to 20 kg.

Pyothorax
Also see Chapters 3 and 37.

Definition
Pyothorax is the presence of exudate within the pleural cavity.

Risk factors
- Failure to place using aseptic technique
  - Not clipping hair
  - Not performing adequate skin disinfection
  - Not wearing sterile gloves
  - Incorrect handling of tube (e.g., allowing the tube to touch a nonsterile surface)
- Ascending infection
  - Tube in place for a prolonged period of time
  - Inappropriate tube management
- Infection caused by underlying disease or thoracotomy or thoracoscopy may be difficult to differentiate from infection as a tube complication.

Diagnosis
See Chapter 3.

Treatment
See Chapter 3.

Outcome
See Chapter 3.

The presence of pyothorax as an iatrogenic hospital-acquired infection may mean infection with multidrug-resistant bacteria, such as methicillin-resistant *Staphylococcus pseudintermedius* (MRSP) or *Staphylococcus aureus* (MRSA), which is more common than other causes of pyothorax. Elimination of pyothorax with these bacteria may be more difficult to achieve, especially with some strains of MRSP that have widespread resistance.

Prevention
- Aseptic technique for tube placement and thoracocentesis, including clipping and aseptic preparation of the skin, and use of sterile gloves, drape, and instruments. A sterile gown is helpful when placing a tube in case the tube touches the forearms, When placing a tube, take care that the tube or wire (if placing using Seldinger technique) does not inadvertently touch nonsterile areas; this is a common problem for personnel not wearing a sterile gown because the long tubes can be hard to handle in an aseptic manner. If this occurs, a new tube is used.
- Keep the tube covered to minimize environmental contamination and patient interference. The tube exit site should be covered with a sterile dressing and the remainder of the tube covered with a bandage. The exit port and gate clamp are placed under the outer layer to allow access for drainage.
- Avoid contamination at drainage. Wash hands before handling the tube, and if possible, wear sterile gloves to drain the tube (Figure 38.6). Use a new syringe for each drainage. Do not allow the end of the tube to touch nonsterile surfaces. If this occurs, the clamp on the end of the tube must be changed.
- Replace three-way taps and clamps on the end of tubing daily.
- The patient should wear a buster collar to prevent licking of the drain.

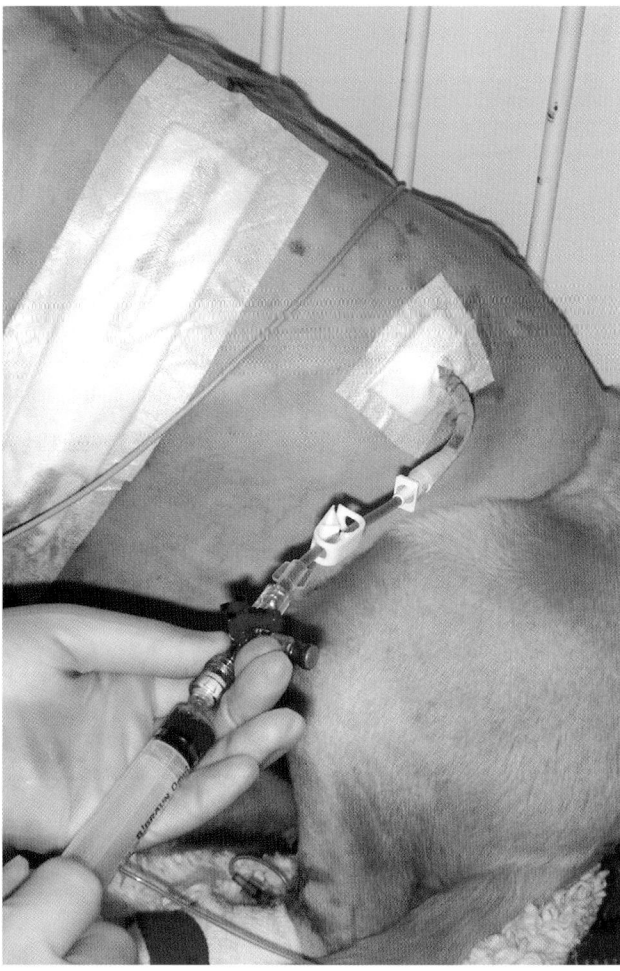

Figure 38.6 Drainage of a chest tube using gloves.

- Assess fluid cytologically every 1 to 2 days that a drain is in place. A change in the neutrophil cytology is suggestive of early infection, meaning proactive measures to treat the infection should be taken.

Pneumothorax
Also see Chapter 37.

Definition
A small amount of air will normally enter the pleural space after the tube is inserted and before the connectors are placed, but it is minimal, and the air is easily removed by tube drainage. Iatrogenic pneumothorax formation occurs because of problems with the tube or errors in drainage.

Risk factors
- Subcutaneous tunnel not created or too large (large-bore tubes)
- Tube connectors not secured properly
- Patient interference (e.g., biting through the tube)
- Inadvertently instilling air rather than draining air or fluid if using a three-way tap and syringe

Diagnosis
See Chapter 37.

Treatment
See Chapter 37.

Outcome
The outcome is usually excellent unless life-threatening pneumothorax has not been noted or managed promptly.

Prevention
- Correct tube placement and management
- Use of small-bore tubes
- Use tube connectors with one-way valves for drainage to prevent inadvertent air instillation
- Prevent patient interference.

Pleural effusion
Also see Chapter 37.

Definition
Pleural effusion is the presence of fluid (exudate, hemorrhage, transudate, modified transudate, chyle) within the pleural cavity.

Risk factors
- Presence of underlying disease
- Hemorrhage and pyothorax: see earlier discussion
- The presence of the tube may incite a reaction caused by mechanical irritation or the presence of foreign material, leading to fluid production. It is usually sterile with a low cell count.

Diagnosis
- Presence of pleural fluid when it is not expected (e.g., after treatment of a vascular anomaly or pneumothorax)
- Diagnosis of fluid production in response to the tube is difficult when the underlying disease produces pleural fluid but may be suggested if fluid is not reducing as expected during the course of treatment.
- Cytology, culture, PCV, and triglycerides to differentiate types of effusion

Treatment
Sometimes it can be hard to know if the fluid is caused by the disease or the tube, and it might require tube removal to differentiate them. Another tube can be placed if it is realized that the first tube was removed too early.

Outcome
Tube removal may lead to resolution of the fluid.

Prevention
Avoid leaving tubes in for longer than necessary.

Pain
Also see Chapter 15.

Definition
Pain may be associated with the presence of a chest tube

Risk factors
Figure 38.7 is an algorithm on tube pain.

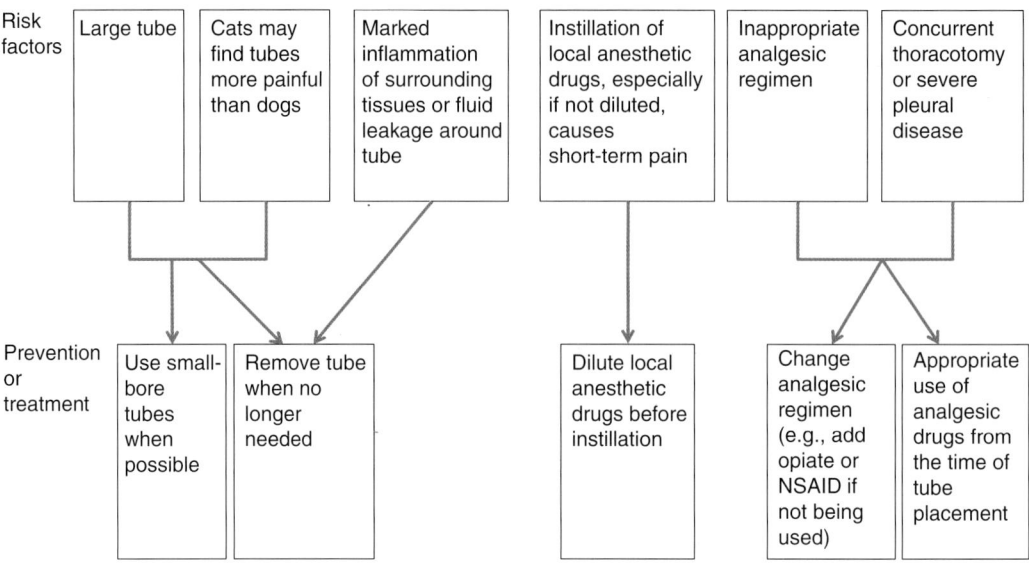

Figure 38.7 Algorithm on tube pain. NSAID, nonsteroidal antiinflammatory drug.

Diagnosis

Diagnosis is obtained through clinical observation.

Treatment

See Figure 38.7.

Outcome

Pain is normally self-limiting with appropriate treatment, but it can have an impact on nutrition and patient well-being.

Prevention

See Figure 38.7.

Relevant literature

Until recently, most thoracostomy tubes were wide-bore tubes, requiring a trocar to place them. Disadvantages to this technique include the need for sedation or anesthesia for placement, difficulty in penetrating the thoracic cavity, and pain associated with the presence of a large tube. Tube placement is not always possible in animals with high chest compliance, necessitating creation of a subcutaneous tunnel and penetration of the pleura with forceps before a trocar or nontrocar type tube can be introduced.

The use of small-bore (14-gauge) wire-guided thoracostomy tubes, placed using the Seldinger technique, allows placement in conscious or lightly sedated animals (Valtolina and Adamantos 2009). Wurtinger *et al.* (2011) described the use of small-gauge catheters (6–8 Fr in dogs; 6 Fr in cats) placed via the Seldinger technique. In a series of 16 cats with pyothorax treated with lavage via a small-gauge catheter, there were no major complications with tube placement and handling, but 2 cats initially had ineffective drainage, leading to surgery or placement of a second drain. Two further cats also had a second drain added, but the reason for this was not clear.

Marques *et al.* (2009) published a retrospective analysis of thoracostomy tube use in 127 dogs and cats. Complications were seen in 22% of animals and are summarized in Tables 38.1 and 38.2. The higher complication rate than noted by Moores *et al.* (2007) was

Table 38.1 Incidence of thoracostomy tube–related complications in 101 dogs

Complication	Number of dogs	Outcome
Discharge around the tube insertion site	9 of 101	
Accidental removal	6 of 101	1 died (tension pneumothorax) 2 tubes replaced 2 tubes did not need replacing
Tube blockage	4 of 101	2 tubes replaced 2 tubes unblocked by flushing
Accidental tube displacement	3 of 101	1 died (tension pneumothorax) 1 tube replaced 1 tube did not need replacing
Air leaking around the tube, causing subcutaneous emphysema	2 of 101	

Source: Data from Marques *et al.* (2009).

Table 38.2 Incidence of thoracostomy tube–related complications in 26 cats

Complication	Number of cats	Outcome
Discharge around the tube insertion site	1 of 26	
Accidental removal	3 of 26	1 tube replaced 2 tubes did not need replacing

Source: Data from Marques *et al.* (2009).

Table 38.3 Incidence of thoracostomy tube–related complications in animals undergoing median sternotomy or intercostal thoracotomy

Complication	Animals affected
Serosanguineous discharge	4 of 84 (5%)
Patient interference	9 of 84 (11%)
Pneumothorax	1 of 84 (1%)

Source: Data from Tattersall and Welsh (2006).

suggested to be attributable to the higher number of animals treated for pleural disease rather than for evacuation of the pleural space after thoracotomy.

In a paper looking at complications associated with lateral thoracotomy (Moores *et al.* 2007), 5 of 72 animals (7%) had thoracostomy tube complications, including leakage of fluid and subcutaneous emphysema. The incidence of short-term (i.e., <14 days postoperatively) complications after thoracotomy was not associated with the duration of thoracostomy tube placement.

In a paper describing outcomes in 98 dogs undergoing median sternotomy or intercostal thoracotomy (Tattersall and Welsh 2006), short-term (<14 days postoperatively) complications were seen in 13 of 64 dogs (22%) that had a thoracostomy tube placed during surgery (Table 38.3). The mean duration of tube use was significantly longer in dogs that had a tube-related complication than those that did not (87 vs. 46 hours). Complications were significantly more likely to occur in dogs with pyothorax as the underlying disease (37%), which may be related to the duration of tube use. One dog died from pneumothorax as a direct result of a thoracostomy tube complication.

Frendin and Obel (1997) originally described small-bore wire-guided chest tube use in 41 animals. Two did not drain because of kinking, either at the thoracic wall or within the pleural cavity, and had to be replaced. One dog was euthanized because sudden, severe pneumothorax, shown to have been caused by the catheter penetrating a lung lobe that was adhesed to the thoracic wall. Valtolina and Adamantos (2009) presented a prospective evaluation of the use of these drains in which complications were seen in 8 of 20 animals (40%). It is possible that the higher complication rate is attributable to the prospective aspect of the study, in which complications are more likely to be noted. Pneumothorax was seen in 8 of the 20 animals after a small-bore tube was placed (mild in 7, moderate in 8), but it is likely that this occurs when placing all tubes and is easily remedied by draining the chest after tube placement. Four animals (20%) had functional complications, including kinking and malpositioning (tubes did not drain fluid if they were positioned caudally rather than cranially). One tube (5%) was removed by the animal. In humans, lower infection rates were seen when small-bore tubes were used in preference to large-bore tubes, and although this has not been assessed in animals, none of the animals reported by Valtolina and Adamantos (2009) developed pyothorax.

References

Boydell, P., Pike, R., Crossley, D., et al. (1997) Horner's syndrome following intrathoracic tube placement. *Journal of Small Animal Practice* 38 (10), 466-467.

Frendin, J., Obel, N. (1997) Catheter drainage of pleural fluid collections and pneumothorax. *Journal of Small Animal Practice* 38 (6), 237-242.

Marques, A.I., Tattersall, J. Shaw, DJ., et al. (2009) Retrospective analysis of the relationship between time of thoracostomy drain removal and discharge time. *Journal of Small Animal Practice* 50 (4), 162-166.

Moores, A.L., Halfacree, Z.J., Baines, S.J., et al. (2007) Indications, outcomes and complications following lateral thoracotomy in dogs and cats. *Journal of Small Animal Practice* 48 (12), 695-698.

Tattersall, J.A., Welsh, E. (2006) Factors influencing the short-term outcome following thoracic surgery in 98 dogs. *Journal of Small Animal Practice* 47 (12), 715-720.

Valtolina, C., Adamantos, S. (2009) Evaluation of small-bore wire-guided chest drains for management of pleural space disease. *Journal of Small Animal Practice* 50 (6), 290-297.

Wurtinger, G., Peppler, C., Schneider, M., et al. (2011) Pyothorax—have we learnt anything in the last 15 years? *Proceedings of the European College of Veterinary Surgeons*, pp. 165-166.

39 Complications After Intercostal and Sternal Thoracotomy

Alison Moores

Anderson Moores Veterinary Specialists, Winchester, Hampshire, UK

Thoracotomy is performed for treatment of intrathoracic disease when other techniques, such as thoracoscopy or interventional radiology techniques, are not appropriate, have failed, are not available, or have been declined by the owner. The most common indications for intercostal thoracotomy, in order of frequency, are vascular anomalies (e.g., patent ductus arteriosus, vascular ring anomaly), lung lobectomy, and esophageal and pericardial diseases (Tattersall and Welsh 2006; Moores et al. 2007). The most common indications for median sternotomy, in order of frequency, are pyothorax, pericardial disease, pneumothorax, mediastinal mass, and pleural effusion (Burton and White 1996; Tattersall and Welsh 2006). Rib resection thoracotomy is rarely performed.

Complications associated with intercostal, rib resection, and median sternotomy techniques are reported in individual case reports and case series for animals undergoing thoracic surgery for a number of indications but are not specific for the approach to the thoracic cavity. A small number of papers have looked specifically at the complications and outcomes in dogs and cats undergoing the surgical approach to the thoracic cavity. In these papers, no death or euthanasia was attributed to the surgical approach.

Excessive wound inflammation, bruising, edema, or swelling

Definition

Inflammation is a normal response to surgical trauma. However in some cases, marked erythema, bruising, and swelling may be associated with the wound (Figures 39.1 and 39.2). Edema is the accumulation of fluid between cells and presents as "pitting" after applying digital pressure. The overall reported incidence is 5% to 8%.

Risk factors

- Thin skin and little subcutaneous fat
- Poor surgical technique (e.g., rough tissue handling, excessive use of diathermy)
- Poor hemostasis
- Underlying clotting disorder
- Failure to create a large enough incision, necessitating excessive traction on wound edges

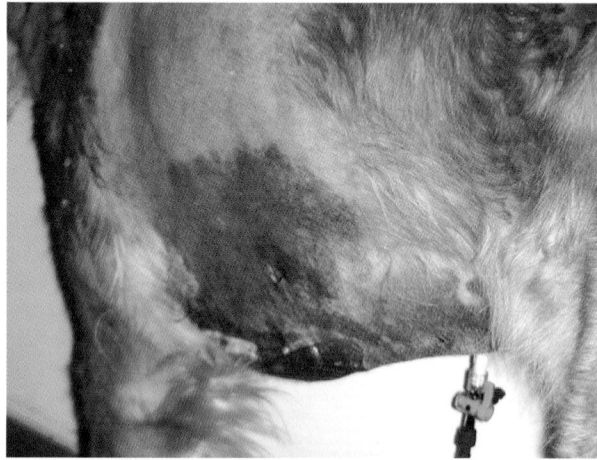

Figure 39.1 Marked bruising after median sternotomy in a thin-skinned dog. Also note a significant amount of hemorrhage on the wound dressing. *Source:* A. Moores, Anderson Moores Veterinary Specialists, Winchester, Hampshire, UK, 2014. Reproduced with permission from A. Moores.

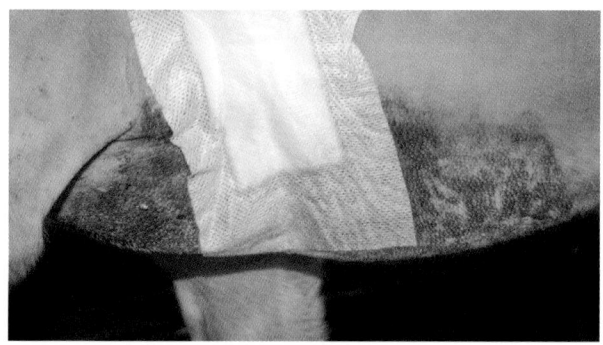

Figure 39.2 Marked ventral bruising after intercostal thoracotomy. There is no discharge on the wound dressing. *Source:* A. Moores, Anderson Moores Veterinary Specialists, Winchester, Hampshire, UK, 2014. Reproduced with permission from A. Moores.

- Wide surgical exposure required (caused by the underlying disease), with increased tension applied to bones or sternebrae and soft tissues during retraction (Figure 39.3)
- Edema may arise from damaged to blood and lymphatic vessels during surgery.

Complications in Small Animal Surgery, First Edition. Edited by Dominique Griffon and Annick Hamaide.
© 2016 John Wiley & Sons, Inc. Published 2016 by John Wiley & Sons, Inc.
Companion website: www.wiley.com/go/griffon/complications

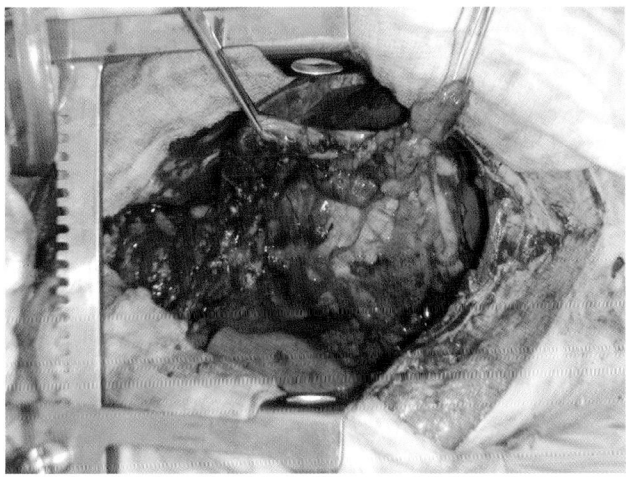

Figure 39.3 Wide exposure of the thoracic cavity during median sternotomy may be a risk factor for postoperative inflammation and bruising. *Source:* A. Moores, Anderson Moores Veterinary Specialists, Winchester, Hampshire, UK, 2014. Reproduced with permission from A. Moores.

Diagnosis

Diagnosis is based on physical examination findings, although it is a subjective diagnosis.

Treatment

No specific treatment is required unless the inflammation progresses to wound discharge, infection, or dehiscence. Pain associated with the inflammation can be managed with additional analgesic drugs and the application of cold compresses.

Outcome

The condition usually resolves without intervention.

Prevention

- Application of Halsted's principles
- Appropriately sized surgical incision

Seroma

Definition

Seroma is defined as an accumulation of sterile serous fluid deep to a wound. The most common location after intercostal thoracotomy is the ventral (i.e., most dependent) part of the wound, where it pools because of gravity (Figure 39.4). After median sternotomy, fluid often accumulates caudal to the thoracic limbs, especially in deep-chested dogs. In some cases, the fluid moves distally down the thoracic limb, leading to limb edema or swelling (Figure 39.5). The overall reported incidence is 11% to 22%.

Risk factors

- Excessive surgical trauma
- Excessive undermining of skin
- Excessive animal movement postoperatively

Diagnosis

- Seroma formation is usually diagnosed on the gross physical appearance of a soft fluid-filled swelling. Rarely, the swelling is

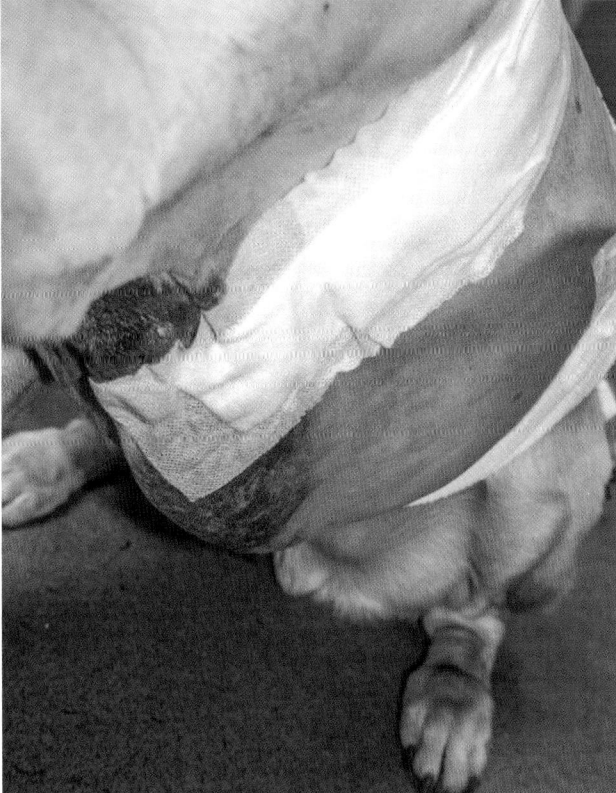

Figure 39.4 Seroma formation in the ventral (i.e., most dependent) part of the wound in a dog after intercostal thoracotomy. *Source:* A. Moores, Anderson Moores Veterinary Specialists, Winchester, Hampshire, UK, 2014. Reproduced with permission from A. Moores.

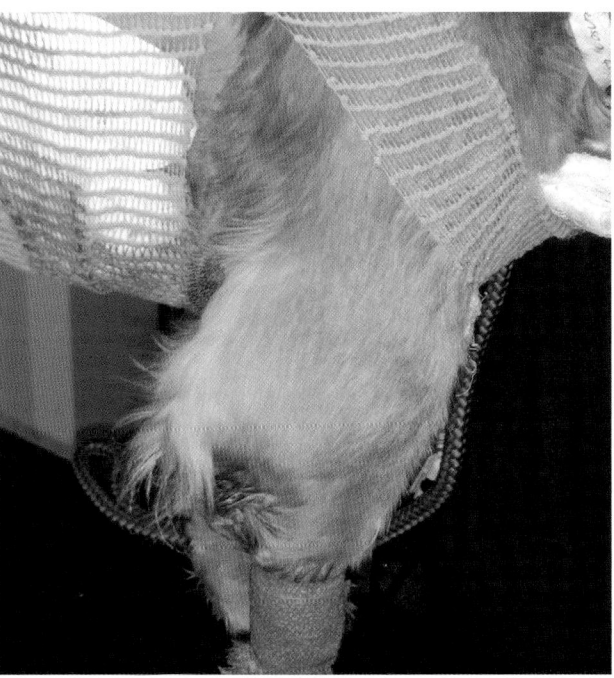

Figure 39.5 Seroma formation in the brachial and elbow region in a dog after median sternotomy. *Source:* D. Anderson, Anderson Moores Veterinary Specialists, Winchester, Hampshire, UK, 2014. Reproduced with permission from D. Anderson.

firmer, if the seroma is deeper than the subcutaneous space, but this is rare as there is little muscle, other than the pectoral muscles, in the ventral aspect of the thorax. It may also become firmer as it becomes more chronic.
- Fine-needle aspiration and cytologic examination

Treatment
Seromas rarely cause discomfort or inhibit wound healing and therefore rarely require treatment. Repeated drainage is avoided because the fluid has a tendency to recur, and there is the risk of iatrogenic infection. Bandaging techniques are difficult to use in this location. Very large seromas may need placement of drains to allow resolution.

Outcome
They usually resolve over a few weeks as the serous fluid is reabsorbed.

Prevention
- Application of Halsted's principles
- Avoid excessive undermining of skin

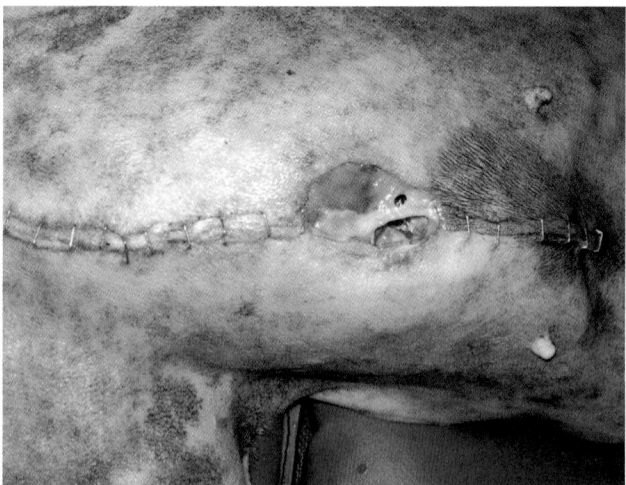

Figure 39.6 Wound dehiscence, necrosis of tissues, and purulent wound discharge affecting a small length of a median sternotomy wound. *Source:* J. Ladlow, University of Cambridge, Cambridge, UK, 2014. Reproduced with permission from J. Ladlow.

Wound discharge, dehiscence, and infection

Definition
Discharge from a wound may be serous, serosanguineous, hemorrhagic, or purulent. Wound dehiscence is breakdown of the surgical wound, may involve part or the entire length of the wound, and may be superficial (skin and subcutaneous tissues) or deep. Deep dehiscence is rare after either median sternotomy or intercostal thoracotomy, but it may accompany sternal osteomyelitis (see later discussion). Infection is usually bacterial and may involve superficial tissues or sternebrae (osteomyelitis). The overall reported incidence is 1% to 8%.

Risk factors
- Serous or serosanguineous wound discharge: underlying seroma, excessive movement, excessive inflammation.
- Hemorrhagic wound discharge: poor surgical hemostasis, laceration of the intercostal or internal thoracic vessels, hemorrhage related to the intrathoracic procedure.
- Purulent wound discharge or infection: poor surgical asepsis, long anesthetic or surgical time, placement of metal implants (median sternotomy wires), poor postoperative wound care (e.g., dirty kennels, allowing the animal to lick the wound, handling the wound with dirty hands).
- Wound dehiscence: infection, animal interfering with the wound, excessive movement

Diagnosis
- Discharge and dehiscence: based on gross appearance (Figure 39.6). The nature of the discharge should be confirmed by cytologic examination.
- Infection: gross appearance, cytologic examination, and aerobic and anaerobic bacteriologic (+/− fungal) culture from a swab or aspirate of deep tissues (to avoid growing surface contaminants) or implants in the case of osteomyelitis.

Treatment
- Serous or serosanguineous wound discharge: No specific treatment is required other than local wound care, assuming the

discharge is mild and does not progress to purulent discharge or dehiscence. The wound should be covered with a sterile dressing, and the animal should be rested and prevented from traumatizing the wound.
- Hemorrhagic wound discharge: No specific treatment is required other than local wound care, assuming there is not marked hemorrhage. If this occurs, particularly if there is also accumulation of blood in the thoracic cavity or it is thought that there is hemorrhage from the intercostal vessels, surgical exploration of the wound may be required to achieve hemostasis.
- Purulent wound discharge or infection: Superficial wounds are treated as other postsurgical wound infections (see Chapter 1). Infections that involve the deeper tissues usually need to opened, lavaged, and have surgical debridement of necrotic material before suturing. They are rarely managed as open wounds because it is difficult to maintain a seal on the thoracic cavity using this technique. Infections that involve the thoracic cavity should be considered pyothorax and should be treated accordingly (see Chapter 3).
- Sternal osteomyelitis: See later discussion.
- Wound dehiscence: See Chapter 9.

Outcome
- Serous or serosanguineous wound discharge: usually resolves with local wound management
- Hemorrhagic wound discharge: Most cases resolve with local wound management or repeat hemostatic techniques.
- Purulent wound discharge or infection: The outcome depends on the depth of infection, health of affected tissues, and causative organism. Superficial infections usually resolve with local wound care and antibiotics. Deep infections and pyothorax carry a more guarded prognosis and may be fatal.
- Wound dehiscence: Superficial wound dehiscence can usually be managed with open wound management techniques or resuturing. However, dehiscence of deep tissues of the thoracic wall is a therapeutic challenge because it may lead to an open thoracic cavity, which leads to an increased risk of death from pneumothorax and ascending infection.

Prevention

- Serous or serosanguineous wound discharge: application of Halsted's principles
- Hemorrhagic wound discharge: See Chapter 12.
- Purulent wound discharge or infection: See Chapter 3.
- Wound dehiscence: See Chapter 9.

Osteomyelitis

Definition

Osteomyelitis is bone inflammation or infection, usually bacterial, caused by direct contamination of the wound with infective organisms. Common aerobic organisms include *Staphylococcus aureus,* other *Staphylococci* species, *Escherichia coli,* β-hemolytic streptococci, *Proteus* spp., *Klebsiella* spp., and *Pseudomonas* spp. Anaerobic organisms are also often present (Cockshutt 2002). Hematogenous (postsurgical) osteomyelitis is probably rare.

Osteomyelitis may be acute, seen in the first 5 to 7 days after surgery and exhibiting signs of wound inflammation and systemic disease. Chronic osteomyelitis may result in discharging sinus tracts, but animals show less marked inflammation and pain. The overall reported incidence of osteomyelitis is 1% to 11%.

Risk factors

No specific data on osteomyelitis of the sternebrae are available. However, risk factors for postsurgical osteomyelitis in orthopedic patients are usually considered to be caused by complications of surgical or aseptic technique.

Diagnosis

- Physical examination: pain, thoracic limb lameness, inflammation, edema or swelling, wound dehiscence, wound discharge (Figure 39.7)
- Radiography or computed tomography Bony changes are seen after 1 to 2 weeks and include bone resorption or lysis, bone production, remodeling, and failure of sternebral healing.
- Wound cytology: Fluid contains degenerate neutrophils +/− intracellular bacteria.
- Bacteriologic (+/− fungal) culture: obtained via needle aspiration of deep tissues to avoid surface contamination

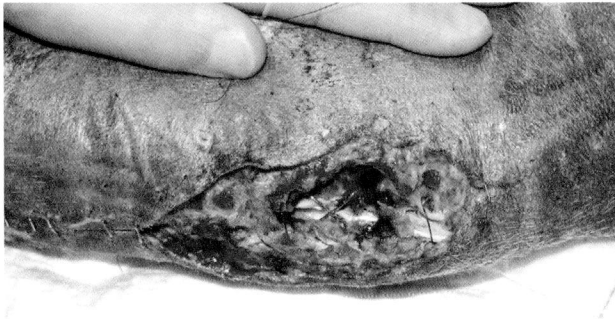

Figure 39.7 Wound dehiscence and necrosis of pectoral muscle, subcutaneous tissues, and skin, with exposure of sternebrae and sternal wires, affecting a large part of a median sternotomy wound. Osteomyelitis was confirmed after positive culture from the deep tissues of the wound. *Source:* V. Lipscomb, Royal Veterinary College, London, 2015. Reproduced with permission from V. Lipscombe.

Treatment

- Broad-spectrum antibiotics to which the most likely causative organisms are susceptible and delivered intravenously initially. They may need to be changed on the base of culture and sensitivity test results. Mild cases may respond to antibiotics alone.
- Surgical debridement and lavage and removal of (metal) implants. Closure of the wound after debridement is preferred to maintain a seal on the thoracic wall. Delayed primary or secondary healing after open wound management may be necessary in severe cases but may be associated with a poor prognosis and risk of death or the need for euthanasia.

Outcome

The condition is potentially fatal, especially if accompanied by wound dehiscence and pneumothorax or pyothorax.

Prevention

- Strict adherence to aseptic technique
- Minimal surgical time
- Careful wound reconstruction

Displaced or fractured sternebrae and fractured ribs

Incidence

- Displaced or fractured sternebrae: 1% to 3%
- Fractured ribs: 2%

Risk factors

- Displaced or fractured sternebrae
  - Inadequate sternal stability
  - Inaccurate sternotomy incision
  - Excessive postoperative movement
- Fractured rib
  - Excessive rib retraction
  - Intercostal sutures pulled too tight

Diagnosis

- May cause localized pain
- There may be no clinical signs, with the diagnosis only made during routine radiography.
- Radiography

Treatment

Treatment is rarely necessary, and fractures can be expected to heal without complications

Outcome

The outcome is usually good.

Prevention

In experimental dogs with median sternotomy wounds closed with wire, there was less sternebral displacement seen on radiographs at 4 weeks after surgery than for median sternotomy wounds closed with suture (Pelsue *et al.* 2002). However, there is no proof this leads to fewer wound displacement or fracture complications in clinical patients.

Wound hemorrhage

Definition

This is excessive hemorrhage from the wound during the intra- or postoperative period. The reported incidence is rare.

Risk factors

- Underlying bleeding disorder
- Bleeding from an intrathoracic procedure
- Intercostal thoracotomy
  - Damage to intercostal vessels on caudal aspect of rib during incision or placement of circumcostal sutures
  - Damage to internal thoracic vessels during extension of incision ventral to costochondral junction
- Sternotomy
  - Failure to ligate or cauterize pectoral muscle vessels
  - Use of a hammer and chisel (rather than saw) in dogs, especially large breeds

Diagnosis

- Clinical signs may be consistent with blood loss (e.g., weak pulses, pale mucous membranes) or presence of blood within the thoracic cavity (e.g., tachypnea; short, shallow breathing pattern).
- Hemorrhage occurring from the wound (Figure 39.8)
- Aspiration of blood via thoracostomy tube or via thoracocentesis

Treatment

- See Chapter 12.
- Significant hemorrhage may require the use of colloid fluid therapy and blood products followed by repeat surgery for hemostasis. Ligation of the intercostal vessels may be required.
- Mild hemorrhage externally from the wound often requires no treatment.

Outcome

- Depends on the degree of hemorrhage; may be life threatening if significant

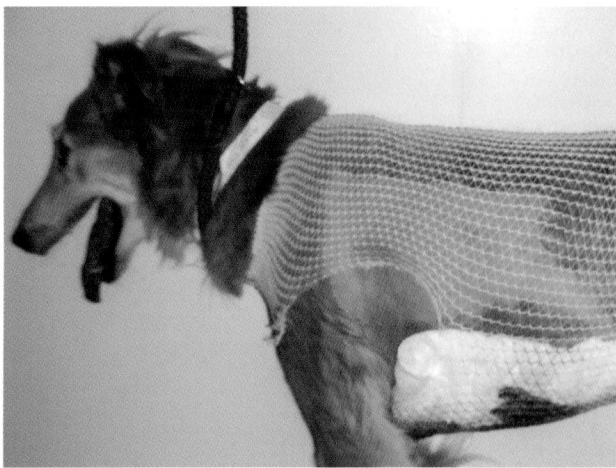

Figure 39.8 Mild to moderate postoperative hemorrhage in a dog after median sternotomy. There was no blood within the thoracic cavity, the hematocrit did not drop, and hemorrhage resolved within 24 hours of surgery. *Source:* A. Moores, Anderson Moores Veterinary Specialists, Winchester, Hampshire, UK, 2014. Reproduced with permission from A. Moores.

Prevention

- Recognition of bleeding disorders
- Careful hemostasis during intrathoracic procedure and monitor for hemorrhage before thoracotomy closure
- Avoid damaging intercostal or internal thoracic vessels

Ipsilateral thoracic limb lameness and neurologic deficits

Definition

- Lameness: pain on the ipsilateral thoracic limb after intercostal thoracotomy or either or both thoracic limbs after median sternotomy
- Neurologic deficits: deficits consistent with brachial plexus injury to thoracic limb(s)
- The overall reported incidence is 2% to 4%.

Risk factors

- Pain from transection or excessive retraction of the latissimus dorsi muscle (Tattersall and Welsh 2006)
- Brachial plexus injury from limb overextension during positioning for surgery

Diagnosis

- Clinical and neurologic examination

Treatment

- Analgesia for pain, but otherwise there is no specific treatment

Outcome

- Usually self-limiting

Prevention

- Manage pain.
- Do not transect latissimus dorsi muscle or apply excessive dorsal retraction unless necessary for increased surgical exposure.
- Avoid pulling the thoracic limbs too far cranially during positioning; keep in a flexed, untied position.

Relevant literature

Animals undergoing median sternotomy have a higher mortality rate than those undergoing intercostal thoracotomy, but this mostly reflects the severity of the underlying disease. Also, animals that survive surgery are significantly younger than those that do not (Tattersall and Welsh 2006, Moores *et al.* 2007). Because 55% of dogs and cats having an intercostal thoracotomy are young animals being treated for vascular anomalies, this helps to explain the lower mortality rate in animals having this surgical approach to the thorax. A total of 45% of animals undergoing median sternotomy died or were euthanized because of either the severity of the underlying disease or the intrathoracic surgical procedure required to treat it compared with 13% of animals having an intercostal thoracotomy (Burton and White 1996; Moores *et al.* 2007).

Ringwald and Birchard (1989) reported complications in 36% of dogs, with half of dogs having postoperative pain. Moores *et al.* (2007) described 70 dogs and 13 cats that had an intercostal thoracotomy, of which only 4 had a rib resection, the majority having one or more intercostal thoracotomies. Eleven animals (13%) died or

Table 39.1 Incidence of short-term complications in animals undergoing lateral thoracotomy

Complication	Percentage of animals affected
Seroma or ventral edema	16 of 72 (22%)
Excessive wound inflammation	6 of 72 (8%)
Ipsilateral thoracic limb lameness	3 (4%)
Wound discharge	3 (4%)

Source: Moore et al., 2007. Reproduced with permission from John Wiley & Sons.

Table 39.2 Incidence of short-term complications in animals undergoing median sternotomy or intercostal thoracotomy

Complication	Percentage of animals affected
Seroma	9 of 84 (11%)
Serosanguineous wound discharge	7 of 84 (8%)
Excessive edema or swelling	4 of 84 (5%)
Wound breakdown	3 of 84 (4%)
Suture reaction	3 of 84 (4%)
Infection	1 of 84 (1%)
Osteomyelitis	1 of 84 (1%)
Displaced sternebrae	1 of 84 (1%)
Thoracic limb lameness	1 of 84 (1%)
Thoracic drain complications	13 of 84 (15%)

Source: Tattersall and Welsh, 2006. Reproduced with permission from John Wiley & Sons.

were euthanized because of their underlying disease. Of the remaining 72 animals that survived to discharge, short-term complications (within 14 days of surgery) occurred in 35 (47%), of which 28 (39%) were attributed to the surgical approach (Table 39.1). Most were considered to be of minor clinical significance. Incidence of complications was not significantly associated with age, species, underlying disease, surgical procedure, duration of surgery, surgeon experience, or duration of thoracostomy tube placement. Long-term complications (>14 days postoperatively) occurred in 3 of 53 (6%) animals available for follow-up, of which two (rib fracture and pyothorax) could be attributed to the surgical approach.

Tattersall and Welsh (2006) described short-term complications (<14 days postoperatively) in 98 dogs undergoing median sternotomy or intercostal thoracotomy. Twenty-one dogs (21%) died or were euthanized within 2 weeks of surgery, of which 1 was because of a complication related to the thoracic drain (pneumothorax). Of the 84 dogs (86%) surviving more than 48 hours, short-term complications were seen in 33 dogs (39%), of which 26 (31%) were associated with the thoracotomy wound (Table 39.2). Complication rates were 71% for median sternotomy and 23% for intercostal thoracotomy. The incidence of complications was not significantly associated with age, duration of surgery, whether the latissimus muscle was transected or retracted, type of thoracic disease, or method of postoperative drainage (thoracostomy tube placement vs. needle thoracocentesis). Although not significant, complications were seen more in dogs with pyothorax as the underlying disease, but this may relate to the surgical approach (median ster-

notomy) or prolonged used of thoracostomy tubes rather than the disease itself.

Burton and White (1996) described complications associated with median sternotomy in 67 dogs and 9 cats. Because of the severity of the underlying disease, only 66% and 63% of animals were alive at 48 hours and 14 days postoperatively, respectively. Of those alive after 14 days, short-term (<14 days postoperatively) complications were seen in 7 dogs (19%), consisting of 3 that needed additional analgesia to the routine protocol, 2 with sternotomy wound hemorrhage, 1 with thoracic limb neurologic deficits, and 2 with wound infection. This complication rate is lower than that reported for median sternotomy by Tattersall and Welsh (2006), which may be because the latter authors included more minor wound complications such as edema, serosanguineous wound discharge, and swelling, which Burton and White (1996) appear not to have done. Burton and White reported long-term (>14 days postoperatively) complications in 8 of 37 dogs (22%) available for follow-up (Table 39.3). There were no complications reported in the cats.

Table 39.3 Incidence of long-term complications in animals undergoing median sternotomy

Complication	Percentage of animals affected
Sternal osteomyelitis +/− recurrent skin swelling	4 of 37 (11%)
Sternal fracture or displacement	1 of 37 (3%)
Leakage of chyle from the wound	1 of 37 (3%)
Wound discharge	1 of 37 (3%)
Delayed skin healing	1 of 37 (3%)

Source: Burton and White 1996. Reproduced with permission from John Wiley & Sons.

References

Burton, C.A., White, R.N. (1996) Review of the technique and complications of median sternotomy in the dog and cat. *Journal of Small Animal Practice* 37 (11), 516-522.

Cockshutt, J.R. (2002) Bone infection. In Sumner-Smith, G. (ed.) *Bone in Clinical Orthopaedics.* Thieme., Stuttgart

Moores, A.L., Halfacree, Z.J., Baines, S.J., et al. (2007) Indications, outcomes and complications following lateral thoracotomy in dogs and cats. *Journal of Small Animal Practice* 48 (12), 695-698.

Pelsue, D.H., Monnet, E., Gaynor, J.S., et al. (2002) Closure of median sternotomy in dogs: suture versus wire. *Journal of the American Animal Hospital Association* 2002, 38 (6), 569-576.

Ringwald, R.J., Birchard, S.J. (1989) Complications of median sternotomy in the dog and literature review. *Journal of the American Animal Hospital Association* 25, 430-434.

Tattersall, J.A., Welsh, E. (2006) Factors influencing the short-term outcome following thoracic surgery in 98 dogs. *Journal of Small Animal Practice* 47 (12), 715-720.

40 Thoracoscopy

Eric Monnet

Small Animal Surgery, Colorado State University, Fort Collins, CO, USA

Thoracoscopy is a minimally invasive technique for viewing the internal structures of the thoracic cavity. The procedure uses a rigid telescope placed through a portal positioned into the thoracic wall to examine the contents of the pleural cavity. When the telescope is in place, either biopsy forceps or an assortment of surgical instruments can then also be introduced into the thoracic cavity through adjacent portals in the thoracic wall to perform various diagnostic or surgical procedures. The minimal invasiveness of the procedure, the rapid patient recovery, and diagnostic accuracy make thoracoscopy an ideal technique over other more invasive procedures.

Despite the advent of newer laboratory tests, such as imaging techniques and ultrasound-directed fine-needle biopsy or aspiration, thoracoscopy remains a valuable tool when appropriately applied in a diagnostic plan. Thoracoscopy may also provide accurate and definitive diagnostic and staging information that would otherwise only be obtained through a surgical thoracotomy. Small animal thoracoscopy has not only developed into a diagnostic tool but more recently has progressed to where it has become a means for minimally invasive surgical procedures.

Interventional thoracoscopy is an emerging surgical technique in veterinary surgery used to perform pericardial window or subtotal pericardiectomy, lung lobectomy, correct vascular ring anomalies, ligate patent ductus arteriosus and the thoracic duct (TD), and help in the treatment of pyothorax. Most of the procedures are performed under thoracoscopy, and some procedures can be performed thoracoscopically assisted.

Thoracoscopy is associated with several complications. Complications can develop during the procedures. Intraoperative complications can be attributable to a lack of visualization, adherence, technical difficulties to perform the procedures, or life-threatening complications (e.g., hemorrhage, desaturation, or interference with ventilation). When the procedure cannot be performed for technical reasons or a life-threatening complication happened, conversion to an open thoracotomy will be required. The conversion rate during thoracoscopy in veterinary surgery is not known because no data are available to evaluate it. The rate of conversion depends on the gravity of the complication, the hemodynamic status of the patient, the equipment available, and the expertise of the surgeon. Because complications can always occur during the procedure, it is important to be always prepared to perform a

thoracotomy. Therefore, the patient has to be prepared (clipped, scrubbed, and draped) as for a thoracotomy. The surgical instruments have to be present in the operating room, and the surgeon has to be able to perform either an intercostal thoracotomy or a median sternotomy.

Complications can also occur during the recovery period. The postoperative complications rate is unknown in veterinary medicine, and it is more likely related to the difficulty of the procedure performed with thoracoscopy.

INTRAOPERATIVE COMPLICATIONS

Lack of visualization

Definition
Lack of visualization is the difficulty or impossibility of observing specific structures in the thoracic cavity.

Risk factors
- Presence of adherences
- Large mass in the lungs
- Severe pleural effusion
- Severe pericardial effusion
- Patient conformation: brachycephalic dogs
- Patient positioning
- Inadequate cannula placement

Diagnosis
During thoracoscopy, it is very difficult to observe the structures of concerns.

Treatment
- Add an extra cannula for a better placement of instruments or endoscope.
- Adherence: Debridement of the adherence can be perform during thoracoscopy, but it will increase the risk of iatrogenic trauma.
- Utilization of retractors: It is always possible to use retractor to help visualize the structures of interest. However, introduction of a retractor requires an extra portal, which then reduces the advantage of thoracoscopy.

Complications in Small Animal Surgery, First Edition. Edited by Dominique Griffon and Annick Hamaide.
© 2016 John Wiley & Sons, Inc. Published 2016 by John Wiley & Sons, Inc.
Companion website: www.wiley.com/go/griffon/complications

- One-lung ventilation (OLV): OLV can be started while in surgery. However, it is better to plan ahead and use it as a preventive measure.
- Insufflation with CO_2: Insufflation of the pleural space to a pressure less than 3 mm Hg can be used as an intraoperative measure to help visualization.

Outcome

- Lack of visualization will result in conversion to an open thoracotomy.
- Increased risk of iatrogenic trauma to intrathoracic structures

Prevention

- **Appropriate positioning of the patient** should be done to use gravity to retract the organs away from the surgical field. Positioning of the patient is extremely important during thoracoscopy because then the surgeon can take advantage of gravity to retract the organs without the need of a specific retractor. If the position is not appropriate, then gravity will interfere with retraction and the motion of organs. It will then be difficult to see the structures of interest. **For a lung lobectomy,** it is useful to place the patient in lateral recumbency in an oblique position. Sand bags are placed on the surgery table to elevate the dorsal part of the thoracic cavity. The lungs and the heart are pulled away from the hilus of the lung, improving its visualization. Also more space is present to allow an easier manipulation of the stapling equipment. Sternal recumbency can be used **for visualization of the dorsal part of the caudal mediastinum and the TD**. This approach is used for the treatment of chylothorax and ligation of the TD.
- **Conformation:** Brachycephalic breeds have a low thoracic depth to width ratio, which makes thoracoscopy difficult almost contraindicated according to the author's experience with brachycephalic dogs. Lack of space and a short long axis of the thorax make thoracoscopy very difficult in these animals. Because the long axis of the thorax is very short, it is difficult to move the camera away from the area of interest and visualize the instruments.
- **Absence of adherence:** Presence of adherence from a previous surgical procedure or from an inflammatory process (pyothorax) increases the complexity of the procedure (Figure 40.1).

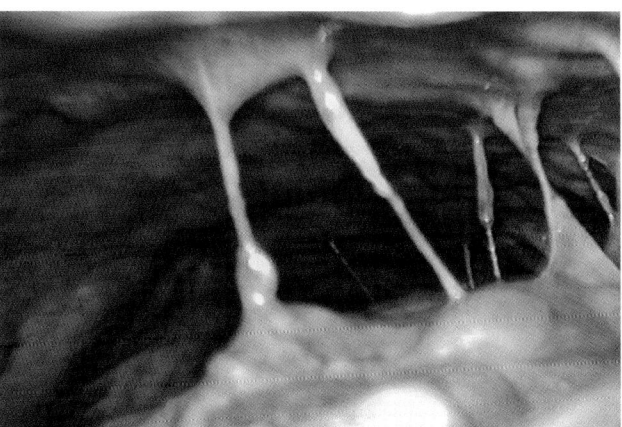

Figure 40.1 Presence of severe adherence in a dog with a chronic pyothorax. The adherence interfered with visualization of the pleural space and mostly the cranial mediastinum.

Adherence can interfere directly with visualization of certain structures or can interfere with manipulation of organs. Also, adherence can increase the risk of iatrogenic trauma of the organ that is adhered to the pleural surface on entry of portals or instruments.
- **OLV** results in atelectasis of the lung lobes that are not ventilated.

Iatrogenic injuries

Definition

Iatrogenic injuries are traumas induced to intrathoracic structures during a surgical procedure. Laceration of the lung parenchyma, laceration of intercostal artery, and puncture or laceration of a major blood vessel are the most common iatrogenic injuries.

Risk factors

- Adherence
- Expertise of the surgeon
- Difficulty of the procedure, which increases the number of cannulas used, the number of instruments used, and the manipulation of organs
- Cannulas
- Instruments used during the procedures
- Electrocautery

Diagnosis

- Air leakage from the surface of the lung parenchyma
- Hemorrhage

Treatment

- Ligation of the bleeding blood vessel with either vascular clips or a vessel sealant device
- Electrocautery or suture placed around a rib to control bleeding from an intercostal vessel
- Lung lobectomy if the laceration in the lung is important.
- Conversion to open thoracotomy

Outcome

Most of the complications are minor and can be controlled during thoracoscopy. However, this depends on the level of expertise of the surgeon. Conversion to an open thoracotomy may be required for the safety of the patient.

Prevention

- Good knowledge of anatomy: Structures are not always well visualized, so it is important to have a good understanding of the three-dimensional anatomy.
- Practice on simulators to improve hand–eye coordination and get used to the loss of depth perception.
- Placement of cannula to protect the intercostal neurovascular pedicle.
- Good technique for placement of cannula under visualization with the endoscope after placement of the first cannula
- After placement of the first cannula, inspection of the pleural space to identify adherence
- Watch the portal site after removal of the cannula. While the endoscope is still in the thoracic cavity at the end of the procedure, each portal site can be inspected for 10 seconds to make sure there is no bleeding from the intercostal artery or vein.
- Visualization of instruments when getting introduced

- Keep instruments in the field of view
- Make sure no electrical arc is getting form between tip of instrument and tissue other than the one that needs to be cauterized.
- Do not activate electrocautery until the target organ is in contact with instrument.
- Eliminate or minimize unnecessary motion of instruments in the thoracic cavity because of the loss of depth perception.
- Manipulate instruments in a close position until the target organ is reached.

Contamination or metastasis of the thoracic wall

Definition
Seeding of the thoracic wall with tumor cells that will lately develop a metastasis.

Risk factor
- Tumor removal

Diagnosis
- Metastasis at the cannula sites several month after surgery

Prevention
- Use of a pouch to retrieve tumor through the thoracic wall

POSTOPERATIVE COMPLICATIONS

Pneumothorax

Definition
Pneumothorax is accumulation of air in the pleural space in the postoperative period that requires drainage.

Risk factor
- Difficulty of the procedure
- Manipulation of instruments

Diagnosis
- Difficulty breathing
- Air removed with the thoracostomy tube for more than 1 hour after surgery

Treatment
- Thoracostomy tube for 24 hours: Air production through the thoracostomy drain seems to persist for at least 6 hours after surgery. The author likes to maintain the patient under continuous suction for 6 hours after surgery.

Prevention
- Visualization of instruments when getting introduced
- Keep instruments in the field of view.
- Eliminate or minimize unnecessary motion of instruments in the thoracic cavity because of the loss of depth perception. Even if the instruments are very blunt, their introduction in the pleural space should always be watched to minimize the risk of trauma to the lungs.
- Manipulate instruments in a close position until the target organ is reached.

Hemorrhage

Definition
Hemorrhage is bleeding caused by trauma to a vascular structure in the thoracic cavity or the chest wall.

Risk factors
- Lack of experience of the surgeon
- Lack of visualization
- Right atrial tumor
- Aggressive manipulation of organ
- Motion of instruments in the thoracic cavity because of the loss of depth perception
- Traumatic placement of cannulas in the intercostal space

Diagnosis
Collection of blood by the thoracostomy tube

Treatment
- Support patient with fluidotherapy or blood transfusion if needed
- Thoracotomy

Prevention
- Provide a good hemostasis during surgery.
- Visualize cannula holes at time of removal of cannula.
- In case of atrial tumor, perform a pericardial window when the patient is stable and not actively bleeding. Clinical signs and echocardiography will help decide if the right atrial tumor stopped bleeding or not.

Relevant literature
One-lung ventilation can be accomplished by either selective intubation of the lungs that can be ventilated or by occluding the main bronchi of the lungs that need to be collapsed (Kudnig et al. 2006; Mayhew et al. 2009). Because OLV induces atelectasis of a lung lobe, it induces a ventilation/perfusion (V/Q) mismatch. The alveoli that are not ventilated induce a low V/Q that will induce a desaturation of the arterial blood that is not responding to oxygen. Therefore, some patients with significant lung pathology may not tolerate OLV. Also, with the patient in lateral recumbency, the dependent lungs that are the only one being ventilated are getting atelectatic under the weight of the heart. Application of positive end-expiratory pressure (PEEP) from 2.5 to 5 cm H_2O can improve the situation by minimizing atelectasis of the dependent lung. It has been shown that application of PEEP in dogs with OLV during thoracoscopy does not interfere with venous return and cardiac output. Therefore, any increase in oxygen saturation observed with application of PEEP will translate in an augmentation of oxygen delivery. It is recommended to start with only 2.5 cm H_2O. If it is not sufficient to improve oxygen saturation, 5 cm H_2O can be used (Kudnig et al. 2006).

There is no equipment specially made for OLV in small animals. Therefore, equipment designed for human patients has to be used. Because the anatomy of the airways in humans are not similar to the anatomy of dogs and cats, adjustments have to be made. An endotracheal tube with an obturator (Univent; Vitaid, Lewiston, NY) (Figure 40.2) can be used in dogs weighing less than 30 kg; however, it is not long enough to reach the mainstem bronchi in larger dogs. An endobronchial blocker (Arndt Endobronchial blocker; Cook Medical, Bloomington, IN) can be used for larger

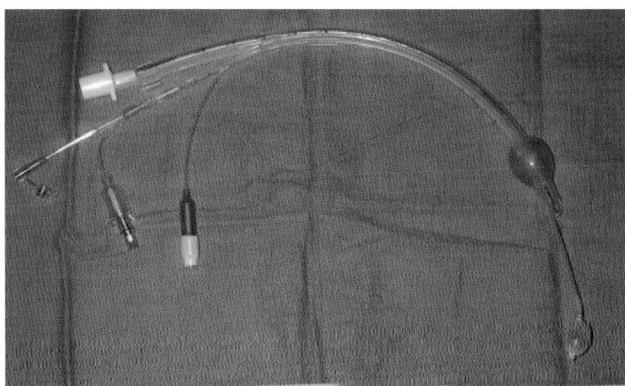

Figure 40.2 Endotracheal tube with its own endobronchial blocker (Univent; Vitaid, Lewiston, NY).

dogs (Figure 40.3). The endobronchial blocker comes with its own delivery system that is connected to a regular endotracheal tube. It can be used in dogs weighing more than 25 kg because it takes a significant amount of space in the endotracheal tube. It is then impossible to advance a bronchoscope to visualize the positioning of the blocker. A dual-lumen tube can be used to selectively ventilated lungs and isolate others. Again, tubes being designed for human patients may be difficult to place in dogs.

One-lung ventilation, especially with an occluder, can fail and lungs will inflate. Then the visualization is seriously compromised, and more likely, the surgery will have to be converted to an open procedure. The occluder can fail because it is not obstructing the bronchi correctly. First, the balloon of the occluder might not be inflated enough letting oxygen going around the balloon during inspiration but not escaping during expiration. Therefore, it is important to inflate correctly the balloon under visualization with bronchoscopy. However, too much insufflation of the balloon can result in iatrogenic damage to the bronchi or displacement of the obturator in the trachea because the balloon is pushed out of the bronchi. Utilization of obturator with an oval-shaped balloon prevents the problem of dislodgment because it is then acting like a wedge. This happens more commonly with the right cranial lung lobe because its bronchus is very proximal. The occluder can also

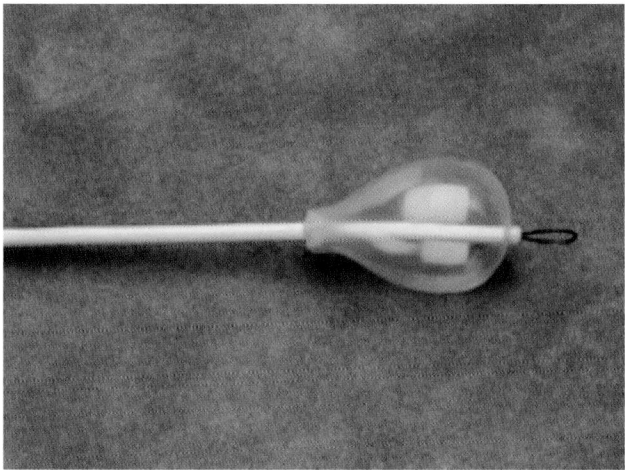

Figure 40.3 Arndt Endobronchial Blocker (Arndt Endobronchial blocker; Cook Medical, Bloomington, IN).

be dislodged during positioning of the patient or during light anesthesia, if the patient starts coughing (Lansdowne *et al.* 2005). The occluder can then be expelled in the trachea, which will result in a complete airway obstruction. It is then very important to monitor the patient with a capnograph because the ventilator will keep triggering however the lungs will not be ventilated. If the trachea is obstructed, the end-tidal CO_2 will fall to 0 mm Hg. It is then paramount to immediately deflate the cuff of the occluder. If the OLV is still required to complete the procedure, the occluder has to be placed back in good location with bronchoscopy. Instead of using an occlusion, selective intubation can be accomplished with double lumen endotracheal tubes that are placed with bronchoscopy. This technique allows ventilation of any lung lobes during the procedure without changing the position of tube (Mayhew *et al.* 2009).

Insufflation of the pleural space has been used to increase the work space and improve visualization during thoracoscopy. The insufflation pressure can interfere with ventilation and induce a severe atelectasis with desaturation of the patient. PEEP cannot be used in this situation because it will be counterproductive by inflating the lungs. To limit the risk of overinflation of the pleural space, it is possible to use a large portal that can let CO_2 escape freely around the instrument.

Iatrogenic injuries to several intrathoracic organs can occur during thoracoscopy. Portals are used to gain access to the pleural space and to protect the intercostal neurovascular pedicle from the instruments that are used during the surgery. Portals are mounted on blunt obturator to minimize the risk of trauma to the intercostal neurovascular pedicle. However, damage to the intercostal neurovascular pedicle can still occur during the placement of a portal (Radlinsky *et al.* 2002; Kudnig *et al.* 2006). The portal usually will provide enough compression of the intercostal artery and vein to prevent bleeding during the procedure. The bleeding will occur after removal of the portal. It is important to observe the portal hole after retrieval of the portal at the end of the surgery while the endoscope is still in the pleural space. If there is a bleeding, it will be controlled with electrocautery or sutures placed around the rib proximal and distal to the bleeding vessel. It might be needed to enlarge the portal hole to place the suture. If portals are not used, the risk of trauma to the intercostal artery and vein is increased each time an instrument is introduced through an intercostal space.

It is also important to always visualize instruments when they are coming in and out of the thoracic cavity to prevent puncture of lung parenchyma that would result in serious pneumothorax in the postoperative period (Jackson *et al.* 1999; Lansdowne *et al.* 2005).

During thoracoscopy and minimally invasive surgery, **the depth perception is compromised**. Also, we can only palpate and move organs with a palpation probe and instruments. Therefore, visualization of certain structures can be very difficult, and iatrogenic damage to organs or blood vessels may occur. When dissecting the mediastinum, during a transdiaphragmatic approach, for example, it is important to localize the internal thoracic artery. Usually one internal thoracic artery is visualized; however, the other one on the other side of the mediastinum is not visible and can be damaged when the dissection of the cranial mediastinum is completed (Figure 40.4). It is then important to have a good three-dimensional understanding of the anatomy. Vascular clips should be present in the instrument tray because they are required to control bleeding from the internal thoracic artery. Vessel sealant device can also be used to control efficiently bleeding from large vessels.

Pericardial effusion is now commonly palliated with a pericardial window, especially when a right atrial hemangiosarcoma is present.

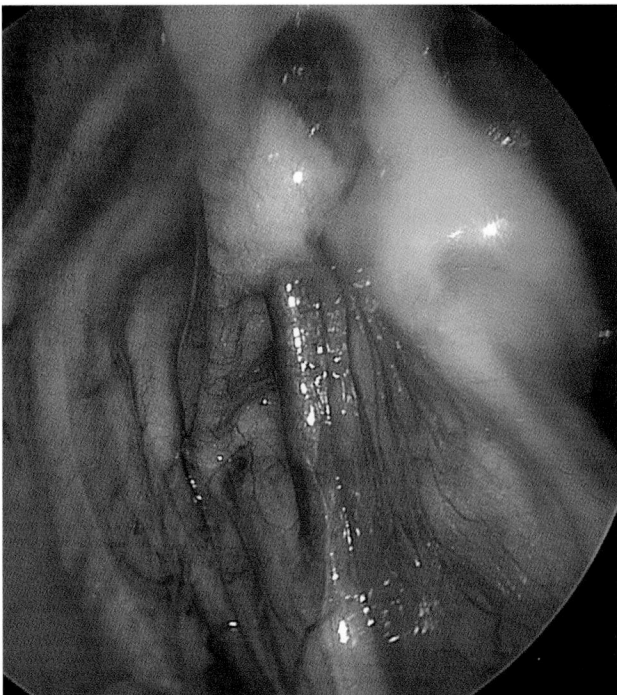

Figure 40.4 The right internal thoracic artery is visible. On the other side of the mediastinum, the left internal thoracic artery is not visible behind the mediastinum.

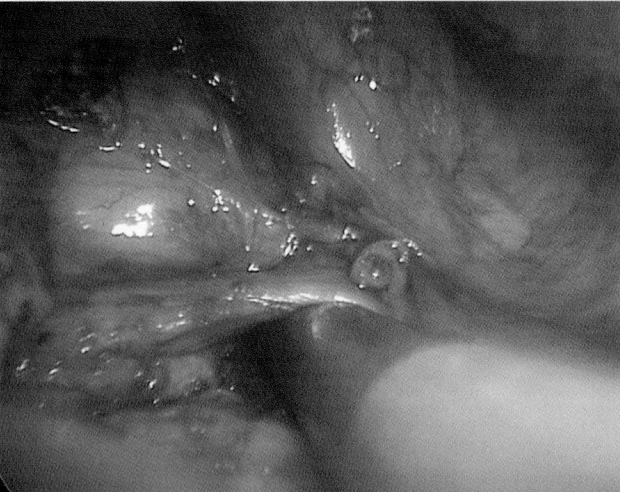

Figure 40.5 The ligamentum arteriosum has been elevated on a palpation probe.

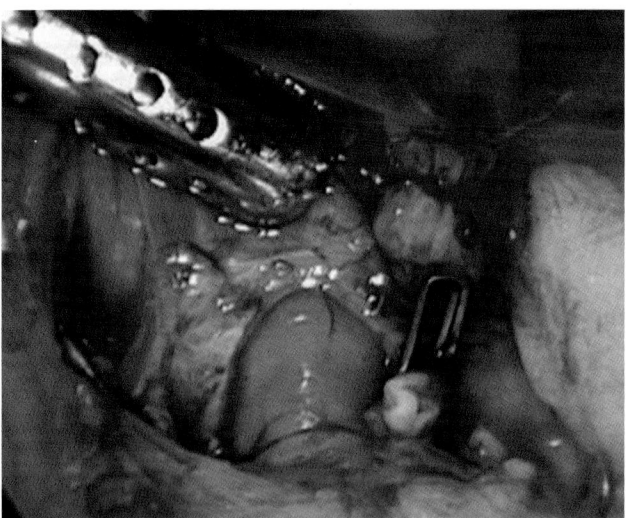

Figure 40.6 The ligamentum arteriosum has been occluded with two vascular clips before its transection.

Iatrogenic injury to the heart can occur during the procedure, especially when the first incision of the pericardium is performed. The right atrial mass can be very large; therefore, to prevent its injury, it is recommended to make the first incision toward the apex of the heart and then extent it toward the heart base when the right atrial mass can be visualized. Also, it is important to grab and pull the pericardium away from the heart when the first incision is performed to prevent any injury to the myocardium or a coronary injury. Iatrogenic transection of a phrenic nerve has been reported during a subtotal pericardectomy with thoracoscopy. It is important to always visualize the phrenic nerve even when only a pericardial window is performed (Jackson *et al.* 1999; Dupré *et al.* 2001; Lansdowne *et al.* 2005).

Persistence of right aortic arches have been corrected thoracoscopically in dogs (MacPhail *et al.* 2001). Correction of persistent right aortic arch with compression of the esophagus by the ligamentum arteriosum can be associated with **intraoperative bleeding** (Figures 40.5 and 40.6). The ligamentum arteriosum can still be perfused at the time of surgery. Therefore, a lack of occlusion of the ligamentum arteriosum before its transection can result in severe bleeding. It requires an immediate conversion to intercostal thoracotomy for control of the hemorrhage.

During the resection of thymoma, right atrial tumors, and lung tumors, it is possible to **seed the thoracic wall with tumor** cells and induce the development of a tumor several weeks or months after surgery (Brisson *et al.* 2006). To prevent contamination of the thoracic wall, it is important to isolate the tumor in a retrieving bag. Retrieving bags are spring-loaded sterile plastic bags that facilitate removal of the tumor because they are made out of strong plastic that can be pulled through small thoracotomy without tearing. It is possible to use sterile surgical gloves to retrieve small tumors. However, because they are spring loaded, it is difficult to place the tissue to retrieve in the sterile glove.

References

Brisson, B.A., Reggeti, F., Bienzle, D. (2006) Portal site metastasis of invasive mesothelioma after diagnostic thoracoscopy in a dog. *Journal of the American Veterinary Medical Association* 229, 980-983.

Dupré , G.P., Corlouer, J.P., Bouvy, B. (2001) Thoracoscopic pericardectomy performed without pulmonary exclusion in 9 dogs. *Veterinary Surgery* 30, 21-27.

Jackson, J., Richter, K.P., Launer, D.P. (1999) Thoracoscopic partial pericardectomy in 13 dogs. *Journal of Veterinary Internal Medicine* 13, 529-533.

Kudnig, S.T., Monnet, E., Riquelme, M., et al. (2006) Effect of positive end-expiratory pressure on oxygen delivery during 1-lung ventilation for thoracoscopy in normal dogs. *Veterinary Surgery* 35, 534-542.

Lansdowne, J.L., Monnet, E., Twedt, D.C., et al. (2005) Thoracoscopic lung lobectomy for treatment of lung tumors in dogs. *Veterinary Surgery* 34, 530-535.

MacPhail, C.M., Monnet, E., Twedt, D.C. (2001) Thoracoscopic correction of persistent right aortic arch in a dog. *Journal of the American Animal Hospital Association* 37, 577-581.

Mayhew, K.N., Mayhew, P.D., Sorrell-Raschi, L., et al. (2009) Thoracoscopic subphrenic pericardectomy using double-lumen endobronchial intubation for alternating one-lung ventilation. *Veterinary Surgery* 38, 961-966.

Radlinsky, M.G., Mason, D.E., Biller, D.S., et al. (2002) Thoracoscopic visualization and ligation of the thoracic duct in dogs. *Veterinary Surgery* 31, 138-146.

41 Bronchial and Pulmonary Surgery

Hervé Brissot

University of Nottingham, Pride Veterinary Centre, Derby, UK

Bronchial and pulmonary surgeries can be associated with severe intra- and postoperative complications that are sometimes delayed by few hours to several weeks from the procedure. Given the very primordial function of these tissues, such complications should be investigated thoroughly because they can quickly become life threatening.

Perioperative bronchopleural fistula

Definition

Unintentional opening of a lobar bronchus (acute bronchopleural fistula) during surgery could make ventilation of the remaining lung difficult because positive-pressure inflation will not be possible. This can lead to life-threatening hypoxemia.

Risk factors

- Incomplete visualization of the lobar hilus
- Poor familiarity with local anatomy
- Undue traction on the hilus structures

Diagnosis

- Direct observation of the air leak during ventilation
- Inability to insufflate the lungs

Treatment

- Immediately stop the leak with a hemostat or digitally. When the leak is controlled, the damaged bronchus is resutured.
- Compared with classic positive-pressure ventilation, high-frequency oscillatory ventilation has proven much more efficient in keeping a high oxygen concentration in the blood in dogs with experimentally induced bronchopleural fistula (Mayer *et al.* 1986).

In cases of severe loss of substance making suture impossible, the defect can be patched with a pericardial or vascularized muscle flap (intercostal, diaphragmatic, or latissimus dorsi muscles) (Nelson and Monnet 2003; Salci *et al.* 2007). When the lobar bronchus cannot be sutured because it is too short or too damaged, an additional lobe can be removed to reach a more suitable place to suture the bronchus.

Outcome

The first emergency is to stop the leak to ensure adequate ventilation. When the leak has been definitively stopped, recovery should be expected.

Prevention

- Gentle dissection of the hilus using fine but not sharp instruments (i.e., hemostats, DeBakey forceps, large sterile cotton buds, Lahey or Waterstones forceps) (Figures 41.1 and 41.2).
- Minimal traction should be applied on the hilus structures to prevent tearing fragile structures.
- Careful use of staplers that can be cumbersome and create undue trauma in the hilus when introduced in the chest.

Perioperative failure to achieve air-thigh seal suture

Definition

This is an inability to achieve a perfect air-thigh seal on the suture line after section of the lung parenchyma (partial lobectomy or

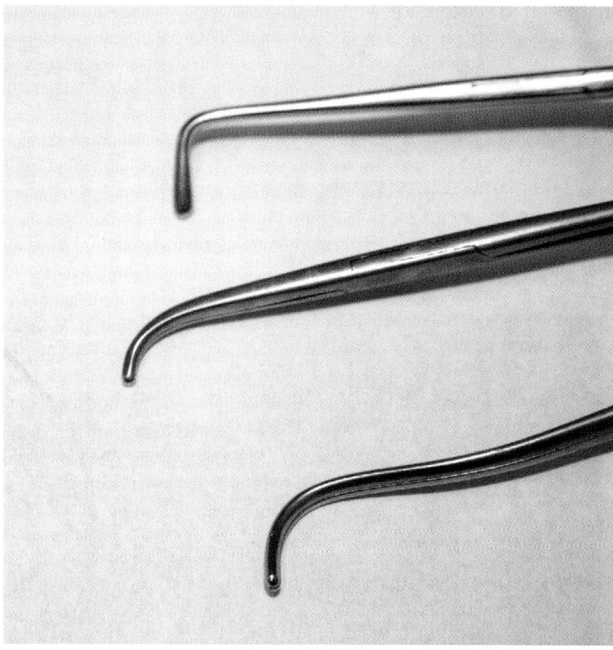

Figure 41.1 Close-up view of the tip of right-angled surgical instruments for hilar dissection.

Complications in Small Animal Surgery, First Edition. Edited by Dominique Griffon and Annick Hamaide.

© 2016 John Wiley & Sons, Inc. Published 2016 by John Wiley & Sons, Inc.

Companion website: www.wiley.com/go/griffon/complications

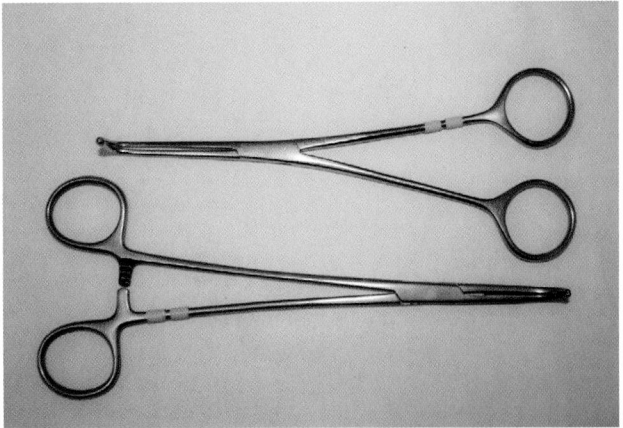

Figure 41.2 Two surgical right angle forceps usually used for hilar dissection. Top, Waterstones forceps (not the absence of ratchet). Bottom, Laheys forceps.

wedge resection) or resection of a lung lobe (lobectomy or pneumonectomy).

Risk factors
- Fragile lung parenchyma (partial lobectomy)
- Improper choice of material (staplers, suture) (Table 41.1)
- Nonlinear parenchymal suture line (wedge resection)
- Incomplete dissection of the lung hilus (lobectomy) and incomplete identification and isolation of the lobar bronchus

Treatment
- If mechanical stapling has failed, it is necessary to understand the origin of the failure, that is, whether it is technical (improper technique was used) or instrumental (stapler failure, inadequate choice of staples). If the suture line is completely inadequate, the staple line could be completely excised for restapling or manual suturing. If air-thigh seal was not achieved because staples failed to achieve full compression, restapling with smaller staples is advised.
- Small bubbles coming from the lung parenchyma, suture, or needle tracts do not require specific attention, and these tracts should seal during the healing process.
- Bigger leaks need additional sutures or additional compression with metallic clips. If adequate stapling has been achieved, systematic oversewing of the stapled lines is not necessary (LaRue et al. 1987).
- When a wedge resection is performed, special attention should be made to check the area where two staple lines will meet. These are potential areas for inadequate air seal. If necessary, additional sutures or clips should be applied.
- If bronchial suture is made manually, placing double-layer sutures to first flatten the lumen and subsequently to close the lumen is advised (Fossum 2007).

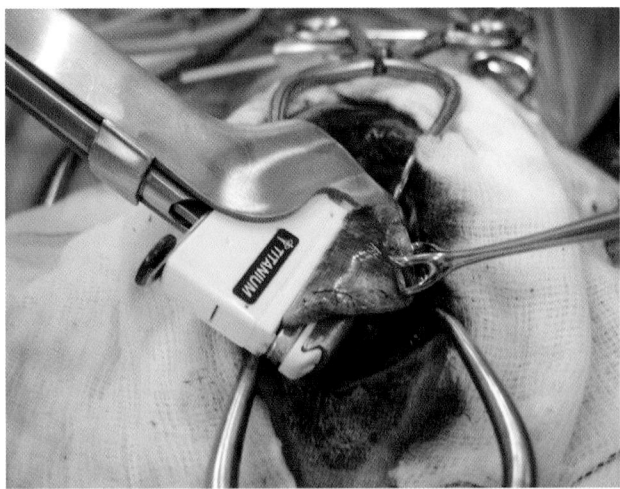

Figure 41.3 Perioperative view of a mechanical partial lung lobectomy. Note the use of a T30 V3 stapler (white cartridge).

- In most cases, stapling of the hilus in small animals should be performed with the vascular TA 30 V3 stapler (Walshaw 1994). Using larger staples is possible to achieve good bronchial suture (Larue et al. 1987).
- When performing partial lobectomy, if air-thigh seal is difficult to achieve because the lung parenchyma appeared fragile or friable, then lung lobectomy is recommended. If lobectomy is not an option because of diffuse parenchymal disease, "sandwiching" the lung parenchyma between two sheets of stronger material (artificial mesh, pericardium) is advised to buttress the sutures or staples to reduce the stain on the fragile parenchyma and improve air-thigh seal (Stammberger et al. 2000).

Outcome
If adequate air seal is achieved perioperatively, recovery should be achieved with minimal complication.

Prevention
- To prevent complication associated with connecting staple lines, an attempt should be made to use one bigger stapler rather than two small ones (Figure 41.3).
- When performing a lobectomy or a pneumonectomy, careful manipulation and dissection of the hilus is recommended. Section of the bronchus should leave enough distance from the median plane to allow rescue and additional suturing if needed.

Perioperative hemorrhage

Definition
Severe hemorrhage generally results from inadvertent damage to the lobar vein and artery during surgery. The subsequent

Table 41.1 Usual mechanical staplers used in lung surgery*

Stapler	Cartridge color	Description	Size staples			Length staple line (mm)	Indications
			Width (mm)	Length open (mm)	Length closed (mm)		
	Green	Two rows	4.0	4.8	2.0	30	Partial lobectomy, wedge resection[†]
	Green	Two rows	4.0	3.5	1.5	53	Partial lobectomy, wedge resection[†]

*Blue and green TA 90 are rarely necessary in small animal surgery.

[†]If the lung parenchyma is so thickened that green staplers are necessary, the clinician could consider performing full lobectomy.

hemorrhage can be severe and associated with rapidly fatal exsanguination.

Risk factors

- Inadequate dissection of the hilus and non identification of the lobar vascularization
- Too restricted an approach
- Infiltration of the hilus
- Using large stapling material in a small chest
- Use of sharp instruments during isolation of the vessels

Treatment

- Immediately stop the hemorrhage with a hemostat or first digitally. Do not try at first to suction the surgical field because life-threatening hemorrhage could be observed very quickly. If direct identification of the bleeder is not quickly achieved, the area is packed with swabs, and pressure is applied. In the meantime, fluid therapy is adapted to compensate for the blood loss, and if compression is efficient, the chest is suctioned to improve visualization. Pressure is then gently released until identification and control of the bleeder are achieved first with hemostats and second with sutures or clips (Figures 41.4 and 41.5).

Outcome

Pulmonary and lobar vessels are highly perfused, and uncontrolled hemorrhage could quickly be life threatening. However, the outcome should be positive providing that blood loss have been controlled and compensated with adequate fluid therapy (including transfusion or administration of blood products).

Prevention

- When a wedge resection is performed, an attempt should be made to use one large stapler rather than two small ones.
- In lobectomy or pneumonectomy, careful dissection of lung hilus and vessels is paramount. As a safety measure, vessel section should be performed as far away as possible from the median plane. During dissection, minimal traction should be applied to allow easy access to vessel as far as possible from the main pulmonary artery or vein to and to ensure easy placement of ligatures. Double ligature of all vessels is indicated, and transfixation of the

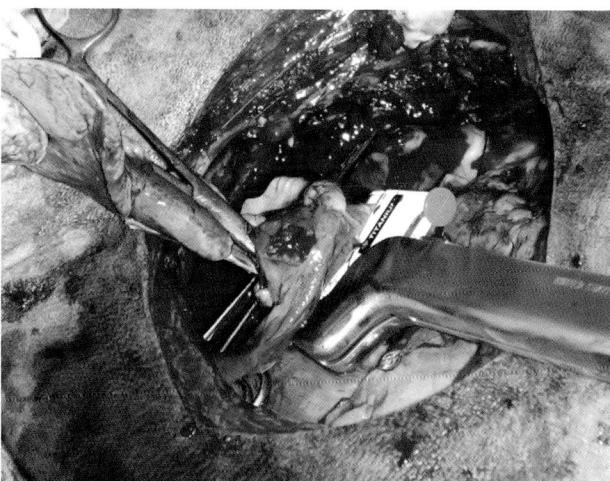

Figure 41.4 Perioperative view of a mechanical lobectomy in a dog with a large chest wall tumor with lung lobe adhesion. Note that the whole hilus is compressed within the stapler at the time of firing.

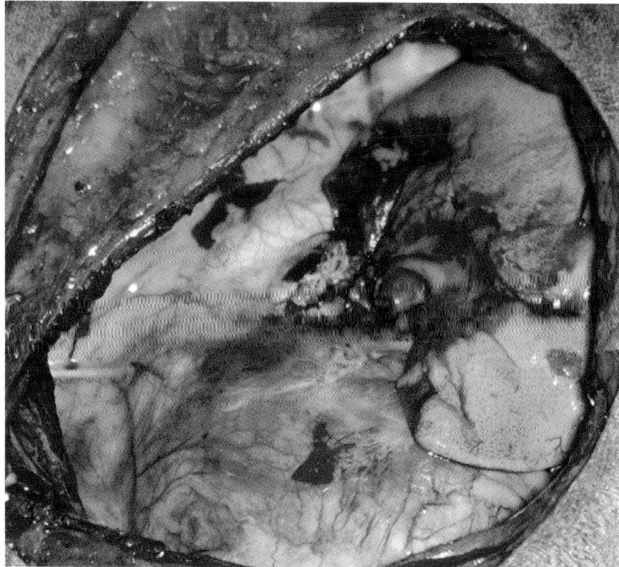

Figure 41.5 Perioperative view after left cranial lung mechanical lobectomy (same dog as in Figure 41.4). Note the empty space left after lobe removal. The stapled hilus is checked for air leakage or local hemorrhage. Note that the bronchus lumen is not oversewn after stapling.

distal aspect of the sectioned artery appears to be a good safety procedure.
- "En-bloc" stapling of the hilus in small animals should be performed with the vascular TA 30 V3 stapler (LaRue *et al.* 1987; Walshaw 1994).
- Using larger staples might be enough to achieve good bronchial suture but might not compress the hilar vessel enough to ensure adequate hemostasis. Incomplete compression of the hilar blood vessels has been observed on several occasions by the author. Therefore, it is advisable to individually suture the vessels before stapling, cranially to the staple line.

Airway obstruction

Definition

Entrapped secretion can spill into the airways as the affected lung tissue is manipulated and can further obstruct the airways bronchus, trachea, or endotracheal tube cranial to the surgical site.

Risk factors

- Pulmonary abscess, tumor with necrotic center.
- Improper manipulation of the fragile tissues.
- Mobilization of the affected lobe before occlusion of the sectioned bronchus

Diagnosis

- Direct observation of secretion within the endotracheal tube.
- Incapacity to insufflate lungs and increased airway pressure.
- Acute drop in end-tidal expiratory CO_2 and decrease in SaO_2.
- Acute hypoxemia and hypercapnia

Treatment

- Suction of the airways via the endotracheal tube or by the surgeon via the bronchial wound

Outcome

When diagnosed and corrected early, the complication should not affect the outcome. Delayed diagnosis and extensive airway occlusion might prevent adequate ventilation and could be fatal.

Prevention

Manipulation of the affected lung should be minimal until complete suture or cross-clamping of the bronchus distal to the anticipated stapled line or suture is done (LaRue *et al.* 1987).

Intraoperative pleural contamination

Definition

Entrapped secretions or necrotic tissues can spill into the pleural cavity as the affected lung tissue is sectioned or manipulated (in case of very fragile or friable tissues).

Risk factors

- Pulmonary abscess, tumor with necrotic centerImproper manipulation of the fragile tissuesMobilization of the affected lobe before occlusion of the bronchus

Treatment

The contaminant should be promptly suctioned. The area should be lavaged with warm sterile saline solution and fully suctioned. One should pay attention to isolate the area from the rest of the cavity with moist swabs.

Outcome

Pleural infection is usually controlled after lavage and thorough removal of the debris from the pleural cavity. In case of neoplastic contamination, the prognosis remains guarded.

Prevention

- Adequate visualization
- Gentle manipulation of the diseased tissues
- Packing of the affected lung with moisten swabs to isolate it from the rest of the pleural cavity
- Cross-clamping the lung parenchyma or bronchus distal to the sutured or staple line before exteriorization or section and removal (LaRue *et al.* 1987)

Postoperative subcutaneous emphysema

Definition

This is subcutaneous accumulation of air at the level of the surgical wound, the neck, or the head.

Risk factors

- Chest drain
- Patient with thin subcutaneous tissue
- Thoracotomy access without muscle-sparing techniques
- Unruly patient

Diagnosis

- Palpation of emphysema (palpation of air bubbles in the subcutaneous tissue)
- Chest radiographs (Figure 41.6)

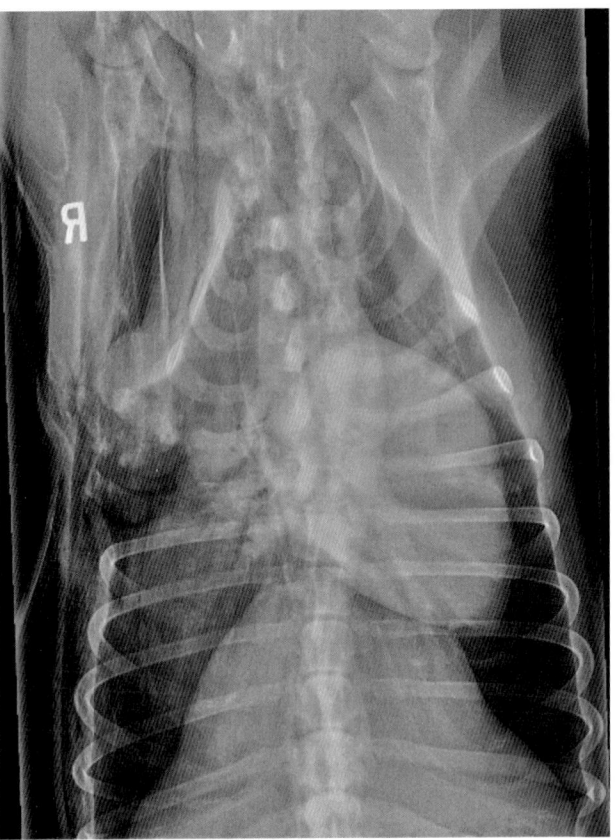

Figure 41.6 Postoperative ventrodorsal chest radiograph in a dog after rupture of a polypropylene mesh. Initially, the dog had rib resection and placement of a mesh to reconstruct the thoracic wall. Note the development of subcutaneous emphysema.

Treatment

- When subcutaneous emphysema is observed after lung surgery, chest radiography is indicated to look for a concomitant pneumothorax. If pneumothorax is confirmed, it should be managed with a chest drain.
- Postoperative air leakage at the level of bronchial sutures can cause a pneumothorax but also a pneumomediastinum. Pneumomediastinum can progress along the trachea up to the neck and head, subsequently causing subcutaneous emphysema. Pneumomediastinum can also result in pneumothorax, which should subsequently be managed with chest drainage.
- Drainage of the subcutaneous air to prevent potential damages to the skin can be done via aspiration through a needle or by creating a surgical wound that is left open.

Outcome

Subcutaneous emphysema should resolve spontaneously after the effusion has resolved, and in any case, it should not require specific treatment if it is localized. If the emphysema is generalized, it can affect the vascular supply of the skin and become complicated with subcutaneous seroma or abscess and skin necrosis.

Prevention

- Control of the air-tight seal at the end of lung or bronchial surgery with a systematic immersion test
- Creation of a long air-thigh seal subcutaneous or submuscular tunnel along the chest drain

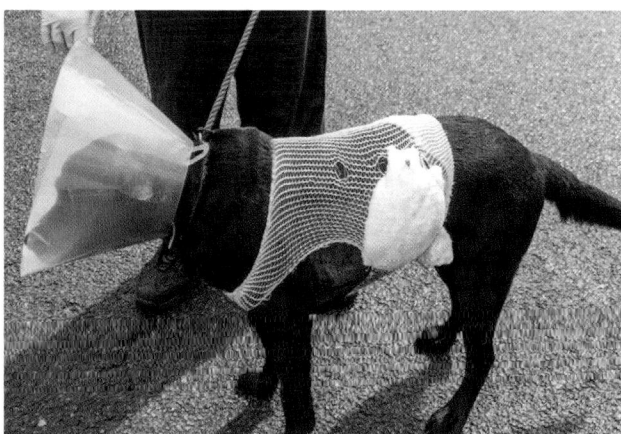

Figure 41.7 Chest drains should be protected with dressings. Systemic use of an Elizabethan collar is recommended to prevent self-mutilation.

- Protection of the surgical wound or drain against any trauma or self-inflicted damage (systematic use of an Elizabethan collar) (Figure 41.7)

Postoperative pulmonary complications

See Chapter 37.

Postoperative cardiac complications

Definition

Postoperative cardiac complications include cardiac arrhythmia.

Risk factors
- Preexisting cardiac condition
- Pneumonectomy

Diagnosis
- Heart auscultation
- Electrocardiography (ECG), echocardiography

Treatment
- Analgesia and electrolytes should be controlled first because pain and electrolyte imbalances can contribute to the development of cardiac arrhythmias (Monnet 2009; Kocaturk et al. 2010).
- Lidocaine (bolus of 1–2 mg/kg intravenously [IV] followed by a constant-rate infusion of 25–100 μg/kg/min) is recommended for the treatment of clinically significant ventricular disorders (Liptak et al. 2004; Monnet 2009; Kocaturk et al. 2010). Digoxin has been successfully used for the treatment of atrioventricular (AV) block and supraventricular tachycardia after lobectomy (Kocaturk et al. 2010).

Outcome

Postoperative atrial and ventricular disturbances are usually successfully treated medically (Liptak et al. 2004; Monnet 2009; Kocaturk et al. 2010). Complete AV blocks can be observed and are associated with a bad prognosis (Kocaturk et al. 2010).

Prevention

Preoperative screening with ECG and echocardiography has been advised to detect silent preoperative conditions (Salci et al. 2007; Kocaturk et al. 2010).

Mediastinal shift

Definition

The absence of pulmonary parenchyma on one side of the mediastinum after a pneumonectomy can cause a mediastinal shift (i.e., deviation of the mediastinum toward the resected side) (Salci et al. 2007).

Diagnosis
- Radiography, computed tomography
- Postoperative regurgitation
- Cardiovascular collapse with abdominal hypertension

Treatment

Postoperative regurgitations can be caused by sigmoid inflexion of the distal thoracic esophagus secondary to mediastinal shift and subsequent disturbance of the normal esophageal motility (Liptak et al. 2004). This has been clinically treated with sucralfate, metoclopramide, and omeprazole.

Outcome

In the report of a dog diagnosed with postpneumonectomy regurgitations secondary to mediastinal shift, medications allowed reduction of the episodes but did not achieved full cure (Liptak et al. 2004).

Prevention

In human medicine, thoracoplasty has been advocated to limit the mediastinal shift. The use of a latissimus dorsi muscle pedicle flap has been recommended to obliterate the pneumonectomy cavity. The well-vascularized muscle ensures adequate filling of the cavity, reenforces bronchial sutures, and decreases the risk of postoperative bronchopleural fistula (Abolhoda et al. 2009).

Postoperative bronchopleural fistula

Definition

This is a delayed healing process at the level of the bronchial stump, resulting in major air leakage from the unhealed stump and formation of a fistula between the bronchus and the pleura.

The fistula is suspected to be the consequence of the devascularization of the bronchial stump at the time of surgery. In absence of adequate vascularization, the healing process is delayed, and eventually some necrosis of the sutured bronchus is observed and the surgical air-thigh seal is lost (Deschamps et al. 1996; Salci et al. 2007; Alloubi et al. 2010). This complication has been reported in 18% of cases of dogs having experimental pneumonectomy (Salci et al. 2007) but never in clinical reports (Liptak et al. 2004, Crawford et al. 2011).

Risk factors
- Devascularization of long bronchial stump
- Excessive compression of bronchial wound

Diagnosis
- Acute severe pneumothorax, up to 3 weeks after pneumonectomy

Treatment

- Prompt thoracic drainage and surgical reexploration
- To ensure successful healing of the airway, the bronchial stump suture could be reinforced (with omental, pericardial, or vascularized muscle flaps based on the intercostal, pectoral, or latissimus dorsi muscles (Deschamps *et al.* 1996; Salci *et al.* 2007; Abolhoda *et al.* 2009).

Outcome

In veterinary medicine, none of the dogs described with such complications survived long enough to have chest drainage and subsequent surgical correction (Salci *et al.* 2007).

Prevention

- Minimum dissection of the bronchial stump to keep the local vascular supply
- Improve local vascular supply in using techniques of suture reinforcement

Acute respiratory distress syndrome and postpneumonectomy pulmonary edema

Definition

Acute lung injury (ALI) has been defined as an initial inflammatory lung injury associated with increased vascular permeability, resulting in development of pulmonary edema without initial pulmonary abnormality or pulmonary hypertension (i.e., noncardiogenic edema). Acute respiratory distress syndrome (ARDS) is defined as the ultimate form of ALI and has been recognized as a severe and often fatal complication (Jordan *et al.* 2000; Duggan and Kavanagh 2005). Postpneumonectomy pulmonary edema (PPPE) is the postoperative development of a generalized, long-lasting, noncardiogenic pulmonary edema after major lung resection. PPPE is the variation of ARDS observed in thoracic surgery (Jordan *et al.* 2000). The main difference with reexpansion pulmonary edema is that PPPE develops in normal lungs without preexisting atelectasis.

Risk factors

- Primary pulmonary insults: smoke inhalation, oxygen toxicity, pneumonia, or drowningConcomitant inflammation (mainly systemic inflammatory response syndrome (SIRS) (Kocaturk *et al.* 2009)
- Pneumonectomy
- Pulmonary exclusion and "one-lung" ventilation
- Extensive mediastinal dissection with damage to lymphatic tissue
- Lung barotraumas, lung reperfusion (Jordan *et al.* 2000)

Diagnosis

- Acute dyspnea, hypoxemia, hypercapnia
- Radiographic observation of diffused noncardiogenic pulmonary edema

Treatment

- Oxygen therapy, mechanical ventilation
- Diuretics and use of IV colloids
- Identification and treatment of any causes of primary ALI (aspiration pneumonia, infection)

Outcome

This well-known complication in human medicine is associated with a high mortality rate.

Prevention

- Identification of risks of ALI or preoperative signs of SIRS
- Minimal use of pulmonary exclusion
- Gentle retraction and packing of the lung parenchyma
- Minimal damages to the mediastinal structures

Respiratory insufficiency

Definition

Respiratory insufficiency is functional incapacity of the residual lung to adequately insure adequate gas exchange.

Causes of respiratory insufficiency can be anatomic (loss of lung parenchyma) or functional (inadequate ventilation, improper diffusion or perfusion [pulmonary edema, lung contusions, pneumonia]).

Risk factors

- Pneumonectomy (higher risk with right pneumonectomy)
- Diffuse lung disease
- Preoperative pulmonary atelectasis and reperfusion edema
- Postpneumonectomy edema
- Fluid overload
- Congestive heart failure

Diagnosis

- Dyspnea
- Hypoxemia and hemoglobin desaturation

Treatment

- Oxygen therapy and if necessary mechanical ventilation
- Sedation in case of a stressed animal
- Analgesia

Outcome

The prognosis remains poor whether the cause of the failure his functional or not. Reversible functional disorder (e.g., fluid-related lung edema) might carry a better prognosis.

Prevention

- Preoperative radiographic observation of compensatory overgrowth of the non to be resected lung is considered a good prognostic factor (Liptak *et al.* 2004) (Figure 41.8).
- Careful monitoring (oxygen saturation, end-tidal expiratory CO_2, ECG, arterial pressure measurement, blood gas analysis) during the perioperative period is paramount for early detection and treatment of complications.

Relevant literature

Cardiovascular complications are the most common and most documented complications observed in human patients after pneumonectomy (Alloubi *et al.* 2010). Postoperative arrhythmias have been reported after lobectomy and pneumonectomy in dogs (Liptak *et al.* 2004; Kocaturk *et al.* 2010). Supraventricular tachycardia and AV blocks are the most frequent abnormalities observed after lobectomy (25% of the cases). Sinus tachycardia and supraventricular tachycardia are the most frequent abnormalities observed after pneumonectomy (25%–75% of cases) (Liptak *et al.* 2004, Kocaturk *et al.* 2010).

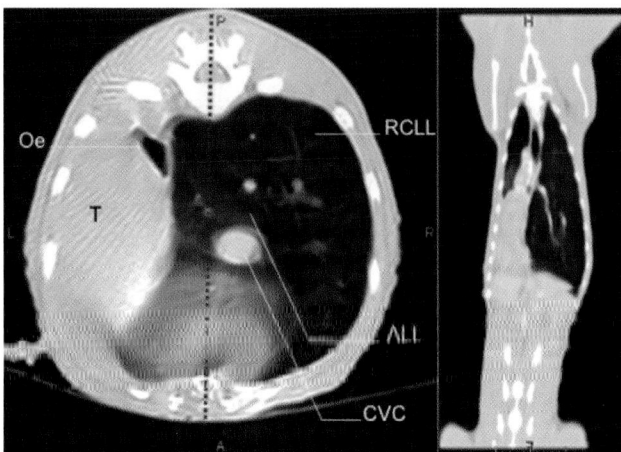

Figure 41.8 Transversal thoracic computed tomography image in a cat affected with a pulmonary adenocarcinoma. The tumor is affecting the hilus of the left lung. Note the overinflation of the right lung and the reduction of the space occupied by the left lung. The cat recovered very well from the left pulmonectomy. ALL, accessory lung lobe; CVC, caudal vena cava; Oe, esophagus; RCLL, right caudal lung lobe; T, tumor.

Postpneumonectomy mediastinal shift is not supposed to resolve with time. However, in cases in which regurgitations were observed, signs resolved a few weeks after the surgery. Mediastinal shift, although present, has not been found to be clinically significant in 27 healthy dogs that underwent experimental pneumonectomy (Salci et al. 2007). In human medicine, mediastinal shift has also been associated with deviation of the caudal vena cava and in severe cases with obstructive kinking of the caudal vena cava with secondary decreased venous return to the heart (Alloubi et al. 2010). This complication has not been reported in clinical veterinary medicine.

Acute respiratory distress syndrome has rarely been reported in veterinary surgery (Parent et al. 1996; Sauvé et al. 2004, Syrjä et al. 2009) but has been reproduced experimentally in dogs, cats, and rodents (Jordan et al. 2000; Kloot et al 2000).

Respiratory insufficiency is a major risk after pneumonectomy if the remaining pulmonary parenchyma fails to achieve immediate full function. It has been reported that the entire left and right lungs represent 42% to 45% and 55% to 58% of the lung parenchyma, respectively. In normal dogs, resection of up to 58% of lung parenchyma has been tolerated provided that the remaining parenchyma is normal (Brugarolas and Takita 1973; Hsai et al. 2001). The risk of postpneumonectomy respiratory failure has been reported to be increased when right pneumonectomy is performed (Nelson and Monnet 2003). The successful case reports might indicate that unilateral progressive disease might induce progressive changes in the opposite lung that would decrease the risk of postoperative respiratory failure (Liptak et al. 2004, Crawford et al. 2011).

Pneumonectomy results in severe reduction of lung parenchyma and acute redirection of blood to the remaining lung. Respiratory failure, increased pulmonary vascular resistance, and cardiac overload are the main complications described with this procedure, which is associated with a high mortality rate (Deschamps et al. 1996; Liptak et al. 2004; Salci et al. 2007).

Lung parenchymal damages can be encountered during manipulation of the lungs or attempt to separate two lobes. Superficial

lacerations usually do not need specific attention, but superficial suture is recommended when substantial air leak is observed. A simple continuous suture with fine monofilament and round needle sutures is usually enough to treat the complication. If necessary, partial lobectomy might be necessary to ensure full control of the leak.

Advanced electric surgical units have been reported as safe for the dissection of lung parenchyma and partial lobectomies and lung biopsies. In a study performed in pigs, the seal achieved with an electrothermal bipolar tissue sealing system (Ligasure TM, Valley Lab, Boulder CO – a division of Covidien Ltd.) was safe for bronchi smaller than 3 mm and vessels smaller than 7 mm (Santini et al. 2006). Similar results have been described in dogs when using t Ultracision Harmonic Scalpel TM (Johnson & Johnson Medical Ltd. – Cincinnati) (Molnar et al. 2004). However, clinical studies in humans showed a high complication rate when lung biopsy were performed with the sole Harmonic scalpel and advised systematic reinforcing maneuvers (i.e., stitches or clips) (Molnar et al. 2008). When using these systems for partial lobectomy, an "immersion test" is still mandatory.

Inadvertent suture of a bronchial blocker has been described during lung lobectomy when selective lung ventilation was performed (Levionnois et al. 2006). To prevent this complication, mobilization of the blocker at the time of bronchial suture is advised.

Acute anaphylactic shock has been reported in a dog after the inadvertent section of a heartworm during lung lobectomy (Carter et al. 2011). The subsequent profound hypotension and severe tachycardia were nonresponsive to the usual therapy (crystalloid bolus, phenylephrine). These eventually resolved after the administration of antihistaminic and dexamethasone.

Postpneumonectomy gastric volvulus has been reported in human medicine. It could be complicated with hiatal herniation and gastric necrosis. The exact mechanism of such complication is unclear, but it is suspected to be the association of different factors such as the change in the diaphragmatic dome and subsequent increased mobility of the gastric fundus, damages to the left phrenic nerve, and potential preexisting hiatal malformation (Thorpe et al. 2011).

Implantation of neoplastic cells on the edges of the surgical wound during thoracoscopic pleural biopsy has been reported (Brisson et al. 2006). Given these evidences, protection of the surgical wound with large abdominal swabs or a surgical drape is warranted to prevent delayed tumoral growth.

References

Abolhoda, A., Bui, T.D., Miliken, J.C., et al. (2009) Pedicled latissimus dorsi muscle flap: routine use in thoracic surgery. *Texas Heart Institute Journal* 36, 298-302.

Alloubi, I., Jougon, J., Delcambre, F., et al. (2010) Early complications after pneumonectomy: retrospective study of 168 patients. *Interactive Cardiovascular and Thoracic Surgery* 11, 162-465.

Brisson, B.A., Reggeti, F., Bienzle, D. (2006) Portal site metastasis of invasive mesothelioma after diagnostic thoracoscopy in a dog. *Journal of the American Veterinary Medical Association* 229 (6), 980-983.

Brugarolas, A., Takita, H. (1973) Regeneration of the lung in the dog. *Journal of Thoracic Cardiovascular Surgery* 65, 187-190.

Carter, J.E., Chanoit, G., Kata, C. (2011) Anaphylactoid reaction in a heartworm-infected dog undergoing lung lobectomy. *Journal of the American Veterinary Medical Association* 238, 1301-1304.

Crawford, A.H., Halfacree, Z.J., Lee, K.C.L., et al. (2011) Clinical outcome following pneumonectomy for management of chronic pyothorax in four cats. *Journal of Feline Medicine and Surgery* 13, 762-767.

Deschamps, C., Pairolero, P.C., Allen, M.S., et al. (1996) Management of postpneumonectomy empyema and bronchopleural fistula. *Chest Surgery Clinics of North America* 6, 519-527.

Duggan M., Kavanagh, B.P. (2005) Pulmonary atelectasis. *Anesthesiology* 102, 838-854.

Fossum, T.W. (2007) Surgery of the lower respiratory system: Lungs and thoracic wall. In Fossum, T.W. (ed.) *Textbook of Small Animal Surgery,* 3rd edn. Mosby/Elsevier, St Louis, pp. 649-657.

Hsia, C.C, Wu, E.Y., Wagner, E., et al. (2001) Preventing mediastinal shift after pneumonectomy impairs regenerative alveolar tissue growth. *American Journal of Physiology - Lung Cellular and Molecular Physiology* 281, L1279-L1287.

Jordan, S., Mitchell, J.A., Quinlan, G.J., et al. (2000) The pathogenesis of lung injury following pulmonary resection. *European Respiratory Journal* 15, 790-799.

Kloot, T.E., Blanch, L., Melynne Youngblood, A., et al. (2000) Recruitment maneuvers in three experimental models in acute lung injury. Effect on lung volume and gas exchange. *American Journal of Respiratory Critical Care Medicine* 161 (5), 1485-1496.

Kocaturk, M., Salci, H., Yilmaz, Z., et al. (2010) Pre- and post-operative cardiac evaluation of dogs undergoing lobectomy and pneumonectomy. *Journal of Veterinary Science* 11 (3), 257-264.

LaRue, S.M., Withrow, S.J., Wykes, P.M. (1987) Lung resection using surgical staples in dogs and cats. *Veterinary Surgery* 16 (3), 238-240.

Levionnois, O.L., Bergadano, A., Shatzmann, U. (2006) Accidental entrapment of an endo-bronchial blocker tip by a surgical stapler during selective ventilation for lung lobectomy in a dog. *Veterinary Surgery* 35, 82-86.

Liptak, J.M., Monnet, E., Dernell, W.S., et al.(2004) Pneumonectomy: four cases studies and a comparative review. *Journal of Small Animal Practice* 45, 441-447.

Mayer, I., Long, R., Breen, P.H., et al. (1986) Artificial ventilation of a canine model of bronchopleural fistula. *Anesthesiology* 64, 739-746.

Molnar, T.F., Szanto, Z., Laszlo, T., et al. (2004) Cutting lung parenchymal using the harmonic scalpel: an animal experiment. *European Journal of Cardiothoracic Surgery* 26 (6), 1192-1195.

Molnar, T.F., Benko, I., Szanto, Z., et al. (2008) Complications alter ultrasonic lung parenchymal biopsy: a strong note for caution. *Surgical Endoscopy* 22 (3), 679-682.

Monnet, E. (2009) Post-thoracotomy management. In Silverstein, D.C., Hopper, K. *Small Animal Critical Care Medicine.* WB Saunders, Philadelphia, pp. 148, 642-644.

Nelson, A.W., Monnet, E. (2003) Lungs. In Slatter, D. (ed.) *Textbook of Small Animal Surgery,* vol 1, 3rd edn. WB. Saunders, Philadelphia, pp 880-889.

Parent, C., King, L.G., Van Winkle, T.J., et al. (1996) Respiratory function and treatment in dogs with acute respiratory distress syndrome: 19 cases (1985-1993). *Journal of the American Veterinary Medical Association* 208 (9), 1, 428-433.

Salci, H., Sami Bayram, A., Ozygit, O., et al. (2007) Comparison of different bronchial closure techniques following pneumonectomy in dogs. *Journal of Veterinary Science* 8 (4), 393-399.

Santini, M., Vicidomini, G., Baldi, A., et al. (2006) Use of electrothermal bipolar tissue sealing system in lung surgery. *European Journal of Cardiothoracic Surgery* 29, 226-230.

Sauvé, V., Parent, C., Seiler, G., et al. (2004) Acute lung injury and acute respiratory distress syndrome in cats: 65 cases (1993-2003). *Journal of Veterinary Emergency and Critical Care* 14 (Suppl. 1), S5.

Stammberger, U., Klepetko, W., Stamasis, G., et al. (2000) Buttressing the staple line in lung volume reduction surgery: a randomized three-centre study. *Annals of Thoracic Surgery* 70, 1820-1825.

Syrjä, P., Saari, S., Rajamäki, M., et al. (2009) Pulmonary histopathology in Dalmatians with familial acute respiratory distress syndrome (ARDS). *Journal of Comparative Pathology* 141 (4), 254-259.

Thorpe, A.C., Foroulis, C.N., Shah, S. (2007) A rare complication of pneumonectomy: hiatal hernia associated with gastric volvulus. *Asian Cardiovascular & Thoracic Annals* 15, 518-520.

Walshaw, R. (1994) Stapling techniques in pulmonary surgery. *Veterinary Clinics of North America: Small Animal Practice* 24 (2), 335-366.

42 Chylothorax

Carolyn A. Burton

Davies Veterinary Specialists, Hertfordshire, UK

In the vast majority of cases, surgical management of chylothorax is performed for treatment of idiopathic chylothorax when medical management has failed to resolve or control the condition. Many known pathological processes can lead to the development of chylothorax, including direct trauma to the thoracic duct (TD) caused by severe external blows to the thorax, iatrogenic injury during thoracic surgery, neoplasia, venous thrombosis, cardiac disease, pericardial disease, fungal granulomas, congenital TD abnormalities, and heartworm disease (Fossum 1993; Campbell et al. 1995; Fossum et al. 2004; Singh and Brisson 2010). There is also a reported association with lung lobe torsion (Neath et al. 2000). In these cases, management is aimed at addressing the underlying disease process together with temporary thoracic drainage. Five cases of surgical management of secondary chylothorax of varying causes have also been reported (Allman et al. 2010), but surgical management is usually reserved for cases in which known causes have been excluded, leaving a diagnosis of idiopathic chylothorax.

In the more recently published case series, the postoperative complication rate after carrying out the animal's first surgery for management of idiopathic chylothorax ranges from 7% to 81%. The most common complication reported was continued chylous pleural effusion, which ranged from 0% to 40% (Fossum et al. 2004; Hayashi et al. 2005; Carobbi et al. 2008; Allman et al. 2010; Stewart 2010; Adrega de Silva and Monnet 2011; Bussadori et al. 2011; McAnulty 2011; Staiger et al. 2011). Sudden death from a variety of known and unknown causes in the first 24 hours to 4 days after surgery was the second most reported complication (0%–33%). The myriad of reported techniques used alone or in combination on only a relative small number of patients together with variable detail of case management documented makes accurate assessment of the true complication rate challenging. All of these case series were able to improve their overall success rates by performing one or more subsequent surgical procedures on the animals with complications.

Continued chylous pleural effusion

Definition

Thoracic drainage is usually continued postoperatively until the accumulation of fluid is less than 2 mL/kg in a 24-hour period. The thoracic drain is then removed. After successful surgical manage

ment of chylothorax, the chylous effusion may stop immediately after ligation, or it may continue for some days before gradually decreasing in volume. In the latter scenario, the assumption is that some "adaption" time is required for new lymphaticovenous anastomoses to form. There is currently no established time point to define when a case is categorized as a postsurgical failure. In practical terms, chylous effusion of sufficient volume that continues beyond 2 weeks after surgery and that requires frequent thoracic drainage to manage dyspnea should be categorized as a surgical failure. Equally, patients with continued lower volume postoperative chylous effusions necessitating intermittent thoracocentesis for weeks and often resulting in loss of body condition are likely to require further management. Some patients have persistent low-volume pleural effusion for months after surgery but are asymptomatic.

Risk factors

The current literature suggests that higher success rates are achieved with a combination of surgical techniques such as combining thoracic duct ligation (TDL) with cisterna chyli ablation (CCA) or TDL or CCA with subtotal pericardectomy (PC).

Diagnosis

Most commonly, chyle is persistently aspirated via the thoracic drain postoperatively. If the thoracic drain has been removed, the animal will represent with clinical signs of tachypnea or dyspnea. Chylous effusion is then confirmed with thoracic radiography, ultrasonography, and thoracocentesis. Analysis of effusion should confirm continued chylous effusion (triglyceride levels in the pleural fluid being greater than in the serum) and exclude concurrent sepsis. If a septic component to the effusion is confirmed, management of pyothorax should be started.

Possible causes for continued chylous effusion postoperatively depend on the surgical technique used during the initial surgery, and they include:

- Failure to stop flow in all branches of the TD during surgery
- Formation of collateral lymphatics or "opening up" of previously nonpatent lymphatic vessels bypassing the TD system, possibly in response to obstruction-induced hypertension within the TD
- Failure of new lymphaticovenous drainage routes to form outside the thoracic cavity
- Intrathoracic leakage of chyle caudal to the obstruction of the TD system

Complications in Small Animal Surgery, First Edition. Edited by Dominique Griffon and Annick Hamaide.

© 2016 John Wiley & Sons, Inc. Published 2016 by John Wiley & Sons, Inc.

Companion website: www.wiley.com/go/griffon/complications

- Thickening of the pericardium causing a postulated increase in right-sided venous pressures, leading to an increase in lymphatic flow through the TD

Further investigation of these causes with lymphangiography can be helpful. Mesenteric lymphangiography or direct injection of water-soluble contrast media into a mesenteric lymph node (particularly the ileocecocolic lymph node) provides good-quality contrast studies. This demonstrates continued flow through the TD system or through any collateral lymphatic vessels bypassing the TD system. These techniques usually require a small celiotomy approach, and fluoroscopic imaging is most helpful to visualize small vessels. Other less invasive techniques have been reported, including percutaneous administration of water-soluble contrast media into the popliteal lymph node (Naganobu *et al.* 2006) and percutaneous ultrasound-guided administration into a mesenteric lymph node (Johnson *et al.* 2009). The less invasive technique of radiographic imaging after popliteal lymph node administration was promising in experimental dogs, but it remains unproven in clinical cases. Imaging of the TD can certainly be improved with mesenteric lymph node administration of water-soluble contrast media and the use of computed tomography (CT) (Esterline *et al.* 2005; Johnson *et al.* 2009). CT may therefore also be useful to improve imaging after percutaneous popliteal lymph node administration, providing a minimally invasive alternative.

Treatment

The current reported techniques for management of chylothorax still fail in some animals. Second surgeries are recommended in these patients because current studies report that they may be successful in many of these animals.

Persistent patency of the thoracic duct or branch of the thoracic duct

Repeat caudal thoracotomy with identification and ligation of the patent branch is possible. In a recent study, 100% of dogs with persistent chylous effusions postoperatively had formation of a large lymphatic branch bypassing the previous TD closure sutures, which was not present or patent during the initial surgery (McAnulty 2011). These ducts or branches may be situated on the left side of the aorta, and a left intercostal thoracotomy may be necessary. In many cases, however, the left side of the aorta can be accessed from the right side by gentle manipulation of the aorta using DeBakey tissue forceps to grasp the aortic adventitial tissue and to rotate the vessel to visualize any branches on the far side.

Visualization of the patent TD or branch of the TD can be improved with administration of methylene blue (0.5 mg/kg of 1% solution; maximum, 10 mg) injected into a mesenteric lymphatic vessel or mesenteric lymph node (Enwiller *et al.* 2003). The toxic effects of methylene blue administration, including Heinz body anemia, pseudocyanosis, increased serum alkaline phosphatase levels, and renal failure are, however, a concern, and minimal doses to obtain visualization of the TD are recommended. Ideally, a postligation lymphangiography should be completed to confirm complete TD occlusion after any ligation.

Formation of intrathoracic collateral lymphatic channels

These channels may not be in the anatomic vicinity of the TD and therefore may not be accessible by the above approach. A consideration at this point would be a CCA to interrupt the flow of chyle into the TD system. CCA should be beneficial in relieving lymphatic hypertension, transiently lessening the drive to form further collateral lymphatics around the region of obstruction of the TD. This would hopefully allow more lymphaticovenous anastomoses to form outside the thoracic cavity. This approach could also be considered when intrathoracic leakage of chyle caudal to the TDL site is suspected. A case has been documented, however, with persisting TD collaterals to the left of the aorta in the absence of the cisterna chyli in a dog after TDL and CCA at the original surgery. These collaterals were leading from an intraabdominal lymphatic plexus. This patient was subsequently successfully managed with ligation of the TD collaterals and ablation of the intraabdominal lymphatic plexus, its regional lymph node, and efferent lymphatic vessels (Staiger *et al.* 2011).

Suspected increased right-sided venous pressure

A subtotal PC has been recommended when it was not performed as part of the original surgery. PC has been successful in resolving persistent postoperative chylous effusions and postoperative nonchylous effusions in several reported cases even when overt thickening or constriction of the pericardium was not apparent. Interestingly, although an increase in right-sided venous pressure is postulated, central venous pressures have been found to be normal in most dogs and to be unaffected by PC in dogs with idiopathic chylothorax (McAnulty 2008, 2011). It is possible that other yet unrecognized mechanisms come into play brought about by performing a PC in these cases.

Unknown reason for surgical failure

In some cases, despite the diagnostic approach described earlier, the reason for surgical failure remains elusive. In these cases, resorting to a repeat surgery using one or more of the alternative techniques to those used during the initial surgery is often performed.

To aid in the postoperative management in these refractory cases, some surgeons place a pleural port for management of postoperative effusions in preference to a thoracic drain (Staiger *et al.* 2011). This allows pain-free intermittent thoracic drainage for weeks after surgery if required and can be used for managing patients on an outpatient basis when low-volume pleural effusion persists. Further surgery is, however, recommended if a significant effusion persists.

Pleuroperitoneal shunts have also been used when TDL failed to resolve idiopathic chylothorax in a study of 10 dogs (Smeak *et al.* 2001). Shunts were placed if thoracocentesis was required weekly or less frequently or usually within 15 days of unsuccessful surgical management of idiopathic chylothorax. After shunt implantation, the number of chamber pumps required per day was initially determined from calculating the mean volume of chyle removed from the pleural space during the 3 to 5 days before shunt implantation and dividing this by the volume of fluid pumped in one pumping cycle. This volume, however, was not completely predictable in successfully managing the effusion, and follow-up radiography before and after pumping was needed in some cases. Careful client training and commitment is required to successfully manage the pleural effusion with a pleuroperitoneal shunt. Approximately half the dogs in the study experienced short-term complications, and 75% of the dogs had long-term complications associated with the shunt, requiring interventions to maintain its use. Most complications were successfully managed, but massive pleural fluid production can overwhelm the capacity of a functional shunt or the absorptive capacity of the abdomen. This study concluded that pleuroperitoneal shunts, although not curative, could offer a reasonable quality of life for dogs with persistent chylous effusion when other techniques have failed.

Outcome

In view of the low case numbers in reported studies of surgical treatment of idiopathic chylothorax and the multitude of techniques used, determining the outcome of revision surgeries is almost impossible. In the author's experience, however, despite some of the highly impressive success rates reported in several studies, there are still some cases of idiopathic chylothorax that defy the statistics and continue to have severe chylous thoracic effusions despite multiple techniques and multiple surgeries being used.

Prevention

- Use a combination of surgical techniques in the initial surgical management of chylothorax (TDL or CCA with PC, TDL with CCA).
- Perform postoperative lymphangiography to confirm the effectiveness or obstruction of flow in the TD.

Continued nonchylous pleural effusion

Definition

This is a nonchylous effusion persisting beyond 2 weeks after surgery and of sufficient volume to require continued thoracic drainage via a thoracostomy tube or intermittent thoracocentesis to manage dyspnea. In some cases, a postoperative chylous effusion changes its character to a persistent nonchylous effusion. A nonchylous effusion is most commonly a serosanguineous, modified transudate in character, but septic pleural effusions are also possible. The cause of the modified transudates is currently unknown. It has been speculated that the effusion may be secondary to chronic pleural inflammation from lymphatic drainage from the head and cranial thorax or from pulmonary lymphatics (Bilbrey and Birchard 1994; Allman *et al.* 2010). This effusion may be present before the initial surgery as a separate entity to the chylous portion of the effusion but persists after the chylous element has stopped. Other undiagnosed etiologies such as intrathoracic neoplasia should also be considered.

Risk factors

Chylous fluid within the thorax causes chronic irritation of the pleural and pericardial surfaces, leading to thickening of these structures. This in turn is postulated to increase systemic venous pressures, hence impeding flow via the lymphaticovenous communications. There are currently no reports stating which patients would be more prone to the development of a persistent nonchylous effusion.

Diagnosis

Diagnosis is made by confirmation of persistent pleural effusion with radiography, ultrasonography, thoracocentesis, or thoracic drainage. Laboratory analysis and cytology of the effusion to rule out ongoing chylous effusion should be carried out. Serum albumin concentrations should also be determined to ensure that hypoalbuminemia is not contributing to the ongoing thoracic effusion.

Treatment

Pyothorax

If analysis of pleural fluid confirms a pyothorax, treatment for pyothorax should be instigated.

Modified transudate

If a transudate or modified transudate is diagnosed, a PC should be considered to minimize systemic venous pressures. Many surgeons consider a PC an essential part of a successful surgical management of idiopathic chylothorax.

In some more problematic cases, a nonchylous effusion persists despite a PC being performed. Symptomatic treatment with antiinflammatory drugs and diuretics is used by many surgeons. In a recent study, the nonchylous effusion resolved in 3 of 5 dogs after the use of a course of antiinflammatory drugs. Four of these dogs had had CCA and TDL and the fifth TDL and PC at the initial surgery. In these dogs, a conventional antiinflammatory decreasing dose regimen of prednisolone over 4 to 6 weeks was used, and the resolution was rapid. One dog that did not respond to this regimen subsequently received a PC. This surgery had no effect on the subsequent volume of effusion (McAnulty 2011). Pleural ports or pleuroperitoneal shunt placement could also be considered for short- or long-term management in the same way as for a persistent chylous effusion.

Outcome

There are isolated reports of resolution of persistent nonchylous effusions after idiopathic chylothorax surgery, but no figures are available to document the success or failure rate.

Prevention

- Combining a PC with the technique to obstruct flow in the TD during the initial surgical technique to manage idiopathic chylothorax maybe helpful in avoiding some postoperative nonchylous effusions. Further studies are needed to confirm or refute this approach.

The management of continued postoperative pleural effusions after idiopathic chylothorax surgery is summarized in Figure 42.1.

Fibrosing pleuritis

Definition

Because chyle is irritant to pleural surfaces, its presence in the pleural cavity leads to inflammation and thickening of the exposed pleura. It is thought that the chronic exposure to the pleura to chyle leads to the development of fibrosing or restrictive pleuritis (FP). This condition is characterized as a thick fibroconnective tissue covering on the visceral pleura of the lungs. This entraps the pulmonary parenchyma thus preventing expansion of the lungs during respiration. In addition to the lungs being unable to expand due to the presence of a pleural effusion, the pleural surface itself acts as a restrictive coating around the lung. Therefore, even when the pleural fluid is removed, the affected lung fields will be unable to expand to fill the pleural cavity.

Risk factors

In one report of 10 cats and 10 dogs treated with idiopathic chylothorax, 3 cats were described as having severe FP, 2 cats moderate FP, and 1 dog mild FP at the time of surgery (Fossum *et al.* 2004). Another study of 15 cats diagnosed 10 of them (67%) as having FP (Suess *et al.* 1994). FP is rarely mentioned as a problem in the papers documenting idiopathic chylothorax in dogs. It would therefore seem that cats were more likely than dogs to have FP at the time of initial surgery. It would seem logical that the more chronic the chylous effusion before diagnosis and treatment, the

Persistent pleural effusion

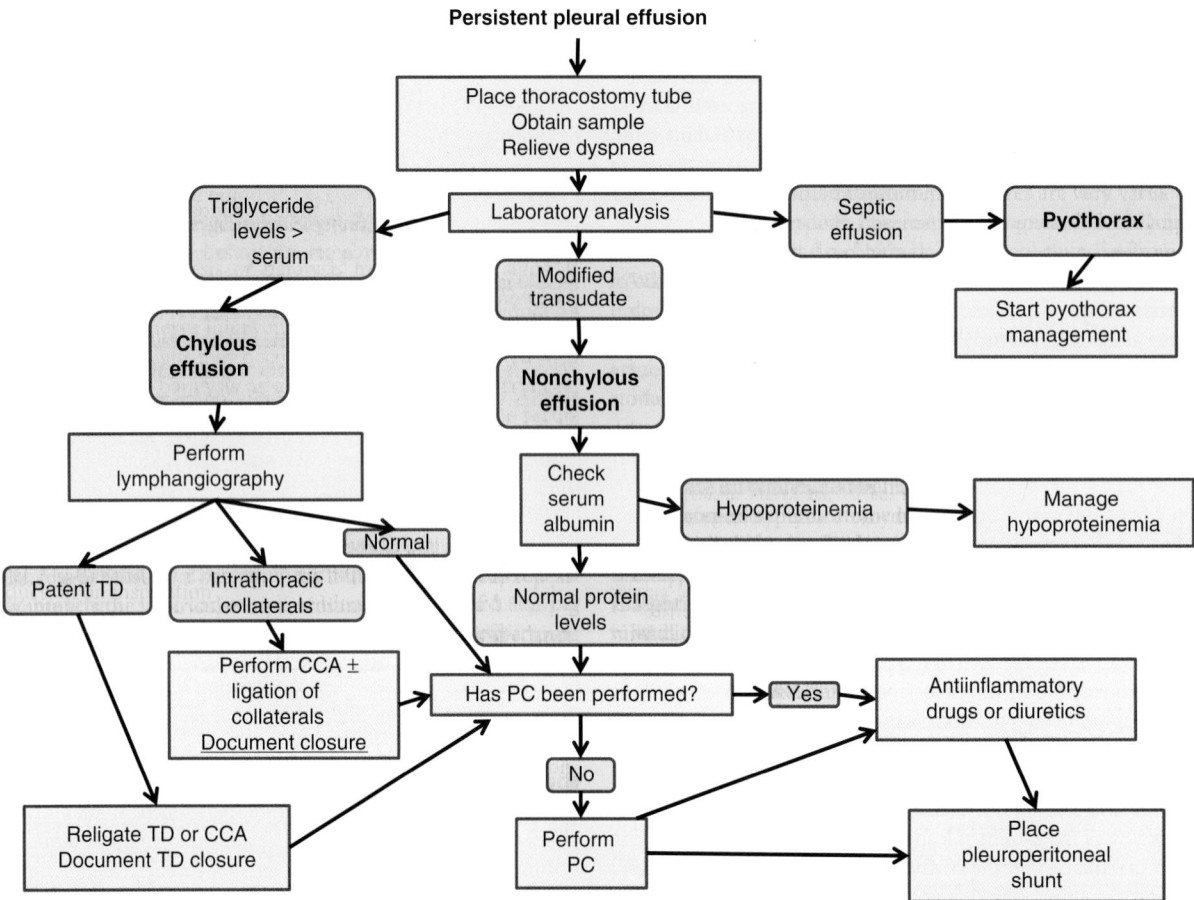

Figure 42.1 Summary of the management of continuing postoperative pleural effusions after surgery for idiopathic chylothorax. CCA, cisterna chyli ablation; PC, pericardectomy; TD, thoracic duct.

more likely FP is to be present. However, severe cases of FP have been seen in animals with very recent onsets of clinical signs. It is not known whether these animals develop FP after only a short duration of a chylous effusion or if a chronic low-volume chylous effusion, not sufficient to give overt clinical signs, has been present for some time.

Diagnosis
The diagnosis is usually confirmed intraoperatively by observation of the lung lobes. When FP is present, the visceral pleural surfaces of the lung are grossly thickened, the lungs are markedly contracted with rounded edges, and they do not expand normally during positive-pressure ventilation. However, the radiographic criteria for diagnosis appear to be reliable if two or more of the following radiographic findings are present:
- Obvious pleural thickening
- Irregular or rounded lung edges
- Persistent lung lobe collapse despite effective thoracic drainage (Suess et al. 1994)

Treatment
Decortication has been described as a treatment option for cases of severe FP but has been associated with high rates of hemorrhage intraoperatively and pneumothorax postoperatively. The pneumothorax then requires thoracic tube placement with intermittent or

continuous drainage to allow the pneumothorax to resolve. In the author's experience, mild to moderate cases of FP resolve over time after successful management of the chylothorax has been carried out with the lung fields gradually reexpanding without resorting to decortication. There are reports, however, of continued decrease in pulmonary function causing dyspnea in cats with FP despite adequate control of their chylous effusions (Suess et al. 1994). Decortication was not performed in these cats.

Outcome
Many of the reported cases of severe FP treated with decortication were successful but had to be combined with aggressive postoperative management of pneumothorax.

Prevention
It is generally thought that early treatment of idiopathic chylothorax is advisable to lessen the risk of FP's forming and progressing.

Postoperative chyloabdomen

Definition
Postoperative chyloabdomen is the accumulation of chylous fluid within the abdomen after surgical management of idiopathic chylothorax. This may occur during the "adaption" period when new

lymphaticovenous anastomoses are being formed, but isolated cases have also been reported as a more long-term problem in some cases.

Risk factors

Risk factors are currently unknown.

Diagnosis

Clinical signs of abdominal distension are suggestive with chylous fluid being confirmed with abdominal ultrasonography and abdominocentesis if necessary.

Treatment and outcome

Generally, no treatment is required. The accumulation of chylous fluid usually resolves over several days. The abdominal cavity appears to be tolerant to chylous fluid accumulation with substantial volumes of fluid having no detrimental consequences. No solution has been described for the isolated cases when long-term chyloabdomen persisted.

Prevention

No information is currently available regarding the incidence of chyloabdomen postoperatively, but it is likely that most dogs have some degree of postoperative chyloabdomen. In the author's experience, its presence does not appear to be detrimental to successful recovery from chylothorax surgery.

Relevant literature

No consensus currently exists regarding the best surgical protocol for idiopathic chylothorax management. TDL alone had initial reported success rates of around 59% in 27 dogs (Birchard and Smeak 1998), 20% in 37 cats (Fossum et al. 1991) and 60% in 11 dogs in a more recent study (McAnulty 2008). En-bloc ligation of the TD and its branches illustrated failure to close all branches of the TD in 7% of normal cadaveric dogs (MacDonald et al. 2008). Combining TDL with PC in one study raised the success rate to 100% in 9 dogs and 80% in 10 cats (Fossum et al. 2004) and in a second study to 100% in 14 dogs (Carobbi et al. 2008), although some of these patients did require more than one surgical procedure to achieve these impressive results. More recent studies have not been able to replicate these high success rates, with a 60% success rate being reported (McAnulty 2011). TDL with or without PC has most commonly been achieved via right lateral thoracotomy, although a median sternotomy approach is also reported (Adrega de Silva and Monnet 2011). Minimally invasive surgery via thoracoscopy for TDL and PC has been reported in 7 dogs with idiopathic chylothorax and had resolution in 88% with the only complication being 1 dog, which was euthanized within 24 hours of surgery with severe systemic inflammatory response syndrome (Allman et al. 2010). TDL combined with CCA in 8 dogs had similar results with resolution of chylothorax in 88% (Hayashi et al. 2005) and 83% in 10 dogs (McAnulty 2011). This technique has also been described using a single approach for TDL and CCA (Staiger et al. 2011). TDL and PC combined with omentalization of the thoracic cavity is reported in 5 dogs and 7 cats with postoperative complications, including pleuritis, respiratory arrest, and serosanguineous effusion, with 5 animals dying within the first month after surgery (Stewart 2010).

Quantifying the success of other treatment modalities for clinical cases of idiopathic chylothorax, including transcatheter embolization of the TD (Pardo et al. 1989; Pardo 1995), pleuroperitoneal shunt placement (Smeak et al. 1987), implantation of diaphragmatic mesh (Peterson et al. 1989), omentalization alone (Williams and Niles 1999; LaFond et al. 2002) or in combination with other techniques (Bussadori et al. 2011), benzopyrone (rutin) administration (Thompson et al. 1999), and pleurodesis (Smeak et al. 1987) alone or in combination with the above techniques is even more difficult than assessing the more mainstream surgical techniques because of the minimal numbers of cases reported. Pleurodesis is, however, not currently recommended by most surgeons.

As can be seen from this summary of the literature, a comparison of the success rates and complications among all the available surgical procedures currently used is challenging for the following reasons:

1 Most studies involve few animals, a reflection of the rarity of the condition.
2 Most studies involve some animals receiving multiple procedures.
3 Many subsequent surgical procedures performed use different techniques than that initially used.
4 Follow-up times for these clinical studies are variable.

It is generally still thought that our lack of understanding of the underlying cause of idiopathic chylothorax hampers our ability to find successful treatments in all cases.

References

Adrega de Silva, C., Monnet, E. (2011) Long-term outcome of dogs treated surgically for idiopathic chylothorax: 11 cases (1995-2009). *Journal of the American Veterinary Medical Association* 239, 107-113.

Allman, D.A., Radlinsky, M.G., Ralph, A.G., et al. (2010) Thoracoscopic thoracic duct ligation and thoracoscopic pericardectomy for treatment of chylothorax in dogs. *Veterinary Surgery* 39, 21-27.

Bilbrey, S.A., Birchard, S.J. (1994) Pulmonary lymphatics in dogs with experimentally induced chylothorax. *Journal of the American Animal Hospital Association* 30, 86-91.

Birchard, S.J., Smeak, D.D. (1998) Treatment of idiopathic chylothorax in dogs and cats. *Journal of the American Veterinary Medical Association* 212, 652-657.

Bussadori, R., Provera, A., Martano, M. (2011) Pleural omentalisation with en bloc ligation of the thoracic duct and pericardectomy for idiopathic chylothorax in nine dogs and four cats. *The Veterinary Journal* 188, 234-236.

Campbell S.L., Forrester S.D., Johnston S.A. (1995) Chylothorax associated with constrictive pericarditis in a dog. *Journal of the American Animal Hospital Association* 206, 1561-1564.

Carobbi, B., White, R.A.S., Romanelli, G. (2008) Treatment of idiopathic chylothorax in 14 dogs by ligation of the thoracic duct and partial pericardectomy. *Veterinary Record* 163, 743-745.

Enwiller, T.M., Radlinsky, M.G., Mason, D.E., et al. (2003) Popliteal and mesenteric lymph node injection with methylene blue for coloration of the thoracic duct in dogs. *Veterinary Surgery* 32, 359-364.

Esterline, M.L., Radlinsky, M.G., Biller, D.S., et al. (2005) Comparison of radiographic and computed tomography lymphangiography for identification of the canine thoracic duct. *Veterinary Radiology and Ultrasound* 46, 391-395.

Fossum, T.W. (1993) Feline chylothorax. *Compendium for Continuing Education for the Practising Veterinarian* 15, 549-567.

Fossum, T.W., Forrester, D., Swenson, C.L. (1991) Chylothorax in cats: 37 cases (1969-1989). *Journal of the American Veterinary Medical Association* 198, 672-678.

Fossum T.W., Mertens, M.M., Miller, M.W., et al. (2004) Thoracic duct ligation and pericardectomy for treatment of idiopathic chylothorax. *Journal of Veterinary Internal Medicine* 18, 307-310.

Hayashi, K., Sicard, G., Gellasch, K., et al. (2005) Cisterna chyli ablation with thoracic duct ligation for chylothorax: results in eight dogs. *Veterinary Surgery* 34, 519-523.

Johnson, E.G., Wisner, E.R., Kyles, A., et al. (2009) Computed tomographic lymphography of the thoracic duct by mesenteric lymph node injection. *Veterinary Surgery* 38, 361-367.

LaFond, E., Weirich, W.E., Salisbury, S.K. (2002) Omentalization of the thorax for treatment of idiopathic chylothorax with constrictive pleuritis in a cat. *Journal of the American Animal Hospital Association* 38, 74-78.

MacDonald, N.J., Noble, P-J.M., Burrow, R.D. (2008) Efficacy of en bloc ligation of the thoracic duct: descriptive study in 14 dogs. *Veterinary Surgery* 37, 696-701.

McAnulty, J. (2008) Comparison of cisterna chyli ablation and pericardectomy with thoracic duct ligation for treatment of chylothorax in dogs: a prospective randomized study. *Proceedings of the 2008 American College of Veterinary Surgery Veterinary Symposium*, p. 22.

McAnulty, J.F. (2011) Prospective comparison of cisterna chyli ablation to pericardectomy for treatment of spontaneously occurring idiopathic chylothorax in the dog. *Veterinary Surgery* 40, 926-934.

Naganobu, K., Ohigashi, Y., Akiyoshi, T., et al. (2006) Lymphography of the thoracic duct by percutaneous injection of iohexol into the popliteal lymph node of dogs: experimental study and clinical application. *Veterinary Surgery* 35, 377-381.

Neath, P.J., Brockman, D.J., King, L.G. (2000) Lung lobe torsion in dogs: 22 cases (1981-1999). *Journal of the American Veterinary Medical Association* 217, 1041-1044.

Pardo, A.D. (1995) Thoracic duct embolization for the treatment of chylothorax. In *Proceedings 5th American College of Veterinary Surgeons Veterinary Symposium*, pp. 552-554.

Pardo, A.D., Bright, R.M., Walker, M.A., et al. (1989) Transcatheter thoracic duct embolization in the dog. An experimental study. *Veterinary Surgery* 18, 279-285.

Peterson, S.L., Pion, P.D., Breznock, E.M. (1989) Passive pleuroperitoneal drainage for management of chylothorax in two cats. *Journal of the American Animal Hospital Association* 25, 569-572.

Singh, A., Brisson, B.A. (2010) Chylothorax associated with thrombosis of the cranial vena cava. *Canadian Veterinary Journal* 51, 847-852.

Smeak, D.D., Gallagher, L., Birchard, S.J., et al. (1987) Management of intractable pleural effusion in a dog with a pleuroperitoneal shunt. *Veterinary Surgery* 16, 212-216.

Smeak, D.D., McLoughlin, M.A., Caywood, D.D. (2001) Treatment of chronic pleural effusion with pleuroperitoneal shunts in dogs: 14 cases (1985-1999). *Journal of the American Veterinary Medical Association* 219, 1590-1597.

Staiger, B.S., Stanley, B.J & McAnulty, J.F. (2011) Single approach to thoracic duct and cistern chyli: experimental study and case series. *Veterinary Surgery* 40, 786-794.

Stewart, K. (2010) Chylothorax treated via thoracic duct ligation and omentalization. *Journal of the American Animal Hospital Association* 46, 312-317.

Suess, R.P., Flanders, J.A. Beck, K.A., et al. (1994) Constrictive pleuritis in cats with chylothorax: 10 cases (1983-1991). *Journal of the American Animal Hospital Association* 30, 70-77.

Thompson, M.S., Cohn, L.A., Jordan, R.C. (1999) Use of rutin for medical management of idiopathic chylothorax in four cats. *Journal of the American Veterinary Medical Association* 215, 345-348.

Williams, J.M., Niles, J.D. (1999) Use of the omentum as a physiologic drain for treatment of chylothorax in a dog. *Veterinary Surgery* 28, 61-65.

43 Esophagoscopy and Esophageal Surgery

Robert J. Hardie

The University of Wisconsin, School of Veterinary Medicine, Department of Surgical Sciences, Madison, WI, USA

Diseases or problems involving the esophagus are relatively common, often requiring esophagoscopy or surgery for diagnosis and treatment. Common diseases or problems of the esophagus include obstructions caused by foreign bodies (Sale and Williams 2006; Gianella *et al.* 2009; Juvet *et al.* 2010) (Figure 43.1); strictures (Adamama-Moraitou *et al.* 2002; Fox *et al.* 2007; Glazer and Walters 2008; Bissett *et al.* 2009); tumors (Ranen *et al.* 2004; Farese *et al.* 2008); vascular ring anomalies; and perforations caused by severe gastric reflux, trauma, or penetrating injury (Adami *et al.* 2011) (Figure 43.2). Less common problems include congenital or acquired diverticula and bronchoesophageal fistula (Pearson *et al.* 1978; Nawrocki *et al.* 2003; Juvet *et al.* 2010; Adami *et al.* 2011).

Esophagoscopy is very useful for determining the location and extent of disease, as well as sampling any potential lesion via endoscopic biopsy techniques. Examination of the entire esophagus depends on whether it is possible to manipulate a scope past a particular lesion. For lesions such as severe strictures or large foreign bodies, it may not be possible to examine the distal portion of the esophagus, and thus the full extent of the disease cannot always be determined. Various therapeutic procedures can also be performed via endoscopy such as removal of foreign bodies, dilation or bougienage of strictures, and submucosal injection of antiinflammatory agents (Lieb *et al.* 2001; Adamama-Moraitou *et al.* 2002; Rousseau

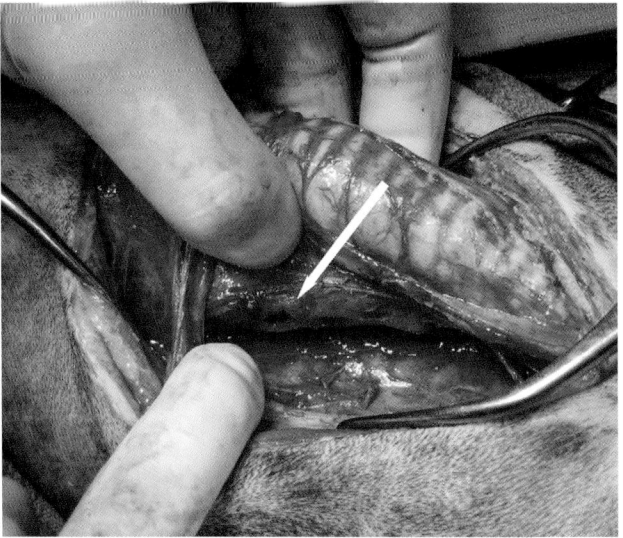

Figure 43.2 Intraoperative image of a perforation in the dorsal aspect of the cervical esophagus (arrow).

et al. 2007; Glazer and Walters 2008; Lieb and Sartor 2008; Bissett *et al.* 2009; Fraune *et al.* 2009; Gianella *et al.* 2009, Juvet *et al.* 2010).

Potential complications associated with endoscopy include intraluminal hemorrhage caused by irritation or excoriation of the mucosa and perforation of the esophagus caused by either direct trauma from the endoscope or excessive insufflation of air. In cases of foreign bodies or strictures, the risk for perforation is likely to be increased because of preexisting damage to the esophagus. Consequences of esophageal perforation include inflammation and infection of the periesophageal tissues, and depending on the location of the perforation, pneumomediastinum, pneumothorax, and subcutaneous emphysema. In addition, severe extraluminal hemorrhage from vessels surrounding the esophagus has been reported as a complication from endoscopic foreign body removal (Cohn *et al.* 2003; Keir *et al.* 2010).

Esophageal surgery typically involves esophagotomy or resection anastomosis for removal of foreign bodies (Figure 43.3), strictures, or tumors. More complicated procedures may involve reconstruction of the esophagus after resection of a diverticulum or dissection and closure of a bronchoesophageal fistula.

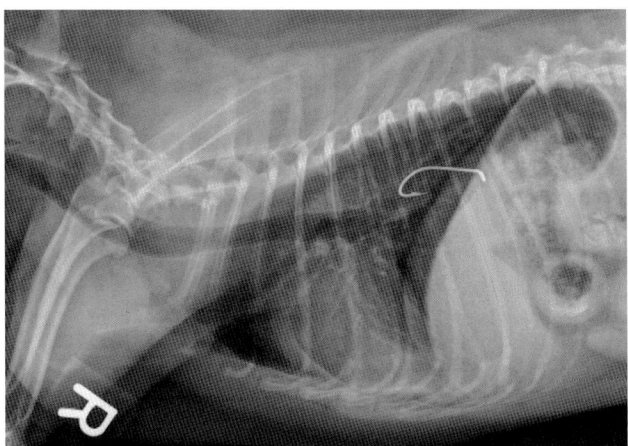

Figure 43.1 Lateral thoracic radiograph of a dog revealing a fishhook foreign body in the caudal thoracic esophagus.

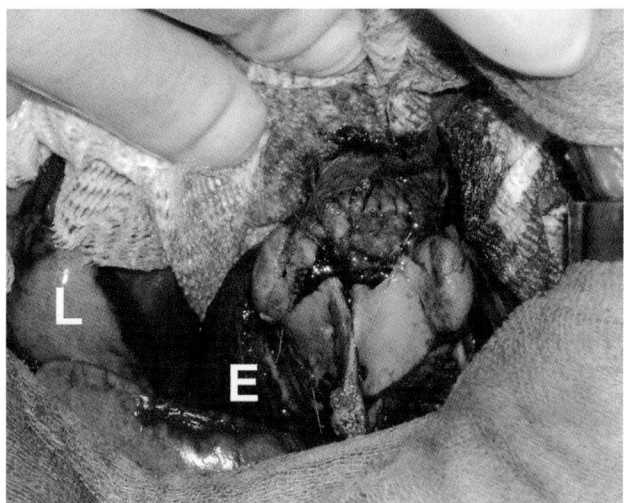

Figure 43.3 Intraoperative image of a bone foreign body in the thoracic esophagus (E) of a dog being removed via longitudinal esophagotomy incision. L, lung.

Potential complications specific to esophageal surgery include hemorrhage, dehiscence, infection, stricture, or rarely development of a diverticulum caused by damage or weakening of the muscular layers of the esophageal wall. The risk for these complications varies depending on the specific disease or lesion being treated; the location, extent, and severity of the lesion; the surgical approach used to access the esophagus; and any other concurrent problems with the animal. In addition, potential complications associated with the approach (i.e., intercostal, median sternotomy, transdiaphragmatic) used for intrathoracic esophageal surgery include hemorrhage, infection, or seroma formation at the surgical site; pneumothorax or subcutaneous emphysema associated with the use of thoracostomy tubes; and postoperative pain and respiratory compromise associated with thoracotomy.

Perforation

Definition

Perforation, rupture, and laceration of the esophagus are all potential complications associated with endoscopic procedures. Damage to the esophageal wall caused by erosion or pressure necrosis from an entrapped foreign body increases the risk for perforation during endoscopy. The type of foreign body and duration of entrapment should also be considered in assessing the risk of perforation (Juvet *et al.* 2010). When damage to the esophagus is identified or suspected, insufflation should be done with caution to minimize the risk of perforation.

Risk factors

- Bone or irregular, sharp foreign bodies
- Prolonged duration (>3 days) of entrapment
- Body weight less than 10 kg
- Degree of local necrosis or inflammation
- Excessive insufflation used during endoscopy
- Excessive volume or pressure used during balloon dilation or bougienage

Diagnosis

- Survey cervical or thoracic radiography looking for evidence of pneumomediastinum, subcutaneous emphysema, or

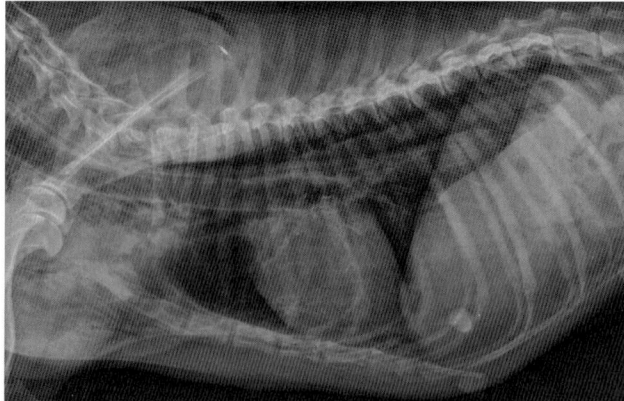

Figure 43.4 Lateral thoracic radiograph of a dog with a perforation of the cervical esophagus revealing subcutaneous emphysema, pneumomediastinum, and increased soft tissue density in the region of the perforation.

pneumothorax or increased soft tissue density surrounding the perforation site (Figure 43.4)
- Contrast esophagography (using iodinated contrast media) looking for evidence of leakage into the periesophageal tissues
- Endoscopy for direct visualization of perforation site

Treatment

Treatment for an esophageal perforation involves surgical debridement and closure of the esophagus in one or two layers using a fine, monofilament, absorbable suture material on a tapered needle (Ranen *et al.* 2004). If performing a two-layer closure, the knots for the first layer should be placed within the lumen of the esophagus and the knots for the second layer outside the lumen. For a very small perforation that has potential to seal spontaneously, conservative management with antibiotic therapy, supportive care, and nothing per os may be appropriate. When it is necessary to bypass the esophagus for a prolonged period of time, placement of a gastrostomy tube may be indicated.

Outcome

The overall prognosis for esophageal perforations is generally guarded but varies considerably based on the underlying condition, the degree of contamination of the periesophageal tissues, the extent of the perforation(s), and the viability of the surrounding esophagus.

Prevention

- Careful assessment of risk factors for perforation before endoscopic examination and attempts to remove foreign bodies
- Avoid excessive insufflation during endoscopic examination
- Avoid excessive manipulation of the scope when visualization of the lumen is impaired

Infection
See Chapter 1.

Stricture

Definition

A stricture is an abnormal narrowing or constriction of the lumen of the esophagus typically caused by excessive damage to the mucosa and submucosa that fails to reepithelialize appropriately during

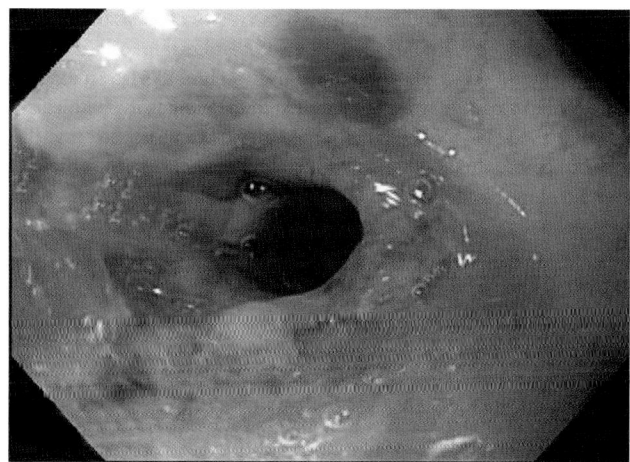

Figure 43.5 Endoscopic image of an esophageal stricture in a dog.

healing, leading to excessive collagen deposition, scarring, poor distensibility, and narrowing of the lumen (Glazer and Walters 2008).

Risk factors
- Excessive mucosal damage caused by prolonged entrapment of a foreign body
- Poor apposition of the mucosa during closure of the esophagus
- Damage or loss of an excessive portion of the circumference of the esophagus leading to narrowing of the lumen despite successful healing of the closure site
- Persistent Gastroesophageal reflux (GER). compromising healing of the esophagus
- Specific risk factors increasing the likelihood of GER include some anesthetic drugs (e.g., propofol), fasting for more than 24 hours, intraabdominal surgical procedures (e.g., ovariohysterectomy), and some oral medications (e.g., tetracycline).

Diagnosis
- Contrast esophagography or fluoroscopy
- Endoscopic examination of the esophagus (Figure 43.5)
- Computed tomography examination of the esophagus (Figures 43.6)

Treatment
- Modified feeding regimen involving soft or liquid diet formulation
- Endoscopic balloon dilation or bougienage (Figure 43.7)
- Endoscopic submucosal injection of corticosteroids (triamcinolone acetonide) around the circumference of a stricture has been described to reduce the degree of fibrosis that occurs during healing (Fraune *et al.* 2009)
- Surgical resection and anastomosis provided the length of the area to be resected is within the range (generally 3–5 cm) that can be safely removed without excessive tension on the anastomosis

Outcome
The overall prognosis for esophageal strictures is variable depending on the extent and degree of the stricture and the ability to dilate the stricture to an adequate diameter to allow for passage of food. Bougienage or balloon dilation generally requires multiple treatments to achieve and maintain adequate luminal diameter. Failure to adequately dilate a stricture typically results in ongoing regurgitation, weight loss, and risk of aspiration pneumonia.

Prevention
- Early diagnosis and treatment of esophageal foreign bodies
- Meticulous surgical technique to ensure proper mucosal apposition during esophagotomy closure or anastomosis
- Appropriate medical management of esophagitis or GER

Diverticulum

Definition
A diverticulum is a pouchlike herniation of the esophageal mucosa through a defect in the muscular and adventitial layers of the esophagus. This has been previously described as the result of esophageal trauma after removal of an entrapped foreign body, severe focal esophagitis caused by GER, and as a congenital defect in dogs.

Risk factors
- Trauma or injury to the esophagus leading to separation or a defect in the muscular and adventitial layers of the esophagus, allowing for dilation or outpocketing of the mucosal layer

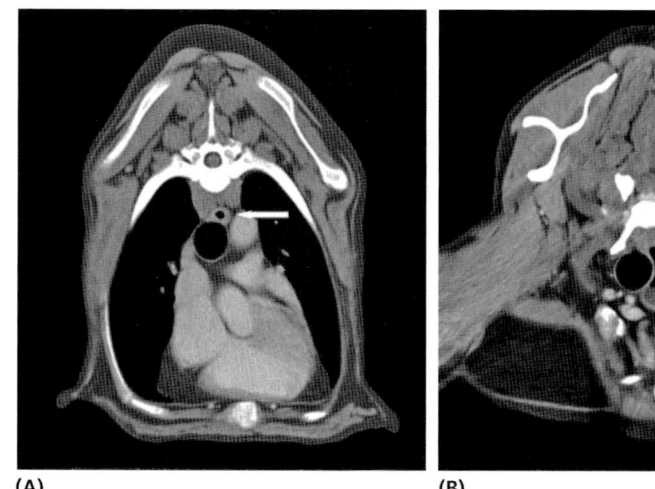
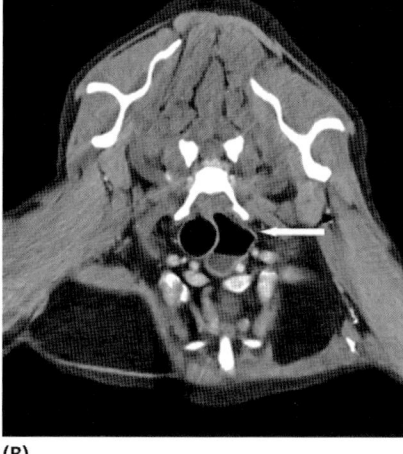
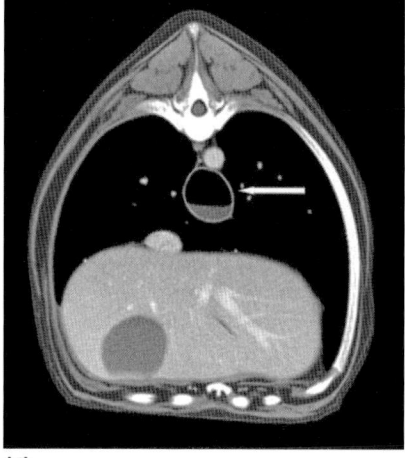

(A) (B) (C)

Figure 43.6 Computed tomography images of a midthoracic esophageal stricture in a dog (white arrow) (**A**). Note the dilation and pooling of fluid in the esophagus cranial (white arrow) (**B**) and caudal (white arrow) (**C**) to the actual stricture.

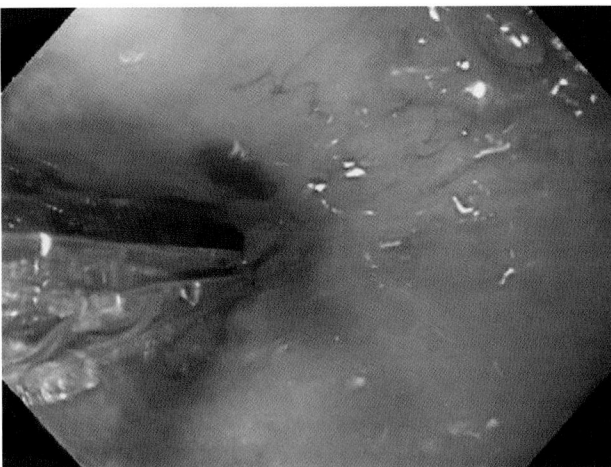

Figure 43.7 Endoscopic image demonstrating placement of a balloon catheter for dilation of an esophageal stricture.

Diagnosis
- Endoscopic examination of the esophagus
- Contrast esophagography or fluoroscopy

Treatment
- Surgical resection of the diverticula and reconstruction of the esophageal wall or resection and anastomosis of the involved area of the esophagus

Outcome
- The overall prognosis is guarded depending on the size and extent of the diverticula and the potential for disruption of normal esophageal motility.

Prevention
- Careful assessment of the risk factors and degree of esophageal injury and avoidance of excessive trauma during endoscopic examination

Relevant literature
Complication rates for various endoscopic procedures such as dilation of strictures and removal of foreign bodies have been described. In a recent study of 20 dogs and 8 cats that underwent bougienage for dilation of esophageal strictures, complications included esophageal perforation (1 cat), aspiration pneumonia (2 dogs), moderate mucosal hemorrhage (11 dogs and 6 cats), and severe mucosal hemorrhage (1 dog) (Bissett *et al.* 2009). The number of perforations, 1 of 28 (3.6%), reported in this study was comparable to previous studies (range, 3.6%–9%) (Harai *et al.* 1995; Melendez *et al.* 1998). In a recent report of 66 dogs with esophageal foreign bodies that underwent endoscopic removal, 10 (15.2%) developed complications, including perforation (*n* = 5), respiratory arrest (*n* = 1), stricture (*n* = 1), periesophageal abscess (*n* = 1), diverticulum (*n* = 1), and pneumothorax and pleural effusion (*n* = 1) (Gianella *et al.* 2009). Of the 10 dogs that developed complications, 4 died, and 2 were euthanized. In another study of 30 dogs that underwent successful removal or dislodgement of foreign bodies from the esophagus, 10 developed complications, including perforation (*n* = 3), aspiration (*n* = 3), vomiting (*n* = 3), and esophageal diverticulum (*n* = 1) (Juvet *et al.* 2010). Two of the 10 dogs ultimately died of progressive complications, resulting in an overall mortality rate of 6.7%.

Postoperative mortality rates for surgical removal of esophageal foreign bodies in dogs have been described in several studies and range from 0% to 57% (Knight 1963; Ryan and Greene 1975; Houlton *et al.* 1985; Spielman *et al.* 1992). In a most recent study involving 14 dogs, the postoperative complication rate was 14% (2 of 14), and the mortality rate was 7% (1 of 14) (Sale and Williams 2006).

References
Adamama-Moraitou, K.K., Rallis, T.S., Prassinos, N.N., et al. (2002) Benign esophageal stricture in the dog and cat: a retrospective study of 20 cases. *Can J Vet Res* 66, 55-59.

Adami, C., Di Palma, S., Gendron, K., et al. (2011) Severe esophageal injuries occurring after general anesthesia in two cats: case report and literature review. *J Am Anim Hosp Assoc* 47, 436-442.

Bissett, S. A., Davis, J., Subler, K., et al. (2009) Risk factors and outcome of bougienage for treatment of benign esophageal strictures in dogs and cats: 28 cases (1995-2004). *J Am Vet Med Assoc* 235, 844-850.

Cohn, L.A., Stoll, M.R., Branson, K.R., et al. (2003) Fatal hemothorax following management of an esophageal foreign body. *J Am Anim Hosp Assoc* 39, 251-256.

Farese, J.P., Bacon, N.J., Ehrhart, N.P., et al. (2008) Oesophageal leiomyosarcoma in dogs: surgical management and clinical outcome of four cases. *Vet Compar Oncol* 6, 31-38.

Fox, E., Lee, K., Lamb, C.R., et al. (2007) Congenital oesophageal stricture in a Japanese shiba inu. *J Small Anim Pract* 48, 709-712.

Fraune, C., Gaschen, F., Ryan, K. (2009) Intralesional corticosteroid injection in addition to endoscopic balloon dilation in a dog with benign oesophageal strictures. *J Small Anim Pract* 50, 550-553.

Gianella, P., Pfammatter, N.S., Burgener, I.A. (2009) Oesophageal and gastric endoscopic foreign body removal: complications and follow-up of 102 dogs. *J Small Anim Pract* 50, 649-654.

Glazer, A., Walters, P. (2008) Esophagitis and esophageal strictures. *Compend Contin Educ for Pract Vet Small Anim Pract* 30, 281-291.

Harai, B.H., Johnson, S.E., Sherding, R.G. (1995) Endoscopically guided balloon dilation of benign esophageal strictures in 6 cats and 7 dogs. *J Vet Intern Med* 9, 332-335.

Houlton, J.E.F., Herrtage, M.E., Taylor, P.M., et al. (1985) Thoracic esophageal foreign bodies in the dog: a review of ninety cases. *J Small Anim Pract* 26, 521-536.

Juvet, F., Pinilla, M., Shiel, R.E., et al. (2010) Oesophageal foreign bodies in dogs: factors affecting success of endoscopic retrieval. *Irish Vet J* 63, 163-168.

Keir, I., Woolford, L., Hirst, C., et al. (2010) Fatal aortic oesophageal fistula following oesophageal foreign body removal in a dog. *J Small Anim Pract* 51, 657-660.

Knight, G.C. (1963) Transthoracic esophagotomy in dogs: a survey of 75 operations. *Vet Rec* 75, 264-266.

Lieb, M.S., Sartor, L.L. (2008) Esophageal foreign body obstruction caused by a dental chew treat in 31 dogs (2000-2006). *J Am Vet Med Assoc* 232, 1021-1025.

Lieb, M.S., Dinnel, H., Ward, D.L., et al. (2001) Endoscopic balloon dilation of benign esophageal strictures in dogs and cats. *J Vet Intern Med* 15, 547-552.

Melendez, L.D., Twedt, D.C., Weyrauch, E.A., et al. (1998) Conservative therapy using balloon dilation for intramural inflammatory esophageal strictures in dogs and cats: a retrospective study of 23 cases (1987-1997). *Eur J Compar Gastroenterol* 3, 31-36.

Nawrocki, M.A., Mackin, A.J., McLaughlin, R., et al. (2003) Fluoroscopic and endoscopic localization of an esophagobronchial fistula in a dog. *J Am Anim Hosp Assoc* 39, 257-261.

Pearson, H., Gibbs, C., Kelly, D.F. (1978) Oesophageal diverticulum formation in the dog. *J Small Anim Pract* 19, 341-355.

Ranen, E., Shamir, M.H., Shahar, R., et al. (2004) Partial esophagectomy with single layer closure for the treatment of esophageal sarcomas in 6 dogs. *Vet Surg* 33, 428-434.

Rousseau, A., Prittie, J., Broussard, J.D., et al. (2007) Incidence and characterization of esophagitis following esophageal foreign body removal in dogs: 60 cases (1999-2003). *J Vet Emerg Crit Care* 17, 159-163.

Ryan, W.W., Greene, R.W. (1975) The conservative management of esophageal foreign bodies and their complications: a review of 66 cases in dogs and cats. *J Am Anim Hosp Assoc* 11, 243-249.

Sale, C.S.H., Williams, J.M. (2006) Results of transthoracic esophagotomy retrieval of esophageal foreign body obstruction in dogs: 14 cases (2000-2004). *J Am Anim Hosp Assoc* 42, 450-456.

Spielman, B.L., Shake, E.H., Garvey, M.S. (1992) Esophageal foreign body in dogs: a retrospective study of 23 cases. *J Am Anim Hosp Assoc* 28, 570-574.

44 Aortic Arch Anomalies

Robert J. Hardie

The University of Wisconsin, School of Veterinary Medicine, Department of Surgical Sciences, Madison, WI, USA

Aortic arch anomalies are developmental abnormalities of the embryonic vessels, including the dorsal and ventral aortas and the six aortic arches. As they develop, the anomalous vessel(s) partially or completely encircle the esophagus and trachea, resulting in various degrees of compression at the level of the heart base.

The various aortic arch anomalies include persistent right aortic arch (PRAA) with a left ligamentum arteriosum, PRAA with left ligamentum arteriosum and aberrant left subclavian artery, PRAA with right ligamentum arteriosum but aberrant left subclavian artery, double aortic arch, left aortic arch with aberrant right subclavian artery, and left aortic arch with persistent right ligamentum arteriosum. PRAA with a "normal" left ligamentum arteriosum is the most common aortic arch anomaly, making up 95% of the cases in dogs.

Breeds of dogs that are overrepresented or are known or suspected to have a genetic predisposition include German shepherds, Irish setters, greyhounds, and German Pinschers (Shires and Liu 1981; Muldoon et al. 1997; Gunby et al. 2004; Philips et al. 2011). Breeds of cats that are overrepresented include Persians and Siamese. Clinical signs result from compression of the esophagus, leading to progressive dilation or megaesophagus, chronic regurgitation, weight loss, poor growth, and aspiration pneumonia. Signs typically develop at the time of weaning onto solid food. Presumptive diagnosis is generally based on a combination of signalment, history, physical examination findings, survey thoracic radiography, and contrast esophagography (Figure 44.1). Treatment involves surgical ligation and transection of the anomalous vessel to relieve compression of the esophagus via thoracotomy or thoracoscopic approach (Figure 44.2).

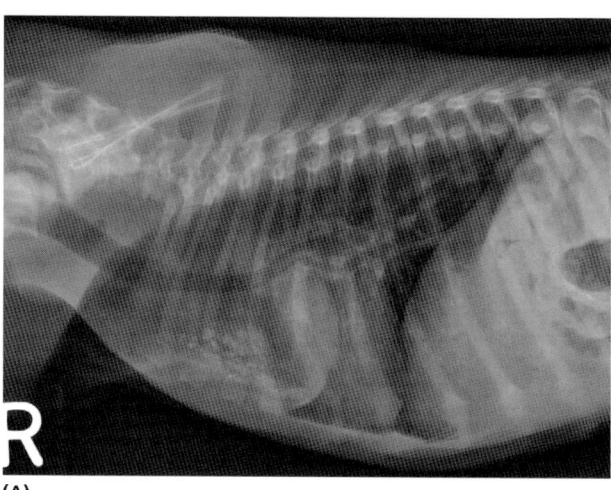

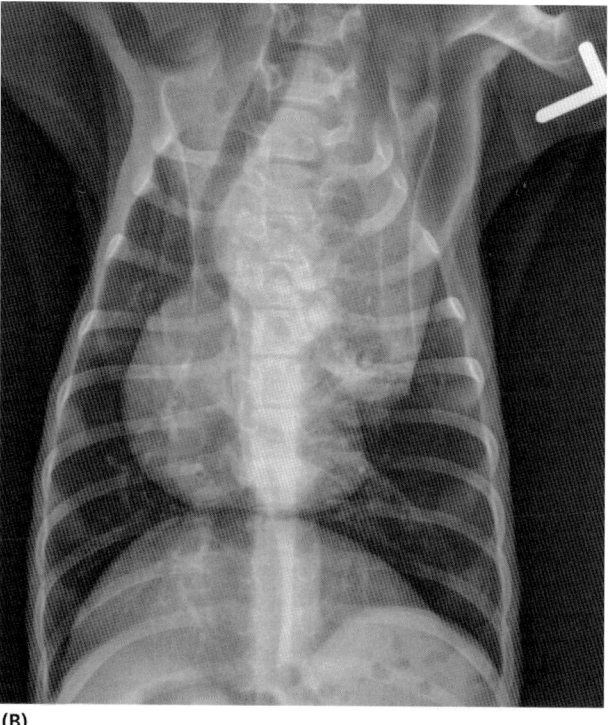

(A) (B)

Figure 44.1 Lateral (**A**) and ventrodorsal (**B**) survey thoracic radiographs demonstrating dilation of the esophagus cranial to the heart base consistent with an aortic arch anomaly. Note the ingesta of mineral opacity within the ventral portion of the esophagus on the lateral view.

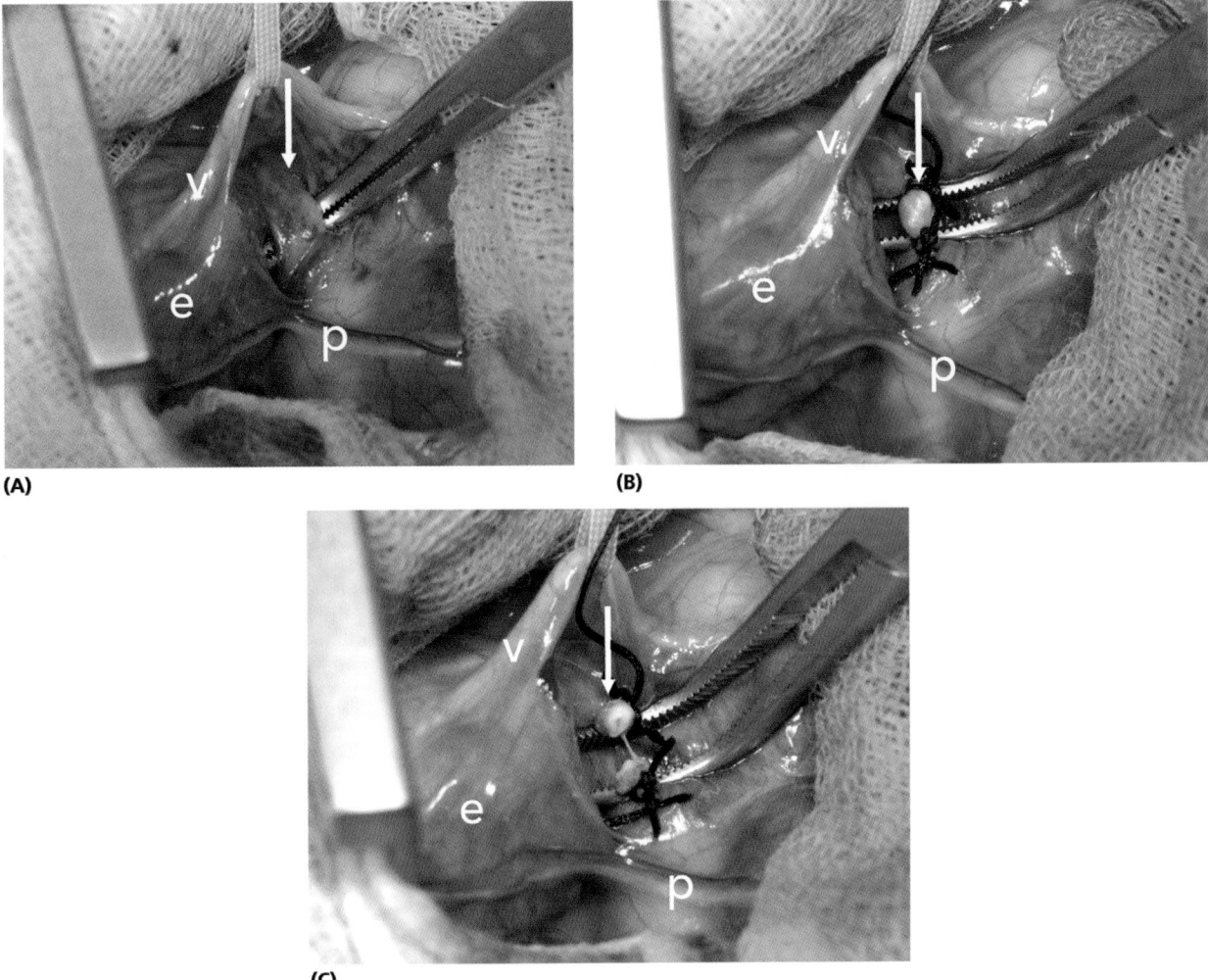

(A)

(B)

(C)

Figure 44.2 Intraoperative photographs demonstrating dissection (**A**) ligation (**B**) and transection (**C**) of the ligamentum arteriosum in a dog with a persistent right aortic arch. Note the white arrow pointing to the ligamentum arteriosum and the esophagus (e), phrenic nerve (p), and vagus nerve (v). *Source:* A. Hamaide, University of Liège, Liège, Belgium, 2014. Reproduced with permission from A. Hamaide.

Complications associated with surgical treatment of aortic arch anomalies appear rare but include those related to the thoracic approach such as hemorrhage, infection, seroma, and problems with thoracostomy tubes (Tattersall and Welsh 2006), as well as those associated with the actual dissection, ligation, and transection of the anomalous vessel, including esophageal perforation; injury to the vagus, phrenic, or recurrent laryngeal nerves; injury to the thoracic duct; or left ventricular hypertension (Ricardo *et al.* 2001; Vianna and Krahwinkel 2004). More important however, are the complications associated with persistent megaesophagus despite correction of the aortic arch anomaly, including regurgitation, weight loss, and aspiration pneumonia.

The short-term prognosis for surgical correction of an aortic arch anomaly is determined by the general health of the individual animal and the degree of dehydration, aspiration pneumonia, or debilitation present at the time of surgery. The long-term prognosis is determined by the degree of improvement in regurgitation and thus the ability to maintain body condition and avoid aspiration pneumonia in the future.

Hemorrhage

See Chapter 12.

Infection

See Chapters 1 and 37.

Aspiration pneumonia

See Chapter 25.

Megaesophagus

Definition

Megaesophagus is local or generalized dilation of the esophagus caused by either structural or functional disease. Megaesophagus caused by aortic arch anomalies occurs as a localized dilation of the cranial thoracic portion of the esophagus because of compression at the level of the heart base. Chronic obstruction leads to progressive esophageal dilation and subsequent disruption of normal peristaltic activity.

Risk factors

- Delayed diagnosis and treatment
- Failure to completely relieve esophageal compression after surgical ligation and transection of the anomalous vessel

Diagnosis

- Survey thoracic radiography
- Contrast esophagography (Figure 44.3)
- Endoscopy may be useful for assessing the condition of the esophageal lumen and aid in determining the presence of either a right or left aortic arch anomaly by detecting arterial pulsation through the wall of the esophagus

Treatment

Treatment involves surgical ligation and transection of the aortic arch anomaly as early as possible after diagnosis to potentially minimize further dilation of the esophagus. After transection of the anomalous vessel, the esophagus should be examined carefully and any remaining fibrous tissue or constrictive bands removed. In addition, passage of an appropriately sized balloon catheter or feeding tube past the affected portion of the esophagus is helpful for confirming that compression has been completely relieved.

Outcome

Megaesophagus typically persists despite surgical correction of the aortic arch anomaly (Shires and Liu 1981). However, there are reports of significant improvement in the degree of megaesophagus and esophageal motility after surgery in dogs.

Prevention

- Early diagnosis and surgical treatment
- Use of gastrostomy tube feeding may potentially reduce the degree of megaesophagus by avoiding accumulation of food and fluid in the cranial esophagus

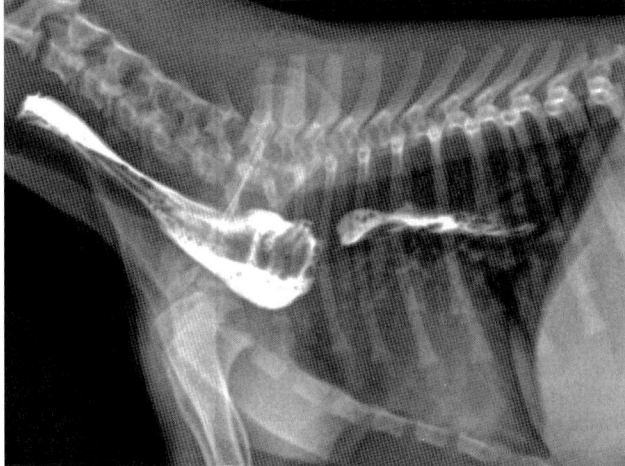

Figure 44.3 Lateral contrast esophagram demonstrating dilation of the cranial esophagus to the level of the heart base consistent with an aortic arch anomaly.

Regurgitation

Definition

Regurgitation is the expulsion or "bringing up" of undigested food from the esophagus generally caused by an obstruction, stricture, or a focal or generalized motility disorder that prevents or delays passage of food into the stomach. Regurgitation is a passive or spontaneous event, different from vomiting, which typically involves active contraction of the abdominal muscles and expulsion of partially digested food and gastric fluid.

Risk factors

- Feeding hard or solid food
- Access to garbage or other sources of inappropriate food
- Feeding excessive amounts of food at one time

Diagnosis

- Direct observation of regurgitation episode
- Evidence of regurgitated undigested food in environment

Treatment

- Feed liquid or a soft food diet.
- Upright feeding or use of a "Bailey chair" to maintain standing posture while eating.
- Gastrostomy tube feeding

Outcome

- Progressive weight loss and poor growth
- Aspiration pneumonia and subsequent respiratory and systemic complications

Prevention

See the Treatment section earlier.

Relevant literature

Persistent right aortic arch is the most common aortic arch anomaly, and thus surgical planning based on that assumption is generally appropriate. However, in one report, 44% of dogs with PRAA had a second anomalous vessel, causing additional compression of the esophagus, so it is important to have a thorough understanding of the anatomy of the various aortic arch anomalies to be able to recognize and potentially treat any anomalous vessel encountered in surgery that might not have been detected preoperatively (Buchanan 2004; Du Plessis *et al.* 2006).

Survey radiographs can be useful for differentiating PRAA from other aortic arch anomalies in dogs. For dogs with PRAA, thoracic radiographs typically reveal left-sided deviation of the trachea cranial to the heart base on the ventrodorsal or dorsoventral view, and in most cases, ventral deviation of the trachea cranial to the heart base on the lateral view (Buchanan 2004). However, if the diagnosis of PRAA is not supported with routine radiography or contrast esophagography, additional diagnostic imaging such as endoscopy, echocardiography, selective angiography, fluoroscopy, thoracoscopy, computed tomography, or magnetic resonance imaging should be considered (Fingeroth and Fossum 1987; Komtebedde *et al.* 1991; Pownder and Scrivani 2008; Henjes *et al.* 2011).

Before surgical correction of an aortic arch anomaly, animals that are significantly underweight or debilitated should be stabilized to minimize perioperative complications. Dehydration and aspiration pneumonia should be treated with intravenous fluids and systemic antibiotics. Also, placement of a gastrostomy tube to provide more consistent nutritional support may be beneficial in some animals (Loughin and Marino 2008).

Currently, there are no clear risk factors for predicting the outcome in dogs with PRAA, and although it seems intuitive that early intervention would improve prognosis, the correlation between the precise timing of surgery and the degree of improvement in esophageal function appears weak.

From various case reports and retrospective studies, it is known that esophageal dilation and motility can improve significantly in dogs treated early (<6 months) (Muldoon et al. 1997; Vianna and Krahwinkel 2004; Christiansen et al. 2007; Moonan et al. 2007). There are also reports of older dogs (>2 years) having positive outcomes despite long-standing esophageal obstruction and dilation (Fingeroth and Fossum 1987; Muldoon et al. 1997; Buchanan 2004; Loughin and Marino 2008). In contrast, there are also reports of persistent regurgitation and little or no improvement in megaesophagus despite early diagnosis and surgical correction (Shires and Liu 1981). In addition, other reasons for lack of improvement in regurgitation despite "successful" correction of a PRAA include failure to thoroughly dissect remaining fibrous bands constricting the esophagus after ligation and transection of the ligamentum arteriosum or failure to recognize and treat a second anomalous vessel such as an aberrant left subclavian artery causing residual compression of the esophagus (Buchanan 2004).

Overall, it appears that most dogs with PRAA are improved after surgery, and the goal of surgery should be to reduce the frequency of regurgitation and potentially allow for a more normal diet and feeding schedule despite the likelihood of persistent megaesophagus. In a retrospective study of 47 dogs that underwent surgery for PRAA, long-term (>6 month) follow-up was available for 25. Of those 25 dogs, 23 (92%) had an excellent outcome, and 2 (8%) had a good outcome based on the owner's perception of improvement in the frequency of regurgitation (Muldoon et al. 1997).

Surgical treatment for other aortic arch anomalies, including double aortic arch (Aultman et al. 1980; Ricardo et al. 2001; Vianna and Krahwinkel 2004; Moonan et al. 2007), left aortic arch with patent right ductus arteriosus (Holt et al. 2000), left aortic arch with right ligamentum arteriosum (Hurley et al. 1993), left aortic arch with aberrant right subclavian artery (Yoon and Jeong 2011), PRAA with left ligamentum arteriosum and aberrant left subclavian artery (House et al. 2005; Kim et al. 2006; Menzel and Distl 2011), PRAA with left patent ductus arteriosus and aberrant left subclavian artery (Christiansen et al. 2007) have been described. These anomalies are obviously much less common than PRAA, and therefore it is difficult to make a general statement about prognosis, but successful outcomes have been described in these individual reports.

Surgical treatment for double aortic arch anomalies can be particularly challenging and requires determining the symmetry (patency) of the two aortic branches, which branch should be preserved, and whether there will be any significant hemodynamic consequences (left ventricular hypertension) after ligation of a patent branch. There are several reports of both successful (Vianna and Krahwinkel 2004; Moonan et al. 2007) and unsuccessful (Aultman et al. 1980; Ricardo et al. 2001) surgical correction of double aortic arch anomalies in dogs, and in these cases, the decision as to which arch to ligate was based on intraoperative visual assessment of the size of the vessels and temporarily occluding each branch while simultaneously assessing femoral pulses. In one dog that died immediately after surgical ligation of the arch with the

"lowest pressure" (left arch), acute left ventricular hypertension was suspected as the cause of death (Ricardo et al. 2001).

A minimally invasive thoracoscopic approach for the successful surgical correction of PRAA in dogs has also been described (Isakow et al. 2000; MacPhail et al. 2001). The procedure was performed with the dog in right lateral recumbency with thoracic cannulas placed in various left intercostal spaces. Selective ventilation of the right lung (left bronchial blockade) was performed in one dog to aid visualization of the esophagus and ligamentum arteriosum. Advantages of this approach compared with conventional intercostal thoracotomy include reduced tissue trauma, reduced postoperative pain, improved visualization of the surgical field because of magnification provided by the scope, and improved body temperature regulation by avoiding opening the thoracic cavity.

References

Aultman, S.H., Chambers, J.N., Verstre, W.A. (1980) Double aortic arch and persistent right aortic arch in two littermates: surgical treatment. *Journal of the American Animal Hospital Association* 16, 533-536.

Buchanan, J.W. (2004) Tracheal signs and associated vascular anomalies in dogs with persistent right aortic arch. *Journal of Veterinary Internal Medicine* 18, 510-514.

Christiansen, K.J., Snyder, D., Buchanan, J.W., et al. (2007) Multiple vascular anomalies in a regurgitating German shepherd puppy. *Journal of Small Animal Practice* 48, 32-35.

Du Plessis, C.J., Keller, N., Joubert, K.E. (2006) Symmetrical double aortic arch in a beagle puppy. *Journal of Small Animal Practice* 47, 31-34.

Fingeroth, J.M., Fossum, T.W. (1987) Late-onset regurgitation associated with persistent right aortic arch in two dogs. *Journal of the American Veterinary Medical Association* 191, 981-983.

Gunby, J.M., Hardie, R.J., Bjorling, D.E. (2004) Investigation of the potential heritability of persistent right aortic arch in greyhounds. *Journal of the American Veterinary Medical Association* 224, 1120-1122.

Henjes, C.R., Nolte, I., Wefstaedt, P. (2011) Multidetector-row computed tomography of thoracic aortic anomalies in dogs and cats: patent ductus arteriosus and vascular rings. *BMC Veterinary Research* 7, 57.

Holt, D., Heldmann, E., Michel, K., et al. (2000) Esophageal obstruction caused by a left aortic arch and an anomalous right patent ductus arteriosus in two German shepherd littermates. *Veterinary Surgery* 29, 264-270.

House, A.K., Summerfield, N.J., German, A.J., et al. (2005) Unusual vascular ring anomaly associated with a persistent right aortic arch in two dogs. *Journal of Small Animal Practice* 46, 585-590.

Hurley, K., Miller, M.W., Willard, M.D., et al. (1993) Left aortic arch and right ligamentum arteriosum causing esophageal obstruction in a dog. *Journal of the American Veterinary Medical Association* 203, 410-412.

Isakow, K., Fowler, D., Walsh, P. (2000) Video-assisted thoracoscopic division of the ligamentum arteriosum in two dogs with persistent right aortic arch. *Journal of the American Veterinary Medical Association* 217, 1333-1336.

Kim, N.S., Alam, M.R., Choi, I.H. (2006) Persistent right aortic arch and aberrant left subclavian artery in a dog: a case report. *Veterinarni Medicina* 51, 156-160.

Komtebedde, J., Koblik, P., Mattoon, J., et al. (1991) Preoperative and postoperative fluoroscopy in dogs with persistent right aortic arch. *Veterinary Surgery* 20, 340.

Loughin, C.A., Marino D.J. (2008) Delayed primary surgical treatment in a dog with persistent right aortic arch. *Journal of the American Animal Hospital Association* 44, 258-261.

MacPhail, C.M., Monnet, E., Twedt, D.C. (2001) Thoracoscopic correction of persistent right aortic arch in a dog. *Journal of the American Animal Hospital Association* 37, 577-581.

Menzel, J., Distl, O. (2011) Unusual vascular ring anomaly associated with a persistent right aortic arch and aberrant left subclavian artery in German pinschers. *Veterinary Journal* 187, 352-355.

Moonan, N., Mootoo, N.F.A., Mahler, S. P. (2007) Double aortic arch with a hypoplastic left arch and patent ductus arteriosus in a dog. *Journal of Veterinary Cardiology* 9, 59-61.

Muldoon, M.M., Birchard, S.J., Ellison, G.W. (1997) Long-term results of surgical correction of persistent right aortic arch in dogs: 25 cases (1980-1995). *Journal of the American Veterinary Medical Association* 210, 1761-1763.

Philips, U., Menzel, J., Distl, O. (2011) A rare form of persistent right aorta arch in linkage disequilibrium with the DiGeorge critical region on CFA26 in German Pinschers. *Journal of Heredity* 51, 568-573.

Pownder, S., Scrivani, P.V. (2008) Non-selective computed tomography angiography of a vascular ring anomaly in a dog. *Journal of Veterinary Cardiology* 10, 125-128.

Ricardo, C., Augusto, A., Canavese, A., et al. (2001) Double aortic arch in a dog (Canis familiaris): a case report. *Anatomia Histologia Embryologia* 30, 379-381.

Shires, P.K., Liu, W. (1981) Persistent right aortic arch in dogs: a long-term follow-up after surgical correction. *Journal of the American Animal Hospital Association,* 17, 773-776.

Tattersall, J.A., Welsh, E. (2006) Factors influencing the short-term outcome following thoracic surgery in 98 dogs. *Journal of Small Animal Practice* 47, 715-720.

Vianna, M.L., Krahwinkel, D.J. (2004) Double aortic arch in a dog. *Journal of the American Veterinary Medical Association* 225, 1222-1224.

Yoon, H.Y., Jeong, S.W. (2011) Surgical correction of an aberrant right subclavian artery in a dog. *Canadian Veterinary Journal* 52, 1115-1118.

45 Thymectomy

Rachel Burrow

Small Animal Teaching Hospital, University of Liverpool, Leahurst, Neston, Wirral, UK

The commonest indication for thymectomy in cats and dogs is in the treatment of thymoma, and less commonly, other thymic neoplasia. Thymomas are uncommon tumors, classified according to their clinical behavior: whereas benign or noninvasive thymomas are encapsulated and do not invade local tissues, malignant or invasive thymomas invade adjacent mediastinal tissues. The indications for performing thymectomy to treat non-neoplastic thymic disease are few. Thymic and thymic branchial cysts have been reported, usually as incidental findings (Zekas and Adams 2002), although they may cause clinical signs associated with cranial vena cava syndrome or pleural effusion if they become large (Liu et al. 1983) or undergo metastatic transformation to carcinoma (Levien et al. 2010). Other potential causes of a thymic mass include thymic abscesses, hyperplasia, or granulomas (Fossum 2007).

There are many case reports of thymectomy to treat neoplastic thymic disease, mostly thymomas, describing management and surgical treatment in cats and dogs (Bellah et al. 1983; Atwater et al. 1994; Zitz et al. 2008), as well as a small case series of thymic branchial cysts of which seven dogs received surgical treatment (Liu et al. 1983). Thymic conditions are uncommon, however, and these retrospective studies of thymectomy present data from a relatively small number of cases collected over many years. A variety of paraneoplastic syndromes have been reported in several case series reviewing thymoma in dogs and cats (Table 45.1). Myasthenia gravis (MG) and megaesophagus are most commonly reported (Bellah et al. 1983; Aronsohn et al. 1984; Klebanow 1992; Atwater et al. 1994; Gores et al. 1994; Smith et al. 2001; Zitz et al. 2008). These are of particular importance because they may increase the risk of complications during anesthesia and influence recovery, surgery, and long-term outcome. Acquired MG has also been diagnosed in association with thymic carcinoma (Stenner et al. 2003) and non-neoplastic disease of the thymus (Malik et al. 1997).

Thymectomy is typically performed via a left intercostal thoracotomy or median sternotomy; the approach is selected to achieve adequate access to the thymus or thymic mass and cranial mediastinum (Bellah and Smith 2003). If intercostal thoracotomy is the chosen approach and inadequate access is achieved, rib resection may be performed (Martin et al. 1986). A thoracoscopic approach has also been described (Mayhew and Friedberg 2008). The potential complications associated with intercostal thoracotomy, median sternotomy, and postoperative thoracostomy tubes are discussed in Chapters 38 and 39.

Table 45.1 Paraneoplastic syndromes identified in case series reporting cats and dogs with thymoma

	Bellah et al. (1983)		Aronsohn et al. (1984)		Atwater et al. (1994)		Gores et al. (1994)		Smith et. al. (2001)		Zitz et al. (2008)	
	Cats	Dogs	Cats	Dogs	Cats	Dogs	Cats	Dogs	Cats	Dogs	Cats	Dogs
Patients (n)	0	22	0	15	0	23	12	0	7	17	9	11†
Paraneoplastic syndrome												
Myasthenia gravis	0	4	0	7	0	7	2*	0	1	1*	1	0
Megaesophagus	0	1	0	0	0	11	0	0	1	3	0	0
Myositis	0	2	0	3	0	0	0	0	0	0	0	0
Hypercalcemia	0	0	0	0	0	2	0	0	0	1	0	1
Arrhythmia	0	0	0	0	0	3	0	0	0	0	0	0
Nonthymic neoplasia	0	7	0	5	0	5	0	0	2	2	0	0
Hyperglobulinemia	0	0	0	0	0	0	0	0	0	2	0	0

*Clinical signs of myasthenia gravis developed at 10 days or longer after surgery.
†Zitz et al. (2008) reported dysphonia in four dogs and regurgitation in two dogs before thymectomy, but these signs were not attributed to a paraneoplastic syndrome.

Intraoperative and early postoperative mortality

Definition

Intraoperative mortality is defined as patient death within the episode of anesthesia induced to achieve thymectomy. The definition of early postoperative mortality varies between clinicians and is usually considered to be death within the 24 hours after completion of surgery and recovery from anesthesia, but it may be considered to be patient death occurring up to 7 days postoperatively.

Risk factors

The commonest causes of death during thymectomy and within 24 hours of surgery include euthanasia, cardiac arrest, and respiratory arrest. The commonest causes of death in the period of 1 to 7 days after surgery are respiratory complications secondary to regurgitation and the development of aspiration pneumonitis or pneumonia.
- Invasive tumor
  - Invasive tumors are considered inoperable, leading to intraoperative euthanasia.
  - Challenging surgery with greater risk of intraoperative hemorrhage and longer surgical and anesthesia times, thus greater risk of complications
  - Risk of thromboembolism, tumor embolism, or air embolism if venotomy or resection and replacement of the cranial vena cava is performed to manage tumor invasion of the cranial vena cava
- Cardiac arrest
  - Increased risk if there is intra- or postoperative hemorrhage, hypoxia, hypotension, other end-stage organ disease, thromboembolism, sepsis, arrhythmia, or cardiac disease
- Respiratory compromise
  - MG
    - Preexisting aspiration pneumonitis or pneumonia or development secondary to intra- or postoperative regurgitation
    - Preexisting weakness of the respiratory muscles. This will be compounded by anesthetic agents, particularly if using neuromuscular blocking agents.
    - Postoperative development of acute fulminating MG
  - Damage to phrenic nerve(s) (see Chapter 37)
  - Damage to recurrent laryngeal nerve(s) (see later discussion)
  - Thromboembolism
  - Poorly controlled postoperative pain
- Concurrent unrelated disease: Thymoma is more common in older patients.

Prevention

- Perform a thorough preoperative assessment of the patient to identify paraneoplastic syndromes or concurrent disease.
- Ensure preoperative treatment or stabilization of paraneoplastic disease or concurrent disease.
  - Perform advanced imaging of the thorax to give more detailed anatomical information about the tumor and allow appropriate planning for potential venotomy or resection and replacement of the cranial vena cava. Although advanced imaging is likely to play a greater part in preoperative assessment regarding tumor resectability with advancements in imaging technology, accurate assessment of resectability of the tumor has remained an intraoperative decision to date.

- If a thymic tumor is considered likely to be inoperable based on preoperative imaging, consider whether medical management or radiotherapy could be a suitable alternative option.
- Perform preoperative blood typing, ensure availability of blood products or alternatives, and perform cross-matching in case of serious intra- or early postoperative hemorrhage.
- Perform meticulous hemostasis throughout surgery and monitor blood loss by measuring that removed by suction and weighing used surgical swabs.
- If third-degree atrioventricular (AV) block (uncommon but can accompany MG) is diagnosed preoperatively, ensure that the facilities are available to perform transvenous pacing if required.
- Perform detailed patient monitoring during anesthesia, especially if neuromuscular junction blockade is used.
- Perform quantitative assessment of neuromuscular function or consider administration of anticholinesterase drugs at completion of surgery.
- Ideally, have facilities or available staffing to ventilate the patient in the event of postoperative respiratory compromise.
- Ensure that postoperative pain is well controlled.

Hemorrhage (see Chapter 12)

Acquired myasthenia gravis

Definition

Acquired myasthenia gravis is failure of neuromuscular transmission at the level of the acetylcholine (Ach) receptor on the muscle membrane. The commonest form of MG is acquired, associated with autoantibody production against the Ach receptors at the postsynaptic membrane, causing inefficient neuromuscular transmission (Inzana 2004). The initiation of autoimmunity remains unclear, but the thymus appears to play a role, and acquired MG is occasionally recognized as a paraneoplastic syndrome occurring secondary to thymoma in cats and dogs. The main concerns associated with MG are the potential risks for megaesophagus and regurgitation, which increase the risk of aspiration pneumonia, and the presence of muscle weakness, which may result in respiratory failure in recovery.

Risk factors

- Thymoma and other thymic disease

Diagnosis

- "Gold standard": demonstration of serum autoantibodies against muscle Ach receptors by radioimmunoassay (Shelton 2009)
- Recognition of clinical signs of focal or generalized neuromuscular weakness; this depends on the specific muscle involvement (Table 45.2)
- Other supportive diagnostic information includes radiographic evidence of megaesophagus or aspiration pneumonia, abnormal fluoroscopic barium swallow study findings, a positive edrophonium or neostigmine test result, and a decrease in the amplitude of the compound muscle action potential in response to repetitive nerve stimulation.

Treatment

- Surgical treatment: removal of underlying cause via thymectomy
- Medical management of MG (Box 45.1)

Table 45.2 Clinical signs of myasthenia gravis associated with muscle weakness, according to muscle group(s) affected

Affected muscle group	Potential associated signs
Limb muscles	• Reluctance or inability to exercise, lethargy, collapse • Stiff thoracic limb gait • Wide-based pelvic stance • Apparent slight protrusion of scapulae when weight bearing (especially cats)
Facial muscles	• Decreased blinking, dropped jaw
Laryngeal muscles	• Dysphonia, laryngeal stridor on stress or exertion
Pharyngeal muscles	• Dysphagia, salivation
Intercostals/diaphragm	• Hypoventilation, respiratory distress
Neck muscles	• Ventroflexion of neck • Eyes positioned dorsally to maintain straight ahead gaze (especially cats)
Esophageal muscle	• Regurgitation

• Treatment of aspiration pneumonia
  ○ Broad-spectrum antibacterial medication ideally chosen on basis of tracheal wash and bacterial culture; avoid antibacterial drugs that may affect the neuromuscular junction
  ○ Oxygen supplementation
  ○ Ventilatory support if severe respiratory distress and respiratory failure is considered a likely complication
  ○ Nebulization

Box 45.1 Medications which have been used in the management of myasthenia gravis in dogs and cats

---

Anticholinesterase agents

• Pyridostigmine, neostigmine
  ○ Usually used as first-line treatment
  ○ Prolong action of Ach at the neuromuscular junction and enhance neuromuscular transmission
  ○ It has been suggested that dogs respond better to anticholinesterase therapy than cats

Immunosuppressive agents

• Corticosteroids
  ○ Can cause initial weakness; a low initial dose is recommended with a gradual increase in dose depending on response
  ○ Can exacerbate regurgitation in dogs with megaesophagus by causing dysphasia and polydipsia and thus increasing the risk of aspiration pneumonia
• Azathioprine
  ○ Can be used if steroids cause worsening of signs or have unacceptable side effects
  ○ Can also be used in combination with steroids if necessary
• Mycophenolate
  ○ Has also been used to treat acquired MG
  ○ A recent study by Dewey et al. (2010) did not support the use of this drug
• Cyclosporine
  ○ Bexfield et al. (2006) reported improvement when used in two dogs with acquired MG, but further study is necessary
• Immunosuppressive drugs can be used to reduce autoantibody production
  ○ Used alone or in combination with anticholinesterase drugs
  ○ The propensity for patients with MG to develop aspiration pneumonia is of concern when using immunosuppressive agents
  ○ Contraindicated in the presence of aspiration pneumonia

Ach, acetylcholine; MG, myasthenia gravis.

• Management of regurgitation and esophagitis
  ○ Intravenous fluid therapy
  ○ Alter feeding regimens (postural feeding, elevation of food and water bowls).
  ○ Consider placement of a gastrostomy tube to facilitate adequate hydration, nutrition, and drug delivery if the patient has severe regurgitation.
  ○ Administer H2 antagonists, proton pump inhibitors, or intestinal mucosal protectants if necessary.

Outcome

A more guarded prognosis is given for cats and dogs with thymoma-associated megaesophagus or MG because of their increased risk of developing respiratory difficulties associated with muscle weakness and aspiration pneumonia secondary to regurgitation in the early and later postoperative periods. The progression of MG is variable and unpredictable; megaesophagus and MG may improve or resolve after thymectomy in some patients, but in others, it may remain unaltered or deteriorate. In addition, MG may actually develop months after surgery in some patients in which it was not evident preoperatively.

Prevention

Consider measuring Ach receptor autoantibodies before general anesthesia and thymectomy to aid identification of those patients without signs of MG that may be at risk of developing MG related respiratory muscle weakness or megaesophagus in the early postoperative period, exacerbated by the stress of anesthesia and surgery.

Metastasis or residual tumor

Definition

Metastasis is dissemination of neoplastic cells to distant secondary sites. Recurrence is gross tumor formation at site of the original tumor, where the original tumor had previously been grossly or microscopically eliminated by treatment.

Risk factors
For metastasis
• Invasive (malignant) tumor?
• Chronicity of thymoma?

For recurrence
• Incomplete resection
  ○ Intimate involvement of tumor with vital structures in the cranial mediastinum such that the surgeon chooses to perform a debulking procedure only
  ○ Invasive, nonencapsulated tumor
• Long-term survival after original surgery? (suggested rather than proven)

Diagnosis
• Computed tomography (CT) scan of thorax +/- abdomen (most sensitive)
• Thoracic radiography (two or three view, inflated)
• Thoracic ultrasonography may be helpful in some cases.
• Abdominal ultrasonography may be helpful in some cases.
• Fine-needle aspirate (or biopsy) and cytologic (or histopathologic) examination of enlarged lymph nodes or suspected metastatic lesion if accessible or appropriate

Treatment

Metastases: palliation of any associated signs

Recurrent disease: surgical (median sternotomy or intercostal thoracotomy and tumor excision)

Practical Tip 45.1

It has been suggested that surgeons performing second surgeries to remove recurrent disease should chose a different surgical approach from the original approach to avoid scar tissue and adhesions that may be present after initial surgery. The approach that is chosen should be that which will allow the best access to the thymic mass with minimal complications, although the above suggestion is also worthy of consideration.

Outcome

Survival of years is possible after second (and third) surgery to remove recurrent noninvasive thymoma.

Hypercalcemia and hypocalcemia

Definition

Hypercalcemia and hypocalcemia are elevation or reduction, respectively, of serum calcium levels beyond the normal reference range. Hypercalcemia occurs uncommonly in association with thymoma in dogs and results from production of a hypercalcemic agent or by production of parathyroid hormone–related protein (PTHrp) by the tumor. Hypocalcemia can occur when the source of PTHrp is removed abruptly before the parathyroid glands, which have received negative feedback from the hypercalcemia, become active and produce parathyroid hormone again.

Risk factors

For hypercalcemia

- Production of a hypercalcemic agent PTHrp by the thymic tumor
- Unrelated causes of hypercalcemia

For hypocalcemia

These are not established for thymectomy of a hypercalcemic patient because this complication is rare but are likely to be as for surgical treatment of other hypercalcemic conditions (e.g., parathyroid adenoma); risk increases with increasing severity and duration of hypercalcemia.

Diagnosis

- Preoperative hypercalcemia: patient demonstrates clinical signs (Table 45.3)

Table 45.3 Clinical signs associated with hypercalcemia

Common	Uncommon
Polyuria	Constipation
Polydipsia	Calcium urolithiasis
Anorexia	Cardiac arrhythmias
Dehydration	Seizures or twitching
Lethargy	Death
Vomiting	
Inappetence	
Weakness	

Table 45.4 Clinical signs associated with hypocalcemia*

Common	Occasional	Uncommon
Muscle tremors	Panting	Polyuria
Rubbing face	Lethargy	Polydipsia
Stiff gait	Anorexia	Hypotension
Altered behavior (restless, hypersensitive, excitable)	Pyrexia	Respiratory arrest
	Prolapsed of nictitans membrane (cats)	Death

*Some of these signs are also common to myasthenia gravis.

- Postoperative hypocalcemia: patient demonstrates clinical signs (Table 45.4)
- Hyper- or hypocalcemia is confirmed by **measuring serum ionized calcium levels**.

Treatment

Preoperative medical treatment of hypercalcemia is indicated if the patient is dehydrated or azotemic or has cardiac arrhythmias, severe neurologic dysfunction, or weakness. However, some of these signs may be caused by other paraneoplastic effects (see earlier).

If hypercalcemia is considered to be contributing to a patient's clinical signs, it can be managed preoperatively as follows:
- Rehydrate the patient and diurese with 0.9% saline intravenous fluid therapy to replace fluid deficits and promote calcium excretion.
- Administer calcitonin.
- Administer furosemide to promote calcium excretion. (Only use this with caution in a patient that is hydrated and receiving supportive intravenous fluid therapy.)

Postoperative hypocalcemia is managed as for that occurring as a complication of thyroidectomy caused by inadvertent removal or devascularization of the parathyroid glands or after removal of functional parathyroid tumors (see Chapters 26 and 27).

Outcome

The presence of preoperative hypercalcemia or the development of postoperative hypercalcemia in dogs and cats undergoing thymectomy to treat thymoma has not been shown to be of prognostic significance in the few cases reported in the veterinary literature. Hypercalcemia generally resolves after thymectomy.

Neurologic complications

Definition

This is involvement of local nerves, either by neoplastic disease or damage during thymectomy. Neurologic injury may be reversible and recover with time.

The location of the recurrent laryngeal and phrenic nerves places them at risk of displacement, extension, or invasion by a thymic mass or damage during thymectomy. The latter can be accidental or inadvertent during resection of the thymic mass, or the nerve(s) may be intentionally resected en bloc with the tumor.

Risk factors

- Invasive tumor
- En-bloc resection of tumor with local nerve

Diagnosis

Phrenic nerve injury (see Chapter 37)

Laryngeal nerve injury (paresis or paralysis)

- Clinical signs
  - Dogs: inspiratory stridor +/- hyperthermia on stress, excitement and exertion, exercise intolerance, dysphonia, dysphagia
  - Cats: tachypnea, dyspnea, weight loss, dysphagia, coughing, lethargy, dysphonia

Unilateral laryngeal paresis or paralysis may not cause signs. If there are other factors causing respiratory compromise, however, unilateral laryngeal nerve injury may become clinically significant. Occasionally, these signs may occur preoperatively associated with idiopathic laryngeal paralysis as a result of MG-related laryngeal muscle dysfunction, or secondary to tumor invasion of the recurrent laryngeal nerves.

- Laryngoscopy with the patient under a light plane of anesthesia: absence of abduction of the arytenoid cartilages(s) at inspiration if laryngeal paralysis is present
- Ultrasonography of the larynx showing failure of arytenoid abduction on inspiration

Treatment

In cases of laryngeal paresis or unilateral paralysis and in patients in which it is considered that laryngeal dysfunction is likely to be temporary and will resolve with time, a respiratory crisis may be averted by cooling the patient, sedation, placing in a cool and calm environment, and giving supplemental oxygen with frequent reassessment.

In dyspneic patients, anesthesia should be induced and the patient intubated, with management options as follows:

- Conservative
  - Cooling the patient if hyperthermic
  - Administration of antiinflammatory drugs if laryngeal swelling or inflammation is present
  - Attempt to recover the patient in a calm and quiet environment

In some patients, particularly those with paresis or unilateral paralysis, this may be adequate. If laryngeal paralysis is bilateral, surgical intervention is often necessary.

- Surgical:
  - Arytenoid lateralization

If laryngeal paralysis is unilateral and the patient is showing clinical signs of laryngeal paralysis, surgery is performed on the paralyzed side of the larynx.

Unilateral surgery is usually adequate to alleviate respiratory distress with bilateral laryngeal paralysis.

After arytenoid lateralization, there is a lifetime risk of aspiration pneumonia, so if the patient has shown preexisting regurgitation, dysphagia, or megaesophagus, this surgical procedure is contraindicated.

  - Permanent tracheostomy (Practical Tip 45.2)
  - Other procedures, including partial arytenoidectomy and transverse cordotomy with cuneiform amputation, are reported for the treatment of laryngeal paralysis and could be considered;

Practical Tip 45.2

Permanent tracheostomy should be considered in patients that are dysphagic or have regurgitation or megaesophagus because a permanent tracheostomy provides a good airway and does not increase the risk of aspiration pneumonia.

---

however, insufficient data are available to recommend these techniques at present.

Outcome

Most studies report a good functional outcome in dogs undergoing an arytenoid lateralization procedure. Reported complication rates after arytenoid lateralization procedures are very variable, but approximately 20% dogs have aspiration pneumonia. Dogs and cats with concurrent dysphagia or megaesophagus are more likely to suffer postoperative morbidity and mortality because of aspiration pneumonia after arytenoid lateralization than patients without these abnormalities. Permanent tracheostomy in dogs is generally associated with a good outcome; there is a much greater risk of stomal occlusion in cats.

Relevant literature

The outcomes of thymectomy in cats and dogs reported in several case series are listed in Table 45.5. Resection of noninvasive thymomas in cats and dogs in the absence of paraneoplastic syndromes is associated with a good long-term outcome. Most morbidity and mortality occur during the operative and early postoperative period and is a result of surgical- or anesthesia-related complications or respiratory complications associated with MG or megaesophagus, regurgitation, and aspiration pneumonia.

The commonest reported causes of **intraoperative death and death within 24 hours of surgery** include euthanasia because the thymoma is considered nonresectable and cardiac and respiratory arrest (Robinson et al. 1974; Aronsohn et al. 1984; Zitz et al. 2008). Complications are most commonly reported for surgical management of invasive thymomas; however, intra- and early postoperative death are also reported for benign thymic tumors (Morini et al. 2009).

The prediction of vascular invasion by cranial mediastinal masses is limited by available imaging techniques. Scherrer et al. (2008) reported that nonangiographic contrast-enhanced CT was significantly less sensitive for detecting vascular invasion of cranial mediastinal masses than surgical evaluation. In this study of cranial mediastinal masses in 25 dogs and 1 cat, of which 16 were thymomas, intra- and early postoperative euthanasia and patient death from surgical- or disease-related problems was significantly higher in patients with vascular invasion. Further advancement of imaging technology is likely to improve the ability to detect vascular invasion, which will aid preoperative surgical planning.

Temporary partial or total occlusion of the cranial vena cava with venotomy, removal of tumor thrombus, and primary repair of the vascular wall has been performed for thymomas with vascular invasion. Hunt et al. (1997) attempted reconstruction of the vena cava using a polytetrafluoroethylene vascular prosthesis, which subsequently thrombosed. Holsworth et al. (2004) successfully replaced the cranial vena cava in a dog with an invasive thymoma and cranial vena cava syndrome using a jugular vein autograft. Experimentally, ligation of the cranial vena cava has resulted in the development of chylothorax (Blalock et al. 1936; Fossum and Birchard 1986), and surgeons should be aware of this potential complication if this vessel is ligated during thymectomy.

The causes of the intraoperative and early postoperative cardiac and respiratory arrests in cats and dogs undergoing thymectomy are unknown or not reported. The commonest non–anesthesia-related reasons for perioperative cardiac arrests in human patients undergoing non–cardiac-related surgery are intraoperative hemorrhage,

Table 45.5 Summary of outcomes of the larger case series of cats and dogs undergoing thymectomy

	Condition	Treatment	Cats	Dogs
Bellah *et al.* (1983)	Thymoma	Thymectomy		5 of 22 dogs presented with cranial vena caval syndrome; all died or were euthanized
				3 of 22 dogs had metastases
				6 of 22 dogs underwent surgery; 4 of 6 dogs survived surgery; 3 of 6 dogs were alive at 1 year; 2 of 6 dogs were alive several years later
Aronsohn *et al.* (1984)	Thymoma	Thymectomy	6 of 15 dogs underwent surgery	
			3 of 6 dogs underwent thymectomy; 1 of these dogs survived surgery but died 4 months after surgery with recurrent disease; 3 of 6 dogs underwent thymic biopsy only	
Gores *et al.* (1994)	Thymoma	Thymectomy	10 of 12 cats survived surgery; 6 of 10 cats were alive after follow up at 6–36 months (mean and median, 21 months); 4 of 10 cats died or were euthanized for unrelated disease at 18–56 months after thymectomy; no cat died or was euthanized as a result of a paraneoplastic syndrome; no cat developed local tumor recurrence or metastases	
Zitz *et al.* (2008)	Thymoma	Thymectomy	8 of 9 cats survived the immediate postoperative period	8 of 11 dogs survived the immediate postoperative period
			2 cats had a recurrence, and survived 3 and 5 years after a second surgery	1 dog had a recurrence and survived 4 years after a second surgery
			Median survival time in cats surviving the immediate postoperative period was 30 months	Median survival time in dogs surviving the immediate postoperative period was 18.5 months
Liu *et al.* (1984)	Thymic branchial cyst	Resection		7 dogs underwent surgery; 3 dogs survived and were clinically normal for 18–36 months.

hypotension, hypoxia, end-stage organ disease, thromboembolic disease, sepsis, and cardiac disease (Jian-xiong *et al.* 2011). It is likely that the reasons are similar in veterinary patients undergoing thymectomy. For cats and dogs with invasive thymomas that survive the early postoperative period, the long-term outcome is good (Zitz *et al.* 2008).

Cardiac arrhythmias, notably third-degree AV block, have been reported in dogs with MG. Third-degree AV block was reported in three dogs with thymoma and megaesophagus by Atwater *et al.* (1994) and in two dogs with thymoma and MG by Hackett *et al.* (1995). AV block was present in three of these dogs at the time of diagnosis, and two dogs developed AV block several months after thymectomy. Although third-degree AV block can be fatal, it has not been reported as a cause of death in dogs with thymoma.

Hemorrhage in the early postoperative period is a well-recognized problem. Gores *et al.* (1994) reported postoperative intrathoracic hemorrhage as the most common complication in 12 cats undergoing thymectomy to treat thymoma; 1 cat died within 3 days of surgery because of persistent intrathoracic hemorrhage, and a further 3 cats required blood transfusions and survived. Similarly, Zitz *et al.* (2008) reported that 6 of 20 cases required blood transfusions after thymectomy.

The other commonest cause of **death in the period of 1 to 7 days after surgery** is respiratory complications, usually secondary to megaesophagus, regurgitation and the development of aspiration pneumonitis or pneumonia (Atwater *et al.* 1994; Hackett *et al.* 1995; Rusbridge *et al.* 1996), and MG-related neuromuscular weakness and hypoventilation.

Acquired MG is reported to occur in up to 47% dogs with thymoma (Aronsohn *et al.* 1984). Although less common, cats with thymoma may also develop megaesophagus and acquired MG (Scott-Moncrieff *et al.* 1990; Zitz *et al.* 2008). Acute fulminant MG, with severe respiratory dysfunction, is uncommon but has been reported as an early postoperative complication after thymectomy in a cat (Meeking *et al.* 2008). It requires prompt

recognition and treatment and is often fatal. Several reports show that veterinary patients with thymoma and acquired MG or megaesophagus have a poor prognosis with a high postoperative morbidity rate because of the risk of aspiration pneumonia (Atwater *et al.* 1994; Rusbridge *et al.* 1996; Taylor 2000). Atwater *et al.* (1994) reported a median survival time of 6 days for 9 dogs with megaesophagus that underwent thymectomy; the potential for resolution of megaesophagus could not be evaluated because no dog with megaesophagus survived long term. However, in the cases more recently reported by Zitz *et al.* (2008), paraneoplastic syndromes were uncommonly recognized and did not affect patient outcome after thymectomy. The recommended treatment for thymoma-related MG is thymectomy, and in many patients, MG resolves after thymectomy (Lainesse *et al.* 1996). However, improvement of megaesophagus postoperatively is variable, and localized MG may become generalized or even develop in patients in which it was not present preoperatively in the months after thymectomy (Atwater *et al.* 1994; Gores *et al.* 1994; Singh *et al.* 2010). Resolution of MG followed by a later recurrence may be associated with regrowth of an incompletely resected thymoma (Lainesse *et al.* 1996; Zitz *et al.* 2008).

Recurrence of thymoma after surgery is variable, and further surgical treatment can result in good long-term survival. Aronsohn *et al.* (1984) reported recurrence 4 months postoperatively in 1 of 6 dogs after thymectomy; this dog died. Breznock (1988) reported recurrence in 3 of 7 dogs, and Zitz *et al.* (2008) reported local recurrence in 1 of 11 dogs and 2 of 9 cats; these latter cases had a long-term survival period of years after a second surgery. Patnaik *et al.* (2003) reported survival at last follow-up of 2520 days in a cat that had undergone two surgeries for recurrent disease; this cat finally developed metastases. Bellah *et al.* (1983), Atwater *et al.* (1994), and Gores *et al.* (1994) reported no recurrence.

Metastasis is reported in association with thymoma but is uncommon (Robinson 1974; Bellah *et al.* 1983; Mitcham *et al.* 1984; Patnaik *et al.* 2003; Moffet 2007).

Hypercalcemia is reported as a paraneoplastic syndrome that can accompany thymoma in cats and dogs; it usually resolves after thymectomy (Mills *et al.* 1985; Squires *et al.* 1986; Harris *et al.* 1991; Day 1997; Foley *et al.* 2000; Zitz *et al* 2008). It was reported in 9% cases in a series of dogs with thymoma reported by Atwater *et al.* (1994), and one dog developed early postoperative **hypocalcemia**.

Phrenic and **laryngeal nerve injuries** are potential complications of thymectomy but are uncommonly recognized clinically. Bellah *et al.* (1983) mentioned resection of a phrenic nerve in one dog undergoing thymectomy but reported no effect on respiration. Gores *et al.* (1994) recognized unilateral laryngeal paralysis 3 weeks after surgery in one cat; this had resolved without treatment at follow-up 32 months later.

References

Aronsohn, M.G., Schunk, K.L., Carpenter, J.L., et al. (1984) Clinical and pathological features of thymoma in 15 dogs. *Journal of the American Veterinary Medical Association* 184, 1355-1362.

Atwater, S.W., Powers, B.E., Park, R.D., et al. (1994) Thymoma in dogs: 23 cases (1980-1991). *Journal of the American Veterinary Medical Association* 205, 1007-1013.

Bellah, J.R., Smith, A.N. (2003) The thymus. In Slatter, D. (ed.) *Textbook of Small Animal Surgery*, vol. 1, 3rd edn. Saunders, Philadelphia, p. 1088.

Bellah, J.R., Stiff, M.E., Russell, R.G. (1983) Thymoma in the dog: two case reports and review of 20 additional cases. *Journal of the American Veterinary Medical Association* 183, 306-311.

Bexfield, N.H., Watson, P. J., Herrtage, M. E. (2006) Management of myasthenia gravis using cyclosporine in 2 dogs. *Journal of Veterinary Internal Medicine* 20, 1487-1490.

Blalock, A., Cunningham, R.S., Robinson, C.S. (1936) Experimental production of chylothorax by occlusion of the superior vena cava. *Annals of Surgery* 104, 359-364.

Breznock, E.M. (1988) Thoracic thymomas and heart base tumours: surgical versus non-surgical treatment. American College of Veterinary Surgeons Scientific Meeting Abstract. *Veterinary Surgery* 17, 30.

Day, M.J. (1997) Review of thymic pathology in 30 cats and 36 dogs. *Journal of Small Animal Practice* 38, 393-403.

Dewey, C.W., Cerda-Gonzalez, S., Fletcher, D.J., et al. (2010) Mycophenolate mofetil treatment in dogs with serologically diagnosed acquired myasthenia gravis: 27 cases (1999-2008). *Journal of the American Veterinary Medical Association* 236, 664-668.

Foley, P., Shaw, D., Runyon, C., et al. (2000) Serum parathyroid hormone related protein concentration in a dog with thymoma and persistent hypercalcaemia. *Canadian Veterinary Journal* 41, 867-870.

Fossum, T.W. (2007) Surgery of the lower respiratory system: pleural cavity and diaphragm. In Fossum, T.W. (ed.) *Textbook of Small Animal Surgery*, 3rd ed. Mosby, St. Louis, p. 926.

Fossum, T.W., Birchard, S.J. (1986) Lymphangiographic evaluation of experimentally induced chylothorax after ligation of the cranial vena cava in dogs. *American Journal of Veterinary Research* 47,967-971.

Gores, B.R., Berg, J., Carpenter, J.L., et al. (1994) Surgical treatment of thymoma in cats: 12 cases (1987-1992). *Journal of the American Veterinary Medical Association* 204, 1782-1785.

Hackett, T.B., Van Pelt, D.R., Willard, M.D., et al. (1995) Third degree atrioventricular block and acquired myasthenia gravis in four dogs. *Journal of the American Veterinary Medical Association* 206, 1173-1176.

Harris, C.L., Klausner, J.S., Caywood, D.D., et al. (1991) Hypercalcaemia in a dog with thymoma. *Journal of the American Animal Hospital Association* 27, 281-284.

Holsworth, I.G., Kyles, A.E., Bailiff, N.L., et al. (2004) Use of a jugular vein autograft for reconstruction of the cranial vena cava in a dog with invasive thymoma and cranial vena cava syndrome. *Journal of the American Veterinary Medical Association* 225, 1205-1210.

Hunt, G., Churcher, R.K., Church, D.B., et al. (1997) Excision of a locally invasive thymoma causing cranial vena caval syndrome in a dog. *Journal of the American Veterinary Medical Association* 210, 1628-1630.

Inzana, K.D. (2004) Paraneoplastic neuromuscular disorders. *Veterinary Clinics of North America: Small Animal Practice* 34, 1453-1467.

Jian-xiong, A.N., Li-Ming, Z., Sullivan, E.A., et al. (2011) Intraoperative cardiac arrest during anesthesia: a retrospective study of 218 274 anesthetics undergoing non-cardiac surgery in a US teaching hospital. *Chinese Medical Journal* 124, 227-232.

Klebanow, E.R. (1992) Thymoma and acquired myasthenia gravis in the dog: a case report and review of 13 additional cases. *Journal of the American Animal Hospital Association* 28, 63–9.

Lainesse, C.M.F, Taylor, S.M., Myers, S.L., et al. (1996) Focal myasthenia gravis as a paraneoplastic syndrome of canine thymoma: improvement following thymectomy. *Journal of the American Animal Hospital Association* 31, 111-117.

Levien, A.S., Summers, B.A., Szladovits, B., et al. (2010) Transformation of a thymic branchial cyst to a carcinoma with pulmonary metastasis in a dog. *Journal of Small Animal Practice* 11, 604-608.

Liu, S., Patnaik, A.K and Burk, R.L. (1984) Thymic branchial cysts in the dog and cat. *Journal of the American Veterinary Medical Association* 182, 1095-1098.

Malik, R., Gabor, L., Hunt, G.B., et al. (1997) Benign cranial mediastinal lesions in three cats. *Australian Veterinary Journal* 75, 183-187.

Martin, R.A., Evans, E.W, August, J.R., et al (1986) Surgical treatment of a thymoma in a cat. *Journal of the American Animal Hospital Association* 22, 347-354.

Mayhew, P.D., Friedberg, J.S. (2008) Video-assisted thoracoscopic resection of noninvasive thymomas using one-lung ventilation in two dogs. *Veterinary Surgery* 37, 756-762.

Meeking, S.A., Prittie, J., Barton, L. (2008) Myasthenia gravis associated with thymic neoplasia in a cat. *Journal of Veterinary Emergency and Critical Care* 18, 177-183.

Mills, J.N., Shaw, S.E., Kabay, M.J.. (1985) The cytopathological features of thymoma in a dog. *JSAP* 26, 176-175

Mitcham, S.A., Clark, E.G., Mills, J.H. (1984) Malignant thymoma with widespread metastases in a dog: case report and brief literature review. *Canadian Veterinary Journal* 5, 280-282.

Moffet, A.C. (2007) Metastatic thymoma and acquired generalized myasthenia gravis in a beagle. *Canadian Veterinary Journal* 48, 91-3.

Morini, M., Bettini, G., Diana, A., et al. (2009) Thymolipoma in two dogs. *Journal of Comparative Pathology* 141, 74-77.

Patnaik, A.K., Lieberman, P.H., Erlandson, R.A., et al. (2003) Feline cystic thymoma: a clinicopathologic, and electron microscopic study of 14 cases. *Journal of Feline Medicine and Surgery* 5, 27-35.

Robinson, M. (1974) Malignant thymoma with metastases in a dog. *Veterinary Pathology* 11, 172-18.

Rusbridge, C., White, R.N., Elwood, C.M., et al. (1996) Treatment of acquired myasthenia gravis associated with thymoma in two dogs. *Journal of Small Animal Practice* 36, 376-380.

Scherrer, W.E., Kyles, A.E., Samii, V.F., et al. (2008) Computed tomographic assessment of vascular invasion and respectability of mediastinal masses in dogs and a cat. *New Zealand Veterinary Journal* 56, 330-333.

Scott-Moncrieff, J.C., Cook, J.R., Lantz, G.C. (1990) Acquired myasthenia gravis in a cat with thymoma. *Journal of the American Veterinary Medical Association* 196, 1291-1293.

Singh, A., Boston, S.E., Poma, R. (2010) Thymoma associated exfoliative dermatitis with post-thymectomy myasthenia gravis in a cat. *Canadian Veterinary Journal* 51, 757-760.

Shelton, G.D. (2009) Treatment of autoimmune myasthenia gravis. In Bonagura, J.D., Twedt, D.C. *Kirk's Current Veterinary Therapy XIV*. Saunders Elsevier, St. Louis, pp. 1108-1111.

Stenner, V.J, Parry, B.W., Holloway, S.A. (2003) Acquired myasthenia gravis associated with a non-invasive thymic carcinoma in a dog. *Australian Veterinary Journal* 81, 543-546.

Taylor, S.M. (2000) Selected disorders of the muscle and the neuromuscular junction. *Veterinary Clinics of North America. Small Animal Practice* 30, 59-75.

Zekas, L.J., Adams, W.M. (2002) Cranial mediastinal cysts in nine cats. *Veterinary Radiology & Ultrasound* 43, 413-418.

Zitz, J.C., Birchard, S.J., Couto, G.C., et al. (2008) Results of excision of thymoma in cats and dogs: 20 cases (1984-2005). *Journal of the American Veterinary Medical Association* 232, 1186-1192.

46 Pericardial Surgery

Daniel J. Brockman
Royal Veterinary College, University of London, Hatfield, Hertfordshire, UK

The indications for pericardial surgery include incision to allow access to the heart for surgical manipulation; and excision (pericardectomy) to treat a range of conditions including neoplastic and idiopathic pericardial effusions, bacterial pericarditis, and chylothorax (Aronson and Gregory 1995; Vicari *et al.* 2001; Ehrhart *et al.* 2002; Fossum *et al.* 2004; Mellanby and Herrtage 2005). Potential complications associated with pericardial surgery include hemorrhage, cardiac tamponade, cardiac herniation, phrenic nerve injury, and recurrence of either pericardial or pleural effusion. Recent advances in surgical equipment such as vessel-sealing devices and harmonic dissection tools, in addition to developments such as minimally invasive techniques, should reduce the incidence of complications associated with surgical pericardial manipulations further (Mayhew 2009).

The pericardium is continuous with the mediastinum and consists of a dense fibrous pericardium that is covered by mesothelium on its pleural and parietal surfaces. The pericardial sac contains a small volume of fluid that lubricates the surfaces of the parietal serous pericardium and the visceral serous pericardium (epicardium). Because of the dense fibrous tissue in the pericardium, it is relatively inelastic, although it can become "stretched" over time, as is seen in dogs with chronic pericardial effusion. A tube of epicardium traverses the base of the heart caudal to the aorta and the pulmonic artery, creating a direct communication, the transverse pericardial sinus, joining the two sides of the pericardial sac. This feature can assist placement of a total cardiac outflow occlusion clamp (see Chapter 47) (Evans and Christensen 1979).

Selecting the correct patient for pericardial surgery and matching that patient with the correct technique is the first step to minimizing both disease-related and technical complications. For example, dogs suspected to have bacterial infective pericarditis are probably best treated by open thoracic exploration and pericardectomy to maximize the ability of the surgeon to identify any underlying cause (e.g., foreign body) and optimize the debridement of infected and diseased tissue while minimizing the risk of iatrogenic phrenic nerve injury (Aronson and Gregory 1995). Alternatively, an aged dog with a chemodectoma at the heart base causing pericardial effusion may be sufficiently palliated by the minimally invasive creation of a pericardial window (Ehrhart *et al.* 2002), but the same procedure may be inferior for the treatment of idiopathic pericardial effusion (Case *et al.* 2013).

Hemorrhage

Definition
See Chapter 12.

Risk factors
- Inflammation of the pericardium causing neovascularization.
- Poor hemostasis
- Coagulopathy

Diagnosis
Ongoing hemorrhage after pericardectomy is typically detected in the immediate postoperative recovery phase by analysis of the quality and quantity of fluid retrieved via the chest drain. Although some bleeding is inevitable, the postoperative care team must evaluate the overall volume and the packed cell volume (PCV) of any fluid produced and compare the latter with the PCV of a contemporaneous sample of peripheral blood while concurrently monitoring other cardiovascular parameters such as blood pressure, heart rate, capillary refill time, urine output, and mucous membrane color, to understand the impact the blood loss is having on the animal.

Treatment
If the impact of hemorrhage is minimal in hemodynamic terms, a more conservative approach can be taken but if the loss is of hemodynamic consequence, blood transfusion and revision surgery to identify the bleeding source should be considered.

Outcome
The outcome is good with appropriate intervention.

Prevention
- Thorough presurgical patient assessment
- Careful attention to hemostasis during surgery

Cardiac tamponade

Definition
Cardiac tamponade, the term used to describe the detrimental effect pericardial fluid accumulation can have on ventricular filling and therefore ventricular ejection, is often the reason for, rather

Complications in Small Animal Surgery, First Edition. Edited by Dominique Griffon and Annick Hamaide.
© 2016 John Wiley & Sons, Inc. Published 2016 by John Wiley & Sons, Inc.
Companion website: www.wiley.com/go/griffon/complications

than a complication of, pericardial surgery. It can only happen postoperatively if there is fluid accumulation inside a sealed pericardium, so this is not a complication of procedures that remove the pericardium or procedures in which the pericardium is left "wide" open, such as is done following cardiac surgery.

Risk factors

- Small openings in the pericardium (e.g., those made during patent ductus arteriosus [PDA] surgery) should be closed to prevent herniation of the left atrial appendage, especially when intrapericardial hemorrhage is unlikely.
- When the pericardium is intact, acute tamponade can develop as a result of even a small volume of effusion or hemorrhage because the pericardium is nondistensible.

Diagnosis

- Affected animals can develop jugular distension in association with poor cardiac output and rapidly progressive systemic hypotension, tachycardia, and prolonged capillary refill time.
- Typically, there are no radiographic abnormalities in affected dogs, but echocardiographic evaluation should reveal a small-volume effusion and the right atrial collapse characteristic of tamponade.

Treatment

- Treatment by pericardiocentesis is challenging because of the small volume of pericardial fluid, so revision surgery, opening of the pericardium, and identification of the source of blood or effusion are required.

Outcome

The outcome is dictated by underlying cause, but resolution of tamponade should be achieved in most patients.

Prevention

- Meticulous attention to hemostasis when the pericardial sac is closed
- When appropriate, leave the pericardium "wide open" (Figure 46.1).

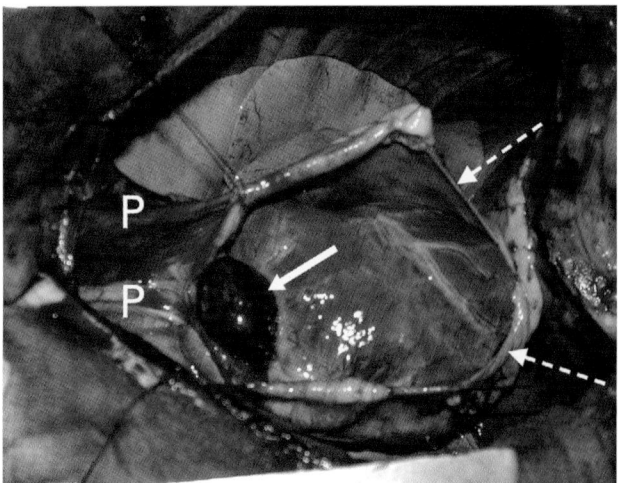

Figure 46.1 Pericardial incision (dotted arrows) made via a sternotomy to reveal a right auricular appendage hemangiosarcoma (solid arrow). After removal of the tumor, such an incision is left wide open to eliminate the risk of subsequent tamponade. Note the close proximity of the phrenic nerves (P).

Cardiac herniation

Definition

Herniation of the heart chamber is rare, but it can interfere with cardiac chamber filling and therefore overall cardiac function.

Risk factor

- Small opening in pericardium

Diagnosis

- Echocardiographic evaluation of the heart

Treatment

- Revision surgery to either open the pericardium completely or to close the pericardium correctly

Outcome

Surgical revision should resolve this complication.

Prevention

In small animal surgery, the surgeon must usually make the decision between making a small hole in the pericardium, which is subsequently closed (e.g., PDA surgery), or making a very large opening and leaving it open (e.g., most other cardiac procedures). The complications associated with leaving the canine pericardium "wide" open seem minimal, and this approach prevents herniation and tamponade, so it is recommended by the author for all situations except PDA surgery.

Phrenic nerve injury

Definition

Phrenic nerve injury is: traumatic, thermal, or electrical injury to the phrenic nerve causing temporary or permanent dysfunction.

Risk factors

In animals with pyothorax, the phrenic nerves are often enveloped in granulation tissue and may be difficult to identify or locate. Dogs and cats undergoing surgical treatment for pyothorax are therefore the most likely to sustain iatrogenic injury to the phrenic nerve.

Diagnosis

- Documented hypoventilation associated with nonexistent diaphragmatic movement (under fluoroscopy)
- Although documented phrenic nerve injury would seem rare (Walsh *et al.* 1999; Case *et al.* 2013), unilateral phrenic nerve injury is well tolerated in adult dogs (Jackson *et al.* 1999), so injury may go unrecognized.

Treatment

- Ventilatory support for a period to determine whether function will be restored

Outcome

- Poor outcome if bilateral injury has occurred (unilateral injury may go unnoticed)

Prevention

- In almost all thoracic operations (except pyothorax), the phrenic nerves can be identified and kept under direct observation or

gently dissected away from the pericardium and protected using atraumatic sutures or silicone "loops."
- Extreme care should be used when using electrocautery or vessel-sealing devices adjacent to the phrenic nerves for fear of inducing thermal or electrical injury.
- Gentle surgical technique is also required to avoid crush or traction injury.

Recurrence of pericardial effusion

Definition
This is recurrence of pericardial effusion after partial pericardectomy

Risk factor
- Sufficient pericardium remaining for adhesions to form between the pericardium and the epicardium

Diagnosis
- Physical examination findings
- Echocardiography to confirm the diagnosis

Treatment
- Open or thoracoscopic removal of as much of the pericardium as is feasible

Outcome
A good outcome should be achieved.

Prevention
The role of "pericardial windows" in the long-term management of pericardial effusion has been questioned in human medicine because of the frequency of recurrence (Olson *et al.* 1995). Recently, a comparison of outcomes after thoracoscopic pericardial window and open surgical pericardectomy in dogs revealed improved long-term results when an open approach was used to treat idiopathic pericardial effusion (Case *et al.* 2013). Case (2013) and others reported that failure of therapy among the thoracoscopic pericardial window group included dogs reported to have a "recurrence of signs." Currently, open pericardectomy might be the preferred technique when long-term survival is anticipated (i.e., idiopathic pericardial disease).

References

Aronson, L.R., Gregory, C.R. (1995) Infectious pericardial effusion in five dogs. *Veterinary Surgery* 24 (5), 402-407.

Case, J.B., Maxwell, M., Aman, A., et al. (2013) Outcome evaluation of a thoracoscopic pericardial window procedure or subtotal pericardectomy via thoracotomy for the treatment of pericardial effusion in dogs. *Journal of the American Veterinary Medical Association* 242 (4), 493-498.

Ehrhart, N., Ehrhart, E.J., Willis, J., et al. (2002) Analysis of factors affecting survival in dogs with aortic body tumors. *Veterinary Surgery* 31 (1), 44-48.

Evans, H.E., Christensen, G,C. (1979) The heart and arteries. In *Miller's Anatomy of the Dog*, 2nd edn. WB Saunders, Philadelphia, pp. 632-756.

Fossum, T.W., Mertens, M.M., Miller, M.W., et al. (2004) Thoracic duct ligation and pericardectomy for treatment of idiopathic chylothorax. *Journal of Veterinary Internal Medicine* 18 (3), 307-310.

Jackson, J., Richter, K.P., Launer, D.P. (1999) Thoracoscopic partial pericardectomy in 13 dogs. *Journal of Veterinary Internal Medicine* 13, 529–533.

Mayhew, K.N., Mayhew, P.D., Sorrell-Raschi, L., et al. (2009) Thoracoscopic subphrenic pericardectomy using double-lumen endobronchial intubation for alternating one-lung ventilation. *Veterinary Surgery* 38 (8), 961-966.

Mellanby, R.J., Herrtage, M.E. (2005) Long-term survival of 23 dogs with pericardial effusions. *Veterinary Record* 156 (18), 568-571.

Olson, J.E., Ryan, M.B., Blumenstock, D.A. (1995) Eleven years' experience with pericardial-peritoneal window in the management of malignant and benign pericardial effusions. *Annals of Surgical Oncology* 2 (2), 165-169.

Vicari, E.D., Brown, D.C., Holt, D.E., et al. (2001) Survival times and prognostic indicators for dogs with heart base masses: 25 cases (1986-1999). *Journal of the American Veterinary Medical Association* 219 (4), 485-487.

Walsh, P.J., Remedios, A.M., Ferguson, J.F., et al. (1999) Thoracoscopic versus open partial pericardectomy in dogs: comparison of postoperative pain and morbidity. *Veterinary Surgery* 28 (6), 472-479.

47 Patent Ductus Arteriosus

Daniel J. Brockman

Royal Veterinary College, University of London, Hatfield, Hertfordshire, UK

Nonsurgical occlusion of patent ductus arteriosus (PDA) using intravascular thrombogenic coils, the Amplatz ductal occluder, or the specifically designed Amplatz canine ductal occluder, using interventional radiology (IR) techniques, has become the most common therapy used in referral practice (Glaus *et al.* 2003; Singh *et al.* 2012; Meijer and Beigerink 2012). As nonsurgical occlusion has evolved, refinements in occluder and delivery system design have meant that surgical ligation of PDA is only considered for either very small or very large animals for which nonsurgical occlusion is not possible for technical reasons (Glaus *et al.* 2003; Singh *et al.* 2012; Meijer and Beigerink 2012). As a consequence, even highly trained surgeons are not practiced at the dissection required for successful surgical ligation of a PDA; in addition, surgery is only ever required for the most challenging patients. Although operative mortality rates of 0% have been reported by individuals highly experienced in cardiac surgery (Bureau *et al.* 2005), for most, the combination of lack of familiarity with the procedure and the challenge associated with patient size means that the risk of a "technical" complication is considerable. Indeed, surgical complications are likely to become more common than they were when surgical ligation was the only treatment.

The anatomic features of the ductus may influence the choice of surgical procedure and therefore influence the complication rate. James Buchanan (Buchanan 1978, 2001) described the anatomy of the ductus arteriosus in a series of animals with naturally occurring PDA. His description of the overall shape of the different forms of ductus and his analysis of the histology of the ductus wall, which suggested that the eccentric distribution of muscular and elastic fibres therein were the cause of failure of the normal closure mechanism, have proved to be definitive studies. These studies also demonstrated that certain regions of the ductus and the section of the aortic wall through which the ductus courses (which Buchanan termed the "ductus aneurysm") were very thin compared with the normal aorta. This finding could explain, in part, the fragility of the ductus or aorta experienced during dissection in some animals. In addition, certain anatomic types of ductus (very short and wide) might be even more challenging to dissect around. Such animals, it is suggested, would be better suited to clamping, division, and oversewing of the cut ends of the ductus (Buchanan 1966).

Ductal occlusion is normally reserved for dogs and cats with "left-to-right" shunting PDA. Animals with "balanced flow" through a PDA and therefore concomitant pulmonary hyperten-sion may also be considered candidates for PDA occlusion, but PDA occlusion is contraindicated in animals with established pulmonary hypertension with permanent "right-to-left" shunting of blood. Although more complications are seen in older dogs with PDA and dogs with more severe left heart dilation (causing severe mitral incompetence or atrial fibrillation), such complications are not usually of a technical surgical nature, and these animals usually still benefit from the occlusion of their ductus (van Israël *et al.* 2003; Bureau *et al.* 2005). IR techniques for PDA occlusion require angiographic evaluation of the abnormal vessel, and this, along with improvements in echocardiographic techniques, allows cardiologists to identify animals that might not be appropriate for intravascular occlusion (by virtue of their duct shape) or for which special surgical considerations might be necessary (short, wide ductus). In addition, as previously mentioned, selection of patients for surgical treatment also depends on patient size (and size of IR delivery systems and devices) in institutions with established cardiac IR programs.

Several surgical techniques that allow the placement of circumferential ductal ligatures have been described in the peer reviewed literature and surgical texts (Buchanan 1966; Jackson and Henderson 1979; Eyster et al. 1976; Eyster 1985). Broadly, these are predominantly extrapericardial dissection (Buchanan 1966), predominantly intrapericardial dissection (Eyster et al. 1976; Eyster 1985), and an indirect approach to encircling the ductus by dissection around the aorta cranial and caudal to the ductus (Jackson and Henderson 1979). The author has no personal experience of the latter technique, so it will not be mentioned further. Both authors of early descriptions of ductus dissection technique (Buchanan 1966 and Eyster 1985) advocated performing maneuvers that would be useful in the event of ductal hemorrhage. Although rarely needed, these maneuvers have formed a routine part of the current author's ritual as preparation in case intraoperative complications develop. These are described later.

Ductus dissection can be performed through a left fourth intercostal space in most animals. Occasionally, a fifth intercostal incision is preferable in cats and some dogs; the evaluation of the position of the ductus relative to the chest wall, based on preoperative radiographs, can assist in this decision. After the chest is opened, the pericardium is opened immediately ventral to the phrenic nerve to provide access to the transverse pericardial sinus; therefore, facilitating the placement of a straight vascular clamp across the ascending aorta and main pulmonary artery

---

Complications in Small Animal Surgery, First Edition. Edited by Dominique Griffon and Annick Hamaide.

© 2016 John Wiley & Sons, Inc. Published 2016 by John Wiley & Sons, Inc.

Companion website: www.wiley.com/go/griffon/complications

trunk to allow temporary total cardiac outflow occlusion in the event of hemorrhage. The author prefers either extrapericardial dissection alone or combined extra- and intrapericardial dissection (very small patients), so no further intrapericardial manipulations are done at this stage. The phrenic nerve and the vagus nerve are dissected free from the pericardium and retracted ventrally using stay sutures or a silicone vessel loop. The recurrent laryngeal nerve is identified and avoided when possible. A right-angled dissection instrument (Mixter or Lahey bile duct forceps) is then used to dissect around the aorta caudal to the ductus but cranial to the first intercostal artery, and either moist umbilical tape or a ¼ inch Penrose drain is placed loosely around the aorta with its ends secured in an artery forceps. Using gentle traction on this aortic noose, the space caudal to the ductus between the aorta, ductus and pulmonary artery trunk can be opened and extended medially by gentle dissection under direct visualization. This dissection is done first because it provides access for the placement of straight ductus clamps, with the tips passing in a caudal to cranial direction across the ductus, to achieve hemostasis if hemorrhage develops during future dissection. This maneuver is facilitated greatly by traction on the aortic noose. Cranial to the ductus, the space between the aortic wall and the ductus can be opened by gentle dissection. In very small animals, this dissection does not always remain extrapericardial, but in larger animals, it should. The preparation caudal to the ductus should give the surgeon a good understanding of the dimensions of the duct and allow gentle passage of a dissection instrument (usually Mixter or Lahey as discussed earlier), either from cranial to caudal or caudal to cranial, to complete the ductus dissection (Figures 47.1 to 47.3).

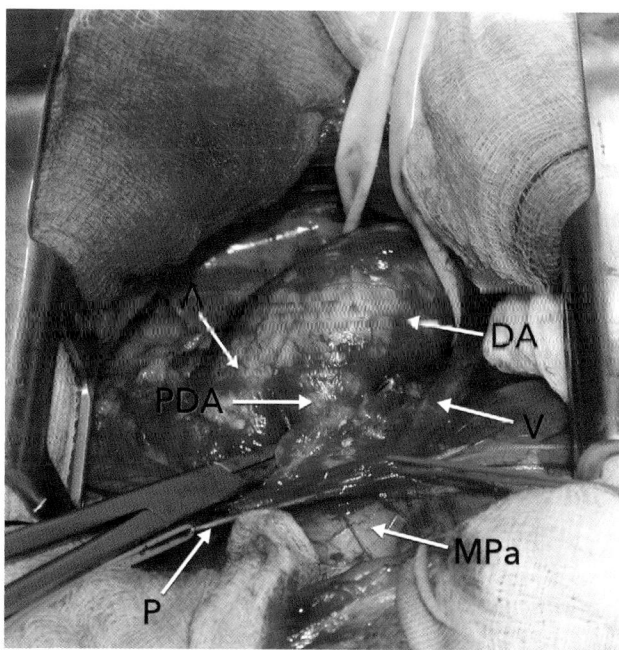

Figure 47.2 The surgical field after dissection of the ductus showing Mixter forceps around the ductus and the silicone loops around the vagus and phrenic nerves along with the Penrose drain around the descending aorta. A, aorta; DA, ductus aneurysm; MPa, main pulmonary artery; P, left phrenic nerve; PDA, patent ductus arteriosus; V, left vagus nerve.

Intraoperative hemorrhage

Definition
Hemorrhage most commonly occurs during dissection of the craniomedial ductus, although the author has also experienced hemorrhage as the ligatures were being tied after an apparently uneventful dissection.

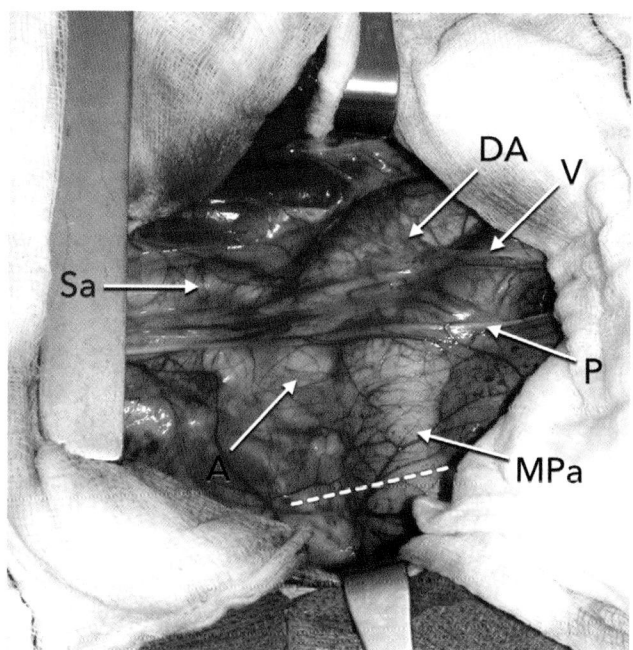

Figure 47.1 Left fourth intercostal thoracotomy with left cranial lung packed caudally showing anatomic landmarks. The dashed line shows the site of pericardial incision to access the transverse pericardial sinus. A, aorta; DA, ductus aneurysm; MPa, main pulmonary artery; P, left phrenic nerve; Sa, left subclavian artery; V, left vagus nerve.

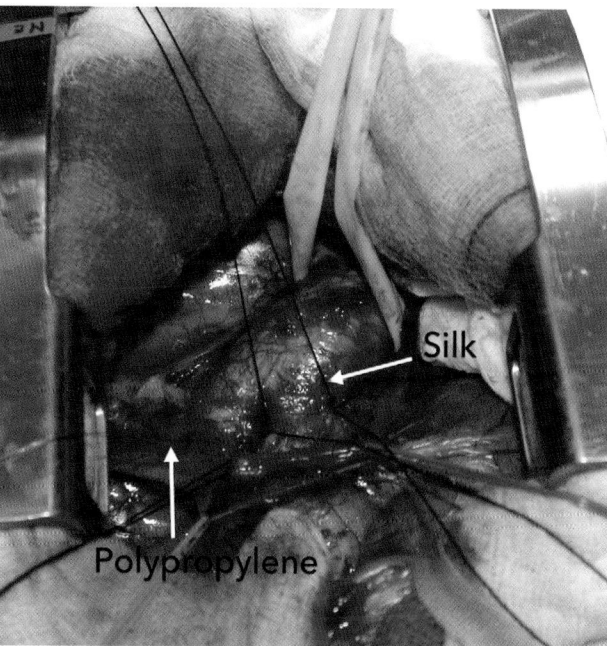

Figure 47.3 The surgical field after placement of two silk and one Prolene suture around the ductus.

Risk factors

- Care must be taken not to continue the dissection "too deep" in relation to the ductus because the right pulmonary arterial branch is vulnerable in this position.
- Similarly, a "shallow" dissection can lead the instrument directly into the medial ductus wall.

Treatment

- Occasionally, when hemorrhage is minimal, a change in the direction of dissection (i.e., changing from cranial to caudal to caudal to cranial) will allow completion of the dissection.
- Hunt (2001) and others have described the clinical use of the temporary total cardiac outflow occlusion, as advocated by Buchanan (1966) and Eyster (1985), either to permit further dissection or to facilitate accurate clamp placement in the event of ductal hemorrhage (Hunt et al. 2001). To achieve this, the pericardial incision made previously is widened if necessary, and a vascular clamp is placed across the aortic and pulmonary artery roots simultaneously with one jaw of the clamp passing across the transverse pericardial sinus and the other passing cranial to the great vessels. In addition, traction on the aortic noose will limit backflow of blood down the aorta and expose the caudal ductus further to facilitate clamp placement, as previously described.
- In more than 25 years performing PDA surgery, the author has only had to do the maneuver described above once but has clamped and oversewn the ductus in more than six animals, including one cat. With ductus clamps in place and hemorrhage under control (Figures 47.4 and 47.5), it is important to create enough room to transect the ductus and oversew the cut ends (hopefully incorporating the iatrogenic tear). This can be achieved either by carefully repositioning the clamps or by placing additional clamps alongside the initial hemostatic clamps, farther away from the intended division site, to create enough room after the primary clamps are removed. The ductus ends can be closed using fine polypropylene suture (4-0 to 6-0 depending on the size of the animal) (Figure 47.6) either in two overlapping rows of simple continuous suture or one continuous horizontal

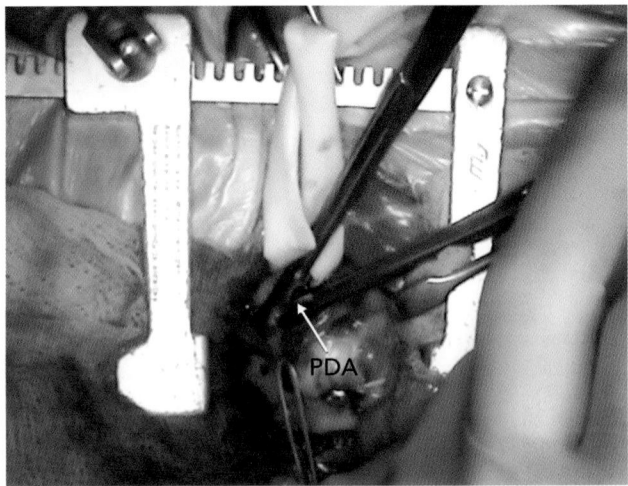

Figure 47.5 The same cat as in Figure 47.4 during ductus (patent ductus arteriosus [PDA]) division.

mattress suture oversewn by a simple continuous suture. Secure knots must be tied at each end and these knots should be augmented by expanded polytetrafluoroethylene (ePTFE) pledgets in large dogs (Figure 47.7). Additional suture material should be ready before the removal of the vascular clamps. If hemorrhage is seen after the clamp is removed, the leak can be either sutured directly or after replacement of the clamp. It is common to see a small amount of leakage adjacent to the suture through suture needle holes, but application of a topical haemostatic (e.g., cellulose, Surgicel, Ethicon, Somerville, NJ) usually facilitates the formation of blood clots that stop this bleeding.

Outcome and Prevention

- Familiarity with ductal anatomy and the dissection techniques required for its isolation will reduce the risk of hemorrhage during attempted surgical closure. The risk that any hemorrhage experienced during dissection will be fatal is reduced when the

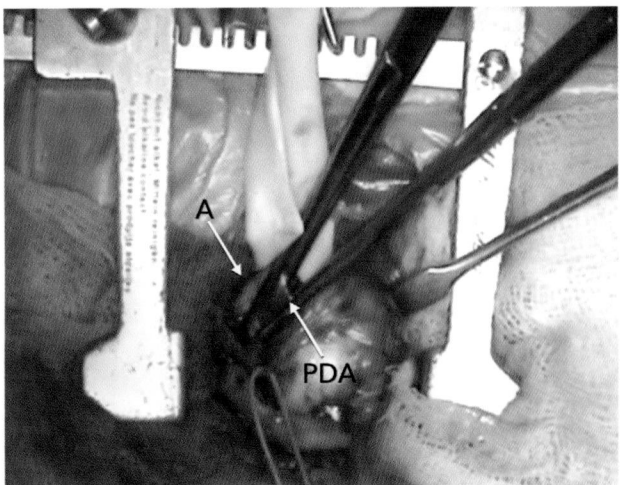

Figure 47.4 The surgical field in a cat after placement of vascular clamps on the ductus (patent ductus arteriosus [PDA]) to control ductal hemorrhage. Blood is able to flow within the aorta (A) and pulmonary arteries around the clamps. Placement was facilitated by traction on the Penrose drain around the descending aorta.

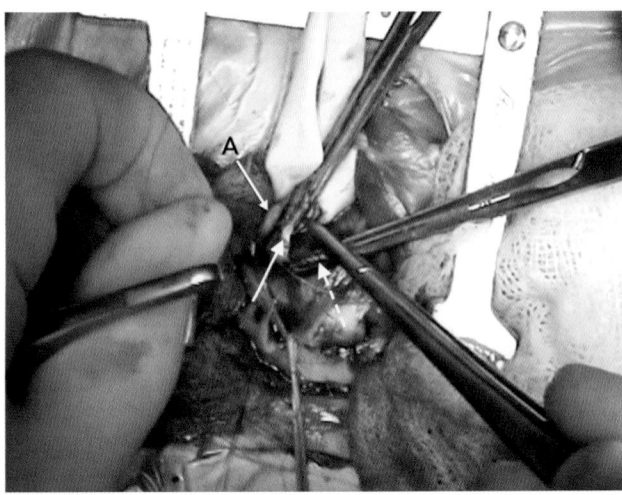

Figure 47.6 The same cat as in Figure 47.4 while 6-0 Prolene sutures are used to oversew the aortic side of the ductus (solid arrow). The pulmonic side is already sutured (dashed arrow). A, aorta.

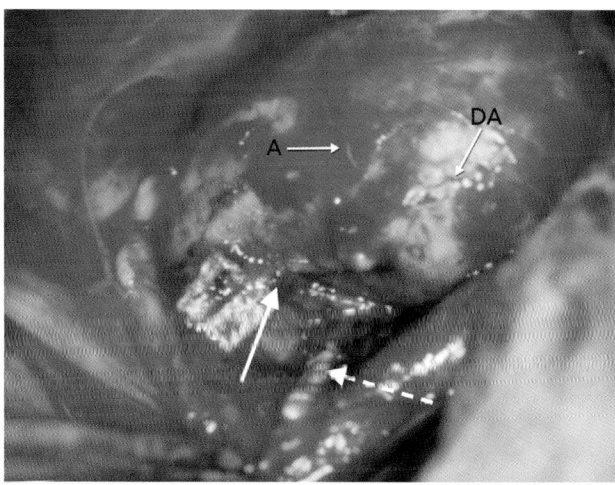

Figure 47.7 Image after "emergency" division and oversew of a canine ductus showing the use of expanded polytetrafluoroethylene pledgets to reinforce the proximal aortic closure (solid line). The pulmonic side has been sutures (dashed line). A, aorta; DA, ductus aneurysm.

surgeon has taken precautionary technical measures, has the relevant instruments, and is prepared for such an eventuality having practiced the techniques required to rescue the operation.

Recanalization of the ductus

Definition
Recanalization is defined as return of blood flow through a previously occluded ductus. It is a technical complication that can be avoided.

Risk factors
The impact of residual flow and "recanalization" of the ductus can be limited by choice of surgical technique (Stanley *et al.* 2003) and choice of suture material.

Diagnosis
- Auscultation
- Echocardiography

Treatment
Treatment will depend on the volume of flow across the ductus, but no treatment or reoperation or device occlusion might be needed.

Outcome
Although the operative risk is potentially higher during reintervention, the outcome is good if complete attenuation is achieved.

Prevention
- If hemorrhage is not experienced during duct dissection, the operation proceeds with the passage of suture material around the ductus. Traditionally, appropriately sized surgical silk was used, and this remains a good choice because of its handling characteristics.
- To reduce the risk of recanalization or limit its effect, the author commonly places a third ligature of polypropylene that is transfixed through the ductus wall and placed between the two

traditional silk ligatures so that if the silk ligatures fail, the ductus will remain constrained by the Prolene and will therefore be unable to "reopen" (see Figure 47.3).
- Alternatively, polypropylene could be used as the primary ligation suture. The aortic suture is typically tied first and is tied such that the machinery murmur disappears and the "thrill" in the pulmonary artery caused by turbulent blood from the ductus is abolished. Use of polypropylene means that even if some flow returns as a result of increased systemic pressure or after atrophy of additional connective tissue inadvertently included in the original ligatures, the flow through the duct should be permanently limited to a hemodynamically insignificant volume.

Recurrent laryngeal nerve injury

Definition and risk factors
The extrapericardial dissection in particular takes place very close to the left recurrent laryngeal nerve, and it can be very difficult to visualize in very small animals. It is impossible to track as it travels cranially after it has passed caudal to the ductus from a left-sided approach. It almost certainly becomes incorporated in the ligatures placed around the ductus in some animals.

Diagnosis
Although this has not been documented in PDA surgical patients, unilateral laryngeal hemiplegia may result.

Outcome
If it does happen, it would seem to be well tolerated.

Prevention
The incidence of postoperative laryngeal impairment is unknown, but dissection techniques that preserve the left recurrent laryngeal nerve will prevent this complication.

Left atrial herniation

Definition and risk factors
Failure to close the pericardial incision or breakdown of the pericardial incision can lead to herniation of the left auricular appendage through the pericardial defect.

Diagnosis
- Echocardiography

Treatment
Treatment consists of reintervention to surgically open or remove the pericardium.

Outcome
A good outcome is expected.

Prevention
- Careful closure of the defect
- Creation of a very large pericardial opening by continuation of the incision ventrally toward the apex of the heart.
- It is more simple and straightforward to carefully repair the incision, avoiding this potential complication.

Ductus aneurysmal rupture

Definition

Fatal postoperative rupture of the ductus aneurysm has been reported (Olsen *et al.* 2002), and the author has witnessed spontaneous aortic rupture in one dog with PDA before surgery that also resulted in death of the patient, but this seems to be a rare event according to studies of PDA treatment (Birchard 1990; Stanley *et al.* 2003; Bureau *et al.* 2005).

Prevention

The factors that cause postoperative ductal aneurysmal rupture are unknown and cannot therefore be avoided.

References

Birchard, S.J. (1990) Results of ligation of patent ductus arteriosus in dogs: 201 cases (1969-1988). *Journal of the American Veterinary Medical Association* 196, 2011-2013.

Buchanan, J. W. (1967) Surgical treatment of congenital cardiovascular diseases. In Kirk, R.W. (ed.) *Current Veterinary Therapy II.* WB Saunders, Philadelphia, pp. 87-103.

Buchanan, J.W. (1978) Morphology of the ductus arteriosus in fetal and neonatal dogs genetically predisposed to patent ductus arteriosus. *Birth Defects Original Article Series* 14 (7), 349-360.

Buchanan, J.W. (2001) Patent ductus arteriosus morphology, pathogenesis, types and treatment. *Journal of Veterinary Cardiology* 3 (1), 7-16.

Bureau, S., Monnet, E., Orton, E.C. (2005) Evaluation of survival rate and prognostic indicators for surgical treatment of left-to-right patent ductus arteriosus in dogs: 52 cases (1995-2003). *Journal of the American Veterinary Medical Association* 227 (11), 1794-1799.

Eyster, G.E. (1985) Basic cardiac procedures. In Slatter, D. (ed.) *Textbook of Small Animal Surgery,* 2nd edn. WB Saunders, Philadelphia, pp. 893-918.

Eyster, G.E., Eyster, J.T., Cords, G.B., et al. (1976) Patent ductus arteriosus in the dog: characteristics of occurrence and results of surgery in one hundred consecutive cases. *Journal of the American Veterinary Medical Association* 168 (5), 435-438.

Glaus, T.M., Martin, M., Boller, M., et al. (2003) Catheter closure of patent ductus arteriosus in dogs: variation in ductal size requires different techniques. *Journal of Veterinary Cardiology* 5 (1), 7-12.

Hunt, G.B., Simpson, D.J., Beck, J.A., et al. (2001) Intraoperative hemorrhage during patent ductus arteriosus ligation in dogs. *Veterinary Surgery* 30 (1), 58-63.

Jackson, W.F., Henderson, R.A. (1979) Ligature placement in closure of patent ductus arteriosus. *Journal of the American Animal Hospital Association* 15, 55-58.

Meijer, M., Beijerink, N.J. (2012) Patent ductus arteriosus in the dog: a retrospective study of clinical presentation, diagnostics and comparison of interventional techniques in 102 dogs (2003-2011). *Tijdschr Diergeneeskd* 137 (6), 376-383.

Olsen, D., Harkin, K.R., Banwell, M.N., et al. (2002) Postoperative rupture of an aortic aneurysmal dilation associated with a patent ductus arteriosus in a dog. *Veterinary Surgery* 31 (3), 259-265.

Singh, M.K., Kittleson, M.D., Kass, P.H., et al. (2012) Occlusion devices and approaches in canine patent ductus arteriosus: comparison of outcomes. *Journal of Veterinary Internal Medicine* 26 (1), 85-92.

Stanley, B.J., Luis-Fuentes, V., Darke, P.G. (2003) Comparison of the incidence of residual shunting between two surgical techniques used for ligation of patent ductus arteriosus in the dog. *Veterinary Surgery* 32 (3), 231-237.

van Israël, N., Dukes-McEwan, J., French, A.T. (2003) Long-term follow-up of dogs with patent ductus arteriosus. *Journal of Small Animal Practice* 44 (11), 480-490.

48 Cardiac Pacemaker Implantation

Rachel Burrow[1] and Sonja Fonfara[2]

[1]Small Animal Teaching Hospital, University of Liverpool, Leahurst, Neston, Wirral, UK
[2]School of Veterinary Sciences, University of Bristol, Langford, Bristol, UK

Cardiac pacemaker implantation is the treatment of choice for symptomatic bradycardia in dogs and cats (Figure 48.1).

In dogs, the first pacemaker implantation was reported by Bonagura in 1968 using an epicardial electrode placed via thoracotomy. For the next 15 to 20 years, this technique was used for treating symptomatic bradyarrhythmias in cats and dogs. Various surgical approaches (intercostal thoracotomy, cranial celiotomy and caudal sternotomy combined, and cranial celiotomy with transdiaphragmatic approach) were developed, all sharing the requirement of access to the heart for epicardial lead placement and generator implantation (Lombard *et al.* 1981; Yoshioka *et al.* 1981; Bonagura *et al.* 1983; Fingeroth and Birchard 1986; Fox *et al.* 1986, 1991). Two methods of electrode attachment were used: (1) suturing and (2) sutureless and screw in. Pacemakers were implanted at various sites, including free within the abdomen, various intermuscular locations over the flank, and at subcutaneous sites. Complications in these retrospective case series were reported in 39% to 100% of patients and included unrelated anesthesia , cardiac-, implant-, and surgery-related problems. Cranial celiotomy with transdiaphragmatic incision is now recommended for epicardial electrode placement; the advantages over other approaches are listed in Box 48.1.

Epicardial electrode placement is still performed in pediatric human patients and cats; development of chylothorax can be associated with transvenous electrode placement in cats (Ferasin *et al.* 2002). In canine patients, a transvenous approach is commonly performed. Usually the electrode is placed via the right jugular vein to avoid possible complications caused by a persistent left cranial vena cava. Endocardial leads can be uni- or bipolar, and they are differentiated into active (screw-tip) and passive (tined-tip) fixation leads (Oyama *et al.* 2001; Wess *et al.* 2006; Johnson *et al.* 2007). Pacemaker generators (PGs) are placed in the subcutaneous tissues of the neck or in the shoulder region.

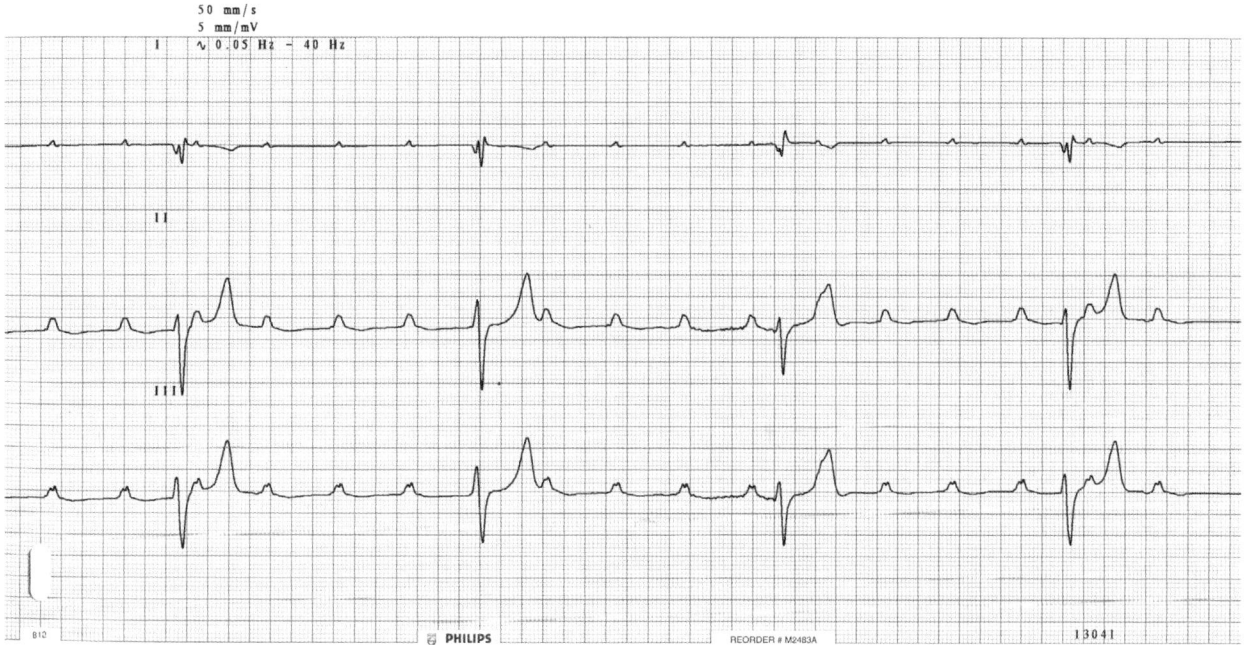

Figure 48.1 Electrocardiographic recording of a third-degree atrioventricular block in a dog presented with lethargy and collapsing episodes.

Complications in Small Animal Surgery, First Edition. Edited by Dominique Griffon and Annick Hamaide.
© 2016 John Wiley & Sons, Inc. Published 2016 by John Wiley & Sons, Inc.
Companion website: www.wiley.com/go/griffon/complications

The procedure can be performed through one incision; a second incision for pacemaker generator implantation is unnecessary.

The cardiac apex lies immediately adjacent to the diaphragm when the patient is positioned in dorsal recumbency, allowing good access to the site for electrode placement.

Pacemaker implantation free within the abdomen or between the internal and transverse abdominal oblique muscles reduces or avoids the risks of seroma, trauma, infection, and delayed wound healing that can accompany implantation in a subcutaneous pocket.

The discomfort for this approach may be less painful than after sternotomy and intercostal thoracotomy.

Most of the complications associated with epicardial and endocardial electrode placement are similar, although their risk factors and treatment may differ. There are also complications specific to each technique of electrode placement associated with the very different surgical approaches. The complications related to these specific surgical approaches are also covered in Chapters 37 to 39. The complications that have been reported in association with pacemaker implantation are listed in Table 48.1.

Table 48.1 Complications reported in association with pacemaker implantation in cats and dogs

Commonly reported	Uncommonly or rarely reported
Seroma or hematoma	Lead failure: lead fracture, insulation break
Lead dislodgement (endocardial > epicardial)	Twiddler's syndrome
Loose connection of lead and generator	Thrombosis or thromboembolism (endocardial)
Exit block	Pulse generator malfunction
Arrhythmias	Ventricular perforation (endocardial)
Infection	Development of congestive heart failure
Migration of pulse generator	Skeletal muscle twitch
	Suture line dehiscence
	Hemorrhage
	Pacemaker syndrome
	Pacemaker rejection
	Neoplasia at generator and electrode implantation sites
	Abscessation
	Pneumonia
	Pneumothorax (epicardial)
	Chylothorax
	Pyothorax (epicardial)
	Endocarditis (endocardial)
	Hemorrhage
	Pericarditis
	Pleuritis
	Air embolism

Ventricular premature complexes and ventricular tachycardia

Definition
Ventricular tachycardia (V-tac) is an abnormally fast heart rate originating from the ventricles.

Risk factors
- Ischemia or hypoxia caused by bradycardia, congestive heart failure (CHF), or anaesthesia
- CHF
- Cardiac diseases (e.g., dilated cardiomyopathy, degenerative valvular disease)
- Increased sympathetic tone
- Infiltrative, inflammatory diseases of the myocardium; myocardial scars
- Electrolyte or acid–base abnormalities
- Systemic inflammatory or infectious diseases
- Stimulation of the myocardium by the electrode
- Oversensing, undersensing, or noise reversion of the pacemaker with pacing during the vulnerable period of the T wave

Diagnosis
Ventricular premature complexes
- Electrocardiography (ECG): presence of ventricular premature complexes (VPCs)

Ventricular tachycardia
- ECG: Tachycardia with wide and bizarre QRS complexes.

Treatment
Ventricular premature complexes
- Treatment might not be necessary.
- If the patient has hemodynamic compromise, class I, II, or III antiarrhythmic medication might be necessary (depending on the case).

Ventricular tachycardia
- Lidocaine bolus followed by constant-rate infusion (CRI)
- Esmolol bolus followed by CRI
- Procainamide, sotalol, amiodarone

Outcome
- Control of arrhythmia with treatment.
- Long-term treatment might be necessary.

Prevention
- Thorough preoperative assessment of patient for noncardiac and cardiac diseases, including complete blood count and serum biochemistry, as well as echocardiography. Some authors recommend investigation for infectious diseases, urinalysis, skin investigation, or bacterial culture if the patient is stable and if pacemaker implantation can be postponed while these investigations or treatment is performed.
- Preoperative treatment of systemic diseases is recommended.
- Oxygenation before and during anaesthesia.
- Prophylactic antibiotherapy before, during, and after pacemaker implantation.
- Careful programming of the pacemaker and regular pacemaker interrogations.

Ventricular fibrillation

Definition
Ventricular fibrillation is turbulent, disorganized electrical activity of the heart resulting in uncoordinated and weak contractions of the ventricular myocardium.

Risk factors
- As for VPC and V-tac
- Induction of anesthesia
- Caused by sensing abnormalities or improper timing of pacing discharges.

Diagnosis
- ECG: irregular, chaotic, deformed ECG deflections that continuously change in shape, magnitude, and direction.

Treatment
- Immediate electrical defibrillation and resuscitation.
- If there is no response, consider vasopressor (epinephrine) and antiarrhythmic agents (lidocaine, amiodarone).

Outcome
- Depends on the success of resuscitation

Prevention
- As for VPC and V-tac

Supraventricular arrhythmias: supraventricular tachycardia and atrial fibrillation

Definition
Tachycardia not originating from the ventricles.

Risk factors
- Dogs with sick sinus syndrome (SSS) or additional degenerative valvular disease might develop supraventricular arrhythmias during the pacemaker placement.
- Atrial fibrillation after atrial lead placement for dual chamber pacemakers.

Diagnosis
- ECG
  - Supraventricular tachycardia: regular narrow QRS complex tachycardia.
  - Atrial fibrillation: irregular narrow QRS complex tachycardia, oscillating baseline, no discernible P waves.
  - In cases of complete atrioventricular block (AVB): a fast atrial rate with slow ventricular rate might be present.

Treatment
- Vagal maneuver
- Class II, III, or IV antiarrhythmic drugs
- Electrical cardioversion
- Treatment of underlying cardiac disease

Outcome
- Long-term treatment might be necessary

Prevention
- Thorough preoperative assessment of patient for noncardiac and cardiac diseases.
- Conservative fluid therapy during pacemaker placement to reduce atrial distension.

Ventricular asystole

Definition
- Absence of ventricular complexes and cardiac output

Risk factors
- Failure of escape rhythm
- Anesthesia
- Electrolyte and acid–base disturbances

Diagnosis
- ECG: no wave forms; straight line on the ECG

Treatment
- Temporary pacing.

Prevention
- Temporary pacing using external pacing patches, or internal temporary pacing lead.

Surgical wound complications

Definition
Healing of the surgical wound is eventful because of reasons other than infection.

Risk factors
- Seroma formation at the PG site or cervical incision (transvenous technique)
  - Excessive dissection for PG placement
  - Failure to close dead space
- Hematoma: inadequate hemostasis
- Skin erosion over the PG
  - Patients with limited subcutaneous fat or thin skin (Figure 48.2)
  - Large PG
  - Subcutaneous placement of the PG
  - Migration of the PG
  - Other surgical wound complications
  - Self-trauma
  - Pacemaker rejection
- Sinus formation: using nonabsorbable multifilament suture material to secure the endocardial electrode
- Migration of the PG
  - Excessively large "bed" for PG
  - Failure to suture the generator in its "pocket"
  - Increasing weight or size of the generator
  - The effects of gravity
  - Seroma or hematoma formation
- Rejection of the pacemaker: rarely reported; risk factors are not established in cats and dogs

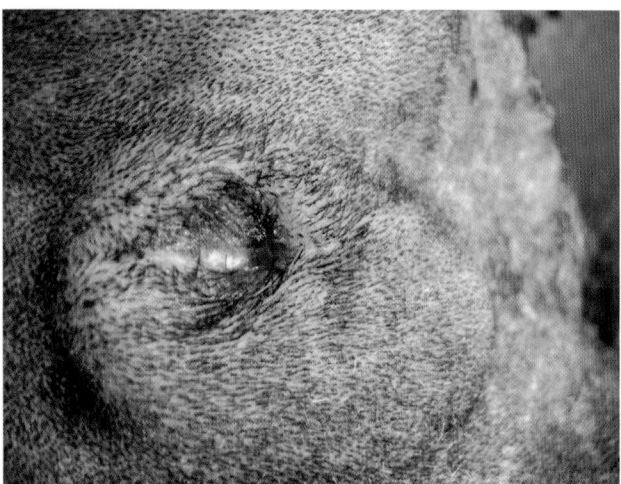

Figure 48.2 Skin erosion and purulent discharge overlying a pacemaker generator that was placed in the subcutaneous tissues of the neck in a patient with little subcutaneous fat. This patient has developed secondary infection associated with the skin erosion.

Diagnosis

- Migration of PG: observation by palpation or on radiographs
- Skin erosion over the PG: observation of skin at the site of generator placement. Bacterial culture and antibacterial sensitivity testing to identify concurrent bacterial infection.
- Sinus formation: discharging sinus
- Rejection of pacemaker
  - Resolution of wound complications on replacement of the pacemaker
  - Bacterial swabs will be sterile unless there is secondary bacterial infection.

Treatment

- Seroma: conservative (avoid aspiration and drainage because this may damage pacemaker lead or result in infection)
Hematoma: conservative (avoid aspiration and drainage as above)
- Skin erosion over the PG
  - For minor skin changes (erythema, superficial erosion), management changes (e.g., removal use of a harness) may be attempted.
  - Appropriate antibacterial therapy if the wound is infected
  - Wound debridement or excision for more extensive lesions
  - PG and lead should be completely replaced at an alternative site if the wound is contaminated or infected
  - If there is no contamination or infection, the generator can be replaced and should be relocated at an alternative site where it can be buried more deeply. The original site of pacemaker implantation is debrided and lavaged, and the wound is closed.
- Sinus formation
  - Antibacterial medications to reduce risk of infection (or to treat concurrent infection)
  - Removal of multifilament suture material; removal of pacemaker system might also be necessary
- Migration of the PG
  - No treatment is required if there are no associated clinical signs and pacemaker interrogation is unremarkable.
  - Surgery to relocate the PG with permanent suture anchorage.

- Rejection of the PG: removal of pacemaker and replacement with a generator of a different manufacturer

Prevention

- Seroma, hematoma, and pacemaker migration
  - Meticulous attention to dissection and hemostasis during implantation of the generator
  - Creation of a pocket of PG size
  - Suture the PG to underlying muscle or tissue.
  - Avoid neck collars.
  - Place a postoperative bandage for PG placement at the neck or thorax to reduce seroma formation.
  - Use monofilament nonabsorbable suture material to secure the lead in the jugular vein.
  - Transdiaphragmatic epicardial lead placement with PG anchored in a pocket between the internal and transverse abdominal muscles reduces the risk of seroma or hematoma formation.

Infection

Definition

Bacterial growth on or in the surgical incision, PG, or lead may occur after bacterial contamination at the time of surgery or secondary to bacterial translocation from a distant site.

Risk factors

- No specific risk factors have been identified in cats and dogs.
- Repeat surgical procedures for pacemaker-related complication (reported in human patients; likely to apply to cats and dogs)
- Non–infection-related surgical wound complication (i.e. hematoma)
- Failure to give prophylactic antibacterial medication
- Increasing duration of the procedure
- Using nonabsorbable multifilament suture material to secure the electrode in the vein

Diagnosis

- Suspect if the patient has a neutrophilia with a left shift
- Surgical incision or pacemaker related complications (e.g., pain, discharging wound, abscessation) (Figure 48.3)
- Recurrent pyrexia, pyothorax, pericarditis (infection associated with epicardial lead)
- Echocardiographic vegetations associated with electrode or heart valves (for endocardial leads)
- Positive bacterial culture of blood
- Positive bacterial culture from the implant or local tissues

Treatment

- Complete implant removal and PG and electrode replacement at another site and appropriate antibacterial medication
- Long-term antibacterial medication if removal of lead and pacemaker has to be delayed and the animal does not show signs of systemic disease

Outcome

Infection can be successfully managed with replacement of pacemaker and electrode and appropriate antibacterial medication treatment. However, if infection of a distant site is present, there is a higher risk of reinfection.

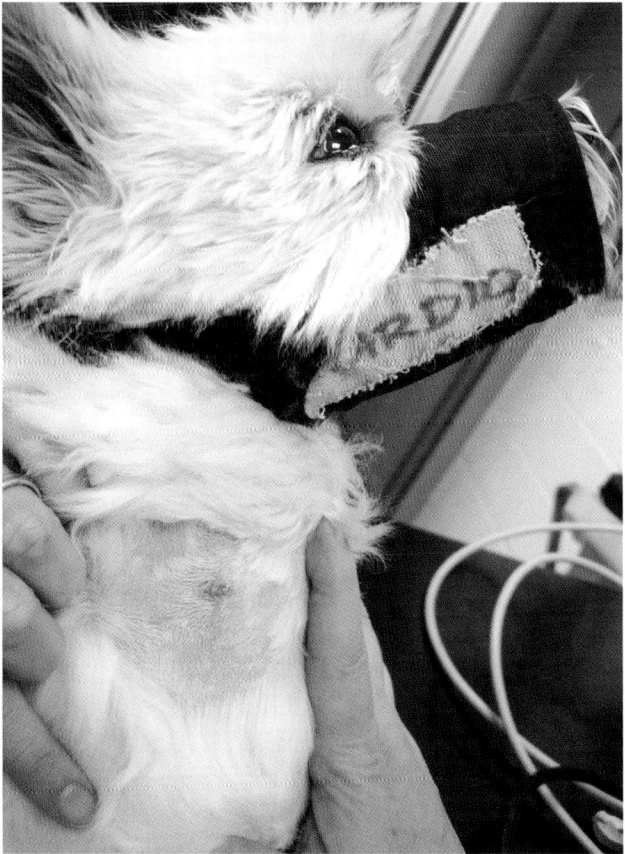

Figure 48.3 Infection, sinus formation, and recurrent purulent discharge that developed as a complication at the site of transvenous electrode placement.

Prevention

- Avoidance of implant- and wound-related complications (see Chapter 1)
- Prophylactic antibacterial medication
- Be vigilant for infections at distant sites (e.g., urinary tract infection, prostatitis, pyoderma, dental-related infections) and treat appropriately if possible before pacemaker placement.

Electrode detachment

Definition

This is separation of the electrode from the endocardial or epicardial surface or detachment of the electrode from the pacemaker with loss of transmission of the generated electrical impulse to the heart.

Risk factors

Epicardial

- Failure to adequately anchor the epicardial lead to the heart
- Connector pin is not completely inserted into the PG; set screw is not tightened
- Tension or traction on the pacing lead
  - No loop of lead
  - Trauma over the implantation site
  - Pacemaker migration (see earlier)
  - Rotation of the PG (Twiddler's or Reel's syndrome) (Figure 48.4)

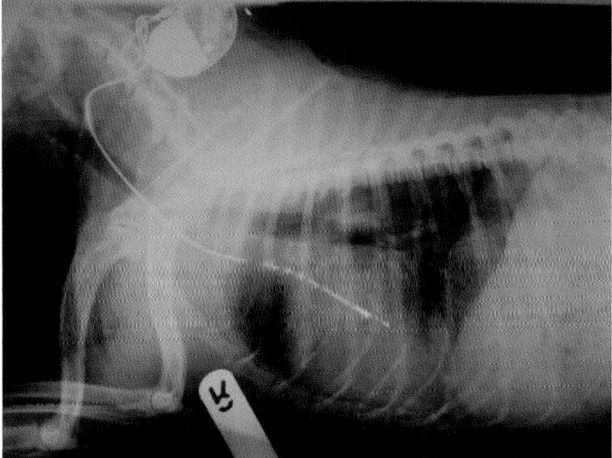

(A)

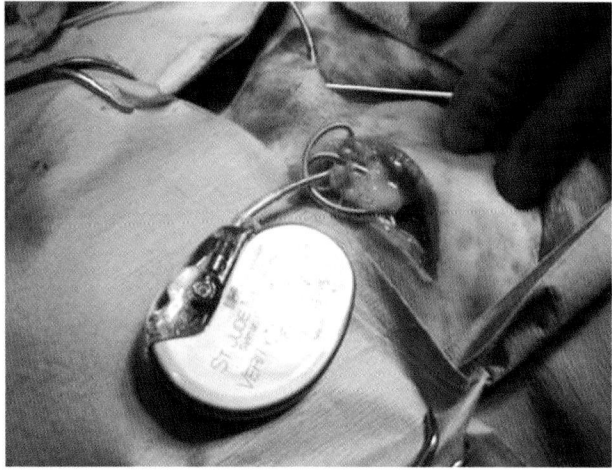

(B)

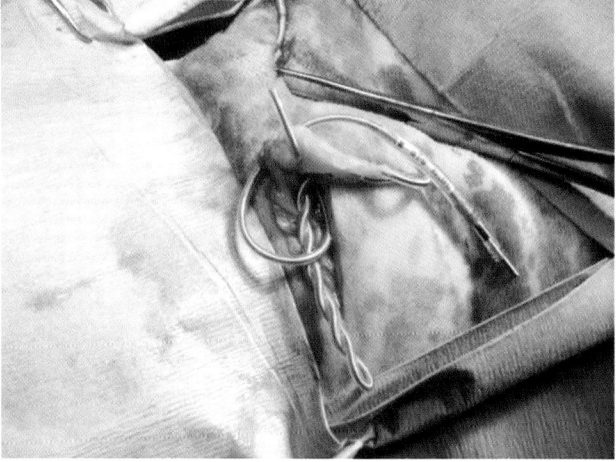

(C)

Figure 48.4 A, Lateral thoracic radiograph showing displacement of the endocardial lead and tight coiling of the lead at the location of the pacemaker. This dog continuously scratched its neck postoperatively, resulting in rotation of the generator and coiling and twisting of the lead (Twiddler's syndrome). **B** and **C**, The same dog underwent surgery to replace the electrode, and the lead was found to be tightly coiled and twisted.

Endocardial

- Improper screwing or lodging of the lead
- Lead sutures are not tightened securely
- Connector pin is not completely inserted into the PG; set screw is not tightened.
- Too little or too much slack of the lead
- Increased activity of the dog
- Movement of the pulse generator (see earlier discussion of epi-cardial lead)
- Tension or traction on the pacing lead as discussed earlier

Diagnosis

- Recurrence of clinical signs
- Bradyarrhythmia
- Malpositioning of the electrode seen on thoracic radiographs (Figure 48.5), fluoroscopy ("macrodisplacement"), or echocardiography
- Minimal displacement ("microdisplacement") of the electrode may not be recognized radiographically.
- ECG: loss of sensing or pacing; V-tac if the dislodged lead repeatedly impacts the ventricular myocardium
- Pacemaker interrogation: high voltage, normal lead impedance, increased capture threshold, loss of capture
- Diaphragmatic stimulation if a dislodged epicardial electrode contacts a phrenic nerve or the diaphragm

Treatment

This is treated with replacement or repositioning of the epicardial or endocardial electrode. If connection within the generator was inadequate, replacement of the lead or pulse generator is necessary.

Outcome

- If the patient develops an escape rhythm lead dislodgement, the patient can be considered as stable until replacement of the lead will restore pacing.

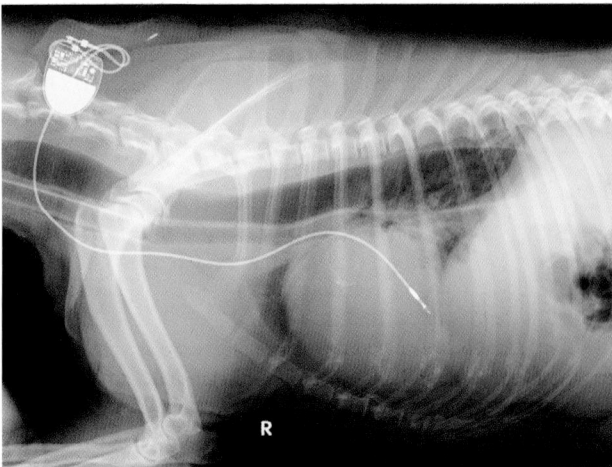

Figure 48.5 Right lateral thoracic radiograph of a dog having undergone transvenous pacemaker and active fixation lead placement, with lead malfunction observed postoperatively. Notice that the pacemaker is placed at the dorsal neck with the lead looped tightly as a "figure of eight" under the generator. In this patient, the electrode has become dislodged.

- Without development of an escape rhythm, immediate pacing is essential.
- If myocardial disease is present, further dislodgements of active leads are possible.

Prevention

Epicardial electrode detachment

- Ensure familiarity with the method of epicardial lead fixation (screw-in or sutured technique).
- When using a transdiaphragmatic approach in deep-chested dogs, placement of a screw-in electrode may be easier than suturing the electrode.
- Leave a loop of lead within the thorax or abdomen.
- Make a snug pocket for the pacemaker and suture the pacemaker to the underlying tissues.
- Ensure secure connection of lead and PG.
- Avoid direct trauma to the implantation site.

Endocardial electrode detachment

- Ensure the electrode is securely anchored at placement.
- Tight placement of sutures around the anchoring sleeve of the lead
- Local anesthetic on the surgery sites to minimize possible post-surgical irritation
- Strict cage rest; consider sedation after the procedure
- Restrict exercise for 4 to 6 weeks after surgery; avoid letting the dog jump or run
- See also points for epicardial leads.

Lead breakage

Definition

Lead breakage is damage of the lead or insulation of the lead, with loss of transmission of the generated electrical impulse to the heart and subsequent loss of pacing.

Risk factors

- External trauma over electrode, lead, or pacemaker implantation site
- Kinking, bending, or damaging of the lead during or after placement
- Drainage of postoperative seromas or hematomas
- Placing sutures directly around the lead; not using the anchoring sleeve
- Attempting jugular blood sampling (endocardial electrodes)
- Neck collars putting pressure or movement on the neck

Diagnosis

- Recurrence of clinical signs
- Bradyarrhythmia
- ECG: loss of pacing
- Lead fracture: increased lead impedance and elevated voltage threshold
- Insulation breakage: low or normal voltage and low impedance
- Complete breakage of a lead or a bent lead may be recognized on thoracic radiographs.

Treatment

- Replacement of the lead

Outcome

- As for lead dislodgement

Prevention

- Careful handling of the lead
- Pacemaker interrogation during the procedure should show adequate pacing and sensing thresholds and lead impedance.
- Place the lead in loose circles under the pulse generator. Avoid coils, tight circles, "figures of eight" (see Figure 48.5), and wrapping the lead around the generator.
- Avoid blood sampling from the jugular vein; avoid neck collars (for endocardial leads)

Electrode fibrosis

Definition

Electrode fibrosis is fibrous tissue formation at the electrode contact with the myocardium.

Risk factors

- Progressive myocardial disease
- Leads with non–steroid-eluting tips

Diagnosis

- Increasing pacing thresholds over time until capture is no longer occurring

Treatment

- Increasing pacing voltage and pulse width to regain capture
- Repositioning or replacing the lead
- Systemic steroids may have some beneficial effects.

Outcome

- As for lead dislodgement

Prevention

- Use of steroid-eluting electrodes
- Pacemaker interrogation at regular intervals and adjustment of pacemaker settings accordingly

Power source depletion or failure

Definition

This is generator malfunction, battery depletion, or damage that results in failure of the pacemaker.

Risk factors

- Placing a used pacemaker (battery depletion)
- Defibrillation or electrical cardioversion
- Magnetic resonance imaging (MRI)
- Cold temperature can cause a drop in battery voltage and resetting of the pacemaker.
- Inadvertent reprogramming or resetting into magnet mode
- Noise reversion caused by tachyarrhythmia
- Improper settings: low voltage, reduced pulse width, increased or reduced sensitivity
- General surgery using electrocautery: Electrocautery might cause resetting or reprogramming of the pacemaker and damage of the pacemaker electronics. The current induced in the lead may cause

internal burns and scarring, creating a higher pacing threshold or exit block.

Diagnosis

- No pacing: no pacing spikes; no or reduced numbers of pacing complexes on the ECG
- Recurrence of clinical signs, bradyarrhythmia
- Noise reversion: inappropriate pacing, which can occur during the vulnerable period of the T wave
- Undersensing or oversensing of the pacemaker
- Pacemaker interrogation reveals improper pacemaker settings.

Treatment

- Reprogramming of the pacemaker
- In case of battery failure or pacemaker failure or damage: generator replacement

Outcome

In case of resetting, reprogramming of the pacemaker will result in a functional pacemaker. Pacemaker replacement will restore pacing in the case of a faulty pacemaker.

Prevention

- Use of new pacemakers
- Careful storage of pacemakers
- Pacemaker interrogation after placement and at regular intervals
- MRI and electrical cardioversion only if necessary. Pacemaker function should be checked after these procedures.
- Avoid electrocautery during surgery.

Skeletal muscle stimulation

Definition

Stimulation of contraction of local skeletal muscle by the electrical activity created by the PG or in the case of lead displacement.

Risk factors

Stimulation of skeletal muscles overlying the generator
- Unipolar lead systems with the generator as anode of the pacing circuit
- Damage to the PG or insulation of the lead, resulting in leakage of voltage

Stimulation of the diaphragm
- Detachment of an epicardial electrode
- Malpositioning of an electrode, resulting in stimulation of a phrenic nerve (epi- and endocardial leads) or diaphragmatic muscle (endocardial electrode).
- Ventricular perforation (endocardial electrode).

Diagnosis

- Muscle twitch at the pacing frequency

Treatment

- No action may be necessary if the patient is not distressed by the muscle twitch. Skeletal muscle will become refractory to the stimulus, and the twitch will resolve after several weeks.
- Reduction in pacing voltage
- Reposition the electrode in the case of malpositioning or detachment of the electrode.
- Replace the damaged generator or damaged lead.

Outcome

Skeletal muscle twitching is generally well tolerated by the patient and usually resolves without treatment (although this depends on the underlying cause).

Prevention

- Avoid using donated PGs that have etching on one surface.
- If using PGs with etching, avoid contact of the etched surface with skeletal muscle.
- Ensure secure and correct positioning of the electrode.
- Avoid damage to the insulation of the lead.
- Place insulating pockets around the generator (human patients).

Thrombosis or thromboembolism

Definition

Thrombosis may result from endothelial injury, circulatory stasis or turbulence, and hypercoagulable state (Virchow's triad). The thrombus can detach and travel in the circulation and may become lodged in a vessel, obstructing further blood flow.

Risk factors

- Cardiac diseases
- Endothelial damage, flow obstruction and turbulence caused by endocardial leads
- Systemic diseases that increase coagulability
- Resterilization of leads, causing damage of the coating or insulation

Diagnosis

Large thrombi can result in flow obstructions, cranial vena cava syndrome, and right-sided CHF. Echocardiography can be used to identify thrombi associated with the electrode.

Treatment

- Aspirin, clopidogrel
- Heparin, or low-molecular-weight heparin
- Ballooning to resolve the obstruction
- Replacement of the lead

Outcome

The outcome depends on the severity of thrombus formation. Small thrombi can be clinically silent, and large thrombi can cause flow obstructions.

Prevention

Long-term anticoagulation treatment after pacemaker implantation is not routinely performed at present.

Right ventricular perforation by the pacing lead

Definition

This is displacement of the endocardial pacing lead, perforating the right ventricular wall.

Risk factors

- Not known in veterinary medicine
- Temporary pacing, corticosteroid use before pacemaker implantation, and use of active fixation leads are reported risk factors in human medicine.

Diagnosis

- Intermittent loss of capture, pacing failure
- Thoracic radiographs showing displacement of the lead
- Diaphragmatic stimulation at pacing rate
- Pacemaker interrogation showing a high capture voltage

Treatment

- Pericardiocentesis in cases of cardiac tamponade
  - Thoracotomy: withdrawal of the lead, but damage of tissues might occur if the lead has become attached to extracardiac structures. Cutting the lead tip might enable a safe removal.
- If the lead tip does not cause complication, a new lead can be placed without extracting the original one. Placement of an epicardial lead might be preferable.

Outcome

- As for lead dislodgment

Prevention

- Because risk factors are not known, prevention is not possible.

Pacemaker syndrome

Definition

This is fatigue, weakness, and occasionally development of CHF in patients with pacemakers.

Risk factors

- VVI pacing.
- Pacing from the right ventricular apex
  - Abnormal sequence of cardiac depolarization, loss of atrioventricular (AV) synchrony: reduced ventricular filling and reduced cardiac output.
- Preexisting cardiac disease

Diagnosis

- Observations obtained by owners
- CHF: physical examination, echocardiography, thoracic radiography

Treatment

- Treatment of heart failure (if present)

Outcome

- In cases of CHF, the prognosis is guarded because no physiological heart rate variation is possible.

Prevention

- Atrial pacing in cases without AVB (e.g. SSS)
- Rate responsive pacing
- Dual-chamber single-lead systems
- Dual-lead dual chamber pacing

Relevant literature

Transvenous placement is now the preferred technique of pacemaker implantation in dogs. Three large studies each including more than 100 dogs report the outcome of transvenous pacemaker implantation in dogs. Major complications were recorded in 13% to 34% patients and are listed in Table 49.2. There was no apparent difference in outcome whether using used or new pacemakers or whether endocardial leads were passive or active (Oyama *et al.* 2001; Wess *et al.* 2006; Johnson *et al.* 2007). Minor complications were recorded in 11% to 31% cases; these were usually treated conservatively and resolved in nearly all cases. An inverse association between complication rate and the number of pacemaker implantations performed by the surgeon was reported (Oyama *et al.* 2001). The two most recent reviews of complications of pacemaker systems using epicardial leads reported major complication rates of 25-28% in dogs, very similar to that reported for transvenous systems, but only 46 dogs were included in these two case series (Oyama *et al.* 2001; Visser *et al.* 2013). A major complication rate was reported in 2 of 5 cats undergoing pacemaker implantation using epicardial leads (Visser *et al.* 2013).

Arrhythmias can be caused by irritation and inflammation associated with electrode placement and are most common in the immediate postoperative period (Sisson *et al.* 1991; Oyama *et al.* 2001; Wess *et al.* 2006; Johnson *et al.* 2007). These typically resolve within days after pacemaker implantation. A small percentage of dogs (6%–13%) die suddenly, and malignant arrhythmias are suspected, which might be caused by pacemaker malfunctions or existing cardiovascular disease (Sisson *et al.* 1991; Oyama *et al.* 2001; Wess *et al.* 2006; Johnson *et al.* 2007).

Surgical wound complications are relatively common after pacemaker implantation. **Seroma** formation within the first 2 weeks of surgery is reported with variable incidence in up to approximately 25% of cases (Darke *et al.* 1989; Fox *et al.* 1991; Sisson *et al.* 1992; Oyama *et al.* 2001; Wess *et al.* 2006; Johnson *et al.* 2007). Seroma and hematoma formation are considered minor complications that resolve without treatment but may cause **pacemaker migration** and predispose to other complications, including discharging sinuses and infection (Darke *et al.* 1989; Fox *et al.* 1991; Johnson *et al.* 2007). Wess *et al.* (2006) suggested that placement of the pulse generator over the thorax instead of the cervical region could result in reduced occurrence of seroma, pulse generator migration, and infection. Pacemaker migration with or without skin erosion occurred in 12.5% cases reported by Sisson *et al.* (1991). It can be accompanied by detachment of the electrode, Twiddler's syndrome (see later discussion), skin ulceration, and pacemaker infection (Fox *et al.* 1991; Johnson *et al.* 2007). In more recent case series, pacemaker migration is not reported.

Infection is considered a serious complication and has been reported in up to 15% of patients undergoing pacemaker implantation (Lombard *et al.* 1981; Bonagura *et al.* 1983; Darke *et al.* 1989; Oyama *et al.* 2001; Wess *et al.* 2006; Fine and Tobias 2007; Johnson *et al.* 2007). Removal of the infected pacemaker system and replacement at a different site with appropriate antibacterial medication is generally associated with a good outcome (Oyama *et al.* 2001; Wess *et al.* 2006; Fine and Tobias 2007; Johnson *et al.* 2007). Antibacterial therapy alone is less successful. Potential predisposing causes of infection have included break in sterility during surgery, suture reaction, hindlimb abscess, and otitis externa (Fine and Tobias, 2007).

Pacemaker rejection is rare and was reported by Yoshioka *et al.* (1981) in 1 of 12 dogs undergoing epicardial electrode placement and was suspected in 1 of 33 dogs receiving a dual-chamber pacemaker undergoing a second intervention (Hildebrandt *et al.* 2009).

Detachment of epicardial electrodes is an uncommon complication with few cases reported (Bonagura *et al.* 1983; Fox *et al.* 1991; Oyama *et al.* 2001).

Electrode dislodgment is the most frequently occurring major complication associated with transvenous pacemaker implantation;

an incidence of 15% to 32.5% is reported (Sisson *et al.* 1991; Oyama *et al.* 2001; Bulmer *et al.* 2006; Wess *et al.* 2006; Johnson *et al.* 2007). Lead detachment occurs most commonly during recovery and in the first days after implantation (Oyama *et al.* 2001; Bulmer *et al.* 2006; Wess *et al.* 2006; Johnson *et al.* 2007; Hildebrandt *et al.* 2009). It may be associated with surgeon experience and increased activity level of the dog (Oyama *et al.* 2001; Wess *et al.* 2006; Johnson *et al.* 2007). No difference in dislodgement was found for active and tined fixation leads (Oyama *et al.* 2001; Wess *et al.* 2006; Johnson *et al.* 2007).

Cardiac perforation is a rarely reported complication in veterinary medicine and might be more frequent with active fixation leads (Oyama *et al.* 2001; Achen *et al.* 2008).

Twiddler's syndrome is an uncommon complication (Fox *et al.* 1991; Oyama *et al.* 2001; Zimmerman and Bright 2004; Johnson *et al.* 2007) that can result in lead detachment. To restore pacing, replacement of the lead is required. Scratching of the neck, rolling on the back, inadequate fixation of the PG or lead, obesity, and seroma formation have been suspected as causes (Zimmerman and Bright 2004; Johnson *et al.* 2007).

Only single cases of epicardial and endocardial **lead breakage** or damage were reported, which are serious complications because they can result in loss of pacing (Lombard *et al.* 1981; Fox *et al.* 1986; Oyama *et al.* 2001; Wess *et al.* 2006).

Electrode fibrosis is a rare complication that can lead to exit block. Furthermore, progression of underlying myocardial disease can result in increased myocardial fibrosis and exit block (Oyama *et al.* 2001; Wess *et al.* 2006; Johnson *et al.* 2007).

Pacemaker failure caused by battery depletion might occur if used pacemakers with short battery lives are implanted (Oyama *et al.* 2001; Johnson *et al.* 2007). Malfunction of the pacemaker can be caused by inappropriate pacemaker settings, changes in electrode-myocardial contact (exit block), resetting, noise reversion or failure of the screw-PG interface through mechanical failure or operator error. (Moise and Estrada 2002; Coleman *et al.* 2012). Treatment of concurrent tachyarrhythmias (Moise and Estrada 2002) and regular interrogations of the pacemaker, with reprogramming if needed, will reduce the risk of pacing during vulnerable periods, which might be the cause for sudden deaths.

Skeletal muscle twitch is considered a minor complication and was recognized in 5% to 12.5% of the cases (Bonagura *et al.* 1983; Fox *et al.* 1986; Sisson *et al.* 1991; Oyama *et al.* 2001). It occurs more frequently with unipolar systems and donated pacemakers with etching on the back to identify that they are not for use in humans. These pacemakers should be implanted with the etched side down to avoid contraction of the overlying musculature (Estrada 2010). Most cases respond to reduction of the pacing voltage (Oyama *et al.* 2001). Furthermore, muscle twitch often resolves with time because the skeletal muscle becomes refractory to the pacing stimulus (Oyama *et al.* 2001).

Cranial and caudal vena cava obstructions caused by pacemaker lead–induced stricture with suspected secondary fibrosis and **thrombosis** are rarely reported (Cunningham *et al.* 2009; Stauthammer *et al.* 2009). Successful treatment included anticoagulant therapy and balloon dilation (Cunningham *et al.* 2009; Stauthammer *et al.* 2009).

Pacemaker syndrome is associated with fatigue, weakness, dizziness, and lethargy in human patients and is therefore difficult to identify in veterinary patients. However, it can be associated with progressive myocardial dysfunction and eventually myocardial failure, which can be caused by loss of normal sequence of ventricular depolarization and AV asynchrony (Oyama *et al.* 2001; Wess *et al.* 2006; Johnson *et al.* 2007).

References

Achen, S.E., Miller, M.W., Nelson, D.A., et al. (2008) Late cardiac perforation by a passive-fixation permanent pacemaker lead in a dog. *Journal of the American Veterinary Medical Association* 233, 1291-1296.

Bonagura, J.D., Helphrey, M.L., Muir, W.W. (1983) Complications associated with permanent pacemaker implantation in the dog. *Journal of the American Veterinary Medical Association* 182, 149-155.

Bulmer, B.J., Sisson, D.D., Oyama, M.A., et al. (2006) Physiologic VDD versus non-physiologic VVI pacing in canine 3rd-degree atrioventricular block. *Journal of Veterinary Internal Medicine* 20, 257-271.

Coleman, A.E., DeFrancesco, T.C., Chanoit, G. (2012) Pacemaker malfunction due to mechanical failure of the lead-header interface. *Journal of Veterinary Cardiology* 14, 519-523.

Cunningham, S.M., Ames, M.K., Rush, J.E., et al. (2009) Successful treatment of pacemaker-induced stricture and thrombosis of the cranial vena cava in two dogs by use of anticoagulants and balloon venoplasty. *Journal of the American Veterinary Medical Association*, 235, 1467-1473.

Darke, P.G., McAreavey, D., Bean, M. (1989) Transvenous cardiac pacing in 18 dogs and one cat. *Journal of Small Animal Practice* 30, 491-499.

Estrada, A. (2010) Artificial pacing of the heart. In Ettinger, S., Feldman, E. (eds.) *Textbook of Veterinary Internal Medicine*, 7th edn. WB Saunders, St. Louis, pp. 1243-1250.

Ferasin, L., van de Stad, M., Rudorf, H., et al. (2002) Syncope associated with paroxysmal atrioventricular block an ventricular standstill in a cat. *Journal of Small Animal Practice* 43, 124-128.

Fine, T., Fine, D.M., Tobias, A.H. (2007) Cardiovascular device infections in dogs: report of 8 cases and review of the literature. *Journal of Veterinary Internal Medicine* 21, 1265-71.

Fingeroth, J.M., Birchard, S.J. (1986) Transdiaphragmatic approach for permanent cardiac pacemaker implantation in dogs. *Veterinary Surgery* 15, 329-333.

Fox et al. (1986) Fox PR, Matthiesen, DT., Purse D., Brown, NO. (1986). Ventral abdominal, transdiaphragmatic approach for implantation of cardiac pacemakers in the dog. *Journal of the American Veterinary Medical Association* 189, 1303-1308.

Fox et al. (1991) Fox, PR., Moise, NS., Woodfield JA., Darke, PG (1991). Techniques and complications of pacemaker implantation in four cats. *Journal of the American Veterinary Medical Association* 199, 1742-53.

Hildebrandt, N., Stertmann, W.A., Wehner, M., et al. (2009) Dual chamber pacemaker implantation in dogs with atrioventricular block. *Journal of Veterinary Internal Medicine* 23, 31-38.

Johnson, M.S., Martin, M.W., Henley, W. (2007) Results of pacemaker implantation in 104 dogs. *Journal of Small Animal Practice* 48, 4-11.

Lombard, C.W., Tilley, L.P., Yoshioka, M.M. (1981) Pacemaker implantation in the dog: survey and literature review. *Journal of the American Animal Hospital Association*, 17, 751-758.

Moise, N.S., Estrada, A. (2002) Noise reversion in paced dogs. *Journal of Veterinary Cardiology* 4, 13-21.

Oyama, M.A., Sisson, D.D., Lehmkuhl, L.B. (2001) Practices and outcome of artificial cardiac pacing in 154 dogs. *Journal of Veterinary Internal Medicine* 15, 229-239.

Stauhammer, C., Tobias, A., France, M., Olson, J. (2009) Caudal vena cava obstruction caused by redundant pacemaker lead in a dog. *Journal of Veterinary Cardiology* 11, 141-145.

Sisson, D., Thomas, W.P., Woodfield, J., Pion, P.D., Luethy, M., DeLellis, L.A. (1991) Permanent transvenous pacemaker implantation in forty dogs. *Journal of Veterinary Internal Medicine* 5, 322-331.

Visser, L.C. Keene, B.W., Mathews, K.G., et al. (2013) Outcomes and complications associated with epicardial pacemakers in 28 dogs and 5 cats, Veterinary Surgery, 42, 544-550.

Wess, G., Thomas, W.P., Berger, D.M., Kittleson, M.D. (2006) Applications, complications, and outcomes of transvenous pacemaker implantation in 105 dogs (1997-2002). *Journal of Veterinary Internal Medicine* 20, 877-884.

Yoshioka, M.M., Tilley, L.P., Harvey, H.J., Wayne, E.S., Lombard, C.W., Schollmeyer, M. (1981) Permanent pacemaker implantation in the dog. *Journal of the American Animal Hospital Association* 17, 746-750.

Zimmerman, S.A., Bright, J.M. (2004) Secure pacemaker fixation critical for prevention of Twiddler's syndrome. *Journal of Veterinary Cardiology* 6, 40-44.

General Abdominal Surgery

49 Celiotomy

Hilde de Rooster

Department of Small Animal Medicine and Clinical Biology, Faculty of Veterinary Medicine, Ghent University, Ghent, Belgium

Abdominal surgeries are common procedures in most companion animal veterinary practices. In the majority of cases, a ventral midline approach is chosen for abdominal procedures. Access to the abdomen can also be obtained by means of a paramedian or a paracostal incision. Occasionally, a combined approach is used.

The abdominal wall consists of four muscle layers, each having a different fiber orientation. From outward to inward, the abdominal muscles are the external abdominal oblique, internal abdominal oblique, rectus abdominis, and transversus abdominis. In the ventral midline, the right and left half of the abdominal wall meet in the linea alba (Hermanson and Evans 1993).

The complication rate after celiotomy is poorly documented in companion animals. In nontraumatized dogs and cats, more than 60% of the postoperative complications after exploratory celiotomy are disease-related (Boothe *et al.* 1992). An incidence rate of "true" incision-related problems as low as 0.18% has been described (Crowe 1978). Morbidity associated with exploration of the abdomen is further decreased by choosing a laparoscopic approach (Schippers *et al.* 1998). The true incidence of iatrogenically induced complications after celiotomy in dogs and cats is difficult to determine. In cats, inflammatory swelling at the ventral midline incision site is a fairly common postsurgical finding (Freeman *et al.* 1987). The condition is self-limiting, and treatment is not necessary. Acute wound breakdown usually occurs 3 to 5 days after surgery. Herniation and evisceration are most likely caused by technical surgical errors during linea alba closure (Smeak 1993). Wound infection occurs in 2.5% to 5.5% of the surgical procedures in dogs and cats (Vasseur *et al.* 1988; Brown *et al.* 1997) and may require a second surgical intervention, especially if the abdominal wall is also involved.

Infections
See Chapter 1.

Peritonitis
See Chapter 4.

Dehiscence
See Chapter 9.

Herniation and evisceration

Definition
An incisional hernia occurs when a surgically closed abdominal fascia loses integrity. Acute incisional hernias occur before or at the time of suture removal. There is a risk of evisceration in the presence of skin dehiscence. Exposed viscera are prone to trauma and self-mutilation. Chronic incisional hernias are diagnosed weeks to years after the original surgical procedure. They rarely cause evisceration because the overlying skin incision has usually fully healed.

Risk factors
Risk factors for herniation ± evisceration are summarized in Table 49.1.

Diagnosis
The diagnosis of herniation is easy to make (Figure 49.1). Herniation without skin disruption, however, should be differentiated from other causes of subcutaneous swelling.

- The most common clinical signs consist of wound swelling or serosanguineous drainage caused by abdominal structure entrapment or fluid accumulation in the subcutaneous space (Figure 49.2).
- It may be possible to palpate the defect in the abdominal wall. The hernia may or may not be reducible. The swelling should be palpated carefully to discern the contents of the hernia.
- Ultrasonography might be useful to evaluate the integrity of the different layers of the abdominal wall and to confirm herniation (Figure 49.3). Ultrasound examination also helps to define the contents of the hernia.

Treatment
Evisceration is a true emergency; whereas acute incisional herniation is a relative emergency, chronic incisional hernia repair can be scheduled as an elective procedure in the majority of cases.

- Cover eviscerated organs with wet towels or sheets, preferably sterile.
- Avoid further contamination and prevent self-mutilation.
- Administer intravenous (IV) fluids, IV broad-spectrum antibiotics, and analgesics.
- Avoid further loss of body warmth.

Complications in Small Animal Surgery, First Edition. Edited by Dominique Griffon and Annick Hamaide.
© 2016 John Wiley & Sons, Inc. Published 2016 by John Wiley & Sons, Inc.
Companion website: www.wiley.com/go/griffon/complications

Table 49.1 Risk factors for herniation or evisceration after celiotomy

Technical errors	Patient factors

Suture pull-out
• Inadequate tissue mass
• Poor holding strength
• Excessive forces
	Impaired collagen remodeling
	• Metabolic disease
	   ○ Diabetes mellitus
	   ○ Hyperadrenocorticism
	   ○ Hypoproteinemia
	   ○ Anemia
	   ○ Fluid or electrolyte imbalances
	• Iatrogenic
	   ○ Corticosteroids
	   ○ Chemotherapy
	   ○ Radiation
	• Extreme age (very young or very old)

Inappropriate suture material • Material properties • Suture breakage	Excessive force on the suture line • Obesity • Ascites • Abdominal tension • Unrestricted activity

Surgical incompetence
• Incorrect placement
• Muscle rather than fascia
• Subcutis instead of fascia
• Excessive space between stitches
• Incorporation of fatty tissues
• Poor knot tying
• Excessive dissection of subcutaneous tissue
	• Immunosuppression
	   ○ Feline immunodeficiency virus
	   ○ Feline leukemia virus

Introduction of infection	Introduction of infection (self-trauma)
Combination of the above	Combination of the above

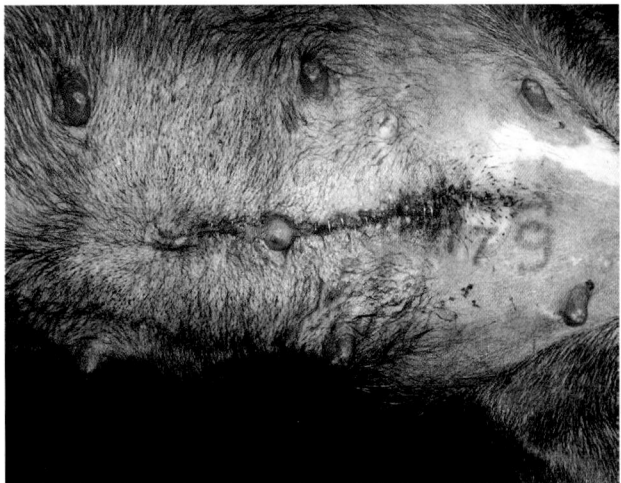

Figure 49.1 Dog presented with evisceration of omental tissue 3 days after routine spaying.

- Prepare for aseptic surgery by avoiding detergents and alcohol solutions.
- Lavage the herniated organs extensively with warm sterile saline outside the abdomen. Antiseptics and soaps should be avoided in lavage of abdominal contents because they predispose to peritonitis.
- Resect devitalized or severely contaminated tissue before reduction.
- Close the abdominal wall temporarily to allow extra surgical preparation if needed.
- Remove the whole previously placed suture line.
- Excise devitalized tissue around the wound margins but avoid unnecessary trimming (Figure 49.4).
- Lavage the abdominal cavity extensively with warm sterile saline.
- Close the rectus abdominis fascia with long-lasting absorbable suture material.
- Use extra mattress or cruciate suture patterns whenever needed.

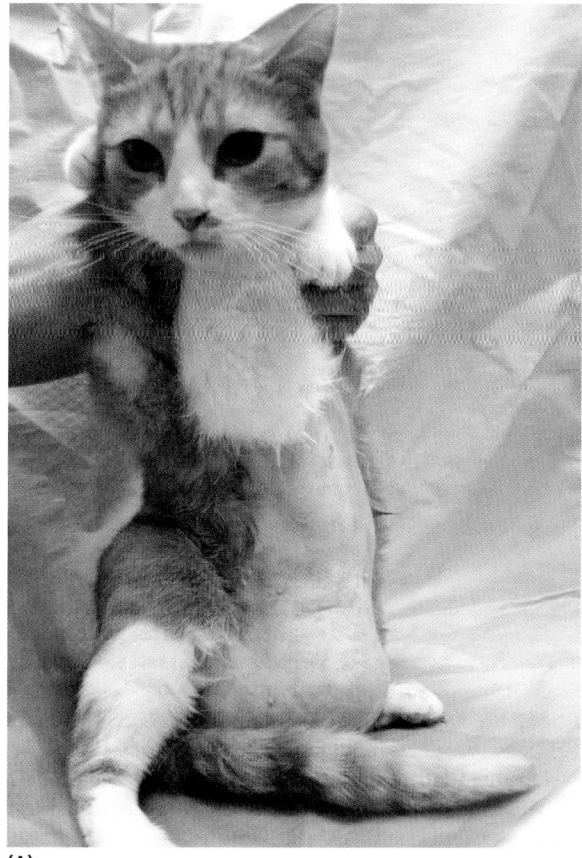

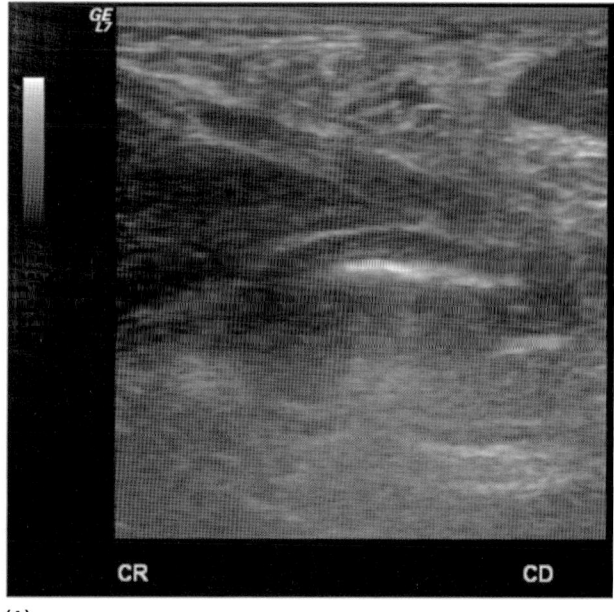

(A)

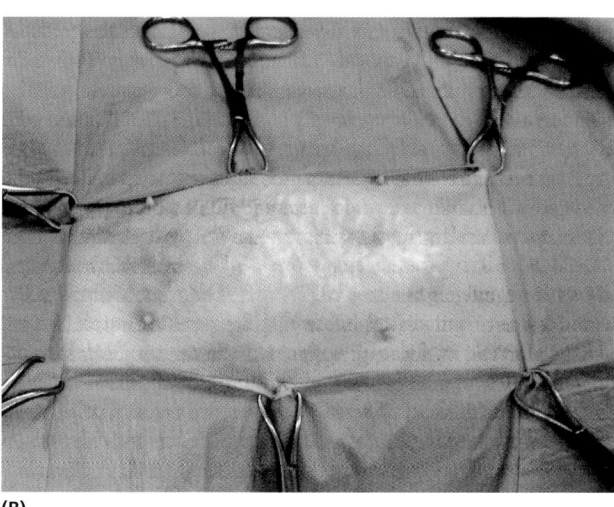

(B)

Figure 49.2 A, Cat presented with a gradually enlarging subcutaneous swelling 2 years after ovariohysterectomy. **B**, In ventral recumbency, a defect in the linea alba could be palpated. Notice the old scars visible on the skin from several previous attempts to close the incisional herniation.

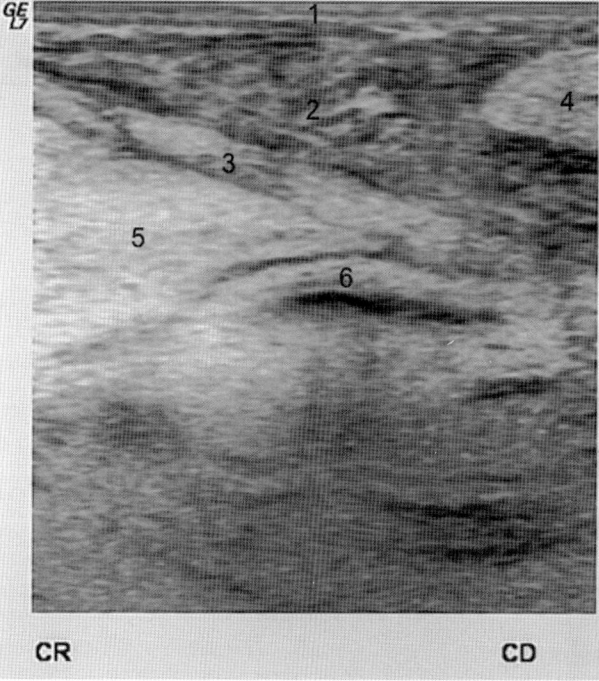

(B)

Figure 49.3 Ultrasonographic image (**A**) and matching schematic image (**B**) of an abdominal hernia in a cat. Left is cranial, and top is ventral. Mesenteric and abdominal fat (2) and the spleen (4) are identified between the skin (1) and the rectus abdominis muscle (3). The liver (5) and the stomach (6) are present within the peritoneal cavity.

• Close the subcutis and skin in routine fashion.
• Control for hypoalbuminemia or signs of peritonitis.
In the absence of skin disruption, a traditional surgical scrub can be used, and temporary closure is not an issue. Debridement of the linea alba is generally not advised because it will lead to an extra delay in the healing process.

Outcome

The outcome of incisional hernias has not been specifically addressed in the literature. The prognosis will vary with the degree of damage and contamination of the herniated viscera. In the majority of cases, the suture line on the linea alba will heal uneventfully if the underlying cause has been addressed.

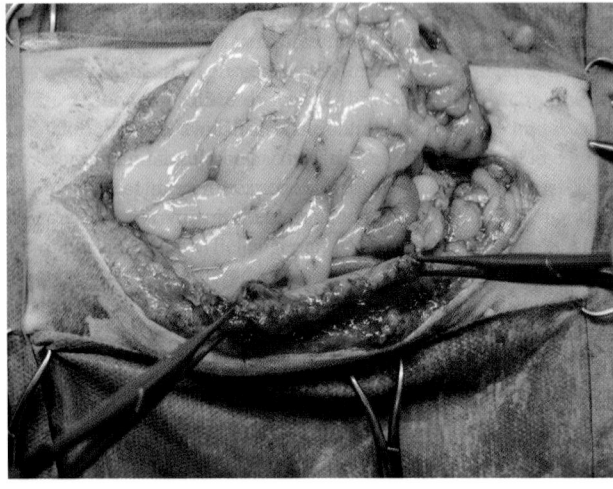 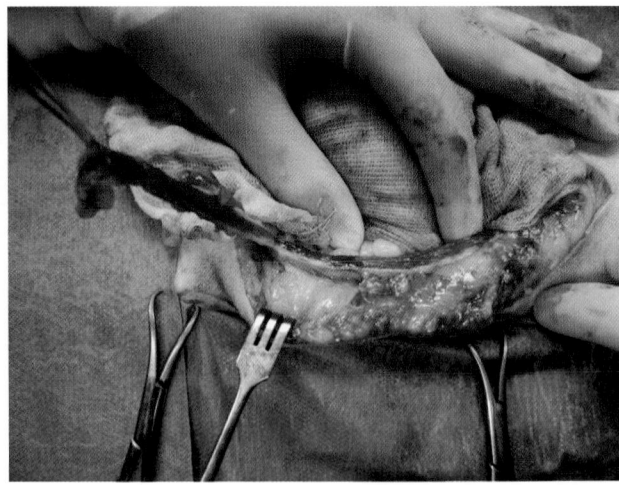

(A)   **(B)**

Figure 49.4 **A** and **B**, Trimming of the wound edges is not routinely performed in hernia repair unless the rim is devitalized or not clean (e.g., if it contains a lot of fatty tissue as in this patient).

Prevention

A good surgical technique will prevent the majority of incisional herniations.
- Identify the linea alba carefully.
- Do not allow fat to become trapped between the suture edges.
- Select long-lasting absorbable monofilament suture of appropriate thickness.
- Check the expiration date of the suture.
- Apply sufficient throws, especially if a continuous suture line is used.
- Add mattress or cruciate sutures whenever fascial tissues appear friable.
- Insist on postoperative restriction of activity.
- Prevent licking and self-mutilation.
- Treat underlying diseases.
- Infrequently, reinforcement of the suture line can be achieved by implementing a prosthetic mesh between the omentum and the body wall (Figure 49.5).

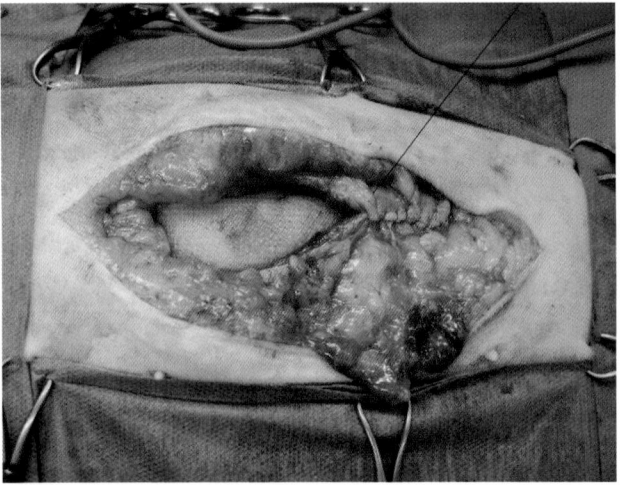

Figure 49.5 In selected cases, the use of a synthetic mesh can be considered. The omentum is nicely spread to cover all abdominal contents, and a Prolene mesh is positioned on top of it. A continuous polydioxanone suture is placed on the rectus sheath, anchoring the prosthesis within the first and the last knot. *Source:* Bellon *et al.*, 2006. Reproduced with permission from Elsevier.

Adhesions

Definition

Adhesions are scar tissue connecting tissues that are not normally connected.

Postoperative adhesions form preferentially with the inner surface of the abdominal wall at the level of the incision or between intraabdominal organs. In selected cases, adhesions may be essentially protective to isolate a local process or to increase vascular supply to injured tissues. Dogs and cats have an efficient balance between fibrinolysis and physiologic fibrin deposition, preventing clinically relevant adhesion formation in most cases.

Risk factors

Surgical manipulations create an imbalance of the fibrinolytic system.
- Serosal trauma
- Ischemia
- Hemorrhage
- Foreign bodies
- Inflammation
- Infection
- Abdominal lavage
- Suturing of the peritoneum

Diagnosis

Clinically irrelevant intraabdominal adhesions will be diagnosed incidentally at the time of repeated exploration of the abdomen (Figure 49.6). During diagnostic laparoscopy, the adhesions may eventually limit an overall view of the abdomen.
- If postoperative adhesions cause obstruction, kinking, or entrapment of abdominal organs, the **clinical signs will be related to the affected organ system**. Being moveable tubular abdominal organs, the small intestines and ureters are most prone to obstruction.
- **Ultrasonographic evaluation** of the complete abdomen is indicated to identify pathologies induced by intraabdominal adhesions. The adhesions themselves can be assessed if free abdominal fluid is present or after instillation of isotonic saline solution into the abdominal cavity.

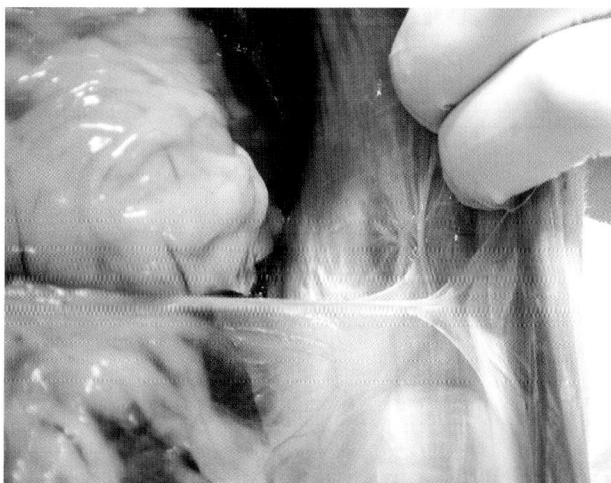

Figure 49.6 Extensive intraabdominal adhesions between the peritoneum and the abdominal organs caused by a previous enterotomy.

- When strangulation is suspected, emergency exploratory celiotomy should be performed (Figure 49.7).

Treatment
- Surgical resection of the adhesions
- Release of entrapped abdominal organ
- Resection of irreversibly damaged tissue
  ∘ Segmental enterectomy
  ∘ Removal of a hydronephrotic kidney
  ∘ Splenectomy, liver lobectomy, and so on

Outcome
Whenever abdominal organs become entrapped, there is a potential risk of necrosis or obstruction. Depending on the affected organ and the severity of the pathology, the condition will vary from reversible to fatal.

Prevention
Postsurgical adhesion formation may be reduced by limiting the causes of peritoneal irritation at the time of celiotomy.

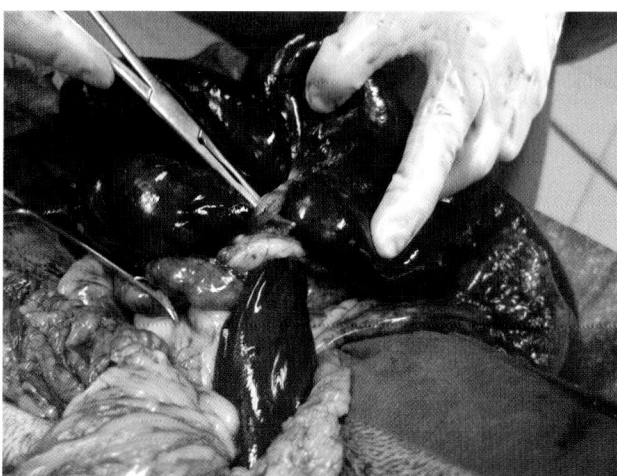

Figure 49.7 Extensive necrosis of the small intestines after entrapment of the intestinal loops behind a fibrous intraabdominal adhesion.

- Handle tissues atraumatically.
- Protect against tissue desiccation.
- Adhere closely to aseptic techniques.
- Control hemostasis.
- Avoid irritating lavage solutions.
- Do not include the peritoneum in the suture line.
- Consider laparoscopy rather than celiotomy.

Iatrogenic abdominal foreign body

Definition
This is unintentionally retained material after celiotomy. The most common iatrogenic abdominal foreign bodies are lint from sponges or towels or an entire surgical sponge remaining inside the patient after closing. Iatrogenic retained material is mostly sterile, but it is likely to induce foreign body granuloma formation that may become a nidus for infection. This reaction is called "textiloma" or "gossypiboma." Surgical instruments and needles are the second most common type of foreign bodies left behind after abdominal surgery.

Risk factors
- Complex or prolonged surgical procedures
- Emergency surgical procedures
- Unexpected change in the course of a surgical procedure
- Troublesome hemostasis
- High body mass
- Use of unusually large number of instruments or sponges
- Use of small-sized sponges

Diagnosis
- The diagnosis of iatrogenic abdominal foreign body is suspected in any patient that has celiotomy in the medical history and present with abdominal complaints.
- The clinical symptoms and the time of presentation relate mainly to the extent of bacterial contamination and the reaction of the body. If symptoms develop early in the postoperative period, they are usually associated with bacterial contamination.
- Commonly, **an abdominal mass can be palpated**. Retained material is often misdiagnosed as an intraabdominal tumor or abscess, especially when the mass is located adjacent to an abdominal organ.
- The **use of medical imaging** is likely to narrow the list of differential diagnosis. Depending on the radiopacity of the retained material, **radiography** may or may not be helpful in diagnosing and locating the retained material. Unfortunately, the radiopaque wire markers in surgical sponges are known to disintegrate and will become less conspicuous with time. Ultrasonography of a textiloma will show poorly echogenic or cystic mass, featuring a hyperechoic area of wavy structures and sharply delineated acoustic shadow. In complex situations, **abdominal** computed tomography will be rewarding to identify a well-defined inhomogeneous hypoattenuating mass.

Treatment
A second exploratory celiotomy is inevitable. The intraabdominal retained material should be removed as soon as the diagnosis is made. The morbidity caused by the foreign body will increase with time, causing further complications such as late infection, migration, and fistulation.

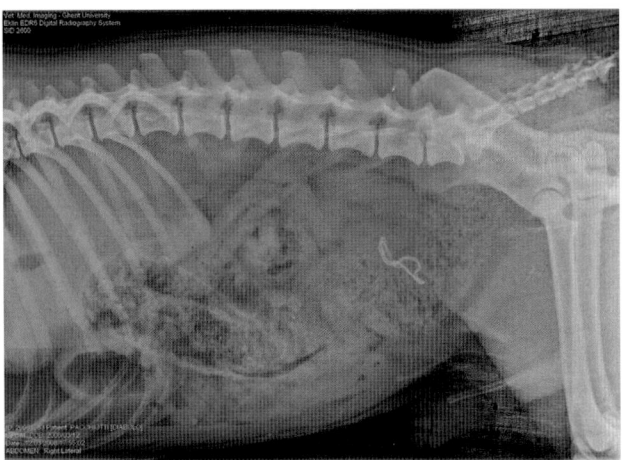

Figure 49.8 Postoperative radiograph in a dog with an incorrect number of sponges recovered after an exploratory celiotomy. The radiopaque wire marker demonstrates the presence of the sponge.

Complete removal of the retained foreign body and the induced granuloma should be attempted. The relation between the lesion and the abdominal organs may necessitate removal of the affected organ. Drainage and omentalization is an alternative to complete removal of an abscess.

Outcome

Complications caused by iatrogenic foreign bodies are frequent, and the morbidity rate can be high. The incited inflammatory reaction may cause obstruction of tubular organs. The prognosis is highly dependent on the degree of bacterial contamination. Sooner or later, sepsis will occur, sometimes leading to death. A poor prognosis is given in cases with malignant transformation of the granulomatous inflammation induced by the foreign body.

Prevention

- Only use sponges with radiopaque wire markers for intraabdominal procedures.
- Count the sponges before the surgical procedure begins.
- Count extra sponges at the time of addition.
- Use sponges that are not prone to linting.
- Tag small sponges by attaching them to an instrument.
- Do not cut surgical sponges.
- Use the minimum number of sponges needed.
- Provide careful hemostasis.
- Thoroughly explore the surgical field.
- Inspect the area surrounding the surgical field.
- Count sponges accurately and repeatedly at the conclusion of the intraabdominal procedure before closure.
- Perform radiography or surgically reexplore whenever there is a suspicion that a sponge or instrument has been left behind (Figure 49.8).

Relevant literature

Postoperative wound infection remains a serious complication after abdominal surgery (Vasseur *et al.* 1988; Brown *et al.* 1997). Wound infection might lead to peritonitis, intraabdominal adhesion, and possibly life-threatening conditions. Exposure of the mesothelial surfaces to air during celiotomy or laparoscopy will cause a subclinical aseptic peritonitis in all cases (Crowe and Bjorling 1993). More severe aseptic peritonitis may occur because of sterile foreign bodies or after surgical contamination (Swann and Hughes 2000).

Incision-related complications after exploratory celiotomy were mentioned in 4% of the patients in a case series of 200 companion animals, but no details on the type or sequela of these problems were provided (Boothe *et al.* 1992).

Swelling at the surgery site is a fairly common postsurgical finding. Extensive undermining of the wound edges might lead to seroma formation and carries a small risk of subsequent skin disruption (Smeak 1993). Certain systemic diseases predispose to impaired wound healing (Smeak 1993).

It is important to **ensure long-lasting repair of the abdominal incision** because it has been shown that only 20% of the tensile strength of the linea alba is regained 3 weeks after celiotomy (Miller 1970). Owing to the modern synthetic absorbable suture materials, closure of the abdominal wall has become much safer. Nevertheless, clear discharge instructions should always be provided to the owner. It is imperative to stress the importance of activity restriction during the first weeks after celiotomy.

The different layers of the abdominal wall do not all need to be sutured after a ventral midline approach. Peritoneum heals rapidly across the incision (Henderson 1993). Available evidence suggests that closure of the peritoneum is not beneficial for wound strength and should be avoided (Rosin and Richardson 1987; Anderson 2005). Inclusion of the muscle component in the sutures is considered to add more pain. The current recommendations are to appose only the fascia of the rectus abdominis muscle. The rectus sheath is composed of an external and internal leaf (Hermanson and Evans 1993) of which only the external leaf needs to be closed (Rosin and Richardson 1987).

There is no experimental or clinical evidence to support the assumption that the use of a continuous suture pattern increases the risk of wound disruption. Furthermore, it is significantly faster than simple interrupted sutures (Crowe 1978). The use of barbed sutures to close the abdominal incision in a continuous suture pattern has recently been described by the author. Theoretically, they combine optimal wound apposition and wound healing with reduced surgery time and complication rate.

There is no controlled veterinary study describing the incidence of **incisional hernias** in companion animals. Herniation, especially eventration, may present as a true emergency. Incisional herniation and evisceration are sporadically mentioned in retrospective studies. There appears to be a correlation between the reason for the surgical access to the abdomen and the risk of dehiscence. It is notable that the few reported cases of evisceration in dogs occurred after elective ovariohysterectomies (Crowe 1978; Boothe *et al.* 1992).

Despite a large number of clinical and experimental studies, the pathophysiology of **postoperative adhesion development** remains controversial. Minimizing mechanical injury to the peritoneal surfaces and reducing the amount of foreign material and blood reduce the incidence of adhesions (Ellis 2007). Available evidence in dogs suggests that inclusion of the peritoneum in the suture repair may predispose to adhesion formation after celiotomy (Anderson 2005). Likewise, less adhesion formation is seen after a laparoscopic approach than after a conventional celiotomy (Schippers *et al.* 1998). The reduced risk might be explained by the smaller peritoneal defects and the decreased manipulation and desiccation of the serosal surfaces.

If fibrin deposition overrules fibrinolysis during the first week after the surgical manipulation, fibrinous adhesions mature to fibrous tissue rather than resolving (Henderson 1993). Adhesion-related complications are common after abdominal surgery in humans (Ellis 2007). The dog is used as a model in various experimental studies on prevention of postoperative intraabdominal adhesion formation in human medicine. The use of heparin or other drugs to reduce fibrin formation and indirectly adhesion formation remains controversial (Akman et al. 2008). However, the balance between fibrinolysis and fibrin formation seems much more efficient in dogs and cats compared with humans and horses, and most of the time, the clinical relevance is negligible (Henderson 1993).

The incidence of intraabdominal **retained foreign bodies** is difficult to determine and is not reported in companion animals. Early detection is often difficult, and the patient may present with vague symptoms for a prolonged period of time. In humans, the reported prevalence varies between 0.3 and 1 per 1000 celiotomies (Stawicki et al. 2009), but this rate is most probably underestimated. It has to be emphasized that; although emergency surgeries are implicated in 30% of cases, approximately 70% of retained material is associated with purely elective surgical procedures.

The suspicion of an intraabdominal foreign body may exist at the time of closure or shortly after. Anesthesia will be extended and the abdomen will need to be reopened. If the foreign body cannot be located by reexploring the abdomen, the patient must be transported to the radiographic unit and brought back to the surgical suite afterward.

If a foreign body is accidentally retained, a classic foreign body granuloma will formed because the body attempts to wall it off. Some granulomas may remain dormant, but others may have serious consequences. In acute presentations, bacterial invasion generally leads to the formation of an intraabdominal abscess and subsequent sepsis. Delayed cases generally present as granulomatous inflammation, a few of which may undergo neoplastic transformation (Miller et al. 2006).

Theoretically, iatrogenic intraabdominal bodies are completely preventable. Guidelines are very efficient in reducing the risk. However, it seems impossible to entirely eliminate the occurrence of retained material. Laparoscopic procedures carry less risk to accidentally leave foreign bodies inside a body cavity.

References

Akman, S., Koyun, M., Gelen, T., et al. (2008) Comparison of intraperitoneal antithrombin III and heparin in experimental peritonitis. Pediatric Nephrology 23 (8), 1327-1330.

Anderson, D.A. (2005) The body wall. In Williams J.M., Niles J.D. (eds.) BSAVA Manual of Canine and Feline Abdominal Surgery, 1st edn. British Small Animal Veterinary Association, Gloucester, UK, pp. 36-57.

Boothe, H.W., Slater, M.R., Hobson H.P., et al. (1992) Exploratory celiotomy in 200 nontraumatized dogs and cats. Veterinary Surgery 21 (6), 452-457.

Brown, D.C., Conzemius, M.G., Shofer, F., et al. (1997) Epidemiologic evaluation of postoperative wound infections in dogs and cats. Journal of the American Veterinary Medical Association 210 (9), 1302-1306.

Crowe, D.T. (1978) Closure of abdominal incisions using a continuous polypropylene suture: Clinical experience in 550 dogs and cats. Veterinary Surgery 7 (3), 74-77.

Crowe, D.T., Bjorling, D.E. (1993) Peritoneum and peritoneal cavity. In Slatter, D. (ed.) Textbook of Small Animal Surgery, vol. 1, 2nd edn. WB Saunders, London, pp. 407-445.

Ellis, H. (2007) Post-operatively intra-abdominal adhesions: a personal view. Colorectal Disease 9 (Suppl. 2), S3-S8.

Freeman, L.J., Pettit, G.D., Robinette, J.D., et al. (1987) Tissue reaction to suture material in the feline linea alba. A retrospective, prospective, and histologic study. Veterinary Surgery 16 (6), 440-445.

Greenfield, C.L., Walshaw, R. (1987) Open peritoneal drainage for the treatment of contaminated peritoneal cavity and septic peritonitis in dogs and cats: 24 cases (1980-1986). Journal of the American Veterinary Medical Association 191 (1), 100-105.

Henderson, R.A. (1993) Adhesion formation. In Bojrab, M.J. (ed.) Disease Mechanisms in Small Animal Surgery, 2nd edn. Lippincott Williams & Wilkins, Philadelphia, pp. 113-117.

Hermanson, J.W., Evans, H.E. (1993) The muscular system. In Evans, H.E. (ed.) Miller's Anatomy of the Dog, 3rd edn. WB Saunders, New York, pp. 258-384.

Miller, J.M. (1970) A new era of non-absorbable sutures. Experimental Medicine and Surgery 28 (3), 274-280.

Miller, M.A., Aper, R.L., Fauber, A., et al. (2006) Extraskeletal osteosarcoma associated with retained surgical sponge in a dog. Journal of Veterinary Diagnostic Investigation 18 (2), 224-228.

Rosin, E., Richardsons, S. (1987) Effect of fascial closure technique on strength of healing abdominal incision in the dog. A biomechanical study. Veterinary Surgery 16 (4), 269-272.

Schippers, E., Tittel, A., Ottinger, A., et al. (1998) Laparoscopy versus laparotomy: comparison of adhesion-formation after bowel resection in a canine model. Digestive Surgery 15 (2), 145-147.

Smeak, D.D. (1993) Abdominal hernias. In Bojrab, M.J. (ed.) Disease Mechanisms in Small Animal Surgery, 2nd edn. Lippincott Williams & Wilkins, Philadelphia, pp. 98-102.

Stawicki, S.P., Evans, D.C., Cipolla, J., et al. (2009) Retained surgical foreign bodies: a comprehensive review of risks and preventive strategies. Scandinavian Journal of Surgery 98 (1), 8-17.

Swann, H., Hughes, D. (2000) Diagnosis and management of peritonitis. Veterinary Clinics of North America: Small Animal Practice 30 (3), 603-615.

Vasseur, P.B., Levy, J., Dowd, E., et al. (1988) Surgical wound infection rates in dogs and cats. Veterinary Surgery 17 (2), 60-64.

50 Laparoscopy

Gilles Dupré[1] and Valentina Fiorbianco[2]

[1]Department für Kleintiere und Pferde, VetMedUni Vienna, Vienna, Austria
[2]Clinica Veterinaria CMV, Varese, Italy

In 1806, Bozzini, an obstetrician from Frankfurt, used a candle light through a tube to examine a patient's urethra and vagina. In 1901, Kelling reported the first laparoscopic examination of a dog cavity. Eighty years later, the introduction of computer chip video camera ignited the development of current laparoscopic surgery. In the late 1980s, Mühe, Mouret, and Dubois successfully realized the first laparoscopic cholecystectomies. They are now considered the pioneers of minimally invasive surgery. In the past 15 years, laparoscopy became the gold standard for many diagnostic and therapeutic procedures in human medicine.

Advantages of laparoscopic surgery

(Table 50.1)
- Reduced surgical trauma and subsequent reduction of postoperative pain and morbidity
- Reduced infection rates and faster recovery (Austin *et al.* 2003; Van Goethem *et al.* 2003; Davidson *et al.* 2004; Devitt *et al.* 2005; Hancock *et al.* 2005; Nickel *et al.* 2007; Monnet *et al.* 2008);
- Magnification and subsequent better visualization of vessels or anatomic structures (Van Goethem *et al.* 2003) or pathological lesions (small metastatic lesions) (Monnet *et al.* 2008)

Disadvantages of laparoscopic surgery

(see Table 50.1)
- Material cost: The need for specific instruments and video tower represents a fair amount of investment.
- Training: Because one deals with completely new surgical methods, training is mandatory.
- Increased duration of surgery (Remedios *et al.* 1997). Because of the technological constraints and need for acquisition of new skills, laparoscopic surgery lasts longer than conventional surgery, at least at the very beginning. However, a reduction in surgical time is usually observed with increased experience (van Nimwegen and Kirpensteijn 2007a). This learning curve considers not only the time to perform a given procedure but also the complication rate. For instance, the time required to perform a laparoscopic ovariohysterectomy in a dog dropped from 120 minutes (Davidson *et al.* 2004) to 21 minutes (Devitt *et al.* 2005). Nowadays, laparoscopic ovariectomies can be performed in less than 33 minutes when using two or one portal and vessel-sealer divider devices (Culp *et al.* 2009; Dupré *et al.* 2009).

Table 50.1 Advantages and disadvantages of laparoscopy in small animals

Advantages	Disadvantages

• Image magnification
• Reduced perioperative pain
• Improved patient recovery
• Lower postoperative morbidity
• Decreased postoperative infection rate
• Surgical trauma reduction
  ○ Surgical stress related factors:
    ▪ Less impairment of metabolism
    ▪ Renal and pulmonary workload
    ▪ Bowel mobility
    ▪ Immune function
  ○ Fewer adhesions?
• Better observation of the ovarian ligament in obese dogs
• Better quality of liver biopsy
• Bleeding control after biopsy (compared with ultrasonography)
• Owner satisfaction
	• Costs
	• Learning curve (time consuming at the beginning)
	• General anesthesia
	• Need for a well-trained team

Major versus minor complications

Major complications are defined as those requiring additional surgery or transfusion. In one human study (Kane and Krejs 1984), laparoscopic liver biopsy led to hemorrhage in 1.3% of patients. Perforation of the gastrointestinal tract requiring an additional procedure occurred in 0.6% of patients. Minor complications occurred in 5.1% of patients and included port site leakage of ascites, cellulitis, hematoma, and wound dehiscence. The overall mortality rate after laparoscopic procedures in this study was 0.49%.

In one veterinary textbook (Twedt and Monnet 2005), the complication rate of laparoscopic procedures was cited as being as low as 2%. Another report (Buote and Kovak 2008) reviewed preoperative, intraoperative, and postoperative factors associated with complication rate in a large population of patients. In this study, there was a significantly increased likelihood of complications in feline patients, older patients, and patients with lower body condition score and weight.

Contraindications of laparoscopic surgery

As laparoscopic surgery becomes more advanced, the absolute contraindications to laparoscopy are diminishing. However, some anatomic changes might preclude the laparoscopic approach or at least

Complications in Small Animal Surgery, First Edition. Edited by Dominique Griffon and Annick Hamaide.
© 2016 John Wiley & Sons, Inc. Published 2016 by John Wiley & Sons, Inc.
Companion website: www.wiley.com/go/griffon/complications

warrant a very conservative approach (Bowers and Hunter 2006; Jones and Jones 2006). These include:

- Pregnancy
- Increased intracranial pressure
- Abnormalities of cardiac output and gas exchange in the lung
- Chronic liver disease and coagulopathy

There are also relative contraindications that preclude the use of a blind approach and require an experienced surgeon and anesthesia team:

- Difficult access to the abdomen because of obliteration of the peritoneal space, organ distension, and potential dissemination or recurrence of cancer
- Reoperation. In humans, in more than 30% of patients with a history of surgery, the bowel or other organs are directly adherent to the abdominal scar, rendering these areas problematic for both open and blind access methods (Miller *et al.* 1993; Halpern 1996; Gersin *et al.* 1998; Halpern 1998; Kumar 1998; Audebert and Gomel 2000; Bowers and Hunter 2006). This might not be true in small animals because abdominal adhesions occur less frequently.

In addition, specific patient conditions might exacerbate the respiratory and cardiovascular side effects of pneumoperitoneum. However, in humans, several studies have confirmed the benefits of laparoscopy in elderly adults, including decreased hospital stay and fewer wound and pulmonary complications (Schwandner *et al.* 1999a).

Complications in laparoscopic surgery may be associated with equipment dysfunction, anesthesia and maintenance of a pneumoperitoneum, entry technique, or surgery itself. After completion of surgery, complications may include hemorrhage, peritonitis, port site incision complications, tumor cell seeding, or adhesion formation.

PERIOPERATIVE COMPLICATIONS

Material dysfunction

Definition

Material dysfunction can occur at any level:

- Video system
- Insufflator
- Light source
- Laparoscopes
- Trocar–cannulas
- Surgical instruments
- Electrosurgical devices

In laparoscopic surgery, the surgeon should rely completely on the quality and reliability of the material at his or her disposal. Any default in the instrumental chain from the scope's extremity to the monitor will result in, at best, a poor image, and at worst, a surgical accident.

Besides, during surgical action, an instrument not acting as it is conceived can have disastrous consequences.

Diagnosis

- Camera or endoscope dysfunction will result in an unsatisfactory image or no image at all.
- Instruments cannot be activated or retrieved.
- In case of an insufflator dysfunction, the abdomen can be overdilated despite an adequate pressure setting (most dangerous situation).

Prevention

The laparoscopic tower should be controlled before the patient is entered. Because of the work at a distance, the surgeon starting to perform laparoscopic surgery should have specific material at his or her disposal:

- Laparoscopic graspers (traumatic and atraumatic), endo-scissors and various sizes of atraumatic retractors
- Suction apparatus and endocoagulation and staplers devices.

Prognosis

In the following instances of instrument dysfunction, the surgeon will have to convert to an open procedure:

- Inability to get an appropriate image
- Lack of adequate instrument
- Obvious insufflator dysfunction

Anesthetic and pneumoperitoneum complications

Definition

Anesthetic complications are usually related to pneumoperitoneum (Marshall *et al.* 1972). The cardiopulmonary effects of carbon dioxide (CO_2) insufflation for the establishment of a pneumoperitoneum have been determined: abdominal insufflation using CO_2 to a pressure of 15 mm Hg for 180 minutes results in significant increases in heart rate, minute ventilation, and saphenous vein pressure and decreases in pH and PaO_2 (Duke *et al.* 1996). Although they were found to be acceptable in healthy, well-ventilated patients, the surgeon should be aware of the respiratory and cardiovascular effects of the pneumoperitoneum.

Respiratory effects

- The absorption of CO_2 across the peritoneal surface may cause hypercarbia and subsequent respiratory acidosis (Duerr *et al.* 2008).
- The transmission of increased intraabdominal pressure raises intrathoracic pressures by 5 to 15 mm Hg. The increased intraabdominal pressure results in a forward displacement of the diaphragm and subsequently decreases lung volumes, decreases compliance, increases resistance, and leads to ventilation–perfusion mismatching and lung atelectasis (Meininger *et al.* 2002). The subsequent cranial displacement of the carina can result in an endobronchial intubation and single-lung ventilation.
- The ventilation problems are exacerbated further when the patient is in a Trendelenburg (head-down) position.

Cardiovascular effects

- Venous return to the heart and cardiac output might decrease in response to peritoneal gas insufflation and compression of the vena cava. On the contrary, in a Trendelenburg position, the increased venous return from the distal or lower extremities and abdomen can subsequently increase the preload.

Diagnosis

End-tidal CO_2 monitoring is essential in the management of the ventilation of patients undergoing laparoscopy. Because the cardiorespiratory effects of the pneumoperitoneum may be exacerbated by the decreased capacity for respiratory compensation (Deveney 2006), hypercarbia or hypoxia might be encountered in patients with a history of preexisting pulmonary or cardiac disease (Halpin and Soper 2006). Arterial monitoring is suggested in these patients.

Treatment

- **Intermittent positive-pressure ventilation** started immediately after the induction and before abdominal insufflation prevents the majority of the side effects induced by the pneumoperitoneum.
- **Positive end-expiratory pressure** helps minimizing the alterations in gas exchange.
- **Hyperventilation** lowers the $PaCO_2$ and raises the pH (Birkett 2006; Deveney 2006).
- **Temporary desinsufflation of the abdomen** (called a "pneumoperitoneum holiday" in humans) (Deveney 2006) usually suffices to handle most pneumoperitoneum-associated complications.

Prognosis

When properly monitored, provided that they are early recognized, anesthetic complications can be easily treated.

Hypothermia and fogging effect

As it enters the abdomen, the temperature of CO_2 is about 20.1°C. In addition, because of convection effects, a net loss of 0.3°C per 60 L of gas insufflated can be observed (Ott 1991). Therefore, gas flow should be kept to a minimum, and leaks around cannulas should be avoided. Also, when the laparoscope with a cold lens is first introduced into the warm, moist abdominal cavity, lens fogging often occurs. For these reasons, heating the insufflation gas is recommended. If a surface wetting agent is used, no lens fogging occurs, and the visual field is usually clear.

OPERATIVE COMPLICATIONS

Entry-related complications

The authors are aware of only a few prospective veterinary studies specifically looking at entry-related complication rates (Desmaizières et al. 2003; Dörner et al. 2009; Fiorbianco et al. 2010).

Definition

Entry-related injuries can occur during creation of the pneumoperitoneum or the secondary portal placement (Bateman et al. 1996); they are very well described in textbooks (Freeman 1999) but more rarely in clinical trials. Because of suspected underreporting, the true incidence of these complications is difficult to access. They include:

- Injury to the abdominal or thoracic wall vasculature
- Injury to intraabdominal or intrathoracic vasculature
- Penetration of solid organs or hollow viscus
- Subcutaneous emphysema, peritoneal tenting, gas embolism, and pneumothorax

The authors are aware of one clinical trial on 40 horses that examined the safety of a variety of trocar placement techniques and found that problems with insufflation or cannula insertion occurred in 12 horses (Desmaizières et al. 2003). In dogs, complications have been reported in few clinical studies and include:

- Intraoperative subcutaneous emphysema (Hardie et al. 1996; Nickel et al. 2007)
- Fatal gas embolism (Gilroy and Anson 1987; Staffieri et al. 2007): Although very rarely reported, a direct injection of gas into the venous system through a Veress needle (VN) did cause gas embolism. Patients became profoundly hypotensive, cyanotic, or bradycardic or developed asystole.

- Spleen injuries (Gilroy and Anson 1987; Hardie et al. 1996; Davidson et al. 2004; Mayhew and Cimino Brown 2007; Nickel et al. 2007; Dupré et al. 2009; Mayhew and Cimino Brown 2009) Several methods to create a pneumoperitoneum have been described. **In the closed methods**, the abdomen is insufflated blindly usually by means of a VN. Alternatively, a direct trocar insertion technique has been also described in which the trocar is inserted in the abdominal cavity without previous insufflation (Mahajan and Gaikwad 2007; van Nimwegen and Kirpensteijn 2007a, 2007b; Vilos et al. 2007). **In the open method**, called the Hasson's technique, a mini-laparotomy is performed, and stay sutures or towel clamps are placed on each side of the incision to lift the abdominal wall and allow the insertion of the Hasson trocar (Kolata and Freeman 1998). Many modifications of the technique have been described (Mayhew and Cimino Brown 2007; Mayhew et al. 2008; Culp et al. 2009).

Even in human medicine, no method has been proven to be totally safe and superior to the others. When considering 42 articles about laparoscopy in dogs and cats, open and closed methods are equally distributed, and complications are infrequently reported (Table 50.2). The spleen is the abdominal organ most frequently reported as injured in studies about laparoscopy (Gilroy and Anson 1987; Hardie et al. 1996; Davidson et al. 2004; Mayhew and Cimino Brown 2007; Nickel et al. 2007; Dupré et al. 2009; Mayhew and Cimino Brown 2009). Davidson and others reported 3 cases of 16 (19%) of spleen injuries caused by first trocar insertion after VN, and Mayhew and others reported spleen lacerations in two cases out of 30 dogs (6.6%) using Hasson's technique and directing the trocar to the right side (Davidson et al. 2004; Mayhew and Cimino Brown 2009). In a study on VN insertion techniques, 3 of 56 patients presented with a spleen laceration, but none of them required conversion to an open surgery (Fiorbianco et al. 2010).

In one study, liver injuries were encountered after intercostal VN insertion in 3 of 56 cases and consisted of liver parenchyma transfixion close to the margin of the right medial lobe. Bleeding related to liver injury was always self-limiting (Fiorbianco et al. 2010). A prospective study of 14,243 laparoscopic procedures performed on human patients documented a 0.18% incidence of trocar-related vascular and visceral injury (Schäfer et al. 2001).

Prevention and treatment

To limit or avoid VN entry-related injuries, the correct intraabdominal position of the tip of the needle should be checked using several tests:

- Aspiration test: A 5-mL syringe is connected to the VN and aspirated. If blood or other fluid is collected, then a vessel, an organ, or an hollow viscus penetration should be suspected.
- Injection-recovery test: Five mL of sterile saline is injected, and no resistance should be felt. When reaspirated, no saline should be retrieved.
- Hanging drop test: One drop of saline is injected in the VN, and the abdominal wall is lifted. When correctly positioned, the saline drop should sink into the needle.
- Low-flow insufflation test: A sudden high pressure is the sign of a misplacement of the VN.

Various locations for VN placement are cited in the literature: retro-umbilical, right caudal abdominal quadrant. An intercostal approach has been recently described (Fiorbianco et al. 2010). In this study, the authors reported only one major complication, a pneumothorax that required a treatment, but no conversion to open surgery was needed. Most of the complications recorded (74%)

Table 50.2 Forty-two laparoscopy clinical studies published in cats and dogs analyzed in order to report the entry method preferences of the authors and the complications encountered*

Reference	Number of animals and procedure	Pneumoperitoneum	Organ injuries
Female dog genital tract			
Fiorbianco et al. (2010)	56 dogs, L-OVE or L-OVH	VN	Injury classification in grades 1, 2, or 3
Dupré et al. (2009)	42 dogs, L-OVE	VN	4 spleen injuries
Culp et al. (2009)	10 dogs L-OVE, 10 dogs OVE	Modified sutureless Hasson's technique	—
Collard (2008)	1 dog, L-OVH (pyometra)	VN	—
van Nimwegen and Kirpensteijn (2007a)	40 dogs, L-OVE	DTI	—
Mayhew and Cimino Brown (2007)	30 dogs, LA-OVH	Modified sutureless Hasson's technique	1 spleen injury caused by trocar insertion
Nickel et al. (2007)	20 L-OVE, 24 OVE + 4 OVH	Open method	1 spleen injury 1 subcutaneous emphysema
Devitt et al. (2005)	10 dogs, OVH; 10 dogs, LA-OVH	VN	—
Hancock et al. (2005)	8 dogs, LA-OVH; 8 dogs, OVH	Hasson's technique	1 spleen injury caused by Babcock forceps
van Nimwegen et al. (2005)	72 dogs, L-OVE	Open method	—
Wenkel et al. (2005)	27 L-OVH + 1 L-OVE	VN Hasson's technique	1 bleeding 1 subcutaneous emphysema (postoperative)
Davidson et al. (2004)	16 dogs, L-OVH; 18 dogs, OVH	VN	3 spleen injuries caused by first trocar
Van Goethem et al. (2003)	103 dogs, L-OVE	Open method	—
Austin et al. (2003)	9 dogs L-OHE	Hasson's technique	—
Remedios et al. (1997)	8 dogs, OVH; 10 dogs, L-OVH	—	Intraabdominal fat affecting view and manipulation
Minami et al. (1997)	2 dogs, LA-OVH (pyometra)	Optical trocar	—
Wildt and Lawler (1985)	8 dogs and 3 cats, L horn occlusion	—	—
van Nimwegen and Kirpensteijn (2007b)	14 cats, L-OVE	DTI	—
Male dog and cat genital tract			
Miller (20043)	10 dogs and 3 cats, LA cryptorchidectomy	Hasson's technique	—
Spinella et al. (2003)	2 dogs, L cryptorchidectomy	VN in the right inguinal region	—
Gallagher and Freeman (1992)	Dogs, L cryptorchidectomy	VN	—
Vannozzi et al. (2002)	1 cat, L cryptorchidectomy	Hasson's technique	—
Salomon et al. (2002)	1 dog, L deferentopexy	VN	—
Dog urinary tract			
Rawlings (2007)	2 dogs, LA cystoscopy and inflammatory polyps removal	Hasson's technique	—
Rawlings et al. (2003)	3 dogs, LA cystoscopy and calculi removal	Hasson's technique	—
Rawlings et al. (2003)	10 dogs, L kidney biopsy	Hasson's technique	—
Rawlings et al. (2002a)	18 dogs, LA cystopexy	Hasson's technique	—
Gastrointestinal tract			
Dujowich (2010)	19 dogs, L control of gastropexy site	VN	—
Mayhew and Cimino Brown (2009)	30 dogs, L gastropexy	Hasson's technique	2 spleen injuries
Mathon et al. (2009)	7 dogs, LA gastropexy	VN	—
Rawlings et al. (2001)	8 dogs, LA gastropexy	Hasson's technique	—
Rawlings et al. (2002b)	23 dogs, LA gastropexy	Hasson's technique	—
Wilson et al. (1996)	4 dogs, L gastropexy	Hasson's technique	—
Hardie et al. (1996)	14 dogs, L gastropexy (stapled)	VN, cranial right side of the abdomen	2 spleen injuries caused by first trocar 2 gastric perforations 8 subcutaneous emphysemas
Hewitt et al. (2004)	15 dogs, LA placement of jejunostomy feeding tube	VN	—
Liver			
Barnes et al. (2006)	20 dogs, LA biopsies	VN	No injuries related to VN of trocar
Mayhew et al. (2008)	6 dogs, L cholecystectomy	Modified sutureless Hasson's technique	—

(Continued)

Table 50.2 (*Continued*)

Reference	Number of animals and procedure	Pneumoperitoneum	Organ injuries
Pancreas			
Webb and Trott (2008)	18 dogs and 13 cats, L diagnosis of pancreatic disease	—	—
Adrenalectomy			
Jimenez Pelaez *et al.* (2008)	7 dogs, L adrenalectomy	VN, paralumbar fossa caudal to the 13th rib	—
Others			
Duerr *et al.* (2008)	23 dogs, pH changes of peritoneal fluid associated with CO_2 insufflation during laparoscopic surgery	VN	—
Miller and Fowler (2006)	2 dogs, L portosystemic shunt attenuation	VN	—
Gilroy and Anson (1987)	1 dog, fatal air embolism	VN, left lateral flank	Spleen injury with secondary embolism (nitrogen gas)

*The studies have been organized based on the anatomic system.

DTI, direct trocar insertion; L, laparoscopic; LA, laparoscopic assisted; OVE, ovariectomy; OVH, ovariohysterectomy; VN, Veress needle.

were considered minimal and included subcutaneous emphysema, falciform tears, and omentum entrapment. In addition, 3 cases of spleen injuries and 3 cases of liver injuries were recorded, but the bleeding was always minimal and self-limiting. No conversion to open surgery was required.

When no VN is used, the first port can be placed after the abdominal wall has been minimally dissected and lifted. Alternatively, screwing trocars (Vilos *et al.* 2007) and self-dilating and "optical" trocars allow direct visualization through each abdominal layer and have been associated with few complications (LeBlanc 2004).

A hollow-viscus penetration warrants an immediate conversion in most of the cases. This complication can occur when portals are placed blindly despite a known gastric or intestinal dilatation.

Prognosis
Any entry-related injury should be considered seriously. Transfixing a liver lobe with a VN is usually harmless, but lacerating the spleen with a sharp trocar might be dangerous and requires prompt conversion.

Tension pneumothorax

Definition
This complication can happen:
- In patients with unknown congenital or iatrogenic diaphragmatic defect (McMahon *et al.* 1993)
- After retroperitoneal dissection during adrenalectomy
- Through inadvertent intrathoracic or transdiaphragmatic insufflation when the VN is placed, as described by some authors, in the last palpable right intercostal space (Fiorbianco *et al.* 2010)

Diagnosis
Pneumothorax can be readily diagnosed through spirometry and capnography. An increased intrathoracic resistance is usually observed.

Treatment
A thoracocentesis should be immediately performed and the chest evacuated.

Prognosis
Surgery can usually be completed provided that intrathoracic pressure is controlled.

Subcutaneous emphysema
Subcutaneous emphysema can occur secondary to subcutaneous insufflation either through the VN or through a port. In a study on intercostal placement of the VN, subcutaneous emphysema occurred exclusively during the first part of the study, verifying the important role of experience even during application of the VN (Fiorbianco *et al.* 2010).

Hemorrhage
Hemorrhage can occur after different events:
- Hemorrhage through an entry point
- Hemorrhage after dissection or organ penetration

Definition
Hemorrhage through an entry point is caused by an inadvertent puncture of an abdominal wall vessel during trocar or VN insertion. It is usually self-limiting in small animals (Hancock *et al.* 2005).

Prevention and treatment
Because it will obscure the view, blood dripping continuously from a port should be controlled. This can be achieved with local cauterization or suture. Alternatively, the port can be replaced, and a special cannula equipped with an inflatable balloon can be applied. Hemorrhage that happens after inadvertent dissection of a major blood vessel warrants an immediate conversion.

When local hemorrhage occurs secondary to an organ penetration (liver, spleen), the following steps should be undertaken before a conversion is planned:
- **Pressure:** Immediate pressure should be applied with a blunt instrument.
- **Suction-irrigation:** The suction-irrigation apparatus should be connected, blood aspirated, the source of hemorrhage visualized, and the bleeding evaluated.
- **Cauterization** (sealing) and application of hemostatic sponges

- **Evaluation of the true blood loss:** Because of the magnification, the actual quantity of blood loss can be overestimated. On the other hand, in small patients, blood flowing away from the camera might not be taken into account. It is then recommended to actually aspirate and calculate the true blood loss. Any doubt about the actual quantity of blood loss warrants an immediate conversion.

Prognosis
In small animal laparoscopic veterinary literature, splenic bleeding has not been associated with a higher conversion rate or to any reported long-term side effects.

Thermal damage
Thermal organ injury may occur after the use of electrosurgical or electrocautery devices (LeBlanc 2004). In humans, occurrence of this complication has been reported to be 0.2%. In veterinary medicine, such complications have not been reported yet. Some basic rules should be respected to minimize their incidence:
- The instrument connected to the electrical power should always remain in the operator's field of view.
- The surgeon should be the only one to activate a foot switch.
- Vessel-sealer devices and bipolar devices should preferably be used.

Conversion
Conversion is not a complication; it is the surgeon's decision. Besides emergent conversions required because of uncontrollable bleeding or rupture of a hollow viscus, factors influencing the conversion rates are usually classified as patient specific, procedure specific, or surgeon specific. Age, obesity, inappropriate case selection, and poor tolerance to the pneumoperitoneum are factors influencing the conversion rate in humans (Rotholtz *et al.* 2008). The conversion rates and risk factors have been specifically calculated for the most common laparoscopic procedures, such as cholecystectomy (1%–10%), colorectal procedures (1%–40%), nephrectomy (5%–14%), adrenalectomy (0%–20%), and splenectomy (1%–18%) (Pandya *et al.* 1999; Schwandner *et al.* 1999b; Tekkis *et al.* 2005; Schak 2007; Rotholtz *et al.* 2008). Belizon and colleagues showed that conversions performed within the first 30 minutes of an operation have a better clinical outcome than conversions performed later in a procedure (Belizon *et al.* 2006; Kovak McClaran *et al.* 2009); therefore, based on his or her progression, each surgeon should set his or her own time limit for conversion.

In a veterinary study, a conversion rate of 23% was found in a population of patients undergoing laparoscopic procedures (Buote and Kovak 2008). In this study, a preoperative finding of a solitary liver tumor or low total protein level and a diagnosis of malignancy were significant risk factors for conversion.

POSTOPERATIVE COMPLICATIONS
After the completion of laparoscopic procedures, reported complications documented in the human literature include postoperative hemorrhage, anastomotic leakage, subcutaneous emphysema, persistent pneumoperitoneum, portal site inflammation, infection, and herniation (Kane and Krejs 1984; McMahon *et al.* 1993). Only a few veterinary studies do report postoperative complications, including subcutaneous cellulitis, respiratory compromise, suture reaction, fever, and bruising (Davidson *et al.* 2004; Jimenez Pelaez *et al.* 2008).

Portal site complications

Herniation and wound complication
Although it has been claimed that the muscular closure of the 5-mm portal is not necessary, herniation of omentum through 5-mm laparoscopic portal sites has been reported in dogs (Freeman 1999). Therefore, it is important to ensure that all abdominal organs and fat are adequately within the abdomen as ports are removed. Fascial layer should be closed under direct visualization.

Portal site metastasis
Portal site metastasis can be caused by direct implantation during sample retrieval, exfoliation of cells during tumor manipulation, and dispersion after CO_2 insufflation (Martinez *et al.* 1995; Brundell *et al.* 2002). To minimize this risk, it is usually recommended to retrieve specimens after putting them in a bag. In a study comparing laparoscopy with laparotomy, there was no evidence of an increase in circulating tumor cells after laparoscopy, but use of specimen retrieval bags for exteriorization of tumor samples was still recommended (Lelievre *et al.* 2004). There is less and less evidence that higher rates of tumor cell implantation occur after laparoscopy.

Pain
It has been demonstrated in humans as well as in small animals that patients undergoing laparoscopic procedures experience less pain and have shorter hospital stays. However, laparoscopic surgery is not a pain-free surgery. Postoperative pain in laparoscopic surgery has been categorized by Joris and others as visceral pain (caused by organ manipulation), abdominal wall pain (caused by the incisions), or shoulder tip pain (caused by distension or diaphragmatic pressure) (Joris *et al.* 1998). The first one happens in the immediate postoperative period, and the last one is delayed (Fichera and Milsom 2006).

Definition
Several factors are likely to contribute to postoperative pain (Mouton *et al.* 1999):
- Localized acidosis
- Peritoneal ischemia
- Distension neuropraxia
- Port size and location
- Anesthetic regimen

The pneumoperitoneum contributes to the postoperative pain because it has an impact on the peritoneal surfaces. The total volume of gas insufflated, rate of insufflation, intraabdominal pressure and temperature, humidity, type of gas used, and volume of residual gas may induce some peritoneal change and thus play significant roles (Fichera and Milsom 2006).

Prevention and treatment
Beside current pain therapies, several methods of pain prevention and control have been advocated in laparoscopic surgery:
- Reduction of number and size of ports
- Local anesthesia preoperative versus postoperative
- Intraperitoneal local anesthetic or saline solution
- Decreased pressure or volume
- Gas removal

Reducing the size and the number of ports is a way to reduce surgical trauma and is a current trend in laparoscopic surgery (Leggett *et al.* 2000; Schwenk *et al.* 2000; Rosin *et al.* 2001). In dogs, a recent study demonstrated the feasibility of single-port laparoscopic ovariectomy and compared the results and complications rates with the two-port approaches (Dupré *et al.* 2009).

Infiltration of the incision sites or of the intraperitoneal cavity with local anesthetics is questioned, but instillation of saline at the end of a procedure is associated with a reduction in postoperative pain and even seems to work better when mixed with local anesthetics. **Removal of residual gas** after surgery has been shown in humans to reduce shoulder tip pain but has a minimal impact on the overall pain experienced. The **total volume of gas** and the **maximal insufflation pressure** have been shown to correlate with the degree of postoperative pain. Then the easiest way to decrease postoperative pain is to limit the insufflation pressure and volume; therefore, gas leakage from around and through the ports should be avoided.

Prognosis

It has been demonstrated that patients undergoing laparoscopic procedures experience less pain and manifest less profound decreases in pulmonary function. In dogs, less perioperative pain (lower pain scores and analgesic supplementation) and surgical stress (cortisol and glucose levels) and better postoperative activity have been demonstrated after laparoscopic procedures (Davidson *et al.* 2004; Devitt *et al.* 2005; Hancock *et al.* 2005; Culp *et al.* 2009).

References

Audebert, A.J., Gomel, V. (2000) Role of microlaparoscopy in the diagnosis of peritoneal and visceral adhesions and in the prevention of bowel injury associated with blind trocar insertion. *Fertility and Sterility* 73 (3), 631–635.

Austin, B., Lanz, O.I., Hamilton, S.M., et al. (2003) Laparoscopic ovariohysterectomy in nine dogs. *Journal of the American Animal Hospital Association* 39, 391-396.

Barnes, R.F., Greenfield, C.L., Schaeffer D.J., et al. (2006) Comparison of biopsy samples obtained using standard endoscopic instruments and harmonic scalpel during laparoscopic and laparoscopic-assisted surgery in normal dogs. *Veterinary Surgery* 35, 243-251.

Bateman, B.G., Kolp, L.A., Hoeger K. (1996) Complications of laparoscopy—operative and diagnostic. *Fertility and Sterility* 66 (1), 30-35.

Belizon, A., Sardinha, C.T., Sher, M.E. (2006) Converted laparoscopic colectomy. What are the consequences? *Surgical Endoscopy* 20, 947-951.

Birkett, D.H. (2006) Pulmonary considerations. In Whelan, R.L., Fleshman, J.W., Fowler, D.L. (eds.) *The SAGES Manual Perioperative Care in Minimally Invasive Surgery.* Springer, New York, pp. 318-325.

Bowers, S.P., Hunter, J.G. (2006) Contraindications to laparoscopy. In Whelan, R.L., Fleshman, J.W., Fowler, D.L. (eds.) *The SAGES Manual Perioperative Care in Minimally Invasive Surgery.* Springer, New York, pp. 25-32.

Brundell, S., Ellis, T., Dodd, T., et al. (2002) Hematogenous spread as a mechanism for the generation of abdominal wound metastases following laparoscopy. *Surgical Endoscopy* 16 (2), 292-295.

Buote, N.J., Kovak, J.R. (2008) Indications and occurrence of conversion from laparoscopy to laparotomy. In *Proceedings of the 5th Annual Meeting of the Veterinary Endoscopic Society*, Keystone, p. 12.

Culp, W.T.N., Mayhew, P.D., Cimino Brown D. (2009) The effect of laparoscopic versus open ovariectomy on post-surgical activity in small dogs. *Veterinary Surgery* 38, 811-817.

Davidson, E.B., Moll, H.D., Payton, M.E. (2004) Comparison of laparoscopic ovariohysterectomy and ovariohysterectomy in dogs. *Veterinary Surgery* 33, 62-69.

Desmaizières, L.M., Martinot, S., Lepage, O.M., et al. (2003) Complications associated with cannula insertion techniques used for laparoscopy in standing horses. *Veterinary Surgery* 32, 501-506.

Deveney, K.E. (2006) Pulmonary Implications of CO_2 Pneumoperitoneum in Minimally Invasive Surgery. In Whelan, R.L., Fleshman, J.W., Fowler, D.L. (eds.) *The SAGES Manual Perioperative Care in Minimally Invasive Surgery.* Springer, New York, pp. 360-365.

Devitt, C.M., Cox, R.E., Hailey, J.J. (2005) Duration, complications, stress, and pain of open ovariohysterectomy versus a simple method of laparoscopic-assisted ovariohysterectomy in dogs. *Journal of the American Veterinary Medical Association* 227 (6), 921-927.

Dörner, J., Dupré, G., Kneissl, S. (2009) Intercostal implantation of Veress needle in canine laparoscopic procedures—a computed tomography and cadaver study [abstract]. *Veterinary Surgery* 38, E2-E3.

Duerr, F.M., Twedt, D.C., Monnet, E. (2008) Changes in pH of peritoneal fluid associated with carbon dioxide insufflation during laparoscopic surgery in dogs. *American Journal of Veterinary Research* 69, 298-301.

Dujowich, M., Keller, M.E., Reimer, S.B. (2010) Evaluation of short- and long-term complications after endoscopically assisted gastropexy in dogs. *Journal of the American Veterinary Medical Association* 236, 177-182.

Duke, T., Steinacher, S.L., Remedios, A.M. (1996) Cardiopulmonary effects of using carbon dioxide for laparoscopic surgery in dogs. *Veterinary Surgery* 25, 77-82.

Dupré, G., Fiorbianco, V., Skalicky, M., et al. (2009) Laparoscopic ovariectomy in dogs: comparison between single portal and two-portal access. *Veterinary Surgery* 38, 818-824.

Fichera, A., Milsom, J.V. (2006) Impact of minimally invasive methods on postoperative pain and pulmonary function. In Whelan, R.L., Fleshman, J.W., Fowler, D.L. (eds.) *The SAGES Manual Perioperative Care in Minimally Invasive Surgery.* Springer, New York, pp. 446-453.

Fiorbianco, V., Skalicky, M., Dörner, J., et al. (2010) Right intercostal insertion of the Veress needle for laparoscopy in dogs. In *Proceedings of the 19th Annual Scientific Meeting of European College of Veterinary Surgeons.*

Freeman, L.J. (1999) Complications. In Freeman, L.J. (ed.) *Veterinary Endosurgery.* Mosby, St. Louis, pp. 92-102.

Gallagher, L.A., Freeman, L.J. (1992) Laparoscopic castration for canine cryptorchidism. *Veterinary Surgery* 21, 411-412.

Gersin, K.S., Heniford, B.T., Arca, M.J., et al. (1998) Alternative site entry for laparoscopy in patients with previous abdominal surgery. *Journal of Laparoendoscopy and Advanced Surgical Techniques* 8 (3), 125-130.

Gilroy, B.A., Anson, L.W. (1987) Fatal air embolism during anesthesia for laparoscopy in a dog. *Journal of the American Veterinary Medical Association* 190 (5), 552-554.

Halpern, N.B. (1996) The difficult laparoscopy. *Surgical Clinics of North America* 76 (3), 603-613.

Halpern, N.B. (1998) Access problems in laparoscopic cholecystectomy: postoperative adhesions, obesity, and liver disorders. *Seminars in Laparoscopic Surgery* 5 (2), 92-106.

Halpin, V.J., Soper, N.J. (2006) Decision to convert to open methods. In Whelan, R.L., Fleshman, J.W., Fowler, D.L. (eds.) *The SAGES Manual Perioperative Care in Minimally Invasive Surgery.* Springer, New York, pp. 296-306.

Hancock, R.B., Lanz, O.I., Waldron, D.R., et al. (2005) Comparison of postoperative pain after ovariohysterectomy by harmonic scalpel-assisted laparoscopy compared with median celiotomy and ligation in dogs. *Veterinary Surgery* 34, 273-282.

Hardie, R.J., Flanders, J.A., Schmidt, P., et al. (1996) Biomechanical and histological evaluation of a laparoscopic stapled gastropexy technique in dogs. *Veterinary Surgery* 25, 127-133.

Hewitt, S.A., Brisson, B.A., Sinclair, M.D., et al. (2004) Evaluation of laparoscopic-assisted placement of jejunostomy feeding tubes in dogs. *Journal of the American Veterinary Medical Association* 225, 65-71.

Jimenez Pelaez, M., Bouvy, B.M., Dupré, G.P. (2008) Laparoscopic adrenalectomy for treatment of unilateral adrenocortical carcinomas: technique, complications, and results in 7 dogs. *Veterinary Surgery* 37, 444-453.

Jones, S.B., Jones, D.B. (2006) Preoperative evaluation of the healthy laparoscopic patient. In Whelan, R.L., Fleshman, J.W., Fowler, D.L. (eds.) *The SAGES Manual Perioperative Care in Minimally Invasive Surgery.* Springer, New York, pp. pp. 3-7.

Joris, J.L., Hinque, V.L., Laurent, P.E., et al. (1998) Pulmonary function and pain after gastroplasty performed via laparotomy or laparoscopy in morbidly obese patients. *British Journal of Anaesthesia* 80 (3), 283-288.

Kane, M.G., Krejs, G.J. (1984) Complications of diagnostic laparoscopy in Dallas: a 7-year prospective study. *Gastrointestinal Endoscopy* 30 (4), 237-240.

Kolata, R.J., Freeman, L.J. (1999) Access, port placement, and basic endosurgical skills. In Freeman, L.J. (ed.) *Veterinary Endosurgery.* Mosby, St. Louis, pp. 44-60.

Kovak McClaran, J., Buote, N.J. (2009) Complications and need for conversion to laparotomy in small animals. *Veterinary Clinics of North America: Small Animal Practice* 39, 941-951.

Kumar, S.S. (1998) Laparoscopic cholecystectomy in the densely scarred abdomen. *The American Journal of Surgery* 64 (11), 1094-1096.

LeBlanc, K.A. (2004) General laparoscopic surgical complications. In LeBlanc, K.A. (ed.) *Management of Laparoscopic Surgical Complications.* Marcel Dekker, New York, pp. 43-62.

Leggett, P.L., Churchman-Winn, R., Miller, G. (2000) Minimizing ports to improve laparoscopic cholecystectomy. *Surgical Endoscopy* 14 (1), 32-6.

Lelievre, L., Paterlini-Brechot, P., Camatte, S., et al. (2004) Effect of laparoscopy versus laparotomy on circulating tumor cells using isolation by size of epithelial tumor cells. *International Journal of Gynecological Cancer*, 14 (2), 229-233.

Mahajan, N.N., Gaikwad, N.L. direct trocar insertion: a safe laparoscopic access. *The Internet Journal of Gynecology and Obstetrics* 8 (2).

Marshall, R.L., Jebson, P.J.R., Davie, I.T., et al. (1972) Circulatory effects of carbon dioxide insufflation of the peritoneal cavity for laparoscopy. *British Journal of Anaesthesia*, 44, 682.

Martinez, J., Targarona, E.M., Balaguée, C., et al. (1995) Port site metastasis. An unresolved problem in laparoscopic surgery. A review. *International Surgery* 80 (4), 313-321.

Mathon, D.H., Dossin, A., Palierne, S., et al. (2009) A laparoscopic natural orifice technique in dogs: mechanical and functional evaluation. *Veterinary Surgery* 38, 967-74.

Mayhew, P.D., Cimino Brown, D. (2007) Comparison of three techniques for ovarian pedicle hemostasis during laparoscopic-assisted ovariohysterectomy. *Veterinary Surgery* 36, 541-547.

Mayhew, P.D., Cimino Brown, D. (2009) Prospective evaluation of two intracorporeally sutured prophylactic laparoscopic gastropexy techniques compared with laparoscopic-assisted gastropexy in dogs. *Veterinary Surgery* 38 (6), 738-46.

Mayhew, P.D., Mehler, S.J., Radhakrishnan, A. (2008) Laparoscopic cholecystectomy for management of uncomplicated gall bladder mucocele in six dogs. *Veterinary Surgery* 37, 625-630.

McMahon, A.J., Baxter, J.N., O'Dwyer, P.J. (1993) Preventing complications of laparoscopy. *British Journal of Surgery* 80 (12), 1593-1594.

Meininger, D., Byhahn, C., Bueck, M., et al. (2002) Effects of prolonged pneumoperitoneum on hemodynamics and acid-base balance during totally endoscopic robot-assisted radical prostatectomies. *World Journal of Surgery*, 26, 1423-1427.

Miller, N.J., Van Lue, S.J., Rawlings, C.A. (2004) Use of laparoscopic-assisted cryptorchidectomy in dogs and cats. *Journal of the American Veterinary Medical Association* 224, 875-878.

Miller, N.J., Fowler, J.D. (2006) Laparoscopic portosystemic shunt attenuation in two dogs. *Journal of the American Animal Hospital Association* 42, 160-164.

Miller, K., Holbling, N., Hutter, J., et al. (1993) Laparoscopic cholecystectomy for patients who have had previous abdominal surgery. *Surgical Endoscopy* 7 (5), 400-403.

Minami, S., Okamoto, Y., Eguchi, H., et al. (1997) Successful laparoscopic assisted ovariohysterectomy in two dogs with pyometra. *Journal of Veterinary Medical Science* 59, 845-847.

Monnet, E., Lhermette, P., Sobel, D. (2008) Rigid endoscopy: laparoscopy. In Lhermette, P. Sobel, D. (eds.) *BSAVA Manual of Canine and Feline Endoscopy and Endosurgery.* Wiley John and Sons, Ames, IA, pp. 158-174.

Mouton, W.G., Bessell, J.R., Otten, K.T., et al. (1999) Pain after laparoscopy. *Surgical Endoscopy* 13 (5), 445-448.

Nickel, R., Stürtzbecher, N., Kilian, H., et al. (2007) Postoperative Rekonvaleszenz nach laparoskopischer und konventioneller Ovariektomie: eine vergleichende Studie. *Kleintierpraxis*, 52, 413-424.

Ott, D.E. (1991) Laparoscopic hypothermia. *Journal of Laparoendoscopic Surgery*, 1, 127.

Pandya, S., Murray, J.J., Coller, J.A., et al. (1999) Laparoscopic colectomy. Indications for conversion to laparotomy. *Archives of Surgery* 134 (5), 471-475.

Rawlings, C.A. (2007) Resection of inflammatory polyps in dogs using laparoscopic-assisted cystoscopy. *Journal of the American Animal Hospital Association* 43, 342-346.

Rawlings, C.A., Foutz, T.L., Mahaffey, M.B., et al. (2001) A rapid and strong laparoscopic-assisted gastropexy in dogs. *American Journal of Veterinary Research* 62, 871-75.

Rawlings, C.A., Howerth, E.W., Mahaffey, M.B., et al. (2002a) Laparoscopic-assisted cystopexy in dogs. *American Journal of Veterinary Research* 63, 1226-1231.

Rawlings, C.A., Mahaffey, M.B., Bement, S., et al. (2002b) Prospective evaluation of laparoscopic-assisted gastropexy in dogs susceptible to gastric dilatation. *Journal of the American Veterinary Medical Association* 221 (11), 1576-1581.

Rawlings, C.A., Mahaffey, M.B., Bersanti, J.A., et al. (2003) Use of laparoscopic-assisted cystoscopy for removal of urinary calculi in dogs. *Journal of the American Veterinary Medical Association* 222, 759-761.

Remedios, A.M., Ferguson, J.F., Walker, D.D., et al. (1997) Laparoscopic versus open ovariohysterectomy in dogs: a comparison of postoperative pain and morbidity. *Veterinary Surgery* 26, 425.

Rosin, D., Kuriansky, J., Rosenthal, R.J., et al. (2001) Laparoscopic transabdominal suspension sutures. *Surgical Endoscopy* 15, 761-763.

Rotholtz, N.A., Laporte, M., Zanoni, G., et al. (2008) Predictive factors for conversion in laparoscopic colorectal surgery. *Techniques in Coloproctology* 12, 27-31.

Salomon, J.F., Cotard, J.P., Viguier, E. (2002) Management of urethral sphincter mechanism incompetence in a male dog with laparoscopic guided deferentopexy. *Journal of Small Animal Practice* 43, 501-505.

Schael, G.W., Capper, M., Krähenbühl, L. (2001) Trocar and Veress needle injuries during laparoscopy. *Surgical Endoscopy* 15 (3), 275-80.

Schwandner, O., Schiedeck, T.H., Bruch, H.P. (1999a) Advanced age: indication or contraindication for laparoscopic colorectal surgery? *Diseases of the Colon Rectum* 42 (3), 356-362.

Schwandner, O., Schiedeck, T.H., Bruch, H. (1999b) The role of conversion in laparoscopic colorectal surgery: do predictive factors exist? *Surgical Endoscopy* 13, 151-156.

Schwenk, W., Neudecker, J., Mall, J., et al. (2000) Prospective randomized blinded trial of pulmonary function, pain, and cosmetic results after laparoscopic vs. microlaparoscopic cholecystectomy. *Surgical Endoscopy* 14 (4), 345-348.

Spinella, G., Romagnoli, N., Valentini, S., et al. (2003) Application of the "extraction bag" in laparoscopic treatment of unilateral and bilateral abdominal cryptorchidism in dogs. *Veterinary Research Communications* 27, 445-447.

Staffieri, F., Lacitignola, L., De Siena, R., et al. (2007) A case of spontaneous venous embolism with carbon dioxide during laparoscopic surgery in a pig. *Veterinary Anaesthesia and Analgesia* 34, 63-66.

Tekkis, P.P., Senagore, A.J., Delaney, C.P. (2005) Conversion rates in laparoscopic colorectal surgery. A predictive model with 1253 patients. *Surgical Endoscopy* 19, 47-54.

Twedt, D.C., Monnet, E. (2005) Laparoscopy: technique and clinical experience. In McCarthy, T.C. (ed.) *Veterinary Endoscopy for the Small Animal Practitioner.* Elsevier. Philadelphia, pp. 357-386.

Van Goethem, B.E., Rosenveldt, K.W., Kirpensteijn, J. (2003) Monopolar versus bipolar electrocoagulation in canine laparoscopic ovariectomy: a nonrandomized, prospective, clinical trial. *Veterinary Surgery* 32, 464-470.

van Nimwegen, S.A., Kirpensteijn, J. (2007a) Comparison of Nd:YAG surgical laser and Remorgida bipolar electrosurgery forceps for canine laparoscopic ovariectomy. *Veterinary Surgery* 36, 533-540.

van Nimwegen, S.A., Kirpensteijn, J. (2007b) Laparoscopic ovariectomy in cats: comparison of laser and bipolar electrocoagulation. *Journal of Feline Medicine and Surgery* 9 (5), 397-403.

van Nimwegen, S.A., van Swol, C.F.P., Kirpensteijn, J. (2005) Neodymium:yttrium Aluminium Garnet surgical laser versus bipolar electrocoagulation for laparoscopic ovariectomy in dogs. *Veterinary Surgery* 34, 353-357.

Vannozzi, I., Benetti, C., Rota, A. (2002) Laparoscopic cryptorchidectomy in a cat. *Journal of Feline Medicine and Surgery* 4, 201-203.

Vilos, G.A., Ternamlan, A., Dempster, J., et al. (2007) Laparoscopic entry: a review of techniques, technologies, and complication. *Le Journal de Gynécologie et Obstétrique du Canada* 193, 433-447.

Webb, C.B., Trott, C. (2008) Laparoscopic diagnosis of pancreatic diseases in dogs and cats. *Journal of Veterinary Internal Medicine* 22, 1263-67.

Wenkel, R., Ziemann, U., Thielebein, J., et al. (2005) Laparoskopische Kastration der Hündin—Darstellung neuer Verfahren zur minimal invasiven Ovariohysterektomie. *TierärtzPraxis* 33, 177-188.

Wildt, D.E., Lawler, D.F. (1985) Laparoscopic sterilization of the bitch and queen by uterine horn occlusion. *American Journal of Veterinary Research* 46, 864-869.

Wilson, E.R., Henserson, R.A., Montgomery, R.D., et al. (1996) A comparison of laparoscopic and belt-loop gastropexy in dogs. *Veterinary Surgery* 25, 221-227.

51 Hiatal Herniorrhaphy

Stephen J. Baines
Willows Veterinary Centre and Referral Service, Solihull, West Midlands, UK

Hiatal herniorrhaphy is performed for the management of symptomatic esophageal hiatal hernia. This disorder may be managed either medically or surgically depending on the nature, severity, and potential causes. Surgery is indicated for animals that do not respond to medical management.

Potential complications include dehiscence of the repair and recurrence of herniation, gastroesophageal reflux (GER), esophageal obstruction, pneumothorax, and aspiration pneumonia. Aspiration pneumonia and massive herniation with gastric tympany are the most common causes of perioperative mortality (Callan *et al.* 1993).

Surgical management of hiatal hernia using sphincter-enhancing techniques has a high rate of failure and frequent complications (Merdan Dhein *et al.* 1980; Ellison *et al.* 1987). The operative mortality rate can be high, up to 64% (Ellison *et al.* 1987), and success rates are not consistently high; in one study, only 25% animals were relieved of all clinical signs (Ellison *et al.* 1987).

However, if surgical closure of the hiatus and fixation of the abdominal organs are performed and if care is taken to identify and correct predisposing conditions, then the prognosis is good (Prymak *et al.* 1989; Bright *et al.* 1990; White 1993; Hardie *et al.* 1998; Lorinson and Bright 1998).

Dehiscence and recurrence

Definition
Dehiscence is partial or complete breakdown of the surgical repair.

Risk factors
Dehiscence may be associated with:
- Poor selection of surgical procedures
- Poor surgical technique: either placement of sutures that are too loose and therefore ineffective or placement of sutures that are placed too tightly, placed with too narrow a tissue bite, or placed so that they do not engage the suture-holding layer
- Poor visualization of the surgical site, usually because of poor surgical exposure
- Poor physical condition of the patient: in a cachexic state with a poor nutritional plane and consequent poor wound healing (Figure 51.1)
- Surgical failure has been attributed to a shortened esophagus and stricture in one case (Bright *et al.* 1990).

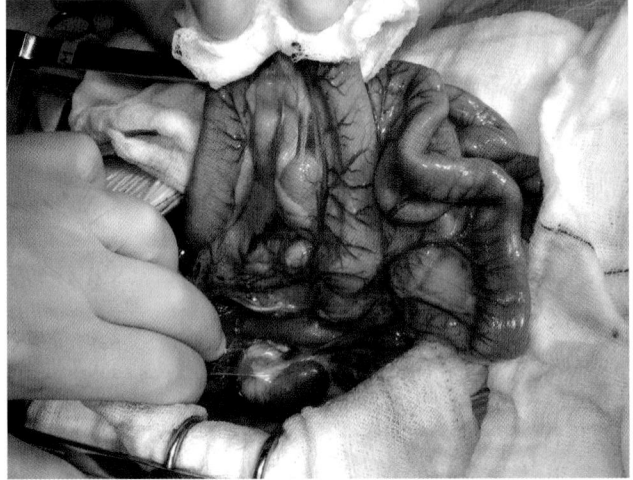

Figure 51.1 Poor physical condition with loss of abdominal fat in a Boston terrier with chronic hiatal hernia.

Diagnosis
- Animals with dehiscence of the surgical wound are likely to show **clinical signs** similar to those exhibited preoperatively. These include salivation, retching, regurgitation or vomiting, dysphagia, coughing, and dyspnea. It is important to differentiate between failure of surgery and recurrence of hiatal herniation and associated GER from persistence of clinical signs after apparently successful surgery caused by either continuing esophagitis or esophageal obstruction (see later discussion).
- As with the initial diagnosis of this clinical condition, **plain radiography; positive contrast esophagography; and, ideally, fluoroscopy** should allow these conditions to be differentiated.
- **Esophagoscopy** is only likely to be useful if sufficient time with adequate treatment has elapsed since the esophagus was last examined so that the presence or absence of the expected improvement in reflux esophagitis may be seen.
- However, in some patients with persistent clinical signs, **surgical exploration** may be needed to provide a diagnosis as to whether the surgical repair is adequate (i.e., is the hiatus of appropriate size and are the pexies still intact?), during which time further surgical procedures to improve the outcome may be performed.

Complications in Small Animal Surgery, First Edition. Edited by Dominique Griffon and Annick Hamaide.
© 2016 John Wiley & Sons, Inc. Published 2016 by John Wiley & Sons, Inc.
Companion website: www.wiley.com/go/griffon/complications

Treatment

True dehiscence of the surgical repair requires a second surgery. However, it is likely that the patient will be in a poorer physical condition than at the first surgery. Hence, more supportive care and more aggressive nutritional support may be needed. Consideration should be given to the likely causes of the surgical failure, and a second surgery should address these to improve the likelihood of a successful outcome (see Prevention below). Long-term medical therapy may still be required in these patients if there is persistence of clinical signs after apparently successful surgery.

Outcome

A poor outcome after the first surgical procedure has been documented in some reports, but no clinical reports have discussed the outcome after a second surgical procedure.

Prevention

Given that a variety of surgical techniques have been described and are used and given that there is some degree of subjectivity in their application, it is difficult to provide an accurate description of the steps needed to perform surgery adequately in all cases. However, the following steps may help to reduce the likelihood of surgical failure:
- Improve exposure and visualization of the surgical site by:
  ◦ Use of a long abdominal incision (xiphoid to umbilicus at least, if not longer)
  ◦ Use of an assistant to manipulate the viscera
  ◦ Transection of the gastrohepatic ligament to allow caudal movement of the stomach
  ◦ Transection of the left triangular ligament to allow medial retraction of the left lateral and left medial liver lobes
- Incise the phrenicoesophageal ligament ventrally to expose the oesophagus, taking care to spare the dorsal and ventral vagal trunks.
- Retract the esophagus into the abdomen so that the gastroesophageal junction is within the abdomen at the completion of the procedure.
- Close the esophageal hiatus by apposing the two diaphragmatic crura ventral to the esophagus to leave an esophageal hiatus of approximately 1 cm (in a small dog) to 2 cm (in a large dog) wide.
- Perform an esophagopexy with simple interrupted sutures between the oesophagus and the diaphragmatic crura.
- Perform a left-sided fundic gastropexy.

General wound healing may be improved by establishing a good nutritional plane, before, and after surgery with enteral feeding (e.g., distal to the esophagus or, if this is not possible, parenteral nutrition).

Gastroesophageal reflux

Definition

Gastroesophageal reflux is the movement of stomach contents into the distal esophagus because of anatomic and functional abnormalities of the stomach, esophagus, and gastroesophageal sphincter.

Risk factors

Risk factors for the development of GER in a patient with hiatal hernia are:
- Too large an esophageal hiatus
- Continuing esophagitis
- Unresolved esophageal motility disorders or megaesophagus (Figure 51.2)
- Continuing gastric hypomotility, which may be related to iatrogenic trauma to the ventral vagus trunk or may be part of gen-

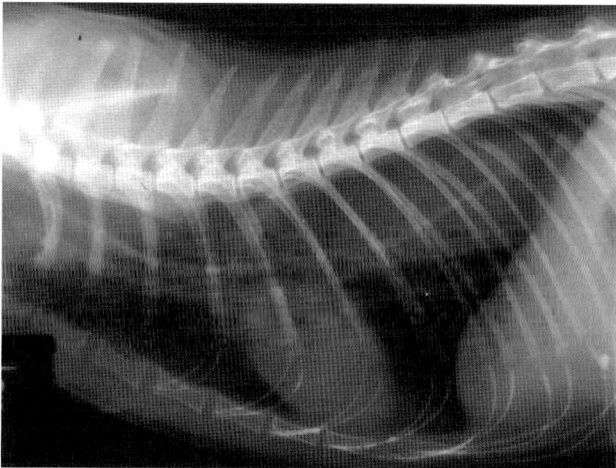

Figure 51.2 Persistence of megaesophagus in a patient with chronic regurgitation associated with hiatal hernia.

eralized gastrointestinal tract hypomotility (Prymak *et al.* 1989; Callan *et al.* 1993).
- Overfeeding, which increases intragastric volume
- Feeding of a high-fat diet, which may delay gastric emptying
- Dehiscence or other failure of the repair

Diagnosis

- The presence of GER is most readily identified using **fluoroscopy** after feeding the patient barium liquid mixed with food.
- **Endoscopy** may be useful if sufficient time has passed since the initial examination and diagnosis.
- **Scintigraphy and continuous pH monitoring** of the distal esophagus may be used to diagnose reflux esophagitis.
- The use of **manometry** to measure lower esophageal sphincter pressure has also been described.

After surgical management of a hiatal hernia, it is important to differentiate between failure of the surgery and persistent hiatal herniation and GER and esophagitis after apparently successful surgery. It is important to realize that hiatal herniation may occur without reflux (Ellison *et al.* 1987; Bright *et al.* 1990; Knowles *et al.* 1990) and that GER may be a normal physiological occurrence in dogs, without esophagitis.

Treatment

Conservative management of GER is generally used preoperatively, and indeed, failure of this management is one indication for considering surgery. This management should be continued postoperatively to treat preexisting esophagitis. In animals with acquired hiatal hernia, the success of the treatment of the predisposing disease should be determined to ensure that this is not a risk factor for continuing reflux.

Conservative or nonsurgical management of GER and esophagitis includes:
- Medical therapy
  ◦ Antacids (e.g., sucralfate)
  ◦ Drugs to reduce gastric acid secretion (e.g., H_2 antagonists or proton pump inhibitors [PPIs])
  ◦ Prokinetic agents (e.g., metoclopramide)
- Feeding practices
  ◦ Feed little and often.
  ◦ Feed in an elevated position.
  ◦ Feed a low-fat diet.

Outcome

In animals with successful surgical management of hiatal hernia, symptomatic GER should be reduced after surgery, either immediately or after 30 days of medical therapy. Persistence of signs beyond this time may indicate that the predisposing factors for the development of an acquired hiatal hernia have not been addressed or that surgery has not been successful.

Prevention

Preoperative conservative management of reflux esophagitis may help to prevent this clinical sign from being apparent in the postoperative period.

Esophageal obstruction

Definition

Esophageal obstruction is an inability of ingested food to move from the esophagus into the stomach through the esophageal hiatus.

Risk factors

Risk factors for esophageal obstruction in surgical patients include:
- Closure of the esophageal hiatus too tightly
- Obstruction of the esophagus with esophagopexy sutures
- Too tight a fundoplication
- Scarring of esophagus after chronic GER

Diagnosis

- Surgery may interfere with function of the lower esophageal sphincter temporarily, leading to an **inability to eructate and/or gastric distension with gas**. More marked mechanical esophageal obstruction will result in the accumulation of ingesta oral to the gastroesophageal junction, with **signs of regurgitation** as before surgery, although the patient may regurgitate larger volumes because less food is likely to enter the stomach.
- **Plain radiographs** may show a large gas-filled stomach.
- **Positive contrast esophagography or fluoroscopy** may demonstrate accumulation of food in the distal esophagus and failure of food boluses to pass into the stomach.

Treatment

Treatment of esophageal obstruction caused by surgical error involves exploring the surgical site again and correcting the reason for the obstruction. This may involve:
- Removing some of the sutures in the hiatus to increase its diameter
- Removing the fundoplication sutures
- Balloon dilation or excision of a distal esophageal scar if chronic

Outcome

If the surgical procedure is modified and performed correctly, then the prognosis should be the same as after initial uncomplicated surgery. However, performing a second surgery soon after the first surgery in a patient likely to have been receiving relatively little food by mouth and likely to have been at increased risk of aspiration pneumonia increases the morbidity and mortality. Animals with scarring of the distal esophagus have a poorer prognosis, and management with balloon dilation may be considered a success if they can tolerate liquid food without regurgitation.

Prevention

Care should be taken with the surgical procedures to avoid causing esophageal obstruction. Fundoplication procedures should be avoided. The placement of a left-sided fundic gastropexy during the first surgery allows the stomach to be deflated in patients that have temporary functional obstruction of the lower esophageal sphincter and consequent interference with eructation and allows feeding of the patients to achieve an adequate nutritional plane and reduce the risk of aspiration pneumonia when there is a more marked obstruction.

Pneumothorax

Also see Chapter 37.

Definition

Pneumothorax is the accumulation of gas, normally atmospheric air, into the pleural space.

Risk factors

Risk factors for the development of pneumothorax after surgical management of hiatal hernia include:
- Division of the phrenicoesophageal junction
- Opening of the esophageal hiatus to retrieve enlarged viscera or a large volume of viscera from the thorax

Diagnosis

- Air entry into the pleural space and loss of the normal subatmospheric intrapleural pressure is normally readily appreciated during surgery, with a loss of the normal concave contour of the abdominal surface of the diaphragm with caudal displacement and loss of tone of the diaphragm.
- If this is not noticed, then problems with ventilation and gas exchange may be noted during anesthesia or on recovery.
- The diagnosis may be made with thoracic radiographs or thoracocentesis.

Treatment

If this complication is identified intraoperatively, the pleural space should be drained at the end of the surgical procedure. The gas may be drained with a large-bore catheter placed through the diaphragm (Figure 51.3). The lungs may be inflated to 10 to 20 cm H_2O during this procedure to aid elimination of the gas, although this increases the risk of barotrauma. If there is any doubt about the nature of the cause or the effectiveness of drainage of the pleural space, then a chest drain may be placed to allow more frequent aspiration of the pleural space and to allow the patient to recover from anaesthesia.

Outcome

Iatrogenic pneumothorax that is recognized and managed appropriately should not influence the outcome of surgery. However, in patients with preexisting respiratory tract disease (e.g., upper respiratory tract obstruction as a predisposing cause), or aspiration pneumonia as a consequence of regurgitation, pneumothorax may be a more serious consequence.

Prevention

Careful dissection at and around the esophageal hiatus may help to prevent this complication. The use of intermittent positive-pressure ventilation in these patients allows successful ventilation with minimal change in the anesthetic management compared with those that are breathing spontaneously.

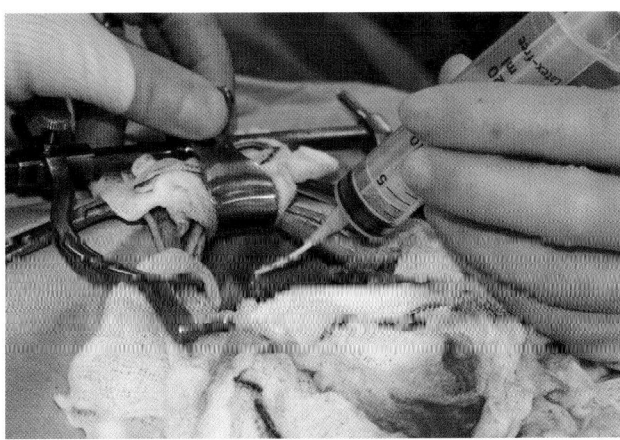

Figure 51.3 Transdiaphragmatic pleurocentesis to manage iatrogenic pneumothorax during surgical management of hiatal hernia.

Relevant literature

The complex nature and interplay of the various pathophysiological events involved in hiatal herniation is reflected in the relatively poor success reported for medical and surgical management. This is hindered by the relatively infrequency of the condition and the tendency to adopt surgical techniques from human medicine, some of which have been found to be inappropriate in small animals.

Gastroesophageal reflux associated with hiatal herniation may be treated medically or surgically. In animals with acquired hiatal hernia secondary to other diseases, these diseases should be treated first before surgical management is considered. In animals with congenital hiatal hernia, surgery is indicated for animals that show no improvement after medical therapy or that have frequent relapses after therapy is stopped.

The most appropriate management of asymptomatic animals with hiatal hernia is unknown (Bright *et al.* 1990). It is not clear whether these animals have a nonprogressive and potentially self-resolving hernia (e.g., as in some young Shar Peis), in which case no therapy would be appropriate, or whether clinical signs associated with the hernia may develop, in which case preventive therapy might be appropriate.

The **aims of therapy** are:
- Amelioration of signs of GER
- Restoration of normal caudal esophageal sphincter function
- Prevention of complications arising from chronic esophagitis (e.g., stricture)
- Prevention of complications arising from regurgitation (e.g., aspiration pneumonia)
- Prevention of complications arising from herniation of abdominal organs (e.g., gastric tympany)

Overview of surgery

From the above, it is apparent that neither surgical nor medical therapy alone is likely to achieve all these aims, and therefore both medical and surgical management are likely to be appropriate in most individuals. It is suggested that medical therapy is instituted initially in all animals (Bright *et al.* 1990; Lorinson and Bright 1998). A decision regarding surgical management is then taken depending on the success of medical therapy. An initial period of medical therapy is indicated in animals destined for surgical management to reduce the signs associated with reflux esophagitis and to allow treatment for aspiration pneumonia.

Medical therapy consists of:
- Establishing a diffusion barrier to peptic mucosal damage (e.g., sucralfate)
- Improving the tone of the caudal esophageal sphincter (e.g., metoclopramide)
- Neutralizing or suppressing gastric acid secretion (e.g., antacids, H_2-blockers, PPIs)
- Decreasing gastric emptying time (e.g., metoclopramide, liquid meals, low fat diet)
- Negating the effect of reduced esophageal tone (e.g., feeding from a height, feeding moist food)
- Removal of predisposing causes (e.g., weight loss if obese, treatment of respiratory disease)

In early reports, medical therapy was regarded as unsuccessful (Gaskell *et al.* 1974; Ellison *et al.* 1987; Prymak *et al.* 1989), but more recent reports conclude that medical therapy may be successful in a proportion of cases (Bright *et al.* 1990; Stickle *et al.* 1992; Lorinson and Bright 1998). One of the reasons for this is that medical therapy is primarily aimed at reducing the clinical signs associated with reflux esophagitis. However, this might not be the main cause of the clinical signs in all animals (Prymak *et al.* 1989; Callan *et al.* 1993).

Although medical therapy may be successful, it does not completely prevent herniation or GER, and long-term complications are possible. These include:
- Aspiration pneumonia from chronic regurgitation
- Esophageal stricture from chronic esophagitis
- Chronic low-grade or massive acute hemorrhage from esophageal ulceration
- Massive herniation of organs from persistence or enlargement of a hernia

Indications for surgical therapy are poorly defined in small animals. In humans, surgery is indicated if:
- Persistent GER is unresponsive to medical therapy
- Esophagitis develops
- Aspiration pneumonia occurs
- A large hernia that interferes with cardiorespiratory function is present

It is likely that similar criteria apply to small animals. Surgery is recommended for animals that do not respond to 30 days of medical therapy, for patients that show frequent relapses after cessation of therapy, or if the clients are unable to comply with the relatively intensive medical regimen (Bright *et al.* 1990; Lorinson and Bright 1998).

Various surgical techniques have been described in the human and veterinary literature and fall into the following categories:
- Sphincter-enhancing techniques
- Closure of the hiatus
- Fixation of the stomach and oesophagus

The surgical principles behind surgical management of any hernia include closure of the hernia ring and fixation of the herniated contents; thus, techniques that achieve these aims are likely to yield success. In humans, closure of the hiatus and gastropexy (Hill technique) are usually combined with a sphincter-enhancing procedure, and long-term follow-up reveals success rates of 80% to 95%. In small animals, sphincter-enhancing techniques are associated with unacceptable intra- and postoperative complications and are no longer recommended.

The surgical technique involves exposure of the abdominal portion of the esophagus and gastroesophageal junction at a cranioventral midline laparotomy. The gastrohepatic ligament, part of the lesser omentum, is incised, and the left lobes of the liver are retracted medially. If the stomach is herniated, it is reduced by caudal retraction. The abdominal portion of the esophagus is further exposed by making a circumferential incision in the phrenico-esophageal ligament, representing the ventral 180 degrees (Prymak *et al.* 1989) or the full 360 degrees (White 1993) of the circumference, taking care to avoid the ventral vagal trunk. The caudal 2 to 3 cm of the esophagus is retracted into the abdomen, and the gastroesophageal sphincter is exposed. Placement of an orogastric tube facilitates identification of the oesophagus.

Sphincter-enhancing techniques

In humans, there is a relatively high incidence of incompetence of the caudal esophageal sphincter. Hence, surgical techniques, such as fundoplication, have been designed to augment this region (Merdan Dhein *et al.* 1980; Miles *et al.* 1988). However, no evidence suggests that this occurs in dogs, and these techniques do not have a rational basis.

Closure of the hiatus

The esophageal hiatus cannot be closed completely because the esophagus still needs to traverse the diaphragm. Partial closure of the hiatus by suturing the two diaphragmatic crura in apposition with simple interrupted sutures has been described (Prymak *et al.* 1989; White 1993). This not only has the effect of partially closing the hiatus but also moves the caudal esophageal sphincter in a dorsocaudal direction if the sutures are placed ventral to the oesophagus. Previous reports have suggested closing the hiatus to a diameter of 1.5 to 2 cm, or the width of one or two fingers, placed alongside the esophagus at the hiatus (Ellison *et al.* 1987; Miles *et al.* 1988). Care is taken to avoid the dorsal and ventral branches of the vagus nerves and esophageal blood vessels.

Fixation of the herniated organs

The abdominal esophagus is fixed in position by esophagopexy. Simple interrupted sutures are placed to anchor the esophagus to the perimeter of the esophageal hiatus. The fundus of the stomach is fixed in position with a left-sided gastropexy. Gastropexy not only physically prevents the stomach from being displaced cranially but also increases caudal esophageal barrier pressure, possibly by increasing longitudinal stretch in the distal oesophagus, which causes reflex contraction and reduction in lumen diameter, thus preventing GER. Stretching of the diaphragmatic crura by gastropexy may also result in an increase in muscle tone at the hiatus.

Similar decision making lies behind the choice of gastropexy technique for hiatal hernia as it does for gastric dilation and volvulus. However, the tube gastrostomy has a number of advantages:
- It is simple and quick to perform.
- It allows deflation of the stomach if gastric tympany occurs.
- It bypasses the esophagus, thus reducing regurgitation.
- It allows feeding of anorectic patients.

Overview of surgery

With such an uncommon condition, it is difficult to compare the results of the various studies directly (Prymak *et al.* 1989; Bright *et al.* 1990; Callan *et al.* 1993; White 1993; Lorinson and Bright 1998). However, the simplest surgery that results in successful resolution of the condition represents the most appropriate choice. The best success rates seem to come from a combination of techniques rather than any single procedure.

In attempting to identify the evidence for a particular method of surgical management, a number of problems are identified:
- Relatively few cases with fewer large studies are reported
- The indications for surgery are not always clearly defined.

- A consistent surgical technique or combination is not always applied to all animals in a report.
- More than one surgical technique is usually applied in one operation.
- The end point of hiatal plication is subjective.
- Some animals with an acquired hernia have had surgery performed to correct the underlying cause and the hernia, with claimed success for surgical management of the hernia (Ellison *et al.* 1987).
- Some asymptomatic animals have had surgery performed, with claimed success for surgical management of the hernia (Bright *et al.* 1990).
- Spontaneous remission of clinical and radiographic signs of hiatal herniation are reported in some young dogs (Stickle *et al.* 1992).
- The definition of "successful" surgical treatment varies from lack of clinical signs to lack of imaging findings.
- There is a relatively short period of follow-up in some reports.

However, the following points can be made:
- Combinations of techniques seem to be more efficacious than single techniques. This is evidenced by the high rate of surgical failure when only one technique is performed (van Sluijs and Happe 1985; Prymak *et al.* 1989; Bright *et al.* 1990) and the failure of the entire procedure if one technique fails.
- Plication of the hiatus and pexy of abdominal organs are the mainstays of surgery.
- Fundoplication techniques have a low rate of success and high rate of morbidity.

References

Bright, R.M., Sackman, J.E., Denovo, C., et al. (1990) Hiatal hernia in the dog and cat—a retrospective study of 16 cases. *Journal of Small Animal Practice* 31 (5), 244-250.

Callan, M.B., Washabau, R.J., Saunders, H.M., et al. (1993) Congenital esophageal hiatal-hernia in the Chinese Shar-Pei dog. *Journal of Veterinary Internal Medicine* 7 (4), 210-215.

Ellison, G.W., Lewis, D.D., Marchevsky, A.M. (1987) Oesophageal hiatal hernia in small animals: literature review and a modified surgical technique. *Journal of the American Animal Hospital Association* 23, 391-400.

Gaskell, C.J., Gibbs C., Pearson, H. (1974) Sliding hiatus hernia with reflux oesophagitis in two dogs. *Journal of Small Animal Practice* 15 (8), 503-509.

Hardie, E.M., Ramirez O. 3rd, Clary, E.M., et al. (1998) Abnormalities of the thoracic bellows: stress fractures of the ribs and hiatal hernia. *Journal of Veterinary Internal Medicine* 12 (4), 279-287.

Knowles, K.E., O'Brien, D.P., Amann J.F., et al. (1990) Congenital idiopathic megaoesophagus in a litter of Chinese Shar-peis: clinical, electrodiagnostic and pathological findings. *Journal of the American Animal Hospital Association* 26, 313-318.

Lorinson, D., Bright, R.M. (1998) Long-term outcome of medical and surgical treatment of hiatal hernias in dogs and cats: 27 cases (1978-1996). *Journal of the American Veterinary Medical Association* 213 (3), 381-384.

Merdan Dhein, C.R., Rawlings, C.A., Rosin, E., et al. (1980) Oesophageal hiatal hernia and eventration of the diaphragm with resultant gastro-oesophageal reflux. *Journal of the American Animal Hospital Association* 16, 517-522.

Miles, K.G., Pope, E.R., Jergens, A.E. (1988) Paraesophageal hiatal-hernia and pyloric obstruction in a dog. *Journal of the American Veterinary Medical Association* 193 (11), 1437-1439.

Prymak, C., Saunders, H.M. Washabau, R.J. (1989) Hiatal hernia repair by restoration and stabilization of normal anatomy. An evaluation in four dogs and one cat. *Veterinary Surgery* 18 (5), 386-391.

Stickle, R., Sparschu, G., Love, N., Walshaw, R. (1992) Radiographic evaluation of esophageal function in Chinese Shar-Pei pups. *Journal of the American Veterinary Medical Association* 201 (1), 81-84.

van Sluijs, F.J., Happe R. (1985) Surgical diseases of the stomach. In Slatter, D.H. (ed.) *Textbook of Small Animal Surgery*, 2nd edn. WB Saunders, Philadelphia, pp. 685-694.

White, R.N. (1993) A modified technique for surgical repair of oesophageal hiatal herniation in the dog. *Journal of Small Animal Practice* 34 (12), 599-603.

52 Diaphragmatic Herniorrhaphy

Stephen J. Baines
Willows Veterinary Centre and Referral Service, Solihull, West Midlands, UK

Traumatic rupture of the diaphragm (RD) is the most common cause of herniation of abdominal organs into the thoracic cavity, representing 77% to 85% of all cases of herniation (Wilson *et al.* 1971; Wilson and Hayes 1986; Boudrieau and Muir 1987).

Young male animals, 1 to 3 years old, are at increased risk for RD (Stokhof 1986; Boudrieau and Muir 1987).

Ruptured diaphragm is caused by blunt abdominal trauma, primarily from road traffic accidents, although kicks, falls and fights have also been implicated (Walker and Hall 1965; Wilson and Hayes 1986; Boudrieau and Muir 1987). Direct trauma from penetrating injuries, (e.g., stab wounds and gunshot wounds) is occasionally seen. Indirect trauma to the abdomen, when the glottis is open, is the most common cause of diaphragmatic rupture. During normal inspiration, the pleuroperitoneal pressure gradient varies from 7 to 20 cm H_2O but may increase to over 100 cm H_2O at peak inspiration. Application of force to the abdomen with the glottis open further increases this gradient, which may lead to RD. If the glottis is closed, the intrathoracic pressure is higher; the pleuroperitoneal gradient is less; and rupture of the lung parenchyma, rather than the diaphragm, is the most likely sequela.

Although blunt, indirect trauma is well recognized as a cause of RD, it must be considered that any trauma sufficient to cause RD will also result in damage to other thoracic and abdominal organs. In fact, after blunt trauma, such as a road traffic accident, RD is considerably less common than other injuries, such as rib fractures, pulmonary contusions, pleural disease (e.g., hemothorax, pneumothorax), and myocardial contusions. Approximately 2% of dogs with long bone fractures have a concomitant RD.

Which abdominal organs become displaced into the thoracic cavity depends on their proximity to the diaphragmatic defect and their mobility. Thus, one or more lobes of the liver are most commonly displaced, being found in the thoracic cavity in approximately 88% of patients with RD. Other organs that can displace into the thoracic cavity after RD, in approximate descending order of frequency, include the small intestine, stomach, spleen, omentum, pancreas, colon, cecum, and uterus. When the right side of the diaphragm tears, the liver, small intestine, and pancreas herniate; in left-sided tears, herniation of the stomach, spleen, and small intestine is more common.

Complications may arise as a result of surgical technique, but pre- and postoperative management of the patient has the greatest influence on the incidence of complications (Levine 1987). The main complications encountered in animals with RD are discussed below. Other complications reported occasionally include gastric ulceration in dogs with chronic ruptures, ascites if there is obstruction to hepatic veins after repositioning of the liver lobes, biliary pleuritis after obstruction or rupture of the extrahepatic biliary tract in the thorax, clostridial intoxication after proliferation of bacteria within the liver, and hepatoencephalopathy after dysfunction of the herniated liver.

Pneumothorax

Also see Chapter 37.

Definition

Pneumothorax is the accumulation of gas, normally atmospheric air, in the pleural space.

Risk factors

Traumatic pneumothorax may be present as a result of the trauma that results in RD or is created during the surgical approach to repair the diaphragm. Risk factors for the development of pneumothorax after diaphragmatic herniorrhaphy include:

- Continued leakage from an intra-thoracic structure (e.g., bronchus or alveoli) damaged at the initial trauma
- Continued leakage from an intrathoracic structure (e.g., bronchus or alveoli) damaged during anaesthesia and surgical repair (e.g., during division of adhesions to the lungs with a chronic rupture or barotrauma during ventilation)
- Failure to close a defect in the diaphragm
- Failure to evacuate the air from the pleural space

Diagnosis

- An abnormal breathing pattern (rapid, shallow breathing) and problems with ventilation and gas exchange may be noted during anaesthesia or on recovery.
- A diagnosis of pneumothorax may be made with thoracic radiography, thoracocentesis, or aspiration of the chest tube.

Treatment

The pleural space should be aspirated by thoracocentesis or via an indwelling chest tube. This should be repeated at regular intervals, depending on the volume of air removed. Reexploration of the abdomen or the chest may be indicated if there is continued leakage of air.

Complications in Small Animal Surgery, First Edition. Edited by Dominique Griffon and Annick Hamaide.
© 2016 John Wiley & Sons, Inc. Published 2016 by John Wiley & Sons, Inc.
Companion website: www.wiley.com/go/griffon/complications

Outcome

Iatrogenic pneumothorax that is recognized and managed appropriately should not influence the outcome of surgery. However, persistence of traumatic pneumothorax may necessitate prolonged thoracic drainage or further investigation of the cause and surgical intervention to repair or remove the source of the leakage.

Prevention

- Careful examination of preoperative radiographs to identify pre-existing pneumothorax, appropriate drainage of the pleural space at the end of the surgical procedure, and meticulous surgical closure of the diaphragm will reduce the risk of postoperative pneumothorax.
- The pleural space should be drained at the end of the surgical procedure. This may be achieved by drainage with a large-bore catheter placed through the diaphragm. The lungs may be inflated to 10 to 20 cm H_2O during this procedure to aid elimination of the gas, although this increases the risk of barotrauma, particularly if there is already traumatic damage to the pulmonary parenchyma. However, a more reliable method is to place a chest drain so that the pleural space can be drained immediately after the surgical procedure and subsequently if needed (e.g., if there is incomplete removal of the air, if there is recurrence of the air) and to allow a more gradual expansion of the lungs.
- Care should be taken when dissecting adhesions between the abdominal viscera and the lungs, particularly if the adhesions are more than 7 to 14 days old (Henderson 1982); it may be more prudent to transect the adhesions through the attached tissue (liver, omentum, attached serosa) to avoid damage to the lungs and leakage of air (Caywood and Lipowitz 1987). More extensive adhesions may require a partial or complete lobectomy.

Hemothorax

Also see Chapters 12 and 37.

Definition

Hemothorax is the presence of blood in the pleural space.

Risk factors

- Bleeding from thoracic structures damaged at the time of the original trauma
- Rupture of viscera (e.g., liver lobes or spleen) that have herniated into the pleural space
- Bleeding from structures damaged during surgical repair, (e.g., lungs, vena cava, phrenic vessels) and from dissection of adhesions
- Preexisting or posttraumatic coagulopathies (e.g., disseminated intravascular coagulation)

Traumatized and malpositioned organs are more likely to rupture than normal viscera that are still in situ. Bleeding from structures damaged during surgical repair may be more likely if surgical access is poor or the defect is sutured without direct visualization. When hepatic tissue is herniated, fibrinolysis may result in hemorrhage, but fibrinolysis may subside after repositioning of the liver (Engen et al. 1974).

Diagnosis

- A diagnosis is made by demonstrating the presence of pleural fluid on **plain radiographs** or **ultrasonography** followed by **thoracocentesis** and obtaining sanguinous fluid with a specific gravity, total protein, packed cell volume, and cytologic picture similar to peripheral blood.
- **Thoracocentesis** may be performed blind in an animal with clinical examination findings indicative of pleural space disease, although in this case, pneumothorax or possibly hydrothorax is more likely. With loss of significant volumes of blood into the pleural space, hypovolemic shock is likely to be appreciated before the volume of blood lost is sufficient to cause dyspnea (Mason et al. 1990).
- **Clinical pathology testing** may be performed to rule out the possibility of a coagulopathy.

Treatment

- The patient is stabilized with intravenous (IV) crystalloids, colloids, or blood products as appropriate. Blood that is removed from the pleural space may be collected into anticoagulant and autotransfusion performed.
- If the hemorrhage persists, then exploration of the abdomen and possibly the thorax is indicated to find the source of bleeding and correct it.

Outcome

The outcome depends on the magnitude and speed of the blood loss, the success of cardiovascular support, and the ability to find and correct the source of bleeding.

Prevention

The tissues should be handled gently at surgery, particularly when repositioning herniated organs. The defect in the diaphragm may need to be enlarged to facilitate this. Adhesions, particularly in animals with a chronic diaphragmatic rupture, should be transected with care, under direct visualization and appropriate hemostasis applied.

Hydrothorax

Definition

Hydrothorax is the presence of fluid (pleural effusion) postoperatively.

Risk factors

- Hydrothorax may be caused by factors that alter the Starling's forces across the pleurae. Any change in the capillary hydrostatic pressure or colloid osmotic pressure across the parietal or visceral pleurae or change in capillary permeability may result in a pleural effusion. This is often caused by dehiscence of the surgical wound, with reherniation of the abdominal viscera, particularly the liver. Herniation of the liver may lead to hydrothorax and ascites in 30% of animals with ruptured diaphragms (Wilson et al. 1971; Creighton and Wilkins 1975).
- It may also be caused by mechanical irritation of the pleura after trauma; the surgical procedure and presence of a chest drain; and, rarely, a lung lobe torsion (Walter 1987).

Diagnosis

- A diagnosis of hydrothorax is relatively straightforward and is made by demonstrating the presence of pleural fluid on **plain radiography** or **ultrasonography** followed by **thoracocentesis** and obtaining serous fluid with a specific gravity, total protein, total cell count, and cytologic picture consistent with a transudate or modified transudate.

- A diagnosis of the cause of hydrothorax may be more difficult to make and, in animals with a large volume of fluid, radiographs may be repeated after drainage of the pleural space to identify any causative lesions and to ensure adequate removal of the fluid.

Treatment

The fluid should be removed for diagnostic and therapeutic purposes. Further thoracocentesis may be required if the effusion and clinical signs related to it return. However, specific treatment of the cause of the effusion is required for its resolution.

Outcome

The outcome depends on the cause of the effusion and the success in managing it.

Prevention

- Prevention of hydrothorax involves all the procedures involved in preventing dehiscence and recurrence of herniation, as well as minimizing trauma to the pleurae during surgery and placement of a chest tube.
- Removal of the chest tube as soon as it is no longer required to evacuate the pleural space of air will reduce an effusion caused by the presence of the tube.

Chylothorax

Also see Chapter 37.

Definition

Chylothorax is defined as the accumulation of chyle in the pleural space.

Risk factors

Chylothorax after RD and its surgical repair is very uncommon. However, trauma to the chest, either accidental or iatrogenic, may result in rupture of the thoracic duct. Herniation of viscera or other pathological processes resulting from trauma (e.g., traumatic pericardial effusion) may increase the pressure in the cranial vena cava and right side of the heart, which may predispose to chylothorax.

Diagnosis

Identification of pleural fluid should prompt thoracocentesis. A diagnosis of chylothorax is made by obtaining fluid that may be milky or serosanguineous with a triglyceride level higher that that in the serum and a predominance of small lymphocytes on cytologic examination, although the cytologic appearance of any pleural effusion may also reflect the previous traumatic episode and postsurgical inflammation.

Treatment

Patients with posttraumatic chylothorax are more likely to respond to conservative management, including drainage, than idiopathic chylothorax. However, persistence of the chylothorax beyond a few weeks may necessitate surgical management with thoracic duct ligation, pericardectomy, thoracic omentalization, and cisterna chyli ablation.

Outcome

The outcome associated with posttraumatic chylothorax that resolves spontaneously is better than for idiopathic chylothorax, which requires surgical intervention.

Prevention

Prompt identification of chylothorax and identification of any predisposing causes are more likely to result in a rapid resolution of the condition.

Pulmonary atelectasis

Definition

Pulmonary atelectasis is partial or complete collapse of one or more lung lobes.

Risk factors

- The presence of intrapleural gas, fluid, or viscera, which causes collapse of the lungs (Figure 52.1)
- Obstruction of the larger conducting airways, either from preexisting disease (e.g., discharge in animals with bronchitis or pneumonia) or the traumatic episode (e.g., hemorrhage)
- Poor ventilation, either when conscious (e.g., caused by pain) or under anaesthesia

Pulmonary atelectasis will persist if the pleural space is not evacuated of fluid, gas, or viscera during the surgical procedure and if the lungs are not reinflated appropriately.

Diagnosis

Thoracic radiographs or computed tomography (CT), ideally after thoracocentesis to remove any concurrent pleural fluid or gas, may allow atelectasis to be suspected and possibly differentiated from other pulmonary parenchymal diseases. Radiographic findings include a focal (often peripheral) or diffuse increase in soft tissue opacity of the lung lobe(s) that may progress to complete collapse, presence of air bronchograms, and a mediastinal shift toward the lesion (Figure 52.2).

Treatment

- Recent pulmonary atelectasis may be reduced or resolved by gentle manual inflation of the lungs with a maximum inflation pressure of 10 to 20 cm H_2O.
- Chronic pulmonary atelectasis may be resolved by gentle application of increasing airway pressure to a maximum of 20 to

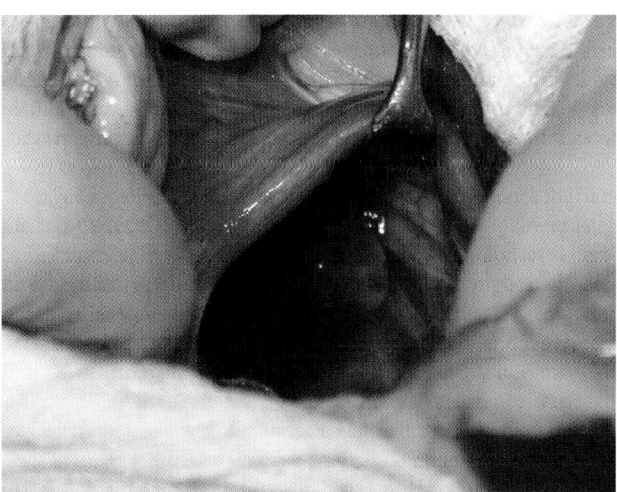

Figure 52.1 Hemothorax and atelectic lung lobes seen during surgery to repair a ruptured diaphragm.

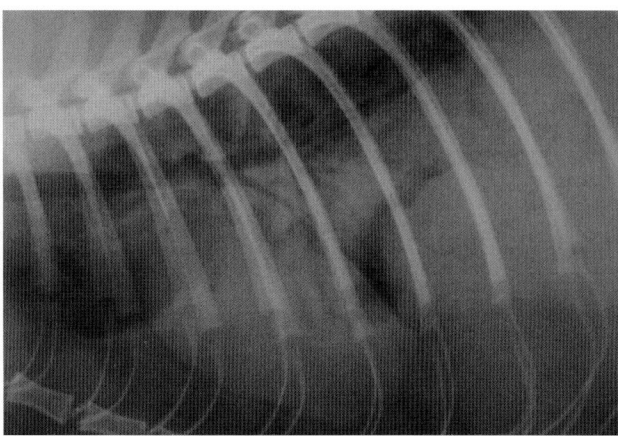

Figure 52.2 Atelectasis of the caudal lung lobe in a patient with a ruptured diaphragm.

30 cm H$_2$O. However, this risks barotrauma, and it may be more appropriate to inflate the lungs to an acceptable level (from a gas exchange point of view), place a thoracostomy tube, and allow the lungs to expand gradually in the postoperative period while retaining control of aspiration of the pleural space with intermittent aspiration or maintenance of a constant negative intrapleural pressure of 10 cm H$_2$O over a few hours.
- Unresponsive atelectasis may be treated with positive-pressure ventilation (PPV) or positive-end-expiratory pressure (PEEP).
- Chronic irreversible atelectasis may require lung lobectomy.

Outcome
Mild atelectasis that can be resolved with expansion of the lungs and evacuation of the lung lobes has a good prognosis. However, chronic atelectasis may persist despite these measures and may have a poor prognosis because of its presence or because of complications arising from attempts to resolve it (e.g., barotrauma and reexpansion pulmonary edema).

Prevention
- Gentle manual inflation of the lungs before closure of the diaphragmatic defect
- Observation of the lung lobes to identify any lobes that do not expand with low inflation pressure
- Gentle handling of the lung lobes during surgery
- Suction of the trachea or bronchi to ensure that there is no obstruction within the conducting airways
- Appropriate drainage of the pleural space (e.g., chest drain).

Other pulmonary lesions: edema, contusions, and pneumonia

Definition
Pulmonary edema is an increase in fluid in the interstitial or alveolar spaces of the lungs. Pulmonary contusion is a contusion (bruise) of the lung parenchyma, with a focal or diffuse increase in blood or other fluids within the lung tissue. Pneumonia is an inflammatory condition of the lung associated with fluid and exudate in the alveoli.

Risk factors
Pulmonary edema has a number of potential causes, including:
- A sudden increase in intrapulmonary pressure when trying to reinflate atelectic lobes
- A sudden decrease in intrathoracic pressure when aspirating gas or fluid from the pleural space postoperatively, particularly in animals with chronically collapsed lungs
- Overinfusion of IV fluids, particularly in animals with preexisting pulmonary contusions

Reexpansion pulmonary edema usually results from an inflammatory response to mechanical injury to the alveolar membrane, mechanical disruption of blood vessels, reperfusion injury to the newly inflated lung, surfactant abnormalities, change in pulmonary artery pressure, and the direct effect of hypoxemia on pulmonary arteries. This complication is more common in cats than dogs.

Pulmonary contusions are caused by trauma, normally blunt trauma, but penetrating trauma (e.g., from a fractured rib) may also be involved. Their severity may be exacerbated by overinfusion of IV fluids. Younger animals with more compliant chest walls are more likely to develop contusions and less likely to get fractured ribs after thoracic trauma. Contusions may involve bleeding and edema initially followed by collapse and consolidation of lung tissue.

Pneumonia may occur after pulmonary contusions, edema, or atelectasis and may be made more likely in patients with abnormal breathing patterns after surgery (e.g., caused by pain and discomfort) or patients with regurgitation or vomiting (e.g., with incarceration of part of the gastrointestinal (GI) tract in the thorax or incompetence of the lower oesophageal sphincter caused by involvement of the esophageal hiatus in the ruptured diaphragm) and subsequent aspiration.

Diagnosis
- Depending on the nature, severity, and extent of the pulmonary lesions, **clinical signs** such as tachypnea, dyspnea, coughing, hypoxemia, and cardiovascular depression may be seen. Depression, anorexia, and pyrexia are more likely with pneumonia.
- Pulmonary rales and rhonchi may be heard on **auscultation**, and in severe cases, pale red fluid or froth may be coughed or be discharged from the nostrils.
- The presence and nature of the pulmonary parenchymal disease can be assessed with **thoracic radiographs or CT**, but any concurrent pleural effusion should be drained before diagnostic imaging to allow an optimum study. The development of clinical signs may precede radiographic changes.
- A **complete blood count** may show evidence of inflammation in animals with pneumonia.
- **Arterial blood gas analysis** may show hypoxemia, hypercapnia, and respiratory acidosis.

Treatment
- Disorders of the pulmonary parenchyma that cause dyspnea or altered gas exchange are emergencies.
- The patient should be maintained in sternal rather than lateral recumbency.
- Treatment may consist of administration of supplementary oxygen (FiO$_2$ of 40%–60%), suction of the airway to remove foam and fluid, PPV, with PEEP as needed, administration of furosemide (1–2 mg/kg IV bolus, repeated every 4–12 hours as required), administration of bronchodilators (e.g., aminophylline 8 mg/kg intramuscularly [IM] every 8 hours in dogs or 4 mg/kg IM every 12 hours in cats), and use of morphine (0.1–0.5 mg/kg IM)

to calm the patient and normalize the volume and frequency of respirations.

- Lung lobectomy may be required for chronic unresponsive disease localized to one or two lung lobes.

Outcome

Mild to moderate pulmonary changes, especially if not associated with dyspnea or hypoxemia, may be associated with a fair to good prognosis. However, severe and widespread involvement of the pulmonary parenchyma, especially if the ventilation–perfusion mismatch does not respond to oxygen therapy, has a guarded to poor prognosis and is a major cause of death after thoracic trauma.

Prevention

- Mechanical ventilation should be performed with care, and high inflation pressures should be avoided.
- Aspiration of the thoracic cavity should be performed with care, and excessive negative pressure should be avoided.
- Use of a thoracic drain minimizes acute changes in intrathoracic pressure and allows chronically atelectic lung lobes to be expanded more gradually.
- Care should be taken to avoid overadministration of IV fluids, which may worsen edema.
- Regular clinical and radiographic assessment of the patient will allow an early diagnosis to be made and improve the outcome.

Lung lobe torsion

Also see Chapter 37.

Definition

This is twisting of a lung lobe, usually the entire lobe, on its pedicle, which results in obstruction of the bronchus and blood vessels.

Risk factors

- Thoracic trauma
- Body conformation
- Presence of a pleural effusion
- Lung lobe collapse
- Altered intrathoracic volume and coughing

Diagnosis

Acute dyspnea, coughing, cardiovascular depression, and possibly thoracic pain may be present, and a serosanguineous effusion may be identified on diagnostic imaging and thoracocentesis. However, differentiating lung lobe torsion from other causes of pleural effusion may be a challenge. In addition, lung lobe torsion may occur postoperatively secondary to a pleural effusion. A focal increase in opacity of a lung lobe and, more specifically, malpositioning and truncation of a gas-filled bronchus may allow a diagnosis of lung lobe torsion.

Treatment

Treatment consists of thoracotomy and lung lobectomy.

Outcome

Lung lobectomy usually results in a rapid resolution of the clinical signs in animals with spontaneous lung lobe torsion. The same may be expected in animals with lung lobe torsion after trauma, although the risk of anesthesia is greater because of the other factors that may affect ventilation and gas exchange such as pain and discomfort, pulmonary atelectasis, pulmonary edema, and pulmonary contusions.

Prevention

Postoperative lung lobe torsion may be prevented by minimizing manipulation of the lung lobes and careful inflation of the lung lobe under direct observation to ensure there is no malpositioning before closure of the diaphragm.

Dehiscence and reherniation

Definition

Dehiscence is the partial or complete breakdown of the surgical repair. Reherniation is the passage of abdominal viscera back into the pleural space.

Risk factors

Dehiscence may be associated with:

- Poor selection of surgical procedure
- Poor surgical technique
- Poor visualization of the surgical site, usually caused by poor surgical exposure
- Poor physical condition of the patient

Dehiscence with reherniation is usually caused by poor surgical technique, which may be:

- Failure to close the entire defect
- Failure to identify more than one defect
- Placement of sutures that are too loose and therefore ineffective
- Placement of sutures that are placed too tightly, placed with too narrow a tissue bite, or placed so that they do hold the tissue in apposition
- Use of suture material that is too small or has too rapid a loss of tensile strength

Poor wound healing and an impaired immune response caused by polytrauma, shock, metabolic disorders, nutritional compromise, or systemic inflammation or infection may also contribute to wound dehiscence. Dehiscence may be more likely with defects in the dorsal or dorsolateral diaphragm because access is more difficult. Dehiscence may be rarely related to surgical site infection, incomplete debridement of the wound margins, and abdominal trauma after herniorrhaphy. Dehiscence has been reported up to 5 months after the initial surgery (Garson *et al.* 1980). Recurrence may also be more likely with chronic ruptures because there may be atrophy of the diaphragm and excessive tension at closure. Although uncommon, multiple defects may be present, and one or more may not be recognized (Levine 1987).

Diagnosis

- Dehiscence of a small part of the wound may not be recognized unless fluid or gas from the abdomen enters the pleural space, but dehiscence of a larger portion of the wound may result in reherniation of abdominal viscera. Strangulation of viscera may be more likely if the viscera reherniate through a smaller defect.
- Animals with dehiscence of the repair and reherniation are likely to show clinical signs similar to those exhibited preoperatively. These include general clinical signs of pleural space disease, such as dyspnea and more specific signs related to the herniated viscus (e.g., gastric tympany, intestinal obstruction or strangulation). Physical examination findings include muffled heart and lung sounds, borborygmi within the chest, and tympany or dullness on percussion, depending on which organs have herniated.
- It is important to differentiate postoperative dyspnea caused by dehiscence and reherniation from other causes, such as persistent

pneumothorax, pleural effusion, pulmonary atelectasis, and pulmonary contusions. As with the initial diagnosis of this clinical condition, plain radiography and ultrasonography should allow these conditions to be differentiated, especially if comparison with preoperative imaging findings is possible.

Treatment

True dehiscence of the surgical repair requires a second surgery. It is likely that the patient will be in a poorer physical condition than at the first surgery; therefore, more supportive care and more aggressive nutritional support may be needed. Consideration should be given to the likely causes of the surgical failure, and a second surgery should address these to improve the likelihood of a successful outcome (see Prevention). During a second surgery, there is a greater likelihood hemorrhage, rupture, infarction, and necrosis of the herniated organs, and surgical excision of some abdominal viscera is more likely. If there is excessive tension at closure, a muscle flap (e.g., transversus abdominis) or synthetic mesh may be used, but this is rarely required (Furneaux and Hudson 1976; Helphrey 1982).

Outcome

For the reasons outlined, the outcome after a second procedure to repair the diaphragmatic defect may be worse than after the first procedure unless a relatively simple cause or error is identified whose correction does not compromise the repair of the defect.

Prevention

- The surgical approach should allow a full and complete inspection of the diaphragm, and maneuvers to improve access should be used to ensure that the entire diaphragm is inspected. These include extending the incision cranially to the xiphisternum or performing a caudal median sternotomy, using of a self-retaining retractor, and making a paracostal incision, although this last manoeuvre is rarely required.
- Suture material of an adequate size (2–3 metric for most cats and dogs) that is either a slowly absorbable (the author's preference) or nonabsorbable material should be used.
- Suturing should usually begin with the dorsal aspect, and the end of the first suture may be used to apply tension to elevate the wound edges into the surgical field.
- Resection of the wound margins should be avoided because this increases the size of the defect and removes fibrous-rich tissue from the edges, which has better suture holding power.
- Excessive tension on the repair should be avoided, and the repair may be omentalized to improve angiogenesis.
- General wound healing may be improved by establishing a good nutritional plane after surgery.

Incarceration of abdominal viscera

Definition

This is herniation of abdominal viscera into the thorax, which becomes entrapped, leading to dilation of the viscus or strangulation of the blood supply (Figure 52.3).

Risk factors

- Herniation of parts of the GI tract into the thoracic cavity may result in dilation of these segments, which then causes compression of the thoracic viscera, especially the lungs and great vessels.

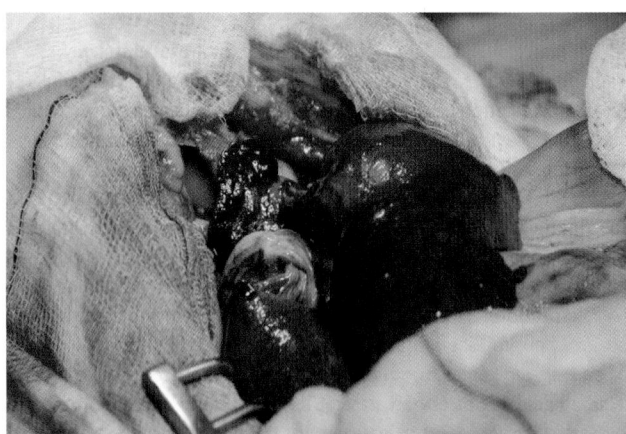

Figure 52.3 Incarceration of the liver in a ruptured diaphragm.

- Compression of the lungs may cause acute, severe dyspnea, which may progress rapidly to cyanosis, and compression of the large veins reduces venous return and therefore cardiac output resulting in shock.
- Compression of the small intestine leads to obstruction, and obstruction of the blood supply to the intestine causes a strangulating obstruction.

Diagnosis

- The animal presents with an acute worsening of its clinical condition associated with severe dyspnea or cardiovascular collapse.
- Tympany may be audible on thoracic auscultation, especially where there is intrathoracic gastric tympany.
- Radiography and ultrasonography should allow a diagnosis of herniation of abdominal viscera, and the acute presentation suggests obstruction, incarceration, or dilation of the affected parts (Figure 52.4).

Treatment

- Dilation of the stomach within the thoracic cavity needs decompression, either by passing an orogastric tube or transthoracic gastrocentesis.
- Surgical exploration of the abdomen, the diaphragm, and possibly the thoracic cavity is indicated as soon as the patient is stable enough for anesthesia. The defect in the diaphragm may have to be enlarged to allow the abdominal contents to be removed.
- Torsion or strangulation of the viscera may necessitate excision of the affected part.

Outcome

The outcome depends of the organs involved and the rapidity and severity of the obstruction or strangulation, as it does for intraabdominal visceral dilation or strangulation. Occurrence of dilation or strangulation within the chest makes treatment of the condition more difficult, however.

Prevention

- Prompt treatment of any animal with a ruptured diaphragm and careful observation during the period of preoperative stabilization are required to prevent an acute exacerbation of the condition.
- Placement of a nasogastric tube is a relatively simple measure that allows the stomach to be decompressed in a conscious animal.

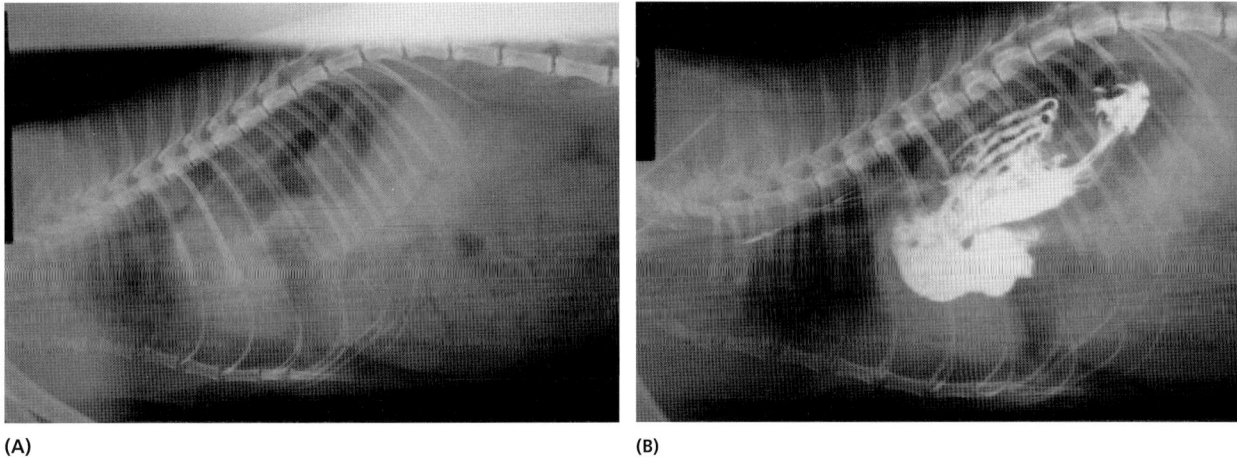

(A) **(B)**

Figure 52.4 A gas-filled viscus (**A**) is present in the caudal dorsal lung field that, on administration of barium (**B**), is noted to be the stomach.

Loss of abdominal domain

Definition

Loss of abdominal domain is defined as a reduction in the intraabdominal volume after a chronic diaphragmatic rupture. With contracture of the muscles of the abdominal wall, the abdominal cavity is then not large enough to accommodate the volume of abdominal viscera that belongs there. This makes abdominal wall closure difficult and may increase intraabdominal pressure excessively, which may impair the function of the abdominal organs (Figure 52.5).

Risk factors

This is more likely with chronic diaphragmatic ruptures and possibly those with herniation of a large volume of abdominal contents (Conzemius *et al.* 1995). The physiological effects of increased abdominal pressure include decreased renal function, hypotension from reduced cardiac output, hypoxia from reduced ventilation and lung compliance, visceral hypoperfusion, acidosis, and increased intracranial pressure.

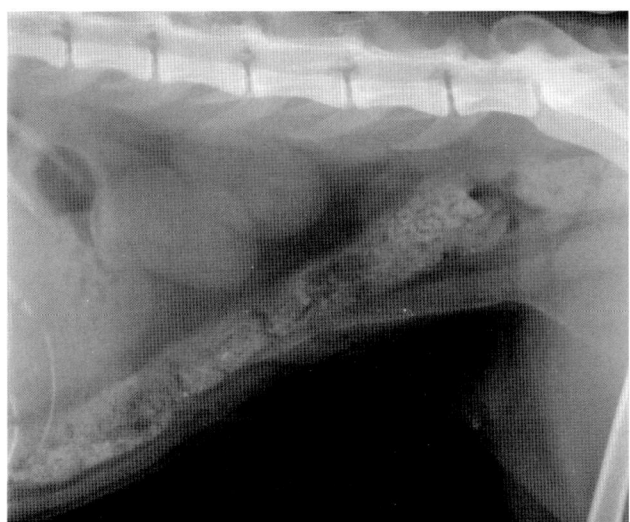

Figure 52.5 Loss of abdominal domain in a patient with chronic diaphragmatic rupture. The patient is also constipated because of ineffective straining with a ruptured diaphragm.

Diagnosis

- This complication is uncommon but clinically apparent when the abdomen is being closed after diaphragmatic herniorrhaphy. If not recognized and not treated, the hemodynamic, hormonal, and visceral changes may be life threatening.
- Measurement of intraabdominal pressure (IAP) after surgery is easily achieved with the use of an indwelling urinary catheter.

Treatment

- The abdomen is closed with care, but if more tension than is normally encountered is appreciated, consideration of the presence of increased abdominal pressure should be considered, and consideration should be given to measuring IAP postoperatively.
- Guidelines for the management of abdominal compartment syndrome are (Drellich 2000):
  - If the IAP is 5 to 10 mm Hg, the patient is monitored.
  - If the IAP is 11 to 20 mm Hg, medical treatment is instituted to reduce IAP.
  - If IAP is greater than 20 mm Hg and the animal has not responded to medical therapy, then surgical decompression is indicated.
- **Medical therapy** involves improving abdominal wall compliance and includes appropriate analgesia, evacuation of intraperitoneal gas or fluid or visceral contents, (e.g., urine or intragastric gas), maintenance of the systemic circulation and organ perfusion with IV fluids, and monitoring of systemic blood pressure and urine output.
- **Surgical therapy** may consist of reduction of the volume of the intraabdominal contents by removal of redundant abdominal viscera (e.g., spleen) or decompression of the abdomen and effective expansion of the intraabdominal volume by using synthetic mesh within the linea alba incision (Conzemius *et al.* 1995), advancement of the diaphragm, creation of relaxing incisions in the external rectus sheath, or leaving the linea alba incision unsutured in the immediate postoperative period.

Outcome

As long as the intraabdominal pressure can be controlled, the prognosis is good. However, the development of abdominal compartment syndrome may be a life-threatening condition.

Prevention

Placement of an indwelling urinary catheter and avoiding gastric distension by feeding little and often and maintaining normal GI motility may help to prevent further elevations in intraabdominal pressure after the abdomen is closed. This condition is prevented in the postoperative period by considering the options for closure listed under Treatment.

Relevant literature

The general prognosis for animals with a ruptured diaphragm (RD) is guarded to fair. The overall survival rate has been reported as 52% to 92% (Wilson et al. 1971; Garson et al. 1980; Stokhof 1986; Boudrieau and Muir 1987; Downs and Bjorling 1987). A significant proportion, up to 15%, of animals die before presentation for anesthesia and surgical correction, and these deaths are generally caused by acute reduction in effective lung volume, hypoventilation, shock, multiple-system organ failure, and cardiac arrhythmias (Wilson et al. 1971; Garson et al. 1980; Boudrieau and Muir 1987). Perioperative death may be caused by inappropriate restraint for examination or other diagnostic intervention, such as radiography and peritoneal or pleural drainage (Wilson et al. 1971; Garson et al. 1980; Stokhof 1986). The other cause of perioperative death is during induction of anesthesia, and any delay in intubation and the establishment of controlled ventilation may have adverse effects (Bednarski 1986). Poor anesthetic management and inadequate ventilation may be implicated in deaths while the patient is anesthetized (Wilson et al. 1971; Garson et al. 1980; Wilson 1992).

The postoperative prognosis for animals has improved over the past 30 to 40 years. In 1980, the survival rate was reported as 52% (Garson et al. 1980), but more recently, the survival to discharge rate is reported as 82% to 89% (Schmiedt et al. 2003; Minihan et al. 2004; Gibson et al. 2005). There is no difference in survival between cats and dogs, between animals with acute or chronic ruptures, or between patients undergoing surgery within 12 and 24 hours. The mortality rate is higher in older animals, with higher respiratory rates and concurrent injuries at presentation (Schmiedt et al. 2003).

Complications may be expected in up to 50% of patients. Life-threatening complications include pneumothorax, organ failure from the initial trauma or as a result of herniation, reexpansion pulmonary edema and hypoxemia, hypothermia, and acute cardiac arrest (Schmiedt et al. 2003; Minihan et al. 2004; Gibson et al. 2005). Postoperative fatal complications may be divided into acute (within 24 hours) and subacute (after 24 hours). Acute fatal complications include hemothorax, pneumothorax, pulmonary edema, shock, pleural effusion, and cardiac dysrhythmias (Walker and Hall 1965; Wilson et al. 1971; Garson et al. 1980; Boudrieau and Muir 1987). Subacute fatal complications include obstruction, strangulation or rupture of the GI tract, or diseases unrelated to herniation of organs (Garson et al. 1980; Boudrieau and Muir 1987). Other complications include postoperative ascites (Helphrey 1982; Downs and Bjorling 1987), gastric ulceration (Willard et al. 1984), oesophagitis, megaesophagus, hiatal hernia, and recurrence of herniation (Pratschke et al. 1998; Joseph et al. 2008).

References

Bednarski, R.M. (1986) Diaphragmatic hernia: anaesthetic considerations. *Seminars in Veterinary Medicine & Surgery: Small Animals* 1, 256-258.

Boudrieau, S.J., Muir, W.W. (1987) Pathophysiology of traumatic diaphragmatic hernia in dogs. *Compendium in Continuing Education for the Practicing Veterinarian: Small Animal Practice* 9, 379-385.

Caywood, D.D., Lipowitz, A.J. (1987) Surgical approaches and techniques for managing pulmonary disease. *Veterinary Clinics of North America Small Animal Practice* 17 (2), 449-467.

Conzemius, M.G., Sammarco, J.L., Holt, D.E., et al. (1995) Clinical determination of preoperative and postoperative intra-abdominal pressures in dogs. *Veterinary Surgery* 24, 195-201.

Creighton, S.R., Wilkins, R.J. (1975) Thoracic effusions in the cat. *Journal of the American Animal Hospital Association* 11, 66-76.

Downs, M.C., Bjorling, D.E. (1987) Traumatic diaphragmatic hernias: a review of 1674 cases. *Veterinary Surgery* 16, 87-87.

Drellich, S. (2000) Intraabdominal pressure and abdominal compartment syndrome. *Compendium in Continuing Education for the Practicing Veterinarian: Small Animal Practice* 22, 764-772.

Engen, M.H., Weirich, W.E., Lund, J.E. (1974) Fibrinolysis in a dog with diaphragmatic hernia. *Journal of the American Veterinary Medical Association* 164 (2), 152-153.

Furneaux, R.W., Hudson, M.D. (1976) Autogenous muscle flap repair of a diaphragmatic hernia. *Feline Practice* 6, 20-24.

Garson, H.L., Dodman, N.H., Baker, G.J. (1980) Diaphragmatic hernia: analysis of 56 cases in dogs and cats. *Journal of Small Animal Practice* 21, 469-481.

Gibson, T.W., Brisson, B.A., Sears, W. (2005) Perioperative survival rates after surgery for diaphragmatic hernia in dogs and cats: 92 cases (1990-2002). *Journal of the American Veterinary Medical Association* 227 (1), 105-109.

Helphrey, M.L. (1982) Abdominal flap graft for repair of chronic diaphragmatic hernia in the dog. *Journal of the American Veterinary Medical Association* 181 (8), 791-793.

Henderson, R.A. (1982) Controlling peritoneal adhesions. *Veterinary Surgery* 11 (1), 30-33.

Joseph, R., Kuzi, S., Lavy, E. (2008) Transient megaoesophagus and oesophagitis following diaphragmatic rupture repair in a cat. *Journal of Feline Medicine and Surgery* 10, 284-290.

Levine, S.H. (1987) Diaphragmatic hernia. *Veterinary Clinics of North America Small Animal Practice* 17, 411-430.

Mason, G.D., Lamb, C.R., Jakowski, R.M. (1990) Fatal mediastinal haemorrhage in a dog. *Veterinary Radiology* 31 (4), 214-216.

Minihan, A.C., Berg, J., Evans, K.L. (2004) Chronic diaphragmatic hernia in 34 dogs and 16 cats. *Journal of the American Animal Hospital Association* 40, 51-63.

Pratschke, K.M., Hughes, J.M.L., Skelly, C., et al. (1998) Hiatal herniation as a complication of chronic diaphragmatic herniation. *Journal of Small Animal Practice* 39 (1), 33-38.

Schmiedt, C.W., Tobias, K.M., Stevenson, M.A.M. (2003) Traumatic diaphragmatic hernia in cats: 34 cases (1991-2001). *Journal of the American Veterinary Medical Association* 222 (9), 1237-1240.

Stokhof, A.A. (1986) Diagnosis and treatment of acquired diaphragmatic hernia by thoracotomy in 49 dogs and 72 cats. *Veterinary Quarterly* 8 (3), 177-183.

Walker, R.G., Hall, L.W. (1965) Rupture of the diaphragm: report of 32 cases in dogs and cats. *Veterinary Record* 77, 830-837.

Walter, P.A. (1987) Non-neoplastic surgical diseases of the lung and pleura. *Veterinary Clinics of North America Small Animal Practice* 17, 359-385.

Willard, M.D., Toal, R.L., Cawley, A. (1984) Gastric complications associated with correction of chronic diaphragmatic hernia in 2 dogs. *Journal of the American Veterinary Medical Association* 184 (9), 1151-1153.

Wilson, D.V. (1992) Anesthesia for patients with diaphragmatic hernia and severe dyspnea. *Veterinary Clinics of North America-Small Animal Practice* 22 (2), 456-459.

Wilson, G.P., Hayes, H.M. (1986) Diaphragmatic hernia in the dog and cat: a 25 year overview. *Seminars in Veterinary Medicine and Surgery: Small Animal* 1, 318-326.

Wilson, G.P., Newton, C.D., Burt, J.K. (1971) A review of 116 diaphragmatic hernias in dogs and cats. *Journal of the American Veterinary Medical Association* 159, 1142-1145.

53 Peritoneal Pericardial Herniorrhaphy

Laura J. Owen
University of Cambridge, Cambridge, UK

Peritoneopericardial diaphragmatic hernia (PPDH) is a common congenital small animal defect that may be associated with cardiac, respiratory, or gastrointestinal signs or may be asymptomatic and an incidental finding. It is more prevalent in the feline population and long-haired cats; in particular, Persians, Himalayans, and Maine Coons are overrepresented (Neiger 1996; Reimer *et al.* 2004; Banz and Gottfried 2010). Weimaraners also appear to be predisposed (Evans and Biery 1980; Banz and Gottfried 2010). The hernia is thought to occur because of failure of development of the septum transversum, arising as a prenatal injury rather than an inherited gene (Bellah *et al.* 1989). Concurrent defects may be present in affected animals, such as a cranioventral abdominal wall defect, umbilical hernia, sternal defect, or intracardiac defect. Surgical correction is the treatment of choice for PPDH in young animals and those with clinical signs relating to the hernia. In older animals or when the PPDH is identified as an incidental finding, conservative management may be an appropriate alternative. In animals treated surgically, reperfusion injury, resulting in hypotension, arrhythmias, and electrolyte or acid–base disturbances is a common complication and one that is potentially fatal (Reimer *et al.* 2004). Other well-recognized complications include cardiac tamponade, the presence of adhesions, pneumothorax, pleural effusion, diaphragmatic atrophy, and hernial recurrence. Patients treated conservatively continue to be at risk of acute decompensation caused by herniation of further abdominal contents or strangulation of organs within the hernia.

Incarceration of abdominal viscera

See Chapter 52.

The liver is the most common organ to become herniated within a PPDH (Figure 53.1) followed by the gallbladder and small intestine (Evans and Biery 1980; Banz and Gottfried 2010). Also reported are the omentum (Figure 53.2), falciform fat, stomach, colon, spleen, and pancreas (Reimer *et al.* 2004; Banz and Gottfried 2010). The containment of these organs within the pericardial sac reduces the likelihood of significant respiratory compromise to the patient compared with a traumatic diaphragmatic rupture; however, a potentially fatal cardiac tamponade may develop because of the increase in intrapericardial pressure and subsequent compression of the right atrium and ventricle (a 5–10 mm Hg rise in intrahepatic pressure can result in significant fluid production (Lipowitz *et al.* 1996).

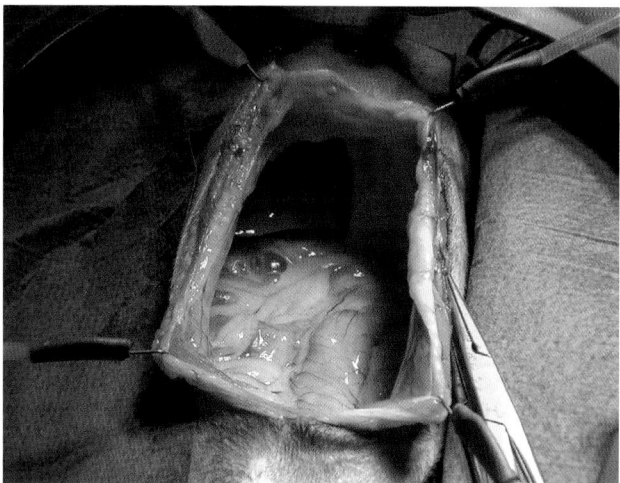

Figure 53.1 Intraoperative view of a peritoneopericardial diaphragmatic hernia in a cat showing a large diaphragmatic defect and herniation of the liver into the pericardial sac. *Source:* A. H. Moore, Bath Veterinary Referrals, Wellsway, Bath. Reproduced with permission from A. H. Moore.

Cardiac tamponade

Definition

Cardiac tamponade is compression of the heart chambers caused by a build-up of pressure within the pericardial sac, most commonly as a result of fluid accumulation; however, with reference to a PPDH, entrapment of air or a large volume of abdominal organs may also be the cause.

Risk factors

See Table 53.1.

Diagnosis

- Preoperative: echocardiography for diagnosis of the tamponade and its cause (fluid or organs)
- Postoperative: lateral thoracic radiography to check for air accumulation within the pericardial sac

Treatment

Cardiac tamponade as a result of fluid accumulation within the pericardial sac or the presence of a cystic structure should be relieved

Complications in Small Animal Surgery, First Edition. Edited by Dominique Griffon and Annick Hamaide.
© 2016 John Wiley & Sons, Inc. Published 2016 by John Wiley & Sons, Inc.
Companion website: www.wiley.com/go/griffon/complications

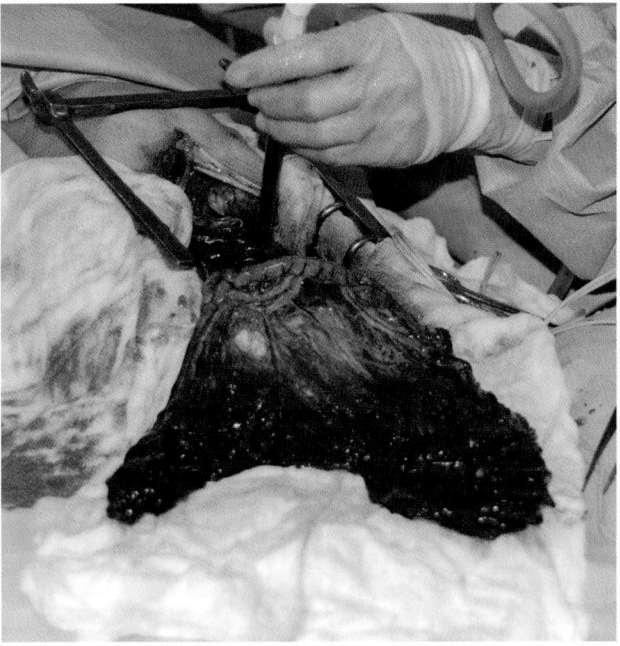

Figure 53.2 Intraoperative view of a peritoneopericardial diaphragmatic hernia in a dog after reduction of the herniated organs showing ischemia of the omentum, which had become strangulated within the hernia. *Source:* J. Demetriou, University of Nottingham, Suffolk, UK. Reproduced with permission from J. Demetriou.

before surgery via pericardiocentesis. This can also be used postoperatively to treat accumulated air causing tamponade.

When the volume of organs is causing the tamponade, celiotomy to reduce the organs back into the peritoneal cavity must be performed as soon as possible.

Outcome

In patients where pericardiocentesis is possible, tamponade is quickly relieved and the patient stabilized. When the volume of organs is causing the tamponade, anaesthesia becomes considerably more risky, and patient mortality may be increased.

Prevention

Accumulated air should always be removed using a needle or catheter placed through the diaphragm just before or just after tightening of the last suture to avoid postoperative air tamponade.

Adhesions

Definition

Adhesions are fibrous bands connecting together previously unconnected tissues or organs. These most commonly form between the

Table 53.1 Pre- and postoperative risk factors for the development of cardiac tamponade associated with peritoneopericardial diaphragmatic hernia

Preoperative	Postoperative
Pericardial fluid caused by incarceration of organs	Accumulation of air after closure of diaphragm
Large volume-entrapped organs	
Bloating of entrapped stomach	
Development of intrapericardial cysts from entrapped fat or liver tissue	

abdominal organs and pericardium; however, adhesions to the myocardium or diaphragm are also possible.

Risk factors

- **Duration of herniation:** Adhesions become more likely with increased duration of herniation. This may be a factor in deciding to manage older patients conservatively when minimal or no clinical signs are present.
- **Herniation of the liver:** The liver is the most commonly herniated organ and the one that appears to form adhesions most readily. This is likely to be attributable to inflammation and necrosis that occur subsequent to malpositioning of the liver lobes, exposing the subcapsular tissue and predisposing to adhesion formation.
- **Previous surgery** resulting in inflammation of abdominal organs (Bellah *et al.* 1989)

Diagnosis

Preoperative diagnosis of adhesions is problematic. Radiographs do not give sufficient contrast to enable adhesions to be identified, and echocardiography is also insensitive. Computed tomography and magnetic resonance imaging have been shown to identify adhesions in human patients, but this has yet to be investigated in dogs or cats (Neiger 1996). Intraoperative diagnosis is usually relied on, and thus the surgeon must be prepared to deal with this possible complication before commencing the procedure.

Treatment

- Improve access to the surgical site, either via further incision of the diaphragm (Figure 53.3) or a median sternotomy. The surgeon must ensure that the patient has been appropriately clipped and prepared and that the equipment is available to allow extension of the surgical incision if necessary.
- Gentle digital or blunt dissection is attempted to break down the adhesions.

Practical Tip 53.1

Use of a Poole suction tip without its outer sheath can also be useful.

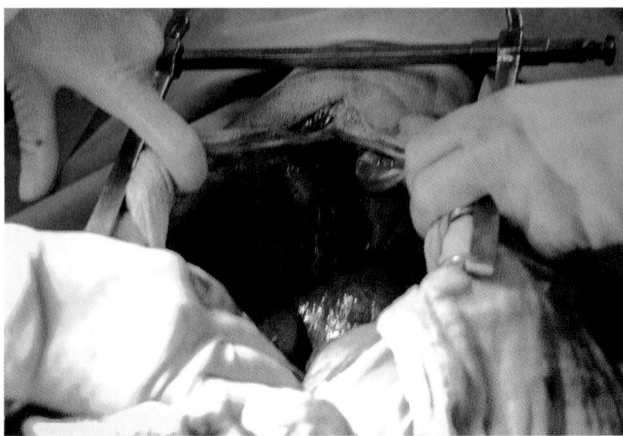

Figure 53.3 Intraoperative view of a peritoneopericardial diaphragmatic hernia in a dog demonstrating extension of the diaphragmatic defect in a dorsal direction to allow reduction of strangulated organs. *Source:* J. Demetriou, University of Nottingham, Suffolk, UK. Reproduced with permission from J. Demetriou.

- Sharp dissection is performed if initial attempts fail. Where attachments are to the pericardium, this tissue is incised cranial to the adhesion to allow the organ to be returned to the abdominal cavity. The pericardium is not sutured. Incision into the pericardium will create an opening into the pleural space and subsequent pneumothorax. Intermittent positive-pressure ventilation will be essential, and the anesthetist should be prepared for this eventuality.
- In rare cases of adhesion to the myocardium, excision of part of an organ (e.g., liver lobectomy) may be required.

Outcome
In the majority of cases, dissection of adhesions is performed uneventfully, and the abdominal organs are returned to the peritoneal cavity. Excessive manipulation of tissue or perforation of organs may cause death in some patients.

Prevention
Early surgery is advised in symptomatic patients. Puppies and kittens are operated on at 8 to 16 weeks of age. Veterinarians should be aware of this risk if advising surgery in older, asymptomatic patients.

Reperfusion injury

Definition
The return of normal circulation to previously ischemic tissues can result in oxidative stress and release of toxins and free radicals. This results in further tissue damage, which may become more widespread and induce systemic inflammatory response syndrome (SIRS).

Risk factors
- Prolonged herniation of tissue
- Herniation of liver lobes

Diagnosis
Development of tachycardia, tachypnea, hyperthermia, hypovolemia, or hypotension postoperatively may indicate SIRS.

Treatment
See Chapter 2.

Intravenous (IV) fluid therapy, IV antibacterial therapy, and oxygen supplementation are the mainstays of treatment of this condition. Careful monitoring of clinical parameters is required, and treatment should be adapted accordingly. Early diagnosis and treatment are vital.

Outcome
Morbidity and mortality are high in patients affected by SIRS.

Prevention
Recognition of liver ischemia and necrosis during surgery and resection of affected lobes may prevent this condition. Careful tissue handling avoids further damage.

Pneumothorax

Definition
Pneumothorax is the presence of air within the pleural cavity, in this instance caused by intraoperative disruption of the pericardial hernial sac or diaphragm.

Risk factors
- Passage of the suture needle into the pleural space during closure of the hernia
- Poor or rough tissue handling
- Additional diaphragmatic incision (to improve access or reduction of organs)
- Presence of adhesions to the pericardium requiring sharp dissection
- Large diaphragmatic defect requiring pericardial flap or free graft for closure

Diagnosis
In most cases, the surgeon will be aware that the pleural space has been entered during the procedure. When this is unknown or uncertain, a postoperative lateral thoracic radiograph can be performed.

Treatment and outcome
See Chapter 37.

Prevention
Careful atraumatic surgical technique can, in many cases, avoid entering the pleural cavity.

Pleural effusion

Definition
Pleural effusion is collection of fluid within the pleural space. Both transudate and chylothorax are associated with PPDH.

Risk factors
See Figure 53.4.

Diagnosis
See Chapter 37.

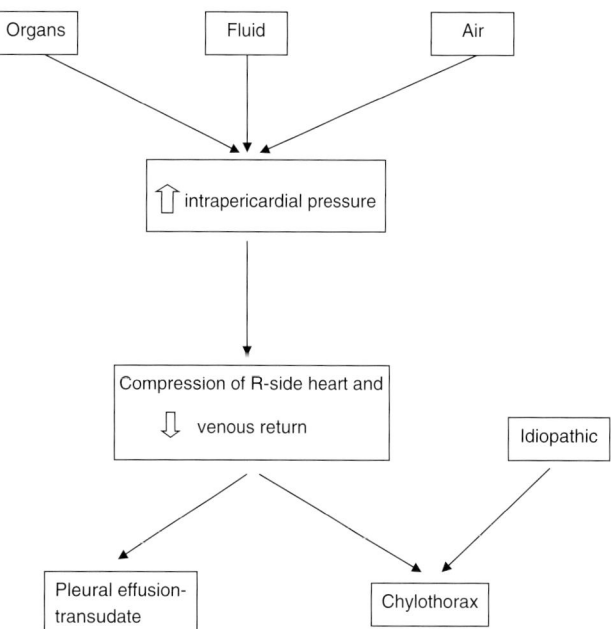

Figure 53.4 Flow chart showing the pathophysiological mechanisms for formation of pleural effusion in patients with peritoneopericardial diaphragmatic hernia.

Treatment

Surgical correction of the PPDH and temporary placement of a thoracostomy tube resolve this complication in most cases. In patients with chylothorax, subtotal pericardectomy and thoracic duct ligation or cisterna chyli ablation may also be indicated.

Outcome

The outcome in patients with pleural effusions is fair, with many effusions being self-limiting; however, the presence of a persistent effusion is a major reason for euthanasia after this surgery.

Hypoventilation

Chapter 52.

Concurrent defects

- Sternal defects, including pectus excavatum
- Intracardiac defects, including ventricular septal defect
- Cranioventral abdominal wall defect
- Umbilical hernia
- Polycystic kidneys
- Pulmonary vascular disease

Risk factors

- Dogs
- Breed (e.g., Persian polycystic kidneys)

Diagnosis

- Physical examination: Be sure to differentiate an umbilical hernia from a cranioventral abdominal wall hernia. The latter is commonly associated with PPDH, but the former is only rarely.
- Radiography
- Echocardiography and ultrasound examination

Practical Tip 53.2

A cardiac murmur heard on auscultation may be caused by the presence of abdominal organs within the pericardial sac rather than an intracardiac defect. Echocardiography is essential to differentiate.

- Contrast imaging studies

Treatment

Sternal and abdominal wall defects are treated surgically at the same time as the PPDH.

Outcome

The prognosis is poorer in patients with concurrent intracardiac defects. Patients with renal or cardiac disease may deteriorate after anesthesia.

Prevention

Careful identification of concurrent defects before surgery ensures that the surgeon and anesthetist are fully prepared and that the owner is aware of any increased risks.

Dehiscence or reherniation

See Chapter 52.

Outcome

Dehiscence and reherniation after PPDH surgery are rare, but because some patients may be asymptomatic, the true prevalence of this complication is unknown.

Prevention

- Surgery should be performed as early as possible (8–16 weeks of age) while the tissues are pliable and easy to manipulate, reducing the tension on the repair.
- When the repair is under tension, consider use of mattress sutures, autogenous flaps (pericardium or transversus abdominis muscle), or synthetic mesh to bridge the defect.

Relevant literature

The largest published retrospective study on PPDH in cats reported an intraoperative complication rate of 38%, of which **hypotension**, likely attributable to reperfusion injury, was the most common (9 of 14 cats) (Reimer *et al.* 2004). A second more recent study reported hypotension to be a complication in only 1 of 31 cats and 1 of 8 dogs (Banz and Gottfried 2010). Surgeon awareness of this potential complication, diligent anesthesia monitoring, careful tissue handling, excision of ischemic tissue, and early detection and treatment of hypotension and arrhythmias in the peri- and postoperative periods may reduce the morbidity associated with this complication.

Adhesions are also reported to occur relatively frequently (9 of 31 cats and 2 of 8 dogs in one study; Banz and Gottfried 2010) They are more likely in older animals (Wallace *et al.* 1992) and when the liver is one of the herniated organs. Ischemia and necrosis of the liver result in exposure of the subcapsular tissues and subsequent development of adhesions to the diaphragm, pericardium, or myocardium. Other abdominal organs are more commonly involved in dogs (Banz and Gottfried 2010). Particular care is taken with adhesions to the myocardium, and it may be safer to excise part of the abdominal organ (usually the liver) than to address the adhesions; indeed, penetration of the ventricle after attempted dissection of adhesions has been reported in one cat (Banz and Gottfried 2010). Excision of part of an organ, usually the liver, may be technically difficult. Surgeons unfamiliar with the anatomy of the liver and inexperienced in its resection should be cautious about undertaking PPDH surgery.

Inability to close the diaphragmatic defect is uncommon but is more likely to occur in older animals. Both the diaphragm and the costal arch lose pliability with age, making it more difficult to manipulate the tissues. In cases with minor degrees of tension, mattress sutures placed between the diaphragm and costal arch may suffice to solve the problem (Bellah *et al.* 1989). In more difficult cases, a pericardial or transversus abdominis flap or synthetic mesh may be required to close the defect (Helphrey 1982; Bellah *et al.* 1989).

Entry into the pleural space occurs rarely in routine cases (Banz and Gottfried 2010). It is important, however, that assisted ventilation is available and that this complication is recognized in a timely fashion, either by the surgeon or anesthetist to enable it to be dealt with. Closure of the defect as a single layer, avoiding dissection at the pericardiodiaphragmatic junction, and careful suture placement minimizes this complication (Wallace *et al.* 1992).

Postoperative complications are common but usually minor. Reimer *et al.* (2004) reported a postoperative complication rate of 78%, with transient postoperative hyperthermia accounting for most of these cases (20 of 37 cats). A second more recent study concurred with this finding (4 of 18 postoperative complications in cats were hyperthermia) (Banz and Gottfried 2010). Major complications in both studies were predominantly respiratory (dyspnea, tachypnea, and hypoventilation), resulting in the deaths of 5 cats. Two of these cats had persistent chylothorax, 1 had refractory pneumothorax, and 2 had presumed acute respiratory distress syndrome.

Transient hyperthermia is a recognized complication of major hepatic surgery in humans (Reimer *et al.* 2004) and thus could be attributed to manipulation and repositioning of the liver in the PPDH cases reported. An alternative theory that the hyperthermia relates to postoperative opioid administration in cats has been put forward by Banz and Gottfried (2010). This complication has not been associated with the development of postoperative infection in these patients and is self-limiting and thus does not require specific treatment.

Pleural effusions occur uncommonly in association with PPDH but are major complications; both transudate and chyle are described (Reimer *et al.* 2004; Schmiedt *et al.* 2009; Banz and Gottfried 2010). Postoperative transudative pleural effusions are reported to be self-limiting after surgical correction of the PPDH (Reimer *et al.* 2004; Banz and Gottfried 2010). Preoperative chylothorax has been reported in one dog and three cats (Kerpsack *et al.* 1994; Reimer *et al.* 2004; Schmiedt *et al* 2009). In the dog, pericardectomy and cisterna chyli ablation were carried out concurrently with PPDH repair, and the effusion rapidly resolved after surgery (Schmiedt *et al.* 2009). In all three feline cases, no additional surgical procedures were performed at the time of the initial surgery beyond PPDH repair, and the effusion remained persistent postoperatively (Kerpsack *et al.* 1994; Reimer *et al.* 2004). In one cat, thoracic duct ligation was subsequently performed, resulting in resolution of the chylothorax (Kerpsack *et al.* 1994). The other two patients did not have further surgery and died or were euthanized within 1 month of PPDH repair (Reimer *et al.* 2004). These reports suggest that in patients with preexisting chylothorax, it is prudent to perform thoracic duct ligation or cistern chyli ablation with or without pericardectomy at the time of PPDH repair.

Long-term follow-up data for PPDH cases are limited but suggest that **recurrence of the hernia** is an uncommon event; reported in 1 of 34 cats (Reimer *et al.* 2004) and 1 of 10 cats (Wallace *et al.* 1992) in two studies. One cat was asymptomatic, with a diagnosis of reherniation made on routine thoracic radiography, and further surgery was not performed (Reimer *et al.* 2004). It is unclear whether clinical signs of reherniation were present in the other cat, but a second surgery was subsequently successful (Wallace *et al.* 1992). Given the potential asymptomatic nature of this condition, this complication may be underdiagnosed.

In addition to recurrence of the hernia, **development of hepatic cysts** (intraabdominal or intrapericardial) is reported in long-term follow-up (Wallace *et al.* 1992; Reimer *et al.* 2004). These cysts have also been documented preoperatively (Weitz 1978; Less *et al.* 2000, Liptak *et al.* 2002; Banz and Gottfried 2010). It is hypothesized that they could be the result of chronic hypoxia of liver tissue and reduced vascular and lymphatic drainage. Intrapericardial cysts associated with herniated omentum or falciform ligament have also been reported (Sisson *et al.* 1993). Resection of the affected tissue has been shown to be curative (Sisson *et al.* 1993; Wallace *et al.* 1992; Reimer *et al.* 2004).

Overall, the **morbidity** associated with surgical correction of a PPDH is considered to be low, with a **mortality rate** ranging from 0% to 14% and the majority of cases resulting in a successful outcome with high owner satisfaction (Bellah *et al.* 1989; Reimer *et al.* 2004; Banz and Gottfried 2010). The complications and mortality rate associated with conservative treatment of this condition are unknown; one text suggests that 75% of asymptomatic or mildly affected cats have a good outcome with conservative treatment (Tobias 2010) but does not give data to corroborate this. When advising clients, it should be remembered that acute and possibly fatal decompensation of a conservatively managed PPDH could occur at any time because of herniation of additional abdominal organs or development of an effusion. Appropriate case selection, recognizing that adhesions and reduced pliability of tissues are more common in older patients and considering referral of these patients to a specialist surgeon, should maximize success.

References

Banz, A.C., Gottfried, S.D. (2010) Peritoneopericardial diaphragmatic hernia: a retrospective study of 31 cats and eight dogs. *Journal of the American Animal Hospital Association* 46, 398-404.

Bellah, J.R., Whitton, D.L., Ellison, G.W., et al. (1989) Surgical correction of concomitant cranioventral abdominal wall, caudal sterna, diaphragmatic and pericardial defects in young dogs. *Journal of the American Veterinary Medical Association* 195 (12), 1722-1726.

Evans, S.M., Biery, D.N. (1980) Congenital peritoneopericardial diaphragmatic hernia in the dog and cat: a literature review and 17 additional case histories. *Veterinary Radiology* 21 (3), 108-116.

Helphrey, M.L. (1982) Abdominal flap graft for repair of chronic diaphragmatic hernia in the dog. *Journal of the American Veterinary Medical Association* 181 (8), 791-793.

Kerpsack, S.J., McLoughlin, M.A., Graves, T.K., et al. (1994) Chylothorax associated with lung lobe torsion and a peritoneopericardial diaphragmatic hernia in a cat. *Journal of the American Animal Hospital Association* 30, 351-354.

Less, R.D., Bright, J.M., Orton, E.C. (2000) Intrapericardial cyst causing cardiac tamponade in a cat. *Journal of the American Animal Hospital Association*, 36, 115-119.

Liptak, J.M., Bissett, S.A., Allan, G.S., et al. (2002) Hepatic cysts incarcerated in a peritoneopericardial diaphragmatic hernia. *Journal of Feline Medicine and Surgery* 4, 123-125.

Lipowitz A.J., Caywood D.D., Newton C.D., et al. (1996) *Complications in Small Animal Surgery, Diagnosis, Management, Prevention*. Williams and Wilkins, A Waverly Company, Baltimore, pp. 336-338.

Neiger, R. (1996) Peritoneopericardial diaphragmatic hernia in cats. *Compendium on Continuing Education for the Practicing Veterinarian* 18 (5), 461-478.

Reimer, S.B., Kyles, A.E., Filipowicz, D.E., et al. (2004) Long-term outcome of cats treated conservatively or surgically for peritoneopericardial diaphragmatic hernia: 66 cases (1987-2002). *Journal of the American Veterinary Medical Association* 224 (5), 728-732.

Schmiedt, C.W., Washabaugh, K.F., Rao, D.B., et al. (2009) Chylothorax associated with a congenital peritoneopericardial diaphragmatic hernia in a dog. *Journal of the American Animal Hospital Association* 45, 134-137.

Sisson, D., Thomas, W.B., Reed, J., et al. (1993) Intrapericardial cysts in the dog. *Journal of Veterinary Internal Medicine* 7, 364-369.

Tobias, K. (2010) Diaphragmatic hernia. In *Manual of Small Animal Soft Tissue Surgery*, 1st Wiley-Blackwell, Ames, IA, pp. 95-102.

Wallace, J., Mullen, H.S., Lesser, M.B. (1992) A technique for surgical correction of peritoneal pericardial diaphragmatic hernia in dogs and cats. *Journal of the American Animal Hospital Association* 28, 503-510.

Weitz, J. (1978) Pericardiodiaphragmatic hernia in a dog. *Journal of the American Veterinary Medical Association* 173 (10), 1336-1338.

54   Perineal Herniorrhaphy

Lynne A. Snow

Southeast Veterinary Specialists, Metairie, LA, USA

Perineal herniorrhaphy is performed to repair a defect of the muscular pelvic diaphragm. Caudal perineal hernias are commonly reported and are the result of a defect between the external anal sphincter, levator ani, and internal obturator muscles. Other hernia locations include dorsal, ventral, and sciatic perineal hernias (Rochat and Mann 1998).

The most common complications after perineal herniorrhaphy are incisional, reported in 5.6% to 45% of cases (Bellenger 1980; Sjollema and van Sluijs 1989; Hosgood *et al.* 1995; Brissot *et al.* 2004; Bongartz *et al.* 2005). Recurrence of herniation is reported in 0% to 15% of cases (Sjollema and van Sluijs 1989; Hosgood *et al.* 1995; Brissot *et al.* 2004; Bongartz *et al.* 2005; Szabo *et al.* 2007). Other potential complications include urinary dysfunction, tenesmus with or without rectal prolapse, fecal incontinence, and sciatic nerve entrapment with suture (Hosgood *et al.* 1995; Bellenger and Canfield 2003).

Recurrence

Definition

Perineal herniorrhaphy is a defect in the muscular pelvic diaphragm on the ipsilateral side of a previously repaired perineal hernia.

Risk factors

- Failure of primary repair
- Progressive deterioration of the perineal muscles
- Tenesmus caused by untreated prostatic disease or constipation
- Intact male (although this has not been definitively proven)
- Repeat herniorrhaphy
- Surgeon inexperience

Diagnosis

- Hernia recurrence may be noted by the owner as a **return of the presenting clinical signs** such as perineal swelling and tenesmus (Figure 54.1).
- **Rectal examination** should be performed during all routine physical examinations after perineal hernia repair because this may diagnose hernia recurrence before a return of clinical signs. If clinical signs have returned, digital rectal examination (DRE) is imperative for definitive diagnosis by palpating a defect in the pelvic diaphragm.

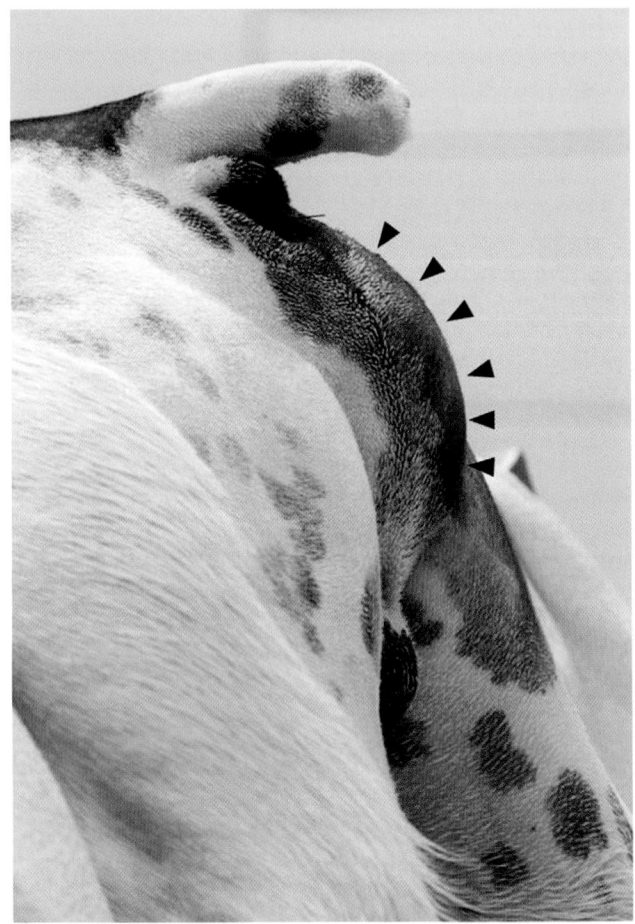

Figure 54.1 Dog with right perineal hernia. Right-sided perianal swelling is noted (arrowheads). The dog is prepared for surgery with an anal purse-sting suture to minimize contamination. *Source:* D. Ogden, Louisiana State University, Baton Rouge, LA, 2014. Reproduced with permission from D. Ogden.

- **Abdominal and perineal ultrasonography and radiography** may be useful to determine the hernia contents.
- If a mass is suspected at the previous hernia site, **fine-needle aspiration** and cytology may be used to differentiate among suture granuloma, steatitis, neoplasia, and hernia recurrence (Figure 54.2).

Complications in Small Animal Surgery, First Edition. Edited by Dominique Griffon and Annick Hamaide.

© 2016 John Wiley & Sons, Inc. Published 2016 by John Wiley & Sons, Inc.

Companion website: www.wiley.com/go/griffon/complications

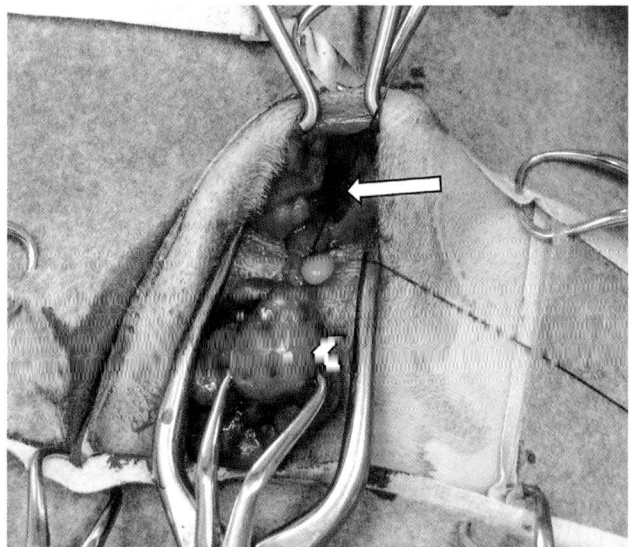

Figure 54.2 Dog with recurrence of perineal hernia 1 year after perineal herniorrhaphy with an internal obturator transposition flap. On examination, the dog had a small 1-cm defect appreciated along the ventral pelvic diaphragm and a firm mass. Upon surgical exploration, the mass was identified as herniated omentum (arrowhead), which was torsed and necrotic. The pelvic diaphragm defect (arrow) resulted from breakdown of the original surgical repair. Suture is seen encircling the pedicle before amputation of the necrotic adipose tissue.

Treatment

Repeated anatomic primary closure may be attempted; however, an improved success rate may be expected by using alternate techniques. Internal obturator transposition is most commonly performed because of minimal morbidity and the ability to close a ventral defect.

Herniorrhaphy with autogenous muscle flaps

- Internal obturator muscle transposition (van Sluijs and Sjollema 1989) (Figure 54.3): The internal obturator muscle flap is useful for decreasing tension on hernia closure at the ventral aspect of the hernia defect.
- Semitendinosus muscle flap (Chambers and Rawlings 1991): The semitendinosus muscle flap is useful for closing a ventral hernia defect when the internal obturator muscle flap has failed or the muscle is atrophied.
- Superficial gluteal muscle transplantation (Spreull and Frankland 1980): The superficial gluteal muscle flap is most useful for closing a dorsal-lateral hernia defect.

Herniorrhaphy with biomaterials

Synthetic, xenographic, or autogenous materials have been used to close perineal hernia defects alone or in combination with autogenous muscle flaps to augment the repair.
- Polypropylene mesh (Szabo et al. 2007): Polypropylene mesh may be used alone or in combination with an internal obturator transposition flap.
- Fascia lata graft (Bongartz et al. 2005): Autogenous fascia lata free graft may be used to close perineal hernia defects when local muscle flaps are inadequate.
- Porcine small intestinal submucosa (Stoll et al. 2002): Porcine small intestinal submucosa has been used in experimentally created perineal hernias with good success.

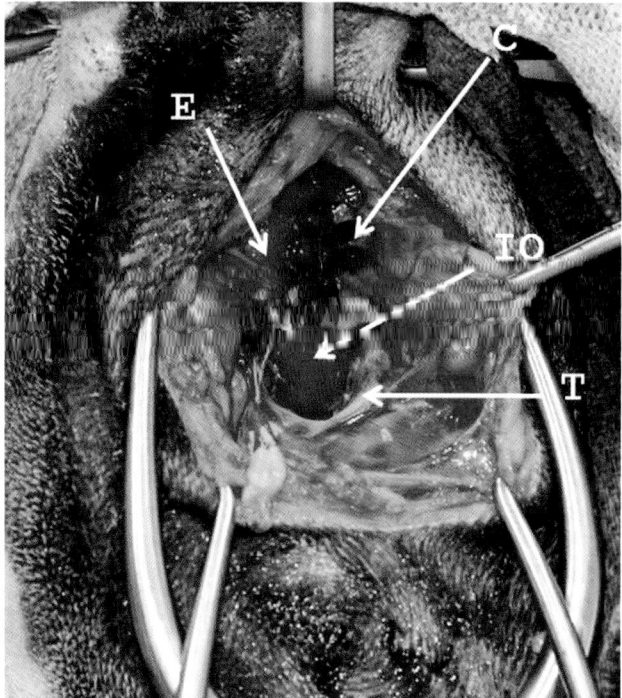

Figure 54.3 Intraoperative image of internal obturator muscle transposition. The internal obturator muscle (IO) is elevated from the ischial tuberosity (T) and sutured to the coccygeal muscle (C) and the external anal sphincter (E). *Source:* D. Ogden, Louisiana State University, Baton Rouge, LA, 2014. Reproduced with permission from D. Ogden.

Consider other techniques to prevent herniation of abdominal contents

- Cystopexy is used when urinary bladder retroflexion is present to permanently fix the urinary bladder in the abdominal cavity.
- Colopexy is used when rectal prolapse accompanies perineal herniation to provide cranial traction on the descending colon.
- Vas deferentopexy is used to prevent retroflexion of the urinary bladder and prostate into the perineal hernia defect (Bilbrey et al. 1990).

Staged repair of perineal hernia may be indicated in animals with complicated perineal hernias (Brissot et al. 2004). Celiotomy is performed first to reduce hernia contents and perform cystopexy, colopexy, or both. Herniorrhaphy is performed 1 to 14 days later. The delay allows the animal to be stabilized in cases of urinary obstruction secondary to a retroflexed bladder.

Outcome

Good to excellent outcomes are reported in 61% to 92% of dogs undergoing surgical treatment for perineal hernia (Brissot et al. 2004; Szabo et al. 2007). Limited information is available regarding resolution of hernia recurrence.

Prevention

The most vulnerable part of the repair is the ventral aspect caused by the broad base of the triangular defect and subsequent tension on the sutures between the external anal sphincter muscle and the internal obturator muscle as well as sutures between the coccygeus muscle and the internal obturator muscle (Robertson 1984). For this reason, internal obturator transposition is often used for herniorrhaphy during the first surgery.

Correct anatomic identification is the most important step in reconstruction to prevent hernia recurrence. The muscle bodies or sacrotuberous ligament used in herniorrhaphy must be correctly identified, allowing sutures placement in healthy tissue to prevent suture pull through. Nonabsorbable suture materials such as nylon or polypropylene should be used if delayed healing is suspected.

Although not proven to be beneficial in preventing recurrence of perineal hernia, castration of intact dogs is recommended at the time of herniorrhaphy (Bellenger and Canfield 2003). In dogs with unilateral perineal herniation, castration has not been shown beneficial in preventing contralateral perineal hernia (Bellenger and Canfield 2003).

Wound infection
See Chapter 1.

Wound seroma

Definition
Wound seroma is a collection of fluid underneath the skin incision accumulated in dead space between tissue planes.

Risk factors
Seromas most commonly develop because of inadequate closure of the subcutaneous tissue and residual dead space from the hernia sac.

Diagnosis
- Seromas are commonly diagnosed in the first 1 to 5 days after surgery. They are soft and fluctuant on palpation.
- Rectal examination is performed to confirm maintenance of the pelvic diaphragm.
- Local ultrasonography may be used to differentiate seroma from hernia recurrence.
- Seroma should be differentiated from surgical site infection by fine-needle aspiration with cytology and culture if indicated.

Treatment
Warm compresses help to open lymphatics and allow seroma drainage. The seroma should *not* be drained repeatedly because doing so may introduce bacteria and lead to infection.

Outcome
Seroma resolution typically occurs over 1 to 2 weeks.

Prevention
Adequate closure of the subcutaneous space will decrease seroma formation. Cold compresses can be used in the initial 24 hours after surgery to decrease inflammation and seroma formation.

Sciatic nerve entrapment

Definition
Sciatic nerve entrapment is suture entrapment of the entire or part of the sciatic nerve during herniorrhaphy.

Risk factors
Sciatic nerve entrapment most commonly occurs when the sacrotuberous ligament is used as the lateral anchoring point for herniorrhaphy (Figure 54.4).

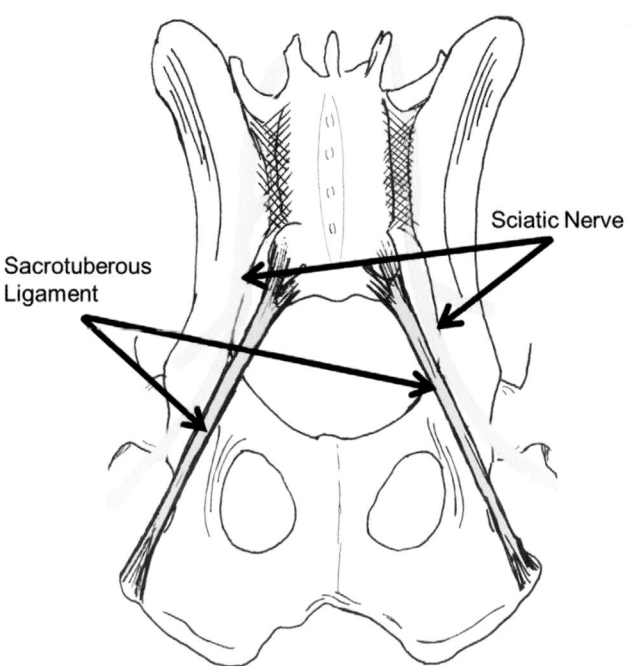

Figure 54.4 Anatomy of the sacrotuberous ligament in relation to the sciatic nerve. The direct cranial position of the sciatic nerve in relation to the sacrotuberous ligament makes the nerve vulnerable to entrapment when encircling the sacrotuberous ligament during herniorrhaphy.

Diagnosis
- Severe pain typically upon anesthetic recovery
- Non–weight-bearing lameness
- Sciatic nerve deficits (Figure 54.5)

Treatment
An immediate caudolateral approach to the hip joint to expose the sciatic nerve is indicated. The offending suture is then carefully removed. The perineal region is only reexplored if hernia recurrence occurs after removal of the offending suture.

Outcome
Sciatic nerve function generally improves over a period of several days to weeks (Bellenger and Canfield 2003). There may be some residual sciatic neuropathy.

Prevention
Sciatic nerve entrapment is most easily avoided by performing herniorrhaphy without incorporating the sacrotuberous ligament if adequate coccygeus muscle is available for herniorrhaphy. If the sacrotuberous ligament must be incorporated into the repair, the needle is directed from lateral to medial while encircling the sacrotuberous ligament (Robertson 1984). This allows the surgeon to palpate the ligament moving it caudally away from the sciatic nerve. In addition, the sciatic nerve may be avoided by using a blunt forceps to pass the suture around the ligament rather than the needle. Alternatively, the suture may be passed through the midsubstance of the ligament rather than encircling the ligament to avoid the sciatic nerve.

Fecal incontinence

Definition
Fecal incontinence is loss of controlled defecation.

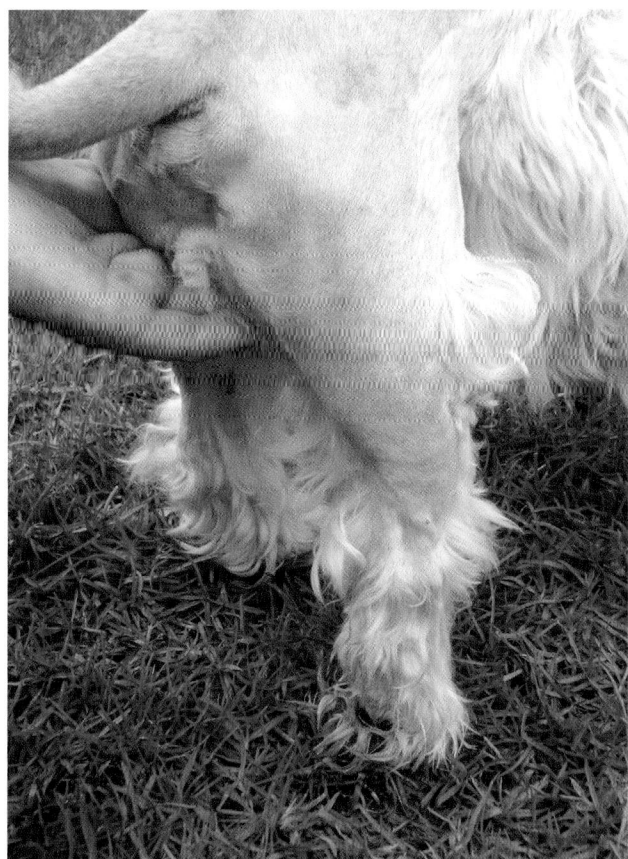

Figure 54.5 Dog with conscious proprioceptive deficit following perineal surgery.

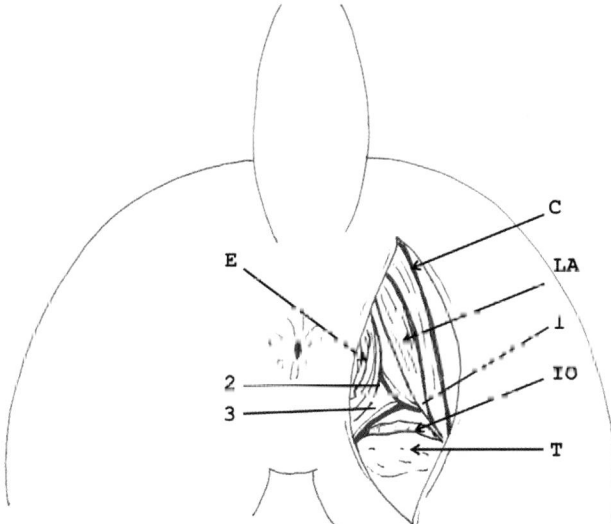

Figure 54.6 Perineal anatomy. Note the vulnerability of the pudendal artery and nerve during perineal herniorrhaphy: external anal sphincter (E), levator ani muscle (LA), coccygeal muscle (C), internal obturator muscle (IO), ischial tuberosity (T), internal pudendal artery and vein and pudendal nerve (1), caudal rectal artery and vein (2), and ventral perineal artery and vein and superficial perineal nerve (3).

Risk factors
• Bilateral herniorrhaphy
• Damage to pudendal or caudal rectal nerves (Figure 54.6)
• Excessive tension on the external anal sphincter
• Tearing or trauma to the external anal sphincter

Diagnosis
Fecal incontinence is diagnosed by witnessing defecation without conscious control. This must be differentiated from diarrhea and urgency incontinence from rectal irritation. Rectal tone and perineal reflex may be decreased in cases of fecal incontinence caused by pudendal nerve damage.

Treatment
There is no effective treatment for reinnervation of the external anal sphincter muscle. Clinical signs may be worsened if diarrhea is present; therefore, diarrhea is treated as indicated.

Outcome
Return of continence depends on the degree of nerve damage. Neuropraxia may resolve over several days to weeks. Permanent unilateral nerve damage may result in incontinence that resolves over several weeks because of reinnervation by the contralateral side (Bellenger and Canfield 2003). Permanent incontinence is the result of severe bilateral nerve damage (Bellenger and Canfield 2003).

Prevention
Careful dissection is used to avoid damage to the pudendal and caudal rectal nerves during herniorrhaphy. Tension on the external anal sphincter is reduced by use of the internal obturator transposition (Robertson 1984).

Rectal prolapse

Definition
Rectal prolapse is protrusion of rectal tissue through the anus to the exterior of the body (Figure 54.7).

Risk factors
• Tenesmus secondary to constipation, diarrhea, prostatic disease, or suture inadvertently placed through the rectal wall (Dieterich 1975)

Diagnosis
• A tubelike mass is noted protruding from the anus.
• DRE differentiates rectal prolapse from prolapsed intestinal intussusception. The digital probe will not pass the anocutaneous junction while a rectal prolapse is being examined. On the contrary, a digital probe will continue along the protruding mass past the anocutaneous junction into the rectum in an animal with a prolapsed intestinal intussusception. Sutures inadvertently penetrating the rectal lumen are identified during examination.
• Ultrasonography is most commonly used to evaluate prostatic disease.
• A fecal sample is obtained to evaluate for parasitism.

Treatment
• Any underlying concurrent conditions are treated appropriately.
• Tenesmus is minimized by feeding a high-fiber, low-residue diet and stool softener for 10 to 14 days after surgery.
• If prolapse is intermittent, it is managed conservatively by keeping the tissue moist and minimizing irritation by preventing licking.

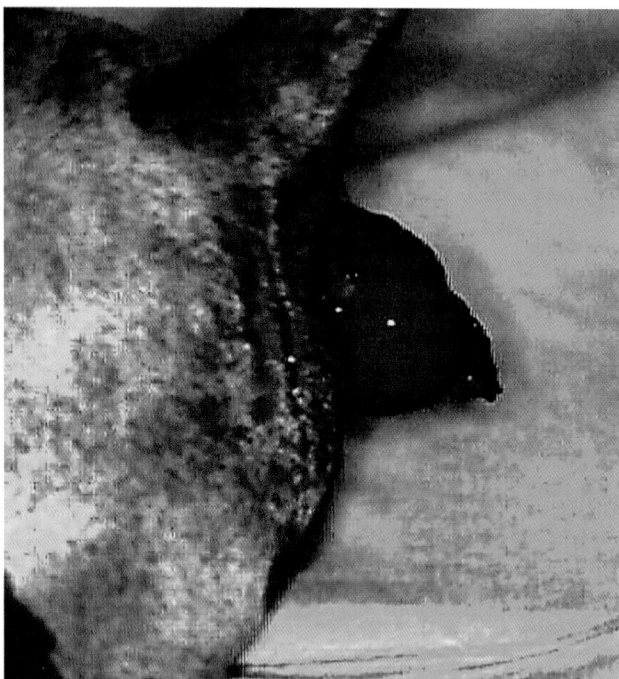

Figure 54.7 Rectal prolapse following perineal herniorrhaphy. *Source:* G. Hosgood, 2014. Reproduced with permission from G. Hosgood.

- If a substantial amount of tissue is prolapsed or prolapse is persistent despite resolution of tenesmus, surgical treatment is warranted:
  - Viable, reducible (Seim 1988): If the prolapsed rectal tissue is viable and reducible, the prolapse is replaced. Hypertonic solution (50% glucose) is used to relieve tissue edema if necessary. A loose purse-string suture is placed around the anus using 2.0 nylon. The suture is removed in 4 to 5 days.
  - Viable, nonreducible or recurrence after removal of purse-string suture (Seim 1988): If the prolapsed tissue is viable but not reducible or prolapse recurs after removal of the purse-string suture, the prolapse is reduced via celiotomy. The rectal prolapse is reduced by gentle cranial traction and manual reduction by an assistant. Left-sided distal descending colopexy may help to prevent recurrence of rectal prolapse.
  - Nonviable or nonreducible by celiotomy (Seim 1988): If the prolapsed tissue is not viable or is unable to be reduced by celiotomy, the prolapsed tissue is amputated.

Outcome

Most rectal prolapses after perineal herniorrhaphy resolve with gentle reduction and treatment of tenesmus. Colopexy resulted in resolution of recurrent rectal prolapse in all 14 animals in one study (Popovitch *et al.* 1994).

Prevention

Prevention of tenesmus by dietary management and appropriate management of any underlying conditions is used to prevent rectal prolapse. A high-fiber diet or the addition of a fiber supplement may minimize tenesmus. Epidural anesthesia may be used to minimize tenesmus in the immediate postoperative period.

Immediate postoperative rectal examination identifies any inadvertent rectal penetration. If rectal penetration is identified, the offending suture is immediately removed.

Anuria and urinary incontinence

Definition

Anuria is the complete lack of urination. Urinary incontinence is urination without conscious control or awareness.

Risk factors

- Retroflexion of the urinary bladder (Figure 54.8)
- Urinary bladder necrosis
- Urinary bladder torsion
- Uroabdomen
- Inadvertent prostatectomy (Sereda *et al.* 2002)

Diagnosis

Careful monitoring of urination after treatment will identify urinary tract malfunction.

- **Serum biochemistry:** Elevations of serum urea and creatinine are seen with urinary obstruction or uroabdomen.
- **Abdominal ultrasonography:** Ultrasonography is used to assess the urinary bladder wall and to determine if free peritoneal fluid is present.
- **Abdominocentesis:** Free peritoneal fluid creatinine concentrations are compared with serum creatinine concentration to confirm the presence of a uroabdomen.
- **Retrograde cystourethrography:** Cystourethrography is used to evaluate patency of the urinary tract and to confirm the location of the urinary bladder. The urinary catheter should be gently advanced retrograde and should not be forced because this may result in urethral tears. Only the tip of the urinary catheter is introduced into the urethra if resistance is felt and contrast is used to highlight any defects of the urinary tract.
  - Loss of urinary tract integrity is diagnosed by identifying free contrast material in the peritoneal cavity.
  - Urethral or trigonal obstruction is identified by the inability of contrast agent to pass into the bladder. Inadvertent prostatectomy may be suspected if a mass was excised at the time of perineal herniorrhaphy. Urinary obstruction may also result if the bladder is torsed during reduction into the abdominal cavity.

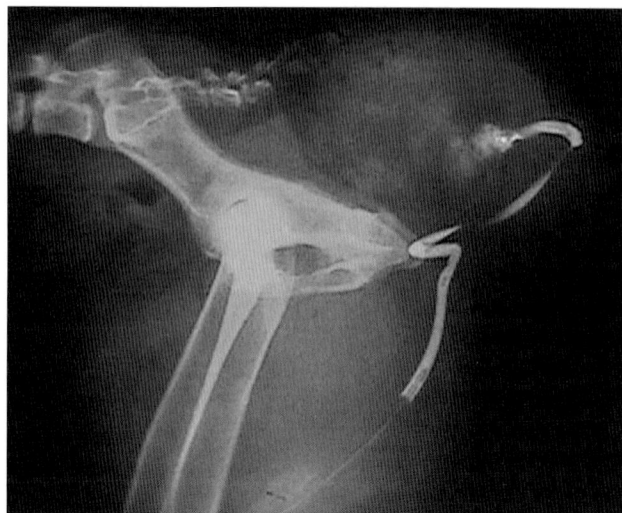

Figure 54.8 Retrograde cystourethrogram of retroflexion of the urinary bladder due to perineal hernia. *Source:* G. Hosgood, 2014. Reproduced with permission from G. Hosgood.

○ Caudal displacement of the urinary bladder into the pelvic canal may result from tearing or stretching of the supporting ligaments of the bladder (Gilley *et al.* 2003). This may result in urinary incontinence caused by a loss of abdominal pressure at the neck of the urinary bladder.

○ Normal cystourethrography findings or identification of a distended urinary bladder is expected in cases of anuria or urinary incontinence caused by neurologic injury or detrusor muscle atony.

Treatment

Treatment depends on the underlying cause.

- Urethral obstruction is investigated by celiotomy. Focal urinary bladder necrosis is treated by partial cystectomy. Complete urinary bladder necrosis is treated by advanced urinary diversion or urinary bladder reconstruction techniques. Inadvertent prostatectomy is treated by resection of any fibrotic tissue present and cystic-urethral anastomosis (Sereda *et al.* 2002). Cystopexy can improve urinary function if the urinary bladder is caudally displaced because of laxity or disruption of the supporting ligaments (Gilley *et al.* 2003).

- Neurologic urinary tract dysfunction may require urinary diversion via a cystostomy tube or urethral catheterization. Bethanechol is used to improve detrusor muscle contraction in dogs with detrusor muscle atony.

Outcome

The prognosis of patients with urinary tract dysfunction depends on the specific cause. The morbidity and mortality of dogs with urinary bladder necrosis, uroabdomen, or prostatectomy may be high. Urinary incontinence caused by neurologic injury typically resolves spontaneously within 1 week, but some animals remain incontinent (Bellenger and Canfield 2003).

Prevention

- Urinary bladder retroflexion is treated immediately by decompression to minimize neurologic injury and detrusor muscle atony. Decompression is performed by urethral catheterization. If catheterization is not possible, the urinary bladder is decompressed by cystocentesis via the perineal region. After being returned to the normal location, the urinary bladder should be evaluated for viability and correct positioning by celiotomy. Cystopexy or vas deferentopexy during the initial surgery may be used to prevent caudal displacement of the bladder if the supporting ligaments have been torn.

- Inadvertent prostatectomy has been reported to cause urethral obstruction after perineal hernia repair. Inadvertent prostatectomy is prevented by precise anatomic identification before excision of any hernia contents. If organ identification is questionable, the hernia should be reduced and celiotomy performed to evaluate the hernia contents. Paraprostatic cysts or other prostatic disease can then be surgically treated via celiotomy with better visualization.

Relevant literature

Recurrence of perineal hernia is reported in 0% to 15% of dogs after herniorrhaphy (Sjollema and van Sluijs 1989; Hosgood *et al.* 1995; Brissot *et al.* 2004; Bongartz *et al.* 2005; Szabo *et al.* 2007).

The most likely location is at the ventral aspect of the hernia caused by increased tension on the repair. The internal obturator muscle transposition was developed to reduce tension on the ventral suture line. The recurrence rate of perineal hernia with this technique has been reported to be 5% in one study (Sjollema and van Sluijs 1989). Other reported complications included wound infection (45%), fecal incontinence (15%), and perineal fistula (7%) (Sjollema and van Sluijs 1989. The semitendinosus muscle flap has been used for augmentation of ventral perineal hernia (Chambers and Rawlings 1991). The semitendinosus muscle flap is useful if the internal obturator transposition has failed or the internal obturator muscle is atrophied. In an experimental model of semitendinosus muscle transposition, there were no gait abnormalities noted; however, muscle atrophy of the transposed semitendinosus muscle was noted on ultrasonography (Mortari *et al.* 2005). The superficial gluteal muscle transposition (Spreull and Frankland 1980) is most useful for closing a dorsal-lateral hernia defect. The use of superficial gluteal transposition and internal obturator transposition together was reported for 44 dogs, and recurrence was noted in 3 of 44 dogs (Raffan 1993). Other reported complications included seroma (5 of 44 dogs), tenesmus (2 of 44 dogs), and iatrogenic urinary bladder torsion (1 of 44 dog) (Raffan 1993).

Interposition of synthetic, allogenic, and autogenous free grafts have been used as primary herniorrhaphy or to augment muscle transposition techniques. Polypropylene mesh was used in combination with internal obturator transposition in 59 dogs with an overall short-term complication rate of 8.7% (Szabo *et al.* 2007). The reported complications in dogs available for follow-up were incisional infection (2 dogs), seroma (3 dogs), and tenesmus (1 dog) (Szabo *et al.* 2007). Long-term follow-up was available for 36 dogs with a recurrence rate of 12.5% (Szabo *et al.* 2007). Interposition of autogenous fascia lata was used to close perineal hernia defects in 12 dogs (Bongartz *et al.* 2005). The most common complication was lameness in 10 dogs, which resolved without specific therapy (Bongartz *et al.* 2005). Other complications reported were rectal prolapse in 2 dogs, which was treated by manual reduction, and seroma in 1 dog (Bongartz *et al.* 2005). Porcine small intestinal submucosa was used to close experimentally created perineal hernias in 12 dogs (Stoll *et al.* 2002). No significant postoperative complications were noted, and the maximum pressure to failure was not significantly different between the porcine small intestinal submucosa and hernias repaired by internal obturator muscle transposition (Stoll *et al.* 2002). The dogs receiving porcine small intestinal submucosa repair had less inflammation and necrosis on histologic examination of the surgery site than was noted in the muscle transposition dogs at 2 weeks (Stoll *et al.* 2002).

Staged repair of perineal hernia with celiotomy to reduce the hernia and perform cystopexy with or without colopexy followed later by herniorrhaphy was performed in 41 dogs with complicated perineal hernias (Brissot *et al.* 2004). In this study, complicated perineal hernias were defined as bilateral perineal hernia, recurrence of perineal hernia, perineal hernia with major rectal dilation, perineal hernia with concurrent prostatic disease, and perineal hernia with urinary bladder retroflexion. Perineal hernia recurrence was seen in 4 of 10 dogs, all within 6 months of the original herniorrhaphy. Other complications included incisional complications in 7 dogs, urine dribbling in 15 dogs (permanent in 7 dogs), tenesmus in 18 dogs (permanent in 4 dogs), and temporary fecal incontinence in 4 dogs (Brissot *et al.* 2004).

References

Bellenger, C.R. (1980) Perineal hernia in dogs. *Australian Veterinary Journal* 56 (9), 434-438.

Bellenger, C.R., Canfield, R.B. (2003) Perineal hernia. In Slatter, D. (ed.) *Textbook of Small Animal Surgery*. WB Saunders, Philadelphia, pp. 487-498.

Bilbrey, S.A., Smeak, D.D., DeHoff, W. (1990) Fixation of the deferent duct for retrodisplacement of the urinary bladder and prostate in canine perineal hernia. *Veterinary Surgery* 19 (1), 24-27.

Bongartz, A., Carofiglio, F., Balligand, M., et al. (2005) Use of autogenous fascia lata graft for perineal herniorrhaphy in dogs. *Veterinary Surgery* 34 (4), 405-413.

Brissot, H.N., Dupre, G.P., Bouvy, B.M. (2004) Use of laparotomy in a staged approach for resolution of bilateral or complicated perineal hernia in 41 dogs. *Veterinary Surgery* 33 (4), 412-421.

Chambers, J.N., Rawlings, C.A. (1991) Applications of a semitendinosus muscle flap in two dogs. *Journal of the American Veterinary Medical Association* 199 (1), 84-86.

Dieterich, H.F. (1975) Perineal hernia repair in the canine. *Veterinary Clinics of North America* 5 (3), 383-399.

Gilley, R.S., Caywood, D.D., Lulich, J.P., et al. (2003) Treatment with a combined cystopexy-colopexy for dysuria and rectal prolapse after bilateral perineal herniorrhaphy in a dog. *Journal of the American Veterinary Medical Association* 222 (12), 1717-1721.

Hosgood, G., Hedlund, C.S., Pechman, R.D., et al. (1995) Perineal herniorrhaphy: perioperative data from 100 dogs. *Journal of the American Animal Hospital Association* 31 (4), 331-342.

Mortari, A.C., Rahal, S.C., Resende, L.A.L., et al. (2005) Electromyographical, ultrasonographical and morphological modifications in semitendinous muscle after transposition as ventral perineal muscle flap. *Journal of Veterinary Medicine. A, Physiology, Pathology, Clinical Medicine* 52 (7), 359-365.

Popovitch, C.A., Holt, D., Bright, R. (1994) Colopexy as a treatment for rectal prolapse in dogs and cats: a retrospective study of 14 cases. *Veterinary Surgery* 23 (2), 115-118.

Raffan, P.J. (1993) A new surgical technique for repair of perineal hernias in the dog. *Journal of Small Animal Practice* 34 (1), 13-19.

Robertson, J.J. (1984) Perineal hernia repair in dogs. *Modern Veterinary Practice* 65 (5), 365-368.

Rochat, M.C., Mann, F.A. (1998) Sciatic perineal hernia in two dogs. *Journal of Small Animal Practice* 39 (5), 240-243.

Seim III, H.B. (1988) Rectal prolapse. In Binnington, A.G., Cockshut, J.R. (eds.) *Decision Making in Small Animal Soft Tissue Surgery*. BC Decker, Philadelphia, pp. 36-37.

Sereda, C., Fowler, D., Shmon, C. (2002) Iatrogenic proximal urethral obstruction after inadvertent prostatectomy during bilateral perineal herniorrhaphy in a dog. *Canadian Veterinary Journal* 43 (4), 288-290.

Sjollema, B.E., van Sluijs, F.J. (1989) Perineal hernia repair in the dog by transposition of the internal obturator muscle: II. Complications and results in 100 patients. *Vet Quarterly* 11 (1), 18-23.

Spreull, J.S.A., Frankland, A.L. (1980) Transplanting the superficial gluteal muscle in the treatment of perineal hernia and flexure of the rectum in the dog. *Journal of Small Animal Practice* 21, 265-278.

Stoll, M.R., Cook, J.L., Pope, E.R., et al. (2002) The use of porcine small intestinal submucosa as a biomaterial for perineal herniorrhaphy in the dog. *Veterinary Surgery* 31 (4), 379-390.

Szabo, S., Wilkens, B., Radasch, R.M. (2007) Use of polypropylene mesh in addition to internal obturator transposition: a review of 59 cases (2000-2004). *Journal of the American Animal Hospital Association* 43 (3), 136-142.

van Sluijs, F.J., Sjollema, B.E. (1989) Perineal hernia repair in the dog by transposition of the internal obturator muscle: I. Surgical technique. *Vet Quarterly* 11 (1), 12-17.

55 Adrenalectomy

Brigitte Degasperi[1] and Gilles Dupré[1]

[1]Department for Companion Animals and Horses, University Clinic for Small Animals, Small Animal Surgery, University of Veterinary Medicine Vienna, Vienna, Austria

The most common indication for adrenalectomy in dogs is the presence of a functional adrenal tumor causing hyperadrenocorticism (Melian *et al.* 2010). Feline hyperadrenocorticism is relatively rare; nevertheless, if detected, adrenalectomy is often preferred over medical management because cats appear to be difficult to manage conservatively (Duesberg *et al.* 1995; Graves 2010). Other reported functional adrenal tumors amenable to surgical excision as primary treatment include pheochromocytoma (Calsyn *et al.* 2010), aldosteronoma (Ash *et al.* 2010), and tumors which produce excessive sex hormones (Millard *et al.* 2009).

General surgical principles, including accurate diagnosis, staging, and stabilization of the debilitated patient before surgery, are of uppermost importance when dealing with adrenal tumors.

Perioperative morbidity and mortality in adrenalectomy patients can be high. In 1986, Scavelli *et al.* reported a 60% mortality rate (15 of 25 patients died, including 7 being euthanized intraoperatively). More recently, this rate has declined to 15.4% (Massari *et al.* 2011) with an open approach (52 dogs, 1 intraoperative and 7 perioperative deaths). In a study on laparoscopic adrenalectomy in dogs for unilateral adrenocortical tumors, Jimenez-Pelaez *et al.* (2008) reported 2 perioperative deaths of 7 cases.

Endocrine surgery is commonly regarded as high-risk surgery (Schwartz 1996; Birchard 2003; Brockman 2006) and should only be performed by a team consisting of experienced surgeons in cooperation with experienced anesthetists.

GENERAL COMPLICATIONS

Intraoperative and early postoperative mortality

Definition
This is euthanasia or unforeseen loss of the patient during surgery or death within a few days thereafter.

Risk factors
- Tumor type
- Tumor size
- Affected side
- Vascular invasion of the vena cava or invasion of nearby organs such as the kidney or liver

- Retraction and manipulation of other organs during surgery
- Preoperative patient condition
- Postoperative hypoadrenocorticism
- Excessive catecholamine production by pheochromocytomas

Treatment and prevention
- Intraoperative manipulation of the adrenal gland should be kept to a minimum. Only pericapsular tissue should be dissected to avoid fragmentation of the fragile adrenal tissue. Adjacent organ manipulation needs to be carried out with special care to try to avoid kidney, liver, and pancreatic damage.
- Every patient undergoing adrenalectomy should be blood typed, and blood products need to be available in case of massive hemorrhage.
- Postoperatively, adrenalectomized patients should be kept in an intensive care unit until regarded as stable. General postoperative care such as analgesia, wound care, antibiotics if needed, oxygen, and infusion are a given. Continuous monitoring of vital and cardiovascular parameters and measures to avoid a hypoadrenocortical crisis need to be installed.

Outcome
Patients surviving the surgical intervention and the postoperative phase may achieve a good long-term outcome even independently of tumor type. Recent studies describe a median survival time between 7 and 35 months (Kyles *et al.* 2003; Jimenez-Pelaez *et al.* 2007; Schwartz *et al.* 2008; Massari *et al.* 2011).

The size of the tumor seems to play a role as masses with a long axis length of more than 5 cm were associated with an 85% shorter survival time (Massari *et al.* 2011).

The presence of metastasis and vein thrombosis at the time of diagnosis carry also a poorer prognosis with a 90% shorter survival time (Massari *et al.* 2011).

Postoperative hypoadrenocorticism

Definition
Postoperative hypoadrenocorticism is a level of glucocorticoids below normal after unilateral adrenalectomy or levels of glucocorticoids and mineralocorticoids below normal after bilateral adrenalectomy.

Complications in Small Animal Surgery, First Edition. Edited by Dominique Griffon and Annick Hamaide.
© 2016 John Wiley & Sons, Inc. Published 2016 by John Wiley & Sons, Inc.
Companion website: www.wiley.com/go/griffon/complications

Risk factors

- Bilateral adrenalectomy
- Excision of functional unilateral adrenal tumors with atrophy of the contralateral gland
- Insufficient prophylactic supplementation with corticosteroids and mineralocorticosteroids during surgery and the early postoperative phase

Diagnosis

- Vomiting, diarrhea, abdominal pain, hypovolemia, and weakness are signs of hypoadrenocorticism.
- Serum chemistry reveals classically hyponatremia and hyperkalemia.
- An adrenocorticotropic hormone (ACTH) stimulation test should be performed before glucocorticoid administration to prove the diagnosis.

Treatment

- Immediate rapid intravenous fluid therapy, preferably with 0.9% normal saline solution, is mandatory to prevent vascular collapse and shock.
- Dexamethasone 0.5 to 2 mg/kg intravenously should be given and repeated every 2 to 6 hours (Feldman and Nelson 2004a).
- Per-oral treatment with prednisone or prednisolone can be initiated when patient stability has been achieved.
- Supplementation of mineralocorticoids with DOCP (desoxycorticosterone pivalate) at a dose of 2.2 mg/kg intramuscularly is initiated.
- After bilateral adrenalectomy, lifelong treatment with both gluco- and mineralocorticoids has to be established.
- After unilateral adrenalectomy, the contralateral gland should assume hormone production in approximately 2 months after surgery. This needs to be monitored by an ACTH test every 2 to 3 weeks.

Outcome

Hypoadrenocorticism is compatible with a normal life, and the prognosis is excellent as long as the owners are well educated about the disease and the special needs of their pets (Feldman and Nelson 2004a).

Prevention

Supplementation of corticosteroids with dexamethasone, prednisolone sodium succinate, or hydrocortisone at the time of anesthetic induction should be given.

Renal and hepatic trauma and pancreatitis

Definition

This is iatrogenic injury to the kidneys, liver, or pancreas or trauma caused by tumor invasion and subsequent resection of the affected organ.

Injury to the pancreas may be caused by manipulation during retraction, especially in right-sided adrenal neoplasia.

Risk factors

- Tumor invasion into the kidney requiring dissection or nephrectomy
- Hepatomegaly; fatty liver infiltration caused by hyperadrenocorticism

- Metastasis
- Inadvertent trauma to vessels or major organs
- Right adrenal gland affected: The right lateral liver lobe may interfere, especially with right-sided adrenalectomy, and retraction might induce bleeding of the friable liver tissue.

Diagnosis and treatment

- Inadvertent ligation of a renal vessel might necessitate nephrectomy.
- In patients with an increased risk of pancreatitis, copious abdominal lavage should be performed. Before abdominal closure, lidocaine (1–2 mg/kg) or bupivacaine (1–2 mg/kg) can be used as a "splash on." After surgery, supportive therapy needs to be installed and tailored to the needs of the individual patient. Appropriate analgesic and fluid therapy, stomach protectants and antiemetics, dietary management (which can vary from nothing by mouth to total parenteral nutrition), and antibiotics are all part of this regimen.

Outcome

Concurrent nephrectomy has been shown to decrease the survival rate. Dogs undergoing a nephrectomy because of invasion of the renal vein or parenchyma were 4.10 times more likely to die in the early postoperative period compared with dogs undergoing only adrenalectomy (Schwartz et al. 2008). However, Massari et al. (2011) found no significant correlation between survival time and additional procedures performed at the time of adrenalectomy.

Prevention

- Gentle manipulation and meticulous dissection help avoid renal and hepatic trauma.
- Preoperative diagnostic imaging might reveal tumor infiltration.

Pulmonary thromboembolism

Definition

Pulmonary thromboembolism (PTE) is occlusion of vessels in the lung caused by thrombi secondary to other disease processes (LaRue and Murtaug, 1990).

Risk factors

- Hyperadrenocorticism and hence high levels of cortisol
- Hypercoagulability
- Other disease processes may induce PTE, including immune-mediated hemolytic anemia, neoplasia, cardiac disease, protein-losing disease (nephropathy or enteropathy), disseminated intravascular coagulation, sepsis, trauma, and recent surgery (Kellihan 2010).

Diagnosis

- Severe dyspnea and intractable respiratory distress raise suspicion of PTE.
- Nonselective angiography (Burns et al. 1981), computed tomography (CT) scan, ventilation/perfusion scintigraphic scan, or magnetic resonance imaging (MRI) may be used as diagnostic tools. Diagnostic procedures that require heavy sedation or anesthesia in respiratory-compromised patients potentially increase the risk of complications.
- The D-dimer test has been shown to be a highly sensitive tool to exclude PTE and in very high concentrations to be a highly specific tool to diagnose PTE (Nelson and Andreasen 2003).

Treatment and prevention

- Cardiovascular supportive care and oxygen are fundamental.
- The underlying disease process needs to be addressed.
- Tissue plasminogen activator, streptokinase (Ramsey *et al.* 1996), and urokinase are thrombolytics, but little experience exists in the treatment of naturally occurring PTE.
- Heparin (100–300 IU/kg subcutaneously every 6–8 hr) or low-molecular-weight heparin (dalteparin 100–150 IU/kg once daily) can be used as anticoagulant therapy (Kellihan 2010).

Outcome

When the diagnosis of PTE is established, it is often late in the course of the disease, and the prognosis is guarded to grave.

SPECIFIC COMPLICATIONS

Complications associated with pheochromocytomas

Definition

Pheochromocytomas originate from the chromaffin cells in the adrenal medulla. They produce excess catecholamines, which can induce hypertension and arrhythmias, creating intraoperative episodes of cardiovascular instabilities.

Risk factors

- Invasion of tumor into vascular system
- Direct intrasurgical manipulation of the tumor

Diagnosis

- Definitive presurgical diagnosis of a pheochromocytoma is not available to date.
- Metabolites of catecholamines such as urine vanillylmandelic acid and metanephrines can be detected in blood or urine, and the concentration can be measured (Feldman and Nelson, 2004b; Kook *et al.* 2007. But tumors secrete in spurts, so positive samples could be missed.
- Practically, the diagnosis of pheochromocytoma is based on episodes of weakness, restlessness, hypertension, collapse, and seizures and the presence of an adrenal mass.
- The definitive diagnosis relies on histologic examination of the adrenal gland.

Prevention

- Patients with a presumptive diagnosis of pheochromocytoma should be prepared for surgery with treatment of the existing hypertension and arrhythmia. The α-blocker phenoxybenzamine should be given for 2 to 3 weeks at a dosage of 0.25 mg/kg twice a day initially. This dosage can be increased until either blood pressure is normalized or if monitoring is not applicable because of episodic hypertension until a maximal dose of 2.5 mg/kg is reached. Surgery should take place 1 to 2 weeks later (Feldman and Nelson 2004b).
- In patients with severe tachycardia, β-blockers should be tried preoperatively (propranolol 0.2–1 mg/kg per os three times a day; atenolol 0.2–1 mg/kg per os once to twice a day). β-Blockers should never be given without pretreatment with α-blockers because severe hypertension could develop after blockade of β-receptor–mediated vasodilation in skeletal muscle (Feldman and Nelson 2004b).

- Anesthetists must be confident in managing such patients, and drugs such as phentolamine, nitroprusside, esmolol, and phenylephrine need to be prepared for immediate therapy of a possible intraoperative hypertensive or hypotensive crisis caused by tumor manipulation and subsequent catecholamine secretion or inadvertent severe bleeding. Surgeons and anesthetists need to have good communication to foresee possible upcoming critical moments during surgery.

Outcome

If surgery is successful and metastasis has not yet occurred, long-term survival is achievable (Gilson *et al.* 1994b). Barthez *et al.* (1997) reported survival times ranging from 1 day to 3.5 years in 17 operated dogs. Gilson *et al.* (1994a) showed a survival time of 3 to 23 months in 4 of 6 operated dogs.

Postoperative persistence or recurrence of hyperadrenocorticism

Definition

This is persistence of signs of hyperadrenocorticism any time after surgery.

Risk factors

- Metastasis
- Incomplete excision of tumor
- Inadvertent fragmentation of tumor during excision
- Unilateral adrenalectomy in case of pituitary-dependent hyperadrenocorticism
- Unilateral adrenalectomy when both glands are tumorous
- Removal of the normal adrenal gland in case of unilateral adrenal tumor

Diagnosis and treatment

- Postoperative ACTH stimulation test shows elevated pre and poststimulation cortisol levels; this can only be performed if dexamethasone was used as perioperative prevention of hypoadrenocorticism; all other corticosteroids will interfere with cortisol levels, and it is warranted to wait a few days.
- Diagnostic imaging should be performed to search for either metastasis or residual tumor.
- If reoperation is suitable, the patient may undergo a second surgery.
- For unresectable tumors or metastasis, medical management with mitotane can be tried at a daily dosage of 50 to 75 mg/kg/day; this dosage may need to be increased. An ACTH stimulation test to evaluate adrenal reserve has to be performed every 10 to 14 days, and glucocorticoid therapy should be instituted (prednisone 0.2 mg/kg/day). Responsiveness of tumors to this therapy may warrant high doses, inducing unwanted side effects (Kintzer and Peterson 1994). Side effects include anorexia, lethargy, weakness, vomiting, and diarrhea, and could be related to hypoadrenocorticism; however, in approximately 50% of dogs, side effects appear to be attributable to direct drug toxicity (Melian *et al.* 2010). Medical treatment with trilostane in one dog with functional adrenocortical neoplasia and in three dogs with hyperadrenocorticism and adrenocortical metastasis, respectively, has been reported (Eastwood *et al.* 2003; Benchekroun *et al.* 2008).

Prevention

- To best prevent recurrence of hyperadrenocorticism after adrenalectomy, a clear diagnosis should be established presurgically. In questionable cases, a ventral midline celiotomy should be used as the approach so both adrenal glands can be examined as well as kidneys, liver, caudal vena cava, and aorta.
- Tumor fragmentation can be avoided by avoiding direct manipulation of the gland, trying to maintain an intact capsule, and grasping only periadrenal tissue. The phrenicoabdominal vein should be ligated just medial and lateral to the gland and not directly over the ventral surface of the gland.
- Resection of tumor thrombi into adjacent vessels such as the phrenicoabdominal vein and the vena cava can be accomplished but needs experienced surgeons and good teamwork with the anesthetists. Temporary inflow occlusion may be necessary.

Central nervous system complications

Pituitary-dependent hyperadrenocorticism (PDH) in dogs is now commonly either treated medically (Melian *et al.* 2010) or surgically with hypophysectomy (Meij *et al.* 1998). In cats, hypophysectomy (Meij *et al.* 2001) or bilateral adrenalectomy is performed because cats do not respond well to medical treatment (Graves 2010).

Definition

Central nervous system (CNS) complications include neurologic signs, including ataxia, seizures, head pressing, or circling any time after bilateral adrenalectomy in patients suffering of PDH.

Risk factors

- PDH treated by bilateral adrenalectomy

Diagnosis

- Diagnostic imaging to confirm continuous growth of the pituitary mass

Treatment

- Radiation therapy

Prevention

- Performing complete hypophysectomy in PDH can prevent CNS complications. Because hypophysectomy is a highly demanding surgical procedure, it is not offered routinely.

Outcome

Radiation therapy is feasible in both dogs and cats. Mayer *et al.* (2006) report improvement of neurologic signs within 2 months in all 5 cats that showed abnormal neurologic signs before treatment. de Fornel *et al.* (2007) report a mean survival time of 22.6 months in 12 dogs with pituitary macrotumors.

COMPLICATIONS ASSOCIATED WITH LAPAROSCOPIC ADRENALECTOMY

Tumor size and invasiveness

Definition

Tumor size, weight, and invasiveness can preclude the use of laparoscopy or necessitate a rapid conversion (Kovak Mc Claran and Buote 2009).

Risk factor

- Invasion of the vena cava precludes the use of laparoscopy.

Diagnosis

Accurate diagnostic imaging techniques are necessary to rule out vena cava invasion (CT, CT angiography, ultrasonography). If this remains unclear, the first step of the laparoscopy is to rule out vena cava invasion.

Treatment

- If an adrenal tumor is too big to be removed laparoscopically, a laparoscopic-assisted removal remains possible. In that case, the tumor and its vascular tributaries can be dissected with the help of the magnification, although a mini-laparotomy is conducted to remove it.
- Because the tumor growth is often associated with a massive necrosis of the adrenal medulla, a close aspiration of the tumor content can shrink it and allow a full-laparoscopic removal (Jimenez-Pelaez *et al.* 2008).

Outcome

It is the surgeon's responsibility to set limits and recognize the cases not amenable to laparoscopic surgery. Conversion should happen early; Belizon and others (2006) showed that conversions performed within the first 30 minutes of the procedure have a better clinical outcome than conversions performed later on.

Complications associated with entry techniques

Definition

Subcutaneous carbon dioxide (CO_2) inflation or inadvertent puncture of the underlying organs can occur during Veress needle or trocar insertion. Alternatively, the portals can be introduced with an open technique.

Risk factors

- Because of the patient's position and condition (Cushing's syndrome), grabbing the muscular part of the abdominal wall might be difficult during an open approach, leading to subcutaneous infusion of CO_2 or secondary cellulitis.
- With a closed approach, because the patient lies in modified lateral recumbency, the Veress needle is implanted retro- or intercostally (but intraabdominally) (Jimenez-Pelaez *et al.* 2008), and therefore hitting a liver lobe (left side) or the spleen (right side) is possible.

Diagnosis

- If the Veress needle transfixes a liver lobe or the spleen, a very local hemorrhage will occur.
- If CO_2 is inflated subcutaneously, the skin will be lifted from the abdominal, wall making the intraabdominal insertion of the portals difficult.

Treatment

After the scope is introduced through another portal, the Veress needle is gently pulled out, and bleeding is controlled.

Outcome

Subcutaneous emphysema resolves spontaneously. Subcutaneous cellulitis around portals has been described (Jimenez-Pelaez *et al.*

2008). Symptomatic treatment with local warm packs was curative in all cases.

Hemorrhage

Definition

The adrenal gland is surrounded by many vessels; numerous arteries supply the gland, and venous drainage is through the adrenal vein. The phrenicoabdominal vein and artery need special attention because of the close intimacy with the adrenal gland. The phrenicoabdominal vein crosses ventrally over the gland, and the phrenico abdominal artery runs dorsally over the gland.

Risk factors

The adrenal vein enters the renal vein on the left side and the caudal vena cava on the right side. A sealing to close to the vena cava or the renal vein can damage these vessels.

Treatment

- Vessel-sealing devices are of great help but should be applied to a maximum of 7-mm vessel diameter; if larger vessels are encountered, hemoclips should be used.
- If major bleeding occurs and immediate suction is not available or does not show the source of hemorrhage, immediate conversion to an open surgery is advised.
- Patients undergoing adrenalectomy should always be blood typed preoperatively, and blood products should be readily available.
- Minor bleeding or minor diffuse bleeding may happen. This type of bleeding is not significant hemodynamically; however, it affects visualization of the surgical field.

Outcome

Late conversion can be detrimental to the patient's life.

Capsule rupture and tumor cell seeding

Definition

Visualization through laparoscopy is excellent, but inadvertent rupture of the glandular capsule may occur because tension is to be exerted to dissect the adrenal gland. In addition, adrenal tumors are often very friable, and tearing of the adrenal cortex and subsequent tumor spread may happen.

Diagnosis

The spillage of the necrotic center will be readily observed during surgery.

Prevention

- When dissecting the adrenal gland, it is recommended to dissect and grasp the immediate surrounding tissue and not the glandular tissue itself.
- Use of blunt instruments such as Babcock forceps is advised (Mayhew 2009).
- To avoid tumor spread during the extraction, the use of a retrieval bag and appropriate port size of 10 mm or greater is recommended.

Outcome

Although it is suspected that gland rupture has no impact on the overall prognosis, it is still recommended to avoid it.

Relevant literature

Adrenalectomy has undergone a great arch of development. Not only have different open approaches been carried out, but more recently, the so-called "keyhole technique" has been applied successfully to this field in veterinary surgery.

In 1977, Johnston the paracostal approach and applied it bilaterally to treat hyperadrenocorticism induced by the pituitary gland. Advantages of this technique are avoidance of tissue trauma to the pancreas and cutaneous incision made in a non–weight-bearing area, which is of importance in classic cushingoid dogs with thin abdominal skin. van Sluijs *et al.* (1995) used this approach to treat adrenal neoplasia in 36 dogs and for Ham *et al.* (2005) compared the results with a group of 43 other dogs consecutively operated by van Sluijs, showing better outcomes compared the first group and hence demonstrating a significant learning curve.

In the current literature, most surgeons use the midline approach, and extend it through a paracostal cut if necessary (Massari *et al.* 2011).

Mortality rates have decreased significantly. Indeed, Massari *et al.* (2011) recently reported a mortality rate of 13.5% (8 of 52 patients); previous rates ranging from 19% to 60% were previously reported (Scavelli *et al.* 1986; van Sluijs *et al.* 1995; Anderson *et al.* 2001; Kyles *et al.* 2003). Through the laparoscopic approach, a mortality rate of 28% (2 of 7) has been reported (Jimenez-Pelaez *et al.* 2008).

Better preoperative preparation of the patient and advances in postoperative intensive care did allow improvement of short-term survival rate after adrenalectomy. Patients with Cushing's disease need to be treated perioperatively with cortisone to avoid a hypoadrenocorticoid crisis after adrenalectomy (Feldman and Nelson 2004a). In the presence of pheochromocytomas, Herrera *et al.* (2008) advices treatment with α-blocking drugs to normalize hypertension because a significant difference in survival between treated and untreated dogs was demonstrated.

Better preoperative diagnosis through different imaging modalities also might contribute to the lower mortality rate. Besso *et al.* (1997) showed that a definitive diagnosis of tumor type cannot be obtained through ultrasound imaging; Kyles *et al.* (2003) showed a 80% sensitivity and a 90% specificity of abdominal ultrasound examination to definitively diagnose a caval thrombus. Improved preoperative visualization of the tumor extent and possible invasion of adjacent tissues help to decrease previously unknown intraoperative findings and may predict the need for more invasive surgeries (Schwartz *et al.* 2008). Currently, no studies describing the use of CT or MRI in all patients are available, but many have used these tools in some patients (Kyles *et al.* 2003; Ash *et al.* 2005; Jimenez-Pelaez *et al.* 2008; Massari *et al.* 2011) and advise to do so regularly (Brockman 2006).

References

Anderson, C.R., Birchard, S.J., Powers, B.E., et al. (2001) Surgical treatment of adrenocortical tumors: 21 cases(1990-1996). *Journal of the American Animal Hospital Association* 37, 93-97.

Ash, R.A., Harvey, A.M., Tasker, S. (2005) Primary hyperaldosteronism in the cat: a series of 13 cases. *Journal of Feline Medicine and Surgery* 7 (3), 173-182.

Barthez, P.Y., Marks, S.L., Woo, J., et al. (1997) Pheochromocytoma in dogs: 61 cases (1984-1995). *Journal of Veterinary Internal Medicine* 11, 272-278.

Belizon, A., Sardinha, C.T., Sher M.E. (2006) Converted laparoscopic colectomy. What are the consequences? *Surgical Endoscopy* 20, 947-951.

Benchekroun, G., De Fornel-Thbaud, P., Lafarge, S., et al. (2008) Trilostane therapy for hyperadrenocorticism in three dogs with adrenocortical metastasis. *Veterinary Record* 163, 190.

Besso, J.G., Penninck, D.G., Gliatto J.M. (1997) Retrospective ultrasonographic evaluation of adrenal lesions in 26 dogs. *Veterinary Radiology and Ultrasound* 38 (6), 448-455.

Birchard, S.J., (2003) Adrenalectomy. In Slatter, D. (ed.) *Textbook of Small Animal Surgery*, vol. 2, 3rd edn. Saunders, Philadelphia, pp. 1694-1700.

Brockman, D.J. (2006) Making adrenalectomy less stressful [abstract]. In *Proceedings of the 16th American College of Veterinary Surgeons Symposium* Rockville, MD: American College of Veterinary Surgeons, pp. 211-212.

Burns, M.G., Kelly, A.B., Hornof, W.J., et al. (1981) Pulmonary artery thrombosis in three dogs with hyperadrenocorticism. *Journal of the American Veterinary Medical Association* 178, 388–393.

Calsyn, J.D., Green, R.A., Davis, G.J., et al. (2010) Adrenal pheochromocytoma with contralateral adrenocortical adenoma in a cat. *Journal of the American Animal Hospital Association* 46 (1), 36-42.

de Fornel, P., Delisle, F., Devauchelle, P., et al. (2007) Effects of radiotherapy on pituitary corticotroph macrotumors in dogs: a retrospective study of 12 cases. *The Canadian Veterinary Journal* 48, 481.

Duesberg, C.A., Nelson, R.W., Feldman, E.C., et al. (1995) Adrenalectomy for treatment of hyperadrenocorticism in cats: 10 cases (1988-1992). *Journal of the American Veterinary Medical Association* 207 (8), 1066-1070.

Eastwood, J.M., Elwood, C.M., Hurley, K.J. (2003) Trilostane treatment of a dog with functional adrenocortical neoplasia. *Journal of Small Animal Practice* 44, 126-131.

Feldman, E.C., Nelson, R.W. (2004a) Hypoadrenocorticism (Addison's disease). In Feldman, E.C., Nelson, R.W. (eds.) *Canine and Feline Endocrinology and Reproduction,* 3rd edn. Saunders, St. Louis, pp. 394-438.

Feldman, E.C., Nelson, R.W. (2004b) Pheochromocytoma and multiple endocrine neoplasia. In Feldman, E.C., Nelson, R.W. (eds.) *Canine and Feline Endocrinology and Reproduction,* 3rd edn. Saunders, St. Louis, pp. 440-463.

Gilson, S.D., Withrow, S.J., Orton E.C. (1994a). Surgical treatment of pheochromocytoma: technique, complications and results in six dogs. *Veterinary Surgery* 23 (3), 195-200.

Gilson, S.D., Withrow, S.J., Wheeler, S.L., et al. (1994b) Pheochromocytoma in 50 dogs. *Journal of Veterinary Internal Medicine* 8 (3), 228-232.

Graves, T.K. (2010) Hypercortisolism in cats (feline Cushing's syndrome). In Ettinger, S.J., Feldman, E.C. (eds.) *Textbook of Veterinary Internal Medicine*, vol. 2, 7th edn. Saunders, Elsevier, St. Louis, pp. 1840-1847.

Herrera, M.A., Mehl, M.L., Kass, P.H., et al. (2008) Predictive factors and the effect of phenoxybenzamine on outcome in dogs undergoing adrenalectomy for pheochromocytoma. *Journal of Veterinary Internal Medicine* 22 (6), 1333-1339.

Jimenez-Pelaez, M., Bouvy, B.M., Dupre, G.D. (2008) Laparoscopic adrenalectomy for treatment of unilateral adrenocortical carcinomas: techniques, complications and results in 7 dogs. *Veterinary Surgery* 37, 444-453.

Johnston, D.E. (1977) Adrenalectomy via retroperitoneal approach in dogs. *Journal of the American Veterinary Medical Association* 170, 1092.

Kellihan, H.B. (2010) Pulmonary hypertension and pulmonary thromboembolism. In Ettinger, S.J., Feldman, E.C. (eds.) *Textbook of Veterinary Internal Medicine*, vol. 2, 7th edn. Saunders, Elsevier, St. Louis, pp. 1138-1141.

Kintzer, P.P., Peterson M.E. (1994) Mitotane treatment of 32 dogs with cortisol-secreting adrenocortical neoplasia. *Journal of the American Veterinary Medical Association* 205, 54.

Kook, P.H., Boretti, F.S., Hersberger, M., et al. (2007) Urinary catecholamine and metanephrine to creatinine ratios in healthy dogs at home and in a hospital environment and in 2 dogs with pheochromocytoma. *Journal of Veterinary Internal Medicine* 21, 388-393.

Kovak McClaran, J., Buote, N.J. (2009) Complications and need for conversion to laparotomy in small animals. *Veterinary Clinics of North America: Small Animal Practice* 39, 941 -951.

Kyles, A.E., Feldman, E.C., De Cock, H.E.V., et al. (2003) Surgical management of adrenal gland tumors with and without associated tumor thrombi in dogs: 40 cases(1994-2001). *Journal of the American Veterinary Medical Association* 223 (5), 654-662.

LaRue, M.J., Murtaug, R.J. (1990) Pulmonary thromboembolism in dogs: 47 cases (1986-1987). *Journal of the American Veterinary Medical Association* 197, 1368-1372.

Massari, F., Nicoli, S., Romanelli, G., et al. (2011) Adrenalectomy in dogs with adrenal tumors: 52 cases (2002-2008). *Journal of the American Veterinary Medical Association* 239, 216-221.

Mayer, M.N., Greco, D.S., LaRue, S.M. (2006) Outcomes of pituitary irradiation in cats. *Journal of Veterinary Internal Medicine* 20 (5), 1151-1154.

Mayhew, P.D. (2009) Advanced laparoscopic procedures (hepatobiliary, endocrine) in dogs and cats. *Veterinary Clinics of North America: Small Animal Practice* 39 (5), 925-939.

Melian, C., Perez-Alenza, M.D., Peterson, M.E. (2010) Hyperadrenocorticism in dogs. In Ettinger, S.J., Feldman, E.C. (eds.) *Textbook of Veterinary Internal Medicine*, vol. 2, 7th edn. Saunders, Elsevier, St. Louis, pp. 1816-1840.

Meij, B.P., Voorhout, G., Van den Ingh, T.S., et al. (1998) Results of transsphenoidal hypophysectomy in 52 dogs with pituitary-dependent hyperadrenocorticism. *Veterinary Surgery* 27, 246.

Meij, B.P., Voorhout, G., Van den Ingh, T.S., et al. (2001) Transsphenoidal hypophysectomy for treatment of pituitary-dependent hyperadrenocorticism in 7 cats. *Veterinary Surgery* 30 (1),72-86.

Millard, R.P., Pickens, E.H., Wells, K.L. (2009) Excessive production of sex hormones in a cat with an adrenocortical tumor. *Journal of the American Veterinary Medical Association* 234 (4), 505-508.

Nelson, O.L., Andreasen, C. (2003) The utility of plasma D-dimer to identify thromboembolic disease in dogs. *Journal of Veterinary Internal Medicine* 17, 830-834.

Ramsey, C.C., Burney, D.P., Macintire, D.K., et al. (1996) Use of streptokinase in four dogs with thrombosis. *Journal of the American Veterinary Medical Association* 209 (4), 780-785.

Scavelli, T.D., Peterson, M.E., Matthiesen D.T. (1986) Results of surgical treatment for hyperadrenocorticism caused by adrenocortical neoplasia in the dog: 25 cases (1980-1984). *Journal of the American Veterinary Medical Association* 189, 1360-1364.

Schwartz, A. (1996) Endocrine Surgery. In Lipowitz, A.J., Caywood, D.D.(eds.) *Complications in Small Animal Surgery* . Williams & Wilkins, Baltimore, pp. 294-309.

Schwartz, P., Kovak, J.R., Koprowski, A., et al. (2008) Evaluation of prognostic factors in the surgical treatment of adrenal gland tumors in dogs: 41 cases (1999-2005). *Journal of the American Veterinary Medical Association* 232 (1), 77-84.

Ter Haar, G., Dierikx, C.M., Veneberg, R.E., et al. (2005) Learning curve in retroperitoneal adrenalectomy; results of 43 adrenalectomies for treatment of adrenocortical tumors [abstract]. In Schramme, M., Tremaine, H., Walmsley J., et al. (eds.) *Proceedings of the European College of Veterinary Surgeons.* European College of Veterinary Surgeons, Lyon, pp. 334-337.

Van Sluijs, F.J., Sjollema, B.E., Voorhout, G., et al. (1995) Results of adrenalectomy in 36 dogs with hyperadrenocorticism. *Vet Quarterly* 17, 113-116.

56 Splenectomy

Paolo Buracco[1] and Federico Massari[2]
[1]Department of Veterinary Science, University of Turin, Grugliasco, Turin, Italy
[2]Clinica Veterinaria Nerviano, Nerviano, Italy

The spleen's shape is tongue like, slightly constricted in the middle, and triangular in transversal section. It lies in the left hypogastrium, grossly oriented dorsoventral and parallel to the greater gastric curvature; its position may change depending on the stomach repletion state. The dorsal and ventral extremities are the head and tail, respectively. Along the hilus, attached to the greater omentum, arteries and nerves enter and veins and lymphatics emerge. The gastrosplenic ligament, part of the greater omentum, connects the spleen to the greater gastric curvature.

Vascularization derives from the splenic artery, a branch of the celiac trunk; intrasplenic arteries lie mainly in the trabeculae. Before reaching the spleen, the splenic artery gives off some branches to the pancreatic left limb, with the latter associated with the gastrosplenic attachment (Tillson 2003). The venous drainage is in form of short venous vessels that form the splenic vein; the latter, after receiving branches from the left stomach, left pancreas, and greater omentum, ultimately empties in the portal vein (Figure 56.1).

The splenic autonomous nervous system is sympathetic only (from the celiac ganglion). Capsule, blood vessels, and trabeculae contract because of α fibers. Spleen relaxation, resulting in organ enlargement, is usually drug induced (e.g., anesthetics, tranquilizers) (Tillson 2003). The spleen has only efferent lymphatics, running along arteries.

The main splenic functions are:
- Storage, concentration, and release of erythrocytes and platelets from megakaryocytes. In asplenic dogs, an increase of about 47% in platelet life span has been described (Dale *et al.* 1996).
- Filtering of blood and destruction of bacteria and old erythrocytes
- Antigen recognition and production of lymphocytes, monocytes, and antibodies

Splenectomy is performed for primary or, less frequently, metastatic malignant tumors, spleen torsion, splenomegaly associated to infiltrative disease, traumatic rupture, and immune-mediated diseases (Horgan *et al.* 2009). Splenectomy may be performed as "open surgery" or laparoscopically (Collard *et al.* 2010).

EARLY POSTOPERATIVE COMPLICATIONS

The rate of early complications ranges from 3.7% to 44%, depending on the complication being investigated. The most common early complication is hemorrhage, associated or not with hemostatic

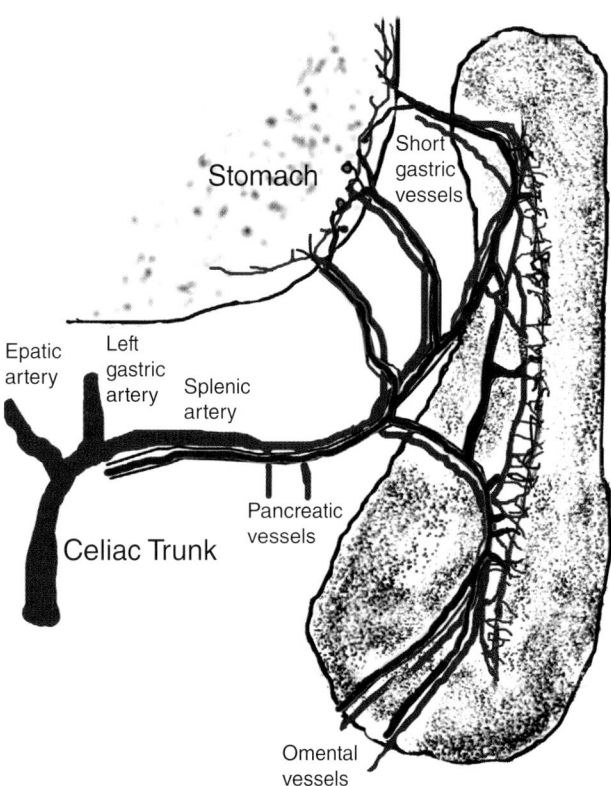

Figure 56.1 Schematic of the splenic vascularization. The splenic artery, after its origin from the celiac trunk, gives off three to five long primary branches as it runs in the greater omentum toward the ventral third of the spleen. The first branch is usually for the left pancreas, further branches are for the proximal part of the spleen, and finally others enter in the gastrosplenic ligament to become short gastric arteries (for the gastric fundus) and left gastroepiploic arteries (for the gastric greater curvature) *Source:* Tillson, 2003. Reproduced with permission from Elsevier.

abnormalities. In one study, it was the most common cause of death in dogs undergoing splenectomy for non-neoplastic causes (Spangler and Kass 1997). Cardiac arrhythmias are commonly reported in dogs with splenic torsion or tumors, with an incidence of about 40% (Marino *et al.* 1994). Early complications also include damage to the left pancreatic lobe and gastric wall because of devascularization and acute infection. Finally, a recent paper reported acute vein

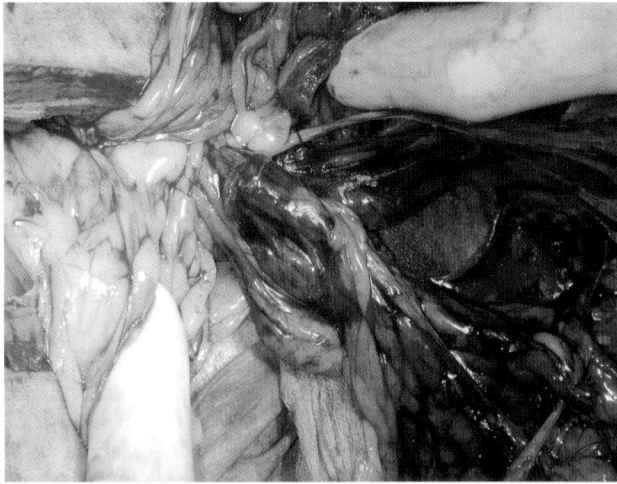

(A)

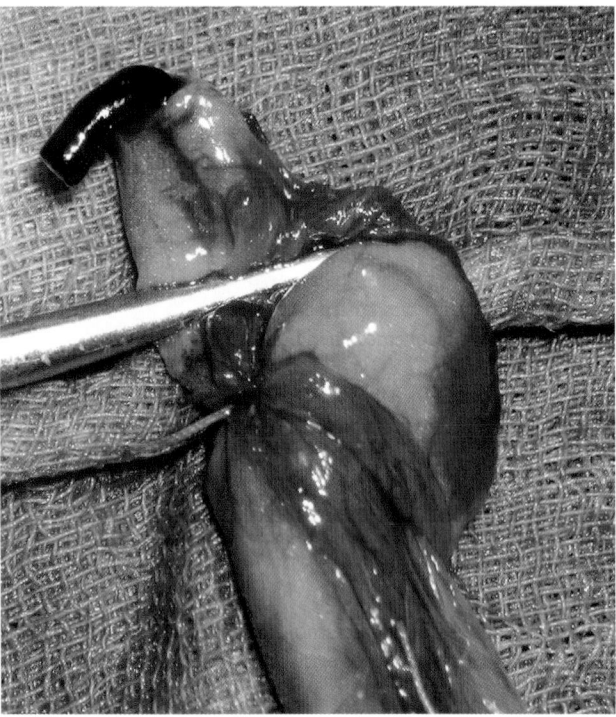

(B)

Figure 56.2. **A**, Intraoperative visualization of splenic vein thrombosis after splenic torsion in a dog. *Source:* Dr. G. Romanelli. Reproduced with permission from Dr. G. Romanelli. **B**, View of a thrombus after splenectomy has been completed.

thrombosis in six dogs, 24 to 48 hours after splenectomy. All dogs died or were euthanized after diagnosis (Figure 56.2) (Beck *et al.* 2005).

Hemorrhage and hemostatic abnormalities
See also Chapter 12.

Definition
This is acute blood loss after splenectomy. Hemorrhage may result from a surgical failure or a hemostatic abnormality.

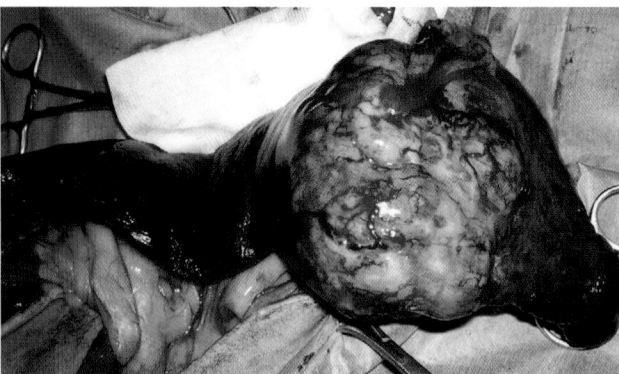

Figure 56.3 Intraoperative view of a splenic liposarcoma in a dog.

Risk factors
- **Surgical failure:** It is usually caused by failure to ligate splenic vessels adequately. It may result from:
  - Poor technique in performing knots (e.g., incorrect tension of the knot) or undersized or oversized suture material
  - Failure to ligate all vessels running in the great omentum
  - Mobilization of vascular clips
  - Incorrect coagulation with sealant devices
- **Hemostatic abnormalities:** Those potentially resulting in post-splenectomy hemorrhage are pathological conditions able to cause endothelial damage or platelet activation or destruction, such as splenic masses (Figure 56.3), infection (Figure 56.4), trauma (usually with rupture), and splenomegaly caused by auto-immune disease. The spleen usually sequesters 30% to 40% of circulating platelets, with up to 90% in splenomegalies secondary to infection or tumor. It has been reported that splenectomy could still be safely performed with a platelet count of 25,000/μL (Kerwin and Mauldin 2003). These disorders may be underestimated preoperatively; laboratory tests should be addressed to

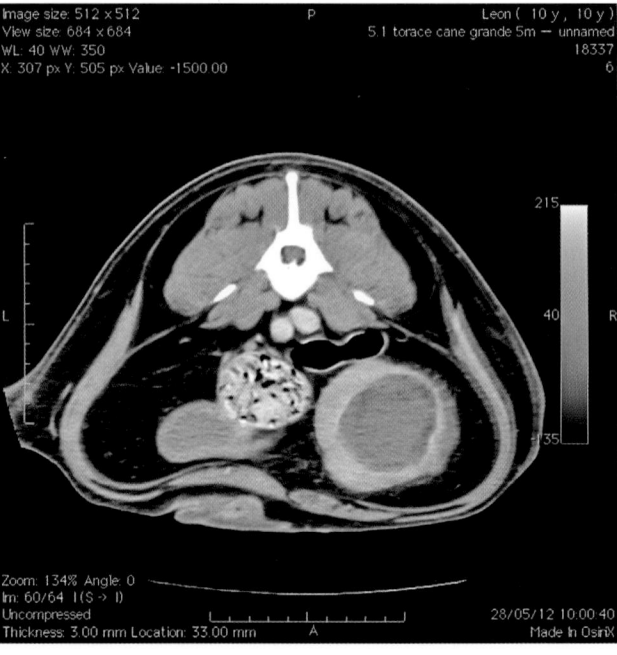

Figure 56.4 Computed tomography scan of the abdomen of a dog with a splenic abscess.

both quantitative (involving platelets) and qualitative (involving coagulation factors) disorders to prevent postoperative bleedings. In a paper, when the activated partial thromboplastin time (aPTT) was prolonged, disseminated intravascular coagulation (DIC) was more common in dogs bearing a malignant tumor (Maruyama *et al.* 2004).

Diagnosis

- Clinical signs vary depending on the amount of blood that is lost. Patients with acute postoperative hemorrhage may die rapidly if not assisted adequately. Dogs may show pale mucous membranes, a weak pulse, tachycardia, hypothermia, and delayed recovering from anesthesia. Abdominal distension is not always evident.
- Hemoabdomen may be confirmed by ultrasound and packed cell volume (PCV) evaluation of the fluid retrieved by abdominocentesis. The PCV of the fluid should be compared with the PCV of the circulating blood. A complete coagulation profile is warranted. Blood being in contact with peritoneal surface for more than 45 minutes does not clot because of peritoneal platelet sequestration (Crowe 1980). Blood that clots after abdominocentesis may indicate an inadvertent organ or vessel puncture (Brockman *et al.* 2000).
- Blood PCV should be routinely monitored in postsplenectomy patients. If PCV continues to decline, ultrasonography or peritoneal lavage is indicated. An abdominal effusion PCV greater than 10% or a peritoneal lavage PCV greater than 2% to 5% is suggestive of acute hemorrhage. Interpretation of peritoneal lavage results is not always easy even though a diagnostic accuracy ranging between 80% and 100% has been reported (Kirby 2003).
- When splenectomy is performed for a highly suspected malignant tumor, a postoperative coagulation profile is advised (platelet count, prothrombin time, aPTT, and plasma fibrinogen) to early detect DIC. In a paper dealing with 164 dogs with malignant tumors of which one third was a hemangiosarcoma (HAS), the reported incidence of DIC was 12.2% (Maruyama *et al.* 2004).

Treatment

- A blood transfusion should start if blood PCV is less than 20% and total proteins are low (Hammond and Pesillo-Crosby 2008); however, these values should be correlated with both the amount of blood loss and the crystalloids already infused.
- When DIC is highly suspected, fresh-frozen plasma concentrate or cryoprecipitate instead of whole blood provides better coagulation factor supplementation and avoids microvascular hemolysis. The role of heparin administration remains unclear, and some authors claim that it may enhance the risk of bleeding (Vlasin 2004).
- Surgery is warranted when clinical conditions deteriorate. After rapid aspiration of the abdominal blood, evaluate the abdomen and clamp with forceps or fingers the splenic artery and vein or any other bleeding vessel to stop hemorrhage. After bleeding is controlled, the whole abdomen is lavaged with warm sterile saline to mobilize blood clots and is aspirated. Then release slowly the forceps, look for the origin of bleeding, and ligate vessel(s) appropriately. It is not indicated to ligate the splenic artery at its origin because both the left pancreatic and gastric branches should be saved. In case of uncontrollable intraoperative hemorrhage, it has been suggested to fill the abdomen with sterile towels and to close it temporarily. A further surgery is planned after 24 to 48 hours,

after patient stabilization (Herold *et al.* 2008). Alternatively, new and very effective sealant products, currently used in human surgery, may also be used (Anderson 2012). Postoperatively, the patient is strictly monitored for, among others, cardiac function, PCV, total protein, and signs of DIC.

Outcome

The prognosis is strictly correlated to the cause of hemorrhage, the timing and quality of intervention, and the patient's preoperative condition.

Cardiac arrhythmias

Definition

Arrhythmias are abnormal rhythms of the heart, causing a less effective cardiac output. Arrhythmias, usually in form of rapid ventricular tachycardia or multifocal ventricular arrhythmia, are reported in dogs undergoing splenectomy for malignant tumors, torsion, and benign splenomegaly.

Risk factors

- **Splenic rupture** (Figure 56.5): In one study, 16 of 23 dogs with rupture and 1 of 17 with no rupture had postoperative arrhythmias (Marino *et al.* 1994).
- **Hemoabdomen** (Minta *et al.* 1993)
- **Anemia**: In two studies, dogs developing arrhythmias had a lower PCV (<35%). It was speculated that anemia and hypovolemia predispose to reperfusion injury (Minta *et al.* 1993; Marino *et al.* 1994).
- **Hypovolemia:** It was found that dogs with mean intraoperative arterial pressure lower than 55 mm Hg for more than 15 minutes were exposed to a greater risk of arrhythmias in the early postoperative period (Minta *et al.* 1993; Marino *et al.* 1994).
- **Myocardial necrosis:** More than 55% of dogs with arrhythmias secondary to spleen lesions have concomitant myocardial necrosis (Minta *et al.* 1993).
- **Splenic torsion** (Figure 56.6): In two studies, arrhythmias developed, respectively, in 100% and 33% of dogs with splenic torsion (Marino *et al.* 1994; Aronsohn *et al.* 2009).

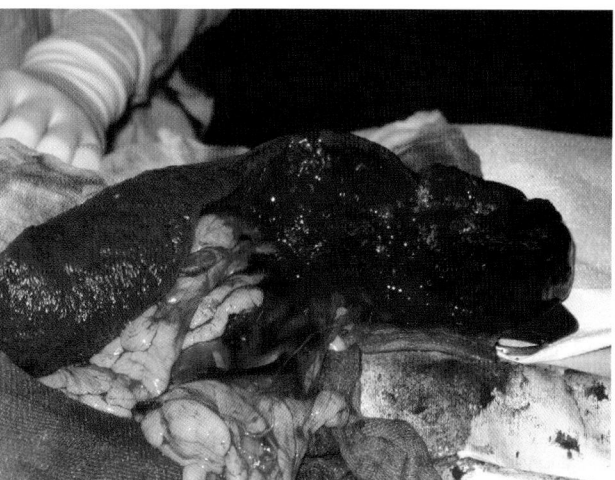

Figure 56.5 Intraoperative view of a posttraumatic ruptured spleen in a dog.

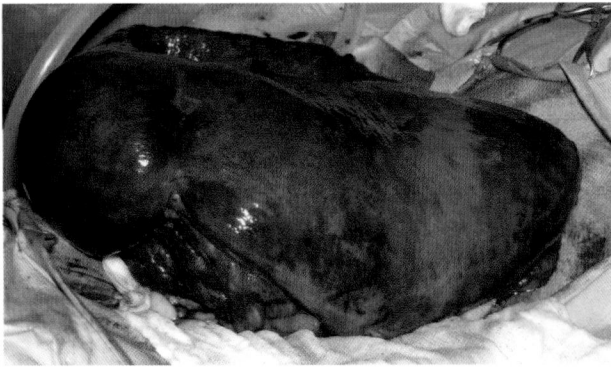

(A)

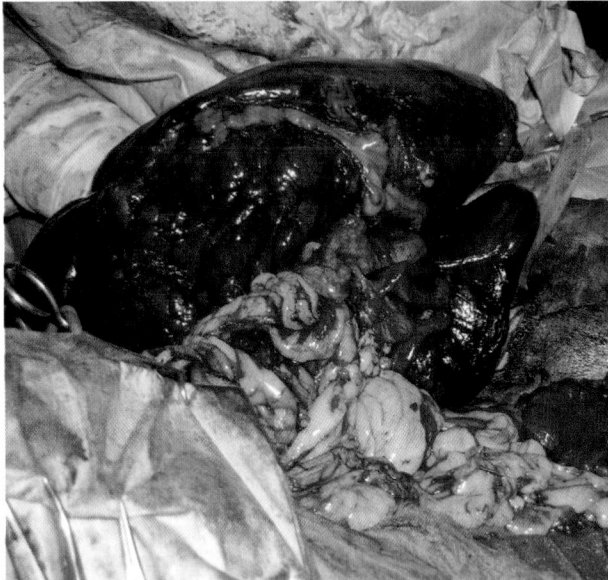

(B)

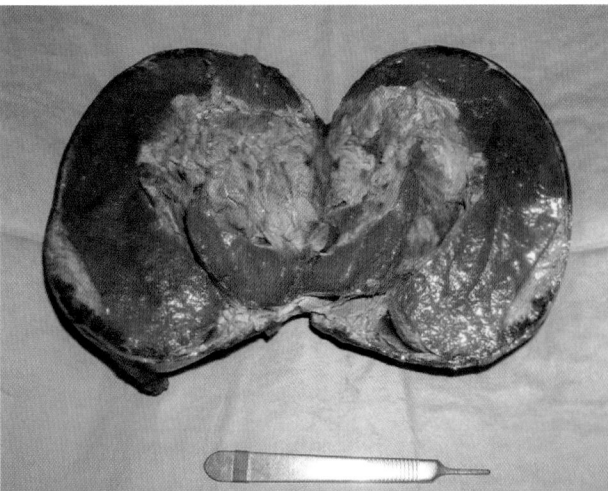

(C)

Figure 56.6 A and **B**, Intraoperative view of a splenic torsion in a dog. **C**, Result of a chronic splenic torsion in another dog.

- **Tumors:** Although previous studies have reported a rate of arrhythmias ranging from 38% to 86% in dogs with HAS, compared with 32% in dogs with hematoma (Knapp *et al.* 1993; Marino *et al.* 1994), a recent study reported a rate of arrhythmias of 44% in dogs with HAS and 86.6% in dogs with hematoma (Aronsohn *et al.* 2009).
- **Heart metastatic HAS:** This was found in 3 of 18 dogs (Minta *et al.* 1993).
- **Local or systemic catecholamine release** (Minta *et al.* 1993)

Diagnosis

- Arrhythmias may cause no **clinical signs**. Symptoms, such as palpitations, slow or irregular cardiac beats, pauses between heartbeats, or chest pain, that are felt by humans are not clinically recognized in animals. The latter may show anxiety, weakness, pulse deficit, and painting. In one study, the mean and median onset of rapid ventricular tachycardia occurred 12 and 5 hours, respectively, after surgery (range, 0–32) (Marino *et al.* 1994); only 3 of 22 dogs with arrhythmias manifested it preoperatively.
- **Electrocardiography** (ECG) may detect ventricular arrhythmias in symptomatic dogs, but continuous monitoring is necessary for subclinical arrhythmias because periodical ECG may fail to detect the alteration. In one study in which results of 1-minute ECG performed every 6 hours were compared with those of continuous 48-hour Holter monitoring, it was found that the latter was able to detect cardiac extrasystoles not detected by ECG. In particular, 1-minute ECG every 6 hours, compared with continuous Holter monitoring, was normal in 29% of dogs with rapid ventricular tachycardia at greater than 3000 ventricular extrasystoles per hour, in 50% of dogs with rapid ventricular tachycardia at 1000 to 3000 ventricular extrasystoles per hour, and in 100% of dogs with 10 to 300 ventricular extrasystoles per hour without rapid ventricular tachycardia (Marino *et al.* 1994).

Treatment

Continuous monitoring is acceptable when neither significant pulse deficit nor clinical signs are evident. No previous study has demonstrated that medical treatment improves survival in asymptomatic dogs. Only symptomatic dogs with no perceptible femoral pulse, multifocal ventricular arrhythmia or tachycardia, and hypoperfusion or preexisting cardiac disease should receive medical therapy. In a recent paper, medical treatment was suggested for patient with hemodynamic instability, multiform ECG complexes, very rapid ventricular tachycardia, or R-on-T complex (Chandler *et al.* 2006). The therapy should consist of lidocaine HCl in bolus (2 mg/kg intravenously; repeat if needed without exceeding 8 mg/kg) followed by lidocaine HCl at constant-rate infusion (CRI) (25–80 µg/kg/min).

Other antiarrhythmic drugs (procainamide HCl at 10 mg/kg as a bolus followed by a CRI of 20 µg/kg/min, oral sotalol HCl at 0.5–2.0 mg/kg twice a day) are considered if patients do not improve with lidocaine HCl. Oxygen administration may increase cardiac performance and favor rhythm normalization.

Outcome

The outcome is usually good for asymptomatic animals. In a study on 60 dogs, 27 developed postsplenectomy arrhythmias, but only 3 needed medical treatment, with good outcomes in all (Aronsohn *et al.* 2009).

Damage to the left pancreatic lobe and gastric wall

Definition

This damage is secondary to left pancreatic ischemia caused by occlusion of splenic vessels directed to this part of the pancreas. Ischemia may evolve in a life-threatening condition. If it is true that this may potentially occur on a pathophysiological point of view, it is also true that, based on the literature and the authors' personal experience, it is rarely appreciated clinically.

Risk factors

- Spleen torsion
- Proximal ligature of the splenic peduncle
- DIC secondary to spleen tumors or, potentially, coagulation abnormalities
- Incorrect surgical manipulation.

Diagnosis

- Just after splenectomy, evaluate the viability of the left pancreatic lobe, paying attention to color variation (from pink to blue). Postoperatively, small ischemic lesions may be asymptomatic.
- Symptomatic patients can show mild abdominal pain up to serious signs of pancreatitis.
- Standard ultrasound and Doppler sonography may potentially detect lesions of the left pancreatic limb and arouse suspicion of vascular impairment.
- In case of pancreatitis, blood tests may reveal leukocytosis and an increase in serum lipase and amylase, elevation of liver enzymes and total bilirubin, hyperlipidemia, azotemia, hypocalcemia, and hyperglycemia.
- Pancreatic lipase immunoreactivity may also be tested; it is 82% sensitive for pancreatitis.
- Peritoneal lavage may be inconclusive because the finding of normal neutrophils postoperatively is usual.
- Continuous monitoring is necessary, and surgery is planned in doubtful situations.

Treatment

A left pancreatectomy is performed if necessary (using either the "fracture" or the "dissection" technique).

Outcome

The outcome is potentially good if the lesion is confined to the left pancreatic limb. Pancreatitis involving the entire gland makes the prognosis worse. Strict monitoring (clinical signs, hemodynamic status, abdominal ultrasonography, laboratory tests) during the early postoperative period is warranted.

Prevention

Diagnosis before abdominal closure helps to avoid a second surgery; thus, an intraoperative histologic evaluation (cryostate) or a cytologic evaluation may help, in uncertain situations, in taking the best decision.

LATE POSTOPERATIVE COMPLICATIONS

Metastatic disease

Definition

The spleen is most frequently affected with primary HAS (Spangler and Kass 1997) and less frequently with other sarcomas, lymphoproliferative disorders, histiocytic sarcoma, and Mast Cell Tumor. The spleen may also be involved with metastases arising from tumors of different origin (e.g., sarcomas, carcinomas, histiocytic sarcoma, Mast Cell Tumor, lymphoma, malignant melanoma) (Figure 56.7).

Diagnosis

- In case of massive spleen involvement or hemoabdomen, clinical signs at presentation may be obvious.
- The abdomen is accurately palpated to detect splenomegaly or abdominal effusion.
- In case of HAS, the possible and concomitant heart involvement resulting in pericardial effusion may cause weakness, a short breathing pattern and jugular pulse, and engorgement.
- Radiography: In case of suspected HAS, the presence of lung metastasis and pericardial effusion should be investigated. Abdominal radiographs may reveal large masses in the craniomedial abdomen or abdominal effusion. Abdominal radiographs are usually not useful to detect metastatic lesions to the spleen.

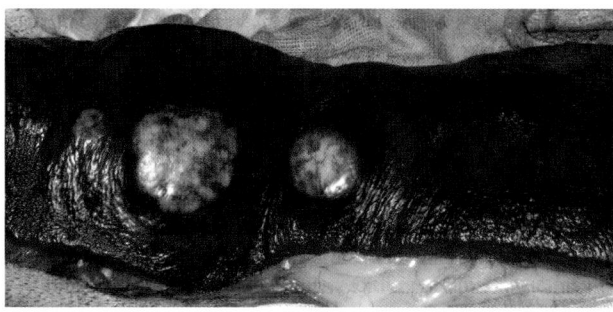

(A)

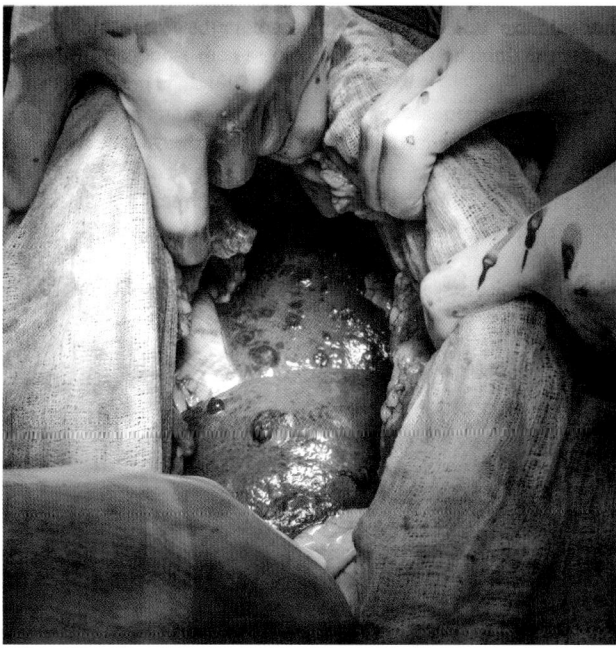

(B)

Figure 56.7 **A**, Intraoperative view of a splenic metastatic lymphoma in a dog. **B**, Intraoperative view of splenic (and hepatic) metastases originating from a primary liver hemangiosarcoma in a dog. *Source:* Dr. G. Romanelli. Reproduced with permission from Dr. G. Romanelli.

- Ultrasonography: At present, it represents the gold standard for diagnosis of splenic lesions, but interpretation may be challenging (Ohlerth *et al.* 2008). Recent efforts aimed at differentiating benign from malignant splenic lesions, but the results are still preliminary (Ohlerth *et al.* 2008; Rossi *et al.* 2008). Multifocal lesions are more suggestive of metastasis. Some tumors (e.g., lymphoma, Mast Cell Tumor) may be primary in the spleen but still nodular; in other instances, they cause splenomegaly.
- Computed tomography (CT): CT provides important information for tumor staging (Owen 1980) because detection of lesions as small as 2 to 3 mm in diameter is possible. A study on CT accuracy in distinguishing benign from malignant splenic lesions in 21 dogs with 24 splenic masses found that malignant tumors (8 of 10 were HAS) had the lowest postcontrast Hounsfield Units (HU) value (40.1), hematoma had an intermediate HU value (62.5), and nodular hyperplasia showed the highest value (90.3) (Fife *et al.* 2004).
- Cytology: Ultrasound-guided fine-needle aspiration may aid in diagnosing the lesion; a coagulation profile is recommended before proceeding. In case of larger masses, aspiration may not be indicated because of the risk of hemorrhage and iatrogenic tumoral spread. It is the authors' opinion that in case of an ultrasonographically heterogenous and localized mass, surgery remains the best option, and in case of splenomegaly (e.g., lymphoma, mastocytoma), cytology may be useful (Stefanello *et al.* 2009).

Treatment

Treatment is influenced by the tumoral histologic type, nature (primary or secondary) and stage. Patients with lymphoma, Mast Cell Tumor, and disseminated histiocytosis are treated with palliative chemotherapy; only isolated lesions may be addressed surgically. Palliative treatment (including chemotherapy) may be instituted for disseminated metastases.

Outcome

The prognosis depends on tumor type, stage, and patient's condition. In case of splenic HAS, a postsplenectomy 1-year survival rate of 6.25% (overall median survival time, 86 days) has been reported (Wood *et al.* 1998). Adjuvant chemotherapy to increase survival is warranted (Thamm 2010). For metastatic or generalized tumors (e.g., lymphoma), the response to medical palliation is variable. Metastatic tumors are usually characterized by shorter survival times than originally disseminated neoplasms.

Gastric dilation and volvulus

See Chapter 57.

Definition

Gastric dilatation and volvulus (GDV) is a life-threatening condition in which the stomach rotates on its axis, more frequently in a clockwise direction. In a recent study, patients with GDV treated also with splenectomy had a worse prognosis than those that had GDV correction only (Mackenzie *et al.* 2010).

Risk factors

- Risk factors for GDV apply also for asplenic dogs.
- The lack of supporting ligaments and the increase of space in the cranial left abdomen in asplenic dogs may potentially predispose

to GDV (Millis *et al.* 1995; Neath *et al.* 1997; Marconato 2006). However, a recent paper dealing with 37 splenectomized dogs followed for 1 postoperative year did not validate this hypothesis even though 1 of these dogs developed GDV after 48 hours from splenectomy (Goldhammer *et al.* 2010). This finding has also been confirmed in a more recent paper (Grange *et al.* 2012). Finally, in a multi-institutional retrospective case-control study on 453 cases published in 2013, the odds of GDV in dogs with a history of previous splenectomy were 5.3 times those of dogs without a history of previous splenectomy. These findings support that prophylactic gastropexy should be considered in dogs undergoing splenectomy, especially if other risk factors for GDV are present (Sartor 2013).

Prevention

Perform a gastropexy at the time of splenectomy, especially in predisposed dogs.

Sepsis

See Chapter 2.

Definition

Sepsis secondary to splenectomy is attributed to the loss of filtering and phagocytic functions of the spleen. This condition is well known in humans. To this regard, Brigden *et al.* (2001) wrote: "Asplenic patients have a long-term susceptibility to serious, potentially life-threatening infections, which may vary in clinical presentation, from mild pneumonia to overwhelming, lethal postsplenectomy infection."

Risk factors

The relative risk for sepsis is 10 times greater in humans undergoing surgery for traumatic splenic rupture and 100 times greater in small children; the risk is also higher in humans who had splenectomy within the previous 2 years, especially for lymphoma or thalassemia (Williams and Kaur 1996). The post-hospitalization mortality rate is greater than 50% (Jones *et al.* 2010), and death may occur early. Reported infections in humans include *Streptococcus pneumonia, Hemophilus influenza, Neisseria meningitidis* (meningococcus), *Capnocytophaga canimorsus, Babesia microti,* and malaria (Brigden *et al.* 2001; Després-Brummer *et al.* 2001; Delanaye *et al.* 2002). Infection is rarely reported in animals and includes *Babesia canis* (Camacho *et al.* 2002), *Mycoplasma hemocanis* (Kemming *et al.* 2004; Sykes *et al.* 2004; Royals *et al.* 2005), and *Haemobartonella canis* (Lester *et al.* 1995).

Diagnosis

The diagnosis is challenging. In a study dealing with asplenic dogs constantly monitored for 10 postoperative days, there were no consistent changes in erythrocyte, leukocyte, and platelet counts; bone marrow samples; biochemistry profile; serum iron; transferrin; and IgM concentrations; 5 of 23 dogs had pyrexia during the first 2 to 5 postoperative days but with no direct correlation with cultures for aerobic bacteria (35% positivity for growth) (Richardson and Brown 1996). As opposed to humans, it appears that clinical signs in asplenic dogs are usually absent and, if present, they are not specific and rarely serious.

Treatment

See Chapter 2.

Outcome

Splenectomy did not enhance or inhibit the recovery of animals in one study (Spangler and Kass 1997). In another report, 1 of 10 dogs died after splenectomy because of *Mycoplasma* infection (Royals *et al.* 2005).

Prevention

In humans, preventive measures include vaccination, antibiotics, and education (even after a minor dog bite) (Williams and Kaur 1996; Jones *et al.* 2010). At present, no preventive measure is taken in asplenic dogs. This reflects the paucity of cases observed, but the condition could be underestimated.

Histopathologic misdiagnosis

Definition

Cytology from fine-needle aspirates, especially in case of sarcoma, may be inconclusive and is rarely performed. In many cases, the final diagnosis depends on histopathology. Unfortunately, in some instances, even histopathology may fail, and immunohistochemistry or other diagnostic procedures are required to further characterize the tumor (Christensen *et al.* 2009).

Risk factors

- Excessive blood contamination (cytology)
- Sampling from a nondiagnostic area (presence of necrosis, blood, or clots) (for both cytology and histology) (Figure 56.8)
- A recent paper concluded that the clinical differentiation between canine splenic HAS from benign lesions (e.g., hematoma) may be helped by the fact that, when dogs with splenic HAS and benign lesions are compared, the latter are characterized by a significantly higher mean mass-to-splenic volume ratio and higher mean splenic weight as a percentage of body weight (Mallinckrodt and Gottfied 2011) (Figure 56.9).
- Technical problems during all the phases of preparation of samples (both for cytology and histology)
- Difficulty to distinguish a very differentiated tumor from normal tissue or, at the opposite, the origin of an undifferentiated tumor type
- In case of a Mast Cell Tumor, it may indeed be challenging to interpret correctly mast cell splenic infiltration (Stefanello *et al.* 2009).
- Misinterpretation

Outcome

Misdiagnosis may not couple with follow-up.

Relevant literature

Hemorrhage was reported in 3.7% to 10% of dogs undergoing splenectomy (Royals *et al.* 2005; Rivier and Monnet 2011). In the first study (Royals *et al.* 2005), splenectomy was performed using an ultrasonic harmonic scalpel. Hemorrhage was intraoperative, likely caused by failure of occlusion of a splenic vein being greater than 6 mm in diameter. No dogs died because of hemorrhage. In the second study (Rivier and Monnet 2011), splenectomy was performed using a vessel sealing device (LigaSure™, Covidien, Minneapolis, MI) (Figure 56.10). No intraoperative bleeding was recorded; nevertheless, 1 of the 27 dogs developed hemoabdomen on the fourth postoperative day.

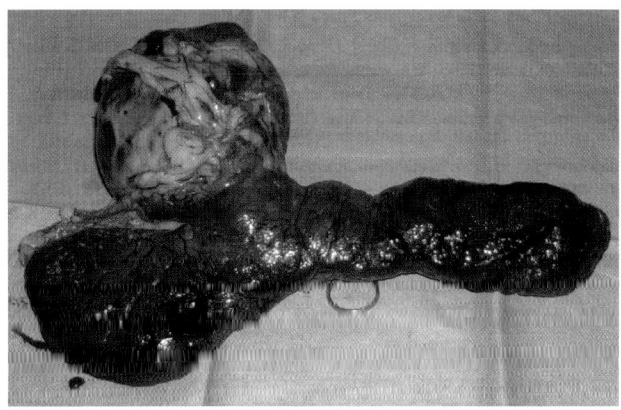

(A)

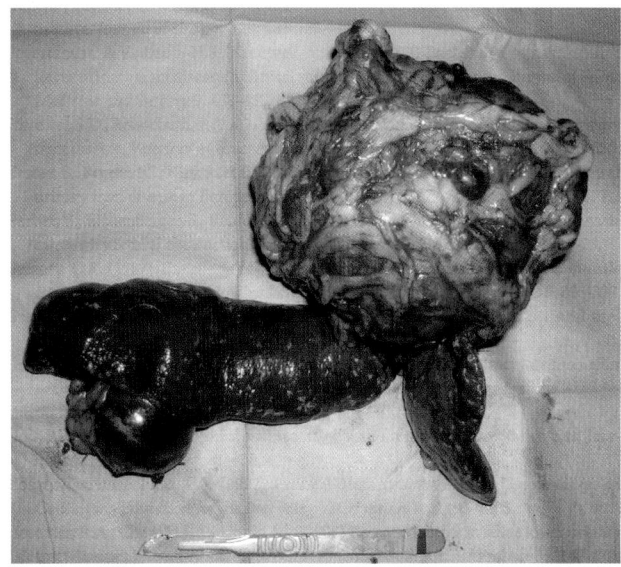

(B)

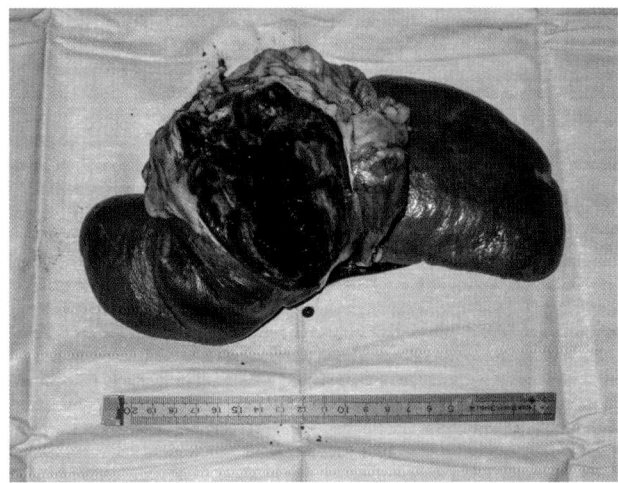

(C)

Figure 56.8 A and **B**, Postoperative views of a splenic hemangioma and hemangiosarcoma, respectively. Macroscopically, they cannot be distinguished. **C**, Postoperative view of the cut surface of a splenic hemangiosarcoma in a dog.

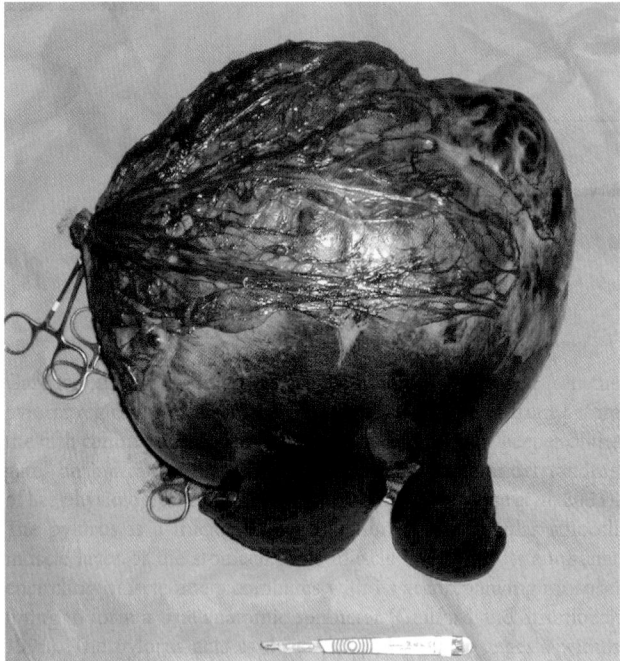

Figure 56.9 Postoperative view of a huge splenic hemangioma. Misdiagnosis may result if only the blood clot or necrosis is sampled.

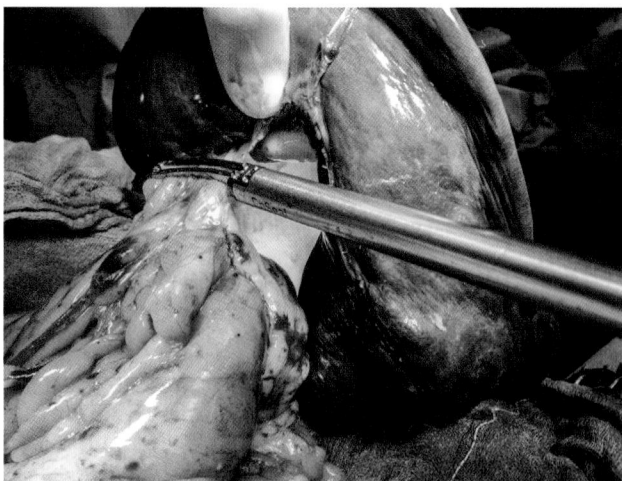

Figure 56.10 Intraoperative view of a splenectomy performed with an vessel sealing device (LigaSure™, Covidien, MI) in a dog. *Source:* Dr. G. Romanelli. Reproduced with permission from Dr. G. Romanelli.

When stapling was used for partial splenectomy, compared with a conventional ligation technique, blood loss was minimal, and both techniques were considered safe (Waldron and Robertson 1995).

In an experimental study in dogs, it was found that splenectomy eliminated exercise-induced polycythemia, with also a 30% reduction in maximal O_2 uptake. The authors concluded that in asplenic dogs, there was an impaired diffusive O_2 transport in the lungs, resulting in a deficit of compensatory mechanism in case of restrictive lung disease or ambient hypoxia (Dane *et al.* 2006). At this point, the clinical implication of this finding is unknown.

Regarding histopathologic diagnosis, one interesting item is the agreement rate between cytologic and histologic findings. In two studies (Brown and Hauser 2007; Christensen *et al.* 2009), the agreement rates were found to be 37.2% and 59%, respectively; in the second study, 2 cases remained undiagnosed, even at histopathology. It is obvious that occasionally, the spleen is removed for nodule(s) that would not have required surgery. Because the differentiation between splenic lesions requiring surgery from those that do not should be realized preoperatively, a major role is given to diagnostic imaging. Apart from radiographs that can only reveal a mass, great efforts are addressed to improve the ability to distinguish benign from malignant splenic lesions. If it is true that standard and contrast-enhanced ultrasonography provided important improvements (Ohlerth *et al.* 2008; Rossi *et al.* 2008), it is also true that, at present, either CT (Fife *et al.* 2004) or magnetic resonance appears more sensitive than ultrasonography. In a study on 8 dogs, both the sensitivity and specificity rates of magnetic resonance in differentiating benign from malignant focal splenic lesions were 100% (Clifford *et al.* 2004).

References

Anderson, D. (2012) Surgical hemostasis. In Tobias, K.M., Johnston, S.A. (eds.) *Veterinary Surgery Small Animal,* 1st edn. Elsevier Saunders, St. Louis, pp. 214-220.

Aronsohn, M.G., Dubiel, B., Roberts, B., et al. (2009) Prognosis for acute non traumatic hemoperitoneum in the dog: a retrospective analysis of 60 cases (2003-2006). *Journal of the American Animal Hospital Association* 45, 72-77.

Beck, J.J., Butler, A., Hackett, T., et al (2005) Acute, fatal portal vein thrombosis following splenectomy in six dogs. In Society of Veterinary Soft Tissue Surgeons, Annual Conference Proceedings.

Brigden, M.L., Pattullo, A., Brown, G. (2001) Practising physician's knowledge and patterns of practice regarding the asplenic state: the need for improved education and a practical checklist. *Canadian Journal of Surgery* 44, 210-216.

Brockman, D.J., Mongil, C.M., Aronson, L.R., et al. (2000) A practical approach to hemoperitoneum in the dog and cat. *Veterinary Clinics of North America: Small Animal Practice* 30, 657-668.

Brown, A.O., Hauser, B. (2007) Correlation between cytopathology and histopathology of the skin, lymph node and spleen in 500 dogs and cats. *Schweizer Archiv fur Tierheilkunde* 149, 249-257.

Camacho, A.T., Pallas, E., Gestal, J.J., et al. (2002) Natural infection by a Babesia microti-like piroplasm in a splenectomised dog. *Veterinary Record* 150, 381-382.

Chandler, J.C., Monnet, E., Staatz, A.J. (2006) Comparison of acute hemodynamic effects of lidocaine and procainamide for postoperative ventricular arrhythmias in dogs. *Journal of the American Animal Hospital Association* 42, 262.

Christensen, N., Canfield, P., Martin, P., et al. (2009) Cytopathological and histopathological diagnosis of canine splenic disorders. *Australian Veterinary Journal* 87, 175-181.

Clifford, C.A., Pretorius, E.S., Weisse, C., et al. (2004) Magnetic resonance imaging of focal splenic and hepatic lesion in the dog. *Journal of Veterinary Internal Medicine* 18, 330-338.

Collard, F., Nadeau, M.E., Carmel, E.N. (2010) Laparoscopic splenectomy for treatment of splenic hemangiosarcoma in a dog. *Veterinary Surgery* 39, 870-872.

Crowe, D.T. (1980) Autotransfusion in the trauma patient. *Veterinary Clinics of North America: Small Animal Practice* 10, 581.

Dale, G.L., Wolf, R.F., Hynes, L.A., et al. (1996) Quantitation of platelet life span in splenectomized dogs. *Experimental Hematology* 24, 518-523.

Dane, D.M., Hsia, C.C., Wu, E.Y., et al. (2006) Splenectomy impairs diffusive oxygen transport in the lung of dogs. *Journal of Applied Physiology* 101, 289-297.

Delanaye, P., Dubois, C., Mendes, P., et al. (2002) Dog bite in a splenectomized patient. *Revue Médicale de Liège* 57, 40-44.

Deprés-Brummer, P., Buijs, J., van Engelenburg, K.C., et al. (2001) Canimorsus sepsis presenting as an acute abdomen in an asplenic patient. *Netherlands Journal of Medicine* 59, 213-217.

Fife, W.D., Samii, V.F., Drost, W.T., et al. (2004) Comparison between malignant and nonmalignant splenic masses in dogs using contrast-enhanced computed tomography. *Veterinary Radiology and Ultrasound* 45, 289-97.

Fossum, T.W. (2007) Surgery of the hemolymphatic system. In Fossum, T.W. (ed.) *Small Animal Surgery*, 3rd edn. Mosby Elsevier, St Louis, MO, pp. 624-634.

Goldhammer, M.A., Haining, H., Milne, E.M., et al. (2010) Assessment of the incidence of GDV following splenectomy in dogs. *Journal of Small Animal Practice* 51, 23-28.

Grange, A.M., Clough, W., Casale, S.A. (2012) Evaluation of splenectomy as a risk factor for gastric dilatation-volvulus. *Journal of the American Veterinary Medical Association* 241, 461-466.

Hammond, T.N., Pesillo-Crosby, S.A. (2008) Prevalence of hemangiosarcoma in anemic dogs with a splenic mass and hemoperitoneum requiring a transfusion: 71 cases (2003-2005). *Journal of the American Veterinary Medical Association* 232, 553-558.

Herold, L.B., Devey, J.J., Kirby, R., et al. (2008) Clinical evaluation and management of hemoperitoneum in dogs. *Journal of Veterinary Emergency and Critical Care* 18, 40-53.

Horgan, J.E., Roberts, B.K., Schermerhorn, T. (2009) Splenectomy as an adjunctive treatment for dogs with immune-mediated hemolytic anemia: ten cases (2003-2006). *Journal of Veterinary Emergency and Critical Care* 19, 254-261.

Jones, P., Leder, K., Woolley, I., et al. (2010) Postsplenectomy infection—strategies for prevention in general practice. *Australian Family Physician* 39, 383-386.

Kemming, G. Messick, J.B., Mueller, W., et al. (2004) Can we continue research in splenectomized dogs? Mycoplasma haemocanis: old problem-new insight. *European Surgical Research* 36, 198-205.

Kerwin, S.C., Mauldin, G.E. (2003) Hemostasis, surgical bleeding and transfusion. In Slatter, D. (ed.) *Textbook of Small Animal Surgery*, 3rd edn. Elsevier Saunders, St. Louis, pp. 44-65.

Kirby, B.M. (2003) Peritoneum and peritoneal cavity. In Slatter, D. (ed.) *Textbook of Small Animal Surgery*, 3rd edn. Elsevier Saunders, St. Louis, pp. 414-445.

Knapp, D.W., Aronsohn, M.G., Harpster, N.K. (1993) Cardiac arrhythmias associated mass lesion of the canine spleen. *Journal of the American Animal Hospital Association* 29, 122-128.

Lester, S.J., Hume, J.B., Phipps, B. (1995) Haemobartonella canis infection following splenectomy and transfusion. *Canadian Veterinary Journal* 36, 444–445.

Mackenzie, G., Barnhart, M., Kennedy, S., et al. (2010) A retrospective study of factors influencing survival following surgery for gastric dilatation-volvulus syndrome in 306 dogs. *Journal of the American Animal Hospital Association* 46, 97-102.

Mallinckrodt, M.J., Gottfried, S.D. (2011) Mass-to-splenic volume ratio and splenic weight as a percentage of body weight in dogs with malignant and benign splenic masses: 65 cases (2007-2008). *Journal of the American Veterinary Medical Association* 239, 1325-1327.

Marconato, L. (2006) Gastric dilatation-volvulus as complication after surgical removal of a splenic haemangiosarcoma in a dog. *Journal of Veterinary Medicine. A, Physiology, Pathology, Clinical Medicine* 53, 371-374.

Marino, D.J., Matthiesen, D.T., Fox, P.R., et al. (1994) Ventricular arrhythmias in dogs undergoing splenectomy: a prospective study. *Veterinary Surgery* 23, 101-106.

Maruyama, H., Miura, T., Sakai, M., et al. (2004) The incidence of disseminated intravascular coagulation in dogs with malignant tumor. *Journal of Veterinary Medical Science* 66, 573-575.

Millis, D.L., Nemzek, J., Riggs, C., et al. (1995) Gastric dilatation-volvulus after splenic torsion in two dogs. *Journal of the American Veterinary Medical Association* 207, 314-315.

Minta, L.K., John, E.R., Helio, S.A., et al. (1993) Ventricular arrhythmias in dogs with splenic masses. *Journal of Veterinary Emergency and Critical Care* 3, 33-38.

Neath, P.J., Brockman, D.J., Saunders, H.M. (1997) Retrospective analysis of 19 cases of isolated torsion of the splenic pedicle in dogs. *Journal of Small Animal Practice* 38, 387-392.

Ohlerth, S., Dennler, M., Rüefli, E., et al. (2008) Contrast harmonic imaging characterization of canine splenic lesions. *Journal of Veterinary Internal Medicine* 22, 1095-1102.

Owen, L.N. (1980) *Classification of Tumours in Domestic Animals.* World Health Organization, Geneva.

Richardson, E.F., Brown, N.O. (1996) Hematological and biochemical changes and results of aerobic bacteriological culturing in dogs undergoing splenectomy. *Journal of the American Animal Hospital Association* 32, 199-210.

Rivier, P., Monnet, E. (2011) Use of a vessel sealant device for splenectomy in dogs *Veterinary Surgery* 40, 102-155.

Rossi, F., Leone, V.F., Vignoli, M., et al. (2008) Use of contrast-enhanced ultrasound for characterization of focal splenic lesions. *Veterinary Radiology and Ultrasound* 49, 154-164.

Royals, S.R., Ellison, G.W., Adin, C.A., et al. (2005) Use of an ultrasonically activated scalpel for splenectomy in 10 dogs with naturally occurring splenic disease. *Veterinary Surgery* 34, 174-179.

Sartor, A.J., Bentley, A.M., Brown, D.C. (2013) Association between previous splenectomy and gastric dilatation-volvulus in dogs: 453 cases (2004–2009). *Journal of the American Veterinary Medical Association* 242, 1381-1384.

Spangler, W.L., Kass, P.H. (1997) Pathologic factors affecting postsplenectomy survival in dogs. *Journal of Veterinary Internal Medicine* 11, 166-171.

Stefanello, D., Valenti, P., Faverzani, S., et al. (2009) Ultrasound-guided cytology of spleen and liver: a prognostic tool in canine cutaneous mast cell tumor. *Journal of Veterinary Internal Medicine* 23, 1051-1057.

Sykes, J.E., Bailiff, N.L., Ball, L.M., et al. (2004) Identification of a novel hemotropic mycoplasma in a splenectomized dog with hemic neoplasia. *Journal of the American Veterinary Medical Association* 224, 1946-1951.

Thamm, D.H. (2007) Miscellaneous tumors. In Withrow, S.J., Vail, D.M. (eds.) *Withrow and MacEwen's Small Animal Clinical Oncology*, 4th edn. Saunders Elsevier, St. Louis, pp. 785-795.

Tillson, D.M. (2003) Spleen. In Slatter, D. (ed.) *Textbook of Small Animal Surgery*, 3rd edn. Elsevier Saunders, St. Louis, pp. 1046-1062.

Vlasin, M., Rauser, P., Fichtel, T., et al. (2004) Disseminated intravascular coagulopathy of the dog. *Acta Veterinaria Brno* 73, 497-505.

Waldron, D.R., Robertson, J. (1995) Partial splenectomy in the dog: a comparison of stapling and ligation techniques. *Journal of the American Animal Hospital Association* 31, 343-348.

Williams, D.N., Kaur, B. (1996) Postsplenectomy care. Strategies to decrease the risk of infection. *Postgraduate Medicine* 100, 195-198.

Wood, C.A., Moore, A.S., Gliatto, J.M., et al. (1998) Prognosis for dogs with stage I or II splenic hemangiosarcoma treated by splenectomy alone: 32 cases (1991-1993). *Journal of the American Animal Hospital Association* 34, 417-21.

Gastrointestinal Surgery

57 Gastric Dilatation and Volvulus and Gastropexies

Zoë Halfacree

The Department of Clinical Science and Services, The Royal Veterinary College, North Mymms, Hertfordshire, UK

Gastric dilatation and volvulus (GDV) is a common life-threatening condition that requires aggressive medical and surgical therapy to achieve a successful outcome. After prompt diagnosis and appropriate management, the prognosis can be good with survival rates approaching 85%. Appropriate management must include a short period of thorough patient stabilization, prompt definitive surgical treatment, and intensive postoperative care (Hosgood, 1994; Brockman *et al.* 1995).

The complication rate associated with this condition is high and careful patient stabilization, thorough intraoperative and postoperative evaluation is essential to improve the chances of survival. A systematic approach is required to achieve early identification and management of postoperative complications (Figure 57.1).

SYSTEMIC COMPLICATIONS

Gastric dilatation and volvulus syndrome is associated with severe changes of cardiovascular, respiratory, and renal physiology in addition to the effects on the gastrointestinal (GI) tract. Systemic complications commonly arise as a result of these pathophysiological changes. Inadequate patient resuscitation and monitoring are likely to exacerbate the severity of these complications.

Hypotension

Definition
Hypotension is defined as a systolic pressure of less than 90 mm Hg and a mean arterial pressure of less than 65 mm Hg. Hypotension noted at any time during management of a patient with GDV is a significant risk factor for death (Beck *et al.* 2006).

Treatment and prevention
Optimal management of dogs with GDV syndrome requires that appropriately aggressive volume resuscitation is instituted at presentation and that ongoing adjustment of intravenous (IV) fluid therapy is performed based on patient monitoring perioperatively Although the protocol for IV fluid therapy should be tailored to individual patient requirements, a rough guide of appropriate management includes:
- Place two large-bore (14–18 gauge) cephalic or jugular IV catheters at presentation.
- A balanced electrolyte solution (compound sodium lactate) is infused as a rate of 90 mL/kg for the first hour. It is most

appropriate for a proportion of this total dose (e.g., 20–25 mL/kg) to be administered as a bolus over 15 minutes and that patient parameters are then reassessed with additional fluid therapy being administered based upon patient response.
- Rapid fluid administration is facilitated by using pressure bags in large dogs.
- After initiation of volume resuscitation, gastric decompression should be achieved by passage of a stomach tube or needle gastrocentesis.
- Intraoperative fluid therapy should be maintained at a high rate (10–20 mL/kg) and supplemented with colloids and blood products as necessary.
- Whole blood or packed red blood cells should be transfused to maintain the packed cell volume (PC) at greater than 22%.
- Use of vasopressor agents is contraindicated before adequate volume resuscitation.

Cardiac arrhythmias

Definition
Cardiac arrhythmias are commonly seen in dogs with GDV syndrome and are generally ventricular in origin, including ventricular premature complexes, which may progress to ventricular tachycardia.

Risk factors
- In recent reports, 40% to 70% of dogs with GDV syndrome are reported to develop cardiac arrhythmias (Brockman *et al.* 1995; Beck *et al.* 2006; Mackenzie *et al.* 2010).
- Cardiac arrhythmias may be noted at the time of presentation or develop 12 to 24 hours postoperatively.
- The presence of preoperative cardiac arrhythmias can be predictive of the requirement for partial gastrectomy or splenectomy (Mackenzie *et al.* 2010).
- Myocardial hypoxia secondary to poor coronary artery perfusion and the effects of hypoventilation and respiratory and metabolic acid–base imbalances exacerbate the proarrhythmic state.

Diagnosis
- Diagnosis is made on thoracic auscultation and peripheral pulse palpation allowing appreciation of pulse deficits.
- Continuous electrocardiography (ECG) is recommended for postoperative monitoring of the dog after surgery for GDV syndrome.

Complications in Small Animal Surgery, First Edition. Edited by Dominique Griffon and Annick Hamaide.
© 2016 John Wiley & Sons, Inc. Published 2016 by John Wiley & Sons, Inc.
Companion website: www.wiley.com/go/griffon/complications

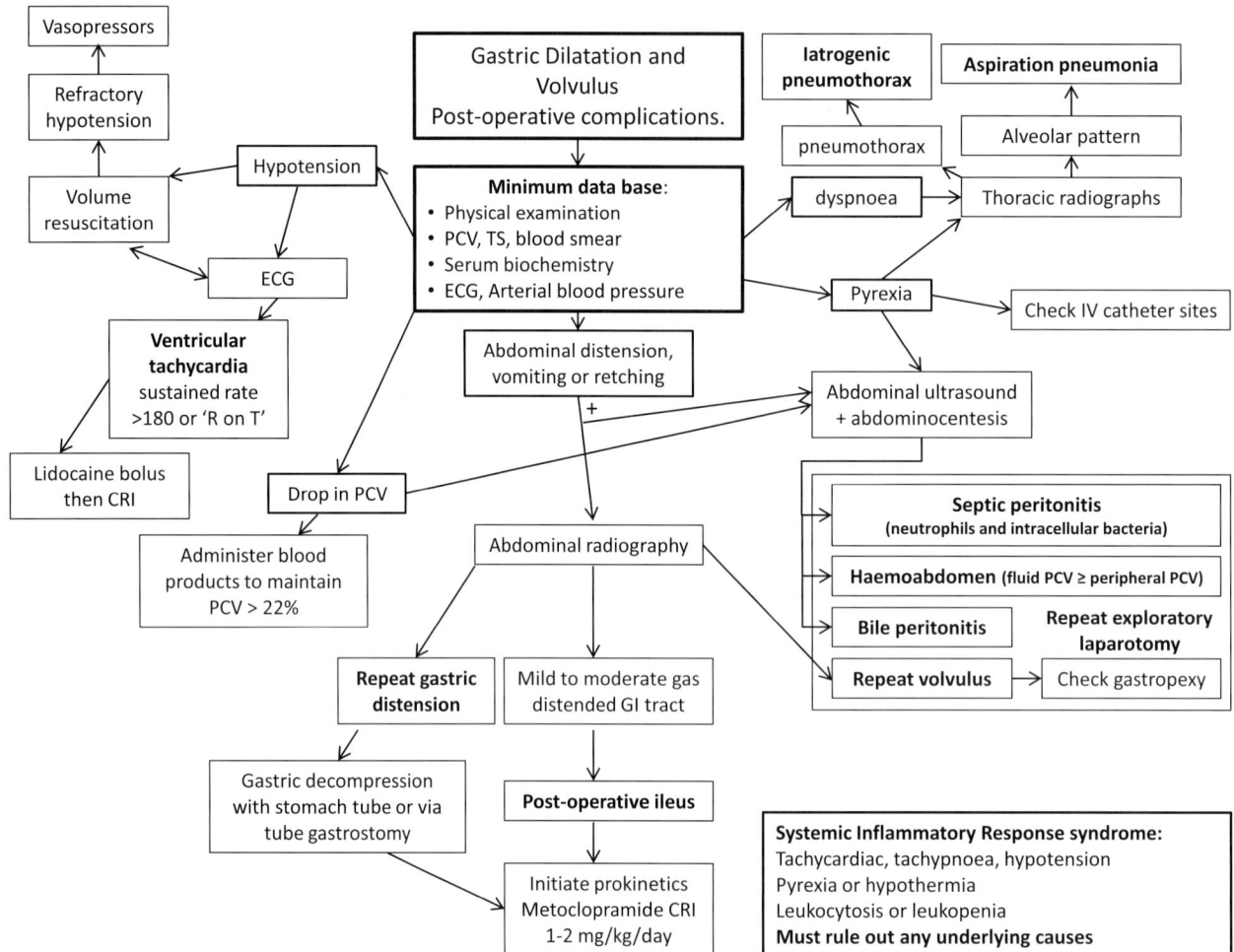

Figure 57.1 An algorithm to aid decision making when monitoring patients with gastric dilatation and volvulus for postoperative complications within the first 5 days after surgery. CRI, constant-rate infusion; ECG, electrocardiography; GI, gastrointestinal; IV, intravenous; PCV, packed cell volume; TS, total solids; US, ultrasonography.

Treatment

Most patients do not require treatment. Treatment of cardiac arrhythmias is only instituted if there are indications that it is hemodynamically significant and affecting tissue perfusion, as determined by arterial blood pressure, peripheral pulse quality, and capillary refill time. Specific indications are:

- Documented hypotension
- Heart rate exceeding 180 beats/min
- R on T phenomenon (superimposition of the QRS complex on the T wave on the ECG)
- Preexisting cardiac disease

Initial treatment of ventricular arrhythmias includes a bolus of lidocaine (1–8 mg/kg IV) followed by a constant-rate infusion (CRI) (0.04–0.08 mg/kg/min) if successful conversion to sinus rhythm is achieved. Boluses of procainamide (0.5–4.0 mg/kg) can be used in dogs that do not respond to lidocaine followed by a CRI (0.04 mg/kg/min) (Brockman *et al.* 1995).

Hypokalemia interferes with the action of lidocaine and procainamide; therefore, serum electrolytes should be measured and supplementation administered as required.

Ensure adequate volume resuscitation is performed before considering antiarrhythmic treatment.

After sustained sinus rhythm, the antiarrhythmic treatment should be stopped. Abrupt cessation is recommended because tapering the dose can lead to a proarrhythmic state.

Outcome

In general, it is reported that the presence of cardiac arrhythmias is associated with increased mortality rates (Beck *et al.* 2006; Mackenzie *et al.* 2010); however, in one study, this was not correlated with outcome (Brockman *et al.* 1995).

Prevention

Although this complication cannot be prevented, attentive fluid resuscitation can optimize tissue perfusion, which may reduce the severity of cardiac arrhythmias.

Sepsis and systemic inflammatory response syndrome

See Chapter 2.

Sepsis or systemic inflammatory response syndrome is a potential complication of GDV syndrome. The most common septic focus is the peritoneal cavity if gastric necrosis or dehiscence has occurred, resulting in septic peritonitis. IV or indwelling urethral catheter sites must always be monitored and managed carefully because they represent an additional site at which infection may become established.

Hypoventilation

Definition

Hypoventilation is reduced ventilation such that hypercapnia ($PaCO_2$ >50 mm Hg) and hypoxia (PaO_2 <50 mm Hg) develop. Hypoventilation may be caused by iatrogenic pneumothorax or may be secondary to severe gastric or abdominal distension (Wingfield *et al.* 1982). Iatrogenic pneumothorax may occur in GDV patients secondary to perforation of the diaphragm during the gastropexy procedure.

Risk factors

Circumcostal gastropexy is the most likely to result in a pneumothorax because a tunnel must be made around the last complete rib, and inadvertent penetration of the diaphragm can occur.

Diagnosis

- Iatrogenic pneumothorax should be detected intraoperatively because of anesthesia monitoring. The surgeon may hear air moving through the circumcostal incision. Inspection of the visceral surface of the diaphragm, confirming a taut diaphragm and absence of pneumothorax, should be performed by the surgeon before abdominal closure.
- Postoperative diagnosis may be achieved by thoracic auscultation, diagnostic and therapeutic thoracocentesis, or demonstration of pleural gas on thoracic radiographs. Blood gas analysis may reveal hypoxia and hypercapnia.

Treatment

- The diaphragmatic defect must be closed as soon as it is noted. This can be achieved by placement of a few simple interrupted sutures. If a significant volume of pneumothorax is present, the pleural space should be drained by transdiaphragmatic thoracocentesis.
- Postoperatively, percutaneous thoracocentesis should be use. Use of a thoracostomy tube should not be necessary.
- Relief of abdominal distension by gastric decompression will improve patient ventilation in addition to improving cardiovascular parameters.

Aspiration pneumonia

See Chapter 25.

Concurrent esophageal dysfunction, as noted by detection of megaesophagus on preoperative thoracic radiography, may predispose to aspiration pneumonia, which is most likely to be detected postoperatively (Figure 57.2).

ABDOMINAL COMPLICATIONS

Gastric necrosis

Definition

Gastric necrosis is loss of viability, and subsequently integrity, of the gastric wall.

Reduced vascular perfusion of the gastric wall occurs because of:
- Occlusion of capillaries caused by high intraluminal pressure
- Avulsion of the short gastric arteries
- Reduced cardiac output

Full-thickness gastric wall necrosis may result in loss of integrity of the gastric wall. Gastric rupture at the time of acute presentation is uncommon; a recent report of 109 cases reported gastric rupture in 4 cases (Buber *et al.* 2007).

Risk factors

Gastric necrosis is reported to occur in 10% to 35% of dogs with GDV (Millis *et al.* 1993; Glickman *et al.* 1998; Beck *et al.* 2006; Mackenzie *et al.* 2010).

Risk factors include:
- Increased duration and severity of clinical signs
- Elevated plasma lactate at presentation. Plasma lactate has been identified as a specific predictive factor for gastric necrosis and survival. de Papp *et al.* (1999) reported that pretreatment plasma lactate greater than 6.0 mmol/L was predictive of the presence of gastric necrosis; however, a subsequent study reported that lactate is not a marker for macroscopic gastric wall necrosis (Green *et al.* 2011).
- Haemostatic profile derangement (greater than one abnormal parameter) is predictive of gastric necrosis (Millis *et al.* 1993).

Diagnosis

The diagnosis of gastric necrosis is made by subjective assessment at the time of surgery, which is based on assessment of the coloration, integrity, and thickness of the gastric wall. It is important that the stomach has been adequately decompressed and derotated so as to allow an accurate assessment after adequate reperfusion and to allow evaluation of all sites, particularly at the cardia (Figure 57.3).

Treatment

Gastric necrosis is addressed by partial gastric resection. This can be performed by hand suturing or by use of a surgical stapling device.
- Isolate the stomach from other abdominal organs using moist laparotomy swabs.
- Stay sutures should be used to manipulate the stomach and aid in assessment of the line of resection.
- Suitable automatic stapling devices include the GI anastomosis (GIA 50 or 90, 3.8 mm) or thoracoabdominal stapler (TA 90, green 4.8-mm or blue 3.4-mm cartridges).
- It is common that more than one cartridge is required. The staple line should be oversewn with a continuous inverting suture; this is particularly important when it has been necessary to overlap staple lines.
- For gastric resection in the region of the cardia, hand suturing may be necessary for precision, and insertion of a stomach tube is recommended to ensure maintenance of an adequate lumen.

Outcome

- In general, dogs with gastric necrosis are reported to have a higher mortality rate.
- Failure to detect gastric necrosis and subsequent gastric perforation resulting in septic peritonitis carries a guarded prognosis (Beck *et al.* 2006).

Prevention

Prevention of gastric necrosis may be achieved by prompt intervention and appropriately aggressive fluid resuscitation, along with gastric decompression, to improve gastric perfusion.

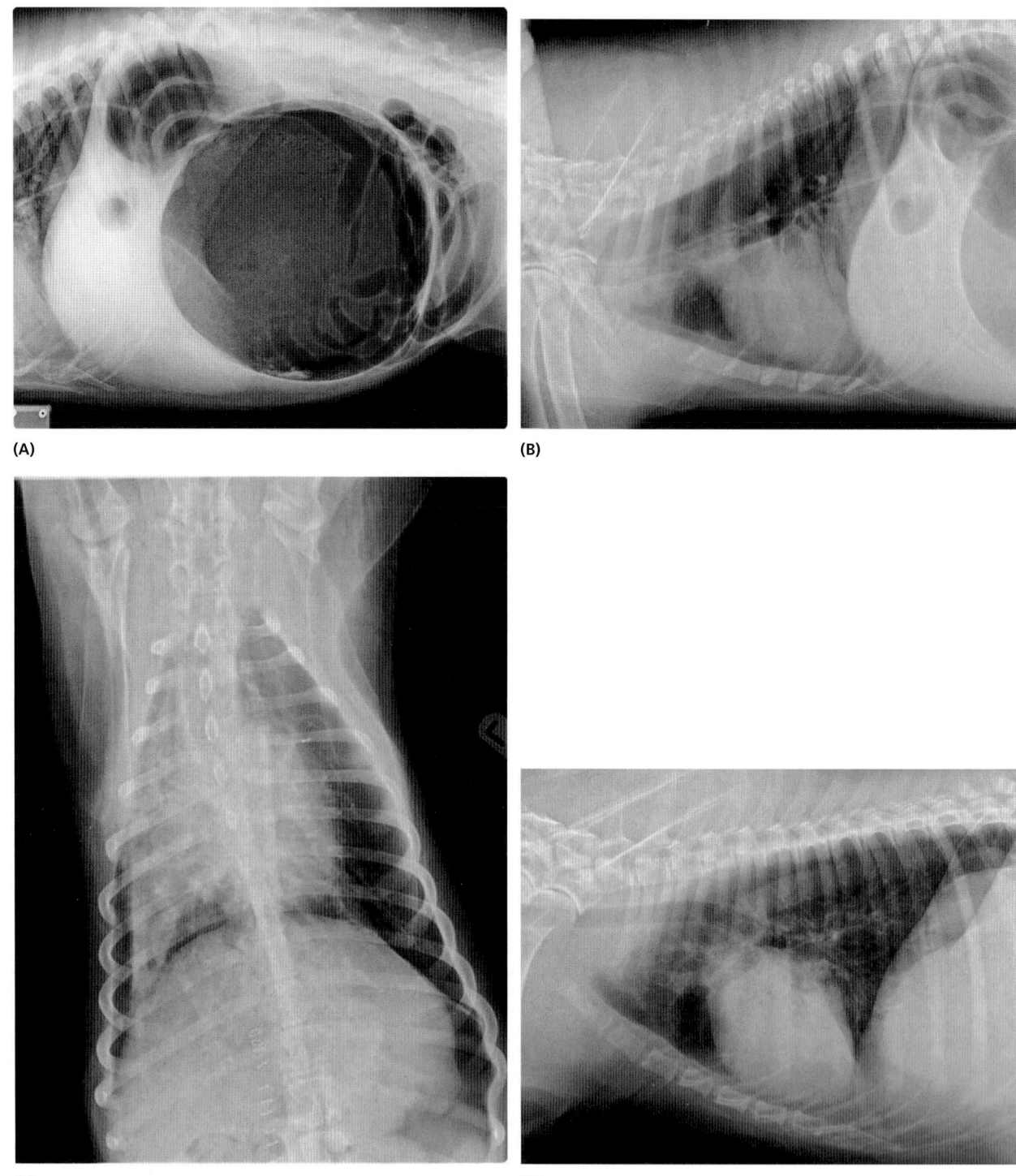

(A)

(B)

(C)

(D)

Figure 57.2 **A** and **B,** Lateral thoracic and abdominal radiography of a 12-year-old Japanese Akita revealed gastric dilatation and volvulus and megaesophagus. **C** and **D,** The dog became tachypneic at 48 hours after surgery, and thoracic radiographs (lateral and ventrodorsal views) revealed an alveolar lung pattern consistent with aspiration pneumonia.

Inadvertent penetration of the gastric lumen

Inadvertent penetration of the gastric lumen may occur upon entering the abdomen because of gastric distension or during elevation of a seromuscular flap when performing a gastropexy. This can be avoided by careful surgical technique. If this complication were to arise, immediate attempts should be made to control leakage of gastric contents by use of suction apparatus and isolation of the perforated area of the stomach from the peritoneal cavity using saline-soaked swabs. The gastric wall can be repaired in two layers (mucosa/submucosa and muscularis/serosa), as appropriate.

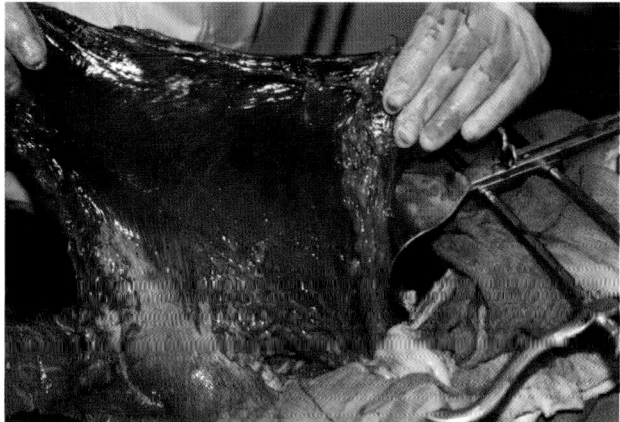

(A)

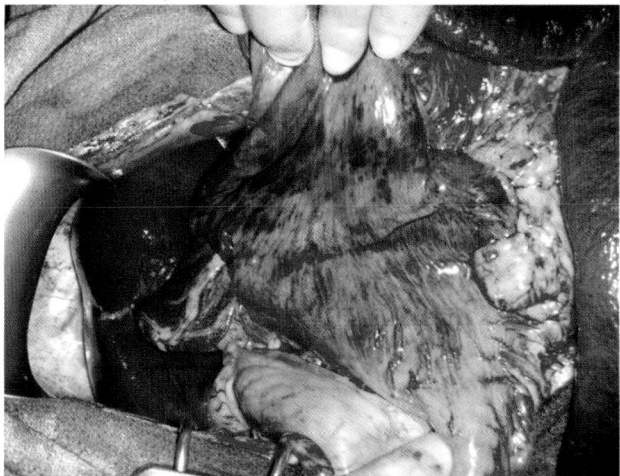

(B)

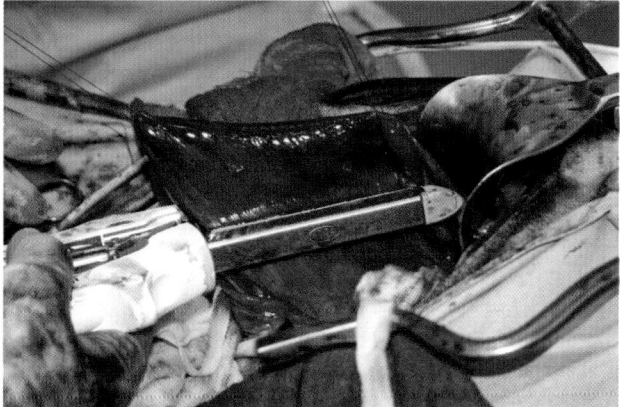

(C)

Figure 57.3 Gastric necrosis is evaluated after full decompression and derotation of the stomach. **A,** A German shepherd with extensive gastric necrosis involving the gastric cardia; this dog was euthanized intraoperatively. Note the sites of avulsion of the short gastric arteries on the greater curvature of the stomach. **B,** A golden Retriever with necrosis of the gastric fundus. **C,** A Dalmatian with gastric necrosis of the fundus undergoing gastric resection using a linear gastrointestinal anastomosis stapler.

Postoperative ileus

Definition
Postoperative ileus is reduced GI motility resulting in gas or fluid distension of the stomach and small intestine. Dogs with GDV experience a disruption of the normal gastric pacemaker activity, resulting in reduced GI motility for around 7 to 14 days postoperatively (Hall 1989; Stampley *et al.* 1992).

Diagnosis
Postoperative ileus may be responsible for vomiting, prolonged inappetence, and abdominal discomfort. Abdominal radiography reveals moderate gas or fluid distension of the stomach and small intestine (Figure 57.4).

Treatment
- Metoclopramide: The dosage for a prokinetic effect is 1 to 2 mg/kg/day intravenously (Woosley 2004).
- Pyloroplasty is not indicated in patients with GDV.

Outcome
Postoperative ileus generally resolves within the first week postoperatively; however, a small number of dogs may continue to have altered GI motility which may predispose them to recurrent bloat. This may represent a preexisting GI motility disorder.

Prevention
Some authors advocate routine use of a metoclopramide infusion postoperatively.

Miscellaneous abdominal injury
The widespread effects on visceral perfusion caused by massive gastric distension and its systemic effects can result in ischemic injury throughout the abdomen, including effects on the spleen, pancreas, and biliary system.

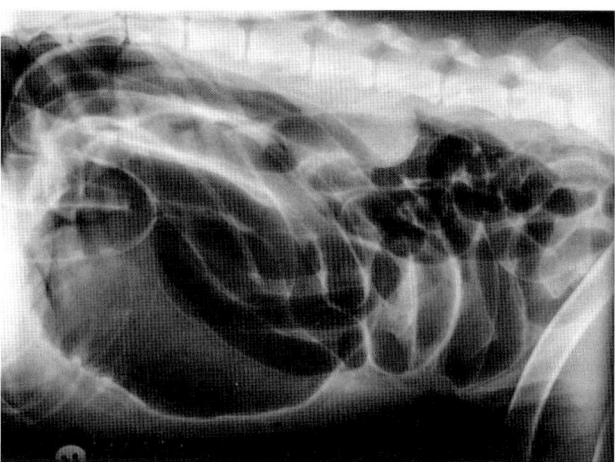

Figure 57.4 A right lateral abdominal radiograph of a 4-year-old female Akita taken 48 hours after surgery for gastric dilatation and volvulus involving derotation and incisional gastropexy. The dog experienced some mild retching and abdominal distension, prompting radiography of the abdomen. The findings are consistent with gaseous distension secondary to postoperative ileus. This resolved within 48 hours with no specific treatment.

The release of a "myocardial depressant factor" caused by ischemic pancreatitis has been implicated in the complex etiopathogenesis of GDV syndrome (Orton and Muir 1983).

Bile peritonitis secondary to ischemic necrosis of the gallbladder fundus has been reported secondary to GDV (Hewitt *et al.* 2005).

Splenic necrosis

Definition

Splenic necrosis is loss of viability of the spleen. Concurrent splenic necrosis may be seen caused by avulsion, torsion, or thrombosis of the splenic vasculature (Figure 57.5). True splenic torsion is seen occasionally.

Diagnosis

Generally, a diagnosis of splenic necrosis is made at the time of exploratory laparotomy. It is recognized as black discoloration of the spleen and loss of pulsation or presence of thrombi within the splenic vasculature.

Treatment

- Splenectomy can be performed using conventional ligatures, a ligate-and-divide staple device, an ultrasonically activated scalpel, or an electrothermal vessel-sealing device.
- Partial splenectomy requires the use of surgical stapling devices and is rarely indicated.
- The spleen should not be derotated before splenectomy to avoid the release of inflammatory mediators and thromboemboli into the circulation.

Outcome

The presence of splenic disease is associated with an increased risk of cardiac arrhythmias (Beck *et al.* 2006; Mackenzie *et al.* 2010).

The need for gastrectomy and concurrent splenectomy is predictive for the development of SIRS and is associated with increased postoperative morbidity and mortality compared with dogs undergoing gastropexy alone or partial gastrectomy (Brourman *et al.* 1996; Beck *et al.* 2006; Mackenzie *et al.* 2010).

Prevention

Prompt diagnosis and intervention may reduce the incidence of splenic necrosis.

Intraabdominal hemorrhage

See Chapter 12.

Definition

Intraabdominal hemorrhage may be seen as a complication of GDV syndrome, both at presentation and postoperatively.

Risk factors

- Avulsion of short gastric arteries (see Figure 57.3A) during volvulus can lead to hemodynamically significant intraabdominal hemorrhage.
- Inadequate hemostasis of the splenic pedicles may lead to hemorrhage after splenectomy.

Diagnosis

Diagnosis is based on documentation of free peritoneal fluid, at the time of surgery or postoperatively via abdominocentesis, with a PCV close to that of the peripheral PCV.

Treatment (see Chapter 12)

- Appropriate intravascular volume replacement with crystalloids, colloids, and blood products is required.
- Blood products should be provided to maintain PCV at greater than 22% and to correct prolongation of coagulation profiles.
- Repeat exploratory laparotomy may be indicated.

Prevention

- Inspect the abdomen and splenic pedicles at the end of surgery for ongoing bleeding.

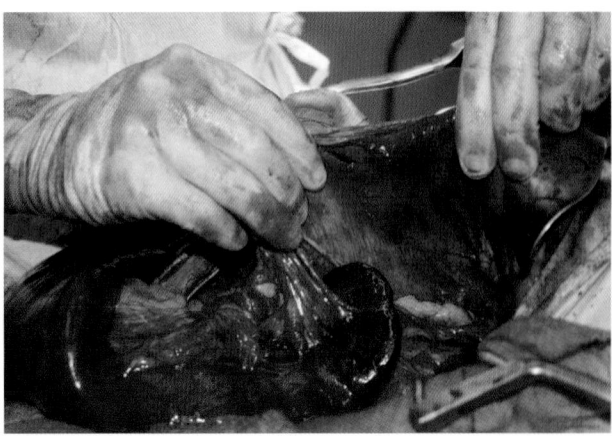

(A)

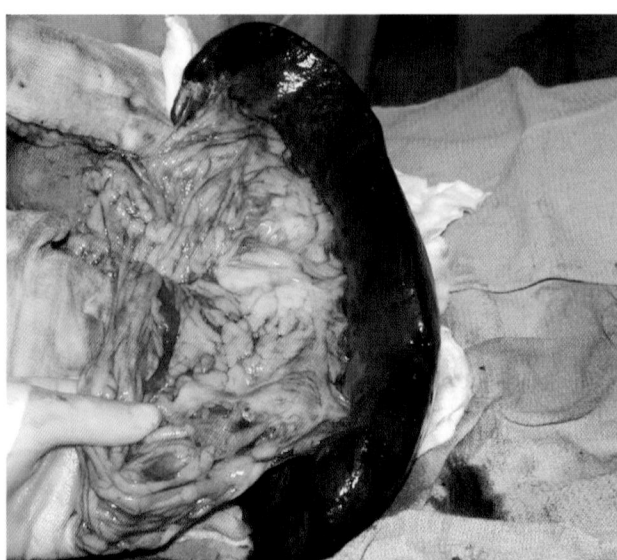

(B)

Figure 57.5 Partial (**A**) or total (**B**) splenic necrosis may occur secondary to gastric dilatation and volvulus and can be identified by engorgement, dark discoloration of the parenchyma, lack of arterial pulsations, and presence of thrombi within the splenic pedicle.

- Ligate avulsed short gastric arteries to avoid postoperative hemorrhage from this site after increased postoperative blood pressure.

Recurrence

Definition
Repeat GDV after a previous episode.

Risk factors
- Previous gastric dilatation or GDV
- The reoccurrence of GDV if gastropexy is not performed is high, around 75% (Meyer-Lindenberg et al. 1993; Glickman et al. 1998; Ward et al. 2003).
- Inappropriate gastropexy (Figure 57.6)

Diagnosis
A diagnosis is made on the basis of repeat abdominal distension and recurrent clinical signs of nonproductive retching or restlessness. Right lateral abdominal radiography is performed to document the presence of GDV.

Prevention and treatment
A gastropexy is a permanent adhesion created between the right body wall and the pyloric antrum, which prevents clockwise rotation and therefore volvulus (Figure 57.7).
- Gastropexy must be performed in all dogs that have had gastric dilatation and GDV.
- Prophylactic gastropexy is advocated in at-risk breeds, including German shepherds, great Danes, bloodhounds, Irish setters, Irish wolfhounds, standard poodles, and Akitas (Glickman et al. 2000; Rawlings et al., 2002; Buber et al. 2007; Green et al. 2011).
- Chronic partial GDV is recognized, for which gastropexy is also required (Paris et al. 2011).

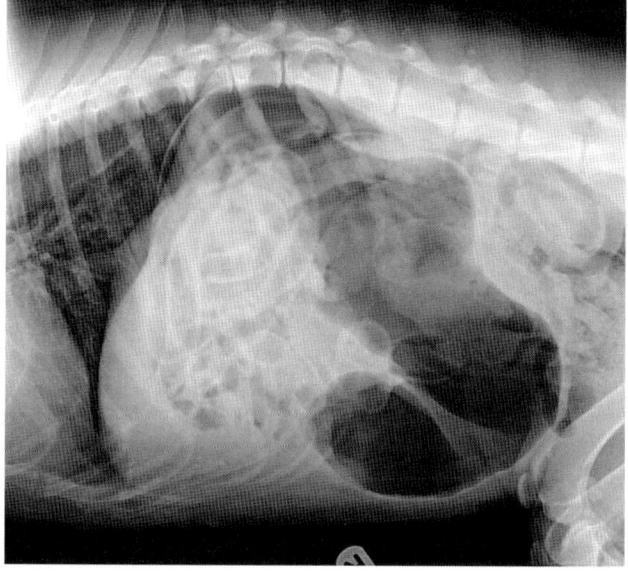

Figure 57.6 A right lateral abdominal radiograph of a 3-year-old German shepherd that had previously had gastric dilatation and volvulus. A gastropexy had been performed but was inappropriately positioned, securing the pyloric antrum to the left body wall. The dog had persistent clinical signs of retching and abdominal discomfort, and surgical revision was performed, after which the dog made a good recovery.

All gastropexy procedures reduce the risk of reoccurrence of GDV to a very low level; however, the relative merits of each different procedure is not clear, and decisions are therefore based on surgeon preference (Table 57.1).

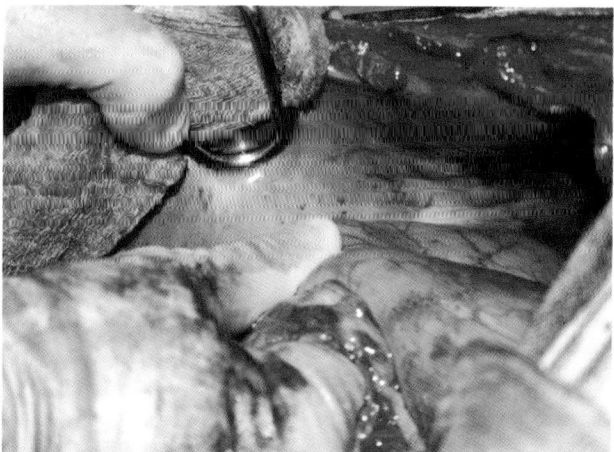

(A)

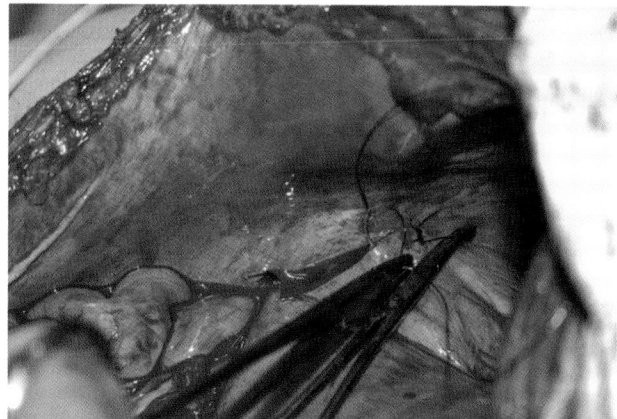

(B)

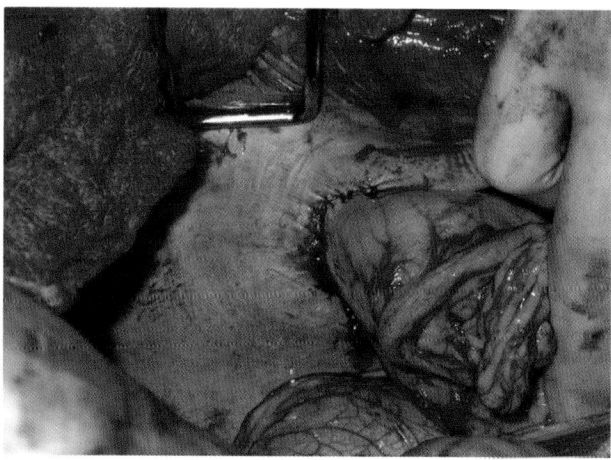

(C)

Figure 57.7 An incisional gastropexy is performed between the pyloric antrum and the right abdominal wall (**A**). After a seromuscular incision on the ventral surface of the pyloric antrum and a corresponding incision in the transversus abdominis caudal to the last rib, the gastropexy is created by suturing the cut edges of the gastric wall to the abdominal wall (**B** and **C**).

Table 57.1 Different gastropexy procedures

Gastropexy	Technique	Advantages	Disadvantages	Comments
Open celiotomy approach (suitable at the time of GDV surgery or for prophylaxis)				
Incorporating	During closure of the linea alba, the suture is passed through the gastric wall at the pyloric antrum.	Quick	Poor adhesion formation increases the risk of recurrence Increased risk of inadvertent gastric perforation at repeat laparotomy	Not recommended
Incisional (muscular) gastropexy	A 3-cm incision is made through the seromuscular portion of the gastric wall at the pyloric antrum. A corresponding incision is made through the transversus abdominis just caudal to the last rib. Two continuous suture lines (polydioxanone) are placed approximating the body wall with the pyloric antrum, along the lines of the incisions (see Fig. 58-7).	Simple technique and reliable adhesion		This technique is favored by the author and is widely used. A single case report documents recurrent GDV caused by stretching of the pexy site (Hammel and Novo 2006).
Tube gastropexy	A tube gastropexy is performed from the pyloric antrum to the right body wall just caudal to the last rib. A purse-string suture is placed in the gastric wall around the exiting tube. Four mattress sutures are placed between the gastric wall and the body wall, securing the gastropexy. Omentum is then wrapped around the tube.	Allows provision of enteral nutrition and gastric decompression if persistent distension occurs	Increased after care and hospitalization Cannot be removed before 7–10 days Risk of patient interference Adhesion is less robust Enters the gastric lumen, increasing the risk of peritoneal contamination and septic peritonitis	Useful for chronic GDV to manage repeat gastric distension
Belt loop gastropexy	A seromuscular flap is elevated from the ventral surface of the pyloric antrum. Two to three branches of the gastroepiploic artery should be incorporated into the base of the flap. This flap is tunneled beneath the transverse abdominis muscle and sutured back into place on the stomach wall.	Simple technique Reliable adhesion		
Circumcostal gastropexy	Two seromuscular flaps are created on the ventral surface of the pyloric antrum, creating an H shape. The last complete rib is identified and exposed, and the cranial flap is then passed around the rib and sutured to the caudal flap creating a strong gastropexy.	Very strong adhesion	Risk of pneumothorax and rib fracture Technically more difficult to perform	Care must be taken to ensure that exposure of the rib does not penetrate the diaphragmatic insertion.
Stapled gastropexy using GIA 50 (AutoSuture)	A 1-cm seromuscular incision is made in the pyloric antrum and through the transverse abdominis muscle caudal to the last rib on the right side of the body wall. Blunt dissection is then used to create a seromuscular tunnel and tunnel in the body wall to accommodate the GIA 50 stapling device. Following activation of the stapler the incisions are closed with a simple continuous suture (Belandria et al. 2009).	Possible increased speed	Increased cost	The increased speed may be negligible given the need to suture the incisions at the site of insertion.
Gastrocolopexy	The transverse colon is sutured to the greater curvature of the stomach over a 10- to 15-cm length after scarification of both serosal surfaces.	Quick Reported to be easy to perform without an assistant (Eggertsdóttir et al. 2001)	Involves suture placement in the colon Involves only scarification of the gastric and colonic serosa, which may not promote as robust and adhesion as the seromuscular flaps	Does not appear superior to other available techniques and is therefore not recommended by the author
Minimally invasive techniques (suitable for prophylaxis only) (Mayhew and Brown, 2009)				
Laparoscopically assisted gastropexy	A laparoscope is inserted to allow exteriorization of the gastric pylorus through a 5-cm incision in the right side of the body wall caudal to the last rib.	Requires only basic laparoscopic skills	Still requires a full-thickness incision through the abdominal wall	All techniques are minimally invasive modifications of the incisional gastropexy with a seromuscular incision made in the pyloric antrum and an incision made through the transverse abdominis muscle of the right body wall.
Total laparoscopic gastropexy with intracorporeal suturing	Three laparoscopic portals are placed, and the pyloric antrum is drawn to the right body wall by passage of a stay suture through the body wall and into the pyloric antrum. Intracorporeal suturing is performed by hand suturing using laparoscopic instruments or by use of a suture-assist device.	Appears to be associated with greater postoperative comfort within 4–5 days postoperatively compared with the laparoscopically assisted technique	Requires greater technical expertise	
Endoscopically assisted gastropexy	The stomach is insufflated via the endoscope, allowing identification of the pyloric antrum at the right body wall and passage of two stay sutures to stabilize the pyloric antrum, allowing a surgical approach through the abdominal wall and a seromuscular incision in the pyloric antrum.	Suitable minimally invasive alternative when laparoscopic equipment or expertise is not available	Requires endoscopic equipment	

GDV, gastric dilatation and volvulus, GIA, gastrointestinal anastomosis.

Relevant literature

The reported mortality rates for dogs experiencing GDV range from 10% to 67% (Glickman *et al.* 1994; Brockman *et al.* 1995; Brourman *et al.* 1996; Glickman *et al.* 1998; de Papp *et al.* 1999; Mackenzie *et al.* 2010). Improved survival rates over time have been attributed to improved facilities and expertise (Ellison 2011). A recent retrospective study reported a postoperative mortality rate of 10% (Mackenzie *et al.* 2010). Reported complication rates associated with GDV remain high (75%); however, prompt recognition and management of serious complications have been attributed to higher survival rates (Beck *et al.* 2006).

Predictors of mortality

Many studies have been published regarding predictors of mortality in dogs with GDV. In general, the prognosis is poorer for dogs that have had a **longer duration of clinical signs** (Buber *et al.* 2007). Dogs that have **signs of depression or are comatose** are 3 and 36 times more likely to die, respectively (Glickman *et al.* 1998). Dogs with **perioperative cardiac arrhythmias** are more likely to die (Mackenzie *et al.* 2010). Dogs with more advanced disease, which required **partial gastrectomy or combined splenectomy and partial gastrectomy**, are also reported to be more likely to die (Brockman *et al.* 1995; Brourman *et al.* 1996; Beck *et al.* 2006; Mackenzie *et al.* 2010). There are studies that provide conflicting evidence; however, Brockman *et al.* (1995) reported that the development of cardiac arrhythmias was not correlated with outcome. Beck *et al.* (2006) reported that partial gastrectomy alone was not associated with a poorer outcome. Buber *et al.* (2007) reported that disseminated intravascular coagulation (DIC) was not an indicator for death. These findings may represent variations in patient population or management but may suggest that optimal management can address these factors and therefore achieve a successful outcome.

Efforts have been made to identify an objective means of patient assessment that may be used at the time of presentation to predict disease severity and survival. **Plasma lactate measurement** has been used to predict gastric necrosis and survival. de Papp (1999) reported that a plasma lactate concentration greater than 6 mmol/L at the time of admission was predictive of gastric necrosis and decreased survival rates. Subsequent studies have evaluated whether serial measurements of plasma lactate concentration, and their response to treatment, has greater predictive value (Zacher *et al.* 2010; Green *et al.* 2011). The findings of Zacher *et al.* supported the guidelines that lower initial levels of plasma lactate were predictive of survival; however, their results indicated that a higher "cut-off" value was appropriate (≤9 mmol/L). Zacher *et al.* also demonstrated that although survival of dogs with a high initial lactate concentration could not be predicted based on the initial lactate concentration alone, evaluation of change in plasma lactate concentration after treatment allowed prediction of survival within this group. Survival rates of dogs with a postresuscitation plasma lactate value of 6.4 mmol/L or less are significantly greater than those in which plasma lactate remains above this cut-off (91% vs. 23%). Green *et al.* (2011) questioned the predictive value of single measurements of plasma lactate; they reported that a decrease in plasma lactate by 50% or more from the initial plasma lactate over a period of 12 hours is predictive of survival.

Recent publications have looked at the use of **plasma myoglobin levels** (Adamik *et al.* 2009) and **urinary 11-dehydrothromboxane B2 excretion** (Baltzer *et al.* 2006) as predictors for survival.

Systemic effects of gastric dilatation and volvulus syndrome

The etiopathogenesis of hypotension and systemic inflammatory response syndrome in dogs with GDV syndrome is a complex interaction between hemodynamic effects and the subsequent release of inflammatory mediators secondary to ischemia. Gastric distension results in increased intraabdominal pressure and collapse of the caudal vena cava, thereby reducing venous return and thus cardiac output. Compromised perfusion to the GI tract and concurrent compression of the hepatic portal vein results in ischemic visceral damage and production of reactive oxygen species (Collard and Gelman 2001) and other cardiodepressive mediators. Cardiac output is further reduced as a result of these humoral cardiodepressant factors ("myocardial depressant factor") and the development of ventricular arrhythmias.

Deteriorating cardiovascular parameters and visceral tissue damage are further exacerbated by the phenomenon of ischemic reperfusion injury (IRI) (Buber *et al.* 2007). In addition, loss of mucosal integrity of the GI tract results in endotoxemia (Davidson *et al.* 1992). IRI and endotoxemia lead to SIRS and the serious consequences of hypotension, acute renal failure, DIC, and cardiac arrhythmias. The systemic distribution of ischemia-induced humoral factors is likely to be increased upon gastric decompression and during fluid resuscitation; therefore, initiation of aggressive fluid therapy before gastric decompression is advocated (Orton and Muir 1983).

Research has been conducted into the use of lidocaine administration to ameliorate the effects of IRI. In experimental studies, dogs treated with IV lidocaine before the ischemic event had reduced gastric histologic damage and cardiac arrhythmias (Pfeiffer *et al.* 1989). Although this appears promising, clinical use may be limited because early intervention is required. In a clinical study, no significant difference in outcome was seen between those dogs that received lidocaine and those that did not (Buber *et al.* 2007); however, further investigations are warranted. There is no clinical evidence to support the use of corticosteroids or flunixin meglumine (Davidson *et al.* 1992).

Intensive patient monitoring is essential perioperatively to assess perfusion status on the basis of physical examination, blood pressure measurement, urine output, and serum biochemistry analysis, with regular adjustments made to ongoing fluid therapy as appropriate. The range of systemic complications that may manifest in GDV syndrome may be ameliorated by prompt intervention and aggressive fluid resuscitation to optimize tissue perfusion.

Abdominal complications

Gastric necrosis initially affects the greater curvature of the gastric fundus and subsequently involves the gastric cardia (Ellison 1993). This distribution likely reflects the effects of regional reduction in gastric perfusion exacerbated by avulsion of the perfusing vessels; however, regional mucosal differences may also predispose certain areas to ulceration (Pfeiffer *et al.* 1989). The gastric body and the pyloric antrum are generally spared; however, regardless of this, a viable stomach cannot be salvaged if extensive necrosis has occurred involving the cardia.

Resection of devitalized tissue is the preferred technique for management of gastric necrosis; however, gastric invagination has been described, in particular for small areas of necrosis (Ellison 2011). Although this technique avoids entering the gastric lumen and has the benefit of reduced surgical time, its use may increase the rate of complications. The release of inflammatory mediators is likely to be greater with retention of tissue undergoing necrosis. Severe gastric ulceration and abdominal hemorrhage have been reported in one dog at the site of previous gastric invagination (Parton *et al.* 2006).

Dogs with gastric necrosis have been reported to have a higher mortality rate (Brourman *et al.* 1996; de Papp *et al.* 1999; Glickman *et al.* 2000; Green *et al.* 2011). However, one more recent study (Beck *et al.* 2006) suggests that although a high postoperative morbidity rate continues to occur, the presence of gastric necrosis may not be an indicator for a higher mortality rate. When facilities and expertise allow optimum management of gastric necrosis and the potential associated complications of peritonitis, DIC, sepsis, and arrhythmias, mortality rates were not increased for patients undergoing partial gastric resection (Beck *et al.* 2006). A previous review of the literature suggested that the use of surgical stapling equipment for partial gastrectomy has reduced mortality rates from 60% to around 10% (Monnet 2003); however other factors are likely to be involved. An increased mortality rate is reported in dogs with necrosis of the cardia (Beck *et al.* 2006); this is likely to reflect the technical difficulty of operating at this site and an increased incidence of intraoperative euthanasia caused by the perceived grave prognosis after resection of the cardia. Lack of detection of gastric necrosis and subsequent gastric perforation lead to septic peritonitis, which carries a guarded prognosis (Beck *et al.* 2006).

Postoperative administration of prokinetic therapy has been advocated after GDV (Hall 1989), and clinical benefits have been reported with administration of metoclopramide (Ellison 1993). However, a clinical study using a metoclopramide CRI failed to demonstrate any difference in outcome (Hall 1996). An experimental study comparing gastroprokinetic agents in dogs demonstrated that metoclopramide and cisapride had prokinetic effects; however, cisapride was more effective (Orihata and Sarna 1994). Cisapride is not widely available after its withdrawal because of the complication of fatal cardiac arrhythmias in humans (Wysowski and Bacsanji 1996); however, mosapride, a newer agent, is an effective gastroprokinetic agent in dogs with no effect on cardiac function (Tsukamoto *et al.* 2011). Although use of this agent may be of benefit for management of gastroparesis in the future, in particular because mosapride selectively enhances the motor activity of the upper GI tract (Mine *et al.* 1997), it is not yet widely approved for use in veterinary species. Historically, pyloric dysfunction was suggested to be responsible for GDV and postoperative gastric atony; however, this has been disregarded, and pyloroplasty is absolutely not indicated for management of GDV (Greenfield *et al.* 1989; van Sluijs and van den Brom 1989).

References

Adamik, N. K., Burgener, I. A., Kovacevic, A. (2009) Myoglobin as a prognostic indicator for outcome in dogs with gastric dilatation and volvulus. *Journal of Veterinary Emergency and Critical Care* 19, 247-53.

Baltzer, W.I., McMichael, M.A., Ruaux, C.G., et al. (2006) Measurement of urinary 11-dehydrothromboxane B_2 excretion in dogs with gastric dilatation-volvulus. *American Journal of Veterinary Research* 67, 78-83.

Beck, J.J., Staatz, A., Pelsue, D., et al. (2006) Risk factors associated with short-term outcome and development of perioperative complications in dogs undergoing surgery because of gastric dilatation-volvulus: 166 cases (1992-2003). *Journal of the American Veterinary Medical Association* 229, 1934-1939.

Belandria, G.A., Pavletic, M.M., Boulay, J.P., et al. (2009) Gastropexy with an automatic stapling instrument for the treatment of gastric dilatation and volvulus in 20 dogs. *Canadian Veterinary Journal* 50, 733-740.

Brockman, D.J., Washabau, R.J., Drobatz, K.J. (1995) Canine gastric dilatation/volvulus syndrome in a veterinary critical care unit: 295 cases (1986 -1992). *Journal of the American Veterinary Medical Association* 207, 460-464.

Brourman, J.D., Schertel, E.R., Allen, D.A., et al. (1996) Factors associated with perioperative mortality in dogs with surgically managed gastric dilatation-volvulus: 137 cases (1988-1993). *Journal of the American Veterinary Medical Association* 208, 1855-1858.

Buber, T., Saragusty, J., Ranen, E., et al. (2007) Evaluation of lidocaine treatment and risk factors for death associated with gastric dilatation and volvulus in dogs: 112 cases (1997-2005). *Journal of the American Veterinary Medical Association* 230, 1334-1339.

Collard, C.D., Gelman, S. (2001) Pathophysiology, clinical manifestations and prevention of ischemia-reperfusion injury. *Anaesthesiology* 94, 1133–1138.

Davidson, J.R., Lantz, G.C., Salisbury, S.K. (1992) Effects of flunixin meglumine on dogs with experimental gastric dilatation-volvulus. *Veterinary Surgery* 21, 113-20.

de Papp, E., Drobatz, K.J., Hughes, D. (1999) Plasma lactate concentration as a predictor of gastric necrosis and survival among dogs with gastric dilatation-volvulus: 102 cases (1995 -1998). *Journal of the American Veterinary Medical Association* 215, 49-52.

Eggertsdóttir, A.V., Stigen, Ø., Lønaas, L., et al. (2001) Comparison of the recurrence rate of gastric dilatation with or without volvulus in dogs after circumcostal gastropexy versus gastrocolopexy. *Veterinary Surgery* 30, 546-551.

Ellison, G.W. (1993) Gastric dilatation volvulus, Surgical prevention. *Veterinary Clinics of North America: Small Animal Practice* 23, 513-531.

Ellison, G.W. (2011) Complications of gastrointestinal surgery in companion animals. *Veterinary Clinics of North America: Small Animal Practice* 41, 915-934.

Glickman, L.T., Glickman, N.W., Pérez, C.M., et al. (1994) Analysis of risk factors for gastric dilatation-volvulus in dogs. *Journal of the American Veterinary Medical Association* 204, 1465-1471.

Glickman, L.T., Lantz, G.C., Shcellenberg, D.B., et al. (1998) A prospective study of survival and recurrence following the acute gastric dilatation-volvulus syndrome in 136 dogs. *Journal of the American Animal Hospital Association* 34, 253-259.

Glickman, L.T., Glickman, N.W., Schellenberg, D. B. (2000) Incidence of and breed-related risk factors for gastric dilatation-volvulus in dogs. *Journal of the American Veterinary Medical Association* 216, 40-45.

Green, T.I., Tonozzi, C.C., Kirby, R., et al. (2011) Evaluation of initial plasma lactate values as a predictor of gastric necrosis and initial and subsequent plasma lactate values as a predictor of survival in dogs with gastric dilatation-volvulus: 84 dogs (2003-2007). *Journal of Veterinary Emergency and Critical Care,* 21, 36-44.

Greenfield, C.L., Walshaw, R., Thomas, M.W. (1989) Significance of the Heineke-Mikulicz pyloroplasty in the treatment of gastric dilatation-volvulus. A prospective clinical study. *Veterinary Surgery* 18, 22-26.

Hall, J.A. (1989) Canine gastric dilatation-volvulus update. *Seminars in Veterinary Medicine & Surgery* 4, 188-193.

Hall, J.A., Solie, T.N., Seim III H.B. et al. (1996) Effect of metoclopramide on fed-state gastric myoelectric and motor activity in dogs. *American Journal of Veterinary Research* 57(11), 1616-1622.

Hammel, S.P., Novo, R.E. (2006) Recurrence of gastric dilatation-volvulus after incisional gastropexy in a Rottweiler. *Journal of the American Animal Hospital Association* 42, 147-150.

Hewitt, S.A., Brisson, B.A., Holmberg, D.A.(2005) Bile peritonitis associated with gastric dilatation-volvulus in a dog. *Canadian Veterinary Journal* 46, 260-262.

Hosgood, G. (1994) Clinical update: gastric dilatation-volvulus in dogs. *Journal of the American Veterinary Medical Association* 204, 1742-1747.

Mackenzie, G., Barnhart, M., Kennedy, S., et al. (2010) A retrospective study of factors influencing survival following surgery for gastric dilatation-volvulus syndrome in 306 dogs. *Journal of the American Animal Hospital Association* 46, 97-102.

Mayhew, P.D., Brown, D.C. (2009) Prospective evaluation of two intracorporeally sutured prophylactic gastropexy techniques compared with laparoscopic assisted gastropexy in dogs. *Veterinary Surgery* 38, 738-746.

Meyer-Lindenberg, A., Harder A., Fehr, M., et al. (1993) Treatment of gastric dilatation-volvulus and a rapid method for prevention of relapse in dogs: 134 cases (1988–1991). *Journal of the American Veterinary Medical Association* 203, 1303-1307.

Millis, D.L., Hauptman, J.G., Fulton, R.B. Jr. (1993) Abnormal hemostatic profiles and gastric necrosis in canine dilatation-volvulus. *Veterinary Surgery* 22, 93-97.

Mine, Y., Yoshikawa, T, Oku, S., et al. (1997) Comparison of effect of mosapride citrate and existing 5-HT₄ receptor agonists on gastrointestinal motility *in vivo* and *in vitro. Journal of Pharmacology and Experimental Therapeutics* 283, 1000-1008.

Monnet, E. (2003) Gastric-dilatation volvulus syndrome in dogs. *Veterinary Clinics of North America: Small Animal Practice* 33, 987-1005.

Orihata, M., Sarna, S.K.(1994) Contractile mechanisms of action of gastroprokinetic agents: cisapride, metoclopramide, and domperidone. *American Journal of Physiology* 266, G665-G676.

Orton, E.C., Muir, W.W. 3rd (1983) Haemodynamics during experimental gastric dilatation-volvulus in dogs. *American Journal of Veterinary Research* 44, 1512.

Paris, J.K., Yool, D.A., Reed, N., et al. (2011) Chronic gastric instability and presumed incomplete volvulus in dogs. *Journal of Small Animal Practice* 52, 651-655.

Parton, A.T., Volk, S.W., Weisse, C. (2006) Gastric ulceration subsequent to partial invagination of the stomach in a dog with gastric dilatation-volvulus. *Journal of the American Veterinary Medical Association* 228, 1895–1900.

Pfeiffer, C.J., Keith, J.C., Cho, C.H., et al. (1989) Gastric and cardiac organoprotection by lidocaine. *Acta Physiologica Hungarica* 73, 129-136.

Rawlings, C.A., Mahaffey, M.B., Bement, S., et al. (2002) Prospective evaluation of laparoscopic assisted gastropexy in dogs susceptible to gastric dilatation. *Journal of the American Veterinary Medical Association* 221, 1576-1581.

Stampley, A.R., Burrows C.F., Ellison G.W., et al. (1992) Gastric myoelectric activity after experimental gastric dilatation and volvulus and tube gastrostomy in dogs. *Veterinary Surgery* 21, 10-14.

Tsukamoto, A, Ohno, K., Maeda, S., et al. (2012) Prokinetic effect of the 5-HT (4) R agonist mosapride on canine gastric motility. *Journal of Veterinary Medical Science* 73, 1635-1637.

van Sluijs, F.J., van den Brom, W.E. (1989) Gastric emptying of a radionuclide-labelled test meal after surgical correction of gastric dilatation-volvulus in dogs. *American Journal of Veterinary Research* 50, 433-435.

Ward, M.P., Patronek, G.J., Glickman, L.T. (2003) Benefits of prophylactic gastropexy for dogs at risk of gastric dilatation-volvulus. *Preventive Veterinary Medicine* 60, 319-329.

Wingfield, W.E., Twedt, D.C., Moore, R.W., et al. (1982) Acid-base and electrolyte values in dogs with acute gastric dilatation-volvulus. *Journal of the American Veterinary Medical Association* 180, 1070-1072.

Woosley, K.P. (2004) The problem of gastric atony. *Clinical Techniques in Small Animal Practice* 19, 43-48.

Wysowksi, D.K., Bacsanji, J. (1996) Cisapride and fatal arrhythmia. *New England Journal of Medicine* 335, 290-291.

Zacher, L.A., Berg, J, Shaw, S.P., et al. (2010) Association between outcome and changes in plasma lactate concentration during presurgical treatment in dogs with gastric dilatation-volvulus. 64 cases (2002-2008). *Journal of the American Veterinary Medical Association* 236, 892-897.

58 Gastric Outflow Procedures

Jeffrey J. Runge

Department of Clinical Studies, School of Veterinary Medicine, University of Pennsylvania, Philadelphia, PA, USA

Gastric outflow procedures are commonly performed on the pyloric region of the stomach. The term *pylorus* dates from before the fifth century and is derived from Greek, meaning "keeper of the gate," an indication that early physicians had some understanding of the physiological function of gastric emptying (Wyse *et al.* 2003). The pylorus is a thickened continuation of the circular smooth muscle layer of the stomach. This muscle layer with its abundant encircling muscle fibers combines with its accompanying mucosal lining to form a true anatomic sphincter (Guilford and Strombeck 1996). The pylorus acts as a "gatekeeper" to keep ingesta within the stomach so that the antrum can grind food into small particles that are titrated through the pylorus into the duodenum (Simpson 2005). Aside from functioning as the "gatekeeper," the pylorus is also responsible for limiting the amount of duodenal-gastric reflux (Happé *et al.* 1982; Sonnenberg *et al.* 1982; Simpson 2005).

The mechanisms of gastric retention and outflow obstruction are varied; the diagnostic evaluation must be thorough and the medical or surgical treatment options chosen appropriately to increase the likelihood of clinical resolution (Ramussen 2003). Gastric outflow obstruction may be caused by pyloric abnormalities, disorders of gastric motility, or extrinsic lesions compressing the outflow tract (e.g., pancreatic, duodenal, or hepatic neoplasia) (Hedlund and Fossum 2007) (Figure 58.1).

Various disease conditions can produce partial or complete obstruction of the gastric outflow tract. Foreign bodies are one of the most common causes of gastric outlet obstruction in dogs and cats. Congenital pyloric stenosis is a condition seen in young animals of the brachycephalic breeds as well as in Siamese cats. The stenosis refers to hypertrophy of the pyloric circular smooth muscle layer. Chronic hypertrophic pyloric gastropathy (CHPH) is the acquired form of pyloric stenosis occurring primarily in middle-aged small breed dogs. Three pathologic categories for CHPH exist: type I cases have circular muscle hypertrophy, type II cases have a combination of muscle hypertrophy and mucosal hyperplasia, and type III cases have only mucosal hypertrophy (Stanton 1993). Hyperplastic pyloric polyps have been reported in French bulldogs with a history of chronic vomiting since weaning (Hedlund and Fossum 2007). Inflammatory diseases caused by eosinophilic gastritis, fungal gastritis, and chronic gastric ulcer disease can produce partial or complete obstruction (Bright 2010). Chronic gastritis from local irritants, infection and infestation, immune reaction, excess histamine, hypergastrinemia (de Brito Galvao *et al.* 2009), or peptide hormone secretion can result in generalized or focal mucosal hypertrophy secondary to the chronic inflammatory stimulus (Ramussen

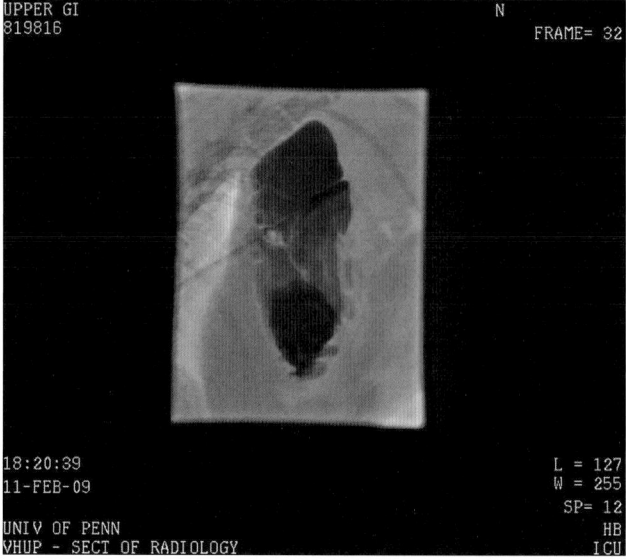

Figure 58.1 Gastrogram under fluoroscopy. This 8-year-old mixed breed dog presented for a 2-month history of vomiting. The patient was administered 20 mL of 50% w/v barium suspension via nasogastric tube. Slow gastric contractions were observed between time 0 and time 1 hour. At 1 hour, the stomach is filled with barium, and there was no barium past the pylorus.

2003). Any neoplasia such as adenocarcinoma (the most common malignant tumor in dogs) or lymphosarcoma (most common in cats) can cause partial or complete obstruction (Swann 2002).

In the approximate order of increasing the gastric outflow tract diameter, surgical options for the treatment of these diseases include the Fredet-Ramstedt pyloromyotomy, Heineke-Mikulicz pyloroplasty, Y-U antral advancement flap pyloroplasty, and gastroduodenostomy (Billroth I) (Pavletic and Berg 1996). Tumors within the pyloric region are treated by gastroduodenostomy or gastrojejunostomy with or without gastric resection (Pavletic and Berg 1996).

Persistence of signs

Definition

The persistence or return of clinical sings indicates failure of the corrective gastric outflow procedure. This is most commonly caused by inadequate selection of the corrective outflow procedure that does

Complications in Small Animal Surgery, First Edition. Edited by Dominique Griffon and Annick Hamaide.
© 2016 John Wiley & Sons, Inc. Published 2016 by John Wiley & Sons, Inc.
Companion website: www.wiley.com/go/griffon/complications

not adequately increase the diameter of the outflow tract (Pavletic and Berg 1996). Poor or inadequate margins after attempts to resect or alleviate obstructive neoplasia can also cause persistence or reoccurrence of signs.

Risk factors
- Inadequate selection of corrective outflow procedure
- Inadequate surgical margins after resection of neoplasia
- Possible suture induced granuloma (Bright 1994)
- Poor surgical technique

Diagnosis
After a corrective gastric outflow procedure has been performed, the return of clinical signs may indicate a failure associated with the surgery. The persistence or return of chronic intermittent vomiting anytime during the postoperative procedure should raise suspicion for a complication. Reflux-associated esophagitis may also be present from chronic vomiting or gastric distension; thus, the history may include regurgitation (Ramussen 2003). For certain procedures, the diagnosis should not be made until several days after surgery because of postoperative intestinal ileus or pancreatitis.

Possible diagnostic tests include:
- Plain film abdominal radiographs (revealing a fluid-filled stomach) (Figure 58.2)
- Upper gastrointestinal (GI) positive contrast study (revealing delayed gastric emptying, filling defects, or a mass effect)
- Abdominal ultrasonography (to assess gastric wall thickness) (Figure 58.3)
- Fluoroscopy
- Gastroscopy (presence of ingesta after a prescribed fast)

Treatment
Pharmacologic therapy with motility enhancers, acid reducers, and mucosal protectants should be combined with dietary modification either concurrently or before a revision surgery. After a Y-U antral flap pyloroplasty, persistent vomiting and the presence of bile in the emesis may suggest the possibility of reflux alkaline

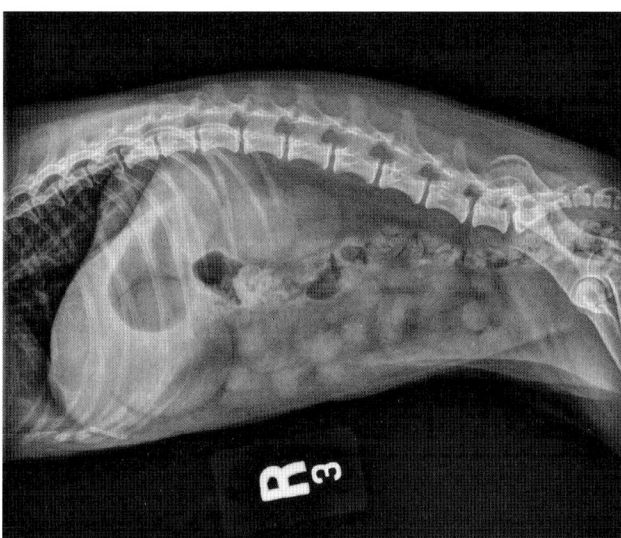

Figure 58.2 Lateral abdominal radiographs. There is large gas and fluid distension of the stomach; the body and antrum appear markedly rounded on the right lateral view.

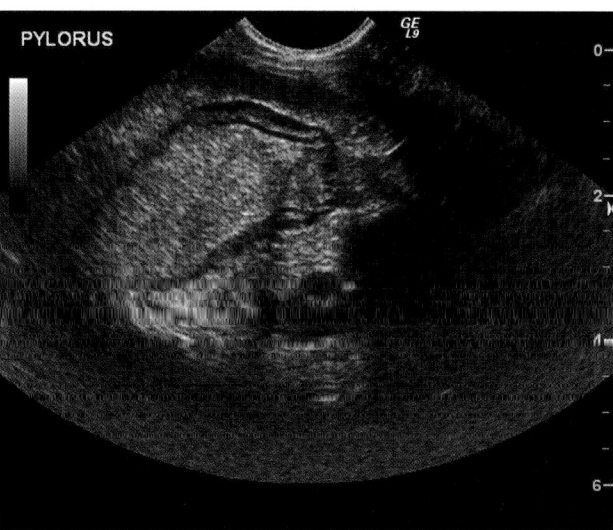

Figure 58.3 Abdominal ultrasonography. Gastric ileus and corrugated proximal duodenum gastroduodenitis with secondary local reactive peritoneal fat.

gastritis secondary to duodenogastric reflux; this condition usually responds to a 2- to 3-week course of metoclopramide, antacids, and sucralfate (Dulish 1993).

Treatment occasionally consists of revising the previous corrective outflow procedure with a more aggressive procedure that will increase the diameter of the gastric outflow tract. Surgical revision options may include Fredet-Ramstedt pyloromyotomy, Heineke-Mikulicz pyloroplasty, Y-U antral advancement flap pyloroplasty, and gastroduodenostomy (Billroth I).

Outcome
The persistence of gastric outflow obstructions occurs more commonly after Fredet-Ramstedt pyloromyotomy or Heineke-Mikulicz pyloroplasty (Pavletic and Berg 1996). Even though Fredet-Ramstedt pyloromyotomy is the simplest and easiest of these procedures, it does not allow inspection or biopsy of the pyloric mucosa and possibly provides only temporary benefit because healing may reduce the diameter of the lumen (Hedlund and Fossum 2007).

Prevention
- An accurate initial diagnosis to determine the location, size, and extent of the lesion is critical for initial preoperative planning.
- Choosing the most appropriate initial corrective procedure to give the maximal outflow tract diameter without unnecessary trauma

Dehiscence
See Chapter 9.

Traumatic pancreatitis

Definition
Traumatic pancreatitis is a syndrome caused by excessive handling and surgical manipulation of the pancreas. Trauma to the pancreas can occur during gastric outflow tract procedures and may result in pancreatitis postoperatively (Cornell and Fischer 2003). Because the right lobe of the pancreas is contained within the mesoduodenum

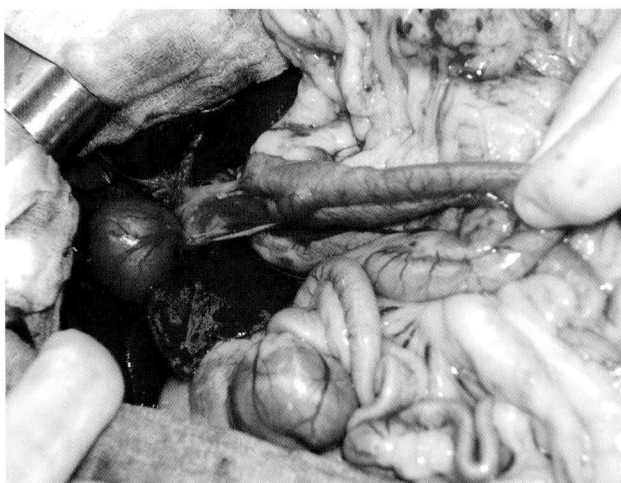

Figure 58.4 Abdominal laparotomy. The surgeon avoids excessive handling of the pancreas intraoperatively to avoid postoperative traumatic pancreatitis.

and is closely associated with the proximal duodenum near the pylorus, there is a risk of inadvertent trauma that typically manifests itself postoperatively. Pancreatitis is usually the end product of activation of zymogens within the pancreatic glandular tissue and subsequent pancreatic autodigestion (Williams and Steiner 2005).

Risk factors
- Excessive manipulation and handling of the pancreas intraoperatively (Figure 58.4)
- Most likely to occur after a gastroduodenostomy

Diagnosis
Suspicion of postoperative traumatic pancreatitis is based on the history and clinical signs. Clinical signs can include lethargy, anorexia, vomiting, abdominal pain, and occasionally diarrhea. No single laboratory test available in veterinary medicine is definitively diagnostic for pancreatitis, but many clinicopathologic findings support or suggest the disease (Cornell and Fischer 2003).

Possible diagnostic tests include:
- Serum amylase and lipase
- Serum trypsin-like immunoreactivity
- Pancreatic lipase immunoreactivity
- Abdominal ultrasonography (highly specific) (Williams and Steiner 2005)
- Computed tomography (the most useful modality in humans) (Williams and Steiner 2005)

Treatment
The classic therapy for acute pancreatitis is maintenance of fluid and electrolyte balance while the pancreas is "rested" and simultaneously withholding food. However, evidence has suggested that parenteral and enteral nutrition have a role in the treatment of pancreatitis.

Management of abdominal pain and prevention of continued vomiting are paramount.

Outcome
Although the outcome of patients with traumatic postoperative pancreatitis has not been specifically addressed within the veterinary literature, generally the outcome is considered good because it is a transient process. However, because of the unpredictable nature of pancreatitis, outcomes are likely variable.

Prevention
- Meticulous and controlled surgical dissection surrounding the pancreas
- Reduce excessive handling and manipulation of the pancreas
- Choice of the most appropriate and least traumatic gastric outflow tract procedure

Biliary obstruction

Definition
Extrahepatic biliary obstruction (EHBO) occurs when the common bile duct stops the normal flow of bile from the liver and gallbladder to the intestine. This complication is most commonly associated with the gastroduodenostomy (Billroth I) gastric outflow tract corrective procedure when the common bile duct is inadvertently ligated. Other causes can include edema from intraoperative handling of the pancreas.

Risk factors
- Inadvertent ligation of the common bile duct during dissection
- Transection of the duodenum aboral to the major duodenal papilla
- Excessive postoperative fibrosis and scar tissue formation near the papilla
- Inadvertent traumatic manipulation of the pancreas

Diagnosis
- Clinical signs may include lethargy, depression, icterus, vomiting, abdominal pain, pyrexia, and dehydration (Martin *et al.* 2003).
- Complete blood count (CBC), serum biochemistry profile, and urinalysis are indicated if dysfunction is suspected (Webster 2005). Blood work abnormalities include increased alanine aminotransferase (ALT), increased alkaline phosphatase (ALP), and increased total bilirubin (hyperbilirubinemia is evident within several hours, and jaundice may be detectable as early as 48 hours) (Tams 1993).
- Diagnostic ultrasonography (the single most useful noninvasive tool)
- Cholangiography (Murphy *et al.* 2007)
- Abdominal exploratory laparotomy

Treatment
Numerous life-threatening metabolic and physiologic derangements induced by EHBO in small animals cause significant morbidity and mortality (Murphy *et al.* 2007). Surgical treatment of the obstruction requires expert judgment in selecting techniques that are the most necessary and beneficial to patients without unnecessarily risking morbidity and mortality (Martin *et al.* 2003). Surgical treatment, by either removal or bypass of the obstruction, is usually indicated for resolution of EHBO. Early cholecystoenterostomy is recommended to establish bile duct patency (by rerouting bile from the gallbladder to the intestine) and to provide relief from the clinical signs. Cholecystoduodenostomy should be performed when biliary obstruction appears to be caused by regional edema or fibrosis or when the common bile duct inadvertently has been sutured (Pavletic and Berg 1996).

Outcome
Diagnosing EHBO before severe metabolic derangements occur is critical in ensuring optimal outcomes with biliary rerouting

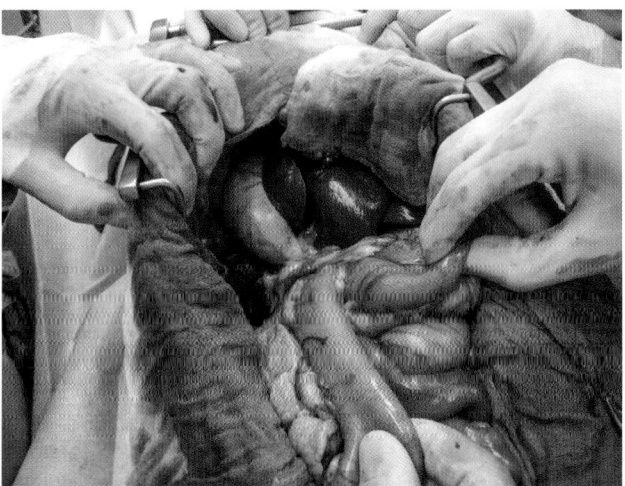

Figure 58.5 Abdominal laparotomy. The surgeon prepares full circumferential exposure of the antral and pyloric region of the stomach and proximal duodenum. By completing this meticulous dissection, the surgeon reduces the chances of inadvertent trauma or ligation of the bile duct.

procedures. Cholecystoduodenostomy, cholecystojejunostomy, and cholecystojejunoduodenostomy are the cholecystenteric surgical procedures used for biliary bypass in small animals (Morrison *et al.* 2008). Survival rates associated with surgery for EHBO range from 41% to 72% (Morrison *et al.* 2008).

Prevention
- Full circumferential exposure of the antral and pyloric regions of the stomach and the proximal duodenum are critical to avoiding inadvertent trauma or ligation of the bile duct (Figure 58.5).
- The bile duct is identified by gently expressing the gallbladder to allow the flow of dark bile to highlight the margins of the duct entering into the duodenum.
- Duodenotomy can be performed and a catheter passed through the papilla to locate the common bile duct.
- A minimum of 1 cm of duodenum is maintained orad to the bile duct aperture.
- If the proximal duodenum and the common bile duct is compromised before surgery, a gastrojejunostomy (Billroth II) with a cholecystoduodenostomy and enzyme replacement are required.

Duodenal reflux

Definition
Duodenogastric reflux gastritis (alkaline reflux gastritis) results from mucosal injury by duodenal contents. This condition is more commonly seen in humans than in small animal patients based on a review of the literature. This type of reflux gastritis usually occurs after surgery that disrupts the protective sphincter function of the pylorus, most commonly after distal gastrectomy (Nath 1984). Duodenogastric reflux has been implicated in the pathogenesis of gastric ulcer and gastritis.

Risk factors
Surgeon should choose a gastric outflow tract procedure that produces a GI opening as close as possible to the size and location of the normal pylorus to minimize the incidence and severity of side effects.

Diagnosis
- Clinical signs include chronic, continuous epigastric pain exacerbated by eating, bilious vomiting, weight loss, iron-deficiency anemia, gastritis, and intragastric bile (Nath 1984).
- Ultrasonography (Agut *et al.* 1996)

Treatment
The primary treatment option is to implement pharmacologic management (Nath 1984):
- Antacids
- H$_2$ antagonists
- Bile salt absorbents
- Metoclopramide
- Synthetic prostaglandins
- Sucralfate

Outcome
Reflux alkaline gastritis secondary to duodenogastric reflux usually responds to a 2- to 3-week course of medical therapy (Ramussen 2003).

Prevention
This complication does not appear to occur commonly in dogs (Pavletic and Berg 1996).

Relevant literature
Different surgical techniques to correct gastric outlet obstructions have been described, and generally the objectives of pyloric surgery are to remove the obstruction and normalize gastric outflow (Sanchez-Margallo *et al.* 2005). **Persistence of signs** after a gastric outflow obstruction is likely to require reoperation. Improperly performed pyloromyotomy and pyloroplasty may lead to a subsequent gastric outflow obstruction (Fossum and Hedlund 2003). Of the commonly used surgical procedures, a Fredet-Ramstedt pyloromyotomy is the simplest and easiest of these procedures. It does not allow inspection or biopsy of the pyloric mucosa and probably only provides temporary benefit because healing may lessen the lumen size.

Because emesis can be a problem after pyloric surgery, it may be advisable to increase the pH of gastric contents perioperatively with H$_2$ receptor antagonists (e.g., cimetidine) to decrease the possibility of esophageal mucosal damage from acidic gastric contents. Use of a motility modifier and antiemetic, such as metoclopramide, may also be beneficial postoperatively (Stanton *et al.* 1987). A recent report compared the effect of laparoscopic and conventional pyloric surgery, in a Ramstedt pyloromyotomy versus a Heineke-Mikulicz pyloroplasty, on complete gastric emptying. This study concluded that pyloromyotomy was a less effective procedure in decreasing complete gastric emptying time than Heineke-Mikulicz pyloroplasty in normal dogs (Sanchez-Margallo *et al.* 2005).

In another report, the recurrence of clinical signs 3 days to 10 months after a Billroth I or a gastrojejunostomy procedure for the removal of neoplasia caused all owners in this retrospective study to elect euthanasia (Nath 1984). Another report evaluating the outcome of pylorectomy and gastroduodenostomy for malignant neoplasia had a good short-term outcome with 75% (18 of 24) of dogs surviving 414 days. It was determined that this procedure is indicated to obtain a histopathologic diagnosis and to increase gastric outflow in dogs with neoplastic or non-neoplastic disease. Long-term survival time is shown to be poor in dogs with malignant neoplasia (Eisele *et al.* 2010). Results of a study evaluating the postoperative changes of the pylorus after gastric outflow surgery suggests that ultrasonography is useful for detecting relevant morphologic changes and postoperative abnormalities in the pyloric sphincter after pyloroplasty (Sanchez-Margallo *et al.* 2003).

After pylorectomy and gastroduodenostomy in dogs, a study reported ultrasonographic evidence of **pancreatitis** in 3 of 24 dogs (12.5%) during the postoperative period (Eisele *et al.* 2010). If damage to the common bile duct occurs, performing a cholecystoduodenostomy or cholecystojejunostomy to alleviate the **biliary obstruction** is necessary. If the pancreatic ducts are inadvertently ligated, supplementation with pancreatic enzymes may be necessary after surgery (Fossum and Hedlund 2003).

Another study reported that although the Y-U pyloroplasty enhanced gastric emptying of solid food in normal dogs, a transient and subclinical increase in **duodenogastric reflux** in the immediate postoperative period was present (Stanton *et al.* 1987). Another study evaluated five different pyloroplasties and gastroenterostomies on complete gastric emptying time of standard commercial canned dog food in normal dogs, as well as other short-term clinical effects. Although none of the procedures significantly altered gastric emptying time, the overall tendency was toward slowing down gastric emptying time. The severity of GI side effects and enterogastric reflux appeared to be related to the size and location of the GI opening (Papageorges and Breton 1987).

References

Agut, A., Wood, A.K., Martin, I.C. (1996) Sonographic observations of the gastroduodenal junction of dogs. *American Journal of Veterinary Research* 57 (9), 1266-1273.

Bright, R.M. (1994) Pyloric obstruction in a dog related to a gastrotomy incision closed with polypropylene. *Journal of Small Animal Practice* 35, 629-632.

Bright, R.M. (2010) Gastric outflow obstruction. In Bojrab, M.J. (ed.) *Mechanisms of Disease in Small Animal Surgery*, 3rd ed. Teton New Media, Jackson WY, pp .158-161.

de Brito Galvao, J.F., Pressler, B.M., Freeman, L.J., et al. (2009) Mucinous gastric carcinoma with abdominal carcinomatosis and hypergastrinemia in a dog. *Journal of the American Animal Hospital Association* 45 (4), 197–202.

Cornell, K., Fischer, J. (2003) Surgery of the exocrine pancreas. In Slatter, D.E. (ed.) *Textbook of Small Animal Surgery*, 3rd edn. WB Saunders, Philadelphia, pp. 752-762.

Dulish, M.L. (1983) Stomach. In Bojrab, M.J. (ed.) *Current Techniques in Small Animal Surgery*, 2nd ed. Lippincott Williams & Wilkins, Baltimore, pp. 157-158.

Eisele, J., McClaran, J.K., Runge, J.J., et al. (2010) Evaluation of risk factors for morbidity and mortality after pylorectomy and gastroduodenostomy in dogs. *Veterinary Surgery* 39 (2), 261-267.

Fossum, T.W., Hedlund, C.S. (2003) Gastric and intestinal surgery. *Veterinary Clinics of North America: Small Animal Practice* 33 (5), 1117-1145, viii.

Guilford, W.G., Strombeck, D.R. (1996) Gastric structure and function In Guilford, W.G. (ed.) *Strombeck's Small Animal Gastroenterology*, 3rd ed. WB Saunders, Philadelphia, p. 239.

Happé, R.P., van den Brom, W.E., van der Gaag, I. (1982) Duodenogastric reflux in the dog, a clinicopathological study. *Research in Veterinary Science* 33 (3), 280-286.

Hedlund, C.S., Fossum, T.W. (2007) Surgery of the stomach. In Fossum, T.W. (ed.) *Small Animal Surgery*, 3rd edn. Mosby, St. Louis, pp. 409-424.

Martin, R.A., Lanz, O.I., Tobias, K.M. (2003) Liver and biliary system. In Slatter, D.E. (ed.) *Textbook of Small Animal Surgery*, 3rd edn. WB Saunders, Philadelphia, pp. 708-726.

Morrison, S., Prostredny, J., Roa, D. (2008) Retrospective study of 28 cases of cholecystoduodenostomy performed using endoscopic gastrointestinal anastomosis stapling equipment. *Journal of the American Animal Hospital Association* 44 (1), 10.

Murphy, S.M., Rodríguez, J.D., McAnulty, J.F. (2007) Minimally invasive cholecystostomy in the dog: evaluation of placement techniques and use in extrahepatic biliary obstruction. *Veterinary Surgery* 36 (7), 675-683.

Nath, B. (1984) Alkaline reflux gastritis and esophagitis. *Annual Review of Medicine* 35, 383-396.

Papageorges, M., Breton, L. (1987) Gastric drainage procedures: effects in normal dogs i. introduction and description of surgical procedures. *Veterinary Surgery* 16 (5), 327-331.

Pavletic, M.M., Berg, J. (1996) Gastric outflow procedures. In Lipowitz, A.J., Newton, C., Caywood, D. (eds.) *Complications in Small Animal Surgery: Diagnosis, Management, Prevention*, 1st ed. Lippincott Williams & Wilkins, Baltimore, pp. 370-373.

Ramussen, L. (2003) Stomach. In Slatter, D.E. (ed.) *Textbook of Small Animal Surgery*, 3rd edn. WB Saunders, Philadelphia, pp. 592-640.

Sánchez-Margallo, F., Soria-Gálvez, F. (2003) Comparison of ultrasonographic characteristics of the gastroduodenal junction during pyloroplasty performed laparoscopically or via conventional abdominal surgery. *American Journal of Veterinary Research* 64 (9), 1099-1104.

Sanchez-Margallo, F.M., Ezquerra-Calvo, L.J., Soria-Galvez, F., et al. (2005) Comparison of the effect of laparoscopic and conventional pyloric surgery on gastric emptying in dogs. *Veterinary Radiology and Ultrasound* 46 (1), 57-62.

Simpson, K.W. (2005) Diseases of the stomach. In Ettinger, S.J., Feldman, E.C. (eds.) *Textbook of Veterinary Internal Medicine*, 6th ed. Elsevier Health Sciences, Philadelphia, pp. 1310-1331.

Sonnenberg, A., Muller-Lissner, S., Schattenmann, G., et al. (1982) Duodenogastric reflux in the dog. *American Journal of Physiology* 242 (6), 603-607.

Stanton, M.L. (1993) Gastric outlet obstruction. In Bojrab, M.J., Smeak, D.D., Bloomberg, M.S. (eds.) *Disease Mechanisms in Small Animal Surgery*, 2nd edn. Lippincott Williams & Wilkins, Philadelphia, pp. 235-236.

Stanton, M., Bright, R.M., Toal, R. (1987) Effects of the Y-U pyloroplasty on gastric emptying and duodenogastric reflux in the dog. *Veterinary Surgery* 16 (5), 392-397.

Swann, H. (2002) Canine gastric adenocarcinoma and leiomyosarcoma: a retrospective study of 21 cases (1986-1999) and literature review. *Journal of the American Animal Hospital Association* 83, 157-164.

Tams, T.R. (1993) Liver disease: surgical considerations. In Bojrab, M.J., Smeak, D.D., Bloomberg, M.S. (eds.) *Disease Mechanisms in Small Animal Surgery*, 2nd edn. Lippincott Williams & Wilkins, Philadelphia, pp. 292-297.

Webster, C.R.L. (2005) History, clinical signs, and physical exam findings in hepatobiliary disease. In Ettinger, S.J., Feldman, E.C. (eds.) *Textbook of Veterinary Internal Medicine*, 6th ed. Elsevier Health Sciences, Philadelphia, pp. 1482-1889.

Williams, D.A., and Steiner, J.M. (2005) Canine exocrine pancreatic disease. In Ettinger, S.J., Feldman, E.C. (eds.) *Textbook of Veterinary Internal Medicine*, 6th ed. Elsevier Health Sciences, Philadelphia, pp. 1482-1889.

Wyse, C.A., McLellan, J., Dickie, A.M., et al. (2003) A review of methods for assessment of the rate of gastric emptying in the dog and cat: 1898-2002. *Journal of Veterinary Internal Medicine* 17 (5), 609-621.

59 Small Intestine Surgery

Jean-Philippe Billet
Centre Hospitalier Veterinaire Atlantia, Nantes, France

Small intestinal surgery is a common procedure for both nonspecialist and specialist veterinarians. The most common procedures of the small intestinal tract in dogs and cats include enterotomy and resection and anastomosis. Surgical goals include diagnosis (e.g., intestinal biopsy), treatment (e.g., foreign body removal, tumor resection), and supportive or preventive management (e.g., jejunostomy tube placement, enteroplication). Potential complications abound, including shock, leakage, ileus, dehiscence, perforation, peritonitis, adhesions, stenosis, obstruction, short bowel syndrome, recurrence, intussusception, and death.

Dehiscence (see Chapter 9)

Peritonitis (see Chapter 4)

Abdominal adhesions (see Chapter 49)

Postoperative intussusception

Definition

Small intestinal intussusception is defined as the invagination of one segment of intestine (intussusceptum) into the lumen of an adjacent segment of intestine (intussuscipiens) (Figure 59.1). Intussusceptions usually occur in the direction of normal peristalsis, from oral to aboral. The intussusceptum invaginates into the intussuscipiens, taking its associated mesentery, vessels, and nerves along with it. This results in venous compression, swelling, obstruction, and subsequent necrosis of the affected segment.

Risk factors
- Puppies and kittens
- The incidence rate of recurrence after surgical reduction or resection ranges from 6% to 27% in dogs and cats.
- Causes of primary intussusception include intestinal parasitism, linear foreign body, viral or nonspecific gastroenteritis, alimentary lymphoma, inflammatory bowel disease, recent previous abdominal or nonabdominal surgery for unrelated disease, and idiopathic.

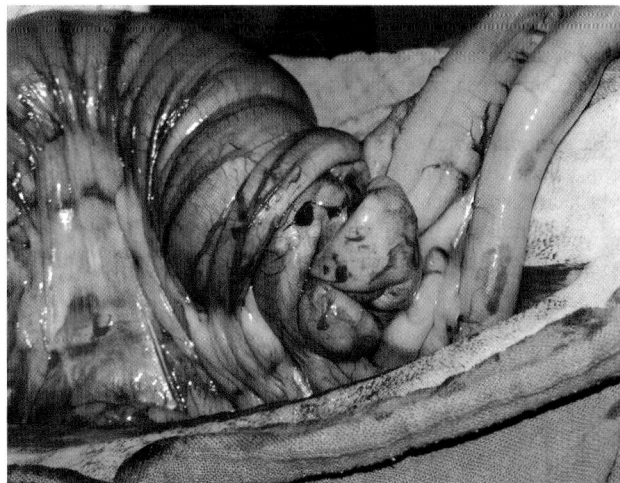

Figure 59.1 Ileocolic intussusception.

Diagnosis
- Postoperative intussusceptions usually manifest within 3 days but can been diagnosed up to 3 weeks after surgery.
- Clinical signs are consistent with a partial or complete obstruction and include intermittent vomiting, inappetence, tenesmus, weight loss, depression, soft stool with bloody mucus, diarrhea, and melena.
- On examination, a cylindrical or sausage-shaped mass can be palpated in the cranial to midabdomen; palpation often elicits pain.
- Ultrasonography is the method of choice. An intussusception appears as a series of concentric rings on the transverse image ("target" effect) (Figure 59.2) or parallel lines on a longitudinal image ("cream slice" effect), reflecting the folded layers of the intestinal wall.

Treatment
The treatment of postoperative intussusception is surgical and involves reduction, resection and anastomosis, or both. Manual reduction is attempted wherever possible; the apex of the intussusceptum is gently milked from within the intussuscipiens combined with gentle traction on the proximal oral segment. Resection and anastomosis, with or without partial reduction, is indicated for

Complications in Small Animal Surgery, First Edition. Edited by Dominique Griffon and Annick Hamaide.
© 2016 John Wiley & Sons, Inc. Published 2016 by John Wiley & Sons, Inc.
Companion website: www.wiley.com/go/griffon/complications

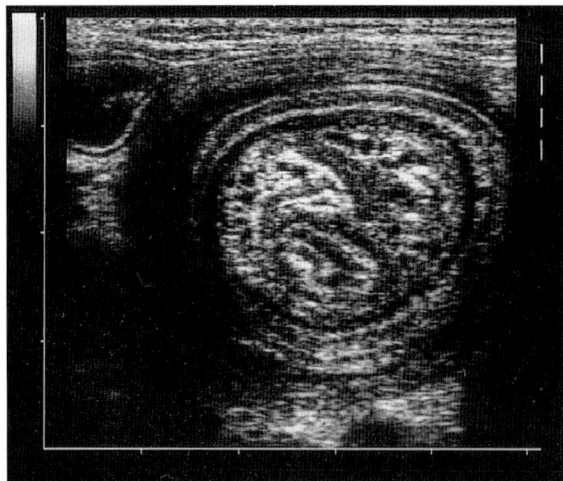

Figure 59.2 Transverse ultrasound image of an intussusception. The multiple eccentric, alternating dark and bright circular bands represent the two layers of bowel wall forming the intussuscipiens. The intussusceptum is located within the intussuscipiens. *Source:* I. Testault. Reproduced with permission from I. Testault.

irreducible intussusceptions or in the presence of nonviable bowel segments. Assessment of bowel viability can be very difficult. The usual standard clinical criteria for viability include color, peristalsis, and arterial pulse in the affected segment. If the status of the segment is in doubt, resection is indicated.

Outcome

Early diagnosis, aggressive fluid therapy, and prompt surgical correction should result in a good prognosis.

Prevention

Enteroplication, which involves the creation of adhesions between adjacent loops of bowel, is recommended for preventing recurrence of intussusception in dogs and cats (Figure 59.3).

Postoperative bowel obstruction

Definition

Postoperative bowel obstruction can be partial or complete and results from intraluminal obstruction, mural thickening, or extraluminal compression.

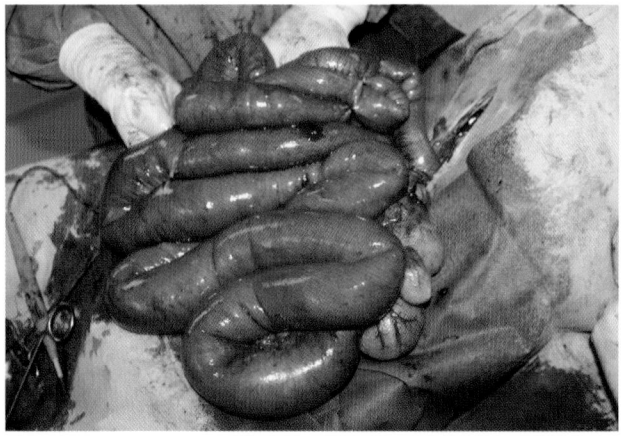

Figure 59.3 Complete enteroplication of the small intestine.

Risk factors

Postoperative bowel obstruction is extremely rare if appropriate abdominal surgical techniques are used.

Intraluminal obstruction

- Intussusception (see earlier)
- Failure to identify and remove multiple intestinal foreign bodies
- The use of staples or nonabsorbable suture material may act as a site of attachment for a foreign body or a bezoar. Such complications are extremely rare but should be considered as an unusual long-term complication of intestinal surgery.

Mural thickening

Certain suture patterns narrow the bowel, causing subsequent partial or complete obstruction.

- Two-layer anastomoses have been shown to generate greater tissue damage and edema, inflammatory response, and loss of collagen content along with delayed healing and higher rates of bowel obstruction than single-layer intestinal closure.
- Inverting suture patterns are associated with a severe inflammatory reaction and increased intraluminal protrusion of tissues, which narrows the intestinal lumen.
- Everting patterns cause less initial narrowing than inverting sutures but are associated with delayed healing, increased adhesion formation, greater anastomotic leakage, and potential stenosis of the anastomosis from extraluminal adhesions and increased fibroplasia.

Extraluminal compression

- Postoperative adhesions
- Bowel entrapment through the laparotomy incision (abdominal herniation): Risk factors include increased intraabdominal pressure because of pain, entrapped fat between the edges of the incision, inappropriate suture material, infection, long-term steroid treatment, and poor postoperative care.
- Bowel entrapment through the mesentery or the omentum (Figure 59.4): Risk factors include aggressive organ manipulation creating tears in the mesentery or the omentum and failure to suture the mesentery after intestinal anastomosis.

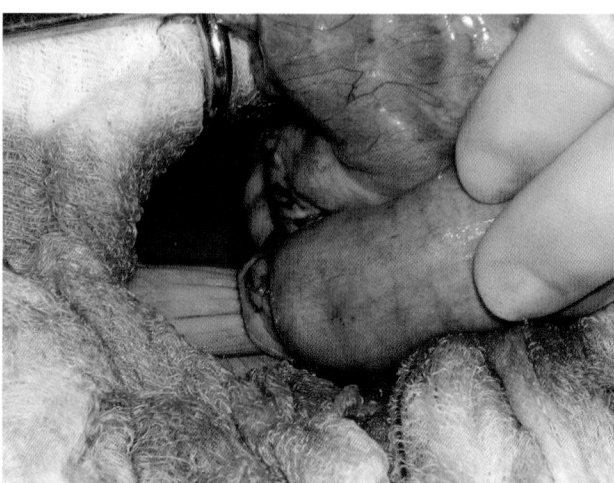

Figure 59.4 Passage of the colon through a mesenteric tear. *Source:* Jane Ladlow, University of Cambridge, Cambridge, UK, 2014. Reproduced with permission from J. Ladlow.

Diagnosis

- Postoperative bowel obstruction can occur immediately after surgery (foreign body still present in the bowel); within 3 to 5 days (abdominal herniation); or several weeks, months, or years after surgery in cases of luminal narrowing or bowel entrapment.
- **Clinical signs** are consistent with a partial or complete intestinal obstruction and commonly include inappetence, anorexia, depression, intermittent vomiting, and hematochezia. The more proximal the obstruction, the more dramatic the vomiting and associated clinical signs.
- Careful abdominal palpation may reveal a focal soft tissue mass and may elicit abdominal pain
- The clinical signs associated with abdominal herniation include swelling, serosanguineous discharge, edema, and inflammation of the abdominal incision.
- **Radiography** does not differentiate intramural, mural, or extramural obstruction and may show moderate or severe dilation of one or several loops of bowel filled with gas or a combination of gas and fluid.
- **On ultrasonography**, segmental or generalized nonuniform dilation of the bowel loops may be seen, and motility will be reduced or absent in the immediate vicinity of an obstruction. Foreign bodies are usually hyperechoic and throw marked acoustic shadows. Segmental narrowing with proximal distention may be seen with scar formation.
- **In case of abdominal herniation**, lateral abdominal radiography and ultrasonography reveal displaced bowel loops in the subcutaneous space between the abdominal wall and the cutis. Ultrasound examination reveals discontinuity of the abdominal wall (Figure 59.5).
- The most consistent ultrasonographic findings with intestinal entrapment are focal abnormalities of one intestinal loop (thickening of the bowel wall and hyperechoic mesentery suggestive of local peritonitis) and abdominal effusion (Swift 2009). These signs are not specific and are indistinguishable from intestinal perforation, infarction, and volvulus.

Treatment

- For intraluminal obstruction, enterotomy or enterectomy is performed on the basis of intestinal viability.

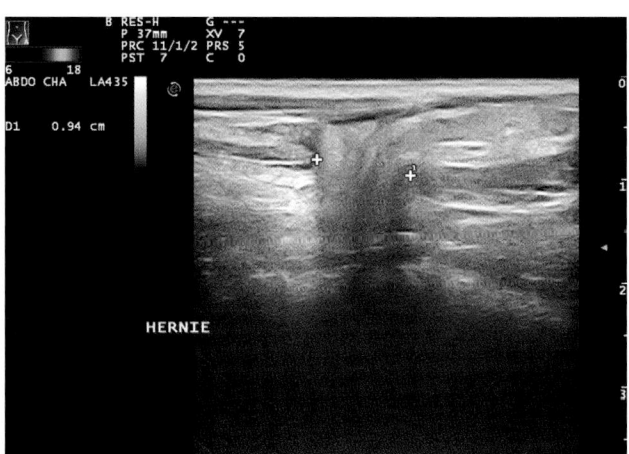

Figure 59.5 Ultrasound image of an abdominal herniation. Discontinuity of the abdominal wall can be observed between the two crosses. *Source:* I. Testault. Reproduced with permission from I. Testault.

- For mural lesions, the affected segment of bowel is removed and an anastomosis performed.
- Early surgical intervention is recommended for patients with evisceration or strangulated hernias. The approach is made over the original incision with care taken not to damage any displaced organs. The full length of the incision is reopened, and incarcerated loops of bowel are lavaged with sterile saline and carefully examined for viability. The loops of bowel are replaced in the abdominal cavity if they are still viable, and nonviable segments are resected and anastomosed. All devitalized tissue and fat is removed from the abdominal wall incision before closure.
- The same approach is used for mesenteric and omental bowel entrapment. Viability is assessed, the affected segment is returned to the abdominal cavity or a resection and anastomosis is performed, and the mesenteric or omental defect is then repaired.

Outcome

- As for primary intestinal obstruction, early diagnosis, appropriate stabilization, prompt surgical treatment, and close postoperative monitoring result in a good prognosis.

Prevention

- When gastrointestinal (GI) surgery is performed, the entire abdominal GI tract should be systematically and routinely examined to ensure no lesions are overlooked.
- The use of an appositional continuous suture pattern is recommended in intestinal surgery. It minimizes mucosal eversion and subsequent adhesion formation, minimizes inversion and tissue overlap, and enables more precise submucosal apposition with minimal stenosis at the anastomosis site.
- Absorbable monofilament suture material such as polydioxanone, polyglyconate, or glycomer 631 is recommended for intestinal closure.
- Successful, durable abdominal wall closures must include the external leaf of the rectus muscle sheath; this layer should be identified before closure, and at least 5 mm of healthy fascia should be incorporated in the suture to ensure adequate anchorage.
- Tears in the mesentery or omentum can be prevented by gentle manipulation and by repairing any iatrogenic defects using a simple continuous absorbable suture pattern.

Short bowel syndrome

Definition

Short bowel syndrome is a state of malabsorption and malnutrition that usually results from extensive small intestinal resection (Box 59.1). It infrequently occurs in dogs and cats.

Risk factors

- Extensive small intestine resection of more than 75% to 80% may result in short bowel syndrome.
- Extensive removal of large intestine associated with removal of the ileocolic valve contributes to the development of more severe chronic diarrhea (favores bacterial overgrowth) and prolongs intestinal transit time.

Diagnosis

The diagnosis must be based on clinical signs as well as remaining intestinal length. The clinical signs depend on the site and extent

Box 59.1 Diseases or conditions that necessitate removal of large segments of the bowel

- Intestinal volvulus
- Linear foreign body
- Intussusception
- Intestinal trauma
- Extensive intestinal neoplasia
- Mesenteric thrombosis/infarction
- Intestinal entrapment
- GI surgical dehiscence
- Fungal infection

GI, gastrointestinal.

of resection, the presence of the ileocolic valve, and the length and adaptive ability of the remaining intestine.

- Animals with short bowel syndrome present with persistent postoperative diarrhea, progressive weight loss, electrolyte imbalances, malabsorption, and subsequent malnutrition.
- Sudan III–stained fecal smears reveal increased fat content.
- Biochemistry findings: dehydration, hyponatremia, hypokalemia, increased urea and creatinine, metabolic acidosis
- Hematology findings: mild normocytic, normochromic, nonregenerative anemia in chronic cases, microcytic anemia if the ileum is removed (cobalamin deficiency)

Treatment (Table 59.1)

- Dietary management: Early oral feeding is recommended because it is one of the most important factors in stimulating and enhancing intestinal hyperplasia. In patients with poor gain weight, total or partial parenteral nutrition is advisable.
- Medical treatment: The aim of medical treatment is to control diarrhea (antidiarrheics, bile salt binders), gastric acid hypersecretion (gastric secretion inhibitors), and bacterial overgrowth (antimicrobials); increase intestinal transit (octreotide); reduce the frequency of defecation (ursodeoxycholic acid); and enhance

intestinal adaptation (growth factors, hormones, octreotide, acid ursodeoxycholic).

- Weekly monitoring of body weight, body condition score, and stool evaluations is useful for assessing the animal's progress and bowel adaptation.

Outcome

The prognosis depends on the response to therapy and the adaptation of the remaining bowel. Some animals may return to a normal diet, but others never respond adequately.

Prevention

Great care should be taken to ensure that only obviously abnormal bowel is resected when more than 50% of the bowel is involved. The ileocolic valve should be preserved wherever possible.

Ileus

Definition

Ileus is the failure of intestinal contents to pass along the intestine.

Risk factors

Postoperative ileus is not as common in dogs as it is in humans.

Postoperative ileus may have a number of causes. Mechanical (or obstructive) postoperative ileus is caused by some physical impediment to the passage of material along the bowel (see the earlier discussion of postoperative bowel obstruction). Functional (adynamic or paralytic) ileus results in loss of peristaltic activity. It may be secondary to:

- Bowel inflammation
- Excessive bowel manipulation
- Peritonitis (see Chapter 4)
- Dehiscence (see Chapter 9)
- Electrolyte imbalance
- Prolonged anesthesia
- Prolonged fasting
- Postoperative pain

Table 59.1 Clinical signs and treatment of short bowel syndrome

Stage	Clinical signs	Treatment Medical	Dietary
Early (first 24–48 hours)	Depressed Massive diarrhea Acute weight loss Electrolyte imbalance	Shock IV fluids Electrolyte restoration	Total or partial parenteral nutrition Early low-fat, highly digestible food (or elemental diet) intake
Intermediate	Bright, alert, active Chronic diarrhea Malnutrition Chronic weight loss Steatorrhea Polyphagia	Antidiarrheic: loperamide (0.1 mg/kg PO bid–tid in dogs, 0.08–0.16 mg/kg PO bid in cats), diphenoxylate (0.1–0.2 mg/kg PO bid– tid in dogs, 0.05–0.1 mg/kg PO bid in cats)	Low-fat and highly digestible food Small meals several times a day Micronutrient supplementation (vitamins, calcium, zinc, magnesium)
		Gastric acid secretion inhibitors: PPIs (omeprazole 0.7 mg/kg PO sid), H₂-receptors blockers (cimetidine 10 mg/kg IV, IM, or PO three times a day or ranitidine 2 mg/kg IV or PO bid– tid in dogs; 2.5 mg/kg IV bid and 3.5 mg/kg PO bid in cats)	
		Bile-salt binding agents: ursodeoxycholic acid (10–15 mg/kg PO), cholestyramine (2 g/dog)	
		Antimicrobials: metronidazole (15 mg/kg PO bid in dogs, 10–25 mg/kg bid in cats), amoxicillin (6–20 mg /kg tid PO), tylosin (7–15 mg/kg PO sid–bid), tetracycline (—20 mg/ kg PO tid), octreotide (10–20 μg/animal SC bid–tid)	
		Parenteral cobalamin supplementation if ileum removed (100–200 μg/day IM in dogs; 50–100 μg/day IM in cats)	
		Pancreatic enzyme supplementation if pancreatic disruption (1–3 tsp/0.45 kg of food)	
Recovery period	Feces more consistent Frequency of defecation decreased Weight gain		Low-fat and highly digestible food

bid, twice a day; IM, intramuscular; IV, intravenous; PO, oral; PPI, proton pump inhibitor; qid, four times a day; SC, subcutaneous; sid, once a day; tid, three times a day.

Diagnosis

- Clinical signs are similar to those of intestinal obstruction and include vomiting, anorexia, depression, abdominal distension, and constipation. Auscultation reveals an absence of normal gut sounds.
- Biochemistry: dehydration with electrolyte imbalance (hyperkalemia, hyponatremia, hypochloremia)
- Radiology: During adynamic ileus, the diameter of the intestine is typically uniform unlike obstructive ileus, in which the intestine can be dilated or normal. The entire length of the tract is involved; loops of bowel are fluid filled with gas present from swallowed air or bacterial fermentation (Figure 59.6). A barium study reveals delayed gastric emptying and slow or no passage of contrast medium along the intestine. Fluid present in the bowel dilutes the barium. Administration of barium may distress the animal and provoke vomiting.
- Ultrasonography: generalized distension of bowel loops, the intestinal lumen is filled with fluid and gas, and motility is reduced or absent

Treatment

- Correct electrolyte imbalances and dehydration.
- Enteral alimentation stimulates parasympathetic tone. If the animal is inappetent, a nasogastric, esophagostomy, or gastrostomy feeding tube should be considered.
- Pain management: buprenorphine (10–20 µg/kg intramuscularly or intravenously [IV] three to four times a day)
- Metoclopramide (0.2–0.4 mg/kg IV tid, 1–2 mg/kg/day constant-rate infusion [CRI] IV) increases the myoelectric and contractile activity of the proximal GI tract.
- Lidocaine CRI IV (20 µg/min) provides prokinetic activity.
- Antimicrobials for bacterial overgrowth: metronidazole (15 mg/kg IV twice a day in dogs or 10–25 mg/kg IV in cats) or amoxicillin (6–20 mg /kg three times day IV)

Outcome

- Uncomplicated ileus usually resolves without aggressive treatment.
- A failure to respond is indicative of mechanical obstruction or septic peritonitis, and surgical exploration is recommended.

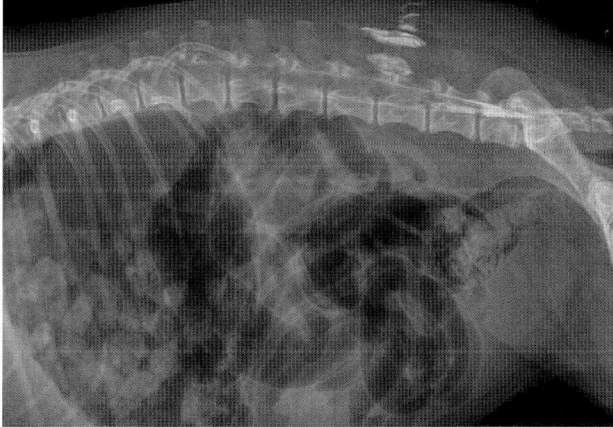

Figure 59.6 Paralytic ileus secondary to prolonged anesthesia. Note the uniformly gas-distended loops of bowel. *Source:* H. Gallois-Bride. Reproduced with permission from H. Gallois-Bride.

Prevention

- Atraumatic surgery
- Reduced surgical time
- Early food intake 12 hours postoperatively
- Perioperative IV fluids
- Perioperative pain management

Relevant literature

Intussusception

Because the predisposing condition that caused intussusception may still be present after surgical correction, recurrence is therefore possible. Predisposing factors to intussusceptions include small intestinal hypermobility secondary to intestinal parasitism, linear foreign body, viral or nonspecific gastroenteritis, alimentary lymphoma, inflammatory bowel disease, and recent previous abdominal or nonabdominal surgery for unrelated disease (Lewis and Ellison 1987; Burkitt *et al.* 2009).

The majority of intussusceptions seen in young animals are considered to be idiopathic (Lewis and Ellison 1987). Whereas the ileocolic junction is the most commonly reported site for intussusception in dogs, enteroenteric intussusceptions are more common in cats (Burkitt *et al.* 2009).

Postoperative intussusception seems to recur more often at a different anatomic location than the primary intussusception irrespective of whether the intussusception was reduced manually or resected at the initial surgery (Levitt and Bauer 1992; Oakes *et al.* 1994).

Perioperative opioid administration has been reported to decrease the rate of intussusception in dogs undergoing renal transplant (McAnulty *et al.* 1989; Klinger *et al.* 1990). The administration of opioids or anticholinergic drugs was not associated with any beneficial effects in terms of recurrence of intussusception in clinical cases (Oakes *et al.* 1994).

The routine use of enteroplication in experimental dogs undergoing renal transplantation is effective and safe (Kyles *et al.* 2003).

In clinical cases, enteroplication decreases recurrence rates but can be associated with serious complications in dogs and cats, such as strangulation, obstruction, foreign body perforation, peritonitis, and recurrence. The reported complication rate after enteroplication is around 19% (Oakes *et al.* 1994; Applewhite *et al.* 2001).

To reduce the incidence of complications, recommendations are (Applewhite *et al.* 2001):

- Plication of the entire small intestine from the duodenocolic ligament to the ileocolic junction
- Ensure that the bends in the intestine are gentle.
- Place the plication sutures at suitable intervals to prevent entrapment and strangulation of other portions of the bowel.
- The anastomotic site should be located at one of the bends in the plicated bowel.
- Plication sutures should be made with absorbable, interrupted sutures; penetrate the submucosal layer; and be placed midway between the mesenteric and antimesenteric borders.

Postoperative intestinal obstruction

- The type of suture material is important in intestinal surgery. Nonabsorbable suture material such as polypropylene or nonabsorbable staples may act as a site of attachment for a foreign body or a trichobezoar (Milovancev *et al.* 2004; Carobbi *et al.* 2009).

Short bowel syndrome

- Intestinal adaptation may take 1 to 2 months. The adaptation begins within a few days of surgery and results in restoration of the absorptive capacity of the intestine through compensatory growth of the remaining intestinal segment and an increase in mucosal surface area. Dilatation, lengthening, and thickening of the intestine are observed along with epithelial cell proliferation in intestinal crypts and migration of cells into intestinal villi.

- In clinical cases, there was no apparent correlation between the percentage of resected bowel and the development of short bowel syndrome (Gorman *et al.* 2006).

- Treatment with keratinocyte growth factor was shown to enhance gut adaptation (increased mucosal thickness, villus length and enzyme activity) in rat models with short bowel syndrome (Johnson *et al.* 2000).

- In humans, intestinal lengthening is the most commonly used method of GI reconstruction for the treatment of short bowel syndrome before intestinal transplantation (Thompson 2008). The Bianchi and serial transverse enteroplasty procedures are the most common surgical procedures used. The Bianchi procedure divides the bowel in two longitudinal halves using the bifurcated mesenteric blood supply before reconnecting the two halves in series with the rest of the small intestine. The serial transverse enteroplasty, procedure staples the bowel into V shapes on alternating sides, decreasing its width and increasing its length. As yet there are no published clinical data concerning the use of surgical techniques to increase intestinal absorption capacity or to increase the absorptive intestinal area in dogs or cats.

References

Applewhite, A.A., Hawthorne, J.C., Cornell, K.K. (2001) Complications of enteroplication for the prevention of intussusception recurrence in dogs: 35 cases (1989–1999). *Journal of the American Veterinary Medical Association* 219, 1415-1418.

Burkitt, J.M., Drobatz, K.J., Saunders, H.M., et al. (2009) Signalment, history, and outcome of cats with gastrointestinal tract intussusception: 20 cases (1986-2000). *Journal of the American Veterinary Medical Association* 234 (6), 771-776.

Carobbi, B., Foale, R.D., White, R.A. (2009) Trichobezoar obstruction after stapled jejunal anastomosis in a dog. *Veterinary Surgery* 38 (3), 417-420.

Gorman, S.C., Freeman, L.M., Mitchell, S.L., et al. (2006) Extensive small bowel resection in dogs and cats: 20 cases (1998-2004). *Journal of the American Veterinary Medical Association* 228 (3), 403-407.

Johnson, W.F., DiPalma, C.R., Ziegler, T.R., et al. (2000) Keratinocyte growth factor enhances early gut adaptation in a rat model of short bowel syndrome. *Veterinary Surgery* 29 (1), 17-27.

Klinger, M., Cooper, J., McCabe, R. (1990) The use of butorphanol tartrate for the prevention of canine intussusception following renal transplantation. *Journal of Investigative Surgery* 3, 229-233.

Kyles, A.E., Gregory, C.R., Griffey, S.M., et al. (2003) Modified noble plication for the prevention of intestinal intussusception after renal transplantation in dogs. *Journal of Investigative Surgery* 16 (3), 161-166.

Levitt, L., Bauer, M. S. (1992) Intussusception in dogs and cats: a review of 36 cases. *Canadian Veterinary Journal* 33, 660-664.

Lewis, D.D., Ellison, G.W. (1987) Intussusceptions in dogs and cats. *Compendium of Continuing Education for Small Animal Veterinarians* 9, 523-533.

McAnulty, J.F., Southard, J.H., Belzer, F.O. (1989) Prevention of postoperative intestinal intussusception by prophylactic morphine administration in dogs used for organ-transplantation research. *Surgery* 105, 494-495.

Milovancev, M., Weisman, D.L., Palmisano, M.P. (2004) Foreign body attachment to polypropylene suture material extruded into the small intestinal lumen after enteric closure in three dogs. *Journal of the American Veterinary Medical Association* 225 (11), 1713-1715.

Oakes, M.G., Lewis, D.D., Hosgood, G., et al. (1994) Enteroplication for the prevention of recurrent intussusceptions in dogs. *Journal of the American Veterinary Medical Association* 205, 72-75.

Swift, I. (2009) Ultrasonographic features of intestinal entrapment in dogs. *Veterinary Radiology and Ultrasound* 50 (2), 205-207.

Thompson, J., Sudan, D. (2008) Intestinal lengthening for short bowel syndrome. *Advances in Surgery* 42, 49-61.

60 Large Intestine Surgery

Jean-Philippe Billet
Centre Hospitalier Veterinaire Atlantia, Nantes, France

Colorectal surgery is often feared because of its high rates of intra- and postoperative complications. The main indications include megacolon, colorectal neoplasia, and rectal prolapse. The most common procedures remain colectomy and anastomosis. Potential complications include leakage, dehiscence, peritonitis, postoperative chronic diarrhea, stricture, fecal incontinence, and recurrence of clinical signs.

Intraoperative contamination of the abdomen

Definition
Spillage of colonic content during surgery can result in rapid and severe peritonitis. The colonic lumen contains high numbers of aerobic and anaerobic bacteria (10^{10} to 10^{11} bacteria per gram of feces), and abdominal contamination can have dramatic consequences.

Risk factors
- Very soft to watery feces present in the colon at the time of surgery
- Poor tissue handling technique and spillage of intestinal contents
- Reuse of contaminated surgical instruments in the abdomen

Diagnosis
- Direct visualization of the spillage
- Bacterial peritonitis (see Chapter 4)

Treatment
- If the spillage is seen during surgery: copious abdominal lavage of the isolated "dirty" site or of the entire abdomen, and preventive placement of a Jackson Pratt or Blake drain
- Parenteral injection of antibiotics with activity against gram-negative aerobes and anaerobes
- Treatment of bacterial peritonitis (see Chapter 4)

Outcome
If appropriate treatment is performed and bacterial peritonitis does not develop, the prognosis is good.

Prevention
- Use of moist laparotomy sponges to isolate the surgical site before entering the colonic lumen

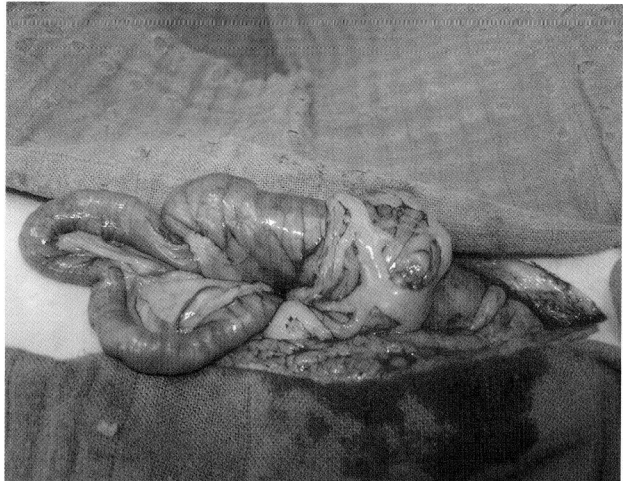

Figure 60.1 Colonic omentalization after colonic resection.

- Gentle tissue handling, accurate mucosal apposition, tension-free closure, preservation of blood supply, and use of atraumatic instruments (Doyen forceps)
- Gently milk out the contents of the segment of colon to be excised.
- Lavage the surgical site.
- Omentalize the surgical site (Figure 60.1).
- Change any contaminated instruments during surgery.
- Avoid routine preoperative enemas because they liquefy the feces and increase the risk of leakage during surgery.

Post–subtotal colectomy diarrhea

Definition
One of the primary complications after subtotal colectomy is chronic diarrhea. This intractable postsurgical diarrhea is the result of small intestine bacterial overgrowth and a lack of water absorption from the colon.

Risk factors
- Removal of the ileocolic junction during subtotal colectomy
- Dogs are more often affected than cats; they do not adapt as well as cats after removal of the ileocolic junction.

Complications in Small Animal Surgery, First Edition. Edited by Dominique Griffon and Annick Hamaide.
© 2016 John Wiley & Sons, Inc. Published 2016 by John Wiley & Sons, Inc.
Companion website: www.wiley.com/go/griffon/complications

Diagnosis

- The diagnosis is based on a history of chronic diarrhea after colectomy. Physical examination may reveal a soiled perianal region.
- Increased defecation
- Water and electrolyte imbalance, loss of body weight (up to 30%)

Treatment

- In cats, without treatment, stool consistency will improve over a 2-month period to semisolid formed stool with ileal adaptation.
- Highly digestible, low-residue diet, short course of antibiotics (metronidazole)
- Adaptation also occurs in dogs but does not resolve diarrhea. Experimentally, the use of an antiperistaltic ileal segment can maintain solid stools (Tuley *et al*. 1976).

Outcome

- Clinical signs improve in cats after 8 weeks, but, soft semiformed or formed stools will remain; weight loss is rare.
- Most dogs survive but will be more or less debilitated from weight loss and massive diarrhea with water and electrolyte depletion.

Prevention

- Preservation of the ileocolic junction in dogs
- Preservation of the ileocolic junction in cats is still controversial; the pros and cons of the chosen technique should be discussed with the owner before surgery.

Rectal incisional dehiscence

Definition

The rectum may be exposed using a ventral, dorsal, rectal pull-through, lateral, or anal approach. The diseased or ruptured rectum is resected or reanastomosed (or both). Spontaneous wound breakdown is one of the most common complications in any rectal surgery.

Risk factors

- Poor surgical site preparation, disruption of the blood supply to the rectal edges, poor suture placement, tension on the sutures
- Systemic factors that increase the risk of dehiscence include hypovolemia, shock, hypoproteinemia, debilitation, and infection.

Diagnosis

- Clinical signs appear within 3 to 5 days of surgery and include depression, fever, excessive discomfort, and perineal swelling.
- The diagnosis is based on clinical signs and rectal examination (Figure 60.2).
- Determination of the exact location of the dehiscence is important. Leakage in the cranial two thirds of the rectum may lead to septic peritonitis, and leakage in the caudal rectum will be more localized and accessible to repair.

Treatment

- Surgical exposure of the dehisced region, thorough lavage of the area, and culture (aerobic and anaerobic) of the surgical site
- Parenteral injection of antibiotics with activity against gram-negative aerobes and anaerobes
- Necrotic, ischemic tissues and the edges of the incision are resected, and the wound is resutured using a simple appositional pattern with minimal tension with an absorbable monofilament suture.

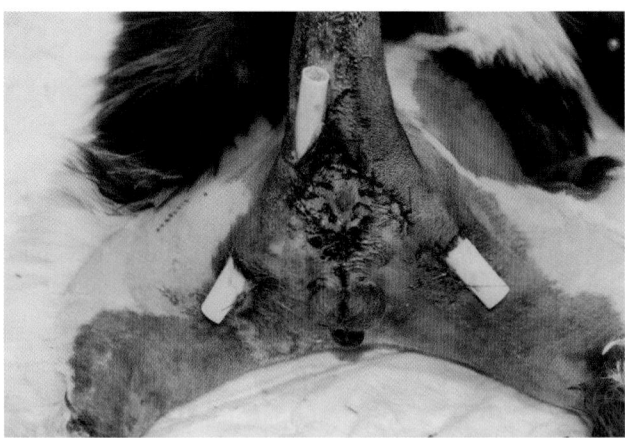

Figure 60.2 Skin dehiscence in a cat with a dorsal rectal tear dehiscence.

- Surgical placement of a suction drain may be necessary and should be placed at a suitable distance from the anastomotic site.
- If contamination is severe, delayed primary closure should be considered. Daily copious lavage of the wound and wet-to-dry bandaging can be an option until healthy granulation tissue appears and closure can be achieved (Figure 60.3).
- Access to the dehisced suture via a rectal pull-through procedure can provide better exposure than the original procedure.
- In very severe cases, intestinal deviation (jejunostomy or colostomy) can be performed temporarily to bypass the rectum until healing is complete.

Outcome

The outcome depends on the location of the wound breakdown. The prognosis is guarded for dehiscence of the cranial two thirds of the rectum. Dorsal dehiscence carries a better prognosis than lateral or ventral breakdown because there is less spillage of fecal matter into the subcutaneous space.

Prevention

- For optimal healing, a monofilament, synthetic, absorbable (polydioxanone, polyglyconate, glycomer 631), appositional suture (simple interrupted or simple continuous) is recommended in

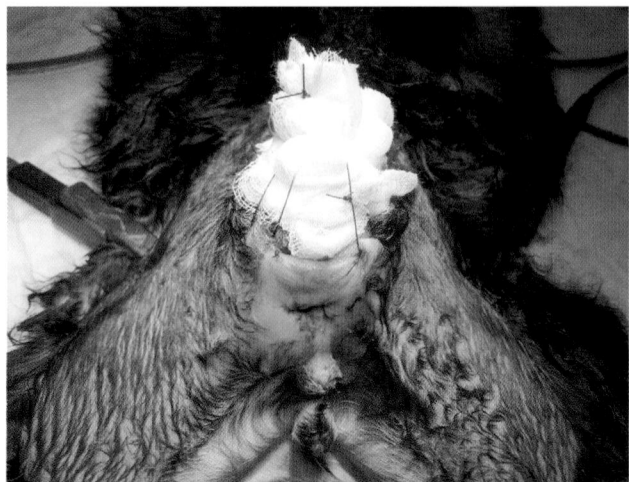

Figure 60.3 A tie-over dressing for delayed primary close of a dorsal rectal tear in a cat.

intestinal surgery. It minimizes eversion, inversion, and tissue overlap and enables more precise submucosal apposition.

- Excessive tension on the suture line should be avoided.
- Careful patient preparation is essential for anorectal surgery. Fecal volume should be minimized during and immediately after surgery. A low-residue, high-calorie diet can be offered 24 to 72 hours before surgery and the animal fasted for 24 hours. Laxatives and warm enemas can be given 24 hours before surgery. Enemas should not be given on the day of surgery to prevent leakage of liquefied fecal matter. During preparation of the surgical site under general anesthesia, any remaining fecal matter present in the rectum is removed manually, and the anal sacs are expressed. The colon is cleaned with swabs impregnated with povidone–iodine solution, these should be wrung out first to avoid liquefied feces. Two to three povidone–iodine swabs are then left in place as cranial as possible in the rectum, and then two to three dry sterile swabs are placed against the povidone–iodine ones and cranial to the surgical site to prevent contamination from any liquid fecal material during surgery. The swabs are removed postoperatively or left to be passed naturally.
- The cranial rectal artery is a branch of the caudal mesenteric artery and is the main blood supply of the rectum. The cranial rectal artery is preserved unless the intrapelvic rectum is removed.
- Parenteral prophylactic antibiotics (first-generation cephalosporins and metronidazole, second-generation cephalosporins) are administered intraoperatively but in no way should they be considered as a substitute for strict cleaning, aseptic intestinal preparation, and surgical technique.

Stricture

Definition

Postoperative luminal narrowing of the rectum or anus can occur after any anorectal and colonic surgery.

Risk factors

- Excessive tension at the anastomosed site from massive intestinal resection
- Use of suture patterns that narrow the intestinal diameter
- Stenosis at the surgical site is most likely when more than half the circumference of the rectum is excised.

Diagnosis

- Clinical signs vary and depend on the degree of narrowing; they may include prolonged tenesmus, dyschezia, hematochezia, passage of ribbonlike feces.
- Secondary megacolon can occur with persistent constipation from the stricture.
- The diagnosis is made by rectal examination and on the basis of the history.
- Contrast radiography may be useful in some cases to determine the extent of the stricture.
- Biopsy of the stricture is indicated in animals with a history of rectal neoplasia to differentiate postoperative stricture from local recurrence.

Treatment

- In mild cases, strictures are managed by digital, balloon dilation, or bougienage or by incision with electrosurgery or laser.

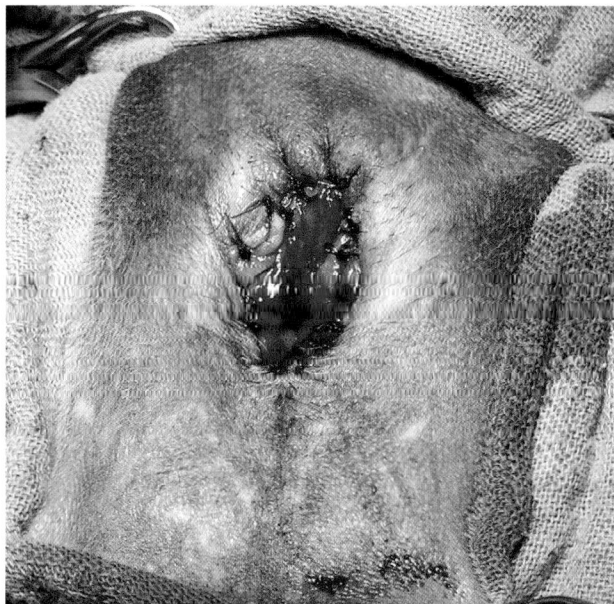

Figure 60.4 Postoperative appearance of a resected anorectal stenosis. Note the simple interrupted appositional sutures between the rectal mucosa and the skin.

- The association of balloon dilation and intralesional triamcinolone injection can also been attempted in dogs with non-neoplastic rectal strictures. A total of 0.5 to 1.0 mL of triamcinolone is injected submucosally in four evenly spaced locations around the stricture before the dilatation procedure.
- If these techniques do not alleviate obstruction or if it recurs, surgical resection of the stenotic segment and rectal anastomosis are indicated (Figure 60.4).

Outcome

The prognosis is good except in the presence of underlying malignant neoplasia (adenocarcinoma), wound dehiscence, infection, or fecal incontinence.

Prevention

- For optimal healing, a monofilament, synthetic, absorbable (polydioxanone, polyglyconate, glycomer 631), appositional suture (simple interrupted or simple continuous) is recommended in intestinal surgery. It minimizes eversion, inversion, and tissue overlap and enables more precise submucosal apposition.
- Gentle manipulation and blunt digital dissection can be performed on the mesorectum to isolate the rectum and reduce tension.

Fecal incontinence

Definition

Fecal incontinence is the inability to retain feces; the two major contributing factors are external anal sphincter function (integrity of both the muscular component and the caudal rectal branch of the pudendal nerve) and reservoir continence. Whereas reservoir-incompetent incontinence develops when the large intestine fails to contain the fecal volume, sphincter-incompetent incontinence is when the sphincter fails to resist fecal propulsion by the large intestine. Fecal incontinence can occur after any anorectal surgery.

Risk factors

- Disruption of the pelvic plexus at the perineal flexure
- Damage to the rectal afferent nerves
- Resection of more than 6 cm of the terminal rectum (leading to disruption of the perineal flexure)
- Resection of the final 1.5 cm of the terminal rectum
- Resection of more than half of the external anal sphincter

Diagnosis

Clinical signs associated with sphincter incontinence are involuntary or unconscious passage of feces. Clinical signs associated with reservoir incontinence are frequent and conscious defecation.

An increase in intraabdominal pressure such as with barking, coughing, or rising from a recumbent position can result in the involuntary passage of feces.

Anorectal lesions can sometimes be detected on physical examination with visual inspection and careful digital palpation.

Treatment

- Medical treatment: The use of a low-residue diet reduces fecal volume and the frequency of defecation. Antidiarrheics such as loperamide promote segmental bowel contractions, thereby decreasing transit time and allowing greater resorption of fecal water.
- Surgical treatment: If the perineal anatomy was disrupted by previous surgery, then initial treatment involves surgical reconstruction of the anal canal, repair of the anal sphincter, and reconstruction of the anal sphincter diameter or of the muscles of continence. Pedicled semitendinosus muscle flaps can be used to reconstruct the anal sphincter muscle. If neurogenic sphincter incontinence is present, sphincter-enhancing procedures can improve clinical signs. A perineal fascial sling or a silicone elastomer sling can be passed around the external anal sphincter to reduce its diameter.

Outcome

Non-neurogenic postoperative sphincter incontinence may be transitory; dietary and medical treatment should be started and continued for 1 month. If no improvement is observed after this time, surgical correction should be attempted. The prognosis is guarded, and long-term follow up is highly recommended.

The prognosis for patients with neurogenic sphincter incontinence is guarded. Sphincter-enhancing procedures may improve clinical signs without total resolution.

Prevention

- Avoid disrupting the pelvic plexus by never removing more than 6 cm of the terminal rectum.
- The final 1.5 cm of the terminal rectum should not be removed.
- The caudal rectal afferent nerve branches should be preserved.
- The external anal sphincter should be identified and preserved wherever possible (at least 50%).

Recurrence of rectal prolapse

Definition

Rectal prolapse is the protrusion of the rectal mucosa from the anus. The degree of prolapse increase with continued straining, varying from a few millimeters to many centimeters.

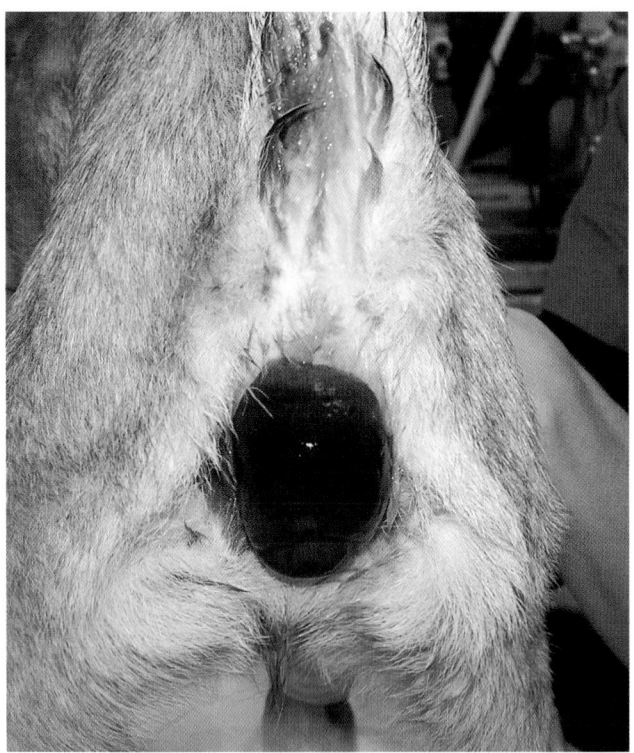

Figure 60.5 Rectal prolapse in a pug puppy.

Risk factors

- History of rectal prolapse
- Endoparasitism and enteritis in young animals
- Tumors and perineal hernia in adult and old dogs
- Any cause of tenesmus (foreign body, dystocia, urolithiasis, constipation, congenital defects, sphincter laxity, prostatic disease)

Diagnosis

Rectal mucosal eversion is obvious on physical examination (Figure 60.5).

Treatment

- The cause of the prolapse should be treated.
- Manual reduction is attempted under general anesthesia. Before digital reduction, the prolapsed portion should be lavaged with a hypertonic solution (30% glucose), massaged, and lubricated (Figure 60.6).
- If the cause is known and has not yet been treated, a purse-string suture can be placed for 3 to 5 days; this is placed in the skin immediately beyond the anocutaneous junction and tied loosely to allow passage of feces (1 cm diameter) (Figure 60.7).
- If the cause is unknown or if treatment with a purse-string suture has failed, abdominal colopexy is performed. The descending colon is exposed via a routine caudal laparotomy and pulled cranially. A nonsterile assistant can determine the reduction of the prolapse by direct visualization. Maintaining mild tension, the descending colon is then sutured to the left ventral abdominal wall 2.5 cm lateral to the linea alba. Two rows of suture are placed parallel to the linea alba, 5 mm apart, using a simple interrupted pattern with absorbable monofilament suture material (2/0 polydioxanone, polyglyconate, or glycomer 631). The sutures

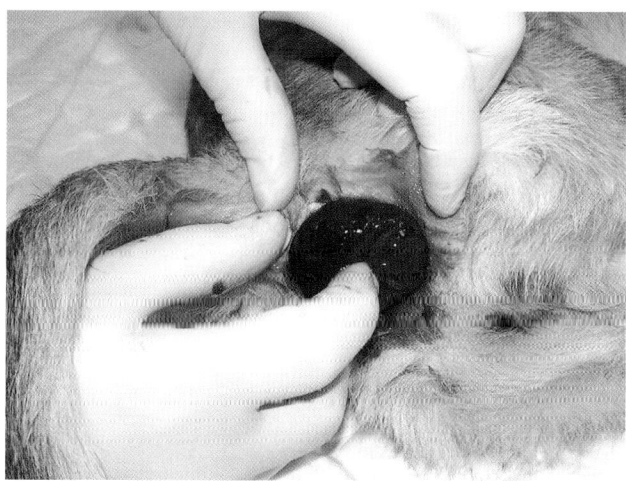

Figure 60.6 Manual reduction of a rectal prolapse.

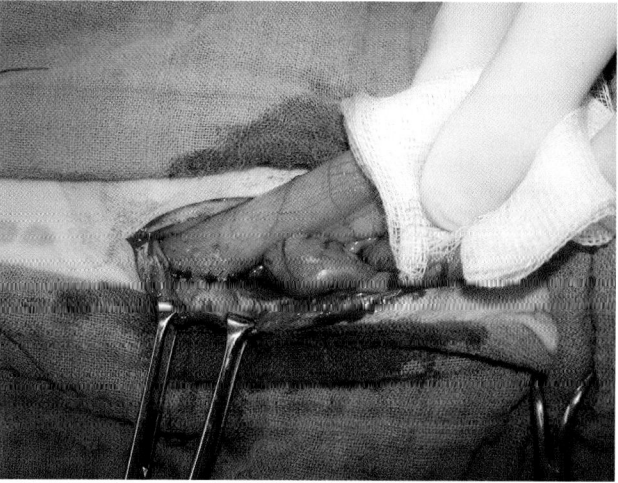

Figure 60.8 The slack is taken out of the descending colon, and simple interrupted sutures are placed between the abdominal wall and the colon to form a colopexy.

are placed through the seromuscular layer of the colon at the antimesenteric border and through the muscle and fascia of the transverse abdominal muscle (Figure 60.8). The colonic serosa and internal fascia of the body wall can be scarified using a scalpel blade between the two rows of suture to enhance adhesions.

- If the rectal prolapse cannot be reduced or if the rectal mucosa is devitalized or necrotic, rectal amputation and anastomosis is performed using a simple interrupted pattern and absorbable monofilament suture material (4/0 polydioxanone, polyglyconate, or glycomer 631).

Outcome

The prognosis is good. Colopexy is an effective surgical treatment for recurrent rectal prolapse.

Prevention

- Identify and treat the underlying cause.
- Perform a preventive colopexy in cases of bilateral perineal hernia with severe colonic deviation.

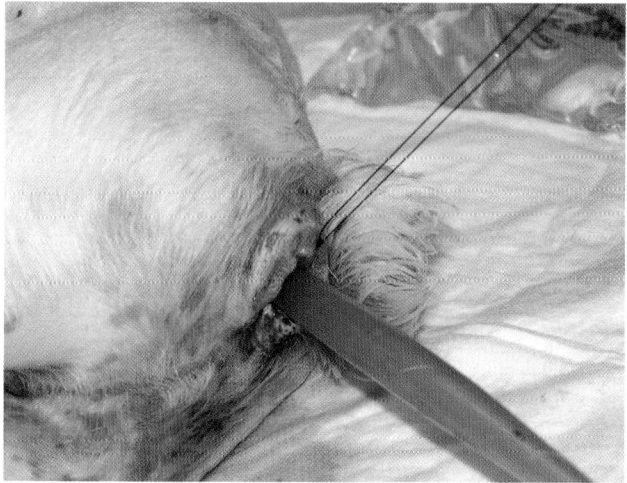

Figure 60.7 Purse-string suture placement to treat rectal prolapse. Note the placement of a suction tip in the rectum to prevent excessive tightening of the suture.

Relevant literature

Animals undergoing large intestinal surgery are not at greater risk for postoperative complications than animals undergoing small intestinal surgery (Wylie and Hosgood 1994).

The value of mechanical cleaning and preoperative antibiotics for colonic surgery has not been proven in veterinary surgery. Enemas are associated with an increased risk of leakage and **gross abdominal contamination**. The use of nonabsorbable oral antibiotics, such as neomycin, is not a generally accepted practice in small animals. The administration of prophylactic perioperative antibiotics at anesthetic induction is also controversial; some veterinary surgeons do not use perioperative antibiotics because surgery in small animals is usually rapid, and spillage is perfectly avoidable.

If the ileocolic junction is resected to treat megacolon, **post-subtotal colectomy diarrhea** occurs secondary to bacterial overgrowth. Experimental studies have shown postoperative increases in ileal villus height, enterocyte height, and enterocyte density, as well as migrating contraction waves propagating beyond the site of anastomosis, signaling recovery of intestinal motility at 8 weeks postoperatively (Bertoy *et al.* 1989; Jimba *et al.* 2002). In cats with idiopathic megacolon, preservation of the ileocolic junction shortens the postoperative recovery period, but it can be more difficult to achieve a tension-free anastomosis, and constipation may recur. Removal of the ileocolic junction in cats has been associated with minimal complications other than soft stools (Rosin *et al.* 1988; Sweet *et al.* 1994).

Rectal dehiscence or stricture formation requires prompt diagnosis and effective treatment.

In extreme or recurrence cases, fecal deviation should be considered. A colostomy or jejunostomy can be performed laparoscopically (Chandler *et al.* 2005). Two techniques have been described in clinical cases, a loop colostomy and an end-on-enterostomy (jejunal or colonic) (Hardie and Gilson 1997; Chandler *et al.* 2005; Tsioli *et al.* 2009). For the first technique, the colon is exteriorized, and a straight plastic loop ostomy rod is placed through the colonic mesentery to block the colon. A longitudinal incision is then made in the colon, and the seromuscular layers are sutured to the skin. After healing, the colostomy site is debrided and closed transversely. In the second technique, the distal portion of the intestine is closed and returned to the peritoneal cavity. A stoma is then created for an end-on-enterostomy. The serosal surface is sutured to the internal abdominal body wall of the left flank and the mucosal layer to the skin. For dogs with a jejunostomy or a colostomy, an adhesive ostomy flange and bag are attached to the stoma, and the ostomy bag is changed every 12 to 18 hours as needed (Hardie and Gilson 1997; Chandler *et al.* 2005). For cats with colostomies, no flange or bag has been used. when wound healing is complete, the stoma site is resected and reanastomosed to the distal portion of intestine (Tsioli *et al.* 2009).

Transanal pull-through rectal surgery for rectal amputation has been feared for complications that include tension at the anastomotic site and **fecal incontinence**. In a retrospective study of 11 dogs treated for colorectal carcinoma using this technique, amputation of more than 6 cm of colon, including the perineal flexure, was not associated with permanent fecal incontinence (Morello *et al.* 2008). Fecal reservoir continence can be lost when anastomosing the colon to the distal 1.5 cm of the rectum; this did not occur in this case series. Incontinence can be transitory with continence being regained within 1 month; a long follow-up period is recommended for these cases.

A semitendinosus muscle transfer flap was used successfully to reconstruct a sphincter in a dog with congenital deficiency of the external anal sphincter (Doust and Sullivan 2003). The muscle was isolated and severed 2 cm from the tibia; its attachment to the ischium, vasculature, and nerve supply were maintained. The muscle was passed ventrally around the rectum and secured dorsally to the levator ani and coccygeus muscles to simulate the external anal sphincter.

Sphincter-enhancing procedures using an implant have been described in dogs (Leeds and Renegar 1981; Dean *et al.* 1988). A strip of fascia harvested from the fascia lata tensor muscle or a strip of polyester-impregnated silicone elastomer can be used to narrow the diameter of the sphincter. Two 4-cm incisions are made on either side of the anus; the incisions are joined by blunt subcutaneous dissection ventral and dorsal to the rectum. The fascia or the elastomer is passed from left to right, dorsal and then ventral to the anus. The ends of the strip are overlapped and tightened around a probe and sutured to itself with a nonabsorbable monofilament suture material. The strip can also be anchored to the left coccygeus

muscle. Experimentally, in bilateral pudendal neurectomized dogs, five of six dogs regained total continence, and one of six dogs regained partial continence using a silicone elastomer sling (Dean *et al.* 1988). A modified fascia strip technique was performed successfully in an iatrogenic neurogenic fecally incontinent dog after anal gland removal (Leeds and Renegar 1981). The fascia strip was passed under the anal orifice and over the base of the tail and then pulled snug and sutured to itself.

References

Bertoy, R.W., MacCoy, D.M., Wheaton, L.G., et al. (1989) Total colectomy with ileorectal anastomosis in the cat. *Veterinary Surgery* 18 (3), 204-210.

Chandler, J.C., Kudnig, S.T., Monnet, E. (2005) Use of laparoscopic-assisted jejunostomy for fecal diversion in the management of a rectocutaneous fistula in a dog. *Journal of the American Veterinary Medical Association* 226 (5) 746-751.

Dean, P.W., O'Brien, D.P., Turk, M.A.M., et al. (1988) Silicone elastomer sling for fecal incontinence in dogs. *Veterinary Surgery* 17, 304-310.

Doust, R., Sullivan, M. (2003) Semitendinosus muscle transfer flap for external anal sphincter incompetence in a dog. *Journal of the American Veterinary Medical Association* 222 (10), 1385-1387.

Hardie, E.M., Gilson, S.D. (1997) Use of colostomy to manage rectal disease in dogs. *Veterinary Surgery* 26 (4), 270-274.

Jimba, Y., Nagao, J., Sumiyama, Y. (2002) Changes in gastrointestinal motility after subtotal colectomy in dogs. *Surgery Today* 32 (12), 1048-1057.

Leeds, E.B., Renegar, W.R. (1981) A modified fascial sling for the treatment of fecal incontinence-surgical technique. *Journal of the American Animal Hospital Association* 17,663-667.

Morello Z., Martano M., Squassino C., et al. (2008) Transanal pull-through rectal amputation for treatment of colorectal carcinoma in 11 dogs. *Veterinary Surgery* 37, 420-426.

Rosin, E., Walshaw, R., Mehlhaff, C., et al. (1988) Subtotal colectomy for treatment of chronic constipation associated with idiopathic megacolon in cats: 38 cases (1979-1985). *Journal of the American Veterinary Medical Association* 193 (7), 850-853.

Sweet, D.C., Hardie, E.M., Stone, E.A. (1994) Preservation versus excision of the ileocolic junction during colectomy for megacolon: a study of 22 cats. *Journal of Small Animal Practice* 35, 358-363.

Tsioli, V., Papazoglou, L.G., Anagnostou, T., et al. (2009) Use of a temporary incontinent end-on colostomy in a cat for the management of rectocutaneous fistulas associated with atresia ani. *Journal of Feline Medicine and Surgery* 11 (12), 1011-1014.

Tuley, R.D., Matolo, N.M., Garfinkle, S.E., et al. (1976) Antiperistaltic bowel segment for prevention of ileoproctostomy diarrhea. *Journal of Surgical Oncology* 8 (1), 67-73.

Wylie, K.B., Hosgood, G. (1994) Mortality and morbidity of small and large intestinal surgery in dogs and cats: 74 cases (1980-1992). *Journal of the American Animal Hospital Association* 30, 469-474.

61 Hepatic and Biliary Tract Surgery

Anne Kummeling

Division of Soft Tissue Surgery, Department of Clinical Sciences of Companion Animals, Faculty of Veterinary Medicine, Utrecht University, Utrecht, The Netherlands

The liver is a large organ that is not only centrally located in the animal's body but also plays a central role in its metabolism. Reasons for surgical intervention of the liver include hepatic injuries, vascular disorders (i.e., portosystemic shunt), local parenchymal disorders such as neoplasia, liver lobe torsion, and diseases of the biliary tract (cholelithiasis, neoplasia, gallbladder rupture and gallbladder mucocele).

Hemorrhage
See Chapter 12.

Bile peritonitis

Definition
Bile peritonitis is inflammation of the peritoneum that develops after leakage of bile into the abdominal cavity. The peritonitis may develop as a sterile inflammation that is characterized by its yellow-brownish discoloration and mild clinical signs. Secondary infection from the gastrointestinal (GI) tract rapidly worsens the clinical signs and prognosis.

Risk factors
- Necrotizing cholecystitis
- Abdominal trauma (blunt or penetrating injuries, surgical procedures)
- Extrahepatic obstructions of the biliary tract (cholelithiasis)
- Infection of the biliary tract

Diagnosis
- Abdominocentesis followed by measurement of bilirubin concentration (elevated compared to serum bilirubin concentration) and cytologic analysis of the fluid
- Abdominal radiography or ultrasonography
- Bacterial culture and testing of sensitivity (most commonly gram-negative bacteria)
- Surgical exploration of the abdominal cavity (Figure 61.1)

Treatment
Surgical intervention is essential to treat the source of bile leakage. Surgical procedures depend on the cause and site of leakage and may consist of cholecystectomy, primary repair of the rupture, or biliary diversion (cholecystoduodenostomy). Additional

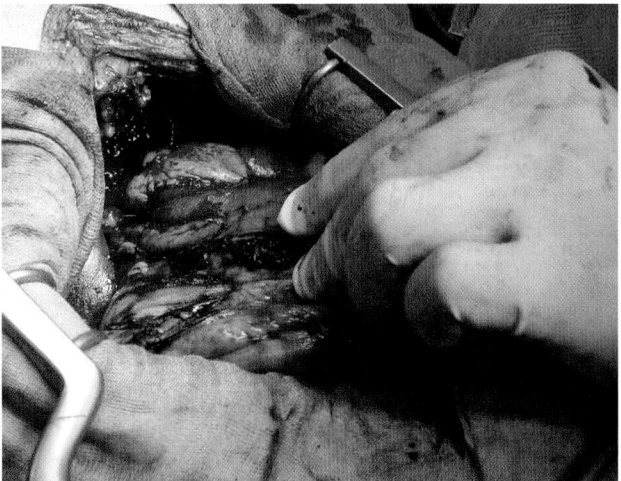

Figure 61.1 Intraoperative appearance of the abdominal cavity and its contents in a dog with a bile peritonitis.

abdominal lavage and open abdominal drainage may be indicated in case of generalized septic bile peritonitis.

Outcome
Animals with sterile bile peritonitis show a much lower mortality rate than those with a septic biliary effusion. The overall survival rate was reported to be 50% in a study of 24 dogs and 2 cats. Distribution of the peritonitis, cause of bile leakage or duration of clinical signs before surgical treatment was not associated with survival and the most common reason for death was euthanasia due to sepsis (Ludwig et al. 1997).

Prevention
Careful surgical handling of tissues during procedures associated with, or next to, the biliary tract is important to prevent postsurgical bile leakage caused by injury or wound dehiscence of the biliary tract.

Hypoglycemia

Definition
Hypoglycemia is defined as low blood glucose levels. Hepatocytes are essential to preserve normal plasma glucose concentrations

---

Complications in Small Animal Surgery, First Edition. Edited by Dominique Griffon and Annick Hamaide.
© 2016 John Wiley & Sons, Inc. Published 2016 by John Wiley & Sons, Inc.
Companion website: www.wiley.com/go/griffon/complications

after surgery because of their role in glucose metabolism with respect to gluconeogenesis, glycolysis, and degradation of insulin. The ability to maintain plasma glucose at a normal level is lost after resection of a large part of the functional liver (e.g., after surgical resection of a large liver tumor or after hepatectomy in animals with existing hepatobiliary disease and dysfunction). Pediatric animals and animals with portosystemic shunting are also more susceptible to postsurgical hypoglycemia, especially after prolonged fasting.

Risk factors
- Extensive liver mass resection
- Pediatric patients
- Portosystemic shunting
- Preexisting hepatic dysfunction
- Fasting or starvation

Diagnosis
Clinical signs may consist of neurologic symptoms such as weakness, seizures, ataxia, and collapse. Hypoglycemia is confirmed by measuring low plasma or serum concentrations (in dogs, <4.2 mmol/L; in cats, <3.4 mmol/L).

Treatment
- Symptomatic treatment consists of administration of glucose by intravenous (IV) administration (5% dextrose 1–5 mL slowly over 10 minutes) followed by oral glucose administration and feeding small meals. The effect is usually rapid after initial treatment. Monitoring of clinical behavior and measuring glucose levels remain important as long as liver function is impaired.
- Seizures can be controlled by diazepam or propofol. Severe central nervous system manifestations may be caused by irreversible lesions and may not respond sufficiently to glucose treatment.
- When secondary cerebral edema is suspected, mannitol administration may be considered.

Outcome
In the veterinary literature, there is little information of outcome after hypoglycemia related to hepatic surgery. Measuring and treating abnormalities in blood glucose levels during and early after hepatic surgery are reported to be effective in human medicine (Brown et al. 1988; Cammu et al. 2009).

Prevention
Glucose levels should be well monitored during and after resection of hepatic tissue, especially in young animals and animals with decreased liver function before surgery.

Hypoalbuminemia

Definition
Hypoalbuminemia is low plasma or serum albumin concentrations.

Risk factors
- Intraoperative blood loss is the most important cause of acute hypoalbuminemia after hepatic surgery. In cats and dogs, the half-life of plasma is long (~8 days), so postoperative hypoalbuminemia usually is not caused by acute hepatic insufficiency (Mathews 2008).
- All animals with preexisting (chronic) hepatic dysfunction may already have low plasma albumin concentrations before surgery and are predisposed to complications related to hypoalbuminemia after surgery.
- Animals with diseases other than hepatic insufficiency that lead to low albumin plasma levels, such as glomerular or GI loss of albumin, are predisposed.
- Fluid therapy may further decrease albumin concentrations.

Diagnosis
- Signs of hypoalbuminemia, such as effusion of fluid in the abdominal cavity and peripheral edema formation, result from decreased colloid osmotic pressure. Edema of multiple organs result in organ dysfunction; for example, pulmonary edema leads to respiratory distress and ultimately to death.
- The diagnosis is confirmed by measuring albumin concentration in plasma or serum.

Treatment
- In dogs and cats, synthetic colloids are usually recommended for treatment of low plasma oncotic pressures.
- Plasma can be considered to correct hypoalbuminemia, but it is difficult to achieve sufficient increases in albumin levels. and colloids are more effective in restoring oncotic pressure. An advantage of plasma is that it can be useful in treating coexisting clotting factor deficiencies.
- In critically ill animals, administration of 25% human serum albumin can be considered (Mathews 2008).

Outcome
Preoperative and postoperative low albumin concentrations are predictors of a poor outcome after hepatic and biliary surgery (Amsellem et al. 2006; Kummeling et al. 2011).

Prevention
Before and after hepatic surgery, plasma or serum albumin should be measured in all animals that are predisposed to hypoalbuminemia. Monitoring of albumin levels after surgery is also important in animals with intraoperative bleeding, postoperative hepatic insufficiency, signs of edema formation, or suspected organ failure.

Hepatic hypofunction

Definition
In animals with postoperative hepatic hypofunction, the liver lacks the ability to maintain its normal metabolic functions after surgery.

Risk factors
- Major hepatic resection
- Hepatic ischemia
- Hepatitis and hepatic or biliary tract infection
- Other (concurrent) hepatobiliary diseases
- Sepsis or disseminated intravascular coagulation (DIC)

Diagnosis
Signs may be variable and depend on the severity and duration of the hepatic hypofunction. Acute signs may result from hypoglycemia, hepatic encephalopathy, and coagulation abnormalities. In animals with hypofunction of the liver, the risk for DIC and multiple organ failure is increased.

Treatment

- The liver has a unique ability for recovery and regeneration. However, in the acute phase, the animal has to be monitored closely (e.g., glucose, electrolyte and albumin concentrations, urine output and coagulation) and supported with careful IV fluid therapy.
- Antimicrobial administration may be needed or considered to prevent and treat septicemia or ascending infections from the intestines.
- During recovery, a specific hepatic diet can be fed.

Outcome

Severe loss of liver function a poor prognosis because most liver functions cannot be replaced artificially, and critical complications can develop while awaiting recovery. However, with good supportive measurements, adequate regeneration of the liver is possible after a loss of up to approximately 70% to 80% of its volume. However, the prognosis for patients with hepatic hypofunction depends on the primary cause.

Prevention

- Before hepatic surgery, the hepatic function of dogs and cats should be assessed to predict the individual risk of postoperative complications, especially in diseased animals.
- After surgery, close monitoring of liver function is important to detect early complications and to be able to provide immediate supportive care.

Hepatic ischemia

Definition

Hepatic ischemia is injury of the hepatocellular tissue and loss of hepatic function caused by lack of sufficient oxygen supply to the cells.

Risk factors

- Preoperative anemia
- Blood loss during surgery
- Severe intraoperative or postoperative arterial hypotension

Diagnosis

See the discussion of hepatic hypofunction.

Treatment

See the discussion of hepatic hypofunction.

Outcome

See the discussion of hepatic hypofunction.

Prevention

- Perioperative monitoring and correction of arterial oxygen saturation and blood pressure (oxygen supply, IV fluids, dobutamine, dopamine)
- Perioperative hematocrit assessment and correction of low levels of circulating erythrocytes by blood transfusion if necessary

Bacterial contamination of the liver and biliary systems

Definition

Biliary tract and hepatic bacterial contamination usually originates from ascending enteric bacteria and can be secondary to an enterobiliary reflux, such as after biliary diversion surgery. Biliary cultures present with a higher contamination rate (30%) than hepatic cultures (7%) in dogs and cats that are evaluated for hepatobiliary disease (Wagner et al. 2007).

Risk factors

- Preoperative bacterial infection of the biliary tract or the liver (e.g., hepatic abscesses)
- Cholestasis (decreased clearance of bacteria by the liver)

Diagnosis

During surgery, samples from the gallbladder, liver, and abdominal fluid can be collected and submitted for anaerobic and aerobic culture.

Treatment

Organisms that are often identified from intraoperative samples in hepatic and biliary tract diseased animals include Enterococcus spp., Escherichia coli, Bacteroides spp., Staphylococcus spp., Streptococcus spp., Clostridium spp., Pasteurella multocida, and Pseudomonas aeruginosa (Amsellem et al. 2006; Buote et al. 2006; Wagner et al. 2007). Antimicrobial treatment based on susceptibility is preferred because sensitivity can be quite variable (Baker et al. 2011).

Outcome

Prevention of postoperative infection by adequate treatment of bacterial contamination will decrease postoperative morbidity and mortality after hepatobiliary surgery.

Prevention

- Prophylactic antimicrobial treatment with extended coverage for aerobic and anaerobic bacteria (e.g., amoxicillin–clavulanate or a fluoroquinolone combined with metronidazole).
- Because resistance occurs regularly, culture and antimicrobial susceptibility should ideally be obtained (Wagner *et al.* 2007).
- Avoid or decrease further contamination from potentially infected sites (e.g., bile or abscesses) by using adequate aseptic techniques or flushing of severely contaminated areas.

Persistent biliary obstruction

Definition

Persistent (or recurrent) biliary obstruction means that normal bile flow through the biliary system into the intestines is still compromised after surgery.

Risk factors

- Residual choleliths or bile sludge in the biliary tract
- Pancreatitis
- Neoplasia
- Stricture formation after healing of biliary tract injuries
- Infection or inflammation of the biliary tract (cholangitis)

Diagnosis

Abdominal ultrasonography in animals with persistent or progressive clinical signs such as icterus, anorexia, vomiting, and lethargy can help to diagnose persistent obstruction. However, presence of air in the abdominal cavity can make visualization of the biliary tract difficult early after surgery.

Treatment

- Another explorative surgery may be needed to confirm and treat the bile tract obstruction. Identification of the common bile duct is improved by passing a catheter into the duct after opening the duodenum (enterotomy) (Figure 61.2).
- To allow better healing of bile duct after injuries, after stricture formation or as a palliative procedure in neoplastic obstructive disease, it is possible to (temporarily) stent the common bile duct, bringing a soft catheter into the duct lumen from the duodenum and suturing it to the duodenal wall (Mayhew *et al.* 2006; Baker *et al.* 2011). Disadvantages may be an increased risk of infection, obstruction, and inflammation caused by a foreign body reaction at the healing site. Morbidity after choledochal stenting may be greater in cats than dogs (Mayhew and Weisse 2008).

Outcome

The overall prognosis for cats and dogs with biliary tract obstruction undergoing cholecystoenterostomy is guarded, but it greatly depends on the primary cause. Malignant diseases usually have a poor prognosis. Adequate surgical technique, perioperative monitoring, and supportive care are critical to improve clinical outcome in other types of biliary obstructions (Mehler et al. 2004; Buote et al. 2006).

Prevention

- Especially before performing a cholecystectomy, patency of the common bile duct should be checked to see if biliary drainage is possible after the procedure.
- Careful suturing of bile duct wounds is important to prevent postoperative stricture formation.
- If an obstruction cannot be removed, a cholecystoenterostomy should be performed.

Cholangitis

Definition

Cholangitis is an inflammation of the biliary system. Usually, cholangitis is caused by an infection from secondary enterobiliary reflux and ascendance of enteric bacteria (Amsellem et al. 2006; Mehler and Bennett 2006). Sometimes the gallbladder and liver parenchyma are also involved (cholangiocystitis and cholangiohepatitis, respectively). In a study of 22 cats with surgical treatment for biliary tract obstruction, postoperative infection appeared to be uncommon; in dogs, this condition is rarely reported (Buote et al. 2006; O'Neill et al. 2006).

Risk factors

- Bacterial contamination of the biliary tract
- Biliary diversion procedures such as cholecystoduodenostomy and cholecystojejunostomy, especially if the postsurgical stoma is relatively too small to easily remove intestinal contamination or contents

Diagnosis

- Postoperative infections can be suspected from clinical and ultrasonographic signs of inflammation or sepsis and should be confirmed by culturing aspirates.
- Clinical signs consist of anorexia, vomiting, and occasionally pyrexia after surgery. Vomiting can also be caused by other causes, such as a localized ileus or pancreatitis as a result of pancreatic ischemia or sepsis (Mehler and Bennett 2006; Papazoglou *et al.* 2008).

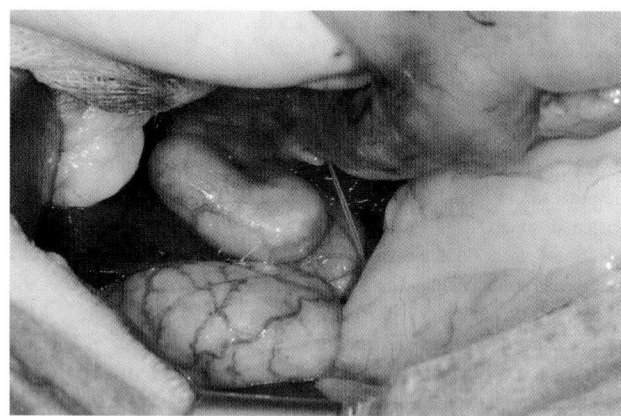

(A)

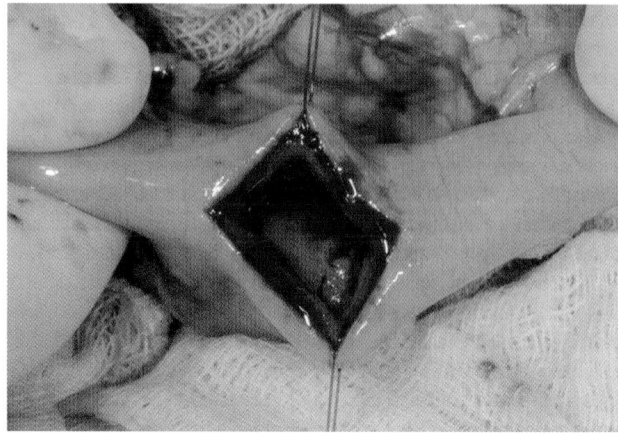

(B)

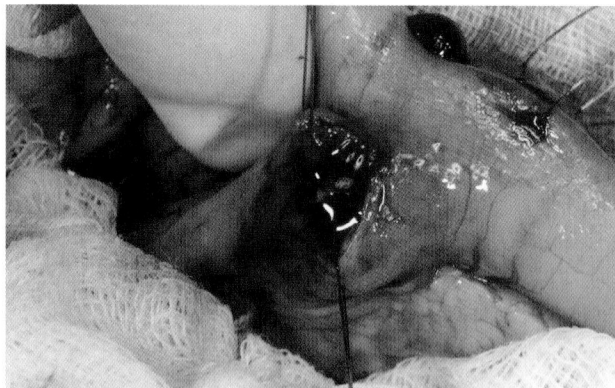

(C)

Figure 61.2 A, Severely dilated extrahepatic biliary tract in a cat with an obstruction of the common bile duct caused by choledocholiths. **B,** A small enterotomy was made in the duodenum to inspect the duodenal papilla and to flush and check patency of the bile duct using a soft catheter. **C,** In this cat, an incision in the common bile duct was made to remove the obstructive calculi. This creates a risk of postoperative dehiscence or stricture formation of the duct. However, the calculi could not be removed with cholecystostomy.

Treatment

- Broad-spectrum antimicrobial treatment, preferably with serial monitoring of bile culture (O'Neill *et al.* 2006)
- Supportive care: parenteral nutrition and IV fluids

- Ursodeoxycholic acid was used in dogs and supports treatment of cholangitis as a choleretic (15 mg/kg orally every 24 hours) (O'Neill *et al.* 2006).

Outcome

Although the primary disease often determines the overall prognosis after hepatobiliary surgery, infection is an important contributing factor to postoperative morbidity and mortality in hepatobiliary surgery. However, with adequate treatment, the prognosis of patients with bacterial cholangitis appears to be good (O'Neill et al. 2006).

Prevention

- See the discussion of bacterial contamination of the liver and biliary systems.
- Creation of a sufficiently wide stoma during biliary diversion procedures

Relevant literature

The liver is unique with respect to its healing capacities and blood supply. Regeneration of hepatic tissue to restore a normal liver function is possible after removal of 70% of the hepatic mass. After hepatectomy, liver volume is rapidly restored to its original size, which depends on body weight and portal blood flow (Michalopoulos 2007). The portal vein collects all venous blood from the stomach, intestines, spleen, and pancreas and normally contributes up to 80% of the total hepatic blood flow. The hepatic artery is only responsible for 20% of the blood flow toward the liver. Healthy hepatic tissue is vulnerable to external trauma because normal liver parenchyma is supported by little fibrous tissue and is well vascularized. Concurrent liver disease can increase risks of surgical complications, for example, by predisposition for pronounced bleeding caused by decreased hepatic production of clotting factors (Kummeling et al. 2006; Prins et al. 2010).

With respect to hepatic surgery, partial or a single lobectomy is one of the most commonly performed procedures. Recently, five different surgical techniques for partial lobectomy were compared with respect to surgical time and blood loss. There was no significant difference in surgical time, but skeletonization and individual clipping of the lobar vessels resulted in more blood loss than the other techniques (thoracoabdominal stapler, LigaSure device, SurgiTie and Ultracision Harmonic Scalpel). However, all of these techniques appear to be safe in small- and medium-sized dogs (Risselada *et al.* 2010).

Extrahepatic biliary tract surgery is associated with a much more guarded outcome in dogs and cats. Several postoperative complications have been described, reflecting the underlying disease (Mehler *et al.* 2004; Amsellem *et al.* 2006; Buote *et al.* 2006). Bile peritonitis is usually caused by rupture in the extrahepatic biliary tract or the gallbladder, which may be traumatic. Bile peritonitis can also result from tissue necrosis caused by inflammation (cholangitis, cholecystitis) and obstruction (cholelithiasis). In dogs, it was reported to be directly associated with surgery, such as after placement of a T-tube in the gallbladder, after manual expression of the gallbladder, after cholecystectomy and cholecystojejunostomy, and even after surgical correction of gastric dilation and volvulus (Ludwig *et al.* 1997; Mehler *et al.* 2004; Hewitt *et al.* 2005). Cholecystectomy and cholecystoduodenostomy are the most common surgical procedures to treat biliary tract problems (Mehler *et al.* 2004). However, choledochotomy and primary repair may be good options in some dogs and cats with extrahepatic biliary tract obstructions or lesions because low complication rates were reported in a pilot study (Baker *et al.* 2011).

Preoperative biliary drainage for patient stabilization has been used to improve outcome after definitive surgical repair of biliary tract disorders. This technique seems to be promising but has not yet been widely used (Lehner and McAnulty 2010).

Besides the complications described in this chapter, other postoperative complications reported after hepatic or biliary surgery include cardiac arrest and postoperative hypotension, which could be caused by prolonged anesthesia, inadequate fluid administration, and sepsis (Mehler *et al.* 2004; Amsellem *et al.* 2006; Buote *et al.* 2006; Papazoglou *et al.* 2008).

References

Amsellem, P.M., Seim III, H.B., MacPhail, C.M., et al. (2006) Long-term survival and risk factors associated with biliary surgery in dogs: 34 cases (1994-2004). *Journal of the American Veterinary Medical Association* 229 (9), 1451-1457.

Baker, S.G., Mayhew, P.D., Mehler, S.J. (2011) Choledochotomy and primary repair of extrahepatic biliary duct rupture in seven dogs and two cats. *Journal of Small Animal Practice,* 52 (1), 32-37.

Brown, T.C.K., Davidson, P.D., Auldist, A.W. (1988) Anaesthetic considerations in liver tumour resection in children. *Pediatric Surgery International* 4 (1), 11-15.

Buote, N.J., Mitchell, S.L., Penninck, D., et al. (2006) Cholecystoenterostomy for treatment of extrahepatic biliary tract obstruction in cats: 22 cases (1994-2003). *Journal of the American Veterinary Medical Association* 228 (9), 1376-1382.

Cammu, G., Vermeiren, K., Lecomte, P., et al. (2009) Perioperative blood glucose management in patients undergoing tumor hepatectomy. *Journal of Clinical Anesthesia* 21 (5), 329-335.

Hewitt, S.A., Brisson, B.A., Holmberg, D.L. (2005) Bile peritonitis associated with gastric dilation-volvulus in a dog. *The Canadian Veterinary Journal* 46 (3), 260-262.

Kummeling, A., Teske, E., Rothuizen, J., Van Sluijs, F.J. (2006) Coagulation profiles in dogs with congenital portosystemic shunts before and after surgical attenuation. *Journal of Veterinary Internal Medicine* 20 (6), 1319-1326.

Kummeling, A., Penning, L.C., Rothuizen, J., et al. (2012) Hepatic gene expression and plasma albumin concentration related to outcome after attenuation of a congenital portosystemic shunt in dogs. *Veterinary Journal* 191 (3), 383-388.

Lehner, C.M., McAnulty, J.F. (2010) Management of extrahepatic biliary obstruction: a role for temporary percutaneous biliary drainage. *Compendium of Continuing Education for Veterinarians* 32 (9), E1-E10.

Ludwig, L.L., McLoughlin, M.A., Graves, T.K., Crisp, M.S. (1997) Surgical treatment of bile peritonitis in 24 dogs and 2 cats: a retrospective study (1987-1994). *Veterinary Surgery* 26 (2), 90-98.

Mathews, K.A. (2008) The therapeutic use of 25% human serum albumin in critically ill dogs and cats. *The Veterinary Clinics of North America, Small Animal Practice* 38 (3), 595-605.

Mayhew, P.D., Weisse, C.W. (2008) Treatment of pancreatitis-associated extrahepatic biliary tract obstruction by choledochal stenting in seven cats. *The Journal of Small Animal Practice,* 49 (3), 133-138.

Mayhew, P.D., Richardson, R.W., Mehler, S.J., et al. (2006) Choledochal tube stenting for decompression of the extrahepatic portion of the biliary tract in dogs: 13 cases (2002-2005). *Journal of the American Veterinary Medical Association* 228 (8), 1209-1214.

Mehler, S.J., Bennett, R.A. (2006) Canine extrahepatic biliary tract disease and surgery. *Compendium on Continuing Education for the Practicing Veterinarian* 28 (4), 302-314.

Mehler, S.J., Mayhew, P.D., Drobatz, K.J., Holt, D.E. (2004) Variables associated with outcome in dogs undergoing extrahepatic biliary surgery: 60 cases (1988-2002). *Veterinary Surgery* 33 (6), 644-649.

Michalopoulos, G.K. (2007) Liver regeneration. *Journal of Cellular Physiology* 213 (2), 286-300.

O'Neill, E.J., Day, M.J., Hall, E.J., et al. (2006) Bacterial cholangitis/cholangiohepatitis with or without concurrent cholecystitis in four dogs. *Journal of Small Animal Practice* 47 (6), 325-335.

Papazoglou, L.G., Mann, F.A., Wagner-Mann, C., Song, K.J.E. (2008) Long-term survival of dogs after cholecystoenterostomy: a retrospective study of 15 cases (1981-2005). *Journal of the American Animal Hospital Association* 44 (2), 67-74.

Prins, M., Schellens, C.J., van Leeuwen, M.W., et al. (2010) Coagulation disorders in dogs with hepatic disease. *Veterinary Journal* 185 (2), 163-168.

Risselada, M., Ellison, G.W., Bacon, N.J., et al. (2010) Comparison of 5 surgical techniques for partial liver lobectomy in the dog for intraoperative blood loss and surgical time. *Veterinary Surgery* 39 (7), 856-862.

Wagner, K.A., Hartmann, F.A., Trepanier, L.A. (2007) Bacterial culture results from liver, gallbladder, or bile in 248 dogs and cats evaluated for hepatobiliary disease: 1998-2003. *Journal of Veterinary Internal Medicine* 21 (3), 417-424.

62 Pancreatic Surgery

Heidi Phillips

Department of Veterinary Clinical Medicine, University of Illinois College of Veterinary Medicine, Urbana, IL, USA

Surgery of the pancreas may be indicated for both exocrine and endocrine diseases and focal and diffuse diseases of the pancreas. The pancreas is in close proximity to adjacent organs and organ systems, including the stomach, duodenum, gallbladder and biliary tree, and spleen. Surgery involving these organ systems may adversely affect the pancreas, and, conversely, surgery of the pancreas may impact surrounding organs.

General complications of pancreatic surgery include inflammation of the pancreas and mesentery, focal or generalized infection, obstruction of associated blood vessels or ducts, and loss of exocrine or endocrine function after loss or fibrous replacement of part or the entire pancreas. The most anticipated complication of pancreatic surgery is postoperative pancreatitis. Although the overall incidence of postoperative pancreatitis has not been reported in dogs and cats, pancreatitis has been reported to develop after both abdominal and nonabdominal surgery. Pancreatic ischemia or congestion resulting from hypotension associated with general anesthesia or from venous outflow occlusion during surgical manipulation in the cranial abdomen may predispose to postoperative pancreatitis. Lack of care in handling the pancreas, its duct system, and peripancreatic tissues also predisposes to postoperative pancreatitis (Matthiesen and Mullen 1990; Yotsumoto et al. 1993; Hess et al. 1999).

Other complications associated with general pancreatic surgery include persistent or recurrent abscessation, obstruction of the common bile duct, peritonitis, hemorrhage, disruption of the blood supply of the pancreas or adjacent organs such as the duodenum, disruption of the pancreatic or biliary duct system, and generalized gastrointestinal (GI) complications (e.g., ileus, inappetence, vomiting, diarrhea). Complications associated with partial or total pancreatectomy include hypoglycemia, hyperglycemia, diabetes mellitus (DM), and exocrine pancreatic insufficiency (EPI).

Historically, in the absence of a minimally invasive and reliable method to diagnose complications related to pancreatic surgery, a diagnosis was made based on a high index of suspicion and supportive data, including blood test results, radiographic and ultrasonographic imaging, and response to treatment. The widespread acceptance of the accuracy of canine and feline pancreatic lipase immunoreactivity (PLI) blood tests and the increased use of advanced imaging techniques permit early and accurate diagnosis of complications associated with pancreatic surgery (Hess et al. 1998; Forman et al. 2004; Whittemore and Campbell 2005; Gaynor 2009).

Postoperative pancreatitis

Definition

Postoperative pancreatitis is an acute, inflammatory disease of the pancreas after surgery ranging in severity from mild, self-limiting, and reversible to severe and irreversible with extensive necrosis and hemorrhage (Steiner 2010). Acute pancreatitis involves activation of zymogen granules to active pancreatic enzymes within the pancreatic tissue, resulting in some degree of pancreatic autodigestion (Glasgow and Mulvihill 2002). Enzymatic activity incites the complement cascade and degranulation of mast cells, leading to inflammatory mediator and free radical release, leukocyte chemotaxis, platelet aggregation, and local ischemia. Local and systemic inflammatory responses disrupt cell membranes, leading to hemorrhage and necrosis of acinar cells, increased capillary permeability, and pancreatic edema (Simpson 1993). Multiorgan failure may develop.

Risk factors

- Hypoperfusion of the pancreas and aggressive handling of the pancreas during surgery: Hypotension associated with general anesthesia, shock, or other comorbidities results in decreased systemic perfusion. Excessive surgical manipulation in the cranial abdomen may result in focal ischemia followed by reperfusion injury to the pancreas. (Matthiesen and Mullen 1990; Cappell 2008).
- History of previous surgery, especially emergency surgery
- Resection of an insulin-secreting β-cell neoplasm (Tryfonidou et al. 1998; Tobin et al. 1999)
- Duodenal or biliary reflux (Matthiesen and Mullen 1990; Yotsumoto et al. 1993)
- Obesity
- Diet (Lem et al. 2008)
- Breed (Steiner 2010)
- Concurrent endocrinopathies such as DM, hypothyroidism, and hyperadrenocorticism (Hess et al. 1999; Gaynor 2009)

Diagnosis

- **History** of anesthesia and surgery or one of the other above risk factors
- **Clinical signs** in dogs include anorexia, vomiting, weakness, depression, and diarrhea. Common clinical findings in cats include lethargy, anorexia, dehydration, and hypothermia.

- **Physical examination** may reveal pyrexia or abdominal discomfort (Williams and Steiner 2000; Williams 2001; Whittemore and Campbell 2005; Mix and Jones 2006; Xenoulis *et al.* 2008).
- The **complete blood count** often shows a neutrophilic leukocytosis with a left shift. Thrombocytopenia is common, and anemia may be seen in cats. Conversely, dehydrated patients may present with an elevated hematocrit caused by hemoconcentration. Serum biochemistry screening may show elevated liver enzymes or hyperbilirubinemia. Patients may be azotemic from prerenal or renal causes. Hyperglycemia reflects stress related increases in endogenous cortisol and catecholamines, especially in cats, or may be caused by overt DM. Hypocalcemia and hypomagnesemia secondary to pancreatic and peripancreatic fat saponification may be noted. Hypoalbuminemia, hypokalemia, hypercholesterolemia, and hypertriglyceridemia are possible. Assessing lipase and amylase levels is of little diagnostic value because neither is pancreas specific, being also produced in the GI tract and liver. Furthermore, both enzymes are excreted via the kidneys; patients with renal failure may show elevations in both enzymes (Whittemore and Campbell 2005; Mix and Jones 2006; Xenoulis *et al.* 2008).
- Although elevations in **trypsin-like immunoreactivity** (TLI) support a diagnosis of pancreatitis, elevations can also be seen with azotemia and GI disease in cats. TLI is normal in some patients with pancreatitis, and it is neither sensitive nor specific for pancreatitis (Steiner 2010; Cornell 2012).
- Species-specific **PLI** assays have been validated for both dogs and cats. PLI testing is highly sensitive and specific for pancreatitis and is not affected by renal disease or glucocorticoid administration (Steiner *et al.* 2003; Forman *et al.* 2004; Cornell 2012).
- **Abdominal radiography** may reveal signs supportive of a diagnosis of pancreatitis. In dogs, radiographic signs of pancreatitis include increased density or loss of detail in the right cranial abdomen, displacement of the descending duodenum to the right with widening of the pyloric angle, and caudal displacement of the transverse colon. In cats, signs include loss of abdominal detail, hepatomegaly, or small intestinal dilatation. (Hess *et al.* 1998; Saunders *et al.* 2002; Whittemore and Campbell 2005; Xenoulis *et al.* 2008).
- **Abdominal ultrasonography** is valuable to identify signs consistent with pancreatitis in dogs, although its value may be diminished in postoperative patients because of pneumoperitoneum. In dogs, the affected pancreas is often of mixed echogenicity; whereas hypoechoic areas are suggestive of pancreatic edema, necrosis, or abscessation, areas of fibrosis may appear hyperechoic (Newman *et al.* 2004) (Figure 62.1). The pancreas may be enlarged and smoothly or irregular marginated. The surrounding mesentery is often hyperechoic. Pancreatic fluid collections such as cysts or peripancreatic abdominal effusion appear anechoic or contain flocculent and echogenic debris. Pancreatic or biliary duct dilation or evidence of thrombosis or infarcts may be seen. All of these findings are less consistently noted in cats (Hess *et al.* 1998; Saunders *et al.* 2002).
- **Cytology** can provide supportive evidence of a diagnosis of postoperative pancreatitis. Ultrasound-guided fine-needle aspiration (FNA) of the pancreas may reveal inflammation, necrosis, or pancreatic infection.
- Laparoscopy can be performed to obtain **biopsy samples** of the right limb or body of the pancreas, which are readily accessible. The value of such a diagnostic should be weighed carefully because additional anesthesia and sample acquisition risk further

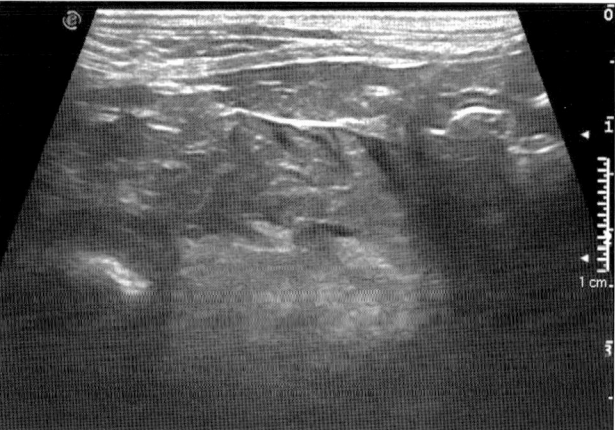

Figure 62.1 Pancreatitis. Note the hyperechoic mesentery adjacent to the pancreas and the lacy appearance of the pancreas from hypoechoic echoes consistent with pancreatic edema. *Source:* Reproduced with permission from Dr. R. O'Brien.

trauma to the pancreas from both anesthetic-induced hypotension and manipulation (Yotsumoto *et al.* 1993; Whittemore and Campbell 2005; Webb and Trott 2008).
- Limited information is available regarding the value of **computed tomography** (CT) in diagnosing pancreatitis. Further studies are needed to determine whether contrast-enhanced, helical CT performed under sedation may prove useful in the diagnosis of postoperative pancreatitis (Forman *et al.* 2004).

Treatment

- Whenever possible, the inciting cause of pancreatitis should be treated specifically. Concerning postoperative pancreatitis, this may not be possible. Postoperative therapeutic regimens should be assessed carefully for any drugs that might be linked to pancreatitis (Steiner 2010).
- **Aggressive fluid therapy** is the mainstay of treatment for pancreatitis because substantial fluid requirements may result from lack of intake, ongoing GI losses or fluid pooling caused by ileus, and third spacing caused by inflammatory responses and hypoproteinemia.
- **Electrolyte or acid–base imbalances** should be identified and corrected early (Whittemore and Campbell 2005; Mansfield 2008).
- **Feeding** nothing by mouth for 3 to 4 days has historically been recommended in all canine cases; however, such restrictions may only be indicated in patients with intractable vomiting. Patients that have received nothing per os (NPO) that have ceased vomiting may tolerate a slow return to full alimentation and begin to receive small amounts of water four to six times daily. A diet rich in carbohydrates and low in fat can be introduced after 24 hours. A dog should be maintained as NPO if vomiting does not cease or returns after the introduction of food. Although a jejunostomy or jejunostomy through gastrostomy (J through G) tube would most effectively bypass the pancreas and associated duct system, gastrostomy, esophagostomy, and nasoesophageal tubes may be placed and utilized in patients that are not vomiting (Whittemore and Campbell 2005; Mansfield 2008; Gaynor 2009).
- **Appropriate analgesia** may also help to decrease circulating levels of catecholamines, ensure comfortable ventilation, and protect against pain-related ileus and hypoperfusion (Whittemore and Campbell 2005; Mansfield 2008). Pure μ-agonist opioid

analgesics such as hydromorphone, methadone, fentanyl, and tramadol can be used in hospitalized patients. Opioids can also be combined with ketamine and local anesthetics such as lidocaine and given as a constant-rate infusion (CRI). Alternatively, α-antagonist medications such as dexmedetomidine or a combination of drugs can be used for pain management.

- **Antiemetics** are useful in treating nausea and vomiting and in preventing recurrence of clinical signs. Dolasetron (0.3–0.6 mg/kg subcutaneously [SC], orally [PO], or intravenously [IV] every 12–24 hours) and ondansetron (0.2 mg/kg PO every 12 hours) are both 5-HT3 antagonists that act centrally at the chemoreceptor trigger zone and medulla oblongata and locally within the GI tract to prevent vomiting. Maropitant is a neurokinin (NK1) agonist and can be given SC (1 mg/kg every 24 hours) or PO (2 mg/kg every 24 hours) (Dowling 2009; Willard 2009; Steiner 2010; Plumb 2011).
- **GI protectants,** including proton pump inhibitors (PPIs), H2 histamine blockers, and sucralfate, can also be given to ameliorate nausea and GI distress associated with pancreatitis (Willard 2009).
- Although studies in humans showed no benefit to patients with pancreatitis given **fresh-frozen plasma** (FFP), other studies have shown that in patients with pancreatitis depleted of α-macroglobulin, death ensues rapidly. The α-macroglobulin provided in FFP may help to scavenge activated digestive enzymes, and FFP is also a source of coagulation factors and albumin (Logan *et al.* 2001).
- The administration of **corticosteroids** has no proven benefit in patients with pancreatitis.
- The administration of **antibiotics** is controversial because no proven benefit has been shown in clinical animals (Gaynor 2009). However, in experimental models of acute pancreatitis, pancreatic infection was shown to occur as a result of bacterial spread from the colon. Other animal studies have shown a decrease in morbidity and mortality in patients treated with oral antibiotics effective against colonic bacteria or IV antibiotics with high pancreatic penetration. Further research is needed to determine whether antibiotic administration to reduce colonic bacterial numbers or protect the pancreas is routinely indicated.
- Debridement or drainage is indicated in patients that develop necrotic mass lesions, peripancreatic or pancreatic fluid accumulations, pancreatic infection, or persistent biliary obstruction (Coleman and Robson 2005; Son *et al.* 2010).

Outcome

The degree to which postoperative pancreatitis affects dogs and cats varies greatly, and dogs or cats with severe pancreatitis can experience complications that can lead to systemic inflammatory responses, multiorgan failure, and death (Ruaux 2000; Whittemore and Campbell 2005; Xenoulis *et al.* 2008). The authors are not aware of any reports discussing the prognosis for patients with postoperative pancreatitis, but many patients with mild to moderate clinical signs that receive appropriate supportive care recover well. Recurrent pancreatitis is possible.

Prevention

- Patients scheduled for anesthetic procedures should be well hydrated. Fluid and electrolyte imbalances should be corrected before anesthetic and surgical procedures whenever possible.
- Drugs that may cause hypotension should be used with caution, and anesthetized patients should be monitored closely and treated for hypotension.

- Surgeons should avoid aggressive handling of the pancreas or excessive manipulation in the cranial abdomen.
- Care should be taken to ligate pancreatic ducts from any portion of the pancreas to be excised.

Persistent or recurrent abscess

Definition

Pancreatic abscess is a circumscribed collection of purulent fluid and necrotic tissue within the pancreatic parenchyma, evident grossly as a firm to friable cavitated mass containing exudates, possibly extending into the adjacent tissues (Salisbury *et al.* 1988; Coleman and Robson 2005; Anderson *et al.* 2008). Most pancreatic abscesses reported in the veterinary literature are considered sterile because many do not culture positive for infecting bacteria (Johnson and Fann 2006; Anderson *et al.* 2008). Pancreatic abscess has not been definitively reported in cats.

Risk factors

- Although described most commonly as a sequela to pancreatitis, pancreatic abscess is reported to occur in only 1.4% to 6.5% of patients with pancreatitis (Coleman and Robson 2005). No additional risk factors have been identified.
- Abscesses may occur throughout the canine pancreas. No predilection for one area of the pancreas has been proven definitively, although one study reported an increased prevalence in the right lobe of the pancreas (Johnson and Fann 2006).

Diagnosis

- **Historical findings** include recent trauma or surgery or a confirmed diagnosis of pancreatitis or DM.
- **Clinical signs** are often nonspecific and include vomiting, weight loss, anorexia, lethargy, diarrhea, and melena.
- An abdominal mass may be palpated on **physical examination,** and the patient may be febrile or icteric.
- **Laboratory testing** often reveals leukocytosis with a left-shifted neutrophilia and signs of toxic change. Lymphopenia and anemia may be present. Patients may show elevations in liver enzyme values, hyperbilirubinemia, hyperglycemia, azotemia, hypocalcemia, and other electrolyte imbalances. PLI test results may be consistent with pancreatitis (Steiner *et al.* 2003).
- On **radiographic evaluation,** loss of abdominal serosal detail caused by generalized pancreatitis and peritonitis may be seen, and gas may be visible within the pancreas.
- **Ultrasonography** often reveals a mass lesion of the pancreas with focal hypoechoic areas suggestive of necrosis (Figure 62.2); abscesses may vary in size, shape, and echogenicity (Coleman and Robson 2005; Johnson and Fann 2006; Anderson *et al.* 2008).
- **FNA** may yield a diagnosis of suppurative inflammation or sepsis.
- Swabs of pancreatic tissue and peritoneal fluid accumulations should be submitted for **aerobic and anaerobic culture and sensitivity.** Although positive pancreatic cultures were obtained in only 15% to 25% of cases, peritoneal fluid cultures from 7 of 12 dogs did yield bacterial growth in one report (Anderson *et al.* 2008). *Escherichia coli, Enterococcus* spp., *Pseudomonas aeruginosa, Streptococcus* spp., *and Staphylococcus epidermidis* were most commonly isolated from patients with pancreatic abscesses.

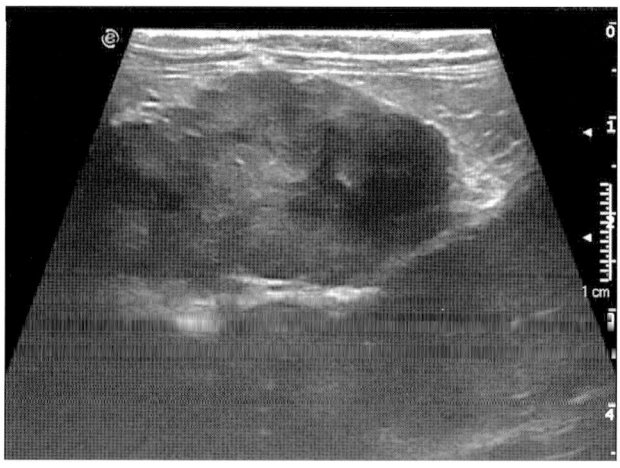

Figure 62.2 Pancreatic mass lesion. Note the mixed echogenicity of the mass and hypoechoic areas possibly indicative of necrosis. Fine-needle aspiration or biopsy is required to distinguish among causes of pancreatic mass lesions. *Source:* Reproduced with permission from Dr. R. O'Brien.

Treatment

- Surgery is recommended to diagnose and treat pancreatic abscesses. Intraoperative decision making is dictated by the location of the abscess and the degree of involvement of surrounding tissue. **Necrosectomy**, or debridement of necrotic tissue, can be performed. Necrosectomy or partial pancreatectomy alone may be sufficient to remove affected tissue. In addition, **partial pancreatectomy** may be performed or combined with duodenal resection and anastomosis or duodenal resection with gastroenterostomy and cholecystoenterostomy in cases of severe extension of disease or significant obstruction to biliary outflow. Patients that undergo necrosectomy benefit from omentalization of the area undergoing debridement and placement of an abdominal drain (Coleman and Robson 2005; Johnson and Fann 2006; Anderson *et al.* 2008; Thompson *et al.* 2009).
- Multiple samples for bacteriologic testing should be procured from the debrided tissue, pancreatic parenchyma, and peritoneal cavity.
- Judicious antibiotic therapy based on culture and sensitivity findings, fluid therapy and maintenance of electrolyte and acid–base balance, and nutritional support should be considered.
- Consideration should be given to feeding tube placement at the time of surgery (Whittemore and Campbell 2005; Mansfield 2008).

Outcome

- The reported survival rate of dogs undergoing surgery for pancreatic abscess ranges from 14 % to 55% (Stimson *et al.* 1998; Coleman and Robson 2005; Johnson and Fann 2006; Anderson *et al.* 2008). In one study of 36 dogs with confirmed purulent material on histopathology of the pancreas, elevated blood urea nitrogen (BUN) and serum alkaline phosphatase activity were associated with a poorer prognosis (Anderson *et al.* 2008).
- The outcome may be dependent on the method of treatment because one study reported 5 of 8 dogs treated with pancreatic debridement, omentalization, and abdominal closure survived, but only 1 of 4 dogs treated by open abdominal drainage survived (Johnson and Fann 2006). Additionally, closed-suction drainage has proven comparable efficacy to open abdominal drainage

and may result in less morbidity (Mueller *et al.* 2001; Staatz *et al.* 2002). In another study of dogs with pancreatic abscess treated by surgery, the method of closure did not influence the outcome (Stimson *et al.* 1998).

- Reported complications include cardiopulmonary arrest, hypoproteinemia, DM, EPI, and septic peritonitis. Some patients may require repeat debridement (Coleman and Robson 2005; Johnson and Fann 2006; Anderson *et al.* 2008).

Prevention

- Because significant risk factors for the development of pancreatic abscess have not been identified, prevention may not be possible.
- In an effort to prevent recurrent pancreatic abscess, surgeons should be careful to thoroughly debride necrotic lesions of the pancreas, perform culture and sensitivity testing on the debrided tissue and abdominal exudate, and treat any clinically significant infection identified. Histopathology of excised tissue may be helpful in identifying an underlying disease process or causative pathogens.

Biliary obstruction

Definition

Obstruction of the common bile duct related to diseases or surgery of the pancreas is termed extrahepatic biliary obstruction (EHBO). An obstruction may cause partial or complete disruption of flow of bile from the gallbladder, cystic duct, and hepatic ducts and may be intermittent or continuous (Mehler and Bennett 2006).

Risk factors

- Common pancreatic-related causes of EHBO include pancreatitis, pancreatic abscess, pancreatic pseudocyst, and pancreatic neoplasia (Cribb *et al.* 1988; Watt 1989; Fahie and Martin 1995; Mehler and Bennett 2006; Mayhew *et al.* 2002).
- Iatrogenic causes include any surgery that involves the right lobe of the pancreas in the area of the common bile duct or major duodenal papilla (Worley *et al.* 2004; Mehler and Bennett 2006).

Diagnosis

- **Clinical signs** include vomiting; inappetence; and lethargy; and physical examination findings such as pale or icteric mucous membranes, generalized icterus, and abdominal pain (Lehner and McAnulty 2010).
- **Serum biochemical evaluation** generally reveals hyperbilirubinemia and elevations of liver enzyme and cholesterol values. Leukocytosis and anemia may also be present.
- Additional evaluation of animals suspected of having pancreatitis or pancreatic-related EHBO should include **urinalysis, urine culture and sensitivity, thoracic radiography, evaluation of venous and arterial blood gases, lactate concentrations, and a complete coagulation profile.** Bilirubinuria may be an early sign of biliary obstruction, often present before clinical signs of icterus. With complete obstructions of the common bile duct, urobilinogen will be absent from the urine. Coagulation abnormalities indicative of disseminated intravascular coagulation (DIC) or hepatic dysfunction are common in patients with pancreatitis and EHBO (Fahie and Martin 1995; Lehner and McAnulty 2010).
- **Abdominal radiography** often shows decreased abdominal detail and an increased density in the right cranial abdominal

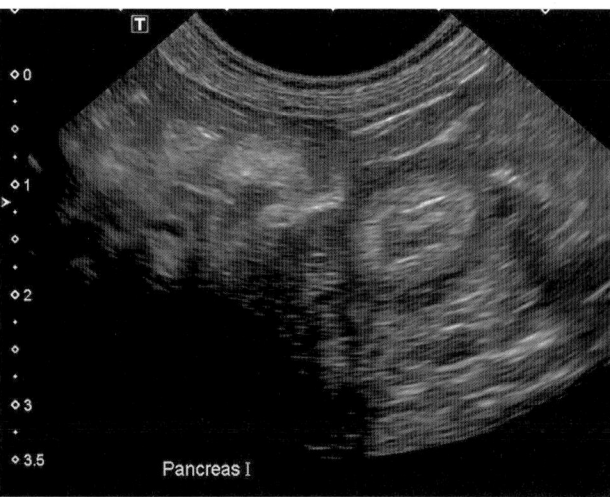

Figure 62.3 Pancreatitis. Note the hyperechoic mesentery adjacent to the pancreas. *Source:* Reproduced with permission from Dr. R. O'Brien.

quadrant associated with pancreatitis or peritonitis, displacement of the descending duodenum to the right with a widened pyloric angle, caudal displacement of the transverse colon, and gastric distension and ileus (Hess *et al.* 1998; Saunders *et al.* 2002; Whittemore and Campbell 2005; Xenoulis *et al.* 2008; Center, 2009).

- **Abdominal ultrasonography** can show a hypoechoic pancreas with hyperechoic adjacent mesentery if pancreatitis is present (Figure 62.3) (Hess *et al.* 1998; Saunders *et al.* 2002). Additionally, common bile duct distension (the normal common bile duct is approximately 2–3 mm in diameter in dogs and cats) would be expected to occur within 48 hours of obstruction and may be severe in cases of complete or near-complete EHBO. Hepatic duct dilatation soon follows, and distension of the intrahepatic bile ducts and gallbladder can also be seen. Choleliths may be seen as radiographic densities on plain radiographs or as shadowing artifacts on ultrasonography when pancreatic disease has resulted in long-standing biliary stasis and precipitation of bile salts and minerals. Serial ultrasonographic evaluation may reveal changes in distension of the biliary tree, although such distension does not necessarily indicate active obstruction; long-term persistence of distension can result from a previous obstructive episode. Moreover, a lack of distension does not preclude a diagnosis of biliary obstruction because chronic inflammation and fibrosis can result in inelasticity of the biliary tree (Herman *et al.* 2005; Kealy and McAllister 2005; Mehler and Bennett 2006; Gaillot *et al.* 2007; Center 2009).
- Bile and any regional fluid accumulations should be sampled via cholecystocentesis and abdominocentesis and **cytology and bacterial culture and sensitivity** performed as indicated (Center 2009).
- Although use of contrast-enhanced CT cholangiopancreatography is considered the gold standard in humans to identify pancreatic necrosis and pancreatic fluid collections, provide functional evaluation of the hepatobiliary system, and identify biliary leakage, this modality has not been used commonly in veterinary medicine for the diagnosis of pancreatic disease and EHBO (Spillman *et al.* 2000; Forman *et al.* 2004).

Treatment

- Treatment of patients with pancreatic-related EHBO depends on the underlying cause and degree of obstruction. Those with partial obstructions may be amenable to supportive care such as fluid therapy, correction of fluid and electrolyte imbalances, nutritional support, antiemetic therapy, and administration of GI protectants and choleretic medications such as ursodeoxycholic acid (15 mg/kg/day divided every 12 hours for both dogs and cats). Medications that aid in the support of liver health and prevention of fibrosis such as S-adenosyl-L-methionine (SAM-e) may be helpful (Gerhardt *et al.* 2001; Mehler and Bennett 2006; Plumb 2011).
- Percutaneous ultrasound-guided cholecystocentesis has been described as a noninvasive method of decompression of the biliary tree for use in patients with temporary or resolving EHBO. Complications associated with this procedure infrequently occur but may include bile leakage and subsequent peritonitis (Herman *et al.* 2005; Center, 2009).
- Near-complete and complete obstructions of the cystic and common bile duct warrant more aggressive intervention and exploratory surgery. Pathophysiologic consequences of EHBO that are particularly relevant to surgical patients include hypotension, decreased myocardial contractility, lack of response to vasopressor agents, acute renal failure, coagulopathy, GI hemorrhage, and delayed wound healing. Sterile or septic bile peritonitis may also result from rupture of a distended biliary tree or from necrotizing cholecystitis (Cribb *et al.* 1988; Watt 1989; Fahie and Martin 1995; Ludwig *et al.* 1997; Mehler *et al.* 2004; Mehler and Bennett 2006).
- Figure 62.4 highlights an algorithm to aid in decision making with regard to surgical treatment of pancreatic-related EHBO. If the gallbladder wall and biliary ducts are healthy, an attempt should be made to alleviate the obstruction via cholecystotomy, choledochotomy, or duodenotomy with or without placement of a choledochal stent. **Cholecystotomy** can be performed to remove bile crystals, mucus, or choleliths from an otherwise healthy gallbladder. **Choledochotomy** is not commonly performed because the wall of the common bile duct is often thin and friable and may be prone to dehiscence. The diameter of the duct may be too narrow to allow for safe incision and closure without risk of stricture or accidental obstruction with suture. However, if a single or few choleliths in the common bile duct are causing obstruction and cannot be flushed retrograde for retrieval by cholecystotomy or normograde for retrieval by sphincterotomy and if the common bile duct is sufficiently dilated, a choledochotomy may be performed. **Antimesenteric duodenotomy** 2 to 6 cm aboral to the pylorus may be performed to evaluate obstructions occurring at the level of the major duodenal papilla or those related to pancreatitis or pancreatic fluid accumulations (Cribb *et al.* 1988; Watt 1989; Fahie and Martin 1995; Ludwig *et al.* 1997; Mehler *et al.* 2004). Choleliths and other obstructions in the distal common bile duct at the papilla may be removed by sphincterotomy, which allows the obstruction to be removed from within the lumen of the duodenum. Duodenotomy also permits placement of a **choledochal stent** to allow for passive flow of bile around the stent. This is indicated when pancreatitis, accumulations of pancreatic fluid, or cholangiohepatitis have led to obstruction of the common bile duct by external compression. Palliation of malignancy is another potential indication for choledochal stenting (Mayhew *et al.* 2006).
- **Cholecystostomy tube placement** provides diversion of bile in cases of temporary obstruction to bile flow as might be expected with many pancreatic diseases. Cholecystostomy tube placement can be accomplished via an open surgical approach, via

Decision-making regarding EHBO

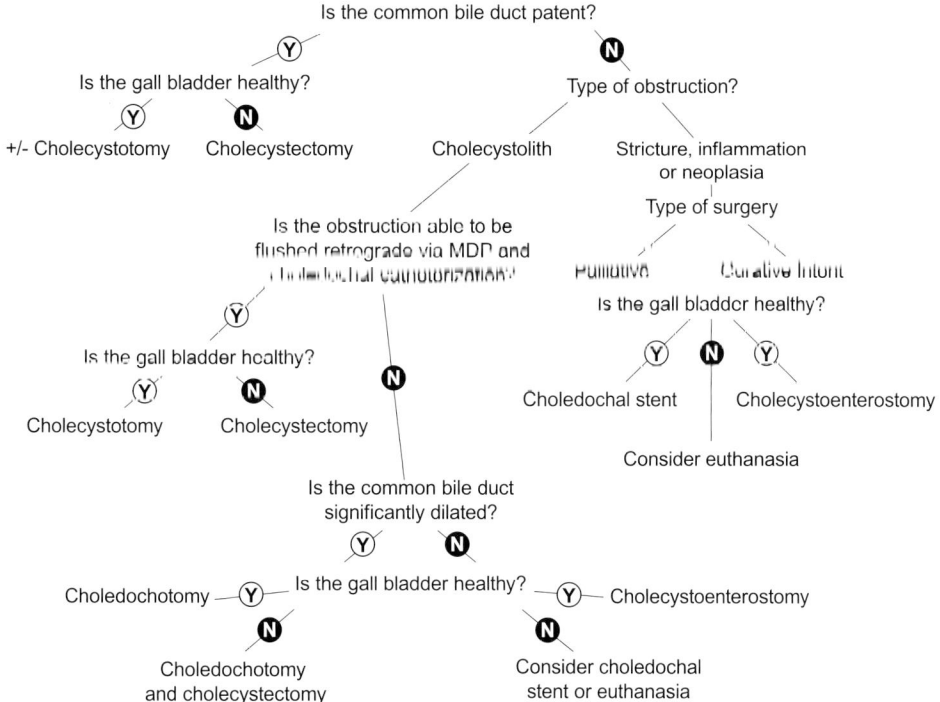

Figure 62.4 Algorithm for decision making with regard to surgical treatment of pancreatic-related extrahepatic biliary obstruction. MDP: major duodenal papilla.

percutaneous placement of a locking loop catheter with ultrasound guidance, or via a laparoscopic-assisted approach (Lehner and McAnulty 2010).

- Provided the gallbladder wall is healthy and the cystic and hepatic ducts are patent, a **cholecystoenterostomy** is indicated when an obstruction of the common bile duct is not able to be relieved by any of the aforementioned procedures or when obstruction would be expected to recur. Cholecystoduodenostomy and cholecystojejunostomy are methods used to reroute the flow of bile from the site of obstruction and into the intestinal lumen (Murphy *et al.* 2007; Papazoglou *et al.* 2008; Center 2009).
- The use of vitamins C and E, silymarin, and SAMe have been advocated to support hepatocytes and protect mitochondria from damage related to cholestasis. Although zinc and ursodeoxycholic acid may have antioxidant capabilities, ursodeoxycholic acid administration may be contraindicated in cases of bile duct obstruction because of the theoretical risk for increased bile flow in the face of obstruction. However, the exact effect of ursodeoxycholic acid on bile flow and biliary distension in patients with partial or complete EHBO has not been demonstrated. Antibiotic therapy should be dictated by the results of bacterial cultures of bile obtained by cholecystocentesis. Empiric therapy should be effective against *Escherichia coli and Enterococcus, Bacteroides, Streptococcus,* and *Clostridium* spp. (Wagner *et al.* 2007).

Outcome

- In the absence of cholelithiasis, patients with pancreatic-related EHBO may respond to supportive care and medical management. However, data evaluating the response of pancreatic disease-induced obstructions of the extrahepatic biliary system are lacking.

- **Cholecystotomy** is not commonly performed, and complications after its performance could include dehiscence or leakage of bile, causing bile peritonitis (Center 2009).
- **Choledochotomy** is also not commonly performed and anecdotally has been associated with a high rate of dehiscence. However, a recent report noted that only 1 of 9 dogs and cats experienced dehiscence of the choledochotomy site. All 9 animals were discharged from the hospital (Baker *et al.* 2011).
- A report of attempted ultrasound-guided cholecystostomy in 6 dogs revealed that placement of indwelling biliary catheters was not successful (McGahan *et al.* 1993). Placement may be more reliable with laparoscopic-assisted placement than with percutaneous placement with ultrasound guidance (Murphy *et al.* 2007). Complications associated with cholecystostomy tubes include premature obstruction and early dislodgement with subsequent bile leakage and bile peritonitis. Recent evidence suggests that successfully placed cholecystostomy tubes should remain in place for 3 to 4 weeks to allow adequate time for catheter tract maturation (Murphy *et al.* 2007; Lehner and McAnulty 2010).
- Complications of cholecystoenterostomy may include vomiting, persistent hypotension, pancreatitis, ileus, dehiscence and septic or bile peritonitis, stricture of the stoma leading to recurrence of clinical signs and ascending cholangiohepatitis, hepatic abscess, gastric ulceration, and hemorrhage. Cholecystoduodenostomy was initially associated with a good success rate in early reports of dogs treated for EHBO associated with pancreatitis (Watt 1989; Fahie and Martin 1995). However, in one recent study evaluating the survival of dogs with EHBO after cholecystoenterostomy, 6 of 15 dogs died within 20 days of surgery from causes related to the surgery or from underlying hepatobiliary or pancreatic disease. The most common cause of death was cardiac arrest

(Papazoglou *et al.* 2008). Although another recent report evaluating variables associated with outcome in dogs undergoing extrahepatic biliary surgery found that the type of surgical procedure performed was not associated with outcome, the authors did find that the highest perioperative mortality rate (50%) occurred in dogs with pancreatic disease-related EHBO (Mehler *et al.* 2004). Cholecystoduodenostomy is preferable to cholecystojejunostomy whenever possible because diversion of bile to sites of the intestine other than the duodenum has been shown to predispose to gastric acid oversecretion and GI ulceration.
- Surgery to treat EHBO has reportedly resulted in mortality rates of 28% to 64% in dogs and 40% to 100% in cats (Fahie and Martin 1995; Ludwig *et al.* 1997; Mayhew *et al.* 2002; Mehler *et al.* 2004). Patients surviving the postoperative period should be monitored carefully for signs of recurrence of EHBO and ascending cholangiohepatitis.

Prevention

Prevention of EHBO after pancreatic surgery may not be possible because the development of postoperative pancreatitis is thought to be common after pancreatic surgery. Because repeat bouts of acute pancreatitis or worsening severity of pancreatitis could result in increased peripancreatic fibrous connective tissue, prevention of postoperative pancreatitis or early diagnosis and treatment may prevent pancreatic surgery-related EHBO.

Septic peritonitis
See Chapter 4.

Hemorrhage
See Chapter 12.

Disruption of blood supply to adjacent organs

Definition
Disruption of the blood supply to adjacent organs during pancreatic surgery can occur because of the close proximity of the duodenum, stomach, omentum, mesentery, and spleen. Disruption of clinical significance would result in infarction or tissue necrosis.

Risk factors
- Tissue swelling and edema as in pancreatitis
- Vascular obstruction caused by neoplastic infiltration
- Disruption caused by vascular dissection or ligation during pancreatectomy or pancreatic biopsy, gastric or duodenal surgery, or splenic surgery (Allen *et al.* 1989; River and Monnet 2011)
- The main blood supply to the left limb of the pancreas is from branches of the splenic artery, hepatic artery, and gastroduodenal artery. Care must be taken during splenic surgery and surgery of the left limb of the pancreas to avoid collateral damage to these organs. The main blood supply to the right limb of the pancreas is from pancreatic branches of the cranial and caudal pancreaticoduodenal arteries that anastomose within the pancreatic tissue. The cranial pancreaticoduodenal artery is a terminal branch of the hepatic artery, and the caudal pancreaticoduodenal artery is a branch of the cranial mesenteric artery. These pancreaticoduodenal vessels also provide branches that supply the duodenum. Because of the proximity and shared blood supply of the right

limb of the pancreas and duodenum, care must be taken during both duodenal and pancreatic surgery to avoid devitalization of either organ (Rosin *et al.* 1972; Papachristou and Fortner 1980; Cobb and Merrell 1984).

Diagnosis
- Disruption in blood supply to the pancreas or an adjacent organ during surgery may be noted by the surgeon because changes to the appearance of the tissue quickly ensue. With obstructions to arterial flow, cyanosis of the organ may be grossly observed with infarcted tissue appearing distinct from well-perfused tissue by a line of demarcation. Swelling and darkening of the tissue may occur in cases of venous occlusion and congestion.
- After surgery, a diagnosis of lack of perfusion to the pancreas or an adjacent organ may be diagnosed by Doppler-assisted ultrasonography or selective or nonselective angiography with fluoroscopy.

Treatment
- Obstruction of the splenic artery or vein or branches requires splenectomy or partial splenectomy (Cornell 2012).
- Apparent disruption of blood supply may not always require treatment. Although duodenal cyanosis was reported to occur routinely with one described technique for partial right limb pancreatectomy, duodenal necrosis did not occur (Papachristou and Fortner 1980).
- When partial or total pancreatectomy is required and the duodenal blood supply cannot be preserved, pancreaticoduodenectomy can be considered (Cornell 2012). Cholecystoenterostomy and gastroenterostomy are required to establish biliary and GI patency, respectively. However, these procedures are associated with significant morbidity and mortality and are not often recommended (Matthiesen 1989; Mehler *et al.* 2004; Amsellem *et al.* 2006; Papazoglou *et al.* 2008).

Outcome
- The prognosis after splenectomy is generally good (Spangler and Kass 1997).
- Additional pancreatic debridement or partial or total pancreatectomy may be needed if portions of the pancreas experience devitalization after surgery. Pancreatic abscess and necrotizing pancreatitis may ensue. After total pancreatectomy, EPI and DM result and must be treated (Rosin *et al.* 1972).
- Patients undergoing cholecystoenterostomy may experience dehiscence and bile peritonitis as well as ascending infection and cholangiohepatitis after surgery. After gastroenterostomy, patients may experience vomiting, nausea, inappetence, diarrhea, weight loss, pancreatitis, and GI ulceration and bleeding. Morbidity and mortality are common after this procedure (Papazoglou *et al.* 2008; Eisele *et al.* 2010).

Prevention
- Surgeons must be intimately familiar with the vascular and relative anatomy of the involved tissues.
- Surgeons should dissect carefully and observe regularly during surgery for any signs of vascular damage to tissues.
- Because the proximity and shared blood supply of the duodenum and pancreas make right limb pancreatectomy or duodenectomy difficult, techniques for pancreatectomy that preserve the duodenal vasculature as much as possible should be used. One technique uses avulsion and blunt dissection of the pancreatic

tissue from the pancreaticoduodenal vessels to maintain blood supply to the duodenum (Cornell 2012). Descriptions of another technique purport a collateral supply to the duodenum from the recurrent duodenal branch of the right gastroepiploic artery, which reportedly provides adequate blood flow to the proximal duodenum after the cranial pancreaticoduodenal artery has been ligated (Cobb and Merrell 1984). A third technique routinely results in cyanosis of the duodenum but does not lead to duodenal necrosis. With this technique, as much duodenal blood supply as possible is maintained by ligation and transection of the anastomotic branches of the cranial and caudal pancreaticoduodenal arteries supplying only pancreatic tissue (Papachristou and Fortner 1990).

Disruption of the duct system and occlusion

Definition

Disruption of the pancreatic duct system is any disturbance in the integrity of the pancreatic ducts such as transection or avulsion that results in pancreatic fluid and enzyme leakage (VanEnkevort 1999; Marchevsky *et al.* 2000; Coleman and Robson 2005; Cornell 2012). Pancreatic pseudocysts may result from pancreatic duct disruption secondary to acute or chronic postoperative pancreatitis or pancreatic trauma (Coleman and Robson 2005). Pseudocysts form as pancreatic enzymes and necrotic tissue collect within or adjacent to the pancreas and become surrounded by inflamed peritoneal, mesenteric, or serosal membranes, which form a thick fibrous, nonepithelialized sac (Figure 62.5) (VanEnkevort 1999; Marchevsky *et al.* 2000). The resultant pseudocyst is usually rich in pancreatic enzymes and sterile. Occlusion of the pancreatic duct system may also occur iatrogenically by ligation or by postoperative pancreatitis-induced edema or necrosis of surrounding pancreatic parenchyma (VanEnkevort 1999; Marchevsky *et al.* 2000; Coleman and Robson 2005).

Risk factors
- Pancreatic biopsy and partial pancreatectomy
- Resection of focal nodular neoplastic disease of the pancreas
- Necrosectomy for pancreatic abscess or necrotizing pancreatitis

Diagnosis
- **Clinical manifestations** of pancreatic pseudocyst include abdominal pain, nausea, vomiting, diarrhea, weight loss, anorexia, fever, ascites, and a palpable abdominal mass. With enlarging pseudocysts, signs of bile duct compression may occur, including icterus. Hemorrhage into the GI tract or peritoneal cavity may occur from erosion of blood vessels in adjacent organs. Pseudocysts that become infected could form abscesses, which may lead to focal or diffuse peritonitis. Pancreatic pseudocyst formation should be suspected if clinical signs of pancreatitis fail to resolve after appropriate treatment or continue after apparent resolution (Coleman and Robson 2005).
- **Abdominal radiography** may reveal a mass lesion in the area of the pancreas, causing displacement of the stomach and colon (VanEnkevort 1999)
- **Ultrasonography** may show anechoic to slightly echoic cystlike lesions with distal acoustic enhancement in the region of the pancreas. Pseudocysts may be solitary or multiple and occur in the left or right lobes or body of the pancreas (Figure 62.6). Pancreatic parenchyma adjacent to the pseudocysts may be hypoechoic and the surrounding omentum and mesenteric fat hyperechoic, findings consistent with concurrent pancreatitis. Evidence of biliary obstruction may be seen (VanEnkevort 1999).
- In humans, **CT** is able to differentiate pseudocysts from other pancreatic mass lesions, including abscess and cystic neoplasia, and may be considered for diagnosis in dogs (Coleman and Robson 2005).
- **Ultrasound-guided aspiration of the pseudocyst** can be both diagnostic and therapeutic, although leakage of luminal contents may occur after aspiration. Pseudocyst fluid is generally thin but may be viscous with necrotic debris. Grossly, the fluid ranges from colorless to blood tinged or even green-tinged when bile pigment is present. **Fluid analysis** may reveal a transudate, modified transudate, or exudate, the latter seen most often in cases of secondary infection. Cytologically, aspirated fluid may be acellular or show a mixed inflammatory response of neutrophils and macrophages in more mature pseudocysts. Scant epithelial cells, fibroblasts, and reactive mesothelial cells may also be present (VanEnkevort 1999). **Bacterial culture** results are negative unless

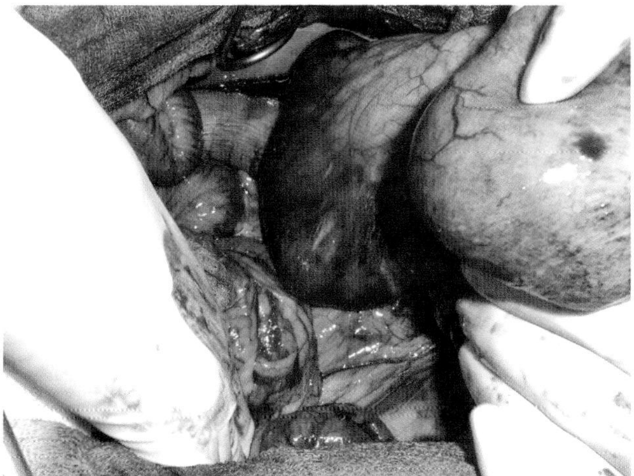

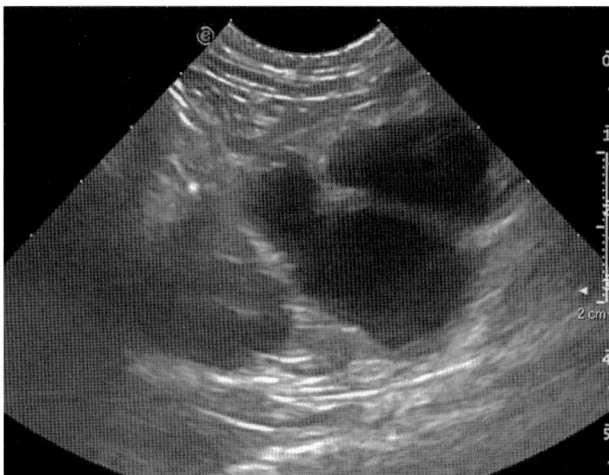

Figure 62.5 Intraoperative photograph of a pancreatic pseudocyst of the left limb of the pancreas. A collection of fluid encased within peritoneal membranes is apparent.

Figure 62.6 Pancreatic pseudocyst. Multiple cysts appear on ultrasonography as anechoic to slightly echogenic areas with distal acoustic enhancement. *Source:* Reproduced with permission from Dr. R. O'Brien.

secondary infection has occurred. **Pancreatic proteolytic enzymatic levels** such as those of amylase and lipase are often elevated in pancreatic pseudocyst fluid up to 3 to 60 times those noted in serum. In humans, a fluid amylase concentration greater than 5000 U/mL has been reported to be 94% sensitive and 74% specific for a diagnosis of pancreatic pseudocyst, helping to differentiate pseudocysts from cystic tumors, which tend to have lower amylase and other proteolytic enzyme concentrations (Coleman and Robson 2005).

Treatment

- Ultrasound-guided or CT-guided percutaneous drainage is simple, minimally invasive, and inexpensive, and few to no procedural complications have been reported in dogs and cats, although repeated aspiration may be required (Smith and Biller 1998).
- Surgical intervention is recommended for cysts that are larger than 3 cm in size, those that have persisted for longer than 6 weeks or are secondarily infected, and those that are causing clinical signs and have failed to resolve spontaneously or with repeated aspiration. Surgical treatment options include cystogastrostomy, cystoenterostomy, excision with omentalization, and external drainage (Marchevsky 2000; Jerram et al. 2004; Coleman and Robson 2005; Cornell 2012). It is recommended that surgical internal drainage be delayed for 6 weeks to allow a fibrous lining to form around the pseudocyst that is durable and amenable to creation of a draining stoma. External drainage can be provided at any time by placement of a closed-suction drain exteriorized lateral to the abdominal incision (Cornell 2012). However, abdominal sepsis has been reported to occur commonly after external drainage (VanEnkevort 1999).
- For excision with omentalization, as much as possible of the cavity wall should be excised. Any adhesions causing compartmentalization of the pseudocyst should be manually or sharply broken down to create a unicompartmental cavity. Excised samples of pseudocyst wall should be submitted for histopathology. After aggressive lavage with sterile saline and suction, the cavity is packed with omentum and the omentum tacked to the pseudocyst wall with several interrupted sutures of 3-0 or 4-0 polydioxanone (Jerram et al. 2004).

Outcome

- Few reports of pancreatic pseudocyst diagnosis and treatment exist in the veterinary literature. Of the reported cases of canine and feline pancreatic pseudocysts treated by ultrasound-guided percutaneous aspiration, surgical excision, or internal or external drainage with or without omentalization, more than 75% of patients were treated successfully and survived. However, frequent complications associated with pseudocyst development include secondary infection, rupture, and hemorrhage (Bellenger et al. 1989; Smith and Biller 1998; VanEnkevort 1999; Jerram et al. 2004; Coleman and Robson 2005).
- Calcification of the pseudocyst, increasing size, lack of reduction in size, and communication with a pancreatic duct are poor prognostic indicators (VanEnkevort 1999; Coleman and Robson 2005).
- In one report evaluating ultrasonographic and clinicopathologic findings in pancreatic pseudocysts in four dogs and two cats, three dogs were able to be managed conservatively with aspiration; leakage of pseudocyst fluid was not noted, and the dogs were clinically normal 1.5 to 4 years after presentation. Both cats died

within 2 months of diagnosis, and the authors concluded that cats may be more susceptible to the effects of concurrent pancreatitis (VanEnkevort 1999).
- The successful management of pancreatic pseudocysts with internal drainage using cystogastrostomy has been described in two dogs (Bellenger et al. 1989). Although internal drainage using endoscopic and surgical cystoenterostomy has shown low recurrence rates and few complications in humans, cystoenterostomy has been associated with higher mortality rates in the few cases reported in the veterinary literature (Coleman and Robson 2005).
- Debridement and omentalization of pancreatic pseudocysts has been reported to be successful and without complication in dogs (Jerram et al. 2004).

Prevention

- Prevention of pancreatic duct disruption or occlusion is best achieved by avoidance of trauma to the pancreatic ducts. It is recommended that the pancreatic duct system and blood vessels to portions of the pancreas to be resected be ligated during surgery to prevent both hemorrhage and the leakage of proteolytic enzymes. In one report comparing the suture fracture technique and the dissection and ligation technique of partial pancreatectomy, both techniques accomplished the aforementioned goals (Allen et al. 1989).
- Pancreatic biopsy should be performed at the distal aspect of the right limb of the pancreas because this area is more readily accessible and distant from the pancreatic duct system, and its vascular supply is not shared by neighboring organs (Cornell 2012). If a nodular neoplasm is to be removed from the pancreas, partial pancreatectomy of the portion of the pancreas containing the nodule and the entire pancreas distal to the nodule should be performed because focal resection, or enucleation, of a proximal nodule may result in disruption of the duct system and blood supply to the distal pancreas.

Decreased gastrointestinal motility

Definition

Decreased GI motility is defined as an increase in GI transit time of ingesta, resulting in decreased gastric emptying and small intestinal stasis (Dowling 2009).

Risk factors

- Disorders of the pancreas, pancreatic surgery, and surgery-related complications
- Infectious and inflammatory conditions such as pancreatitis and peritonitis can cause primary myenteric neuronal or gastric smooth muscle dysfunction and incoordination, resulting in decreased gastric propulsion and gastroparesis (Guilford 1990).
- Electrolyte and acid–base imbalances resulting from vomiting, diarrhea, and inappetence can cause secondary delayed gastric emptying (Washabau 2003).
- Anesthetic and pain medications such as cholinergic antagonists, adrenergic agonists, and opioid receptor agonists contribute to decreased GI motility (Washabau 2003; Dowling 2009).

Diagnosis

- **Clinical signs** such as excessive salivation, licking of lips, eructation, inappetence, vomiting, or regurgitation may be indicative of decreased gastric emptying and small intestinal ileus.

- **Physical examination findings** may include signs of nausea or pain on abdominal palpation or lack of borborygmus on abdominal auscultation.
- **Abdominal radiography** shows a gas or ingesta-distended stomach and intestinal loops dilated with gas.
- **Abdominal ultrasonography** readily identifies lack of GI peristalsis and may help to characterize any underlying pancreatic-related causes.

Treatment

- Treatment of the underlying primary cause
- Because serotonin-laden enterochromaffin cells in the GI tract serve as sensory transducers that coordinate enteric neurotransmission, serotonergic drugs may be used to treat intestinal myenteric disorders. Antagonism of the 5HT-3 serotonin receptor inhibits nausea and induction of vomiting caused by suppression of visceral hypersensitivity. Conversely, agonism of the 5HT-4 serotonin receptor responsible for acetylcholine-dependent–enhanced neurotransmission promotes propulsive peristaltic and secretory activity. Metoclopramide is a peripheral 5HT-3 receptor antagonist and 5HT-4 receptor agonist and acts to coordinate esophageal, gastric, pyloric, and duodenal peristaltic activity. However, metoclopramide is also a dopaminergic antagonist; antagonism of dopamine receptors may not be desirable in patients with pancreatitis. Metoclopramide may be given PO or SC at dosages of 0.2 to 0.4 mg/kg every 8 hours or as a slow IV infusion at a rate of 0.01 to 0.02 mg/kg/hr or 1 to 2 mg/kg/day (Dowling 2009; Plumb 2011).
- Ranitidine is a histamine-2 receptor antagonist that inhibits gastric acid secretion in dogs and cats. Its inhibition of acetylcholinesterase also results in prokinetic activity. Ranitidine administered at a dose of 1 to 2 mg/kg PO, SC, or IV inhibits gastric acid secretion and promotes gastric emptying (Dowling 2009; Willard 2009; Plumb 2011). Famotidine is also a histamine-2 receptor antagonist but does not inhibit acetylcholinesterase activity and therefore does not exhibit prokinetic activity. Its ability to inhibit gastric acid secretion, however, warrants its use in cases with pancreatic-related GI disease. It may be administered PO, SC, or IV at a dosage of 0.25 to 0.5 mg/kg every 12 to 24 hours (Willard 2009; Plumb 2011).
- Although not prokinetic, specific 5HT-3 receptor antagonists such as ondansetron and dolasetron may be used to manage GI distress in patients with pancreatic-related disturbances (Steiner 2010).
- Other GI protectants without prokinetic activity may be considered for their positive effects of decreasing gastric acid production and protection of the gastric mucosal barrier. These include PPIs such as omeprazole (0.7–1 mg/kg PO every 24 hours) and esomeprazole (0.7 mg/kg IV every 24 hours), prostaglandin analogs such as misoprostol (2–5 µg/kg PO every 6–12 hours), and locally acting barrier medications such as sucralfate (0.25–1g PO every 6–12 hours) (Plumb 2011).
- A route for enteral feeding should be provided unless contraindicated. If a patient is unwilling to take food by mouth, a nasoesophageal or esophagostomy tube may be placed during the same anesthetic as the primary surgery or after surgery. Consideration should be given to the placement of a gastric tube (G-tube), jejunostomy tube (J-tube), or J-through G tube at the time of initial surgery (Mansfield 2008).

Outcome

Disorders of GI motility are common in dogs and cats with pancreatic disease. The outcome depends on resolution of the underlying pancreatic-related disorder. However, untreated, decreased GI motility negatively impacts the patient by contributing to vomiting and regurgitation, which in turn contribute to electrolyte and acid–base disturbances. Gastric and intestinal stasis also prolong hospitalization; impair the clinician's ability to provide adequate nutrition via alimentation; and may contribute to secondary infectious complications such as aspiration pneumonia, small intestinal bacterial overgrowth, absorption of endotoxin, and even septicemia (Washabau 2003; Dowling 2009; Willard 2009).

Prevention

- Early and judicious use of GI protectants and prokinetic agents
- Close monitoring of the postoperative patient after surgery for pancreatic-related disease allows for early recognition of symptoms of ileus and appropriate and timely intervention.

Diabetes mellitus after pancreatectomy

Definition

Diabetes mellitus is a collection of conditions in which there is a deficiency of the pancreatic islet cell–produced hormone insulin or there is insensitivity to insulin. Absolute or relative insulin deficiency leads to increased hepatic gluconeogenesis and glycogenolysis; decreased tissue uptake and utilization of glucose; and accumulation of glucose in the bloodstream, or hyperglycemia. Although insulin-dependent DM, type I DM, is most common in dogs, type II DM, for which insulin resistance is the postulated mechanism of hyperglycemia, is more common in cats (Nelson 2010; Reusch 2010).

Risk factors

- Although the true incidence of DM after pancreatic surgery or after pancreatitis is unknown, one report documented the development of DM in 3 of 37 dogs treated with medical or surgical management for acute necrotizing pancreatitis (Thompson et al. 2009). An association between acute necrotizing pancreatitis and DM has also been shown in cats, especially with progression to chronic nonsuppurative pancreatitis (Whittemore and Campbell 2005; Xenoulis et al. 2008).
- Complete pancreatectomy has not been commonly performed in clinical dogs and cats; therefore, definitive data on the development of DM after complete pancreatectomy are lacking (Cornell and Fischer 2003; Cornell 2012). It is proposed that EPI may develop when more than 80% to 90% of pancreatic tissue is resected (DiMagno 1973; Kyles 2003).

Diagnosis

- **Clinical signs** attributable to hyperglycemia and glucosuria, such as polydipsia, polyuria, and polyphagia, often accompanied by weight loss
- Although no absolute **value of hyperglycemia** is diagnostic for DM in dogs or cats, repeated blood glucose levels of greater than 180 to 200 mg/dL in dogs and greater than 200 to 250 mg/dL in cats should prompt concern and further investigation (Hoenig 2002). Stress hyperglycemia is common in cats and can induce hyperglycemia as significant as 400 to 500 mg/dL (Laluha et al. 2004). Repeated measurements may help to ensure accuracy, although many cats remain stressed while hospitalized. **Serum fructosamine measurements** may be helpful (Reusch 2010).
- Urine reagent test strips allow for **assessment of glucosuria and ketonuria**. Documenting persistent hyperglycemia concurrent

with glucosuria is imperative in making an accurate diagnosis of DM because both hyperglycemia and glucosuria may occur independently in patients that do not have true DM.

Treatment

- The goals of therapy are to eliminate the clinical signs of polyuria, polydipsia, polyphagia, and weight loss.
- Although normalizing blood glucose is a worthy goal, normalization may not be possible, and hypoglycemic crises may occur with overzealous focus on maintaining blood glucose values within the reference range.
- A multimodal approach to therapy produces the best results, with attention to consistent and accurate insulin therapy and feeding and medication schedules, prevention and control of concurrent disorders that may cause hyperglycemia and promote insulin resistance, and diet and exercise (Reusch 2010; Steiner 2010).

Outcome

- Routine blood and urine testing is necessary.
- Complications include hypoglycemia and neuroglycopenia; cataract and blindness; pancreatitis; recurrent infections, especially of the skin and urinary tract; neuropathy; nephropathy; and diabetic ketoacidosis.
- Median survival time (MST) for most dogs diagnosed with DM is 2 to 3 years from the time of diagnosis, with increased mortality rate observed during the first 6 months after diagnosis. During this time, life-threatening ketoacidosis, renal failure, or pancreatitis is more common (Steiner 2010).
- The outcome largely depends on the underlying cause of DM; in patients with concurrent pancreatic disorders such as pancreatitis or those having undergone partial or total pancreatectomy, the prognosis is likely more grave than for patients with other causes of DM.

Prevention

- Prevention of DM associated with pancreatectomy for β-cell neoplasia or other significant pancreatic disease may not be possible. Loss of pancreatic tissue by inflammation and replacement with fibrous tissue, acute necrotizing pancreatitis, resection by partial or total pancreatectomy, or damage to pancreatic ducts or blood supply may be unavoidable in treatment of various pancreatic conditions.
- Prevention should focus on obtaining an accurate diagnosis of pancreatic disease, adequate preoperative stabilization of surgical patients, gentle handling of the pancreas and cranial abdominal organs during surgery, accurate hemostasis, resection of only as much pancreatic tissue as necessary, and ligation of only the blood supply and pancreatic ducts of the portion of tissue to be resected.
- Patients should undergo close observation for recurrence or worsening of hyperglycemia; development of glucosuria or ketonuria; and clinical signs of concurrent inflammatory, infectious, endocrine, or neoplastic disorders.

Exocrine pancreatic insufficiency

Definition

Exocrine pancreatic insufficiency is a syndrome characterized by severe weight loss, loose stools, and other GI disturbances that occurs because of insufficient synthesis or secretion of pancreatic enzymes. All pancreatic digestive enzymes or only a single enzyme may be lacking (Xenoulis et al. 2007).

Risk factors

- Acute necrotizing or chronic pancreatitis
- Neoplastic pancreatic duct obstructions
- Inflammation
- Accidental ligation
- Partial or complete pancreatectomy

Diagnosis

- The most common **clinical sign** is weight loss, often accompanied by an increased appetite and loose stools. Patients may exhibit flatulence and borborygmus, coprophagia, and pica (Westermarck and Wiberg 2003).
- **Serum testing of TLI** is the gold standard, being highly sensitive and specific for the diagnosis of EPI. Patients that have EPI, however, may demonstrate normal TLI test results in two situations, that is, when a single enzyme deficiency is present or when the pancreatic duct system is obstructed (Steiner et al. 2006).
- Additional testing can be performed to rule out the above two scenarios. A serum assay for the **measurement of canine- or feline-specific PLI** can be performed. The test is highly species specific and sensitive and measures the mass concentration of pancreatic lipase in serum (Steiner et al. 2003; Xenoulis et al. 2007).
- A fecal assay for **pancreatic elastase** has also been developed but is not yet widely used (Spillman et al. 2001).
- **Abdominal ultrasonography** should be performed to assess for the presence of a mass effect in the area of the pancreatic duct(s), potentially causing obstruction.

Treatment

- Exocrine pancreatic enzyme replacement therapy: Although tablets and capsules are also available, the most popular and effective treatment uses dried, powdered extract from beef or pork pancreas. One teaspoon of dried extract per 10 kg of patient body weight is given each meal. Alternatively, fresh, raw bovine, porcine, ovine, or game species' pancreata may replace dried pancreatic extract at a dose of 30 to 90 g of raw pancreas per 1 tsp of dried powdered supplement. However, because raw pancreata may contain life-threatening parasite infestations, use of the dried extract supplement is preferred (Westermarck and Wiberg 2003).
- Experimental and retrospective studies have failed to show a benefit to the convention of feeding a low-fat diet to patients with EPI; restriction of dietary fat may predispose to deficiencies of fat-soluble vitamins A, D, E, and K and the development of associated clinical signs (Batchelor et al. 2007).
- Cobalamin deficiency may accompany EPI and contributes to a worse prognosis; supplementation of cobalamin is imperative for these patients.
- A high-quality maintenance diet low in fiber should be fed.
- Treatment for obstructive disease should be pursued in patients with obstruction of the pancreatic duct system.
- Patients should be rigorously monitored for ongoing weight loss, vitamin and other nutritional deficiencies, stool quality, and quality of life.

Outcome

- Spontaneous resolution of EPI is very rare; lifelong therapy is expected to be required. With appropriate management and attention, many dogs with EPI can achieve a normal life expectancy (Steiner 2010).

- Concurrent cobalamin deficiency may impact outcome and survival negatively; therefore, all patients diagnosed with EPI should undergo evaluation of serum cobalamin levels.
- Concurrent DM may be noted in patients with chronic or significant pancreatitis or requiring extensive pancreatic resection (Pairent *et al.* 1969; Simpson *et al.* 1991; Wasserman *et al.* 1993).

Prevention

- Iatrogenic EPI may be a consequence of adequate resection of diseased tissue in cases requiring pancreatectomy (DiMagno 1973; Kyles 2003).
- However, care should be taken in handling the pancreas and in maintaining adequate perfusion during surgery and anesthetic procedures to prevent postoperative pancreatitis.
- Care should be taken to avoid accidental ligation of the pancreatic duct system or other injury to the pancreas.

Perioperative hypoglycemia

Definition

Perioperative hypoglycemia is defined as a blood glucose level less than normal (60 mg/dL) during the hospitalization period of insulinoma resection surgery (Dunn *et al.* 1992).

Risk factors

- Poor medical management of hypoglycemic patients before anesthesia or the persistence of severe hypoglycemia despite adequate medical management (Kyles 2003; Cornell 2012)
- Patients with concurrent endocrine disorders such as hypoadrenocorticism or hypopituitarism or those with concurrent conditions such as liver disease, sepsis, malnutrition, or pregnancy may be at increased risk for perioperative hypoglycemia (Hess 2010).
- A small or fasted patient may also be at greater risk of hypoglycemia.

Diagnosis

Serial serum or whole-blood glucose monitoring should be performed every 15 minutes to 1 to 2 hours during the perioperative period to ensure adequate glycemic control (Hess 2010).

Treatment

- During acute hypoglycemic crises, dextrose may be given as an IV bolus, as a CRI, or both; however, dextrose administration may trigger insulin release and cause worsening hypoglycemia. Dextrose may be given as a bolus at a dose of 0.25 to 0.5 g/kg diluted 1:3 with sterile 0.9% saline and given slowly over 5 to 10 minutes. A CRI of 2.5% to 5% dextrose may be administered in sterile water or saline. Dextrose can be administered in concentrations up to 10%; concentrations higher than 5%, however, must be given via a central vein by placement of a central venous catheter to avoid causing peripheral venous phlebitis (Kraje 2003; Hess 2010).
- If dextrose administration fails to restore euglycemia, dexamethasone (0.1 mg/kg every 12 hours) or the synthetic somatostatin analogue, octreotide (10–50 mcg SC every 8–12 hours) may be administered IV (Kraje 2003; Polton *et al.* 2007; Cornell 2012).
- If persistent hypoglycemia and neuroglycopenia result in tremor or focal or grand mal seizures, sedation with diazepam or propofol may be required (Polton *et al.* 2007).

- Glucagon may be given as a CRI (5–13 ng/kg/min +/− 10% dextrose infusion); if successful, clinical signs and hypoglycemia may resolve within 1 hour. Similar to dextrose, however, glucagon administration may trigger insulin secretion and lead to persistent hypoglycemia. Patients receiving dextrose and glucagon should be monitored carefully (Fischer *et al.* 2000).

Outcome

Patients with perioperative hypoglycemia are generally well managed by a combination of the methods described with intensive care and monitoring. Long-term resolution of hypoglycemia depends on patient variables, method of treatment, and response to therapy.

Prevention

- Fasting of hypoglycemic patients should be avoided.
- Drugs that may induce hypoglycemia should be avoided; these include the oral hypoglycemic sulfonylurea, and salicylates, β-agonists or antagonists, angiotensin-converting enzyme inhibitors, antibiotics such as tetracyclines, and tricyclic antidepressants (Hess 2010).
- Placement of a central venous catheter is highly recommended and permits intensive perioperative blood pressure monitoring, drawing of repeated samples for blood glucose and other testing, and administration of high concentrations of dextrose if required.

Persistent hypoglycemia

Definition

Persistent hypoglycemia is defined as a blood glucose level lower than 60 mg/dL with or without clinical signs in a well-nourished, nonfasted patient after surgery to resect an insulin-secreting β-cell neoplasm (Figure 62.7) (Dunn *et al.* 1992).

Risk factors

- Incomplete resection of the primary tumor or metastatic lesions
- Recurrence of the primary tumor
- Spread of metastases.

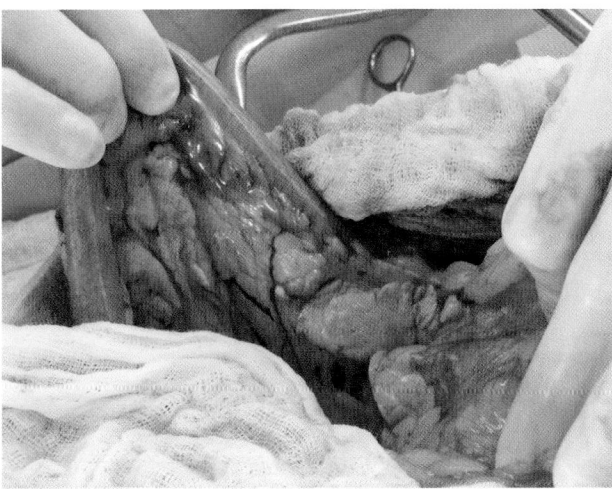

Figure 62.7 Intraoperative photograph of a pancreatic mass lesion of the right limb of the pancreas. Histologic evaluation revealed an insulin-secreting β-cell neoplasm of the pancreas, insulinoma.

Diagnosis

- Recognition of associated **clinical signs**, coupled with **confirmation of hypoglycemia** (<60 mg/dL) **and concurrent hyperinsulinemia** (>20–26 µU/mL) raises the index of suspicion for persistence of an insulin-secreting β-cell neoplasm (Dunn *et al.* 1992; Kyles 2003; Cornell 2012).
- **Abdominal ultrasonography** may be a useful tool to confirm and characterize a pancreatic lesion and assess for the presence of any suspect metastatic lesions, but it may lack sensitivity, especially in the postoperative patient (Robben *et al.* 2005).
- Recent information suggests **abdominal CT** may be useful in localizing an insulinoma lesion (Figure 62.8) (Iseri *et al.* 2007).

Treatment

- The treatment of choice for insulinoma is surgical resection of as much gross tumor as possible, including the primary tumor and suspected metastases (Tryfonidou *et al.* 1998; Tobin *et al.* 1999; Polton *et al.* 2007; Cornell 2012).
- When surgery has failed to resolve hypoglycemia, medical therapy options can be divided into those that are cytotoxic to insulin-secreting neoplastic β cells and those that help to control hypoglycemia (Hess 2010).
- Patients should be fed small, frequent meals of a diet rich in complex carbohydrates and proteins; simple sugars should be avoided because of their tendency to cause insulin release.
- Prednisone may be given as described earlier.
- Diazoxide (10–40 mg/kg/day divided every 8–12 hours) is a benzothiadiazine derivative that prevents depolarization of β cells and causes decreased exocytosis of secretory vesicles containing insulin. It also increases blood glucose concentrations by increasing gluconeogenesis and glycogenolysis and decreasing tissue uptake of glucose. Dosing should begin at the lower end of the dose range and be increased incrementally according to response to therapy (Leifer *et al.* 1986).

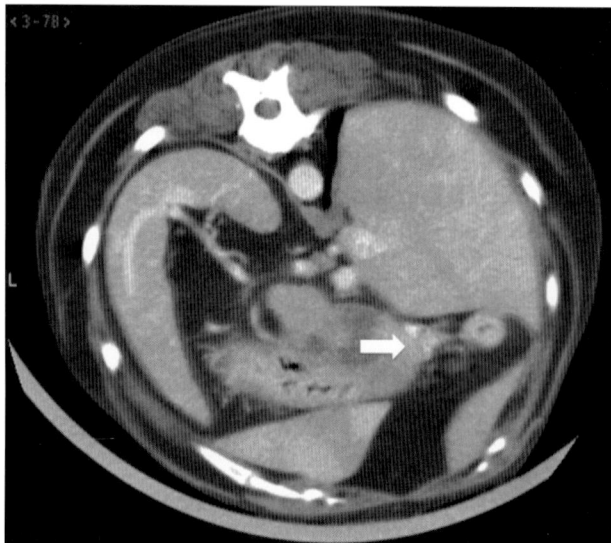

Figure 62.8 Abdominal computed tomography arterial phase image. Note the uptake of contrast at the level of the midpancreas in the left limb (white arrow). This area was found to correspond with a mass lesion of the pancreas at surgery, which was diagnosed on histopathology as insulinoma. *Source:* Reproduced with permission from Dr. R. O'Brien.

- Octreotide is a somatostatin analogue that inhibits insulin secretion by binding to somatostatin receptor subtypes on neoplastic insulin-secreting β cells. Response to therapy is variable in dogs, but administration showed no side effects in one study of 12 dogs. Additional studies are needed to determine efficacy and risk (Kraje 2003; Polton *et al.* 2007; Cornell 2012).
- Streptozocin is a nitrosurea antibiotic with selective cytotoxicity for β cells of the pancreas and metastatic lesions. It has been administered at a dosage of 500 mg/m² every 3 weeks. Administration is coupled with intensive diuresis of the patient with 0.9% saline for several hours before, during, and after treatment because streptozocin is nephrotoxic and reported to cause renal failure in dogs and cats (Kraje 2003). Dogs may also experience vomiting during administration. Use of streptozocin cannot be advocated at this time because studies confirming its efficacy are currently lacking; the median duration of normoglycemia in dogs with insulinoma treated with streptozocin was not significantly different than that of control dogs treated surgically or otherwise. It is unclear if streptozocin may be more efficacious in patients whose disease has been diminished by surgery. Other side effects of its administration include DM, neuroglycopenia and associated signs, azotemia, neutropenia, and elevations in alanine aminotransferase (Hess 2010).

Outcome

Dogs with persistent postoperative hypoglycemia showed a median survival time of 90 days compared with dogs that became normoglycemic or hyperglycemic after surgery (MST, 680 days) (Tryfonidou 1998). Recurrent hypoglycemia occurs in 52% to 100% of dogs, with a median time to recurrence of 60 days. The duration of normoglycemia is longer in dogs with stage I disease (14 months) compared with dogs with stage II or III disease (20 days) (Polton *et al.* 2007; Cornell 2012).

Prevention

- The duration of normoglycemia appears to depend on several patient parameters and on the method of treatment. Dogs treated with conservative management exhibit significantly shorter survival times (MST, 74 days) compared with dogs treated by partial pancreatectomy (MST, 381 days) (Tobin *et al.* 1999).
- The type of surgery appears to influence the outcome; dogs that underwent enucleation of the mass within the pancreas fared worse (MST 11.5 months) than dogs that underwent partial pancreatectomy (MST, 17.9 months) (Mehlhaff *et al.* 1985).
- Additionally, dogs that underwent partial pancreatectomy and postoperative treatment with prednisone lived longer (MST, 1316 days) than dogs treated by partial pancreatectomy alone (MST, 785 days) (Polton *et al.* 2007).

References

Allen, S.W., Cornelius, L.M., Mahaffey, E.A. (1989) A comparison of two methods of partial pancreatectomy in the dog. *Veterinary Surgery* 18 (4), 274-278.

Anderson, J.R., Cornell, K.K., Parnell, N.K., et al. (2008) Pancreatic abscess in 36 dogs: a retrospective analysis of prognostic indicators. *Journal of the American Animal Hospital Association* 44, 171-179.

Amsellem, P.M., Seim, H.B., MacPhail, C.M., et al. (2006) Long-term survival and risk factors associated with biliary surgery in dogs: 34 cases (1994-2004). *Journal of the American Veterinary Medical Association* 229 (9), 1451-1457.

Baker, S.G., Mayhew, P.D., Mehler, S.J. (2011) Choledochotomy and primary repair of extrahepatic biliary duct rupture in seven dogs and two cats. *Journal of Small Animal Practice*, 52, 32-37.

Batchelor, D.J., Noble, P.J., Taylor, R.H., et al. (2007) Prognostic factors in canine exocrine pancreatic insufficiency: prolonged survival is likely if clinical remission is achieved. *Journal of Veterinary Internal Medicine* 21, 54-60.

Bellenger, C.R., Ilkiw, J.E., Malik, R. (1989) Cystogastrostomy in the treatment of pancreatic pseudocyst/abscess in two dogs. *Veterinary Record* 125, 181-184.

Cappell, M.S. (2008) Acute pancreatitis: etiology, clinical presentation, diagnosis, and therapy. *Medical Clinics of North America* 92, 889-923.

Center, S.A. (2009) Diseases of the gallbladder and biliary tree. *Veterinary Clinics of North America Small Animal Practice* 39, 543-598.

Cobb, L.F., Merrell, R.C. (1984) Total pancreatectomy in dogs. *Journal of Surgical Research* 37, 235-240.

Coleman, M., Robson, M. (2005) Pancreatic masses following pancreatitis: pancreatic pseudocysts, necrosis, and abscesses. *Compendium on Continuing Education for the Practicing Veterinarian* 27, 147-154.

Cornell, K. (2012) Pancreas. In Tobias, K.T., Johnston, S.A. (eds.) *Veterinary Surgery Small Animal*. Elsevier Saunders, St. Louis, pp. 1659-1673.

Cornell, K., Fischer, J. (2003) Surgery of the exocrine pancreas. In Slatter, D. (ed.) *Small Animal Surgery*. Saunders, Philadelphia, pp. 752-762.

Cribb, A.E., Burgener, D.C., Reimann, K.A. (1988) Bile duct obstruction secondary to chronic pancreatitis in seven dogs. *Canadian Veterinary Journal* 29, 654-657.

DiMagno, E.P., Go, V.L.W., Summerskill, W.H.J. (1973) Relations between pancreatic enzyme outputs and malabsorption in severe pancreatic insufficiency. *New England Journal of Medicine* 288, 813-815.

Dowling, P.M. (2009) Motility disorders. In Silverstein, D. (ed.) *Small Animal Critical Care*. Elsevier Saunders, St. Louis, pp. 562-565.

Dunn, J.K., Heath, M.K., Herrtage, M.E., et al. (1992) Diagnosis of insulinoma in the dog: a study of 11 cases. *Journal of Small Animal Practice* 33, 514-520.

Eisele, J., McClaran, J.K., Runge, J.J., et al. (2010) Evaluation of risk factors for morbidity and mortality after pylorectomy and gastroduodenostomy in dogs. *Veterinary Surgery* 39, 261-267.

Fahie, M.A., Martin, R.A. (1995) Extrahepatic biliary tract obstruction: a retrospective study of 45 cases (1983-1993). *Journal of the American Animal Hospital Association* 31 (6), 478-482.

Fischer, J.R., Smith, S.A., Harkin, K.R., et al. (2000) Glucagon constant-rate infusion: a novel strategy for the management of hyperinsulinemic-hypoglycemic crisis in the dog. *Journal of the American Animal Hospital Association* 36, 27-32.

Forman, M.A., De Cock, H.E.V., Hergesell, E.J., et al. (2004) Evaluation of serum pancreatic lipase immunoreactivity and helical computed tomography versus conventional testing for the diagnosis of feline pancreatitis. *Journal of Veterinary Internal Medicine* 18, 807-815.

Gaillot, H.A., Penninck, D.G., Webster, C.R.L., et al. (2007) Ultrasonographic features of extrahepatic biliary obstruction in 30 cats. *Veterinary Radiology and Ultrasound* 48, 439-447.

Gaynor, A.R. (2009) Acute pancreatitis. In Silverstein, D. (ed.) *Small Animal Critical Care*. Elsevier Saunders, St. Louis, pp. 537-541.

Gerhardt, A., Steiner, J.M., Williams, D.A., et al. (2001) Comparison of the sensitivity of different diagnostic tests for pancreatitis in cats. *Journal of Veterinary Internal Medicine* 15, 329-333.

Glasgow, R.E., Mulvihill, S.J. (2002) Liver, biliary tract, and pancreas. In O'Leary, J.P. (ed.) *The Physiologic Basis of Surgery*. Lippincott Williams and Wilkins, Philadelphia, pp. 523-530.

Guilford, W.G. (1990) The enteric nervous system—function, dysfunction, and pharmacological manipulation. *Seminars in Veterinary Medicine and Surgery (Small Animal)* 5, 46-56.

Herman, B.A., Brawer, R.S., Murtaugh, R.J., et al. (2005) Therapeutic percutaneous ultrasound-guided cholecystocentesis in three dogs with extrahepatic biliary obstruction and pancreatitis. *Journal of the American Veterinary Medical Association* 227 (11), 1782-1785.

Hess, R.S. (2010) Insulin-secreting islet cell neoplasia. In Ettinger, S.J., Feldman, E.C. (eds.) *Textbook of Veterinary Internal Medicine,* 7th edn. Elsevier Saunders, St. Louis, pp. 1779-1782.

Hess, R.S., Kass, P.H., Shofer, F.S., et al. (1999) Evaluation of risk factors for fatal acute pancreatitis in dogs. *Journal of the American Veterinary Medical Association* 214 (1), 46-51.

Hess, R.S., Saunders, H.M., VanWinkle, T.J., et al. (1998) Clinical, clinicopathologic, radiographic, and ultrasonographic abnormalities in dogs with fatal acute pancreatitis: 70 cases (1986-1995). *Journal of the American Veterinary Medical Association* 213 (5), 665-670.

Hoenig, M. (2002) Comparative aspects of diabetes mellitus in dogs and cats. *Molecular and Cellular Endocrinology* 197, 221-229.

Iseri, T., Yamada, K., Chijiwa, K., et al. (2007) Dynamic computed tomography of the pancreas in a normal dog and in a dog with pancreatic insulinoma. *Veterinary Radiology and Ultrasound* 48 (4), 328-331.

Jerram, R.M., Warman, C.G., Davies, E.S.S, et al. (2004) Successful treatment of a pancreatic pseudocyst by omentalisation in a dog. *New Zealand Veterinary Journal* 52 (4), 197-201.

Johnson, M.D., Fann, F.A. (2006) Treatment for pancreatic abscesses via omentalization with abdominal closure versus open peritoneal drainage in dogs: 15 cases (1994-2004). *Journal of the American Veterinary Medical Association* 228 (3), 397-402.

Kealy, J.K., McAllister, H. (2005) *Diagnostic Radiology and Ultrasonography of the Dog and Cat*, 4th edn. Elsevier Saunders, St. Louis, p. 478.

Kraje, A.C. (2003) Hypoglycemia and irreversible neurologic complications in a cat with insulinoma. *Journal of the American Veterinary Medical Association* 223 (6), 812-814.

Kyles, A.E. (2003) Surgery of the endocrine system. In In Slatter, D. (ed.) *Small Animal Surgery*. Saunders, Philadelphia, pp. 1724-1736.

Laluha, P., Gerber, B., Laluhova, D., et al. (2004) Stresshyperglykämie bei kranken Katzen: Eine retrospektive Studie über 4 Jahre. *Schweiz Arch Tierheilkd* 146, 375-383.

Lehner, C.M., and McAnulty, J.F. (2010) Management of extrahepatic biliary obstruction: a role for temporary cutaneous biliary drainage. *Compendium on Continuing Education for the Practicing Veterinarian* 32 (9), E1-E10.

Leifer, C.E., Peterson, M.E., Matus, R.E., et al. (1986) Insulin-secreting tumor: diagnosis and medical and surgical management in 55 dogs. *Journal of the American Veterinary Medical Association* 188, 60-64.

Lem, K.Y., Fosgate, G.T., Norby, B., et al. (2008) Associations between dietary factors and pancreatitis in dogs. *Journal of the American Veterinary Medical Association* 233 (9), 1425-1431.

Logan, J.C., Callan, M.B., Drew, K., et al. (2001) Clinical indications for use of fresh frozen plasma in dogs: 74 dogs (October-December 1999). *Journal of the American Veterinary Medical Association* 218, 1449-1455.

Ludwig, L.L., McLoughlin, M.A., Graves, T.K., et al. (1997) Surgical treatment of bile peritonitis in 24 dogs and 2 cats: a retrospective study (1987-1994). *Veterinary Surgery* 26, 90-98.

Mansfield, C. (2008) Acute pancreatitis in the dog- current approach to management. In *Proceedings, 33rd Congress of the World Small Animal Veterinary Association*. Dublin, Ireland, August 20-24, pp. 371-372.

Marchevsky, A., Yovich, J.C., Wyatt, K.M. (2000) Pancreatic pseudocyst causing extrahepatic biliary obstruction in a dog. *Australian Veterinary Journal* 78 (2), 99-101.

Matthiesen, D.T. (1989) Complications associated with surgery of the extrahepatic biliary system. *Problems in Veterinary Medicine* 1, 295-313.

Matthiesen, D., Mullen, H. (1990) Problems and complications associated with endocrine surgery in the dog and cat. *Problems in Veterinary Medicine* 2, 627-667.

Mayhew, P.D., Holt, D.E., Washabau, R.J. (2002) Pathogenesis and outcome of extrahepatic biliary obstruction in cats. *Journal of Small Animal Practice* 43 (6), 247-253.

Mayhew, P.D., Richardson, R.W., Mehler, S.J., et al. (2006) Choledochal tube stenting for decompression of the extrahepatic portion of the biliary tract in dogs: 13 cases (2002-2005). *Journal of the American Veterinary Medical Association* 228 (8), 1209-1214.

McGahan, J.P., Phillips, H.E., Nyland, T., et al. (1993) Sonographically guided percutaneous cholecystostomy performed in dogs and pigs. *Radiology* 149, 841-843.

Mehler, S.J., Bennett, R.A. (2006) Canine extrahepatic biliary tract disease and surgery. *Compendium on Continuing Education for the Practicing Veterinarian* 28, 302-314.

Mehler, S.J., Mayhew, P.D., Drobatz, K., et al. (2004) Variables associated with outcome in dogs undergoing extrahepatic biliary surgery: 60 cases (1988-2002). *Veterinary Surgery* 33, 644-649.

Mehlhaff, C.J., Peterson, M.E., Patnaik, A.K., et al. (1985) Insulin-producing islet cell neoplasms: surgical considerations and general management in 35 dogs. *Journal American Animal Hospital Association* 21, 607–612.

Mix, K., Jones, C. (2006) Diagnosing acute pancreatitis in dogs. *Compendium on Continuing Education for the Practicing Veterinarian* 28, 226-234.

Mueller, M.G., Ludwig, L.L., Barton, L.J. (2001) Use of closed-suction drains to treat generalized peritonitis in dogs and cats: 40 cases (1997-1999). *Journal of the American Veterinary Medical Association* 219 (6), 789-794.

Murphy, S.M., Rodriguez, J.D., McAnulty, J.F. (2007) Minimally invasive cholecystotomy in the dog: evaluation of placement technique and use in extrahepatic biliary obstruction. *Veterinary Surgery* 36, 675-683.

Nelson, R.W. (2010) Canine diabetes mellitus. In Ettinger, S.J., Feldman, E.C. (eds.) *Textbook of Veterinary Internal Medicine,* 7th edn. Elsevier Saunders, St. Louis, pp. 1782-1796.

Newman, S., Steiner, J.M., Woosley, K., et al. (2004) Localization of pancreatic inflammation and necrosis in dogs. *Journal of Veterinary Internal Medicine* 18, 488-493.

Pairent, F.W., Trapnell, J.E., Howard, J.M. (1969) The treatment of pancreatic exocrine insufficiency: the effects of pancreatic ductal ligation and oral pancreatic enzyme supplements on fecal lipid excretion in the dog. *Annals of Surgery* 170 (5), 737-746.

Papachristou, D.N., Fortner, J.G. (1980) A simple method of pancreatic transplantation in the dog. *American Journal of Surgery* 139, 344-347.

Papazoglou, L.G., Mann, F.A., Wagner-Mann, C., et al. (2008) Long-term survival of dogs after cholecystoenterostomy: a retrospective study of 15 cases (1981-2005). *Journal of the American Animal Hospital Association* 44, 67-74.

Plumb, D.C. (2011) *Plumb's Veterinary Drug Handbook,* 7th edn. John Wiley and Sons, Hoboken, NJ.

Polton, G.A., White, R.N., Brearly, M.J., et al. (2007) Improved survival in a retrospective cohort of 28 dogs with insulinoma. *Journal of Small Animal Practice* 48, 151-156.

Reusch, C. (2010) Feline diabetes mellitus. In Ettinger, S.J., Feldman, E.C. (eds.) *Textbook of Veterinary Internal Medicine,* 7th edn. Elsevier Saunders, St. Louis, 1796-1816.

Robben, J.H., Pollak, W.E.A., Kirpenstein, J., et al. (2005) Comparison of ultrasonography, computed tomography, and single-photon emission computed tomography for the detection and localization of canine insulinoma. *Journal of Veterinary Internal Medicine* 19, 15-22.

Rosin, E., Campos, R., Moberg, A.W., et al. (1972) Technique for total pancreatectomy of the dog. *American Journal of Veterinary Research* 33, 1299-1302.

Ruaux, C.G. (2000) Pathophysiology of organ failure in severe acute pancreatitis in dogs. *Compendium on Continuing Education for the Practicing Veterinarian* 22, 531-542.

Salisbury, S., Lantz, G., Nelson, R. (1988) Pancreatic abscess in dogs: six cases (1978-1986). *Journal of the American Veterinary Medical Association* 193, 1104-1108.

Saunders, H.M., VanWinkle, T.J., Drobatz, K., et al. (2002) Ultrasonographic findings in cats with clinical, gross pathologic, and histologic evidence of acute pancreatic necrosis: 20 cases (1994-2001). *Journal of the American Veterinary Medical Association* 221 (12), 1724-1730.

Simpson, K.W. (1993) Current concepts of the pathogenesis and pathophysiology of acute pancreatitis in the dog and cat. *Compendium of Continuing Education for the Practicing Veterinarian* 15, 247-253.

Simpson, K.W., Simpson, J.W., Morton, D.B., et al. (1991) Effect of pancreatectomy on plasma activities of amylase, isoamylas, lipase, and trypsin-like immunoreactivity in dogs. *Research in Veterinary Science* 51 (1), 78-82.

Smith S.A., Biller, D.S. (1998) Resolution of a pancreatic pseudocyst in a dog following percutaneous ultrasonographic-guided drainage. *Journal of the American Animal Hospital Association* 34, 515-522.

Son, T.T., Thompson, L., Serrano, S., et al. (2010) Surgical intervention in the management of severe acute pancreatitis in cats: 8 cases (2003-2007). *Journal of Veterinary Emergency and Critical Care* 20 (4), 426-435.

Spangler, W.L., Kass, P.H. (1997) Pathologic factors affecting post-splenectomy survival in dogs. *Journal of Veterinary Internal Medicine* 11, 166-171.

Spillman, T., Litzlbauer,H., Moritz, A., et al. (2000) Computed tomography and laparoscopy for the diagnosis of pancreatic disease in dogs. *Proceedings of the 18th ACVIM Forum.* Seattle, June 12-15, pp. 485-487.

Spillman, T., Wittker, A., Teigelkamp, S., et al. (2001) An immunoassay for canine pancreatic elastase 1 as an indicator for exocrine pancreatic insufficiency in dogs. *Journal of Veterinary Diagnostic Investigation* 13, 468-474.

Staatz, A.J., Monnet, E., Seim, H.B. (2002) Open peritoneal drainage versus primary closure for the treatment of septic peritonitis in dogs and cats: 42 cases (1993-1999). *Veterinary Surgery* 31, 174-180.

Steiner, J.M. (2010) Canine pancreatic disease. In Ettinger, S.J., Feldman, E.C. (eds.) *Textbook of Veterinary Internal Medicine,* 7th edn. Elsevier Saunders, St. Louis, pp. 1695-1704.

Steiner, J.M., Rutz, G.M., Williams, D.A. (2006) Serum lipase activities and pancreatic lipase immunoreactivity concentrations in dogs with exocrine pancreatic insufficiency. *American Journal of Veterinary Research* 67, 84-87.

Steiner, J.M., Teague, S.R, Williams, D.A. (2003) Development and analytic validation of an enzyme-linked immunosorbent assay for the measurement of canine pancreatic lipase immunoreactivity in serum. *Canadian Journal of Veterinary Research* 67, 175-182.

Stimson, E.L., Espada, Y., Moon, M., et al. (1998) Pancreatic abscess in nine dogs [abstract]. *Journal of Veterinary Internal Medicine* 9, 202.

Thompson, L.J., Seshadri, R., Raffe, M.R. (2009) Characteristics and outcomes in surgical management of severe acute pancreatitis: 37 dogs (2001-2007). *Journal of Veterinary Emergency and Critical Care* 19 (2), 165-173.

Tobin, R.L., Nelson, R.W., Lucroy, M.D., et al. (1999) Outcome of surgical versus medical treatment of dogs with beta cell neoplasia: 39 cases (1990-1997). *Journal of the American Veterinary Medical Association* 215 (2), 226-230.

Tryfonidou, M.A., Kirpensteijn, J., Robben, J.H. (1998) A retrospective evaluation of 51 dogs with insulinoma. *The Veterinary Quarterly* 20, S114-S115.

VanEnkevort B.A., O'Brien R.T., Young, K.M. (1999) Pancreatic pseudocysts in 4 dogs and 2 cats: ultrasonographic and clinicopathologic findings. *Journal of Veterinary Internal Medicine* 13, 309-313.

Wagner, K.A., Hartmann, F.A., Trepanier, L.A. (2007) Bacterial culture results from liver, gallbladder, or bile in 248 dogs and cats evaluated for hepatobiliary disease: 1998-2003. *Journal of Veterinary Internal Medicine* 21, 417-424.

Washabau, R.J. (2003) Gastrointestinal motility disorders and gastrointestinal prokinetic therapy. *Veterinary Clinics of North America Small Animal Practice* 33, 1007-1028.

Wasserman, D.H., Johnson, J.L., Bupp, J.L., et al. (1993) Regulation of gluconeogenesis during rest and exercise in the depancreatized dog. *American Journal of Physiology* 265, E51-E60.

Watt, P.R. (1989) Surgical relief of biliary obstruction secondary to chronic pancreatitis. *Australian Veterinary Practitioner* 19 (4), 208-213.

Webb, C.B., Trott, C. (2008) Laparoscopic diagnosis of pancreatic disease in dogs and cats. *Journal of Veterinary Internal Medicine* 22, 1263-1266.

Westermarck, E., Wiberg, M. (2003) Exocrine pancreatic insufficiency in dogs. *Veterinary Clinics of North America Small Animal Practice* 33, 1165-1179.

Whittemore, J.C., Campbell, V.L. (2005) Canine and feline pancreatitis. *Compendium on Continuing Education for the Practicing Veterinarian* 27, 766-776.

Willard, M.D. (2009) Gastrointestinal protectants. In Silverstein, D. (ed.) *Small Animal Critical Care.* Elsevier Saunders, St. Louis, pp. 775-777.

Williams, D.A. (2001) Exocrine pancreatic disease and pancreatitis. In Ettinger, S.J., Feldman, E.C. (eds.) *Textbook of Veterinary Internal Medicine: Diseases of the Dog and Cat,* 5th edn. WB Saunders, Philadelphia, pp. 1345-1355.

Williams, D.A., Steiner, J.M. (2000) Canine pancreatitis. In Bonagura, J.D. (ed.) *Kirk's Veterinary Therapy XIII.* WB Saunders, Philadelphia, p. 1308.

Worley, D.R., Hottinger, H.A., Lawrence, H.J. (2004) Surgical management of gallbladder mucoceles in dogs: 22 cases (1999-2003). *Journal of the American Veterinary Medical Association* 225 (9), 1418-1422.

Xenoulis, P.G., Fradkin, J.M., Rapp, S.W., et al. (2007) Suspected isolated pancreatic lipase deficiency in a dog. *Journal of Veterinary Internal Medicine* 21, 1113-1116.

Xenoulis, P., Sichodolski, J., Steiner, J.M. (2008) Chronic pancreatitis in dogs and cats. *Compendium on Continuing Education for the Practicing Veterinarian* 30, 166-180.

Yotsumoto, F., Manabe, T., Ohshio, G., et al. (1993) Role of pancreatic blood flow and vasoactive substances in the development of pancreatitis. *Journal of Surgical Research* 55, 531-536.

63 Portosystemic

Barbara Kirby

Section of Veterinary Clinical Studies, School of Veterinary Medicine University College Dublin, Dublin, Ireland

Portal vascular anomalies (PVAs) in dogs and cats include congenital or acquired macrovascular portosystemic shunts (PSS), portal venous hypoplasia (formerly known as microvascular dysplasia), hepatic arteriovenous malformation, and noncirrhotic portal hypertension with portal vein atresia (Webster 2010).

Congenital portosystemic shunts (CPSS) are the most common PVA managed surgically. CPSS are most frequently diagnosed in purebred dogs, with familial relationships in Irish wolfhounds, Yorkshire terriers, and Cairn terriers documented (Ubbink *et al.* 1999; Tobias and Rohrbach 2003; van Straten *et al.* 2005). In Irish wolfhounds, breeding trials have confirmed a hereditary basis considered most likely polygenic (van Steenbeek *et al.* 2009). Breed predispositions are known in Australian cattle dogs, Maltese terriers, miniature schnauzers, dachshunds, pugs, bichon frises, havanese, dandie Dinmont terriers, and Bernese mountain dogs, among others. CPSS also occur occasionally in nonpredisposed breeds and mixed-breed dogs.

Portal vascular anomalies are less common in cats relative to dogs. CPSS occur most frequently in mixed-breed cats, but Persians and Himalayans are overrepresented.

Suspicion of CPSS in dogs and cats is based on typical clinical signs. The diagnosis is most often based on typical hematology and biochemistry abnormalities, including elevated fasting ammonia or elevated fasting and postprandial bile acid levels. The presence of a macrovascular CPSS is most often confirmed by abdominal ultrasonography or computed tomography (CT) angiography and surgery.

Most clinicians recommend a period of medical management for stabilization before elective surgical treatment of the shunt vessel. Surgery is not useful in management of acute hepatoencephalopathy secondary to CPSS. Surgery is considered the preferred treatment of CPSS over long-term medical management because the probability of survival is significantly lower in medically treated dogs with extrahepatic CPSS than in surgically treated dogs (Greenhalgh *et al.* 2010).

Complication rates in the surgical management of CPSS vary widely. Comparison of complication rates among different reports is exceedingly difficult because definitions of short- and long-term complications, inclusion and exclusion criteria, surgical techniques, and outcome measures vary. In addition, both cats and dogs are included in many reports, and both intrahepatic and extrahepatic shunts of various types are included in some reports. In most reports, small case numbers weaken the evidence and make comparison between individual techniques and reports impossible.

About 67% to 75% of CPSS are extrahepatic. Complication rates of 9% to 50% are reported for surgical management of extrahepatic portosystemic shunts (EHPSS) with good to excellent outcomes in 80% to 85% of these cases.

About 25% to 33% of CPSS are intrahepatic (Berent and Weisse 2010). Intrahepatic portosystemic shunt (IHPSS) complication rates are generally higher than reported for EHPSS. Mortality rates of 0% to 77% have been reported with good to excellent outcomes reported in 75% to 100% of dogs treated with various techniques.

Complete acute suture attenuation is reported in 32% to 52% of EHPSS and 15% of IHPSS in dogs. Complication rates reported after partial or complete suture attenuation are 9% to 50% with mortality rates of 2% to 10% and good to excellent outcome in 80% to 85% (Berent and Weisse 2010). Criteria to determine the end point of suture attenuation vary.

Gradual progressive shunt attenuation by ameroid constrictor, cellophane banding, and hydraulic occlusion have been reported. Ameroid constrictor complication rates of 10% to 20%, mortality rates of 0% to 17%, and good to excellent outcomes in 94% of dogs are reported. Good to excellent outcomes were reported despite continued blood flow through the shunt in 21% of dogs in one study (Berent and Weisse 2010). Cellophane band complication rates of 10% to 13%, mortality rates of 3% to 9%, and good to excellent outcomes in 84% of dogs are reported (Berent and Weisse 2010).

For IHPSS, a complication rate of 55% and mortality rate of 27% is reported for cellophane banding; intraoperative complication rate of 0%, postoperative complication rate of 20%, and mortality rate of 0% are reported for ameroid constrictor (Bright *et al.* 2006); an intraoperative complication rate of 20%, surgical revision rate of 30%, and mortality rate of 0% are reported for hydraulic occlusion (Adin *et al.* 2006); and an intraoperative complication rate of 15% and mortality rate of 10% are reported for percutaneous transvenous coil embolization (Weisse *et al.* 2006). However, in one study comparing partial suture ligation with ameroid constrictor in IHPSS in dogs, there was a significant difference in long-term outcome, with a recommendation against use of ameroid ring constrictor on the left hepatic vein for management of left-divisional IHPSS (Mehl *et al.* 2007).

Cats with CPSS are generally considered to have a higher complication rate and poorer outcome than dogs (Berent and Weisse 2010). In a retrospective study of 9 cats with EHPSS, there was a 3-year survival rate of 66% (Cabassu *et al.* 2011). Perioperative complication rates for cats with EHPSS were 37% after suture

Complications in Small Animal Surgery, First Edition. Edited by Dominique Griffon and Annick Hamaide.

© 2016 John Wiley & Sons, Inc. Published 2016 by John Wiley & Sons, Inc.

Companion website: www.wiley.com/go/griffon/complications

ligation, 8% to 77% after ameroid constrictor placement, and 20% after cellophane banding. Cats are reported with a high frequency of neurologic signs before and after surgery, with 8% to 22% affected by seizures and 44% affected with central blindness, although the latter is usually transient. In a retrospective study of 25 cats with CPSS, the reported intraoperative complication rate was 0%, but 60% developed postattenuation neurologic complications between 12 and 72 hours after surgery (Lipscomb et al. 2009). Long-term outcomes for cats with EHPSS are worse than dogs with 33% to 66% of cats with persistent abnormal liver function test results and 57% with evidence of persistent shunting. Good to excellent long-term outcome by technique is reported as 75% for suture ligation, 25% to 75% after ameroid constrictor placement, and 100% after cellophane banding, although only 5 cats were included in the cellophane banding group. Separate outcome reports for feline IHPSS are not available, with the exception of a retrospective study involving 6 cats (White et al. 1996). Thirteen of 49 cats included in a retrospective study of long-term outcomes and complications of CPSS had IHPSS, but results were not reported separately for the IHPSS and EHPSS cats (Lipscomb et al. 2007).

Tivers et al. assessed the evidence base for management of EHPSS and concluded that there is a lack of evidence of short- and long-term outcomes that precludes recommendation of one treatment over another (Tivers et al. 2012). Perioperative mortality rates were reported in 11 articles for suture ligation (2%–28.8%), 2 articles for ameroid constrictors (7.1%–16.7%), and 4 articles for cellophane banding (0%–9.4%). Several studies comparing 2 different surgical techniques (suture ligation versus ameroid constrictor and suture ligation vs. cellophane banding) found no statistically significant differences.

The period of follow-up in most reports of outcome in surgical management of CPSS is short. Recurrence of clinical signs can occur many years after seemingly successful surgery. In addition, outcome measures are not standardized and most frequently include clinical assessment or biochemical testing only. Persistent shunting, acquired multiple EHPSS, and other complications are often not evaluated in an adequately long period of follow-up.

Large, well-designed, multi-institutional randomized prospective clinical trials separating canine and feline CPSS and intrahepatic and extrahepatic CPSS, stratified by treatment with well-defined long-term follow-up are required.

Prognostic factors

To date, few prognostic indicators have been identified. Age at diagnosis and treatment, preoperative neurologic status, and presence of urolithiasis have been shown not to influence outcome. Packed cell volume and total proteins (TP) were identified as prognostic indicators for long-term survival, whereas body weight, TP, albumin, and BUN were identified as indicators for short-term outcome in dogs with IHPSS (Papazoglou et al. 2002). There is no identified ideal time to perform surgery after diagnosis. Hypothermia is reported as an early predictor of postoperative death in toy breeds (Bostwick and Twedt 1995). Attempts to preoperatively identify individual patients that will tolerate acute complete suture ligation have not identified predictors.

In a prospective case series of 17 dogs with single EHPSS aimed at establishing criteria for optimal degree of shunt narrowing and predicting outcome, Szatmári et al. (2004) identified establishment of hepatopetal flow in the shunt vessel and in the portal vein cranial to the shunt and maintenance of hepatofugal flow caudal to the

shunt as the end point of shunt attenuation. Portal flow direction was reported to be more closely associated with outcome than other variables. A portal vein congestion index calculated from the cross-sectional area divided by the time-averaged mean velocity determined by Doppler ultrasonography was predictive of outcome, with a more than 3.6 times increase of congestion index associated with poor outcome and less than 3.6 times increase associated with a good outcome in this study (Szatmári et al. 2004).

In a retrospective study of hepatic portal vascularity assessed via intraoperative mesenteric portography in 25 cats undergoing surgical attenuation of CPSS (21 EHPSS and 4 IHPSS cats), median portovenogram grades assigned after temporary shunt occlusion were significantly higher in cats that did not have postoperative neurologic complications, had better clinical response, and had reduced fasting and postprandial bile acid concentrations at follow-up. Postocclusion intraoperative mesenteric portovenogram grade was considered a potential indicator of postattenuation neurologic complications in cats (Lipscomb et al. 2009).

Hypotension

Systemic hypotension is a common problem during anesthesia and surgery for CPSS and is often multifactorial. Direct arterial pressure monitoring via arterial catheterization is recommended. Most animals with CPSS are predisposed to hypothermia under anesthesia because of immaturity; low body mass index; heat loss to the external environment, including wide and prolonged exposure of the peritoneal cavity; and other factors with hypotension occurring secondarily. Measures to prevent hypothermia are paramount. Surgical manipulations for exposure and isolation of the shunt vessel may directly interfere with flow in the caudal vena cava and venous return to the heart. Manipulation or temporary occlusion of the shunt may result in severe portal hypertension and acute systemic hypotension. Acute hypotension and hemorrhagic shock can be expected in animals that have severe intraoperative bleeding. Acute, severe systemic hypotension may also result from a vagal shock reaction; this phenomenon may occur more frequently in cats (Brovida and Rothuizen 2010).

Regardless of the cause of systemic hypotension, aggressive treatment to maintain mean arterial blood pressure above 50 mm Hg is recommended. Maintenance of circulating volume by administration of intravenous (IV) crystalloid or colloid fluids plus blood products if required, administration of α-adrenergic drugs such as dopamine or dobutamine in support of blood pressure, and specialist anesthetic management to minimize the cardiovascular effects of anesthetic and analgesic drugs are critically important.

Hypoglycemia

Hypoglycemia occurs commonly in dogs with CPSS, particularly small breeds. Hypoglycemia appears to be an infrequent problem in cats with CPSS. Hypoglycemia may occur before, during, or after surgery for CPSS. Hypoglycemia is reported in up to 35% of dogs with CPSS and is considered to result from impaired hepatic glucose production, decreased hepatic glycogen stores, or reduced responsiveness to glucagon. Poor muscle mass and low body fat are also implicated in predisposing dogs with CPSS to hypoglycemia. Hypoglycemia results when less than 30% of normal hepatic function remains.

Presurgical fasting of animals with CPSS may result in hypoglycemia with no apparent clinical signs or may result in profound hypoglycemia with exacerbation of clinical signs of hepatic encephalopathy. In the author's surgical practice, a maximum period of preanesthetic fasting of 8 hours is recommended. Despite this relatively short period of fasting, nearly 100% of CPSS cases are hypoglycemic at the time of IV catheterization before anesthesia induction. IV dextrose supplementation is initiated at the first evidence of low blood glucose and continued based on serial glucose determination well into the postoperative period until the animal has resumed eating and maintains normoglycemia. Other concurrent conditions, including internal parasites, diarrhea, hypothermia, and poor diet, may increase the risk of hypoglycemia.

Postoperative hypoglycemia (blood glucose <60 mg/dL) was reported in 44% of dogs with EHPSS managed surgically, with approximately one third of these dogs failing to respond to dextrose supplementation. Some of these animals responded to supraphysiologic glucocorticoid administration (dexamethasone 0.1–0.2 mg/kg IV once) and were considered to have a relative glucocorticoid insufficiency (Holford et al. 2008). Relative adrenal insufficiency has been correlated with refractory hypotension in dogs with sepsis.

Another study showed no significant differences in preoperative adrenocorticotropic hormone (ACTH) stimulation test results between dogs with CPSS undergoing surgical shunt attenuation and normal dogs undergoing elective ovariohysterectomy (OVH). In the postoperative period, the CPSS dogs had significantly higher baseline cortisol levels than the OVH dogs. There was no correlation between ACTH response and postoperative hypoglycemia or prolonged anesthetic recovery (Holford et al. 2008).

Hemorrhage

Intraoperative bleeding is most commonly considered a complication of surgery for IHPSS, although the specific incidence of intraoperative hemorrhage in CPSS surgery is rarely reported. Regardless of shunt type, morphology, and planned surgical procedure, preoperative coagulation profile, platelet count and assessment of platelet function, and blood typing are routinely recommended. Crossmatch is required in animals with a history of previous transfusion. Transfusion, when required, should ideally be provided with fresh whole blood or fresh packed red blood cells because ammonia levels rise progressively during storage of blood (Waddell et al. 2001) and may contribute to postoperative neurologic complications.

A prolonged partial thromboplastin time has been reported in 39 dogs with CPSS, although this finding was not associated with bleeding tendencies in any of the dogs (Niles et al. 2001). Coagulation profiles were reported in a prospective study of 34 dogs with CPSS and 39 healthy dogs (Kummeling et al. 2006). Platelet counts were lower; activity of factors II, V, VII, and X were lower; activity of factor VIII was higher; and activated partial thromboplastin time and prothrombin time were prolonged in the CPSS dogs compared with normal dogs. Increased coagulation time abnormalities were documented immediately after surgery. Hemostasis normalized after surgery in dogs without persistent shunting but remained abnormal in dogs with persistent shunting. Average platelet count decrease of 27% has been reported in dogs that have undergone acute shunt ligation (Kummeling et al. 2004).

Severe gastrointestinal (GI) ulceration and bleeding have recently been reported as the most common causes of long-term morbidity and mortality in a group of dogs with IHPSS (Weisse et al. 2006; Berent and Tobias 2012). The pathophysiologic mechanism of gastric ulceration in IHPSS is unknown. Suggested etiologies include abnormal gastric wall vasculature or unidentified

gastric varices, increased blood flow through gastric arteries, and gastric inflammation. Increased gastric perfusion has been documented in dogs with IHPSS compared with normal dogs by dynamic CT (Zwingenberger and Shofer 2007). Lifelong antacid therapy with omeprazole and sucralfate is highly recommended in dogs with IHPSS. The mortality rate from hemorrhage associated with GI ulceration decreased from 25% to 3.2% after the introduction of lifelong antacid therapy in one group of dogs (Berent and Weisse 2010).

Hypoalbuminemia

Hypoalbuminemia is a common biochemical abnormality in dogs with CPSS but is rarely reported in cats with CPSS. In puppies being managed medically for CPSS before surgery, it is important to recognize that hepatic diets do not provide adequate protein levels for growth and must be supplemented with high-quality, high-bioavailability protein to prevent precipitous declines in serum albumin levels before surgery. Supplementation of hepatic diets with cottage cheese or egg whites is recommended in all growing puppies, particularly large and giant breeds.

Hypoalbuminemia in preoperative CPSS is rarely associated with peripheral edema or ascites, although these clinical signs are sometimes seen in the postoperative period, particularly in animals that develop severe ascites presumably secondary to portal hypertension. Hypoalbuminemia in CPSS patients has important implications for anesthetic management, particularly in the dose and duration of action of drugs that are bound to serum albumin. Albumin-bound drugs should be avoided when feasible.

Animals with severe hypoalbuminemia may develop postoperative hyponatremia. Monitoring of serum electrolytes is critical in the postoperative period because postoperative seizures and coma may develop when serum sodium fall below 120 mEq/L (Berent and Tobias 2012).

Hypoalbuminemia may also be associated with delayed wound healing and increased wound dehiscence, although this does not appear to be a common complication in CPSS. Use of nonabsorbable suture materials may be considered for prolonged wound support, although in the author's opinion, nonabsorbable suture materials are not required.

Ascites

Ascites is a rare preoperative clinical finding in CPSS. Ascites is more commonly seen in animals with multiple acquired EHPSS and liver failure.

Rates of development of ascites postoperatively in CPSS are not specifically reported. Accumulation of free peritoneal fluid is a common consequence of portal hypertension (Brovida and Rothuizen 2010). Postoperative ascites in CPSS is most often transient and does not require specific treatment, although maintenance of colloid osmotic pressure through administration of synthetic colloids, plasma, or albumin may be beneficial in minimizing peritoneal fluid accumulation in the perioperative period.

Portal hypertension

Acute, severe portal hypertension is a potentially fatal complication of surgical management of CPSS with a 2% to 14% incidence of portal hypertension reported with acute suture ligation (Berent and Tobias 2012). Fatal portal hypertension has also been reported in association with perioperative portal vein thrombosis in CPSS, although this complication appears to be exceedingly rare.

Intraoperative monitoring for signs of portal hypertension is considered an integral part of the surgical decision-making process in CPSS. Signs of portal hypertension include cyanosis of the intestines and pancreas, intestinal hypermotility, and prominent mesenteric arteriolar pulsations and venule congestion. Vital parameter changes relative to immediate preocclusion measurements in serious portal hypertension include a greater than 15% increase in heart rate and a greater than 15% decrease in mean arterial pressure (Szatmári et al. 2004). Criteria for pre- and postattenuation portal pressure changes vary, but most recommendations are for a maximum increase in portal pressure of 10 cm H_2O or final portal pressure below 20 to 23 cm H_2O. To date, there is no single criterion or group of measurable criteria that can predict a safe attenuation end point and prevent development of portal hypertension. Most surgeons use a combination of subjective and objective criteria to determine the attenuation end point. Some surgeons strive to apply gradual occluding devices without any initial occlusion of the shunt vessel, with shunt closure expected in 2 to 5 weeks with ameroid constrictor (Tobias 2007) and 8 to 12 weeks with cellophane banding (Monnet 2007).

In the first 24 hours after surgery for CPSS, regardless of surgical procedure and implants chosen, the patient should be monitored closely for clinical signs of acute severe portal hypertension. These signs include restlessness, severe abdominal pain, sudden or persistent systemic hypotension, and clinical signs of hypovolemic shock. In some animals, abdominal distention may be prominent. A rapid assessment for other acute perioperative complications of shunt attenuation should be made, including assessment for hypoglycemia and hemorrhage. Ultrasonography may be useful in diagnosis of portal vein thrombosis. Treatment involves immediate return to surgery to release the ligature or attenuating implant on the shunt vessel or remove the thrombus. The prognosis is guarded.

Status epilepticus

Status epilepticus is a devastating complication of surgery for CPSS, with postoperative seizures reported in 3% to 18% of dogs and 8% to 22% of cats (Berent and Tobias 2012). The incidence of seizures is not associated with hypoglycemia, hyperammonemia, or attenuation technique (Berent and Tobias 2012). To date, there are no pre- or perioperative predictors of postoperative status epilepticus, although there may be a trend for increased incidence in older dogs, in cats and small breed dogs with EHPSS, and in animals with preoperative seizures. The cause of postoperative status epilepticus is currently unknown. Proposed pathophysiologic mechanisms include decreased endogenous inhibitory central nervous system benzodiazepine agonist levels and imbalances in excitatory and inhibitory neurotransmitters (Heldmann et al. 1999). Elevated blood levels of endogenous benzodiazepine receptor ligand have been documented in peripheral and portal blood of dogs with CPSS (Aronson et al. 1997).

Various preoperative anticonvulsants have been used in an attempt to prevent postoperative status epilepticus, including phenobarbital, potassium bromide, and levetiracetam (Tisdall et al. 2000; Mehl et al. 2005; Fryer et al. 2011). To date, levetiracetam has proven successful in preventing this complication in one study (Fryer et al. 2011). In this retrospective study of preoperative anticonvulsant treatment, Fryer et al. (2011) describe 126 dogs with EHPSS with (42 dogs) or without (84 dogs) treatment with levetiracetam at a dosage of 20 mg/kg orally every 8 hours for a

minimum of 24 hours before surgical attenuation of their shunt using ameroid constrictor. Postoperative seizures were reported in 0% of the levetiracetam treatment group and in 5% of the group without levetiracetam treatment. None of the dogs experiencing postoperative seizures survived to discharge from the hospital. The authors concluded that preoperative treatment with levetiracetam significantly decreased the risk of postoperative seizures and death (Fryer et al. 2011). A large randomized prospective clinical trial of this treatment would be invaluable.

Status epilepticus most frequently occurs between 12 and 80 hours after surgery. Initial clinical signs may include abnormal vocalization or restlessness, acute blindness, ataxia, facial twitching, and muscle fasciculations. Typically, there is a rapid progression to generalized motor seizures and status epilepticus. Seizures are typically nonresponsive to anticonvulsant drug treatment, including IV diazepam and midazolam. Control of seizure activity is most often accomplished by bolus administration of IV propofol followed by propofol constant-rate infusion. Adjunctive treatment with phenobarbital, mannitol, and medetomidine CRI has been reported (Berent and Tobias 2012; Heidenreich and Kirby 2012).

Postattenuation seizures or status epilepticus differs from seizures associated with preoperative hepatoencephalopathy in that the former results in structural damage to the brain, including cortical necrosis and polioencephalomalacia, but the latter does not cause structural abnormalities in the brain. The prognosis for animals that develop postattenuation seizures or status epilepticus is poor with an approximately 50% mortality rate by death or euthanasia. Survivors generally have some degree of neurologic dysfunction or seizure activity, requiring lifelong anticonvulsant therapy.

Urinary tract calculi

Urinary tract calculi are commonly associated with PSS in dogs and cats. Increased urinary excretion of ammonia and uric acid has been documented in dogs with PSS, resulting from a failure of hepatic conversion of uric acid to allantoin (Hardy 1989). Fifty percent of dogs and 15% of cats with PVA have ammonium biurate crystalluria (Webster 2010). Calculi in PSS are most often ammonium biurate or ammonium magnesium phosphate and can occur anywhere in the urinary tract (kidneys, ureters, bladder, urethra). The presence of urinary tract calculi can be confirmed by radiographs because most are radiopaque or by sonography.

Calculi can be removed at the time of CPSS surgery, most commonly when they are located in the urinary bladder. Calculi can also be removed during a separate surgical procedure. Dissolution of renal calculi in dogs with CPSS after surgical correction of the shunt has been reported. Cystic calculi can also be managed medically with combined treatment with reduced purine diet, allopurinol 10 mg/kg every 8 hours orally, and urinary alkalinization by administration of oral sodium bicarbonate (Grauer 1993).

The occurrence of ammonium biurate urolithiasis has been reported years after apparently successful shunt occlusion (Cabassu et al. 2011). Late occurrence or recurrence or ammonium biurate urolithiasis warrants investigation of the animal for shunting of portal flow through the original shunt vessel or development of multiple EHPSS.

Portal vein thrombosis

Portal vein thrombosis is a rare, but usually fatal, postoperative complication of CPSS in dogs and cats. Three of 6 cats in a retrospective study of portal vein thrombosis had evidence of CPSS, with occurrence of the thrombus 10 days after ameroid constrictor placement in 1 cat (Rogers *et al.* 2008).

Evaluation of protein C activity in cats and dogs with CPSS has been recommended (Toulza *et al.* 2006; Rogers *et al.* 2008). Decreased protein C activity has been documented in canine CPSS with normalization of protein C activity after restoration of hepatic perfusion by shunt ligation (Toulza *et al.* 2006). Normal hepatic perfusion and gut-derived factors in portal blood are needed to maintain normal hepatic production of protein C.

Clinical signs of portal vein thrombosis are those of acute severe portal hypertension. Treatment involves emergency surgical removal of the thrombus. Treatment with low–molecular-weight heparin (dalteparin 100–125 IU/kg every 12–24 hours in cats), which selectively inhibits factor Xa, may prevent clot formation with minimal effect on clotting time and may be warranted preoperatively. There are no reports of the efficacy of dalteparin in the prevention of portal vein thrombosis in CPSS.

Persistent elevation of serum bile acids

Persistent elevation of serum bile acids does not necessarily correlate with clinical outcome after shunt attenuation. Potential causes of persistently elevated bile acids include persistent shunting in the original shunt vessel by failure of complete shunt attenuation or recannulation, presence of a second shunt vessel, concurrent hepatic microvascular dysplasia, and development of multiple acquired PSS (Worley and Holt 2008). Establishment of a specific diagnosis in animals with persistently elevated serum bile acids may require imaging the portal vascular system via operative mesenteric portography or CT angiography, exploratory surgery or laparoscopy, or liver biopsy. Multiple acquired extrahepatic shunts can be small and difficult to identify with portography and CT angiography.

Multiple extrahepatic shunts

The development of acquired multiple EHPSS is most commonly diagnosed in animals surgically treated for CPSS that are investigated for persistent elevation of serum bile acids postoperatively. Burton and White (2001) described 10 of 36 dogs and cats with single EHPSS that were investigated for persistent bile acid elevation 1 to 6 months after surgical attenuation of their shunt vessels and found persistent shunting in the original shunt vessels in 6 of 10 and multiple acquired EHPSS in addition to persistent shunting in the original shunt vessels in 4 of 10. Multiple acquired EHPSS are reported in 17% of dogs treated with ameroid constrictor (Berent and Weisse 2010) and 18.6% of dogs with elevated shunt fraction 6 weeks after cellophane banding (Landon *et al.* 2008).

Acquired multiple EHPSS are believed to form as a result of sustained intrahepatic or prehepatic portal hypertension through enlargement of extrahepatic rudimentary vessels that normally contain no blood flow (Brovida and Rothuizen 2010). There is considerable controversy surrounding the rate of rise, magnitude, and duration of portal hypertension necessary for acquired multiple EHPSS to develop. This contributes to ongoing controversy over whether or not CPSS should be acutely attenuated at all.

Device-associated complications

The incidence of device or implant-associated complications, including acute and chronic infection, in surgical treatment of CPSS appears to be low. Failure to achieve complete occlusion of EHPSS or IHPSS using all devices designed for gradual shunt occlusion (ameroid ring, cellophane band, hydraulic occluder) has been reported. There is anecdotal evidence of failure of ameroid ring constrictors as a result of dislodgement of the ameroid key, which has now been replaced with a stainless steel key. There is also anecdotal evidence of failure of cellophane banding caused by loss of the hemostatic clips securing the bands, which prompted a mechanical study resulting in recommendation for alternate side placement of four clips for security of the band (McAlinden *et al.* 2010).

Specific device-associated complications have been reported in 4 of 10 dogs with hydraulic occluder attenuation of IHPSS, prompting changes in the manufacturing of the device or removal of the device (Adin *et al.* 2006).

Septic complications

In the author's surgical practice, a variety of septic complications, including septic arthritis, discospondylitis, septic peritonitis, and bacterial endocarditis, have been seen in animals with CPSS before or after surgical management of their shunts. Vertebral physitis and epiphyseal sequestration has been reported in a dog with CPSS (Walker *et al.* 1999). These may represent coincidental comorbidity, particularly in light of the young age of many of these animals. Alternatively, animals with shunting of portal blood directly into the systemic circulation, bypassing the hepatic sinusoids, may be at increased risk of septic complications because portal blood contains bacteria in normal animals. However, in a study of 12 clinically normal dogs and 15 dogs with CPSS, portal bacteremia was found in only one dog with CPSS (Swalec Tobias and Besser 1997).

References

Adin, C.A., Sereda, C.W., Thompson, M.S., et al. (2006) Outcome associated with use of a percutaneously controlled hydraulic occluder for treatment of dogs with intrahepatic portosystemic shunts. *Journal of the American Veterinary Medical Association* 229, 1749-1755.

Aronson, L.R., Gacad, R.C., Kaminsky-Russ, K., et al. (1997) Endogenous benzodiazepine activity in the peripheral and portal blood of dogs with congenital portosystemic shunts. *Veterinary Surgery* 26, 189-194.

Berent, A.C., Tobias, K.M. (2012) Hepatic vascular anomalies In Tobias, K.M., Johnston, S.A. (eds.) *Veterinary Surgery Small Animal*, vol. 2. Elsevier Saunders, St. Louis, pp. 1624-1658.

Berent, A.C., Weisse, C. (2010) Hepatic vascular anomalies In Ettinger, S.J., Feldman, E.C. (eds.) *Textbook of Veterinary Internal Medicine: Diseases of the Dog and the Cat*, vol. 1, 7th edn. Saunders Elsevier, St. Louis, pp. 1649-1672.

Bostwick, D.R., Twedt, D.C. (1995) Intrahepatic and extrahepatic portal venous anomalies in dogs: 52 cases (1982-1992). *Journal of the American Veterinary Medical Association* 206, 1181-1185.

Brovida, C., Rothuizen, J. (2010) World Small Animal Veterinary Association (WSAVA) Guidelines. In Ettinger, S.J., Feldman, E.C. (eds.) *Textbook of Veterinary Internal Medicine: Diseases of the Dog and the Cat*, vol. 1, 7th edn. Saunders Elsevier, St. Louis, pp. 1609-1612.

Burton, C.A., White, R.N. (2001) Portovenogram findings in cases of elevated bile acid concentrations following correction of portosystemic shunts. *Journal of Small Animal Practice* 42, 536-540.

Cabassu, J., Seim, 3rd H.B., MacPhail, C.M., et al. (2011) Outcomes of cats undergoing surgical attenuation of congenital extrahepatic portosystemic shunts through cellophane banding: 9 cases (2000-2007). *Journal of the American Veterinary Medical Association* 238, 381-393.

Fryer, K.J., Levine, J.M., Peycke, L.E., et al. (2011) Incidence of postoperative seizures with and without levetiracetam pretreatment in dogs undergoing portosystemic shunt attenuation. *Journal of Veterinary Internal Medicine* 25, 1379-1384.

Grauer, G. (1993) Medical treatment of canine uroliths. In Slatter, D. (ed.) *Textbook of Small Animal Surgery*, vol 2, 2nd edn. WB Saunders, Philadelphia, pp. 1488-1495.

466 Section 7 General Abdominal Surgery

Greenhalgh, S.N., Dunning, M.D., McKinley, T.J., et al. (2010) Comparison of survival after surgical or medical treatment in dogs with a congenital portosystemic shunt. *Journal of the American Veterinary Medical Association* 236, 1215-1210.

Hardy, R.H. (1989) Diseases of the liver and their treatment. In Ettinger, S.J. (ed.) *Textbook of Veterinary Internal Medicine: Diseases of the Dog and Cat,* 3rd edn. WB Saunders, Philadelphia, pp. 1499-1525.

Heidenreich, D., Kirby, B. (2012) Successful treatment of refractory seizures with phenobarbital, propofol, and medetomidine following congenital portosystemic shunt attenuation. *Veterinary Surgery* 41, E11-E12.

Heldmann, E., Holt, D.E., Brockman, D.J., et al. (1999) Use of propofol to manage seizure activity after surgical treatment of portosystemic shunts. *Journal of Small Animal Practice* 40, 590-594.

Holford, A.L., Tobias, K.M., Bartges, J.W., et al. (2008) Adrenal response to adrenocorticotropic hormone in dogs before and after surgical attenuation of a single congenital portosystemic shunt. *Journal of Veterinary Internal Medicine* 22, 832-838.

Kummeling, A., van Sluijs, F.J., Rothuizen, J. (2004) Prognostic implications of the degree of shunt narrowing and of the portal vein diameter in dogs with congenital portosystemic shunts. *Veterinary Surgery* 33, 17-24.

Kummeling, A., Teske, E., Rothuizen, J., van Sluijs, F.J. (2006) Coagulation profiles in dogs with congenital portosystemic shunts before and after surgical attenuation. *Journal of Veterinary Internal Medicine* 20, 1319-1326.

Landon, B.P., Abraham, L.A., Charles, J.A. (2008) Use of transcolonic portal scintigraphy to evaluate efficacy of cellophane banding of congenital extrahepatic portosystemic shunts in 16 dogs. *Australian Veterinary Journal* 86,169-179.

Lipscomb, V.J., Jones, H.J., Brockman, D.J. (2007) Complications and long-term outcomes of the ligation of congenital portosystemic shunts in 49 cats. *Veterinary Record* 160, 465-470.

Lipscomb, V.J., Lee, K.C., Lamb, C.R., et al. (2009) Association of mesenteric portovenographic findings with outcome in cats receiving surgical treatment for single congenital portosystemic shunts. *Journal of the American Veterinary Medical Association* 234, 221-228.

McAlinden, A.B., Buckley, C.T., Kirby, B.M. (2010) Biomechanical evaluation of different numbers, sizes, and placement configurations of ligaclips required to secure cellophane bands. *Veterinary Surgery* 39, 59-64.

Mehl, M.L., Kyles, A.E., Hardie, E.M., et al. (2005) Evaluation of ameroid ring constrictors for treatment for single extrahepatic portosystemic shunts in dogs: 168 cases (1995-2001). *Journal of the American Veterinary Medical Association* 226, 2020-2030.

Mehl, M.L., Kyles, A.E., Case, J.B., et al. (2007) Surgical management of left-divisional intrahepatic portosystemic shunts: outcome after partial ligation of, or ameroid ring constrictor placement on, the left hepatic vein in twenty-eight dogs (1995-2005). *Veterinary Surgery* 36, 21-20.

Monnet, E. (2007) Portosystemic shunt: why I use cellophane banding. *Proceedings 2007 American College of Veterinary Surgeons Veterinary Symposium*, pp. 231-232.

Niles, J.D., Williams, J.M., Cripps, P.J. (2001) Hemostatic profiles in 39 dogs with congenital portosystemic shunts. *Veterinary Surgery* 30, 97-104.

Papazoglou, LG, Monnet, E, Seim III, HB. (2002) Survival and prognostic indicators for dogs with intrahepatic portosystemic shunts: 32 cases (1990-2000). *Veterinary Surgery* 31, 561-570.

Rogers, C.L., O'Toole, T.E., Keating, J.H., et al. (2008) Portal vein thrombosis in cats: 6 cases (2001-2006). *Journal of Veterinary Internal Medicine* 22, 282-287.

Swalec Tobias, K.M., Besser, T.E.(1997) Evaluation of leukocytosis, bacteremia, and portal vein partial oxygen tension in clinically normal dogs and dogs with portosystemic shunts. *Journal of the American Veterinary Medical Association* 211, 715-718.

Szatmári, V., van Sluijs, F.J., Rothuizen, J., et al. (2004) Ultrasonographic assessment of hemodynamic changes in the portal vein during surgical attenuation of congenital extrahepatic portosystemic shunts in dogs. *Journal of the American Veterinary Medical Association* 224, 395-402.

Tisdall, P.L., Hunt, G.B., Youmans, K.R., et al. (2000) Neurological dysfunction in dogs following attenuation of congenital extrahepatic portosystemic shunts. *Journal of Small Animal Practice* 41, 539-546.

Tivers, M.S., Upjohn, M.M., House, A.K., et al. (2012) Treatment of extrahepatic congenital portosystemic shunt in dogs—what is the evidence base? *Journal of Small Animal Practice* 53, 3-11.

Tobias, K.M. (2007) PSS-why I use ameroid constrictors. *Proceedings 2007 American College of Veterinary Surgeons Veterinary Symposium*, pp. 229-230.

Tobias, K.M., Rohrbach, B.W. (2003) Association of breed with the diagnosis of congenital portosystemic shunts in dogs: 2,400 cases (1980-2002). *Journal of the American Veterinary Medical Association* 223, 1636-1639.

Toulza, O., Center, S.A., Brooks, M.B., et al. (2006) Evaluation of plasma protein C activity for detection of hepatobiliary disease and portosystemic shunting in dogs. *Journal of the American Veterinary Medical Association* 229, 1761-1771.

Ubbink, G.J., van de Broed, J., Myes, H.P., et al. (1999) Prediction of inherited portosystemic shunts in Irish wolfhounds on the basis of pedigree analysis. *American Journal of Veterinary Research* 59, 1553-1556.

van Steenbeek, F.G., Leegwater, P.A.J., van Sluijs, F.J., et al. (2009) Evidence of inheritance of intrahepatic portosystemic shunts in Irish wolfhounds. *Journal of Veterinary Internal Medicine* 23, 950-952.

van Straten, G., Leegwater, P.A.J., de Vries, M., et al. (2005) Inherited congenital extrahepatic portosystemic shunts in Cairn terriers. *Journal of Veterinary Internal Medicine* 19, 321-324.

Waddell, L.S., Holt, D.E., Hughes, D., et al. (2001) The effect of storage on ammonia concentration in canine packed red blood cells. *Journal of Veterinary Emergency and Critical Care* 11, 23-26.

Walker, M.C., Platt, S.R., Graham, J.P., et al. (1999) Vertebral physitis with epiphyseal sequestration and portosystemic shunt in a Pekingese dog. *Journal of Small Animal Practice* 40, 525-528.

Webster, C.R.L. (2010) History, clinical signs, and physical findings in hepatobiliary disease. In Ettinger, S.J., Feldman, E.C. (eds.) *Textbook of Veterinary Internal Medicine: Diseases of the Dog and the Cat,* vol. 1, 7th edn. Saunders Elsevier, St. Louis, pp. 1612-1634.

Weisse C., Solomon J. A., Berent A., et al. (2006) Percutaneous transvenous coil embolization (PTCE) of canine intrahepatic portosystemic shunts: experience in 33 dogs. In *24th Annual ACVIM Forum Proceedings,* Louisville, KY, p. 783.

White, R.N., Forster-van Hijfte, M.A., Petrie, G., et al. (1996) Surgical treatment of intrahepatic portosystemic shunts in six cats. *Veterinary Record* 139, 314-317.

Worley, D.R., Holt, D.E. (2008) Clinical outcome of congenital extrahepatic portosystemic shunt attenuation in dogs aged five years and older: 17 cases (1992-2005). *Journal of the American Veterinary Medical Association* 232, 722-727.

Zwingenberger, A.L., Shofer, F.S. (2007) Dynamic computed tomographic quantitation of hepatic perfusion in dogs with and without portal vascular anomalies. *American Journal of Veterinary Research* 68, 970-974.

Surgery of the Urinary Tract

64 General Complications

Anne Kummeling

Division of Soft Tissue Surgery, Department of Clinical Sciences of Companion Animals, Faculty of Veterinary Medicine, Utrecht University, Utrecht, The Netherlands

Retroperitoneal and peritoneal urine leakage

Definition

Retroperitoneal and peritoneal urine leakage is urine leaking from a defect in the urinary tract, including the bladder, into the peritoneal cavity or into (retroperitoneal) tissues surrounding the kidneys and urinary tract. Urine leakage can result from trauma, improper suture technique, tissue necrosis, or dehiscence of sutured wounds in the urinary tract after urologic surgery. Another possibility is that existing defects in the urinary tract are missed during surgical exploration.

Risk factors

- Trauma, including traumatic catheterization, palpation, or manual expression of the bladder
- Urinary tract obstruction
- Infection

Diagnosis

- Analyses of time-matched testing of creatinine or potassium concentrations in aspirated peritoneal or retroperitoneal fluid and plasma. Although animals with urine leakage may be azotemic and hyperkalemic, the measured concentrations are expected to be higher in the aspirated fluid than the plasma. Urea readily diffuses from peritoneal cavity to the blood, which makes it less useful in diagnosis.
- The exact location of leakage can be visualized using contrast diagnostic imaging.

Treatment

- Intravenous (IV) prophylactic broad-spectrum antimicrobial treatment should be started after the aspirated fluid is sampled for culture.
- After surgical exploration of the suspected location of the leakage, the defect should be closed. Necrotic tissue should be removed, and only healthy tissue should be sutured, preferably with monofilament suture material and without tension on the wound edges. If this is not possible (e.g., after laceration of a ureter), reimplantation of the intact part of the ureter into the bladder or unilateral nephrectomy may be considered.

Outcome

In general, the prognosis is favorable when the defect can be repaired. Leaking infected urine into the abdomen can result into a generalized septic peritonitis, but this complication is rarely seen if the leakage is stopped and the infection is treated appropriately.

Prevention

- Careful palpation and handling of tissue
- Proper suture techniques
- Adequate treatment of urinary tract obstructions and infections

Renal failure

Definition

Renal failure means a decline in renal function, usually by acute tubular damage caused by ischemic injury (decreased renal perfusion) with or without toxic injury (e.g., aminoglycosides, nonsteroidal antiinflammatory drugs [NSAIDs]).

Risk factors

- Decreased mean arterial blood pressure during surgery (hypotension, decreased cardiac output)
- Dehydration
- Treatment with potential nephrotoxic drugs (aminoglycosides, NSAIDs)
- Preexisting renal disease
- Prolonged anesthesia and surgery times
- Anemia or severe hemorrhage
- Fever, septicemia, shock, or multiple organ disease
- Performing a nephrotomy (a nephrotomy a temporary and moderate reduction of the renal function)
- Performing a unilateral nephrectomy (decreasing the total number of functional nephrons)

Diagnosis

- An early sign of renal injury may consist of decreased urine production (normal output is ~1–2 mL/kg/hr), but polyuria can also result from acute renal dysfunction.
- Other signs are sudden glucosuria, proteinuria, and increasing azotemia.

Treatment

- When a decrease in renal function is suspected, the first step is to eliminate or treat any potential cause or contributing factors

Complications in Small Animal Surgery, First Edition. Edited by Dominique Griffon and Annick Hamaide.

© 2016 John Wiley & Sons, Inc. Published 2016 by John Wiley & Sons, Inc.

Companion website: www.wiley.com/go/griffon/complications

for further renal injury. Provided that cardiovascular function is normal, renal insufficiency is managed by IV fluid administration in combination with close monitoring of urinary output (using an indwelling urinary catheter and sterile collection system) and preferably with monitoring of the central venous pressure. Rehydration and increased diuresis help correct potential fluid deficits, protect against additional tubular injury, and facilitate excretion of toxic substances.

- Correction of electrolytes and, if necessary, administration of diuretics (e.g., furosemide or mannitol) to increase urine production have been assumed to be beneficial.
- Measurements of body weight and hematocrit can help to prevent overhydration.
- After severe bleeding or anemia, a whole-blood transfusion or administration of packed red blood cells is helpful.
- Colloid solutions may be needed for volume expansion, but there is evidence that high-molecular-weight starch solutions may promote renal injury (Cowgill and Langston 2011).

Outcome

Acute renal damage is not always reversible. Survival rates vary from 20% to 60% (Cowgill an Langston 2011). Early supportive treatment can help in the repair of damaged tubules, but the long-term outcome also depends on the underlying cause, degree of renal recovery, and progression to chronic renal insufficiency.

Prevention

- In animals with an increased risk of renal failure, screening of plasma or serum electrolytes, total protein, albumin, urea, and creatinine concentrations is important to evaluate kidney function before surgery.
- Intraoperative monitoring of urine output and mean arterial pressure is essential for early recognition of potential problems in renal functioning.
- Medical treatment of hypotension and sufficient fluid administration intravenously before and during anesthesia can prevent renal ischemic injuries.

Urinary tract infection

Definition

Urinary tract infection (UTI) is bacterial colonization and growth in the urinary tract.

Risk factors

- Bacterial contamination during surgery
- Residual urine in the urinary tract because of bladder atony, ureterocele, or mechanical or functional obstructions
- Foreign body material in the urinary tract (presence of catheters or nonabsorbable suture material)
- Presence of necrotic or damaged tissue, such as by (iatrogenic) trauma
- Presence of uroliths
- Feline perineal urethrostomy

Diagnosis

Bacteria can often be found in the urine sediment in UTIs, but an infection is more reliably diagnosed by culturing urine. Urine for culture should be collected in a sterile manner, such as by cystocentesis.

Treatment

- Antimicrobial treatment is preferably instituted based on testing of bacterial sensitivity. Depending on the anatomic localization (lower urinary tract or renal infections), treatment can be continued for days to 6 weeks, respectively.
- Primary causes and risk factors such as uroliths or foreign materials should be removed or treated as well. It is good practice to repeat urine culturing to 10 days after antimicrobial treatment is discontinued.
- In case of pyelonephritis, it is advisable to check the urine for bacterial growth during antimicrobial treatment as well.

Outcome

In general, the prognosis is good with appropriate treatment.

Prevention

- Proper aseptic technique and careful handling of tissues
- Prevention or adequate handling of causes and risk factors

Hemorrhage

See Chapter 12.

Hematuria

Definition

Hematuria is the presence of an increased number of erythrocytes in the urine by blood loss from the kidney or the lower urinary tract. Blood in voided urine can also originate from the female genital organs, vagina, prepuce, or prostate.

Risk factors

- Infection or inflammatory diseases
- Trauma or traumatic handling of tissue during surgery
- Residual uroliths or (bladder) polyps
- Indwelling catheters
- Coagulopathies, platelet disorders, and disseminated intravascular coagulation
- Neoplastic diseases

Diagnosis

- A positive reaction of a urine dipstick heme pigment test is indicative of hematuria.
- The diagnosis is confirmed by detection of an increased number of intact erythrocytes in the examination of the urine sediment. Reference values depend on the urine collection method.
- Other causes of reddish discoloration of the urine are hemoglobinuria and myoglobinuria.
- Further assessment of the animal should be aimed at identifying the localization and cause of the hematuria. For example, the finding of casts in the urine that are partly composed of erythrocytes indicates renal bleeding or inflammation.
- Concurrent dysuria is often seen in patients with lower urinary tract disorders.
- Diagnostic imaging techniques that can be useful to locate bleeding are ultrasonography, contrast radiography or computed tomography scanning, and endoscopic examination.

Treatment

- Treatment depends on the severity and the primary cause of the hematuria. If hematuria is caused by tissue trauma during surgery

(c.g., after nephrotomy, renal biopsies, bladder and urethral surgery, or endoscopic procedures), it should resolve spontaneously within 1 week. After surgery involving the corpus spongiosum or penis or after urethral prolapse resection, bleeding from the wound may be expected for a longer period (up to 2 weeks).
- As in all surgical patients, it is important to provide sufficient postoperative analgesic medication.
- Antimicrobials are started if there is evidence of infection, but otherwise they are preferably only used prophylactically (up to 24 hours).
- When hematuria persists or is severe, further examination and, if possible, (local) treatment of the cause are needed to stop the bleeding. Depending on the cause, surgical intervention may be necessary.

Outcome

The outcome may be good when hematuria is adequately monitored and treated if necessary. It is important to realize that blood clots can lead to urinary tract obstructions.

Prevention
- Careful tissue handling and proper suture technique
- Assess and treat potential risk factors (Figure 64.1).
- Avoid indwelling catheters after surgery if they are not really needed.
- In procedures such as scrotal urethrostomy and urethral prolapse resection in dogs or perineal urethrostomy in cats, it is important to minimize trauma to cavernous tissues, to carefully appose mucosa to skin (e.g., by using simple continuous sutures), and to avoid wound trauma after surgery by the animal itself or by cleaning the wound edges.

Recurrence of uroliths

Definition

This is newly formed uroliths in the urinary tract after (surgical) urolith removal. Incomplete urolith removal is actually not defined as a real recurrence and should be considered as a postoperative complication by an inadequate technique (pseudo-recurrence).

Risk factors
- Inadequate flushing or inspection of the urinary tract during (surgical) removal of uroliths (pseudo-recurrence)
- Concurrent UTI
- Breed, gender, and age predispositions
- Underlying (metabolic) disorders
- Hypercalcemia
- Urine pH
- Dietary factors or intake of calculogenic agents, such as ethylene glycol (calcium oxalate) and allopurinol in combination with a purine-rich diet (xanthine)

Diagnosis
- Diagnostic imaging (radiographic contrast studies or ultrasonography)
- Endoscopic inspection of the urethra and bladder.

Treatment

Uroliths can be removed by medical dissolution, voiding urohydropropulsion, endoscopy, lithotripsy or surgery, depending on the composition and size of the stones, available equipment, and gender and size of the animal.

Outcome
- Usually stones can be removed with good short-term outcome, but unfortunately, uroliths frequently show recurrence, especially when no preventive treatment is instituted after initial stone removal.
- Urolith or plug formation obstructing a ureter often occurs in combination with renal failure and more often results in serious postoperative complications (see Chapter 67).
- Unfortunately, the incidence of upper urinary tract uroliths (calcium oxalate) in cats seems to have increased during the past years, parallel with an increase of feline calcium oxalate uroliths in general (Osborne *et al.* 2009).

Prevention
- To avoid pseudo-recurrence, postoperative diagnostic imaging is important to confirm that all uroliths are removed (Figure 64.2).

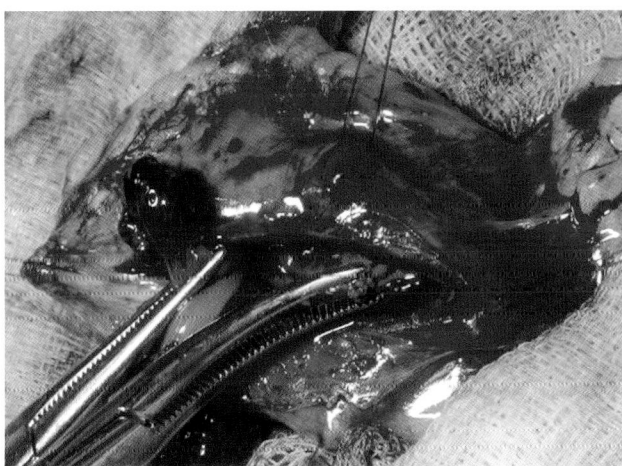

Figure 64.1 View into the bladder of a dog after a ventral cystotomy. Besides the uroliths that were detected with radiography, this dog also developed multiple polyps in the bladder. If a polyp is missed during surgical removal of the stones, persistent hematuria after surgery may occur.

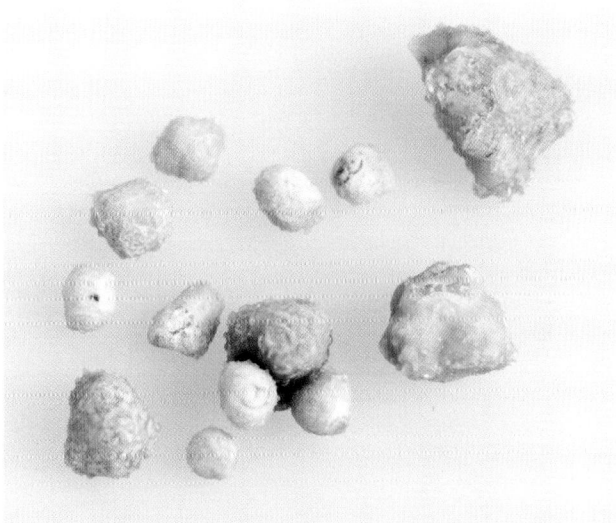

Figure 64.2 Multiple calcium oxalate stones surgically removed from the bladder and the urethra in a male dog. A urolith is often not alone.

- Stimulation of water consumption by feeding high-moisture diets (i.e., canned food or adding extra water to the food): Increased water intake will decrease mineral concentrations in the urine and increase voiding of crystals.
- Dietary and pharmacological measures: Specific medical protocols and diets have been developed to reduce the risk of new urolith formation in dogs and cats. Therefore, determination of the composition of removed uroliths is essential. Use of diuretics or addition of supplemental sodium chloride to stimulate thirst should be avoided because of potential adverse effects (Ulrich *et al.* 2009).
- Treatment of underlying disorders if possible (chronic UTIs, hypercalcemia, metabolic disorders such as congenital portosystemic shunts)
- Repeated urinalysis and diagnostic imaging for early detection of infection or stone recurrence. Small stones may be easily removed by voiding urohydropropulsion in female dogs and cats.

Relevant literature

Renal and ureteral surgery potentially bears a greater potential risk for intraoperative and postoperative complications than lower urinary surgery, such as renal dysfunction and ureteral obstruction. As a consequence, perioperative monitoring and care may be more challenging, and patients are more often referred to specialized practices (Tobias 2011a). As long as a proper technique is used, bladder and urethra often show rapid healing because of a rich blood supply and rapid mucosal regeneration. Therefore, lower urinary tract surgery such as cystotomy and urethrostomy are commonly performed in general practice (Tobias 2011b). Although surgical removal of uroliths from the bladder usually is reported to be a safe and an effective procedure, **failure to remove all uroliths** apparently occurs in a substantial percentage of patients. In a group of 44 dogs, incomplete removal after cystotomy was reported in 20% of the animals (Grant *et al.* 2010). Postsurgical diagnostic imaging to ensure complete urolith removal is therefore considered as a standard of patient care (Ulrich *et al.* 2009; Grant *et al.* 2010). **Real recurrence rates of uroliths** have been decreased by instituting specific preventive protocols but can not be eliminated completely. Recurrence of uroliths in cats is reported to vary from 7% with calcium oxalate stones to 13% in cats with ammonium urate stones. These recurrence rates do not count uroliths recurring within 6 months after the first stone removal because these were designated as incomplete urolith removal. Cats with struvite stones appeared to show even lower recurrence rates (nearly 3%), possibly because of effective preventive management of struvite stone formation. In 94% of the cases, the composition of recurrent stones was identical to that of the initial stone, meaning that the composition of the first stone may be used as a predictor of the composition of newly formed stones (Albasan *et al.* 2009). In dogs with compound uroliths, which represent nearly 9% of canine uroliths, prevention is usually aimed at minimizing the recurrence of minerals that formed the center of the stones (Ulrich *et al.* 2009).

References

Albasan, H., Osborne, C.A., Lulich, J.P., et al. (2009) Rate and frequency of recurrence of uroliths after an initial ammonium urate, calcium oxalate, or struvite urolith in cats. *Journal of the American Veterinary Medical Association* 235 (12), 1450-1455.

Cowgill, L.D., Langston, C. (2011) Acute kidney insufficiency. In Bartges, J., Polzi, D.J. (eds.) *Nephrology and Urology of Small Animals,* 1st ed. Blackwell Publishing, Chichester, UK, pp. 472-523.

Grant, D.C., Harper, T.A., Werre, S.R. (2010) Frequency of incomplete urolith removal, complications, and diagnostic imaging following cystotomy for removal of uroliths from the lower urinary tract in dogs: 128 cases (1994-2006). *Journal of the American Veterinary Medical Association* 236 (7), 763-766.

Osborne, C.A., Lulich, J.P., Kruger, J.M., et al. (2009) Analysis of 451,891 canine uroliths, feline uroliths, and feline urethral plugs from 1981 to 2007: perspectives from the Minnesota Urolith Center. *The Veterinary Clinics of North America, Small Animal Practice* 39 (1), 183-197.

Tobias, K. (2011a) Renal and ureteral surgery. I n Bartges, J., Polzi, D.J. (eds.) *Nephrology and Urology of Small Animals,* 1st ed. Blackwell Publishing, Chichester, UK, pp. 472-523.

Tobias, K. (2011b) Renal and ureteral surgery. I n Bartges, J., Polzi, D.J. (eds.) *Nephrology and Urology of Small Animals,* 1st ed. Blackwell Publishing, Chichester, UK, pp. 835-853.

Ulrich, L.K., Osborne, C.A., Cokley, A., et al. (2009) Changing paradigms in the frequency and management of canine compound uroliths. *The Veterinary Clinics of North America, Small Animal Practice* 39 (1), 41-53.

65 Complications Specific to Lithotripsy

Joseph W. Bartges,[1] Amanda Callens,[1] and India Lane[2]

[1]Department of Small Animal Clinical Sciences, Veterinary Teaching Hospital, College of Veterinary Medicine, The University of Tennessee, Knoxville, TN, USA
[2]Office of Academic Affairs and Student Success, The University of Tennessee, Knoxville, TN, USA

Laser lithotripsy via cystoscopy

Laser lithotripsy is minimally invasive, intracorporeal fragmenting of uroliths by laser energy. In veterinary medicine, a holmium:yttrium-aluminum-garnet (Ho:YAG) laser is used typically, which is a solid-state pulsed laser emitting light in the infrared wavelength range of 2100 nm (Grasso and Chalik 1998; Wollin and Denstedt 1998). It is performed via cystoscopy using a rigid cystoscope in female dogs and cats and a flexible cystoscope in male dogs. This allows visualization of the uroliths and provides a means of continuous sterile fluid irrigation. Laser energy is delivered via a quartz fiber ranging in size from 200 to 1000 μm that is passed through the working channel of the cystoscope. The fiber is placed in contact with the stone surface using the aiming beam. Fragmentation of uroliths occurs through a photothermal effect involving a thermal drilling process (Chan et al. 1999; Vassar et al. 1999). The 2100-mm wavelength of the Ho:YAG laser is absorbed in less than 0.5 mm of fluid; therefore, it fragments uroliths safely with minimal risk of urothelial damage. It also combines tissue cutting and coagulation properties (Wollin and Denstedt 1998). Stone fragments are retrieved using retrieval devices such as baskets or graspers or by voiding urohydropropulsion. There are several reports of Ho:YAG lithotripsy in small animal urology (Zerbib et al. 1988; Davidson et al. 2004; Adams et al. 2008; Grant et al. 2008; Bevan et al. 2009; Lulich et al. 2009).

In addition to the more than 250 canine and feline cases reported in the veterinary literature (Davidson et al. 2004; Adams et al. 2008; Grant et al. 2008; Bevan et al. 2009; Lulich et al. 2009), the authors have performed laser lithotripsy in more than 150 cases. We summarize the complications reported in the literature and from our experience. They are presented as complications occurring during the procedure and complications occurring after the procedure.

COMPLICATIONS OCCURRING DURING THE PROCEDURE

Potential complications occurring during the procedure may involve the patient or the equipment. Many patients with urocystoliths have clinical signs of lower urinary tract disease (e.g., pollakiuria, stranguria, hematuria); therefore, it is difficult to discern complications occurring because of the urocystoliths and complications occurring because of the procedure.

Cystoscopy-associated trauma to bladder and urethra

Cystoscopy may result in damage to the urethral or bladder wall, particularly when using rigid cystoscopes. In our experience, the trauma is usually superficial and most often occurs at the bladder neck because of the dorsal recumbent position of the patient and the angled view that rigid cystoscopes provide (Figure 65.1). Trauma may result in hemorrhage that can obscure visualization, making completion of the procedure difficult. The urethra may also be traumatized with rigid cystoscopes. Typically, this results in linear hemorrhages or mucosal tears. A urethral tear has been described in one female dog in one study (Adams et al. 2008). Cystoscopy-associated trauma is minimized by performing the procedure using gentle and controlled technique. Undue force can result in trauma, including perforation.

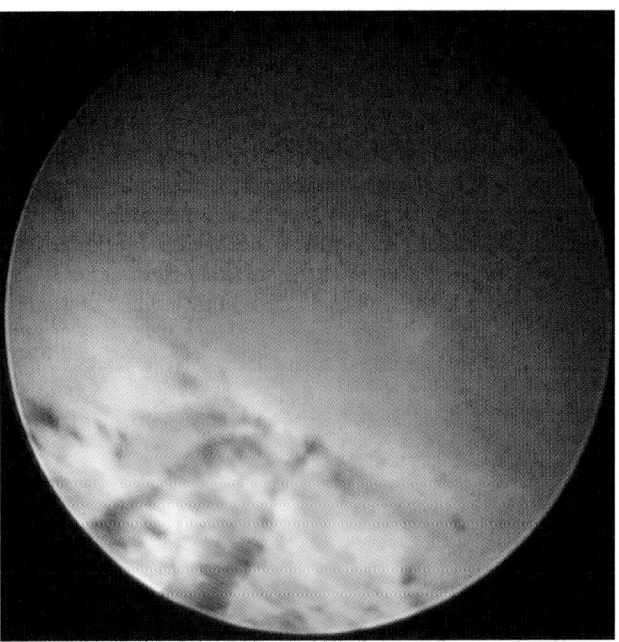

Figure 65.1 Linear mucosal trauma on caudal dorsal urinary bladder from a 2.7-mm, 30-degree, 18-cm rigid cystoscope in a female dog.

Laser-associated trauma to the bladder or urethra

Trauma to the urothelium of the bladder or urethra may occur from accidental contact with the laser fiber while the laser is turned on. Usually, this results in a small mucosal irregularity that often does not bleed because of coagulation provided by laser energy (Figure 65.2). In one experimental study of male dogs, laser-induced trauma to the urethral urothelium occurred in 30% of the cases (Davidson *et al.* 2004). Perforation caused by accidental contact of the laser with the bladder or urethral wall may occur, but it is rare. There must be long enough close or direct contact for perforation to occur or severe disease of the bladder or urethral wall. It has been reported to occur in 0% (Grant *et al.* 2008; Lulich *et al.* 2009) to 1.4% (Adams *et al.* 2008) of cases, and we have observed it in one of our cases. Perforation is prevented by maintaining good visualization cystoscopically and by avoiding contact of the laser fiber with the urothelium. If perforation occurs and is small, place an indwelling urinary catheter for 1 to 3 days. Closure of the perforation is verified by performing a contrast cystogram before removing the indwelling urinary catheter. If the perforation is large, surgical correction may be required. Urothelial trauma may also occur from the laser fiber even when the laser is not operated because of the sharp end of the quartz fiber contacting the mucosal surface. This may result in a circular to linear excoriation of the urothelium and hemorrhage. Theoretically, perforation can occur, but it has not been observed.

Trauma caused by retrieval and passage of uroliths and fragments

Fragmentation of uroliths often results in small pieces with sharp edges. As these fragments are retrieved either through use of retrieval instruments or by voiding urohydropropulsion, they may damage the urothelium. Urolith fragments may also embed in the urethral wall during retrieval, resulting in a mucosal tear (Figure 65.3). Retrieval instruments used for uroliths include three-

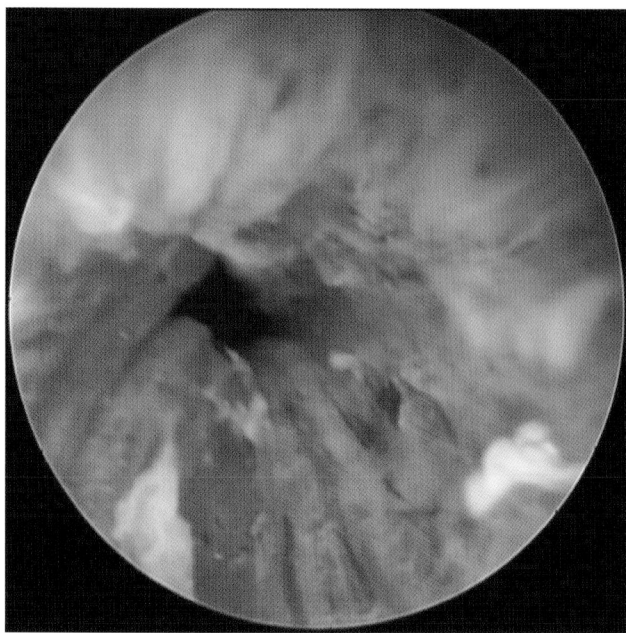

Figure 65.3 Urethral urothelial trauma induced from retrieving urocystoliths fragments by retrieval instruments and voiding urohydropropulsion.

or four-prong graspers and stone baskets. These instruments may grasp the mucosa as well as uroliths or urolith fragments, resulting in tearing of the urothelium or removal of larger pieces of urothelium as traction is applied on the retrieval instrument (Figure 65.4).

Incomplete fragmentation and removal (failure)

Incomplete removal of uroliths or urolith fragments has been reported to occur in 8% to 60% of male dogs and 0% to 9% of female

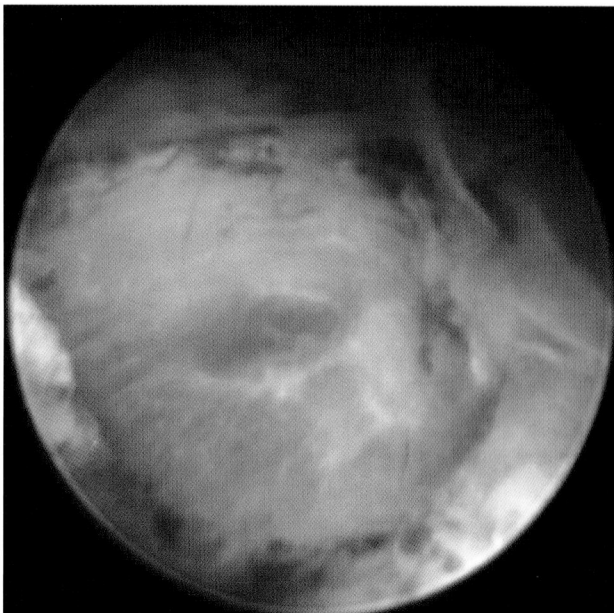

Figure 65.2 Laser-induced trauma to bladder urothelium in a female dog undergoing laser lithotripsy. The submucosa is exposed, but hemorrhage is minimal.

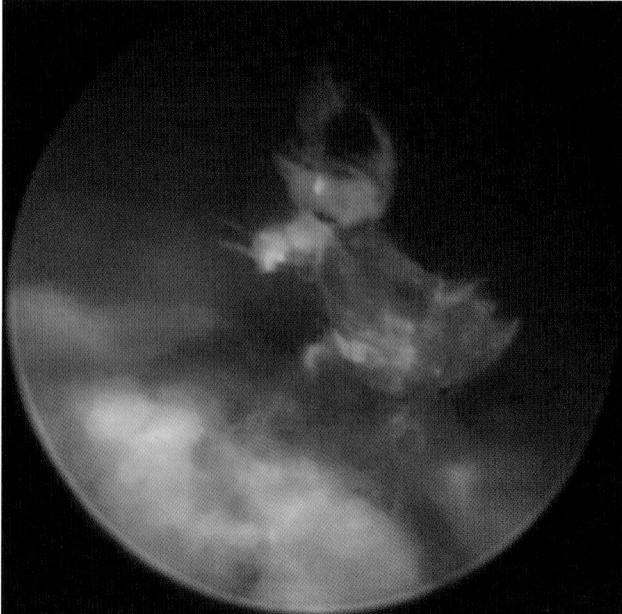

Figure 65.4 Urinary bladder mucosal trauma induced by retrieving urocystoliths fragments with a basket retrieval instrument.

dogs (Davidson *et al.* 2004; Adams *et al.* 2008; Grant *et al.* 2008; Bevan *et al.* 2009; Lulich *et al.* 2009). This may occur because of inadequate visualization caused by hemorrhage or by an inability to fragment the urolith into small enough fragments to be retrieved. There is no difference between laser lithotripsy management of uroliths and cystotomy with incomplete urolith retrieval occurring in 10% of patients managed by laser lithotripsy and 14% of patients managed by cystotomy (Bevan *et al.* 2009).

Length of procedure

The length of time required to perform laser lithotripsy is variable depending on whether the patient is a male or female, the ease of cystoscopy, the number and size of uroliths, and degree of visualization. In our experience, the procedure typically takes 30 to 40 minutes in females but has been reported to take as long as 6 hours (Lulich *et al.* 2009). Reported median procedural times range from 59 to 179 minutes (Adams *et al.* 2008; Grant *et al.* 2008; Lulich *et al.* 2009); however, the reported range in one study was 15 to 225 minutes (Grant *et al.* 2008), and in another study, it was 35 to 439 minutes (Adams *et al.* 2008). Median procedure time is shorter in dogs with only urocystoliths compared with dogs with urocystoliths and urethroliths and is significantly longer in males than females (Lulich *et al.* 2009).

Complications involving the cystoscope

Although not described in published reports, damage to the cystoscope may occur during the procedure. Damage may occur to a rigid cystoscope if bending occurs to the telescope and sheath and the Hopkins rod lens system breaks. When this occurs, the image appears white, similar in appearance to milk glass. Damage to the tip of a rigid scope may also occur if the laser is activated while the tip is within the sheath or near the end of the telescope. This results in a black appearance to the image (Figure 65.5). When performing urethrocystoscopy with a flexible scope, similar damage may occur. Flexible urethrocystoscopes are approximately 2.2 mm in diameter, and while digital video flexible scopes are available; most flexible urethrocystoscopes are fiberoptic. Overinsertion or overflexion of the flexible urethrocystocope may result in broken fibers that appear as black dots in the

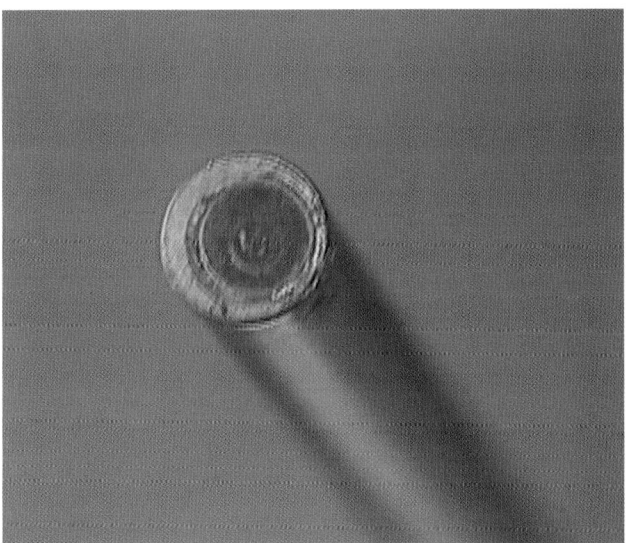

Figure 65.5 Laser-induced damage to the distal end of a 2.7-mm, 30-degree, 18-cm rigid cystoscope. The telescope is charred along the edge.

honeycomb appearance that is normally visualized. Flexible nephroureteroscopes used for urethrocystoscopy in male dogs have a ceramic tip that protects them from damage by the laser; however, other flexible scopes do not have ceramic tips, and damage may occur to the end of the flexible urethrocystocope by the laser.

COMPLICATIONS OCCURRING AFTER THE PROCEDURE

Patients undergoing laser lithotripsy may experience complications after the procedure is completed either from the procedure itself or from the preexisting inflammation or infection associated with urocystoliths.

Lower urinary tract clinical signs

Many patients exhibit signs of lower urinary tract disease characterized as pollakiuria, stranguria, inappropriate urination, or hematuria. Clinical signs may occur in 50% to 88% of patients in the first 24 hours after the procedure (Davidson *et al.* 2004; Grant *et al.* 2008; Lulich *et al.* 2009). Usually, these signs are self-limiting and resolve within 72 to 96 hours. There are several strategies for treating postprocedural clinical signs. We routinely administer a nonsteroidal antiinflammatory drug (Metacam, meloxicam; Boehringer Ingelheim Vetmedica, St. Joseph; 0.1 mg/kg orally every 24 hours) for 3 days beginning on the night of the procedure. Additionally, patients typically receive an opioid, such as buprenorphine or hydromorphone, at the end of the procedure.

Urethral obstruction

Patients may experience urethral obstruction, which may occur after the procedure caused by urethral spasm, edema, or inflammation. In one report, urethral obstruction occurred in a male dog because of a blood clot (Bevan *et al.* 2009). If urethral obstruction occurs, an indwelling urinary catheter is typically required for 1 to 2 days. This occurs uncommonly and has been reported in approximately 0% to 6.5% of the cases (Adams *et al.* 2008; Grant *et al.* 2008; Bevan *et al.* 2009; Lulich *et al.* 2009). The authors have not had urethral obstruction occur.

Urinary tract infection

Bacterial urinary tract infection (UTI) may occur in patients that have undergone laser lithotripsy for uroliths. In many of these patients, the infection was present before the procedure. In one study, 13% of dogs had leukocyturia before the procedure, but this increased to 47% of dogs on the day after the procedure; 1% had a culture-proven bacterial UTI (Lulich *et al.* 2009). In another study, 32% of dogs had a positive bacterial culture results before the procedure, and 12% had an iatrogenic bacterial UTI after the procedure (Grant *et al.* 2008). Patients with a culture-proven bacterial UTI or those with additional preexisting conditions that increase risk for iatrogenic bacterial UTI (e.g., diabetes mellitus, hyperadrenocorticism, hypothyroidism) should receive antimicrobial therapy after the procedure for at least 14 days with the antimicrobial agent used based on sensitivity results. In patients that do not have a bacterial UTI before the procedure, use of antimicrobial agents after the procedure is controversial. Some clinicians administer a broad-spectrum antimicrobial agent for 3 to 5 days after the procedure,

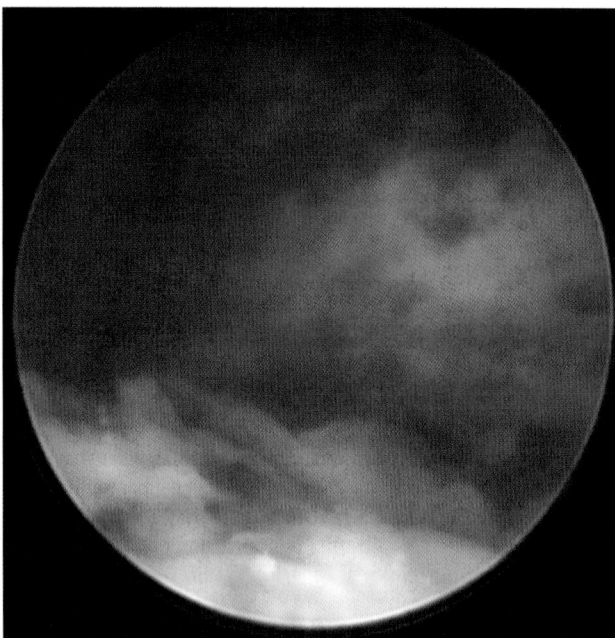

Figure 65.6 Cystoscopic view of white plaques and cystitis caused by iatrogenic *Corynebacterium urealyticum* urinary tract infection in a female dog with insulin-dependent diabetes mellitus and hyperadrenocorticism 5 days after laser lithotripsy for *Staphylococcus*-associated struvite urocystoliths. At the time of the first procedure, a single dose of parenteral ampicillin had been administered, but additional postprocedural enteral antimicrobial agent administration was not.

but others do not. We routinely administer ampicillin (22 mg/kg intravenously) at the end of the procedure but do not routinely continue antimicrobial therapy unless the patient has a culture-proven bacterial UTI before the procedure or has additional risks for iatrogenic bacterial UTI (Figure 65.6). In our experience, iatrogenic bacterial UTI occurs in approximately 1 of 1000 cystoscopic procedures in patients with a negative aerobic bacteriological culture results before the procedure.

EXTRACORPOREAL SHOCK-WAVE LITHOTRIPSY

Extracorporeal shock-wave lithotripsy (ESWL), in which high-amplitude sound waves are generated outside the body and focused on a hard surface, has been applied primarily to fissure and fragment nephroliths and ureteroliths in dogs and humans. Shock waves (SWs) can be effective against bladder stones and nonurinary stones (gallstones, salivary stones). In human medicine, adaptation of SW treatment revolutionized the treatment of urolithiasis in the 1980s (Chaussy 1980). Since that time, SW modalities, endosurgical techniques, percutaneous techniques, and combinations of these minimally invasive procedures have made open surgery of the urinary tract uncommon in humans. SW lithotripsy, laser lithotripsy, and interventional radiologic techniques have now been applied to urinary disorders in dogs, cats, and horses, so a similar transformation is occurring in veterinary medicine (Lulich *et al.* 2008). ESWL still requires the most costly and bulky equipment, limiting the number of patients that can be treated with this modality.

Application of SW lithotripsy requires a source to generate SWs, a method for focusing the SW onto a target, and a method for transmitting (or "coupling") the SW to the patient. SWs are generated by electrohydraulic, electromagnetic, or piezoelectrical energy sources. With extracorporeal methods, SW are generated outside the body and reflected to converge on the patient's urolith. Similar to ultrasound waves, SWs readily travel through fluid or soft tissue until they reach the "hard" acoustic surface of the urolith. Energy reflection, creation of tensile stresses at stone interfaces, generation of cavitation bubbles at the stone surface and in microcracks, and dynamic fatigue lead to fragmentation with repeated SW (Preminger 1991). Theories of fragmentation have expanded from simple reflection on the proximal and distal surfaces to "squeezing" effects brought about by shearing forces at multiple surfaces and corners (Rasweiller *et al.* 2011).

Extracorporeal shock-wave lithotripsy is typically described as a low-risk procedure, especially when compared with open surgical manipulation of the kidneys and ureters. Generally, healthy dogs with normal kidney function tolerate a typical SW dose well (Lulich *et al.* 2008). However, SWs are inherently impactful on tissue, and urolith fragments are not completely harmless. In a recent series of more than 3000 human patients, an overall complication rate of 36.3% was recorded (Salem *et al.* 2010), but this included mild, self-limiting complications such as nausea, pain, and hematuria. In dogs, severe pain or lasting hematuria is rare. ESWL is contraindicated in animals with uncontrolled coagulopathy, hypertension, pregnancy, or concurrent intraabdominal disease (e.g. chronic pancreatic, biliary or hepatic disease).

Incomplete fragmentation

Definition
Incomplete fragmentation is residual fragments larger than 2 mm in size, or symptomatic fragments of any size. Note that even small ("clinically insignificant") residual fragments can serve as a nidus for urolith recurrence in stone-forming individuals (Osman 2005; Tan and Wong 2005).

Risk factors
- Urolith composition: Calcium oxalate and struvite uroliths are more amenable to fragmentation than urate uroliths. Cystine uroliths are the most resistant; ESWL is not recommended for this stone type in dogs.
- Urolith size: Uroliths larger than 2 cm in their greatest diameter are more difficult to fragment and often require multiple treatments.
- Species: Calcium oxalate uroliths in cats are more resistant to SW fragmentation.
- Urolith location: Positioning of the focal zone for optimal SW application is more difficult with nephroliths in the right kidney (because of cranial position) and with distal ureteroliths (pelvic location, superimposition of other structures).
- Lithotriptor features, including power, depth of penetration, and size of focal zone, affect effectiveness (typically termed "efficiency" of treatment). Dry lithotripters with smaller focal zones have higher retreatment rates.
- SW dose and efficiency: A full SW dose, with each SW impacting the target area, is essential for effective fragmentation of nephroliths. Accurate targeting becomes even more critical when treating ureteroliths.

Diagnosis
Survey radiographs and ultrasound examination of the urinary system are typically performed 1 day after the procedure and then at regular intervals (every 3 to 4 weeks), depending on the number and size of fragments seen on day 1 and other patient characteristics.

Treatment

Smaller fragments may ultimately move out of the renal pelvis or ureter with time. When large residual fragments (or a resistant urolith) persist for several months, retreatment is considered. A second ESWL treatment may be needed in about one third of patients with nephroliths. Occasionally, surgical intervention may be necessary for refractory ureteroliths.

Outcome

One or two ESWL treatments are usually sufficient for most common uroliths in dogs. Residual fragments, regardless of size, can speed recurrence of uroliths by serving as a nidus for regrowth.

Prevention

Appropriate SW focus and application, dose (power and number of shocks), and frequency of application can maximize fragmentation. The quality of coupling the SW source to the patient is important for dry lithotripters; large amounts ("mounds") of bubble-free ultrasound gel are needed between the patient and the coupling cushion. SWs are usually initiated at low power settings, with the power increased slowly to the most effective level (usually 13–18 kV). Although this "ramping" or "voltage-stepping" protocol was primarily created to improve patient comfort and procedure tolerance, it also effects optimal urolith fragmentation by slowly creating small dustlike particles. Higher SW power is also required as the treatment proceeds because fragments overly each other and create increasing attenuation. Additionally, slow frequency of application (30–60 SW/min) is now recommended for more effective and safer treatment (Argyropoulos and Tolley 2007; Rassweiler *et al.* 2011). Fragmentation has been considered complete in humans when only clinically insignificant (<2 mm) fragments remain visible. Based on veterinary experience, even smaller fragments are desired in small animal patients to facilitate passage of all debris along the ureter.

Steinstrasse and ureteral obstruction

Definition

This is partial or complete obstruction created by urolith fragments migrating singly or in series down the ureter. Steinstrasse, or "stone street," refers to a line of fragments positioned along most of the ureter.

Risk factors

- Large stone size with multiple fragments
- Large fragment size
- Ureteral inflammation or stricture
- Species: cats with very small ureteral lumens

Diagnosis

Serial survey abdominal radiographs and ultrasonographic examination of the urinary system are routinely performed after the procedure. Additional imaging may be needed to determine the degree of obstruction in some cases. Note that obstruction of a single ureter may not cause clinical signs in a patient with a functional contralateral kidney.

Treatment

- After lithotripsy treatment, a 2- to 4-day period of diuresis is continued to promote passage of stone fragments. Mild

diuresis and tincture of time are usually sufficient for management of fragments.
- The use of pharmacologic aids to promote fragment passage is enticing but unproven; α-blocking agents, amitriptyline, or anti-inflammatory agents help relax the ureter and facilitate passage of fragments.
- Ureteral stents, placed with fluoroscopic and cystoscopic assistance, have become more common in veterinary urology and can be left in place to keep the ureter open while fragments advance down the ureter. In human patients, stents are preplaced for larger nephroliths.
- Alternatively, a temporary nephrostomy tube can be placed to provide urine drainage while an obstruction is addressed.

Outcome

Ureteral fragments in dogs, fortunately, are rarely completely obstructive and eventually move into the urinary bladder, obviating the need for aggressive treatments. Occasionally, a ureteral fragment will require further fragmentation by ESWL. In cats, obstruction by urolith fragments is more likely to be associated with significant morbidity and mortality and necessitate immediate attention.

Prevention

- Appropriate SW regimens designed to produce small particulate fragments (see the earlier discussion of incomplete fragmentation)
- Consider staging treatments for large or refractory bilateral nephroliths to avoid bilateral ureteral obstruction.
- Avoid ESWL for very large nephroliths.
- Ensure adequate postprocedural diuresis.

Kidney injury

Definition

Shock waves are inherently traumatic to renal tissue and primarily cause focal vascular damage that is SW dose dependent. Acute kidney injury with tubular, interstitial, and functional damage is also possible. Perirenal or retroperitoneal fluid has been observed, suggesting edema and subcapsular hemorrhage (Siems *et al.* 1999). One of the authors has managed a cat with retroperitoneal urine accumulation secondary to a ureteral tear after ESWL treatment of a ureterolith. Transient macroscopic or microscopic hematuria is common after treatment. An acute drop in glomerular filtration rate (GFR) is likely in the treated kidney during and immediately after SW application but usually does not affect the patient's clinical status. Minor increases in serum creatinine may be observed (Adams and Senior 1999). As with any other insult that may injure or cause nephron loss, long-term renal impairment, fibrosis, or a delayed decline in function is possible after ESWL. A significant long-term impact on renal function is not common in humans; however, the long-term effects of ESWL have not been well studied in dogs or cats. In a small number of dogs followed by the author, GFR as assessed by nuclear scintigraphy declined within the first month after ESWL and rebounded within a few months after treatment in all dogs (Lane 2003).

Risk factors

- Species: Cat kidneys appear to be more susceptible to SW damage.
- Preexisting renal disease or decreased renal function
- Preexisting pyelonephritis

- SW dose: Application of greater than 1500 to 2000 high-power SW is more likely to cause significant trauma.
- Lithotriptor features: The type of renal and perirenal trauma varies based on lithotriptor type and focal zone. Whereas larger focal zones allow SW impact on a larger amount of tissue, lithotriptors with high-intensity, small focal zones tend to create more severe focal damage.

Diagnosis

Postprocedural monitoring of hematocrit, serum creatinine, urinalysis, abdominal radiographs, and ultrasonographic examination of the urinary system is essential.

Treatment

- Fluid administration is usually sufficient.
- Blood product or more aggressive management of the consequences of acute kidney injury could be necessary in rare circumstances.

Outcome

Macroscopic or microscopic hematuria resolves within 1 to 2 days. Reduced renal function usually returns to pretreatment measures within a few weeks; increased azotemia returns to baseline in a few days. Rare patients may develop chronic progressive kidney disease requiring ongoing monitoring and management.

Prevention

- Appropriate patient selection: Measure coagulation parameters and blood pressure. (ESWL is contraindicated in patients with untreated coagulopathy or hypertension.) Ideally, estimation of GFR.
- Appropriate SW protocol (see the earlier discussion of incomplete fragmentation) Damage to the kidney can be minimized by limiting the SW dose as much as possible and the rate at which SW are applied. Frequencies of approximately 1 SW per second (60 Hz) or 1 SW per 2 seconds (30 Hz) are recommended based on human and animal studies (Gilitzer et al. 2009; Anglada-Curado et al. 2012). Conservative, staged SW protocols should be followed in patients with known preexisting decreased renal function.
- Follow the "do no harm" principle Avoid unnecessary ESWL for silent (asymptomatic and static) nephroliths.

Infection or urosepsis

Definition

Urinary stones often coexist with UTI, either as infection-induced (struvite) stones or by harboring bacteria within stone layers. The microvascular trauma and stone disruption that occurs with ESWL can release bacteria into urine or the bloodstream. In human patients, infections manifest as bacteriuria or relapse of prior infection (D'Addessi 2012). More severe and symptomatic infection (pyelonephritis, urosepsis) is observed in up to 10% of human patients (Salem et al. 2010) but is uncommon in dogs and cats.

Risk factors

- Infection-induced struvite urolithiasis
- Large stone burden
- Recurrent UTI
- Renal disease or trauma
- Persistent *Escherichia coli* infection
- Additional instrumentation (catheters, stents, cystoscopies)

Diagnosis

- Urinalysis and urine culture

Treatment

- Appropriate antimicrobials (for UTI) and supportive care (for sepsis)

Outcome

Usually favorable. Persistent *E. coli* infections are possible and may never be fully eradicated. Recurrent active infections are likely if fragmentation is incomplete. Residual fragments in the kidney may provide a nidus for harboring infection.

Prevention

- UTI should be managed and sterile urine obtained before performing ESWL.
- Continuing antimicrobial treatment during the posttreatment phase is important while fragments are migrating.
- Appropriate prophylactic antimicrobial treatment is recommended for patients that have a history of UTI or large or suspected struvite uroliths or have undergone additional urinary tract instrumentation (e.g., catheterization, cystoscopy, stent placement).

Injury to surrounding tissue

Definition

Trauma from SW energy can affect surrounding tissues, including the pancreas, lungs, liver, spleen, and gastrointestinal (GI) structures. The pancreas appears to be most sensitive in dogs. The GI effects of SW application in humans usually manifest as nausea and vomiting. More severe injury occurs in rare cases, including mucosal erosions, bleeding, and perforation; severe effects have been associated with high SW doses (Maker and Layke 2004). In dogs, mild, transient diarrhea occasionally occurs after ESWL. The authors are unaware of acute pulmonary, hepatic, or splenic complications in dogs or cats despite their small size compared with human patients.

Risk factors

- Small patient size
- SW application to the right kidney
- Improper shielding or positioning
- High SW dose
- Preexisting chronic pancreatic disease?
- Other risk factors for acute pancreatitis

Diagnosis

- Clinical signs such as vomiting, lethargy, and fever as well as typical clinicopathologic findings and indicators of pancreatic inflammation
- Abdominal sonography can be supportive.

Treatment

- Supportive and nutritional support for acute pancreatitis and its complications

Outcome

- Variable depending on the severity and type of inflammation.
- May be fatal

Prevention

- Appropriate positioning for ESWL treatment
- Use narrow SW focal zone if feasible.

Arrhythmias and other anesthetic complications

Definition

Ventricular premature contractions can be observed during treatment, presumably as a result of the SW on heart muscle or cardiac conduction.

Risk factors

- Unknown; arrhythmias may simply be a result of anesthetic agents

Diagnosis

- Electrocardiographic (ECG) monitoring is essential during SW application.

Treatment

- Stop application of SW.
- Administer antiarrhythmic agents.
- Review anesthetic management.

Outcome

- Usually transient but can be fatal

Prevention

- Assess pretreatment ECG.
- Gate SW with ECG.

Relevant literature

Procedural complications are rare during ESWL treatment. Fatal arrhythmia, possibly secondary to SW, was described in one dog treated with the Human Model 3 (HM-3) (Adams 2006). By gating SW to the refractory period using ECG monitoring, induced arrhythmias are minimized in human patients. The author has observed a transient ventricular arrhythmia in one cat during ESWL application. The procedure was aborted, but we do not routinely gate the SW as others may. Although it was not a direct complication of SW application, iohexol contrast nephropathy has been described in one dog in which iohexol administration was used to facilitate positioning during ESWL (Adams and Goldman 2011).

Immediately after the procedure, **manageable pain**, **mild bruising** at the treatment site, and microscopic or macroscopic **hematuria** are common transient complications. In humans, severe pain and site trauma, including the occasional abdominal hematoma, are possible. Severe "colicky" pain is quite rare in small animals (Adams and Goldman 2011). Other potential complications of lithotripsy for nephroliths include **obstructive ureteral fragments**, **damage to the kidney** (parenchymal hemorrhage or subcapsular hematoma), **reduced renal function**, or **damage to other organs** secondary to SW application (Adams 2006; Lulich *et al.* 2008. Transient hematuria, a transient or progressive decrease in renal function, retroperitoneal fluid accumulation, ureterectasia, pain, diarrhea, and ureteral obstruction by urolith fragments have been observed in dogs (Siemens *et al.* 2003; Lane 2004). Fragmentation or movement of a ureterolith can create a more lodged stone even if the uretero-

lith was nonobstructive initially. Adams (2006, 2011) estimates 10% of treated dogs experience transient obstruction in the ureter; some require retreatment of the ureteral fragment.

Renal function as measured by serum creatinine concentration is not altered in most dogs. Concurrent pyelonephritis or renal failure, although considered an indication for pursuing treatment of nephroliths, may increase the risk of SW-induced renal injury in dogs and cats. In 4 dogs in a series of 116, serum creatinine rose transiently (48 hours) after ESWL; these dogs had known preexisting renal failure (Adams 2006).

Although small body size is not a contraindication, a greater percentage of the kidney is exposed to SW injury in patients or species with small kidneys (Blomgren *et al.* 1997, Willis *et al.* 1999). Acute pancreatitis has been described as a consequence of right kidney ESWL treatment in two small (<5 kg) dogs, with fatal complications in one dog (Daugherty *et al.* 2004).

These short-term complications can be minimized by ensuring the health and suitability of the patient for anesthesia and SW treatment, staging treatment of bilateral uroliths when appropriate, ensuring appropriate SW dosage and application, shielding other organs from SW during treatment, ensuring adequate diuresis and monitoring post treatment, and providing prompt treatment of obstructive fragments. The place of ureteral stents in ESWL protocols is still uncertain, but the expanding application and experience with stents in dogs and cats offers a minimally invasive tool for preventing posttreatment obstruction (Berent 2011; Berent *et al.* 2012).

Incomplete fragmentation necessitating retreatment is relatively common. The reported retreatment rate for canine nephroliths varies with machines, ranging from 30% (Adams 1999) to 50% (Lane 2003). In several reports, Adams has reported overall success in approximately 85% of dogs treated with the HM-3 lithotriptor. Calcium oxalate and struvite uroliths are most amenable to fragmentation. In 5 dogs with urate or xanthine stones, lithotripsy was effective in only 2 dogs (Adams 2006).

Treatment of large stones is also difficult, requiring high SW dose and longer anesthetic time to create adequate fragmentation. Additionally, large fragments may be expected, leading to the increased likelihood or ureteral obstruction by stone fragmentation after ESWL.

Ureteroliths pose technical challenges: they are more difficult to image and focus, are not in contact with as much fluid as stones in the renal pelvis, have less room for fragments to fall away, and may be imbedded in the ureteral wall. A higher SW dose may be required to sufficiently fragment ureteroliths. Using an aggressive treatment approach (mean, 2600 SW at 14–19 kV) and a lithotripter with a small, high-pressure focal zone, one of the authors had good success (>90%) in fragmenting ureteroliths in dogs (Lane 2005).

In cats, ESWL treatment of uroliths has been limited by disappointing results and unique features of feline urolithiasis. Adams (1999) observed significant renal trauma (renal hemorrhage and functional impairment) in a small number of healthy cat kidneys treated with the HM-3 lithotriptor, as well as insufficient fragmentation of upper tract uroliths in five clinically affected cats. In addition, transient or permanent worsening of renal function occurred in several cats. Although promising results were obtained in a small group of healthy cats treated with a dry lithotriptor (Gonzales *et al.* 2002), fragmentation of nephroliths or ureteroliths to the size needed to pass through the extremely small ureteral lumen still poses a considerable challenge.

Feline uroliths also are more difficult to fragment. In an ex vivo study, significantly less breakage was observed in feline stones than

Box 65.1 Methods to Minimize Extracorporeal shock-Wave Lithotripsy Complications

> Treat only symptomatic or obstructive nephroliths or ureteroliths.
>
> Assess patient pretreatment for compromised renal function, hypertension, infection, and cardiac disease.
>
> Treat urinary tract infections.
>
> Avoid lithotripsy for large stone burdens.
>
> Maximize efficiency of each shock wave to reduce the total dose.
>
> Use slow pulse frequency.
>
> Be prepared to retreat or stent ureteral fragments.
>
> Monitor urinary system carefully posttreatment.
>
> Ensure that surgical intervention or repeat extracorporeal shock-wave lithotripsy treatment is readily available for obstructive fragments.

in canine uroliths after the same SW dosage (100 SW at 20kV) (Adams *et al.* 2003). The number and size of nephroliths (or the finding of multiple, concurrent nephroliths, ureteroliths, and cystoliths) makes lithotripsy impractical for stone disease in many cats.

Lithotripsy of ureteroliths in cats poses similar, but magnified, challenges compared with those encountered in dogs. We reported progressively improving results in several feline ureteroliths treated with ESWL (Lane 2005) and experienced an approximately 50% success rate (complete fragmentation and passage) after one or two treatments. Short-term interim morbidity (reobstruction, slow passage of fragments or debris, ureteral tear) can be highly stressful. Surgical intervention, stent placement, or dialysis support may be necessary to salvage incompletely fragmented ureteroliths.

Methods to minimize ESWL complications are listed in Box 65.1.

References

Adams, L.G. (2006) Lithotripsy using shock waves and lasers. In 24th Annual American College of Veterinary Internal Medicine Forum, Louisville, KY, pp. 439-441.

Adams, L.G., Goldman, C.K. (2011) Extracorporeal shock wave lithotripsy. In Bartges, J., Polzin, D.J. (eds.) *Nephrology and Urology of Small Animals*. Wiley-Blackwell, Ames, IA, pp. 340-348.

Adams, L.G., Senior, D.F. (1999) Electrohydraulic and extracorporeal shock-wave lithotripsy. *Veterinary Clinics of North America: Small Animal Practice* 29, 293-302.

Adams, L.G., Williams, J.C. Jr., McAteer, J.A., et al. (2005) In vitro evaluation of canine and feline urolith fragility by shock wave lithotripsy. *American Journal of Veterinary Research* 66, 1651-1654.

Adams, L.G., Berent, A.C., Moore, G.E., Bagley, D.H.. (2008) Use of laser lithotripsy for fragmentation of uroliths in dogs: 73 cases (2005-2006). *Journal of the American Veterinary Medical Association* 232 (11), 1680-1687.

Anglada-Curado, F.J., Campos-Hernandez, P., Anaya-Henares, F., et al. (2012) Extracorporeal shock wave lithotripsy for distal ureteral calculi; improved efficacy using low frequency. *International Journal of Urology* 20 (2), 214-219.

Argyropoulos, A.N., Tolley, D.A. (2007) Optimizing shock wave lithotripsy in the 21st century. *European Urology* 57, 344-354.

Berent, A.C. (2011) Ureteral obstructions in dogs and cats: a review of traditional and new interventional diagnostic and therapeutic options. *Journal of Veterinary Emergency and Critical Care* 21, 86-103.

Berent, A.C., Weisse, C.W., Todd, K.L., et al. (2012) Use of lockin-loop pigtail nephrostomy catheters in dogs and cats: 20 cases (2004-2009). *Journal of the American Veterinary Medical Association* 241, 348-357.

Bevan, J.M., Lulich, J.P., Albasan, H., Osborne, C.A. (2009) Comparison of laser lithotripsy and cystotomy for the management of dogs with urolithiasis. *Journal of the American Veterinary Medical Association* 234 (10), 1286-1294.

Blomgren, P., Connors, B., Lingeman, J., et al. (1997) Quantitation of shock wave lithotripsy-induced lesion in small and large pig kidneys. *Anatomical Record* 249, 341.

Chan, K.F., Vassar, G.J., Pfefer, T.J., et al. (1999) Holmium:YAG laser lithotripsy: a dominant photothermal ablative mechanism with chemical decomposition of urinary calculi. *Lasers in Surgery and Medicine* 25 (1), 22-37.

Chaussy, C., Brendel, W., Schmidt, E. (1980) Extracorporeally induced destruction of kidney stones by shock waves. *Lancet* 2, 1265.

D'Addessi, A., Vittori, M., Racioppi, M., et al. (2012) Complications of extracorporeal shock wave lithotripsy for urinary stones: to know and to manage them—a review. *The Scientific World Journal* 2012:619820.

Daugherty, M., Adams, L.G., Baird, D.K., et al. (2004) Acute pancreatitis in two dogs associated with shock wave lithotripsy. *Jouranl of Veterinary Internal medicine* 18, 441.

Davidson, E.B., Ritchey, J.W., Higbee, R.D., et al. (2004) Laser lithotripsy for treatment of canine uroliths. *Veterinary Surgery* 33 (1), 56-61.

Gilitzer, R., Neisius, A., Wollner, J. (2009). Low-frequency extracorporeal shock wave lithotripsy improves renal pelvic stone disintegration in a pig model. *BJU International* 103:1284-1288.

Gonzales, A., Labato, M., Solano, M., et al. (2002) Evaluation of the safety of extracorporeal shock-wave lithotripsy in cats (abstr). *Journal of Veterinary Internal Medicine* 16, 376.

Grant, D.C., Were, S.R., et al. (2008) Holmium: YAG laser lithotripsy for urolithiasis in dogs. *Journal of Veterinary Internal Medicine* 22 (3), 534-539.

Grasso, M., Chalik, Y. (1998) Principles and applications of laser lithotripsy: experience with the holmium laser lithotrite. *Journal of Clinical Laser Medicine and Surgery* 16 (1), 3-7.

Lane, I. (2003) Dry extracorporeal shock-wave lithotripsy. In 21st Annual American College of Veterinary Internal Medicine Forum, Charlotte, NC, pp. 775-776.

Lane, I. (2004) Lithotripsy: an update on urologic applications in small animals. *Veterinary Clinics of North America: Small Animal Practice* 34, 1011-1025.

Lane, I. (2005) Extracorporeal shock-wave lithotripsy for ureteroliths in dogs and cats. In 23rd Annual American College of Veterinary Internal Medicine Forum, Baltimore, pp. 13-14.

Lane, I. Labato, M., Adams, L.G. (2006) Lithotripsy. In August, J. (ed.) *Consultations in Feline Internal Medicine*, 5th edn. Elsevier, Philadelphia, pp. 407-414.

Lulich, J.P., Adams, L.G., Grant, D., et al. (2008) Changing paradigms in the treatment of uroliths by lithotripsy. *Veterinary Clinics of North America: Small Animal Practice* 39, 143-160.

Lulich, J.P., Osborne, C.A., Albasan, H., et al. (2009) Efficacy and safety of laser lithotripsy in fragmentation of urocystoliths and urethroliths for removal in dogs. *Journal of the American Veterinary Medical Association* 234 (10), 1279-1285.

Maker, V., Layke, J. (2004) Gastrointestinal injury secondary to extracorporeal shock wave lithotripsy: a review of the literature since its inception. *Journal of the American College of Surgeons* 198, 128-135.

Preminger, G. (1991) Shock wave physics. *American Journal of Kidney Disease* 17, 431-435.

Osman, M., Alfano, Y., Kamp, S., et al. (2005) Five-year-follow-up of patients with clinically insignificant residual fragments after extracorporeal shockwave lithotripsy. *European Urology* 47, 860-864.

Rassweiler, J.J., Knoll, T., Kohrmann, K.U., et al. (2011) Shock wave technology and application: an update. *European Urology* 59, 784-796.

Salem, S., Mehrsai, A., Zartab, H., et al. (2010) Complications and outcomes following extracorporeal shock wave lithotripsy: a prospective study of 3,241 patients. *Urological Research* 38, 135-142.

Siemens, J., Adams, L.G., et al. (1999) Ultrasound findings in 14 dogs following extracorporeal shock-wave lithotripsy for treatment of nephrolithiasis [abstract]. *Veterinary Radiology and Ultrasound* 40, 662.

Skolarikos, A., Alivizatos, G., delaRosette, J. (2006) Extracorporeal shock wave lithotripsy 25 years later: complications and their prevention. *European Journal of Urology* 50, 981-990.

Tan, Y., Wong, M. (2005) How significant are clinically insignificant residual fragments following lithotripsy? *Current Opinion in Urology* 15, 127-131.

Vassar, G.J., Chan, K.F., Teichman, J.M., et al. (1999) Holmium: YAG lithotripsy: photothermal mechanism. *Journal of Endourology* 13 (3), 181-190.

Willis, L., Evan, A.P., Connors, B.A., et al. (1999) Relationship between kidney size, renal injury and renal impairment induced by shock wave lithotripsy. *Journal of the American Society of Nephrology* 10, 1753.

Wollin, T.A., Denstedt J.D. (1998) The holmium laser in urology. *Journal of Clinical Laser Medicine and Surgery* 16 (1), 13-20.

Zerbib, M., Steg, A., Moissonier, P., et al. (1988) Effects of pulsed dye laser lithotripsy on tissues. Experimental study in the canine ureter. *Urologic Clinics of North America* 15 (3), 547-550.

66 Renal Transplantation

Andrew Kyles

Blue Pearl Veterinary Partners, New York, NY

Renal transplantation is an established treatment for end-stage renal failure in cats. Short- and long-term complications are relatively frequent. The perioperative mortality rate (i.e., death before discharge from the hospital) is reported as 23% to 29% (Mathews and Gregory 1997; Schmiedt et al. 2008). Schmiedt et al. (2008) reported that 14 of 60 cats (23%) died before discharge, with the cause of death including cardiopulmonary arrest (9 cats), hemorrhage (2), chronic heart failure (1), pulmonary thromboembolism (1), and unknown (1). Several factors were identified that increased the risk of death before discharge, including increased preoperative serum blood urea nitrogen (BUN) and creatinine concentrations, increased left ventricular wall thickness on preoperative echocardiography, and duration of intraoperative hypotension (Schmiedt et al. 2008). Cats that died before discharge were also more likely to receive Hetastarch and to have experienced significant hemorrhage or a thromboembolic event (Schmiedt et al. 2008).

After renal transplantation in cats, the reported 6-month and 3-year survival rates are 59% to 65% and 40% to 42%, respectively, with a median overall survival time of 613 days (Adin et al. 2001; Schmiedt et al. 2008). Increased recipient age has been associated with reduced overall survival times (Adin et al. 2001; Schmiedt et al. 2008). Schmiedt et al. (2008) estimated the median survival time of transplant recipients younger than 5 years was 1423 days compared with 613 days for cats between 5 and 10 years and 150 days for cats older than 10 years.

Schmiedt et al. (2008) compared survival in a group of consecutively operated feline renal transplant recipients and a control group of nonoperated cats with chronic renal failure. Transplant recipients survived significantly longer, with a median survival time of 613 days (95% confidence interval [CI] 131–1095 days) compared with a median survival time in control cats of 270 days (95% CI 153–387 days). However, if age is considered as a covariant, the significance is lost. It is difficult to compare nonrandomized groups of transplanted versus nontransplanted cats with chronic renal failure because of difficulties matching the severity of azotemia or proteinuria, occurrence of comorbid conditions (some of which would have precluded transplantation), inability to account for the time that transplanted cats were medically treated before transplantation, and differences in owners' expectations and desire to pursue therapy. The authors did conclude that renal transplantation appeared to prolong survival time.

Renal transplantation is rarely performed in dogs.

PERIOPERATIVE COMPLICATIONS

Vascular complications

Intraoperative hemorrhage can be encountered when the vascular occlusion clamps are removed after completion of the arterial and venous anastomoses. Hemorrhage is controlled by pressure or the addition of additional simple interrupted sutures. Reapplication of the occlusion clamp should be avoided, if possible, because this will result in substantial damage to the allograft, but it is sometimes necessary to control hemorrhage.

Postoperative hemoabdomen is an uncommon complication. It was the reported cause of death in 1 of 61 (1.6%) (Adin et al. 2001) and 2 of 60 (3.3%) (Schmiedt et al. 2008) cats in two case series. Management of severe, ongoing abdominal bleeding requires fluid resuscitation and blood transfusion before laparotomy, with the likelihood of requiring removal or replacement of the allograft.

Postoperative renal torsion was observed in 4 of 19 cats in which the renal allograft was sutured to the abdominal wall (Mathews and Gregory 1997). Modification of the technique using a ventrally based peritoneal-transversus abdominis flap for the nephropexy has largely eliminated this complication. Renal torsion was not observed in consecutively operated cats using the muscle-flap technique.

Hind limb ischemia is associated with the technique of end-to-end iliac to renal allograft arterial anastomosis. Ipsilateral hind leg complications were reported in 8 of 66 cats (12%) using this technique, including pain, hypothermia of the limb, edema, and paresis or paralysis (Mathews and Gregory 1997). One cat required hindlimb amputation (Mathews and Gregory 1997). Hindlimb ischemia appears to occur in some cats after ligation of the external iliac artery, presumably because of a lack of collateral blood supply. Because of this complication, the recommended technique has been modified to a side-to-end renal artery to postrenal aorta technique. Bernsteen et al. (1999) compared the two techniques in research cats and reported that 5 of 8 cats with the end-to-end technique developed neuropraxia and lameness that resolved within 4 days (Bernsteen et al. 1999). There was no significant difference in the surgical or warm ischemia times nor in the postoperative serum creatinine and BUN concentrations or allograft ultrasonographic appearance between the two techniques (Bernsteen et al. 1999).

Renal vascular thrombosis is uncommon in feline renal allograft recipients. Schmiedt et al. (2008) reported complete graft thrombosis as a cause of graft failure in 2 of 60 cats (3.3%). Both cats required a second renal transplantation.

Complications in Small Animal Surgery, First Edition. Edited by Dominique Griffon and Annick Hamaide.

© 2016 John Wiley & Sons, Inc. Published 2016 by John Wiley & Sons, Inc.

Companion website: www.wiley.com/go/griffon/complications

Ureteral complications

Ureteroneocystostomy is technically challenging in cats because of the small size of the feline ureter (0.4 mm in diameter at the level of the bladder). Thus, ureteral complications, particularly **ureteral obstruction**, occur relatively frequently after feline renal transplantation. Several techniques for ureteroneocystostomy have been described. The original technique in feline transplantation was the "drop-in" technique, in which the ureter was inserted into a small opening in the bladder and secured with a single transmural suture (Gregory et al. 1996). This technique was associated with complications, including granuloma formation at the ureterovesicular junction, which can cause varying degrees of ureteral obstruction, and hemorrhage from the ureteral artery (Gregory et al. 1996). This technique was replaced by a mucosal apposition technique (modified Leadbetter-Politano technique) in which the mucosa of the ureter and bladder were apposed with sutures to prevent exposure of the submucosal tissue to urine to minimize inflammation and reduce granuloma formation (Gregory et al. 1996). This technique is an intravesical technique, which involves a ventral cystotomy and eversion of the bladder mucosa. In cats, this results in substantial swelling of the bladder, making accurate suturing of the ureteroneocystostomy difficult. The mucosal apposition technique has itself been replaced by an extravesical technique (modified Lich Gregoir technique), which is technically easier and may be associated with reduced risk of extravasation of urine and bleeding. In a research study, the extravesical technique was associated with a reduced postoperative peak serum creatinine concentration (mean +/− standard deviation [SD] of 4.9 +/− 3.3 mg/dL vs. 9.4 +/− 2.4 mg/dL), faster decrease in serum creatinine concentration, and faster resolution of renal pelvic dilation on ultrasonographic examination compared with the intravesical technique, although the improvement did not reach statistical significance ($P = 0.11$ for creatinine concentration and $P = 0.14$ for pelvic dilation) (Mehl et al. 2005). The ureteral papilla implantation technique provides a further modification to prevent ureteral obstruction (Hardie et al. 2005). This technique involves removing the ureteral papilla with a 2- to 3-mm margin of bladder from the donor and implanting into the recipient bladder using a double-layered, extravesical technique. In research cats, this technique resulted in transient elevation in serum creatinine concentration in 3 of 5 cats (Hardie et al. 2005).

Ureteral obstruction can result in an **elevated serum creatinine concentration** after renal transplantation in the immediate postoperative period. Abdominal ultrasonographic examination may show renal pelvic dilation and swelling at the ureteroneocystostomy site, which supports the diagnosis. Other causes of postoperative azotemia should be excluded. The condition generally responds to conservative management. Failure to respond and progressive pelvic and ureteral dilation necessitate revision ureteroneocystostomy.

Uroabdomen is an infrequent postoperative complication after renal transplantation. The most likely site of urine extravasation is the ureteroneocystostomy site. Surgery is indicated for the management of postoperative uroabdomen.

Delayed graft function

In humans, delayed graft function is generally defined as the need to perform hemodialysis within 1 week of transplantation. The incidence is 22% to 29%. Delayed graft function in human renal transplant recipients is associated with an increased incidence of acute rejection, poor long-term graft function, and reduced survival. The high incidence in humans likely relates to prolonged ischemia and suboptimal donor conditions, which are not pertinent to cats. There is no established definition of delayed graft function in cats. Approximately 40% of cats are reported to have a serum creatinine concentration above the reference range the day after surgery (Mehl et al. 2006). Delayed graft function has been defined as a serum creatinine concentration above 3 mg/dL 3 days after surgery in a feline renal recipient in which other causes of an elevated creatinine concentration, such as ureteral obstruction, uroabdomen, graft thrombosis, and cyclosporine toxicity, have been ruled out (Schmiedt et al. 2008). Based on this definition, delayed graft function was observed in 5 of 60 cats (8.3%) (Schmiedt et al. 2008). Delayed graft function is likely caused by acute tubular necrosis secondary to ischemia and reperfusion injury or severe graft hypoperfusion after reperfusion. Mehl et al. (2006) evaluated delayed graft function by performing autotransplantation in research cats without ureteral transection and reimplantation compared with research cats in which extravesicular ureteroneocystostomy without vascular surgery was performed to try to evaluate the relative contributions of vascular injury and ureteral obstruction to impaired graft function immediately after surgery. The mean (+/− SD) serum creatinine concentration peaked 1 to 2 days after surgery at 3.2 (+/− 0.8) mg/dL and returned to the reference range by 6 days after autotransplantation compared with a peak of 4.9 (+/− 3.3) mg/dL after ureteral surgery (Mehl et al. 2006). The authors concluded that both ischemic injury and ureteral obstruction likely contribute to impaired allograft function in the immediate period after transplantation (Mehl et al. 2006). Minimizing ischemic injury, such as reducing ischemic time and using preservative solution to flush the allograft after donation, may reduce delayed graft function. Poor immediate graft function may also be caused by thromboembolism and allograft infarction, which has also been documented in research cats after autotransplantation (Bernsteen et al. 1999).

Cats with poor immediate allograft function should be evaluated ultrasonographically. Allografts with delayed graft function should have minimal renal pelvic dilation (a sign of ureteral obstruction), good graft perfusion, and a normal resistive index (Mehl et al. 2006; Schmiedt et al. 2008). In most cases, the graft will eventually function, although this may take several weeks. In the interim, these patients should be treated supportively, including, potentially, the need for dialysis. Severe, prolonged delayed graft function and graft nonfunction are indications for retransplantation.

Hypertension and congestive heart failure

Severe hypertension occurs relatively frequently in the immediate postoperative period after transplantation. The reported rate of severe hypertension, defined as a systolic blood pressure greater than 160 mm Hg, was 30% (9 of 30 cats) (Schmiedt et al. 2008) and, when defined as greater than 170 mm Hg, was 33% (20 of 60) (Adin et al. 2001) and 62% (21 of 34) (Kyles et al. 1999). Potential contributors to postoperative hypertension include preoperative renal dysfunction causing persistent activation of the renin–angiotensin system and uremic vasculitis, perioperative fluid and blood administration, stress response to surgery, graft ischemia and reperfusion causing release of vasoactive mediators, and intra- and postoperative pain. Current recommendations for the management of postoperative hypertension include hourly monitoring of blood pressure for at least 48 hours after surgery. Severe hypertension is treated with hydralazine (2.5 mg/cat subcutaneously [SC]) and intractable hypertension with acetylpromazine (0.05 mg/kg SC).

Congestive heart failure (CHF) has been reported in the immediate postoperative period in 7 of 60 allograft recipients (12%), of which 3 died (Schmiedt et al. 2008). Echocardiographic examination of all potential renal allograft recipients should be performed before surgery and cats with significant cardiac dysfunction excluded. Cats with chronic renal failure commonly have some degree of myocardial hypertrophy secondary to hypertension, and specific exclusion criteria are lacking. Potential causes of postoperative CHF include exacerbation of preexisting cardiac problems and aggressive fluid therapy, particularly in patients with impaired postoperative graft function. Cats that develop postoperative CHF should be treated with a reduction of the rate of administration of intravenous (IV) fluids and diuretics, and the use of positive inotropes should be considered.

Neurologic complications

Neurologic complications are a common cause of morbidity and mortality in the immediate postoperative period. Gregory et al. (1997) reported postoperative neurologic complications in 12 of 57 allograft recipients (21%) starting 1 hour to 5 days after transplantation. Seven of 12 cats survived; 3 had multiple episodes of seizures, 1 had a seizure followed by coma, 1 had disorientation and cardiac arrest, 1 had a single seizure, and 1 experienced blindness and ataxia (Gregory et al. 1997). Five of 12 cats died, all of which experienced either a seizure or disorientation, followed by coma (Gregory et al. 1997). Adin et al. (2001) reported postoperative neurologic complications in 9 of 61 cats (15%), of which 6 experienced seizures and 3 experienced nystagmus and obtundation. Two cats died (Adin et al. 2001).

There are many potential causes for postoperative neurologic complications, and the etiology may be multifactorial. These causes include a preexisting central nervous system problem, infection, and uremic encephalopathy. High cyclosporine concentrations, particularly when associated with low cholesterol or magnesium concentrations, and use of recombinant erythropoietin have been associated with postoperative neurologic complications in humans, but there does not appear to be similar associations in cats (Gregory et al. 1997; Wooldridge and Gregory 1999). Thromboembolic complications and seizures have been reported in research cats undergoing autotransplantation (Bernsteen et al. 1999; Mehl et al. 2006) and may occur in feline renal allograft recipients. Kyles et al. (1999) reported that treating severe postoperative hypertension was associated with a significant reduction in the prevalence of postoperative seizures and neurologic complication–related deaths and hypothesized a role for hypertensive encephalopathy. Adin et al. (2001) reported an association between the preoperative serum creatinine and BUN concentrations and postoperative neurologic complications. The authors hypothesized that rapid correction of the hyperosmolar state after transplantation could results in cerebral edema (a mechanism similar to dialysis dysequilibrium) (Adin et al. 2001). Postoperative neurologic complications were not observed in any of 11 cats that received preoperative hemodialysis. The authors recommended preoperative dialysis in cats with serum creatinine and BUN concentrations greater than 8 mg/dL and 100 mg/dL, respectively (Adin et al. 2001).

Hemolytic uremic syndrome

Hemolytic uremic syndrome (HUS) is an uncommon, serious complication of cyclosporine therapy in human transplant recipients. The syndrome results from the formation of glomerular and renal arteriolar platelet and fibrin thrombi (thrombotic microangiopathy). This results in thrombocytopenia, hemolysis, anemia, and a rapid deterioration in renal function. The diagnosis is normally confirmed on renal biopsy, which shows the presence of microthrombi and resulting renal cortical necrosis. A number of cats with presumed HUS have been described, all of which died (Aronson and Gregory 1999; Adin et al. 2001). Potential therapy includes a discontinuation or reduction of cyclosporine administration and initiation of alternative immunosuppression, such as azathioprine.

LONG-TERM COMPLICATIONS

After renal transplantation, lifelong immunosuppressive therapy is needed to maintain the allograft and prevent rejection. In cats, the standard immunosuppressive protocol consists of microemulsified cyclosporine (initial dose, 3–5 mg/kg orally [PO] twice a day) and prednisolone (initial dose, 1 mg/kg PO twice a day, reducing to 0.5–1 mg/kg PO once a day by 1 month after surgery).

Ketoconazole (10 mg/kg PO once daily) can be used to reduce cyclosporine clearance, allowing once-daily cyclosporine dosing. Ketoconazole should be discontinued if there is an elevation in liver enzyme activity. Many of the complications observed after discharge from the hospital are a result of too little immunosuppression (rejection) or too much immunosuppression (infection, diabetes mellitus, neoplasia). The whole-blood concentration of cyclosporine is periodically monitored. The target trough (C12) concentration for the first month is 500 ng/mL, reducing to 250 ng/mL by 3 months after surgery (Mehl et al. 2003).

Allograft rejection

Acute or active allograft rejection was diagnosed in 13% to 26% of cats (8 of 60 [Schmiedt et al. 2008] and 12 of 46 [Mathews and Gregory 1997]). In one study, allograft rejection was reported as the commonest cause of death in feline renal allograft recipients, occurring in 19% (23 of 122) of cats in which the cause of death was established (Kadar et al. 2005).

Acute rejection is suspected in renal allograft recipients when the serum creatinine concentration increases by more than 1 mg/dL. Other potential causes should be ruled out, such as prerenal azotemia (e.g., volume depletion, cardiac insufficiency), renovascular disease (e.g., renal arterial stenosis), renal parenchymal disease (e.g., recurrent or de novo renal disease, HUS, cyclosporine nephrotoxicity, acute pyelonephritis, oxalosis [Gregory et al. 1993] or lymphoma), and postrenal azotemia caused by urinary obstruction or extravasation.

Clinical signs include lethargy, depression, loss of appetite, and vomiting; sometimes acute rejection is suspected based on routine blood work in the absence of clinical signs. Mathews and Gregory (1997) reported no clinical signs associated with episodes of presumed rejection in 5 of 19 rejection episodes. In research cats, acute rejection does not produce consistent clinical signs other than a decrease in rectal temperature (Kyles et al. 2002). Acute rejection is associated with low whole-blood cyclosporine concentrations and poor owner compliance in administration of medications and cyclosporine monitoring. Allograft rejection often occurs relatively early after transplantation; in one study, the median time to acute rejection was 64 days (range, 21–251 days) (Schmiedt et al. 2008).

Renal biopsies have not been used routinely for the diagnosis of allograft rejection in cats because of a concern about the effect of the biopsy procedure on allograft function. Biopsies have often been reserved for cats with suspected allograft rejection that failed to respond to therapy. Ultrasound-guided biopsy of the renal cortex, without perforation of the corticomedullary junction, has been shown to produce mild lesions and minimal effect on glomerular filtration rate and effective renal blood flow (Minkus et al. 1994; Drost et al. 2000) and is likely to be a safe technique for obtaining biopsies from feline renal allografts. Histologically, acute allograft rejection in humans and cats differs significantly; feline renal allograft rejection is characterized primarily by severe, predominantly lymphocytic, interstitial inflammation (DeCock et al. 2004).

Acute rejection requires immediate therapy with IV cyclosporine (6.6 mg/kg once daily over 4–6 hours), corticosteroids, and fluids.

Infection

Postoperative infections are relatively common in immunosuppressed feline renal allograft recipients (Bernsteen et al. 1999; Griffin et al. 2003; Kadar et al. 2005; Nordquist and Aronson 2008; Schmiedt et al. 2008). Postoperative infections were diagnosed in 25% to 37% of cats (43 of 169 [Kadar et al. 2005] and 22 of 60 [Schmiedt et al. 2008]) and are reported as the second most common cause of death in feline renal allograft recipients, resulting in death in 14% (17 of 122) of cats in which the cause of death was established (Kadar et al. 2005). Cats with concurrent diabetes mellitus have a significantly higher risk of developing an infection after renal transplantation (Kadar et al. 2005).

Infection is often reported relatively early after transplantation; in two studies, the median time to diagnosis of infection of 40 days and 2.5 months (Kadar et al. 2005; Schmiedt et al. 2008). In one study, 12 of 26 infections occurred before discharge; the median time to infection in the 14 cases of infection diagnosed after discharge was 575 days (range, 134–1192 days) (Schmiedt et al. 2008). Bacterial infections are the most common, accounting for 53% to 65% of infections (25 of 47 [Kadar et al. 2005] and 16 of 26 [Schmiedt et al. 2008]). The most common bacterial infections observed were urinary tract infections (UTIs) and infections associated with gastrostomy and esophagostomy feeding tubes and jugular catheters (Kadar et al. 2005; Schmiedt et al. 2008). Viral infections were the second most common, accounting for 28% to 35% of infections (13 of 47 [Kadar et al. 2005] and 9 of 26 [Schmiedt et al. 2008]). Upper airway infection was the most common viral infection observed. In most cats with upper airway infection, the signs developed close to the time of transplantation and were particularly severe (Kadar et al. 2005). Fungal infections accounted for 4% to 13% of infections (1 of 26 [Schmiedt et al. 2008] and 6 of 47 [Kadar et al. 2005]). Fungal infections included Cryptococcus, Candida, Microsporum canis, and Cladosporidium spp. Protozoal infections accounted for 6% of infections (3 of 47) (Kadar et al. 2005). Toxoplasmosis is the most commonly diagnosed protozoal infection, described as causing diffuse interstitial pneumonia in 3 cats 3 weeks to 6 months after transplantation (Bernsteen et al. 1999) and localized to the allografted kidney and ureter in one cat (Nordquist and Aronson 2008).

In cats with infections, appropriate medical therapy should be initiated. Aminoglycosides and trimethoprim–sulfonamide drugs should be avoided because they are nephrotoxic in combination with cyclosporine. Many drugs alter cytochrome P-450 activity and thus affect cyclosporine metabolism. Cyclosporine concentration should be carefully monitored and adjusted.

Screening of potential feline recipients and donors should include serologic testing for feline leukemia virus and feline immunodeficiency virus and assays for IgG and IgM antibodies against *Toxoplasma gondii*. *Toxoplasma* seropositive cats can be successfully managed after transplantation with lifelong clindamycin therapy (Kadar et al. 2005). Potential recipients with pyelonephritis or bacterial cystitis are treated with appropriate antimicrobial agents based on bacterial culture and sensitivity testing. Two negative urine bacterial culture results should be obtained before transplantation. Cats with suspected pyelonephritis should have a cyclosporine challenge test before transplantation and have negative urine culture results after a minimum of 7 days of cyclosporine therapy.

Posttransplant diabetes mellitus

Posttransplant diabetes mellitus (PTDM) has been reported in 14% (26 of 187) of cats that survived 30 days after transplantation (Case et al. 2007). The median time to diagnosis was 287 days (range, 31 days–10.7 years). The incidence of PTDM has been reported as 66 cases per 1000 cat years at risk compared with 18 cases per 1000 cat years at risk for a control group of nontransplanted cats with chronic renal failure (Case et al. 2007). Cats that underwent transplantation were 5.4 (95% CI 3.5–8.0) times as likely to develop diabetes mellitus as were control cats with chronic renal failure (Case et al. 2007). The mortality rate in cats with PTDM was 2.4 (95% CI 1.2–4.8) times the rate in cats that did not develop PTDM (Case et al. 2007).

Posttransplant diabetes mellitus is associated with the administration of glucocorticoids, which antagonize the effects of insulin, and cyclosporine, which is toxic to the pancreatic β cells. In one study, 5 of 8 cats with PTDM had resolution of diabetes mellitus after discontinuation of glucocorticoid administration or a reduction in the dosage of prednisone (Case et al. 2007). A reduction in the cyclosporine dose should also be considered.

Neoplasia

De novo malignant neoplasia has been reported in 9.5% to 18% (9 of 95 [Wooldridge et al. 2002] and 18 of 60 [Schmiedt et al. 2009]) of cats after renal transplantation. The median time to diagnosis of neoplasia was reported as 9 months and 1020 days (Wooldridge et al. 2002; Schmiedt et al. 2009). Cats that underwent transplantation were 6.1 (95% CI 1.8–20.4) times as likely to develop malignant neoplasia as were control cats with chronic renal failure (Schmiedt et al. 2009). In one study, the median time to diagnosis of neoplasia was 9 months after transplantation and the median survival time was 14 months after transplantation in cats that developed a neoplasm compared with 22 months in cats that died of other causes (Wooldridge et al. 2002). In another study, the median survival time in cats that developed a malignant neoplasm was 1020 days (range, 19–2915 days), which was not significantly different from the survival time in cats that did not develop neoplasia (1146; range, 19–2915 days) (Schmiedt et al. 2009). In the same two studies, the number of cats with lymphoma was 36% to 44% (4 of 11 [Schmiedt et al. 2009] and 4 of 9 [Wooldridge et al. 2002]). However, lymphoma is common in cats, and it is unclear if there is an increased risk of lymphoma after renal transplantation.

The mechanism for posttransplant malignant neoplasia is unclear. Potential causes include chronic antigenic stimulation, infection, impaired immune surveillance, cyclosporine-mediated oncogenesis (e.g., because of induction of transforming growth factor β), and cyclosporine-mediated promotion of DNA mutations.

MISCELLANEOUS LONG-TERM COMPLICATIONS

Urolith recurrence

Calcium oxalate urolithiasis was considered a relative contraindication for transplantation because of concern regarding formation of uroliths within the allograft. In one study, recurrence was observed in 5 of 18 cats that survived to discharge (Aronson et al. 2006). However, no significant difference ($P = 0.67$) was detected in survival time between cats with a history of calcium oxalate urolithiasis and a control group of transplanted cats without uroliths (Aronson et al. 2006). Four of 5 cats with urolith recurrence had small calcium oxalate stones attached to the 8-0 nylon suture used to perform the ureteroneocystostomy (Aronson et al. 2006). Use of an absorbable suture for the ureteroneocystostomy is recommended.

Retroperitoneal fibrosis

Retroperitoneal fibrosis was identified as a cause of ureteral obstruction in 4 cats 6 weeks to 5 months after transplantation (Aronson 2002). The cause is unknown. All 4 cats responded to surgical removal of the scar tissue, and there was no reported recurrence of ureteral obstruction.

Renal allograft rupture

A single case of renal allograft rupture is reported in a feline allograft recipient 3 months after transplantation (Palm et al. 2010). The proposed etiology is interstitial and medullary edema caused by acute rejection, acute tubular necrosis, vascular thrombosis, urinary tract obstruction, or UTI, which results in an increased pressure within the graft and subsequent cortical and capsular ischemia.

References

Adin, C.A., Gregory, C.R., Kyles, A.E., et al. (2001) Diagnostic predictors of complications and survival after renal transplantation in cats. *Veterinary Surgery* 30, 515-521.

Aronson, L.R. (2002) Retroperitoneal fibrosis in four cats following renal transplantation. *Journal of the American Veterinary Medical Association* 221, 984-989.

Aronson, L.R., Gregory, C. (1999) Possible hemolytic uremic syndrome in three cats after renal transplantation and cyclosporine therapy. *Veterinary Surgery* 28, 135-140.

Aronson, L.R., Kyles, A.E., Preston, A., et al. (2006) Renal transplantation in cats with calcium oxalate urolithiasis: 19 cases (1997-2004). *Journal of the American Veterinary Medical Association* 228, 743-749.

Bernsteen, L., Gregory, C.R., Aronson, L.R. (1999a) Acute toxoplasmosis following renal transplantation in three cats and a dog. *Journal of the American Veterinary Medical Association* 201, 1123-1126.

Bernsteen, L., Gregory, C.R., Pollard, R.E., et al. (1999b) Comparison of two surgical techniques for renal transplantation in cats. *Veterinary Surgery* 28, 417.

Case, J.B., Kyles, A.E., Nelson, R.W., et al. (2007) Incidence of and risk factors for diabetes mellitus in cats that have undergone renal transplantation: 187 cases (1986-2005). *Journal of the American Veterinary Medical Association* 230, 880-884.

DeCock, H.E.V., Kyles, A.E., Griffey, S.M., et al. (2004) Histopathologic findings and classification of feline renal transplants. *Veterinary Pathology* 41, 244-256.

Drost, W.T., Henry, G.A., Meinkoth, J.H., et al. (2000) The effects of a unilateral ultrasound-guided renal biopsy on renal function in healthy sedated cats. *Veterinary Radiology & Ultrasound* 41, 57-82.

Gregory, C.R., Olander, H.J., Kochin, E.J., et al. (1993) Oxalate nephrosis and renal sclerosis after renal transplantation in a cat. *Veterinary Surgery* 22, 221-224.

Gregory, C.R., Lirtzman, R.A., Kochin, E.J., et al. (1996) A mucosal apposition technique for ureteroneocystostomy after renal transplantation in cats. *Veterinary Surgery* 25, 13-17.

Gregory, C.R., Mathews, K.G., Aronson, L.R., et al. (1997) Central nervous system disorders after renal transplantation in cats. *Veterinary Surgery* 26, 386-392.

Griffin, A., Newton, A.L., Aronson, L.R., et al. (2003) Disseminated *Mycobacterium avium* complex infection following renal transplantation in a cat. *Journal of the American Veterinary Medical Association* 222, 1097-1101.

Hardie, R.J., Schmiedt, C., Phillips, L., et al. (2005) Ureteral papilla implantation as a technique neoureterocystostomy in cats. *Veterinary Surgery* 34, 393-398.

Kadar, E., Sykes, J.E., Kass, P.H., et al. (2005) Evaluation of the prevalence of infections in cats after renal transplantation: 169 cases (1987-2003). *Journal of the American Veterinary Medical Association* 227, 948-953.

Kyles, A.E., Gregory, C.R., Wooldridge, J.D., et al. (1999) Management of hypertension controls postoperative neurologic disorders after renal transplantation in cats. *Veterinary Surgery* 28, 436-441.

Kyles, A.E., Gregory, C.R., Griffey, S.M., et al. (2002) Evaluation of the clinical and histologic features of renal allograft rejection in cats. *Veterinary Surgery* 31, 49-56.

Mathews, K.G., Gregory, C.R. (1997) Renal transplants in cats: 66 cases. *Journal of the American Veterinary Medical Association* 211, 1432-1436.

Mehl, M.L., Kyles, A.E., Craigmill, A.L., et al. (2003) Disposition of cyclosporine after intravenous and multi-dose oral administration in cats. *Journal of Veterinary Pharmacology and Therapeutics* 26, 349-354.

Mehl, M.L., Kyles, A.E., Pollard, R., et al. (2005) Comparison of 3 techniques for ureteroneocystostomy in cats. *Veterinary Surgery* 34, 114-119.

Mehl, M.L., Kyles, A.E., Reimer, S.B., et al. (2006) Evaluation the effects of ischemic injury and ureteral obstruction on delayed graft function in cats after renal autotransplantation. *Veterinary Surgery* 35, 341-346.

Minkus, G., Reusch, C., Horauf, A., et al. (1994) Evaluation of renal biopsies in cats and dogs: histopathology in comparison with clinical data. *Journal of Small Animal Practice* 35, 465-472.

Nordquist, B.C., Aronson, L.R. (2008) Pyogranulomatous cystitis associated with Toxoplasma gondii infection in a cat after renal transplantation. *Journal of the American Veterinary Medical Association* 232, 1010-1012.

Palm, C.A., Aronson, L.R., Mayhew, P.D. (2010) Feline renal allograft rupture. *Journal of Feline Medicine and Surgery* 12, 330-333.

Schmiedt, C.W., Holzman, G., Schwarz, T., et al. (2008) Survival, complications and analysis of risk factors after renal transplantation in cats. *Veterinary Surgery* 37, 683-695.

Schmiedt, C.W., Grimes, J.A., Holzman, G., et al. (2009) Incidence and risk factors for development of malignant neoplasia after feline renal transplantation and cyclosporine-based immunosuppression. *Veterinary Comparative Oncology* 7, 45-53.

Wooldridge, J.D., Gregory, C.R. (1999) Assessment of total and ionized magnesium levels in feline renal transplant recipients. *Veterinary Surgery* 28, 31-37.

Wooldridge, J.D., Gregory, C.R., Mathews, K.G., et al. (2002) The prevalence of malignant neoplasia in feline renal-transplant recipients. *Veterinary Surgery* 31, 94-97.

Ureteral Surgery

Stéphanie Claeys and Annick Hamaide

Department of Clinical Sciences (Companion Animals and Equids), School of Veterinary Medicine, University of Liège, Liège, Belgium

Various types of surgical procedures may be performed on the ureters in dogs and cats. Ureterotomy can be performed at any level of the ureter and may be indicated in case of ureteral obstruction caused by ureterolithiasis. Ureteroneocystostomy consists of reimplantation of the distal ureter in the bladder after resection of the distal ureteral portion. It is indicated in case of distal ureteral obstruction (e.g., ureterolithiasis, neoplasia) or in case of extramural ectopic ureter. Ureteroureterostomy consists of the resection of a portion of the ureter and reapposition by end-to-end anastomosis. It is technically challenging and may be indicated in selected cases in which the proximal portion of the ureter cannot be reimplanted into the bladder. Neoureterostomy is performed, with or without trigonal reconstruction, to correct intramural ectopic ureters.

Recently, the placement of ureteral stents has gained popularity, especially in case of ureteral obstruction in cats. Placement of a nephrostomy tube and a subcutaneous ureteral bypass are also novel salvage procedures indicated in case of ureteral obstruction in dogs and cats.

Surgery of the ureter is associated with a high incidence of complications. The most common complication is the development of uroabdomen because of urine leakage from the ureteral incision. In a study of 101 cats, uroabdomen was reported in 16% of the cats that survived the surgery (Kyles *et al.* 2005). The second most common complication is ureteral obstruction, which has been described in 5% of the cats treated with ureterotomy and 11% of the cats treated with neoureterocystostomy for ureterolithiasis (Kyles *et al.* 2005).

Undiagnosed ureteral obstruction eventually causes the development of hydroureter and hydronephrosis and finally loss of renal function. Stricture formation is another reported complication after ureterotomy. Its true incidence is unknown in dogs and cats.

Postoperative residual incontinence is a potential complication after correction of ectopic ureters by neoureterocystostomy or neoureterostomy.

Ureteral stricture

Definition

A stricture is an abnormal narrowing of a hollow structure, usually caused by scar tissue.

Risk factors

- Any ureteral surgery may cause stricture at the surgical site.
- The small size of the ureter, especially in cats and small dogs, may predispose to stricture formation.
- Passage of ureteroliths may cause mucosal injury and subsequent stricture.
- The use of temporary stenting catheters to allow healing of the ureter over the stent is controversial because they may increase fibrosis and the risk of stricture.
- Excessive tension after ureteral anastomosis
- Excessive tissue trauma during surgery

Diagnosis

- Postoperative ureteral stricture may result in obstruction of the ureter with its associated clinical signs. **Clinical signs** are often nonspecific in cats (inappetence, lethargy, and weight loss). Signs of uremia may also be present such as polyuria, polydipsia, vomiting, and anorexia. Dogs with ureteral obstruction are more frequently presented with micturition disorders (incontinence, stranguria, pollakiuria, hematuria, polyuria), abdominal pain, and systemic signs (anorexia, vomiting, lethargy, and weight loss). In cats, stricture may be evident as early as 5 days after ureterotomy or may be diagnosed months to years after surgery (Zaid *et al.* 2011).
- Imaging of the ureter is required to identify the cause of the obstruction, especially to differentiate recurrent ureterolithiasis from postoperative stricture.
- **Abdominal radiography** may be used to rule out the presence of radiopaque calculi.
- **Abdominal ultrasonography** allows detection of ureteral and renal pelvic dilatation and localization of the obstruction (Figure 67.1). Hyperechoic periureteral tissue was also identified around the area of the stricture in 6 of 10 cats with a stricture (Zaid *et al.* 2011).
- **Ultrasonographic-guided percutaneous antegrade pyelography** provides good visualization of the renal pelvis and ureter and allows localization of the obstruction (Rivers *et al.* 1997; Adin *et al.* 2003).
- **Retrograde ureteropyelography** is performed via cystoscopy and fluoroscopy by cannulating the ureterovesicular junction. It is less invasive than antegrade pyelography because needle access is not needed, which eliminates the risk of bleeding or urinary leakage through the renal parenchyma if a ureteral obstructive lesion persists (Berent 2011).

Complications in Small Animal Surgery, First Edition. Edited by Dominique Griffon and Annick Hamaide.
© 2016 John Wiley & Sons, Inc. Published 2016 by John Wiley & Sons, Inc.
Companion website: www.wiley.com/go/griffon/complications

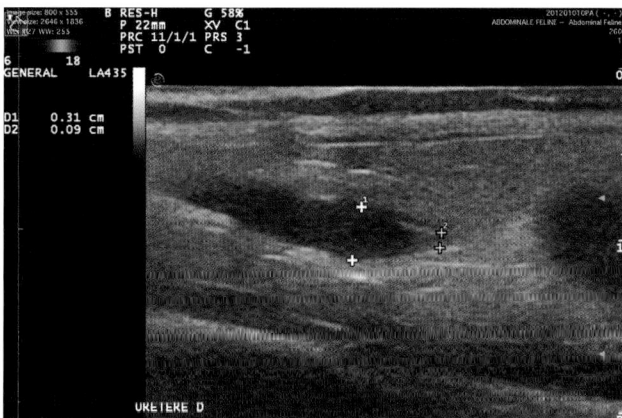

Figure 67.1 Longitudinal ultrasound image of a feline ureter showing dilated ureter (0.31 cm) proximal to the site of obstruction. Ureteral stricture is suspected because of the absence of an intraluminal structure associated with acoustic shadowing (mineralized calculi). *Source:* G. Bolen. Reproduced with permission from G. Bolen.

- **Intravenous excretory urography** may be performed, but it is often not useful in case of ureteral obstruction because of the poor opacification of the affected kidney and ureter and the potential risk of nephrotoxicity of the contrast media.
- **Renal scintigraphy** (technetium Tc-99m diethylenetriamine pentaacetic acid scintigraphy) allows measurement of the glomerular filtration rate (GFR) of individual kidneys. The GFR of an obstructed kidney is reduced, and the return to function of the kidney after obstruction relief cannot be predicted by scintigraphy. Measurement of the GFR of the opposite kidney may help deciding if a nephrectomy of the obstructed kidney is a potential option.

Treatment
- Animals with ureteral obstruction often present with concurrent renal disease and azotemia. They should therefore be stabilized before any invasive treatment. Fluid therapy should be initiated immediately. Severe azotemia should be treated before definitive surgery with hemodialysis if available or with drainage of urine via a nephrostomy tube (Hardie and Kyles 2004). A nephrostomy tube allows rapid and effective relief of the ureteral obstruction and allows evaluation of the remaining renal function before definitive ureteral surgery (Berent 2011).
- **Nephrostomy tubes** may be placed surgically or percutaneously under ultrasound or fluoroscopic guidance. They require dilatation of the renal pelvis. Tube dislodgement and urinary leakage were common reported complications with Foley or red rubber catheters. Locking-loop pigtail catheters are associated with fewer complications and are therefore recommended (Berent *et al.* 2009; Berent 2011).
- **Ureteronephrectomy** should only be performed if the kidney is grossly infected or the ureter is so damaged that it can not be salvaged (Mathews 2012). Patients should be nonazotemic with a normal GFR of the opposite kidney. Treatment of the ureteral disease should always be recommended when possible because patients often have, or may develop in the future, chronic kidney disease, especially cats, and some patients may be at risk of developing obstruction in the opposite ureter (in the case of ureterolithiasis).

- **Partial ureterectomy and ureteroneocystostomy** (implantation of the distal ureter into the bladder) may be performed when the stricture is located in the distal two thirds of the ureter.
- Strictures located closer to the kidney may be treated by **ureteral resection-anastomosis** (ureteroureterostomy) if the tension will be excessive after ureteroneocystostomy. The procedure is technically more difficult than ureteroneocystostomy and is associated with a higher incidence of postoperative ureteral obstruction (Hardie and Kyles 2004). Spatulation of the distal ureter may be needed to overcome the disparity in diameter between the dilated proximal ureter and the normal distal ureter, especially in cats and small dogs (Mathews 2012).
- Tension on the ureteroneocystostomy or ureteroureterostomy should be avoided and may be reduced by moving the kidney caudally (renal descensus) or by pexying the apex of the urinary bladder to the caudal pole of the kidney (nephrocystopexy) or to the iliopsoas muscle (psoas cystopexy).
- **Ureteral stenting** is a less invasive alternative to traditional surgeries. Ureteral stents may be placed cystoscopically in a retrograde manner (in dogs and, when possible, in female cats) or in an antegrade manner through the renal pelvis percutaneously or surgically. In cats, stents are usually placed surgically antegrade (via pyelocentesis), retrograde (via a cystotomy), or both (via ureterotomy).
- Placement of a **subcutaneous ureteral bypass** (SUB) device is a novel option for cats with ureteral obstruction secondary to postoperative stricture. This procedure involves placement of a locking-loop pigtail nephrostomy catheter and a locking-loop cystostomy catheter that are connected using a subcutaneous access port. The SUB is considered a salvage procedure for cats in which traditional treatments have failed or are contraindicated (Berent *et al.* 2010; Berent 2011; Horowitz *et al.* 2013).

Outcome
The prognosis after relief of a ureteral obstruction depends on the chronicity and degree of obstruction, the therapeutic options available, and postoperative management. Outcomes reported in the literature after various treatments are presented in the relevant literature section below.

Clinicians cannot predict postdecompression outcome based on admitting parameters, and relieving the obstruction does not address the preexisting renal disease.

Prevention
- Ureteral surgery should be performed under magnification (in cats and small dogs) by experienced surgeons.
- Delicate atraumatic surgical technique, preserving the ureteral blood supply, is mandatory.
- Adequate suture material (5-0 to 8-0 monofilament) should be used.
- In case of ureterolith, retropulsion of the calculi in the renal pelvis should be initially attempted because pyelolithotomy is often safer and simpler than ureterotomy.
- The use of temporary stenting catheters after ureteral surgery is controversial because they may predispose to stricture.
- Ureterotomy incisions should be performed in the proximal dilated portion of the ureter.
- Longitudinal ureterotomies are usually closed longitudinally but may also be closed transversally to preserve luminal diameter.
- Avoid tension at the surgical site.
- Spatulation of the ureter is recommended because it increases the circumference of ureteral anastomosis.
- Short- and long-term postoperative monitoring by ultrasonography is recommended to allow early detection of a potential stricture.

Uroabdomen

Definition

Leakage of urine into the peritoneal cavity is a commonly reported complication after ureteral surgery. Causes include dehiscence of a sutured incision, ureteral necrosis or avulsion from the urinary bladder after ureteroneocystostomy, ureteral tear during stent placement, and leakage from a nephrostomy tube used for pre- or postoperative management.

Risk factors

- Poor surgical technique
- Inadequate suture material or pattern
- Presence of a nephrostomy tube

Diagnosis

- Abdominocentesis and fluid analysis
- Positive contrast study results if needed

Treatment

- Patient stabilization
- Thorough abdominal lavage
- Broad-spectrum antibiotherapy if needed (in case of associated urinary tract infection [UTI])
- Ureterotomy incisions may heal by second intention if urine is drained via a nephrostomy tube or evacuated from the abdomen using an abdominal drain. Uroabdomen was reported in 5 cats after ureterotomy; 2 of these cats had urine drained via nephrostomy tubes and healed without further surgery (Kyles *et al.* 1998).
- Revision of the dehisced ureteral suture
- Reimplantation of the ureter in the urinary bladder in case of avulsion
- Ureteral stenting and SUB are new interventional options available in case of failed ureteral surgery.
- Urine leakage after ureteral stenting (from a ureterotomy incision or from a ureteral tear created during stent placement) may resolve spontaneously within a few days or may be managed with a closed-suction drain (Berent *et al.* 2014).
- Ureteronephrectomy if the ureter cannot be salvaged; the animal should be nonazotemic with a normal GFR to the opposite kidney.

Outcome

The outcome of uroabdomen is usually favorable if the defect can be closed. Revision ureteral surgery may, however, be challenging. Uroabdomen was observed in 14 of 88 (16%) cats after ureteral surgery (Kyles *et al.* 2005). Three cats were euthanized without further treatment, and 11 cats had a second surgery. The mortality rate in cats that underwent a second surgery because of uroabdomen was 27% (3 of 11).

New interventional procedures are now part of the therapeutic options available and may be alternatives when traditional surgery fails.

Prevention

- Atraumatic surgical technique
- Use adequate suture material (5-0 to 8-0 monofilament) and pattern. Closure of ureterotomy incisions using a simple continuous pattern is recommended to ensure a watertight seal.
- A nephrostomy tube may be used to divert urine after ureteral surgery. They are usually not required after a properly performed ureterotomy.

- If a nephrostomy tube is used (for pre- or postoperative management), a locking-loop pigtail nephrostomy tube is recommended. If the tube is placed surgically, a nephropexy should be performed to decrease the risk of leakage (Berent 2011).
- An abdominal closed-suction drain may be placed during the initial surgery to allow detection of urine leakage and help palliate the clinical signs in the event of postoperative uroabdomen.

Incontinence

Also see Chapter 71.

Definition

Urinary incontinence is defined as an involuntary leakage of urine. A postoperative incontinence rate of 27% to 78% has been reported after correction of ectopic ureters, either by ureteroneocystostomy or by neoureterostomy, with or without trigonal reconstruction (Stone and Mason 1990; McLaughlin and Miller 1991; Holt and Moore 1995; Mayhew *et al.* 2006; Ho *et al.* 2011; Reichler *et al.* 2012; Noël and Hamaide 2014).

Postoperative incontinence is frequently attributable to functional anomalies of the urethra (Lane *et al.* 1995; Koie *et al.* 2000) but it may also be caused by recanalization of the distal ureteral segment (Stone and Mason 1990; McLaughlin and Miller 1991).

Risk factors

- Presence of concurrent urethral sphincter mechanism incompetence (USMI)
- The effect of neoureterostomy without trigonal reconstruction, allowing the distal ureteral remnant to interfere with normal sphincter function at the level of the bladder neck, is questionable.
- The effect of concurrent removal of gonads on postoperative incontinence is still debatable (Reichler *et al.* 2012; Noël and Hamaide 2014).
- The presence of UTI is not a risk factor per se, but it may worsen the clinical signs of incontinence.
- Recanalization of the distal ureteral remnant is possible after ureterocystostomy with simple ligation.
- Nonidentified ureteral branches
- Hypoplastic bladder
- Vestibulovaginal stenosis (Figure 67.2)

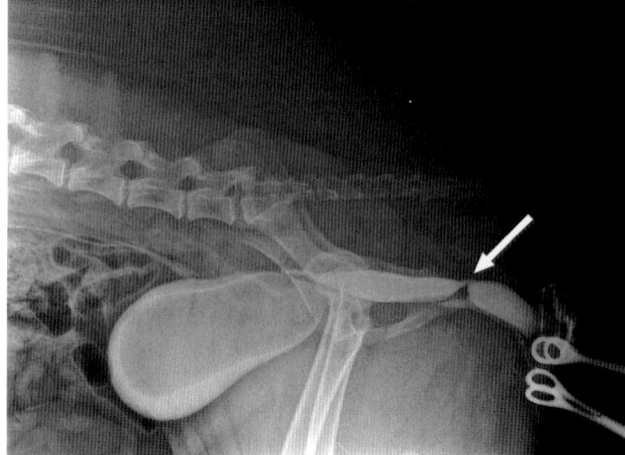

Figure 67.2 Vaginourethrogram (right lateral recumbency) in an incontinent female dog suspected of urethral sphincter mechanism incompetence. Note the vestibulovaginal stenosis (white arrow).

Diagnosis

- Urinary incontinence may be present immediately after the surgical correction of ectopic ureters or may recur months after the initial surgery (Noël and Hamaide 2014).
- Depending on the cause of urinary incontinence, **clinical signs** could slightly differ. Clinical signs of USMI have been described (see Chapter 71). In case of recanalization of the distal ureteral segment, continuous dribbling of urine might be present. In the presence of a hypoplastic bladder, frequent micturition episodes can accompany urine leakage.
- **Urine culture and antibiogram** are mandatory to confirm the presence of UTI.
- **Diagnostic imaging techniques** (ultrasonography, positive contrast studies, computed tomography) will help to identify the cause of residual incontinence (also see Chapter 71).
- **Postoperative urodynamic investigation** (urethral pressure profile and cystometry) might help to diagnose the presence of USMI or the presence of a hypoplastic bladder.

Treatment

- Treatment of any concurrent UTI with adequate antibiotherapy is mandatory.
- If USMI is identified, treatment may be medical or surgical (see Chapter 71).
- In case of recanalization of the distal ureteral remnant, surgical correction should be performed as soon as possible. The distal remnant is either religated or dissected from the urethral wall.
- Hypoplastic bladder is often the result of bilateral ectopia, leading to disuse atrophy and possibly short-term postoperative incontinence. It is therefore often reversible after successful surgical repair and may not be a cause of long-term incontinence (McLaughlin and Miller, 1991).
- Vestibulovaginal stenosis may need surgical correction or bougienage.

Outcome

The outcome varies depending on the cause of the postoperative incontinence. In case of recanalization of the distal remnant, reintervention should solve the problem. The outcome might be less favorable if the postoperative incontinence is attributable to concurrent USMI. Various studies have shown that 30% to 50% of the dogs with postoperative incontinence may regain continence after medical or surgical management (Lane *et al*. 1995; Ho *et al*. 2011; Reichler *et al*. 2012; Noël and Hamaide 2014).

Prevention

- Ligation of the distal ureteral segment with nonabsorbable suture material, double ligation, or ligation and transection may prevent recanalization (Mc Laughlin and Miller 1991).
- Preoperative urodynamic evaluation might help identifying dogs with concurrent functional anomalies of the urinary tract.
- Although dissection of the intramural distal ureteral remnant has not been identified in the current literature as a predictive factor for postoperative incontinence, it is the author's opinion that the procedure should be favored because it probably decreases part of the risk of sphincter incompetence.
- Colposuspension performed during the surgical correction of ectopic ureters in dogs with a pelvic bladder might be helpful (Noël and Hamaide 2014).
- Correction of anatomic vaginal abnormalities

Relevant literature

Ureteral stricture is a commonly reported complication of ureteral surgery (Snyder *et al*. 2005; Zaid *et al*. 2011; Fossum 2013). The true incidence of postoperative ureteral stricture is, however, unknown because postoperative imaging is not always performed in the absence of clinical signs. Postoperative ureteral stricture was identified in 1 of 16 dogs treated surgically for ureteral calculi (Snyder *et al*. 2005). Stricture was diagnosed 1 month after the initial surgery, and a nephroureterectomy was required because of severe hydronephrosis. Zaid *et al*. (2011) reported 10 cases of feline ureteral stricture among which 4 were secondary to a previous ureterotomy at the site of the stricture. Another cat of the study developed a stricture after ureteral reimplantation for correction of the first stricture. Fifty percent of those cases had a surgical cause for their stricture, so stricture should be considered an important short- or long-term complication of ureteral surgery (Zaid *et al*. 2011). Healing of the ureter occurs by fibrous tissue replacement. When 5-cm ureteral defects were experimentally created in dogs and were left to heal over a stent, the healed segment was covered with urothelium but was narrow, and the wall consisted of fibrous tissue (Kuzaka *et al*. 1996).

Nephrostomy catheters may be used preoperatively to stabilize the patient by relieving the obstruction. They may also be used to divert the urine from the ureteral surgical site postoperatively. They have, however, been associated with a high rate of complications (46% of the 24 cats that had a nephrostomy tube placed in a study of 153 cats), including urinary leakage, poor drainage, and tube dislodgment (Kyles *et al*. 2005). Locking-loop pigtail nephrostomy catheters are associated with fewer complications and have been used successfully in 11 cats (13 kidneys) and 3 dogs (3 kidneys) (Berent *et al*. 2009). Ten were placed surgically, and 6 were placed percutaneously under ultrasound or fluoroscopic guidance. Complications included UTI (4 of 16) and accidental tube dislodgement (1 of 16). Whereas percutaneous placement is recommended in dogs, surgical placement is recommended in cats because of the mobility of the feline kidney and greater risk of leakage without a surgical nephropexy (Berent 2011; Berent and Weisse 2013). This procedure is reserved for animals that have renal pelvises larger than 10 mm because of the size of the loop on the catheter.

Treatment options for ureteral stricture include traditional surgical techniques and new interventional procedures. Strictures located in the distal two thirds of the ureter may be treated by partial ureterectomy and ureteroneocystostomy. Various techniques for ureteroneocystostomy have been described and are divided into intravesical techniques, which require a cystotomy (mucosal apposition technique), and extravesical techniques (modified Lich Gregoir technique). The mucosal apposition technique is commonly used in dogs. It was also described in cats after renal transplantation, and no obstruction was observed postoperatively (Gregory *et al*. 1996). The modified Lich-Gregoir technique (extravesical procedure using simple interrupted sutures) is, however, preferred in cats, especially if the degree of ureteral dilatation is minimal, because it is associated with reduced postoperative ureteral obstruction (Mehl *et al*. 2005).

The outcome after treatment of ureteral stricture has not been commonly reported. Most of the literature reports outcome after different treatments of ureteral obstruction, among which only few cases are secondary to postoperative stricture.

Zaid *et al*. (2011) reported 10 cases of feline ureteral stricture among which 4 were secondary to previous ureterotomy. Six cats had a stent placed, 2 had traditional surgery, and 2 did not have any intervention. All patients survived to discharge, and 7 of the 8 treated cats had decrease in serum creatinine concentration and renal pelvic parameters preceding discharge. The median survival time was longer than 294 days (range, 14 to >858 days).

In a study of 153 cats with ureteral calculi, 89 had a ureteral surgery (Kyles *et al.* 2005). The postoperative complication rate and perioperative mortality rate were 31% and 18%, respectively. The 12-month survival rate after medical treatment was 66% versus 91% after surgical treatment. Persistent ureteral obstruction was observed in 5 cats after surgery (3 of 27 cats after ureteroneocystostomy and 2 of 70 cats after ureterotomy). Postoperative **uroabdomen** occurred in 14 cats (16%). Uroabdomen was more frequent in cats that had a nephrostomy tube placed (25%) than in cats that did not (12%). The cats that underwent a second surgery because of uroabdomen had a mortality rate of 27%. Urine leakage was observed with similar frequency after ureterotomy and ureteroneocystostomy. In dogs, a study of 16 cases of ureteral obstructions treated surgically reported a median survival time of 904 days (range, 2–1876) (Snyder *et al.* 2005). Two dogs required a second surgery, including 1 case of stricture.

The outcome after ureteral stenting was recently reported in a study of 69 cats (Berent *et al.* 2014). A stricture (secondary to previous surgery or circumcaval ureter) was present in 22 of 79 (28%) ureters. The perioperative mortality rate was 7.5%, and the median survival time was 498 days (range, 2 to >1262 days). Patients with a ureteral stricture were found more difficult to stent and were more likely to have reobstructions (37%) than patients without a stricture (9.8%). Berent *et al.* (2014) therefore recommend placement of a SUB device instead of a ureteral stent in cats with suspected ureteral stricture. Uroabdomen associated with the procedure was diagnosed in 5 patients (7%): 2 had leakage from a tear during stent placement, 2 from the ureterotomy incision, and 1 from the stay suture in the urinary bladder.

Placement of a SUB device is a new functional option under investigation for cats in which traditional treatments have failed or are contraindicated (Berent 2011; Berent and Weisse 2013; Horowitz *et al.* 2013). The procedure has been reported in 19 cats (20 ureters) and 2 dogs, most commonly for proximal ureteral strictures (Berent *et al.* 2010; Berent *et al.* 2011). Thirteen of the 21 patients were still alive with the longest one surviving 717 days with a patent SUB. No device was seen to encrust or obstruct long term, and they were all well tolerated. The SUB is considered a salvage procedure because complications may be severe if they occur.

Predictors of outcome have been evaluated in 41 cats treated either by ureteral stenting or by a SUB device (Horowitz *et al.* 2013). Predictors associated with a decreased overall survival time were a higher presenting blood urea nitrogen, higher creatinine at hospital discharge, and overhydration during hospitalization. Cats with International Renal Interest Society stage 1 and 2 kidney disease (vs. stage 3 and 4) at 3 and 6 months postprocedure lived longer. No admitting parameter was associated with survival to discharge, making it difficult to predict patient outcome before ureteral decompression.

Regardless of the treatment option chosen in case of ureteral obstruction, the timing of intervention is very important for renal recovery. In normal dogs, a near-complete return of renal function was observed after relief of a complete obstruction of 4 days, a 46% recovery of GFR was noted by 4 months after correction of an obstruction of 14 days, and little recovery was seen after 40 days of obstruction (Vaughan and Gillenwater 1971; Vaughan *et al.* 1973; Fink *et al.* 1980).

Postoperative incontinence is a serious complication described after surgical correction of ectopic ureters. A postoperative incontinence rate of 27% to 78% has been reported after correction of ectopic ureters (Stone and Mason 1990; McLaughlin and Miller 1991; Holt and Moore 1995; Mayhew *et al.* 2006; Ho *et al.* 2011; Reichler *et al.* 2012; Noël and Hamaide 2014), with an additional 7% to 28% of dogs becoming continent with medical or surgical treatment (or both) (McLaughlin and Miller 1991; Mayhew *et al.* 2006; Noël and Hamaide 2014).

Residual incontinence is commonly the result of concurrent USMI in dogs affected with ectopic ureters (Lane *et al.* 1995; Koie *et al.* 2000). Some authors believe that USMI may result from interference between the urethral sphincter and the distal intramural ureteral remnant (Holt *et al.* 1982; Dean and Bojrab 1988; McLoughlin and Chew 2000). This was the rationale for developing the technique of neoureterostomy with trigonal reconstruction (McLoughlin and Chew 2000) in which the entire distal ureteral remnant is dissected free from the urethral wall. Leaving the distal remnant can also be a cause of recurrent UTI or recanalization. However, comparisons of neoureterostomy with and without trigonal reconstruction (ligation of the distal remnant) did not show any significant difference in postoperative incontinence rates (Mayhew *et al.* 2006; Ho *et al.* 2011). It is therefore still debatable whether or not ligation of the intramural distal ureteral remnant would increase the likelihood of postoperative incontinence compared with complete dissection of the remnant.

Reichler *et al.* (2012) reported a fair prognosis after correction of ectopic ureters with only resection of the intravesicular ectopic ureter. The use of this technique resulted in resolution of incontinence in 72% of dogs and could therefore be an acceptable alternative to complete dissection of the ureteral remnant.

The role of preoperative urodynamic investigation to predict continued postoperative urinary incontinence in dogs affected with ectopic ureters has been evaluated (Lane *et al.* 1995; Mayhew *et al.* 2006). Urodynamic evaluation in 9 dogs with ectopic ureters revealed functional anomalies of the bladder or urethra in 8 dogs (Lane *et al.* 1995). Mayhew *et al.* (2006) reported a lower maximal urethral pressure in dogs that remained incontinent postsurgically compared with dogs that achieve continence.

Preliminary results on 42 dogs with ectopic ureters showed that a preoperative diagnosis of pelvic bladder does not appear to be a predictive factor for postoperative incontinence (Noël and Hamaide 2014). On the other hand, colposuspension performed during surgical correction of ectopic ureters in dogs diagnosed with a pelvic bladder did appear to be predictive of long-term continence (Noël and Hamaide 2014).

Predictive factors for postoperative incontinence have been investigated. Intramural versus extramural, left versus right sided, unilateral versus bilateral, the presence of hydroureter, and the presence of UTI were not associated with postoperative incontinence (McLaughlin and Miller 1991; Ho *et al.* 2011; Reichler *et al.* 2012; Noël and Hamaide 2014). Reichler *et al.* (2012) also reported the same rate of postoperative incontinence in male and female dogs.

Urinary tract infection is not proven to increase the rate of incontinence, but it may cause detrusor instability or urethral instability, which cause incontinence, or it can just worsen the signs of incontinence (Reichler *et al.* 2012).

The possible role of the concurrent removal of the gonads during surgical correction of ectopic ureters on the postoperative incontinence rate is still under investigation. Removal of the gonads results in a decrease in maximal urethral pressure and therefore might increase the risk of postoperative incontinence in dogs with ectopic ureters (Reichler *et al.* 2012). However, neutering was not a predictive factor for postoperative incontinence in a preliminary study on 42 dogs with ectopic ureters (Noel and Hamaide 2014).

References

Adin, C.A., Herrgesell, E.J., Nyland, T.G., et al. (2003) Antegrade urography in cats with suspected ureteral obstruction: 11 cases (1995-2001). *Journal of the American Veterinary Medical Association* 222, 1576-1581.

Berent, A.C. (2011) Ureteral obstructions in dogs and cats: a review of traditional and new interventional diagnostic and therapeutic options. *Journal of Veterinary Emergency and Critical Care* 21, 86-103.

Berent, A.C., Weisse, C. (2013). Urinary diversion techniques. In Monnet, E. (ed.) *Small Animal Soft Tissue Surgery*, Wiley-Blackwell, Ames, IA, pp. 600-614.

Berent, A.C., Weisse, C., Bagley, D (2010) The use of a subcutaneous ureteral bypass device for feline ureteral obstructions: 15 cases [abstract]. *Veterinary Surgery* 39, E26-E62.

Berent, A.C., Weisse, C., Bagley, D. (2011) The use of a subcutaneous ureteral bypass device for ureteral obstruction in dogs and cats [abstract]. *Journal of Veterinary Internal Medicine* 25, 632-767.

Berent, A.C., Weisse, C., Solomon, J., et al. (2009) The use of locking-loop pigtail nephrostomy catheters in dogs and cats (abstract). *Veterinary Surgery* 38, E26.

Berent, A.C., Weisse, C., Todd, K., et al. (2014) Technical and clinical outcomes of ureteral stenting in cats with benign ureteral obstruction: 69 cases (2006-2010). *Journal of the American Veterinary Medical Association* 244 (5), 559-576.

Dean, P.W., Bojrab, M.J. (1988) Canine ectopic ureter. *Compendium of Continuing Education for the Practicing Veterinarian: Small Animal Practice* 10, 146-157.

Fink, R.L., Caridis, D.T., Chimile, R., et al. (1980) Renal impairment and its reversibility following variable periods of complete ureteral obstruction. *Australian and New Zealand Journal of Surgery*, 50, 77-83.

Fossum, T.W. (2013) Surgery of the kidney and ureter. In Fossum, T.W. (ed.) *Small Animal Surgery*, 4th edn. Elsevier, St. Louis, pp. 705-734.

Gregory, C.R., Lirtzman, R.A., Kochin, E.J., et al. (1996) A mucosal apposition technique for ureteroneocystostomy after renal transplantation in cats. *Veterinary Surgery* 25, 13-17.

Hardie, E.M., Kyles, A.E. (2004) Management of ureteral obstruction. *Veterinary Clinics of North America Small Animal Practice* 34, 989-1010.

Ho, L.K., Troy, G.C., Waldron, D.R. (2011) Clinical outcomes of surgically managed ectopic ureters in 33 dogs. *Journal of the American Animal Hospital Association* 47, 196-202.

Holt, P.E., Gibbs, C., Pearson, H. (1982) Canine ectopic ureter: a review of twenty-nine cases. *Journal of Small Animal Practice* 23, 195-208.

Holt, P.E., Moore, A.H. (1995) Canine ureteral ectopia: an analysis of 175 cases and comparison of surgical treatments. *Veterinary Record* 136, 345-349.

Horowitz, C., Berent, A., Weisse, C., et al. (2013) Predictors of outcome for cats with ureteral obstruction after interventional management using ureteral stenting or a subcutaneous ureteral bypass device. *Journal of Feline Medicine and Surgery* 15 (12), 1052-1062.

Koie, H., Ymaya, Y., Sakai, T. (2000) Four cases of lowered urethral pressure in canine ectopic ureter. *Journal of Veterinary Medical Science* 62, 1221-1222.

Kuzaka, B., Szymanska, K., Borkowski, A., et al. (1996) Restoration of the continuity of dog ureter after resection of its 5 cm middle segment. *British Journal of Urology* 77, 342-346.

Kyles, A.E., Stone, E.A., Gookin, J., et al. (1998) Diagnosis and surgical management of obstructive ureteral calculi in cats: 11 cases (1993-1996). *Journal of the American Veterinary Medical Association* 213 (8), 1150-1156.

Kyles, A.E., Hardie, E.M., Wooden, B.G., et al. (2005) Management and outcome of cats with ureteral calculi: 153 cases (1984-2002). *Journal of the American Veterinary Medical Association* 226, 937-944.

Lane, I.F., Lappin, M.R., Seim, H.B. Evaluation of results of preoperative urodynamic measurements in nine dogs with ectopic ureters. *Journal of Veterinary Medical Association* 206, 1348-1357.

Mathews, K. (2012) Ureters. In Tobias, K.M., Johnston, S.A. (eds.) *Veterinary Surgery Small Animal*. Elsevier Saunders, St. Louis, pp. 1962-1977,

Mayhew, P.D., Lee, K.C.L., Gregory, S.P., et al. (2006) Comparison of two surgical techniques for management of intramural ureteral ectopia in dogs: 36 cases (1994-2004). *Journal of the American Veterinary Medical Association* 229, 389-393.

McLaughlin, R., Miller, C.W. (1991) Urinary incontinence after surgical repair of ureteral ectopia in dogs. *Veterinary Surgery* 20, 100-103.

McLoughlin, M.A. and Chew, D.J. (2000) Diagnosis and surgical management of ectopic ureters. *Clin Tech Small Anim Pract.* 15(1), 17-24.

Mehl, M.L., Kyles, A.E., Pollard, R., et al. (2005) Comparison of 3 techniques for ureteroneocystostomy in cats. *Veterinary Surgery* 34, 114-119.

Noël, S., Hamaide, A. (2014) Surgical management of ectopic ureters: clinical outcome and prognostic factors for long-term continence. In *BSAVA Congress 2014 Scientific Proceedings: Veterinary Programme*, Birmingham, UK, p. 576.

Reichler, I.M., Specker, C.E., Hubler, M., et al. (2012) Ectopic ureters in dogs: clinical features, surgical techniques and outcome. *Veterinary Surgery* 41, 515-522.

Rivers, B.J., Walter, P.A., Polzin, D.J. (1997) Ultrasonographic-guided, percutaneous antegrade pyelography: technique and clinical application in the dog and cat. *Journal of the American Animal Hospital Association* 33, 61-68.

Snyder, D.M., Steffey, M.A., Mehler, S.J., et al. (2005) Diagnosis and surgical management of ureteral calculi in dogs: 16 cases (1990-2003). *New Zealand Veterinary Journal* 53, 19-25.

Stone, E.A., Mason, L.K. (1990) Surgery of ectopic ureters: types, method of correction, and postoperative results. *Journal of the American Animal Hospital Association* 26, 81.

Vaughan, E.D. Jr., Gillenwater, J.Y. (1971) Recovery following complete chronic unilateral ureteral occlusion: functional, radiographic, and pathologic alterations. *Journal of Urology* 106 (1), 27-35.

Vaughan, E.D. Jr., Sweet, R.E., Gillenwater, J.Y. (1973) Unilateral ureteral occlusion: pattern of nephron repair and compensatory response. *Journal of Urology* 109 (6), 979-982.

Zaid, M.S., Berent, A.C., Weisse, C., et al. (2011) Feline ureteral strictures: 10 cases (2007-2009). *Journal of Veterinary Internal Medicine* 25, 222-229.

68 Surgery of the Urinary Bladder

Annick Hamaide

Department of Clinical Sciences (Companion Animals and Equids), School of Veterinary Medicine, University of Liège, Liège, Belgium

Surgery of the urinary bladder is a common procedure in small animal practice. Procedures of the urinary bladder in dogs and cats include cystotomy, partial cystectomy, placement of a cystostomy tube, and cystopexy.

Main indications for cystotomy are removal of uroliths, repair of bladder rupture (Figure 68.1), repair of ectopic ureters, and biopsy of bladder masses. Main indications for partial cystectomy include resection of bladder tumor or polyp, excision of a patent urachus or a bladder diverticulum, and bladder necrosis. Placement of a temporary cystostomy tube may be indicated whenever urine diversion is required, for example, to stabilize a patient with lower urinary tract obstruction, in case of bladder or urethral trauma, or after bladder or urethral surgery. Long-term cystostomy tubes may be indicated in patients with obstructive bladder neck or urethral neoplasia and in patients with neurogenic bladder atony. Cystopexy may be recommended in patients with displacement of the bladder into a perineal hernia to prevent recurrence of bladder retroflexion.

Complications after surgery of the urinary bladder include, but are not limited to, urine leakage, hematuria, recurrence of uroliths, urinary tract infection (UTI), small bladder volume, and tumor recurrence. Additional complications reported after the placement of a cystostomy tube include inadvertent tube removal, fistula formation after tube removal, urine leakage around the tube, inflammation at the tube exit site, tube obstruction, breakage of the mushroom tip during removal, breakage of sutures anchoring the tube to the skin, and possibly rectal prolapse secondary to straining (Beck *et al.* 2007).

Urine leakage

Definition

Leakage and accumulation of urine into the peritoneal cavity (also called *uroabdomen* or *uroperitoneum*) can occur after any surgery of the urinary bladder. Urine leakage can result from dehiscence of a sutured wound, necrosis of the bladder wall, or postoperative trauma to the urinary bladder. Peristomal urine leakage or leakage of urine from the antireflux valve has also been described after cystostomy tube placement (Stiffler *et al.* 2003; Beck *et al.* 2007).

Risk factors
- Poor surgical technique (traumatic tissue handling)
- Inadequate suture material
- Inadequate suture pattern
- Postoperative urethral obstruction leading to increased urinary bladder pressure
- Bladder neoplasia
- Bladder wall necrosis (Figure 68.2)

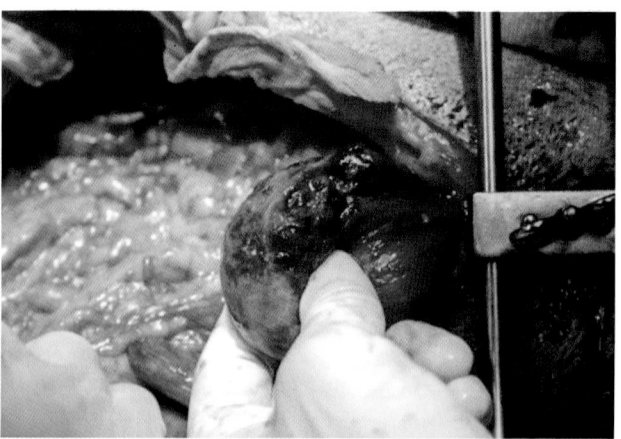

Figure 68.1 Intraoperative view of an iatrogenic rupture of the bladder (on the ventral aspect) caused by excessive pressure during external bladder expression.

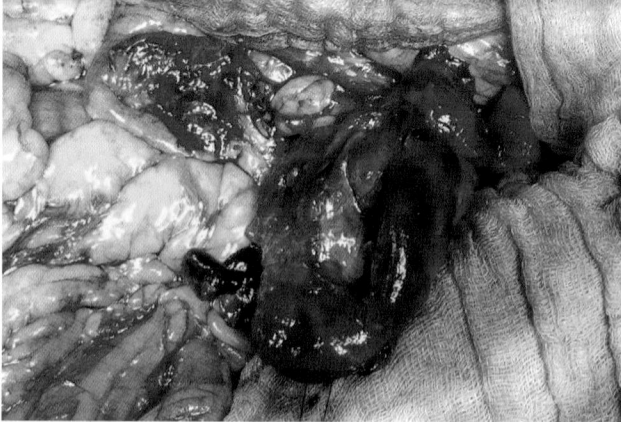

Figure 68.2 Intraoperative view of bladder necrosis (ventral aspect) after partial cystectomy and ureteroneocystostomy performed for removal of a transitional cell carcinoma in a dog. The dog presented with uroabdomen 3 days after the initial procedure.

Complications in Small Animal Surgery, First Edition. Edited by Dominique Griffon and Annick Hamaide.
© 2016 John Wiley & Sons, Inc. Published 2016 by John Wiley & Sons, Inc.
Companion website: www.wiley.com/go/griffon/complications

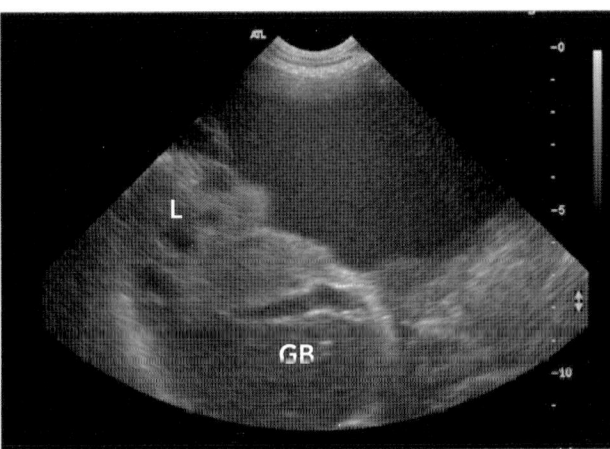

Figure 68.3 Ultrasonographic image of a dog presented with uroabdomen. A large amount of intraabdominal fluid is present around the liver lobes. GB, gallbladder; L, liver.

- Presence of UTI (especially with *Proteus* spp.)
- Postoperative trauma (traumatic catheterization or manual expression of the urinary bladder)
- Presence of a cystostomy tube
- Early removal of a cystostomy tube
- For peristomal urine leakage: loose purse-string suture in the bladder, inadequate decompression of the bladder, or placement of a small cystostomy tube compared with the size of the mature cystocutaneous fistula (Stiffler *et al.* 2003)

Diagnosis
- **Clinical signs** may be vague in animals with uroperitoneum.
- **Ultrasonography** will confirm the presence of abdominal fluid (Figure 68.3).
- **Positive contrast studies** to identify the location of the leakage (Figure 68.4)
- **Abdominocentesis and fluid analysis** will confirm the presence of urine.
- **Bacteriological culture and antibiogram** of the fluid

Treatment
- Patient stabilization
- Relief of the urethral obstruction if present

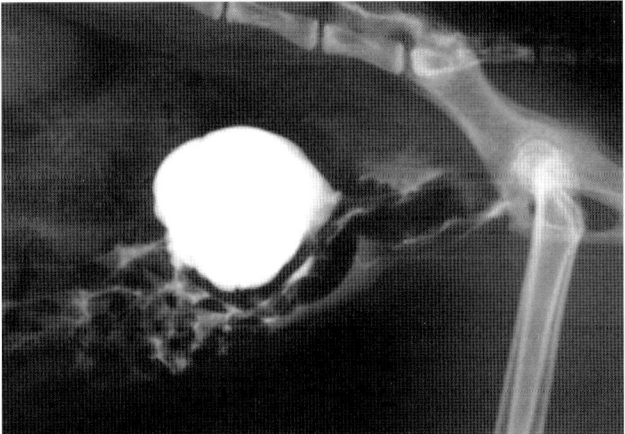

Figure 68.4 Positive contrast cystography in a dog with bladder rupture demonstrating leakage of contrast material into the abdominal cavity.

- In case of urine leakage caused by postoperative urethral obstruction, placement of an indwelling urinary catheter for 7 to 10 days might be sufficient to allow a minor break in bladder sutures to heal.
- Revision surgery includes debridement of necrotic parts followed by suturing of healthy wound edges without tension, preferably using monofilament resorbable material in a single-layer appositional suture pattern. Accurate needle placement in the submucosal layer is mandatory.
- Omentalization of the incision site
- Thorough abdominal lavage
- Broad-spectrum antibiotherapy if needed (in case of associated UTI)
- Valve replacement in case of urine leakage from the antireflux valve of the cystostomy tube
- Debridement of the fistula in case of persistent cystocutaneous fistula
- Peristoma urine leakage will resolve spontaneously in most cases.

Outcome
The presence of uroabdomen should be diagnosed and addressed as soon as possible. In general, the outcome is favorable if the defect can be closed. However, leakage of infected urine into the abdomen can result in generalized septic peritonitis, although this is rarely encountered if infection is treated appropriately.

In a study on complications after cystostomy tube placement in 76 cases (37 dogs and 39 cats), persistent peritoneal urine leakage was reported in one cat and lead to euthanasia.

Peristomal urine leakage usually ceases within 24 hours. It may, however, predispose the animal to UTI (Stiffler *et al.* 2003).

Prevention
- Use of adequate suture material: Polydioxanone, polyglyconate, and glycomer 631 are acceptable in the presence of sterile urine and *Escherichia coli*–contaminated urine (Greenberg *et al.* 2004).
- Avoid exposure of suture material that degrades via hydrolysis to urine containing *Proteus* spp. (Greenberg *et al.* 2004).
- Use of appropriate suture pattern: An appositional single-layer suture pattern for cystotomy or partial cystectomy closure is safe and effective (Thieman-Mankin *et al.* 2012).
- Accurate needle placement through the strength-holding submucosal layer of the bladder
- Omentalization or serosal patch may be used in case of a diseased bladder.
- Placement of a urinary catheter during the postoperative period if any urethral obstruction is expected (i.e., caused by postoperative inflammation)
- Performing a cystopexy during cystostomy tube placement could prevent leakage of urine into the peritoneum in case of early or inadvertent removal of the tube (Beck *et al.* 2007).
- The size of the cystostomy tube should match the size of the mature cystocutaneous fistula to prevent peristomal urine leakage.

Hematuria
See Chapter 64.

Recurrence of uroliths
See Chapter 64.

Small bladder volume

Definition
This is decreased bladder capacity after subtotal cystectomy. The bladder is no more able to store appropriate volumes of urine.

Risk factors
- Resection of more than 70% of bladder tissue
- Resection of the trigone area
- Inflammation
- Infection
- Bladder fibrosis
- Neoplasia

Diagnosis
- **Clinical signs** of increased frequency of urination (pollakiuria) or possibly unvoluntary urine leakage (urinary incontinence) will be present.
- **Urinalysis and urine culture** will rule out inflammation and infection.
- During **contrast cystography**, only a small volume of contrast is required to fill the bladder.
- **Cystometry** is useful to determine whether the bladder capacity is normal.

Treatment
- If present, UTI should be treated appropriately based on the antibiogram results.
- In rare cases in which the bladder does not regain normal capacity after a subtotal cystectomy, antimuscarinic molecules acting on bladder smooth muscle to improve bladder storage can be administered, with oxybutynin being the molecule most commonly used. In dogs, gastrointestinal upset and ptyalism can be encountered at higher dosages and usually resolve at lower doses.
- Autologous bladder augmentation techniques have been described in single case reports in dogs, including colonic seromuscular augmentation cystoplasty (Pozzi et al. 2006), ileocystoplasty (Schwarz et al. 1991), or the use of a rectus abdominis muscle flap (Savicky and Jackson 2009).
- Porcine small intestinal submucosa (SIS) has been used in humans as an extracellular matrix scaffold for bladder regeneration. In dogs, porcine SIS has been used successfully in experimental dogs in a 40% cystectomy model (Kropp et al. 1996; Zhang et al. 2006). Clinical use of porcine SIS for bladder augmentation after subtotal cystectomy has not been reported in dogs or cats.

Outcome
In most cases, the urinary bladder in dogs regains normal size and function in 4 to 6 months after resection of 70% to 90% of the bladder (Schwarz et al. 1991; Stone et al. 1996; Cornell 2000). Therefore, bladder augmentation techniques are very seldom needed in veterinary medicine.

In an experimental dog model, bladder capacity was still decreased by 72% at 9 months after cystectomy of more than 90% of the bladder (Zhang et al. 2006). Similarly, the use of porcine SIS was not successful in a 90% cystectomy dog model, suggesting that the extent of the bladder injury is important.

Prevention
- Appropriate treatment of UTI if present
- Resection of no more than 70% of bladder volume

- Preservation of the dorsal neurovascular pedicle of the trigone area

Tumor recurrence

Definition
Transitional cell carcinoma (TCC) is the most common type of bladder neoplasia in dogs and cats (Schwarz et al. 1985; Norris et al. 1992; Knapp et al. 2000). Tumor recurrence (or tumor regrowth) is a frequent complication after partial cystectomy for removal of bladder neoplasia, and a recurrence rate as high as 90% has been reported after surgical resection of bladder TCC followed by chemotherapy (Stone et al. 1996). Indeed, TCC is highly invasive and has a predilection for the trigone area (Knapp et al. 2000). At the time of diagnosis, local extension to the bladder neck is also frequent. Even if wide macroscopic margins can be obtained during partial cystectomy, obtaining clean margins at histopathology is unlikely.

Tumor seeding probably also plays an important role in tumor recurrence of bladder TCC (Stone et al. 1996; Knapp et al. 2000; Wilson et al. 2007). Indeed, new lesions can be observed distant from the original site during recurrence. Contamination of the abdominal incision site by tumoral cells and development of TCC of the abdominal wall is a possible complication after cystotomy or partial cystectomy for bladder TCC removal (Saulnier-Troff et al. 2008; Higuchi et al. 2013).

Risk factors
- Large tumor size
- Invasive TCC
- Tumor invading the trigone area and the bladder neck
- Presence of clusters of tumor cells distant from the primary site
- Inadequate surgical technique, leading to contamination of surrounding tissues
- In case of TCC, surgical resection without any adjuvant therapy

Diagnosis
- Recurrence of clinical signs (hematuria, pollakiuria, dysuria)
- Ultrasonography
- Contrast imaging studies (cystography, vaginourethrography)
- Computed tomography or magnetic resonance imaging
- Cytology (via transurethral catheter aspiration or brush cytology)
- Histology (biopsy via cystoscopy or cystotomy)

Treatment
- Palliative control of clinical signs with nonsteroidal antiinflammatory drugs (i.e., piroxicam)
- Antibiotherapy if UTI is also present
- Palliative placement of a cystostomy tube in case of urethral obstruction
- In case of TCC, additional surgery in case of tumor recurrence will most likely be ineffective in controlling the tumor locally. It is therefore not recommended by the author.
- Poor local tumor control and high morbidity have been reported with intraoperative radiation therapy (Withrow et al. 1989). Radiotherapy associated with a laparoscopically implanted tissue expander has been described in two dogs with TCC (Murphy et al. 2008).

Outcome

In case of benign bladder tumors, the outcome is good if wide excision can be achieved (Burnie and Weaver 1983). Unfortunately, in case of TCC, the patient is likely to die from the disease, whatever treatment modality is chosen. A study on 85 dogs with TCC in which the cause of death was known showed that 61% of dogs died because of the primary tumor, 14% died from metastatic disease, and 25% died of non–tumor-related causes (Knapp *et al.* 2000).

Prevention

- Early diagnosis and treatment because survival time can be increased when TCC is confined to the mucosa (Stone *et al.* 1996)
- If partial cystectomy is performed in case of TCC, it should always be combined with adjuvant chemotherapy.
- After excision of a TCC, the surgeon should change gloves and instruments before closure of the abdominal wall to avoid contamination by tumor cells.

Relevant literature

The urinary bladder is one of the most rapidly healing organs in the body and regains nearly 100% of normal tissue strength in 14 to 21 days (Bellah 1989; Degner and Walshaw 1996). **Urine leakage**, although infrequent, is the most common described complication after surgery of the urinary bladder. A recent study comparing the short-term complications between dogs and cats undergoing appositional single-layer or inverting double-layer cystotomy closure did not find any significant difference with regard to the prevalence of minor or major complications (Thieman-Mankin *et al.* 2012). One animal in each group (2 of 144 animals) did develop dehiscence and postoperative uroabdomen. The authors concluded that an appositional single-layer suture pattern for cystotomy closure was a safe and effective procedure with minimal risk of urine leakage.

For effective repair of bladder wounds or incisions, a suture material that maintains acceptable tensile strength through 21 days should be used (Greenberg *et al.* 2004). Monofilament suture is recommended because it causes less tissue drag than multifilament suture, and fewer bacteria adhere to monofilament suture compared with multifilament suture (Lipscomb 2012). A study evaluating the tensile strengths of four monofilament absorbable suture materials (polydioxanone, poliglecaprone 25, polyglyconate, and glycomer 631) found a reduction in tensile strength for all materials in infected and noninfected urine specimens over time (Greenberg *et al.* 2004). Polyglyconate and polydioxanone had superior tensile strengths in sterile neutral and *E. coli*–inoculated urine, and polydioxanone retained the greatest tensile strength throughout the study period. All four suture materials disintegrated before day 7 in *Proteus mirabilis*–infected urine. They concluded that polydioxanone, polyglyconate, and glycomer 631 are acceptable suture material for urinary bladder closure in the presence of sterile and *E. coli*–infected urine. However, exposure of any suture material that degrades via hydrolysis to urine contaminated with *Proteus* spp. should be minimized (Greenberg *et al.* 2004).

In a study on complications after cystostomy tube placement in 76 cases (37 dogs and 39 cats), persistent peritoneal urine leakage leading to euthanasia was reported in 1 cat, and urine leakage around the tube was reported in 7 animals (Beck *et al.* 2007).

In a study on the use of low-profile cystostomy tubes in 4 dogs and 1 cat, leakage of urine from the antireflux valve was noted in 3 dogs and 1 cat, which necessitated the replacement of the valve in 3 of the patients (Stiffler *et al.* 2003). In the same study, transient and self-limiting peristomal urine leakage was reported in 2 dogs.

The exact percentage of bladder that may be excised in dogs and cats without resulting in long-term **small bladder volume** is unknown. In human surgery, more than 75% of the bladder (excluding the trigone) may be excised and regained normal bladder capacity within 3 months (Peacock 1984). After partial cystectomy, bladder capacity increases by mucosal regeneration and remodeling of scar tissue, combined with hypertrophy and proliferation of smooth muscle and distension of the remaining bladder wall (Peacock 1984). It has been previously stated as mandatory to keep the trigone area intact because the regenerating cells arise from the epithelium of the terminal ureters and urethra (Wishnow *et al.* 1989). However, en bloc removal of the trigone area and proximal urethra with preservation of the dorsal neurovascular pedicles (Figure 68.5) in dogs with bladder neoplasia did not lead to urinary incontinence or small bladder volume (Saulnier-Troff *et al.* 2008).

In human surgery, besides the traditional enterocystoplasty techniques, various materials are used as a scaffold for bladder regeneration. Recently, tissue engineering to produce bladder tissue using autologous cells has been successfully used in experimental dogs after subtotal cystectomy (Kwon *et al.* 2008; Watanabe *et al.* 2011).

In case of TCC, the frequency of **tumor recurrence** and metastatic disease is high after surgical resection alone. Even after obtaining wide surgical margins (>1 cm), it is very unlikely to obtain clean margins at histology. New lesions can also be observed distant from the initial tumor site. Therefore, surgery should be considered as a palliative procedure and should be combined to other treatment modalities. Reported survival times in dogs after partial cystectomy and adjuvant chemotherapy range from 2 to 19 months (Stone *et al.* 1996; Saulnier-Troff *et al.* 2008). More than 90% of these dogs experienced local recurrence or distant metastasis. In a study on cats with TCC, 6 of 8 cats that underwent partial cystectomy and adjuvant chemotherapy had tumor recurrence,

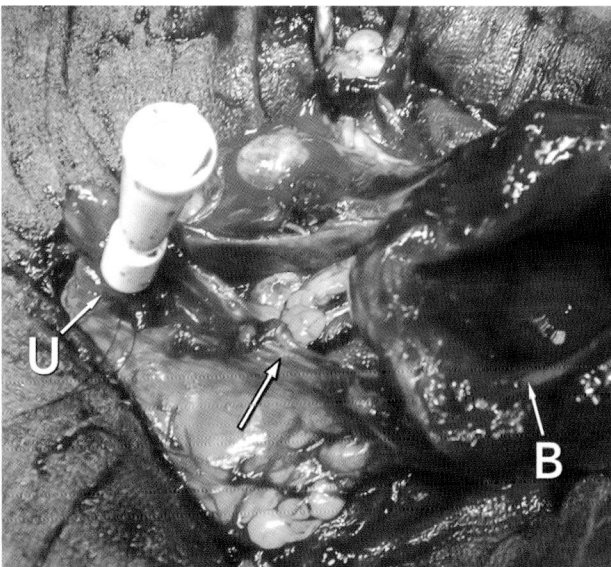

Figure 68.5 Intraoperative view during resection of the trigone area and proximal urethra (U), in a dog with transitional cell carcinoma. The bladder (B) neck, including the trigone area, and the proximal urethra have been removed. The arrow shows the preserved dorsal neurovascular pedicle. The urinary catheter is inserted into the urethra in a normograde fashion.

and the median disease-free period was 89 days (range, 61–1545 days) (Wilson *et al.* 2007).

In a study of 76 cases (37 dogs and 39 cats), a complication rate of 49% was reported after **placement of a cystostomy tube** (Beck *et al.* 2007). In this study, complications included inadvertent tube removal, fistula formation after tube removal, urine leakage around the tube, inflammation at the tube exit site, hematuria, tube obstruction, breakage of mushroom tip during removal, breakage of sutures anchoring the tube to the skin, and possibly rectal prolapse. Apart from these complications, recurrent or persistent UTI was identified in 86% of the animals postoperatively (Beck *et al.* 2007).

References

Beck, A.L., Grierson, J.M., Ogden, D.M., et al. (2007) Outcome of and complications associated with tube cystostomy in dogs and cats: 76 cases (1995-2006). *Journal of the American Veterinary Medical Association* 230 (8), 1184-1189.

Bellah, J.R. (1989) Wound healing in the urinary tract. *Seminars in Veterinary Medicine and Surgery (Small Animal)* 4, 294-303.

Burnie, A.G., Weaver, A.D. (1983) Urinary bladder neoplasia in the dog: a review of seventy cases. *Journal of Small Animal Practice* 24, 129.

Cornell, K.K. (2000) Cystotomy, partial cystectomy, and tube cystostomy. *Clinical Techniques in Small Animal Practice* 15, 11-16.

Degner, D.A., Walshaw, R. (1996) Healing response of the lower urinary tract. *Veterinary Clinics of North America: Small Animal Practice* 26, 197-206.

Greenberg, C.B., Davidson, E.B., Bellmer, D.D., et al. (2004) Evaluation of the tensile strengths of four monofilament absorbable suture materials after immersion in canine urine with or without bacteria. *American Journal of Veterinary Research* 65 (6), 847-853.

Higuchi, T., Burcham, G.N., Childress, M.O., et al. (2013) Characterization and treatment of transitional cell carcinoma of the abdominal wall in dogs: 24 cases (1985-2010). *Journal of the American Veterinary Medical Association* 242 (4), 499-506.

Knapp, D.W., Glickman, N.W., DeNicola, D.B., et al. (2000) Naturally-occurring canine transitional cell carcinoma of the urinary bladder: a relevant model of human invasive bladder cancer. *Urologic Oncology* 5, 47.

Kropp, B.P., Ripp, M.K., Badylak, S.F., et al. (1996) Regenerative urinary bladder augmentation using small intestinal mucosa: urodynamic and histopathologic assessment in long-term canine bladder augmentations. *Journal of Urology* 155, 2098.

Kwon, T.G., Yoo, J.J., Atala, A. (2008) Local and systemic effects of a tissue engineered neobladder in a canine cystoplasty model. *Journal of Urology* 179 (5), 2035.

Lipscomb, V.J. (2012) Bladder. In Tobias, K.M., Johnston, S.A. (eds.) *Veterinary Surgery Small Animal*, vol. 2, 1st edn. Elsevier Saunders, St. Louis, pp. 1978-1992.

Murphy, S., Gutiérrez, A., Lawrence, J., et al. (2008) Laparoscopically implanted tissue expander radiotherapy in canine transitional cell carcinoma. *Veterinary Radiology & Ultrasound* 49 (4), 400.

Norris, A.M., Laing, E.J., Valli, V.E., et al. (1992) Canine bladder and urethral tumours: a retrospective study of 155 cases (1980-1985). *Journal of Veterinary Internal Medicine* 6, 145.

Peacock, E.E. (1984) Healing and repair of peritoneum and viscera. In Peacock, E.E. (ed.) *Wound Repair,* 3rd ed Saunders, Philadelphia, p. 438.

Pozzi, A., Smeak, D.D., Aper, R. (2006) Colonic seromuscular augmentation cystoplasty following subtotal cystectomy for treatment of bladder necrosis caused by bladder torsion in a dog. *Journal of the American Veterinary Medical Association* 229 (2), 235-239.

Saulnier-Troff, F.G., Busoni, V., Hamaide, A. (2008) A technique for resection of invasive tumours involving the trigone area of the bladder in dogs: preliminary results in two dogs. *Veterinary Surgery* 37, 427.

Savicky, R.S., Jackson, A.H. (2009) Use of a rectus abdominis muscle flap to repair urinary bladder and urethral defects in a dog. *Journal of the American Veterinary Medical Association* 234 (8), 1038.

Schwarz, P.D., Greene, R.W., Patnaik, A.K. (1985) Urinary bladder tumours in the cat: a review of 27 cases. *Journal of the American Animal Hospital Association* 21, 237.

Schwarz, P.D., Egger, E.L., Klause, S.E. (1991) Modified "cup-patch" ileocystoplasty for urinary bladder reconstruction in a dog. *Journal of the American Veterinary Medical Association* 198 (2), 273.

Stiffler, K.S., McCrackin Stevenson, M.A., Cornell, K.K., et al. (2003) Clinical use of low-profile cystostomy tubes in four dogs and a cat. *Journal of the American Veterinary Medical Association* 223 (3), 325-329.

Stone, E.A., George, T.F., Gilson, S.D., et al. (1996) Partial cystectomy for urinary bladder neoplasia: surgical technique and outcome in 11 dogs. *Journal of Small Animal Practice* 37, 480-485.

Thieman-Mankin, K.M., Ellison, G.W., Jeyapaul, C.J., et al. (2012) Comparison of short-term complication rates between dogs and cats undergoing appositional single-layer or inverting double-layer cystotomy closure: 144 cases (1993-2010). *Journal of the American Veterinary Medical Association* 240 (1), 65-68.

Watanabe, E., Yamato, M., Shiroyanagi, Y., et al. (2011) Bladder augmentation using tissue-engineering autologous oral mucosal epithelial cell sheets grafted on demucosalized gastric flaps. *Transplantation,* 91 (7), 700-706.

Wilson, H.M., Chun, R., Larson, V.S., et al. (2007) Clinical signs, treatments, and outcome in cats with transitional cell carcinoma of the urinary bladder: 20 cases (1990–2004). *Journal of the American Veterinary Medical Association* 231, 101.

Wishnow, K.I., Johnson, D.E., Grignon, D.J., et al. (1989) Regeneration of the canine urinary bladder mucosa after complete surgical denudation. *Journal of Urology* 141 (6), 1476.

Withrow, S.J., Gilette, E.L., Hoopes, P.J., et al. (1989) Intraoperative irradiation of 16 spontaneously occurring canine neoplasms. *Veterinary Surgery* 18, 7.

Zhang, Y., Frimberger, D., Cheng, E.Y., et al. (2006) Challenges in a larger bladder replacement with cell-seeded and unseeded small intestinal submucosa grafts in a subtotal cystectomy model. *BJU International* 98 (5), 1100.

69 Urethrostomy in Male Dogs

Joshua Milgram

Veterinary Teaching Hospital, Koret School of Veterinary Medicine, Rehovot, Israel

Urethrostomy is a surgical procedure in which a permanent diversion of urine is created by suturing the penile mucosa to the skin subsequent to exposure of the urethral lumen (McLoughlin 2011). Meticulous soft tissue handling is essential for a successful surgical outcome (McLoughlin 2011).

Recommended anatomic locations for the creation of an urethrostomy differ between dogs and cats; however, the complications are common to both species. Complications associated with urethrostomy include stricture formation, hemorrhage, dehiscence, urine leakage, perineal hernia, urinary or fecal incontinence, rectal prolapse, and ascending urinary tract infection (UTI) (Smith and Schiller 1978; Johnson and Gourley, 1980; Gregory and Vasseur 1983; Scavelli 1989; Dean et al. 1990; Bilbrey et al. 1991; Griffin and Gregory 1992; Smeak 2000; Bjorling 2003; Wood et al. 2007).

The majority of complications can be avoided with a combination of meticulous surgical technique and attentive postoperative management. The best results are achieved by adhering to surgical techniques that promote primary healing of the surgical site and prevent wound disruption in the postoperative period. Accurate apposition of the tissues and tension free closure (Bjorling 2003), prevention of self-trauma and oral contamination, and recommended wound care and removal of all suture material at 10 to 14 days are the keys to surgical success (McLoughlin 2011).

Hemorrhage

Definition
- Active or spontaneous hemorrhage from the surgical site or hemorrhage associated with urination (Burrow et al. 2011)
- Adequate hemostasis from the cavernous tissues of the penis can be a challenge both intraoperatively and postoperatively.

Risk factors
- Location of the urethrostomy. Scrotal urethrostomy is the preferred site in dogs because relatively less cavernous tissue is incised during the approach, which results in less intraoperative and postoperative hemorrhage (Fossum 2007).
- Poor surgical technique. Failure to adequately seal the corpus spongiosum and oppose the skin and mucosa when suturing (Newton and Smeak 1996).
- Patient with an excitable disposition

Diagnosis
- Active postoperative hemorrhage or hemorrhage associated with urination, 0.2 days and 3.1 days, respectively (Newton and Smeak 1996) and for up to 21 days postoperatively (Burrow et al. 2011).

Treatment
Conservative management is recommended. Hemorrhage is unlikely to be severe enough to warrant surgical revision or blood transfusion (Burrow et al. 2011).

Outcome
Prolonged bleeding from the surgical site can delay wound healing with resultant dehiscence (Newton and Smeak 1996; Smeak 2000; Bjorling 2003). It can also result in excessive bruising and hematoma formation (Burrow et al. 2011).

Prevention
- A continuous suture pattern with closely spaced bites that oppose the skin and mucosa and seal the corpus spongiosum by passing through the penile mucosa and tunica albuginea (Newton and Smeak 1996)
- No difference in postoperative hemorrhage was found between the use of continuous or simple interrupted suture patterns (Burrow et al. 2011).
- Sealing the corpus spongiosum is recommended regardless of the suture pattern used (Newton and Smeak 1996; Burrow et al. 2011).
- Judicious use of sedatives in selected patients

Urine leakage

Definition
- Leakage of urine from the urethra into the subcutaneous tissues after urethrostomy

Risk factors
- Suturing of tissue under tension
- Failure to oppose the urethral mucosa to the skin

Diagnosis
- Clinical diagnosis can be challenging.
  ○ The anatomic location of the site of leakage determines the location of the urine accumulation. Leakage in the ischial part of the urethra results in urine accumulation in the subcutaneous tissues of the perineum, thighs, or inguinal region.

Complications in Small Animal Surgery, First Edition. Edited by Dominique Griffon and Annick Hamaide.

© 2016 John Wiley & Sons, Inc. Published 2016 by John Wiley & Sons, Inc.

Companion website: www.wiley.com/go/griffon/complications

- Leakage of urine into the subcutaneous tissues results in edema, cellulitis, and bruising that can progress to tissue necrosis.
- Retrograde positive contrast urethrogram.

Treatment
- Revision of the urethrostomy
- Aspiration of subcutaneous fluid
- Placement of active or passive drains
- Urinary diversion with a cystostomy tube
- Conservative management

Outcome
- Peristomal skin necrosis
- Necrosis of the skin of the perineum or hindlimbs
- Considered to be a predisposing factor for stricture of the stoma

Prevention
- Adequate mobilization of tissue and tension free apposition of the mucosa and skin
- Meticulous surgical technique

Urethral stricture

Definition
- Narrowing of the urethral stoma/lumen to the extent that normal urine flow is prevented

Risk factors
- Postoperative hemorrhage and hematoma formation
- Subcutaneous urine leakage
- Wound dehiscence
- Excessive tension on sutures placed between the urethral mucosa and the skin
- Self-induced trauma
- Subsequent to partial penile amputation (Boothe 2003)

Diagnosis
- Clinical signs of stranguria
- A visibly narrowed urethral stoma on physical examination
- Diagnosis confirmed with positive contrast urethrogram

Treatment
- Balloon dilatation of the urethral stricture followed by temporary urethral stenting (Bjorling and Petersen 1990; Bennett *et al.* 2005; Powers *et al.* 2010)
- Minimally invasive placement of a urethral stent
- Surgical revision of the urethrostomy
- Permanent urinary diversion proximal to the stricture

Outcome
- The prognosis after surgical intervention is less favorable (Boothe 2000; Bjorling 2003; Anderson *et al.* 2006) in case of:
  - Multiple sites of urethral stricture
  - A stricture longer than 2 to 3 cm
- Permanent urinary diversion, if possible, may be the best way to avoid further complications (Wood *et al.* 2007).

Prevention
- Precise apposition of urethral mucosa to the skin
- Tension-free apposition of urethral mucosa to the skin

- Select anatomic location and technique associated with lower complication rates when possible
- Prevent self-induced trauma.

Urinary tract infection
See Chapter 64

Urine scalding

Definition
- Inflammation, maceration, and necrosis of the peristomal skin as a result of chronic skin contact with urine (McLoughlin 2011)

Risk factors
- Site of urethrostomy
- Urinary incontinence

Diagnosis
- Observation of peristomal skin irritation, dermatitis, or skin necrosis (Baines *et al.* 2001)

Treatment
- Clipping the hair around the stoma (McLoughlin 2011)
- Protection of the skin by topical application of a petroleum jelly or antibiotic ointment to the skin surrounding the stoma (Baines *et al.* 2001; McLoughlin 2011)
- Systemic antibiotic therapy if severe ulceration or maceration of the peristomal skin is present (McLoughlin 2011)
- Debridement of necrotic or chronically ulcerated peristomal skin and creation of a new stoma (McLoughlin 2011)

Outcome
- Spontaneous resolution is possible, particularly when a new posture is adopted during urination (Smith 1993).
- Severe peristomal skin necrosis may lead to euthanasia (Baines *et al.* 2001).

Prevention
- Scrotal urethrostomy is the ideal location in dogs because it minimizes urine contact with the skin and resultant urine scalding.
- Procedures that are less likely to compromise continence should be selected.

Relevant literature
Permanent damage of the distal urethra may require long-term urinary diversion by urethrostomy. Urethrostomy is indicated to divert urine in instances of permanent pathology and to prevent recurrent obstructions with uroliths in predisposed individuals (Bleedom and Bjorling 2012). In male dogs, urethrostomy can be performed at prescrotal, scrotal, perineal, subpubic (Bernarde and Viguier 2004; Liehmann *et al.* 2010) and prepubic locations; in female dogs, it is limited to a prepubic location (Bleedom and Bjorling, 2012). Scrotal urethrostomy is preferred because the urethra in this region is superficial, wide and has relatively less cavernous tissue, which results in less postoperative hemorrhage (McLoughlin 2011; Bleedom and Bjorling 2012).

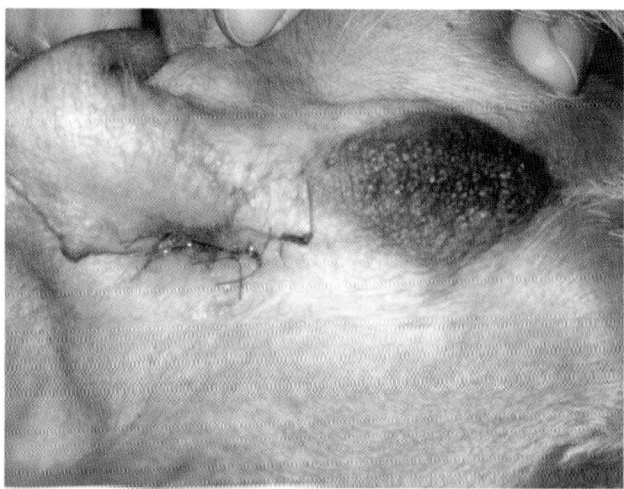

Figure 69.1 Prepubic urethrostomy in a male dog. Note the slight amount of urine scalding at the stoma (Courtesy of Annick Hamaide).

The most common complication of scrotal urethrostomy is hemorrhage (Newton and Smeak 1996; Bjorling 2003; Fossum 2007; Burrow *et al.* 2011). A continuous suture pattern that both seal the corpus spongiosum and oppose the mucosa and skin was shown to decrease the duration of postoperative hemorrhage (Newton and Smeak 1996); however, postoperative hemorrhage has been reported to persist for 21 days (Burrow *et al.* 2011). The current recommendation is that emphasis should be placed on accurate suture placement rather than suture pattern (Bleedom and Bjorling 2012). Postoperative hemorrhage is usually self-limiting and may last from 3 to 21 days (Newton and Smeak 1996; Burrow *et al.* 2011). Surgical revision has been recommended for hemorrhage that persists for more than 10 to 14 days (Bleedom and Bjorling 2012); however, this is rarely necessary (Burrow *et al.* 2011).

Intermittent urine scalding, recurrent UTIs, and recurrent obstruction from struvite calculi have a reported incidence of 20% in case of scrotal urethrostomy (Newton and Smeak 1996). Stricture is rare and in most instances can be avoided with meticulous surgical technique and attentive postoperative care.

Prepubic urethrostomy is performed as a salvage procedure when none of the standard urethrostomy procedures can be performed. This technique has been used successfully in several case reports (Katayama *et al.* 2012; Vnuk *et al.* 2014). Although the urethra is usually significantly shortened by this procedure, urinary continence is maintained if the sphincter and innervation are preserved.

Complications associated with the prepubic urethrostomy procedure are incontinence, urine scalding (particularly with incontinence) (Figure 69.1), stricture of the stoma, or kinking or compression of the urethra as it passes across the abdominal wall (Bleedom and Bjorling, 2012). The potential for recurrent infection with this procedure has also been reported.

References

Anderson, R.B., Aronson, L.R., Drobatz, K.J. et al. (2006) Prognostic factors for successful outcome following urethral rupture in dogs and cats. *Journal of the American Animal Hospital Association* 42, 136-146.

Baines, S. J., White, R. S. (2001) Prepubic urethrostomy: a long-term study in 16 cats. *Veterinary Surgery* 30, 107-113.

Bennett, S. L., Edwards, G. E., Tyrrell, D. (2005) Balloon dilation of a urethral stricture in a dog. *Australian Veterinary Journal* 83, 552-554.

Bernarde, A., Viguier, E. (2004) Transpelvic urethrostomy in 11 cats using an ischial ostectomy. *Veterinary Surgery* 33, 246-252.

Bilbrey, S.A., Birchard, J, Smeak, D.D. (1991) Scrotal urethrostomy: a retrospective review of 38 dogs (1973-1988). *Journal of the American Animal Hospital Association* 27, 560-564

Bjorling, D.E. (2003) Surgery of the urethra. In Slatter, D.H. (ed.) *Textbook of Small Animal Surgery*, 3rd edn, WB Saunders, Philadelphia, pp. 1638-1651.

Bjorling, D.E., Petersen, S. W. (1990) Surgical techniques for urinary tract diversion and salvage in small animals. *Compendium on Continuing Education for the Practicing Veterinarian* 12, 1699-1709.

Bleedom, J.A., Bjorling, D. E. (2012) Urethra. In Tobias, K M., Johnston, S.A. (eds.) *Veterinary Surgery—Small Animal*, 1st edn. Elsevier, St. Louis, pp. 1993-2010.

Boothe, H.W. (2000) Managing traumatic urethral injuries. *Clinical Techniques In Small Animal Practice* 15, 35-39.

Boothe, H.W. (2003) Penis, prepuce and scrotum. In Slatter, D.E. (ed.) *Textbook of Small Animal Surgery*, 3rd edn. WB Saunders, Philadelphia, pp. 1531-1541.

Burrow, R.D., Gregory, S.P., Giejda, A.A. et al. (2011) Penile amputation and scrotal urethrostomy in 18 dogs. *Veterinary Record* 169, 657-663.

Dean, P.W., Hedlund, C.S., Lewis, Dd. et al. (1990) Canine urethrotomy and urethrostomy. *Compendium on Continuing Education for the Practicing Veterinarian* 12, 1541-1554.

Fossum, T.W. (2007) Surgery of the bladder and urethra. In Fossum, T.W. (ed.) *Small Animal Surgery*, 3rd edn. Mosby, St. Louis, pp. 663-685.

Gregory, C.R., Vasseur, P.B. (1983) Long-term examination of cats with perineal urethrostomy. *Veterinary Surgery* 12, 210-212.

Griffin, D.W., Gregory, C.R. (1992) Prevalence of bacterial urinary tract infection after perineal urethrostomy in cats. *Journal of the American Veterinary Medical Association* 200, 681-684.

Johnson, M.S., Gourley, I.M. (1980) Perineal hernia in a cat: a possible complication of perineal urethrostomy. *Veterinary Medicine, Small Animal Clinician* 75, 741-743.

Katayama, M., Okamura, Y., Kamishina, H. et al. (2012) Urinary diversion via preputial urethrostomy with bilateral pubic-ischial osteotomy in a dog. *Turkish Journal of Veterinary & Animal Sciences* 36, 730-733.

Liehmann, L.M., Doyle, R.S., Powell, R.M. (2010) Transpelvic urethrostomy in a Staffordshire bull terrier: a new technique in the dog. *Journal of Small Animal Practice* 51, 325-329.

McLoughlin, M.A. (2011) Complications of Lower urinary tract surgery in small animals. *Veterinary Clinics of North America-Small Animal Practice* 41, 889-913.

Newton, J.D., Smeak, D.D. (1996) Simple continuous closure of canine scrotal urethrostomy: results in 20 cases. *Journal of the American Animal Hospital Association* 32, 531-534.

Powers, M.Y., Campbell, B.G., Weisse, C. (2010) Porcine small intestinal submucosa augmentation urethroplasty and balloon dilation of a urethral stricture secondary to inadvertent prostatectomy in a dog. *Journal of the American Animal Hospital Association* 46, 358-365.

Scavelli, T.D. (1989) Complications associated with perineal urethrostomy in the cat. *Problems in Veterinary Medicine*, 1, 111-119.

Smeak, D.D. (2000) Urethrotomy and urethrostomy in the dog. *Clinical Techniques in Small Animal Practice* 15, 25-34.

Smith, C.W. (1993) Surgical diseases of the urethra. In Slatter, D. (ed.) *Textbook of Small Animal Surgery*, 2nd edn. WB Saunders, Philadelphia.

Smith, C.W., Schiller, A.G. (1978) Perineal urethrostomy in cat—retrospective study of complications *Journal of the American Animal Hospital Association* 14, 225-228.

Vnuk, D., Bottegaro, N.B., Slunjski, I., et al. (2014) Prepubic urethrostomy opening within a prepuce in a dog: a case report. *Veterinarni Medicina* 59, 107-111.

Wood, M. W., Vaden, S., Cerda-Gonzalez, S., Keene, B. 2007. Cystoscopic-guided balloon dilation of a urethral stricture in a female dog. *Canadian Veterinary Journal-Revue Veterinaire Canadienne* 48, 731-733.

70 Feline Perineal Urethrostomy

Joshua Milgram

Veterinary Teaching Hospital, Koret School of Veterinary Medicine, Rehovot, Israel

Perineal urethrostomy (PU), a surgical procedure for the treatment of penile urethral obstruction and trauma in male cats, was first reported in 1963 (Carbone 1963). The modifications of this technique (Christensen 1964; Wilson and Harrison 1971; Yeh and Chin 2000) are the commonly used surgical methods for the treatment of urethral obstruction in male cats.

The urethra of a male cat is divided into four anatomically discrete sections, preprostatic, prostatic, postprostatic, and penile urethra. The order of the sections, based on increasing internal diameter is, penile urethra (0.7 mm), postprostatic urethra at the level of the bulbourethral glands (1.3 mm), and preprostatic urethra (2.0 mm) (Cullen *et al.* 1983). The diameter of the urethra at the level of the bulbourethral glands is almost double the diameter of the penile urethra and provides adequate luminal diameter (1.3 mm) for the creation of a permanent stoma (Wilson and Harrison 1971; Phillips and Holt 2006). Failure to dissect cranially to this level results in the creation of stoma with a smaller diameter that is predisposed to stricture formation.

Although perineal urethrostomy is usually a successful procedure when performed correctly, numerous serious complications have been reported, including stricture formation and recurrent obstruction, bacterial urinary tract infection (UTI), sterile cystitis, subcutaneous urine leakage at the surgical site, urinary and fecal incontinence, rectal prolapse, rectourethral fistula formation, and perineal hernia (Smith and Schiller 1978; Gregory and Vasseur 1983; Gregory 1987; Scavelli 1989; Griffin and Gregory 1992; Hosgood and Hedlund 1992).

Hemorrhage

See Chapter 12.

Wound dehiscence

See Chapter 9.

Subcutaneous urine leakage

Definition

- Leakage of urine into the subcutaneous tissues of the perineum and hindlimbs
- Occurred in 25% of cats in one study (Bass *et al.* 2005)

Risk factors

- Rupture of the postprostatic urethra may be caused by blunt or penetrating trauma, but iatrogenic trauma when attempting retrograde urethral catheterization is more common (Ladlow 2014).
- Inadequate mucocutaneous apposition caused by:
  - Excessive tension on the suture line
  - Technical error: misidentification of the urethral mucosa and failure to oppose the skin and mucosa

Diagnosis

- Rupture of the postprostatic urethra may result in a fluctuant swelling of the perineum and the dorsum around the tail base (Ladlow 2014).
- Marked hyperemia, pain, edema, and bruising of the perineal area and hindlegs immediately after performing a PU (Figure 70.1)
- Pain during and after urination (Ladlow 2014)
- Dehiscence of stoma (Ladlow 2014)
- Necrosis and sloughing of the peristomal skin

Treatment

- Aspiration of the subcutaneous fluid (Holt 1989; Clarke and Findji 2011)
- Placement of a small closed-suction drain (Holt 1989; Clarke and Findji 2011)

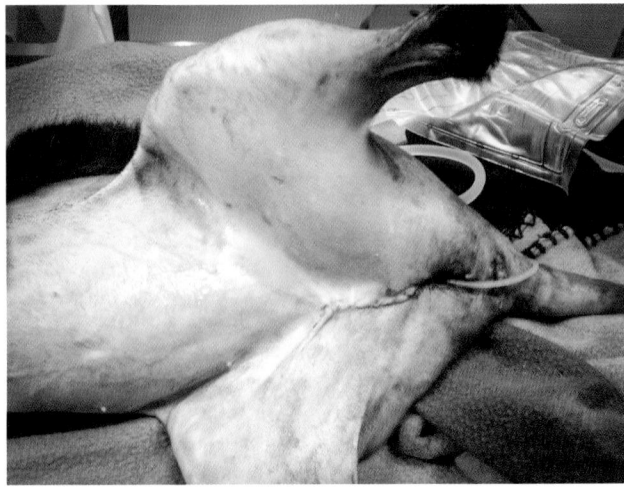

Figure 70.1 A cat with subcutaneous leakage of urine after a transpelvic urethrostomy. Note the swelling and edema present in the perineal region and thighs (Courtesy of Annick Hamaide).

Complications in Small Animal Surgery, First Edition. Edited by Dominique Griffon and Annick Hamaide.

© 2016 John Wiley & Sons, Inc. Published 2016 by John Wiley & Sons, Inc.

Companion website: www.wiley.com/go/griffon/complications

- Urinary diversion with a cystostomy tube (Ladlow 2014)
- Conservative management (Bass *et al.* 2005)

Outcome
- Necrosis of skin of the perineum or hindlimbs
- Considered to be a predisposing factor for stricture of the stoma

Prevention
- Atraumatic retrograde urethral catheterization
- Meticulous surgical technique

Urinary incontinence

Definition
- Urinary incontinence is the loss of voluntary control of urination, resulting in leakage of urine from the urinary system to the exterior of the body.
- Urinary incontinence is occasionally seen postoperatively after perineal urethrostomy but is usually temporary (Smith and Schiller 1978; Gregory and Vasseur 1983; Scavelli 1989).

Risk factors
- Excessive dorsal dissection with damage to the pelvic plexus
- Excessive removal of the urethra with retention of inadequate length of urethra (Ladlow 2014)
- Intraoperative damage to the pudendal nerve during the surgery
- Bladder damage during an obstructive episode

Diagnosis
- Diagnostic tests should be undertaken as needed to distinguish between urinary incontinence and other causes of dysuria.
- These tests include urinalysis and culture, as well as ultrasonography and positive contrast studies of the lower urinary tract.
- Urodynamic examination (urethral pressure profile and cystometry) may confirm the diagnosis if needed.

Treatment
- Medical treatment is adapted depending on the etiology of the urinary incontinence. In case of damage to the urethral sphincter, the administration of α-adrenergic agents (e.g., phenylpropanolamine) may be attempted. If bladder dysfunction is suspected or diagnosed, a urinary catheter should be left in place for at least 10 days, while parasympathicomimetic agents are administered.
- When the urinary incontinence is not responsive to medical management, endoscopic injection of submucosal urethral bulking agents has been attempted to improve the continence with limited success.

Outcome
- In most cases, spontaneous recovery may be expected.
- The prognosis for recovery is guarded in case of irreversible nerve damage.

Prevention
- Avoid excessive dissection of the tissues dorsal to the penis.
- Avoid removal of excessive urethral length.

Urinary tract infection
See Chapter 64.

Urethral stricture

Definition
- Most commonly used to describe postoperative narrowing of the urethral stoma

Risk factors
- Insufficient dissection of the urethra to the level of the bulbourethral glands
- Excessive tension on sutures placed between the urethral mucosa and the skin
- Subcutaneous urine leakage
- Suture pattern: No difference was found between the use of a simple continuous pattern of absorbable material and a simple interrupted closure of nonabsorbable material to close a perineal urethrostomy (Agrodnia *et al.* 2004). However, a simple continuous pattern of absorbable material has been associated with a higher incidence of complications in cats referred for revision of perineal urethrostomy (Bleedorn and Bjorling 2012).
- Surgeon experience has been reported to be a contributing factor to stricture formation (Smith and Schiller 1978). However, in a later report, no difference was found between supervised residents and senior staff surgeons (Bass *et al.* 2005).
- Postoperative use of urethral catheters (Smith and Schiller 1978)
- Self-induced trauma (Smith and Schiller 1978)

Diagnosis
- History of treatment, in the immediate postoperative period, for clinical signs consistent with urine leakage (hyperemia of the surgical site, edema and bruising of the perineal area and hindlegs).
- Clinical signs include complaints of stranguria, urinary incontinence, vocalization on urination, inappropriate urination, hematuria, dyschezia, bruising of the perineum, licking at the urethral stoma, vomiting, and weight loss (Phillips and Holt 2006).
- A visible narrowed urethral stoma on physical examination (Figure 70.2).

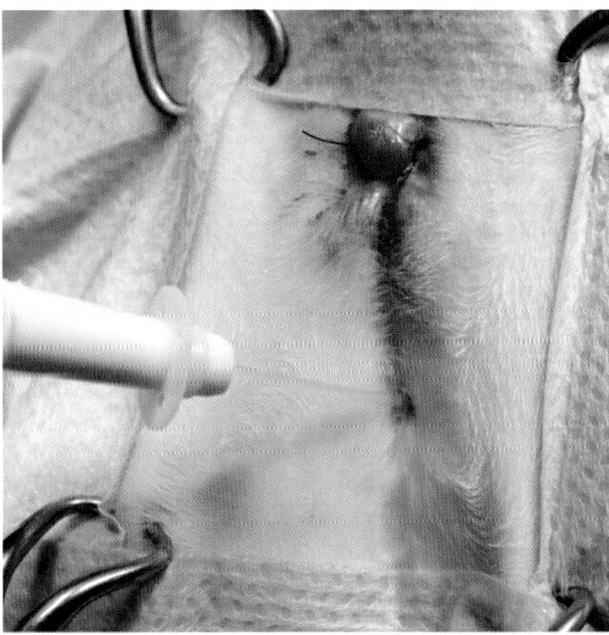

Figure 70.2 Stricture (pinpoint opening) after to a perineal urethrostomy in a cat (Courtesy of Annick Hamaide).

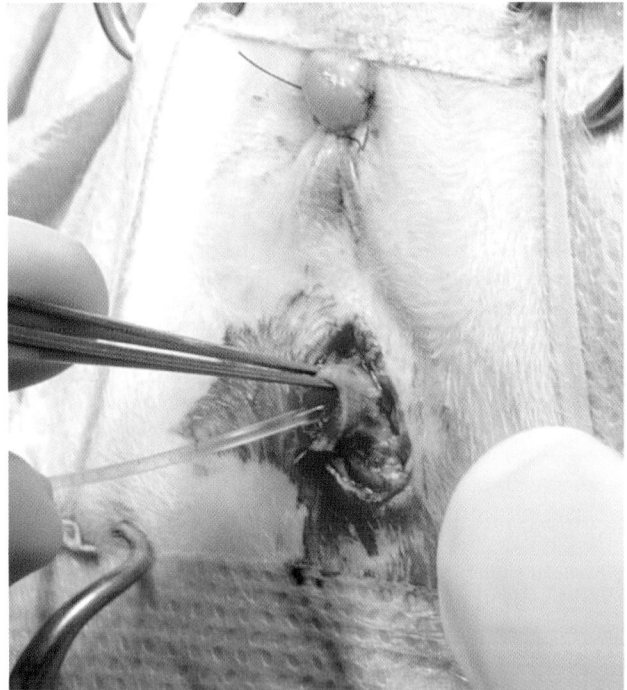

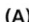
(A)

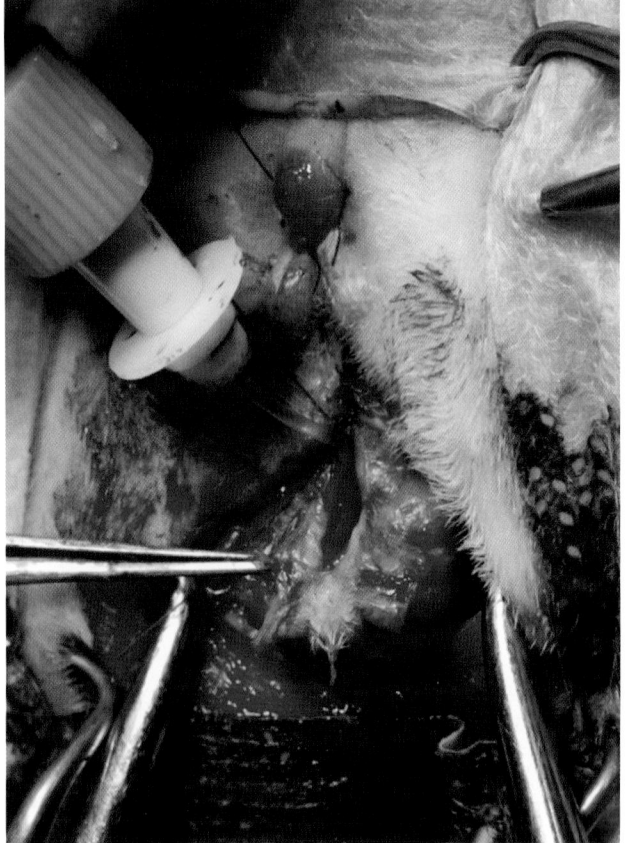
(B)

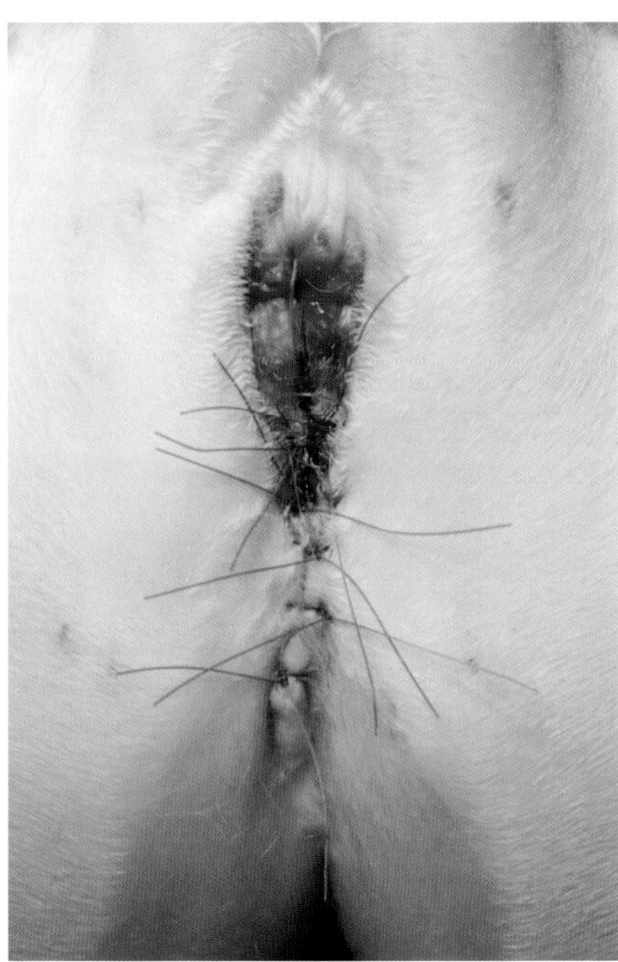
(C)

Figure 70.3 Surgical revision of a stricture consecutive to a perineal urethrostomy (the same cat as in Figure 70.2). **A,** An elliptical incision is made around the stenotic stoma and periurethral tissues are dissected. **B,** The urethral remnant is dissected up to the bulbourethral glands. The first suture is placed at the apex. **C,** The new urethral stoma is created (Courtesy of Annick Hamaide).

- Ultrasonography and positive contrast urethrocystogram might be necessary to exclude other causes of stranguria.

Treatment

- Revision of the stenotic stoma is generally possible because the most common cause is incomplete dissection of the urethra.
- The surgical approach is similar to that for a standard perineal urethrostomy. An elliptical incision is made around the stenotic stoma, and the urethra is undermined and mobilized as in the standard surgical approach. If a technical error is encountered (e.g., failure to cut the crura of the penis), it is corrected during the revision surgery. After the urethra has been adequately mobilized, the urethra is exposed and sutured depending on the technique being used (Figure 70.3).
- Positioning in dorsal recumbency may be advantageous because it allows the surgeon to perform a cystotomy, if required, without the need to reposition the animal. In addition, dorsal recumbency simplifies the conversion to a prepubic or subpubic urethrostomy if the revision of the PU fails.

Outcome

Revision of the structure has a good prognosis, particularly if the cause of the stricture was inadequate dissection of the urethra.

Prevention

- It is important to cut the pelvic attachments of the urethra to allow adequate mobilization of the urethra.
- Mobilize the urethra until the bulbourethral glands are at the level of the skin incision.
- Precise apposition of urethral mucosa to the skin
- Tension-free apposition of urethral mucosa to the skin
- Self-induced trauma should be prevented.

Relevant literature

Perineal urethrostomy has been reported to result in a long-term disease-free outcome for the majority of cats. The procedure is well accepted by clients, and the majority of clients consider their cats to have a good quality of life (Bass *et al.* 2005; Corgozinho *et al.* 2007; Ruda and Heiene 2012). In one study, however, the authors concluded that although the rate of reobstruction was low in the operated group (20%) compared with the nonoperated group (36%) of cats, there was no reduction in the recurrence of clinical signs of feline lower urinary tract disease between the operated (50%) and the nonoperated (51%) groups of cats (Gerber *et al.* 2008).

The most frequently reported complication of PU is recurrent UTI. There is a wide reported incidence of UTI associated with PU, which may vary from symptomatic to asymptomatic or self-limiting (Smith and Schiller 1978; Gregory and Vasseur 1983; Griffin and Gregory 1992; Baines *et al.* 2001; Bass *et al.* 2005; Corgozinho *et al.* 2007; Gerber *et al.* 2008). A wide reported incidence of UTI has also been reported in cats with feline lower urinary tract disease that were not treated surgically (Gerber *et al.* 2005; Hostutler *et al.* 2005; Eggertdottir *et al.* 2007; Forrester and Roudebush 2007; Kruger *et al.* 2009; Sævik *et al.* 2011; Segev *et al.* 2011; Westropp and Buffington 2010).

References

Agrodnia, M.D., Hauptman, J.G., Stanley, B.J. (2004) A simple continuous pattern using absorbable suture for perineal urethrostomy in the cat: 18 cases (2000-2002). *Journal of the American Animal Hospital Association* 40, 479.

Baines, S.J., Rennie, S., White, R.A.S. (2001) Prepubic urethrostomy: a long-term study in 16 cats. *Veterinary Surgery* 30, 107-113.

Bass, M., Howard, J., Gerber, B. (2005) Retrospective study of indications for and outcome of perineal urethrostomy in cats. *Journal of Small Animal Practice* 46, 227-231.

Bleedorn, J.A., Bjorling, D.E. (2012) Urethra. In Tobias, K.M. Johnston, S. (eds.) *Veterinary Surgery Small Animal*. WB Saunders, St. Louis.

Carbone, M. (1963) Perineal urethrostomy to relieve urethral obstruction in the male cat. *Journal of the American Veterinary Medical Association* 143, 34-39.

Christensen, N.R. (1964) Preputial urethrostomy in the male cat. *Journal of the American Veterinary Medical Association* 145, 903-8.

Clarke, B.S., Findji, L. (2011) Bilateral caudal superficial epigastric skin flap and perineal urethrostomy for wound reconstruction secondary to traumatic urethral rupture in a cat. *Veterinary Comparative Orthopedics and Traumatology* 24, 142-145.

Corgozinho, K.B., De Souza, H.J.M., Pereira, A.N., et al. (2007) Catheter-induced urethral trauma in cats with urethral obstruction. *Journal of Feline Medicine and Surgery* 9, 481-486.

Cullen, W.C., Fletcher, T.F., Bradley, W.F. (1983) Morphometry of the male feline pelvic urethra. *Journal of Urology* 129, 186-189.

Eggertdottir, A.V., Lund, H.S., Krontveit, R., et al. (2007) Bacteria in cats with feline lower urinary tract disease: a clinical study of 134 cases in Norway. *Journal of Feline Medicine and Surgery* 9, 458-465.

Forrester, S.D., Roudebush, P. (2007) Evidence-based management of feline lower urinary tract disease. *Veterinary Clinics of North America Small Animal Practice* 37, 533-538.

Gerber, B., Boretti, F.S., Kley, S., et al. (2005) Evaluation of clinical signs and causes of lower urinary tract disease in European cats. *Journal of Small Animal Practice* 46, 571-577.

Gerber, B., Eichenberger, S., Reusch, C.E. (2008) Guarded long-term prognosis in male cats with urethral obstruction. *Journal of Feline Medicine and Surgery* 10, 16-23.

Gregory, C.R. (1987) The effects of perineal urethrostomy on urethral function in male cats. *Compendium on Continuing Education for the Practicing Veterinarian* 9, 895-899.

Gregory, C.R., Vasseur, P.B. (1983) Long-term examination of cats with perineal urethrostomy. *Veterinary Surgery* 12, 210-212.

Griffin, D.W., Gregory, C.R. (1992) Prevalence of bacterial urinary tract infection after perineal urethrostomy in cats. *Journal of the American Veterinary Medical Association* 200, 681-684.

Holt, P.E. (1989) Hindlimb skin loss associated with urethral rupture in two cats. *Journal of Small Animal Practice* 30, 406-409.

Hosgood, G., Hedlund, C.S. (1992) Perineal urethrostomy in cats. *Compendium on Continuing Education for the Practicing Veterinarian* 14, 1195-1205.

Hostutler, R.A., Chew, D.J., Dibartola, S.P. (2005) Recent concepts in feline lower urinary tract disease. *Veterinary Clinics of North America Small Animal Practice* 35, 147-170.

Kruger, J.M., Osborne, C.A., Lulich, J.P. (2009) Changing paradigms of feline idiopathic cystitis. *Veterinary Clinics of North America Small Animal Practice* 39, 15-40.

Ladlow, J.F. (2014) Urethra. In Langley-Hobbs, S.J., Demetriou, J.L., Ladlow, J.F. (eds.) *Feline Soft Tissue and General Surgery*. Elsevier, Philadelphia.

Phillips, H., Holt, D.E. (2006) Surgical revision of the urethral stoma following perineal urethrostomy in 11 cats: (1998-2004). *Journal of the American Animal Hospital Association* 42, 218-222.

Ruda, L., Heiene, R. (2012) Short- and long-term outcome after perineal urethrostomy in 86 cats with feline lower urinary tract disease. *Journal of Small Animal Practice* 53, 693-698.

Sævik, B., Trangerud, C., Ottesen, N., et al. (2011) Causes of lower urinary tract disease In Norwegian cats. *Journal of Feline Medicine and Surgery* 12, 410-417.

Scavelli, T. (1989) Complications associated with perineal urethrostomy in the cat. *Problems in Veterinary Medicine* 1, 111-119.

Segev, G., Livne, H., Ranen, E., et al. (2011) Urethral obstruction in cats: predisposing factors, clinical, clinicopathological characteristics and prognosis. *Journal of Feline Medicine and Surgery* 13, 101-108.

Smith, C.W., Schiller, A.G. (1978) Perineal urethrostomy in cat—retrospective study of complications. *Journal of the American Animal Hospital Association* 14, 225-228.

Westropp, J. L., Buffington, T.C.A. (2010) Lower urinary tract disorders in cats. In Ettinger, S.J. (ed.) *Textbook of Veterinary Internal Medicine*, 7th edn. WB Saunders, St Louis.

Wilson, G.P., Harrison, J.W. (1971) Perineal urethrostomy in cats. *Journal of the American Veterinary Medical Association* 159, 1789-1793.

Yeh, L.H., Chin, S.C. (2000) Modified perineal urethrostomy using preputial mucosa in cats. *Journal of the American Veterinary Medical Association* 216, 1092-1095.

Surgery of the Reproductive Tract

71 Ovariectomy and Ovariohysterectomy

Annick Hamaide
Department of Clinical Sciences (Companion Animals and Equids), School of Veterinary Medicine, University of Liège, Liège, Belgium

Elective ovariectomy (OVE) and ovariohysterectomy (OVH) are routinely performed in companion animal practice and are indicated to prevent pregnancy and undesirable behavior or vaginal discharge during estrus, as well as to decrease the incidence of mammary tumors and pyometra.

OVE and OVH are also performed to treat ovarian or uterine diseases such as ovarian or uterine tumors, pyometra, uterine torsion, and uterine prolapse or uterine rupture and to prevent recurrence of vaginal hyperplasia. These procedures are also indicated in patients with endocrine diseases to prevent hormonal changes.

The incidence of complications after elective OVH or OVE is high and has been reported to be between 12% and 31.5% (Berzon 1979; Pollari and Bonnett 1996; Pollari et al. 1996; Burrow et al. 2005).

Short-term complications include hemorrhage, vaginal bleeding, wound infection or dehiscence, seroma formation, anesthesia complications, uterine stump abscess, tracheitis, pancreatitis, and tissue reaction to suture material that may lead to the formation of granulomas or draining tracts (Dorn and Swist 1977; Berzon 1979; Spackman et al. 1984; Campbell 2004; Davidson et al. 2004; Burrow et al. 2005).

Long-term complications include ovarian remnant syndrome, uterine stump pyometra, pyometra, fistulous tracts or stump granuloma formation, ureteral injury, obstipation, uretero-, vesico-, or enterovaginal, as well as vaginoperitoneal fistula formation, urinoma, colonic obstruction, pyelonephritis, urinary incontinence, and weight gain (Pearson 1973; Dorn and Swist 1977; Berzon 1979; Pearson and Gibbs 1980; Spackman et al. 1984; Tidwell et al. 1990; Wallace 1991; Ewers and Holt 1992; Grassi et al. 1994; McEvoy 1994; Kyles et al. 1996; Pollari and Bonnett 1996; Coolman et al. 1999; Gopegui et al. 1999; Mehl and Kyles 2003; Ragni 2005; Holt et al. 2006; Kanazono et al. 2009; Demirel and Acar 2012).

Although traditional OVH and OVE involve surgical removal of the ovaries or uterus through a median celiotomy, laparoscopic OVH and OVE offer a minimally invasive surgical option for clients that resist traditional OVH or OVE for their pets. Advantages of laparoscopic OVH and OVE include decreased pain, less risk of dehiscence and hemorrhage, and shortened hospitalization and convalescence (Davidson et al. 2004). Complications described with laparoscopic OVH include minor splenic hemorrhage, minor pedicle hemorrhage, intermittent vaginal hemorrhagic discharge, and suture reaction (Davidson et al. 2004).

Hemorrhage
Also see Chapter 12.

Definition
Intraabdominal hemorrhage can arise from the ovarian pedicles, uterine vessels, or uterine wall. Hemorrhage rarely occurs from vessels that accompany the suspensory ligament or within the broad ligament.

Risk factors
- Large breed dogs
- Obese dogs
- Inadequate exteriorization of the ovaries by insufficient breakage of the suspensory ligament
- Insufficient length of the laparotomy incision
- Inadequate placement of ligatures on the ovarian pedicles or the uterus
- Performing OVE or OVH during the estrous phase because of the increased vascularity of the genital tract (Pearson 1973)
- Presence of coagulopathies
- Performing an OVH rather than an OVE has additional risk for bleeding from the uterine vessels near the cervix.

Diagnosis
- Bleeding may be directly recognized during surgery.
- Development of hemoabdomen postoperatively
  - Presence of clinical signs of hypovolemic shock
  - Presence of hemorrhage from the abdominal wound
  - Ultrasonography (Figure 71.1)
  - Abdominocentesis and fluid analysis

Treatment
- If hemorrhage is recognized during the procedure, the laparotomy incision should be extended to better visualize the sources of the bleeding, and the failing ligature should be carefully replaced.
- If hemorrhage is recognized postoperatively, stabilization of the patient by conservative treatment should be attempted and includes placement of a semicompressive body bandage and appropriate fluid therapy.
- If hemorrhage cannot be controlled by conservative treatment, a laparotomy should be performed. At opening, each ligature should be checked to determine the origin of the hemorrhage, and the failing ligature(s) should be carefully replaced.

Complications in Small Animal Surgery, First Edition. Edited by Dominique Griffon and Annick Hamaide.
© 2016 John Wiley & Sons, Inc. Published 2016 by John Wiley & Sons, Inc.

Companion website: www.wiley.com/go/griffon/complications

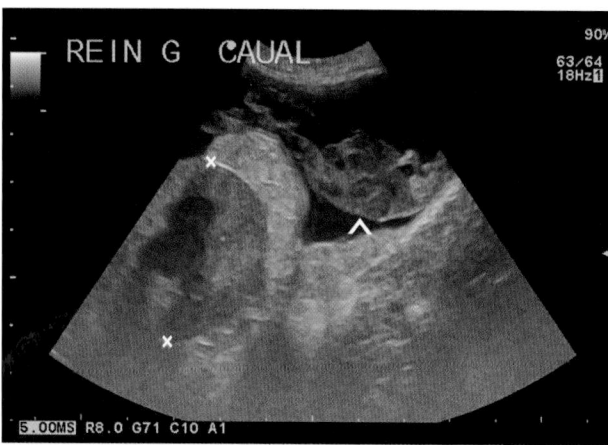

Figure 71.1 Longitudinal ultrasound image of the caudal pole of the left kidney (asterisk) in a female dog with an history of neutering showing an heterogenous mass (^) caudal to the left kidney surrounded by fluid containing hyperechoic foci consistent with an hematoma associated to a peritoneal hemorrhage.

Outcome

Although hemorrhage has been previously recognized as the most common cause of death after OVH in large breed dogs (Pearson 1973), adequate surgical technique and careful placement of ligatures should prevent this complication.

Prevention

- The laparotomy incision should allow good visualization of ovarian sites (and uterine body in case of OVH).
- Before laparotomy closure, ligatures should be checked for presence of bleeding.
- OVE or OVH should always be performed during the anestral phase.

Vaginal bleeding

Definition

This is significant frank hemorrhage from the vagina resulting from erosion of one of the uterine vessels. Vaginal bleeding has been reported in 11 of 72 dogs (15%) 4 to 16 days after OVH (Pearson 1973).

Risk factors

- Use of nonabsorbable multifilament ligatures around the uterine body
- Infection caused by surgical contamination
- Use of infected suture material
- Use of transfixing ligatures entering the lumen of the uterus or the cervix
- Transection of the uterine horns during OVE

Treatment

- Vaginal tamponade (van Goethem *et al.* 2006)
- Exploratory celiotomy if bleeding becomes severe. In this case, the uterine vessels should be individually religated, and the uterine stump should be resected closer to the cervix.

Outcome

The outcome is usually favorable.

Prevention

- Avoid contamination during surgery.
- Avoid the use of nonabsorbable suture material on the uterus.
- Avoid penetration into the uterine lumen at the level of the cervix or at the level of the uterine horns (during OVE).

Ovarian remnant syndrome

Definition

Ovarian remnant syndrome (ORS) after OVE or OVH is caused by residual ovarian tissue that becomes functional (Pearson 1973). Revascularization of the residual ovarian tissue can develop even though the ovarian pedicle has been ligated (Fingland 1998). A uterine stump pyometra can develop if the uterus or part of it is still present.

It appears that dogs are more often affected by ORS than cats (Ball *et al.* 2010).

Risk factors

- Inadequate exposure and exteriorization of the ovaries (Berzon 1979): Ovarian remnants are more frequent on the right side because the right ovary is located more cranially and is therefore more difficult to exteriorize.
- Insufficient length of the laparotomy incision (Miller 1995)
- Obese animals with large amount of adipose tissue at the ovarian pedicle
- In cats, ovarian remnants are found more commonly after OVE or OVH performed through a flank incision (Stone *et al.* 1993; Demirel and Acar 2012).

Diagnosis

- Clinical signs may not be recognized until years after OVE or OVH (Ball *et al.* 2010).
- Persistent signs of estrus can be present if a functional ovarian cyst or neoplasm develops in the residual ovarian tissue.
- **Clinical signs** include vulvar swelling, sanguinous vulvar discharge, attraction to male dogs, receptivity to mating, lactation during false pregnancy, and aggressive behavior (especially in cats).
- **Vaginal cytologic examination** can be helpful and may show predominance of cornified epithelial cells. However, in queens, a smear with normal anestrus characteristics does not rule out ORS (Wallace 1991; Pineda 2003).
- **Hormonal assay** (measurement of estrogen-estradiol, progesterone, or luteinizing hormone [LH] levels) is not helpful in confirming ORS. A more reliable diagnosis can be obtained by the use of hormone stimulation tests (Wallace 1991; England 1997).
- **Abdominal ultrasonography** may show ovarian remnant tissue resembling a mass or hypoechoic mass or a cystic structure (Ball *et al.* 2010) (Figure 71.2).
- **Exploratory laparotomy**

Treatment

- Treatment consists of surgical removal of the residual ovarian tissue. The laparotomy incision should be of sufficient length. Both ovarian pedicles should be resected, and the excised tissue should be sent for histopathologic examination.

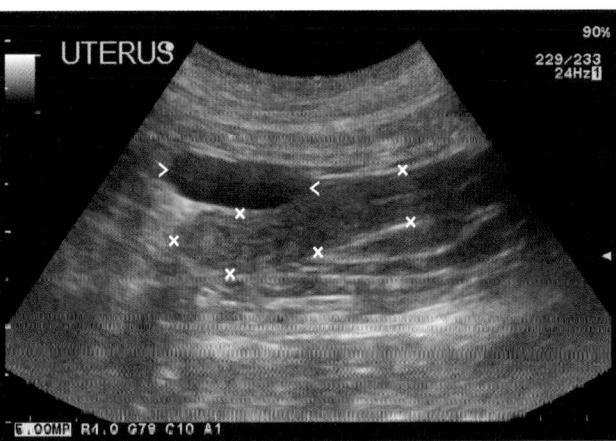

Figure 71.2 Longitudinal ultrasound image of the left uterine horn (asterisk) in a neutered female dog with history of recurrent heat. Adjacent to the uterine horn is a well-delineated anechoic oval-shape imaged (^) with distal acoustic enhancement (cyst) consistent with remnant ovarian tissue.

• Surgical exploration should be performed when the animal is in proestrus, estrus, or diestrus because follicles or corpora lutea in the ovarian tissue and prominence of ovarian blood vessels may make the identification of ovarian tissue easier (Wallace 1991; Perkins and Frazer 1995).

Outcome

Surgical removal of residual ovarian tissue results in resolution of clinical signs (Ball *et al.* 2010).

Prevention

• Adequate exposure and exteriorization of both ovaries
• Laparotomy incision of sufficient length
• After resection of the ovaries, complete excision should be confirmed by palpation of the tissue being excised and by opening of the ovarian bursa.

Pyometra and uterine stump pyometra

Definition

Pyometra is a diestral disorder resulting from interaction of bacteria with an abnormal endometrium that is subjected to pathological changes caused by an exaggerated response to progesterone stimulation (Nelson and Feldman 1986). Pyometra (after OVE) or uterine stump pyometra (after OVH) can develop if residual endometrial tissue is stimulated by endogenous progesterone (in case of incomplete ovarian tissue removal) or by exogenous progesterone (Kyles *et al.* 1996).

Risk factors

• Incomplete removal of the ovaries and development of ORS (see earlier discussion)
• Administration of progestational drugs

Diagnosis

• **History** may include signs of estrus in the preceding 8 to 10 weeks or previous use of progestational drugs.

• **Clinical signs** include lethargy, depression, inappetence, a serosanguineous to mucopurulent vaginal discharge, polyuria, polydipsia, and vomiting.
• **Hematology and biochemistry profiles** may show neutrophilia with a left shift, nonregenerative anemia, hyperglobulinemia, azotemia, and increased alkaline phosphatase.
• **Abdominal ultrasonography** will confirm the presence of enlarged uterine horns or a fluid-filled mass in the caudal portion of the abdomen.

Treatment

• Preoperative stabilization of the patient with administration of intravenous fluids and broad-spectrum antibiotherapy
• During exploratory laparotomy, any remaining ovarian tissue should be removed. The uterine vessels should be ligated, and the pus-filled residual uterine tissue should be excised at the level of, or including, the cervix.
• In the presence of massive adhesions between the uterine stump and the lower urinary tract, en bloc resection of the uterine stump could cause damage to the distal ureters or the neurovascular supply to the bladder. In case of nonresectable uterine stump abscess, drainage of the stump and omentalization has been reported (Campbell 2004).

Outcome

To obtain a favorable outcome, it is crucial to recognize the condition early and to address it adequately as soon as possible. The outcome of pyometra or stump pyometra may be fatal, especially in queens (Demirel and Acar 2012).

Prevention

Pyometra (in case of OVE) or uterine stump pyometra (in case of OVH) is prevented by complete removal of the ovaries.

Ovarian or uterine stump granuloma and sinus tracts

Definition

This is inflammation and ovarian and uterine stump granuloma formation in response to ligatures of nonabsorbable suture material, poor aseptic technique, or the presence of excessive devitalized tissue (Kyles *et al.* 1996). Granulomas can cause massive adhesions involving the small intestine, colon, bladder, mesentery, and omentum. Ovarian granulomas can involve the caudal pole of the kidney and constrict the proximal ureter, causing hydronephrosis (Kanazono *et al.* 2009) (Figure 71.3). Uterine stump granulomas can obstruct the distal ureters (Kyles *et al.* 1996).

Risk factors

• Use of nonabsorbable suture material (nylon, silk, linen, nonsurgical self-locking nylon bands) (Pearson 1973; Werner *et al.* 1992; Boza *et al.* 2010)
• Poor aseptic technique
• Excessive residual devitalized tissue

Diagnosis

• **Clinical signs** include dyschezia, constipation, vomiting, dysuria, pollakiuria, and incontinence.
• **Sinus tracts**, caused by the inflammation response to suture material, may develop years after surgery (Pearson 1973). The

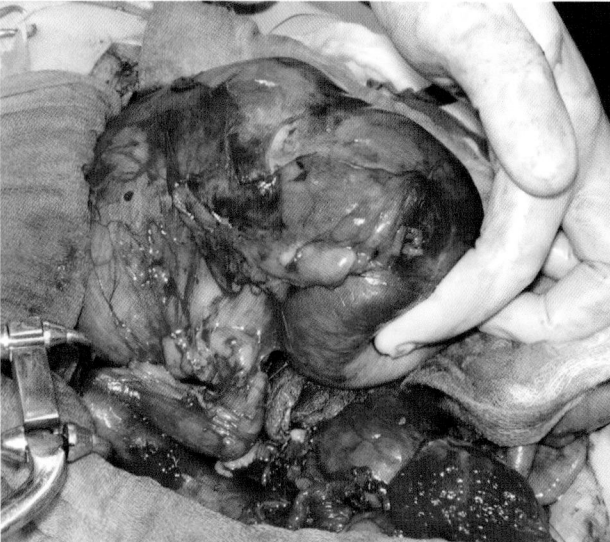

Figure 71.3 Intraoperative view showing right hydronephrosis and hydroureter caused by the presence of an ovarian granuloma in a dog. A nephrectomy is being performed.

tract extends from the granuloma through the surrounding tissues to the skin. A soft, painful swelling appears below the skin, with intermittent drainage of serosanguineous fluid or pus. Whereas ovarian granulomas are associated with sublumbar sinuses, uterine stump granulomas are associated with sinus tracts in the precrural, inguinal, or medial thigh regions (Kyles *et al.* 1996) (Figure 71.4).
- **Bacteriologic culture**
- **Fine-needle aspiration or biopsy**
- **Abdominal ultrasonography**

Treatment
- Successful treatment consists of excision of the stump granuloma via a midline laparotomy. The offending ligature is usually embedded in reactive tissues. Removal of the sinus tract is worthless.

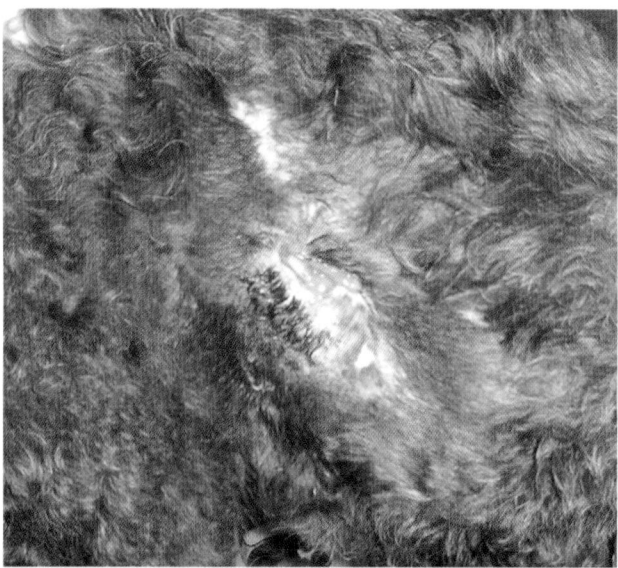

Figure 71.4 Chronic fistular tract caused by the presence of an ovarian pedicle granuloma in a 10-year-old female spayed Bouvier.

- In case of severe hydronephrosis, a nephrectomy should be performed.
- In case of extensive adhesions to the small intestine causing obstruction, an enterectomy may be needed.
- Great care should be taken when dissecting uterine stump granulomas, especially with extensive adhesions to the bladder, ureters, or colon. In these cases, removal of the ligature only is preferable.

Outcome
The outcome is usually favorable after the offending nonabsorbable suture material is removed.

Prevention
- Careful tissue handling
- Minimal residual devitalized tissue
- Aseptic technique
- Use of synthetic absorbable suture materials
- Braided nonabsorbable suture material (silk, nylon, linen) and nonsurgical self-locking nylon bands should be avoided (Pearson 1973; Werner *et al.* 1992; Boza *et al.* 2010).

Iatrogenic injury to the urinary tract

Definition
Because of the close relationship with the ovarian arteries or the uterine body, the proximal or distal part of the ureter may be inadvertently lacerated or included in the ovarian or the uterine pedicle ligature during OVE or OVH. Inadvertent ligation of the bladder neck has also been reported (Ewers and Holt 1992).

Risk factors
- Inadequate exteriorization of the ovaries
- Ligature of the ovarian pedicle too close to its base
- Inadequate exposure of the caudal pole of the kidney (Kyles *et al.* 1996)
- Distension of the bladder. An distended bladder displaces the trigone cranially and increases the risk of inadvertent ligature of the distal ureter (Kyles *et al.* 1996).

Diagnosis
- In case of laceration of a ureter:
  - Uroperitoneum will develop postoperatively and will be confirmed by abdominocentesis and fluid analysis.
  - An excretory urography will confirm the site of the leakage.
- In case of bilateral ureteral obstruction by ligatures:
  - Anuria and postrenal azotemia will develop postoperatively.
  - Excretory urography and abdominal ultrasonography will confirm the ureteral obstruction.
- In case of unilateral ureteral obstruction:
  - The diagnosis is often delayed because azotemia will not develop in a otherwise healthy animal.
  - Clinical signs are much more subtle and might include reduced urine production or signs of abdominal pain (Kyles *et al.* 1996).
  - Abdominal ultrasonography may reveal nephromegaly caused by hydronephrosis or renal abscess, as well as the site of ureteral obstruction.
  - Excretory urography will allow detection of the site of obstruction only if renal function is still present on the affected side.
- Ligation of a ureter at the uterine body can result in the formation of a ureterovaginal fistula (MacCoy 1988). A sudden onset of

urinary incontinence occurs soon after the OVH. The diagnosis is made by excretory urography or retrograde vaginourethrography.

Treatment

- Surgical exploration is mandatory after the diagnosis of ureteral damage is confirmed.
- In case of laceration of a ureter, ureteral resection and anastomosis or a ureteroneocystostomy or a nephrectomy will be required.
- Total ureteral obstruction for more than 4 weeks has been associated with a complete loss of kidney function on the affected side (Wilson 1977). In case of severe unilateral hydronephrosis or renal abscessation, a nephrectomy is mandatory.
- In case of partial obstruction or if renal function is not yet affected by the ureteral obstruction, the ligature should be removed and the ureter evaluated. Ureteral stricture is at great risk to develop. Severe ureteral damage or stricture formation requires ureteral resection and anastomosis, ureteroneocystostomy, or nephrectomy. In selected cases, placement of a ureteral stent might be an option.
- A ureterovaginal fistula is treated by ligation of the fistula and ureteroneocystostomy.

Outcome

- The outcome is grave in case of unrecognized bilateral ureteral obstruction.
- In case of ureteral laceration or unilateral obstruction by a ligature, the outcome will depend on the type of procedure and the expertise of the surgeon.

Prevention

- The ureters and the uterus should be carefully identified during the surgery.
- The bladder should be expressed before surgery or drained during the surgery because bladder distension results in cranial displacement of the trigone and decreased exposure of the uterine body.

Urinary incontinence

Definition

Urinary incontinence is defined as involuntary leakage of urine. Urethral sphincter mechanism incompetence (USMI) is the most common cause of urinary incontinence in adult spayed bitches (Holt 1985a; Krawiec 1989), with an incidence ranging from 4.5% (Thrusfield 1985) to 18% to 20% (Arnold et al. 1989).

Urethral sphincter mechanism incompetence is a multifactorial condition associated with a decreased urethral resistance. Urine leakage occurs when the intraabdominal pressure rises, such as during recumbency or barking (Holt 2008).

Risk factors

- Low urethral tone
- Intrapelvic position of the bladder neck
- Neutering
- Urethral length
- Breed
- Body size
- Docked tail
- Obesity
- Age

Diagnosis

- The diagnosis of USMI is commonly made by exclusion of other causes of urinary incontinence.
- **Clinical signs** include urine leakage during sleep or periods of excitement. Micturition episodes are usually normal. Clinical signs may develop a few weeks to several years after spaying, most commonly after 2 to 3 years (Holt 1985a; Arnold et al. 1989).
- **Urine culture and antibiogram** are mandatory because secondary urinary tract infections (UTIs) are usually present.
- **Ultrasonography** will help eliminating other potential causes of incontinence such as ectopic ureters, urolithiasis, or neoplasia, for example
- **Vaginourethrography** is helpful in bitches with USMI to assess the position of the bladder neck and the length of the urethra (Figure 71.5).
- **Urodynamic investigation** (urethral pressure profile and cystometry) allows the measurement of urethral resistance and bladder compliance. It might be helpful to determine the exact cause of the urinary incontinence and to monitor response to treatment. Unfortunately, its access is limited to specialized institutions.

Treatment and outcome

Medical treatment

- Treatment of any concurrent UTI with adequate antibiotherapy is mandatory.
- **α-Adrenergic agonists**
  - Administration of **phenylpropanolamine** (PPA) is successful in treating USMI in up to 90% of the female patients. Recommended dosages range from 1 to 1.5 mg/kg once, twice, or three times a day.
  - **Ephedrine** could be useful in the treatment of refractory urinary incontinence involving detrusor instability. Complete response has been observed in 74% of treated bitches, and continence improvement was noted in another 24% of the dogs (Arnold et al. 1989).
- **Estrogens:** Long-acting synthetic estrogen preparations, such as estradiol and diethylstilbestrol, should not be used because they are associated with bone marrow depletion (Osborne et al. 1980; Krawiec 1989). Estriol is a short-acting natural estrogen compound with fewer side effects. Continence is achieved in 65% of treated bitches (Mandigers and Nell 2001).

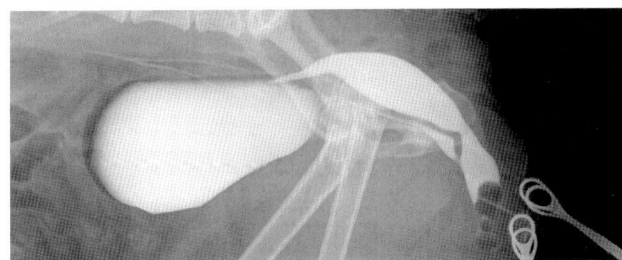

Figure 71.5 Vaginourethrogram (right lateral view) in a female dog diagnosed with urethral sphincter mechanism incompetence. An intravenous pyelography was performed before the vaginourethrography and showed normal ureteral openings at the trigone area. Note the rounded appearance of the caudal pole of the bladder.

- **Gonadotropin-releasing hormone (GnRH) analogues:** The administration of GnRH analogues could be suitable for patients showing side effects after treatment with α-adrenergic agents or if α-adrenergic agents are contraindicated. In recent studies, complete continence was achieved in 50% of the dogs (Reichler *et al.* 2003; 2006).
- **Miscellaneous:** In selected cases, agents such as duloxetine, oxybutynin, imipramine, or flavoxate, which are used in human medicine and have an effect on the bladder, could also be used in dogs.

Surgical treatment

Several surgical techniques have been developed to restore continence in dogs affected with USMI.

- **Colposuspension** consists in the fixation of the vagina to the prepubic tendon on each side (Holt 1985c) (Figure 71.6). The overall reported success rate for complete continence with colposuspension alone (Holt 1990; Marchevsky *et al.* 1999) or with addition of medical treatment (Rawlings *et al.* 2001) varies between 40% and 50%, and an additional 40% of the patients are greatly improved.

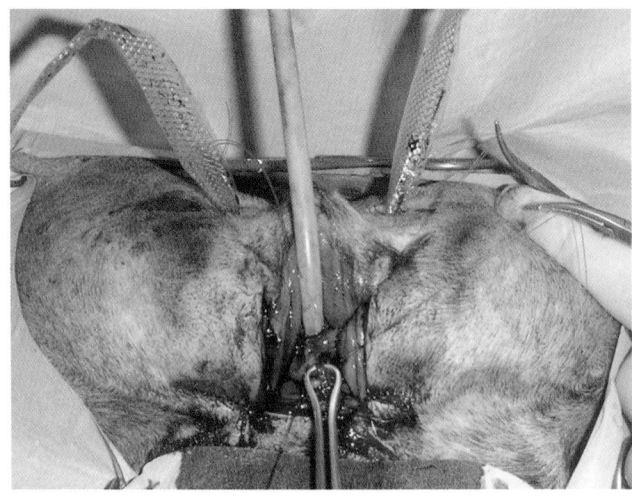

Figure 71.7 Intraoperative view of a transobturator vaginal tape inside-out showing the placement of the polypropylene tape between the urethra and the vagina through an episiotomy incision. The dog is placed in dorsal recumbency.

- **Urethropexy** consists in the fixation of the urethra to the ventral abdominal wall at the level of the cranial pubic brim. The reported outcome in 100 bitches was fairly similar to outcome reported with colposuspension (White 2001). Combined urethropexy and colposuspension has recently been described in 30 bitches with USMI (Martinoli *et al.* 2014). At a median follow-up period of 39.5 months, this technique resulted in complete continence in 70% of the bitches.
- **Urethral submucosal collagen injections** consist of endoscopic injections of collagen in three submucosal sites of the proximal urethra (Arnold *et al.* 1996; Barth *et al.* 2005). The overall success rate is 75% (Barth *et al.* 2005).
- Placement of a **static hydraulic artificial urethral sphincter** is another option to treat USMI in dogs and results in a significant postoperative improvement in the continence score (Delisser *et al.* 2012; Currao *et al.* 2013; Reeves *et al.* 2013).
- Among the previously described sling procedures (Muir *et al.* 1994; Nickel *et al.* 1998), the technique of **transobturator vaginal tape inside-out** (TVT-O) is the least invasive because it does not require an abdominal approach (Claeys *et al.* 2010) (Figure 71.7). At a mean follow-up time of 11.3 months, six of the seven bitches treated were continent (Claeys *et al.* 2010).

Relevant literature

Hemorrhage has been reported to be the most common complication after OVH (79%) in dogs weighing more than 25 kg; it was only reported in 2% of the dogs weighing less than 25 kg (Berzon 1979). Hemorrhage is also the most common cause of death after OVH in large breed dogs (Pearson 1973).

In obese animals, the large amounts of abdominal fat make exteriorization of the ovaries and ligation of the ovarian pedicles more difficult (Burrow *et al.* 2005).

In a study on complications after OVH performed by final year students on 142 bitches (Burrow *et al.* 2005), hemorrhage occurred intraoperatively in 9 dogs (6.4%). In 7 of them, hemorrhage was arising from the right ovarian pedicle. The right ovary is located more cranially in the abdomen than the left one and may be more difficult

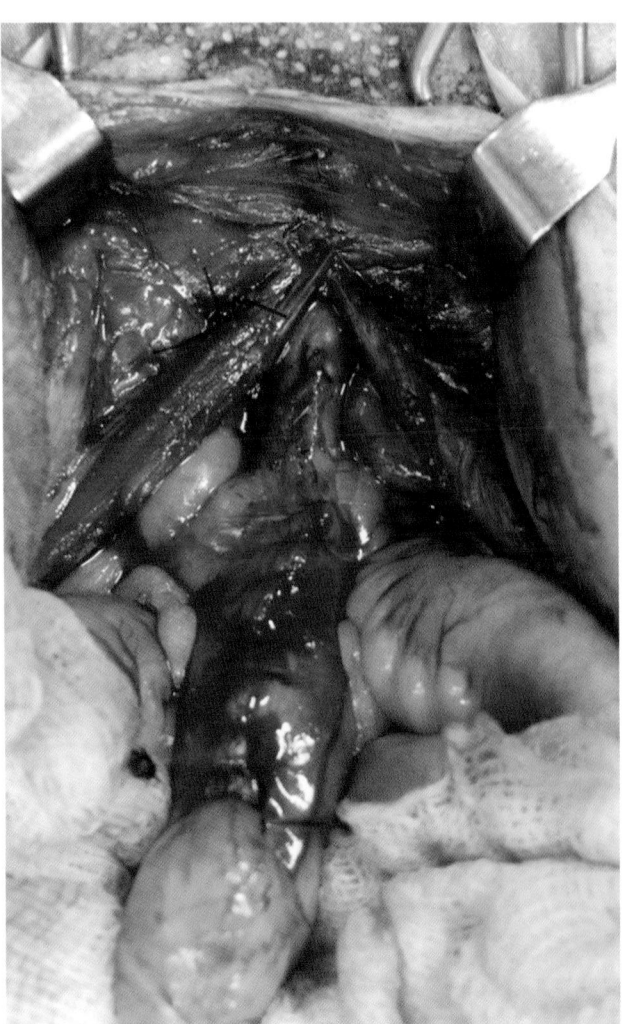

Figure 71.6 Intraoperative view showing a colposuspension performed in a female dog. Two interrupted sutures of nonresorbable suture material have been placed on each side of the urethra between the vagina and the prepubic tendon.

to exteriorize properly, particularly if the suspensory ligament is not correctly broken or if the laparotomy incision is too short (Burrow *et al*, 2005). In that study, hemorrhage from the wound occurred in 4 of 142 bitches postoperatively. In 3 of these bitches, application of a body bandage was sufficient to stop the bleeding; in the fourth dog, exploratory celiotomy was required and revealed that subcutaneous vessels were bleeding (Burrow *et al*. 2005).

Persistent postoperative hemorrhage that required surgical exploration and administration of bovine hemoglobin glutamer has been reported after OVH in one dog diagnosed with a tickborne coagulopathy (Davidson *et al*. 2004).

Ovarian remnant syndrome has been reported in 12 of 72 dogs (17%) with complications after OVH (Pearson 1973). In Okkens' study (1981b), residual ovarian tissue was observed in 43% of the dogs after OVH (47 of 109 animals). Sixteen of these dogs had bilateral, 25 had right-sided, and 6 had left-sided residual ovarian tissue. Ovarian remnants tend to be more frequently located on the right side because the right ovary is located in a more cranial and deeper location, which makes its exteriorization more difficult (Pearson 1973; Wallace 1991).

This was recently confirmed by Ball and collaborators (2010), who described 21 cases of ORS (19 dogs and 2 cats). In this study, ovarian remnants were found in typical locations for ovaries and were not considered to be ectopic tissue. The authors concluded that a surgical error during OVH was the cause of the ORS. Seven of these 21 animals had neoplasms of the reproductive system. These animals showed longer intervals between the OVH and the diagnosis of recurrent estrus than did animals without neoplasms (Ball *et al*. 2010).

Ovarian remnant syndrome might be more frequent in dogs than cats (Ball *et al*. 2010). One reason could be the anatomic difference because dogs typically have deeper abdominal cavities, which makes it more challenging to exteriorize both ovaries.

Ovarian remnant syndrome and uterine stump pyometra have recently been described in three queens (Demirel and Acar 2012). In two of these queens, remnants of ovarian tissue were found in the area of the right ovary. A left flank OVH had been performed in these queens and may have limited the access to the right ovary, thereby increasing the risk of incomplete resection.

Pyometra or uterine stump pyometra may occur in dogs and cats after incomplete removal of the uterus. However, progesterone is an essential factor in the occurrence of pyometra. OVE was not associated with pyometra in any of the 72 dogs after a mean follow-up time of 10 years (Janssens and Janssens 1991). This finding corroborates with results obtained by Okkens and collaborators (1997). In this study, none of the 69 bitches that underwent OVE had signs of endometritis or pyometra. On the other hand, the same authors reported that 19 of 55 dogs (35%) that underwent OVH did have stump pyometra associated with residual ovarian tissue (Okkens *et al*. 1981b).

This further emphasizes, if needed, that OVE will not increase the chance for development of pyometra compared with OVH, and that, when correctly performed, OVH or OVE will prevent the development of pyometra later in life (van Goethem *et al*. 2006).

Granulomas were observed at the level of the uterine stump in 8 of 55 dogs (15%) with gynecologic complications after OVH (Okkens *et al*. 1981b). In another study, Okkens and collaborators (1981a) reported granuloma at the ovarian pedicle in 1 patient (6%) and at the uterine stump in 5 patients (28%).

Historically, nonabsorbable ligatures were routinely used to perform OVH, and Pearson (1973) reported 37 dogs (of 72) with uterine stump granulomas, of which 27 had sinus formation. A chronic partial ureteral obstruction by an ovarian pedicle granuloma presumably caused by the use of silk was recently reported (Kanazono *et al*. 2009). Treatment consisted of an end-to-side ureteral anastomosis.

The use of synthetic absorbable suture material as a routine should decrease the incidence of ovarian or uterine stump granulomas.

Despite the proximity of the ureters with the urogenital tract, few studies have reported **ureteral injury** secondary to OVE or OVH (Kyles *et al*. 1996; Gopegui *et al*. 1999; Mehl and Kyles 2003). In Okkens' study (1981a) on 109 dogs, ligation of the ureter at the ovarian pedicle was reported in 2 dogs (2%), and ureter ligation at the uterine body was reported in 3 dogs (2.7%). However, it is likely that this complication is more common but goes unrecognized because unilateral ureteral obstruction would not cause azotemia in an otherwise healthy animal (Adin 2011). Indeed, the ureters travel in the retroperitoneal space caudal to the kidney, where they are at risk of being inadvertently traumatized or ligated during OVE or OVH. The distal ureter is closely associated with the uterine body and therefore is also at risk of being incorporated in the uterine ligature during OVH, especially when the bladder is distended.

The chance of injury to the proximal ureter is identical between OVE and OVH, but distal ureteral ligation is inexistent during OVE (van Goethem 2006).

USMI is a multifactorial condition associated with a significant decreased urethral resistance compared with continent dogs (Rosin and Barsanti 1981; Richter and Ling 1985; Holt 1988). A hyperactive bladder may also contribute to USMI (Nickel 1998).

Bladder neck position and urethral length may play roles in the development of USMI. The pelvic bladder is a frequent radiographic finding in incontinent bitches and is generally associated with a shorter urethra (Holt *et al*. 1984; Holt 1985a, 1985b). The pelvic position of the bladder neck could alter the pressure transmission between the bladder and urethra (Holt 1985b).

A relationship between neutering and USMI exists because 90% of the bitches with USMI are spayed (Holt 1985a; Krawiec 1989), and up to 20% of the spayed bitches may develop urinary incontinence (Arnold *et al*. 1989). However, the relationship between USMI and the age of spaying is controversial. A lower rate of incontinence has been reported in bitches spayed before the first estrus cycle (Holt 1985a; Arnold *et al*. 1989; Stöcklin-Gautschi *et al*. 2001). However, a recent case-control study found no significant association between early spaying and incontinence, although there was a tendency that early spayed bitches were less likely to be incontinent (de Bleser *et al*. 2011). A recent systematic review of peer-reviewed English analytic journal articles concluded that the evidence is neither consistent nor strong enough to make firm recommendations on the effect of neutering or age of neutering on the risk of USMI (Beauvais *et al*. 2012).

Neutering is associated with structural modifications within the bladder and urethra such as a decrease in smooth muscle, an increase in the volume of vascular urethral plexus, an increased proportion of collagen, and a decrease in striated fibers (Augsburger and Cruz-Orive 1995; 1998; Ponglowhapan *et al*. 2008a). Excessive collagen deposit and decreased muscle volume could impair the functional integrity of the lower urinary tract.

The urethral length is shorter in spayed female dogs than intact female dogs (Wang *et al*. 2006).

Neutering is also associated with urethral functional modifications. OVE induces a significant decrease in urethral resistance (Nickel 1998; Reichler *et al*. 2004; Salomon *et al*. 2006). Different hypotheses have been proposed, such as adhesions between the bladder neck and uterine stump or damage to the lower urinary tract supporting structures at the time of surgery. These hypotheses are now obsolete (Holt 1990), and no significant difference was observed between the percentage of dogs developing USMI after OVE or OVH (Arnold *et al.* 1989). Estrogen deficiency is the most widespread explanation for the development of USMI. However, no significant difference is observed between the endogenous estrogen concentration of continent bitches in anestrus and spayed incontinent bitches (Richter and Ling 1985). The role of gonadotrophins in the development of USMI has been suggested because OVE induces a chronic increase in follicle-stimulating hormone (FSH) and LH (Reichler *et al.* 2003). However, no relationship between the increased gonadotrophin concentration and decreased values of maximal urethral pressure has been demonstrated (Reichler *et al.* 2004, 2006). Prostaglandins may play a role in micturition. Prostaglandin receptors and expression of cyclooxygenase-2 (COX-2) in the canine urinary tract are decreased in gonadectomized dogs (Ponglowhapan *et al.* 2009). Moreover, the expression of FSH and LH receptors in the lower urinary tract is decreased in gonadectomized female dogs (Ponglowhapan *et al.* 2008b). A possible relation could exist between the variation in expression of LH and FSH receptors and COX-2 after neutering.

Large and giant breeds are at risk for USMI. Principal affected breeds include Dobermans, old English shepherd dogs, Rottweilers, Weimaraners, Springer spaniels, and Irish setters (Holt 2008). Bitches weighing more than 10 kg could be 3.7 times more likely to be incontinent than smaller dogs (de Bleser *et al.* 2011).

Older bitches are more likely to be incontinent than younger animals (de Bleser *et al.* 2011). Furthermore, it has been showed that urethral resistance in older continent bitches was decreased compared with middle-aged continent animals (Hamaide *et al.* 2005).

Tail docking has been suggested as a possible etiologic factor (Holt and Thrusfield 1993). In a recent study, docked bitches were 3.8 times more likely to be incontinent than undocked bitches (de Bleser *et al.* 2011).

Finally, obesity can worsen urinary incontinence. The retroperitoneal fat can displace the caudal peritoneum cranially so that the bladder neck is displaced in an extraperitoneal position (Holt 1985b).

Phenylpropanolamine induces a contraction of the bladder neck and proximal urethra by acting on the α-adrenergic receptors (Ek 1978). Administration of PPA in bitches with USMI results in continence in 75% (Arnold *et al.* 1989) to 90% of the patients (Richter and Ling 1985; White and Pomeroy 1989; Claeys *et al.* 2011). However, a decreased urethral response associated with recurrence of incontinence can be observed after prolonged administration of PPA (White and Pomeroy 1989). Recommended dosages range from 1 to 1.5 mg/kg twice or three times a day. However, the administration of a single daily dose of PPA (1.5 mg/kg) can achieve long-term continence in 90% of cases (Claeys *et al.* 2011).

Side effects include hypertension, restlessness, anxiety, and tachycardia (Krawiec 1988; Carofiglio *et al.* 2006; Noël *et al.* 2010). Therefore, PPA should be administered cautiously to dogs with concurrent cardiovascular diseases (Vick *et al.* 1994; Carofiglio *et al.* 2006; Noël *et al.* 2010).

Ephedrine is a mixed-acting sympathomimetic drug whose efficacy is slightly less predictable than PPA. An experimental study on continent beagle dogs showed that the administration of ephedrine could improve urethral function and bladder compliance, probably by acting on the β adrenergic receptors located in the bladder dome (Noël *et al.* 2012).

Side effects include restlessness, hypertension, excitability, and tachycardia (Krawiec 1988; Carofiglio *et al.* 2006).

Estrogens increase the number and the responsiveness of α-adrenergic receptors to sympathetic stimulation (Creed 1983). Studies in humans and rats indicate that estrogens increase bladder capacity (Fleischmann *et al.* 2002). Minor associated side effects include swelling of the vulva, attractiveness of males, and metrorrhagia (Mandigers and Nell 2001).

Reichler and collaborators (2003) used **GnRH analogues** to downregulate gonadotrophins in ovariectomized incontinent bitches. The subcutaneous application of GnRH analogues (deslorelin 4.7 mg/kg) did increase bladder compliance. Treatment was associated with a decrease in FSH and LH plasmatic concentrations, and no side effects were observed.

During **colposuspension**, the bladder is relocated in an intraabdominal position (Holt 1990), and the urethral length is increased (Holt 1990; Rawlings *et al.* 2001). Postoperative complications include increased frequency of micturition, tenesmus, and pain during first defecation.

Urethropexy relocates the bladder neck into a more cranial position and may also increase urethral resistance. Postoperative complications include an increased frequency of micturition, dysuria, and anuria that is spontaneously resolved within 2 weeks (White 2001).

Urethral submucosal collagen injection is an alternative in the treatment of patients with USMI. More than one treatment might be required. In a recent study on 31 dogs, whereas the mean duration of continence in dogs not needing additional medical treatment was 16.5 months, the mean duration of continence in dogs needing additional medical therapy was 5.2 months (Byron *et al.* 2011).

Placement of **static hydraulic artificial urethral sphincter** in dogs with USMI has been evaluated in three recent studies (Delisser *et al.* 2012; Currao *et al.* 2013; Reeves *et al.* 2013). In Delisser and colleagues' study (2012), complete continence was achieved in 36.4% of the 11 dogs, with a median follow-up time of 13 months. Reported complications included dysuria, bacterial cystitis, urinary retention, hematuria, pain, and seroma. Currao and coworkers (2013) reported a continence rate of 33%, with a median follow-up time of 32 months. They encountered urethral obstruction in 3 of their 18 dogs. Finally, Reeves and coworkers (2013) reported partial urethral obstruction in 2 of 27 dogs.

Transobturator vaginal tape inside-out is widely used in human medicine to treat stress incontinence in women (de Leval 2003). It has been extrapolated to dogs to develop a minimally invasive procedure for the treatment of USMI. Short-term results are encouraging with 6 of 7 bitches being continent and no postoperative complications encountered (Claeys *et al.* 2010).

References

Adin, C.A. (2011) Complications of ovariohysterectomy and orchiectomy in companion animals. *Veterinary Clinics of North America: Small Animal Practice* 41, 1023-1039.

Arnold, S., Arnold, P., Hubler, M., et al., (1989) Incontinentia urinae bei der kastrietem hunden: haufigkeit und rassedisposition. *Schweizer Archiv fur Tierheilkunde* 131, 259-263.

Arnold, S., Hubler, M., Lott-Stolz, G., et al. (1996) Treatment of urinary incontinence in bitches by endoscopic injection of glutaraldehyde cross-linked collagen. *Journal of Small Animal Practice* 37, 163-168.

Augsburger, H., Cruz-Orive, L. (1995) Stereological analysis of the urethra in sexually intact and spayed female dogs. *Acta Anatomica* 154, 135-142.

Augsburger, H., Cruz-Orive, L. (1998) Influence of ovariectomy on the canine striated external urethral sphincter (M. urethralis): a stereological analysis of slow and fast twitch fibres. *Urological Research* 26, 417-422.

Ball, R.L., Birchard, S.J., May, L.R., et al. (2010) Ovarian remnant syndrome in dogs and cats: 21 cases (2000-2007). *Journal of the American Veterinary Medical Association* 236, 548-553.

Barth, A., Reichler, I.M., Hubler, M., et al. (2005) Evaluation of long-term effects of endoscopic injection of collagen into the urethral submucosa for treatment of urethral sphincter incompetence in female dogs: 40 cases (1993-2000). *Journal of the American Veterinary Medical Association* 226, 73-76.

Beauvais, W., Cardwell, J.M., Brodbelt, D.C. (2012) The effect of neutering on the risk of urinary incontinence in bitches—a systematic review. *Journal of Small Animal Practice* 53, 198-204.

Berzon, J.L. (1979) Complications of elective ovariohysterectomies in the dog and cat at a teaching institution: clinical review of 853 cases. *Veterinary Surgery* 8, 89-91.

Boza, S., Lucas, X. Zarelli, M., et al. (2010) Late abscess formation caused by silk suture following hysterectomy in a female dog. *Reproduction in Domestic Animals* 45 (5), 934-936.

Burrow, R., Batchelor, D., Cripps, P. (2005) Complications observed during and after ovariohystectomy of 142 bitches at a veterinary teaching hospital. *Veterinary Record* 157, 829-833.

Byron, J.K., Chew, D.J., McLoughlin, M.L. (2011) Retrospective evaluation of urethral bovine cross-linked collagen implantation for treatment of urinary incontinence in female dogs. *Journal of Veterinary Internal Medicine* 25 (5), 980-984.

Campbell, B.G. (2004) Omentalization of a nonresectable uterine stump abscess in a dog. *Journal of the American Veterinary Medical Association* 224, 1799-1803.

Carofiglio, F., Hamaide, A., Farnir, F., et al. (2006) Evaluation of the urodynamic and hemodynamic effects of orally administered phenylpropanolamine and ephedrine in female dogs. *American Journal of Veterinary Research* 67, 723-730.

Claeys, S., de Leval, J., Hamaide, A. (2010) Transobturator vaginal tape inside out for treatment of urethral sphincter mechanism incompetence: preliminary results in 7 female dogs. *Veterinary Surgery* 39 (8), 969-979.

Claeys, S., Rustichelli, F., Noël, S., et al. (2011) Clinical evaluation of a single daily dose of phenylpropanolamine in the treatment of urethral sphincter mechanism incompetence in the bitch. *Canadian Veterinary Journal* 52 (5), 501-505.

Coolman, B.R., Manfra Marretta, S., Dudley, M.B., et al. (1999) Partial colonic obstruction following ovariohysterectomy: a report of three cases. *Journal of the American Animal Hospital Association* 35, 169-172.

Creed, K. (1983) Effect on hormones on urethral sensitivity to phenylephrine in normal and incontinent dogs. *Research in Veterinary Science* 34, 177-181.

Currao, R.L., Berent, A.C., Weisse, C., et al. (2013) Use of a percutaneously controlled urethral hydraulic occluder for treatment of refractory urinary incontinence in 18 female dogs. *Veterinary Surgery* 42 (4), 440-447.

Davidson, E.B., Moll, H.D., Payton, M.E. (2004) Comparison of laparoscopic ovariohysterectomy and ovariohysterectomy in dogs. *Veterinary Surgery* 33, 62-69.

de Bleser, B., Brodbelt, D.C., Gregory, N.G., et al. (2011) The association between acquired urinary sphincter mechanism incompetence in bitches and early spaying: a case-control study. *The Veterinary Journal* 187 (1), 42-47.

de Gopegui, R.R., Espada, Y. and Majo, N. (1999) Bilateral hydroureter and hydronephrosis in a nine-year-old female German shepherd dog. *Journal of Small Animal Practice* 40, 224-226.

de Leval, J. (2003) Novel surgical technique for the treatment of female stress urinary incontinence: transobturator vaginal tape inside-out. *European Urology* 44, 724-730.

Delisser, P.J., Friend, E.J., Chanoit, G.P., et al. (2012) Static hydraulic urethral sphincter for treatment of urethral sphincter mechanism incompetence in 11 dogs. *Journal of Small Animal Practice* 53 (6), 338-343.

Demirel, M.A., Acar, D.B. (2012) Ovarian remnant syndrome and uterine stump pyometra in three queens. *Journal of Feline Medicine and Surgery* 12, 913-918.

Dorn, A.S., Swist, R.A. (1977) Complications of canine ovariohysterectomy. *Journal of the American Animal Hospital Association* 13, 720-724.

Ek, A. (1978) Adrenergic innervation and adrenergic mechanisms. A study of the human urethra. *Acta Pharmacologica et Toxicologica* 43, 35-40.

England, G.C. (1997) Confirmation of ovarian remnant syndrome in the queen using hCG administration. *Veterinary Record* 141, 309-310.

Ewers, R.S., Holt, P.E. (1992) Urological complications following ovariohysterectomy in a bitch. *Journal of Small Animal Practice* 33, 236-238.

Fingland, R.B. (1998) Ovariohysterectomy. In Bojrab, M.J. (ed.) *Current techniques in small animal surgery*, 4th ed. Williams & Wilkins, Baltimore, pp. 489-496.

Fleischmann, N., Christ, G., Sclafani, T., et al. (2002) The effect of ovariectomy and long-term estrogen replacement on bladder structure and function in the rat. *Journal of Urology* 168, 1265-1268.

Grassi, F., Romagnoli, S., Camillo, F., et al. (1994) Iatrogenic enterovaginal fistula following hysterectomy. *Journal of Small Animal Practice* 35, 32-34.

Hamaide, A.J., Verstegen, J.P., Snaps, F.R., et al. (2005) Influence of the estrous cycle on urodynamic and morphometric measurements of the lower portion of the urogenital tract in dogs. *The American Journal of Veterinary Research*, 66, 1075-1083.

Holt, P.E. (1985a) Urinary incontinence in the bitch due to sphincter mechanism incompetence: prevalence in referred dogs and retrospective analysis of sixty cases. *Journal of Small Animal Practice* 26, 181-190.

Holt, P. (1985b) Importance of urethral length, bladder neck position and vestibulovaginal stenosis in sphincter mechanism incompetence in the incontinent bitches. *Research in Veterinary Science*, 39, 364-372.

Holt, P. (1985c) Urinary incontinence in the bitch due to sphincter mechanism incompetence: surgical treatment. *Journal of Small Animal Practice* 26, 237-246.

Holt, P. (1988) "Simultaneous" urethral pressure profilometry: comparison between continent and incontinent bitches. *Journal of Small Animal Practice* 29, 761-769.

Holt, P. (1990) Long term evaluation of colposuspension in the treatment of urinary incontinence due to incompetence of the urethral sphincter mechanism in the bitch. *Veterinary Record* 127, 537-542.

Holt, P. (2008) Urinary Incontinence. In Holt, P. (ed.) *Urological Disorders of the Dog and Cat: Investigation, Diagnosis and Treatment*. Manson Publishing: London, pp. 134-159.

Holt, P., Thrusfield, M. (1993) Association in bitches between breed, size, neutering and docking and acquired urinary incontinence due to incompetence of the urethral sphincter mechanism. *Veterinary Record* 133, 177-180.

Holt, P., Gibbs, C., Lathman, J. (1984) An evaluation of positive contrast vaginourethrography as a diagnostic aid in the bitch. *Journal of Small Animal Practice* 25, 531-549.

Holt, P.E., Bohannon, J. and Day, M.J. (2006) Vaginoperitoneal fistula after ovariohysterectomy in three bitches. *Journal of Small Animal Practice* 47, 744-746.

Janssens, L.L.A., Janssens, G.H.R.R. (1991) Bilateral flank ovariectomy in the dog—surgical technique and sequelae in 72 animals. *Journal of Small Animal Practice* 32, 9.

Kanazono, S., Aikawa, T., Yoshigae, Y. (2009) Unilateral hydronephrosis and partial ureteral obstruction by entrapment in a granuloma in a spayed dog. *Journal of the American Animal Hospital Association* 45, 301-304.

Krawiec, D.R. (1988) Urinary incontinence in dogs and cats. *Modern Veterinary Practice* 1, 17-24.

Krawiec, D. (1989) Diagnosis and treatment of acquired urinary incontinence. *Companion Animal Practice* 69, 17-24.

Kyles, A.E., Aronsohn, M. and Stone, E.A. (1996) Urogenital Surgery. In Lipowitz, A.J., Caywood D.D., Newton, C.D., Schwartz, A. (eds.) *Complications in Small Animal Surgery*, 1st edn. Williams & Wilkins, Baltimore, pp. 496-503.

Kyles, A.E., Douglass, J.P., Rottman, J.B. (1996) Pyelonephritis following inadvertent excision of the ureter during ovariohysterectomy in a bitch. *Veterinary Record* 139, 471-472.

MacCoy, D.M., Ogilvie, G., Burke, T. et al. (1988) Postovariohysterectomy ureterovaginal fistula in a dog. *Journal of the American Animal Hospital Association* 469-471.

Mandigers, P., Nell, T. (2001) Treatment of bitches with acquired urinary incontinence with oestriol. *Veterinary Record* 22, 764-767.

Marchevsky, A.M., Edwards, G.A., Lavelle, R.B., et al. (1999) Colposuspension in 60 bitches with incompetence of the urethral sphincter mechanism. *Australian Veterinary Practitioner* 29, 2-8.

McEvoy, F.J. (1994) Iatrogenic renal obstruction in a dog. *Veterinary Record* 135, 457-458.

Mehl, M.L., Kyles, A.E. (2003) Ureteroureterostomy after proximal ureteric injury during an ovariohysterectomy in a dog. *Veterinary Record* 153, 469-470.

Miller, D.M. (1995) Ovarian remnant syndrome in dogs and cats: 46 cases (1988-1992). *Journal of Veterinary Diagnostic Investigation* 7, 572-574.

Muir, P., Goldsmid, S.E., Bellenger, C.R., (1994) Management of urinary incontinence in five bitches with incompetence of the urethral sphincter mechanism by colposuspension and a modified sling urethroplasty. *Veterinary Record* 134, 38-41.

Nelson, R.W., Feldman, E.C. (1986) Pyometra. *Veterinary Clinics of North America: Small Animal Practice* 16, 561-576.

Nickel, R. (1998) Studies on the function of the urethra and the bladder in continent and incontinent female dogs (PhD thesis). Utrecht University, Utrecht, The Netherlands, pp. 11-126.

Nickel, R.F., Wiegand, U., Van Den Brom, W.E., (1998) Evaluation of a transpelvic sling procedure with and without colposuspension for treatment of female dogs with refractory urethral sphincter mechanism incompetence. *Veterinary Surgery* 27, 94-104.

Noël, S., Cambier, C., Baert, K., et al. (2010) Combined pharmacokinetic and urodynamic study of the effects of oral administration of phenylpropanolamine in female Beagle dogs. *The Veterinary Journal* 184, 201-207.

Noël, S., Massart, L., Hamaide, A. (2012) Urodynamic and haemodynamic effects of single oral administration of ephedrine of phenylpropanolamine in continent female dogs. *The Veterinary Journal* 192, 89-95.

Okkens, A.C., van de Gaag, I., Biewenga, W.J., et al. (1981) Urological complications following ovariohysterectomy in dogs. *Tijdschrift voor Diergeneeskunde* 106, 1189-1198.

Okkens, A.C., Dieleman, S.J., van de Gaag, I. (1981) Gynaecologische complicaties na ovariohysterectomy bij de hond ten gevolge van: 1. het incompleet verwijderen van de ovaria en 2. Een ontsteking van de uterus-cervix stomp. *Tijdschrift voor Diergeneeskunde* 106, 1142-1158.

Okkens, A.C., Kooistra, H.S., Nickel, R.F. (1997) Comparison of long-term effects of ovariectomy versus ovariohysterectomy in bitches. *Journal of Reproduction and Fertility*, 51 (Suppl.), 227-231.

Osborne, C., Oliver, J., Polzin, D. (1980) Non-neurogenic urinary incontinence. In Kirk, R. (ed.) *Current Veterinary Therapy VII. Small Animal Practice.* WB Saunders, Philadelphia, pp. 1128-1136.

Pearson, H. (1973) The complications of ovariohysterectomy in the bitch. *Journal of Small Animal Practice* 14, 257-266.

Pearson, H., Gibbs, C. (1980) Urinary incontinence in the dog due to accidental vagino-ureteral fistulation during hysterectomy. *Journal of Small Animal Practice* 21, 287-291.

Perkins, N.R., Frazer, G.S. (1995) Ovarian remnant syndrome in a Toy Poodle: a case report. *Theriogenology*, 44, 307-312.

Pineda, M.H. (2003) Reproductive patterns in cats. In Pineda, M.H., Dooley, M. (eds.) *McDonald's Veterinary Endocrinology and Reproduction*, 5th edn. Iowa State Press, Ames, IA, pp. 505-522.

Pollari, F.L., Bonnett, B.N. (1996) Evaluation of postoperative complications following elective surgeries of dogs and cats at private practices using computer records. *Canadian Veterinary Journal* 37, 672-678.

Pollari, J.L., Bonnett, B.N., Barnsey, S.C., et al. (1996) Postoperative complications of elective surgeries in dogs and cats determined by examining electronic and paper medical records. *Journal of the American Veterinary Medical Association* 208, 1882-1886.

Ponglowhapan, S., Church, D., Khalid, M. (2008a) Differences in the proportion of collagen and muscles in the canine lower urinary tract with regard to gonadal status and gender. *Theriogenology* 70, 1516-1524.

Ponglowhapan, S., Church, D., Khalid, M. (2008b) Differences in the expression of luteinizing hormone and follicle-stimulating hormone receptors in the lower urinary tract between intact and gonadectomised male and female dogs. *Domestic Animal Endocrinology* 34, 339-351.

Ponglowhapan, S., Church, D.B., Khalid, M. (2009) Expression of cyclooxygenase-2 in the canine lower urinary tract with regard to the effects of gonadal status and gender. *Theriogenology* 71 (8), 1276-1288.

Ragni, R.A. (2005) Pyometra in a bitch following unusual sterilisation. *Journal of Small Animal Practice* 46, 39-40.

Rawlings, C., Barsanti, J.A., Mahaffey, M.B., et al. (2001) Evaluation of colposuspension for treatment of incontinence in spayed female dogs. *Journal of the American Veterinary Medical Association* 219, 770-775.

Reichler, I., Hubler, M., Jöchle, W., et al. (2003) The effect of GnRH analogs on urinary incontinence after ablation of the ovaries in dogs. *Theriogenology* 60, 1207-1216.

Reichler, I., Pfeiffer, E., Piché, C., et al. (2004) Changes in plasma gonadotrophin concentrations and urethral closure pressure in the bitch during the 12 months following ovariectomy. *Theriogenology* 62, 1391-1402.

Reichler, I., Wolfgang, J., Piché, C., et al. (2006) Effect of long acting GnRH analogue or placebo on plasma LH/FSH, urethral pressure profiles and clinical signs of urinary incontinence due to sphincter mechanism incompetence in bitches. *Theriogenology* 66, 1227-1236.

Reeves, L., Adin, C., McLoughlin, M., et al. (2013) Outcome after placement of an artificial urethral sphincter in 27 dogs. *Veterinary Surgery* 42 (1), 12-18.

Richter, K., Ling, G. (1985) Clinical response and urethral pressure profile changes after phenylpropanolamine in dogs with primary sphincter incompetence. *Journal of American Veterinary Medical Association* 187, 605-611.

Rosin, A., Barsanti, J. (1981) Diagnosis of urinary incontinence in dogs: role of the urethral pressure profile. *Journal of American Veterinary Medical Association* 178, 814-822.

Ruiz de Gopegui et al. 1999

Salomon, J-F., Goriou, M., Dutot, E., et al. (2006) Experimental study of urodynamic changes after ovariectomy in 10 dogs. *Veterinary Record* 159, 807-811.

Spackman, C.J.A., Caywood, D.D., Johnston, G.R., et al. (1984) Granulomas of the uterine and ovarian stump: a case report. *Journal of the American Animal Hospital Association* 20, 449-453.

Stöcklin-Gautschi, N., Hässig, M., Reichler, M., et al. (2001) The relationship of urinary incontinence to early spaying in bitches. *Journal of Reproduction and Fertility* 57 (Suppl.), 233-236.

Stone, E.A., Cantrell, C.G., Sharp, N.J.H. (1993) Ovary and uterus. In Slatter, D. (ed.) *Textbook of Small Animal Surgery*. WB Saunders, Philadelphia, p. 13.

Tidwell, A.S., Ullman, S.L., Schelling, S.H. (1990) Urinoma (para-ureteral pseudocyst) in a dog. *Veterinary Radiology*, 31, 203-206.

Thrusfield, M. (1985) Association between urinary incontinence and spaying in bitches. *Veterinary Record* 116, 695.

Van Goethem, B.E.B.J., Schaefers-Okkens, A., Kirpensteijn, J. (2006) Making a rationale choice between ovariectomy and ovariohysterectomy in the dog: a discussion of the benefits of either techniques. *Veterinary Surgery* 35, 136-143.

Vick, J., Weiss, L., Ellis, S. (1994) Cardiovascular studies of phenylpropanolamine. *Archives Internationales de Pharmacodynamie et Thérapie* 327, 13-24.

Wallace, M.S. (1991) The ovarian remnant syndrome in the bitch and queen. *Veterinary Clinics of North America: Small Animal Practice* 21, 501-507.

Wang, K., Samii, V., Chew, D., et al. (2006) Vestibular, vaginal and urethral relationship in spayed and intact normal dogs. *Theriogenology* 66, 726-735.

Werner, R.E., Straughan, A.J. and Vezin, D. (1992) Nylon cable band reactions in ovariohysterectomized bitches. *Journal of the American Veterinary Medical Association* 200, 64.

White, R., Pomeroy, C. (1989) Phenylpropanolamine: An alpha-adrenergic agent for the management of urinary incontinence in bitch with urethral sphincter mechanism incompetence. *Veterinary Record* 125, 478-480.

White, R.N. (2001) Urethropexy for the management of urethral sphincter mechanism incompetence in the bitch. *Journal of Small Animal Practice* 42, 481-486.

Wilson, D.R. (1977) Renal function during and following obstruction. *Annual Review of Medicine* 3.

72 Pyometra

Kathryn Pratschke

Northeast Veterinary Referrals, Northumberland, UK

Pyometra (uterine inflammation with accumulation of purulent material within the uterus) is the most severe form of endometritis and has been reported in up to 25% of all unspayed female dogs before 10 years of age in Scandinavian countries (Egenvall *et al.* 2001). The incidence in cats is unknown. It typically occurs during or after a period of progesterone dominance, although prior exposure to estrogen is also thought to be essential (Pretzer 2008). The etiology and pathogenesis are complex, likely involving both hormonal and bacterial elements. Large age- and breed-related differences have been reported with respect to occurrence; for example within Scandinavian canine populations, Rottweilers, collies, golden retrievers, Labrador retrievers, and German shepherd dogs are considered at-risk breeds. The majority of cases occur in animals around 7 to 9 years of age, but pyometra has also been recorded in both very young (younger than 1 year) and very old patients (13–20 years) in dogs and cats (Kenney *et al.* 1987; Hagman *et al.* 2011). Although a variety of organisms have been cultured in cases with pyometra, the most commonly seen is *Escherichia coli*. Pyometra, especially closed cervix pyometra (Figure 72.1) is a potentially life-threatening illness that may be associated with systemic sepsis, endotoxic shock, and a systemic inflammatory response syndrome (SIRS)

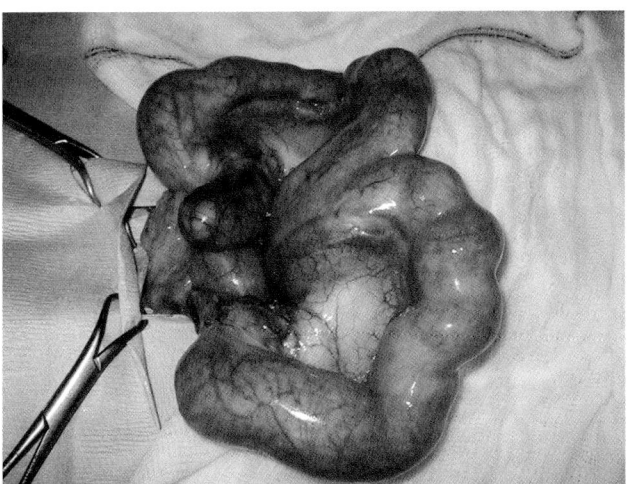

Figure 72.1 Closed cervix pyometra results in a potentially life-threatening condition with profound systemic effects. The degree of distension of the uterus does not necessarily influence the severity of the clinical signs, although clearly rupture is more likely with more fluid accumulation.

leading to organ failure. Renal compromise is commonly seen in dogs with pyometra, although this appears to be a rare occurrence in cats. The treatment of choice is ovariohysterectomy (OVH) as soon as possible, allowing for patient stabilization, although there has been a recent report of successful medical management in dogs with milder disease (England *et al.* 2011). Reported complications of pyometra include peritonitis and sepsis, uterine stump abscess, wound infections, renal disease, anemia, anorexia, icterus, splenic infarction, and thromboembolic disease.

Systemic complications

Definition
Although pyometra specifically affects the genitourinary system, it can have profound systemic effects.

Risk factors
- The immunologic profile in bitches has been shown to change with pyometra, with inhibition of mitogen-driven lymphocyte proliferation being the characteristic feature. Sera from 34 affected bitches in one study also showed higher levels of immunoglobulins, lysozyme, and circulating immune complexes, leading to the conclusion that pyometra is associated with both a significant inflammatory response and immune suppression (Faldyna *et al.* 2001).
- Virulence factors associated with *E. coli* involve the capsule (resistance to phagocytosis); cell wall lipopolysaccharide (endotoxin release), pili (allow attachment to mucous membranes); and extracellular products such as cytokines, hemolysins, aerobactin, and mucopolysaccharide (Gyles 1993). Production of cytotoxic necrotizing factor may also contribute to the virulence of *E. coli* in pyometra in bitches (Dhaliwal *et al.* 1998).
- Many dogs with pyometra have concurrent urinary tract infection (UTI), and it has been suggested in the past that subclinical UTI with *E. coli* was linked to pyometra in bitches. Studies in the past 10 years have shown that pyometra is caused by *E. coli* that originates from the normal flora of the affected dog rather than by spread between animals of specific clones with higher ability to affect the uterus (Hagman *et al.* 2002). There is also evidence that the *E. coli* isolates from both urinary tracts and uteri of animals with pyometra and concurrent UTI are identical (Hagman *et al.* 2002).

Complications in Small Animal Surgery, First Edition. Edited by Dominique Griffon and Annick Hamaide.

© 2016 John Wiley & Sons, Inc. Published 2016 by John Wiley & Sons, Inc.

Companion website: www.wiley.com/go/griffon/complications

- Endotoxins and inflammation are both factors that can result in myocardial damage. Cardiac-specific troponin I (cTnI) is a protein expressed at high concentrations only in the myocardium. When cardiac myocytes are damaged, cTnI leaks into the circulation and can be measured in the bloodstream (Schober *et al.* 2002). In a study of 46 dogs with pyometra, 37 of which showed signs consistent with SIRS, the authors concluded that mild to moderate increases in cTnI appeared to be common in dogs with pyometra both before and after surgery; however, the clinical importance was uncertain (Pelander *et al.* 2008).
- Endotoxemia may also be associated with sepsis and developing SIRS and is believed to be responsible for many of the clinical signs associated with pyometra. If the uterus ruptures and the purulent contents leak to the peritoneal cavity, then septic peritonitis may ensue with a resulting poor prognosis (Figure 72.2).

Diagnosis

- **Clinical signs** associated with pyometra in dogs typically include purulent vaginal discharge (in open cervix pyometra), anorexia, depression, lethargy, vomiting, diarrhea, and polyuria and polydipsia. In cats, very much the same clinical signs are seen but often at a lower intensity, and polyuria and polydipsia have not been so much noted (Kenney *et al.* 1987).
- **Hematology** will often identify the presence of normochromic normocytic anemia and leucocytosis with a left shift and increased numbers of band neutrophils. Patients may also be hyperproteinemic and hyperglobulinemic. In cats, hypokalemia may be seen, but azotemia was documented in only 12% of 183 cats in the only large study of feline pyometra to date (Kenney *et al.* 1987). A study from 1988 in dogs suggested that a higher percentage have azotemia, although this finding has not been consistent in all studies (Stone *et al.* 1988; Maddens *et al.* 2010). Proteinuria may be present in dogs although it is not clear whether this is also the case in cats. If the patient is septic then hypoglycemia, metabolic acidosis, hyperlactatemia, hypothermia, and coagulation abnormalities may be seen.
- **Diagnostic imaging** may be used to help confirm a diagnosis of pyometra; abdominal ultrasonography is generally more helpful than radiography.

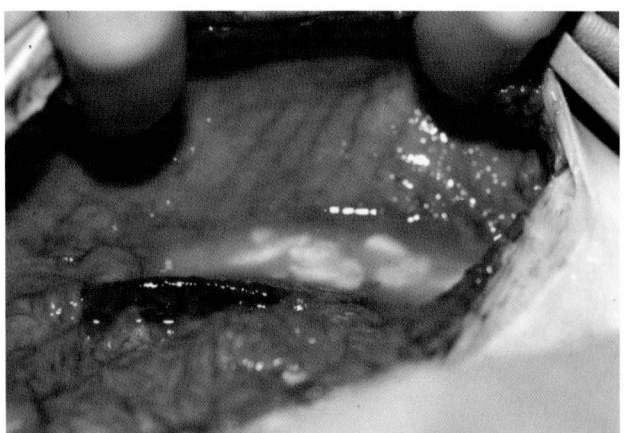

Figure 72.2 If the uterus ruptures in a patient with pyometra, then generalized septic peritonitis will result, requiring aggressive and intensive management.

Treatment, outcome, and prevention

- **Intensive intravenous (IV) fluid therapy** should be provided with balanced electrolyte solutions supplemented as necessary if patients are severely hypokalemic or hypoglycemic. Ideally, a urinary catheter should be placed connected to a closed collection system so that fluid therapy can be titrated to effect based on physiological variables and urine output.
- **Broad-spectrum antibiotics** should be administered intravenously, using drugs such as second-generation cephalosporins (e.g., cefuroxime 30 mg/kg every 6–8 hours), amoxicillin–clavulanate (20–30 mg/kg every 6–8 hours), metronidazole (15 mg/kg by slow infusion every 12 hours), and enrofloxacin (5 mg/kg every 24 hours).
- **Serial lactate measurements** may be of use in assessing the response to resuscitation, although one-off measurements are of little clinical use.
- **Specific antiendotoxic therapy** is controversial. Previous recommendations have included flunixin meglumine and corticosteroids; however, flunixin carries the risk of adversely affecting renal function, particularly in a hypotensive anesthetized patient, and is rarely if ever used any more. Corticosteroids were previously held to be of benefit if given before the onset of endotoxemia or within the first 60 minutes; however, meta-analyses have shown no benefit but possibly a detrimental effect. Subsequent to this, low-dose steroids were trialed and gave promising results in animal models and smaller clinical studies in humans; however, this beneficial effect has not been maintained in larger studies and meta-analyses, and there is still no consensus regarding whether to use them or not (Batzofin *et al.* 2011).
- When signs of icterus and elevated alkaline phosphatase are present, these are almost always attributable to intrahepatic cholestasis (cholestasis of sepsis). They do not require specific treatment beyond correction of fluid deficits and OVH. The same is true where metabolic acidosis exists, whether with or without respiratory alkalosis.
- The anemia typically seen with pyometra is normochromic and normocytic in nature and reflects bone marrow suppression from inflammation. The anemia usually resolves after the pyometra has been treated, but before surgery, the hematocrit should be monitored to assess whether the use of blood products is indicated.
- Septic peritonitis may result from rupture of the uterus, although it has also been seen documented in a dog with an intact uterus but an ovarian bursa abscess (Van Israel *et al.* 2002). A full discussion of peritonitis can be found in Chapter 4.

Persistent azotemia

Definition

Azotemia is defined as increased concentrations of urea and creatinine (and other nonproteinaceous nitrogenous substances) in the blood. However, urea is synthesized in the liver from ammonia and production can be increased by high dietary protein uptake, hemorrhage in the upper gastrointestinal (GI) tract, and catabolic states that cause breakdown of body proteins as well as in response to renal dysfunction. Creatinine production is relatively constant, so an increase in creatinine is a more reliable indicator of decreased renal excretion than is the case with urea.

Risk factors

- Prerenal azotemia may be seen in any condition that adversely affects blood flow to the kidneys, including hypovolemia, hypotension, endotoxemia or sepsis, all of which may be present with pyometra.

- Renal azotemia is associated with nephron loss or damage and is diagnosed when azotemia is persistently associated with isosthenuria or minimally concentrated urine. In the clinical setting, it can be very difficult to differentiate prerenal from true renal azotemia.
- In older patients, there may be increased risk of prerenal azotemia caused by cardiac disease as well as the possibility of preexisting glomerular changes such as sclerosis.
- Anesthesia is known to reduce renal blood flow and therefore worsens any prerenal or renal insufficiency present.

Diagnosis

A combination of clinical history, physical examination, serum biochemistry findings, and urinalysis has been the mainstay of diagnosis of renal compromise in the majority of clinical cases.

Whether cats have similar renal problems to dogs with pyometra is unclear. There are only limited studies regarding the phenomenon of pyometra in cats, but one study of 183 cats found that only 12% were azotemic and 9% had polyuria and polydipsia, and no postoperative problems with renal dysfunction were documented (Kenney *et al.* 1987). Whether cats are genuinely less predisposed to renal injury with pyometra or it has been insufficiently investigated remains uncertain.

Treatment

- The mainstay of treatment for azotemia and renal injury is IV fluid therapy, and preoperative correction of fluid, electrolyte, and acid–base imbalances is mandatory. If true renal azotemia is present, then this tends not to respond to fluid therapy alone, and this may help to differentiate the origin.
- If urine output does not improve in response to fluid therapy, then cautious volume expansion can be tried while physiological variables are monitored. If this is unsuccessful, then diuretics, vasodilators, or both can be administered (Table 72.1).
- Based on the fact that up to 69% of dogs with pyometra have been reported to also have UTI, it is advisable to obtain a urine sample during surgery and submit it for bacterial culture.

Uterine stump abscess

Definition

Uterine stump abscess, stump pyometra, and persistent infection of the uterine stump involve localized infection, which may be associated with foreign body reaction to multifilament suture material

(Spackman *et al.* 1984), unusual bacterial infections such as *Brucella canis* (Dillon and Henderson 1981), or poor surgical technique (Stone 2003).

Risk factors

- Uterine stump abscess, persistent infections of the uterine stump, and stump pyometra (there is much overlap among these three conditions) have been typically listed in the veterinary literature as potential complications of pyometra. However, a review of the currently available literature shows limited evidence to support this assumption. It is probably more correct to consider these conditions as potential complications of OVH because uterine stump abscess has almost invariably been documented after a routine neutering procedure.
- In one case when uterine stump abscess was described specifically as a postpyometra complication, the animal was actually undergoing revision surgery to resect an area of splenic infarction and the uterine stump abscess within 4 days of the initial OVH for pyometra. At such a short time interval after the first surgery, it is likely that this represented an incompletely performed uterine body resection at the first procedure (i.e., inappropriate surgical technique rather than a true uterine stump abscess) (Wheaton *et al.* 1989).
- Use of multifilament suture material has been documented as a potential cause of uterine stump abscess or granuloma and is anecdotally well recognized as a cause of persistent infection at both uterine and ovarian ligation sites. The use of nonsurgical self-locking nylon ties should also be avoided.
- It is important to ensure that excessive devitalized tissue does not remain distal to the ligature because this may predispose to infection or granuloma (Figure 72.3).

Diagnosis

- The diagnosis is usually based on a combination of clinical signs, laboratory evaluation, and diagnostic imaging.
- Typical clinical signs are similar to those seen with pyometra and include vaginal discharge, lethargy depression, vomiting, polyuria and polydipsia, and inappetence.

Table 72.1 Drugs that may be used to treat poor urine output in patients with renal injury associated with pyometra

Drug	Administration
Furosemide	2 mg/kg IV followed 1 hour later by 4 mg/kg IV if there is no diuresis
	May be combined with dopamine (see below)
Mannitol	0.25–0.5 g/kg IV infusion given over 5–10 minutes
	N.B.: contraindicated if patient is anuric and has not been rehydrated
Dopamine	2–10 µg/kg/min as a CRI
	Dopamine must be diluted in normal saline to the appropriate concentration, and accurate dosing is very important because higher concentrations (>10 µg/kg/min) are associated with increased reduced renal and peripheral blood flow. If cardiac arrhythmias arise, then the dose should be decreased and the infusion stopped.

CRI, constant-rate infusion; IV, intravenous,.

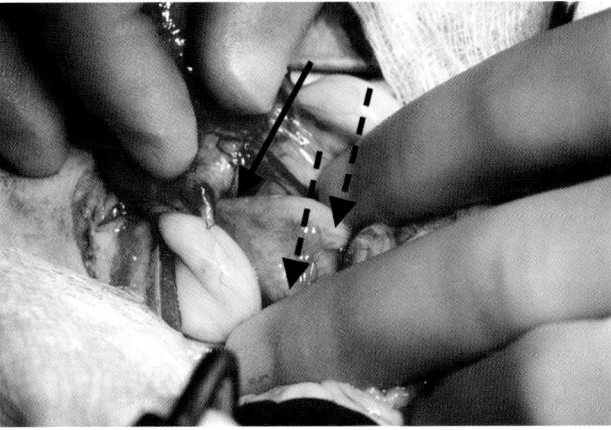

Figure 72.3 One of the factors that may predispose to formation of stump pyometra or uterine stump abscess is failure to complete ovariohysterectomy correctly. This figure shows a cat that has had the uterine stump and first portion of both right and left uterine horns left in situ after routine spaying. The arrow indicates the uterine body and the arrows, and dashed lines indicate the uterine horns. Histology on the uterine body subsequently identified cystic endometrial hyperplasia, which may be a precursor to pyometra.

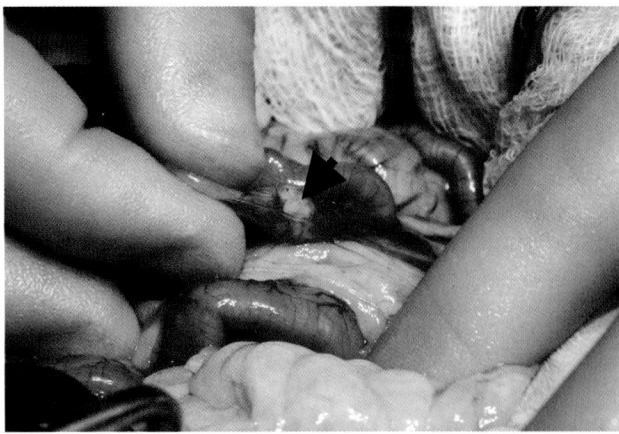

Figure 72.4 Photograph, taken from the same patient as Figure 72.3, showing an ovarian remnant, indicated by the arrowhead. Histology subsequently identified a cystic ovarian carcinoma.

- Hematology and biochemistry may show a leucocytosis, elevated alkaline phosphatase, and azotemia similar to those seen with pyometra.
- Diagnostic imaging can confirm a soft tissue opacity mass or lesion in the caudal abdomen between the bladder and colon. Ultrasound examination is more useful than radiography for assessment of this condition.

Treatment

The patient should be stabilized as previously described for pyometra before surgery. The goal of surgery is to carefully break down any adhesions present to allow resection of the uterine stump to the level of the cervix. Both ovarian stumps should be very carefully assessed to rule out the possibility of ovarian remnant syndrome as a cause for the uterine stump abscess or stump pyometra (Figure 72.4). If any additional tissue is resected, it should be submitted for histology to confirm the presence or absence of ovarian tissue.

Peritonitis and sepsis

See Chapters 2 and 4.

Relevant literature

Historically, it has been assumed that the cause of renal damage secondary to pyometra in dogs was an immune-complex glomerulonephritis. However, when this was specifically evaluated in one study (Bartoskova *et al.* 2007), there were no increased levels of circulating immune complexes in dogs with pyometra compared with healthy dogs. In other studies, only tubulointerstitial lesions were seen or even no histologic abnormalities at all (Stone *et al.* 1988). A study of renal histomorphometry in dogs with pyometra in 2007 documented interstitial inflammation and tubular atrophy as being pronounced features in dogs with pyometra. Glomerular sclerosis, on the other hand, was seen in both the control group and the pyometra group and was considered an age-related change rather than true pathology related to the pyometra (Heiene *et al.* 2007). These findings were supported by a more recent study using urinary biomarkers including albumin, immunoglobulin

G, retinol-binding protein, and *N*-acetyl-β-D-glucosaminidase to assess renal function (Maddens *et al.* 2010). These authors found that *E. coli* pyometra induced transient glomerular and tubular dysfunction in dogs, but the changes had all resolved by recheck 6 months after surgery. Interestingly, in this study, the serum parameters for renal dysfunction did not differ significantly in 17 dogs with pyometra compared with healthy, dogs although the results for biomarkers were different. Based on the biomarkers used, the authors concluded that pyometra had an adverse effect on the nephron at several levels, not just glomerular. Two of the 25 dogs in this study developed renal failure and were euthanized; the values for both the routine serum markers and the urinary biomarkers were among the highest in the pyometra group in these cases. A study in 2011 evaluating renal injury in dogs with pyometra concluded that dogs with pyometra and urine protein:creatinine ratios greater than 1.0 or high ratios of urinary biomarkers were likely to have clinically relevant renal histologic lesions and would require monitoring after OVH (Maddens *et al.* 2011). The role of pyometra-associated pathogenic mechanisms in causing or exacerbating focal and segmental glomerulosclerosis in dogs is not currently understood.

It is, of course, better to avoid a uterine stump abscess or stump pyometra rather than treat it. This is best done through thorough knowledge of the relevant surgical anatomy and careful application of the chosen neutering technique (Ragni 2005; Van Goethem *et al.* 2006). In addition to complete removal of both ovaries, if OVH is to be performed, then both uterine horns and the entire uterine body should be removed and the uterine ligature placed just cranial to the cervix; this can be trickier in cats, particularly from a flank approach. The use of multifilament suture materials and nonsurgical self-locking nylon ties should be avoided because they have been associated with granuloma and inflammation (Boza *et al.* 2010). It is also important to ensure that excessive devitalized tissue does not remain distal to the ligature.

There has been much anecdotal discussion regarding whether to use a Parker-Kerr oversew (or a similar technique) on the uterine stump in cases with pyometra. Again, a review of the available literature suggests that there is little evidence behind the original suggestion to use this technique. The Parker-Kerr suture was described in 1908 by Drs. Edward Mason Parker and Harry Kerr as part of a new technique for intestinal anastomosis, which reduced the risk of spillage from the intestinal tract during the procedure, and it has since then been described for use in several other surgeries involving the GI tract in humans, as well as in animals. The main source for the recommendations to use the Parker-Kerr suture for infected uterine stumps appears to be an unreferenced statement in a textbook describing fundamental veterinary surgical techniques published in 1987. As such, the recommendation to use a Parker-Kerr suture on the uterine stump in dogs and cats with pyometra cannot really be substantiated and current clinical opinion favors careful surgical technique to ensure that the appropriate tissues are resected, the use of sterile saline lavage, and omentalization of the uterine stump to reduce the risk of adhesions forming.

References

Bartoskova, A., Vitasek, R., Leva, L., et al. (2007) Hysterectomy leads to fast improvement of haematological and immunological parameters in bitches with pyometra. *Journal of Small Animal Practice* 48, 564-568.

Batzofin, B.M., Sprung, C.L., Weiss, Y.G. (2011) The use of steroids in the treatment of severe sepsis and septic shock. *Best Practice & Research Clinical Endocrinology & Metabolism* 25, 735-743.

Boza, S., Lucas, X., Zarelli, M., et al. (2010) Late abscess formation caused by silk suture following hysterectomy in a female dog. *Reproduction in Domestic Animals* 45, 934-936.

Dhaliwal, G.K., Wray, C., Noakes, D.E. (1998) Uterine bacterial flora and uterine lesions in bitches with cystic endometrial hyperplasia (pyometra). *Veterinary Record* 143, 659-661.

Dillon, A.R., Henderson, R.A. (1981) Brucella canis in a uterine stump abscess in a bitch. *Journal of the American Veterinary Medical Association* 178 (9), 987-988.

Egenvall, A., Hagman, R., Bonnett, B.N., et al. (2001) Breed risk of pyometra in insured dogs in Sweden. *Journal of Veterinary Internal Medicine* 15, 530-538.

England, G.C.W., Freeman, S.L., Russo, M. (2007) Treatment of spontaneous pyometra in 22 bitches with a combination of cabergoline and cloprostenol. *Veterinary Record* 160, 293-296.

Faldyna, M., Laznicka, A., Toman, M. (2001) Immunosuppression in bitches with pyometra. *Journal of Small Animal Practice* 42, 5-10.

Gyles, C.L. (1993). Escherichia coli. In Gyles, C.L. Thoen, C.O. (eds.) *Pathogenesis of Bacterial Infections in Animals* Iowa State University Press, Ames, IA, pp. 164-187

Hagman, R., Kuhn, I. (2002) Escherichia coli strains isolated from the uterus and urinary bladder of bitches suffering from pyometra, comparison by restriction enzyme digestion and pulsed field gel electrophoresis. *Veterinary Microbiology*, 84, 143-153.

Hagman, R., Lagerstedt, A.-S., Hedhammar, A., et al. (2011). A breed-matched case-control study of potential risk-factors for canine pyometra. *Theriogenology* 75, 1251-1257.

Heiene, R., Kristiansen, V., Teige, J., et al. (2007) Renal histomorphology in dogs with pyometra and control dogs, and long term clinical outcome with respect to signs of kidney disease. *Acta Veterinaria Scandinavica* 49, 13.

Kenney, K.J., Matthiesen, D.T., Brown, N.O., et al. (1987) Pyometra in cats: 183 cases (1979-1984). *Journal of the American Veterinary Medical Association* 191 (9), 1130-1132.

Maddens, B., Daminet, S., Smets, P., et al. (2010) Escherichia coli pyometra induces transient glomerular and tubular dysfunction in dogs. *Journal of Veterinary Internal Medicine* 24, 1263-1270.

Maddens, B., Heiene, R., Smets, P., et al. (2011) Evaluation of kidney injury in dogs with pyometra based on proteinuria, renal histomorphology, and urinary biomarkers. *Journal of Veterinary Internal Medicine* 25, 1075-1083.

Pelander, L., Hagman, R., Häggström, J. (2008) Concentrations of cardiac troponin I before and after ovariohysterectomy in 46 female dogs with pyometra. *Acta Veterinaria Scandinavica* 50, 35.

Pretzer, S.D. (2008) Clinical presentation of canine pyometra and mucometra: a review. *Theriogenology* 70, 359-363.

Ragni, R. (2005) Pyometra in a bitch following unusual sterilization. *Journal of Small Animal Practice* 46, 39-40.

Schober, K.E., Cornand, C., Johnston, G.R. et al. (2002) Serum cardiac troponin I and cardiac troponin T concentrations in dogs with gastric dilatation-volvulus. *Journal of the American Veterinary Medical Association* 221, 381-388.

Spackman, C.J., Caywood, D., Johnston, G.R., et al. (1984) Granulomas of the uterine and ovarian stumps: a case report. *Journal of the American Animal Hospital Association* 20, 449-453.

Stone, E.A., Littman, M.P., Robertson, J.L., et al. (1998) Renal dysfunction in dogs with pyometra. *Journal of the American Veterinary Medical Association* 193, 457-464.

Stone, E.A. (2003) Ovary and uterus. In Slatter, D. (ed.) *Textbook of Small Animal Surgery*. WB Saunders, Philadelphia, pp. 1487-1502.

Van Goethem, B., Schaeffers-Okkens, A., Kirpensteijn, J. (2006) Making a rational choice between ovariectomy and ovariohysterectomy in the dog: a discussion of the benefits of either technique. *Veterinary Surgery* 35, 136-143.

Van Israel, N., Kirby, B., Munro, E.A.C. (2002) Septic peritonitis secondary to unilateral pyometra and ovarian bursal abscessation in a dog. *Journal of Small Animal Practice* 43, 452-455.

Wheaton, L.G., Johnson, A.L., Parker, A.J., et al. (1989) Results and complications of surgical treatment of pyometra: a review of 80 cases. *Journal of the American Animal Hospital Association* 25, 563-568.

Bart Van Goethem

Small Animal Medicine and Clinical Biology, Faculty of Veterinary Medicine, Ghent University, Ghent, Belgium

Reviews indicate that 60% to 80% of dystocia cases require surgery and that only 20% to 40% can be successfully treated by various combinations of medical therapy and manipulation (Münnich and Küchenmeister 2009). Traditional hysterotomy is the treatment of choice for canine and feline dystocia. When the owner expresses no desire for the pet's future reproduction, the dam or queen is often spayed (ovariohysterectomy [OVH]) after delivering the neonates from the hysterotomy incision. En bloc OVH followed by rapid removal of neonates from the gravid uterus is a valid alternative that decreases anesthetic times (Robbins and Mullen 1994).

Systemic disturbances and positional complications

Definition
When the decision for surgery is made, the dam has often endured hours of intensive labor and is physiologically compromised. Abnormalities can include physical exhaustion, dehydration, acid–base disorders, hypotension, hypocalcemia, and hypoglycemia. Supine hypotension syndrome is thought to occur from compression of the gravid uterus on the caudal vena cava, thus reducing venous return.

Risk factors
- Hypovolemia and hypotension are the most common complications during anesthesia.
- En bloc OVH results in increased blood loss through the removal of the gravid uterus with engorged blood vessels.
- Hypocalcemia (eclampsia) is most commonly seen in small dogs, first whelpings, and dogs with large litter sizes.

Diagnosis
- Laboratory tests before surgery include hematocrit, total plasma protein concentration, urine specific gravity, and blood urea nitrogen, and glucose concentrations. Other tests that may be indicated based on the clinical situation are complete blood count, blood calcium concentration, and blood gas analysis.
- Supine hypotension syndrome should be suspected in case of sudden decrease in blood pressure after positioning in dorsal recumbency.
- Hypocalcemia is diagnosed by measuring ionized calcium levels (<6 mg/dL) in combination with typical signs as a stiff gait,

trembling, twitching, seizures, tachycardia, panting, and hyperthermia. Cats may also display hyperexcitability, hypersensitivity, or flaccid paralysis.

Treatment
- Vigorous intravenous (IV) fluid therapy with a balanced electrolyte solution is instituted at a minimum of 10 mL/kg/hr.
- When the animal is hypoglycemic, a 2.5% dextrose solution is more appropriate.
- Blood or blood replacements can be given.
- IV antibiotics are administered if the fetuses are known to be dead and decomposing or if uterine infection is established.
- Hypocalcemia is treated with an infusion of 10% calcium gluconate at 0.5 to 1.5 mL/kg and active cooling for seizure-induced hyperthermia. Oral calcium carbonate supplementation is continued afterward.

Outcome
Maternal mortality rates for cesarean section in dogs and cats vary from 0% to 4%, the latter owing to the emergency nature and the patient's stressed condition at the time of surgery.

Prevention
- Physiological abnormalities are stabilized or corrected before induction of anesthesia.
- Continued perioperative fluid therapy at 20 L/kg/hr is essential to counteract vasodilatation and hypotension.
- A 10- to 20-degree left or right lateral tilt is used in women to prevent compression of the caudal vena cava.
- Recurrence of hypocalcemia is prevented by bottle feeding and early weaning of the neonates.

Hemorrhage

Definition
There may be as much as twice the blood loss with a cesarean section compared with normal parturition. This partly attributable to the increased cardiac output, blood pressure, and venous distensibility. Severe uterine hemorrhage can be caused by uterine vessel tears secondary to obstetric trauma, inherited or acquired coagulopathies, uterine or vaginal masses, subinvolution of placental sites, cystic endometrial hyperplasia–pyometra complex, uterine serosal

Complications in Small Animal Surgery, First Edition. Edited by Dominique Griffon and Annick Hamaide.
© 2016 John Wiley & Sons, Inc. Published 2016 by John Wiley & Sons, Inc.
Companion website: www.wiley.com/go/griffon/complications

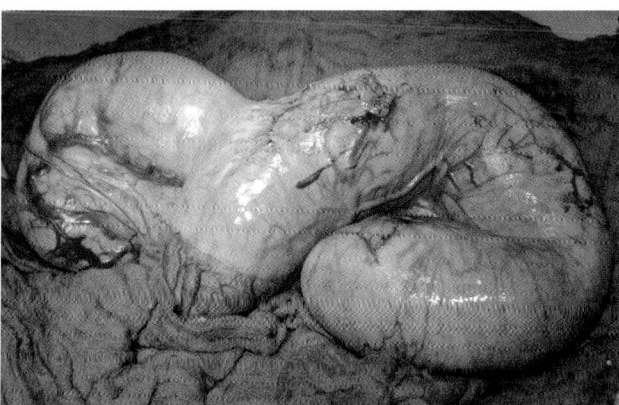

Figure 73.1 Enlarged and fragile uterine vessels in a gravid queen.

inclusion cysts, and uterine torsion. Extrauterine causes are ruptured uterine vessels, persistent hemorrhage from the uterine wall incision or the abdominal wall, and distended mammary gland vessels.

Risk factors
- The hematocrit in the normal periparturient dog decreases to approximately 30%.
- The placenta should not be forcefully extracted when it does not readily separate from the uterus or bleeds excessively.
- Uterine vessels are at risk for inadvertent trauma when manipulated because of the weight of the uterine horns and hormone-induced ligamentous laxity.
- Enlarged uterine vessels on the expanded uterine horns are susceptible to iatrogenic trauma during the surgical procedure (Figure 73.1).

Diagnosis
- Clinical signs, such as tachycardia, tachypnea, anorexia, weakness, or altered mentation.
- Serial hematocrit measurements, ultrasonography, or abdominocentesis will confirm the diagnosis.

Treatment
- In case of mild but persistent postpartum intrauterine hemorrhage in an otherwise clinically normal animal, oxytocin (1–5 IU intramuscularly or intravenously) may be given to hasten resolution by promoting uterine involution.
- Severe anemia is an indication for packed red blood cell transfusion.
- Persistent hemorrhage requires an emergency OVH.

Outcome
Most causes of uterus-related hemorrhage are cured by OVH. The outcome will benefit from early detection and appropriately aggressive fluid therapy.

Prevention
- Attention to careful surgical technique is important.
- Gentle peristaltic motion is used to bring the fetus to the incision site, and it is exteriorized only with moderate traction.
- Anemic patients benefit from the return of uterine blood to the peripheral circulation caused by oxytocin-induced involution of the uterus after hysterotomy.
- Studies in women showed that single-layer closure of the uterus was associated with a statistically significant reduction in mean blood loss (Dodd *et al.* 2008) (Figure 73.2).

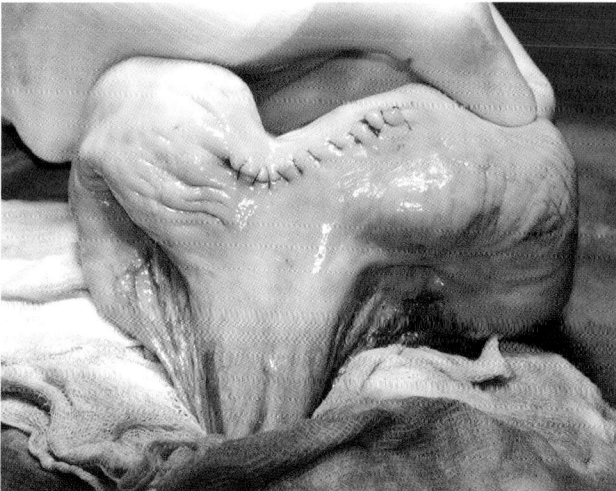

Figure 73.2 Single-layer appositional closure for a horizontal hysterotomy incision for cesarean section in a cat.

Incisional complications

Definition
Improper suturing of the uterine wall can lead to wound dehiscence, with the potential for peritonitis and death, or it might lead to uterine scarring, which may prevent future placentation, or uterine adhesions, which may interfere with uterine motility (Figure 73.3). Inappropriate suturing of the stretched abdominal wall can lead to abdominal herniation. Neonates can injure the skin incision site during nursing.

Risk factors
- The linea alba is often stretched thin and the abdomen distended, so care is taken not to incise underlying organs during the celiotomy incision.
- Accidental laceration of the fetus is possible when incising the uterine wall.

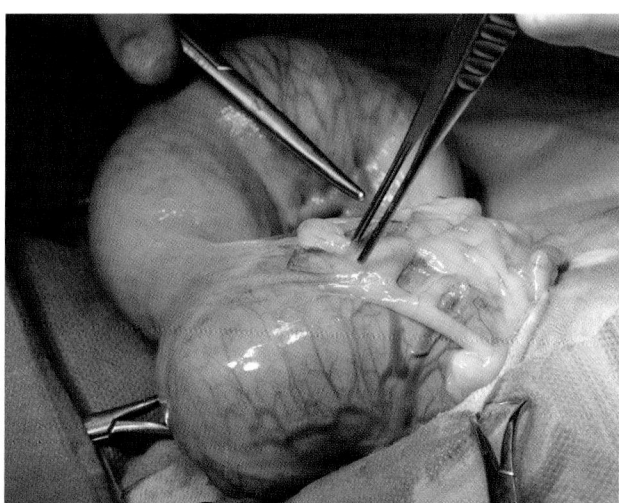

Figure 73.3 Omental adhesions to the uterine body as a result of a previous cesarean section.

Diagnosis

- Iatrogenic lacerations are noticed perioperatively.
- Abdominal wall herniation can be diagnosed on palpation, radiography, or ultrasonography.
- Uterine wound dehiscence leading to peritonitis is diagnosed by ultrasonography and abdominocentesis.

Treatment

- Iatrogenic lacerations of the uterine wall can almost always be repaired. Tears resulting from obstructive dystocia are more irregular, and the edges often need trimming to permit uncomplicated healing. Unrepairable lesions are cured by OVH.
- Peritoneal contamination is treated by extensive rinsing of the abdomen and IV antibiotic therapy.
- In case of wound dehiscence, the edges are evaluated, trimmed if deemed necessary, and closed with appropriate suture material.
- The skin incision can be protected from offspring-induced trauma with a polyurethane film bandage.

Outcome

Uterine wound dehiscence can lead to potentially fatal septic peritonitis.

Prevention

- Opening the uterine wall with a careful stab incision and lengthening it with scissors prevents trauma to the neonate.
- If uterine sutures are carefully placed and knots buried, adhesion formation is minimal.
- Subcuticular sutures are preferred over skin sutures to prevent irritation of the suture line by nursing neonates.
- With proper uterine closure, dogs with dystocia caused by fetal malposition or malformation can have subsequent normal vaginal deliveries.
- Studies in women showed that single-layer closure of the uterus was quicker than a two-layer closure and was associated with a statistically significant reduction in postoperative pain (Dodd et al. 2008).

Infectious complications

Definition

Endometritis is a bacterial infection of the uterus that is generally seen within the first 3 to 7 days. Potential causes are retained fetuses or placentas, abortions (Figure 73.4), uterine trauma secondary to dystocia or obstetric manipulation, and ascending infection from the vaginal canal. Mastitis is a postpartum complication that results from bacterial infection of the mammary glands. Incisional complications such as swelling, infection, seroma, self-trauma, or dehiscence occur in 5% of clean-contaminated and 12% of contaminated surgeries.

Risk factors

- Surgical clipping performed in the awake animal to decrease anesthetic time is associated with a higher risk for postoperative surgical site infection (Brown et al. 1997).
- Thorough palpation of the uterus and vagina is necessary to prevent leaving a fetus behind in the pelvic canal.
- A break in surgical technique or abdominal contamination with septic uterine contents may result in postoperative peritonitis.

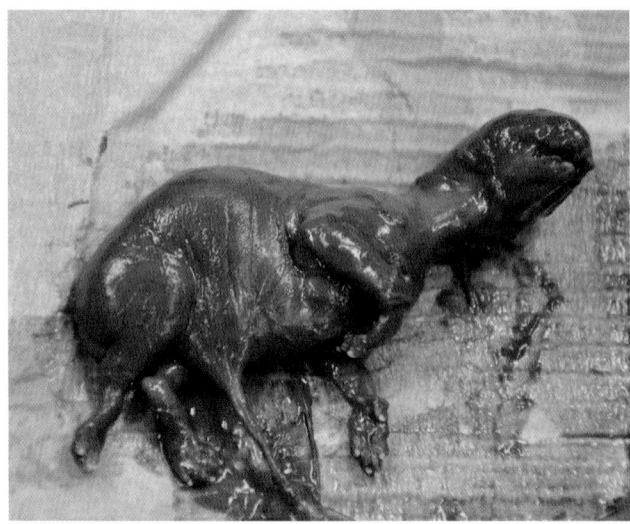

Figure 73.4 In case of fetal death and putrefaction, ovariohysterectomy is advocated because it minimizes the chance of peritoneal contamination. *Source:* Julius Liptak, Alta Vista Animal Hospital, Ottawa, Ontario. Reproduced with permission from Julius Liptak.

Diagnosis

- An odorless, dark red-brown to serous uterine discharge (lochia) is expected for 4 to 6 weeks postpartum. A foul-smelling discharge together with fever, lethargy, anorexia, vomiting, diarrhea, poor lactation, and neglect of offspring are typical signs of endometritis.
- Blood analysis, radiography, and ultrasonography will confirm the diagnosis.
- Mastitis is characterized by swollen and painful mammary glands; purulent, stringy, hemorrhagic, or grey milk; and systemic illness.
- Wound dehiscence with purulent discharge suggests surgical site infection. Cytology smears and bacterial culture should be performed.

Treatment

- Endometritis is treated aggressively with IV fluids and broad-spectrum antibiotics. After stabilization, OVH is the treatment of choice. In breeding animals without signs of sepsis, evacuation of the uterus' contents can be attempted with prostaglandins.
- Mastitis treatment consists of broad-spectrum antibiotics supplemented with frequent stripping of the milk, warm compresses, and hydrotherapy. Fluctuating abscess pockets are surgically drained, and large ruptured abscesses are treated as open wounds or with mastectomy.

Outcome

Postpartum endometritis and mastitis are considered potentially life threatening and make early weaning unavoidable. Endometritis results in OVH, and mastitis may necessitate mastectomy.

Prevention

- Careful surgical technique is needed to prevent any break in asepsis.
- Abdominal contents are inspected for any signs of contamination and then lavaged with 100 to 200 mL/kg body weight of warm saline.
- The uterine serosa and incision should be wiped clean in preparation for closure.
- Studies in humans show a lower rate of postoperative endometritis when placentas are allowed to pass naturally versus being removed at the time of surgery (Ayzac et al. 2008).

Uterine prolapse

Definition
Uterine prolapse is a rare postpartum complication reported more commonly in cats than in dogs. It is generally only seen during or immediately after parturition because the cervix must be open for prolapse to occur.

Risk factors
• Severe tenesmus during partus (dystocia) or immediately afterward

Diagnosis
If the uterus prolapses into the cranial vagina, nonspecific signs of abdominal pain and straining may be noted. In case of complete uterine prolapse, a large mass of tissue protrudes visibly through the vaginal orifice, with varying degrees of tissue edema, ulceration, and necrosis. Symptoms of hemorrhagic shock frequently develop as a result of ovarian or uterine vessel rupture.

Treatment
• Treatment consists of lubricating the exposed tissues while the animal receives IV fluids to correct shock. Blood transfusion (in case of severe hemorrhage) and antibiotic therapy (when tissue necrosis is seen) can be instituted. Manual reduction of the prolapse is performed under general anesthesia when the animal is stable. A dorsal episiotomy may facilitate reduction. Oxytocin is given to promote uterine involution and therefore prevent recurrence. Ultrasonography or laparoscopy can be used to ensure proper positioning of the uterine horns and integrity of the uterine vessels.
• When manual reduction is unsuccessful, surgical reduction may be necessary. After reduction, the uterus may then be pexied to the abdominal wall to prevent recurrence.
• Signs of hemorrhagic shock indicate rupture of the uterine vessels during prolapse and necessitate emergency celiotomy.

Outcome
In acute or subacute situations, manual reduction is often successful. OVH is indicated for chronic cases. Ruptured uterine vessels are life threatening.

Prevention
• When involution of the uterus is not already evident after closure of the hysterotomy incision, oxytocin supplementation should be started.

Agalactia

Definition
Normal milk flow after cesarean section usually occurs within 24 hours.

Risk factors
• Dehydration.
• Hypovolemia.
• Postoperative pain.

Diagnosis
• Clinical examination and blood tests are performed to evaluate hydration status.
• Postoperative pain scores are used to evaluate sufficient analgesia.

Treatment
In cases of hypovolemia, fluid therapy is prolonged after cesarean section. When vomiting prevents oral intake, antiemetic therapy should be instituted. Appropriate analgesic therapy is given for a few days postoperatively. Oxytocin can be given to stimulate milk production.

Outcome
Correcting the underlying cause is most often curative.

Prevention
• The dam's milk production is not affected by OVH because prolactin and cortisol are responsible for maintaining lactation.
• To promote early suckling from the neonates, the surgical site should be washed with warm water to remove residual antiseptic solution.

Complications associated with neonates

Definition
Neonatal care starts when the amniotic sac is opened and the fetus exteriorized. Neonates are extremely susceptible to hypoxemia and hypothermia at this time. The neonate should also be inspected for obvious birth defects such as palatoschisis, atresia ani, and limb deformities (Figure 73.5). With appropriate care, neonatal survival after cesarean section is higher compared with vaginal birth (respectively 92% vs. 86%) (Moon *et al.* 2000).

Risk factors
• Sixty percent of cesarean sections are performed on an emergency basis.
• Large litters (more than four pups).

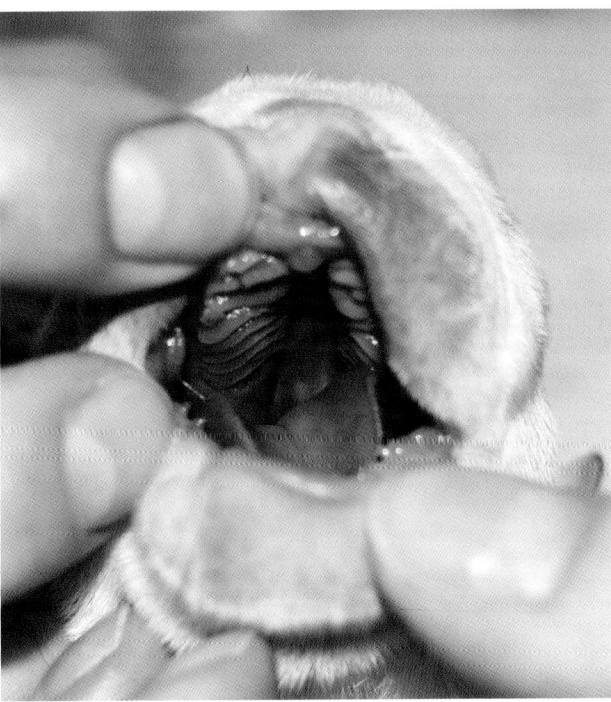

Figure 73.5 The presence of palatoschisis can cause severe problems during nursing with malnourishment, chronic rhinitis, and pneumonia as possible consequences.

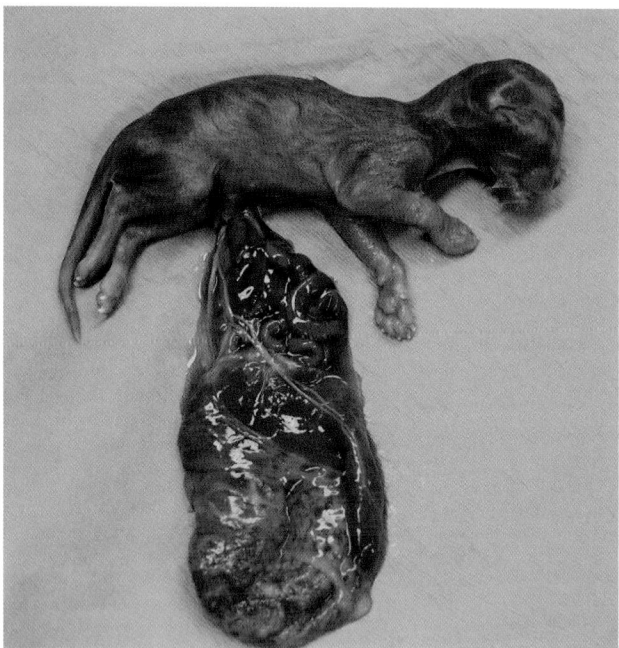

Figure 73.6 Kitten in which intestines remain outside of the abdomen because of a defect in the development of the muscles of the abdominal wall (omphalocele).

- Brachycephalic bitch.
- The presence of naturally delivered or deformed puppies (Figure 73.6).
- Poor anesthetic choices (xylazine, thiopental, ketamine).
- Swinging the neonate in a downward arc to promote fluid removal from the respiratory tract by centrifugal force is discouraged because of the potential for cerebral hemorrhage as a result of concussive injury.
- During en bloc OVH, the time between clamping the uterus and opening the amniotic sacs should be as short as possible to decrease hypoxemic time for the neonates.

Diagnosis

Fetal depression in neonates is caused by hypoxia associated with dystocia and depression from medications given to the dam during cesarean section. The neonate responds to hypoxia by decreasing heart rate, respiratory rate, and movements (Smith 2012). Bradycardia in newborns is defined as a heart rate less than 80 beats/min, and the initial respiratory rate is 10 to 18 breaths/min (Traas 2008). When puppy vigor was assessed 2 minutes after delivery from cesarean section, spontaneous breathing was seen in 85%, moving in 73%, and vocalizing in 60% of the puppies (Moon-Massat 2002).

Treatment

- Amniotic fluids are vigorously wiped away to clean the neonate and to stimulate respiration. The oral cavity and nostrils should be cleared of fluids with gentle suction or cotton swabs.
- Oxygen is administered if cyanosis or respiratory depression is present.
- If the neonate is still not responding, anesthetics should be reversed (naloxone 0.1 mg/kg if the dam received opioid analgesics).
- If spontaneous respiration is still not evident, artificial respiration by catheter intubation or gentle mouth-to-mouth resuscitation is instituted.

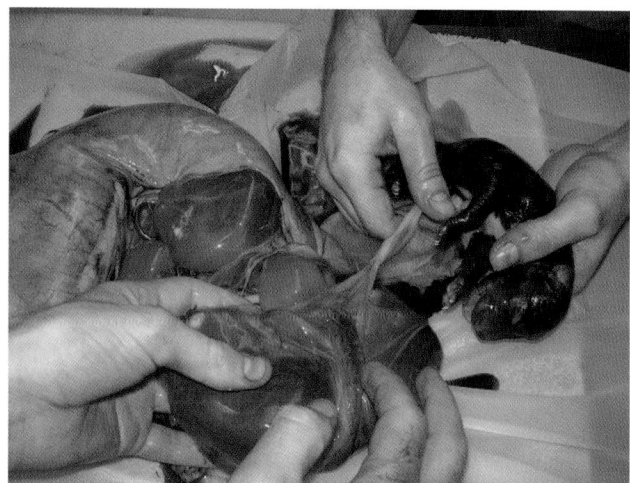

Figure 73.7 During en bloc ovariohysterectomy, multiple assistants are required for simultaneous resuscitation of the neonates.

- In case of bradycardia, epinephrine can be administered at a dose of 0.1 to 0.3 mg/kg IV.
- When no heartbeat can be detected, cardiac massage is instituted.

Outcome

Neonatal survival rates of 90% in queens and 70% in bitches are reported in animals not severely compromised at the time of cesarean section (Moon et al. 1998). Survival rates after en bloc OVH are 40% for cats and 75% for dogs (Robbins and Mullen 1994). With protracted dystocia and poor physical condition of the dam, survival rates as low as 10% to 25% are reported (Moon et al. 1998).

Prevention

- Resuscitation efforts are provided in the following order: warmth, airway, breathing, circulation, and drugs.
- Ideally, one assistant should be available for each neonate, although one person can care for two or three neonates at a time if the neonates are healthy.
- During en bloc OVH, multiple assistants are needed for simultaneous neonatal resuscitation (Figure 73.7).
- The neonate's umbilical cord clamp is removed after several minutes, and ligation is only indicated when hemorrhage persists.
- To facilitate acceptance by the mother, some vaginal or placental fluids can be smeared onto the neonates' fur.

Relevant literature

Supine hypotension syndrome is a cause of shock and bradycardia in human patients positioned in dorsal recumbency. Several studies in pregnant dogs could not detect any positional influence on systemic blood pressure (Abitbol 1978; Probst and Webb 1983; Probst et al. 1987). Satisfactory collateral circulation and the uterus bicornus in dogs and cats with gravid horns located lateral to the vena cava are possible explanations.

Rupture of the uterus is associated with faulty obstetric technique, gross uterine dilatation caused by excessive fetal size, or dystocia (Jutkowitz 2005). Rupture has also been reported to occur after cesarean section when an intrauterine pessary was placed in combination with a postoperative oxytocin drip (Bomzon 1977).

Although routinely administered as a respiratory stimulant in veterinary neonates, doxapram is banned for this use in human neonates (Perlman *et al.* 2010). Studies in goats and humans have shown doxapram to decreases cerebral blood flow; therefore, it could be harmful in vulnerable hypoxic newborns (Miletich *et al.* 1976; Roll and Horsch 2004). The effectiveness as a respiratory stimulant is furthermore decreased in case of cerebral hypoxemia, so it is unlikely to be helpful in an apneic newborn (Jutkowitz 2005).

In one study, en bloc OVH (Robbins and Mullen 1994) was associated with decreased neonatal survival for dogs and cats compared with recent reviews on traditional hysterotomy (Moon *et al.* 2000). Reported postoperative complications were anemia necessitating blood transfusion (12% of all cats), bladder rupture (1%), and death (1%). It remains, however, a feasible technique with benefits as decreased anesthetic time for the mother, scant to no postoperative lochial discharge, and population control in pets unable to reproduce naturally (Bebchuk and Probst 1998).

In human obstetric surgery, the old adage "once a cesarean section, always a cesarean section" no longer holds true for patients with the low hysterotomy incisions. In fact, patients with development of a low segment scar only had a 1% risk for uterine rupture during subsequent labor (Martin *et al.* 1997). No veterinary studies exist to date on complications of vaginal birth after cesarean section. Dogs that needed more than one cesarean section have been found to hardly have any visible uterine scars from the previous surgery, and normal deliveries have been documented even in dogs bred at the next estrus after cesarean section (Traas 2008). Therefore, the current opinion is that dogs with cesarean section after dystocia for fetal malposition or fetal malformation can have normal vaginal deliveries subsequently.

References

Abitbol, M.M. (1978) Inferior vena cava compression in the pregnant dog. *American Journal of Obstetrics & Gynecology* 130 (2), 194-198.

Ayzac, L., Caillat-Vallet, E., Girard, R., et al. (2008) Decreased rates of nosocomial endometritis and urinary tract infection after vaginal delivery in a French surveillance network, 1997-2003. *Infection Control and Hospital Epidemiology* 29 (6), 487-95.

Bebchuk, T.N., Probst, C.W. (1998) Cesarean section. In Bojrab, M.J. (ed.) *Current Techniques in Small Animal Surgery*, 4th edn. Williams & Wilkins, Baltimore, pp. 496-502.

Bomzon, L. (1977) Rupture of the uterus following caesarean section in a bitch. *South Africa Veterinary Record* 101, 38.

Brown, D.C., Conzemius, M.G., Shofer, F., et al. (1997) Epidemiologic evaluation of postoperative wound infections in dogs and cats. *Journal of the American Veterinary Medical Association* 210 (9), 1302-1306.

Dodd, J.M., Anderson, E.R., Gates, S. (2008) Surgical techniques for uterine incision and uterine closure at the time of caesarean section. *Cochrane Database Systematic Reviews* 16 (3), CD004732.

Jutkowitz, L.A. (2005) Reproductive emergencies. *Veterinary Clinics of North America: Small Animal Practice* 35, 397-420.

Martin, J.N., Perry, K.G., Roberts, W.E., et al. (1997) The case for trial of labor in the patient with a prior low-segment vertical cesarean incision. *American Journal of Obstetrics & Gynecology* 177 (1), 144-148.

Miletich, D.J., Ivankovich, A.D., Albrecht, R.F., et al. (1976) The effects of doxapram on cerebral blood flow and peripheral hemodynamics in the anesthetized and unanesthetized goat. *Anesthesia & Analgesia* 55, 279-285.

Moon, P.F., Erb, H.N., Ludders, J.W., et al. (1998) Perioperative management and mortality rates of dogs undergoing cesarean section in the United States and Canada. *Journal of the American Veterinary Medical Association* 213 (3), 365-369.

Moon, P.F., Erb, H.N., Ludders, J.W., et al. (2000) Perioperative risk factors for puppies delivered by cesarean section in the United States and Canada. *Journal of the American Animal Hospital Association* 36 (4), 359-368.

Moon-Massat, P.F., Erb, H.N. (2002) Perioperative factors associated with puppy vigor after delivery by cesarean section. *Journal of the American Animal Hospital Association* 38 (1), 90-96.

Münnich, A., Küchenmeister U. (2009) Dystocia in numbers—evidence-based parameters for intervention in the dog: causes for dystocia and treatment recommendations. *Reproduction in Domestic Animals* 44 (2), 141-147.

Perlman, J.M., Wyllie, J., Kattwinkel, J., et al. (2010) Part 11: neonatal resuscitation: 2010 International Consensus on Cardiopulmonary Resuscitation and Emergency Cardiovascular Care Science with Treatment Recommendations. *Circulation* 19, 122 (16 Suppl. 2), S516-S538.

Probst, C.W., Webb, A.I. (1983) Postural influence on systemic blood pressure, gas exchange, and acid/base status in the term-pregnant bitch during general anesthesia. *American Journal of Veterinary Research* 44 (10), 1963-1965.

Probst, C.W., Broadstone, R.V., Evans, A.T. (1987) Postural influence on systemic blood pressure in large full-term pregnant bitches during general anesthesia. *Veterinary Surgery* 16 (6), 471-473.

Robbins, M.A., Mullen, H.S. (1994) En bloc ovariohysterectomy as a treatment for dystocia in dogs and cats. *Veterinary Surgery* 23 (1), 48-52.

Roll, C., Horsch, S. (2004) Effect of doxapram on cerebral blood flow velocity in preterm infants. *Neuropediatrics* 35 (2), 126-129.

Smith, F.O. (2012) Guide to emergency interception during parturition in the dog and cat. *Veterinary Clinics of North America: Small Animal Practice* 42, 489-499.

Traas, A.M. (2008) Surgical management of canine and feline dystocia. *Theriogenology* 70 (3), 337-342.

74 Orchiectomy

Bart Van Goethem

Small Animal Medicine and Clinical Biology, Faculty of Veterinary Medicine, Ghent University, Ghent, Belgium

Orchiectomy in cats and prepubertal dogs is performed by a scrotal incision. In adult dogs, a prescrotal incision (standard technique), scrotal ablation (pendulous scrotum), perineal approach (concurrent perineal surgery), or parapreputial incision (cryptorchid dogs) is made (Crane 1998).

Serious complications after orchiectomy are rare, but may include scrotal swelling and bruising, hemorrhage, scrotal hematoma, abscess, granuloma, incisional problems (swelling, seroma formation, cellulitis, infection, automutilation, dehiscence), urinary incontinence, endocrine alopecia, behavioral changes, and eunuchoid syndrome (Boothe 2003).

Most complications associated with orchiectomy can be prevented by using good surgical technique, including gentle tissue handling, good hemostasis, and aseptic technique (Hedlund 2007).

Scrotal inflammation and swelling

Definition

Minor bruising and swelling are part of the normal inflammatory reaction caused by surgical trauma to the tissues. Swelling of the scrotum is caused by the accumulation of edematous fluids filling up dead space in the scrotum. The scrotal skin is very susceptible to trauma, both sharp and blunt, and easily develops contact dermatitis. The characteristic severe erythema causes intense pruritus that may promote relentless automutilation (Figure 74.1).

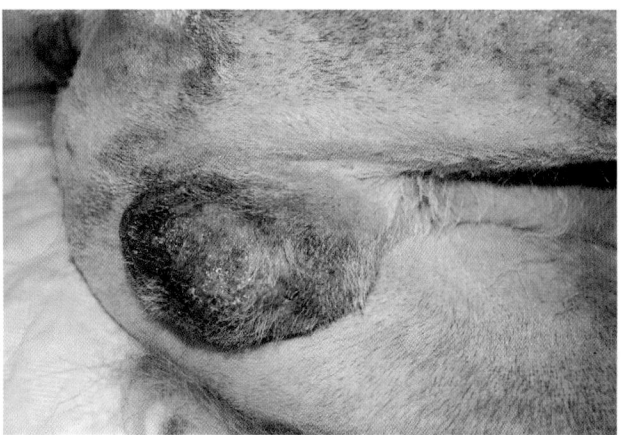

Figure 74.1 Typical signs of scrotal contact dermatitis in a dog.

Risk factors

- Prolonged contact between skin antiseptics and the scrotum.
- The Trendelenburg position during perineal orchiectomy promotes gravitational run down of antiseptics toward the scrotum.
- Overzealous amounts of antiseptic solution will lead to pooling in the inguinal region with possible contact to the scrotum.
- Opening the parietal vaginal tunic (open canine orchiectomy) more commonly leads to the development of bruising and swelling of the scrotum.
- Perineal orchiectomy, because of anatomical reasons, favors open castration.
- Older dogs with pendulous scrotums are at risk for postoperative problems.

Diagnosis

Scrotal swelling is evidenced by a nonfluctuating filled aspect. The primary lesions of contact dermatitis are patches of erythema, macules, and papules with serous exudation followed by formation of crusts, excoriation, and hyperpigmentation.

Treatment

Swelling after open castration can be limited by exercise restriction, cold packs, and prevention of automutilation with an Elizabethan collar or protective suit and, when necessary, sedation. The application of petroleum jelly–based products on a swollen scrotum will prevent further skin abrasion from the thighs. In cases of severe scrotal dermatitis with skin necrosis, scrotal ablation is indicated (Figure 74.2).

Outcome

This complication is mostly self-limiting or can be managed conservatively. However, severe cases may need scrotal ablation.

Prevention

- Unless a scrotal ablation or incision is planned, clipping is limited to the prescrotal region because trauma to the scrotum and medial thighs with clippers encourages automutilation.
- The use of chlorhexidine instead of povidone–iodine solutions is advocated.
- Towel clamps are placed at some distance to avoid injury to the scrotum.
- Careful attention to hemostasis is important.

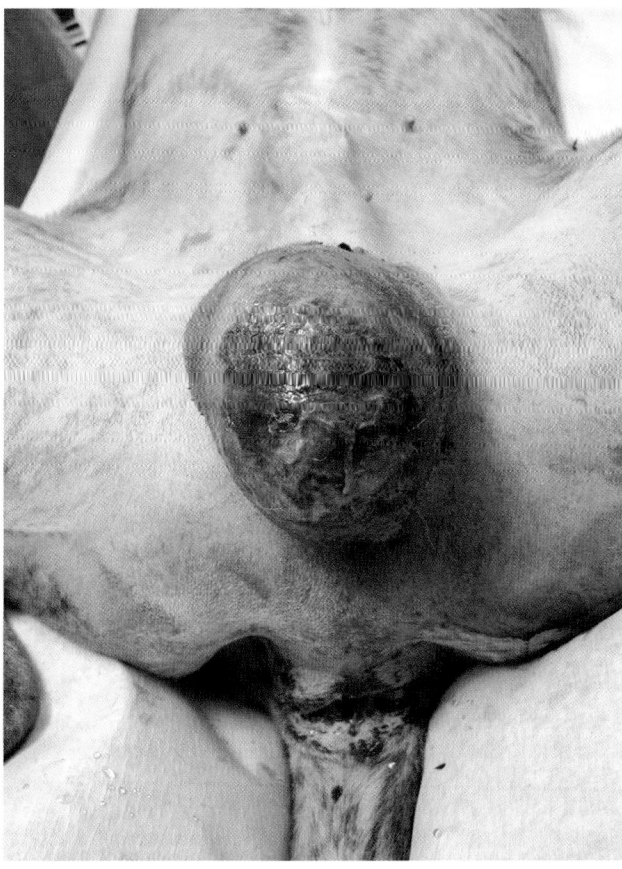

Figure 74.2 Extensive scrotal swelling leading to scrotal skin necrosis.

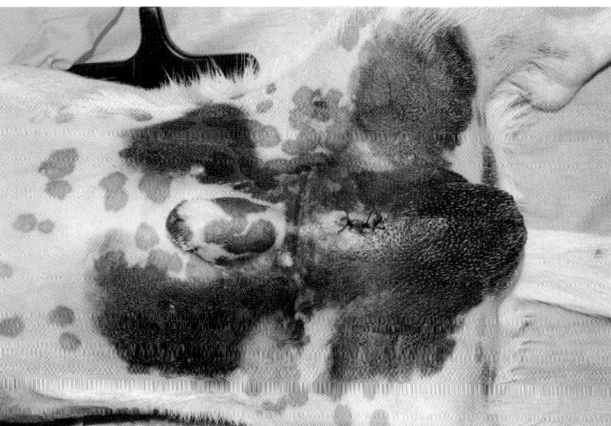

Figure 74.3 Ligature slippage resulting in bleeding from the spermatic cord. The minor scrotal hematoma but intense inguinal discoloration suggests location of the bleeding vessel close to the inguinal canal.

- Potential dead space is ablated by closing the subcutaneous layers with care taken to incorporate connective tissue surrounding the retractor penis muscle.
- Scrotal ablation may be preferred over prescrotal orchiectomy in older dogs.

Hemorrhage

Definition

Scrotal hemorrhage in cats may occur if testicular vessels tear during exposure or if the knot fails. Hemorrhage in dogs most often occurs from bleeding subcutaneous and septal vessels. Accumulation of blood in the scrotum leads to scrotal hematoma. Poorly ligated vascular pedicles can also result in scrotal hemorrhage, but additionally, they can retract through the inguinal canal and bleed intraabdominally.

Risk factors

- Ligature slippage in cats, resulting in unligated vessels, leads to surgical site hemorrhage but rarely causes significant intraabdominal bleeding.
- Performing an open castration has the risk of additional bleeding from vessels on the parietal vaginal tunic.
- When a closed castration is performed, retraction of the cremaster muscle can cause suture slippage.
- Trauma to penile cavernous tissue, during dissection for scrotal ablation or trauma of the periurethral tissue may lead to severe subcutaneous bleeding.

Diagnosis

- Scrotal hemorrhage in the cat causes bleeding from the surgical site.
- In dogs, it is clinically evident by a firm swelling of the scrotum (hematoma), the skin turns reddish purple, and a serosanguineous discharge from the incision line can be observed (Figure 74.3). Dogs are often uncomfortable.
- Intraabdominal hemorrhage can be suspected from serial hematocrit measurements, abdominal ultrasonography, or abdominocentesis.

Treatment

- Scrotal hemorrhage in cats is treated by enlarging the scrotal incision in an attempt to find the dropped vessel. Occasionally, it can be grasped blindly with a hemostat, but often the cord retracts enough to prevent retrieval. If the vessel cannot be found, conservative treatment is first initiated by placing firm pressure on the inguinal area and scrotal regions for 5 to 15 minutes. In combination with postoperative sedation, this often resolves the problem. If, however, significant anemia develops, the vessel should be located through an abdominal incision and ligated.
- Minor scrotal hemorrhage in dogs is often treated successfully with sedation and local pressure. Severe or continued scrotal hemorrhage requires revision surgery to ligate the bleeding cord and evacuate the hematoma. When a large scrotal hematoma is present, scrotal ablation is warranted to allow identification and ligation of the spermatic cords (Figure 74.4).
- Hemorrhage after orchiectomy in dogs may be serious, particularly if it occurs within the abdomen and goes unnoticed. Treatment consists of ligation of the bleeding spermatic cord, intravenous fluid therapy, and possibly blood transfusion. The intraabdominal spermatic cord is approached through a caudal median celiotomy or laparoscopic technique and ligated (suture), sealed (energy based device) or clamped (staples) (Koenraadt 2014).

Outcome

Patients with hemorrhage often respond to conservative management. Large scrotal hematomas should be resected by scrotal ablation. Intraabdominal bleeding, when left untreated, can be life threatening.

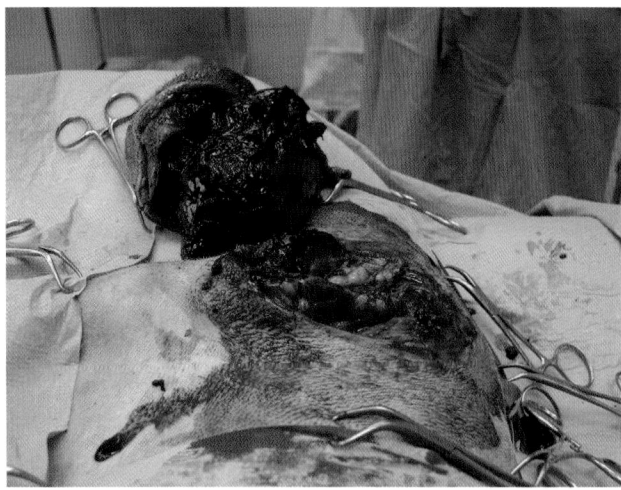

Figure 74.4 Scrotal ablation and removal of a large hematoma was needed to localize the bleeding vessel.

Prevention

- In dogs weighing less than 20 kg, a closed castration technique is used, thus avoiding hemorrhage from large blood vessels on the vaginal tunic.
- To avoid slippage, when the cremaster muscle contracts, the hemostatic ligature is transfixed through the spermatic cord with care taken not to perforate vascular structures.
- In dogs weighing more than 20 kg, an open castration technique is used because vascular ligations directly on the vessels are more secure.
- Whereas small spermatic cords are double ligated with encircling sutures of absorbable monofilament material, spermatic cords larger than 5 mm in diameter are ligated with at least one transfixing or encircling suture.
- Control during the release of the cord is important because the vessels shorten and dilate as tension on them is released. Any ligature slippage will probably occur at this time. If bleeding occurs, the vessels or cord can be immediately retrieved for further attention if it is still held by thumb forceps.

Surgical site inflammation and infection

Definition

Surgical site infection is the term used to prevent confusion between the infection of a surgical incision and the infection of a traumatic wound. Most surgical site infections are superficial, but even so, they contribute greatly to the morbidity and sometimes even mortality associated with surgery. Scrotal granulomas can be caused by large amounts of foreign material (long suture ends) or abundant necrotic tissue (Figure 74.5).

Risk factors

- When the scrotal skin incision in a cat is made too large, the vaginal tunic can prolapse through the open incision site, resulting in granuloma formation, and impaired second intention healing.
- Skin sutures that are placed too tight will attract the patient's attention and promote automutilation, resulting in premature suture removal.
- After prepubertal orchiectomy premature removal of skin sutures is a common complication. However, the frequency of surgical site infections is low.

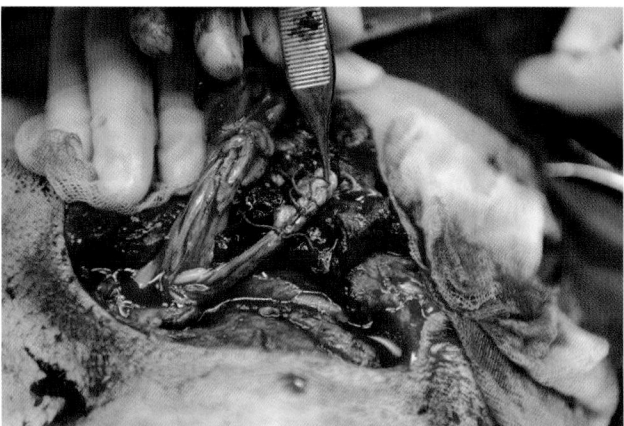

Figure 74.5 Scrotal incision and closure with interrupted cruciate sutures, resulting in complicated wound healing.

- Care should be taken to avoid incising the scrotal sac because this may result in severe edema of the scrotum and inflammation of the skin (Figure 74.6).

Diagnosis

Clinical signs of postoperative infection in cats might be indistinct, including anorexia and perineal pain. Infected surgical sites can be swollen and erythematous with variable degrees of wound dehiscence and drainage or accumulation of purulent material.

Treatment

Most cats respond to oral antibiotics and do not need additional wound drainage. A prolapsed vaginal tunic is treated by resection of the granuloma and debridement of the skin edges.

Limited areas of wound dehiscence are treated with antiseptic ointment and an Elizabethan collar and are left to heal by second intention. Antibiotics are indicated when systemic signs of infection are present (e.g., pyrexia). Infection after orchiectomy in dogs usually necessitates local irrigation and drainage and the institution of parenteral antimicrobial treatment. Revision surgery to shorten the spermatic cord and remove previous suture material in case of a granuloma is curative. Infected suture material should be removed to prevent persisting fistulae.

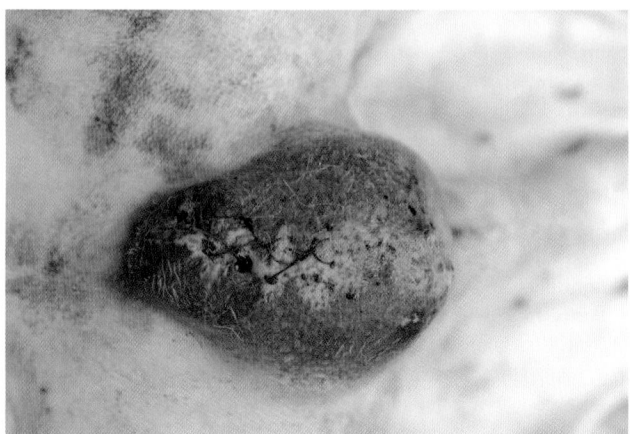

Figure 74.6 Scrotal granuloma caused by abundant suture material and necrotic tissue from the spermatic cord stump.

Outcome
Minor wound complications are treated by topical measures. Major wound abscessation or infection with multiresistant bacteria will require prolonged local (irrigation and drainage) and parenteral antimicrobial therapy.

Prevention
- The risk of infection is reduced by atraumatic and aseptic surgical technique and by closing all dead space.
- Closed castration in cats and limiting the length of the scrotal skin incision prevent prolapse of the vaginal tunic. Limiting the incision length too much, however, results in inadequate drainage and an increased chance of infection.
- Placement of intradermal sutures in prepubertal orchiectomy lowers the chance of premature suture removal by the patient.
- In adult dogs, knots from the subcutaneous suture line are buried and skin sutures are placed loosely or buried intradermally.
- After scrotal ablation all dead space must be carefully closed.
- Correctly sized resorbable monofilament suture material decreases the risk for suture related complications.

Urethral trauma

Definition
The anatomical presence of the urethra at the site of skin incision for prescrotal, scrotal ablation, or perineal orchiectomy can lead to iatrogenic urethral damage in case of inappropriate technique. Local bleeding or urinary leakage will result in wound healing complications.

Risk factors
- During the scrotal ablation technique, curvilinear incisions are made on both sides of the scrotum. Any trauma to the urethra must be avoided during this dissection.
- Because it is more difficult to displace the testes in a direction caudal to the scrotum, care should be taken not to damage the urethra when making the skin incision for a perineal orchiectomy.

Diagnosis
During micturition, urine might leak from the surgical wound (Figure 74.7). Extensive skin discoloration can be present because of urea-induced subcutaneous and dermal tissue damage. Urethral catheterization and flushing with saline or performing a retrograde urethrogram will confirm the diagnosis.

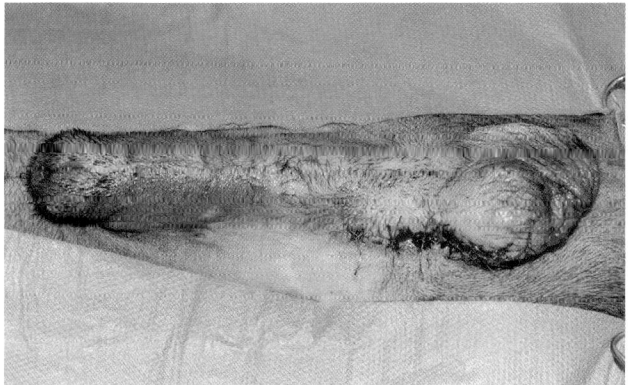

Figure 74.7 Complicated wound healing after inaccurate placement of the skin incision and perforation of the urethra.

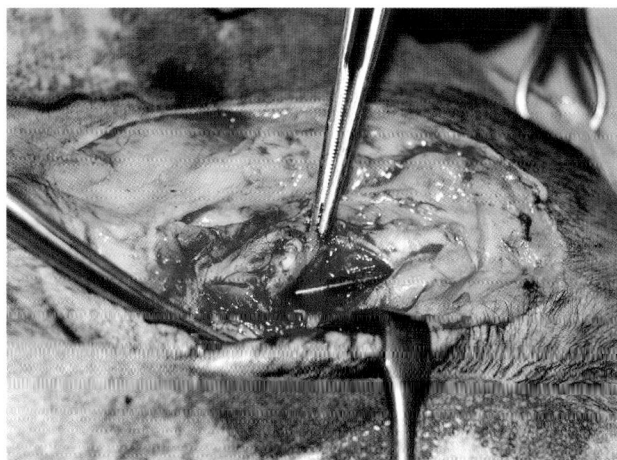

Figure 74.8 Resection of devitalized tissue and view of the defect of the urethral wall after inadvertent laceration during prescrotal orchiectomy.

Treatment
Minor damage to the urethra can often be repaired by suturing the urethra over a urinary catheter (Figure 74.8). When left unnoticed, the resulting inflammatory reaction and sometimes extensive skin reaction at the level of the prescrotal urethra will necessitate conversion to a scrotal urethrostomy. Perineal urethral damage is reconstructed when possible; failure to do so may lead to prepubic urethrostomy.

Outcome
Second intention healing or urethral reconstruction is successful in acute situations and when minimal trauma is present. Conversion to scrotal ablation and urethrostomy is sometimes necessary.

Prevention
- During the prescrotal orchiectomy technique, the testis is pushed cranially, and the skin incision and dissection of subcutaneous tissues is performed directly over the testis to protect the underlying urethra.
- Perineal orchiectomy patients should preoperatively receive a urinary catheter for easy identification of the urethra.

Complications associated with removal of cryptorchid testes

Definition
Retained testicles can be located in the prescrotal area, inguinal area, inguinal canal, and abdominal cavity. Removal of the retained testicle is recommended because of continued hormone production, increased risk for neoplasia, and testicular torsion.

Complications encountered after cryptorchid surgery include swelling, parapreputial seroma, wound dehiscence, infection, iatrogenic damage to the urethra, and even inadvertent prostatectomy (Figure 74.9).

Risk factors
- Swelling commonly occurs at the surgical site, particularly in active dogs that have undergone parapreputial incisions.
- When the surgical approach is too small, proper identification of the retained testicle is not possible, and continued blind exploration will result in iatrogenic damage.

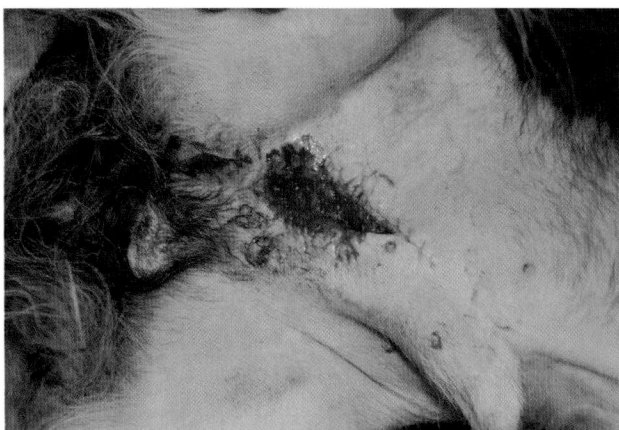

Figure 74.9 Wound dehiscence after infection of a parapreputial incision.

- The use of spay hooks to blindly locate a retained abdominal testicle has been associated with iatrogenic ureteral damage.

Diagnosis
- Cats with retained testes will continue to display penile barbs.
- Cryptorchid testes are frequently small, soft, and proportionally misshapen. Locating extraabdominal ectopic testes by palpation is not always possible. Large inguinal fat pads and the presence of the inguinal lymph node may obscure the testis.
- Ultrasonography is highly sensitive for detecting retained testes, particularly when they are neoplastic or located inguinally.
- Cryptorchidism can also be diagnosed by measuring increased blood testosterone concentrations after stimulation with gonadotropin-releasing hormone or human chorionic gonadotropin.
- Exploratory laparoscopy can visualize the inguinal ring to determine if the testicle has exited the abdomen.

Treatment
Parapreputial seromas can take several weeks to resorb spontaneously (Figure 74.10). Placement of an active drain will give sooner resolution. Wound dehiscence and infection are treated with local (debridement, topic antibiotic or antiseptic ointment) and, when indicated, systemic measures (parenteral antibiotics). Iatrogenic

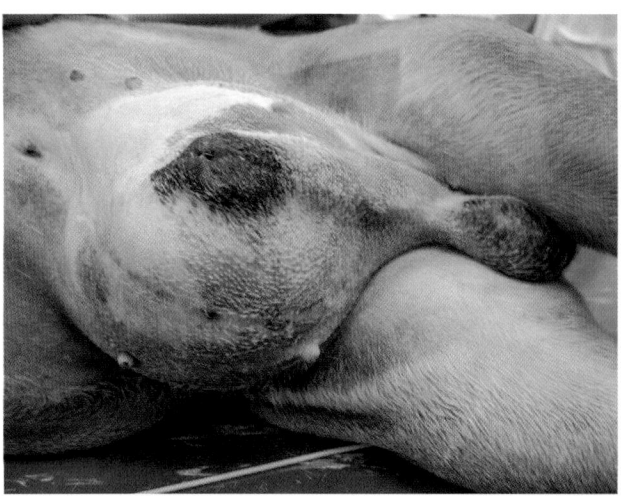

Figure 74.10 Development of a huge seroma after parapreputial surgery.

damage to the urethra requires fluid therapy in case of azotemia, abdominocentesis or drainage of the uroabdomen, and reconstructive surgery as soon as the patient is stable.

Outcome
Seromas can be left to resolve spontaneous or can be drained. Wound dehiscence and infection has a favorable prognosis when superficial. End-to-end anastomosis of the urethra after inadvertent prostatectomy does not lead to urinary incontinence in the absence of prostatic disease.

Prevention
- If a prepubertal pup or kitten is a unilateral or bilateral cryptorchid, it is advisable to delay orchiectomy until the testes can be palpated in the scrotum or until the animal is 5 to 8 months of age.
- The skin incision to remove an inguinal or prescrotal located ectopic testis is made directly over the testis.
- When the location of the testis is uncertain, the initial skin incision should be parapreputial in dogs and on the caudal ventral midline in cats. This allows examination of the superficial inguinal ring. If the testicle is not found, an abdominal incision is made.
- To limit seroma formation and steatitis, it is essential to avoid damage to the inguinal fat pad and to carefully prevent dead space during closure.

Relevant literature
The popularity of orchiectomy is reflected by an epidemiologic study in the United States that found 82% of all cats and 64% of dogs to be castrated (Trevejo *et al.* 2011).

Apart from numerous beneficial effects, which are often the reason for the procedure, gonadectomy may also have an unwanted impact on other conditions. In both dogs and cats, it is the most commonly reported risk factor for the development of obesity (10 times increased risk). It is, however, not a mandatory consequence and is prevented with an appropriate diet, feeding regimen, and exercise regimen (Robertson 2003). Epidemiologic studies have looked at the difference between castrated and intact dogs and have found castrated dogs to be at an increased risk for the development of prostatic neoplasms (2.4–4.3 times the risk), urinary tract transitional cell carcinoma (2–4 times the risk), osteosarcoma (1.3–2.0 times the risk), and both cardiac and splenic hemangiosarcoma (2.4 times the risk). Also, cranial cruciate ligament rupture, hypothyroidism, and urinary incontinence are more prevalent in gonadectomized dogs than in sexually intact dogs (Kustritz 2007). The cause and relation of these findings remains unclear.

The scrotal skin in dogs is thinner and therefore more susceptible to trauma or irritants than other skin. Scrotal contact dermatitis may already result from single contact with an antiseptic solution (Cerundolo and Maiolino 2002).

Surgical exploration of scrotal hemorrhage is reserved for severe or ongoing cases (Boothe 2003). One case report, however, describes the formation of an arteriovenous fistula after slippage of a single applied ligature in a closed orchiectomy. The conservatively managed scrotal hematoma allowed blood from the arteries to pass directly into the vein. Because the fistula gradually increased in size, surgical resection became necessary (Aiken *et al.* 1993).

To decrease patient morbidity, a mini-celiotomy was advocated to remove abdominal cryptorchid testes (Kirby 1980). The decreased visualization, however, resulted in several severe complications, including ureteral and urethral trauma caused by the use of a spay

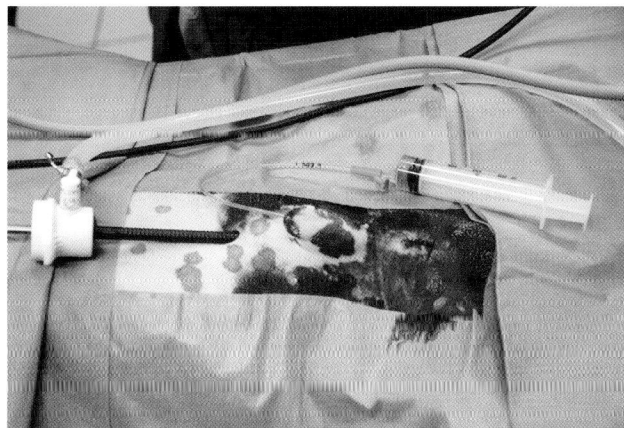

Figure 74.11 Laparoscopic exploration of the caudal abdomen and both inguinal rings to verify the site of bleeding. Introduction of a second instrument cannula allowed the placement of vascular clips on the hemorrhaging spermatic cord.

hook and one case of hemiprostatic urethral avulsion (Bellah *et al.* 1989). Another author described the inadvertent removal of the prostatic gland, instead of the ectopic testes, in four dogs (Schulz *et al.* 1996). Currently, minimal invasive surgery (laparoscopy) is the preferred technique because it offers all the advantages of a minimal laparotomy without the disadvantages of poor visibility and exposure of the abdomen (Miller *et al.* 2004). The same laparoscopic technique can also be used to explore the inguinal canal in case of intraabdominal or scrotal hemorrhage and to ligate the bleeding vessel (Figure 74.11).

Testicular tumors occur commonly in older dogs, especially in cryptorchid testes. Current prevalence at time of death is estimated at 27%, with 50% interstitial cell tumors, 42% seminomas, and 8% Sertoli cell tumors (Grieco *et al.* 2008). Dogs with testicular neoplasia should be properly staged and monitored for myelotoxicity, particularly if anemia or feminization is present.

Myelotoxicity usually resolves within 2 to 3 weeks after tumor removal but can also be fatal despite appropriate therapy (Sontas *et al.* 2009).

References

Aiken, S.W., Jakovljevic, S., Lantz, G.C., et al. (1993) Acquired arteriovenous fistula secondary to castration in a dog. *Journal of the American Veterinary Medical Association* 202 (6), 965-967.

Bellah, J.R., Spencer, C.P., Salmeri, K.R. (1989) Hemiprostatic urethral avulsion during cryptorchid orchiectomy in a dog. *Journal of the American Animal Hospital Association* 25, 553-556.

Boothe, H.W. (2003) Testes and epididymis. In Slatter, D. (ed.) *Textbook of Small Animal Surgery*, 3rd edn. Saunders, Philadelphia, pp. 1521-1530.

Cerundolo, R., Maiolino, P. (2002) Cutaneous lesions of the canine scrotum. *Veterinary Dermatology* 13, 63–66.

Crane, S.W. (1998) Orchiectomy of descended and retained testes in the dog and cat. In Bojrab, M.J. (ed.) *Current Techniques in Small Animal Surgery*, 4th edn. Williams & Wilkins, Baltimore, pp. 517-523.

Grieco, V., Riccardi, E. Greppi, G.F., et al. (2008) Canine testicular tumours: a study on 232 dogs. *Journal of Comparative Pathology* 138, 86-89.

Hedlund, C.S. (2007) Surgery of the reproductive and genital systems In Fossum, T.W. (ed.) *Small Animal Surgery*, 3rd edn. Mosby, St. Louis, pp. 714-729.

Kirby, F.D. (1980) A technique for castrating the cryptorchid dog or cat. *Veterinary Medicine* 75 (4), 632.

Kustritz, M.V. (2007) Determining the optimal age for gonadectomy of dogs and cats. *Journal of the American Veterinary Medical Association* 11, 1665-1675.

Koenraadt, A., Stegen, L., Bosmans, T., et al. (2014) Laparoscopic treatment of persistent inguinal haemorrhage after prescrotal orchiectomy in a dog. *Journal of Small Animal Practice* 55(8), 427-430.

Miller, N.A., Van Lue, S.J., Rawlings, C.A. (2004) Use of laparoscopic-assisted cryptorchidectomy in dogs and cats. *Journal of the American Veterinary Medical Association* 6, 875-878.

Robertson, I.D. (2003) The association of exercise, diet and other factors with owner-perceived obesity in privately owned dogs from metropolitan Perth, WA. *Preventive Veterinary Medicine* 58, 75-83.

Schulz, K.S., Waldron, D.R., Smith, M.M., et al. (1996) Inadvertent prostatectomy as a complication of cryptorchidectomy in four dogs. *Journal of the American Animal Hospital Association* 32 (3), 211-214.

Sontas, H.B., Dokuzeylu, B., Turna, O., et al. (2009) Estrogen-induced myelotoxicity in dogs: A review. *Canadian Veterinary Journal* 50 (10), 1054-1058.

Trevejo, R., Yang, M., Lund, E.M. (2011) Epidemiology of surgical castration of dogs and cats in the United States. *Journal of the American Veterinary Medical Association* 238, 898-904.

Prostatic Cyst and Abscess Drainage

Henry L'Eplattenier
VRCC Veterinary Referrals, Laindon, Essex, UK

Cavitary lesions of the prostate include prostatic cysts, paraprostatic cysts, and abscesses. Small cysts are often seen in conjunction with benign prostate hyperplasia (BPH) and are usually not clinically significant. Larger cysts can be caused by retention of prostatic fluid secondary to occlusion of secretory ducts in dogs with BPH or squamous metaplasia of the prostate induced by estrogens. Paraprostatic cysts have no connection to the parenchyma of the prostate and are attached to the prostatic capsule (Freitag *et al.* 2007). The pathophysiological mechanism of the formation of large prostatic cysts and paraprostatic cysts is not entirely clear (Basinger 2003).

Prostatic abscesses develop either as a consequence of prostatitis or if prostatic cysts become infected (Freitag *et al.* 2007). Dogs with prostatic abscesses are usually systemically ill and can show signs of lethargy, fever, and anorexia (Basinger 2003). Treatment should not be delayed and should include aggressive fluid therapy, intravenous (IV) antibiotherapy, and surgery to avoid the risk of peritonitis, sepsis, and shock.

Surgical treatment of cavitary lesions of the prostate include marsupialization (Basinger 2003), percutaneous drainage under ultrasonographic control (Boland *et al.* 2003), and omentalization during celiotomy (White and Williams 1995; Bray *et al.* 1997; White 2000; Basinger 2003; Freitag *et al.* 2007). Marsupialization involves the formation of a stoma in the wall of the caudal abdomen to allow drainage of the contents. Because of postoperative morbidity, more frequent complications, and the need for a second surgical procedure to close the stoma, this procedure is now rarely used, and the current procedure of choice for management of cavitary lesions of the prostate is omentalization (Freitag *et al.* 2007). Omentalization of the prostate is performed via a caudal midline celiotomy. The cysts or abscesses are incised on either side of the prostate, the cavities are drained, and separations between cavities are broken down digitally to ensure that all fluid is removed from the prostate. Then all cavities are copiously flushed with sterile saline, and finally the omentum is pulled through the prostate (if necessary around the urethra) and sutured to the prostatic capsule (White and Williams 1995; Bray *et al.* 1997; Freitag *et al.* 2007).

Systemic complications

Definition

Peritonitis, sepsis, shock, and death are complications in the surgical treatment of prostatic abscesses. Septic peritonitis, sepsis, and shock caused by rupture of a prostatic abscess were present in one third of the 92 dogs included in one study (Mullen *et al.* 1990), and the mortality rate was 21%. The organisms most commonly reported to cause suppurative prostatitis and prostatic abscesses are *Escherichia coli* and occasionally *Staphylococcus* spp. and *Proteus* spp. Contamination of the peritoneal cavity with bacteria causes a cascade of events leading to septic peritonitis. Cytokines such as interleukin-1 and tumor necrosis factor-α are released and initiate many events, leading to the mobilization of polymorphonuclear leukocytes and an increase in vascular permeability and vasodilatation, which in turn cause fluid and albumin to accumulate in the peritoneal cavity. As albumin decreases in the intravascular space, more fluid moves into the extravascular space because of the reduced oncotic pressure. The resulting reduction in circulating blood volume leads to decreased cardiac output and poor tissue perfusion associated with shock. In addition, sepsis may be associated with coagulation abnormalities characterized by a procoagulant state combined with decreased fibrinolytic activity, leading to disseminated intravascular coagulation and the formation of microvascular thromboemboli, which can further reduce tissue perfusion. If left untreated, these processes can lead to multiple-organ dysfunction syndrome (MODS), which includes respiratory distress, pulmonary thromboembolism, pleural effusion, renal failure, gastrointestinal hypoperfusion, vomiting, diarrhea, and neurologic infarction (Culp and Holt 2010).

Risk factors

Septic peritonitis can either be caused by the rupture of a prostatic abscess before surgery or can result from severe contamination of the peritoneal cavity with pus from the prostate during surgery. However, severe complications associated with sepsis and MODS can still develop even after removal of the source of infection.

Diagnosis

- Peritonitis should be suspected in animals that are depressed and lethargic after surgery and animals that are cardiovascularly unstable.
- The diagnosis of septic peritonitis after surgery for prostatic abscess is centered on ultrasonography to confirm presence of peritoneal effusion and analysis of peritoneal fluid. The presence of increased numbers of neutrophils ($>10,000 \times 10^6$/L) and macrophages with intra- or extracellular bacteria is indicative of septic peritonitis. Neutrophils may look degenerate (cell or nuclear swelling, nuclear fragmentation, eosinophilic nuclear chromatin) (Culp and Holt 2010) (Figure 75.1).

Complications in Small Animal Surgery, First Edition. Edited by Dominique Griffon and Annick Hamaide.
© 2016 John Wiley & Sons, Inc. Published 2016 by John Wiley & Sons, Inc.
Companion website: www.wiley.com/go/griffon/complications

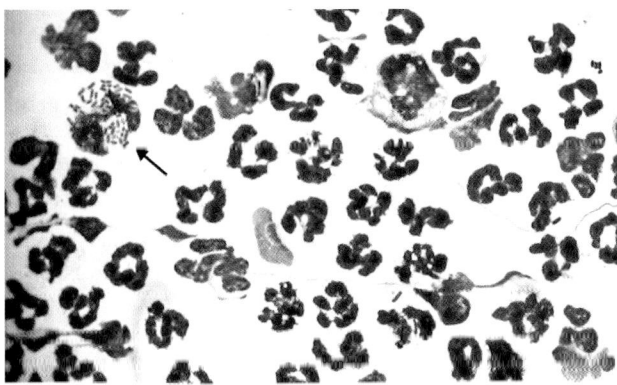

Figure 75.1 Septic peritonitis. Cytology of abdominal fluid showing large numbers of neutrophils and macrophages, including some with intracellular bacteria (arrow). *Source:* Courtesy of Laurent Findji.

- The concentration of glucose and lactate in the blood and the peritoneal fluid can be compared to confirm the presence of peritonitis as shown in Table 75.1 (Bonczynski *et al.* 2003).
- Packed cell volume, total protein and albumin, electrolytes, and coagulation parameters (prothrombin time, partial thromboplastin time, thrombocyte count) should be determined in septic patients because these parameters may require corrective treatment as part of management.

Treatment
- Septic patients should be managed with aggressive IV fluid therapy, including transfusion of blood products (e.g., fresh-frozen plasma or whole blood) in cases of severe hypoalbuminemia and coagulation abnormalities.
- Broad-spectrum antibiotics should be administered intravenously. If culture and sensitivity test results are not known, empirical therapy should be initiated combining, for example, a penicillin with a fluoroquinolone (Culp and Holt 2010).
- If peritonitis was already present before surgery for prostatic abscess, the abdomen should be copiously flushed with several liters of sterile saline during surgery. All fluid should be removed using an appropriate suction device.
- Open peritoneal drainage should be considered because it allows effective removal of remaining peritoneal fluid and creates an environment where anaerobic bacteria are less likely to prosper. Disadvantages of open abdominal drainage include the requirement for postoperative monitoring and support in an intensive care unit, the possible evisceration of abdominal organs, the risk of nosocomial infections, and excessive fluid and protein loss.
- Enteral nutrition should be resumed as soon as possible postoperatively to meet the enormous metabolic needs of the patients, including the massive loss of protein into the peritoneal fluid. If necessary, an esophagostomy or gastrostomy tube should be placed.
- See Chapter 4 for a detailed review of the treatment of septic peritonitis

Table 75.1 Comparison of peritoneal fluid and peripheral blood

Glucose	Peritoneal fluid	<	Peripheral blood	Difference ≥20
Lactate		>		Difference ≥2.0 mmol/L

Outcome
In one study of 92 dogs with prostatic abscessation treated with multiple Penrose drains, 18 of 29 dogs that developed septic peritonitis and shock died or were euthanized in the immediate postoperative period (Mullen *et al.* 1990), indicating a mortality rate of 62% for this complication. In another study of 19 dogs treated with omentalization of prostatic abscesses, only one dog presented with septic peritonitis before surgery and was successfully managed with open peritoneal drainage (White and Williams 1995). No dogs developed peritonitis postoperatively.

Prevention
- To prevent rupture of a prostatic abscess and development of a septic peritonitis, surgery to drain and omentalize the abscess should be undertaken without delay.
- During surgery, moistened laparotomy sponges should be placed around the prostate to contain any leakage of prostatic fluid.
- The prostate should be carefully examined, and all fluid-filled pockets should be opened (using blunt or digital dissection) and appropriately emptied using a suction device to avoid subsequent contamination of the peritoneal cavity.
- If contamination has occurred, lavage of the peritoneal cavity with copious amounts of sterile saline is necessary.

Peripheral edema

Definition
Swelling and edema can develop in the hindlimbs, inguinal area, and scrotum as a consequence of prostatic abscesses and after prostatic surgery. The problems can be exacerbated by hypoproteinemia secondary to septic peritonitis, which causes a low oncotic pressure or can be caused by obstruction of vascular or lymphatic vessels.

Risk factors
- Hypoproteinemia secondary to septic peritonitis
- Extensive enlargement of the prostate causing reduced venous and lymphatic return from the hind limbs.

Treatment, outcome, and prevention
No specific treatment is required, and the problems usually subside after the initiating factor has resolved. Hypoproteinemia is managed with a combination of fluid therapy, transfusion of blood products, and early nutrition support, as discussed under Systemic complications.

Prostatic abscess or cyst recurrence

Definition
Drainage and omentalization of prostatic cysts and abscesses does not always resolve the problem completely, and there are cases in which cysts or abscesses can reappear. Recurrence can occur as soon as a few days after the original operation and up to more than 1 year later.

Risk factors
- Inadequate drainage of fluid from the prostate
- Incomplete breakdown of all fluid-filled cavities in the prostate
- Persistence of underlying prostate pathology (BPH, prostatitis)

Diagnosis

The most effective way of diagnosing recurrence of abscesses and cysts is by ultrasound scan of the prostate. A first ultrasound recheck should be performed 3 to 5 days after surgery to diagnose short-term recurrence. Then a second scan about 1 month after surgery is recommended. In the absence of clinical signs, a routine ultrasound scan should be performed every 3 to 4 months for the first year.

Treatment

- Recurrent cysts and abscesses are treated by redraining them. If possible, partial prostatectomy and removal of larger portions of the abscess or cyst walls can improve drainage of the fluid and enlarge the contact area provided by omentalization (Figure 75.2).
- Antibiotic treatment should be adapted to the results of culture and sensitivity and continued for an extended period of time (usually 4 weeks after discharge from the hospital).

Outcome

With adequate surgical and medical treatment, recurrence of abscesses and cysts usually resolves after the second surgical procedure. When abscesses and cysts are emptied by ultrasound-guided percutaneous drainage, recurrence is more frequent, and multiple (up to four) drainage procedures are often necessary, but long-term resolution can be obtained (Boland *et al.* 2003).

Prevention

- Thorough exploration of the prostate parenchyma to discover and drain all pockets of fluid: Use of hypodermic needles and syringes to probe the prostatic parenchyma can aid in detecting any residual fluid-filled cavities.
- Appropriate antibiotic treatment based on results of culture and sensitivity and of appropriate duration (at least 4 weeks)
- Choice of antibiotic with sufficient penetration into the prostatic parenchyma (e.g., trimethoprim–sulfamethoxazole, quinolones)

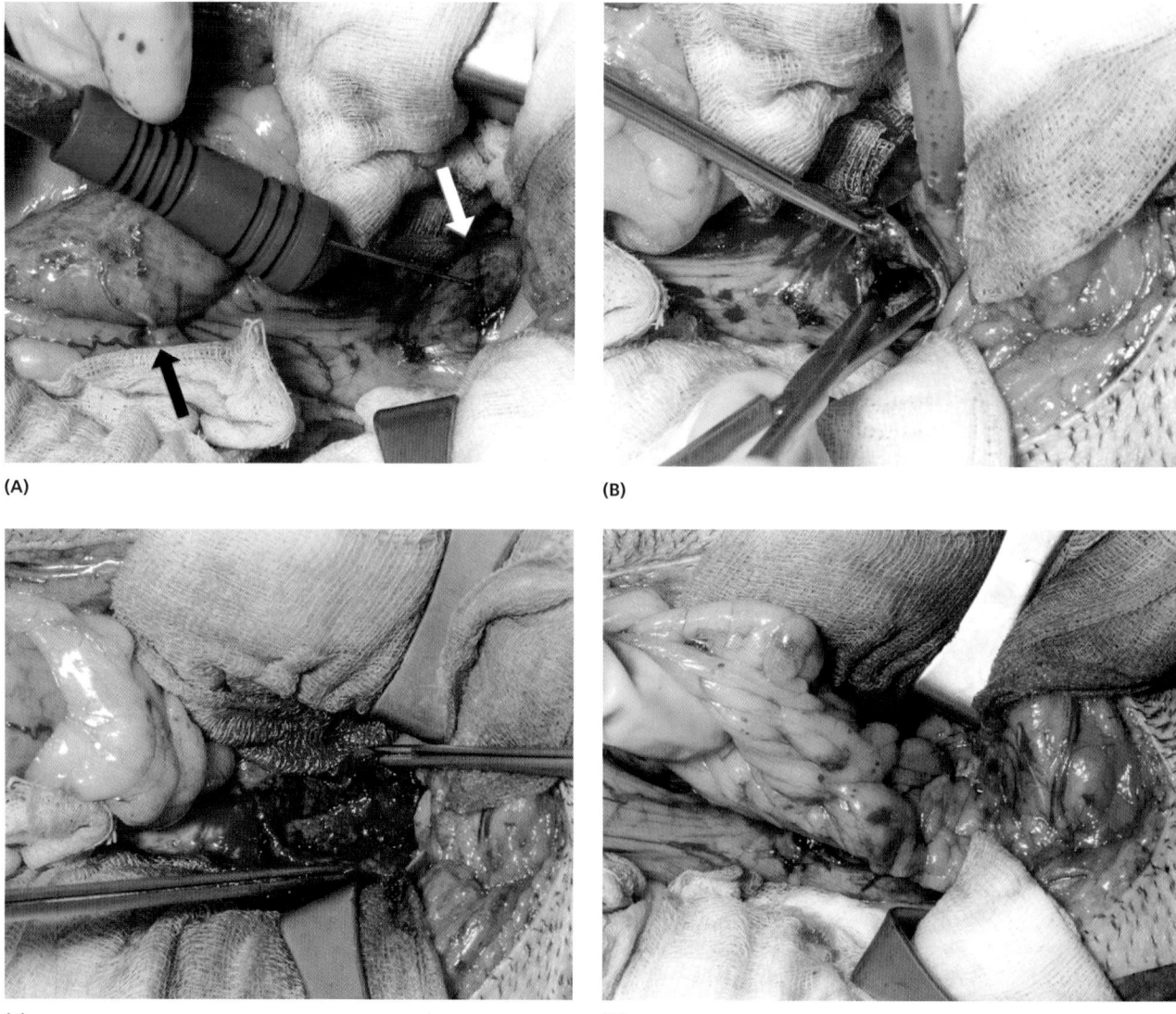

(A)

(B)

(C)

(D)

Figure 75.2 Cyst resection and omentalization. **A,** Intraoperative photographs showing the prostate (white arrow) and the bladder (black arrow). Fluid is being aspirated from a cyst in the prostate using a hypodermic needle attached to a surgical suction device. **B,** Dissection and removal of the wall of the cyst. **C,** Most of the cyst wall has been removed to allow maximum contact of the omentum with the prostate parenchyma. **D,** Omentum has been placed over the prostate parenchyma and maintained in place with sutures.

- Castration or initiation of medical treatment at the time of surgery to induce involution of the prostate and resolution of underlying conditions (e.g., BPH)

Urinary incontinence

Definition
Urinary incontinence is a clinical sign characterized by unconscious leakage of urine out of the urethra. Incontinence is sometimes dependent on the position of the dog (e.g., exacerbated in lateral recumbency). Incontinence is caused either by the inability of the bladder sphincter successfully close the bladder during the filling and storage phase or by bladder atony whereby the bladder is unable to empty completely and the overfilled bladder overflows, allowing urine to leak. It is important to distinguish between these two situations because their medical management is different.

Risk factors
The integrity of the innervation to the bladder trigone and prostatic urethra is necessary to maintain normal bladder and urethral sphincter function. The hypogastric, pelvic, and pudendal nerves divide into multiple branches as they approach the bladder neck and prostate, forming a nervous plexus, which is located within the lateral umbilical ligament, dorsolaterally on either side of the bladder and prostate. With cysts or abscesses located in this dorsolateral area of the prostate, the risk of iatrogenic damage to the neural supply to the bladder neck is increased. It has also been suggested that chronic traction of very large prostatic cysts on the prostate and bladder neck can compromise neural components of the bladder neck and cause postoperative urinary incontinence (Bray et al. 1997).

Some dogs are continent immediately after surgery but develop urinary incontinence several months after surgery, suggesting that postoperative incontinence is not always directly related to the surgical procedure.

Diagnosis
- Differentiation of urethral sphincter incompetence and overflow incontinence can made by palpation or catheterization of the bladder after voiding. If there is a large volume of residual urine in the bladder or if the bladder is permanently distended without the dog attempting to void, incontinence is related to bladder atony and caused by urine overflowing. If necessary, an ultrasound scan can confirm the degree of bladder filling.
- Urinalysis including culture and sensitivity is recommended in all cases of urinary incontinence because incontinence can predispose the urinary tract to infection, and, inversely, urinary tract infection (UTI) can exacerbate urinary incontinence.
- Urethral pressure profiles and electromyography may help identify the underlying cause of urinary incontinence (Gookin et al. 1996).

Treatment
- Medical treatment for urethral sphincter incompetence consists of α-adrenergic drugs such as phenylpropanolamine (1-1.5 mg/kg p.o. every 8-12 hours)
- Medical treatment for bladder atony consists of cholinergic drugs such as bethanechol chloride (5-25 mg/dog p.o. every 8 hours) or carbachol (0.03 mg/kg p.o. every 8 hours). An indwelling urinary catheter attached to a closed urine collection system helps keep the bladder empty and prevents over-distention of the bladder wall.

- Antibiotics are used to control UTI based on the results of urine culture and sensitivity tests.

Outcome
The outcome is directly related to the damage caused to the innervations of the bladder trigone and prostate. Whereas treatment of prostatic abscesses with drain placement caused long-term persistence of incontinence in 25% of dogs (Mullen et al. 1989), omentalization of prostatic abscesses and cysts did not cause any long-term incontinence, and all dogs that were incontinent postoperatively were successfully managed medically or the incontinence resolved without treatment (White and Williams 1995; Bray et al. 1997).

Prevention
Avoiding damage to the dorsolateral portion of the prostate and lateral umbilical ligaments during surgery is the single most important factor in preventing postoperative urinary incontinence (Glennon and Flanders 1993).

Urinary retention

Definition
Urinary retention is the inability to void urine caused by atony of the bladder wall. An inability of the detrusor muscle to contract can be combined with malfunction of afferent pathways triggering the voiding reflex when the bladder is full. Therefore, the dog makes no attempts to urinate even though the bladder is very full.

Risk factors
- Similar to urinary incontinence, iatrogenic damage to the innervations of the bladder trigone will increase the risk of bladder atony.
- Urinary retention can also be a complication of epidural anesthesia using long-lasting local anesthetic agents or opioids (Baldini et al. 2009).

Diagnosis
- History of absent attempts to urinate
- Physical examination revealing an overdistended bladder on abdominal palpation with or without overflow incontinence
- Catheterization of the bladder is easy, ruling out mechanical urethral obstruction and reveals a large volume of residual urine in the bladder.
- Ultrasound scan revealing an overdistended bladder
- Urinalysis, including culture and sensitivity, is recommended in cases of urinary retention because the presence of large amounts of residual urine in the bladder can predispose to the development of UTIs.
- Urethral pressure profiles and cystometry may help identify bladder atony (Gookin et al. 1996).

Treatment
- Medical treatment for bladder atony consists of cholinergic drugs such as bethanechol chloride (5–25 mg/dog orally [PO] every 8 hours) or carbachol (0.03 mg/kg PO every 8 hours). An indwelling urinary catheter attached to a closed urine collection system helps keep the bladder empty and prevents overdistention of the bladder wall.
- Antibiotics are used to control UTI based on the results of urine culture and sensitivity tests.

Outcome

The outcome is directly related to the damage caused to the innervations of the bladder trigone and prostate. Treatment of prostatic cysts with omentalization only caused short-term urinary retention, which responded well to medical management (White and Williams 1995; Bray *et al.* 1997).

Prevention

See Urinary incontinence.

Relevant literature

The treatment of cavitary lesions of the prostate by omentalization reduces the period of hospitalization and postoperative care and is associated with fewer complications than other surgical techniques such as marsupialization and drainage with dependant Penrose drains. Omentalization is therefore now recommended as surgical treatment of choice for prostatic abscesses and cysts (White and Williams 1995; Bray *et al.* 1997; White 2000; Basinger 2003; Freitag *et al.* 2007). Most notably, the incidence of **systemic complications,** including perioperative death from sepsis, is markedly lower. In a study of 92 dogs with prostatic abscesses treated with multiple Penrose drains, 33% of dogs developed septic shock after surgery. Three dogs died during surgery, and 15 others were euthanized in the immediate postoperative period as a result of sepsis (16.3% mortality rate) (Mullen *et al.* 1990). Although patient numbers are smaller, two studies describing omentalization did not show any perioperative deaths. In a study of 19 dogs with prostatic abscesses, only one dog (5.2%) had septic peritonitis secondary to preoperative rupture of the prostatic abscess. This dog was successfully managed with abdominal lavage and open peritoneal drainage (White and Williams 1995). Direct comparison between these studies should be undertaken with care because differences in mortality rates can reflect differences in the population of patients studied (e.g., percentage of dogs with preoperative abscess rupture) as well as improvement in the diagnosis and management of serious systemic complications (e.g., use of open peritoneal drainage). In a study describing omentalization for the management of prostatic cysts in 18 dogs, none of the patients developed any systemic complications (Bray *et al.* 1997).

Edema of the hind limbs, scrotum, or inguinal area is reported as a complication regardless of the surgical technique used to manage prostatic abscesses (Mullen *et al.* 1990; White and Williams 1995). Edema is presumably caused by obstruction of the lymphatic flow or venous return and resolves without any specific treatment (White and Williams 1995).

Recurrence of the abscess or cyst is more common when treated with ultrasound-guided percutaneous drainage only compared with surgical drainage. In one study, 6 of 13 dogs treated with ultrasound-guided percutaneous drainage required more than one procedure, and some dogs required up to four (Boland *et al.* 2003). Of 19 dogs with abscesses treated with omentalization, only 1 (5%) developed a recurrence (White and Williams 1995). This compares very positively with techniques used previously because treatment of prostatic abscesses with multiple dependent Penrose drains was reported to carry an 18% rate of recurrence (Mullen *et al.* 1990). Of 18 dogs treated with omentalization for prostatic cysts, none developed recurrence of the cysts (Bray *et al.* 1997). These results confirm the superiority of the technique of omentalization of prostatic

cysts and abscesses. Because of the characteristics of the omentum (lymphatic drainage, induction of local vascularization, phagocytic function and removal of bacterial contamination, promotion of local adhesions) (Bray *et al.* 1997; White 2000), the risk of recurrence of abscesses and cysts can best be prevented by maximizing the surface of omentum placed into the cyst or abscess to be drained.

Similar to other postoperative complications, the incidence of **urinary incontinence** is also reported to be lower when prostatic cysts and abscesses are treated with omentalization compared with placement of Penrose drains or marsupialization. Incontinence occurred postoperatively in 16.6% of dogs with prostatic cysts treated with omentalization (Bray *et al.* 1997) and in 5% of dogs with prostatic abscesses treated with omentalization (White and Williams 1995). In all dogs, incontinence resolved spontaneously or after treatment. In dogs with prostatic abscesses treated with Penrose drains, long-term urinary incontinence remained a problem in 25% of dogs (Mullen *et al.* 1989); however, with more careful placement of the drains to avoid damaging the innervations of the bladder trigone and prostate, the same technique was shown to cause only short-term incontinence and in only 17.6% of dogs (Glennon and Flanders 1993).

Urinary retention is an uncommon complication reported only in one dog in one study (Bray *et al.* 1997). In this study, it represented a 5% incidence. The complication was only seen in the immediate postoperative period and responded to medical management.

References

Baldini, G., Bagry, H., Aprikian, A., et al. (2009) Postoperative urinary retention: anesthetic and perioperative considerations. *Anesthesiology* 110, 1139-1157.

Basinger, R.R., Robinette, C.L., Hardie, E.M., et al. (2003) Prostate. In Slatter, D. (ed.) *Textbook of Small Animal Surgery*, 3rd edn. Saunders, Philadelphia, pp. 1542-1557.

Boland, L.E., Hardie, R.J., Gregory, S.P., et al. (2003) Ultrasound-guided percutaneous drainage as the primary treatment for prostatic abscesses and cysts in dogs. *Journal of the American Animal Hospital Association* 39, 151-159.

Bonczynski, J.J., Ludwig, L.L., Barton, L.J., et al. (2003) Comparison of peritoneal fluid and peripheral blood pH, bicarbonate, glucose, and lactate concentration as a diagnostic tool for septic peritonitis in dogs and cats. *Veterinary Surgery* 32, 161-166.

Bray, J.P., White, R.A., Williams, J.M. (1997) Partial resection and omentalization: a new technique for management of prostatic retention cysts in dogs. *Veterinary Surgery* 26, 202-209.

Culp, W.T.N., Holt, D.E. (2010) Septic peritonitis. *Compendium of Continuing Education for the Practicing Veterinarian* 32, E1-E15.

Freitag, T., Jerram, R.M., Walker, A.M., et al. (2007) Surgical management of common canine prostatic conditions. *Compendium of Continuing Education for the Practicing Veterinarian* 29, 656-658, 660, 662-663 passim; quiz 673.

Glennon, J.C., Flanders, J.A. (1993) Decreased incidence of postoperative urinary incontinence with a modified Penrose drain technique for treatment of prostatic abscesses in dogs. *The Cornell Veterinarian* 83, 189-198.

Gookin, J.L., Stone, E.A., Sharp N.J. (1996) Urinary incontinence in dogs and cats. Part II. Diagnosis and management. *Compendium of Continuing Education for the Practicing Veterinarian* 18 (5), 525-540.

Mullen, H.S., Matthiesen, D.T., Scavelli, T. (1989) Abscessation of the prostate gland treated with a multiple drain technique: an evaluation of postoperative complications and long-term results in 92 dogs. *Veterinary Surgery* 18, 70-71.

Mullen, H.S., Matthiesen, D.T., Scavelli, T.D. (1990) Results of surgery and postoperative complications in 92 dogs treated for prostatic abscessation by a multiple Penrose drain technique. *Journal of the American Animal Hospital Association* 26, 369-379.

White, R.A. (2000) Prostatic surgery in the dog. *Clinical Techniques in Small Animal Practice* 15, 46-51.

White, R.A., Williams, J.M. (1995) Intracapsular prostatic omentalization: a new technique for management of prostatic abscesses in dogs. *Veterinary Surgery* 24, 390-395.

76 Prostatectomy

Henry L'Eplattenier
VRCC Veterinary Referrals, Laindon, Essex, UK

Prostatectomy can be either total or partial. Total prostatectomy is rarely performed because it is a technically demanding procedure (White 2000; Freitag *et al.* 2007) and commonly results in postoperative complications, including death (Vlasin *et al.* 2006) and urinary incontinence (Basinger *et al.* 1989; Goldsmid and Bellenger 1991). Total prostatectomy is indicated for selected cases of prostatic tumors that are small and confined to the prostatic parenchyma (Liptak 2010).

Partial prostatectomy can be performed as part of the surgical procedure to manage prostatic abscesses and cysts or as a palliative treatment for prostatic carcinoma. Various techniques of partial prostatectomy for the treatment of prostatic abscesses and cysts have been described. These include partial prostatectomy using a Nd:YAG (neodymium-doped yttrium aluminium garnet) laser (Hardie *et al.* 1990) and intracapsular subtotal prostatectomy using electrocoagulation (Harari and Dupuis 1995) or an ultrasonic aspirator (Rawlings *et al.* 1994; Rawlings *et al.* 1997). Partial prostatectomy techniques for the treatment of prostate carcinoma include transurethral resection using an electrosurgical loop (Liptak *et al.* 2004) and intracapsular subtotal prostatectomy using either an Nd:YAG laser (L'Eplattenier *et al.* 2006) or electrocautery (Vlasin *et al.* 2006). In dogs, all prostatic tumors reported are malignant, and the majority have been reported to be adenocarcinomas (Theilen and Madewell 1979; Cooley and Waters 2001). In some cases, transitional cell carcinomas are seen originating from the collecting ducts of the prostate. Canine prostate carcinomas are very malignant tumors, and metastases are commonly present at the time of diagnosis. The main sites of metastatic spread are the sublumbar lymph nodes lungs and skeletal system, particularly the lumbar vertebrae, pelvis, and femur (Bell *et al.* 1991; Cornell *et al.* 2000). Therefore, partial prostatectomy alone is only a palliative procedure when used for the management of prostatic neoplasia, and further treatment is necessary to control both local recurrence and metastatic spread of the tumor. Techniques described to try to control local progression of the disease and used in conjunction with partial prostatectomy include radiotherapy (Liptak *et al.* 2004), local injections of interleukin-2 (IL-2) (L'Eplattenier *et al.* 2006), and photodynamic therapy (L'Eplattenier *et al.* 2008).

Systemic complications

Definition

Serious systemic complications such as uncontrolled bleeding, shock, acute renal failure, and hypoproteinemia have been reported after both partial and total prostatectomy procedures for the treatment of prostate cancer. In the studies in which such complications were reported, they led to death or euthanasia of the patients within the first 2 weeks after surgery (L'Eplattenier *et al.* 2006; Vlasin *et al.* 2006). Intraoperative hemostasis is a challenge regardless of the technique used, and particularly larger blood vessels located in the prostatic capsule can be difficult to ligate or cauterize.

In addition, when prostatectomy is performed as a treatment for prostatic abscesses, septic peritonitis and septic shock can develop as described in Chapter 75.

Risk factors
- Inadequate hemostasis during surgery
- Preexisting clotting disorder such as disseminated intravascular coagulation (DIC)

Diagnosis
- Regular physical examination, including temperature, respiration rate, heart rate, pulse quality, blood pressure, mucous membranes, and capillary filling time
- Laboratory tests, including packed cell volume, total protein, albumin, kidney parameters, electrolytes, clotting parameters, and thrombocyte count
- Imaging of the caudal abdomen to detect evidence of continued hemorrhage (usually with an ultrasound scan)

Treatment
- Aggressive intravenous fluid therapy to ensure cardiovascular stability and correct electrolyte disturbances
- Transfusion of blood products: whole blood, plasma or packed red blood cells, depending on the requirement for platelets, clotting factors or red blood cells, respectively, and for the correction of hypoproteinemia
- Medical treatment of acute kidney failure if present

Complications in Small Animal Surgery, First Edition. Edited by Dominique Griffon and Annick Hamaide.
© 2016 John Wiley & Sons, Inc. Published 2016 by John Wiley & Sons, Inc.
Companion website: www.wiley.com/go/griffon/complications

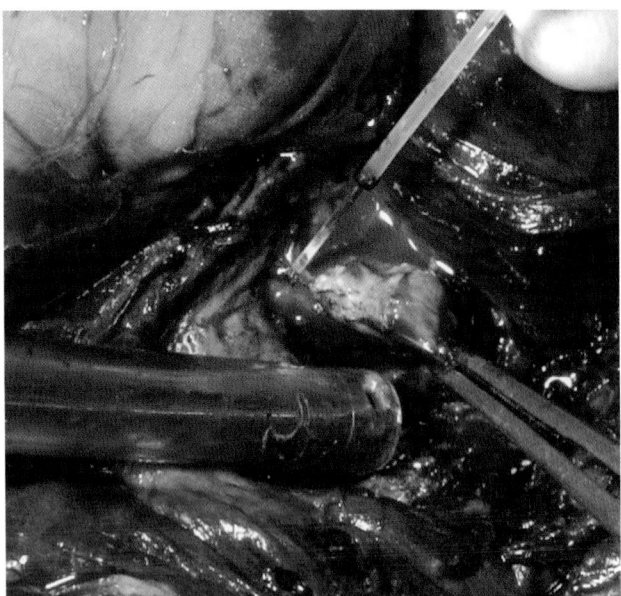

Figure 76.1 Partial prostatectomy. Portions of prostatic parenchyma are dissected and removed using an Nd:YAG (neodymium-doped yttrium aluminium garnet) laser to ensure hemostasis. Note the coagulation of the tissue surface where the laser tip has been in contact with the tissue.

Outcome

The prognosis for dogs developing postoperative systemic complications after partial or total prostatectomy is poor, and many dogs are euthanized or die in the first 2 weeks after surgery.

Prevention

- Meticulous hemostasis using an effective device such as electrocautery, laser, or ultrasonic aspirator (Figure 76.1)
- Early detection of preexisting clotting disorders such as DIC and initiation of treatment before surgery

Urinary incontinence

See Chapter 75.

Tumor recurrence

Definition

Complete excision of neoplastic tissue in the prostate is hardly ever achieved; therefore, tumor recurrence or metastatic spread is to be anticipated in the weeks or months after surgery. Even cases treated with total prostatectomy rarely result in clean margins because carcinoma tissue has frequently already penetrated the urethra at the time of surgery and has started to grow beyond the limits of the prostate.

Tumor-related complications that occur shortly after surgery are usually due to the fact that surgery was inadequate in addressing the clinical signs of the dog. For example, an intracapsular subtotal prostatectomy alone is not indicated to manage dogs with severe stranguria caused by urethral stenosis and invasion of the carcinoma tissue into the lumen of the urethra.

By definition, with partial prostatectomy, neoplastic tissue is left behind, and additional measures are necessary to prevent or slow down further growth. Such reported measures include local injections of IL-2 (L'Eplattenier *et al.* 2006) and photodynamic therapy (L'Eplattenier *et al.* 2008). In addition, systemic administration of nonsteroidal antiinflammatory drugs is thought to be of potential benefit because of their inhibitory effect on cyclooxygenase-2 (Sorenmo *et al.* 2004; L'Eplattenier *et al.* 2006).

Risk factors

- Presence of stranguria preoperatively
- Cancer extending into the bladder neck or further

Diagnosis

- Recurrence of clinical signs related to prostate cancer: straining to defecate, stranguria, lameness, or back pain in the case of metastases to the lumbar spine or ilium
- Regular ultrasound scans are indicated to monitor any postoperative changes.
- Contrast urethrogram to evaluate the length and degree of urethral stenosis

Treatment

Stenting the urethra may be considered in cases of severe stenosis of the prostatic urethra causing straining to urinate. In cases in which tumor regrowth causes straining to defecate, palliative administration of stool softeners (e.g., lactulose) can alleviate the clinical signs.

Outcome

All dogs develop clinical signs associated with tumor regrowth and are eventually euthanized. The longest survival times reported are 8 or 9 months (Liptak *et al.* 2004; L'Eplattenier *et al.* 2006).

Prevention

No treatment report to date has been successful in curing prostate cancer and preventing local recurrence.

Relevant literature

One of the main reasons why total prostatectomy is rarely performed is the incidence of postoperative **urinary incontinence**. Reported rates of incontinence range from 30% (Goldsmid and Bellenger 1991; Liptak 2010) to 90% (Basinger *et al.* 1989) and 100% (Hardie *et al.* 1984; Vlasin *et al.* 2006). Urinary incontinence is much less common when performing a partial prostatectomy, provided the dorsal prostatic capsule with its associated neurovascular structure is preserved. In one study describing ablation of the prostate capsule and prostate tissue using an Nd:YAG laser, all four dogs with prostatic disease became incontinent (Hardie *et al.* 1990). Partial prostatectomy with preservation of the prostatic capsule has not been associated with postoperative incontinence (Rawlings *et al.* 1994, 1997; L'Eplattenier *et al.* 2006; Vlasin *et al.* 2006; L'Eplattenier *et al.* 2008).

Systemic complications can occur after partial as well as total prostatectomy. In one study, 3 of 10 dogs undergoing total prostatectomy developed life-threatening complications and had to be euthanized within 2 weeks after surgery (Vlasin *et al.* 2006). In another report, 2 of 6 dogs undergoing partial prostatectomy died intraoperatively (Hardie *et al.* 1990). Partial prostatectomy techniques that preserve the prostatic capsule can also result in serious complications and euthanasia within days after surgery. This occurred in 2 of 11 dogs in one study (Vlasin *et al.* 2006) and 1 of 8 dogs in another study (L'Eplattenier *et al.* 2006).

No treatment for prostate cancer in dogs has been shown to successfully cure the patient and prevent **tumor recurrence**. In some cases, the surgical procedure fails to resolve the clinical signs, and the dogs are euthanized soon after surgery. This was the case in 2 of 8 dogs in one study. These dogs presented with severe stranguria caused by prostate cancer (L'Eplattenier *et al.* 2006). Total prostatectomy has been reported as a possible treatment option for selected cases in which the tumor is small and confined to the prostate (Liptak 2010); however, the number of patients included in the report was very small, and no conclusions can be drawn on the ability of this technique to prevent tumor recurrence.

References

Basinger, R.R., Rawlings, C.A., Barsanti, J.A., et al. (1989) Urodynamic alterations associated with clinical prostatic disease and prostatic surgery. *Journal of the American Animal Hospital Association* 25, 385-392.

Bell, F.W., Klausner, J.S., Hayden, D.W., et al. (1991) Clinical and pathologic features of prostatic adenocarcinoma in sexually intact and castrated dogs: 31 cases (1970-1987). *Journal of the American Veterinary Medical Association* 199, 1623-1630.

Cooley, D.M., Waters, D. J. (2001) Tumors of the male reproductive system. In Withrow, S.J., MacEwen, E.G. (eds.) *Small Animal Clinical Oncology,* 3rd edn. Saunders, Philadelphia, pp. 637-648.

Cornell, K.K., Bostwick, D.G., Cooley, D., et al. (2000) Clinical and pathologic aspects of spontaneous canine prostate carcinoma: a retrospective analysis of 76 cases. *Prostate* 45, 173-83.

Freitag, T., Jerram, R.M., Walker, A.M., et al. (2007) Surgical management of common canine prostatic conditions. *Compendium of Continuing Education for the Practicing Veterinarian* 29, 656-658, 660, 662-663 passim; quiz 673.

Goldsmid, S.E., Bellenger, C.R. (1991) Urinary incontinence after prostatectomy in dogs. *Veterinary Surgery* 20, 253-256.

Harari, J., Dupuis, J. (1995) Surgical treatments for prostatic diseases in dogs. *Seminars in Veterinary Medicine and Surgery (Small Animal)* 10, 43-47.

Hardie, E.M., Barsanti, J.A., Rawlings, C.A. (1984) Complications of prostatic surgery. *Journal of the American Veterinary Medical Association* 20, 50-56.

Hardie, E.M., Stone, E.A., Spaulding, K.A., et al. (1990) Subtotal canine prostatectomy with the neodymium: yttrium-aluminum-garnet laser. *Veterinary Surgery* 19, 348-355.

L'Eplattenier, H.F., Klem, B., Teske, E., et al. (2008) Preliminary results of intraoperative photodynamic therapy with 5-aminolevulinic acid in dogs with prostate carcinoma. *The Veterinary Journal* 178, 202-207.

L'Eplattenier, H.F., Van Nimwegen, S.A., Van Sluijs, F.J., et al. (2006) Partial prostatectomy using Nd:YAG laser for management of canine prostate carcinoma. *Veterinary Surgery* 35, 406-411.

Liptak, J.M. (2010) Total prostatectomy. European College of Veterinary Surgeons, 19th Annual Conference, Helsinki, Finland, ECVS.

Liptak, J.M., Brutscher, S.P., Monnet, E., et al. (2004) Transurethral resection in the management of urethral and prostatic neoplasia in 6 dogs. *Veterinary Surgery* 33, 505-516.

Rawlings, C.A., Crowell, W.A., Barsanti, J.A., et al. (1994) Intracapsular subtotal prostatectomy in normal dogs: use of an ultrasonic surgical aspirator. *Veterinary Surgery* 23, 182-189.

Rawlings, C.A., Mahaffey, M.B., Barsanti, J.A., et al. (1997) Use of partial prostatectomy for treatment of prostatic abscesses and cysts in dogs. *Journal of the American Veterinary Medical Association* 211, 868-871.

Sorenmo, K.U., Goldschmidt, M.H., Schofer, et al. (2004) Evaluation of cyclooxygenase-1 and cyclooxygenase-2 expression and the effect of cyclooxygenase inhibitors in canine prostatic carcinoma. *Veterinary Comparative Oncology* 2, 13-23.

Theilen, G.H., Madewell, B.R. (1979) Tumors of the urogenital tract. In Theilen, G.H. (ed.) *Veterinary Cancer Medicine.* Lea & Febiger, Philadelphia.

Vlasin, M., Rauser, P., Fichtel, T., et al. (2006) Subtotal intracapsular prostatectomy as a useful treatment for advanced-stage prostatic malignancies. *Journal of Small Animal Practice* 47, 512-516.

White, R.A. (2000) Prostatic surgery in the dog. *Clinical Techniques in Small Animal Practice* 15, 46-51.

Plastic and Reconstructive Surgery

77 Open Wounds

Davina Anderson

Anderson Moores Veterinary Specialists, Winchester, UK

Open wound healing in cats and dogs is largely very efficient. Factors affecting open wound healing are poorly documented, and there is little data supporting the use of any of the commonly advocated wound management systems or protocols. However, the principles of wound management appear to be consistent across most species, with removal of necrotic or contaminated tissues, maintenance of a moist environment, and prevention of ongoing inflammation being key to the promotion of normal healing of open wounds. What data are available suggest that wound healing is different in cats versus dogs, and these patients may present with different complications.

Chronic open wounds are associated with a unique combination of proteinases that are thought to interfere with the normal process of epithelialization and contraction, and it seems logical that removal of these proteinases should be helpful in encouragement of normal healing.

Incomplete healing or delayed healing

Definition

Open wound healing is regarded as being complete when there is continuity of epithelial cover over the skin deficit being treated. However, it is difficult to define at what point in the process of healing a wound might be considered "delayed." The time frame of healing of an open wound depends on the location of the wound, the depth of tissue loss, the presence of infection or contamination, and the cause of the wound. For example, a simple abrasive injury incurring partial skin loss with little contamination and the preservation of adnexal structures such as hair follicle roots would be expected to epithelialize within a few days. However, full-thickness abrasion involving loss of subcutaneous tissue with heavy tissue contamination would heal very slowly and may cause systemic consequences that could delay healing (Bohling *et al.* 2006) (Figure 77.1).

Granulation tissue is expected to be established in a healthy wound within 3 to 5 days in dogs and slightly later in cats (Bohling *et al.* 2004). Thereafter, contraction starts, which achieves up to about 50% closure if healing proceeds normally. Contraction ceases either when the tension in the surrounding skin counters the pull of myofibroblasts in the wound, or when the wound bed becomes fibrotic and immovable. Contraction in wounds may continue for up to 42 days, but the remaining deficit must be covered by epithelialization. Wounds close faster in younger animals, and contraction

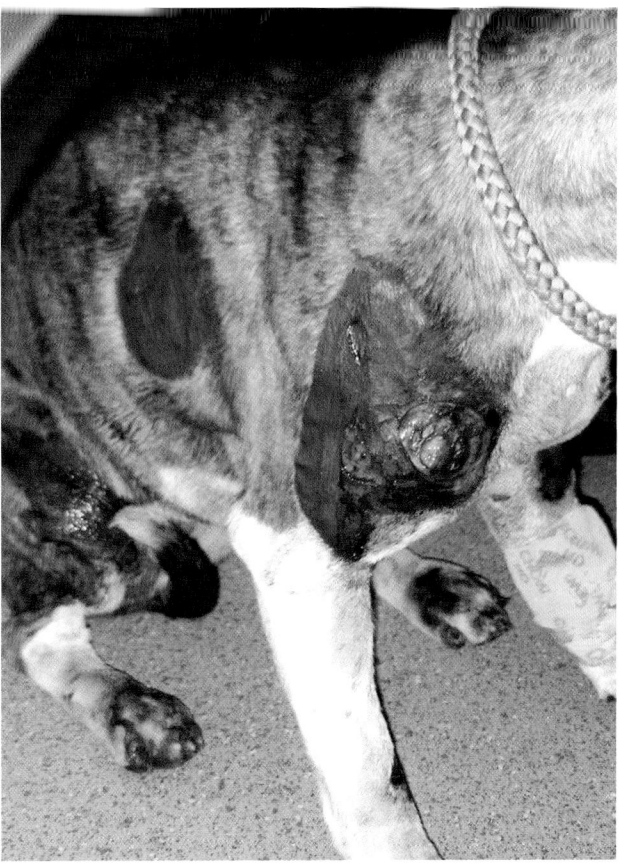

Figure 77.1 The cause of the wound will affect the time frame for normal or "expected" healing. A greater degree of tissue loss or contamination means a longer expected time frame. This wound was a result of abrasions on the road after a road traffic accident. *Source*: A. Moores, Anderson Moores Veterinary Specialists, Winchester, Hampshire, UK, 2014. Reproduced with permission from A. Moores.

is swifter and more effective in younger animals, resulting in more cosmetic and functional scars.

Wounds that fail to contract or in which epithelialization is absent should be evaluated for delayed healing. The granulation tissue bed may be pale and avascular or even proud of the surrounding epithelial edge. Epithelialization fails when there is repeated surface

Complications in Small Animal Surgery, First Edition. Edited by Dominique Griffon and Annick Hamaide.
© 2016 John Wiley & Sons, Inc. Published 2016 by John Wiley & Sons, Inc.
Companion website: www.wiley.com/go/griffon/complications

trauma, desiccation, or chemical irritation (e.g., antiseptic lavage or ointments). Other common signs are wounds that are painful or have signs of inflammation in the skin surrounding the wound such as edema, erythema, pain, or exudation.

A combination of these processes of failure is seen in "pocketed wounds." In this circumstance, the granulation tissue may be healthy, but the skin edges fail to adhere to the underlying tissue; this scenario is often seen in axilla or inguinal wounds. The epithelial cells cannot migrate across the wound because the skin edge is rolled underneath into the pocket. The contraction cannot occur because it curls the skin edge into the pocket, and healing stops. These wounds are best treated with excision and surgical intervention (e.g., thoracodorsal flap with omentalization is recommended for feline axilla wounds) (Lascelles *et al.* 1998).

Risk factors

- Open wound healing is delayed by any factor that perpetuates inflammation. This includes foreign material in the wound, infection (by noncommensal organisms), necrosis or thrombosis, poor blood supply, poor wound management that results in maceration of the wound caused by inflammatory exudate retention at the wound surface, or wound management that results in desiccation of surface tissues and damage to the granulation tissue, excessive motion at the wound site (e.g., over joint surfaces), or self-molestation. Some wound dressing products can cause wound healing to be delayed if they are used inappropriately. The commonest cause of damage to the wound surface is self-trauma by the patient, and this is particularly noticeable in patients that lick their sutures.
- Intrinsic failure of wound healing is rare but is occasionally seen in patients with collagen linking abnormalities (Ehlers-Danlos syndrome) and wounds that have residual tumors such as sarcoma or mast cell tumor within the granulation tissue.
- Systemic conditions may also affect wound healing, although this is less well documented in animals than it is in humans, and the chronic distal limb wounds seen in human diabetic or cardiovascular patients are not recognized in veterinary surgery. Hypothyroidism, hyperadrenocorticism, cachexia, and malnutrition are known to affect open wound healing.
- Less well documented are factors such as pain, stress, and protein-losing conditions that appear (anecdotally) to have an effect on wound healing.
- Systemic and topical medications can also affect wound healing either by direct inhibition of proliferating cells (e.g., topical antiseptics) or by inhibition of normal cell populations (e.g., corticosteroids, radiotherapy, some chemotherapeutic drugs)

Diagnosis

- The wound must be assessed closely and objectively.
  - Look at texture and color of the granulation tissue. (Remember that granulation tissue is naturally slightly paler in the cats.)
  - Look at the edges of the wound and determine if there are signs of epithelialization.
  - Look at the skin surrounding the wound and determine if there are cardinal signs of inflammation in these tissues (i.e., swelling, erythema, pain, and heat).
- Measure the wound daily with photographs or templates and determine if there is ongoing contraction or progress, particularly with epithelialization at the edges because this is an indication of wound health.
- Assess the dressing each time it is removed for signs of infection, excessive exudate, or odor.

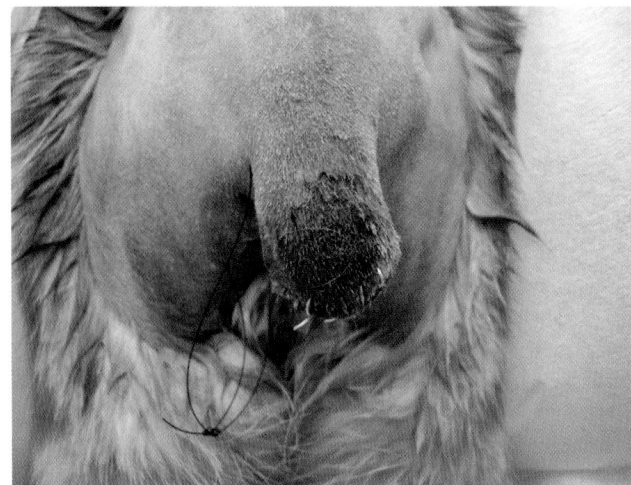

Figure 77.2 Necrosis of the skin after amputation of a cat's tail after a traumatic injury. Ultrasound examination confirmed the loss of blood supply to the distal vertebra, and this had led to skin necrosis and wound healing failure of the overlying repair. The wound healed after removal of the necrotic vertebra and skin.

- Identify possible foreign or necrotic material; radiography, diagnostic ultrasonography, or other investigation may be necessary.
- Evaluation of the vascular supply to the area may be very useful, especially with the extremities such as the distal limbs or tail wounds. Angiography may not be necessary because ultrasonography using color-flow Doppler may be sufficient to demonstrate loss of blood flow to the affected area (Figure 77.2).
- Review the clinical condition and status of the patient, monitoring vital parameters on each visit (temperature, pulse, respiratory rate, and body weight).
- Tissue samples should be taken for histology to screen for neoplastic disease as well as culture for unusual organisms. Culture results should be interpreted with caution. Infected granulation tissue has a "melting" appearance, and the wound may be enlarging at each dressing change. However, a surface swab of a wound may produce a positive culture of normal commensal or nosocomial organisms that are not necessarily limiting wound healing and do not justify antibiotic therapy. Acid-fast organisms such as *Nocardia* and *Actinomyces* spp. are sometimes cultured from chronic wounds, especially those associated with foreign material sequestration. Multidrug-resistant organisms associated with purulent exudate and enlarging wound surface area are more likely to be significant (e.g., methicillin-resistant *Staphylococcus aureus* (or other multiresistant organisms).

Treatment (Figure 77.3)

- The source of the inflammation must be resolved; this may not be possible if it is secondary to orthopedic implants (e.g., with traumatic wounds of the distal limb). However, other foreign material or necrotic tissue (e.g., sequestra, grass or thorns, glass or gravel fragments) may be removed surgically.
- The wound should be assessed and dressed regularly to allow prompt removal of exudate-soaked dressings, which may perpetuate inflammation of the wound and surrounding tissue.
- Infected or contaminated wounds benefit from debridement. This may be carried out surgically or using topical dressings. Adherent dressings, debriding gels, pastes, and myiasis are all useful to remove infected material, inflammatory exudate, and necrotic

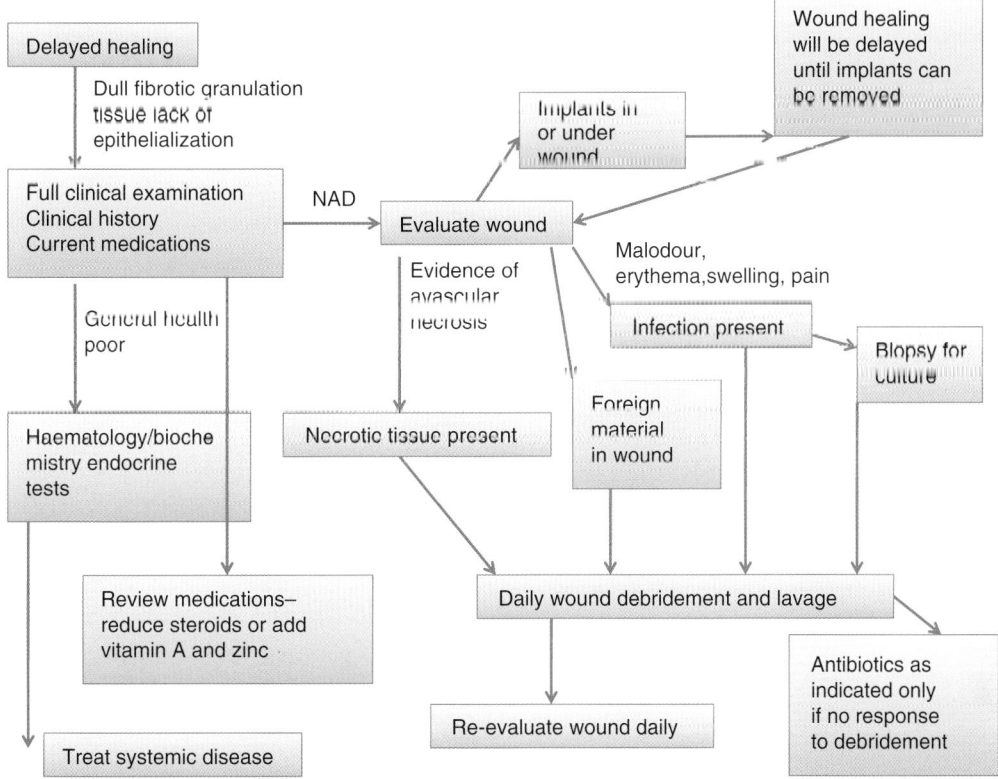

Figure 77.3 Algorithm for management of delayed wound healing.

tissue while preserving healthy tissue. This treatment may also reactivate chronic granulation tissue by removing enzymes (met-alloproteinases) found in chronic open wounds.

- Negative-pressure wound therapy has been described to manage large open wounds that are healing slowly or when healing appears to be delayed (Ben-Amotz *et al.* 2007; Guille *et al.* 2007; Ubbink *et al.* 2008). Very large skin deficits that are not suitable for surgical closure may be difficult to manage well because of the logistical problems of applying wound dressings. The dressings and apparatus are adherent to the adjacent skin and provide wound protection while subatmospheric pressure is also applied across the wound, usually at about -75 to -125 mm Hg. There are no published data proving the benefits of this treatment in clinical situations in humans or animals, but anecdotal reports suggest that it improves perfusion, stimulates granulation tissue, reduces edema, and decreases bacterial colonization. The removal of exudate from the wound alone, however, is likely to improve wound healing, contraction, and epithelialization. The technique is contraindicated in the presence of hemorrhage or coagulopathy.

Outcome

The wound should be monitored on a daily basis to determine the response to treatment. The prognosis should be good with adequate wound management and investigations. However, discussion with the owner regarding surgical reconstruction of the skin deficit (skin grafts or skin flaps and other techniques) may be appropriate.

Prevention

- Prevention of delayed healing depends on adequate wound assessment and management in the first instance. Some wounds,

such as those over joints or near orifices or circumferential skin deficits of the distal limb, are not suitable for healing by second intention (Figure 77.4). Delaying dressing changes to weekly or twice weekly is likely to be a false economy, and regular dressing changes are very important in the health of the wound, the welfare of the patient, and the normal progression of healing.

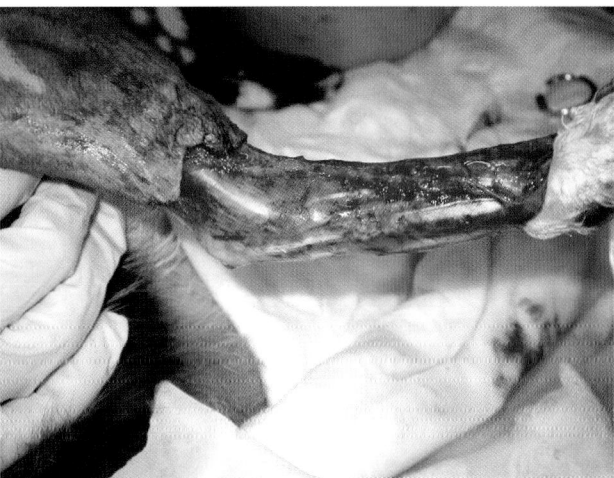

Figure 77.4 Circumferential skin loss on the extremities will not heal satisfactorily by open wound management and should be prepared for reconstruction techniques. This cat had a distal skin avulsion and this wound was surgically debrided and managed with dressings for 7 days until the granulation tissue was sufficiently established to receive a full-thickness free skin graft.

- The commonest cause of delayed healing or wound infection is inadequate debridement and lavage. All wounds should be thoroughly lavaged using sterile isotonic solutions and debrided at the first and subsequent inspections until granulation tissue is well established.
- Investigating the cause of delayed healing should follow a standard protocol involving laboratory tests, critical appraisal of wound management to date, home care, history, and clinical examination:
  ◦ Biopsy.
  ◦ Culture, polymerase chain reaction, or acid-fast stains of tissue samples.
  ◦ Surface cytology and Gram stains may be useful pending culture.
  ◦ Detailed review of history of the wound management protocol and home care.
  ◦ Possible causes: systemic disease, neoplasia, viral infection (in cats), acid-fast organisms, multidrug-resistant organisms or nosocomial infection, foreign material (implants, foreign body, hair, grass material), treatments (steroids, chemotherapy, radiotherapy), adverse drug reactions (e.g., nonsteroidal anti-inflammatory drugs), self-trauma, inflammation, poor wound management, or iatrogenic damage to the wound surface.
- Adequate treatment
  ◦ The wound should be cleaned and lavaged with sterile isotonic fluids at each dressing change. This allows removal of the inflammatory fluids as well as surface bacteria, debris, and remnants of wound dressing material. Clinical notes should record the nature of the exudate, the appearance and measurement of the wound surface area, and the response to treatment so far. Dressings used to debride the wound should not remain in place for longer than 24 hours, and in very exudative wounds may be changed twice daily to prevent maceration of the wound surface.
  ◦ Wounds that are infected may benefit from debriding dressings or treatment, and resolution of infection may occur spontaneously after debridement without the use of antibiotics (e.g., use of wet-to-dry dressings over 12–24 hours). Wounds overlying orthopedic implants may have to be managed as open wounds until the implants can be removed (Figures 77.5 and 77.6).
  ◦ Surgical debridement can be very useful to restimulate normal healing processes and to speed up removal of necrotic material and exudate. Tangential tissue removal with a scalpel blade under sterile conditions together with repeated lavage is an important tool. Reconstruction procedures should be considered, particularly for wounds of the distal limb or near orifices, where functional compromise may occur if the wound contracts. Wounds on the thoracic or abdominal wall may have to be reconstructed with synthetic mesh or muscle flaps to achieve adequate strength.

Scar formation

Definition

Scar formation is inevitable and is a normal process in the healing of any skin wound other than in the embryo where scarring does not occur. However, the degree to which scarring occurs varies, and although it is considered a normal end stage of the healing process, in some circumstances, scarring may cause complications in terms of tissue function caused by stenosis, stricture, contracture, or cicatrization (distortion caused by fibrosis or scarring).

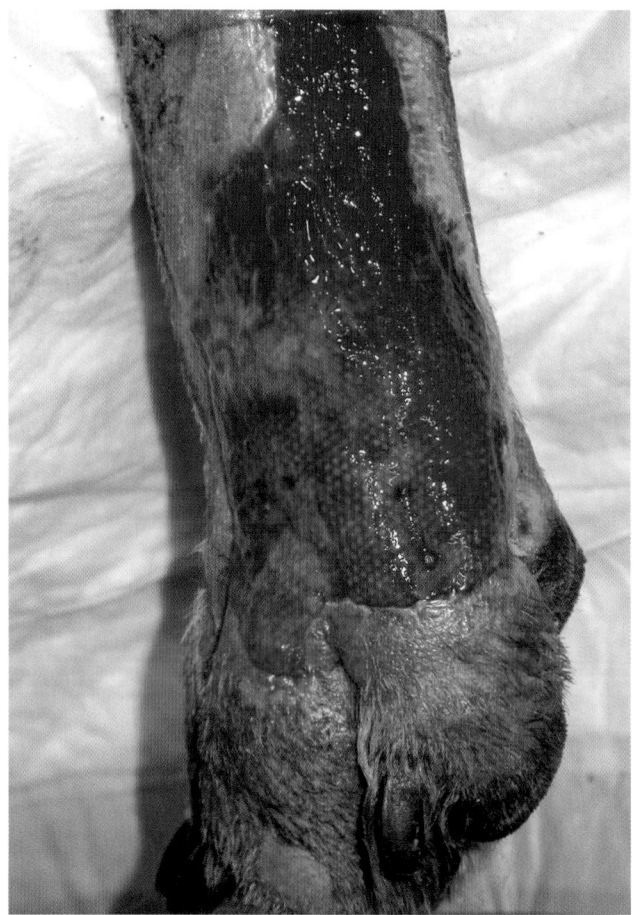

Figure 77.5 A shear injury on the carpus of a dog that had been treated with bandaging for 7 days. On presentation, the foot was swollen, non–weight bearing, and highly exudative with a positive culture for pseudomonas. The wound was lavaged and dressed with a debriding dressing (dry-to-dry) overnight, resulting in complete resolution of the clinical signs of inflammation. No antibiotics were used to resolve the infection.

Risk factors

- Extensive tissue loss, particularly over extremities, the flexure aspect of joints, or near orifices, may increase the risk of the normal scar process causing complications (Figure 77.7).
- The depth of tissue loss also contributes to scarring and contracture; partial-thickness loss of epithelial tissue is not associated with significant functional scarring.

Diagnosis

Early scar tissue is easily identified by the nature of the inflexible thick banding of pale tissue. In the early stages of scar formation, the scar may be erythematous and is sometimes hypersensitive. With normal remodeling, the scar becomes less noticeable and less sensitive and in haired animals (e.g., dogs and cats), the haired skin often hides the scar. A scar that gradually becomes thicker and less malleable, culminating in contraction of the adjacent tissues in a concentric fashion, potentially causes complications.

Soft tissue scarring must be differentiated from functional contracture of muscles such as may be seen with prolonged flexure of a limb or "tie down" of a muscle over a malunion of a fracture site.

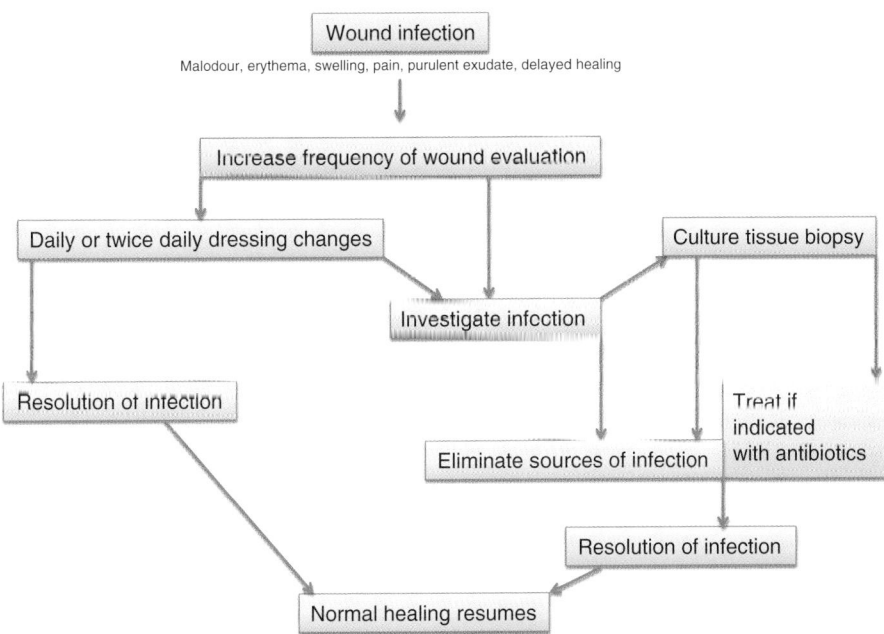

Figure 77.6 Algorithm for management of an infected open wound.

Treatment

- Scars may be resected and reconstructed in such as fashion as to lengthen the scar and release the tension. In severe scarring such as in Figure 77.8, release of the scar to allow normal function raises the challenge of reconstruction of the skin deficit because allowing the wound to heal by second intention again will only allow the regeneration of the same scar tissue. It is important to understand the cause of the scarring to avoid recurrence of the same problem.
- In specific circumstances, surgical technique failure may the cause of the scarring (e.g., stenosis of urethrostomy sites).
- "Z-plasty" has been described in which lines are cut along the scar in a Z shape and the wound reconstructed to lengthen the original scar and release the tension along the line of the scar. This and other procedures are technically very demanding and require considerable experience to make them work well.

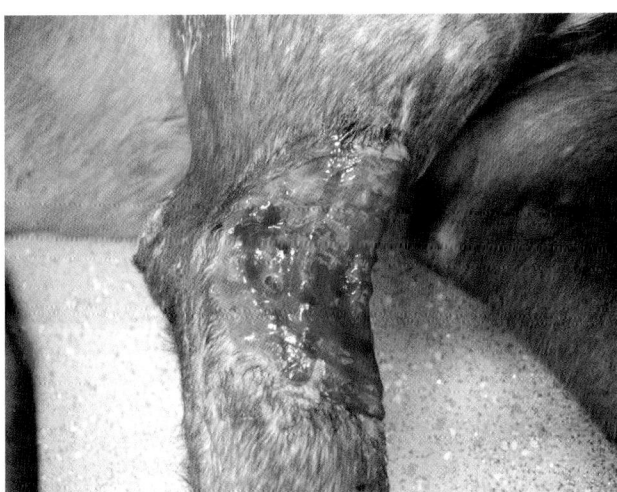

Figure 77.7 Tissue loss over joints cannot be allowed to heal by second intention because the contraction and scarring may result in compromise of function.

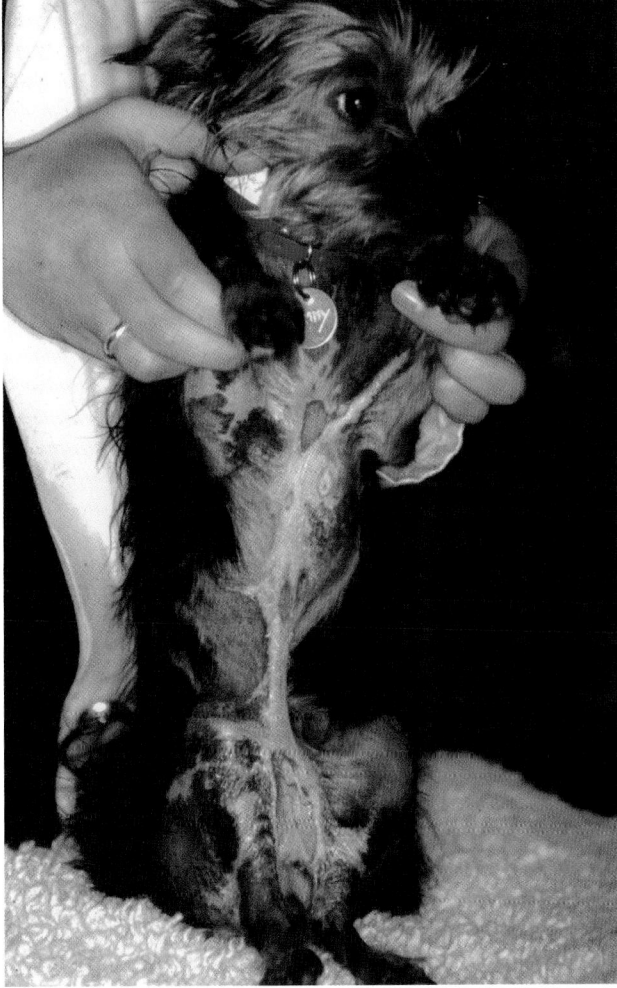

Figure 77.8 This Yorkshire terrier sustained full-thickness burns in hot water. The skin deficits healed by second intention but resulted in severe cicatrization of the limbs and craniocaudal contracture along the ventral abdomen.

Outcome

The outcome depends on the location of the scar. Minor scarring may be managed with physiotherapy and tension exercises (Figure 77.9), but major scars may require surgery to release the scar to improve function, and the prognosis may be guarded depending on

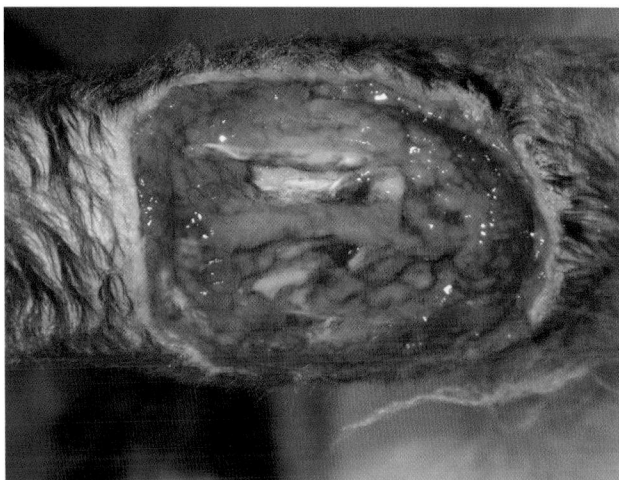

(A)

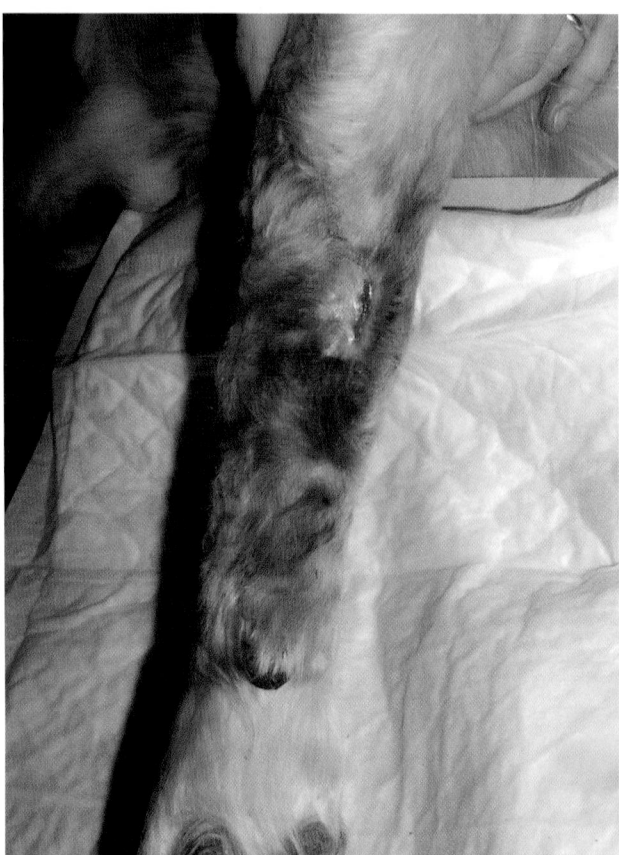

(B)

Figure 77.9 A and **B**, A large wound dehiscence after a tumor removal on the palmar aspect of the distal forelimb was managed as an open wound and healed in 7 weeks. However, it resulted in contracture of the underlying flexor tendons because of scarring and required extensive physiotherapy to regain normal limb function.

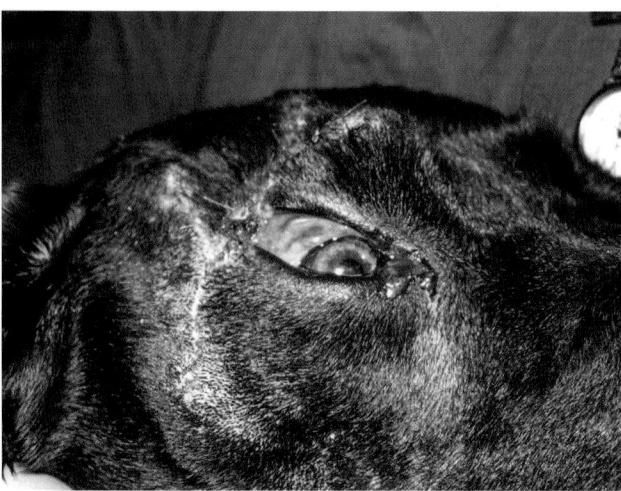

Figure 77.10 This Labrador retriever had a neoplastic lesion removed from the lateral aspect of the canthus. The skin deficit was reconstructed with a rotational temporal skin flap, but 1 week after surgery, contracture was apparent, and the scar had to be released and reconstructed.

the success of the revision surgery (Figure 77.10). Multiple attempts to resolve functional scarring will increase the risk of progressive dysfunction, and this requires considerable surgical expertise.

Prevention

The decision to allow a wound to heal by second intention should be based on the assessment of whether the wound is likely to cause complications in the event of scarring. Wounds can contract by up to 30% and will contract regardless of the lines of tension and mobility. Thus, an open wound over a flexure surface or adjacent to an orifice is unlikely to heal without contracture and scarring with functional consequences. These types of wounds should be very closely monitored or closed with a surgical procedure. Silicone dressings have been described for softening of keloid scars in humans but have not been described in veterinary patients.

Infection (see Chapter 1)

Wound dehiscence (see Chapter 9)

Hematoma and seroma

Definition

Hematoma is an accumulation of blood or blood clot within a surgical or traumatic wound trapped under the skin or within other soft tissues. A seroma is an accumulation of fluid (transudate) also trapped in a similar circumstance within the soft tissues. Generally, the size of a hematoma or seroma is limited by the tension of the associated fascial planes, which provides pressure to limit further fluid leak into the cavity. Thus, seromas or hematomas around the subcutaneous area of the neck in dogs and cats, where the skin may be loose, can become very large indeed, but swelling may be limited in other areas where the skin is more closely attached to the underlying fascia.

Patients with a coagulopathy may be at risk of hematoma formation despite no apparent bleeding at the time of surgical closure. Patients with a fibrinolytic defect will bleed at 24 to 48 hours postoperatively and may present with a very large painful hematoma

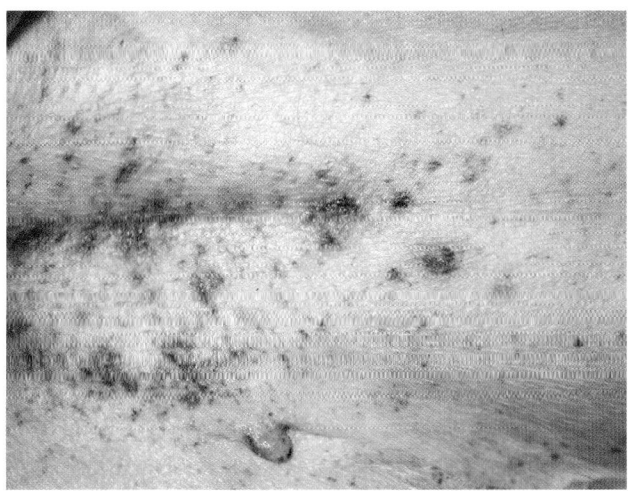

Figure 77.11 This dog was being prepared for surgery after preoperative chemotherapy. Clipping and skin preparation caused petechiation of the skin, and the dog was found to be thrombocytopenic.

2 to 3 days after neutering or other elective surgery. The diagnosis is made difficult because of normal laboratory clotting test results.

Risk factors

Surgical procedures that result in incomplete hemostasis or large areas of dead space are more at risk of fluid accumulation in the postoperative period. For example, thyroidectomy in dogs may involve considerable dissection of a very vascular tissue within an area of very loose tissue; thus, postoperatively, there is a high risk of hematoma formation. Mastectomy is frequently associated with postoperative seroma formation because it is difficult to close the dead space along the ventral abdomen, particularly in the inguinal area. Some preoperative treatments may cause coagulopathies such as chemotherapeutic protocols or antithyroid medication that then increase the risk of postoperative hematoma formation (Figure 77.11).

Diagnosis

- Early wound monitoring in the recovery period often identifies swelling or hemorrhage underneath the wound at a very early stage.
- Progressive postoperative swelling over the first 4 to 5 days is likely to be a seroma.
- Hematomas tend to form acutely in the first 12 to 24 hours after surgery unless there is delayed bleeding related to a coagulopathy.

Treatment (Figure 77.12)

- In the very early stages postoperatively when swelling is identified, gentle pressure using cold packs may reduce the development of the swelling. The cold packs should not be below 0°C, which could cause hypothermic damage to the overlying skin. After discharge from the veterinary hospital, increased activity at home may cause further enlargement of the swelling, and owners can be advised to continue cold pack therapy for 1 to 3 days.
- As the fluid-filled cavity stabilizes, percutaneous needle drainage may be helpful, particularly if there is concern that the swelling may occlude other structures such as impinging on the pharynx. The area is prepared for aseptic treatment, and a sterile needle is placed into the seroma; a suction apparatus may be useful to treat large seromas, but gravitational drainage may be adequate. However, there is a risk of introducing infection with percutaneous drainage, and without adjunctive pressure or cold packing, the fluid may recur. In this situation, placement of a surgical drain may be necessary.

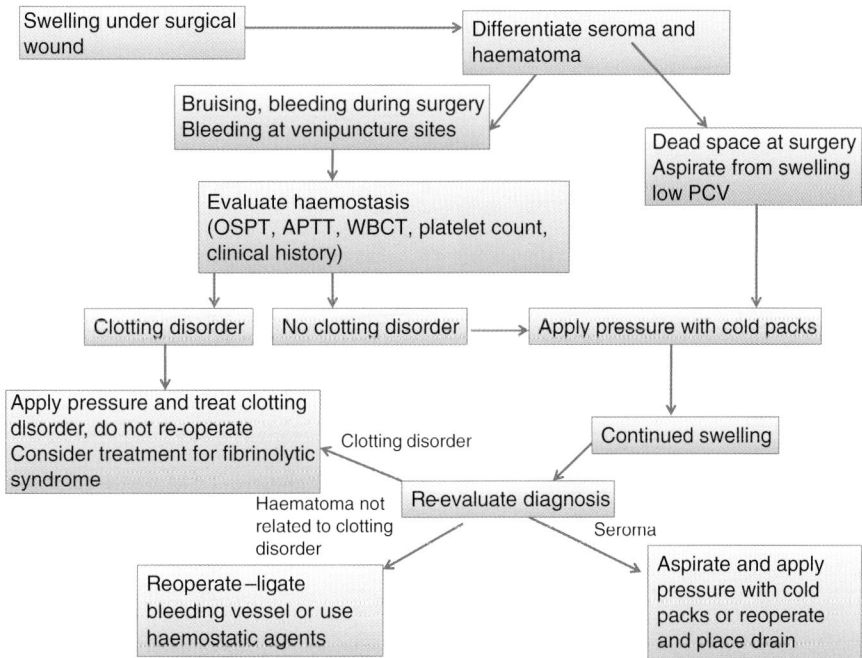

Figure 77.12 Algorithm for the treatment of postoperative seroma.

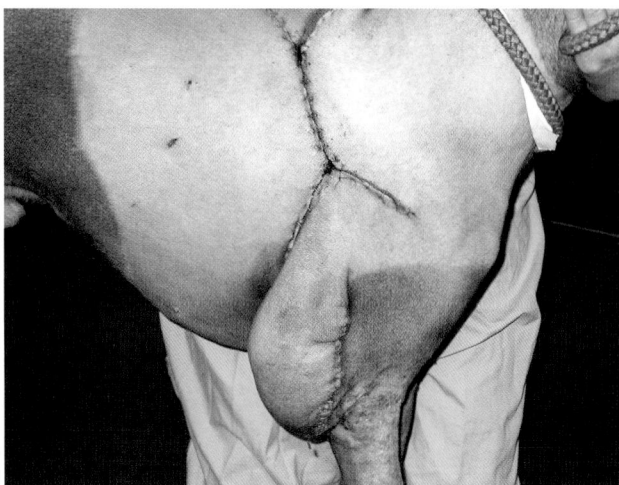

Figure 77.13 A large seroma underneath a thoracodorsal axial pattern flap that was used to reconstruct a wound on the caudal aspect of the elbow.

Outcome

Providing the seroma is carefully managed, most gradually resolve, although they can take some weeks in the cervical area of loose-skinned dogs or underneath large surgical resections (Figure 77.13). Hematomas also eventually resolve, although in cases with a coagulopathy, there is also the risk that they will recur or be life threatening.

Prevention

- Surgical hemostasis and closure of dead space are very important with regard to prevention of these complications and cannot be substituted with attempts to treat them postoperatively. If diffuse bleeding is present, it is important to stabilize this before closure. Depending on the surgical access to the bleeding site, various techniques may be used, such as lavage with cold sterile fluids, pressure with swabs soaked in cold sterile isotonic fluids, diluted adrenaline solution, simple tamponade, or the use of topical hemostatics (e.g., collagen or gelatin foam) (Figure 77.14).
- Large areas of dead space should either have a light bandage placed before recovery to hold the dead space closed or a passive

or active drain placed to allow the fluid to drain in the postoperative period until the tissues adhere and the dead space is closed naturally (Figure 77.15). Some surgeries, such as reconstruction of inguinal and prepubic wounds, and axillary trauma are known to carry a high risk of postoperative seroma formation. Surgical planning should include the use of a drain or omentalization of the dead space to help prevent seroma formation in the postoperative period.

Relevant literature

Wound healing in dogs and cats is for the most part very efficient, and complications are more likely to be associated with patient interference, surgical technique, or poor wound management. Scarring, contracture, and distortion caused by fibrosis are infrequently reported in the veterinary literature and described in surgical textbooks or single case reports. Contracture of muscles associated with fracture repair is a well-known phenomenon (Pavletic 1999;

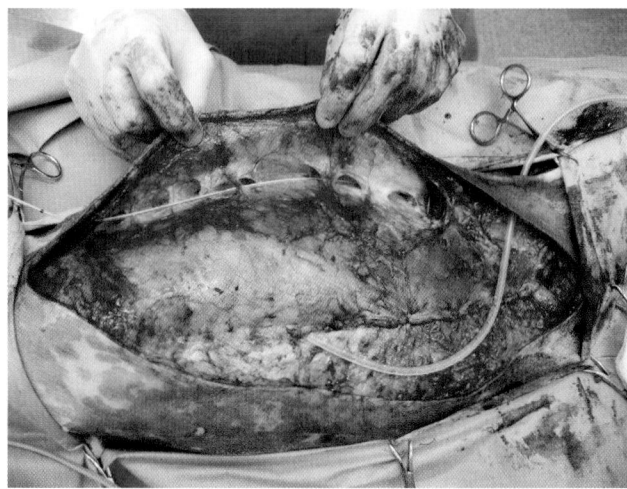

(A)

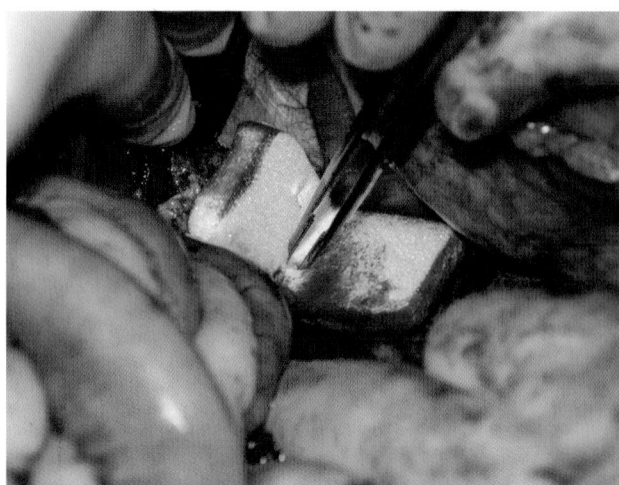

Figure 77.14 A piece of gelatin foam is placed over the dissection site of a liver lobectomy to provide adjunctive hemostasis.

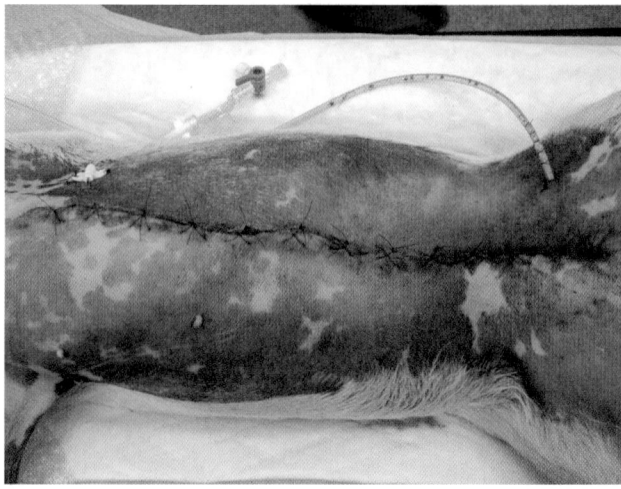

(B)

Figure 77.15 A and B, A complete left-sided mastectomy was performed, and before closure, a wound catheter for infusion of bupivacaine was placed (laterally on the upper side of the image), and a suction drain was placed caudally (lower side and on the right of the image).

Moores and Sutton 2009; Westermeyer *et al.* 2009; Pavletic 2010; Hosgood 2012). Seromas are one of the common reported complications of surgeries, and the incidence varies from 10% to 30% depending on the type of surgery (Lascelles *et al.* 1998; Aper and Smeak 2005; Hammell *et al.* 2006; Matiasek *et al.* 2006; Ritter *et al.* 2006; Talaat *et al.* 2006; Tattersall and Walsh 2006).

References

Aper, R.L., Smeak, D.D. (2005) Clinical evaluation of caudal superficial epigastric axial pattern flap reconstruction of skin defects in 10 dogs. *Journal of the American Animal Hospital Association* 41 (3), 185-192.

Ben-Amotz, R., Lanz, O.I., Miller, J.M., et al. (2007) The use of vacuum-assisted closure therapy for the treatment of distal extremity wounds in 15 dogs. *Veterinary Surgery* 36, 684.

Bohling, M.W., Henderson, R.A., Swaim, S.F., et al. (2004) Cutaneous wound healing in the cat: a macroscopic description and comparison with cutaneous wound healing in the dog. *Veterinary Surgery* 33 (6), 579-587.

Bohling, M.W., Henderson, R.A., Swaim, S.F., et al. (2006) Comparison of the role of the subcutaneous tissues in cutaneous wound healing in the dog and cat. *Veterinary Surgery* 35 (1), 1-12.

Guille, A.E., Tseng, L.W., Orsher, R.J. (2007) Use of vacuum-assisted closure for management of a large skin wound in a cat. *Journal of the American Veterinary Medical Association* 230, 1669.

Hammell, S.P., Hottinger, H.A., Novo, R.E. (2006) Postoperative results of unilateral arytenoid lateralization for treatment of idiopathic laryngeal paralysis in dogs: 39 cases (1996-2002). *Journal of the American Veterinary Medical Association* 228 (8), 1215-1220.

Hosgood, G. (2012) Open Wounds. In Tobias, K., Johnston, S. (eds.) *Veterinary Surgery Small Animal*, vol. 2, 1st ed. Elsevier Saunders, St Louis, pp. 1210-1220.

Lascelles, B.D.X., Davison, L., Dunning, M., et al. (1998) Use of omental pedicle grafts in the management of non-healing axillary wounds in 10 cats. *Journal of Small Animal Practice* 39 (10), 475-480.

Matiasek, L.A., Platt, S.R., Dennis, R., et al. (2006) Subfascial seroma causing compressive myelopathy after cervical dorsal laminectomy. *Veterinary Radiology and Ultrasound* 47 (6), 581-584.

Moores, A.P., Sutton, A. (2009) Management of quadriceps contracture in a dog using a static flexion apparatus and physiotherapy. *Journal of Small Animal Practice* 50 (5), 251-254.

Pavletic, M.M. (1999) *Atlas of Small Animal Reconstructive Surgery*, 2nd edn. WB Saunders Philadelphia.

Pavletic, M.M. (2010) *Atlas of Small Animal Wound Management and Reconstructive Surgery*. Wiley Blackwell, Ames, IA.

Ritter, M.J., von Pfeil, S.B.J., Stanley, B.J., et al. (2006) Mandibular and sublingual sialoceles in the dog: a retrospective evaluation of 41 cases using the ventral approach for treatment *New Zealand Veterinary Journal* 54 (6), 333-337.

Talaat, M.B., Kowaleski, M.P., Boudrieau, R.J. (2006) Combination tibial plateau leveling osteotomy and cranial closing wedge osteotomy of the tibia for the treatment of cranial cruciate ligament-deficient stifles with excessive tibial plateau angle. *Veterinary Surgery* 35 (8), 729-739.

Tattersall, J.A., Welsh, E. (2006) Factors influencing the short-term outcome following thoracic surgery in 98 dogs. *Journal of Small Animal Practice,* 47 (12), 715-720.

Ubbink, D.T., Westerbos, S.J., Nelson, E.A., et al. (2008) A systematic review of topical negative pressure therapy for acute and chronic wounds. *British Journal of Surgery* 95, 685.

Westermeyer, H.D., Tobias, K.M., Reel, D.R. (2009) Head and neck swelling due to a circumferential cicatricial scar in a dog. *Journal of the American Animal Hospital Association* 45 (1), 48-51.

78 Reconstructive Flaps

Stéphanie Claeys
Small Animal Surgery, Department of Clinical Sciences (Companion Animals and Equids), Faculty of Veterinary Medicine, University of Liège, Liège, Belgium

Reconstructive surgery is commonly performed to correct congenital defects and to repair acquired defects that occur secondary to trauma or removal of neoplasms. A pedicle graft (or skin flap) is a segment of skin and subcutaneous tissue with a vascular attachment moved from one area of the body to another. They can be classified as rotating (rotation, transposition, interpolation, or skinfold flaps) or advancement flaps (single or bipedicle). A pedicle graft incorporating a direct cutaneous artery and vein into its base is termed an axial pattern flap. Axial pattern flaps have a better perfusion than pedicle grafts, which receive their blood supply from subdermal plexus alone. Direct or indirect distant flaps are constructed at a distant location from a skin defect involving almost exclusively the middle to lower extremities. Compound flaps involve the elevation and transfer of flaps that incorporate skin with other tissues, including muscle, mucosa, fat, bone, and cartilage. Free flaps may also be used by dividing the major supplying artery and vein and reestablishing circulation by microvascular anastomosis to an artery and vein at the recipient site. They require an operating microscope and are therefore limited to specialty practice.

Regarding the technique used, maintaining adequate blood flow through the flap is the most critical factor in determining the success or failure of the procedure.

Ischemia and necrosis

Definition
Ischemia is a restriction in blood supply with resultant damage or dysfunction of tissue. Ischemia of a flap may induce necrosis, which is defined as the premature death of cells and living tissue.

Risk factors
- Inadequate blood supply is the most common cause of flap necrosis. It is usually the result of combined arterial and venous occlusion.
- Excessive tension can interfere with circulation in the flap and result in necrosis of a part or the totality of the flap. Tension also retards wound healing.
- Underlying hematoma or seroma secondary to dead space can interfere with circulation because of pressure beneath the flap.
- Traumatic surgical technique may contribute to flap necrosis.
- Improper bandaging techniques inducing excessive pressure on the flap can reduce circulation in the flap and contribute to necrosis.
- Self-trauma to the flap (Figure 78.1)
- Infection

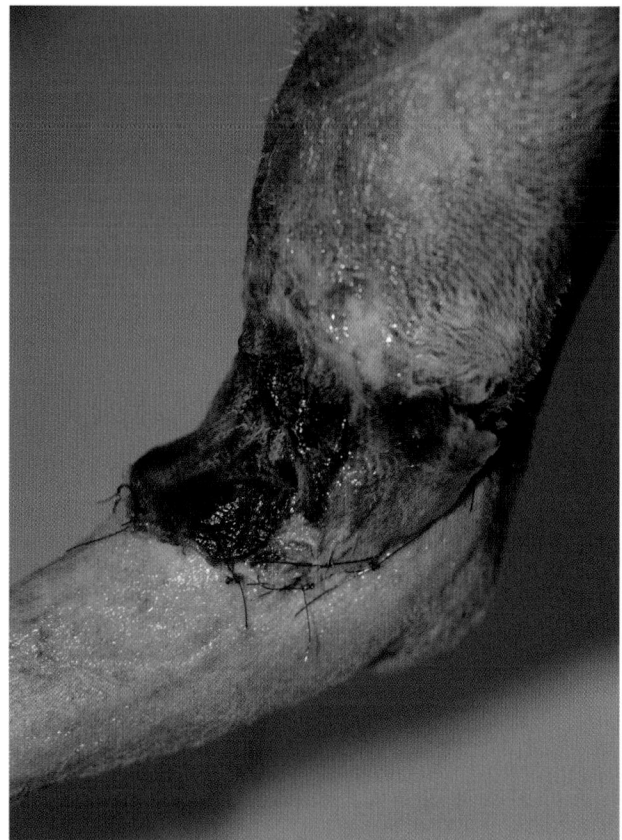

Figure 78.1 Inguinal flank fold flap damaged because of self-trauma. The distal necrotic portion of the flap was debrided, and the flap was reelevated and advanced into the remainder of the defect. *Source:* Julius Liptak, Alta Vista Animal Hospital, Ottawa, Ontario. Reproduced with permission from Julius Liptak.

Diagnosis
- Skin flaps should be examined periodically in the days after transfer. Changes in color should be interpreted with caution because contused skin often survives if no additional circulatory compromise occurs. Color change is indicative of a circulatory problem or inflammation. Flaps with severe circulatory obstruction pass through changes in color from red to lavender, to deep purple, and finally to black after 2 to 6 days (Figures 78.2 and 78.3). Portions of flaps may pass from red to lavender with eventual

Complications in Small Animal Surgery, First Edition. Edited by Dominique Griffon and Annick Hamaide.
© 2016 John Wiley & Sons, Inc. Published 2016 by John Wiley & Sons, Inc.
Companion website: www.wiley.com/go/griffon/complications

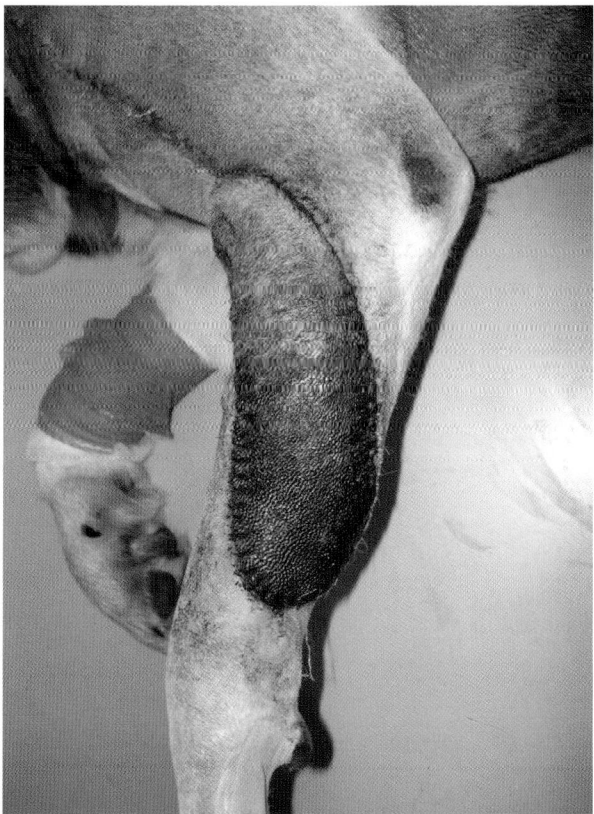

Figure 78.2 Distal necrosis of a superficial brachial axial pattern flap after excision of an antebrachial hemangiopericytoma (4 days postoperatively). The superficial brachial artery is relatively small and at greater risk for surgical trauma. The necrotic portion of the flap was debrided, and the defect was left to heal by second intention at the owner's request.

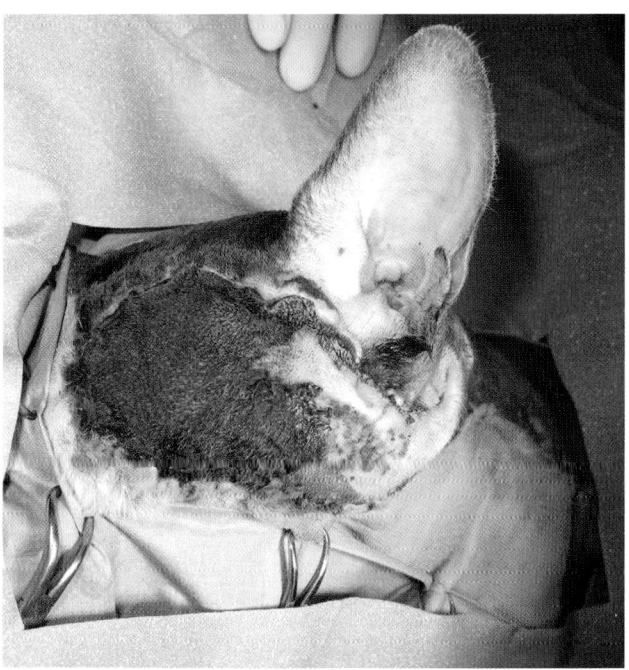

Figure 78.3 Distal necrosis of a caudal auricular axial pattern flap after excision of a recurrent eyelid soft tissue sarcoma. The necrotic skin was debrided, and the flap was advanced into the defect with minimal tension. *Source:* Julius Liptak, Alta Vista Animal Hospital, Ottawa, Ontario. Reproduced with permission from Julius Liptak.

resolution without necrosis. Subjective criteria such as color changes, warmth, pain sensation, and bleeding may be inaccurate and should therefore not be used to predict outcome.

- Various objective techniques have been described to assess flap circulation, such as disulphide blue and patent blue dye, assessment of pH and hematocrit of blood obtained by stab incision in the flap, and laser Doppler blood flow measurements. Cost and interpretation of these techniques limit their clinical use in veterinary medicine.

- Fluorescein dye has been used to assess flap circulation and to predict flap survival in various species. Fluorescein is administered intravenously, and the flap is illuminated with an ultraviolet lamp. It is simple and safe. A yellow to green fluorescence is demonstrated in areas of adequate circulation. Areas without adequate circulation do not fluoresce and may undergo necrosis. Areas of spotty fluorescence indicate poor circulation, but such areas may survive. The fluorescence pattern may not be clear, and predicting flap survival based on fluorescein may not be accurate because nonfluorescent areas may also survive.

Treatment

- The ability to salvage a failing flap is influenced by the cause and the duration of the compromise. Various methods have been studied in experimental animals and humans to prevent necrosis when circulatory compromise is present (e.g., hyperbaric oxygen, thrombolytic drugs, vasodilators, corticosteroids, prostaglandin inhibitors, hypothermia). These techniques are not very practical and therefore are not routinely used in veterinary medicine in clinical situations. Preventing circulatory compromise is therefore critical.

- When necrosis is evident, excision of necrotic tissue should be performed (Figures 78.4 to 78.6). Clear demarcation should be evident between nonviable and viable skin. Necrotic skin usually results in infection and delayed healing. Small areas of necrosis may be left to slough spontaneously if no infection is present.

- Depending on the size of the defect left after excision of necrotic tissue, variable options are possible. Small defects may be left to heal by second intention. Larger defects may be closed primarily or may require another flap procedure or a skin graft.

Outcome

Given the difficulty of salvaging a failing flap, necrosis may not be avoided when circulatory compromise is well established and irreversible. The entire flap will, however, usually not undergo necrosis. Most of the time, part of the pedicle graft will survive. Variable closure techniques can then be used to cover the defect.

Prevention

- Flap procedures should be planned carefully, with the blood supply as a primary consideration.

- Keep flaps as short as possible to assure optimal perfusion to the distant extremity, especially when using subdermal plexus flaps.

- Large flaps should include a direct cutaneous artery and vein whenever possible.

- The size of the flap should be sufficient to cover the defect without undue tension.

- Undermine skin below the panniculus muscle when present to preserve the subdermal plexus and direct cutaneous vessels.

- Consider a "delay procedure" if there is a concern regarding the flap circulation if transferred in a single stage. Flap transfer is delayed 18 to 21 days after initial creation, which improves circulation and survival.

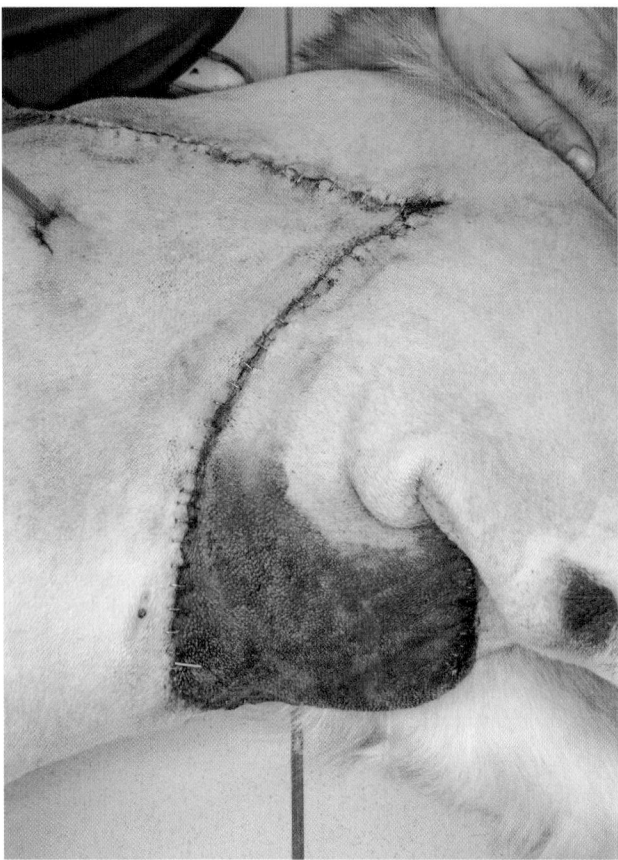

Figure 78.4 Use of a thoracodorsal axial pattern flap after excision of a ventrolateral chest wall soft tissue sarcoma. Note the deep purple coloration of the distal portion of the flap 1 day after surgery. *Source:* Julius Liptak, Alta Vista Animal Hospital, Ottawa, Ontario. Reproduced with permission from Julius Liptak.

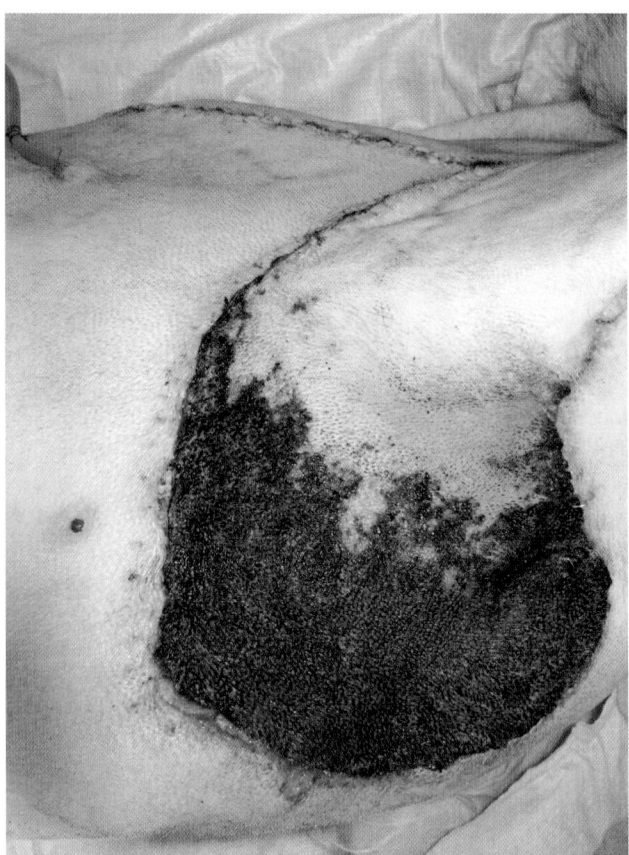

Figure 78.5 The same dog as in Figure 78.4, 3 days after surgery. Note the black coloration of the distal portion of the flap consistent with necrosis. A clear demarcation is evident between viable and nonviable skin. *Source:* Julius Liptak, Alta Vista Animal Hospital, Ottawa, Ontario. Reproduced with permission from Julius Liptak.

- Avoid kinking and twisting of the flap pedicle.
- Avoid sharply angled borders of the flap. Rounded extremities are preferable.
- Use skin hooks, stay sutures, or Adson-Brown forceps to manipulate the flap and limit tissue trauma.
- Respect adequate hemostasis and asepsis.
- Place a closed-suction drain if seroma formation is anticipated postoperatively.
- If a soft-padded bandage is used, it should be placed without excessive compression.
- Soft-padded bandages should be used if a flap is placed over a pressure area such as the elbow. Pressure-induced necrosis may indeed occur over the olecranon in these cases. Deep bedding and strict rest are also recommended in these cases.
- Damage to the flap by self-trauma is easily avoided by using an e-collar or by covering the flap with a bandage.

Hematoma and seroma

Definition

A hematoma is a pocket or localized collection of blood usually in liquid form within the tissue. A seroma is a pocket of clear serous fluid that may develop after surgery. It is composed of plasma seeping out after rupture of small blood vessels. Inflammation also contributes to the fluid.

Risk factors

- Presence of dead space under the flap: This is particularly true with large local or axial pattern flaps where considerable dissection is performed.

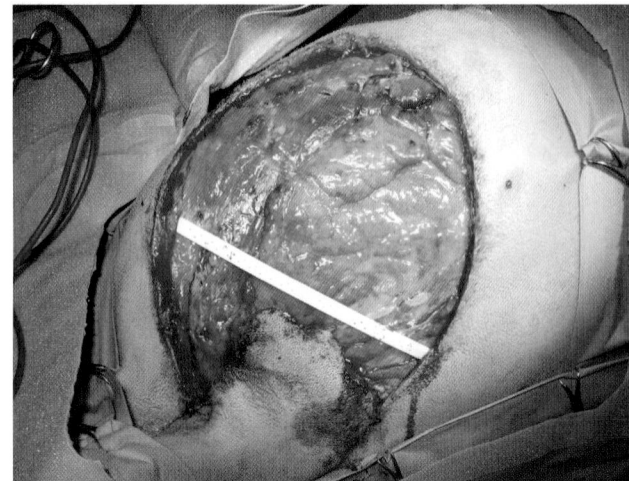

Figure 78.6 The same dog as in Figures 78.4 and 78.5. The necrotic skin has been debrided surgically. The defect was then closed by advancing the remaining flap. *Source:* Julius Liptak, Alta Vista Animal Hospital, Ottawa, Ontario. Reproduced with permission from Julius Liptak.

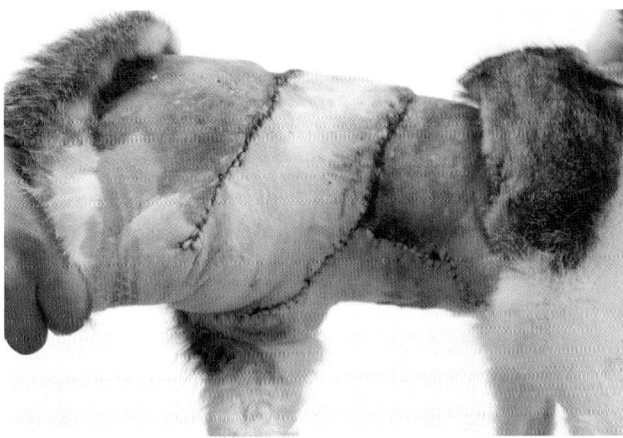

Figure 78.7 Use of a caudal superficial epigastric axial pattern flap in a cat after excision of an injection site sarcoma of the right flank. Note the presence of inguinal seroma postoperatively secondary to dead space. *Source:* Jean-Philippe Billet, Centre Hospitalier Veterinaire Atlantia, Nantes, France. Reproduced with permission from Jean-Philippe Billet.

- Large reconstructive procedures involving the thigh or inguinal areas are especially prone to seroma formation (Figure 78.7).
- Traumatic surgical technique
- Inadequate hemostasis
- Areas of excessive mobility

Diagnosis
- Swelling will be present.
- Fine-needle aspiration of the fluid will confirm the nature of the liquid accumulated below the flap: Aspiration will also differentiate accumulation of fluid below the flap from edema.
- Changes in color may appear if circulatory compromise occurs secondary to the pressure induced by the hematoma or seroma.

Treatment
Small seromas usually self-resolve. Early detected mild accumulation of fluid may also be treated conservatively by aspiration with a sterile hypodermic needle followed by placement of a soft-padded bandage. Placement of a closed suction drain may be necessary in case of recurrence or if the amount of fluid is important. Passive drains (Penrose) are not recommended because of the increased risk of contamination and infection.

Outcome
Collection of fluid under the flap can interfere with its blood supply and predispose it to necrosis. It also inhibits the influx of phagocytic cells into the area, increasing the risk of infection.

Seromas and hematomas are easily avoided by placing a closed-suction drain at the time of surgery (Figure 78.8). Early and adequate drainage should prevent skin necrosis.

Prevention
- Atraumatic surgical technique
- Adequate hemostasis
- Limit dead space as much as possible.
- Closed-suction drain may be placed for the first 2 to 4 days if postoperative accumulation of fluid is likely because of important dead space (e.g., large local or axial pattern flaps). Passive drains should be avoided because of the increased risk of contamination.

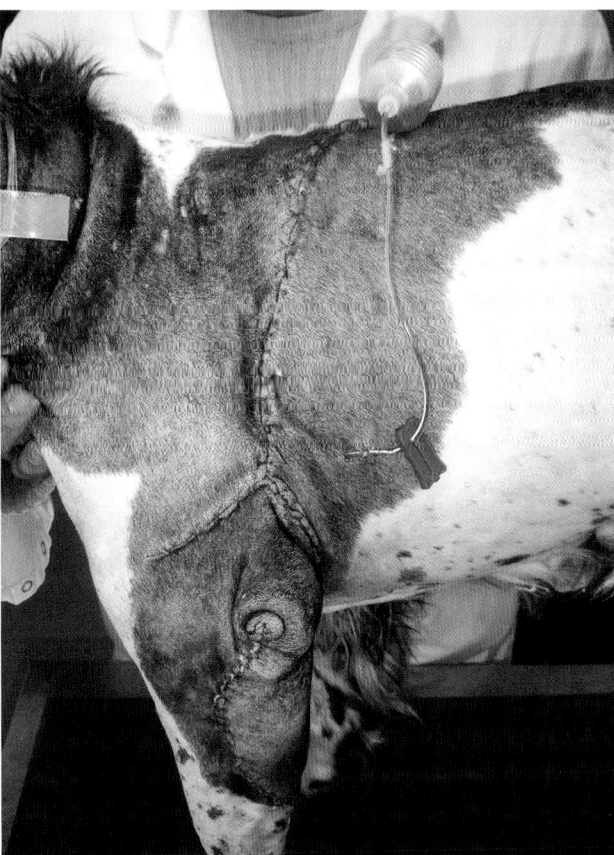

Figure 78.8 Thoracodorsal axial pattern flap used to cover a caudal antebrachial wound. A closed-suction drain was placed intraoperatively to prevent seroma formation.

- Drains should be used with caution in oncologic cases because their exit at the site distant from the primary surgical site may increase the size of any resection or radiation therapy treatment if margins are incomplete or recurrence occurs.
- Soft-padded bandages should be used in areas of excessive motion to maintain as much contact as possible between the flap and underlying tissue. Excessive compression should, however, be avoided to prevent circulatory compromise.

Inadequate flap immobilization

Definition
Inadequate flap immobilization can be defined as excessive mobility of the flap over underlying tissue. Skin flaps have, however, an inherent blood supply and do not require a bandage for their early revascularization unlike free grafts. Furthermore, bandages could compromise circulation to the flap if improperly applied.

Risk factors
- Inadequate or absent bandage over a flap covering a flexion surface such as the carpus or tarsus
- Absence of a bandage to cover distant direct flaps; bandages should be used in these flaps to immobilize the elevated extremity
- Inadequate restriction of movements or exercise of the animal postoperatively

Diagnosis

Excessive mobility of the flap in flexion areas may increase the risk of seroma formation and dehiscence. It may also cause excessive tension in some areas of the flap, which can interfere with circulation in the flap and induce necrosis.

Treatment

As mentioned previously, bandages should be used only in selected cases. If excessive motion or trauma of the flap is identified, proper soft-padded bandage (potentially reinforced with splints) should be placed as soon as possible. Treatments of seroma and circulatory compromise were described earlier.

Outcome

The outcome depends on the damages caused by the excessive motion. Outcomes of seroma and circulatory compromise were described earlier.

Prevention

- Use adequate soft-padded bandage to immobilize flaps covering a flexion surface (e.g., carpus, tarsus).
- Use adequate soft-padded bandage to cover local and axial pattern flaps placed in areas where excessive motion is anticipated and when large dead space has been created.
- Use a bandage to support the elevated extremity when using a distant direct flap.
- Soft-padded bandages should be used if a flap is placed over a pressure area such as the elbow. Pressure-induced necrosis may indeed occur over the olecranon in these cases.
- Bandages may be reinforced with splints if needed.
- Excessive compression should be avoided in all cases.
- Movements of the animal should be strictly restricted during the postoperative period.

Edema

Definition

Edema is an increased interstitial fluid in the flap caused by increased secretion of fluid in the interstitium or impaired removal of this fluid (impaired venous or lymphatic drainage).

Risk factors

- Excessive tension
- Excessively long flap causing impaired drainage of the extremity
- Kinking or twisting of the flap pedicle
- Underlying hematoma or seroma
- Inflammation or infection
- Traumatic surgical technique

Diagnosis

- Swelling of the flap will be present (Figures 78.9 and 78.10).
- Fine-needle aspiration can be performed to differentiate edema from seroma or hematoma.

Treatment

Moist warm compresses may be applied over the flap to reduce edema. A soft-padded bandage may also be applied.

Severe venous obstruction may lead to necrosis. Treatment associated with necrosis has been described earlier.

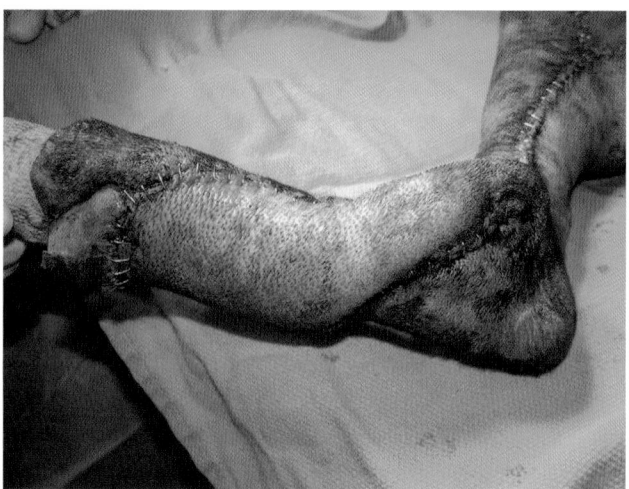

Figure 78.9 Immediate postoperative view of the use of a reverse saphenous conduit flap in a dog. *Source:* Julius Liptak, Alta Vista Animal Hospital, Ottawa, Ontario. Reproduced with permission from Julius Liptak.

Outcome

Edema usually resolves over time. It may, however, lead to flap necrosis if venous obstruction persists or is associated with arterial occlusion.

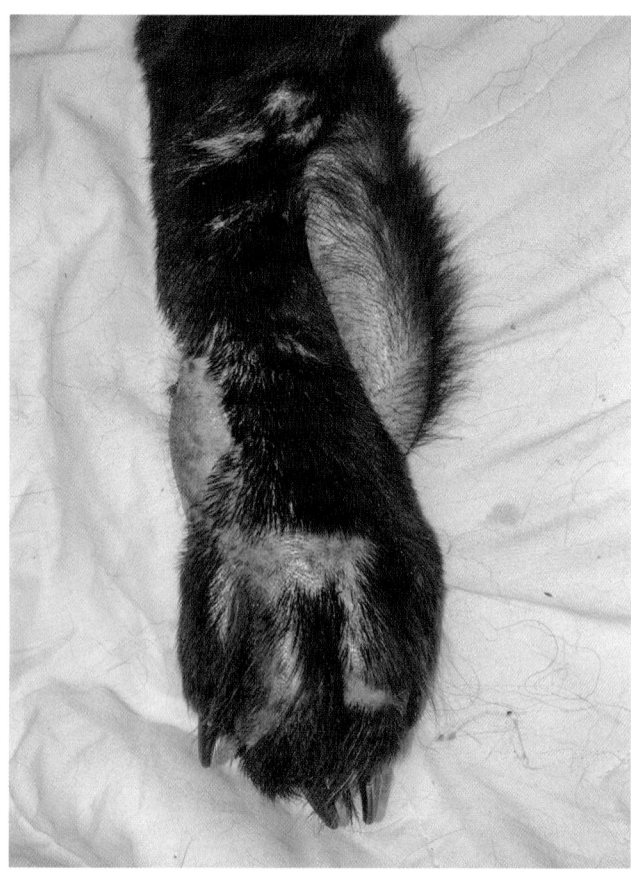

Figure 78.10 The same dog as in Figure 78.9 showing edema of the flap 1 month after surgery. Edema was most likely secondary to reverse blood flow and abnormal venous return. *Source:* Julius Liptak, Alta Vista Animal Hospital, Ottawa, Ontario. Reproduced with permission from Julius Liptak.

Prevention

- Keep flaps as short as possible to assure optimal perfusion and drainage to the distant extremity.
- Large flaps should include a direct cutaneous artery and vein whenever possible.
- The size of the flap should be sufficient to cover the defect without undue tension.
- Avoid kinking or twisting of the flap pedicle.
- Use skin hooks, stay sutures, or Adson-Brown forceps to manipulate the flap and limit tissue trauma.
- Respect adequate hemostasis and asepsis.
- If a soft-padded bandage is used, it should be placed without excessive compression.

Infection

See Chapter 1.

Relevant literature

The most common postoperative complication after a reconstructive flap procedure consists of **ischemia and necrosis** of a part or the totality of the flap. Guidelines for skin flap development and transfer have been largely described in textbooks (Pavletic 1998, 2003, 2010) and should be followed to maximize the chances of flap survival. The survival of reconstructive flaps is variable and has been reported in different experimental and clinical studies. It should be noted that the area of flap survival may not be as great in clinical cases as in experimental studies (Moores 2009). Greater flap necrosis in clinical cases may be related to greater rotation of the flap, movement of the flap during joint flexion, or pressure necrosis (Moores 2009). Conversely, it may sometimes be possible to harvest longer flaps than those described in the literature.

The survival of axial pattern flaps in general is high. A mean survival area of 73.3% was reported for omocervical axial pattern flaps, 84.7% for thoracodorsal axial pattern flaps, and 85.7% for deep circumflex iliac axial pattern flaps in a study of 15 dogs (Pavletic 1981). In the same study, survival areas of flaps incorporating a direct cutaneous artery and vein were significantly higher (95.1%) compared with the areas of flaps dependent only on the subdermal plexus (53.43%). Flap survival of caudal superficial epigastric flaps were 91% in a clinical series (Trevor *et al*. 1992), 100% in a case report using bilateral flaps (Mayhew and Holt 2003), and almost 100% in another case series of 10 dogs (Aper and Smeak 2005). Clinically, partial flap necrosis seems to be a frequent complication of thoracodorsal axial pattern flaps. A survival of 98% of the flap was reported in 2 animals in a clinical study (Trevor *et al*. 1992). In another clinical study of 10 dogs, however, only 3 dogs had complete flap survival; partial necrosis of the distal flap, ranging from 2% to 53% (mean, 21%) of the flap surface area, occurred in 7 dogs (Aper and Smeak 2003). Six dogs required surgical management of the skin necrosis, resulting in successful resolution in 5 dogs. The wound healed by second intention in 2 dogs. **Edema** and bruising of the distal portion of the flap was also noted in 8 dogs; distal flap necrosis subsequently occurred in 7 of them. Use of cranial superficial epigastric axial pattern flap resulted in an 87% to 100% area of flap survival in experimental dogs (Sardinas *et al*. 1995). Caudal auricular axial pattern flaps were used in 5 clinical cases in dogs and cats with a mean survival area of 99% (Trevor *et al*. 1992). Superficial temporal axial pattern flaps resulted in a mean survival area of 98% in cats and 93% in dogs (Fahie and Smith 1997; Fahie and

Smith 1999). An axial pattern flap based on lateral caudal arteries of the tail resulted in 78% survival in an experimental study in dogs (Saifzadeh *et al*. 2005). Axial pattern flaps based on the superficial brachial artery and the genicular artery resulted, respectively, in mean survival lengths of 98% and 89% in experimental dogs (Kostolich and Pavletic 1987; Henney and Pavletic 1988). Reverse saphenous conduit axial pattern flaps raised in experimental dogs and cats resulted in 100% survival in both (Pavletic *et al*. 1983; Cornell *et al*. 1995).

In a clinical study using random skin flaps based on subdermal plexus in 15 dogs, a mean flap survival of 89% was reported (de Carvalho Vasconcellos *et al*. 2005).

Seroma formation has been reported in 2 of 19 flaps in a clinical study of axial pattern flaps (Trevor *et al*. 1992) and in 2 of 10 dogs after thoracodorsal axial pattern flaps (Aper and Smeak 2003). Seroma resulted in flap survival in 1 dog and distal flap necrosis in the other in that study.

Omental pedicle grafts have been combined with thoracodorsal axial pattern flaps for the reconstruction of chronic nonhealing axillary wounds in 10 cats (Lascelles and White 2001). Complete healing occurred in all cats despite the need for a second surgery in 2 of them (1 for donor site dehiscence and 1 for flap dehiscence). Omentalization of chronic axillary wound has also been combined with omocervical axial pattern flap in a cat (Gray 2005). Omentalization of chronic wounds may aid healing by increasing vascularity via angiogenic factors released by the omentum, by absorbing tissue fluid, and by filling dead space (Goldsmith *et al*. 1967; Zhang *et al*. 1997; Lascelles and White 2001). Omentum may therefore replace a drain in wounds where dead space is present and fluid accumulation anticipated, decreasing the risk of ascending contamination.

Microvascular free tissue transfer involves the harvest of any autogenous tissue or combination of tissues with a consistent vascular pedicle from a donor site and its transfer to a recipient site with microvascular anastomosis of the donor artery and vein to an artery and vein at the recipient site. Free flaps are useful for one-stage reconstruction of difficult defects resulting from trauma or ablative cancer surgery, correction of congenital defects, osteomyelitis, nonunion fractures, and segmental bone loss (Fowler *et al*. 1998). Vascular occlusion (thrombosis) is the primary reason for free flap loss, with venous occlusion being more common than arterial occlusion (Novakovic *et al*. 2009). The majority of flap failures occur within the first 48 hours. Early recognition and rapid reexploration are crucial to maximize the chances of flap salvage (Novakovic *et al*. 2009). Development of flap congestion is consistent with venous insufficiency. Arterial flow is best assessed by Doppler monitoring (Fowler *et al*. 1998). Outcomes and complications after microvascular reconstructive procedures were evaluated in a retrospective clinical study of 57 consecutive cases (Fowler *et al*. 1998). Donor tissues were variable. A total of 53 flaps (93%) survived. A significant relationship was found between flap failure and level of assistant surgeon experience, enhancing the fact that both primary and assistant surgeons should be practiced in microvascular technique. Latissimus dorsi flaps were significantly more likely to fail than other flaps.

Radiation therapy combined with surgery is becoming more common for management of veterinary cancer patients. Reconstructive flaps may therefore be performed either after or before radiation therapy. Tolerance of cutaneous and mucosal flaps placed into a radiation therapy field has been evaluated clinically in 26 dogs (Séguin *et al*. 2005). Radiation therapy was performed either preoperatively or postoperatively. In a third group of dogs, a flap was performed as a salvage procedure for management of complications or local tumor recurrence after radiation therapy. Complications (necrosis, local infection, dehiscence, or ulceration) were observed in 77% of the dogs. A dose per fraction of 4 Gy compared with 3 Gy was prognostic for increased severity of complications. The authors found that placing a cutaneous or mucosal flap into a radiation therapy field led to a successful outcome in 85% of the dogs but was associated with substantial morbidity. Using a flap to correct a complication or failure of radiation therapy was more likely to result in a complication, but planned preoperative irradiation increased the severity of the complications compared with postoperative irradiation.

References

Aper, R.L., Smeak, D.D. (2003) Complications and outcome after thoracodorsal axial pattern flap reconstruction of forelimb skin defects in 10 dogs, 1989-2001. *Veterinary Surgery* 32, 378-384.

Aper, R.L., Smeak, D.D. (2005) Clinical evaluation of caudal superficial epigastric axial pattern flap reconstruction of skin defects in 10 dogs (1989-2001). *Journal of the American Animal Hospital Association* 41, 185-192.

Cornell, K., Salisbury, K., Jakovljevic, S., et al. (1995) Reverse saphenous conduit flap in cats: an anatomic study. *Veterinary Surgery* 24, 202-206.

de Carvalho Vasconcellos, C.H., Matera, J.M., Zaidan Dagli, M.L. (2005) Clinical evaluation of random skin flaps based on the subdermal plexus secured with sutures or sutures and cyanoacrylate adhesive for reconstructive surgery in dogs. *Veterinary Surgery* 34, 59-63.

Fahie, M.A., Smith, M.M. (1997) Axial pattern flap based on the superficial temporal artery in cats: an experimental study. *Veterinary Surgery* 26, 86-89.

Fahie, M.A., Smith, M.M. (1999) Axial pattern flap based on the cutaneous branch of the superficial temporal artery in dogs: an experimental study and case report. *Veterinary Surgery* 28, 141-147.

Fowler, J.D., Degner, D.A., Walshaw, R., et al. (1998) Microvascular free tissue transfer: results in 57 consecutive cases. *Veterinary Surgery* 27, 406-412.

Goldsmith, H.S., de Los Santos, R., Beattie, E.J. (1967) Relief of chronic lymphedema by omental transposition. *Annals of Surgery* 166, 573-584.

Gray, M.J. (2005) Chronic axillary wound repair in a cat with omentalisation and omocervical skin flap. *Journal of Small Animal Practice,* 46, 499-503.

Henney, L.H., Pavletic, M.M. (1988) Axial pattern flap based on the superficial brachial artery in the dog. *Veterinary Surgery* 17, 311-317.

Kostolich, M., Pavletic, M.M. (1987) Axial pattern flap based on the genicular branch of the saphenous artery in the dog. *Veterinary Surgery* 16, 217-222.

Lascelles, B.D., White, R.D. (2001) Combined omental pedicle grafts and thoracodorsal axial pattern flaps for the reconstruction of chronic, nonhealing axillary wounds in cats. *Veterinary Surgery* 30, 380-385.

Mayhew, P.D., Holt, D.E. (2003) Simultaneous use of bilateral caudal superficial epigastric axial pattern flaps for wound closure in a dog. *Journal of Small Animal Practice* 44, 534-538.

Moores, A. (2009) Axial pattern flaps. In Williams, J., Moores, A. (eds.) *BSAVA Manual of Canine and Feline Wound Management and Reconstruction*, 2nd edn. British Small Animal Veterinary Association, Gloucester, UK, pp. 100-143.

Novakovic, D., Patel, R.S., Goldstein, D.P., et al. (2009) Salvage of failed free flaps used in head and neck reconstruction. *Head and Neck Oncology* 1, 33.

Pavletic, M.M. (1981) Canine axial pattern flaps, using the omocervical, thoracodorsal, and deep circumflex iliac direct cutaneous arteries. *American Journal of Veterinary Research* 42, 391-406.

Pavletic, M.M. (1998) Skin grafting techniques. In Bojrab, M.J. (ed.) *Current Techniques in Small Animal Surgery*, 4th edn. Williams & Wilkins, Baltimore, pp. 585-603.

Pavletic, M.M. (2003) Pedicle grafts. In Slatter, D. (ed.) *Textbook of Small Animal Surgery*, vol. 1, 3rd edn. Saunders, Philadelphia, pp. 292-321.

Pavletic, M.M. (2010) *Atlas of Small Animal Wound Management and Reconstructive Surgery*, 3rd edn. Wiley-Blackwell, Ames, IO

Pavletic, M.M., Watters, J., Henry, R.W. (1983) Reverse saphenous conduit flap in the dog. *Journal of the American Veterinary Medical Association* 182, 380-389.

Saifzadeh, S., Hobbenaghi, R., Noorabadi, M. (2005) Axial pattern flap based on the lateral caudal arteries of the tail in the dog: an experimental study. *Veterinary Surgery* 34, 509-513.

Sardinas, J.C., Pavletic, M.M., Ross, J.T., et al. (1995) Comparative viability of peninsular and island axial pattern flaps incorporating the cranial superficial epigastric artery in dogs. *Journal of the American Veterinary Medical Association* 207, 452-454.

Séguin, B., McDonald, D.E., Kent, M.S., et al. (2005) Tolerance of cutaneous or mucosal flaps placed into a radiation therapy field in dogs. *Veterinary Surgery* 34, 214-222.

Trevor, P.B., Smith, M.M., Waldron, D.R., et al. (1992) Clinical evaluation of axial pattern flaps in dogs and cats: 19 cases (1981-1990). *Journal of the American Veterinary Medical Association* 201, 608-612.

Zhang, Q.X., Magovern, C.J., Mack, C.A., et al. (1997) Vascular endothelial growth factor is the major angiogenic factor in omentum: mechanism of the omentum-mediated angiogenesis. *Journal of Surgical Research* 67, 147-154.

79 Skin Grafting

Stéphanie Claeys

Small Animal Surgery, Department of Clinical Sciences (Companion Animals and Equids), Faculty of Veterinary Medicine, University of Liège, Liège, Belgium

A free skin graft is a segment of dermis and epidermis that is completely detached from its original location and transferred to a recipient site. In veterinary medicine, grafts are exclusively autografts (i.e., donor and recipient are the same patient). Free grafts are primarily indicated for reconstruction of full-thickness skin defects on the extremities. They are usually used when the defect cannot be repaired by other reconstruction techniques such as primary closure, flaps, and so on.

Free grafts are classified according to the graft thickness or the graft design. Free grafts may be harvested as full- or split-thickness grafts. Split-thickness grafts contain a variable depth of the upper dermal layers and epidermis. They are harvested with razor blades, graft knives, or a dermatome. They take more readily than full-thickness grafts, but they lack durability and proper hair growth, and they are more susceptible to secondary graft contraction (Pavletic 2010). Full-thickness grafts contain the entire dermal layer with the epidermis. They are robust and retain all the adnexal dermal elements that are essential for the ultimate functional and cosmetic success of the graft (White 2009).

Grafts may completely cover the wound (sheet grafts) or may be used as partial-coverage grafts to increase the surface area of epithelialization within the wound (punch, pinch, stamp, strip, and mesh grafts).

Regarding the technique used, free grafts lack a vascular attachment upon transfer to the recipient bed. They must first survive through plasmatic imbibition (absorption of fluids and cells into the graft by capillary action). Graft vessels will then anastomose with recipient vessels (inosculation), and new capillaries will later grow into the graft. In addition, fibrous connective tissue forms to hold the graft securely in place.

Complications are mainly related to the presence of material between the graft and recipient bed that will delay or prevent graft revascularization, resulting in graft necrosis. Motion between the graft and the recipient bed will have the same effect.

Inadequate graft preparation

Definition

This is poor preparation of the segment of skin harvested at the donor site.

Risk factors

- Insufficient removal of hypodermal tissue in full-thickness grafts. Any hypodermal adipose tissue interposed between the dermis and recipient bed may impede plasmatic imbibition, inosculation, and revascularization of the graft.
- Removal of the hypodermal layer with a scalpel blade may damage the dermal layer.
- Desiccation of the graft caused by a delay between harvest of the graft and application to the wound
- Inadequate size of the graft compared with the recipient wound: Whereas a graft made too small will be too stretched over the recipient bed, an excessively large graft may form folds that lack proper bed contact. Both cases will cause improper contact between the graft and the recipient bed, preventing good graft revascularization.
- Insufficient numbers of full-thickness incisions in mesh grafts, resulting in insufficient drainage of the fluid produced by the recipient wound

Diagnosis

Inadequate graft preparation may result in graft failure if insufficient hypodermal tissue is removed, for example, or if insufficient meshing result in accumulation of fluid between the graft and recipient bed. Nonviable grafts appear white or black and separate from the wound bed. Failure may imply the whole graft or only a portion of the harvested skin.

Treatment

Guidelines for grafting techniques should be followed to adequately prepare the segment of harvested skin and avoid failure. Graft salvage is impossible in most cases. Nonviable grafts are removed from the wound when necrosis is well established.

Outcome

Inadequate graft preparation may lead to graft failure. Superficial graft necrosis may sometimes occur, but hair follicles and cutaneous adnexa in the deep portion of the graft may survive and help epithelialization of the wound.

Prevention

- Hypodermal adipose tissue should be removed completely in full-thickness grafts to improve vascular access to the dermis. The

Complications in Small Animal Surgery, First Edition. Edited by Dominique Griffon and Annick Hamaide.

© 2016 John Wiley & Sons, Inc. Published 2016 by John Wiley & Sons, Inc.

Companion website: www.wiley.com/go/griffon/complications

bases of the hair follicles should be visible if the graft has been properly prepared.

- Avoid removal of the hypodermal layer with a scalpel blade; the use of fine scissors is preferred.
- The graft should be placed on the recipient wound as soon as possible after collection. If not immediately applied, the graft should be placed in saline-soaked gauze pads to avoid desiccation.
- Grafts should be collected under strict aseptic conditions. Some surgeons also recommend presoaking the graft in antibiotic solution before application to reduce infection.
- To adequately determine the size of the graft to be harvested, create a template of the wound using, for example, the paper from a package of sterile surgical gloves. The paper is applied to the wound, cut to its shape, and placed over the recipient site to determine the size of the required donor skin.
- A sufficient number of perforations should be performed in mesh grafts to allow drainage. Skin grafts can be meshed by making handmade stab incisions with a scalpel blade or by using an expansion unit.

Inadequate preparation of the graft bed

Definition
This is poor preparation of the graft recipient site before graft application.

Risk factors
- Presence of debris or infection on the recipient site: Bacteria may cause dissolution of fibrin attachments, and exudate accumulation may separate the graft from its bed.
- Presence of stratified squamous epithelial surfaces
- Exposed bone, cartilage, tendon, and nerve (Figure 79.1)
- Irradiated tissues
- Avascular fat
- Crushing injuries
- Hypertrophic or long-standing granulation tissue
- Chronic ulcers

Diagnosis
Inadequate preparation of the graft bed may result in graft failure, which is characterized by a black or white coloration and separation of the graft.

Treatment
Careful preparation of the graft bed is very important to maximize graft take. Salvage of a failing graft is impossible in most cases. Nonviable portions of the graft should be resected as soon as apparent.

Outcome
Inadequate preparation of the graft bed may lead to graft failure. Superficial graft necrosis may sometimes occur, but hair follicles

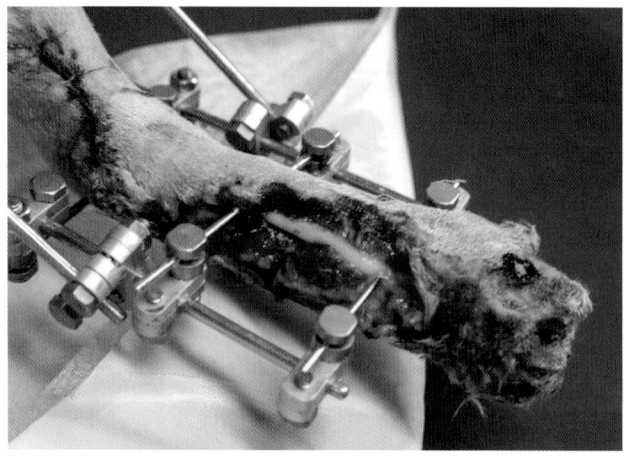

(A)

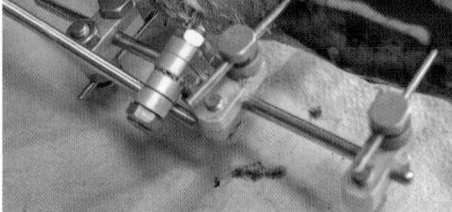

(B)

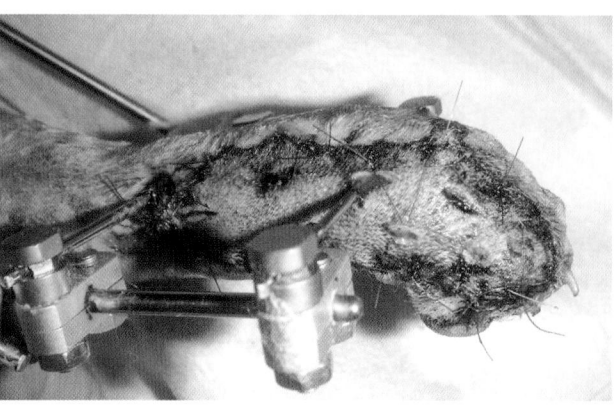

(C)

Figure 79.1 Traumatic wound of the hind limb in a cat. **A**, The initial wound bed is inadequate for grafting because of exposed bone, necrotic tissue, and absence of granulation tissue. **B**, Three weeks of wound management was required to obtain a healthy granulating bed. Exposed bone required a few more days to be covered by granulation tissue. **C**, A partially meshed full-thickness free graft was applied to the wound with complete graft survival (picture taken 2 days after grafting).

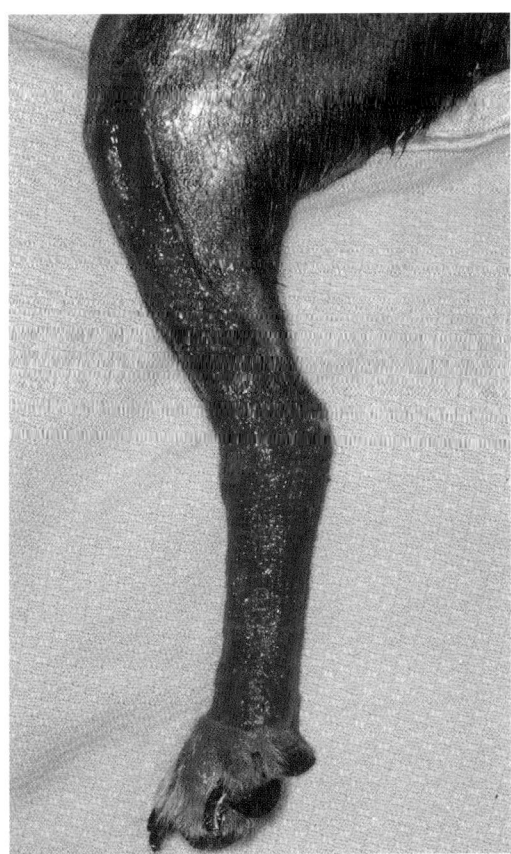

Figure 79.2 Healthy fresh granulation tissue ideal for grafting. A free meshed skin graft was used to cover the defect with complete graft survival. *Source:* Julius Liptak, Alta Vista Animal Hospital, Ottawa, Ontario. Reproduced with permission from Julius Liptak.

and cutaneous adnexa in the deep portion of the graft may survive and help epithelialization of the wound.

Prevention
- Suitable recipients sites include healthy granulation tissue, fresh surgical wounds, or surgically clean wounds.
- Healthy pink granulation tissue is an ideal recipient bed because it contains a large amount of vascular capillaries (Figure 79.2).
- The grafting procedure should be delayed until debris and infection are eliminated from the wound. Infected wounds should be thoroughly lavaged, debrided, and properly bandaged until healthy granulation tissue is present.
- The grafting procedure should be performed under strict aseptic conditions.
- Topical antibiotics should be used to cover the recipient bed after healthy granulation tissue is present. Systemic antibiotics are also recommended before surgery and for 1 postoperative week.
- Skin grafts should be performed as soon as possible to benefit from the vascular support of newly formed granulation tissue. Long-standing granulation tissue contains fewer capillaries and more connective tissue.
- Chronic or hypertrophic granulation tissue, chronic ulcers, or crushed tissue should be completely resected and properly bandaged to create fresh granulation tissue.
- If epithelialization is present at the periphery of the wound, the wound edges should be excised.

Hematoma and seroma

Definition
A hematoma is a localized collection of blood usually in liquid form within the tissue. A seroma is a pocket of clear serous fluid composed of plasma seeping out after rupture of small blood vessels.

Fluid will be produced by the recipient site during the first few days until adherence is complete. This fluid provides nourishment for the graft tissues, but its excessive accumulation can also separate the graft from the recipient wound, breaking down the fibrin seal and ultimately causing graft failure.

Risk factors
- Traumatic surgical technique
- Inadequate hemostasis of the recipient bed
- Insufficient meshing of the graft preventing adequate drainage
- Absence of a drain underneath a sheet graft (complete wound coverage)
- Grafts placed over fresh wounds are more prone to development of hematomas or seromas than grafts placed over granulation tissue.
- Excessively large grafts may form folds that lack contact with the recipient bed and may move over the wound, increasing the risk of fluid accumulation.

Diagnosis
Accumulation of fluid underneath the graft may be recognized during bandage changes. Swelling will be present. If unrecognized early, fluid will cause separation of the graft from the recipient site, and mobility of the graft will be visible. This will ultimately lead to graft failure characterized by a black or white coloration of the graft.

Treatment
If accumulation of fluid is noticed during inspection of meshed grafts, gentle pressure may be applied with cotton buds over mesh openings to remove the fluid. Alternatively, fluid may be aspirated with a fine hypodermic needle.

Outcome
Fluid accumulation should be detected early and removed as soon as possible. Undetected fluid accumulation will otherwise lead to graft separation and failure. Prevention is again very important.

Prevention
- Atraumatic surgical technique
- Good preparation of the recipient wound, which should be free of any debris and infection
- Adequate hemostasis of the recipient wound: Time should be allowed for natural hemostatic processes to occur, and vascular oozing should be controlled before graft application. Some authors recommended using diluted epinephrine to control hemorrhage.
- A closed-suction drain should be placed under sheet grafts for complete coverage of the wound (unmeshed).
- An opportunity for drainage (drains or meshing) should be provided if excessive exudation is anticipated, such as after application of a graft over a fresh wound.
- Grafts should be of adequate size to fit the recipient wound and should be sutured in place under a little tension to improve wound contact.

Infection (see Chapter 1)

Inadequate graft immobilization

Definition

Immobilization is essential for graft take. Movement between the graft and the recipient bed can interfere with the development of the fibrin seal, preventing adherence of the graft and ingrowth of new capillaries from the recipient bed. This may delay or even prevent graft take.

Risk factors

- Insufficient number of sutures placed at the periphery or through the graft
- Inadequate or insufficient bandaging placed over the graft
- Inadequate restraint of the animal during bandage changes
- Inadequate restriction of activity postoperatively

Diagnosis

Movement of the graft over the recipient wound may be visible. If unrecognized, graft instability will lead to failure of revascularization and graft necrosis characterized by a black or white coloration.

Treatment

Prevention of graft movement is essential because graft movement will rapidly lead to graft failure, and a failing graft is usually impossible to salvage.

Outcome

Minor movement of the graft during the first 24 hours does not necessarily lead to graft failure. Subsequent movement will, however, prevent revascularization by ingrowth of new capillaries and will lead to graft necrosis.

Prevention

- A sufficient number of sutures should be placed at the periphery of the graft to minimize movement.
- Sutures may be placed through the holes of meshed grafts to increase stability.
- Adequate bandaging technique is essential for graft take. A non- or low-adherent contact layer should be used to prevent the bandage from sticking to the graft during bandage changes. An antibiotic ointment is commonly added to reduce bacterial contamination and prevent desiccation of the graft. Skin staples or sutures may be used to help maintaining the contact layer over the grafted area. An absorbent intermediate layer (gauze sponges and cotton) is then applied to immobilize the graft against the recipient bed, absorb exudates, and limit movement of the limb. An outer elastic layer is then applied to protect the bandage.
- Additional immobilization is commonly required, especially for skin grafts applied over or close to a joint surface. Various types of splints may be added to the bandage. A spica splint is recommended for grafts applied to the proximal portions of the limb.
- Tie-over bandages may be useful in some areas such as the inner thighs.
- Dressings should not be changed too frequently frequently to avoid movement of the graft, but accumulation of exudates should also be avoided. The first bandage change is usually performed after 48 to 72 hours to avoid disturbing early revascularization of the graft. The contact layer should be removed carefully to avoid lifting the graft during removal. If the dressing adheres to the graft, it can be softened with warm saline and gently pulled. Alternatively, the dressing may be left on the graft, and antibiotic ointment may be added on top of it. The frequency of subsequent bandage changes depends on the type of graft and the amount of exudates produced. Bandage changes are commonly timed every 2 to 4 days. Daily changes may be needed if infection is present or if the bandage becomes soiled with feces or urine.
- Adequate restraint of the patients is required during bandage changes to avoid trauma to the graft. Animals should be sedated or even anesthetized if needed.
- Animals should be confined and activity restricted to short leash walks outside to urinate and defecate. Restriction of the activity is particularly important during the first 48 hours.

Tissue ischemia

Definition

Ischemia is a restriction in blood supply with resultant damage or dysfunction of tissue. Graft ischemia will lead to necrosis and graft failure. Ischemia may be caused by failure of plasmatic imbibition, inosculation, or ingrowth of new capillaries.

Risk factors

- Inadequate removal of hypodermal tissue during graft preparation
- Poorly vascularized recipient bed (long-standing or hypertrophic granulation tissue, irradiated tissue, exposed bone)
- Inadequate drainage, causing excessive accumulation of fluid underneath the graft
- Inadequate immobilization of the graft
- Excessively tight bandages

Diagnosis

Grafts are pale when initially placed on the recipient bed. They will then appear cyanotic and edematous from day 1 to day 3 as plasmatic imbibition peaks (Figure 79.3). Blue coloration is then normal at this point. A reddish tinge will then appear by 72 to 96 hours. The entire graft should be less edematous and pinker by postoperative day 7 or 8 if survival is complete.

- Graft ischemia is indicated by the persistence of white areas (Figure 79.4). These will ultimately necrose and slough (Figure 79.5). Necrosis is characterized by a black coloration and separation of the graft from the wound bed.

Treatment

Areas of necrosis should be resected as soon as recognized. The wound can be left to heal by second intention or be treated by another grafting procedure (after obtaining a healthy granulation bed) or any other reconstructive technique when possible.

Outcome

Salvaging an ischemic graft is often impossible. Prevention is therefore essential. As stated previously, partial-thickness take of the graft is sometimes observed. The epidermis may then slough, but the underlying viable dermis reepithelializes from adnexa in the dermis.

Prevention

- See the above recommendations for proper graft and recipient bed preparation, adequate drainage, and bandaging techniques.

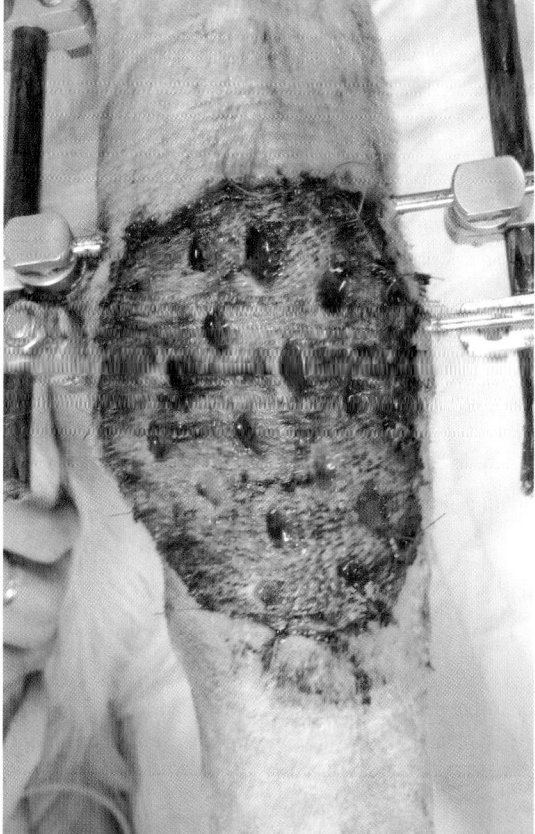

(A)

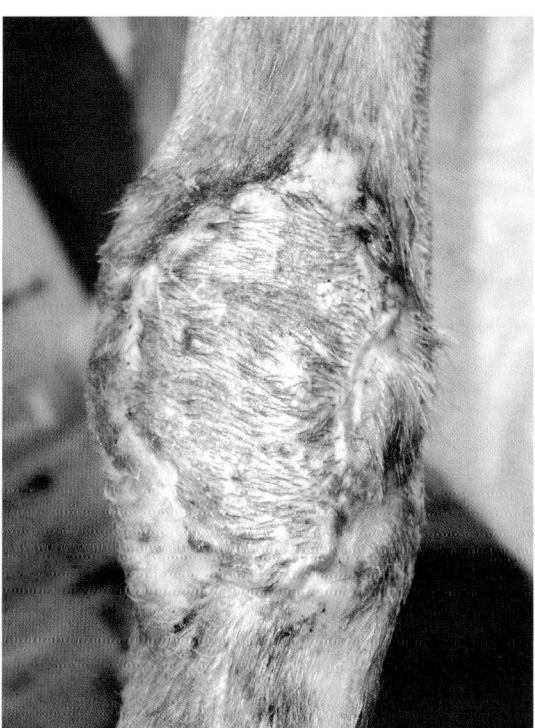

(B)

Figure 79.3 Free meshed graft over the carpus of a dog. **A**, Two days after surgery. Note the normal cyanotic appearance of the graft caused by plasmatic imbibition. **B**, Fourteen days after grafting: complete graft survival is noted as well as hair regrowth.

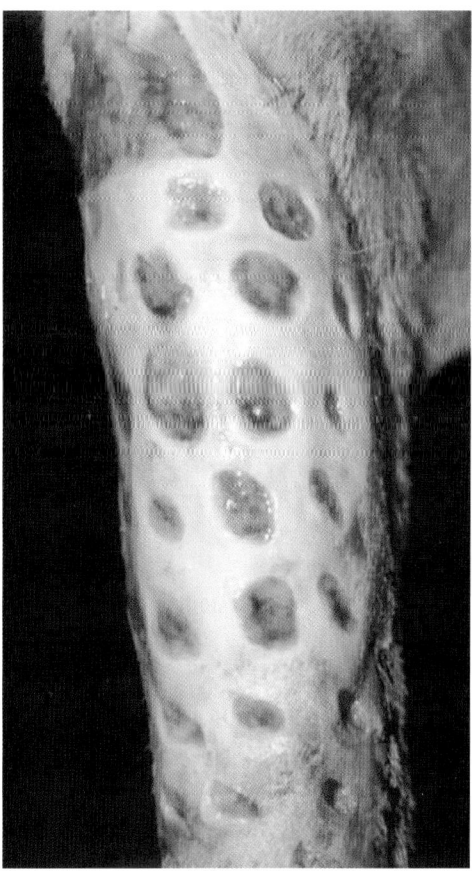

Figure 79.4 Complete failure of a free meshed skin graft. Note the white ischemic appearance of the graft. No secondary healing is observed in the open mesh areas. *Source:* Julius Liptak, Alta Vista Animal Hospital, Ottawa, Ontario. Reproduced with permission from Julius Liptak.

Lack of reinnervation

Reinnervation of grafts depends on the type and thickness of the graft, the amount of scar tissue formation, and the innervation of surrounding tissue. Return of sensation is better in full-thickness grafts than in split-thickness grafts. Animals may show signs of paresthesia as grafts reinnervate (at about 3 weeks), which may manifest as licking at the graft. The graft may be covered by a bandage for an additional week, or an Elizabethan collar may be used until paresthesia subsides.

Cosmetic defects

Definition

These are unsatisfactory cosmetic results after a grafting procedure.

Risk factors

- Split-thickness grafts contain fewer adnexal structures than full thickness grafts. Hair regrowth is therefore sparse and less cosmetic.
- Extensively meshed grafts, even if full thickness, will heal with a greater proportion of epithelialized tissue within the created holes. The cosmetic result will therefore be less satisfactory because epithelialized areas contain no adnexal structures.
- Strip, punch, and pinch grafts give the worst cosmetic results because they heal with large areas of epithelialization. Hair regrowth will therefore be patchy.

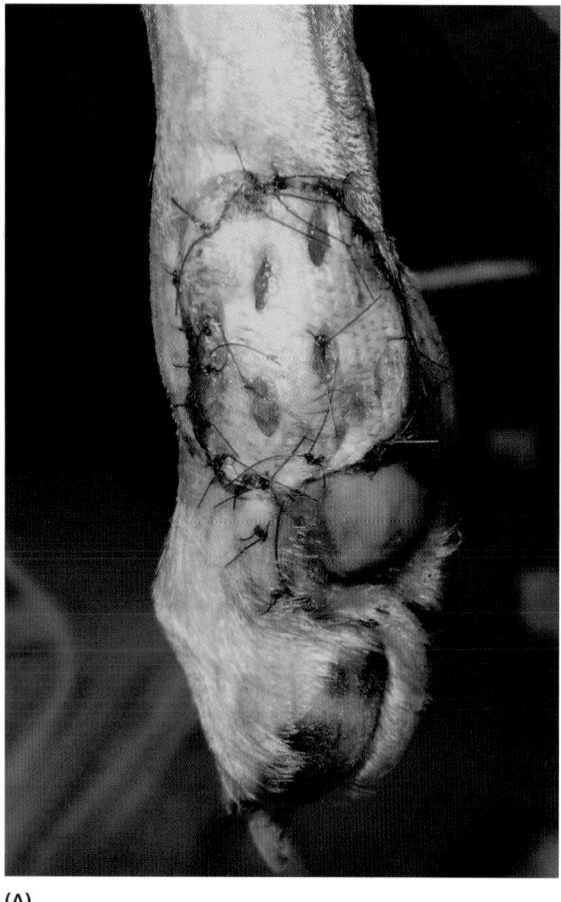

(A)

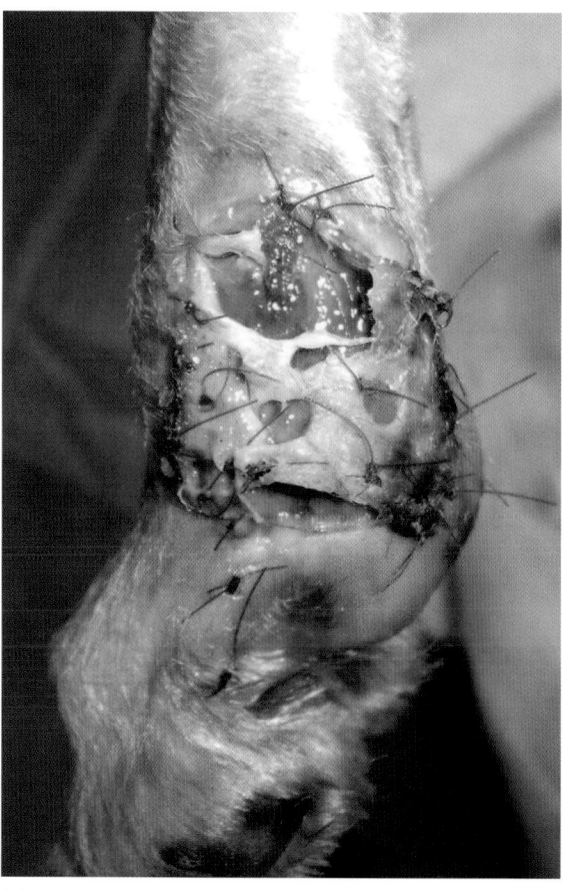

(B)

Figure 79.5 Free meshed skin graft applied to the distal extremity of a dog. **A**, Two days after surgery. Note the abnormal pale coloration of the graft. The graft should be cyanotic at that point because of plasmatic imbibition. **B**, Six days after surgery: complete graft failure is observed with sloughing of the graft. The underlying granulation tissue seems pale (long-standing), which may have caused graft failure. More than 2 weeks of wound management was indeed required because of abundant initial necrotic tissue. Graft movement may be another explanation.

- Damage to hair follicle bases during hypodermal tissue removal may cause sparse hair regrowth.
- Inadequate match between the donor skin and the skin surrounding the recipient site (different hair direction, color, and so on)

Diagnosis
Hair regrowth is usually noticed 2 to 3 weeks after grafting (see Figure 79.3). Some grafts may never regrow hair despite good functional results (Figure 79.6). Epithelialized skin will be more fragile and lack hair growth.

Treatment
No treatment is required. Although the cosmetic appearance may be an important factor, the functional result should be the primary goal.

Outcome
Some grafts may never regrow hair despite good functional results. Epithelialized skin will be more fragile and lack hair growth. An inadequate match between the grafted and the surrounding skin is not of primary importance. A different color or direction of hair may be less cosmetic but is of little importance compared with the functional result of the graft.

Prevention
- Prefer full-thickness grafts to split-thickness grafts whenever possible.
- Unmeshed grafts are more cosmetic than meshed grafts. They, however, do not provide drainage and expansion. Avoid extensively meshed grafts whenever possible.
- Strip, punch, and pinch grafts should be used only if absolutely needed, and owners should be informed of their poor cosmetic result.
- Matching the appearance of the donor skin to that of the surrounding recipient site should be attempted whenever possible, although this is not of primary importance.

Relevant literature
Free skin grafts are separated from their blood supply when transferred to their recipient site. Their survival depends on the reestablishment of a vascular supply from the recipient bed. Complications after grafting procedures are mainly related to inadequate preparation of the graft bed or the recipient site, inadequate bandaging techniques causing movement of the graft, and the accumulation of fluid underneath the graft, all of which may ultimately lead to graft

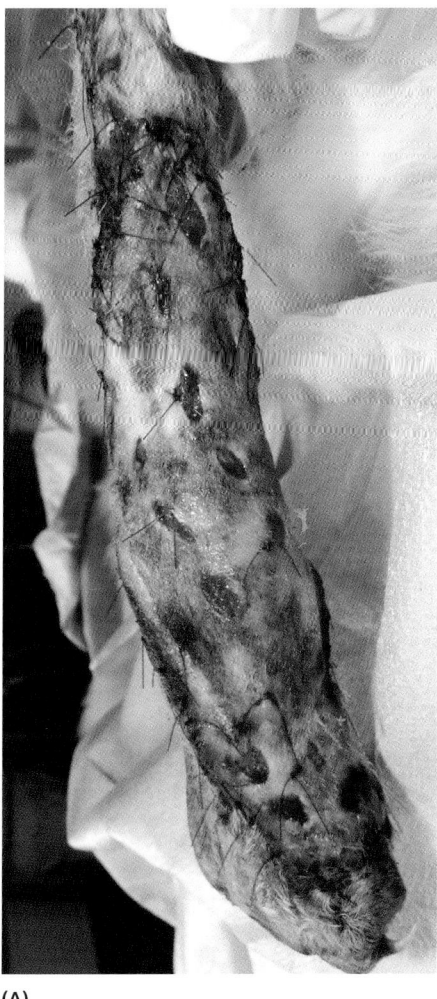 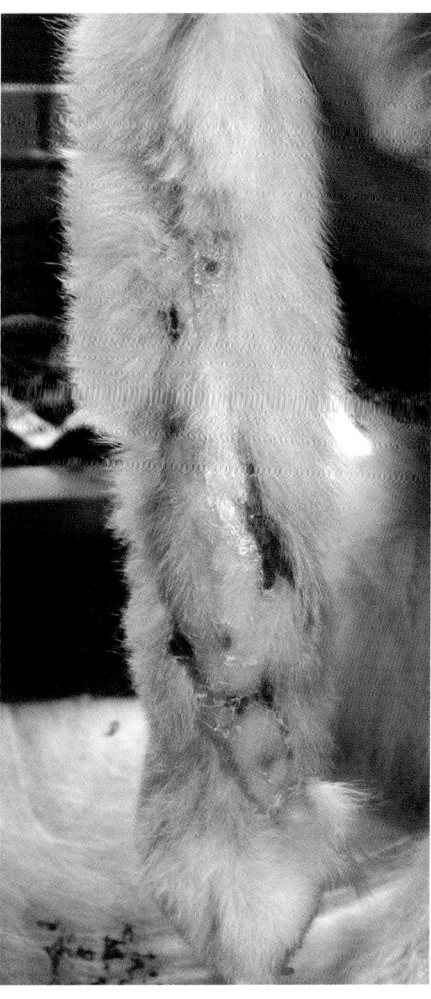

(A)   (B)

Figure 79.6 Free meshed skin graft covering the right front limb of a cat. **A**, Six days after surgery. **B**, Six weeks after surgery. Although graft take was complete, only very sparse hair regrowth is visible.

ischemia and failure. Recommendations for grafting procedures are widely available in the literature (Pope 1990; Probst 1990; Swaim 1990; Pope 1998; Swaim 2003; White 2009; Pavletic 2010). Principles of skin grafting should be followed to maximize graft take and minimize complications.

Limited data are, however, available in the literature regarding the success rates and complications of varying grafting procedures in companion animals.

Survival of unexpanded partial thickness mesh grafts was evaluated in 9 dogs and 1 cat presented with wounds of the distal extremity (van Zuilen and Kirpensteijn 1995). Graft take approached 100% in 5 cases, 95% in 1 case, 90% in 2 cases, 75% in 1 case, and 30% in 1 case. The overall percentage take reported in this study was 88%.

Split-thickness skin grafts are usually considered to take more easily than full-thickness grafts. One study, however, showed that full-thickness grafts tended to have a greater viability and contracted more than split-thickness grafts in dogs, although no significant differences were found (Bauer and Pope 1986). In this study, graft viability of both types of skin grafts was evaluated 10 days after surgery. The mean graft viabilities for full- and split-thickness grafts placed on fresh recipient beds were 81% and 55%, respectively.

Full- and split-thickness grafts placed on granulating beds had mean viabilities of 58% and 47%, respectively.

Adjunct treatments that may improve the survival of free skin grafts have been investigated. The effect of deferoxamine and hyperbaric oxygen on free autogenous full-thickness skin grafts was evaluated in dogs (Hosgood *et al.* 1995). The authors did not recommend their clinical use because hyperbaric oxygen appeared detrimental to the viability of free skin grafts, and deferoxamine-10% hydroxyethyl pentafraction starch failed to improve their survival.

The use of vacuum assisted closure (VAC) therapy has been reported to improve **immobilization** of free skin grafts on their recipient bed on distal extremities in dogs (Ben Amotz *et al.* 2007). VAC therapy is the intermittent or continuous application of negative pressure to a specialized wound dressing to help promote wound healing. In this study, VAC therapy was used after full-thickness mesh grafts in 9 dogs to immobilize the graft–wound bed interface immediately after surgery. Petroleum-impregnated gauze was applied over the graft before the foam was placed, and 75 mm Hg of continuous suction pressure was applied. Graft viability was assessed after 72 hours by removing the VAC. All grafts survived. The mean VAC time was 9.7 days. This study describes an adjunctive method of securing skin grafts to the wound bed. The application of continuous negative pressure dressing allows uniform distribution of pressure and apposition between the graft and the bed, even in case of an irregular surface. It immobilizes the graft tissue interface, reducing graft failures caused by movement. The dressing also provides continuous removal of wound fluids, preventing hematoma and seroma formation. Graft desiccation is also prevented by the occlusive nature of the VAC dressing.

Wound drainage and **cosmetic appearance** of four types of full-thickness skin grafts were evaluated in 12 dogs (Pope and Swaim 1986a, 1986b). The techniques evaluated were a sheet graft, continuous low-level suction, piecrust incisions, and nonexpanded mesh graft. In the first part of the study, the amount of wound drainage was quantified for the first 10 postoperative days (Pope and Swaim 1986a). Results showed that significantly more fluid was removed by continuous low-level suction than the other techniques. Meshing allowed more drainage than the piecrust or sheet grafts but was not as effective as low-level suction. Piecrust incisions had no significant effect on drainage. In the second part of the study, they evaluated graft survival on the 10th postoperative day and hair growth 3 months postoperatively (Pope and Swaim 1986b). The mean survival rate for all grafts was 90%. No statistical differences in categories of hair growth were detected within types or between types of grafts, and all types exhibited a significantly greater area of acceptable (normal or moderate hair growth) than nonacceptable hair growth (sparse or none).

References

Bauer, M.S., Pope, E.R. (1986) The effect of skin graft thickness on graft viability and change in original graft area in dogs. *Veterinary Surgery* 15, 321-324.

Ben-Amotz, R., Lanz, O.J., Miller, J.M., et al. (2007) The use of vacuum-assisted closure therapy for the treatment of distal extremity wounds in 15 dogs. *Veterinary Surgery* 36, 684-690.

Hosgood, G., Hodgin, E.C., Strain, G.M., et al. (1995) Effect of deferoxamine and hyperbaric oxygen on free, autogenous, full-thickness skin grafts in dogs. *American Journal of Veterinary Research* 56, 241-247.

Pavletic, M.M. (2010) *Atlas of Small Animal Wound Management and Reconstructive Surgery*, 3rd edn. Wiley-Blackwell, Ames, IO.

Pope, E.R. (1990) Mesh skin grafting. *Veterinary Clinics of North America. Small Animal Practice* 20 (1), 177-187.

Pope, E.R. (1998) Mesh skin grafting. In Bojrab, M.J (ed.) *Current Techniques in Small Animal Surgery*, 4th edn. Williams & Wilkins, Baltimore, pp. 603-607.

Pope, E.R., Swaim, S.F. (1986a) Wound drainage from under full-thickness skin grafts in dogs. Part I. Quantitative evaluation of four techniques. *Veterinary Surgery* 15, 65-71.

Pope, E.R., Swaim, S.F. (1986b) Wound drainage from under full-thickness skin grafts in dogs. Part II. Effect on cosmetic appearance. *Veterinary Surgery* 15, 72-78.

Probst, C.W. (1990) Grafting techniques and failures in small animal surgery. *Problems in Veterinary Medicine* 2 (3), 413-423.

Swaim, S.F. (1990) Skin grafts. *Veterinary Clinics of North America. Small Animal Practice* 20 (1), 147-175.

Swaim, S.F. (2003) Skin grafts. In Slatter, D. (ed.) *Textbook of Small Animal Surgery*, vol. 1, 3rd edn. WB Saunders, Philadelphia, pp. 321-338.

Van Zuilen, C.D., Kirpensteijn, J. (1995) Distal extremity mesh grafts in nine dogs and one cat. *Vet Quarterly* 17 (Suppl.), S9-S10.

White, R.A.S. (2009) Free skin grafting. In Williams, J. Moores, A. (eds.) *BSAVA Manual of Canine and Feline Wound Management and Reconstruction*, 2nd edn. British Small Animal Veterinary Association, Gloucester, UK, pp. 144-158.

80 Anal Sac Excision

Lynne A. Snow
Southeast Veterinary Specialists, Metairie, LA, USA

Anal sac excision is performed to treat chronic or recurrent anal sacculitis and anal sac neoplasia and to assist in the management of perianal fistulas. Anal sacculitis is diagnosed in approximately 12.5% of dogs (Halnan 1976a). Treatment options include conservative therapy such as flushing of the duct and antibiotics or surgical excision (Halnan 1976b). Historically, chemical ablation of the anal sacs with infusion of cetrimide and formaldehyde (Halnan 1976b) was proposed but is not recommended because of devastating complications associated with extravasation of caustic materials and the development of extensive soft tissue wounds (Figure 80.1).

Long-term complications are reported in 15% of dogs after anal sac excision for non-neoplastic disease (Hill and Smeak 2002).

The most commonly reported long-term complication associated with anal sac excision is persistent infection or fistula formation reported in 6.3% (6 of 95 dogs) of dogs (Hill and Smeak 2002).

Fecal incontinence is reported in 2.1% (2 of 95 dogs) of dogs after anal sac excision for anal sacculitis (Hill and Smeak 2002), but a smaller study of 25 dogs reported an incidence as high as 8% (2 of 25 dogs) (Halnan 1976b). Up to 33% of dogs undergoing anal sac adenocarcinoma excision experienced fecal incontinence in one report of 32 dogs (Aronson 2003). Fecal incontinence is reported in 4% to 29% of dogs treated for anal furunculosis by fistula excision and anal sacculectomy (Aronson 2003; Milner 2006). The high occurrence of incontinence in these dogs may be related to extensive dissection necessitated by concurrent muscle damage associated with the primary disease.

Anal stricture is an uncommon complication of anal sac excision with a reported incidence of 3.2% (3 of 95 dogs), all of which had open anal sacculectomy (Hill and Smeak 2002). Anal stricture was reported in 13% (6 of 48 dogs) of dogs treated for anal furunculosis by fistula excision and anal sacculectomy, which is likely attributable to concurrent disease in these dogs (Milner 2006).

Persistent infection and drainage

Definition
Infection may manifest as excessive wound drainage or incisional dehiscence within the first 2 weeks after surgery. A long-term complication after anal sac excision is chronic persistent infection, which typically presents as a fistulous tract with purulent discharge (Figure 80.2).

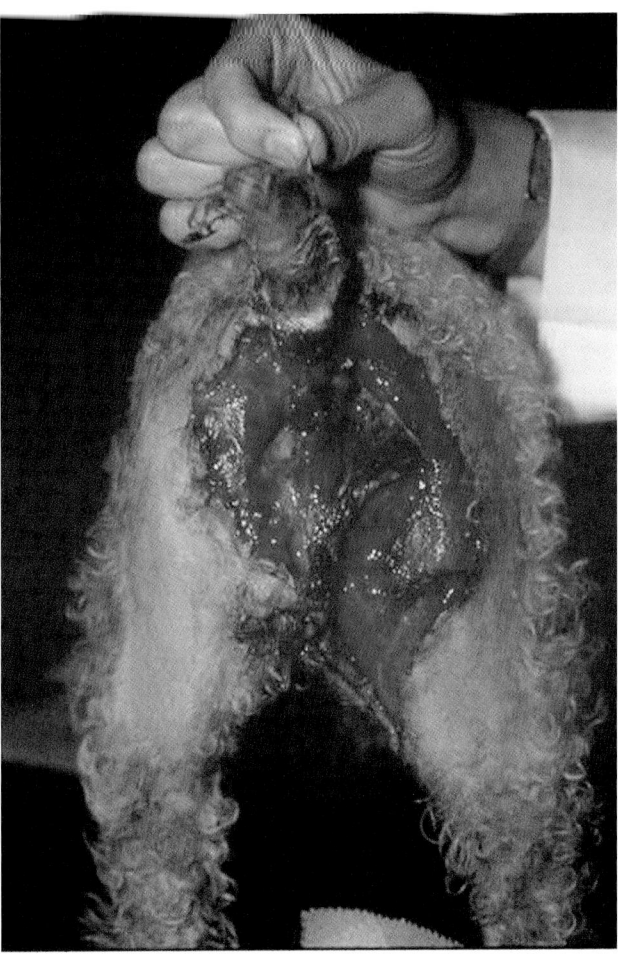

Figure 80.1 Dog with extensive perianal wound after use of formaldehyde for anal sac ablation. *Source:* G. Hosgood, 2014. Reproduced with permission from G. Hosgood.

Risk factors
- Short term. Contamination at the time of surgery may lead to infection in the initial postoperative period. Contamination may arise from the anal sac or from fecal contamination.
- Long term: The most common cause of fistulous tract formation after anal sac excision is retained anal sac epithelium or anal sac duct (Figures 80.3 and 80.4).

Complications in Small Animal Surgery, First Edition. Edited by Dominique Griffon and Annick Hamaide.
© 2016 John Wiley & Sons, Inc. Published 2016 by John Wiley & Sons, Inc.
Companion website: www.wiley.com/go/griffon/complications

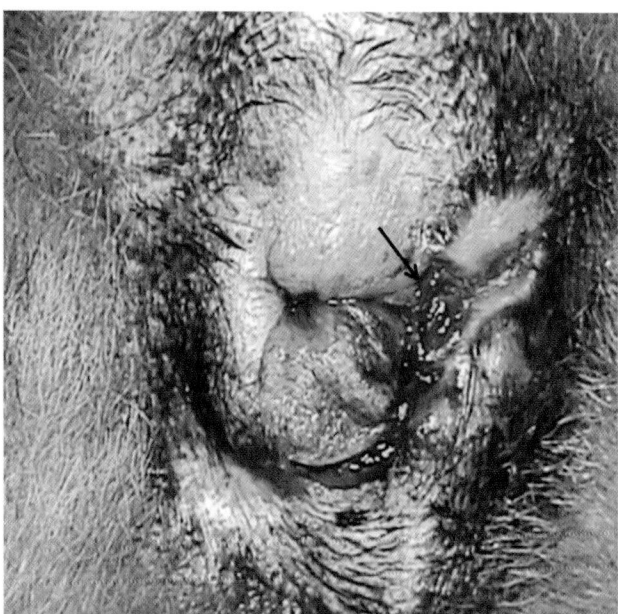

Figure 80.2 Dog with fistulous tract after anal sac excision. The fistula (arrow) developed 2 weeks after anal sac excision. Resolution of fistula was achieved with en-bloc excision. *Source:* G. Hosgood, 2014. Reproduced with permission from G. Hosgood.

Diagnosis

- The presumptive diagnosis of persistent anal sac epithelium is often made on the history of recent anal sac excision and the presence of a fistula.
- Fistulography may be useful if there is concern that the fistula may involve the rectum or other perianal structures.
- When a persistent infection is suspected, wound tissue culture and sensitivity testing is indicated to confirm the presence of bacterial colonization and facilitate selection of appropriate antibiotic therapy.

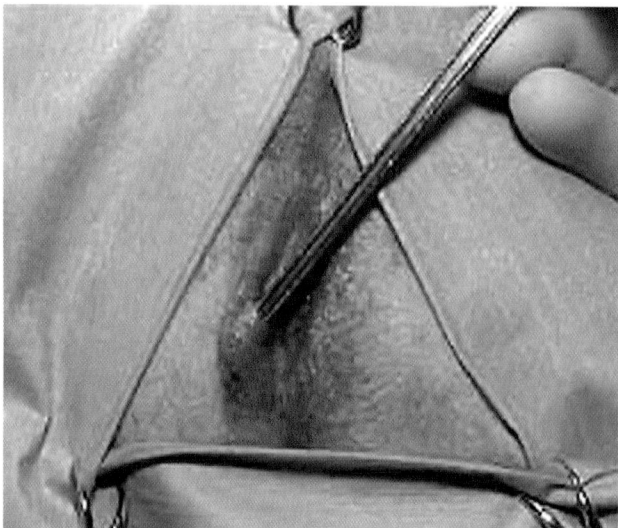

Figure 80.3 Probe placed in anal sac duct to identify the location of the anal sac. The entire anal sac duct and orifice should be excised to prevent fistula formation. *Source:* G. Hosgood, 2014. Reproduced with permission from G. Hosgood.

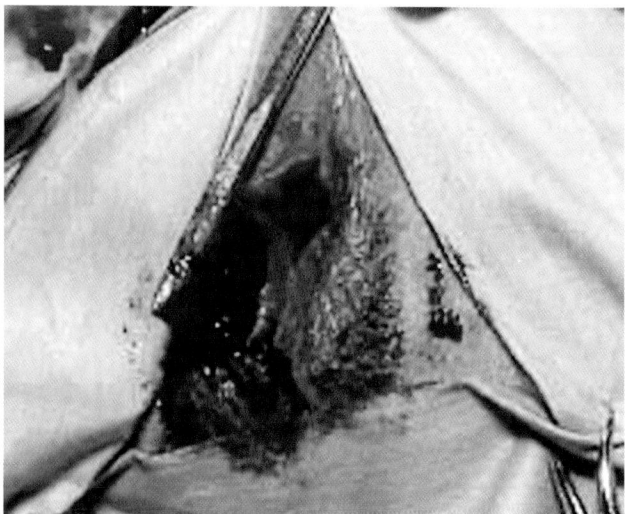

Figure 80.4 Incision along axis of anal sac. The outer surface of the anal sac is visualized. *Source:* G. Hosgood, 2014. Reproduced with permission from G. Hosgood.

Treatment

Wound infection caused by contamination at the time of surgery is treated with appropriate antibiotics based on culture and sensitivity testing results. If the infection does not resolve or recurs after discontinuation of appropriate antimicrobials, the area should be explored for residual epithelial tissue. Incomplete excision of the anal sac or its duct is suspected if a fistulous tract develops after the initial incision has healed. In these dogs, the area must be delicately explored to ensure removal of all remaining epithelial tissue or the tissue removed en bloc. The excised tissue should be submitted for culture and sensitivity testing and histopathology.

Outcome

Fistulous tracts should resolve with excision of all remaining epithelial tissue. Surgical excision of residual epithelial tissue is technically demanding. There is an increased risk of bleeding and nerve damage, resulting in partial or complete fecal incontinence (Marretta and Matthiessen 1989; MacPhail 2008).

Prevention

Anal sac excision is delayed for several days to 2 weeks after anal sac rupture to allow inflammation and infection to resolve. If surgery is attempted during this acute inflammatory phase, the excessive friability of the anal sac may increase the risk of incomplete epithelial excision and secondary fistula formation (Marretta and Matthiessen 1989). Delayed surgery also improves identification of tissue layers and decreases the amount of contamination because the bacterial load will be reduced after treatment with appropriate antimicrobials. Perioperative antibiotics effective against gram-negative and anaerobic bacteria are indicated because the perianal region is easily contaminated with fecal material during surgery. Fecal contamination is decreased by packing the distal rectum with gauze sponges.

Closed anal sac excision is recommended to minimize direct contamination at the time of surgery. Various techniques have been described to aid in identification of the anal sac to help facilitate complete excision. Instillation of a potentially caustic or irritating substance such as silicone sealant (Frye *et al.* 1970), melted paraffin,

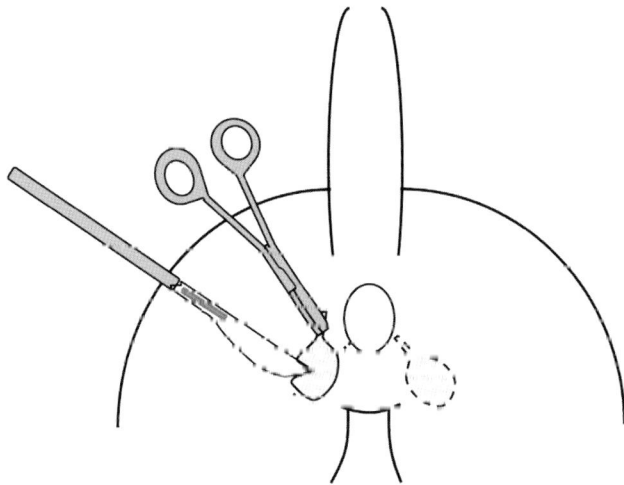

Figure 80.5 Scalpel blade technique for anal sac excision due to anal sacculitis. With a probe in the anal sac (see Fig 80.3), the skin and external anal sphincter are incised along the axis of the duct to expose the outer surface of the anal sac (see Fig 80.4). A small elliptical incision is made around the anal sac duct orifice and the duct dissected. The duct is grasped with a hemostatic forceps. The external anal sphincter muscle is scraped away from the outer surface of the anal sac using a #15 scalpel blade. This allows the entire outer surface to be visualized during dissection without excessive trauma to the external anal sphincter or other surrounding soft tissues. The anal sac remains closed throughout the procedure. The incision is closed with several deep sutures and a subdermal layer *Source:* G. Hosgood, 2014. Reproduced with permission from G. Hosgood.

and dental acrylic are not recommended because this may lead to complications if the anal sac integrity is compromised. A Foley catheter (Downs and Stampley 1998) or string can be instilled into the anal sac, but this may be difficult to do in small dogs.

One technique to ensure complete excision of the anal sac is by semi-open dissection, beginning at the duct. The skin and external anal sphincter are incised along the axis of the sac to expose the outer surface of the anal sac. The opening of the duct is isolated and grasped with hemostatic forceps. Dissection follows down the duct to the anal sac. A small scalpel blade is used to push the external anal sphincter off the outer surface of the sac (Hosgood 2011) (Figure 80.5). This provides excellent visualization of the outer anal sac surface with minimal trauma to the surrounding soft tissues.

Fecal incontinence

Definition
Fecal incontinence is loss of controlled defecation.

Risk factors
- External anal sphincter trauma
- Caudal rectal nerve damage
- Excessive soft tissue trauma during surgical dissection

Diagnosis
- Fecal incontinence is diagnosed by witnessing defecation without conscious control. This must be differentiated from diarrhea and urgency incontinence secondary to rectal irritation.
- Anal tone and perineal reflex may be decreased in cases of fecal incontinence because of caudal rectal nerve damage or

inflammation. Perianal skin sensation is evaluated by application of an external stimulus. If sensation is decreased or absent, caudal rectal nerve damage is suspected.
- Electromyography may be used to confirm loss of innervation to the external anal sphincter muscle.

Treatment
Inflammation from surgical dissection is treated with nonsteroidal antiinflammatory drugs. Surgical inflammation generally resolves in 5 to 10 days with return of continence. There is no effective method of reinnervation of the external anal sphincter muscle. A low-bulk diet is used to produce a firm formed stool (Marretta and Matthiessen 1989). Frequent walks, especially after meals, should be encouraged to minimize accidents in the house (Marretta and Matthiessen 1989).

Outcome
Incontinence caused by external anal sphincter muscle trauma will resolve spontaneously over 1 to 2 weeks if less than 50% of the external anal sphincter is damaged (MacPhail 2008). Unilateral nerve damage typically causes a transient fecal incontinence, which may last from several days up to 2 weeks (MacPhail 2008). Incontinence persisting for more than 3 to 4 months is considered permanent (Marretta and Matthiessen 1989).

Prevention
Careful dissection with gentle tissue handling is required for anal sac excision. The caudal rectal nerve is located cranial to the anal sac, and deep dissection is minimized to avoid inadvertent nerve damage (Marretta and Matthiessen 1989).

Anal stricture

Definition
Anal stricture is circumferential narrowing or stenosis of the anus resulting from deposition and contracture of fibrous tissue.

Risk factors
- Open anal sac excision
- Excessive trauma to the anal mucosa or external anal sphincter
- Chemical ablation of anal sacs
- Previous anal sac abscess rupture and formation of perirectal stricture (Walshaw 1983).

Diagnosis
- Anal stricture is suspected in an animal that develops tenesmus several weeks after anal sac excision. Upon digital rectal examination, a constricting band at the site of anal sac excision is palpated.
- Abdominal radiographs may be normal or confirm obstipation by identifying impacted fecal material in the colon (Webb *et al.* 2007).
- Colonoscopy can be used to directly visualize the constriction if more extensive disease is suspected.

Treatment
Treatment for anal stricture depends on the severity of stricture. Clinical signs associated with a small stricture may be alleviated by administration of a stool softener and a high-fiber diet. Anal stricture over a large area may require more aggressive treatment. Surgical excision of the constricting band or reconstructive techniques

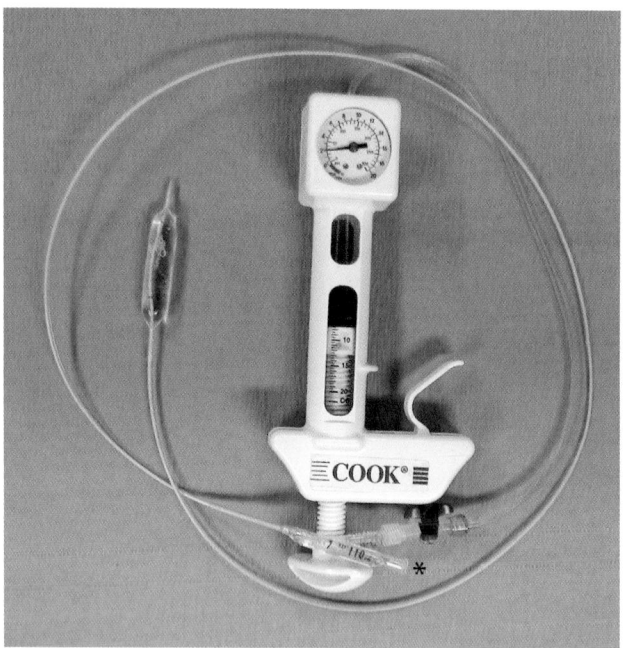

Figure 80.6 Balloon dilation catheter and pump. The length of the stricture is measured and an appropriate length balloon chosen. A guidewire is placed across the stricture through the portal (asterisk). When in the correct location, the balloon is dilated by injecting water using the inflation device to the desired pressure.

may be attempted; however, the risk of recurrence is considered high (Marretta and Matthiessen 1989). Balloon dilation or bougienage may be used to increase the anal diameter and alleviate tenesmus (Marretta and Matthiessen 1989). Results of balloon dilation (Figure 80.6) and intralesional triamcinolone injection of rectal strictures have been promising with 12 out of 15 dogs having resolution of rectal stricture caused by non-neoplastic conditions (Webb *et al.* 2007).

Outcome

Complete resolution of anal stricture is rare. Clinical signs may be alleviated with a combination of balloon dilation and dietary management.

Prevention

Careful dissection with delicate tissue handling is required for anal sac excision. Surgeon experience decreases the incidence of anal stricture. Closed anal sac excision is recommended to minimize rectal and external anal sphincter trauma.

Relevant literature

Anal sac excision may be performed via an open approach in which the anal sac is opened and the epithelial lining visualized. There is increased risk of contamination, but dissection may be easier. Alternatively, a closed approach is used in which the anal sac is not opened, thus containing the contents and minimizing contamination. A study involving 95 dogs undergoing anal sac excision for non-neoplastic conditions compared the incidence of long-term complications by either open or closed techniques (Hill and Smeak 2002). The overall complication rate was 15% (14 of 95 dogs). Of these, 11.6% (11 of 14 dogs with complications) were in dogs in which anal sacculectomy was performed by an open approach compared with 3.2% (3 of 14 dogs with complications) in dogs in which a closed approach was used (Hill and Smeak 2002). The development of fistulous tracts was the most common complication with a reported incidence of 6.3% (Hill and Smeak 2002). Other complications were fecal incontinence in 2 dogs (2.1%) and anal stricture in 3 dogs (3.2%) (Hill and Smeak 2002). Age, weight, type of anal sac disease, and whether the wound was closed were not associated with the incidence of complications (Hill and Smeak 2002).

References

Aronson, L. (2003) Rectum and anus. In Slatter, D. (ed.) *Textbook of Small Animal Surgery*, 3rd edn. WB Saunders, Philadelphia, pp. 682-708.

Downs, M.O., Stampley, A.R. (1998) Use of a Foley catheter to facilitate anal sac removal in the dog. *Journal of the American Animal Hospital Association* 34 (5), 395-397.

Frye, F.L., Hoeft, D.J., Cucuel, J.P., et al. (1970) Silicone sealant for preoperative packing of canine anal sacs. *Journal of the American Veterinary Medical Association* 156 (8), 1030-1031.

Halnan, C.R. (1976a) The frequency of occurrence of anal sacculitis in the dog. *Journal of Small Animal Practice* 17 (8), 537-541.

Halnan, C.R. (1976b) Therapy of anal sacculitis in the dog. *Journal of Small Animal Practice* 17 (10), 685-691.

Hill, L.N., Smeak, D.D. (2002) Open versus closed bilateral anal sacculectomy for treatment of non-neoplastic anal sac disease in dogs: 95 cases (1969-1994). *Journal of the American Veterinary Medical Association* 221 (5), 662-665.

Hosgood, G. (2011) Personal communication. Murdoch University Veterinary Hospital, Murdoch University, Murdoch, WA, Australia.

MacPhail, C. (2008) Surgical views: anal sacculectomy. *Compendium of Continuing Education for the Practicing Veterinarian* 30 (10), 530-535.

Marretta, S.M., Matthiessen, D.T. (1989) Problems associated with the surgical treatment of diseases involving the perianal region. *Problems in Veterinary Medicine* 1 (2), 215-242.

Milner, H.R. (2006) The role of surgery in the management of canine anal furunculosis: a review of the literature and a retrospective evaluation of treatment by surgical resection in 51 dogs. *New Zealand Veterinary Journal* 54 (1), 1-9.

Walshaw, R. (1983) Anal sac disease. In Bojrab, M.J. (ed.) *Current Techniques in Small Animal Surgery*. WB Saunders, Philadelphia, pp. 196-201.

Webb, C.B., McCord, K.W., Twedt, D.C. (2007) Rectal strictures in 19 dogs: 1997-2005. *Journal of the American Animal Hospital Association* 43 (6), 332-336.

81 Feline Onychectomy

Ameet Singh and Brigitte A. Brisson
Department of Clinical Studies, University of Guelph, Guelph, Ontario, Canada

Onychectomy, or surgical amputation of the third phalanx (P3) is an elective surgical procedure performed on the forelimbs of cats to eliminate destructive or harmful scratching behavior. It is also indicated for treatment of nail bed neoplasia or paronychia. Several onychectomy techniques have been described, including guillotine amputation of P3 with nail shears (Resco) and disarticulation of P3 with scalpel blade dissection, a carbon dioxide (CO_2) laser or a radiofrequency (RF) unit with or without the use of a tourniquet. After removal of P3, the surgical site is closed using suture or surgical tissue adhesive or left open to heal by second intention. Bandages can be applied postoperatively based on surgeon preference.

Both short- and long-term complications have been described after onychectomy in cats; however, long-term complications are poorly described (Patronek 2001). Short-term complications include hemorrhage, pain, neuropraxia or ischemic injury secondary to tourniquet application, digital pad trauma, lameness, and non–weight bearing (Tobias 1994; Patronek 2001). Long-term complications include infection or osteomyelitis, nail regrowth, chronic pain syndrome, development of a palmigrade stance, lameness, and protrusion of the second phalanx (P2) (Tobias 1994; Patronek 2001). In a retrospective study performed on cats undergoing onychectomy at a teaching institution, short-term complications were associated with the use of a scalpel blade for onychectomy, and long-term complications were associated with guillotine onychectomy (Tobias 1994). In that study, 50% of cats had at least one or more complications immediately after surgery (Tobias 1994). The use of CO_2 laser for onychectomy has been advocated because it has been suggested that the precise vaporization of soft tissues limits hemorrhage and inflammation and reduces early postoperative pain compared with traditional techniques (Holmberg and Brisson 2006; Robinson *et al.* 2007).

Infection

See Chapter 1.

Pain and lameness

Definition

This is reluctance to ambulate or place weight on the onychectomized limbs as if walking on hot coals. Neurologic deficits or tissue injury may be apparent and secondary to ischemic injury

or compression effect from tourniquet or forelimb bandages. Cats with chronic pain syndrome may also exhibit behavioral changes such as increased aggression, inappropriate urination, licking or chewing at their paws, anorexia, and aversion to having their paws touched.

Risk factors

- Retained bone fragments of P3
- Inadequate perioperative analgesia
- Prolonged tourniquet application
- Use of tissue adhesive for wound closure
- Flexor tendon contracture
- Excessive or traumatic tissue manipulation during surgery
- Iatrogenic digital pad trauma
- Bandage complications
- Infection or osteomyelitis
- Nail regrowth
- Arthritis

Diagnosis

The owner should be carefully questioned and a thorough history obtained to determine the cat's behavior before and after onychectomy. The most common physical examination finding is pain or discomfort upon palpation of the distal aspects of the digits. Additional physical examination findings may include:

- Soft tissue swelling at the distal aspect of the digits
- Digital pad trauma
- Exposed P2
- Permanent flexion of the digits
- Radial nerve deficits
- Nail regrowth

Examination of the digits will provide evidence for infection, trauma, or exposed P2. If permanent flexion of the digits is present, contracture of the flexor tendons is diagnosed. A complete neurologic examination should be performed to eliminate a neurologic cause of pain or lameness. If neurologic deficits are present, electrodiagnostic testing may be indicated for neurolocalization of the lesion. Radiographs should be performed to rule out the presence of retained bone fragments of P3. Chronic postsurgical pain as a result of inadequate perioperative analgesia is diagnosed when other causes have been ruled out. Chronic pain is likely the most common reason for a persistent long-term lameness in onychectomized cats (Robertson and Lascelles 2010).

Treatment

- If bone fragments of P3 are discovered radiographically, surgical removal should be performed. Conservative management of retained fragments of P3 is not recommended because resolution of lameness without removal is unlikely.
- Permanent digit flexion secondary to contracture of the flexor tendon requires surgical tendonectomy of the involved digits. An approach is made to the palmar surface of the digit to allow for an approximate 5-mm tendonectomy of the flexor tendon (Cooper *et al.* 2005). A thorough understanding of regional anatomy is required before tendonectomy for flexor tendon contracture.
- A neuroma is a tangled web of regenerating neuronal fibers mixed with connective tissue that can grow after onychectomy and is thought to contribute to chronic postsurgical pain of neuropathic origin (Mathews 2008). After it is diagnosed, chronic postsurgical pain must be treated aggressively.
- The major pathophysiological event in onychectomized cats with chronic pain is peripheral and central sensitization. Peripheral sensitization is the reduced threshold of peripheral nociceptors that can occur from exposure to inflammatory mediators. Prolonged stimulation of peripheral nociceptors can result in altered neuronal activity in the dorsal horn of the spinal cord, leading to central sensitization (also known as the "wind-up" phenomenon) (Mathews 2008). Activation of N-methyl-D-aspartate (NMDA) receptors is thought to be a critical event in the development of central sensitization or wind-up, and treatment with an NMDA receptor antagonist (amantadine) is recommended. A multimodal approach to analgesia should be performed in addition to the use of an NMDA receptor antagonist for its spinal cord modulatory ability. An example protocol for the treatment of chronic pain in cats is:

  Amantadine (3–5 mg/kg orally [PO] every 24 hours for 3 weeks)

  Meloxicam (0.01–0.03 mg/kg PO every 24 hours long term as necessary) (Carroll *et al.* 2005; Gunew *et al.* 2008)

  Buprenorphine (0.01–0.02 mg/kg transmucosal (buccal) every 12 hours for 3–7 days)

  +/− Gabapentin (10 mg/kg PO every 12 hours for 7–14 days) Environmental enrichment

Outcome

The prognosis of cats treated surgically for retained fragments of P3 or permanent contracture of the flexor tendons is good, but a report in the literature on a large series of cats with these complications is lacking. A report on outcome for the treatment of cats with chronic pain after onychectomy is also lacking from the literature because this complication is underrecognized and not widely reported. With early and aggressive treatment including spinal cord modulation with NMDA receptor antagonists, it is expected that most cats will have a reduction in pain and improved limb function and behavioral response. However, response is variable in each cat with some requiring weeks to months before medications can be discontinued (Robertson and Lascelles 2010).

Prevention

- A thorough knowledge of regional anatomy, meticulous dissection, and gentle soft tissue manipulation is required to reduce inflammation at the sites of onychectomy.
- A CO_2 laser may be the preferred method for onychectomy, especially in adult cats. It has been reported that this technique reduces inflammation and neuroma formation and improves weight bearing and comfort level in the early postoperative period.
- An additional advantage of onychectomy using a CO_2 laser is that a tourniquet and postoperative bandaging are not required. This eliminates the potential for ischemic injury and neurologic deficits to the forelimbs.
- A multimodal approach to perioperative analgesia should be undertaken. A fentanyl transdermal patch should be applied 18 to 24 hours before surgery. Premedication can be achieved with an α_2 agonist and an opioid. A presurgical four-point block of the pes with bupivacaine (1 mg/kg per forelimb) can be performed to disrupt nociceptive signaling in branches of the median, ulnar, and radial nerves. A nonsteroidal antiinflammatory drug (NSAID) can be administered at the time of induction to prevent the spinal "wind-up," assuming contraindications are not present. Postoperative analgesia should include an opioid with or without gabapentin. If preoperative administration of an NSAID was not performed, it should be given postoperatively.

Nail regrowth

Definition

This complication occurs when the germinal epithelium of the ungual crest of P3 is incompletely removed during onychectomy. Persistent germinal epithelial cells are allowed to regenerate deformed nails, which have also been termed *scurs*.

Risk factors

- Inadequate removal of the germinal epithelium of the ungual crest of P3
- Excessive dissection and aggressive tissue handling during surgery
- Use of the guillotine technique for onychectomy

Diagnosis

- Careful examination of the paw will reveal deformed nails protruding from the distal aspect of the digits (Figure 81.1).
- Radiography should be performed to determine whether retained bone fragments of P3 are also present.

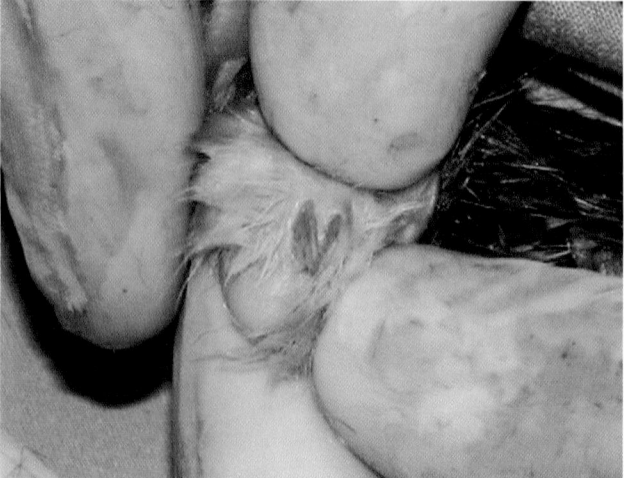

Figure 81.1 Typical nail regrowth, also known as scurs, consisting of a deformed nail protruding from the distal aspect of the digit 1 year after declaw procedure.

Treatment

When regrowth has been diagnosed, surgical exploration and removal of the regrown nail with or without bone fragments should be performed. Careful evaluation of all digits by palpation and radiography will determine which digits require surgical exploration. An aggressive approach to perioperative analgesia (see earlier) should be undertaken because it has been the authors' experience that surgical exploration of regrown nails can involve excessive dissection and tissue manipulation. Nail regrowth can be an extremely painful condition, and affected cats likely have some component of peripheral and central sensitization.

Surgical removal can be performed with a CO_2 laser; however, blade dissection may be the technique of choice because it allows the surgeon to follow the contour of the regrown nail with or without any bone fragment. Using a CO_2 laser for removal of regrown nails may lead to an increased incidence of collateral thermal damage. The surgeon should use caution during surgery along with meticulous tissue handling to prevent excessive tissue trauma.

Outcome

Most cats undergoing surgical removal of regrown nails make a full recovery. Aggressive perioperative analgesia will prevent these cats from having chronic pain syndrome postoperatively.

Prevention

- Ensure complete removal of the germinal epithelium of the ungual crest of P3.
- Perform blade dissection or CO_2 laser onychectomy because the guillotine technique may result in an increased risk of nail regrowth.

Relevant literature

The **infection** rate after onychectomy has been found to occur in as many as 11.6% (Tobias 1994) of cases which is much higher than the 4.7% reported infection rate for clean procedures in small animal surgery (Brown *et al.* 1997). The higher rate associated with onychectomy is likely a result of breaks in asepsis during surgery, excessive tissue dissection, and the challenge associated with protecting the surgical sites from contamination postoperatively. One retrospective study found that infection was associated with the guillotine technique and the use of cyanoacrylate adhesive for wound closure (Tobias 1994). The authors speculated that nail shears used for guillotine onychectomy crush tissues compromising vascular supply to the region and create a larger surgical wound, predisposing to infection (Tobias 1994). In the same study, infection was not associated with the type of antiseptic solution used for preparation of the surgical site or hair length (Tobias 1994). The literature fails to specifically examine other factors that could influence infection after onychectomy, including the influence of aseptic technique, postoperative bandages, CO_2 laser for onychectomy, material used in the litterbox postoperatively, and leaving the surgical wound open to heal by second intention.

Pain and lameness after onychectomy is a debilitating complication for the patient and can cause significant emotional stress for the pet owner. Most recent literature regarding feline onychectomy has focused on the use of CO_2 laser and its potential for reducing pain and lameness compared with traditional blade dissection. Evaluating pain in cats after surgery can be difficult (Robertson and Lascelles 2010). An objective method of limb function after onychectomy has been reported using pressure platform gait analysis (Romans *et al.*

2004). Using this method for gait analysis, cats having onychectomy performed with CO_2 laser had significantly improved limb use and function in the first 2 days postoperatively compared with cats having onychectomy with blade dissection (Robinson *et al.* 2007). In the same study, when cats were evaluated after the initial 48 hours postoperatively, no significant differences were found (Robinson *et al.* 2007). The improved limb function in the early postoperative period with the use of CO_2 laser for onychectomy has been corroborated in other studies (Mison *et al.* 2002; Holmberg and Brisson 2006). The underlying mechanism for improved limb function after CO_2 laser onychectomy has yet to be determined.

Disadvantages associated with the use of CO_2 laser are the purchase and maintenance costs of the equipment and the safety precautions and training required for all personnel involved with its use. Although the use of CO_2 laser in veterinary surgery is growing, it not a common piece of equipment found in general practice. The time associated with safety training and equipment purchase cost may be prohibitive for some veterinary surgeons. RF units are not as expensive as a CO_2 laser and do not require special safety measures. RF was compared with CO_2 laser for performing onychectomy in cats (Burns *et al.* 2011). This study found that RF was a suitable alternative to CO_2 laser for onychectomy; however, it was associated with more inflammation and hemorrhage that required postoperative bandages (Burns *et al.* 2011). Clinical trials using RF are required to evaluate limb function and pain compared with CO_2 laser (Burns *et al.* 2011).

As onychectomy is a painful procedure, pain/lameness can be prevented by using a multi-modal approach to perioperative analgesia. Failure to do so may lead to chronic pain syndrome (Robertson and Lascelles 2010). Several analgesic management regimes for onychectomy have been evaluated in the literature. Transdermal administration of fentanyl (25 mg/hr patch applied 18–24 hours preoperatively) has been shown to provide adequate analgesia after onychectomy in cats and is equivalent in its analgesic efficacy to postoperative administration of butorphanol (0.2 mg/kg at the time of sedation, immediately after extubation, and every 4 hours for 12 hours postoperatively) (Franks *et al.* 2000; Gellasch *et al.* 2002). The benefit of transdermal fentanyl is that continuous analgesia is provided without multiple injections (Gellasch *et al.* 2002). No significant difference in pain or complications using subjective pain scores was found when buprenorphine (0.01 mg/kg intramuscular [IM]) was used alone compared with buprenorphine and a four-point regional nerve block of bupivacaine (1 mg/kg of 0.75% solution) (Curcio *et al.* 2006). The authors of this study stated that buprenorphine alone likely masked any beneficial effect of the regional nerve block (Curcio *et al.* 2006). In another study, buprenorphine (0.01 mg/kg IM) showed the greatest analgesic efficacy compared with oxymorphone (0.05 mg/kg IM) and ketoprofen (2 mg/kg IM) in cats undergoing onychectomy or onychectomy and sterilization (Dobbins *et al.* 2002). Objective measurement of gait analysis revealed significantly improved limb function after onychectomy when fentanyl was administered transdermally (25-mg patch applied 12 hours preoperatively) compared with irrigation of the surgical wound with bupivacaine (1 mL of 0.75% bupivacaine) after onychectomy (Romans *et al.* 2005). In the same study, administration of butorphanol (4 mg/kg IM every 4 hours for 24 hours postoperatively) also led to improved limb function compared with irrigation of the wound with bupivacaine but was not significantly different than transdermal fentanyl analgesia (Romans *et al.* 2005). It is interesting to note that irrespective of analgesic protocol cats did not regain normal limb function up to 12 days after onychectomy

(Romans *et al.* 2005). This suggests that multimodal analgesic techniques should be undertaken and postoperative analgesia should be provided for at least 12 days postoperatively (Romans *et al.* 2005).

Regrowth of the nail occurred in 7.4% of cases in one study and was associated with the use of the guillotine technique (Tobias 1994). The use of nail shears for guillotine onychectomy requires blind ostectomy of P3 increasing the risk of leaving a portion of the ungual crest. This complication can be avoided by ensuring complete removal of the ungual crest and P3 regardless of technique used for onychectomy.

Feline onychectomy is a controversial procedure that remains commonly performed in veterinary practice in North America. When performing onychectomy, the veterinary surgeon must use meticulous surgical technique and an aggressive approach to perioperative analgesia in an attempt to limit complications associated with this procedure. The long-term outcome of onychectomized cats is poorly described in the literature. The lack of reported complications given the procedure is performed commonly in general practice is likely indicative that onychectomy is well tolerated in domestic cats.

References

Brown, D.C., Conzemius, M.G., Shofer, F., et al. (1997) Epidemiologic evaluation of postoperative wound infections in dogs and cats. *Journal of the American Veterinary Medical Association* 210, 1302-1306.

Burns, S.M., Howerth, E.W., Rawlings, C.A., et al. (2010) Comparison of the carbon dioxide laser and the radiofrequency unit for feline onychectomies. *Journal of the American Animal Hospital Association* 46, 375-384.

Carroll, G.L., Howe, L.B., Peterson, K.D. (2005) Analgesic efficacy of pre-operative administration of meloxicam or butorphanol in onychectomized cats. *Journal of the American Veterinary Medical Association* 226, 913-919.

Cooper, M.A., Laverty, P.H., Soiderer, E.E. (2005) Bilateral flexor tendon contracture following onychectomy in 2 cats. *Canadian Veterinary Journal* 46, 244-246.

Curcio, K., Bidwell, L.A., Bohart, G.V., et al. (2006) Evaluation of signs of post-operative pain and complications after forelimb onychectomy in cats receiving buprenorphine alone or with bupivacaine administered as a four-point regional nerve block. *Journal of the American Veterinary Medical Association* 228, 65-68.

Dobbins, S., Brown, N.O., Shover, F.S. (2002) Comparison of the effects of buprenorphine, oxymorphone hydrochloride, and ketoprofen for post-operative analgesia after onychectomy or onychectomy and sterilization in cats. *Journal of the American Animal Hospital Association* 38, 507-514.

Franks, N.J., Boothe, H.W., Taylor, L., et al. (2000) Evaluation of transdermal fentanyl patches for analgesia in cats undergoing onychectomy. *Journal of the American Veterinary Medical Association* 217, 1013-1020.

Gellasch, K.L., Kruse-Elliot, K.T., Osmond, C.S., et al. (2002) Comparison of transdermal administration of fentanyl versus intramuscular administration of butorphanol for analgesia after onychectomy in cats. *Journal of the American Veterinary Medical Association* 220, 1020-1024.

Gunew, M.N., Menrath, V.H., Marshall, R.D. (2008) Long-term safety, efficacy and palatability of oral meloxicam at 0.001-0.03 mg/kg for treatment of osteoarthritic pain in cats. *Journal of Feline Medicine and Surgery* 10, 235-241.

Holmberg, D.H., Brisson, B.A. (2006) A prospective comparison of post-operative morbidity associated with the use of scalpel blades and lasers for onychectomy in cats. *Canadian Veterinary Journal* 47, 162-163.

Mathews, K.A. (2008) Neuropathic pain in dogs and cats: if only they could tell us if they hurt. *Veterinary Clinics of North America: Small Animal Practice* 38, 1365-1414.

Mison, M.B., Bohart, G.H., Walshaw, R., et al. (2002) Use of carbon dioxide laser for onychectomy in cats. *Journal of the American Veterinary Medical Association* 221, 651-653.

Patronek, G.J. (2001) Assessment of claims of short- and long-term complications associated with onychectomy in cats. *Journal of the American Veterinary Medical Association* 219, 932-937.

Robertson, S.A., Lascelles, B.D.X. (2010) Long term pain in cats: how much do we know about this important welfare issue? *Journal of Feline Medicine and Surgery* 12, 188-199.

Robinson, D.A., Romans, C.W., Gordon-Evans, W.J., et al. (2007) Evaluation of short-term limb function following unilateral carbon dioxide laser or scalpel onychectomy in cats. *Journal of the American Veterinary Medical Association* 230, 353-358.

Romans, C.W., Conzemius, M.G., Horstman, C.L., et al. (2004) Use of pressure platform gait analysis in cats with and without bilateral onychectomy. *American Journal of Veterinary Research* 65, 1276-1278.

Romans, C.W., Gordon, W.J., Robinson, D.A., et al. (2005) Effect of post-operative analgesic protocol on limb function following onychectomy in cats. *Journal of the American Veterinary Medical Association* 227, 89-93.

Tobias, K.S. (1994) Feline onychectomy at a teaching institution: a retrospective study of 163 cases. *Veterinary Surgery* 23, 274-280.

Neurologic Surgery

General Complications

Belinda Comito

Veterinary Specialty Center, Buffalo Grove, IL, USA

Clinical surgical complications are wide ranging. This chapter covers peripheral nerve damage (iatrogenic), urine scalding, and decubital ulcers. Other complications such as urinary tract infections seizures, incontinence, and gastrointestinal perforations are covered in other chapters (see index).

Neuropraxia

Definition

Neuropraxia is defined as a peripheral nerve injury causing transient loss of nerve conduction without axonal disruption. Demyelination may or may not occur (Figure 82.1).

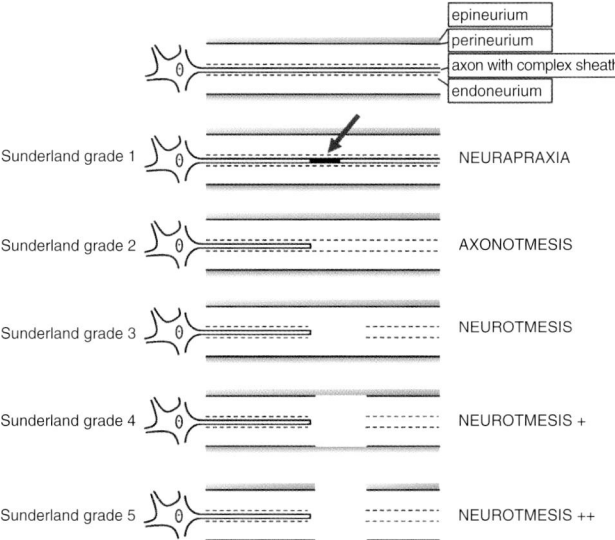

Figure 82.1 Sunderland grades of peripheral nerve injury. Grade 1: Neuropraxia defined as transient loss of nerve conduction without axonal disruption (noted by red arrow). Grade 2: Axonotmesis defined as disruption of the axonal structure. Grades 3 to 5: Neurotmesis (increasing severity noted by the + in the diagram) based on the degree of injury to the supporting structures of the nerve. *Source:* Deumens *et al.*, 2010. Reproduced with permission from Elsevier.

Risk factors

- Traumatic neuropathies:
  - Traction injury (brachial plexus injury)
  - Fractures or luxations (pelvic or humeral)
  - Iatrogenic (pelvic surgeries, injection injury of the sciatic nerve)
  - Osteofacial compartment syndrome

Diagnosis

Localization of peripheral nerve injury is based on clinical signs. Neurogenic muscle atrophy should not be present, and autonomous zones of cutaneous sensation are helpful in localizing the peripheral nerve involved. Patients with neuropraxia generally have intact nociception, and the presence of motor and proprioception deficits is variable. Electrodiagnostic studies (electromyography, motor and nerve conduction velocities) allow for assessment of peripheral nerve function but should be performed at least 7 days after the injury.

Treatment

Spontaneous recovery is expected within 1 to 2 weeks of the injury, but if demyelination has occurred, recovery may take longer. If surgical iatrogenic trauma has occurred, surgical revision may be indicated (e.g., removal of an intramedullary pin).

Prevention

Iatrogenic injury to peripheral nerves can be avoided with careful surgical technique and proper knowledge of the anatomy.

One of the most common iatrogenic nerve injuries consists of sciatic nerve damage during pelvic surgery. To prevent this complication, avoiding extravasation of cement and intraoperative saline irrigation have been suggested during total hip replacement. During triple pelvic osteotomy, a Hohman retractor may be used to retract the sciatic nerve dorsally and protect it during osteotomy of the dorsal third of the ilium. This maneuver remains controversial because it may decrease the risk of neurotmesis with the saw blade but may increase the risk of neuropraxia caused by retraction of the nerve.

Axonotmesis

Definition

Axonotmesis is peripheral nerve injury that disrupts the axonal structure and separates the axon from the neural body. The endoneurium and Schwann cell remain intact, allowing axonal regrowth (Figure 82.1).

Complications in Small Animal Surgery, First Edition. Edited by Dominique Griffon and Annick Hamaide.

© 2016 John Wiley & Sons, Inc. Published 2016 by John Wiley & Sons, Inc.

Companion website: www.wiley.com/go/griffon/complications

Risk factors

- Traumatic neuropathies:
  - Traction injury (brachial plexus injury)
  - Fractures or luxations (pelvic or humeral)
  - Iatrogenic (pelvic surgeries, injection injury of the sciatic nerve)

Diagnosis

The diagnosis is based on localization of the peripheral nerve injury based on clinical signs. Assessing cutaneous sensation of autonomous zones and electrodiagnostic testing (electromyography, sensory and motor nerve conduction velocities) may be most helpful in identifying the peripheral neuropathy. Electrodiagnostics should be performed at least 7 days after the injury. Patients with axonotmesis are expected to have motor, proprioceptive, and nociceptive dysfunction with neurogenic muscle atrophy. Recently, magnetic stimulation was used as a diagnostic and prognostic tool in brachial nerve trauma and sciatic nerve injury.

Treatment

Recovery from axonotmesis depends on on how far the axonal injury occurred from the target muscle, the degree of muscle contraction, and muscle atrophy. Physical therapy should be implemented to limit the degree of muscle contraction and atrophy. Surgical revision should be considered in iatrogenic surgical trauma when indicated.

Prevention

Iatrogenic injury to peripheral nerves can be avoided with careful surgical technique and proper knowledge of the anatomy. One of the most common iatrogenic nerve injuries consists of sciatic nerve damage during pelvic surgery. To prevent this complication, avoiding extravasation of cement and intraoperative saline irrigation have been suggested during total hip replacement. During triple pelvic osteotomy, a Hohman retractor may be used to retract the sciatic nerve dorsally and protect it during osteotomy of the dorsal third of the ilium. This maneuver remains controversial because it may decrease the risk of neurotomesis with the saw blade but may increase the risk of neuropraxia caused by retraction of the nerve.

Neurotomesis

Definition

Neurotomesis is complete severance of the nerve, including the axon, Schwann cells, and supporting connective tissues. Neurotomesis is the most severe nerve injury because axonal regrowth cannot occur (see Figure 82.1).

Risk factors

- Traumatic neuropathies:
  - Traction injury (brachial plexus injury)
  - Fractures or luxations (pelvic or humeral)
  - Iatrogenic (pelvic surgeries, injection injury of the sciatic nerve)
  - Osteofacial compartment syndrome

Diagnosis

Patients with neurotomesis have complete loss of motor, proprioceptive, and pain sensation and have neurogenic muscle atrophy. The diagnosis is made based on clinical signs, including assessment of cutaneous sensation of autonomous zones and electrodiagnostic testing (electromyography, sensory and motor nerve conduction velocities). Electrodiagnostics should be performed at least 7 days after the injury. Recently, magnetic stimulation was used as a diagnostic and prognostic tool in brachial nerve trauma and sciatic nerve injury.

Treatment

Surgical intervention including nerve anastomosis or nerve grafts may be attempted. Absent nociception is a poor prognostic indicator. Peripheral neuropathies may cause paresthesia or hyperesthesia, leading to self-mutilation in which case amputation should be considered.

Prevention

Iatrogenic injury to peripheral nerves can be avoided with careful surgical technique and proper knowledge of the anatomy. One of the most common iatrogenic nerve injuries consists of sciatic nerve damage during pelvic surgery. To prevent this complication, avoiding extravasation of cement and intraoperative saline irrigation have been suggested during total hip replacement. During triple pelvic osteotomy, a Hohman retractor may be used to retract the sciatic nerve dorsally and protect it during osteotomy of the dorsal third of the ilium. This maneuver remains controversial because it may decrease the risk of neurotomesis with the saw blade but may increase the risk of neuropraxia due to retraction of the nerve.

Urine scalding

Definition

Urine scalding is skin irritation secondary to contact with urine.

Risk factors

- Nonambulatory, severely debilitated, or incontinent patients

Diagnosis

Urine scald is diagnosed based on skin irritation in the inguinal area, discoloration of the fur from urine staining, and should be suspected in non-ambulatory, debilitated, or incontinent patients (see Figure 82.2).

Treatment

- Clean the affected area using warm water and mild shampoo.
- Thoroughly dry the area.
- Apply moisture-barrier ointment and cornstarch baby powder after cleansing.

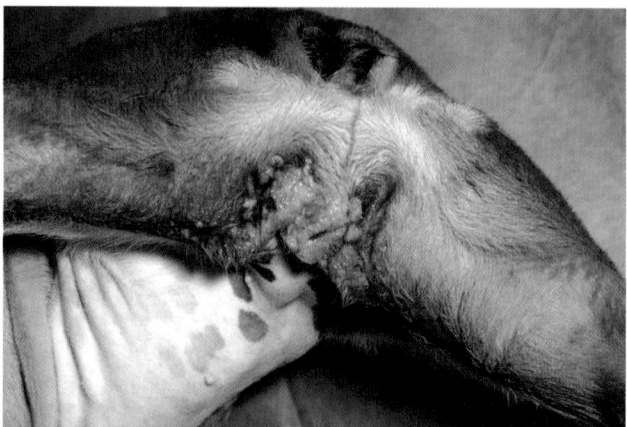

Figure 82.2 Patient with severe urine scald. *Source:* D. Griffon, Western University of Health Sciences, Pomona, CA, 2014. Reproduced with permission from D. Griffon.

Prevention

- Use of hygiene pads or diapers
- Keep the patient clean and dry
- Change bedding frequently when soiled.
- Bladder expression and urinary catheterization every 6 to 8 hours

Decubital ulcers

Definition

Decubital ulcers are skin wounds that develop over bony prominences. Decubital ulcers are most severe when deep tissue loss has led to bone exposure.

Risk factors

- Recumbent patients who are unable to rotate or shift positions and do not have proper bedding.

Diagnosis

The diagnosis is based on history (recumbent patient) and clinical appearance of the wound over a bony prominence:

- Grade I: dark thickened skin without subcutaneous exposure
- Grade II: exposed subcutaneous tissue
- Grade III: ulceration to the deep facial layers
- Grade IV: loss of deep tissue with bone exposure

See Figure 82.3.

Treatment

Treatment depends on the severity of the ulcer. Management should include clipping the wound, lavaging and debriding ischemic tissue, antibiotics (systemic, topical), and wet-to-dry bandages. In some cases, primary closure or cutaneous flaps may be appropriate. Elevation of pressure points by using doughnuts and appropriate bedding is recommended in all patients with decubital ulcers.

Prevention

- Use of appropriate bedding: soft pads, waterbeds, egg crate mattresses, trampoline beds
- Frequent turning of the patient (every 4–6 hours)
- Pressure point massage to promote circulation
- Intermittent assisted standing with the patient; sling walking
- Hydrotherapy

Relevant Literature

Neuropraxia causes temporary loss of nerve function with little to no axonal damage or supportive connective tissues (Años 2004; Olby *et al.* 2005; Dewey and Cerda-Gonzalez 2008). Spontaneous recovery generally occurs within 2 weeks of injury, but demyelination will delay recovery (Años 2004; Olby *et al.* 2005; Dewey and Cerda Gonzalez 2008). Recovery is typically complete (Anos 2004). **Axonotmesis** refers to peripheral nerve injury that disrupts the axonal structure and separates the axon from the neural body (Años 2004; Olby *et al.* 2005; Dewey and Cerda-Gonzalez 2008). The endoneurium and Schwann cell act as scaffolding, allowing axonal regrowth to occur (Años 2004; Olby *et al.* 2005; Dewey and Cerda-Gonzalez 2008). Axonal regrowth occurs approximately 1 mm/day (Uchida *et al.* 1993). If the injury occurs far from the target muscle, contracture and atrophy may limit recovery by the time muscle reinnervation has occurred (Olby *et al.* 2005). **Neurotomesis** is the most severe peripheral nerve injury because severance of

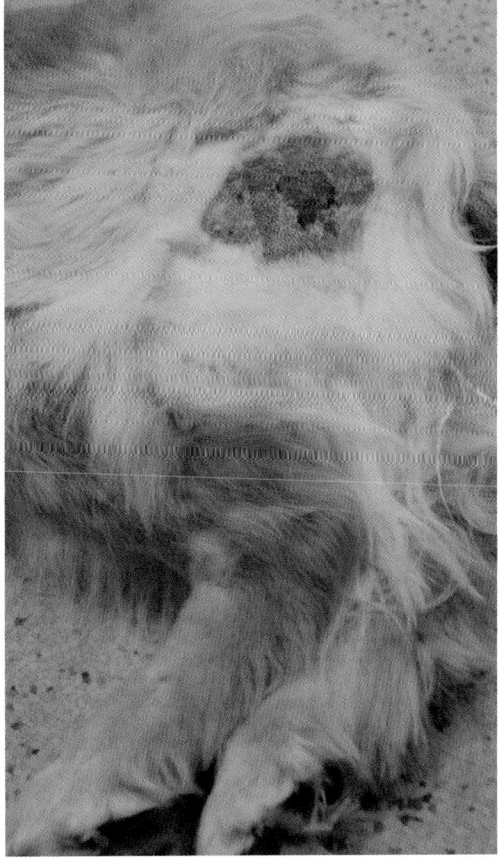

(A)

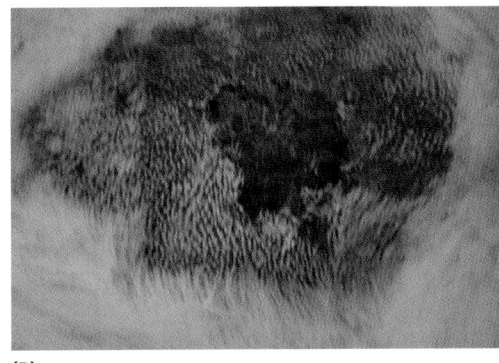

(B)

Figure 82.3 **A**, Patient with pressure sore over the femur. **B**, Close-up view.

the axons, Schwann cells, and supportive connective tissues has occurred (Anos 2004; Olby *et al.* 2005; Dewey and Cerda-Gonzalez 2008). Patients with neurotomesis are expected to have complete motor, proprioceptive, and nociceptive dysfunction (Dewey and Cerda-Gonzalez 2008). Loss of pain sensation is a negative prognostic indicator (Faissler *et al.* 2002; Olby *et al.* 2005; Dewey and Cerda-Gonzalez 2008; Van Soens *et al.* 2009), and if pain sensation remains absent 2 weeks after the initial injury, recovery of motor function is guarded (Olby *et al.* 2005).

Electrodiagnostics, clinical signs, and cutaneous sensation are helpful in identifying the location of the peripheral nerve injury.

Electrodiagnostics should not be performed until at least 7 days after the injury (Años 2004), although spontaneous electrical activity in denervated muscles may be present as early as 5 days after the injury. Magnetic stimulation of the radial and sciatic nerves with absence of a muscular evoked potential has been associated with a poor outcome in patients with brachial plexus trauma and sciatic nerve injury (Van Soens *et al.* 2009, 2010).

Sciatic nerve dysfunction is a reported complication in orthopedic surgery. Iatrogenic sciatic neuropraxia was identified in 19 of 1000 patients undergoing total hip replacement (Andrews *et al.* 2008). Patient age and length of surgery were significantly associated with development of neuropraxia, and all patients made a full recovery with variable recovery rates (Andrews *et al.* 2008). In a study of iatrogenic sciatic nerve injury, 25 of the 27 patients developed sciatic dysfunction secondary to pelvic orthopedic surgery (Forterre *et al.* 2007). Of the 27 patients, 13 made a full recovery, 7 showed clinical improvement, and 7 remained unchanged (Forterre *et al.* 2007).

Surgical treatment of a peripheral nerve injury depends on the underlying cause and severity of the injury. Surgical approaches may include nerve anastomosis, nerve external neurolysis, and nerve grafts. Nerve grafts should be considered when the neural defect length is more than five times the nerve diameter (Granger *et al.* 2006), and grafted nerve segments should be similar in width to the injured nerve (Dewey and Cerda-Gonzalez 2008). A cutaneous saphenous nerve graft has been used successfully to surgically treat one dog with peroneal and tibial nerve injuries (Granger *et al.* 2006). Physical therapy to help prevent muscle contracture and atrophy is generally recommended regardless of whether surgery is performed.

Complete brachial plexus avulsions carry a poor prognosis for functional recovery of the limb (Dewey and Cerda-Gonzalez 2008). Patients with a brachial plexus avulsion should be given time to determine if limb function will return before considering amputation unless self-mutilation is evident.

Urine scald is a concern in all nonambulatory, debilitated, or incontinent patients. Absorptive pads and diapers are useful in limiting the amount of urine contact with the skin (Shearer 2011). Hair should be kept trimmed, but overzealous clipping should be avoided over common pressure points to prevent decubital ulcers (Sherman and Olby 2004; Shearer 2011). When urine or fecal material come into contact with skin, the patient should be washed with warm water and mild shampoo when (Shearer 2011) (Figure 82.4). After

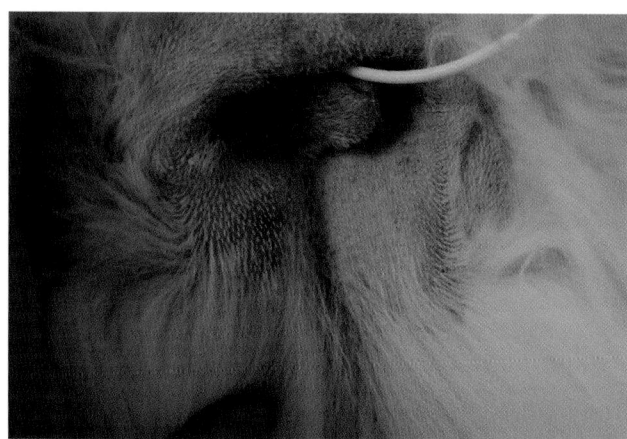

Figure 82.5 Patient with indwelling urinary catheter placed. Notice the perivulvular erythema. The catheter was placed to help prevent urine scald.

the skin is thoroughly dried, a moisture barrier ointment and baby powder should be applied (Shearer 2011). Soiled bedding should be changed immediately. Bladder expression or intermittent catheterization every 6 to 8 hours may aid in nursing care (Drum 2010). Indwelling catheters should be used at the clinician's discretion, and proper aseptic techniques should be practiced. (Figure 82.5)

Decubital ulcers develop when the soft tissues are compressed between a bony prominence and the surface a patient is in contact with (Swaim *et al.* 1997). The compression of soft tissue leads to circulation obstruction, causing ischemic necrosis of the tissue and ultimately ulcer formation (Swaim *et al.* 1997, Sherman and Olby 2004). Decubital ulcers are graded in severity from least to most severe (Swaim *et al.* 1997; Tefend and Dewey 2008). (See the descriptions of the grades under Diagnosis.) Medical and surgical treatment are case dependent based on the severity of the wound. Medical treatment includes doughnut placement over bony prominences, wound lavage, antibiotics (systemic, topical), and wet-to-dry bandages (Figure 82.6) (Swaim *et al.* 1997; Tefend and Dewey 2008). Surgical treatment entails wound debridement, primary wound closure, or creation of a cutaneous or myocutaneous flap (Swaim *et al.* 1997; Tefend and Dewey 2008). Severe decubital ulcers may take a

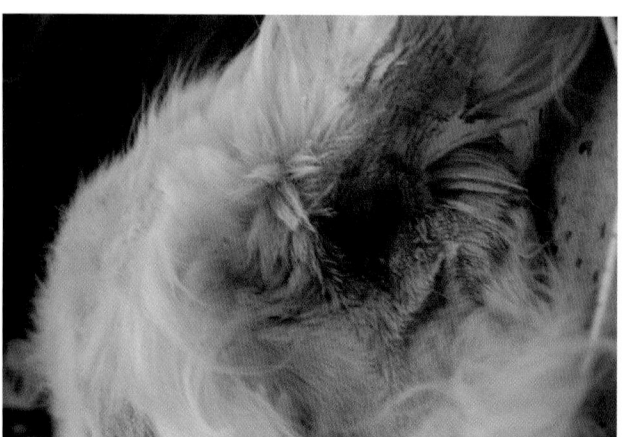

Figure 82.4 This picture depicts a patient with severe fecal staining secondary to fecal incontinence.

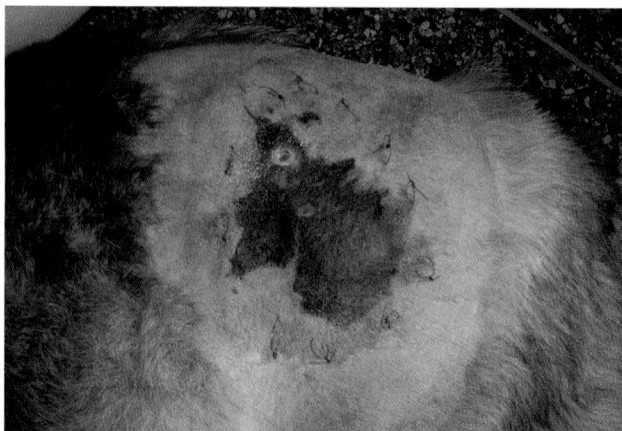

Figure 82.6 A decubital ulcer during treatment. The tissue in the center is necrotic. Stay sutures are placed to aid in bandage changes.

long time to heal (Drum 2011) and could ultimately result in patient euthanasia depending on the severity. Prevention of decubital ulcers is far easier than treatment, and there is no excuse for poor nursing care in the clinical setting. Good nursing care is essential should include patient rotation, appropriate bedding, daily sling support, and pressure point massage (Sherman and Olby 2004).

References

Andrews, C.M., Liska, W.D., Roberts, D.J. (2008) Sciatic neurapraxia as a complication in 1000 consecutive canine total hip replacements. *Veterinary Surgery* 37, 254-262.

Añor, S. (2004) Monoparesis. In Platt, S.R., Olby, N.J. (eds.) *BSAVMA Manual of Canine and Feline Neurology*, 3rd edn. British Small Animal Veterinary Association, Gloucester, UK, pp. 369-370.

Drum, G.W., Corda Gonzalez, S. (2008) Disorders of the peripheral nervous system. In Dewey, C.W. (ed.) *A Practical Guide to Canine and Feline Neurology*, 2nd edn. Wiley-Blackwell, Ames, IA, pp. 452-455.

Drum, M.G. (2010) Physical rehabilitation in the neurologic patient. *The Veterinary Clinics of North America: Small Animal Practice* 40 (1), 181-193.

Faissler, D., Cizinaukas S., Jaggy, A. (2002) Prognostic factors for functional recovery in dogs with suspected brachial plexus avulsion. *Journal of Veterinary Internal Medicine* 16, 370.

Forterre, F., Tomek, A., Rytz, U., et al. (2007) Iatrogenic sciatic nerve injury in eighteen dogs and nine cats (1997-2006). *Veterinary Surgery* 36, 464-471.

Granger, N., Moissonnier, P., Fanchon, L., et al. (2006) Cutaneous saphenous nerve graft for the treatment of sciatic neurotmesis in a dog. *Journal of the American Veterinary Medical Association* 229 (1), 82-86.

Olby, N., Halling, K.B., Glick, T.R. (2005) Rehabilitation for the neurologic patient. *The Veterinary Clinics of North America: Small Animal Practice* 35 (6), 1389-1409.

Shearer, T.S. (2011) Managing mobility challenges in palliative and hospice care patients. *The Veterinary Clinics of North America: Small Animal Practice* 11, 609-617.

Sherman, J., Olby, N.J. (2004) Nursing and rehabilitation of the neurologic patient. In Platt, S.R., Olby, N.J. (eds.) *BSAVMA Manual of Canine and Feline Neurology*, 3rd edn. British Small Animal Veterinary Association, Gloucester, UK, pp. 397-398.

Swaim, S.F., Hanson, R.R., Coates, J.R. (1997) Decubitus ulcers in animals. In Parish, L.C., Witkowski, J.A., Crissey, J.T. (eds.) *The Decubitus Ulcer In Clinical Practice*. Springer, New York, pp. 217-238.

Tafend, R.M., Dewey, C.W. (2008) Nursing care and physical therapy for patients with neurologic disease. In Dewey, C.W. (ed.) *A Practical Guide to Canine and Feline Neurology*, 2nd edn. Wiley-Blackwell, Ames, IA, pp. 466-483.

Uchida, Y., Sugimura, M., Onaga, T., et al. (1993) Regeneration of crushed and transected sciatic nerves in young dogs. *Journal of the Japanese Veterinary Medical Association* 46, 775.

Van Soens, I., Struys, M.M., Bhatti, S.F., et al. (2009) Magnetic stimulation of the radial nerve in dogs and cats with brachial plexus trauma: a report of 53 cases. *The Veterinary Journal* 182, 108-113.

Van Soens, I., Struys, M.M.R.F., Van Ham, L.M.L. (2010) Muscle potentials evoked by magnetic stimulation of the sciatic nerve in unilateral sciatic nerve dysfunction. *Journal of Small Animal Practice* 51, 275-279.

83 Practical Guide to Myelographic Complications

Belinda Comito
Veterinary Specialty Center, Buffalo Grove, IL, USA

Myelography

Myelography is an imaging modality used to identify the location and extent of lesions affecting the spinal cord. Myelography requires subarachnoid injection of contrast medium, causing opacification of the subarachnoid space (Robertson and Thrall 2011). Myelography was the primary modality for investigating spinal cord abnormalities before the increased availability of magnetic resonance imaging (MRI) and computed tomography (CT) imaging. Myelograms are performed at the level of the cerebellomedullary cistern or between two lumbar vertebrae (de Lahunta and Glass 2009). Myelography is an invasive but relatively safe diagnostic procedure, but side effects and complications may arise from the contrast medium or from direct penetration into the spinal cord or brainstem (da Costa *et al.* 2011). Newer contrast agents have reduced neurotoxicity (Widmer *et al.* 1992). Iohexol is the most common contrast agent currently used (da Costa *et al.* 2011).

Seizures

Definition

Generalized seizures are the most common postmyelographic complication. Contrast agents may cause neurotoxicity and leptomeningeal irritation and are epileptogenic. However, fewer complications are reported with the use of the newer contrast agents. Postmyelographic seizures may manifest as generalized or partial seizures.

Risk factors

- Contrast agent: Metrizamide is no longer used for myelography because of the high incidence of seizures. Newer agents such as iohexol, iopamidol, and iomeprol are considered safer because the lower risk of postmyelographic seizures.
- Rapid injection of contrast medium
- Patient size (weighing >22 kg)
- Site of injection: Injection in the cerebellomedullary cistern is more prone to complications than lumbar injection.
- Volume of contrast (>8 mL)
- Location of the lesion
- Breed (Dobermans, Rottweilers)

Diagnosis

Postmyelographic seizures generally occur within the first hour of anesthetic recovery. Recurring seizures may occur 4 to 12 hours after regaining consciousness, but this is relatively rare (Adams and Stowater 1981).

Treatment

- Administration of diazepam (0.5 mg/kg dose, intravenous [IV])

Outcome

Patients with postmyelographic seizures respond to administration of diazepam. Recurrence of seizures beyond the first 24 hours has not been reported. Long-term seizure disorders have not been reported as a result of myelography, and patients do not require anticonvulsant therapy.

Prevention

- Use nonionic contrast agents: iohexol, iopamidol, iomeprol
- Use the lowest concentration of contrast medium that still allows for diagnostic quality images
- Inject a volume of contrast agent ranging between 0.3 and 0.45 mL/kg, without exceeding a total volume of 8 mL
- Avoid multiple injections.
- Perform lumbar myelography.
- Maintain head elevation during cervical myelography.

Meningitis

Definition

Meningitis is inflammation of the spinal cord and brain meninges.

Risk factors

Injection of contrast medium into the subarachnoid space leads to a chemical reaction in the leptomeninges.

Diagnosis

The diagnosis of postmyelographic meningitis is not specific. An elevated white blood cell (WBC) count in cerebrospinal fluid (CSF) can be seen in any patient undergoing myelography, including patients who do not experience neurologic deterioration. The WBC count in the CSF may remain elevated for up to 10 days after uncomplicated myelography. For this reason, CSF should always be collected before injection of contrast agents (Figure 83.1).

Treatment

Generally, chemically induced meningitis or myelitis will improve within 1 to 3 days of the procedure. If neurologic dysfunction persists or becomes progressive and other causes such as postoperative worsening or expected disease progression have been excluded, administration of prednisone should be initiated (0.5–1.0 mg/kg/day).

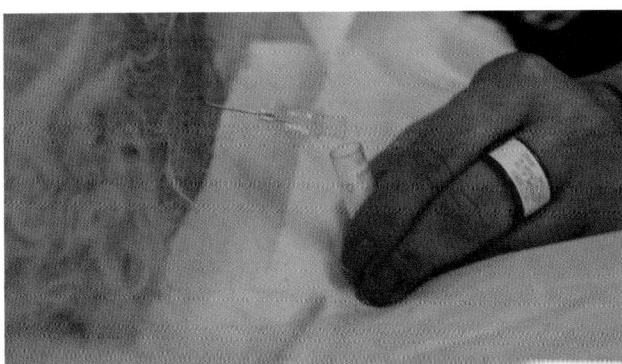

(A)

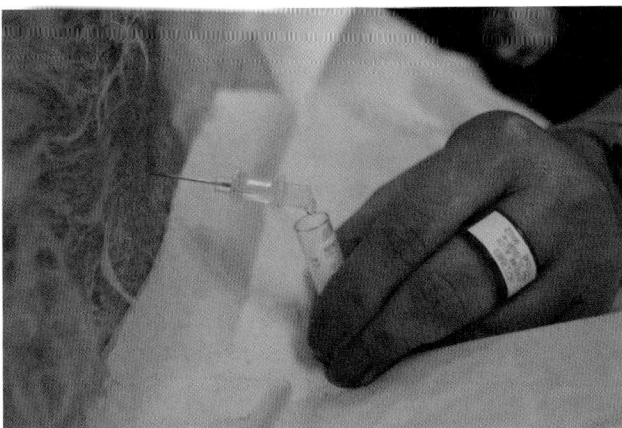

(B)

Figure 83.1 Collection of cerebrospinal fluid (CSF). **A**, After placement of a spinal needle, a sterile container is maintained in position. **B**, CSF is allowed to passively flow for collection. Approximately 0.5 to 1 mL should be collected for analysis. If the fluid appears hemorrhagic, fluid should be collected in an ethylenediaminetetraacetic acid (EDTA) tube. Fluid collected in an EDTA tube cannot be used for bacterial culture.

Outcome

Most patients with worsening of neurologic signs will return to their premyelographic neurologic status within a few days of the procedure.

Prevention

Consider alternative imaging modalities that do not require injection of contrast medium into the subarachnoid space. If injection of contrast medium is required, use contrast agents with minimal neurotoxicity. Myelography should be avoided in patients in which primary inflammatory disease is considered as a likely diagnosis.

Neurologic deterioration

Definition

Neurologic deterioration may be caused by the contrast agent injected into the subarachnoid space or by physical trauma resulting from the placement of the needle in the nervous tissue. Neurologic signs may vary from transient worsening to death.

Risk factors

• Repeated attempts at injecting contrast medium in the subarachnoid space

Box 83.1 Supportive care for patients with neurologic conditions*

Rotate recumbent patients every 4–6 hours.
Provide appropriate bedding.
Encourage patients to move supported by slings or carts.
Keep patients clean and dry.
Bladder care: manual expression, catheterization
Physical therapy: underwater treadmill, range of motion activities

*These measures are important to promote neurologic recovery and prevent concurrent morbidities.

• Incorrect injection site during lumbar myelography can lead to iatrogenic spinal cord damage. Lumbar myelography should not be performed in locations cranial to L4 to L5.
• Injection of contrast agent in the cerebellomedullary cistern
• Incorrect needle size
• Excessive manipulation of the patient during the procedure (Adams and Stowater 1981)

Diagnosis

The diagnosis is made based on deterioration of the neurologic status after anesthetic recovery. In patients undergoing myelography and surgery under one anesthetic event, the cause of neurologic deterioration cannot be determined. If iatrogenic trauma has occurred after injecting at the cerebellomedullary cistern, clinical signs referable to the brainstem will be present. These may include obtundation, vestibular signs, inability to rise, paresis, cessation of respiration, or sudden death.

Treatment

Mild deterioration from lumbar myelography is typically transient, lasting from 24 hours to 1 to 3 weeks (Kirberger and Wrigley 1993); however, more severe neurologic signs may persist. Treatment options are limited to supportive care.

Outcome

Neurologic deterioration from lumbar myelography is transient, and most patients return to their neurologic baselines. Iatrogenic trauma during cerebellomedullary cisternal taps carries a much more guarded prognosis, depending on the severity of neurologic deficits, but patients may make a functional recovery with supportive care (Box 83.1).

Prevention

• To prevent postmyelographic neurologic deterioration, avoid multiple injections and cisternal injection.
• To minimize the risk of lumbar puncture, use fluoroscopic guidance and 22-gauge needles for injection of contrast medium and limit the location of puncture to L5 to L6 in small dogs (weighing <22 kg) and cats and L4 to L5 or L5 to L6 in larger dogs (weighing >22.7 kg) unless fluoroscopic guidance is used (Packer et al. 2007) (Figures 83.2 and 83.3).

Damage to the spinal cord

Definition

Damage to the spinal cord during myelography occurs if the needle is inserted into the spinal cord parenchyma or if contrast medium is injected into the spinal cord parenchyma.

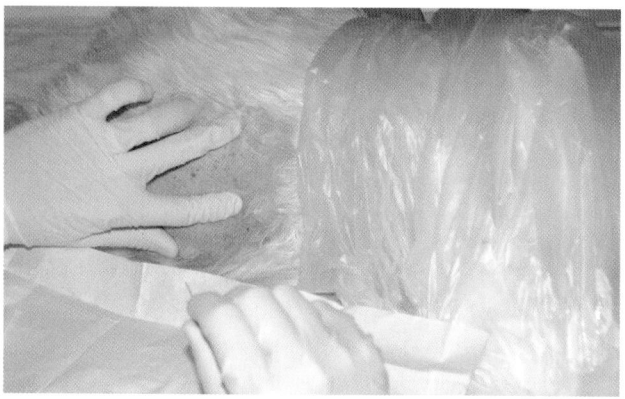

(A)

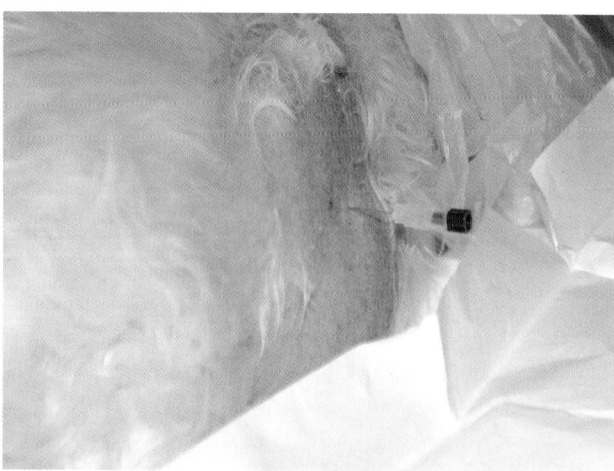

(B)

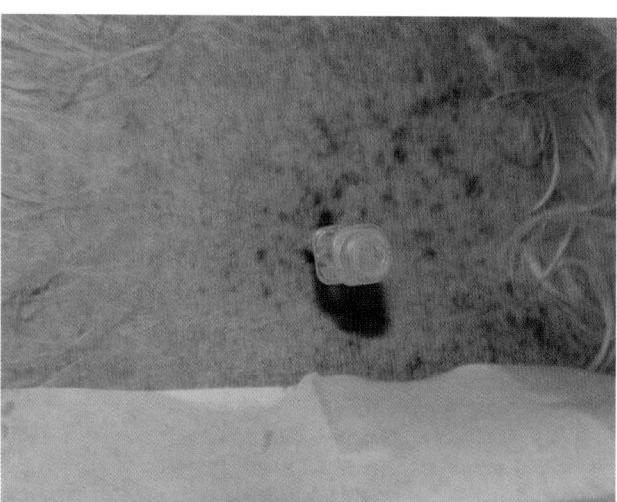

(C)

Figure 83.2 Identification of landmarks relevant to lumbar anatomy. **A,** The iliac crests are palpated and the dorsal spinous process cranial to those is identified as the sixth lumbar (L6) vertebra. **B,** The spinal needle is advanced cranial to the dorsal spinous process of L6 with the stylet in place. **C,** The stylet is removed, and the hub is checked for cerebrospinal fluid.

Risk factors
- Insertion of a needle and injection of contrast medium during lumbar or cervical myelography

Diagnosis
Spinal cord damage can be observed on histopathology or MRI. Iatrogenic widening of the central canal caused by injection of contrast during myelography has been associated with worsening of neurologic signs and can be identified on the myelography images. A presumptive diagnosis can be made based on increased severity of clinical signs after the procedure. The criteria for increased severity depend on the baseline premyelographic neurologic examination results.

Treatment
There is no treatment to reverse spinal cord damage. For patients with neurologic deterioration, treatment is limited to supportive care (see Box 83.1).

Outcome
Patients may make a full recovery, especially if damage is limited to the lumbar spinal cord.

Prevention
- Use fluoroscopic guidance during lumbar myelography to confirm the correct anatomic site and needle placement (Figure 83.3).

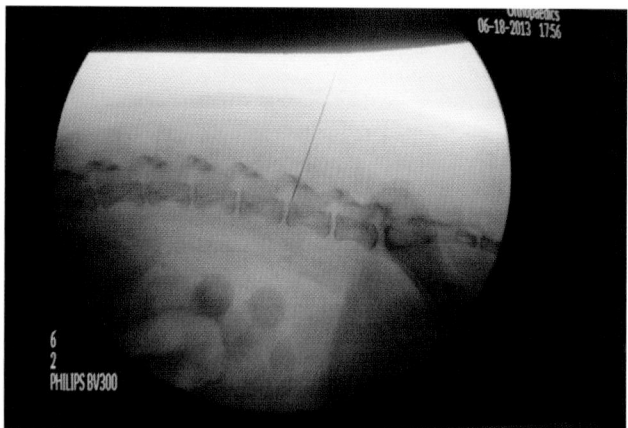

(A)

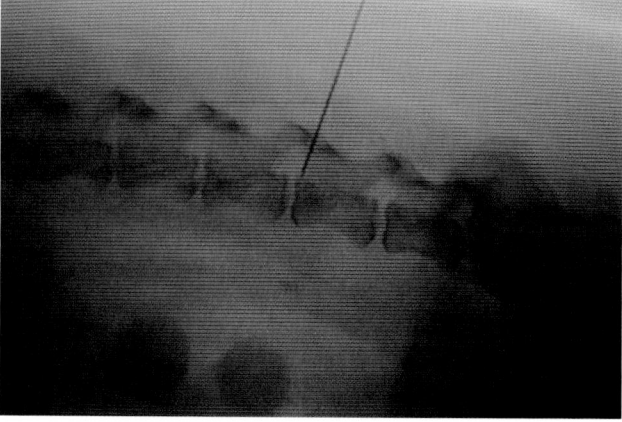

(B)

Figure 83.3 Fluoroscopic guidance during myelography. **A,** Fluoroscopy can be used to verify the placement of the spinal needle. **B,** Close-up view of the needle at between the fifth and sixth lumbar vertebrae.

- In patients undergoing cervical myelography, the clinician should have a working knowledge of the anatomy to ensure correct needle placement and avoid iatrogenic trauma.
- Damage to the spinal cord could be avoided by choosing a less invasive imaging modality such as MRI or CT scan.

Magnetic resonance imaging gadolinium toxicity

Definition
Intravenous gadolinium-based contrast agents are widely used in patients undergoing MRI. Adverse effects are rare and include anaphylactoid reactions, bradycardia, tachycardia, hypotension, and hypertension (Pollard *et al.* 2008; Girard and Leece 2010; Smith 2010). Nephrogenic systemic fibrosis, a severe adverse effect associated with gadolinium-based contrast agents, has been reported in humans with preexisting renal disease (Pollard *et al.* 2008) but has not been reported in veterinary medicine (Smith 2010).

Risk factors
All patients are at risk for an anaphylactoid reaction, but patients with atopic dermatitis are at a higher risk.

Patients with renal impairment may be at risk for developing nephrogenic systemic fibrosis, but this has not been reported in animals.

Diagnosis
Anaphylactic reactions are diagnosed based on the rapid onset of hypotension and tachycardia and periorbital, labial, or facial edema within 10 to 15 minutes of contrast administration.

Treatment
Treatment for anaphylactic reactions depends on the clinical signs manifested by the patient. Edema can be treated using chlorphenamine (maximum dose, 0.4 mg/kg IV), IV fluid bolus (10 mL/kg IV), and methylprednisolone (10 mg/kg IV) (Girard and Leece 2010). Tachycardia and hypotension can be treated using an IV fluid bolus and decreasing the inhalational anesthetic concentration. If the patient does not respond, the procedure should be aborted, and appropriate therapy should be instituted to correct the cardiovascular abnormalities.

Outcome
Patients will make a full recovery with early diagnosis and treatment. Side effects secondary to edema improve within several hours of treatment.

Prevention
Anaphylactoid reactions occur without prior exposure to gadolinium-based contrast agents. Opioids may cause histamine release and should be avoided in the premedication protocols of patients identified as high risk. High-risk patients, such as those with preexisting atopic dermatitis, may benefit from preanaesthetic medications such as H1 or H2 receptor antagonists or corticosteroids (Girard and Leece 2010). A thorough medical history must be obtained before the procedure.

Patients with preexisting renal disease should be adequately hydrated and on appropriate fluid rates during and after the procedure. The benefits of contrast studies should be weighed against their risks in patients with renal impairment (Smith 2010).

Relevant literature

Generalized **seizures** are the most common complications resulting from myelograms (Adams and Stowater 1981). The development of second and third generation contrast agents has greatly decreased the risk of seizures (Widmer *et al.* 1992). The incidence of myelogram-related seizures reported in the literature ranges from less than 10% (Allan and Wood 1988; Fatone *et al.* 1997) to 21.4% (Barone *et al.* 2002). However, the incidence dropped to 3% in the most recent study with the largest patient population (da Costa *et al.* 2011). There are conflicting reports in the literature regarding the pathogenesis of these seizures. The following factors were reported as contributing to the development of seizures in several studies: total volume of contrast medium administered (Adams and Stowater 1981; Allan and Wood 1998; Barone *et al.* 2002; da Costa *et al.* 2011), injection into the cerebellomedullary cistern (Allan and Wood 1998; Barone *et al.* 2002; da Costa *et al.* 2011), presence of a cervical lesion (da Costa *et al.* 2011), and patient weight (Adams and Stowater 1981; Barone *et al.* 2002; da Costa *et al.* 2011). However, Lexmaulova *et al.* did not find a correlation between the incidence of seizures and the volume of contrast injected or weight of the patient. Instead, this study identified paraplegic patients with thoracolumbar lesions subjected to lumbar myelography as predisposed to seizures (Lexmaulova *et al.* 2009).

Controversy also surrounds the causal relationship between seizures and duration of anesthesia (Widmer *et al.* 1992; Barone *et al.* 2002; Lexmaulova *et al.* 2009; da Costa *et al.* 2011), anesthetic protocol (da Costa *et al.* 2011), concentration of contrast medium (da Costa *et al.* 2011), breed (Barone *et al.* 2002; da Costa *et al.* 2011), and type of lesion (Barone *et al.* 2002; Lexmaulova *et al.* 2009; da Costa *et al.* 2011). Despite these conflicting reports, several recommendations have emerged from the literature to reduce the risk of seizures such as injecting contrast at a slow, steady rate (Court *et al.* 1990; Barone *et al.* 2002); use of the lowest concentration of contrast medium available (da Costa *et al.* 2011); elevating the patient's head when injecting at the cerebellomedullary cistern (Barone *et al.* 2002); careful monitoring during anesthesia recovery (Barone *et al.* 2002); use of the 0.3- to 0.45-mg/kg contrast dosing range without exceeding a total volume of 8 mL (Adams and Stowater 1981; da Costa *et al.* 2011); avoiding multiple injections (da Costa *et al.* 2011); and preferential injection of contrast medium into the lumbar region (Adams and Stowater 1981; Barone *et al.* 2002; da Costa *et al.* 2011).

Aseptic meningitis is a rare complication of myelography (Barone *et al.* 2002; Packer *et al.* 2007; Isreal *et al.* 2009). Contrast agents induce leptomeningeal irritation (Wright and Clayton 1981) and alter CSF interpretation (Carakostas *et al.* 1983; Wheeler and Davies 1985). An increase in neutrophils and large mononuclear cells with an elevated WBC count have been reported in dogs receiving older contrast agents such as metrizamide (Carakostas *et al.* 1983). An increase in the WBC count has been reported up to 10 days after iohexol myelography (Carroll *et al.* 1997). In one study, CSF analysis and histologic evaluation of the meninges were consistent with a neutrophilic response to iopamidol and a mononuclear response to metrizamide, without deterioration of neurologic status (Spencer *et al.* 1982). These alterations justify the timing of CSF collection before rather than after injection of contrast medium. Myelography should be avoided if meningitis or myelitis is a primary differential.

Deterioration of premyelographic neurologic status is the second most common complication of myelography (Adams and Stowater 1981). Transient worsening of clinical signs is well described in the literature (Funkquist 1962, Adams and Stowater

1981; Kirberger and Wrigley 1993; Barone *et al.* 2002; Robertson and Thrall 2011; De Decker *et al.* 2011). In a recent prospective study, 3 of 22 dogs undergoing myelography without subsequent surgery had more pronounced ataxia or paraparesis after myelography. These neurologic changes were transient in 2 of the 3 dogs (De Decker *et al.* 2011). Rare complications include fatal subarachnoid hemorrhage after lumbar myelography (Packer *et al.* 2007), asystole (Carroll *et al.* 1997), irreversible progression of signs leading to euthanasia (Allan and Wood 1988), death from acute subdural brainstem and cervical spinal cord hemorrhage related to needle placement (Adams and Stowater 1981), and hematomyelia after lumbar puncture for CSF analysis (Platt *et al.* 2005). Neurologic deterioration may occur regardless of the injection site. Kishimoto *et al.* (2004) suggested that lumbar myelography leads to microscopic parenchymal changes in the spinal cord even if neurologic deterioration is not present. However, iatrogenic damage from needle placement at the cisternal level carries a higher risk of severe and clinically relevant complications compared to lumbar puncture (Olby *et al.* 1994).

Histopathologic evidence of **spinal cord damage** has been reported secondary to lumbar myelography (Kishimoto *et al.* 2004). These microscopic changes include hemorrhage, gliosis, and axonal degeneration (Kishimoto *et al.* 2004). Direct trauma from the spinal needle and chemical toxicity from the contrast agent have been implicated as causes of these changes (Carlisle *et al.* 1995; Kishimoto *et al.* 2004). Direct trauma from the spinal needle may occur if lumbar myelography is not performed at the correct site. Lumbar myelography may be technically more challenging than cisternal myelography, but iatrogenic damage from needle placement at the cisternal level carries a higher risk of severe complications (Olby *et al.* 1994). Vital structures of the central nervous system are located close to the atlanto-occipital space, and inadvertent trauma may cause severe, irreversible damage. Sudden death, secondary to extensive acute subdural hemorrhage involving the brainstem, and cranial cervical spinal cord from iatrogenic trauma have been reported (Adams and Stowater 1981). Iatrogenic brainstem injury after cerebellomedullary cistern puncture should be suspected in patients with cranial nerve dysfunction, vestibular signs, mentation changes, or tetraparesis after myelography (Luján Feliu-Pascual *et al.* 2008). Supportive treatment has been advocated and can lead to recovery (Luján Feliu-Pascual *et al.* 2008).

Gadolinium-associated toxicity has been reported in veterinary medicine. A recent report identified three cases of anaphylactoid reactions during an 18-month period in which 1500 dogs received IV gadolinium-based contrast (Girard and Leece 2010). All three dogs made complete recoveries despite variations in clinical signs and treatment approaches. Recognition of edema may be delayed because patient access is restricted during the MRI study (Girard and Leece 2010). The diagnosis of anaphylactoid reaction may be delayed until the process has become severe enough to cause tachycardia and hypotension (Girard and Leece 2010). Because anaphylactoid reactions are relatively rare, precautions do not need to be taken with preanesthetic medications unless the patient is identified as high risk (Girard and Leece 2010). Prophylactic administration of antihistaminic or corticosteroids is limited to patients with preexisting atopy or other allergic disease. In humans with preexisting renal disease, administration of gadolinium-based contrast agents is associated with nephrogenic systemic fibrosis, a life-threatening skin disease (Pollard *et al.* 2008, Smith 2010). Although this syndrome has not yet been reported in animals, administration of contrast agent warrants careful consideration in patients with renal impairment (Smith 2010).

References

Adams, W.M., Stowater, J.L. (1981) Complications of metrizamide myelography in the dog: a summary of 107 clinical case histories. *Veterinary Radiology* 22 (1), 27-34.

Allan, G.S., Wood, A.W. (1988) Iohexol myelography in the dog. *Veterinary Radiology* 29 (2), 78-82.

Barone, G., Ziemer, L.S., Shofer, F.S., et al. (2002) Risk factors associated with development of seizures after use of iohexol for myelography in dogs: 182 cases (1998). *Journal of the American Veterinary Medical Association* 220 (10), 1499-1502.

Carakostas, M.C., Gossett, K.A., Watters, J.W., et al. (1983) Effects of metrizamide myelography on cerebrospinal fluid analysis in the dog. *Veterinary Radiology* 24 (6), 267-270.

Carlisle, C.H., Pass, M.A., Lowndes, H.E., et al. (1995) Toxicity of the radiographic contrast medium iopamidol, iohexol and metrizamide to cell cultures. *Veterinary Radiology & Ultrasound* 36 (3), 207-211.

Carroll, G.L., Keene, B.W., Forrest, L.J. (1997) Asystole associated with iohexol myelography in a dog. *Veterinary Radiology & Ultrasound* 38 (4), 284-287.

Court, M.H., Dodman, N.H., Norman, W.M. (1990) Anaesthesia and central nervous system disease in small animals. Part II: anaesthetic management for specific diseases and procedures. *British Veterinary Journal,* 146 (4), 296-308.

da Costa, R.C., Parent, J.M., Dobson, H. (2011) Incidence of and risk factors for seizures after myelography performed with iohexol in dogs: 503 cases (2002-2004). *Journal of the American Veterinary Medical Association Journal of the American Veterinary Medical Association* 238 (10), 1296-1300.

De Decker, S., Gielen, I.M.V.L., Duchateau, L., et al. (2011) Intraobserver, interobserver, and intermethod agreement for results of myelography, computed tomography-myelography, and low-field magnetic resonance imaging in dogs with disk-associated wobbler syndrome. *Journal of the American Veterinary Association* 238 (12), 1601-1608.

de Lahunta, A., Glass, E. (2009) *Veterinary Neuroanatomy and Clinical Neurology,* 3rd edn. Saunders Elsevier, St. Louis.

Fatone, G., Lamagna F., Pasolini, M.P., et al. (1997) Myelography in the dog with nonionic contrast media at different iodine concentrations. *Journal of Small Animal Practice* 38, 292-294.

Funkquist, B. (1962) Thoraco-lumbar myelography with water-soluble contrast medium in dogs I. Technique of myelography; side-effects and complications. *Journal of Small Animal Practice* 3, 53-66.

Girard, N.M., Leece, E.A. (2010) Suspected anaphylactoid reaction following intravenous administration of a gadolinium-based contrast agent in three dogs undergoing magnetic resonance imaging. *Veterinary Anaesthesia and Analgesia* 37, 352-356.

Isreal, S.K., Levine, S.M., Kerwin, S.C., et al. (2009) The relative sensitivity of computed tomography and myelography for identification of thoracolumbar intervertebral disk herniations in dogs. *Veterinary Radiology & Ultrasound* 50 (3), 247-252.

Kishimoto, M., Yamada, K., Ueno, H., et al. (2004) Spinal cord effects from lumbar myelographic injection technique in the dog. *The Journal of Veterinary Medical Science* 66 (1), 67-9.

Kirberger, R.M., Wrigley, R.H. (1993) Myelography in the dog: review of patients with contrast medium in the central canal. *Veterinary Radiology & Ultrasound* 43 (4), 253-258.

Lexmaulova, L., Zatloukal, J., Proks, P., et al. (2009) Incidence of seizures associated with iopamidol or iomeprol myelography in dogs with intervertebral disk disease: 161 cases (2000-2002). *Journal of Veterinary Emergency and Critical Care* 19 (6), 611-616.

Luján Feliu-Pascual, A., Garosi, L., Dennis, R., et al. (2008) Iatrogenic brainstem injury during cerebellomedullary cistern puncture. *Veterinary Radiology & Ultrasound* 49 (5), 467-471.

Olby, N.J., Dyce, J., Houlton, J.E.F. (1994) Correlation of plain radiographic and lumbar myelographic findings with surgical findings in thoracolumbar disc disease. *Journal of Small Animal Practice* 35, 345-350.

Packer, R.A., Bergman, R.L., Coates, J.R., et al. (2007) Intracranial subarachnoid hemorrhage following myelography in two dogs. *Veterinary Radiology & Ultrasound* 48 (4), 323-327.

Platt, S.R., Dennis, R., Murphy, K., et al. (2005) Hematomyelia secondary to lumbar cerebrospinal fluid acquisition in a Dog. *Veterinary Radiology & Ultrasound* 46 (6), 467-471.

Pollard, R.E., Puchalski, S.M., Pascoe, P.J. (2008) Hemodynamic and serum biochemical alterations associated with intravenous administration of three types of contrast medium in anesthetized dogs. *American Journal of Veterinary Research* 69, 1268-1273.

Robertson, I., Thrall, D.E. (2011) Imaging dogs with suspected disc herniation: pros and cons of myelography, computed tomography, and magnetic resonance. *Veterinary Radiology & Ultrasound* 52 (1), S81–S84.

Smith, J.A. (2010) Hazards, safety, and anesthetic considerations for magnetic resonance imaging. *Topics in Companion Animal Medicine* 25 (2), 98–106.

Spencer, C.P., Chrisman, C.L., Mayhew, I.G., et al. (1982) Neurotoxicologic effects of the nonionic contrast agent iopamidol on the leptomeninges of the dog. *American Journal of Veterinary Research* 43 (11), 1958–1962.

Widmer, W.R., Blevins, W.E., Jakovljevic S., et al. (1992) Iohexol and iopamidol myelography in the dog: a clinical trial comparing adverse effects and myelographic quality. *Veterinary Radiology & Ultrasound* 33 (6), 327–333.

Wheeler, S.J., Davies, J.V. (1985) Iohexol myelography in the dog and cat: a series of one hundred cases, and a comparison with metrizamide and iopamidol. *Journal of Small Animal Practice* 26, 247–256.

Wright, J.A., Clayton, D.G. (1981) Metrizamide myelography in sixty eight dogs. *Journal of Small Animal Practice* 22, 415–435.

84 Ventral Slot and Fenestration

Wanda Gordon-Evans
Wisconsin Veterinary Referral Center, Waukesha, WI, USA

A ventral slot is a ventral surgical approach to the spinal canal through the vertebral body and disk. This technique is most commonly used to relieve compressive disk lesions. Ventral fenestration consists of incising the vertebral disks to remove the nucleus pulposus in an effort to decrease the risk of future compression at that site. Ventral slot procedures are performed almost exclusively in the cervical region. Although complications are rare, they may be severe and include hypotension, cardiac arrhythmias, and respiratory distress. These complications are only relevant in the cervical area. Rarely, ventral slots may be performed at other locations in cases of diskospondylitis unresponsive to antibiotics. Fenestration may be performed in any area of the spine. Whereas a ventral approach is typically used in the cervical region, thoracolumbar fenestration is performed through a dorsolateral approach. Complications associated with fenestration are less common than with ventral slot and tend to be less severe.

Hemorrhage
See Chapter 12.

Definition
Hemorrhage is copious discharge of blood from vessels. More specifically, hemorrhage occurring from the venous sinus can result in significant impairment of visualization, leading to other complications.

Risk factor
• Preoperative aspirin use

Diagnosis
• Visualization of blood welling up from the ventral slot during surgery

Treatment
If still attempting to remove the disk:
• Gel foam placed in the slot: Direct pressure for 2 to 10 minutes.
• Saline in slot and wait for 2 to 10 minutes before suctioning
• Simultaneous suctioning of the slot while attempting disk removal
• Abandoning disk removal
If all disk has been removed or abandoned, any of the following methods can be used before closure:
• Free fat graft
• Gel foam in slot
Blood transfusion (see Chapter 12) may be required in rare cases.

Outcome
The outcome depends on the severity and if the disk can still be removed from the canal. If surgery has to be abandoned before disk removal, pain and neurologic deficits will likely remain.

Prevention
The approach is very important in avoiding the venous sinus. The widest safe zone is at the disk on the midline. Tracking with the bur to the right or left of the midline increases the chances of puncturing the sinus. Careful and gentle removal of disk with atraumatic instruments minimizes the risk of traumatizing the sinus.

Horner's syndrome
See Chapter 23.

Hypotension

Definition
Hypotension is an abnormally low blood pressure (mean blood pressure <60 to 70 mm Hg or systolic blood pressure <90 mm Hg).

Risk factors
• Anesthesia (most common), cervical spinal trauma, manipulation of the vagus nerve, hemorrhage, arrhythmia

Diagnosis
• Direct or indirect measurement of blood pressure

Treatment
Remove the cause (i.e., decrease anesthetic inhalant, reduce retraction on vagus nerve, replace blood volume as needed) or in refractory cases, administer vasopressors to support blood pressure (Table 84.1).

Outcome
The outcome depends on the cause and response to treatment. Hypotension can be fatal with severe spinal cord trauma.

Prevention
• Delicate dissection and retraction during the approach and removal of disk material
• Careful balance of anesthetic analgesia and inhalant drugs

Complications in Small Animal Surgery, First Edition. Edited by Dominique Griffon and Annick Hamaide.
© 2016 John Wiley & Sons, Inc. Published 2016 by John Wiley & Sons, Inc.
Companion website: www.wiley.com/go/griffon/complications

Table 84.1 Treatments for hypotension

Drug	Dose	Route
Hypotension		
Dobutamine	2–10 µg/kg/hr	IV
Dopamine	2–10 µg/kg/hr	IV
Bradyarrhythmia		
Glycopyrrolate	0.005–0.011 mg/kg	IV, IM, or SC
Atropine	0.02 mg/kg	IV, IM, or SC
Ventricular tachycardia		
Lidocaine	2–4 mg/kg	IV
	25–80 µg/kg/hr	IV

IM, intramuscular; IV, intravenous; SC, subcutaneous.

Cardiac arrhythmias

Definition
Cardiac arrhythmias are abnormal heart rhythms.

Risk factors
- Vagus nerve manipulation: bradyarrhythmias, typically sinus bradycardia
- Spinal cord manipulation: tachyarrhythmias from pain or direct sympathetic nerve stimulation, ventricular premature complexes
- Anesthesia

Diagnosis
- Electrocardiography (ECG)

Treatment
Treatment is initiated when the arrhythmia affects blood pressure, is indicative of pain, or predisposes to ventricular fibrillation (not typically associated with ventral slot).
- Tachyarrhythmia: pain medication and maintenance of an appropriate anesthetic plain.
- Bradyarrhythmia (second-degree atrioventricular block): Parasympatholytic (Table 84.1) drugs may be used to treat bradycardia.
- Ventricular premature complexes: Treat only if the rate is greater than 180 beats/min (ventricular tachycardia) or is affecting blood pressure (see Table 84.1)

Outcome
If anesthetic drugs are contributing to the cause, recovery from anesthesia often resolves the problem.

Prevention
- Delicate dissection and retraction of neurologic structures during approach and removal of disk material
- Anesthetic monitoring with appropriate balance of drugs
Vertebral instability or subluxation

Definition
- Vertebral instability or subluxation is a decrease in the capacity of the vertebral stabilizing system to maintain a physiologic range of motion without neurologic dysfunction, deformity, or pain.

Risk factors
- Ventral slot
- Ventral fenestration

- Preexisting instability (i.e., cervical spondylomyelopathy)
- Caudal cervical spine

Diagnosis
- Clinical signs include failure to meet expectations in terms of recovery: loss of function, failure to regain function, and prolonged postoperative pain
- Evidence of subluxation on radiographs of the surgical area
- Advanced imaging is indicated to rule out other causes of dysfunction (disk herniation at other sites, inadequate removal of disk) and confirm the subluxation.

Treatment
- Reduction and ventral stabilization
- Methods of stabilization include vertebral body plating or pins and polymethylmethacrylate (PMMA).

Outcome
There should be improvement with surgical stabilization, but stress increases at adjacent disks and may lead to other ruptures (domino effect; see Chapter 87).

Prevention
Keep the ventral slot less than one third of the length vertebral bodies above and below the slot. The overall ratio of slot width to the vertebral body width should be less than 0.5 (Figure 84.1).

Respiratory distress
Penetration of the chest and pneumothorax during thoracolumbar fenestration.

Definition
Respiratory distress is a clinical inability to adequately ventilate or oxygenate.

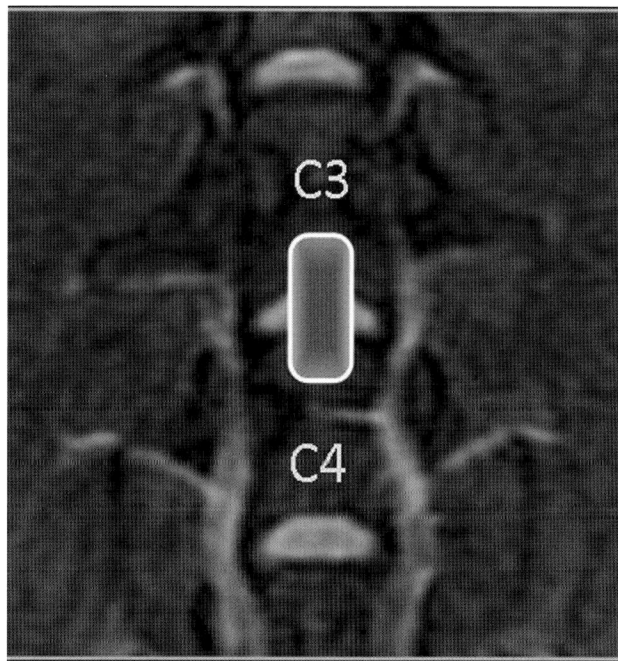

Figure 84.1 Ventral slot size recommendations. The inverted cone method is shown below. The slot spans one third or less of each vertebra length and half the vertebral width.

Risk factors

Cervical spinal trauma (especially between C2 and C4), anesthesia, iatrogenic injury to spinal cord or vagus nerve or branches (recurrent laryngeal nerve)

Diagnosis

Clinical signs:
- Dyspnea
- Tachypnea
- Collapse
- Blue mucous membranes
- Stridor

Diagnostic tests:
- SpO$_2$ less than 95 mm Hg
- PaCO$_2$ greater than 45 mm Hg

Treatment

- Supportive care as needed: oxygen, ventilation, or both

Outcome

The outcome is guarded depending on the cause.
- Vagus neuropraxia: good
- Recurrent laryngeal neuropraxia: guarded
- Spinal trauma: fair with prolonged supportive care (including ventilation)
- Anesthetically induced: excellent

Prevention

- Delicate dissection and retraction of neurologic structures during approach and removal of disk material
- Anesthetic monitoring with appropriate balance of drugs

Iatrogenic spinal injury

Definition

Iatrogenic spinal injury is injury caused by surgery or the surgeon.

Risk factors

- Cervical location
- Inappropriate visualization (e.g., hemorrhage)

Diagnosis

It is often difficult to ascertain whether the injury results from spinal trauma at the time of the disk extrusion or from anesthetic effects. However, iatrogenic injury must be the top differential when profound neurologic deficits appear after surgery and the effects persist after anesthetic recovery.

Treatment

- Time and supportive care
- Consider advanced imaging to confirm adequate disk removal and spinal decompression.

Outcome

The outcome depends on the dysfunction and level of injury. See cardiac arrhythmias, respiratory distress, hypotension, Horner's syndrome (Chapter 23).

Prevention

- Delicate dissection and retraction of neurologic structures during approach and removal of disk material (Figure 84.2)

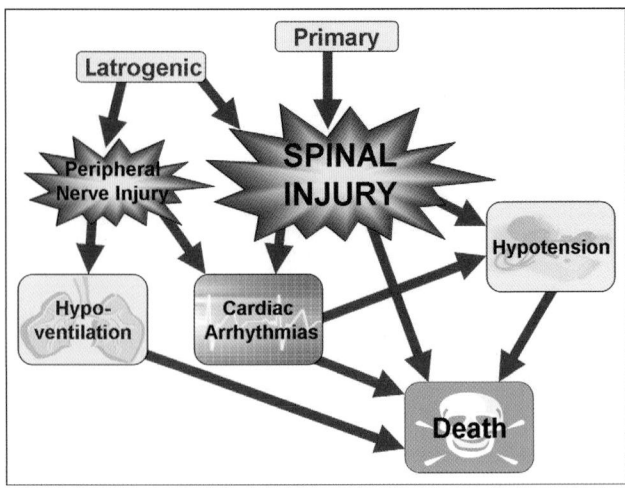

Figure 84.2 Relationship of complications.

Death

Definition

Death is cessation of all biologic functions often marked by cardiac or pulmonary arrest followed by the absence of brain activity.

Risk factors

Cardiac arrest causing death is predisposed by cardiac arrhythmias, hypotension, and high vagal tone. These all can be caused by the primary spinal trauma in the cervical region and anesthesia.

Diagnosis

- Often detected by electrocardiography combined with cessation of pulse and blood pressure
- Technically, death may not be declared until after cardiopulmonary resuscitation (CPR) has failed.

Treatment

Cardiac and respiratory arrest may be treated with CPR techniques, but death cannot be treated.

Outcome

Anesthetic or vagal causes of arrest may respond to CPR that has been promptly initiated.

Prevention

- Delicate dissection and retraction of neurologic structures during approach and removal of disk material
- Appropriate monitoring of anesthetic depth, hypotension, ventilation, and ECG allows for appropriate preventive measures.

Hematoma formation

See Chapter 86.

Postoperative disk disease

Definition

This is spinal compression caused by the presence of herniated disk material resulting from inadequate removal or further extrusion of disk material at the same site. In this case, nucleus pulposus exits the center of the disk through a rent in the annulus fibrosus, causing concussion or compression of the spinal cord.

Risk factors
- Fenestration
- Overactivity
- Steroid use (see Prevention)
- Inadequate removal of herniated disk
- Technical error in localization of the surgical site

Diagnosis
Magnetic resonance imaging (MRI) is preferred, but compression can be detected via computed tomography (CT) with or without contrast. CT can detect the difference between a hematoma and further disk extrusion, especially if the disk is mineralized. MRI is more sensitive than CT at differentiation among hematoma, neoplasia, and disk extrusion using multiple sequences and contrast enhancement.

Treatment
- Conservative therapy, including rest and analgesia or surgical intervention (Figure 84.3)

Outcome
The prognosis is good with surgical intervention when central perception of pain is present.

Prevention
- Accurate localization of the surgical site over the determined site of compression
- Appropriate removal of disk: Accurate localization of the ventral slot over the midline and respecting appropriate dimensions are essential to avoid hemorrhage and preserve visualization. Extruded disk material is gently removed with a curette until the spinal cord become visible through the ventral slot.
- Fenestration is designed to remove nonextruded nucleus pulposus and prevent further extrusion. However, this procedure may cause further disc extrusion because of the pressure exerted on the nucleus pulposus during the approach. Creating an adequate window and scooping the contents in an outward direction may help

to mitigate this risk. Fenestration can be considered (despite the risks) in dogs with other degenerative disks in the surgical area.
- Strict rest postoperatively is the only noncontroversial preventive measure.
- The benefits of perioperative prednisone have been challenged. Theoretically, the antifibrotic effects of steroids may reduce the scar tissue repair of the annulus, allowing further extrusion. (Mann *et al.* 2007).

Diskospondylitis

Definition
Diskospondylitis is infection of the vertebral endplates and disk.

Risk factors
- Surgical approach to the spine
- Other sites of infection (e.g., teeth, urinary tract infection [UTI])

Diagnosis
Possible clinical signs include back pain and varying neurologic dysfunction from no deficits to nonambulatory paraplegic. Dogs with diskospondylitis often have concurrent UTIs.
- Complete blood count, chemistry, urinalysis, and urine culture are diagnostics that can aid in determining severity of systemic infection and appropriate antibiotic treatment.
- If urine culture results are negative, aspirates of the boney lesions with fluoroscopic, CT, or MRI guidance can be cytologically analyzed and cultured to determine the best choice of antibiotics or antifungal medications.
- MRI is the most sensitive method.
- Radiography can be used, but lysis of the vertebral endplates may not be evident radiographically at the onset of clinical signs.

Treatment and outcome
See Figure 84.3.

Prevention
- Aseptic technique during surgery
- Treatment of concurrent infections
- The preventive effects of perioperative antibiotherapy remain unclear.

Recurrence and pain
See Chapters 14 and 87.
These are also symptoms of other complications such as instability or diskospondylitis.

Relevant literature
Cervical disc disease accounts for 15% of intervertebral disc extrusions in dogs (Cherrone *et al.* 2004). An early study reported a complication rate of 15% (Smith *et al.* 1997). However, the inverted cone technique may help decrease the possibility of subluxation or excessive hemorrhage (Goring *et al.* 1991; Da Costa 2010). Arguably, the most common complication (~20%) of ventral slot surgery consists of venous sinus **hemorrhage,** which rarely requires blood transfusion but is often significant enough to impair visualization and occasionally prompt the surgeon to abort the procedure (McCartney 2007). Residual postoperative spinal compression results more

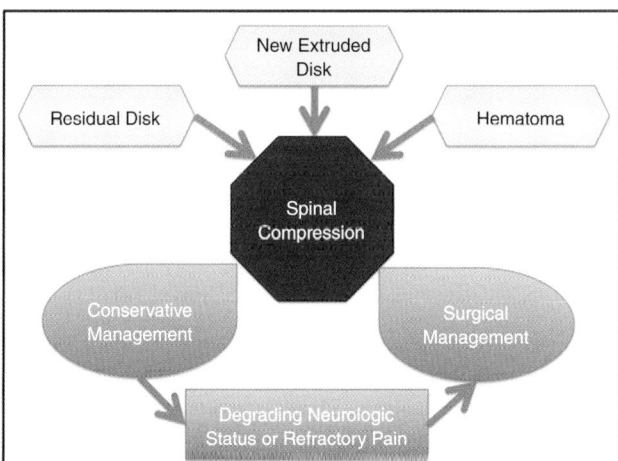

Figure 84.3 Algorithm for residual compression.

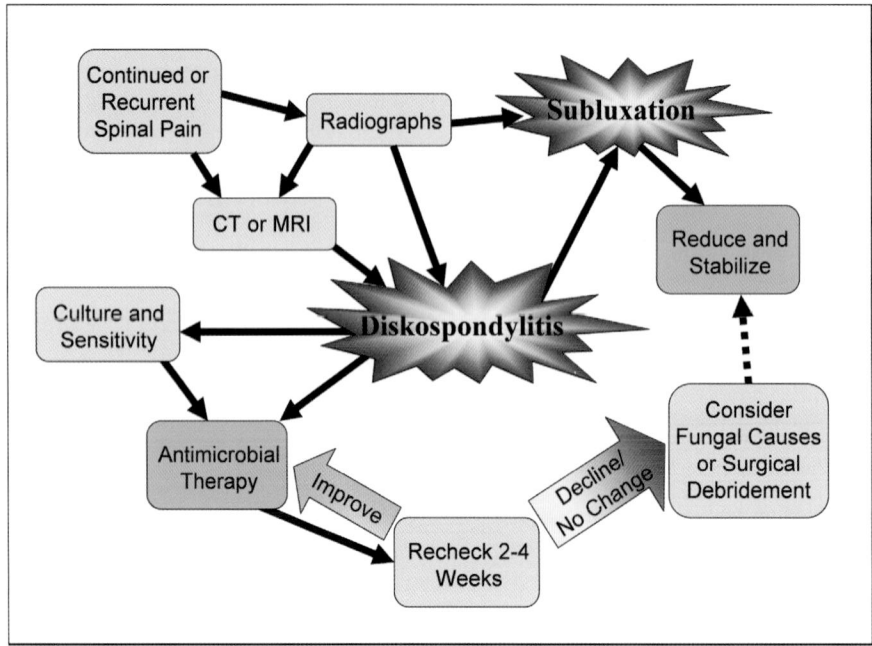

Figure 84.4 Diagnosis and treatment algorithm for diskospondylitis. CT, computed tomography; MRI, magnetic resonance imaging.

commonly from incomplete disk removal, although one case of hematoma causing spinal cord compression has been reported after a ventral slot (Seim and Prata 1982). Modifications have been suggested with and without common adoption in an effort to minimize the risk of penetrating the vertebral sinus (McCartney 2007). The modified cone ventral slot provided for a smaller opening into the vertebral canal, which may allow avoidance of the venous sinuses. McCartney (2007) suggested a slanted slot modification that requires a smaller breech of the vertebral canal compared with standard ventral slot techniques. In a retrospective report, the slanted slot group had less intraoperative hemorrhage, but this technique limits the amount of disk retrievable from the caudal aspect of the disk and thus has not been widely put to use.

Spinal cord trauma in the cervical area can be life threatening, requiring hemodynamic or ventilatory support (or both) (Kube *et al.* 2003; Beal *et al.* 2001). **Bradycardia** is 2.5 times more likely, and ventricular premature complexes are 3.5 times more likely in patients with spinal compression localized to the cervical region (Stauffer 1988). Supportive care including ventilation can lead to a successful recovery. In a retrospective study, 9 of 14 dogs requiring ventilatory support recovered neurologic function (Beal *et al.* 2001). These dogs must likely sustained surgical trauma to the spinal cord, although trauma to the vagus nerve or recurrent laryngeal nerve during the surgical could carry respiratory or hemodynamic consequences.

Instability is a complication that has generated extensive experimental research, leading to multiple proposed solutions such limiting slot size, articular facet arthrodesis, grafting the vertebral defect after decompression, pins and PMMA stabilization, and vertebral body plating (Adamo *et al.* 2007; Fitch *et al.* 2000; Fauber *et al.* 2006; Lemarie *et al.* 2000; Koehler *et al.* 2005). Biomechanically, ventral slots and fenestrations increase range of motion in extension (McCartney 2007; Koehler *et al.* 2005). It is hypothesized that the instability created at surgery is transient and that secondary systems stabilize the spine postoperatively in vivo (Crisco *et al.* 1990).

However, the reported rates of postoperative subluxations reach up to 8% to 10% of operated dogs (Cherrone *et al.* 2004; Lemarie *et al.* 2000; Fitch *et al.* 2000). Fitch *et al.* (2000) report that ventral slot provides a better outcome (as measured by return to ambulation) when combined with stabilization with an allograft block inserted into the slot or pins in adjacent vertebral bodies with bridging PMMA. However, stabilization of a vertebral space increases the stress placed on spaces cranial and caudal to the stabilized site. This stress may expedite degeneration and predispose to a domino effect, in which clinical signs of spinal compression originate from adjacent disks (Lemarie *et al.* 2000; Koehler *et al.* 2005; Adamo *et al.* 2007). Although domino lesions have been reported in up to 30% of dogs with vertebral fusion, it is unknown whether the disk degeneration is attributable to the domino effect or the dog's underlying disease.

Diskospondylitis is a potential complication of any surgery involving intervertebral disks, including fenestration or ventral slot. Among dogs with diskospondylitis, 3.3% have a history of vertebral surgery, and 2.4% have had other surgeries (Burkert *et al.* 2005). The rate of diskospondylitis as a complication disk surgery is unknown. Diskospondylitis may contribute to instability, thereby requiring additional surgical intervention.

References

Adamo, P.O., Kobayashi, H., Markel, M., et al. (2007) In vitro biomechanical comparison of cervical disk arthroplasty, ventral slot procedure, and smooth pins with polymethylmethacrylate fixation at treated and adjacent canine cervical motion units. *Veterinary Surgery* 36, 729-741.

Beal, M.W., Paglia, D.T., Griffin, G.M., et al. (2001) Ventilatory failure, ventilator management, and outcome in dogs with cervical spinal disorders: 14 cases (1991-1999). *Journal of the American Veterinary Medical Association* 218 (10), 1598-1602.

Burkert, B.A., Kerwin, S.C., Hosgood, G.L., et al. (2005) Signalment and clinical features of diskospondylitis in dogs: 513 cases (1980-2001). *Journal of the American Veterinary Medical Association* 227 (2), 268-275.

Cherrone, K.L., Dewey, C.W., Coates, J.R., et al. (2004) A retrospective comparison of cervical intervertebral disk disease in nonchondrodystrophic large dogs versus small dogs. *Journal of the American Animal Hospital Association* 40, 316-320.

Crisco, J.J., Panjabi, M.M., Wang, E., et al. (1990) The injured canine cervical spine after six months of healing: an in vitro three-dimensional study. *Spine* 15, 1047-1052.

Da Costa, R.C. (2010) Cervical spondylomyelopathy (Wobbler syndrome) in dogs. *Veterinary Clinics of North America: Small Animal Practice* 40, 881-913.

Fauber, A., Wade, J., Lipka, A., et al. (2006) Effect of width of disk fenestration and a ventral slot on biomechanics of the canine C5-C6 vertebral motion unit. *American Journal of Veterinary Research* 67, 1844-1848.

Fitch, R.B., Kerwin, S.C. ,Hosgood, G. (2000) Caudal cervical intervertebral disk disease in the small dog: Role of distraction and stabilization in ventral slot decompression. *Journal of the American Animal Hospital Association* 36, 68-74.

Goring, R.L., Beale, B.S., Faulkner, R.F. (1991) The inverted cone decompression technique: a surgical treatment for cervical vertebral instability "wobbler syndrome" in Doberman Pinschers. *Journal of the American Animal Hospital Association* 27 (4), 403-409.

Koehler, C.L., Stover, S.M., LeCouteur, R.A., et al. (2005) Effect of a ventral slot procedure and of smooth or positive-profile threaded pins with polymethylmethacrylate fixation on intervertebral biomechanics at treated and adjacent canine cervical vertebral motion units. *American Journal of Veterinary Research* 66, 678-687.

Kube, S., Owen, T., Hanson, S. (2003) Severe respiratory compromise secondary to cervical disk herniation in two dogs. *Journal of the American Animal Hospital Association* 39, 513-517.

Lemarie, R.J., Kerwin, S.C., Partington, B.P., et al. (2000) Vertebral subluxation following ventral cervical decompression in the dog. *Journal of the American Animal Hospital Association* 36, 348-358.

Mann, F.A., Wagner-Mann, C.C., Dunphy, E.D., et al. (2007) Recurrence rate of presumed thoracolumbar intervertebral disc disease in ambulatory dogs with spinal hyperpathia treated with anti-inflammatory drugs: 78 cases (1997-2000). *Journal of Veterinary Emergency and Critical Care* 17, 53-60.

McCartney, W. (2007) comparison of recovery times and complication rates between a modified slated slot and the standard ventral slot for the treatment of cervical disc disease in 20 dogs. *Journal of Small Animal Practice* 48, 498-501.

Seim H.B. and Prata R.G. (1982) Ventral decompression for the treatment of cervical disk disease in the dog: a review of 54 cases. *Journal of the American Animal Hospital Association* 18, 233.

Smith, B.A., Hosgood, G., Kerwin, S.C. (1997) Ventral slot decompression for cervical intervertebral disc disease in 112 dogs. *Australian Veterinary Practitioner* 27 (2), 58-64.

Stauffer, J.L., Gleed, R.D., Short, C.E., et al. (1988) Cardiac dysrhythmias during anesthesia for cervical decompression in the dog. *American Journal of Veterinary Research* 49, 1143-1146.

85 Dorsal Laminectomy

Wanda Gordon-Evans
Wisconsin Veterinary Referral Center, Waukesha, WI, USA

A dorsal laminectomy is a surgical approach selected to manage numerous neurologic abnormalities, including spinal malformations such as stenosis, neoplasia, intervertebral disk disease, subarachnoid cysts, and cervical spondylopathy. Indications and complications may vary depending on the disease process, anatomic location, and type of laminectomy performed. The epidemiology of complications for dorsal laminectomies has not been specifically studied in veterinary medicine, and most knowledge derives from human medicine, case reports, anecdotal reports, and extrapolation of experimental studies.

After cervical dorsal laminectomy, postoperative worsening of neurologic status has been reported in up to 70% of dogs with cervical spondylopathy and in 36% of dogs with dural masses (De Risio et al. 2002; Forterre et al. 2007). The incidence of other types of complications remains undocumented in the literature.

Complications tend to be influenced by the type of dorsal laminectomy and seem to correlate with the extent of bone removal. Dorsal laminectomies have been classified as Funkquist type A, Funkquist type B, and a modified dorsal laminectomy (Figure 85.1). The most aggressive laminectomy is a Funkquist type A, which involves bilateral resection of both the articular facets and partial removal of the pedicle. Type B laminectomy preserves the majority

of the cranial articular facets and pedicles. A Funkquist type B laminectomy is less likely to allow the formation of a laminectomy membrane across the exposed spinal cord. This procedure theoretically minimizes the destabilization of the vertebral column but provides a narrower exposure to the spinal cord than a Funkquist type A laminectomy. The Funkquist type B dorsal laminectomy has consequently been modified to improve the exposure while minimizing the risk of constrictive fibrosis: the cranial articular facets are preserved on each side, but the pedicles are undercut with a high-speed burr. It should be noted that postoperative formation of a laminectomy membrane has been reported in dogs, but the incidence of this complication remains unknown (De Risio et al. 2002).

Pain
See Chapter 14

Seroma formation

Definition
A seroma is a mass of serum localized within a tissue or organ. Although a seroma may form after dorsal laminectomy, this

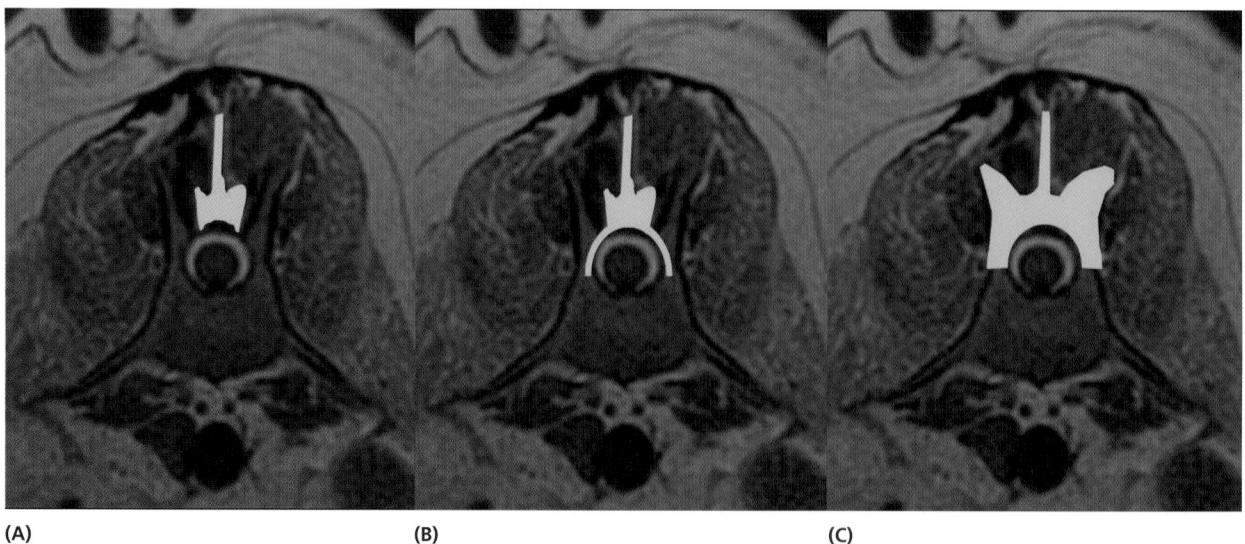

(A)   **(B)**   **(C)**

Figure 85.1 Types of dorsal laminectomies. Axial magnetic resonance imaging slice of a lumbar vertebra where the shaded area represents the area of bone removal. **A,** Funkquist type B. **B,** Modified dorsal laminectomy. **C,** Funkquist type A.

Complications in Small Animal Surgery, First Edition. Edited by Dominique Griffon and Annick Hamaide.
© 2016 John Wiley & Sons, Inc. Published 2016 by John Wiley & Sons, Inc.
Companion website: www.wiley.com/go/griffon/complications

complication rarely bears clinical significance. Potential secondary problems include compression of the spinal cord by the seroma or infection of the seroma leading to abscessation or myelitis.

Risk factors

The most common cause of seroma is the presence of dead space due to suboptimal closure of tissue layers. Motion may also contribute to seroma formation. The risk of infection increases with fine needle aspirates of the fluid. Seroma formation is more common after cervical procedures because of the thickness of the soft tissues covering the dorsal aspect of the spine in that region. The motion of the scapula on each side of the surgical site may also act as a predisposing factor.

Diagnosis

A tentative diagnosis is based on the detection during physical examination of a soft or fluctuant, nonpainful mass over the surgery site (Figure 85.2). Seromas tend to develop in the early postoperative phase and are not associated with obvious signs of inflammation. A definitive diagnosis is based on cytological examination of a fine-needle aspirate. The need to confirm the diagnosis should, however, be weighed against the risk of bacterial seeding during fine-needle aspirate. The decision to proceed should be based on an evaluation of the clinical relevance of the seroma in terms of failure to respond to conservative treatment or concurrent clinical signs. Advanced imaging (magnetic resonance imaging) may be repeated if the presence of a seroma is suspected within deep tissues (Figure 85.3).

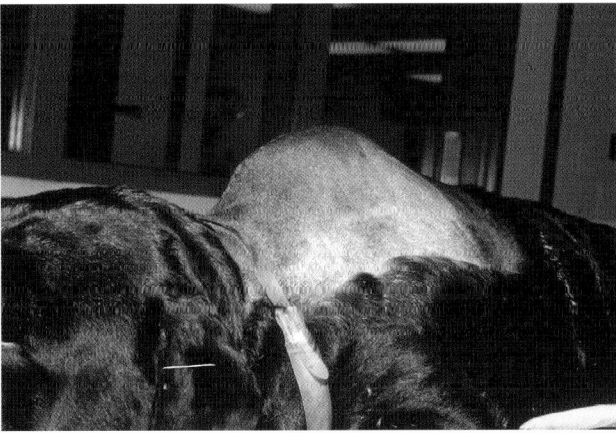

Figure 85.2 Seroma after cervical dorsal laminectomy in a Rottweiler. The seroma failed to respond to treatment consisting of aspiration, compression bandage, and cage rest for 1 week. *Source:* D. Griffon, Western University of Health Sciences, Pomona, CA, 2014. Reproduced with permission from D. Griffon.

Treatment

Most seromas are managed conservatively initially. Strict rest is recommended to limit motion of tissues adjacent to the surgical site. Warm compresses are applied two to three times daily to encourage drainage. Local compression can usually not be achieved with bandages because of the location of the surgical site. Seromas

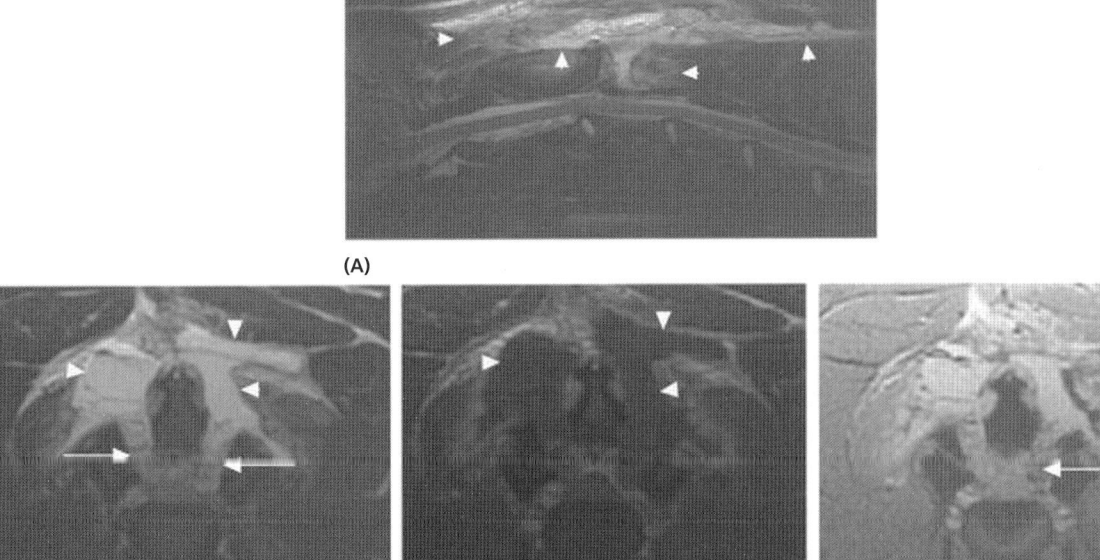

(A)

(B)   (C)   (D)

Figure 85.3 Appearance of a subfascial seroma on magnetic resonance imaging. Subfascial seroma admixed with a small amount of blood and soft tissue causing dorsoventral compression of the spinal cord. Postoperative midline sagittal (**A**) T2-weighted (T2W) images of the cervical spine and transverse T2W (**B**), postcontrast T1-weighted T1W (**C**) and T2*W gradient echo (**D**) at the level of C2 to C3 (T2W Time Repitition (TR) = 3800 ms, Time Echo (TE) = 81.4 ms; T1W TR = 420 ms, TE = 10.8 ms; T2*GEW TR = 400 ms, TE = 15 ms, flip angle = 20 degrees). Soft tissue planes dorsal to the cranial cervical spine are disrupted (arrowheads in **A**) and several pockets of material appearing hyperintense to muscle on T2W (arrowheads in **B**) and iso- to hypointense on T1W (arrowheads in **C**) are present. A material of mixed intensity, consistent with soft tissue, fluid and hemorrhage has filled the bony defect and is causing dorsal cord compression (arrows in B and D). *Source:* Matiasek *et al.*, 2006. Reproduced with permission from John Wiley & Sons.

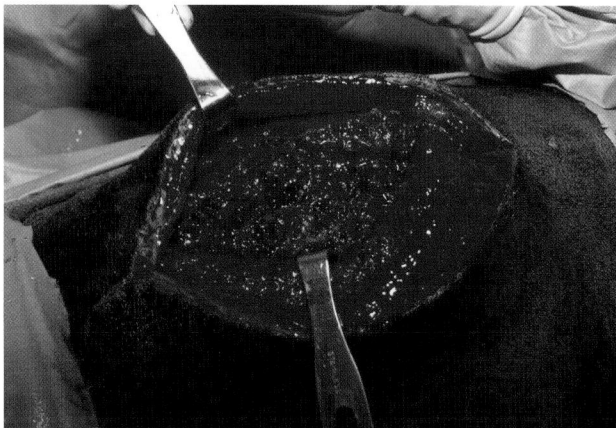

Figure 85.4 Intraoperative view of a seroma after cervical dorsal laminectomy. The seroma shown in Figure 85.2 is debrided before obliteration of dead space and wound drainage. *Source:* D. Griffon, Western University of Health Sciences, Pomona, CA, 2014. Reproduced with permission from D. Griffon.

in the cervical region may benefit from a figure-of-eight bandage applied around the forelimb with additional padding placed over the surgical site. Drainage can be performed but is not recommended because of the risk of bacterial contamination and propensity to reform. Surgical treatment is rarely necessary but may be considered for large seromas that fail to respond to conservative management or recur. In these cases, treatment includes surgical debridement of the membrane surrounding the seroma and occlusion of dead space (Figure 85.4). Occlusion of dead space typically requires thorough apposition of tissue layers and wound drainage. Penrose drains are best avoided because of the risk of ascending contamination and the inability to place the drain along planes of gravity around the spine. Instead, closed active drainage is preferred (Figure 85.5). A bandage should be maintained over the surgical site until removal of the drain, usually within 3 to 5 days.

Outcome

The prognosis is excellent. Most seromas are self-resolving over time, but warm compresses may speed resorption of the serum.

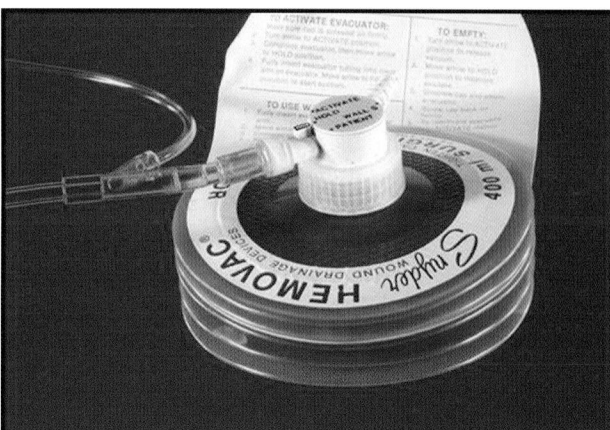

Figure 85.5 Example of a drain used for closed active wound drainage. This type of drainage relies essentially on negative pressure and limits the risk of ascending contamination compared with a Penrose drain. *Source:* D. Griffon, Western University of Health Sciences, Pomona, CA, 2014. Reproduced with permission from D. Griffon.

Prevention

- Thorough apposition of tissue layers during closure of the surgical site
- Postoperative exercise restriction

Vertebral instability

Definition

Vertebral instability is a decrease in the ability of vertebral supporting structures to maintain the physiologic stability of the spine. This loss of biomechanical properties becomes clinically significant when a normal range of motion cannot be maintained without neurologic dysfunction, deformity, or pain. This instability may translate into chronic micromotion, exacerbating disk degeneration or subluxation (rare).

Risk factors

- Suspected preoperative instability
- Dorsal laminectomy over three or more continuous sites
- Bilateral removal of articular facets

Diagnosis

It is extremely difficult to document abnormal motion as a cause of disk degeneration, but subluxation can be detected by computed tomography or radiography. A tentative diagnosis is based on recurrence of clinical signs localized to a site of previous extensive dorsal laminectomy. The decision to pursue advanced imaging in these cases depends on the severity of signs.

Treatment

- Conservative management: external coaptation, pain medications, steroids or nonsteroidal antiinflammatory drugs (NSAIDs)
- Surgical fusion of the vertebrae is rarely performed as a second surgery unless subluxation is documented.

Outcome

The outcome is variable and not well reported.

Prevention

Preventive measures aim at preserving supporting structures of the spine while allowing adequate visualization of the spinal cord. The steps most commonly taken to prevent postoperative motion-induced disk degeneration include:
- Preservation of articular facets
- Postoperative exercise restriction

In the rare cases in which extensive dorsal laminectomy is required over consecutive spaces, stabilizing procedures may be performed during the initial surgery to prevent subsequent instability. These procedures include:
- Placement of screws across the articular facets
- Fixation bridging affected vertebrae via locking plate and screws
- Fixation bridging affected vertebrae via placement of pins and polymethyl methacrylate (Figures 85.6 and 85.7)

Iatrogenic spinal or nerve root injury

Definition

This is injury to the spinal cord or nerve roots caused by surgery or the surgeon.

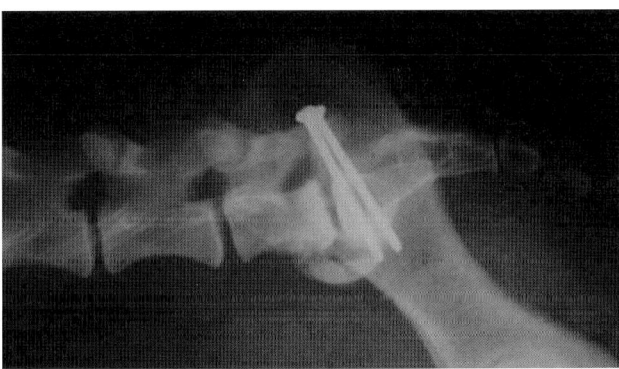

Figure 85.6 Postoperative radiograph after dorsal laminectomy at the lumbosacral junction and transarticular facet screw stabilization. *Source:* Hankin *et al.*, 2012. Reproduced with permission from John Wiley & Sons.

Risk factors
- Cervical spondylomyelopathy
- Ventral lesions that require manipulation of the spinal cord
- Surgery extending over multiple consecutive vertebrae
- Concurrent durotomy

Diagnosis
Iatrogenic spinal injury can be diagnosed at the time of surgery as in the case of a rhizotomy. However, in most cases, iatrogenic trauma is a differential for deterioration of neurologic status in the immediate to early postoperative phase (see Table 88.1). Other differentials include:
- Incorrect location of the surgical site
- Postoperative spinal instability
- Progression of the disease process
- Missed diagnosis of concurrent presurgical disease
- Postoperative hemorrhage and hematoma
- Myelomalacia
- Presence of a new spinal disease

It is often difficult to differentiate between iatrogenic injury and other causes of postoperative deterioration, especially progression of disease. Advanced imaging should be repeated in patients

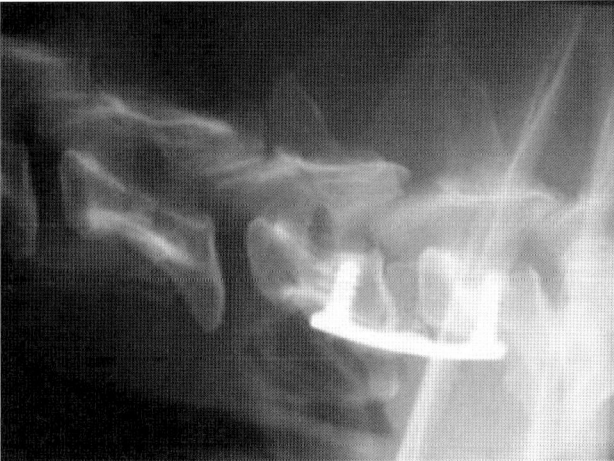

Figure 85.7 Postoperative radiograph after cervical dorsal laminectomy and locking plate stabilization. *Source:* Trotter, 2009. Reproduced with permission from John Wiley & Sons.

with severe deterioration of neurologic signs (loss of deep pain) or failure to respond to postoperative medical treatment. In both instances, the goal is to rule out the presence of any lesion that may benefit from a second surgery.

Treatment
The treatment of patients with postoperative worsening of neurologic signs caused by iatrogenic trauma is limited to medical management (see Table 88.2):
- NSAIDs or steroids may help decrease inflammation
- Pain management
- Supportive care

Outcome
The outcome varies with the disease process and degree of injury.

Prevention
- Careful dissection and gentle treatment of the spinal cord and associated structures (Figure 85.8).
- Good visualization of the surgical site: focused surgical lighting, retraction of tissues, thorough hemostasis with bipolar cautery, surgical assistance and use of magnification

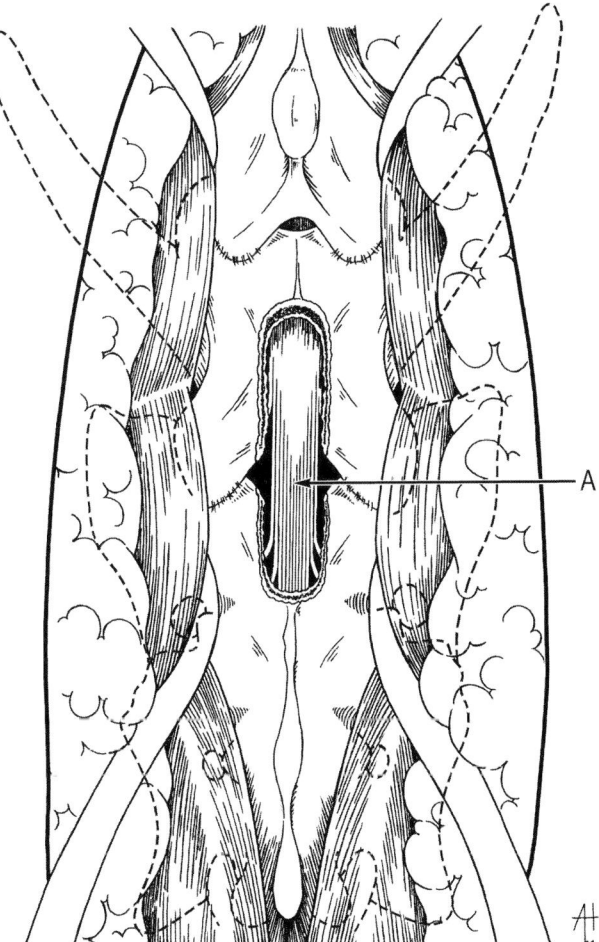

Figure 85.8 Dorsal laminectomy at the lumbosacral junction. Note the location of the nerve roots. *Source:* Coates *et al.*, 2002. Reproduced with permission from Elsevier.

- Methylprednisolone sodium succinate (30 mg/kg once) has been advocated to help protect the spinal cord from further injury. However, there is no clinical evidence in the literature to support the use of steroids preoperatively.

Laminectomy membrane formation

Definition
This is a constrictive band of scar tissue forming over the laminectomy site and causing recurring signs of spinal compression several weeks to months after surgery.

Risk factor
- Funkquist type A dorsal laminectomy

Diagnosis
Patients with clinically relevant laminectomy membrane formation experience a recurrence of neurologic signs localized over the previously operated area. This complication tends to occur late in the postoperative phase. Laminectomy membrane formation should be differentiated from disease progression, spinal instability, and the presence of new lesions in sites adjacent to the previous surgical site. The diagnostic approach to these cases requires advanced imaging. Evidence of a dorsal compression over the previous surgical site is consistent with the formation of a laminectomy membrane. The diagnosis is confirmed during surgical exploration.

Treatment
Treatment requires surgical removal of the constrictive band of tissue. This surgery is delicate because adhesions are commonly found between the laminectomy membrane and the underlying dura. The previous surgical site is approached, and surrounding soft tissues are carefully elevated from the affected vertebra. One edge of the laminectomy membrane is incised along the vertebra with a #11 surgical blade. The membrane is gently elevated from the dura with sterile, moistened Q-tips. After excision, a gelatin film or sponge may be placed to avoid recurrence.

Outcome
Surgical decompression is usually effective provided that iatrogenic trauma can be avoided.

Prevention
- Avoid dorsal laminectomy if possible.
- Funkquist type A dorsal laminectomy is not recommended.
- Placement of a gelatin film or sponge or a cellulose mesh over the laminectomy site
- The use of a fat graft over the site is controversial. Free fat grafts have been found to create some initial compression in the cervical area and have been hypothesized to cause some of the postoperative decline in neurologic status.

Relevant literature
Seromas have been reported in dogs after dorsal laminectomy, including a case report of a seroma causing postoperative compression of the spinal cord (Matiasek et al. 2006). Although there have been claims that all dorsal laminectomies are more prone to seromas, they have only been reported in the cervical area, with a rate ranging from 6% to 18% (Rossmeisl 2005; De Risio et al. 2002).

Most of the knowledge regarding instability after dorsal laminectomy derives from biomechanical testing of cadaver specimen rather than from in vivo data. Based on this evidence, dorsal laminectomies produce more **vertebral instability** than hemilaminectomies, and preserving the integrity of articular facets plays a crucial role in minimizing postoperative instability (Smith and Walter 1988; McKee 1992). Indeed, Meij et al. (2007) reported that postoperative instability in flexion and extension at L7 to S1 was eliminated if the articular facets were left intact. It has been hypothesized that over time, postoperative micromotion, although grossly undetectable, could contribute to the progression of clinical signs or recurrence. This theory is difficult to prove but has led to some surgeons advocating stabilization after dorsal laminectomy of the lumbosacral and cervical areas (De Risio et al. 2002).

Formation of a **laminectomy membrane** after dorsal laminectomy is problematic in humans but rare in dogs (De Risio et al. 2002; Da Costa et al. 2006; Da Costa 2010). In the past, fat grafts were advocated to prevent dural adhesions and formation of a laminectomy membrane, but these have fallen out of favor (Da Costa 2010). Recent literature proposes fat grafts as contributors to declining postoperative neurologic status by acting as a space-occupying structure, thereby creating immediate postoperative compression of the exposed spine (Da Costa et al. 2006). Alternatively, the devascularized fat graft may undergo fibrosis, thereby adhering to the spinal cord in the long term. A cellulose membrane has less detrimental effects than a fat graft but may still not be better than no graft (Da Costa et al. 2006). Instead, prevention of the laminectomy membrane may not be necessary (Da Costa 2010).

The majority of the literature addressing complications of dorsal laminectomy focuses on a **postoperative decline in neurologic status**. The incidence of this complication ranges from 36% in the thoracolumbar area to 70% in the cervical area (De Risio et al. 2002; Forterre et al. 2007; Da Costa 2010). The decline in status can be transient or permanent, but most dogs improve if given enough time. The average time to improvement approximates 3.6 months after cervical dorsal laminectomy (De Risio et al. 2002; Da Costa 2010). In the meantime, the decline in neurologic function is severe enough to warrant postoperative ventilation in 4.9% of operated dogs (Beal et al. 2001). Of those, 71% survived (Beal et al. 2001). Although iatrogenic injury can be a cause of postoperative decline, other potential causes include fat graft compression, reperfusion injury, transient postoperative instability, and complications related to myelography (Da Costa 2010).

In the lumbosacral area, deterioration of the neurologic status immediately after surgery does not typically occur. However, dogs with urinary or fecal incontinence preoperatively are less likely to improve after surgery (De Risio et al. 2001; Linn et al. 2003). The success rate for dorsal laminectomy in the lumbosacral area has been reported to reach up to 79%. However, recurrence is common, reported in 54.5% of dogs, as a result of progression of the disease or potentially secondary to instability (Linn et al. 2003).

References
Beal, M.W., Paglia, D.T., Griffin, G.M., et al. (2001) Ventilatory failure, ventilator management, and outcome in dogs with cervical spinal disorders: 14 cases (1991-1999). *Journal of the American Veterinary Medical Association* 218 (10), 1598-1602.
Da Costa, R.C. (2010) Cervical spondylomyelopathy (Wobbler syndrome) in dogs. *Veterinary Clinics of North America: Small Animal Practice* 40, 881-913.
Da Costa, R.C., Pippi, N.L., Graca, D.L., et al. (2006) The effects of free fat graft or cellulose membrane implants on laminectomy membrane formation in dogs. *The Veterinary Journal* 171 (3), 491-9.

De Risio, L., Sharp, N.H., Olby, N.J., et al. (2001) Predictors of outcome after dorsal decompressive laminectomy for degenerative lumbosacral stenosis in dogs: 69 cases (1987-1997). *Journal of the American Veterinary Medical Association* 219, 624-628.

De Risio, L., Muñana, K., Murray, M., et al. (2002) Post-operative recovery and long term follow-up in 21 dogs undergoing dorsal laminectomy for caudal cervical spondylomyelopathy. *Veterinary Surgery* 31, 418-427.

Forterre, F., Spreng, D., Rytz, U., et al. (2007) Thoracolumbar dorsolateral laminectomy with osteotomy of the spinous process in 14 dogs. *Veterinary Surgery* 36, 458-463.

Hankin, EJ, Jerram, RM, Walker, AM, et al. (2012) Transarticular facet screw stabilization and dorsal laminectomy in 26 dogs with degenerative lumbosacral stenosis with instability. *Veterinary Surgery* 41 (5), 611-619.

Linn, L.L., Bartels, K.E., Rochat, M.C., et al. (2003) Lumbosacral stenosis in 29 military working dogs: epidemiologic findings and outcome after surgical intervention (1990-1999). *Veterinary Surgery* 32, 21-29.

Matiasek, L.A., Platt, S.R., Dennis, R., et al. (2006) Subfascial seroma causing compressive myelopathy after cervical dorsal laminectomy. *Veterinary Radiology & Ultrasound* 47 (6), 581-584.

McKee, W.M. (1992) A comparison of hemilaminectomy and dorsal laminectomy for the treatment of thoracolumbar disc protrusion in dogs. *Veterinary Record* 130, 296-300.

Meij, B.P., Suwankong, N., Van der veen, A.J., et al. (2007) Biomechanical flexion-extension forces in normal canine lumbosacral cadaver specimens before and after dorsal laminectomy-discectomy and pedicle screw-rod fixation. *Veterinary Surgery* 36, 742-751.

Rossmeisl J.H. Jr, Lanz O.I., Inzana K.D., Bergman R.L. (2005) A modified lateral approach to the canine cervical spine: procedural description and clinical application in 16 dogs with lateralized compressive myelopathy or radiculopathy. *Veterinary Surgery* 34, 436-44.

Smith, G.K., Walter, M.C. (1988) Spinal decompressive procedures and dorsal compartment injuries: comparative biomechanical study in canine cadavers. *American Journal of Veterinary Research* 49, 266-273.

Trotter, EJ. (2009) Cervical spine locking plate fixation for treatment of cervical spondylotic myelopathy in large breed dogs. *Veterinary Surgery* 38 (6), 705-718.

86 Hemilaminectomy

Wanda Gordon-Evans
Wisconsin Veterinary Referral Center, Waukesha, WI, USA

Hemilaminectomy is designed to relieve compression of the spinal cord and is most commonly indicated in the treatment of intervertebral disk extrusion, protrusion, and masses that develop extradurally and ventrally in the thoracolumbar spine. The surgical procedure is largely successful at restoring ambulation in dogs with conscious pain perception. Surgical complications are rare with appropriate technique and care during surgery. Many of the spinal surgeries share identical types of complications.

Seroma

See Chapter 85.

Iatrogenic spinal injury

See Chapter 85.

Laminectomy membrane

See Chapter 85.

Hematoma formation

Definition

This is a blood clot that forms because of hemorrhage. The clinical significance of this complication depends on the size of the hematoma and resulting compression on the spinal cord.

Risk factors

Most hematomas associated with hemilaminectomies result from a disruption of the longitudinal vertebral venous sinuses. These sinuses extend in a craniocaudal direction along the ventral floor of the vertebral canal (Figure 86.1). The trajectory deviates laterally over each intervertebral space. Risk factors for this complication include:
- Excessive ventral extension of the hemilaminectomy, usually combined with excision of the accessory process in the lumbar region (Figure 86.2)
- Presence of adhesions between extruded intervertebral disk material and structures ventral to the spinal cord
- Curettage of hypertrophied dorsal vertebral ligament in Hansen type II disk disease
- Poor visualization of the surgical site

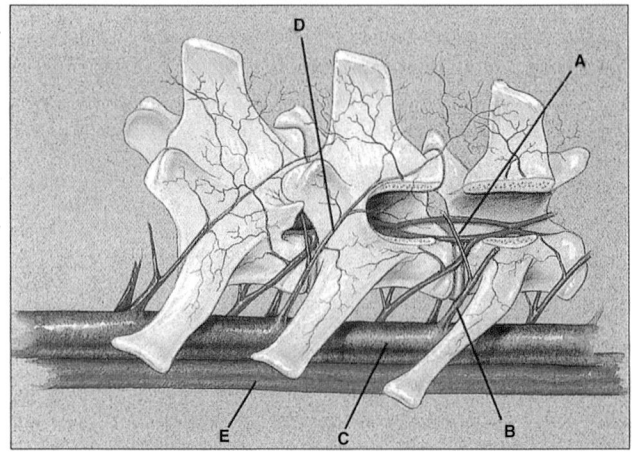

Figure 86.1 The lumbar spine is supplied by spinal branches (**A**) of the lumbar arteries (**B**), which arise from the aorta (**C**). Each lumbar artery also gives rise to a nutrient vessel that enters the vertebral body. A dorsal branch runs caudally behind the articular process of the musculature (**D**). The lumbar internal vertebral venous plexus drains into major veins of the abdomen (**E**), mainly the azygous vein and the caudal vena cava. Note the location of vertebral venous sinuses. *Source:* Sharp and Wheelan, 2005. Reproduced with permission from Elsevier.

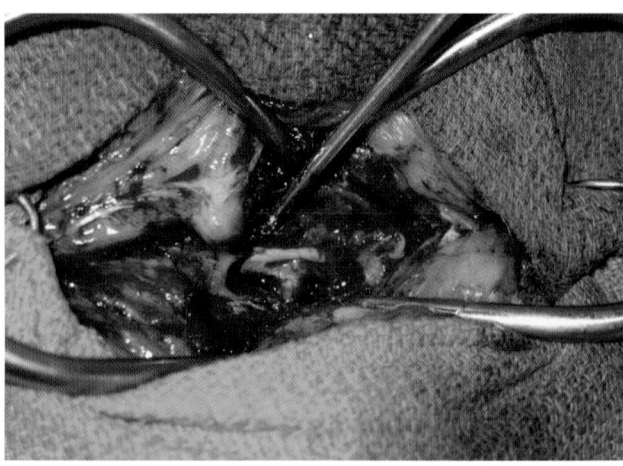

Figure 86.2 Intraoperative view of a hemilaminectomy on the left side of lumbar vertebrae 6 and 7. Note the position of the nerve root, surrounded by disk material. *Source:* D. Griffon, Western University of Health Sciences, Pomona, CA, 2014. Reproduced with permission from D. Griffon.

Complications in Small Animal Surgery, First Edition. Edited by Dominique Griffon and Annick Hamaide.
© 2016 John Wiley & Sons, Inc. Published 2016 by John Wiley & Sons, Inc.
Companion website: www.wiley.com/go/griffon/complications

Table 86.1 Differential diagnosis for declining neurologic status

Short term	Incorrect space addressed
	Residual disk present
	New or more disk extruded
	Hematoma
	Myelomalacia
	Concurrent fibrocartilaginous embolus
	Progression of spinal disease
	Instability
	Iatrogenic injury
Long term	Laminectomy membrane
	Fat pad compression
	Recurrence or new neurologic problem

Diagnosis

Hematoma formation is a differential for worsening of neurologic signs in the immediate postoperative phase. Other differentials for acute postoperative deterioration of neurologic signs are listed in Table 86.1. Evidence of extradural compression can be detected on myelogram or computed tomography (CT) myelography, but magnetic resonance imaging (MRI) can distinguish hematoma from other causes.

Treatment

Unless the patient has lost deep pain after surgery, patients with postoperative worsening of neurologic signs are initially managed medically (Table 86.2). Advanced imaging is indicated if deep pain is no longer present postoperatively or if the neurologic status fails to improve with medical management. If a compressive lesion, such as a hematoma, is identified, exploration of the surgical site is indicated to relieve the compression. Removal of the hematoma should be meticulous and, if possible, the hematoma that is direct contact with the initial source of hemorrhage (usually the ventral venous sinus) should be preserved. If hemorrhage recurs during removal of the hematoma, hemostasis should be achieved before closure. A combination of hemostatic techniques may be required including bipolar cauterization, compression, and hemostatic agent such as gelatin sponges.

Outcome

- Conservative: unknown
- Surgical decompression: good when conscious pain perception is present

Table 86.2 Medical management of the postoperative neurologic patient

Pain management	Multimodal therapy (NSAID or steroid, opioid, gabapentin)
Exercise restriction	No running, jumping, or playing or stairs; short assisted walks on leash
Supportive care	Express or catheterize the bladder if the patient is unable to control urination
	Maintain clean and dry skin to prevent urine and fecal scald
	Rotate every 4 hours if the patient is unable
	Well-padded bedding
Physical therapy	Range of motion, massage, electric stimulation, balancing exercises, hydrotherapy

NSAID, nonsteroidal antiinflammatory drug.

Prevention

The following measures should be considered to avoid rupture of the longitudinal vertebral venous sinuses:
- Limit the extent of the hemilaminectomy ventrally, preserving the accessory process of lumbar vertebrae.
- Maintain good visualization of the surgical site through focused surgical lighting, retraction of tissues with self-retaining retractors (e.g., Weitlaner retractors), thorough hemostasis with bipolar cautery, surgical assistance, and use of magnification.
- Gentle dissection of adhesions surrounding extruded disk material: A moistened Q-tip or nerve root retractor may be used to peel off adhesions from structures ventral to the spinal cord.
- Careful curettage of hypertrophied dorsal vertebral ligament in Hansen type II disk disease: The location of the vertebral sinus deviates laterally along the ventral floor of the vertebral canal at each intervertebral space. Limiting curettage to the median floor of the vertebral canal limits the risk of laceration of the venous sinus.

Recurrence

Definition

This is postoperative extrusion or protrusion of intervertebral disk material, causing clinical signs (Figure 86.3). The extrusion may occur at a previously operated site, although a new site is more commonly involved.

Risk factors

- Presence of multiple calcified disks on preoperative imaging studies (Figure 86.4)
- Administration of steroids
- Conservative management of intervertebral disk disease: 50% recurrence rate (Mann *et al.* 2007)
- Breed predisposition (Dachshunds)

Diagnosis

Clinical signs include pain with or without neurologic dysfunction. The severity of the neurologic dysfunction can be anywhere from very minor proprioceptive deficits to the absence of conscious pain perception. Imaging studies are indicated if signs are significant enough to warrant surgery or if medical management fails to alleviate clinical signs. Whereas myelography or CT myelography will show compression, MRI can distinguish disk from hematoma (Figure 86.5).

Treatment

- Conservative: see Table 86.2
- Surgical decompression

Outcome

- Conservative: depends on the level of dysfunction
- Surgical decompression: good outcome when conscious pain perception is present, although owners are often reluctant to pursue a second surgery

Prevention

- Although highly controversial, fenestration of adjacent disk spaces or those calcified may prevent recurrence.
- Laser disk ablation (Bartels *et al.* 2003)
- Controlled physical activity excluding jumping (although this has not been scientifically evaluated)

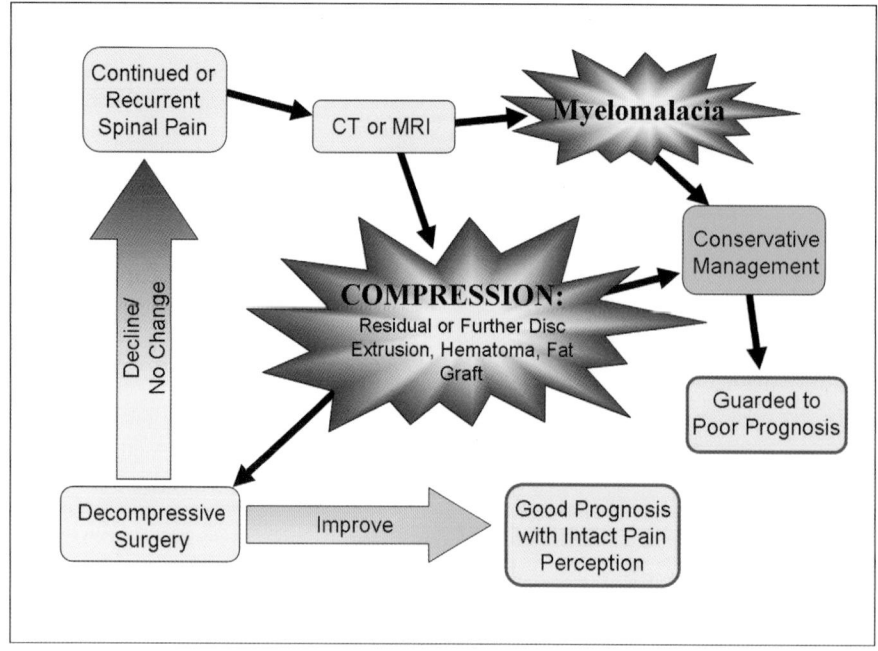

Figure 86.3 Algorithm for static or declining postoperative neurologic status. CT, computed tomography; MRI, magnetic resonance imaging.

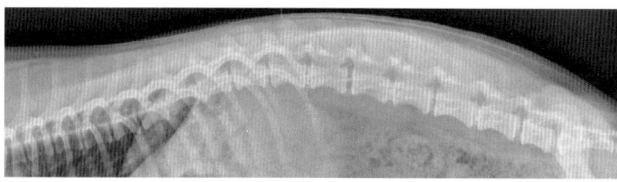

Figure 86.4 Radiographic appearance of calcified intervertebral disks in the thoracolumbar spine.

Further disk extrusion

See the section above on recurrence and Chapter 84.

Decubital ulcers

See Chapter 82.

Urine scalding

See Chapter 82.

Myelomalacia

Definition

Myelomalacia is softening of the spinal cord. The clinical affect is dysfunction or interruption of nerve transmission in the area. It can be focal or quite severe and ascend or descend from the site of injury, eventually causing death.

Risk factor

• Severe spinal cord injury

This complication affects 10% of dogs with absent pain sensation (Scott and McKee 1999; Olby *et al.* 2003).

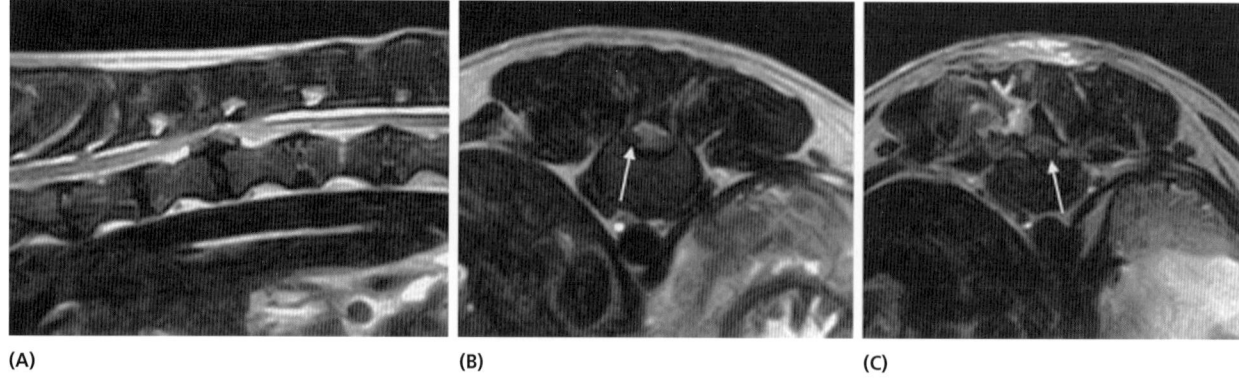

(A) (B) (C)

Figure 86.5 Postoperative magnetic resonance image (MRI) in a dog with abnormal recovery after hemilaminectomy. T2-weighted fast-spin echo sequences, sagittal, and transverse planes. **A** and **B,** Presurgical MRI with hypointense disc material dorsal to the intervertebral disc space T11 to T12, which is located on the right side in the transverse plane (arrow). **C,** Postsurgical MRI after right sided hemilaminectomy; the hypointense material is displaced to the left side in the vertebral canal (arrow). *Source:* Forterre *et al.*, 2010. Reproduced with permission from John Wiley & Sons.

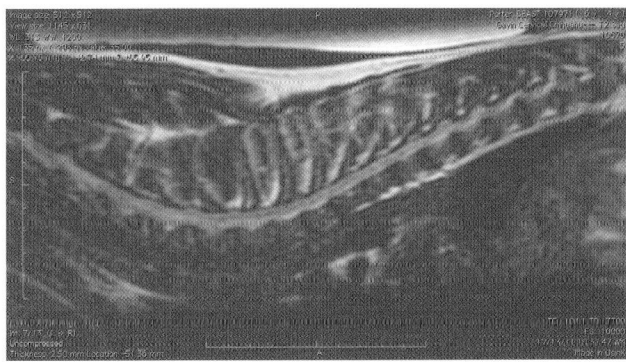

Figure 86.6 Magnetic resonance image of a dog with myelomalacia. T2 sagittal image of the cervicothoracic spine in a dog whose neurologic status declined after a T13 to L1 hemilaminectomy.

Diagnosis

Clinical signs include depression, anorexia, hypotension, and progression to lower motor neuron deficits in all four limbs. Movement of the cutaneous trunci muscle reflex cutoff point cranially is an early indicator of ascending myelomalacia (Muguet-Chanoit *et al.* 2012). MRI is the most accurate method of diagnosing myelomalacia (Figure 86.6) followed by CT and then myelography.

Treatment

There is no treatment for myelomalacia. Humane euthanasia should be considered if the condition is ascending and descending from the site of injury.

Outcome

The prognosis is poor for recovery, and most dogs progress to death.

Prevention

No methods are available for prevention.

Relevant literature

Many of the potential complications such as decubital ulcers and urine scald are likely a result of spinal trauma rather than a specific complication of the surgery. However, **surgical exacerbation of neurologic status and absence of postoperative improvement** are arguably the most significant complications associated with hemilaminectomy, resulting from iatrogenic trauma, myelomalacia, hematoma formation, or residual disk compression and (Griffiths 1972; Levine and Caywood 1984; Dhupa *et al.* 1999; Forterre *et al.* 2010). In a large retrospective study, 5.8% of dogs treated via hemilaminectomy failed to improve after surgery (Forterre *et al.* 2010). Of those, one dog was diagnosed with a hematoma, two with myelomalacia, and seven with residual or new disk extrusion (Forterre *et al.* 2010). Dogs diagnosed with compressive lesions responded favorably to a second decompressive surgery (Forterre *et al.* 2010).

Formation of a **laminectomy membrane** has been speculated as a cause of recurrent clinical signs but has not been confirmed after hemilaminectomies. Nonetheless, free fat grafts are routinely placed over hemilaminectomy sites to theoretically prevent formation of a laminectomy membrane or other adhesions to the dura. In an experimental study, fat grafts placed at hemilaminectomy sites prevented adhesions without causing any morbidity (Shimizu *et al.* 2009). The authors also claimed that the degree of postoperative compression of the spinal cord was not influenced by the size of grafts tested in the study (Shimizu *et al.* 2009).

Recurrence of pain or compression at the surgical site or adjacent site has been reported in 19.2% of dogs treated via hemilaminectomy with 4% to 10% of those patients undergoing a second surgery (Mayhew *et al.* 2004). Dachshunds and dogs with preoperative evidence of mineralization of intervertebral disks seemed predisposed to recurrence (Mayhew *et al.* 2004). Fenestration may be of use to prevent recurrence in high-risk dogs (Brisson *et al.* 2004; Forterre *et al.* 2008). Please see Chapter 86 for a more detailed discussion. Laser disk ablation has been shown in a retrospective clinical study to decrease the incidence of recurrence to 3.4% with less morbidity than fenestration.

Instability of the spine has also been hypothesized to reach clinical relevance after hemilaminectomy over multiple adjacent vertebrae. One author suggested that hemilaminectomies could be performed in up to five consecutive vertebrae without inducing clinical evidence of instability (Jerram and Dewey 1999). In a biomechanical evaluation of cadaver spines with three consecutive hemilaminectomies, the stiffness of specimens decreased within the neutral zone without concurrent increase in range of motion (Corse *et al.* in 2003). However, fenestration in addition to the hemilaminectomy may destabilize the spine to some degree (Jerram *et al.* 1999).

References

Corse, M.R., Renberg, W.C., Friis, E.A. (2003) In vitro evaluation of biomechanical effects of multiple hemilaminectomies on the canine lumbar vertebral column. *American Journal of Veterinary Research* 64, 1139-1145.

Bartels, K.E., Higbee, R.G., Bahr, R.J. (2003) Outcome of and complications associated with prophylactic percutaneous laser disk ablation in dogs with thoracolumbar disk disease: 277 cases (1992-2001). *Journal of the American Veterinary Medical Association* 222, 1733-1739.

Brisson, B.A., Moffatt, S.L., Swayne, S.L., et al. (2004) Recurrence of thoracolumbar intervertebral disk extrusion in chondrodystrophic dogs after surgical decompression with or without prophylactic fenestration: 265 cases (1995-1999). *Journal of the American Veterinary Medical Association* 224, 1808-1814.

Dhupa, S., Glickman, N., Waters, D.J. (1999) Reoperative neurosurgery in dogs with thoracolumbar disk disease. *Veterinary Surgery* 28, 421-428.

Forterre, F., Konar, M., Spreng, D., et al. (2008) Influence of intervertebral disk fenestration at the herniation site in association with hemilaminectomy on recurrence in chondrodystrophic dogs with thoracolumbar disc disease: a prospective MRI study. *Veterinary Surgery* 37, 399-405.

Forterre, F., Gorgas, D., Dickomeit, M., et al. (2010) Incidence of spinal compressive lesions in chondrodystrophic dogs with abnormal recovery after hemilaminectomy for treatment of thoracolumbar disc disease: a prospective magnetic resonance imaging study. *Veterinary Surgery* 39, 165-172.

Griffiths, I.R. (1972) The extensive myelopathy of intervertebral disc protrusions in dogs ("the ascending syndrome"). *Journal of Small Animal Practice* 13, 425-438.

Jerram, R.M., Dewey, C.W. (1999) Acute thoracolumbar disk extrusion in dogs— Part II. *Compendium* 21, 1037-1045.

Levine, S.H., Caywood, D.D. (1984) Recurrence of neurological deficits in dogs treated for thoracolumbar disk disease. *Journal of the American Animal Hospital Association* 20, 869-894.

Mann, F.A., Wagner-Mann, C.C., Dunphy, E.D., et al. (2007) Recurrence rate of presumed thoracolumbar intervertebral disc disease in ambulatory dogs with spinal hyperpathia treated with anti-inflammatory drugs: 78 cases (1997-2000). *Journal of Veterinary Emergency and Critical Care* 17, 53-60.

Mayhew, P.D., McLear, R.C., Ziemer, L.S., et al. (2004) Risk factors for recurrence of clinical signs associated with thoracolumbar intervertebral disk herniation in dogs: 229 cases (1994-2000). *Journal of the American Veterinary Medical Association* 225, 1231-1236.

Muguet-Chanoit, A.C., Olby, N.J., Lim, J.H., et al. (2012) The cutaneous trunci muscle reflex: a predictor of recovery in dogs with acute thoracolumbar myelopathies caused by intervertebral disc extrusions. *Veterinary Surgery* 41, 200-206.

Olby, N., Levine, J., Harris, T., et al. (2003) Long-term functional outcome of dogs with severe injuries of the thoracolumbar spinal cord: 87 cases (1996-2001). *Journal of the American Veterinary Medical Association* 222 (6), 762-769.

Scott, H.K., McKee, W.N. (1999) Laminectomy for 34 dogs with thoracolumbar intervertebral disk disease and loss of deep pain perception. *Journal of Small Animal Practice* 40, 417-422.

Shimizu, J., Koga, M., Kishimoto, M., et al. (2009) Effect of an autogenous free fat graft on hemilaminectomy defects in dogs. *The Journal of Veterinary Medical Science* 71, 1291-1294.

87 Ventral Cervical Fusion

Wanda Gordon-Evans
Wisconsin Veterinary Referral Center, Waukesha, WI, USA

Indications for ventral cervical fusion include cervical spondylomyelopathy, spinal fracture or luxation, and atlantoaxial (AA) subluxation or instability. Ventral cervical fusion is most often performed with pins or screws with polymethylmethacrylate (PMMA). Plate fixation may be an alternative option, including the more recent use of locking plates and unicortical screws. In general, complications after ventral cervical fusion result most commonly from the underlying disease, the surgical approach, iatrogenic spinal injury, or implant failure. Implant failure is the most common and most researched complication of ventral cervical fusion. The clinical significance of implant failure may range from incidental findings to catastrophic failure. Other general complications are common to spinal surgical procedures such as ventral decompression, dorsal laminectomy, and hemilaminectomy. These procedures share similar complications associated with surgical approaches. Ventral decompression is often combined with a ventral vertebral fusion, and conversely, fusion has been advocated by some in candidates for ventral decompression.

Death
See Chapter 84.

Hypotension
See Chapter 84.

Cardiac arrhythmias
See Chapter 84.

Respiratory distress
See Chapter 84.

Iatrogenic spinal injury
See Chapter 84.

Horner's syndrome
See Chapter 23.

Instability or subluxation
See Chapter 85.

Urine scald
See Chapter 82.

Decubital ulcers
See Chapter 82.

Implant failure and migration

Definition
This is failure to maintain rigid fixation or appropriate segment alignment and apposition as a result of implant loosening, bending, breaking, or migration (Figure 87.1).

Risk factors
- Improper size or placement of implants
- Improper bone cement handling
- Incomplete removal of cartilage (AA luxation)

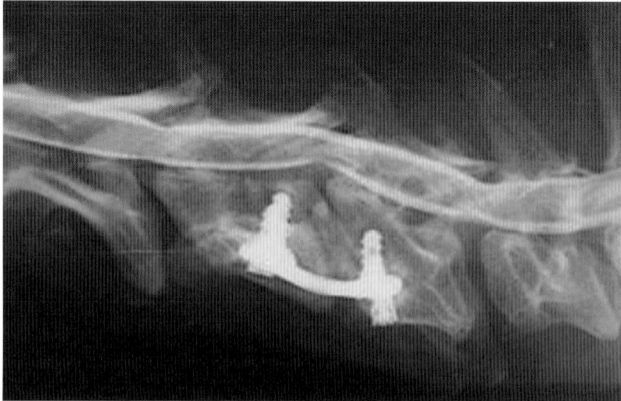

Figure 87.1 Implant failure after ventral cervical fusion (Bergman *et al.* 2008) Lateral myelogram of the cervical spine 591 days after surgery in a 10-year-old male Doberman pinscher. Pseudoarthrosis and severe ventral extradural spinal cord compression are noted at C5 to C6, and mild compression of the spinal cord is evident at C6 to C7.

Complications in Small Animal Surgery, First Edition. Edited by Dominique Griffon and Annick Hamaide.
© 2016 John Wiley & Sons, Inc. Published 2016 by John Wiley & Sons, Inc.
Companion website: www.wiley.com/go/griffon/complications

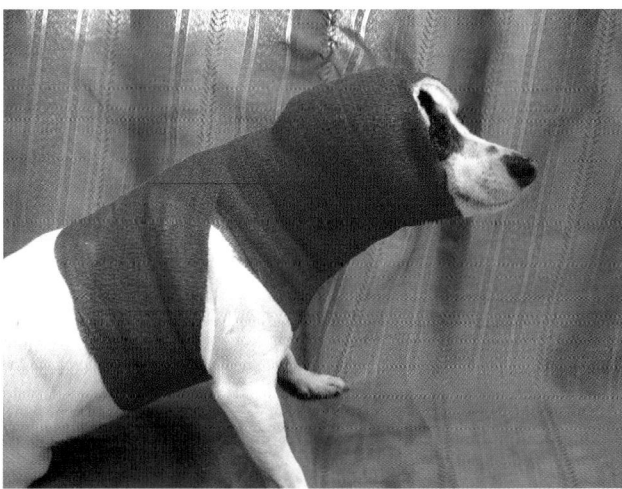

Figure 87.2 External coaptation after ventral cervical fusion.

Diagnosis

Radiographs of the surgical site should be examined for evidence of implant failure (loosening, breakage, migration), decreased diameter of the spinal canal, and loss of apposition of bony structures. Stress radiographs are contraindicated because motion of the surgical site may lead to spinal injury by defective implants or spinal instability.

Treatment

The treatment is based on the severity of clinical signs along with an estimation of the risk for deterioration and disastrous consequences. The severity of clinical signs, location of the implant relative to nervous structures, estimated instability of the spine, and risk for further neurologic damage are first evaluated. The potential benefits from surgery against the risk of inducing further damage must be weighed when deciding between surgical revision or conservative treatment.

- Conservative management is generally indicated when implant failure does not appear to create clinical signs: external coaptation (Figure 87.2), pain medications (see Chapter 4) steroids or nonsteroidal antiinflammatory drugs. Dorsal reduction and further stabilization is considered in cases of implant failure and protracted pain or worsening neurologic status.

- Removal of migrating implants may be safely performed if bony fusion is complete. Removal is indicated if the path of migration is potentially dangerous or causing clinical signs.

Outcome

The outcome of implant failure postventral cervical fusion has not been well reported but appears to vary, depending on the severity of clinical signs.

Prevention

- Careful placement of implants with optimal bone purchase while avoiding important structures
- Pins have been advocated over screws to counteract bending forces.
- Grafting the ventral slot or the articular surface of the AA joint may accelerate bone healing, thereby decreasing the risk of fatigue failure of the implants.
- Postoperative external coaptation (see Figure 87.2)
- Owner compliance with exercise restriction and bandage care

Continued degeneration or recurrence of clinical signs

Definition

Declining neurologic status postoperatively either after temporary postoperative clinical improvement or immediately after surgical intervention.

Risk factors

- Caudal cervical spondylomyelopathy
- Concurrent decompressive procedures such as ventral slot or dorsal laminectomy
- Implant failure or subluxation
- Domino effect: The relatively high stiffness of the operated vertebrae increase the stress placed on adjacent intervertebral spaces, thereby predisposing them to degeneration and herniation.
- Bicortical screws or pins carry a risk of inadvertent penetration into the spinal canal during placement (Figure 87.3), as well as postoperative loosening and migration into the spinal canal.

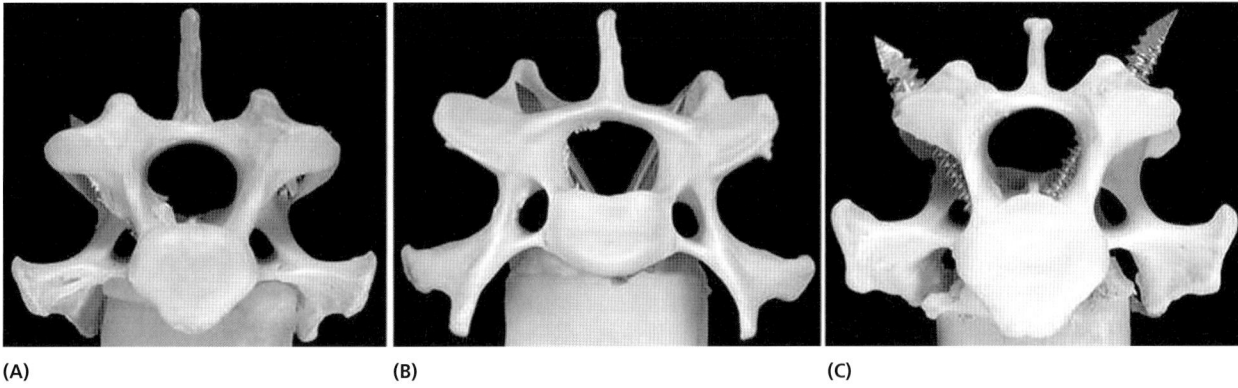

(A)   (B)   (C)

Figure 87.3 Iatrogenic damage associated with pin placement (Kochler et al. 2005) Photographs illustrating the pin positions observed in cadaveric specimens of cervical vertebral columns of 14 dogs after a ventral slot procedure and pin–polymethylmethacrylate fixation with smooth or positive profile threaded (PPT) pins. **A,** Optimal pin positioning. **B,** Protrusion of smooth pins into the vertebral foramen. **C,** Protrusions of PPT pins into the transverse and spinal foramina.

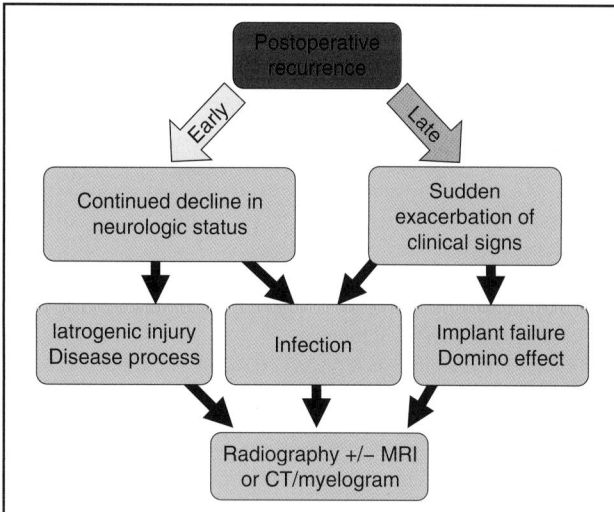

Figure 87.4 Differential diagnoses for recurrence of clinical signs after ventral cervical fusion. CT, computed tomography; MRI, magnetic resonance imaging.

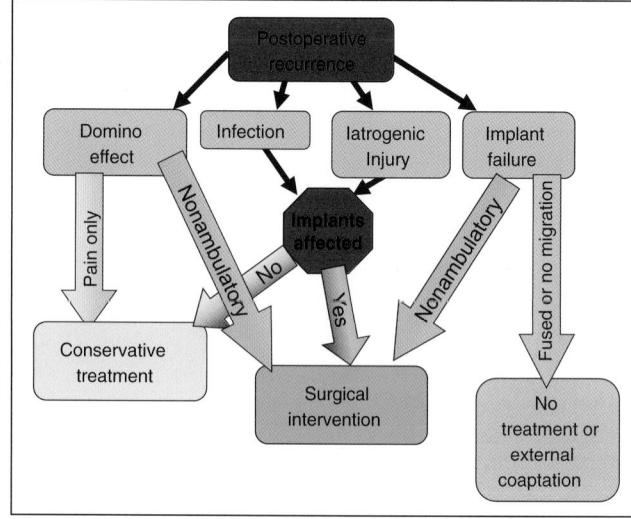

Figure 87.5 Algorithm for treatment of recurrence or progression of neurologic signs after ventral cervical fusion.

Diagnosis

The goal of the diagnostic approach in patients with postoperative worsening or recurrence of clinical signs is to identify the cause of the complication (Figure 87.4) and evaluate the potential for improvement with revision surgery.

Unfortunately, magnetic resonance imaging cannot be used unless the implants have been removed because of artifact creation. In most instance, computed tomography or myelography is necessary (Table 87.1).

Treatment

The decision-making process to manage dogs with recurrence or continued deterioration of signs is largely influenced by the severity of signs, the ability to identify an underlying cause, and the likelihood of surgery to address the cause (Figure 87.5).

- Conservative management with pain management and exercise restriction is generally selected as the first line of action in dogs whose signs are limited to pain and when no evidence of implant failure can be detected.
- Surgical intervention depending on cause and owner's willingness to pursue additional surgery (see Table 87.1)

Outcome

Most dogs improve postoperatively over time even when extensive supportive care is necessary (e.g., ventilatory support)

Prevention

- Fenestration of adjacent discs may help decrease the possibility of a domino effect.
- Preoperative administration of methyl prednisolone sodium succinate (30 mg/kg intravenously) may help to decrease perioperative iatrogenic damage.
- Locking plates require unicortical screws, thereby decreasing the risk of iatrogenic nerve trauma.

Relevant literature

The literature for ventral cervical stabilization focuses essentially on the treatment of cervical spondylomyelopathy or AA subluxation. In general, the purpose of stabilizing the segments is to promote fusion. Complication rates have been reported to range anywhere from 26% to 53% when all techniques proposed for the treatment of AA luxation are combined (Thomas et al. 1991; Schulz et al. 1996; Sanders et al. 2004). The two most common complications are implant failure or migration and recurrence or deterioration of signs. Most preventive strategies are designed to prevent implant-related complications by limiting the risk of iatrogenic damage, improving the stability of implants, and accelerating bone healing.

Fixation via ventral pins, screws, and PMMA is associated with complications in 26% to 42% of operated dogs (Platt et al. 2004; Sanders et al. 2004). Those consist mainly of **implant failure or migration**, which is responsible for 18% to 25% of the complications. In other studies, 20% to 40% percent of pins were reported to migrate without PMMA (Thomas et al. 1991; Beaver et al. 2001). In general, the risk of pin migration is reduced when PMMA is used to stabilize the vertebra across the disk space. Placement of a bone graft between the cervical vertebrae has been recommended to accelerate healing and therefore decrease the risk of fatigue failure of implants. Although fixation methods have not been directly compared, autografting has been reported to promote cervical fusion in dogs treated with locking plate fixation (Steffen et al. 2011). Although screw loosening was reported in 40% of cases, all progressed to fusion

Table 87.1 Diagnostic approach to persistence or recurrence of clinical signs

Etiology	Diagnostic test	Treatment
Implant failure	Radiography	See implant failure section
Adjacent disk degeneration or compression	CT myelography* +/- stress views	Surgical decompression
Progression of primary disease	CT myelography* +/- stress views	Surgical decompression +/- stabilization of new lesion if it is compressive or dynamically compressive

*MRI may be chosen if implants have been removed.

without further surgery except for a case of pseudoarthrosis (Steffen *et al.* 2011).

Declining neurologic status or peripheral nerve injury accounts for up to 80% of the remaining complications (Schulz *et al.* 1996; Sanders *et al.* 2004). The two main differentials for this complication include iatrogenic trauma, progression of the preoperative myelopathy, and the domino effect. Placement of pins can cause iatrogenic trauma. In a study of canine cadavers, 41% of pins penetrated in the spinal canal or foramina, but clinical significance of this finding could not be ascertained because of the nature of the study (Agnello *et al.* 2010). Ventral plate fixation with a locking plate is biomechanically similar to pins and PMMA and screws do not require bicortical purchase, which is arguably safer than pins and PMMA (Koehler *et al.* 2005; Agnello *et al.* 2010). In one study, clinical signs resulting from peripheral nerve injury, including Horner's syndrome and laryngeal paralysis, accounted for 40% of the complications (Sanders *et al.* 2004). In another study, fatal aspiration pneumonia was listed as a complication; however, the reason for aspiration was attributed to iatrogenic laryngeal paralysis (Platt *et al.* 2004). This scenario is less likely with ventral cervical fusion for cervical spondylomyelopathy because in these cases, the approach is typically more caudal, thus making it easier to avoid the recurrent laryngeal nerve.

Recurrent pain or neurologic dysfunction is often attributed to the domino effect or degeneration of adjacent intervertebral disks. This complication is reported in 2.5% to 22% of dogs undergoing cervical fusion (Trotter 2009; Steffen *et al.* 2011). Fusion of one intervertebral disk space may increase the stress placed on adjacent disk spaces even under physiologic loading (Lemarie *et al.* 2000; Koehler *et al.* 2005; Adamo *et al.* 2007).

References

Adamo, P.O., Kobayashi, H., Markel, M., et al. (2007) In vitro biomechanical comparison of cervical disk arthroplasty, ventral slot procedure, and smooth pins with polymethylmethacrylate fixation at treated and adjacent canine cervical motion units. *Veterinary Surgery* 36, 729-741.

Agnello, K.A., Kapatkin, A.S., Garcia, T.C., et al. (2010) Intervertebral biomechanics of locking compression plate monocortical fixation of the canine cervical spine. *Veterinary Surgery* 39 (8), 991-1000.

Beaver, D.P., Ellison, G.W., Lewis, D.D., et al. (2000) Risk factors affecting the outcome of surgery for atlantoaxial subluxation in dogs: 46 cases (1978-1998). *Journal of the American Veterinary Medical Association* 216, 1104-1109.

Bergman, R.L., Levine, J.M., Coates, J.R., et al. (2008) Cervical spinal locking plate in combination with cortical ring allograft for a one level fusion in dogs with cervical spondylotic myelopathy. *Veterinary Surgery* 37 (6), 530-536.

Koehler, C.L., Stover, S.M., LeCouteur, R.A., et al. (2005) Effect of a ventral slot procedure and of smooth or positive-profile threaded pins with polymethylmethacrylate fixation on intervertebral biomechanics at treated and adjacent canine cervical vertebral motion units. *American Journal of Veterinary Research* 66, 678-687.

Lemarie, R.J., Kerwin, S.C., Partington, B.P., et al. (2000) Vertebral subluxation following ventral cervical decompression in the dog. *Journal of the American Animal Hospital Association* 36, 348-358.

Platt, S.R., Chambers, J.N., Cross, A. (2004) A modified ventral fixation for surgical management of atlantoaxial subluxation in 19 dogs. *Veterinary Surgery* 33, 3493-3454.

Sanders, S.G., Bagley, R.S., Silver, G.M., et al. (2004) Outcomes and complications associated with ventral screws, pins, and polymethyl methacrylate for atlantoaxial instability in 12 dogs. *Journal of the American Animal Hospital Association* 40, 204-210.

Schulz, K.S., Waldron, D.R., Grant, J.W., et al. (1996) Biomechanics of the thoracolumbar vertebral column of dogs during lateral bending. *American Journal of Veterinary Research* 57 (8), 1228-1232.

Steffen, F., Voss, K., Morgan, J.P. (2011) Distraction–fusion for caudal cervical spondylomyelopathy using an intervertebral cage and locking plates in 14 dogs. *Veterinary Surgery* 40 (6), 743-752.

Thomas, T.B., Sorjonen, D.C., Simpson, S.T. (1991) Surgical management of atlantoaxial subluxation in 23 dogs. *Veterinary Surgery* 20, 409-412.

Trotter, E.J. (2009) Cervical spine locking plate fixation for treatment of cervical spondylotic myelopathy in large breed dogs. *Veterinary Surgery* 38 (6), 705-718.

88 Vertebral Fracture Repair

Wanda Gordon-Evans
Wisconsin Veterinary Referral Center, Waukesha, WI, USA

Urine scald

See Chapter 82.

Decubital ulcers

See Chapter 82.

Nonunion

See Chapter 99.

Malunion

See Chapter 100.

Delayed union

See Chapter 98.

Iatrogenic spinal injury

See Chapter 85.

Spinous process fracture

Definition

This is a fracture of a dorsal or transverse spinous process. Fractures of dorsal spinous processes are most commonly associated with spinal plating or spinal stapling. Fractures of transverse processes are rare complications of spinal stapling.

Risk factors

This complication generally results from fixation of implants to spinous processes:

- Spinal process plating: Plates are applied on each side of spinal processes, extending over two or three vertebrae cranial and caudal to the injured vertebra.
- Metal plates: Fixation to the spinal processes is achieved via bolts placed through predrilled holes. Hole diameter and overtightening of the bolts predispose the spinous processes to fracture

- Plastic plates: The friction grip surface of the plates is positioned against the right and left aspects of each spinous process. Bolts placed between the spinous processes maintain stability. Residual instability, motion of the plates, and bone erosion in contact with bolts predispose the spinous processes to fracture
- Spinal stapling: One or several stainless steel pins are fixed to the spinous processes via wiring in small dogs (weighing <10 kg). Hole and wire diameter, as well as body weight may predispose spinous processes to fractures

With all techniques, excessive postoperative exercise and motion will increase the stress placed on spinous processes.

Diagnosis

The goal of the diagnostic approach is to confirm the presence of a fracture and evaluate its clinical relevance.

- History may be insidious because this complication may not affect the neurologic status of the patient.
- Swelling, pain, and crepitus may be noted on palpation of the surgical site.
- Radiography: Orthogonal projections of the surgery site allow definitive diagnosis. Fractures are usually simple but may affect several contiguous spinous processes. Radiographs should be thoroughly reviewed for evidence of migration or instability of the repair.

Treatment

- Conservative treatment with enforced exercise restriction and analgesia is usually recommended if the neurologic status is unchanged.
- Surgical revision with vertebral body stabilization is indicated in cases with a change in neurologic status and should be considered in dogs with fractures of multiple spinous processes and questionable spinal stability.

Outcome

The prognosis is generally good in dogs with unchanged neurologic status. A prognosis has not been established in cases with fractures severe enough to compromise the entire fixation and affect neurologic function. In these cases, the prognosis depends on the severity of the recurrent spinal cord injury and the owners' willingness to continue care.

Prevention

Plates should be placed as close to the base of the spinous processes as possible. Overall, spinal process plating and spinal stapling have become historical means of fixation and have been replaced by bio mechanically superior techniques.

Implant failure or migration

Definition

This is loss of implant fixation. This complication varies in nature and clinical relevance with the type of fixation chosen (Table 88.1).

Risk factors

- Improper size or number of implants (eight pins recommended for pins and polymethylmethacrylate [PMMA] constructs)
- Screws may be more prone to breakage than pins, but pins may be more prone to migration.
- Negative end-threaded pins are predisposed to breakage compared with positive threaded pins.
- Instability of the fracture
- Diameter of PMMA

Diagnosis

- Physical examination: Suspect implant failure with sudden decline in neurologic status.
- Radiography: displacement or migration of implants along with loss of reduction (Figure 88.1)

Treatment

- Conservative if no change in neurologic status
- Change in neurologic status: Consider alternative stabilization (see Figure 88.1).
- Migrating implants should be removed when causing clinical signs, typically after healing is complete.

Outcome

- The prognosis is good if implant failure occurs as an incidental finding without exacerbation of clinical signs.
- The prognosis is guarded to good after removal of migrating implants or surgical revision of an unstable implant depending on the severity of neurologic decline and the owner's willingness to continue management.

Prevention

- Optimal implant placement: Pins should angle away from the fracture in an eight-pin construct with PMMA and toward the fracture in a four-pin and PMMA construct. Vertebral body plates should span two adjacent vertebral bodies unless a mid-body fracture requires spanning three spaces (see Figure 88.1).
- Choosing appropriate technique for animal size (e.g., spinal stapling is not recommended for dogs weighing >10 kg or if modified with tension bands >20 kg)

Table 88.1 Type of fixation based on fracture location

Location	Method of fixation
AA	Dorsal wires or ventral pins or screws and PMMA
Cervical	Ventral with pins or screws and PMMA or locking plate
Thoracolumbar	Dorsal pins or screws and PMMA, locking plate, dorsal spinal stapling (<10 kg), external fixator
Lumbosacral	Dorsal pins or screws and PMMA, external fixator

AA, atlantoaxial; PMMA, polymethylmethacrylate.

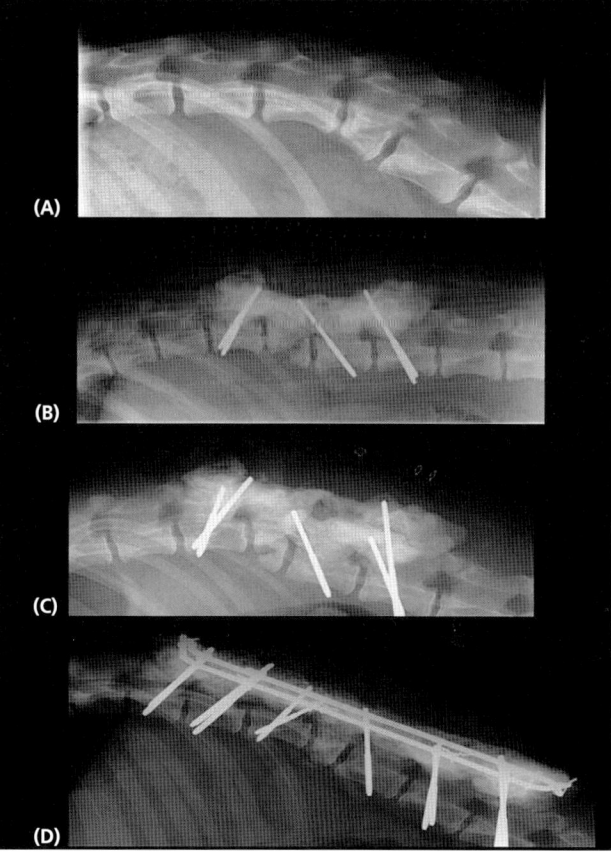

Figure 88.1 Implant failure after repair of a compression fracture of the second lumbar vertebra in a 7-month-old boxer. **A,** Preoperative lateral radiograph of the thoracolumbar spine. The second lumbar vertebra is displaced dorsally, compressing the spinal cord. **B,** Radiograph obtained immediately after dorsal spinal decompression (the cranial lamina of L3 and the caudal lamina of L2 were removed), and placement of 3/32 inch positive profile pins on both sides of L1 and L4 and on the right side of L3. Pins were embedded in polymethylmethacrylate (PMMA). A fracture was found at the base of the left transverse process of L3. **C,** Radiograph obtained 2 weeks after surgery. Loss of reduction consistent with a fracture of the cement. Crepitus and pain were noted on physical examination of the surgical site. **D,** Radiograph obtained 1 month after revision of the surgical repair of the lumbar fracture. Pins were added in the vertebrae adjacent to the previous repair and connected to Steinman pins embedded in PMMA on each side of the spine. The patient's neurologic status is improved, and the fracture is healing. *Source:* D. Griffon, Western University of Health Sciences, Pomona, CA, 2014. Reproduced with permission from D. Griffon.

Seroma

See Chapter 85.

Hemorrhage

See also Chapters 12, 84 and 86.

Definition

Bleeding may occur secondary to the original trauma. Although uncommon, iatrogenic damage to the aorta, vena cava, or vertebral artery may occur during pin placement depending on the location of the fracture.

Risk factors
- Pins or screw and PMMA fixation
- Vertebral body plating
- External fixator fixation

Diagnosis
- Hypovolemic shock
- Decrease in packed cell volume
- Sudden death
- Necropsy

Treatment
Control or stop hemorrhage
- Pressure (bone wax, hemostat, Gelfoam)
- Cautery
- Ligation
Depending on clinical signs
- Fluid boluses
- Blood transfusion

Outcome
The prognosis varies from good depending on the severity of vascular injury.

Prevention
Follow guidelines in terms of landmarks and direction of pins recommended for each level of the spine.
- Fluoroscopic guidance of pin placement
- Use blunted trocar pins (Figure 88.2).

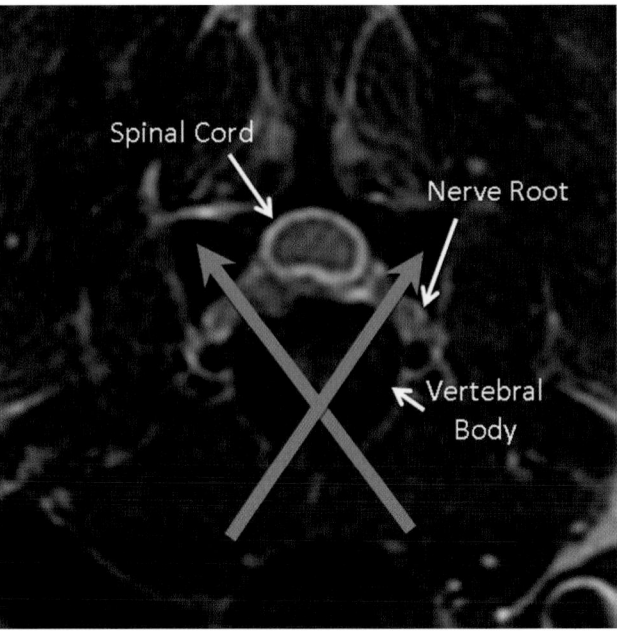

Figure 88.3 Appropriate landmarks relative to the midline and direction of pins placed during ventral cervical fixation. This figure highlights the importance and difficulty of avoiding nerve roots.

- Appropriate pin or screw directionality (Figures 88.1, 88.2, 88.3, 88.4)
- Controlled use of power equipment
- Sharp drill bit or pins decrease the force placed on the bone–pin interface and allow a quicker stop after the far cortex.
- Use of locking plates because they do not require the transcortex for rigid fixation (Table 88.2).

Table 88.2 Angles and landmarks recommended for placement of pins during vertebral fracture repair

Vertebra	Angle in degrees from vertical axis	Starting Landmark
C1	45–60 degrees	Caudal ventral median line
C2–C7	33–45 degrees	Ventral median line
T10	20–25 degrees	Base of accessory process
T11–T12	25–35 degrees	Base of accessory process
T13	40–45 degrees	Base of accessory process
L1–L6	55–65 degrees	Junction of pedicle and transverse process
L7	Parallel to sagittal plane	Base of cranial articular process
S1	5 degrees relative to sagittal plane	Just behind cranial auricular surface

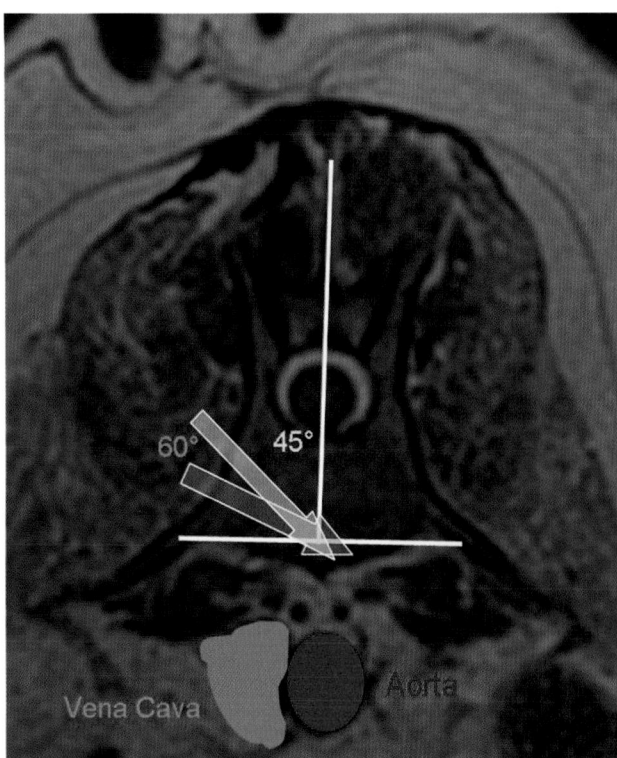

Figure 88.2 Appropriate landmarks relative to the transverse processes and direction of pins placed during dorsal fixation of a lumbar vertebra.

C, cervical vertebrae; L, lumbar vertebrae; S, sacral vertebra; T, thoracic vertebrae.
Source: Data from Watine *et al.*, 2006.

Spinal compression caused by soft tissues

Definition
Postoperative compression of the spinal cord after fracture repair may result from the presence of soft tissues, such as soft callous, hematomas, nucleus pulposus, annulus fibers (from intervertebral disk rupture or hypertrophy), or hypertrophy of the dorsal annular ligament caused by instability. However, these complications are not well described in the literature.

Risk factor
Residual vertebral instability

Diagnosis
Spinal cord compression may be detected on myelogram or computed tomography myelography, but magnetic resonance imaging is more sensitive and can potentially be used to distinguish causes of compression.

Treatment
Decompressive surgery should be considered in cases with deteriorating or unsatisfactory neurologic signs, consistent with the presence of a compressive lesion on advanced imaging.

Outcome
The prognosis depends on the severity of signs, the ability to detect a compressive lesion responsible for the signs, and the ability to treat the underlying cause. The prognosis is fair to good in cases with conscious pain perception, if decompression can be accomplished without destabilization of the spine.

Prevention
Accurate reconstruction of the fracture with rigid fixation may help reduce dorsal annular ligament hypertrophy or soft callous compression.

Relevant literature
Overall implant complications have been reported in 14% of surgically stabilized vertebral fractures (Bruce 2008). These were largely attributed to pin migration in fractures stabilized with pins and PMMA (Bruce 2008). Other methods of stabilization such as Lubra plating are associated with a higher incidence of second surgeries (30% of cases) because of demineralization and an increased likelihood of implant migration or dorsal spinous process fracture (Krauss 2012).

Fixation via pins or screws augmented with PMMA probably remains the most versatile method for surgical management of spinal fractures (Lanz et al. 2000; Weh 2007; Pike et al. 2012). This technique can be used in all sizes of dogs and in most areas of the vertebral column. Most reports of complications associated with this type of vertebral fracture fixation deal with **implant failure** or **migration** (Jeffery 2010). Based on experimental studies of cadaver thoracolumbar specimens, eight-pin constructs are recommended over four pins because of their biomechanical superiority (Garcia et al. 1994). Modifications of the technique include the use of screws or threaded pins to reduce the rate of implant pullout. However, these constructs are generally weaker and predisposed to break at the thread pin interface (Bagley et al. 2000). Migration may be

decreased by notching or bending pins before application of the PMMA (Bagley et al. 2000).

Spinal stapling is recommended for dogs weighing less than 10 kg unless tension bands are added to the construct. If tension bands are added, dogs weighing less than 20 kg may be treated with this technique, resulting in a complication rate of 16% (Voss and Montavon 2004). This adjunct fixation improves the strength of the construct and decreases the risk of **iatrogenic** damage to major vessels or nerves; however, one third of the complications reported were related to pain caused by imprecise placement of the implant (Voss and Montavon 2004). The remainder of the complications was attributed to **implant failure** within the first postoperative week (Voss and Montavon 2004).

Newer methods of spinal fracture stabilization include extraskeletal fixation and vertebral body plating with locking plates. Although the use of external fixators with or without internal fixation has been reported in the past, more recent studies have addressed the strength of these constructs and propensity for complications (Shores et al. 1988; Lewis et al. 1989). External fixation using arches was as strong as the 8 pins and PMMA construct previously advocated (Walker et al. 2002). Wheeler et al. (2002) expanded on the safety of pin placement, describing fewer complications and improved percentage of bone purchase in cadaver specimen, when Steinman pins were placed from T10 to L7 under closed fluoroscopic guidance compared with an open approach. Complications from **iatrogenic** vascular, pulmonary, or nervous trauma occurred in 2.9% of pins in the lumbar area when an open approach was used compared with

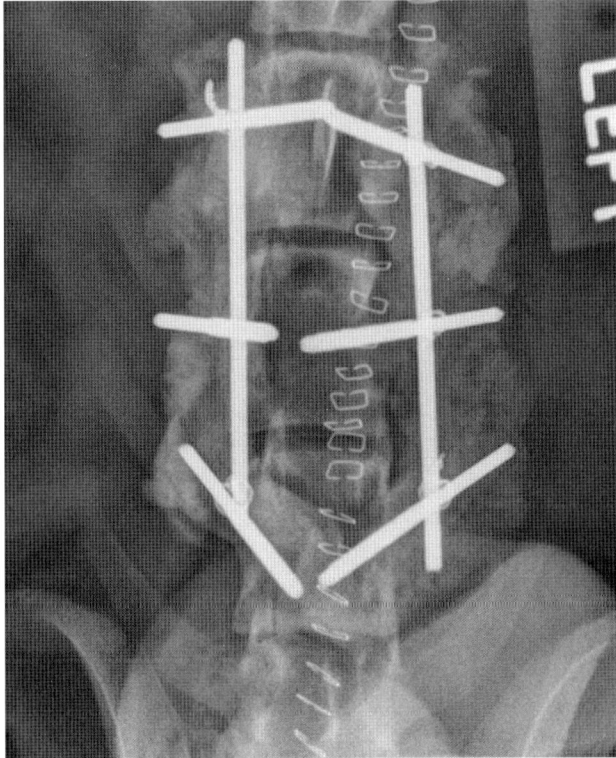

Figure 88.4 Use of blunted trocar pins (INTERFACE NP [No Point], IMEX Veterinary Products, Longview, TX) may prevent iatrogenic damage during placement through the transcortex of vertebrae. *Source:* D. Griffon, Western University of Health Sciences, Pomona, CA, 2014. Reproduced with permission from D. Griffon.

no trauma in the fluoroscopic group (Wheeler *et al.* 2002). In the thoracic area, complications were more dramatic with an incidence of 42% after an open approach versus 10% under fluoroscopic guidance (Wheeler *et al.* 2002). These results were confirmed in vivo, with satisfactory recovery of neurologic function in five dogs with thoracolumbar or lumbar fractures treated by closed fluoroscopic-assisted spinal arch external fixation. Based on their results, the authors concluded that this surgical technique resulted in satisfactory reduction and stabilization of spinal fractures, with few complications (Wheeler *et al.* 2007).

Locking plates have recently been introduced in veterinary medicine and are rapidly gaining popularity. These are particularly appealing for spinal plate fixation because their expected biomechanical advantage and decreased risk of penetration associated with monocortical screws (Jeffery 2010). One biomechanical study in seven cadavers confirmed the feasibility of stabilizing the cervical spine with a locking compression plate over the ventral surface of vertebrae without penetration of the transcortex (Agnello *et al.* 2010). This approach provides an alternative to pins or screws and PMMA fixation for cervical fractures. In the thoracolumbar and lumbar spine, the string-of-pearl plates combine locking technology with versatility in terms of length (cut to length) and contouring (three dimensional). Plates may be placed on each side of the spine, thereby improving the stiffness of the construct. However, further clinical evaluation of locking plates is required to determine the rate and types of complications associated with their application (see Chapter 107).

References

Agnello, K.A., Kapatkin, A.S., Garcia, T.C., et al. (2010) Intervertebral biomechanics of locking compression plate monocortical fixation of the canine cervical spine. *Veterinary Surgery* 39, 991-1000.

Bagley, R.S., Silver, G.M., Connors, R.L., et al. (2000) Exogenous spinal trauma: surgical therapy and aftercare. *Compendium* 22, 218-229.

Bruce, C.W., Brisson, B.A., Gyselinck, K. (2008) Spinal fracture and luxation in dogs and cats. *Veterinary and Comparative Orthopaedics and Traumatology* 21, 280-284.

Garcia, J.N., Milthorpe, B.K., Russell, D., et al. (1994) Biomechanical study of canine spinal fracture fixation using pins or bone screws with polymethylmethacrylate. *Veterinary Surgery* 23(5), 322-329.

Jeffery, N.D. (2010) Vertebral fracture and luxation in small animals. *Veterinary Clinics of North America: Small Animal Practice* 40, 809-828.

Krauss, M.W., Theyse, L.F.H., Tryfonidou, M.A. et al. (2012) Treatment of spinal fractures using Lubra plates. *Veterinary and Comparative Orthopaedics and Traumatology* 25, 326-331.

Lanz, O., Bergman, R., Shell, L. (2000) Managing spinal fractures and luxations in dogs. *Veterinary Medicine* Nov, 868-876.

Lewis, D.D., Stampley, A., Bellah, J.R., et al. (1989) Repair of sixth lumbar vertebral fracture-luxations, using transilial pins and plastic spinous-process plates in six dogs. *Journal of the American Veterinary Medical Association* 194(4), 538-542.

Pike, F.S., Kumar, M.S., Boudrieau, R.J. (2012) Reduction and fixation of cranial cervical fracture/luxations using screws and polymethylmethacrylate (PMMA) cement: a distraction technique applied to the base of the skull in thirteen dogs. *Veterinary Surgery* 41, 235-247.

Shores, A., Nichols, C., Koelling, H.A., et al. (1988) Combined Kirshner-Ehmer apparatus and dorsal spinal plate fixation of caudal lumbar fractures in dogs: biomechanical properties. *American Journal of Veterinary Research* 49, 1979-1982.

Voss, K., Montavon, P.M. (2004) Tension band stabilization of fractures and luxations of the thoracolumbar vertebrae in dogs and cats: 38 cases (1993-2002). *Journal of the American Veterinary Medical Association* 225, 78-83.

Walker, T.M., Welch, W.A.P. (2002) External fixation of the lumbar spine in a canine model. *Veterinary Surgery* 31, 181-188.

Watine, S., Cabassu, J.P., Catheland, S., et al. (2006) Computed tomography study of implantation corridors in canine vertebrae. *Journal of Small Animal Practice* 47, 651-657.

Weh, J.M., Kraus, K.H. (2007) Use of a four pin and methylmethacrylate fixation in L7 and the iliac body to stabilize lumbosacral fracture–luxations: a clinical and anatomic study. *Veterinary Surgery* 36, 8.

Wheeler, J.L., Cross, A.R., Rapoff, A.J. (2002) A comparison of the accuracy and safety of vertebral body pin placement using a fluoroscopically guided versus an open surgical approach: an in vitro study. *Veterinary Surgery* 31, 468-474.

Wheeler, J.L., Lewis, D.D., Cross, A.R., et al. (2007) Closed fluoroscopic-assisted spinal arch external skeletal fixation for the stabilization of vertebral column injuries in five dogs. *Veterinary Surgery* 36, 5.

89 Craniotomy and Craniectomy

Belinda Comito
Veterinary Specialty Center, Buffalo Grove, IL, USA

Surgical approaches to the brain are chosen based on the location of the lesion and the goals of the surgical procedure (Bagley 2003). *Craniotomy* is defined as partial removal of the skull to access the intracranial space with replacement of bone (Bagley 2003). *Craniectomy* is defined as partial removal of the skull to access the intracranial space without replacement of bone (Bagley 2003). The most common indications for intracranial surgery include removal or debulking of brain tumors, tissue biopsy, and depressed skull fractures; stabilizing intracranial pressure (ICP); and placement of ventriculoperitoneal shunts. The surgical approach or combination of approaches depends on the tumor size, location, and degree of invasiveness (Talarico and Dewey 2012). A list of surgical approaches can be found in Table 89.1.

Hemorrhage
See Chapter 2.

Urine Scalding
See Chapter 84.

Seizures
See Chapter 85.

Subcutaneous Emphysema
See Chapter 3.

Pneumonia
See Chapter 3.

Table 89.1 Common surgical approaches to intracranial structures

Approach	Accessible anatomy
Transfrontal	Olfactory bulbs, rostrolateral frontal lobes
Rostrotentorial	Lateral parietal, temporal, occipital lobes
Suboccipital	Caudal cerebellum, caudodorsal brainstem, craniodorsal spinal cord

Source: Data from Sturges and Dickinson (2004).

Iatrogenic peripheral nerve injury

Definition
This is injury to a cranial nerve(s) caused by a surgical procedure. Injury to the cranial nerve(s) may occur as the result of nerve retraction to gain exposure to the tumor (Forterre *et al.* 2009) or on the initial surgical approach (Klopp *et al.* 2000; Bagley 2003). The severity of injury may vary from neuropraxia to neurotmesis (see Chapter 84).

Risk factors
- Surgical approach: Surgical approaches to the ventral brainstem may cause iatrogenic damage to cranial nerves IX, X, XI, and XII (Klopp *et al.* 2000) (Table 89.2).
- Muscle dissection: Careful temporalis muscle dissection allows preservation of the mandibular branch of the trigeminal nerve (Bagley 2003) (Table 89.2).
- Nerve retraction: Reversible facial nerve paralysis has been reported (Forterre *et al.* 2009) (Table 89.2)

Diagnosis
Diagnosing iatrogenic cranial nerve trauma relies on accurate neurologic examinations before and after surgery. The presence of new cranial nerve deficits after surgery should heighten the clinician's suspicion that iatrogenic trauma has occurred. Cranial nerve deficits are dependent on the location of the surgical procedure.

Treatment
No treatment is available.

Outcome
Cranial nerve deficits may resolve, usually within 3 weeks of the injury in case of neuropraxia or persist in case of neurotmesis.

Prevention
- Clinicians should be aware of the anatomy and innervation of the head to avoid iatrogenic damage.
- Preserve nervous structures during muscle dissection.

Complications in Small Animal Surgery, First Edition. Edited by Dominique Griffon and Annick Hamaide.
© 2016 John Wiley & Sons, Inc. Published 2016 by John Wiley & Sons, Inc.
Companion website: www.wiley.com/go/griffon/complications

Table 89.2 Clinical signs associated with iatrogenic injury to peripheral nerves

Cranial nerve	Clinical signs of injury
V (mandibular branch of trigeminal nerve)	Unilateral muscle atrophy Reduced jaw tone, dropped jaw (if bilateral) Possible enophthalmus Protrusion of the third eyelid
VII (facial nerve)	Facial palsy Reduced to absent palpebral reflex Reduced tear production
IX and X (glossopharyngeal, vagal nerves)	Dysphagia Absent gag reflex Reduced pharyngeal tone Inspiratory stridor Voice changes
XI (accessory nerve)	Trapezius muscle atrophy
XII (hypoglossal nerve)	Difficulty prehending Deviation of the tongue to the side of injury

Source: Klopp *et al.*, 2000. Reproduced with permission from John Wiley & Sons.

- Gentle retraction of nerves: A long loop of moist Penrose drain may be placed around nerves and loosely clamped to facilitate retraction and identification of the nerve during surgery.

Iatrogenic brain injury

Definition

This is trauma to the brain tissues as a direct result of the surgical procedure. Increased ICP and brain tissue herniation may occur as the result of edema, ischemia, and hemorrhage from iatrogenic trauma.

Risk factors

- Limited surgical approach
- Manipulation or inadequate retraction of brain parenchyma may lead to hematoma formation
- Inability to distinguish normal cortical tissue from the surgical lesion

Diagnosis

Accurate assessment of the patient's neurologic status before and immediately after surgery is essential. The diagnosis is made presumptively based on progression or change in the patient's neurologic status immediately after surgery. Clinical signs include seizures, mentation changes (obtundation, coma), absent gag reflex, pupillary changes (anisocoria, miosis, mydriasis), reduced oculovestibular reflex, reduced pupillary light reflex, gait abnormalities (ataxia, paresis), absent menace response, and nystagmus. Patients may have a Cushing's response, which is identified clinically as high blood pressure and a low heart rate (Tefend and Dewey 2008). Postoperative magnetic resonance imaging (MRI) may show brain herniation, increased edema in the tissue as a result of tissue manipulation, or hemorrhage.

Treatment

Treatment goals are aimed at reducing ICP. Medical therapy should be instituted immediately in patients with neurologic deterioration. Medications used to reduce ICP are mannitol (0.5–1.0 g/kg intravenously [IV] administered over 15–20 minutes) and dexamethasone SP (0.25 mg/kg IV). The mannitol dosing can be repeated if a patient responds to administration. Postoperative

seizures should be treated with diazepam (0.5 mg/kg IV), and anticonvulsant therapy should be started. Anticonvulsant options include phenobarbital (2–4 mg/kg IV every 12 hours) or levetiracetam (20 mg/kg IV every 8 hours). Caution should be used in using high doses of phenobarbital or loading the medication. Loading or high doses of phenobarbital can make it difficult to distinguish between neurologic deterioration and medication side effects. Care should be taken to elevate the patient's head and avoid compression of the jugular veins. If neurologic signs do not improve, MRI should be repeated. If the MRI shows a compressive lesion, such as a hematoma, decompression is warranted (Sturges and Dickinson 2004).

Outcome

The outcome depends on the patient's response to treatment. If a surgically correctable lesion can be identified on the MRI, a full recovery is possible (Sturges and Dickinson 2004). Patients that are unresponsive to aggressive medical management with severe, progressive neurologic deterioration have a poor prognosis.

Prevention

The surgeon should have a well-thought-out surgical plan and use the surgical approach that allows for best visualization of the lesion; however, the location of the lesion ultimately dictates the amount of exposure. Appropriate exposure allows for adequate visualization of the lesion and lessens the amount of manipulation and retraction of brain tissue. Use of an ultrasonic aspirator has been shown to limit the amount of iatrogenic damage to brain tissue (Figure 89.1).

Increased intracranial pressure

Definition

The skull is a rigid compartment containing brain parenchyma, blood, and cerebrospinal fluid (CSF). The brain parenchyma, blood, and CSF exert pressure within the skull referred to as ICP. The rigidity of the cranial envelope implies that any volume increase of one component must be compensated by shrinking of another component. If the change in volume cannot be fully compensated for, ICP will rise. Normal ICP is between 5 and 12 mm Hg in cats and dogs (Dewey and Fletcher 2008). ICP and mean arterial blood pressure affect cerebral perfusion pressure (CPP). The CPP dictates cerebral blood flow, thereby controlling oxygenation and nutrient availability. ICP may be measured directly with a fiberoptic ICP monitoring device, but expense limits the clinical application. Indirect measurement of ICP relies on monitoring the patient's neurologic status. Clinically, increased ICP can be recognized by altered mentation, Cushing's reflex (bradycardia, systemic hypertension), pupillary size, and reduced pupillary light reflex (Packer *et al.* 2011).

Risk factors

- Overmanipulation of brain tissue results in parenchymal swelling and edema, leading to increased parenchymal volume and subsequent increased ICP.
- Poor hemostasis leading to secondary hematoma formation
- Inappropriate patient positioning: head overflexed; occlusion of the jugular veins
- Anesthetic risks
  - Inappropriate ventilation
  - Inadequate pain control

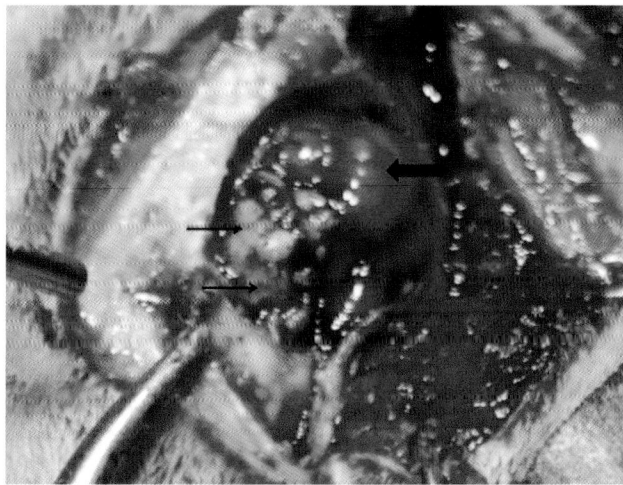

(A)

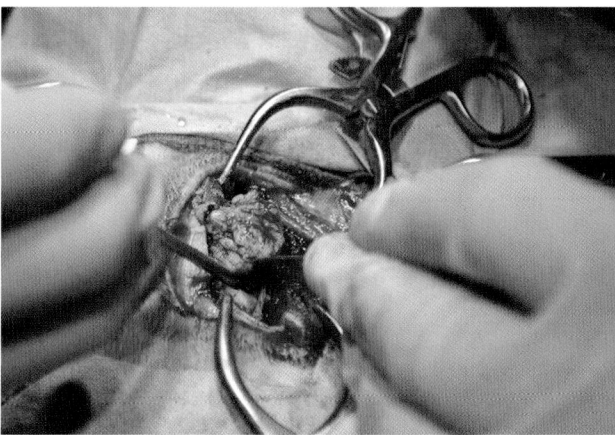

(B)

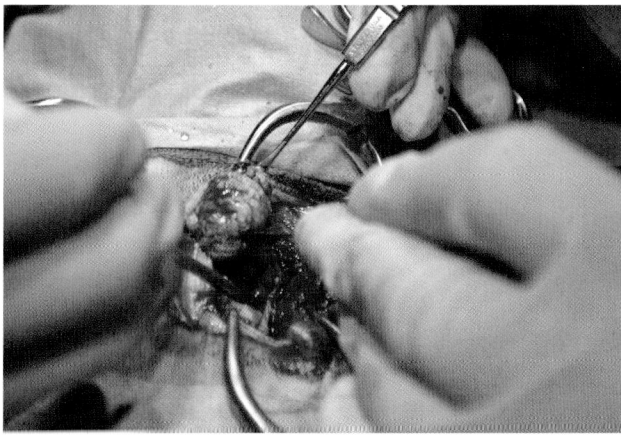

(C)

Figure 89.1 Prevention of iatrogenic trauma during excision of an intracranial meningioma. **A,** Intraoperative appearance of a meningioma. Distinguishing between cortical tissue and lesion is important to avoid iatrogenic brain injury. The cortical tissue (block arrow) is hyperemic secondary to compression from the meningioma. The meningioma (arrows) is well demarcated, fibrous, and firm. Cortical tissue may remain compressed after removal of the mass. **B,** Dissection of the meningioma. A dissection plane is carefully created between the mass and the underlying cortical tissue. **C,** Appearance of the meningioma after dissection.

- ○ Inability to maintain appropriate mean arterial blood pressure
- ○ Poor body temperature regulation: hyperthermia or hypothermia
- ○ Inability to maintain normocapnia and adequate oxygenation

Diagnosis

Increased ICP is most often diagnosed based on clinical signs such as altered mentation or consciousness, bradycardia, systemic hypertension, pupillary size or response to light, or decreased to absent oculocephalic reflexes. Fiberoptic ICP monitoring devices have been used intraoperatively. Intraoperative use has allowed for monitoring ICP trends, allowing the surgeon to determine the effects of surgical manipulation on ICP (Bagley *et al.* 1995).

Treatment

Medical therapy should be instituted immediately in patients with neurologic deterioration. Medications used to reduce ICP include mannitol (0.5–1.0 g/kg IV administered over 15–20 minutes) and dexamethasone SP (0.25 mg/kg IV). The administration of mannitol can be repeated if a patient initially responds to the medication. Postoperative seizures should be treated with diazepam (0.5 mg/kg IV) and should prompt initiation of anticonvulsant therapy. Options for this therapy include phenobarbital (2–4 mg/kg IV every 12 hours) or levetiracetam (20 mg/kg IV every 8 hours). Caution should be used when using high doses of phenobarbital or loading the medication. Loading or high doses of phenobarbital can make it difficult to differentiate neurologic deterioration from side effects of the medication. Care should be taken to elevate the patient's head and avoid compression of the jugular veins.

Prevention

Patients with intracranial disease are at risk for increased ICP. Anesthetic recommendations include:
- Avoid premedications that will induce vomiting.
- Preoxygenate for 5 to 10 minutes.
- Induce anesthesia with propofol.
- Consider constant-rate infusions to limit inhalant agents.
- Administer mannitol (0.5–1 g/kg IV over 10–15 minutes).
- Administer injectable short-acting corticosteroids.
  - ○ Dexamethasone SP (0.25 mg/kg IV).
  - ○ Methylprednisolone sodium succinate (30 mg/kg IV).
- Maintain appropriate ventilation.
- Maintain mean arterial blood pressures (80–100 mm Hg).
- Maintain normocapnia (35–45 mm Hg).
- Maintain normothermia.
- Maintain adequate blood oxygenation.

Surgical recommendations
- Ensure proper positioning of the patient before surgery.
- Avoid overmanipulation or rough tissue handling (Figure 89.2).
- Maintain proper hemostasis.

Outcome

Patients with increased ICP are at risk for brain herniation, which happens when brain structures move from their normal anatomic compartments (Walmsley *et al.* 2006). Patients manifesting clinical signs associated with increased ICP have a poor prognosis (Packer *et al.* 2011).

Coma

Definition
Patients that are comatose are unresponsive to repeated noxious stimuli.

Risk factors
- Iatrogenic brain injury
- Increased ICP
- Brain herniation

Diagnosis
Serial neurologic examinations are recommended upon recovery from anesthesia with emphasis placed on level of consciousness, pupillary reflexes, and motor activity (Platt *et al.* 2001). Level of consciousness is impaired by abnormal function of the cerebral cortex or by interference of signal transmission by the brainstem or ascending reticular activating system in the brainstem (Sande and West 2010). Comatose patients are unresponsive to repeated noxious stimuli. A patient's level of consciousness may also impact motor activity (Platt *et al.* 2001; Sande and West 2010). Patients with damage to the reticular activating system at the level of the midbrain will be comatose with decerebrate rigidity (Sande and West 2010). Decerebrate rigidity is defined as opisthotonus with hyperextension of all four limbs (Sande and West 2010). Pupillary reflexes are an essential part of the neurologic examination. Fixed, mydriatic pupils are a negative prognostic indicator (Platt *et al.* 2001; Sande and West 2010) and in the presence of other cranial nerve deficits are suggestive of brain herniation (Walmsley *et al.* 2006). (Figure 89.3)

Treatment
Treatment is aimed at reducing ICP (see Increased intracranial pressure).

Outcome
Comatose patients have a poor prognosis.

Prevention
Avoid iatrogenic trauma during surgery by minimizing tissue handling and using gentle retraction (Figure 89.2).

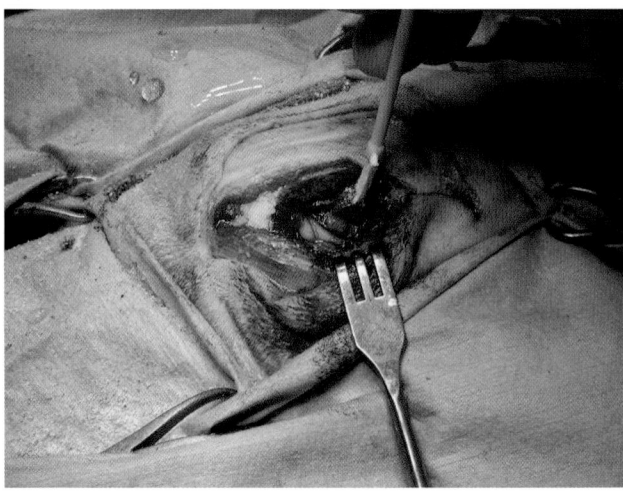

Figure 89.2 Proper tissue handling to avoid iatrogenic trauma during intracranial surgery. Gentle retraction and hemostasis facilitate identification of margins between normal and abnormal tissues. (Courtesy of Karen Kline.)

Relevant literature
Iatrogenic peripheral nerve damage occurs as a result of the surgical approach to access the intracranial space. Care should be taken when performing a lateral rostrotentorial approach to avoid damaging the facial nerve when the skin incision is made (Bagley 2003). Careful temporalis muscle dissection allows preservation of the mandibular branch of the trigeminal nerve (Bagley 2003). Meningiomas, the most common tumor in cats, are described as having a predilection for the skull base region (Forterre *et al.* 2009). A suprazygomatical temporobasal surgical approach to expose these lesions in the ventral lateral aspect of the cerebrum have been used to minimize soft tissue damage (Forterre *et al.* 2009). This approach requires retraction of the facial nerve, causing a reversible facial nerve paralysis (Forterre *et al.* 2009). The proximity of the lesion to the cranial nerves puts patients at an increase risk for iatrogenic trauma, but it can be difficult to distinguish iatrogenic trauma from the original disease process in some cases (Bagley *et al.* 1997).

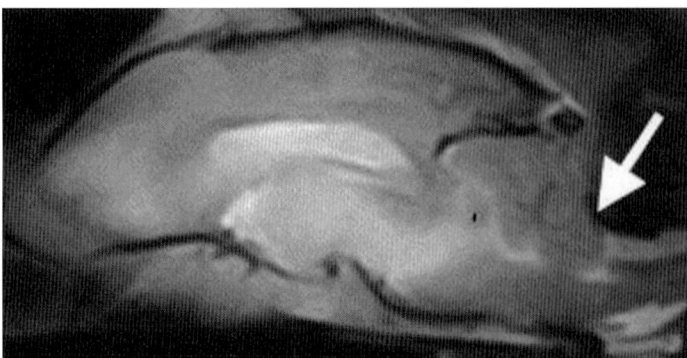

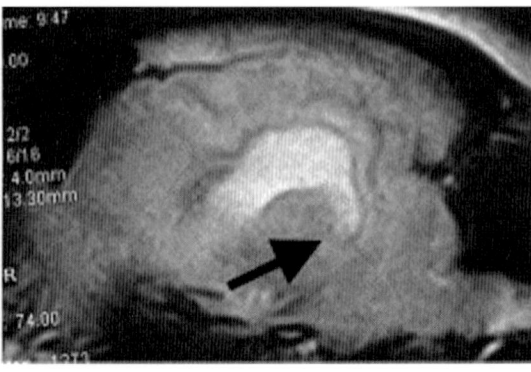

(A)

(B)

Figure 89.3 T2-weighted sagittal magnetic resonance image of caudal transtentorial and foramen magnum herniation. **A,** The caudal part of the cerebellum is entering the foramen magnum (white arrow) and the fourth ventricle is almost obliterated. **B,** Additional features of caudal transtentorial herniation: The caudal margin of the lateral ventricle is depressed ventrally and caudally (black arrow), implying caudoventral displacement of the cerebral cortex. (Reproduced with permission from Walmsley, G.L., Herrtage M.E., Dennis, R., et al. (2006) The relationship between clinical signs and brainstem herniation associated with rostrotentorial mass lesions in the dog. *The Veterinary Journal* 172, 258-264. Copyright 2005, with permission from Elsevier.)

Iatrogenic brain injury is a possible complication of craniotomies or craniectomies. The most common factors associated with this complication include manipulation of brain tissue, poor visualization of the lesion because of a limited surgical approach, and aggressive retraction of brain tissue (Bagley 2003). Distinguishing abnormal from normal brain tissue can be difficult. The use of ultrasonic aspirators improves the extent of tumor resection and prolongs survival times (Greco et al. 2006).

Increased ICP can be a consequence of intracranial surgery. In the Monroe-Kellie theory, the skull consists of a rigid compartment containing brain tissue, blood, and CSF (Sande and West 2010). An increase in ICP occurs when one component expands in volume without compensatory shrinkage of other components (Sande and West 2010). During intracranial surgery, excessive parenchymal manipulation can lead to brain swelling and edema, thereby increasing ICP (Bagley 2003). Hyperventilation, mannitol, and steroid administration have been used to reduce ICP. Leaving the skull open has been proposed as a strategy to control ICP and brain swelling after lateral rostrotentorial craniectomy (Bagley 2003). ICP may be monitored directly with a fiberoptic ICP monitoring device (Bagley et al. 1997); however, cost and the fragility of the equipment affect its clinical application in veterinary medicine (Packer et al. 2011). Clinical signs associated with increased ICP may not be evident until a patient recovers from anesthesia. Signs may include pupil abnormalities, mentation alteration, bradycardia, hypertension, absent pupillary light reflexes, and oculocephalic reflexes (Platt et al. 2001; Packer et al. 2011).

Level of consciousness is an important assessment in patients with intracranial disease both before and after surgery. Assessment of level of awareness, motor activity, and brainstem reflexes should be performed (Platt et al. 2001). **Comatose** patients are unresponsive to repeated noxious stimuli. Decerebrate posture characterized by opisthotonus and rigid extension of all four limbs may be present in a comatose patient (Sande and West 2010). Patients with fixed, mydriatic pupils have a poor prognosis (Platt et al. 2001; Sande and West 2010). Brain herniation, caused by increased ICP, can cause changes in the level of awareness. There are five types of herniations: subfalcine, rostral and caudal transsternorial, foramen magnum, and herniation through a craniotomy defect (Walmsley et al. 2006).

The two most common and clinically significant types are caudal transtentorial herniation and foramen magnum herniation, which then lead to brainstem compression (Walmsley et al. 2006). The prognosis is poor in comatose patients. Treatment should be aimed at reducing ICP, but clinical signs may be irreversible.

References

Bagley, R.S. (2003) Brain. In Slatter, D. (ed.) *Textbook of Small Animal Surgery*, vol. 2, 3rd edn. Elsevier Health Sciences, London, pp. 1163-1172.

Bagley, R.S., Keegan, R.D., Greene, S.A., et al. (1995) Intraoperative monitoring of intracranial pressure in five dogs with intracranial lesions. *Journal of the American Veterinary Association* 5, 588-591.

Bagley, R.S., Harrington, M.L., Pluhar, G.E., et al. (1997) Acute unilateral transverse sinus occlusion during craniectomy in seven dogs with space occupying intracranial disease. *Veterinary Surgery* 26, 195-201.

Dewey, C.W., Fletcher, D.J. (2008) Head trauma management. In Dewey, C.W. (ed.) *A Practical Guide to Canine and Feline Neurology*. Wiley-Blackwell, Ames, IA, p. 223.

Forterre, F., Jaggy, A., Rohrbach, H., et al. (2009) Modified temporal approach for a rostro-temporal basal meningioma in a cat. *Journal of Feline Medicine and Surgery* 11, 510-513.

Greco, J.J., Aiken, S.A., Berg, J.M., et al. (2006) Evaluation of intracranial meningioma resection with a surgical aspirator in dogs: 17 cases (1996-2004). *Journal of the American Veterinary Association* 229 (3), 394-400.

Klopp, L.S., Simpson, S.T., Sorjonen, D.C., et al. (2000) Ventral surgical approach to the caudal brain stem in dogs. *Veterinary Surgery* 29, 533-542.

Packer, R.A., Simmons J.P., Davis, N.M., et al. (2011) Evaluation of an acute focal epidural mass model to characterize the intracranial pressure-volume relationship in healthy beagles. *American Journal of Veterinary Research* 72, 103-108.

Platt, S.R., Radaelli, S.T., McDonnell, J.J. (2001) The prognostic value of the modified Glasgow coma scale in head trauma in dogs. *The Journal of Veterinary Internal Medicine* 15, 581-584.

Sande, A., West, C. (2010) Traumatic brain injury: a review of pathophysiology and management. *Journal of Veterinary Emergency and Critical Care* 20 (2), 177-190.

Sturges, B.K., Dickinson, P.J. (2004) Principles of neurosurgery. In Platt, S.R., Olby, N.J. (eds.) *BSAVA Manual of Canine and Feline Neurology*, 3rd edn. British Small Animal Veterinary Association, Gloucester, UK, pp. 363-364.

Talarico, L.R., Dewey, C.W. (2012) Intracranial neoplasia. In Tobias, K.M., Johnston, S.A. (eds.) *Veterinary Surgery Small Animal*, vol 1. Elsevier Saunders, St. Louis, p. 513.

Tefend, M.B., Dewey, C.W. (2008). Nursing care and physical therapy for patients with neurologic disease. In Dewey, C.W. (ed.) *A Practical Guide to Canine and Feline Neurology*. Wiley-Blackwell, Ames, IA, p. 581.

Walmsley, G.L., Herrtage M.E., Dennis, R., et al. (2006) The relationship between clinical signs and brainstem herniation associated with rostrotentorial mass lesions in the dog. *The Veterinary Journal* 172, 258-264.

90 Intracranial Shunt Placement

Belinda Comito
Veterinary Specialty Center, Buffalo Grove, IL, USA

Placement of intracranial shunts is recommended in patients with hydrocephalus when neurologic signs fail to respond to medical therapy or worsen over time (Coates *et al.* 2006; Thomas 2010; Shihab *et al.* 2011; Figure 90.1). *Hydrocephalus* is defined as an increase in cerebrospinal fluid (CSF) volume in the ventricular system within the cranial cavity (Dewey 2002; Shihab *et al.* 2011). The term *congenital hydrocephalus* refers to cases in young patients when an underlying cause is not identified (Figure 90.2). The term acquired *hydrocephalus* refers to cases when an underlying etiology is identified (Dewey 2002) (Figure 90.3). Examples of acquired hydrocephalus include infectious or inflammatory disorders, intracranial hemorrhage, and neoplasia (Dewey 2002). Hydrocephalus may occur in the absence of clinical signs (Vite and Cross 2011). The clinician must therefore correlate the location of the lesion with the examination findings (Vite and Cross 2011) because the presence of ventriculomegally alone does not constitute a surgical indication (Thomas 2010).

Every attempt should be made at identifying and treating the underlying cause of hydrocephalus (Thomas 2010). Shunt placement should be considered as a palliative measure in cases with hydrocephalus of unknown origin or in those with acquired hydrocephalus and an unsatisfactory response to treatment (Coates *et al.* 2006;

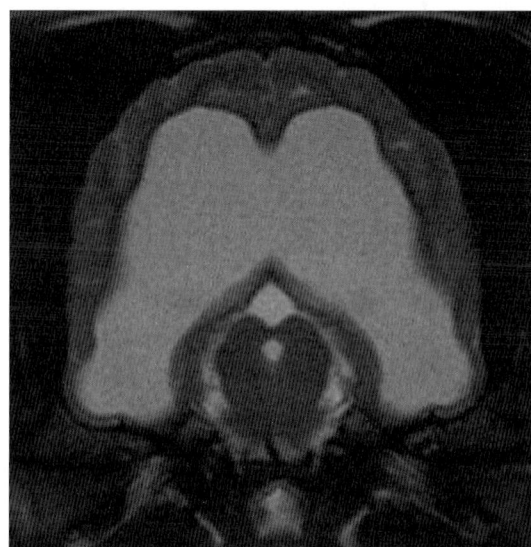

(A)

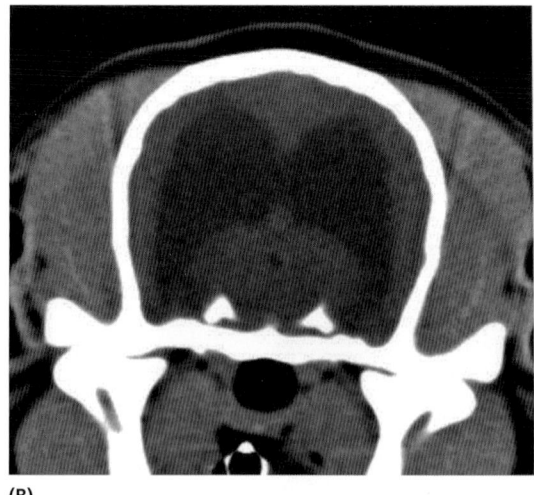

(B)

Figure 90.2 Congenital hydrocephalus. **A,** Magnetic resonance image of a patient with congenital hydrocephalus. Note the ventricular distension caused by fluid, with limited parenchymal content at the periphery. *Source:* Shihab *et al.*, 2011. Reproduced with permission from John Wiley & Sons. **B,** Computed tomography scan of a patient with congenital hydrocephalus. Note the presence of dilated lateral ventricles. *Source:* Biel *et al.*, 2013. Reproduced with permission from American Veterinary Medical Association.

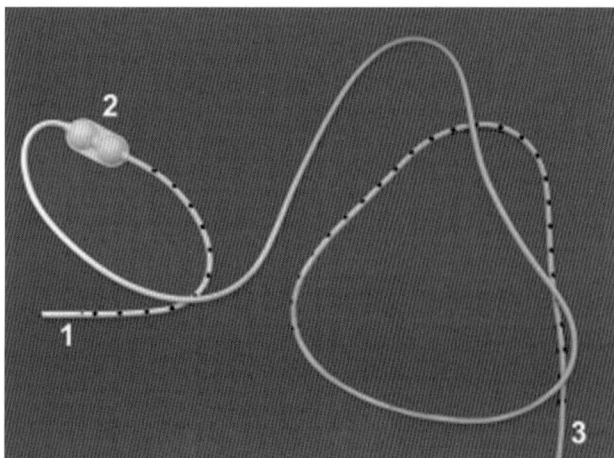

Figure 90.1 Ventriculoperitoneal shunt. 1, Ventricular end. 2, Access port and reservoir. 3, Distal end (Uni-Shunt with Reservoir; Codman). *Source:* Thomas, 2010. Reproduced with permission from Elsevier.

Complications in Small Animal Surgery, First Edition. Edited by Dominique Griffon and Annick Hamaide.
© 2016 John Wiley & Sons, Inc. Published 2016 by John Wiley & Sons, Inc.
Companion website: www.wiley.com/go/griffon/complications

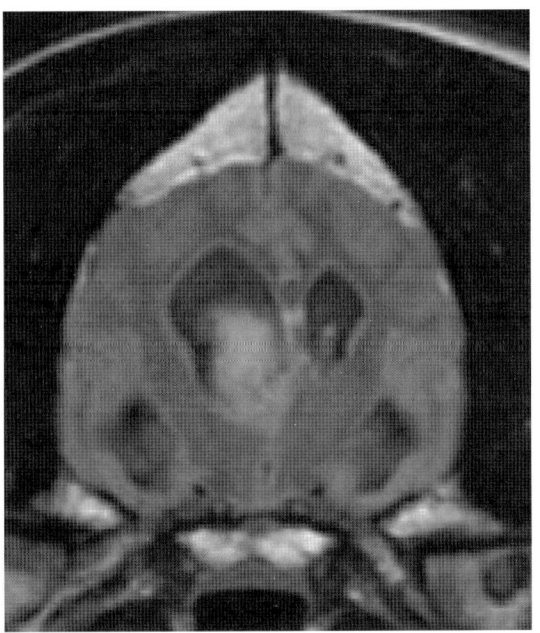

Figure 90.3 Obstructive hydrocephalus: Magnetic resonance image of a patient with obstructive hydrocephalus. The lateral ventricles are dilated secondary to a space-occupying mass in the right lateral ventricle. *Source:* de Stefani *et al.*, 2011. Reproduced with permission from John Wiley & Sons.

Shihab *et al.* 2011). Shunt placement is aimed at reducing intracranial pressure (ICP), improving patient neurologic status, and minimizing damage to the brain (de Stefani *et al.* 2011). In these cases, a shunt is placed to divert CSF from the ventricles into another body cavity (Thomas 2010). In veterinary medicine, ventriculoperitoneal (VP) shunts are most commonly used (Dewey 2002; Hasegawa *et al.* 2005; Kitagawa *et al.* 2005; Kim 2006; Shihab *et al.* 2011).

Infection
See Chapter 1.

Undershunting

Definition
Undershunting is defined as an inability of a shunt to maintain the ICP within normal range (5–12 mm Hg), generally because of an obstruction of CSF flow through the shunt (Thomas 2010). Undershunting may therefore result from blockage, disconnection, or kinking of the shunt (Kitagawa *et al.* 2008). Blockage may be localized to the level of the ventricular catheter, valve, or distal tubing (Figures 90.4 to 90.6). The nature of the obstruction may relate to the accumulation of debris, blood, protein, choroid plexus, intraparenchymal placement, gliosis, or infection (de Stefani *et al.* 2011). Other causes of undershunting include misplacement or migration of the ventricular catheter or incorrect placement of the distal tubing into the subcutaneous tissue.

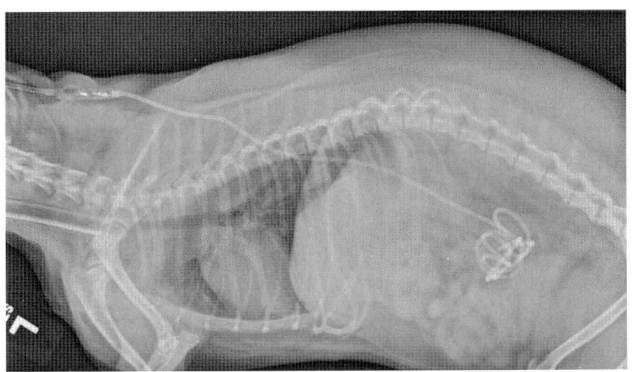

(A)

(B)

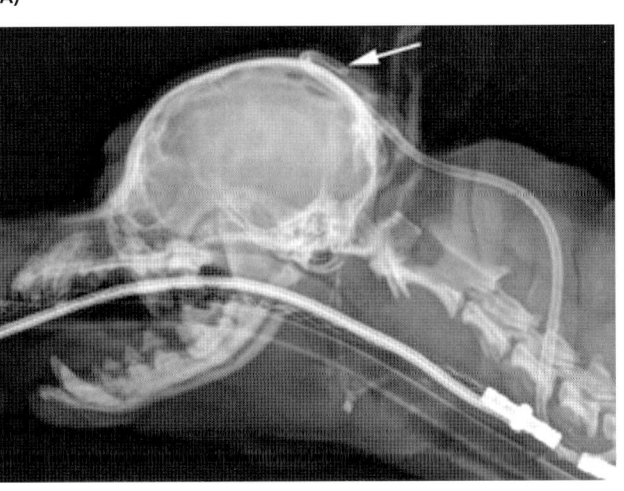

(C)

Figure 90.4 Postoperative radiographic appearance of ventriculoperitoneal shunts. **A** and **B,** Lateral radiographs illustrating the normal path of a shunt. (Courtesy of Stephanie Thomovsky.) **C,** Migration of a ventricular catheter (arrow) caused by improper immobilization of the catheter to adjacent tissues. *Source:* Thomas, 2010. Reproduced with permission from Elsevier.

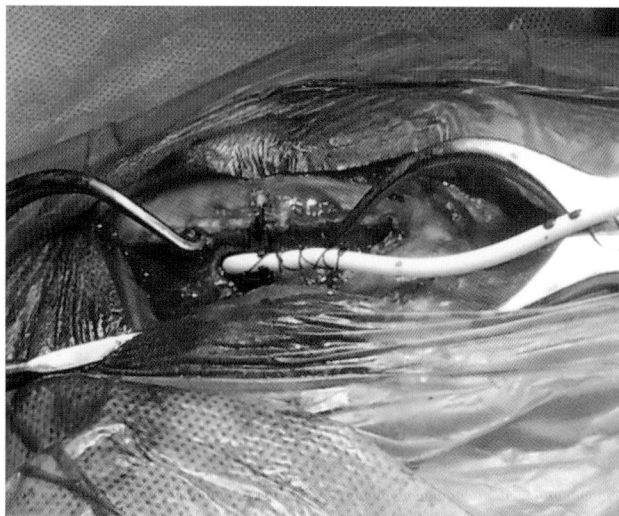

Figure 90.5 Intraoperative image illustrating proper immobilization of a ventricular catheter. *Source:* Reproduced with permission from L. Marni.

Risk factors

- Improper placement of the ventricular catheter
- Improper placement of the distal tubing into the subcutaneous tissue instead of into the abdomen
- Acquired hydrocephalus (Figure 90.7)
- Poor aseptic technique during surgery (Figure 90.8)

Diagnosis

Undershunting should be suspected in patients in which initial postoperative improvement is followed by deterioration of clinical signs. Magnetic resonance imaging (MRI) and computed tomography (CT) scans are often performed in the immediate postoperative period to confirm proper placement of the shunt; however, CT scans require less time to complete the study and are often used after surgery (Figure 90.9). If neurologic deterioration occurs, repeating the CT or MRI is indicated. Repeating the imaging allows for comparison of ventricular size; enlargement of ventricles is suspicious for obstruction. In patients without appreciable ventricular enlargement shunt, obstruction can be diagnosed by inserting a

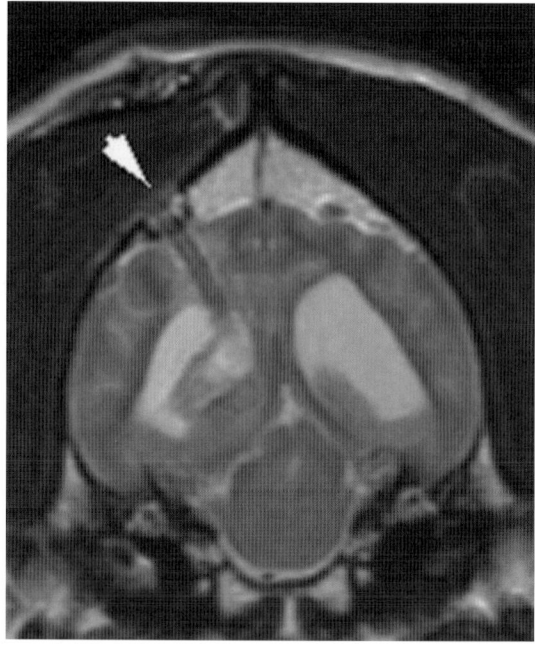

Figure 90.7 Undershunting after placement of a ventriculoperitoneal shunt. The ventricular catheter (white arrow) seems embedded in the ventricular mass, explaining undershunting of cerebrospinal fluid. *Source:* de Stefani *et al.*, 2011. Reproduced with permission from John Wiley & Sons.

needle into the reservoir and blocking the distal tubing (Thomas 2010). If CSF cannot be collected, the ventricular portion of the shunt is blocked (Thomas 2010). Postoperative radiographs allow identification of misplacement, migration, or disconnection of the shunt (Thomas 2010) (see Figure 90.4). Injection of nonionic iodinated contrast agent into the shunt reservoir to check for patency may also be performed (da Rocha Filgueiras *et al.* 2009; Thomas 2010) (Figure 90.10).

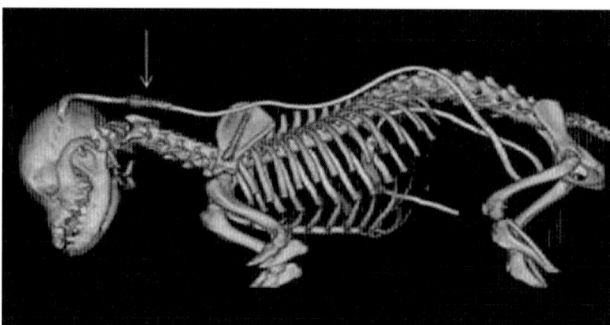

Figure 90.6 Reconstructed three-dimensional computed tomographic appearance of a ventriculoperitoneal shunt placement 20 days after proper placement. The arrow points to a Codman Hakim Precision Valve containing a small synthetic ruby ball controlling cerebrospinal fluid flow while mitigating the risk of long-term obstruction. *Source:* da Rocha Filgueiras *et al.*, 2009. Reproduced with permission from John Wiley & Sons.

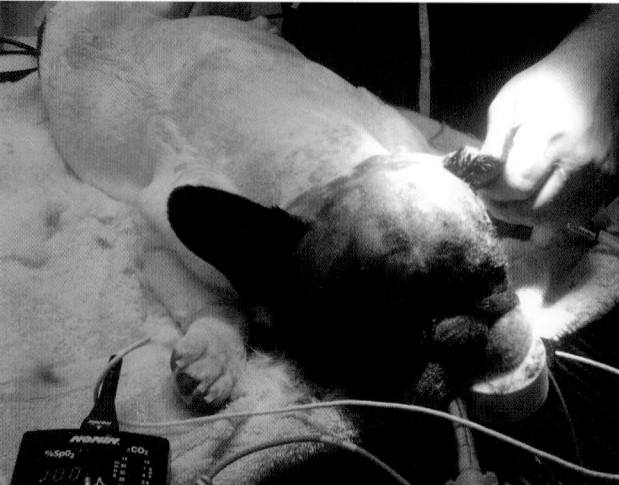

Figure 90.8 Aseptic preparation before placement of a ventriculoperitoneal shunt. Preparation should extend from the site of the ventricular catheter placement to the site of the peritoneal incision. *Source:* Reproduced with permission from L. Marni.

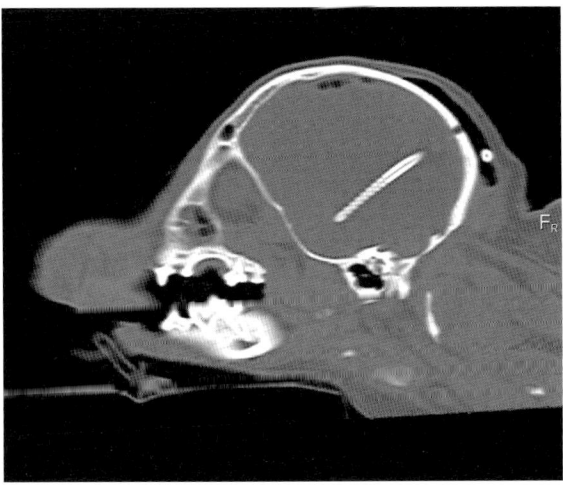

Figure 90.9 Postoperative confirmation of ventricular catheter placement via computed tomography. *Source:* S. Thomovsky, Purdue University, West Lafayette, IN. Reproduced with permission from S. Thomovsky.

Treatment

Treatment of undershunting depends on the underlying cause. The goal is to reestablish CSF flow through the shunt apparatus. Migration, disconnection, or misplacement of the shunt in the immediate postoperative period requires surgical revision. Migration or misplacement of the shunt requires placement of the shunt into the lateral ventricle. Migration may occur if the shunt

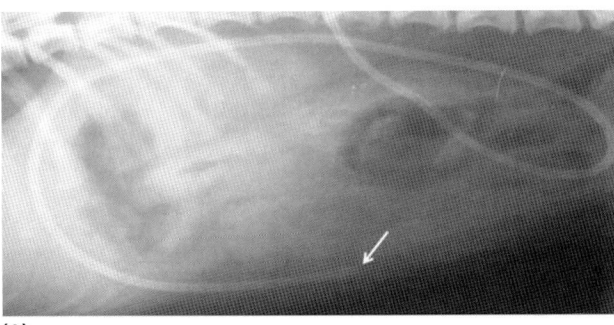

(A)

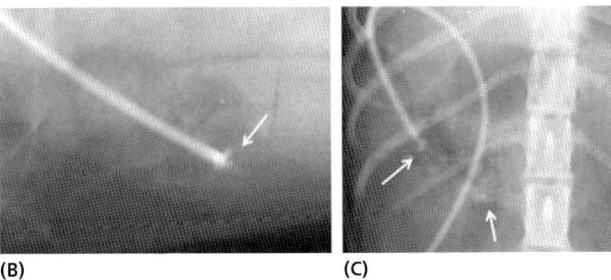

(B)   (C)

Figure 90.10 Postoperative verification of the patency of a ventriculoperitoneal shunt. A lateral radiograph of the abdomen (**A**) is obtained before a noniodinated contrast agent is injected into the shunt. The presence of contrast in the abdomen is subsequently verified via radiography (**B** and **C**), confirming patency of the shunt. *Source:* da Rocha Filgueiras *et al.*, 2009. Reproduced with permission from John Wiley & Sons.

has not been properly anchored. Disconnection occurs if the shunt components have not been properly secured. Shunt replacement may be indicated in cases with infection or physical blockage of the shunt by debris, glial tissue, or choroid plexus. Treatment with antibiotics is warranted in patients diagnosed with an infection.

Outcome

Success rates for VP shunt implantation have varied, but several studies report a success rate of approximately 75% (Coates *et al.* 2006, Biel *et al.* 2013). The majority of patients improve; however, many continue to have residual clinical signs. Patients are at risk for developing seizures, and patients with preexisting seizures may not have resolution with shunt placement. Patients with severe hydrocephalus can experience an improvement, but full resolution of clinical signs should not be expected (Coates *et al.* 2006; Biel *et al.* 2013). Most complications are likely to develop within the first 3 months of surgery. (Biel *et al.* 2013). Reported long-term survival times are variable. In a recent study of 36 animals, 20 were alive after 18 months with the longest follow-up period being 9.5 years (Biel *et al.* 2013).

Prevention

Undershunting is a complication inherent to shunt placement and may develop despite adherence to surgical technique and preventive measures. Postoperative radiographs and MRI or CT scan ensure proper placement in the immediate postoperative period.

Overshunting

Definition

Overshunting is defined as an excessive outflow of CSF after VP shunt placement. Overshunting of CSF leads to overdraining of CSF, causing a sudden drop in ICP, leading to cerebral collapse, pain, subdural hematoma formation, or subdural fluid accumulation (Kitagawa *et al.* 2005; Thomas 2010; Shihab *et al.* 2011) (see Figure 90.11), 90.11 is a picture of subdural fluid accumulation. Patients with severe ventriculomegaly and thin cerebral cortexes are reportedly predisposed to overshunting (Coates *et al.* 2006; Biel *et al.* 2013) (see Figure 90.12), 90.12 is a picture of severe ventriculomegaly. Ventricular shunts with and without pressure valves exist. The ventricular pressure valves allow ventricular pressures to be maintained within preset ranges with the goal of preventing overdrainage of CSF (da Rocha Filgueiras *et al.* 2009). Medium pressure valves work closest to the normal ICP of dogs (da Rocha Filgueiras *et al.* 2009). Low-pressure valves or valveless ventricular shunts have reportedly been associated with overdrainage of CSF (da Rocha Filgueiras *et al.* 2009); however, valve-free catheter systems are less expensive and have been used in veterinary medicine (Biel *et al.* 2013).

Risk factors

- Patients with thin cerebral cortexes and severe ventricular enlargement (Figure 90.12)
- Use of shunt catheters without a valve system or use of low-pressure valves may lead to overshunting.

Diagnosis

Overshunting is an uncommon complication of VP shunt placement. Repeat advanced imaging such as MRI or CT is recommended to detect collapse of the brain, decreased ventricular size, and accumulation of subdural hemorrhage.

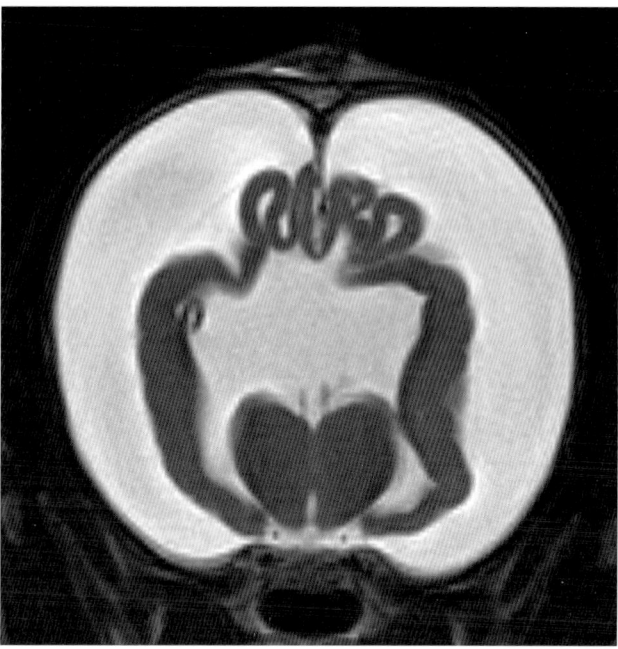

Figure 90.11 Magnetic resonance image of subdural fluid accumulation 9 days after ventriculoperitoneal shunt placement. *Source:* Reproduced with permission from Kitagwa Masato.

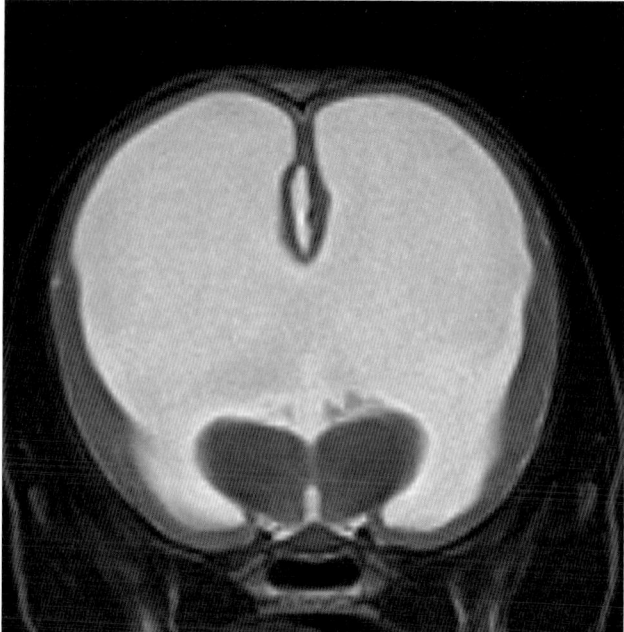

Figure 90.12 Magnetic resonance image showing severe dilation of the lateral ventricles and a thin cerebral cortex. *Source:* Reproduced with permission from Kitagwa Masato.

Treatment

Overshunting may manifest as pain (Shihab *et al.* 2011), neurologic deterioration, or peracute death. In some patients, MRI or CT imaging may be consistent with overshunting, but neurologic signs are not present, or neurologic progression is not evident (Kitagwa *et al.* 2005). Placement of medium- to high-pressure VP systems should be considered in patients with low-pressure valves or valveless systems when overdrainage is confirmed. Unfortunately, peracute death is one of the more common manifestations of overdrainage of CSF.

Outcome

Overshunting may or may not be clinically significant. Clinical signs may range from pain to peracute death. Patients that manifest pain may have spontaneous resolution of clinical signs (Shihab *et al.* 2011). Shunt revision is not recommended in patients with evidence of overshunting on MRI or CT scans without corresponding neurologic deterioration.

Prevention

Patients with severe ventricular dilation and thin cerebral cortexes are at highest risk for overshunting (Coates *et al.* 2006; Biel *et al.* 2013). Placement of medium- or high-pressure valves is recommended in these patients (Thomas 2010; Biel *et al.* 2013).

Seizures

Definition

Seizures are a common presenting complaint in patients with hydrocephalus but are not a commonly reported complication of VP shunt placement.

Risk factors

Patients with seizures before VP shunt placement may have persistent seizures after surgery. Placement of a VP shunt may cause

compression of the cerebral cortex (Hasegawa *et al.* 2005) or cause direct cortical injury (Biel *et al.* 2013), leading to the development of seizures in patients without a previous seizure history.

Diagnosis

A diagnosis of seizures is based on observation or history of seizures.

Treatment

Treatment with anticonvulsants should be initiated in patients with a history of seizures before VP shunt placement. Phenobarbital is the anticonvulsant of choice based on review of the literature, but the efficacy of newer anticonvulsants has not been evaluated. Phenobarbital treatment is initiated at doses ranging from 2 to 4 mg/kg orally every 12 hours. Resolution of preexisting seizure activity may not occur after surgery; therefore, anticonvulsant therapy should not be immediately discontinued. Recurrence of seizure activity after shunt implantation has been reported 3 to 22 months after surgery (Biel *et al.* 2013). Persistent or recurrent seizure activity can negatively impact a patient's quality of life and as a result may lead to the decision of euthanasia. Therefore, the decision to discontinue anticonvulsant therapy should only be made only after careful consideration. Surgical revision should be considered in patients with cerebral cortex compression secondary to shunt placement.

Prevention

Anticonvulsants should be used to reduce the frequency and severity of seizures.

Relevant literature

Success rates for VP shunt implantation have varied. Several studies report a success rate of approximately 75% (Coates *et al.* 2006; Biel *et al.* 2013). A recent study showed that 25% of patients were free of clinical signs (Biel *et al.* 2013). The majority of patients improve, but many continue to have residual clinical signs. Patients with severe hydrocephalus can experience an improvement, but full resolution of clinical signs should not be expected (Coates *et al.* 2006; Biel *et al.* 2013). Patients with preexisting seizures may not resolve with shunt placement. Most complications are likely to develop within the first 3 months of surgery. Recent studies have shown 22% postoperative complication rate (Biel *et al.* 2013) and 25% failure rate (Shihab *et al.* 2011). Reported long-term survival times are variable. In a recent study of 36 animals, 20 were alive after 18 months with the longest follow-up period being 9.5 years (Biel *et al.* 2013).

Undershunting is the most common complication encountered after placement of intracranial shunts in dogs. This complication results from blockage, disconnection, or kinking of the VP shunt (Kitagawa *et al.* 2000). The most frequent complication of VP shunt placement is blockage of CSF flow through an intact shunt (Thomas 2010). Intact shunt catheters may become occluded from several causes, including choroid plexus, gliosis, blood, protein, intraparenchymal placement, or infection (Thomas 2010; de Stefani *et al.* 2011). Migration and disconnection may also prevent proper CSF flow (Thomas 2010). Repeat MRI, CT, or radiography to check the positioning of the ventricular catheter, tapping of the shunt, and measurement of ventricular catheter pressure may be used to diagnose shunt obstruction (Thomas 2010). Injection of nonionic iodinated contrast agent into the shunt reservoir to check for patency may also be performed (da Rocha Filgueiras *et al.* 2009; Thomas 2010). Patients with VP obstruction generally require surgical revision of the shunt.

Overshunting secondary to VP shunt placement leads to brain collapse, decreased ventricular size, and accumulation of subdural hemorrhage or fluid (Kitagawa *et al.* 2005; Shihab *et al.* 2011). This complication is less prevalent than undershunting and is not always clinically significant or is reported as an incidental finding on longitudinal evaluation of postoperative MRIs. However, Shihab *et al.* (2011) recently reported pain 10 to 18 days after shunt placement in four dogs suspected of overshunting. Two dogs had spontaneous resolution of clinical signs, and two were euthanized for persistent pain and neurologic deterioration, respectively. The suspected pathogenesis is related to overdrainage of CSF causing intracranial hypotension related to the use of a low-pressure valve catheter system (Shihab *et al.* 2011) Overshunting has been related to the type of shunts placed, specifically with the type of valve used to maintain ventricular pressures within preset ranges (da Rocha Filgueiras *et al.* 2009; Thomas 2010). It has been suggested that the use of low-pressure valves may lead to overshunting (da Rocha Filgueiras *et al.* 2009; Thomas 2010). Patients with large ventricles are at risk for overshunting when low-pressure valves are used because of sudden overdrainage and size reduction of ventricles, leading to collapse of the cerebral cortex, and tearing of blood vessels between the dura and brain, leading to subdural blood or fluid accumulation (Thomas 2010).

Seizures are not a common complication of VP shunt placement (da Rocha Filgueiras *et al.* 2009; Shihab *et al.* 2011). In a recent study, 33% of patients had preexisting seizures before shunt placement (Biel *et al.* 2013). A mild episode of seizures episode without recurrence was reported in 1 of 12 dogs undergoing shunt placement (Shihab *et al.* 2011). Recurrence of seizure activity has been reported after surgery in patients that had been seizure free between 3 and 22 months (Biel *et al.* 2013). However, a case report described severe generalized seizures resulting in the death of a dog with combined hydrocephalus, syringohydromyelia, and ventricular cyst (Hasegawa *et al.* 2005), and one dog developed status epilepticus and died after shunt implantation (Biel *et al.* 2013). Placement of the shunt may not be effective in altering the seizure pattern in patients, and persistence of seizures should be discussed with clients before surgery (da Rocha Filgueiras *et al.* 2009). Anticonvulsants should not be immediately discontinued after surgery (Hasegawa *et al.* 2005). The variable time frame reported for recurrence of seizure after surgery complicates the decision-making process regarding the best timing for discontinuing therapy. In patients that are tolerating the medication and do not have severe side effects, medication should be continued indefinitely.

References

Biel, M., Kramer, M., Forterre, F., et al. (2013) Outcome of ventriculoperitoneal shunt implantation for treatment of congenital internal hydrocephalus in dogs and cats: 36 cases (2001-2009). *Journal of the American Veterinary Medical Association* 242, 948-958.

Coates, J.R., Axlund T.W., Dewey, C.W., et al. (2006) Hydrocephalus in dogs and cats. *Compendium of Continuing Education for Practicing Veterinarians* 28, 136-146.

da Rocha Filgueiras, R., de Souza Martins, C., de Almeida, R.M., et al. (2009). Long-term evaluation of a new ventriculoperitoneal shunt system in a dog. *Journal of Veterinary Emergency and Critical Care* 19 (6), 523-528.

de Stefani, A., de Risio L., Platt, S., et al. (2011) Surgical technique, postoperative complications and outcome in 11 dogs treated for hydrocephalus by ventriculoperitoneal shunting. *Veterinary Surgery* 40, 183-191.

Dewey, C.W. (2002) External hydrocephalus in a dog with suspected bacterial meningoencephalitis. *Journal of the American Animal Hospital Association* 38, 563-567.

Hasegawa, T., Taura, Y., Kido, H. (2005) Surgical management of combined hydrocephalus, syringohydromyelia, and ventricular cyst in a dog. *Journal of the American Animal Hospital Association* 41, 267-272.

Kim, H., Itamoto, K., Watanabe, M., et al. (2006) Application of ventriculoperitoneal shunt as a treatment for hydrocephalus in a dog with syringomyelia and Chiari I malformation. *Journal of Veterinary Science* 7 (2), 203-206.

Kitagawa, M., Kanayama, K., Sakai, T. (2005) Subdural accumulation of fluid in a dog after the insertion of a ventriculoperitoneal shunt. *The Veterinary Record* 156, 206-208.

Kitagawa, M., Ueno, H., Watanabe, S., et al. (2008) Clinical improvement in two dogs with hydrocephalus and syringohydromyelia after ventriculoperitoneal shunting. *Australian Veterinary Journal* 86, 36-42.

Shihab, N, Davies, E, Kenny, P.J., et al. (2011) Treatment of hydrocephalus with ventriculoperitoneal shunting in twelve dogs. *Veterinary Surgery* 40, 477-484.

Thomas, W.B. (2010) Hydrocephalus in dogs and cats. *Veterinary Clinics of North America: Small Animal Practice* 40, 143-159.

Vite, C.H., Cross, J.R. (2011) Correlating magnetic resonance findings with neuropathology and clinical signs in dogs and cats. *Veterinary Radiology & Ultrasound*, 52 (Suppl. 1), S23-S31.

Management of Fractures and Osteotomies: Perioperative Complications

91 Inadequate Fracture Reduction

Ann Johnson

College of Veterinary Medicine, University of Illinois, Champaign, IL, USA

Definitions

Failure to anatomically reconstruct a reducible fracture particularly an articular fracture, or failure to achieve normal limb alignment after indirect fracture reduction and stabilization of a nonreducible fracture are complications that should be addressed either during surgery or immediately after the initial surgery if there is an anticipated long-term problem.

A two- or three-piece fracture in which anatomic reduction before implant placement has been unsuccessful may be predisposed to slower healing because of the strain concentration at the gap in the fracture (Rahn 2002). Articular fractures in which anatomic reduction before an implant placement has been unsuccessful are predisposed to degenerative joint disease (DJD) (Boudrieau and Kleine 1988; Matis 2005; see Chapter 18).

Bones with nonreducible fractures treated with indirect reduction (distraction of the ends of the fractured long bone that uses the pull of the soft tissues to realign the fragments) must be carefully realigned using available anatomic references (Johnson 2003). Common problems include angular malalignments such as valgus deformity, which is a deviation of the distal end of a bone or limb away from the midline when the proximal portion is held in an anatomically correct position. Conversely, varus deformity is a deviation of the distal end of a bone or limb toward the midline when the proximal portion is held in an anatomically correct position. Recurvatum and procurvatum are also angular malalignments in the craniocaudal plane, but they seem to have less clinical significance unless severe. Additionally, rotational malalignment, when the distal end of a long bone is rotated out of the sagittal plane of the proximal end of the long bone, and translational malalignments, when the distal end of the bone is out of the sagittal plane, may occur.

Risk factors

- Articular fractures, particularly comminuted fractures
- Comminuted fractures treated with bridging fixation techniques
- Poor plate contouring causing malalignment
- Poor attention to the relationship of anatomic structures during surgery
- Closed reduction and biologic fracture stabilization
- Minimally invasive plate fixation
- External fixation (especially in the plane perpendicular to the frame)

Diagnosis

The diagnosis of inadequate fracture reduction is made after scrutiny of the postoperative orthogonal radiographs. Multiple additional views may be needed to assess articular fracture reduction (Figure 91.1). Joint palpation during range of motion may detect articular surface incongruity.

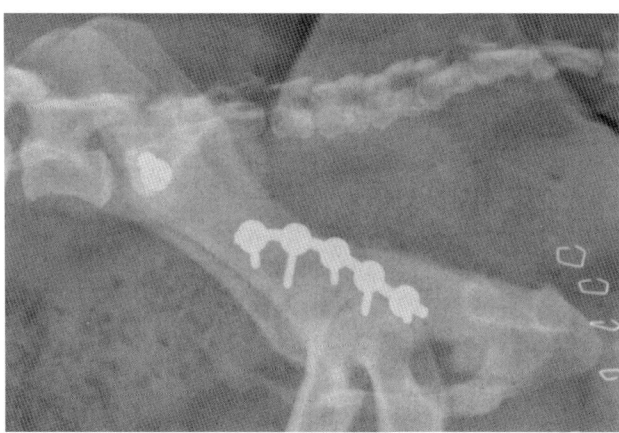

(A)

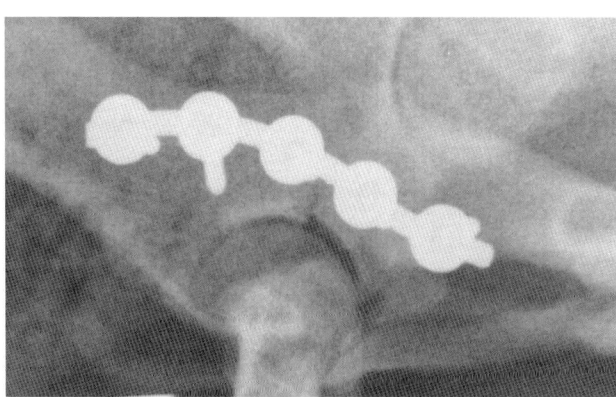

(B)

Figure 91.1 **A,** Lateral view of a stabilized acetabular fracture. **B,** Positioning the dog with the normal leg abducted gives an unobstructed view of the articular surface of the acetabulum.

The diagnosis of inadequate bone alignment is made after carefully scrutinizing orthogonal radiographs of the affected bone, which include the joint above and below the fractured bone. For evaluation of a radius and tibia, the animal should be positioned to achieve true cranial caudal and lateral images of the proximal joint. For evaluation of the femur and humerus, the animal should be positioned to achieve true cranial caudal and lateral views of the distal joint. Often, similar images of the contralateral bone may be used as a normal image for comparison. Varus and valgus malalignment is detected by evaluating the relationship of the proximal and distal joint surfaces to each other on the cranial caudal views. Recurvatum and procurvatum malalignment are detected by evaluating the relationship of the proximal and distal joint surfaces to each other on the lateral views. Complex measurements and calculations may be used to determine angular deformity in comparison to reference values (Fox *et al.* 2006; Dismukes *et al.* 2007; Tomlinson *et al.* 2007; Dismukes *et al.* 2008). Translational malalignment can be observed on radiographs. Finally, bone length can be evaluated by comparing the lengths of the lateral radiographic images of the affected and contralateral bones.

Rotational malalignment is diagnosed both by physical examination and radiographic evaluation. The relationship of anatomic structures should be evaluated to detect rotational malalignment between limb segments. For example, when the femur is held parallel to the table with the patella facing craniad, the greater trochanter should be palpable on the lateral aspect of the femur and should be approximately 90 degrees to the patella (Figure 91.2). When the stifle is then rotated internally and externally, the trochanter should move equidistant cranially and caudally before meeting resistance from the pelvis. Lateral radiographs of the femur should show the femoral head in slight anteversion in relationship to a true lateral view of the stifle. Similarly, the radiographs of the radius and tibia are evaluated to determine the relationship of the joints. To determine rotational alignment physically, the limb is held loosely in the sagittal plane, and the joints are flexed. The long bones of the limb should remain in the sagittal plane during flexion. Rotation of one bone out of plane indicates rotational malalignment (Figure 91.3).

Treatment

Although it is tempting to accept poor reduction or malalignment after a long surgical procedure, it is best to correct serious problems at this time rather than adopt a "wait and see" attitude (Figure 91.4).

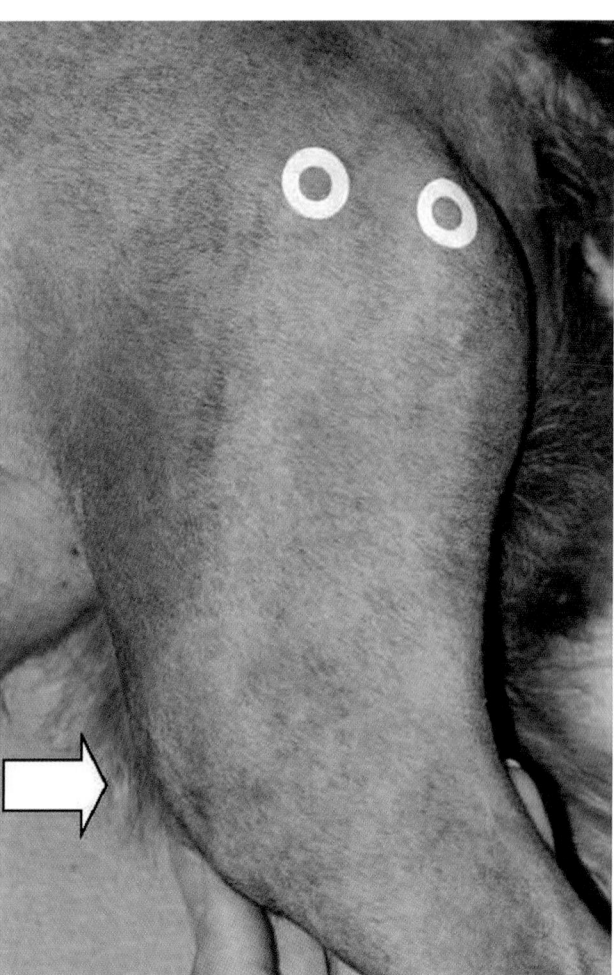

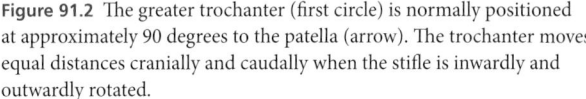

Figure 91.2 The greater trochanter (first circle) is normally positioned at approximately 90 degrees to the patella (arrow). The trochanter moves equal distances cranially and caudally when the stifle is inwardly and outwardly rotated.

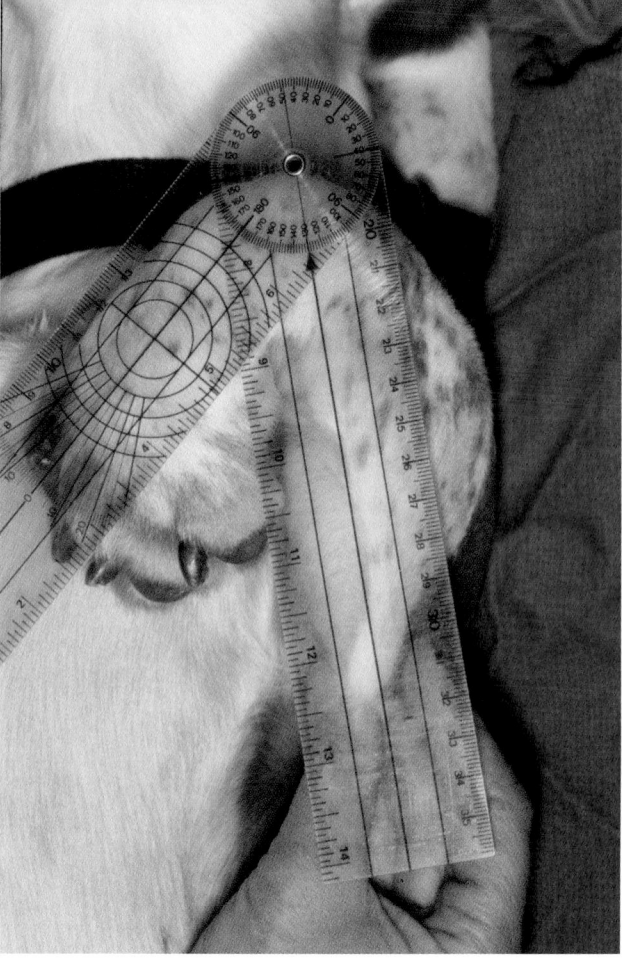

Figure 91.3 Degrees of rotation may be estimated by flexing the elbow and carpus and using a goniometer to measure the angle formed by the paw and the ulna at the carpus.

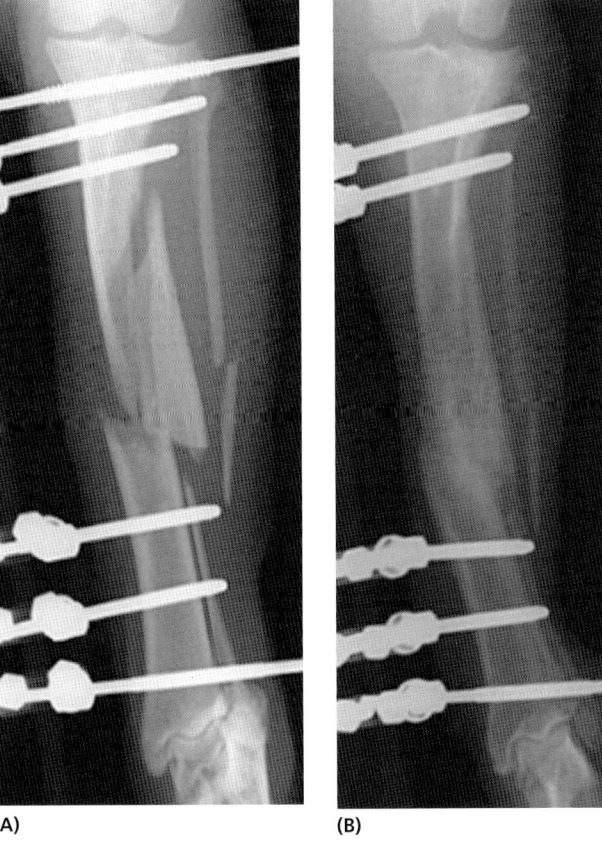

(A)   **(B)**

Figure 91.4 **A,** Postoperative radiograph of a tibia with a valgus deformity. This could have been corrected at this time to restore normal alignment. **B,** Radiograph of the healed tibia with the deformity uncorrected.

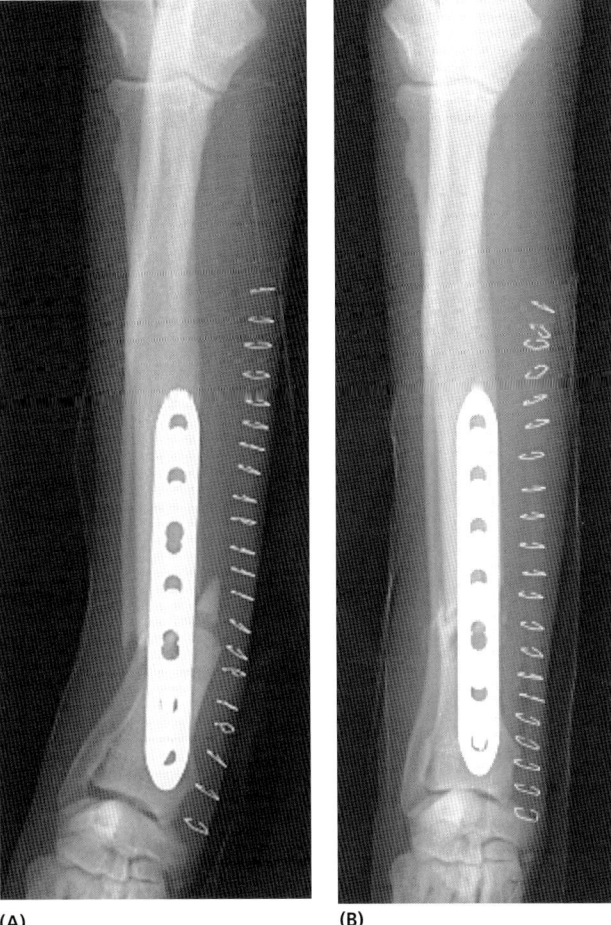

(A)   **(B)**

Figure 91.5 **A,** Postoperative radiograph of a radius with a valgus deformity. **B,** The dog was returned to surgery, and radial alignment was restored.

This approach is especially relevant to intraarticular fractures. The goal traditionally set for anatomic reduction of articular fractures is to achieve a gap of less than 1 mm between articular surfaces to avoid postoperative osteoarthritis (see Chapter 18). In these cases, poor reduction must be assessed with physical examination, and the surgeon must determine whether reoperation would improve reduction. If so, the correction should be made shortly after the initial surgery (Figure 91.5). Similarly, a judgment call must be made as to the degree of acceptable angular and rotational malalignment. Visible malalignment of the limb is generally an indication for correction.

External fixators may be manipulated to correct some deformities caused by malalignment. For angular deformities, loosen clamps on pins penetrating the distal portion of the fractured bone and manipulate the bone segment to restore alignment. For rotational deformities, some correction may be obtained by derotating the distal segment and positioning the pins penetrating the distal portion of the fractured bone on the opposite side of the connecting bar. Fractures treated with interlocking nails, plates, or screws generally must be reoperated to correct the reduction or deformity. The surgeon has to decide if reoperation will improve the outcome. Occasionally, the bone stock is limited for repositioning screws, or the comminution is too severe to improve articular reduction.

Outcome

The prognosis after correction of fracture reduction or bone alignment is similar to that of an uncomplicated fracture. However, reoperating may further compromise vascularity, delaying healing, increasing the opportunity for infection, or both.

Prevention

- Careful preoperative planning
- Careful attention to anatomic structure relationships during surgery
- Critical assessment of articular surface alignment during surgery
- Intraoperative imaging

Relevant literature

The goal of treatment in intraarticular fractures is to obtain anatomic restoration of the articular surface and stable internal fixation. DJD is predicted as the outcome after inadequate reduction of articular fractures. Most of the information in the literature relates to the coxofemoral joint. When caudal one third acetabular fractures treated conservatively were evaluated radiographically 6 to 67 months after injury, most dogs had moderate to severe DJD in the affected hips (Boudrieau and Kleine 1988). The long-term prognosis after acetabular fractures treated surgically depends on the anatomic reconstruction of the articular surface. The reported frequency of arthrosis ranges between 60% and 90%, and the frequency of lameness ranges between 20% and 40% (Matis 2005). Presumably, this outcome can be related to all joints treated for fractures; however, a literature review of 36 articles that were critically analyzed related to intraarticular injuries of distal radius, acetabulum, distal femur, and tibial plateau in humans concluded that factors other than just the extent of articular displacement affect the management of articular fractures. Different joints and even different areas of the same joint appeared to have different tolerances for posttraumatic articular step-offs (Giannoudis *et al.* 2010).

Failure to realign a bone properly can lead to altered appearances and in severe cases affect function. Limb alignment and joint angles have been documented for normal dogs, and these values can be useful for determining if postoperative alignment is correct, especially with bilateral injuries (Dismukes *et al.* 2007; Tomlinson *et al.* 2007; Dismukes *et al.* 2008). Additionally, this information is used to realign bones after corrective osteotomy (Fox *et al.* 2006).

References

Boudrieau, R.J., Kleine, L.J. (1988) Nonsurgically managed caudal acetabular fractures in dogs: 15 cases (1979-1984). *Journal of the American Veterinary Medical Association* 15 (6), 701-705.

Dismukes, D.I., Fox, D.B., Tomlinson, J.L., et al. (2008) Determination of pelvic limb alignment in the large-breed dog: a cadaveric radiographic study in the frontal plane. *Veterinary Surgery* 37 (7), 674-682.

Dismukes, D.I., Tomlinson, J.L., Fox, D.B., et al. (2007) Radiographic measurement of the proximal and distal mechanical joint angles in the canine tibia. *Veterinary Surgery* 36 (7), 699-704.

Fox, D.B., Tomlinson, J.L., Cook, J.L., et al. (2006) Principles of uniapical and biapical radial deformity correction using dome osteotomies and the Center of Rotation of Angulation Methodology in dogs. *Veterinary Surgery* 35, 67–77.

Giannoudis, P.V., Tzioupis, C., Papathanassopoulos, A., et al. (2010) Articular step-off and risk of post-traumatic osteoarthritis. Evidence today. *Injury* 41 (10), 986-995.

Johnson, A.L. (2003) Current concepts in fracture reduction. *Veterinary and Comparative Orthopaedics and Traumatology* 16, 59-66.

Matis, U. (2005) Fractures of the acetabulum. In Johnson, A.L., Houlton, J.E.F., Vannini, R. (eds.) *AO Principles of Fracture Management in the Dog and Cat.* Thieme, New York, pp. 178-191.

Rahn, B.A. (2002) Bone healing: histologic and physiologic concepts. In Smith, S. (ed.) *Bone in Clinical Orthopedics*, 2nd ed. Thieme, New York, pp. 287-325.

Tomlinson, J., Fox, D., Cook, J.L., et al. (2007) Measurement of femoral angles in four dog breeds. *Veterinary Surgery* 36 (6), 593-598.

92 Improper Implant Placement

Ann Johnson

College of Veterinary Medicine, University of Illinois, Champaign, IL, USA

Definition

Implants that are inappropriately placed and fail to stabilize the fracture, impair soft tissues, invade the joint, or impede physeal function lead to serious complications in short- and long-term fracture management. These problems must be addressed either during or immediately after surgery.

Examples of improper implant placement requiring intervention include:

- Intramedullary (IM) pins that miss the distal medullary canal
- IM pins that penetrate the joint
- IM pins that are not driven far enough distally to seat in the metaphysis
- External fixator fixation pins that penetrate excessive muscle, nerves, or vessels
- External fixator fixation pins that do not penetrate the far cortex and are needed to provide the minimum number of cortices of purchase above and below the fracture
- Plates that are not long enough to provide three screws or six cortices of purchase above and below the fracture
- Nonlocking plate screws that do not penetrate the far cortex and are needed to provide the minimum of six cortices of purchase above and below the fracture
- Plates poorly contoured causing angular deformities
- Implants that interfere with physeal function such as screws, plate, cross pins, tension bands, or external fixator bridging the physis
- Interlocking nails that are not penetrated and secured by the bone screw (Figure 92.1).

Risk factors

- Poor technical skills
- Poor surgical approach and visualization of the bone
- Inadequate preoperative radiographs
- Inadequate postoperative radiographs
- Closed reduction and stabilization
- Swollen soft tissues adjacent to the fracture

Diagnosis

The diagnosis of improper implant placement is made after scrutiny of the postoperative orthogonal radiographs. Multiple additional views may be needed to assess implant position. Careful critical

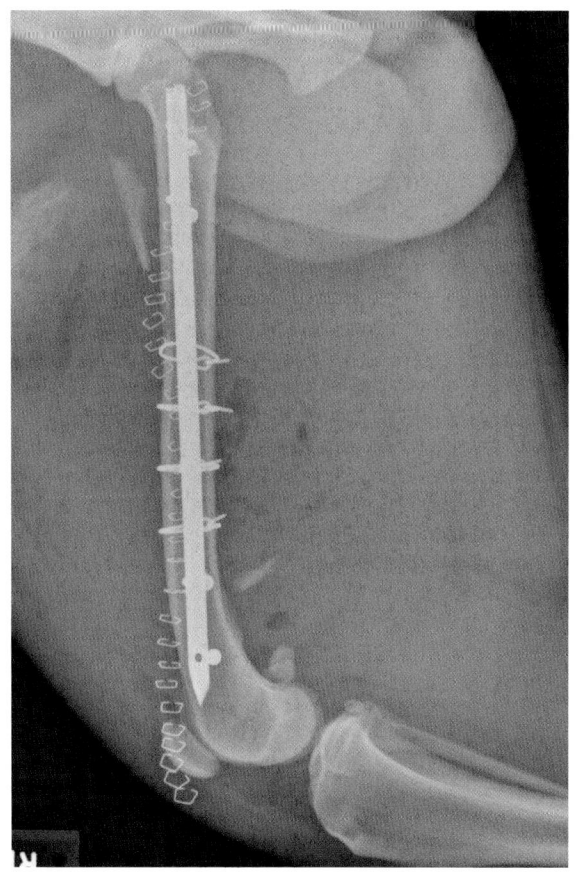

Figure 92.1 Improper penetration of a screw into an interlocking nail. The most distal screw is not engaging the interlocking nail on these postoperative radiographs, requiring immediate revision.

scrutiny of the images is necessary for identifying implant-related complications. Joint palpation during range of motion maneuvers may detect implants penetrating the articular surface or crossing the joint. Poorly placed implants that do not affect the outcome, such as short screws through a plate where there are more than enough cortices purchased for stability, do not need to be removed. Similarly, overly long implants that do not interfere with joints or vital structures are often safe to leave in place (Figure 92.2). Although

Complications in Small Animal Surgery, First Edition. Edited by Dominique Griffon and Annick Hamaide.
© 2016 John Wiley & Sons, Inc. Published 2016 by John Wiley & Sons, Inc.
Companion website: www.wiley.com/go/griffon/complications

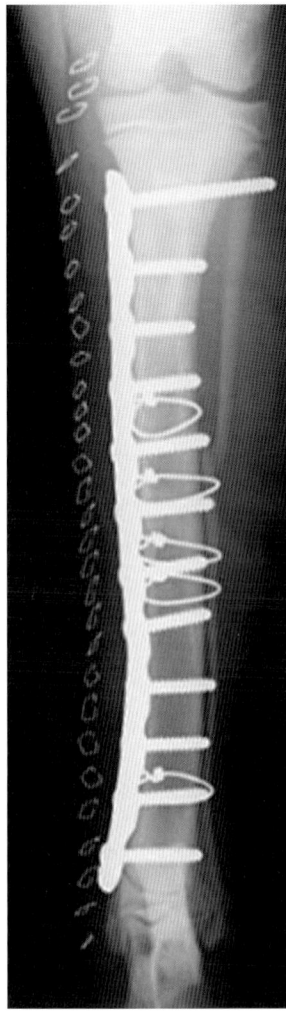

Figure 92.2 Although the proximal screw is overly long, it does not interfere with joints or vital structures and is left in place.

it is tempting to accept poorly placed implants with the potential for impaired function, stability, or appearance after a long surgical procedure, it is best to correct the problem at this time rather than adopt a "wait and see" attitude.

Treatment

The decision to revise the positioning of an implant depends on the clinical relevance of the poor placement in terms of bone healing and overall function of the limb (Figure 92.3)

Treatment is best done immediately and consists of repositioning, removing, or replacing the offending implant(s). IM pins that miss the distal medullary canal must be redirected, which requires a return to the operating room and aseptic conditions. IM pins that penetrate the joint can often be retracted (Figure 92.4). IM pins that are not driven far enough distally to seat in the metaphysis can be driven farther if the excess pin has not been cut before the problem has been identified. In either case, the area surrounding the extension of the pin from the soft tissues, and the pin must be kept sterile. The pin is secured with a pin chuck and either withdrawn or advanced appropriately. It is helpful to measure the distance needed for pin movement and place a marker on the pin to use as a guide for movement.

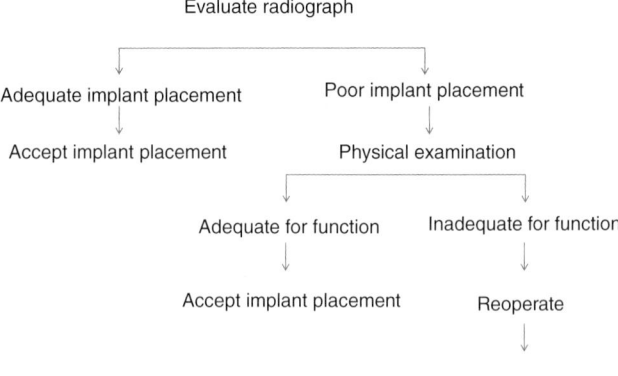

Figure 92.3 Algorithm for the management of poor placement of implants.

Fixation pins or wires that invade either a joint or the fracture must be replaced, avoiding these areas. Fixator pins that do not fully penetrate the far cortices or alternatively penetrate excessive muscle on the far side of the bone should be either driven farther or retracted into the appropriate position. Excessive manipulation of the pin may lead to premature pin loosening. Fixation pins occasionally penetrate adjacent vessels, although this complication is

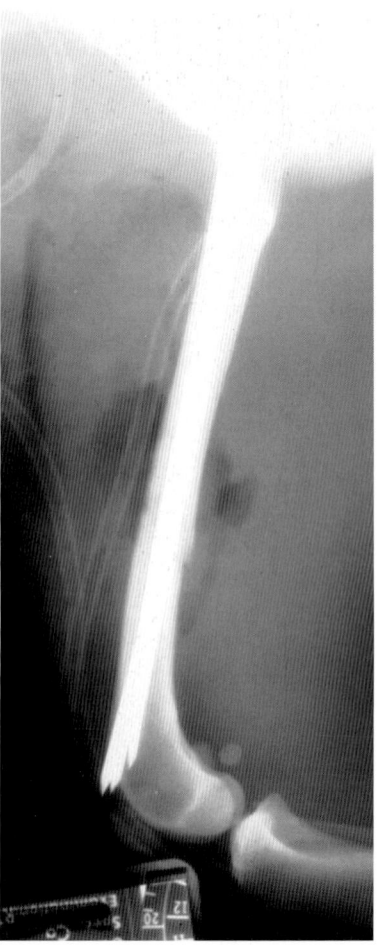

Figure 92.4 Improper intramedullary (IM) pin placement in the femur. The IM pins are penetrating the articular surface and must be retracted.

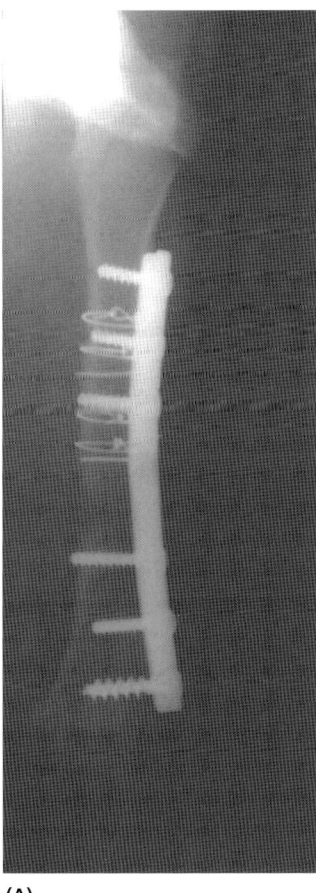 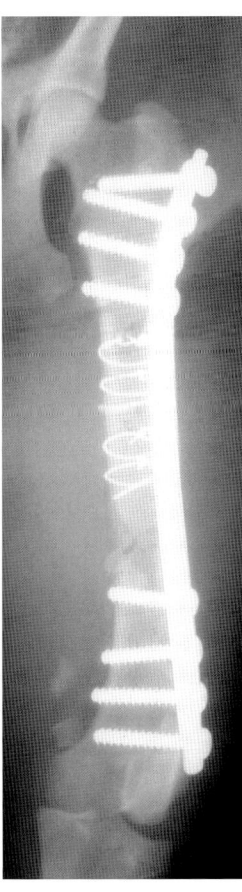

(A)   **(B)**

Figure 92.5 **A,** The femoral fracture was initially stabilized with a bone plate that is too short and bone screws that do not penetrate both cortices. **B,** The dog was returned to surgery, and the implants were replaced.

usually noted some time after surgery. Persistent bleeding from a pin site is treated with pin removal and pressure. Occasionally, surgical exploration and ligation of the vessel are required.

Plates and screws inappropriately applied must be replaced. Short plates are replaced with plates of appropriate length. Traditional plate screws (nonlocking) that do not penetrate the far cortex are also replaced with screws of appropriate length (Figure 92.5). Poorly contoured plates are recontoured and replaced. Similarly, bone screws that miss the hole in an interlocking nails should be replaced.

Implants that interfere with physeal function such as screws across the physis or a plate or external fixator bridging the physis should be repositioned if there is potential for physeal growth.

Outcome

The prognosis after correction of implant placement is identical to that of an uncomplicated fracture. However, reoperating may further compromise vascularity, delaying healing or increasing the opportunity for infection.

Prevention

- Careful preoperative planning
- Careful attention to detail during surgery
- Intraoperative evaluation of limb alignment based on palpation of bony landmarks and joints

- Intraoperative evaluation of the range of motion of joints adjacent to the fracture
- Intraoperative radiographs or fluoroscopy
- Use a locking plate if bicortical penetration of three screws on each side of the fracture will lead to joint penetration or affect function (e.g., distal humeral fractures).

Relevant literature

Improper IM pin placement can cause articular damage, irritate soft tissues, and affect bone development in immature animals. Retrograde pin placement results in invasion of the articular surface in the tibia, and to a lesser extent the humerus, and should be avoided in the tibia and used cautiously in the humerus (Dixon *et al.* 1994; Sissener *et al.* 2005). Retrograde pin placement in feline tibias does not interfere with the articular surface but does skewer the patellar tendon (Payne *et al.* 2005). Placement of an IM pin close to the femoral head in immature dogs may cause coxa vara development of the femoral neck. Improper use of IM pins results in instability at the fracture and ultimately migration of the pin (Johnson 2013).

External fixator pins must be placed through safe corridors to avoid major nerves and vessels and excessive soft tissue damage (Marti and Miller 1994a, 1994b). Blunt-tipped pins used with predrilling techniques minimize soft tissue irritation. Care should be taken to drive the pin to the appropriate position rather than driving it too far and then pulling back because this method of insertion weakens the bone–implant interface. Descriptions of the optimal numbers of pins and appropriate placement of fixation pins in the bone are available (Johnson 2013).

Descriptions of proper plate and screw application are also available (Johnson 2013). Most complications resulting from improper implant placement involve misdirection of bone screws. For example, a significant percentage of screws stabilizing iliosacral luxations in cats were either malpositioned or exited the sacrum ventrally (Shales *et al.* 2010). Fluoroscopically guided screw placement improves visualization of the implant location during surgery (Tonks *et al.* 2008). Similarly, bone screws used with interlocking nails may be misdirected despite the use of a jig (Díaz-Bertrana *et al.* 2005).

By necessity, implants invade the physis when stabilizing Salter I and II fractures. Research has shown that whereas smooth implants may traverse perpendicular to the normal physis with minimal effect, threaded implants impede growth (von Pfeil *et al.* 2009). However, most traumatized physes are irreversibly damaged and appear to lose function regardless of implant placement (Johnson *et al.* 1994). Premature physeal closure has varying effects on the animal depending on physis location and growth potential. Whereas animals with stabilized distal femoral physeal fractures may have a significantly shortened bone, animals with physeal fractures of the distal humerus have no deformity or clinically relevant length discrepancy regardless of implant penetration of the physis (Berg *et al.* 1984; Lefebvre *et al.* 2008).

References

Berg, R.J., Egger, E.L., Konde, L.J., et al. (1984) Evaluation of prognostic factors for growth following distal femoral physeal injuries in 17 dogs. *Veterinary Surgery* 13, 172-180.

Díaz-Bertrana, M.C., Durall I., Puchol, J.L., et al. (2005) Interlocking nail treatment of long-bone fractures in cats: 33 cases (1995-2004). *Veterinary and Comparative Orthopaedics and Traumatology* 18 (3), 119-126.

Dixon, B.C., Tomlinson, J.L., Wagner-Mann, C.C. (1994) Effects of three intramedullary pinning techniques on proximal pin location and articular damage in the canine tibia. *Veterinary Surgery* 23, 448-453.

Johnson, A.L. (2013) Fundamentals of orthopedic surgery and fracture management. In Fossum, T.W. (ed.) *Small Animal Surgery,* 4th edn. Elsevier Mosby, St. Louis, pp. 1033-1105.

Johnson, J.M., Johnson, A.L., Eurell, J.A. (1994) Histological appearance of naturally occurring canine physeal fractures. *Veterinary Surgery* 23 (2), 81-86.

Lefebvre, J.B., Robertson, T.R.A., Baines S.J., et al. (2008) Assessment of humeral length in dogs after repair of Salter-Harris type IV fracture of the lateral part of the humeral condyle. *Veterinary Surgery* 37, 545–551.

Marti, J.M., Miller, A. (1994a) Delimitation of safe corridors for the insertion of external fixator pins in the dog 1: hindlimb. *Journal of Small Animal Practice* 35 (1), 16-23.

Marti, J.M., Miller A. (1994b) Delimitation of safe corridors for the insertion of external fixator pins in the dog 2: forelimb. *Journal of Small Animal Practice* 35 (2), 78-85.

Payne, J., McLaughlin, R., Silverman, E. (2005) Comparison of normograde and retrograde intramedullary pinning of feline tibias. *Journal of the American Animal Hospital Association* 41 (1), 56-60.

Shales, C., Moores, A., Kulendra, E., et al. (2010) Stabilization of sacroiliac luxation in 40 cats using screws inserted in lag fashion. *Veterinary Surgery* 39 (6), 696-700.

Sissener T.R., Jones E., Langley-Hobbs S.J. (2005) Effects of three intramedullary pinning techniques on pin location and articular damage in the canine humerus. *Veterinary and Comparative Orthopaedics and Traumatology* 18 (3), 153-156.

Tonks, C.A., Tomlinson J.L., Cook J.L.(2008) Evaluation of closed reduction and screw fixation in lag fashion of sacroiliac fracture-luxations. *Veterinary Surgery* 37 (7), 603-607.

von Pfeil, D.J., DeCamp, C.E. (2009) The epiphyseal plate: physiology, anatomy, and trauma. *Compendium on Continuing Education for the Practicing Veterinarian* 31 (8), E1-E11.

93 Limb Shortening

Ann Johnson

College of Veterinary Medicine, University of Illinois, Champaign, IL, USA

Definition

Limb shortening after diaphyseal fracture is generally secondary to loss of bone length in the fractured bone, which can be caused by bone loss in open comminuted fractures, bone resorption in nonunions, or uncorrected bone segment overriding. Physeal closure after injury in immature animals also causes limb shortening, which is often combined with angular and rotational deformity. The surgeon must make the decision regarding the clinical significance of the resultant limb shortening. Functionally, most dogs and cats do well with short limbs because they compensate by extending the elbow or stifle (Franczuszki *et al.* 1987) and occasionally benefit from compensatory growth of adjacent long bones after premature physeal closure (Schulz and Davidson 1999) (Figure 93.1).

Risk factors

- Severely comminuted fractures
- Nonunions
- Chronic untreated overriding fractures
- Premature physeal closure after fracture

Diagnosis

The diagnosis of limb shortening is made during physical evaluation, especially if the limb is short enough to cause the animal difficulty ambulating. However, orthogonal radiographs are necessary to identify the etiology of the short limb. In general, radiographs are made of the affected bone and the contralateral bone for length comparisons. Lateral radiographic views are most accurate for measuring length of the femur, humerus, and tibia. Cranial caudal views may be used of the radius and metacarpals or metatarsals. Similar landmarks are identified on the affected and contralateral bone and length measurements made. Subtracting the affected bone length from the contralateral bone length determines the amount of bone shortening. Often bone shortening is combined with angular deformities. Accurate evaluation of the deformity is needed to determine treatment.

Treatment

The treatment is based on the animal's function and appearance. If the animal adequately compensates for length discrepancy and

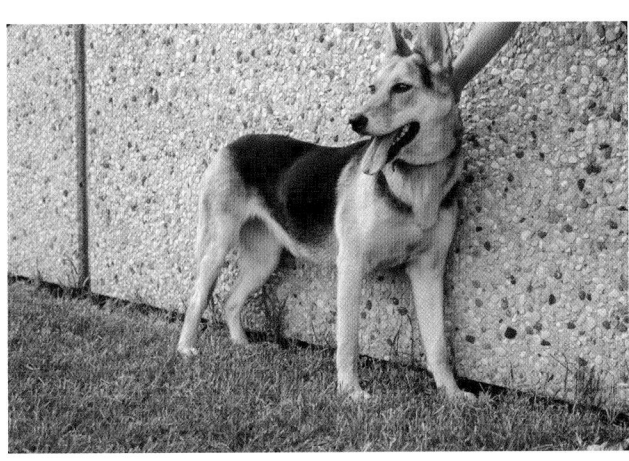

(A)

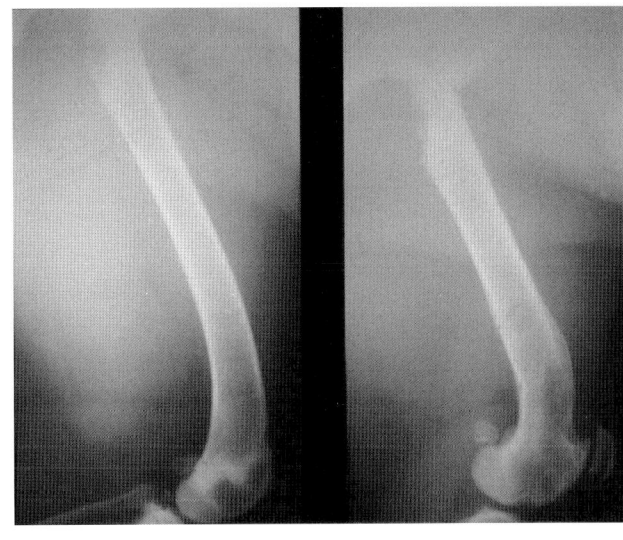

(B)

Figure 93.1 A, German shepherd dog 6 months after a distal femoral physeal fracture treated when the dog was 4 months of age. **B,** Although there is a significant length discrepancy between femurs, the dog was functional and not treated for the problem.

Complications in Small Animal Surgery, First Edition. Edited by Dominique Griffon and Annick Hamaide.
© 2016 John Wiley & Sons, Inc. Published 2016 by John Wiley & Sons, Inc.
Companion website: www.wiley.com/go/griffon/complications

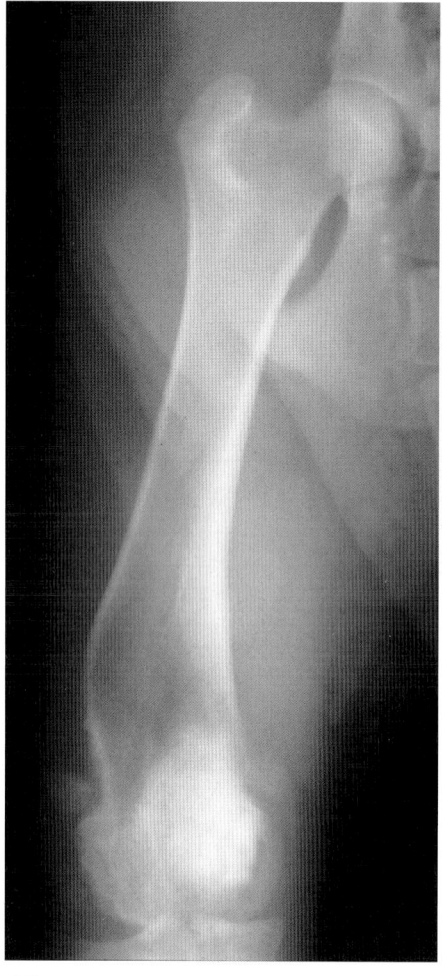

(A)

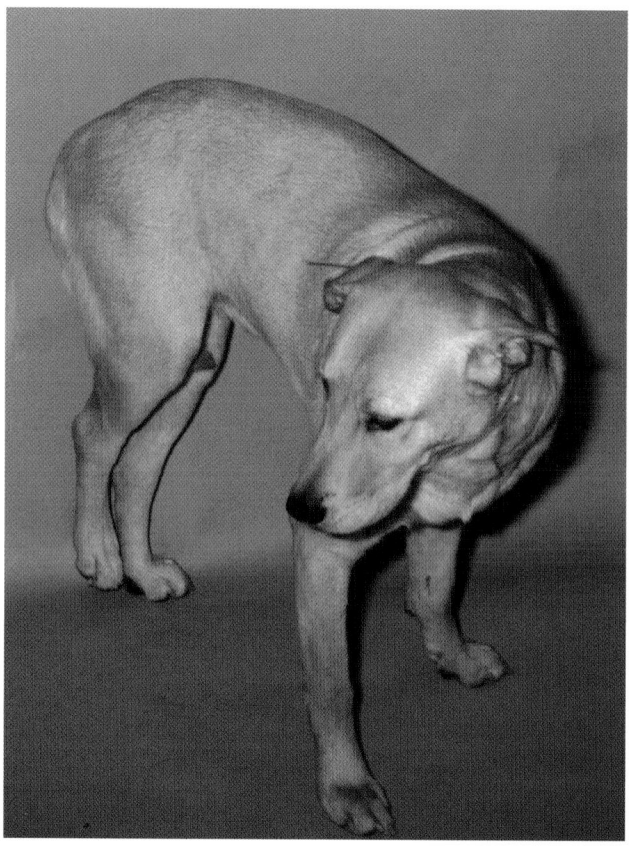

(B)

Figure 93.2 Premature closure of a fractured distal femoral physis. **A,** Combined angular deformity and length discrepancy are noted on preoperative radiographs. **B,** Preoperative appearance of the dog: the abnormal stance was associated with severe lameness.

is functional, no treatment is necessary (see Figure 93.1). If function is a problem, a corrective osteotomy should be performed (Figure 93.2). The osteotomy chosen will depend on the deformity. Lengthening osteotomies may be one-stage or continuous procedures. One-stage correction is often used when correcting a concurrent angular deformity (Figure 93.3). However, the length discrepancy is usually minimally affected (Quinn *et al.* 2000) Whereas one-stage length correction is limited by the soft tissues, continuous distraction overcomes this limitation and provides for new bone formation during distraction osteogenesis. With distraction osteogenesis, bone lengthening can be achieved unifocally or bifocally (Figure 93.4). Unifocal lengthening occurs when a single osteotomy is created in the bone. Bifocal bone lengthening occurs when two osteotomy sites are created in the bone, effectively doubling the rate of distraction.

Growing animals with premature physeal closure in either the radius or ulna may be treated initially with an ostectomy and fat graft of the affected bone to allow unrestricted growth of the unaffected bone. A corrective osteotomy is usually necessary after growth has ceased to obtain the final result.

Outcome

The outcome depends on function at time of diagnosis and treatment options. The ability to restore the length of the bone is best when dealing with acute overriding or comminuted fractures. Chronic limb shortening results in adaptation of soft tissues that will ultimately limit the ability to lengthen the limb. If the dog is functional at diagnosis, then the outcome will be good. If surgery is needed, appearance and function are generally improved, but the prognosis for return to normal should be guarded (see Figure 93.4). The amount of length that may be regained ultimately depends on the ability of soft tissues to adapt to the elongation. Gradual distraction improves this adaptation, but contracture of adjacent joints may develop during treatment. In humans, the outcome is improved if lengthening does not exceed 20% of the bone length (Aston *et al.* 2009). Adjusting the location of the osteotomy relative to adjacent joints and placement of an intramedullary nails have been used to prevent complications. Severe shortenings may be treated by staged lengthening. In veterinary medicine, the goal of the treatment is to reduce limb length discrepancy within the compensatory range for small animals while avoiding

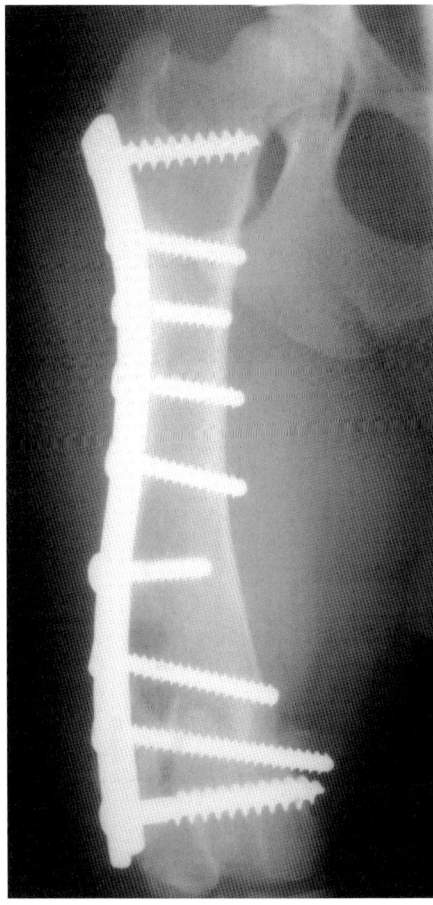

(A)

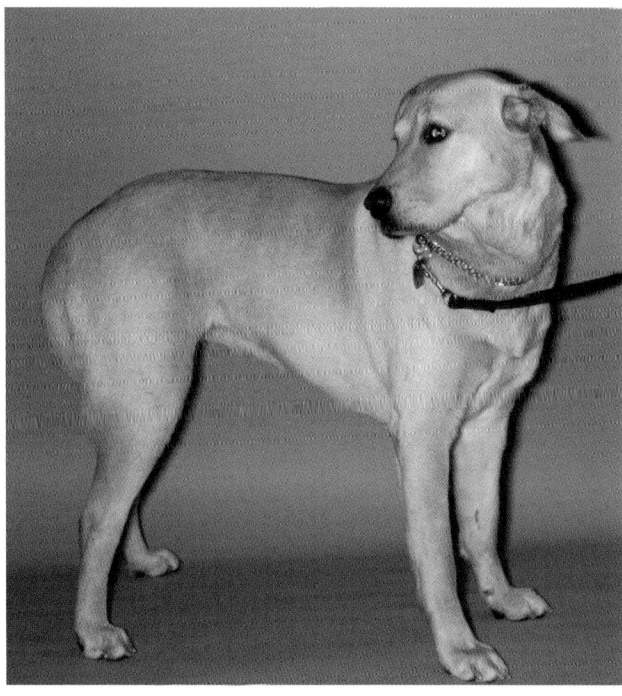

(B)

Figure 93.3 Treatment of the limb shortening and angulation illustrated in Figure 93.2. **A,** Radiograph of the femur after an open wedge osteotomy was used to correct the varus deformity and improved the length of the bone. **B,** Postoperative appearance of the dog with regained function of the limb.

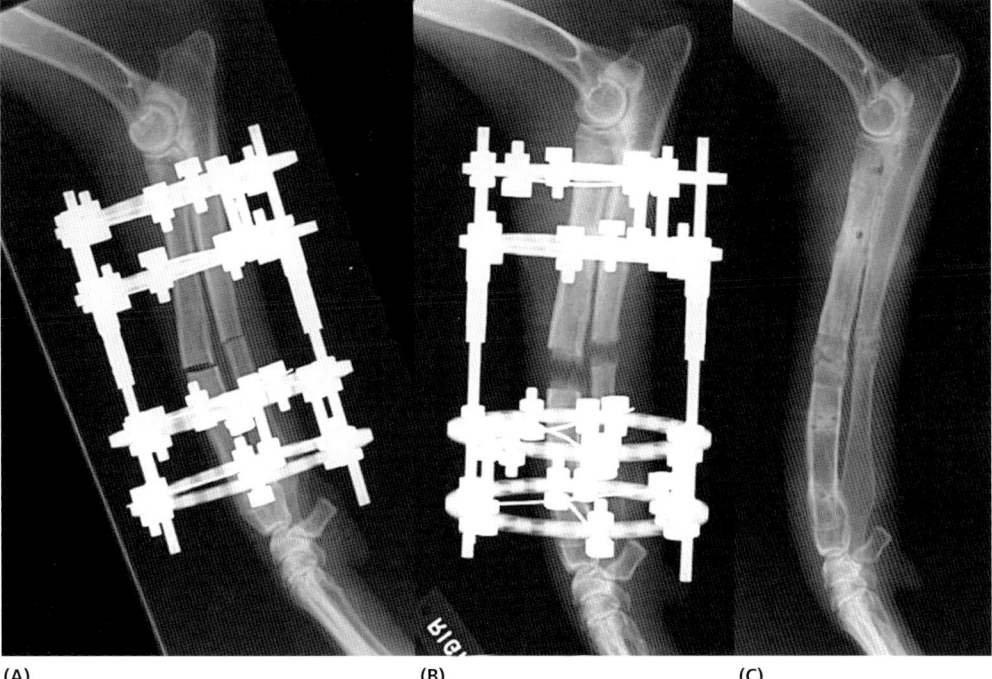

(A)   (B)   (C)

Figure 93.4 Treatment of a dog with premature closure of the distal radial growth plate with distraction osteogenisis. **A,** Postoperative radiographs after acute correction of the rotational and angular deformity followed by placement of an Ilizarov apparatus. **B,** Gradual distraction leads to regenerate bone formation 3 weeks after initial surgery. **C,** Removal of the apparatus at 6 weeks and placement of a splint to complete the consolidation.

complications such as soft tissue contracture and reduced motion of adjacent joints.

Prevention

- Attention to reestablishing bone length during fracture repair
- Other causes of bone shortening such as untreated malunions, nonunions, and physeal injury may not have been preventable depending on type of injury and owner decisions.

Relevant literature

Most of the relevant literature regarding limb shortening discusses treatment of growth deformities caused by physeal injury or congenital defects using the principles established by Ilizarov for distraction osteogenesis (Ferretti 1991; Stallings *et al.* 1998). The most frequent use of the technique is treating antebrachial deformities although it is applicable to other bones (Marcellin-Little *et al.* 1998; Lewis *et al.* 1999; Theyse *et al.* 2005; Wendelburg *et al.* 2011). Physeal fractures of the distal femur can result in limb length discrepancy and angular deformity, affecting ambulation. Corrective osteotomy with lengthening can restore function (Wendelburg *et al.* 2011). Distraction techniques have also been used to treat radial hemimelia and agenesis and to lengthen metatarsals (Rahal *et al.* 2005; McKee and Reynolds 2007; Hancock *et al.* 2003).

Circular external fixators are commonly used for stabilization because of the flexibility in construction and ease of access during distraction but are best used on bones below the elbow and stifle. Hybrid fixators have been combined with interlocking nails to achieve continuous distraction of the femur; however, the complications were significant (Wendelburg *et al.* 2011).

References

Aston, W.J., Clader, P.R., Baker, D., et al. (2009) Lengthening of the short femur using the Ilizarov technique: a single surgeon series. *Journal of Bone & Joint Surgery* 91 (7), 962-967.

Ferretti, A. (1991) The application of the Ilizarov technique to veterinary medicine. In Maiocchi, A.B., Aronson, J. (eds.) *Operative Principles of Ilizarov*. Williams & Wilkins, Baltimore, pp. 551-575.

Franczuszki, D, Chalman, J.A., Butler, H.C., et al. (1987) Postoperative effects of experimental femoral shortening in the mature dog. *Journal of the American Animal Hospital Association* 23, 429-435.

Hancock, R.B., Cook, J.L., Tomlinson, J.L. (2003) Distraction osteogenesis for treatment of premature physeal closure and shortening of the third and fourth metatarsals of a dog. *Journal of the American Animal Hospital Association* 39 (1), 97-103.

Lewis, D.D., Radasch, R.M., Beale, B.S., et al. (1999) Initial clinical experience with the IMEX TM circular external skeletal fixation system, part II: use in bone lengthening and correction of angular and rotational deformities. *Veterinary and Comparative Orthopaedics and Traumatology* 12, 118-127.

Marcellin-Little, D.J., Ferretti, A., Roe, S.C., et al. (1998) Hinged Ilizarov external fixation for correction of antebrachial deformities. *Veterinary Surgery* 27, 231-245.

McKee, W.M., Reynolds, J. (2007) Ulnocarpal arthrodesis and limb lengthening for the management of radial agenesis in a dog. *Journal of Small Animal Practice* 48 (10), 591-595.

Quinn, M.K., Ehrhart, N., Johnson, A.L., et al. (2000) Realignment of the radius in canine antebrachial growth deformities treated with corrective osteotomy and bilateral (Type II) external fixation. *Veterinary Surgery* 29, 558-563.

Rahal, .S.C, Volpi, R.S., Ciani, R.B., et al. (2005) Use of the Ilizarov method of distraction osteogenesis for the treatment of radial hemimelia in a dog. *Journal of the American Veterinary Medical Association* 226 (1), 65-68.

Schulz, K.S., Davidson, E. (1999) Compensatory humeral overgrowth in a dog. *Veterinary and Comparative Orthopaedics and Traumatology* 12, 92-96.

Stallings, J.T., Lewis, D., Welch, R., et al. (1998) An introduction to distraction osteogenesis and the principles of the Ilizarov method. *Veterinary and Comparative Orthopaedics and Traumatology* 11, 59-67.

Theyse, L.F., Voorhout, G., Hazewinkel, H.A. (2005) Prognostic factors in treating antebrachial growth deformities with a lengthening procedure using a circular external skeletal fixation system in dogs. *Veterinary Surgery* 34 (5), 424-435.

Wendelburg, K.M., Lewis, D.D., Sereda, C.W., et al. (2011) Use of an interlocking nail-hybrid fixator construct for distal femoral deformity correction in three dogs. *Veterinary and Comparative Orthopaedics and Traumatology* 24 (3), 236-245.

94 Implant Failure

Ann Johnson

College of Veterinary Medicine, University of Illinois, Champaign, IL, USA

Definition

Implant failure can be defined as either failure of the bone–implant surface, resulting in implant motion and loss of fracture stability or by mechanical failure of the implant such as bending or breaking. Implant failure can precipitate serious complications in fracture management if failure occurs before adequate bone healing. In some patients, these problems can be anticipated and avoided by adequate fracture planning preoperatively, good technical skills during surgery, and critical review of the radiographs immediately after surgery. However, the problems are addressed in most patients as they are discovered.

Examples of implant failure defined by loss of the bone–implant integrity include loose and migrating intramedullary (IM) pins, Kirschner wires, and external fixation pins. Smooth implants secure the bone by frictional hold and are susceptible to forces generated by motion. IM pins that inadequately stabilize a fracture often loosen at the pin–bone interface and migrate in response to fracture motion, which in turn causes more instability at the fracture (Johnson 2013) (Figure 94.1). Likewise, weight bearing generates forces on an external fixator, increasing the strain environment around smooth external fixator pins and, to a lesser extent, threaded external fixator pins, resulting in bone resorption and implant instability (Palmer *et al.* 1992) (Figure 94.2). Infection also causes bone resorption around implants (Figure 94.3).

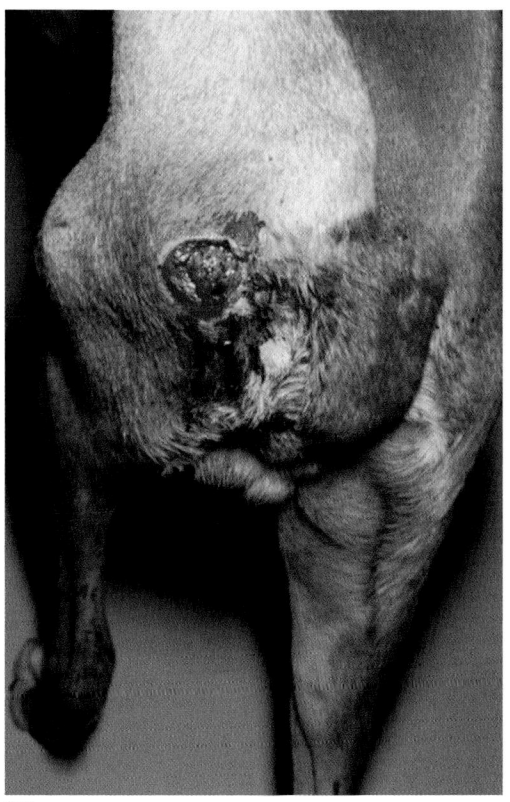

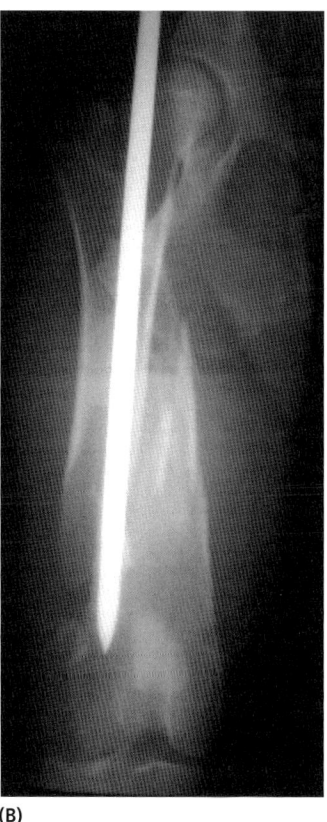

(A) (B)

Figure 94.1 Wound created by an intramedullary pin migrating from the femur. **A**, Gross photo. **B**, Radiograph.

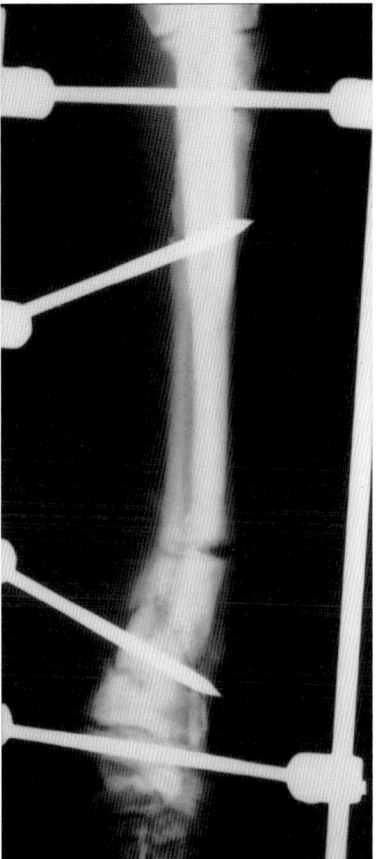
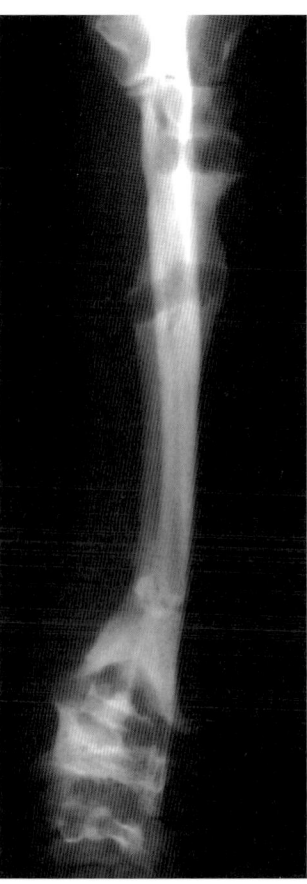

Figure 94.2 Pin track osteolysis occurring with smooth external fixator pins and a minimally constructed frame.

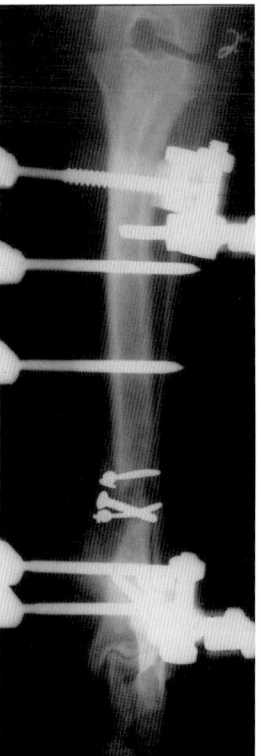
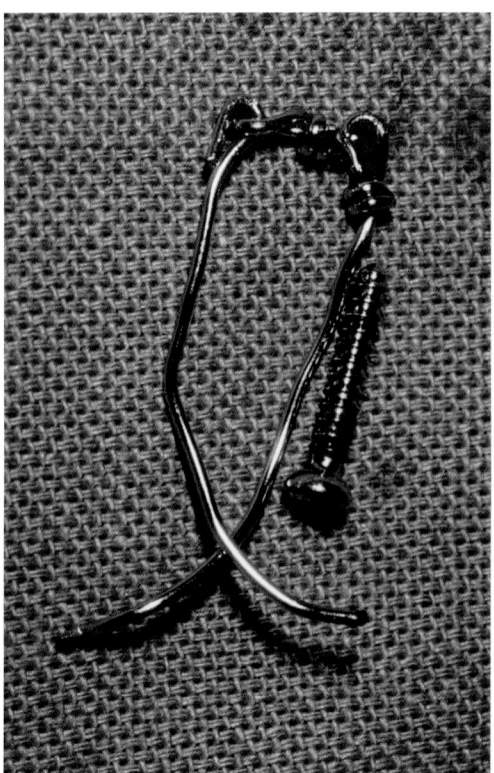
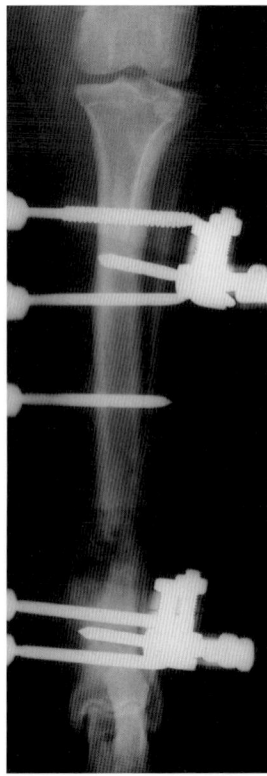

Figure 94.3 Osteomyelitis in the tibial diaphysis resulted in bone resorption and loose implants at the fracture site. The loose implants were removed and a cancellous bone graft added. Note the fixation frame was stable and left in place.

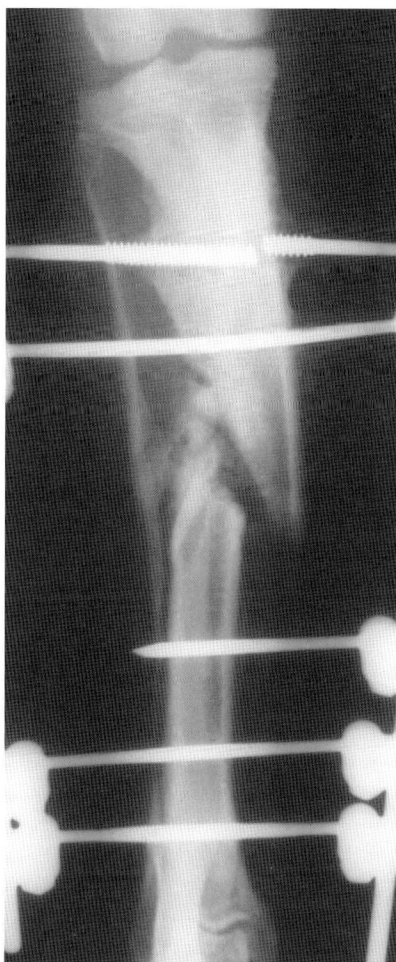

Figure 94.4 Broken external fixator pin resulting from an overactive dog and a fixator that did not have enough pin support in the proximal segment.

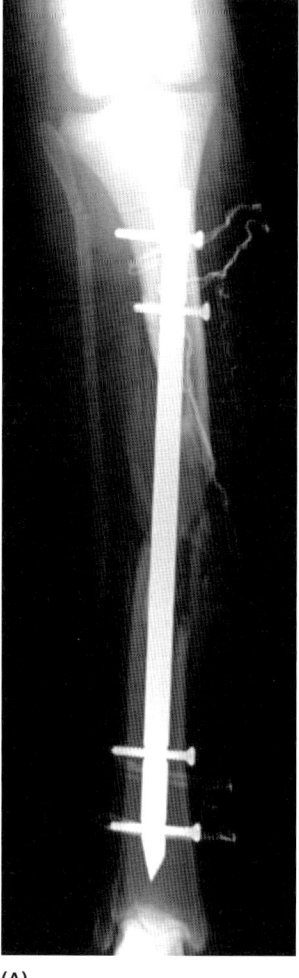
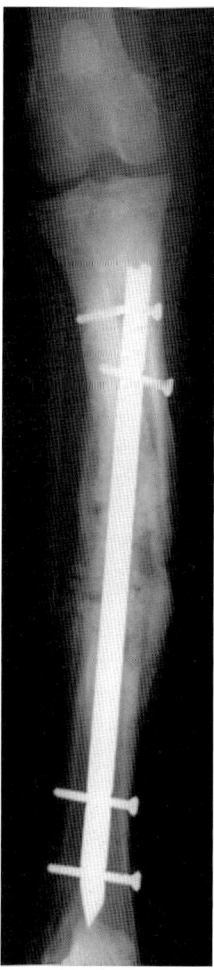

(A)   **(B)**

Figure 94.5 Postoperative (**A**) and 15-week follow-up (**B**) radiographs of a comminuted tibial fracture in a Great Pyrenees dog that was not confined after surgery. Although the proximal screw broke, the fracture healed. The malalignment was present on the postoperative radiograph and not subsequent to screw failure.

Mechanical failure of implants may occur when the implant is subjected to an acute catastrophically high load but more often results from cyclic load causing fatigue failure of the implant when fracture healing is delayed (Goh et al. 2009). Most implant failures occur at weak areas of the implant or implant construct. For example, threaded IM pins or fixation pins may break if the stress is concentrated area at the junction of the thread and shaft (Figure 94.4). Bone screws used to secure an interlocking nail can fail if the animal is overactive as the screw is weaker than the nail (Figure 94.5). Bone screws securing a plate may break at the head and shaft junction if load is too great, particularly the 3.5-mm cortex screws used with the 3.5 broad plate (Figure 94.6). Bone screws used as lag screws without plate support may break if there is delayed healing (Figure 94.7). Bone plates fail either by plastic deformation when subjected to a high loads soon after surgery or fatigue when subjected to chronic excessive cyclic loads occurring when healing is delayed (Goh et al. 2009). Bone plate and interlocking nail failure generally occur at a screw hole in an area of the implant located near or over the fracture (Figure 94.8).

Risk factors

General risk factors for implant failure
- Fixation not adequate mechanically for the fracture or the patient
- Overactive patient
- Poor owner compliance

Risk factors for implant loosening
- Fractures fixed solely with IM pins or Kirschner wires
- External fixators secured with smooth fixation pins
- External fixators that are minimally constructed
- Bone screws securing a plate to the ilium after triple pelvic osteotomy
- Infection

Risk factors for implant breaking
- End threaded IM pins with the thread pin junction located at the fracture or Ellis pins used in external fixators
- Bridging plates
- Humeral condylar fractures stabilized by a bone screw in dogs with incomplete ossification

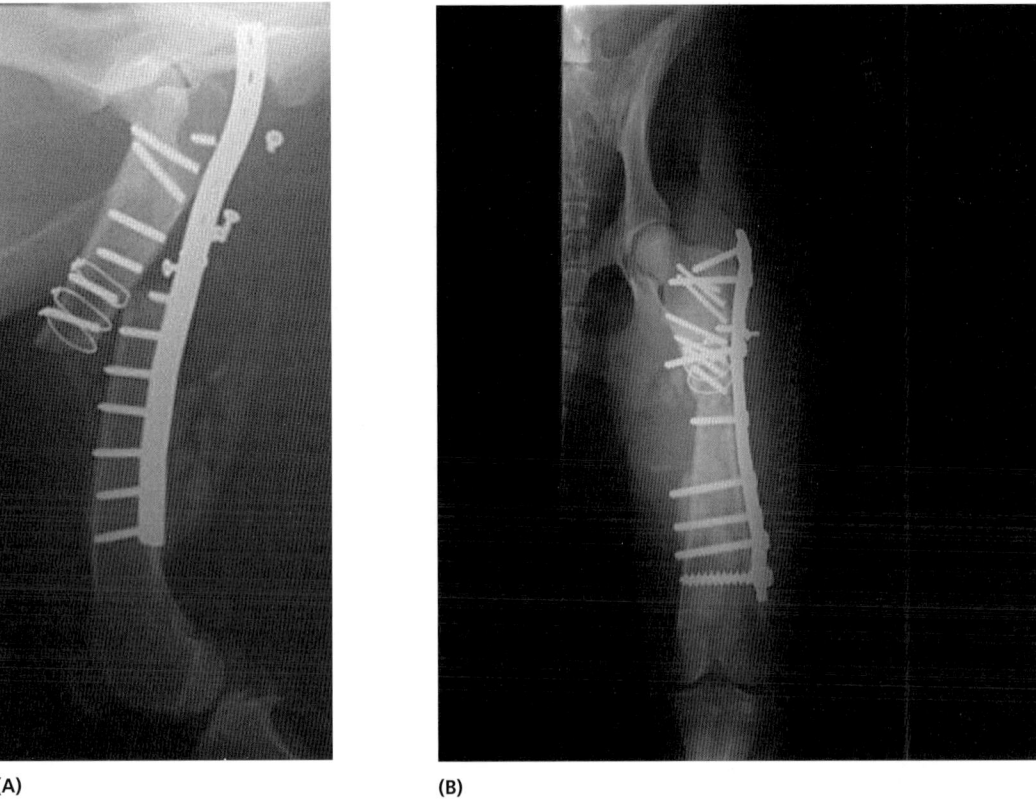

(A)   (B)

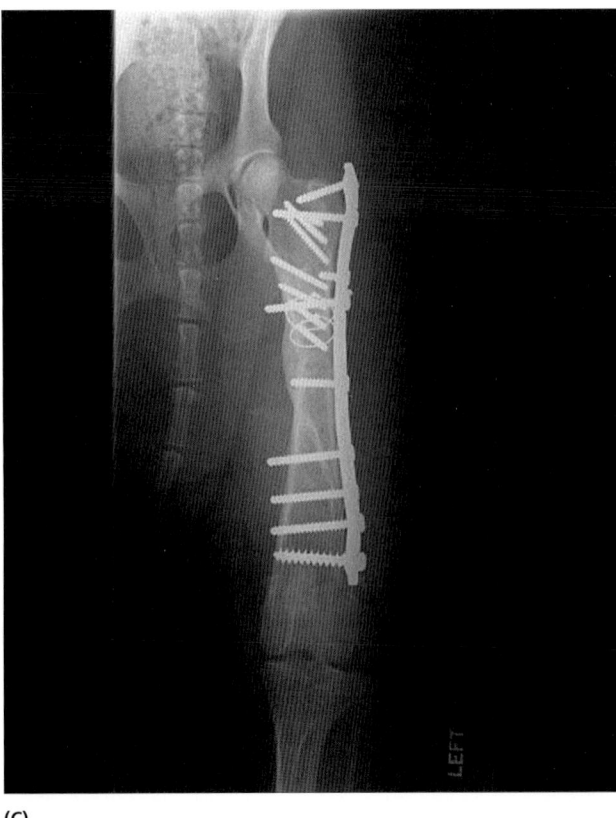

(C)

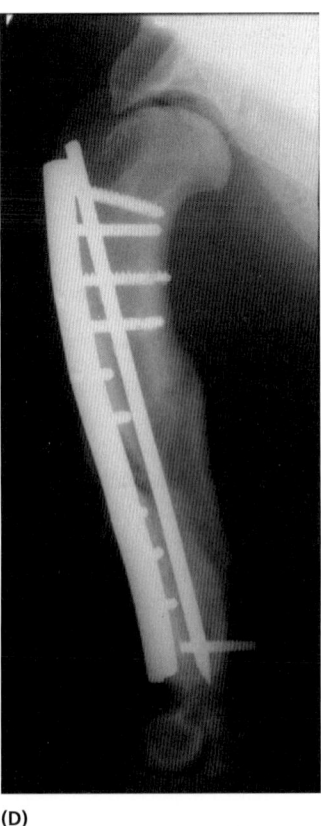

(D)

Figure 94.6 A, Failed 3.5-mm cortex bone screws occurring 2 weeks after surgery. **B**, The 3.5 broad plate was replaced with a 4.5 narrow plate and larger screws. Loose implants were removed, but the shafts of the broken screws were left in place. **C**, The fracture was healed in 12 weeks. **D**, Another broken 3.5-mm cortex screw in a 3.5 broad plate. However, the fracture had healed by the time the problem was discovered, and the implants were not disturbed.

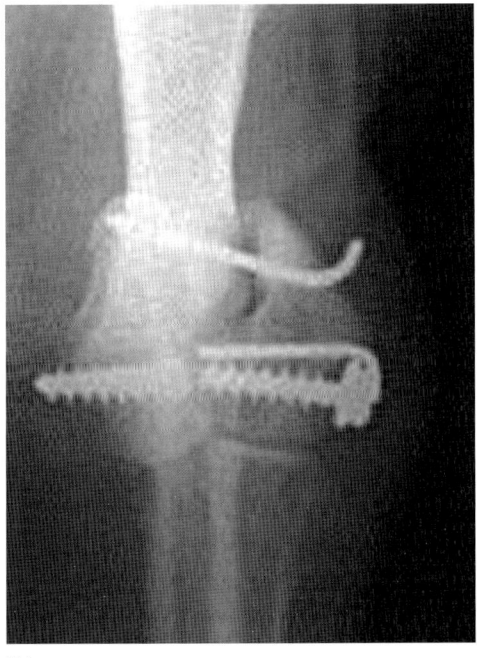

(A)

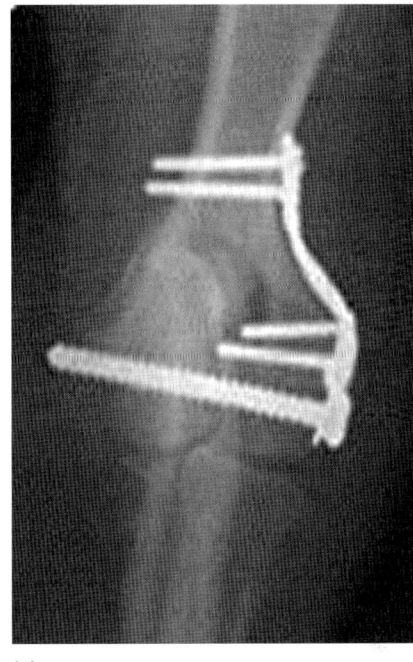

(C)

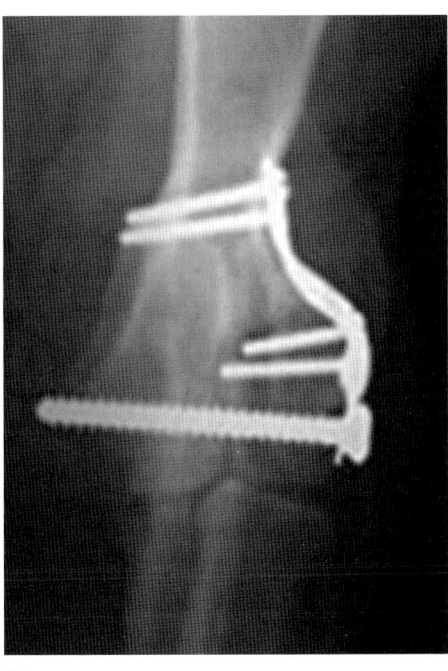

(B)

Figure 94.7 **A**, Failure of a 3.5 cancellous bone screw and Kirschner wire used to stabilize a humeral condylar fracture. **B**, The failed implants were removed and the fracture stabilized with a 3.5-mm cortex screw (larger core) and a small plate. **C**, The fracture is healed at 12 weeks after surgery

Diagnosis

Implant failure is suspected when an animal presents with acute loss of limb function soon after fracture fixation. Additional evidence garnered with physical examination includes limb misalignment, implants protruding from the skin, the loss of or loose external fixation, and palpable fracture instability. Joint palpation during range of motion maneuvers may detect migrating implants penetrating the articular surface or crossing the joint. The diagnosis of implant failure is made after scrutiny of orthogonal radiographs of the

affected bone. Although most failed implants are easily observed, in some cases, multiple additional views may be needed to fully assess implant integrity. Occasionally, follow-up radiographs reveal loose or failed implants even though the fracture is healed and the animal is functional. Examples include pin track osteolysis in external fixators (see Figure 94.2) and internal implants that apparently failed as the fracture healed (see Figure 94.9) or are imbedded in bone without interfering with joints or vital structures (see Figure 94.5 and Figure 94.6).

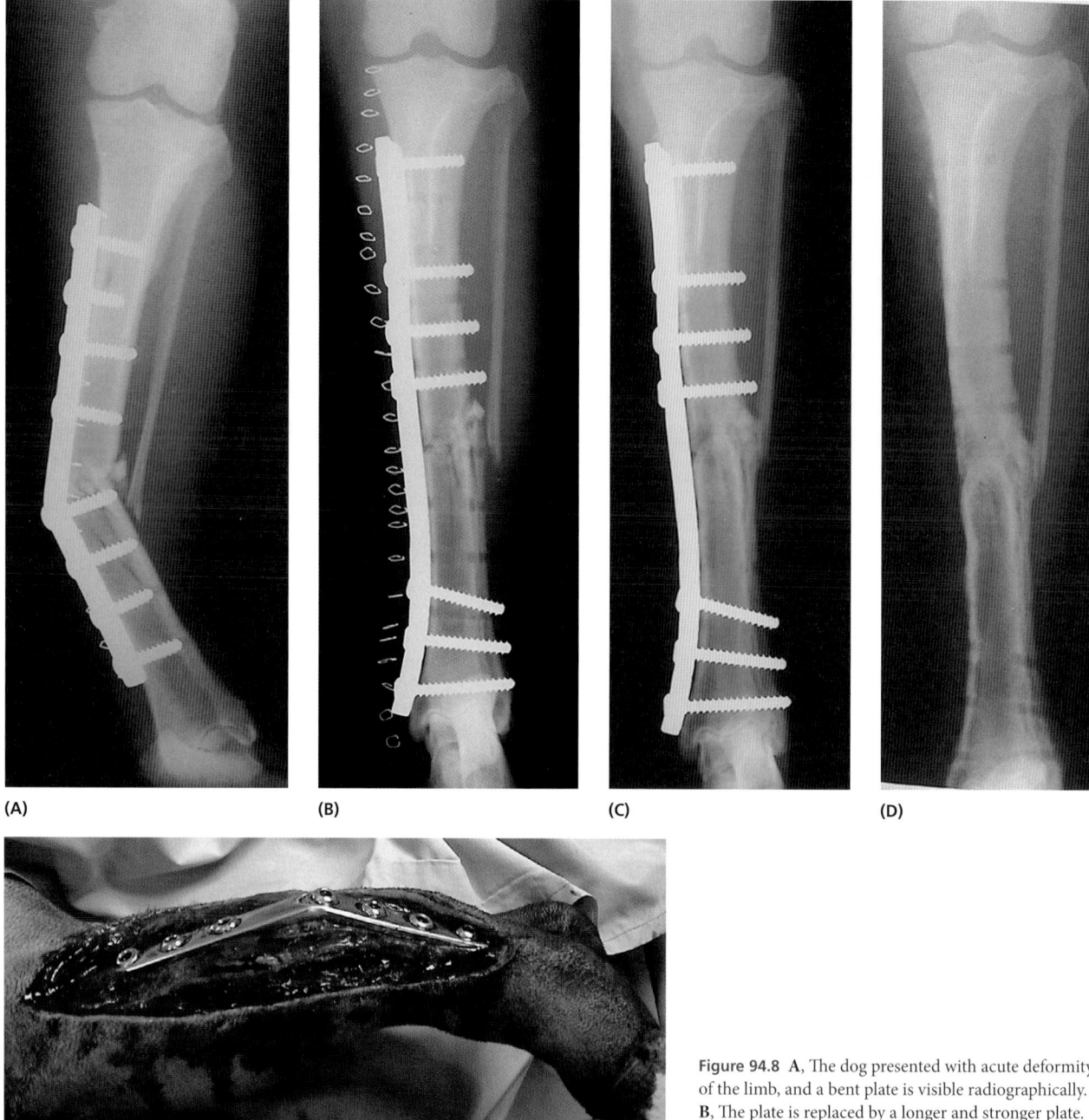

(A)   (B)   (C)   (D)

(E)

Figure 94.8 **A**, The dog presented with acute deformity of the limb, and a bent plate is visible radiographically. **B**, The plate is replaced by a longer and stronger plate. **C**, The fracture is healing at 6 weeks. **D**, The plate was removed at 16 weeks after surgery. **E**, Note that the plate has bent at a screw hole adjacent to the fracture.

Treatment

If the fracture has healed and the failed implant is not interfering with soft tissues or function, then no treatment is required (beyond removal of an external fixator). However, if implant failure has resulted in fracture instability, treatment consists of replacing the affected implant(s) to restore stability and promote bone union. Migrating IM pins or broken pins are removed and the fracture realigned if needed and generally stabilized with a plate. Loose external fixators are replaced if more stability is needed to encourage fracture healing. Broken plates are removed and replaced as are failed bone screws. However, when segments of the screws are buried in bone, the excessive trauma needed to retrieve them is not warranted

unless they are infected. Osteomyelitis is treated as necessary (see Chapter 5) as is nonunion or malunion resulting from the failed implant (see Chapters 94 and 99))

Outcome

The prognosis after implant failure is generally good, especially if the fracture is healed when the implant failure is diagnosed. Even if implant failure has contributed to fracture instability, the prognosis remains good if the fracture can be adequately stabilized and bone healing stimulated with a bone graft. However, care must be taken because reoperating may further compromise vascularity, delaying healing or increasing the opportunity for infection.

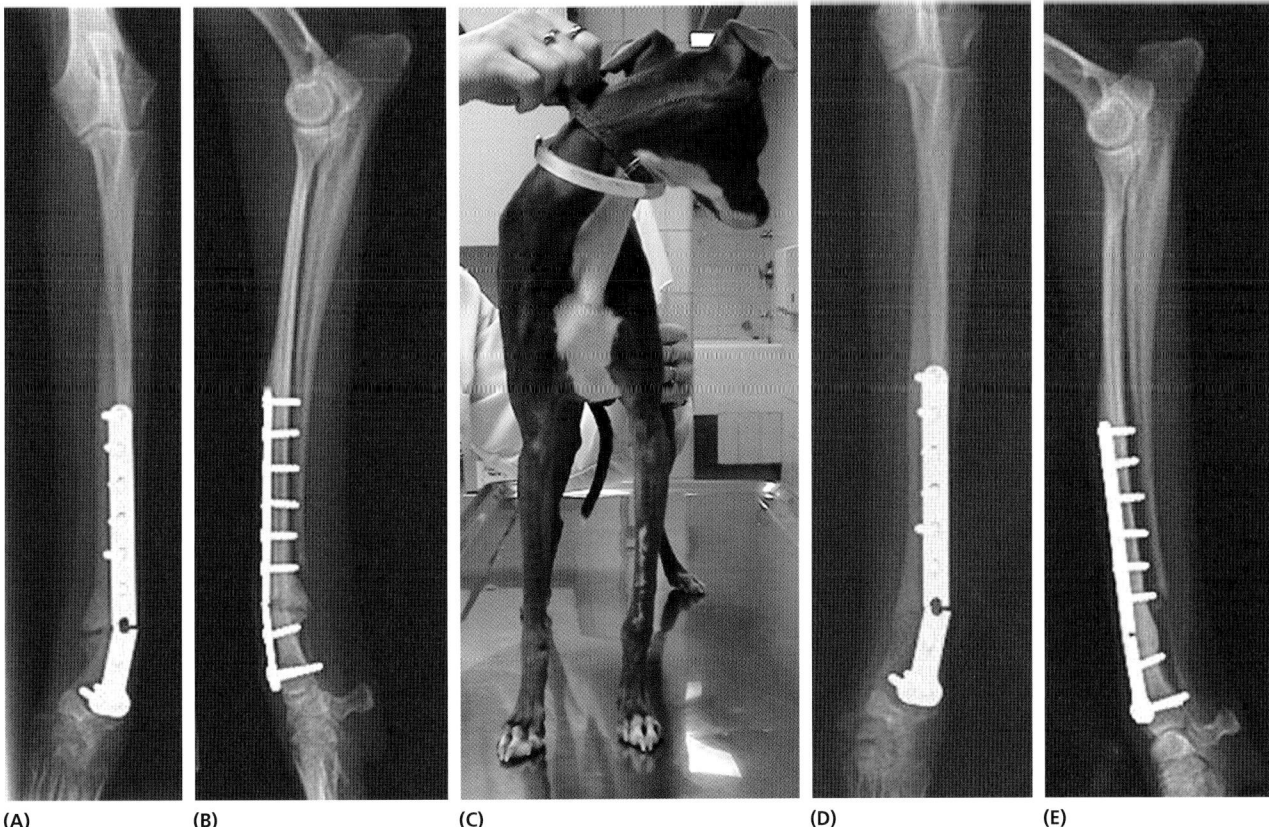

(A)   **(B)**   **(C)**   **(D)**   **(E)**

Figure 94.9 A and **B,** Follow-up radiographs made 4 weeks after surgery show a broken plate. The fracture was stable on palpation, and the dog was weight bearing. **C,** Despite the malalignment, which was not as evident grossly, the decision was made to leave the implant in place. **D** and **E,** Twelve weeks after surgery, the fracture is healed.

Prevention

Implant failure may be minimized by accurately assessing the fracture and the patient and choosing implants appropriate for the mechanical and biologic environment. Additionally, the use of negative-profile threaded pins and smooth pins should be minimized. Critical evaluation of postoperative radiographs to assess the potential for complications is helpful. Good client communication regarding postoperative fracture management is also essential to minimize implant failure.

Relevant literature

Accurate patient fracture assessment, good decision making, and fracture planning will minimize the implant failure. Accurately assessing the mechanical needs of the patient and the fracture allows the surgeon to estimate the strength of the implant to be used. Accurately assessing the biology of the fracture and the patient allows the surgeon to predict the rate of healing and subsequently how long the implants must function (Johnson 2013). If the predicted mechanical load is high (large active dogs with nonreconstructable fractures), the implant will have to carry most, if not all, of the load of weight bearing until callus forms. If, in addition, the animal is older and there is significant soft tissue damage, healing may be delayed, causing reliance on the implant integrity for a long time (Johnson 2013) These animals require strong implants that are secured to the bone with threads. Reliance solely on smooth

implants; minimally constructed fixators; or small, short plates leads to implant failure.

Pin migration occurs most commonly when a single IM pin is used to stabilize a femoral diaphyseal fracture in an adult dog. The IM pin poorly resists axial load and is only effective when a reduced transverse fracture line helps resist axial load. However, the IM pin is secured only by the friction generated in the few areas where pin and bone contact, making it susceptible to torsional forces, causing micromotion at the pin–bone interface, bone resorption, and subsequent pin migration (Dallman *et al.* 1990; Johnson 2013).

Pin track osteolysis and external fixator pin loosening are apparently unavoidable when smooth fixation pins are used exclusively (Johnson and Schaeffer 2008). Pin design, insertion technique, and cyclic implant loading may conspire to create a high strain environment at the pin–bone interface, causing bone resorption and pin loosening. Adding threaded fixation pins to the frame increases the stability, but it is not until all fixation pins used are threaded that the incidence of pin track osteolysis decreases (Johnson and Schaeffer 2008). Although premature pin loosening may cause patient morbidity and fracture instability, leading to delayed or nonunion (Palmer et al. 1992) in many animals, the fracture heals despite pin loosening, and removal of the fixator solves the problem.

Loosening followed by migration commonly affects bone screws securing the cranial portion of the plate to the ilium over the sacroiliac joint after triple pelvic osteotomies and is attributed to the effect of the micromotion of the sacroiliac joint (Simmons *et al.* 2004). This outcome may be minimized by using one of two approaches. One group of investigators found that screws that sufficiently engaged the sacrum were less likely to loosen (Whelan *et al.* 2004). Another group of investigators discovered that cancellous bone screws used to secure the cranial portion of the plate to the ilium without sacral engagement were associated with the lowest frequency of loosening (Doornink *et al.* 2006).

Although pins may bend if subjected to a high load, more often they fatigue after repeated loads. End-threaded IM pins with the thread cut from the core of the pin fail at the threaded–nonthreaded shaft junction, especially if that area is located at the fracture. Negative-profile end-threaded fixation pins also fail at the threaded–nonthreaded shaft junction despite attempts to protect the weak junction within the medullary canal (Palmer and Aron 1990). Positive-profile threaded pins are more resistant to failure but can break at the bone–pin interface with sufficient loads (Palmer *et al.* 1992).

Bone screws also fail if the load is sufficient. Cancellous bone screws have a smaller core-to-thread ratio and are susceptible to failure if unsupported by a plate, especially with delayed healing. The 3.5-mm cortex screws used with 3.5 broad plates appear to be more susceptible to failure as the weak link in the construct. Failed bone screws used to treat incomplete ossification of the humeral condyle have been examined and are thought to be fatigued by chronic micromotion of the condyle (Charles *et al.* 2009).

Plates are susceptible to plastic deformation or breakage early in the postoperative period or fatigue failure over time (Goh *et al.* 2009). The eccentrically placed plate is subjected to cyclic bending and is particularly susceptible to failure at a screw hole adjacent to the fracture gap (Hammel *et al.* 2006). Despite being placed in the medullary canal, interlocking nails are also susceptible to failure if an inadequately sized nail is used or the screw hole is adjacent to the fracture (Aper *et al.* 2003).

References

Aper, R.L., Litsky, A.S., Roe, S.C., et al. (2003) Effect of bone diameter and eccentric loading on fatigue life of cortical screws used with interlocking nails. *American Journal of Veterinary Research* 64, 569-573.

Charles, E.A., Ness, M.G., Yeadon, R. (2009) Failure mode of transcondylar screws used for treatment of incomplete ossification of the humeral condyle in 5 dogs. *Veterinary Surgery* 38, 185-191.

Dallman, M.J., Martin, R.A., Self, B.P., et al. (1990) Rotational strength of double pinning techniques in repair of transverse fractures of femurs in the dog. *American Journal of Veterinary Research* 51 (1), 123-127.

Doornink, M.T., Nieves, M.A., Evans, R. (2006) Evaluation of ilial screw loosening after triple pelvic osteotomy in dogs: 227 cases (1991-1999). *Journal of the American Veterinary Medical Association* 229, 535-541.

Goh, C.S, Santoni, B.G., Puttlitz, C.M., et al. (2009) Comparison of the mechanical behaviors of semicontoured, locking plate–rod fixation and anatomically contoured, conventional plate–rod fixation applied to experimentally induced gap fractures in canine femora. *American Journal of Veterinary Research* 70, 23-29.

Hammel, S.P., Pluhar, E.G., Novo, R.E., et al. (2006) Fatigue analysis of plates used for fracture stabilization in small dogs and cats. *Veterinary Surgery* 35, 573-578.

Johnson, A.L. (2013) Fundamentals of orthopedic surgery and fracture management. In Fossum, T.W. (ed.) *Small Animal Surgery,* 4th edn. Elsevier Mosby, St. Louis, pp. 1033-1105.

Johnson, A., Schaeffer, D.J. (2008) Evolution of the treatment of canine radial and tibial fractures with external fixators. *Veterinary and Comparative Orthopaedics and Traumatology* 21, 26-261.

Palmer, R.H., Aron, D.N. (1990) Ellis pin complications in seven dogs. *Veterinary Surgery* 19, 440-445.

Palmer, R.H., Hulse, D.A., Hyman, W.A. (1992) Principles of bone healing and biomechanics of external skeletal fixation. *Veterinary Clinics of North America: Small Animal Practice* 22, 45-68.

Roush, J.K., Manley, P.A. (1992) Mini plate failure after repair of ilial and acetabular fractures in nine small dogs and one cat. *Journal of the American Animal Hospital Association* 28, 112.

Simmons, S., Johnson, A.L., Schaeffer, D.J. (2001) Risk factors for implant failure after triple pelvic osteotomy. *Journal of the American Animal Hospital Association* 39, 269-273.

Whelan, M.F., McCarthy, R.J., Boudrieau, R.J., et al. (2004) Increased sacral screw purchase minimizes screw loosening in canine triple pelvic osteotomy. *Veterinary Surgery* 33, 609-614.

95 Premature Physeal Closure After Fracture

Ann Johnson

College of Veterinary Medicine, University of Illinois, Champaign, IL, USA

Definition

Trauma causing loss of blood supply to or crushing of the growing cells of the physis may induce endochondral ossification of the physis earlier than normal for the size of the animal and location of the physis. Any fractured physis is subject to premature closure because the growing cells appear to be traumatized in most Salter-Harris fractures in dogs (Johnson *et al.* 1994). Cone-shaped physes such as the distal ulnar physis are susceptible to crushing caused by trauma elsewhere in the bone (von Pfeil and DeCamp 2009). Physeal closure may be complete, with simultaneous calcification of all parts of the physis, or partial, affecting one area of the physis. Premature physeal closure causes a range of abnormalities, including shortening, angulation, and rotation of the long bone. The clinical significance depends on the age of the animal and the location of the injury. In a paired bone system such as the radius and ulna, premature closure of a physis can also result in incongruity of the adjacent joints.

Risk factors

- Fracture of the diaphysis of the radius and ulna in a growing dog
- Fracture of a physis
- Penetration of the physis with an implant
- Bridging the physis with a plate or external fixator

Diagnosis

Physeal closure is a functional diagnosis of abnormal growth and therefore cannot be diagnosed at the time of injury. However, this complication may be suspected based on epidemiologic data. Indeed, any immature animal is at risk for premature closure of a fractured physis. Additionally, any immature dog with a radial and ulnar diaphyseal fracture is also at risk for premature closure of the distal ulnar physis. In these cases, timely reevaluations allow the surgeon to recognize the complication early and in some cases circumvent the outcome with an ostectomy.

The diagnosis of premature physeal closure may be made during physical evaluation if the affected limb is grossly shorter or deformed. However, it is preferable to identify physeal closure as a complication after fracture early, before serious deformities have occurred. This is particularly true for distal ulnar physeal closures. Serial radiographs are currently the best method for early detection of premature physeal closure after fracture. Rapidly growing dogs should be radiographed 2 weeks after fracture. Orthogonal radiographs should be made of the affected bone(s), including the joint above and below the bone, and the contralateral corresponding area for comparison. The physis is evaluated for the presence of mineralization within the cartilage. The normal functioning physis is radiolucent. A completely ossified physis is obviously nonfunctional; however, a lucent physis is not necessarily functional. A physis that has slowed or ceased functioning will still be radiolucent until endochondral ossification is complete. Length discrepancy between the affected bone and its contralateral counterpart is the first indication of premature physeal closure. Lateral radiographic views are most accurate for comparing length. Similar landmarks are identified on the affected and contralateral bone to measure the length of each bone. Subtracting the affected bone length from the contralateral bone length gives an estimate of the amount of bone shortening. Any shortening of the affected bone should raise an index of suspicion for premature physeal closure (Figure 95.1).

Complete physeal closures are relatively easy to identify. Partial physeal closures are more problematic, and computed tomography or magnetic resonance imaging may be useful for determining the extent of the partial physeal closure (Figure 95.2).

Implants with the potential to impede physeal growth are identified on the postoperative radiographs, and action should be taken to remove or replace the implant if the animal has significant growth potential. Examples include placement of a plate used to stabilize a diaphyseal or metaphyseal fracture over the adjacent physis with one screw on either side of the physis or similar placement of external fixator pins. Smooth pins crossing the physis perpendicularly will not impede growth unlike threaded implants crossing or otherwise invading the physis.

After premature physeal closure has been identified, the diagnostic approach should focus on assessing its clinical significance and planning surgical treatment. Assessing the clinical significance of a physeal closure takes into consideration the patient's age at diagnosis, abnormal gait, and radiographic signs. Preoperative radiographic planning (Figure 95.3) is designed to assess:

- Length discrepancy between the affected and contralateral bone: This measurement guides the decision making in terms of indication and modality for length correction.
- Severity of limb deviations in each of the following planes: cranio-caudal, mediolateral, and transverse (rotation). This measurement guides the selection of treatment modality and assists in the planning of corrective osteotomies.

Complications in Small Animal Surgery, First Edition. Edited by Dominique Griffon and Annick Hamaide.

© 2016 John Wiley & Sons, Inc. Published 2016 by John Wiley & Sons, Inc.

Companion website: www.wiley.com/go/griffon/complications

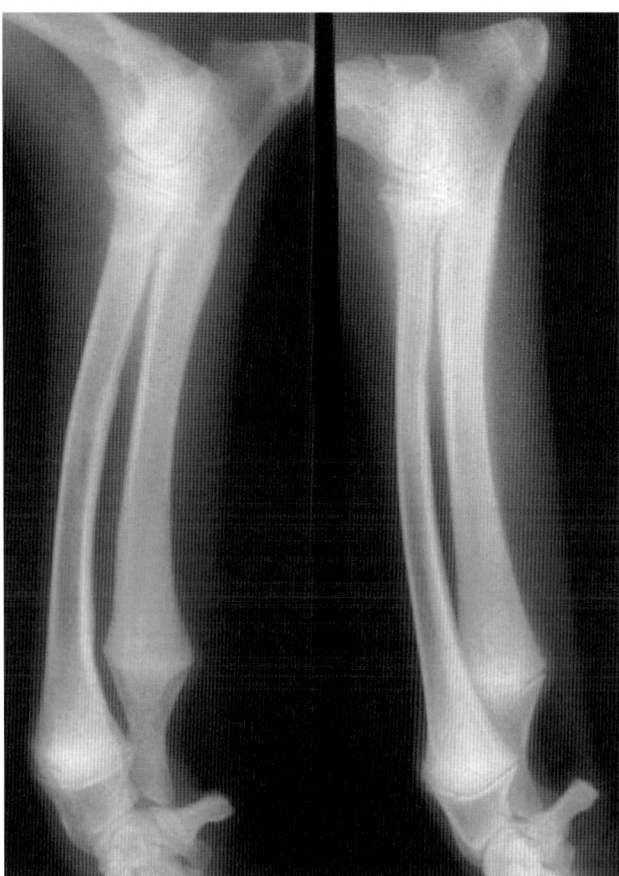

Figure 95.1 Premature closure of a distal ulnar physis. Lateral radiographs of the affected bone and the contralateral bone allow observation of physeal lucency and length measurements for comparisons.

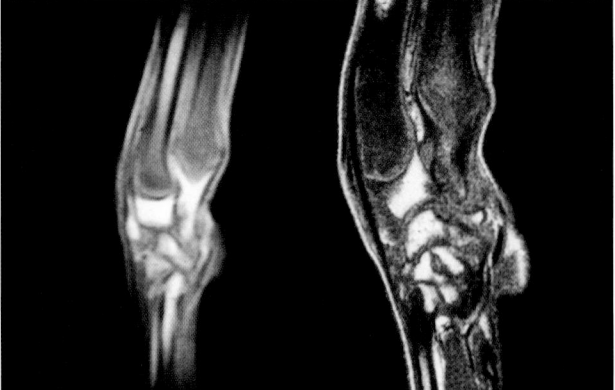

Figure 95.2 Magnetic resonance imaging may be beneficial for visualizing physeal bridging with bone. **A,** The normal limb. **B,** Closure of the distal ulnar physis.

The location of the point of maximum deformity along the bone. This point, localized in reference to a joint, should coincide with the location of a proposed corrective osteotomy. Two points of deviations are occasionally identified, requiring double-level corrections.

Treatment

Treatment depends on the location of the injury and the age of the dog (Figure 95.4). Dogs with minimal growth remaining or minimal deformity do not need treatment. Immature dogs with physeal closure in a paired bone system where the unaffected bone can carry the load of weight bearing are candidates for ostectomy of the affected bone to achieve as much naturally induced limb length as possible. Dogs with complete closure of a physis in a single bone such as the femur are candidates for limb lengthening if the deformity affects the dog's function.

Growing animals with premature physeal closure in either the radius or ulna may be treated initially with an ostectomy and fat graft of the affected bone to allow unrestricted growth of the unaffected bone. Dogs presenting with premature closure of the distal ulnar physis are treated with ulnar ostectomy, and an autogenous fat graft is placed to prevent premature bone bridging the ostectomy gap (Figure 95.5). Dogs presenting with complete premature closure of the radial physes can be treated with a radial ostectomy

and autogenous fat graft. Dogs with concurrent angular and rotational deformity may require a corrective osteotomy after growth has ceased to obtain the final cosmetic result.

Partial closure of the physis is treated by resection of the bone bridging the physis and placement of an autogenous fat graft to prevent ossification. The bone bridge is identified with reconstructed imaging and localized by placing hypodermic needles at the periphery of the bridge. The needles easily penetrate physeal cartilage and do not penetrate bone (VanDeWater and Olmstead 1983) (Figure 95.6).

Dogs with complete closure of the physis in a single bone such as the femur or tibia (the fibula is not large enough the bear weight as a paired bone system) or with premature physeal closure in both the radius and ulna may be monitored until most growth is complete and the effect of shortening on function can be assessed. Functionally, most dogs and cats do well with short limbs because they compensate by extending the elbow or stifle (see Chapter 95). Angular deformities are more problematic. If function is a problem, a lengthening osteotomy may be indicated. Angular deformities require a corrective osteotomy. Lengthening osteotomies may be one-stage or continuous procedures. One-stage length correction is limited by the restraining soft tissues but can be stabilized with internal fixation. Continuous distraction overcomes the soft tissue limitations and provides new bone formation with distraction osteogenesis. Bone lengthening can be achieved unifocally or bifocally. Unifocal lengthening occurs when a single osteotomy is created in the bone. Bifocal bone lengthening involves two osteotomy sites in the bone, effectively doubling the rate of distraction (Stallings *et al.* 1998). Some very young dogs are treated with continuous distraction as they grow.

Outcome

The prognosis after any ostectomy is guarded until there is radiographic evidence of physeal function in the unaffected bone (i.e., evidence of bone lengthening on serial radiographs). If the ipsilateral radial physes are functioning normally and there is growth potential, increased length and decreased angulation of the affected limb will occur after an ulnar ostectomy. There will be no change in rotational deformity. Owners should be warned that the dog may require a corrective osteotomy after it reaches maturity, particularly if the deformity is severe. Similarly, radial ostectomy will allow increased limb length if the ulnar physis is functional. After radial

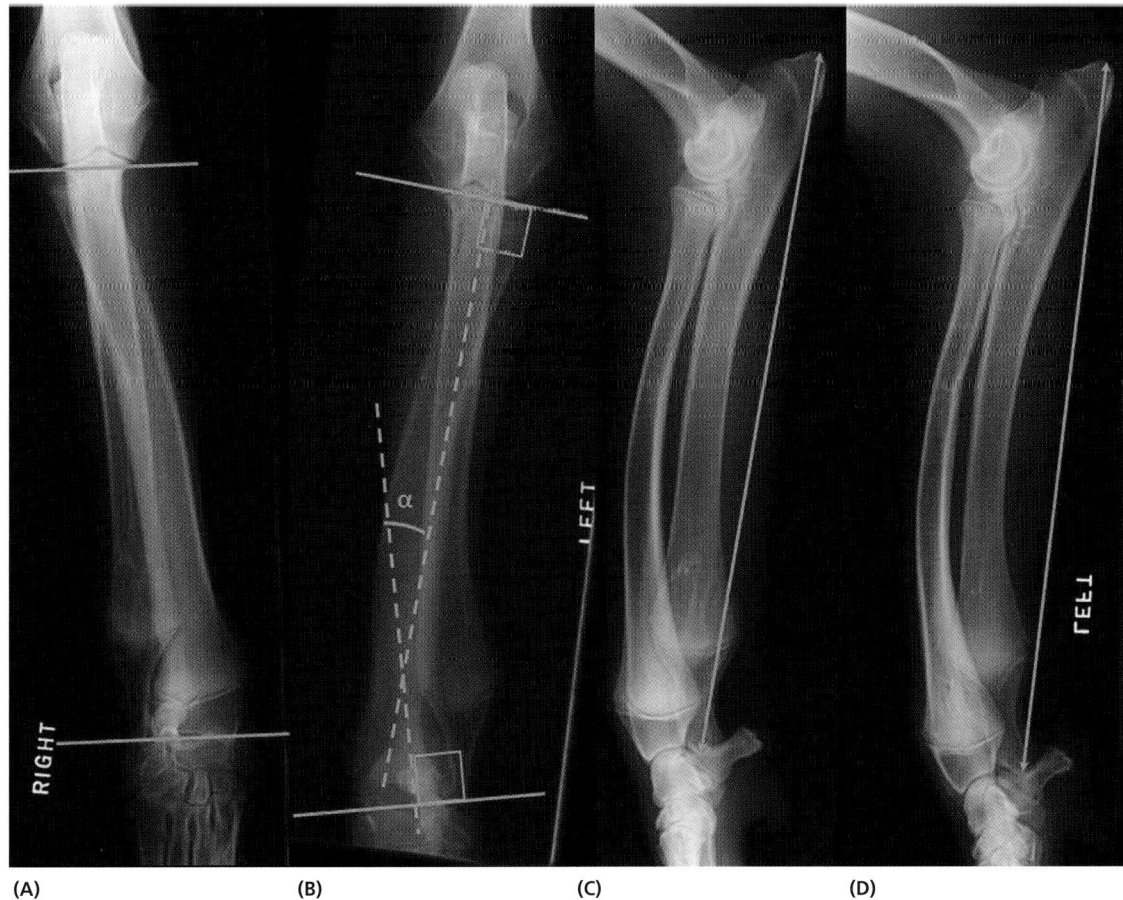

(A) (B) (C) (D)

Figure 95.3 Preoperative assessment of a dog with premature closure of the distal ulnar growth plate and radius valgus. **A,** Anteroposterior (AP) radiograph of the contralateral limb. The joint surfaces of the elbow and carpus are parallel with each other. **B,** AP view of the affected radius. The point of maximum angulation is located at the intersection of the proximal and distal axes of lines perpendicular to the joint surfaces. The angle of mediolateral angulation is measured. **C** and **D,** Mediolateral projections of the affected and contralateral limbs are used to assess length discrepancy.

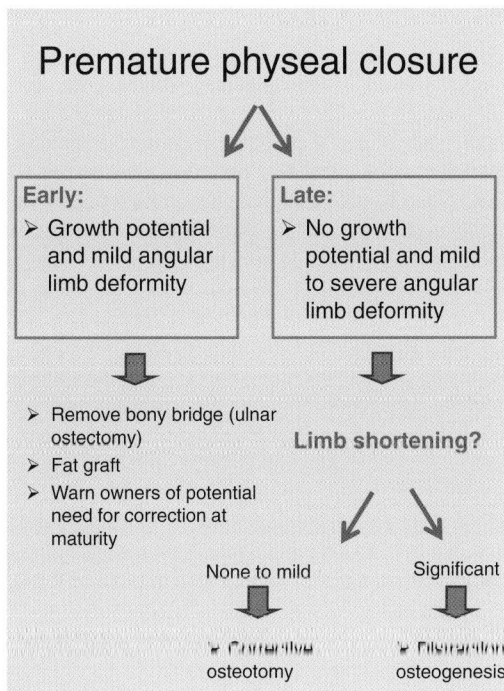

Figure 95.4 Algorithm for treatment of premature physeal closure.

ostectomy, the ulna will hypertrophy in response to increased load of weight bearing as will the radius in a dog with an ulnar ostectomy. Complications may occur after ostectomy, including bone bridging, synostosis of the radius and ulna, disuse osteoporosis, and carpal hyperextension (Van Vechten and Vasseur 1993). Dogs with asymmetrical complete closure of the physis may develop degenerative joint disease of the adjacent joint.

The outcome after corrective osteotomies including continuous distraction is generally successful in correcting angular and rotational deformity but not in completely correcting length discrepancies. Osteoarthritis of adjacent joints may develop, ultimately affecting function (Theyse *et al.* 2005).

Prevention

- Trauma-related premature closures cannot be prevented but if observed early can be managed in paired bones to avoid major deformity.
- Ulnar ostectomy may be considered as part of the initial surgical repair of a radial fracture in young dogs, especially if the fracture resulted from a traumatic event likely to generate compression (e.g., jumping off a height) (Figure 95.7).
- Implant-related premature closures are avoided by careful implant selection and placement.

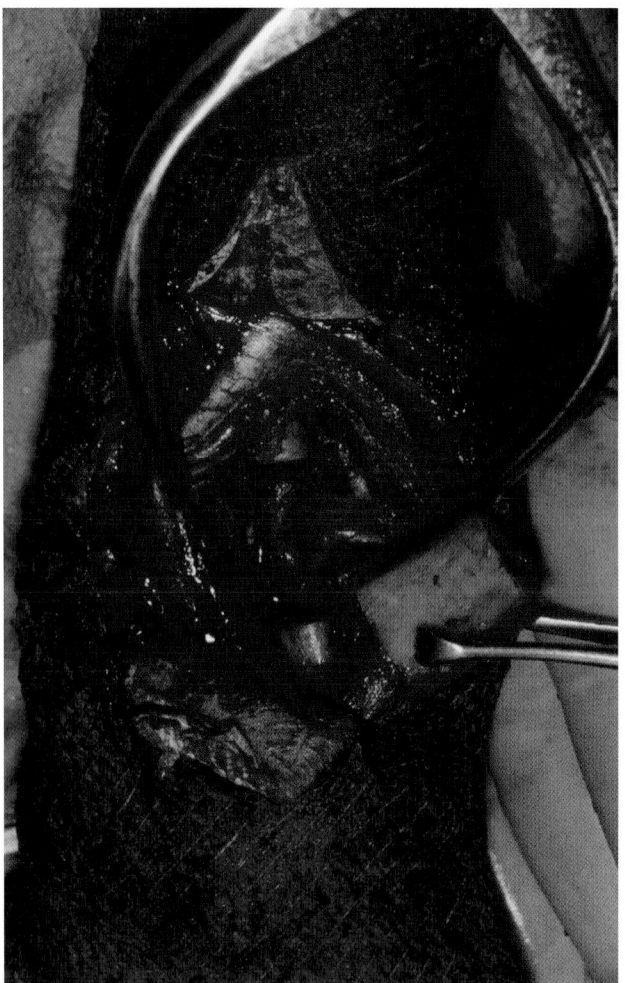

(A)

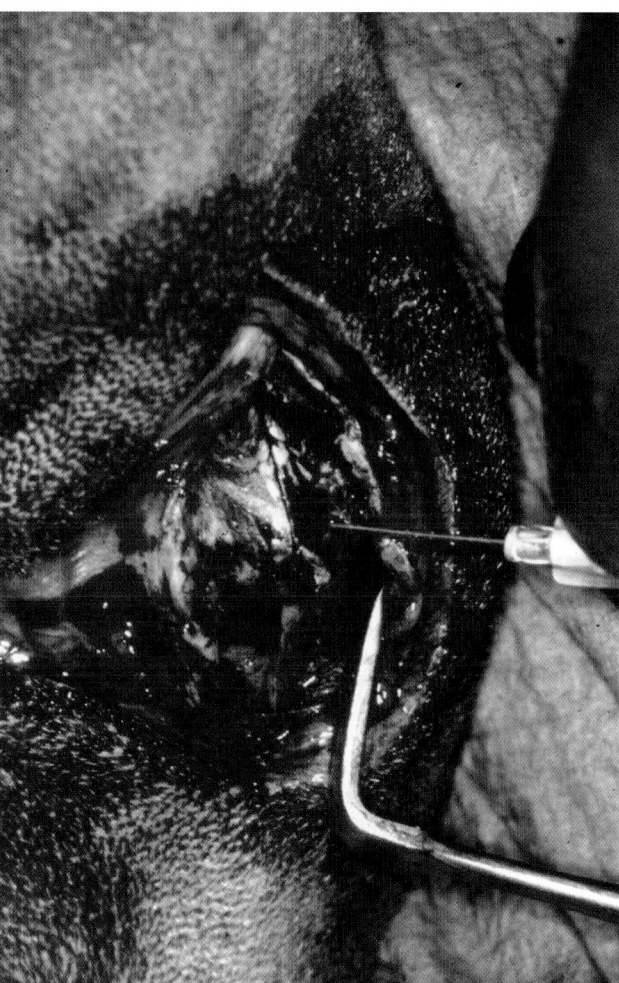

Figure 95.6 The extent of the bone bridging a physis can be identified with a hypodermic needle.

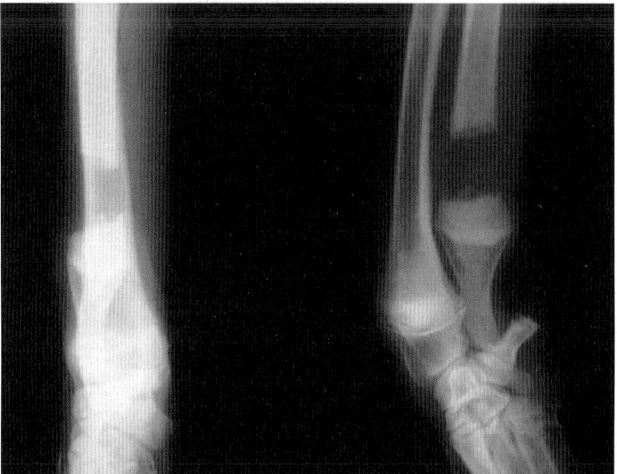

(B)

Figure 95.5 **A,** An ulnar ostectomy is performed to release the restraint of the ulna on radial growth. The bone and surrounding periosteum are removed, and the site is filled with autogenous fat. **B,** Postoperative radiograph.

Relevant literature

The Salter and Harris classification scheme for physeal fractures is based on radiographic and histologic appearances and used to predict prognosis for growth in pediatric patients. Whereas fracture types I through III have been given a good prognosis for continued growth, types IV and V are typically considered to have a poor prognosis for continued physeal function. However, realistically, most canine Salter I and II fractured physes close after fracture. Histologic evaluation of naturally occurring canine physeal fractures showed damage to the zone of growing cells in all cases (Johnson *et al.* 1994). The prognosis for physeal function should be guarded until radiographic evidence of function is obtained by observing increased bone length over time. Nevertheless, all efforts should be made during physeal fracture repair to encourage any possible function of the physis by minimizing surgical trauma during reduction and carefully selecting smooth implants crossing the physis.

Premature physeal closure in a single bone in a growing animal can cause sufficient shortening of the bone to affect function. Although the distal femoral physis appears to close after fracture, the effect on function is variable and depends on the age of the animal. Most dogs can compensate for femoral length loss and still function normally by extending the stifle. Additionally, an overgrowth of the adjacent tibia has been reported after distal femoral physeal fracture (Wagner *et al.* 1987). Salter-Harris type IV fractures of the humeral condyle did not cause shortening of the humerus; instead there was an overall mild overgrowth of the bone (Lefebvre *et al.* 2008). The

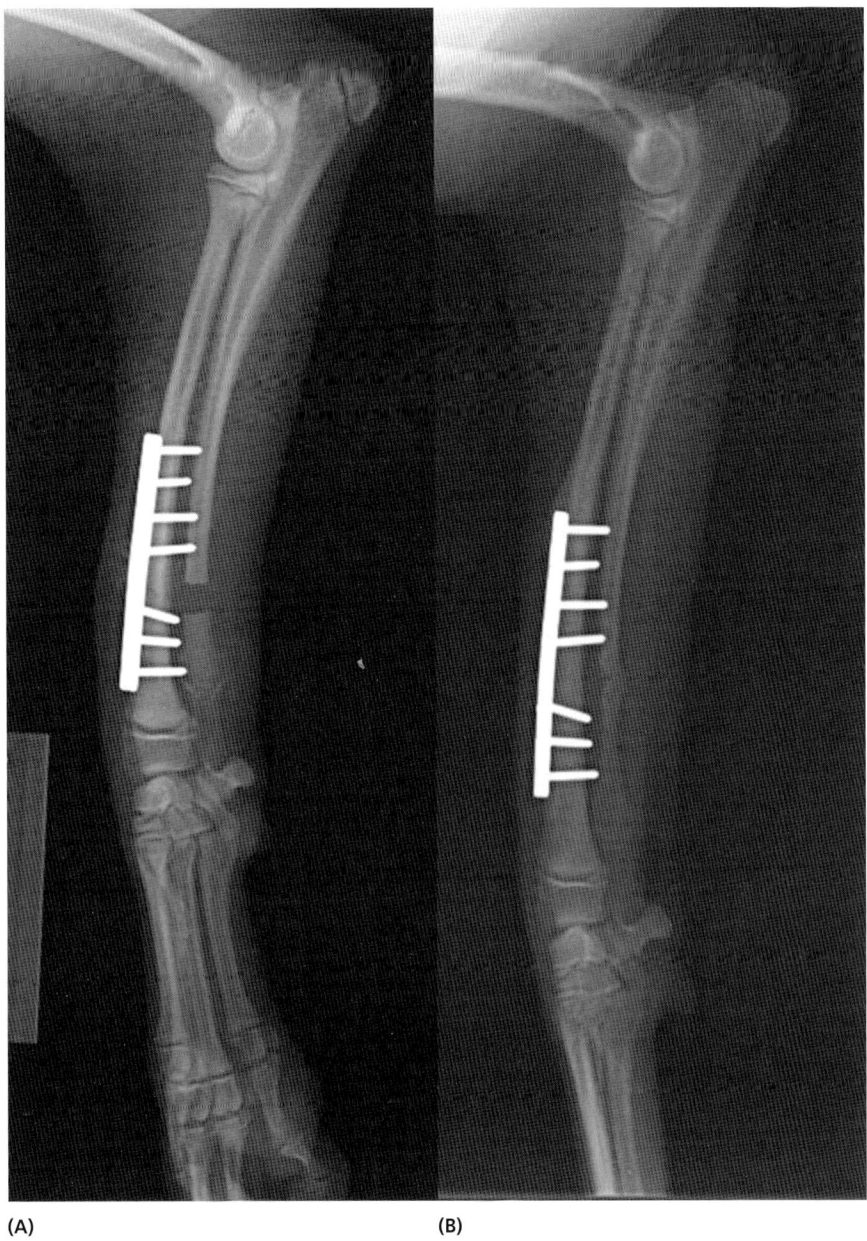

(A)   **(B)**

Figure 95.7 Preventive ulnar ostectomy in a young Italian greyhound treated for a distal radial fracture secondary to jumping off a deck. **A,** The radial fracture healed uneventfully, **B,** and no shortening or angulation of the limb was present at maturity. *Source:* D. Griffon, Western University of Health Sciences, Pomona, CA, 2014. Reproduced with permission from D. Griffon.

phenomenon of bone overgrowth has been reported for the tibia after femoral fractures and for the humerus after antebrachial shortening in dogs (Schaefer *et al*. 1995; Clements *et al*. 2004). Theories for overgrowth include decreased pressure on the physis, resulting in increased growth plate function, and increased vascularity with subsequent overstimulation of growth (Lefebvre *et al*. 2008).

Forelimb angular deformities in mature dogs resulting from premature physeal closure are generally treated with osteotomies designed to correct alignment of the bone, but these corrective osteotomies do little to restore length (Quinn *et al* 2000). The principles established by Ilizarov for distraction osteogenesis are used to treat animals with functional problems related to premature physeal closure and length (Ferretti 1991; Stallings *et al*. 1998). Although the most frequent application deals with antebrachial deformities,

other bones may also be treated with this method (Marcellin-Little *et al*. 1998; Lewis *et al*. 1999; Theyse *et al*. 2005; Wendelburg *et al*. 2011). Treating limb length discrepancy and angular deformity of the distal femur affecting ambulation with corrective osteotomy with lengthening can restore function (Wendelburg *et al*. 2011).

References

Clements, D.N., Gemmill, T.J., Clarke, S.P., et al. (2004) Compensatory humeral overgrowth associated with antebrachial shortening in six dogs. *Veterinary Record* 154, 531-532.

Ferretti, A. (1991) The application of the Ilizarov technique to veterinary medicine. In Maiocchi, A.B., Aronson, J. (eds.) *Operative Principles of Ilizarov*. Williams & Wilkins, Baltimore, pp. 551-575.

Johnson, J.M., Johnson, A.L., Eurell, J.C. (1994) Histologic appearance of naturally occurring canine physeal fractures. *Veterinary Surgery* 23, 81-86.

Lefebvre, J.B., Robertson, T.R., Baines, S.J., et al. (2008) Assessment of humeral length in dogs after repair of Salter-Harris type IV fracture of the lateral part of the humeral condyle. *Veterinary Surgery* 37, 545-551.

Lewis, D.D., Radasch, R.M., Beale, B.S., et al. (1999) Initial clinical experience with the IMEX TM circular external skeletal fixation system, part II: use in bone lengthening and correction of angular and rotational deformities. *Veterinary and Comparative Orthopaedics and Traumatology* 12, 18-127.

Marcellin-Little, D.J., Ferretti, A., Roe, S.C., et al. (1998) Hinged Ilizarov external fixation for correction of antebrachial deformities. *Veterinary Surgery* 27, 231-245.

Quinn, M.K., Ehrhart, N., Johnson, A.L., et al. (2000) Realignment of the radius in canine antebrachial growth deformities treated with corrective osteotomy and bilateral (Type II) external fixation. *Veterinary Surgery* 29, 558-563.

Schaefer, S.L., Johnson, K.A., O'Brien, R.T. (1995) Compensatory tibial overgrowth following healing of closed femoral fractures in young dogs. *Veterinary and Comparative Orthopaedics and Traumatology* 8, 159-162.

Stallings, J.T., Lewis, D., Welch, R., et al. (1998) An introduction to distraction osteogenesis and the principles of the Ilizarov method. *Veterinary and Comparative Orthopaedics and Traumatology* 11, 59-67.

Theyse, L.F., Voorhout, G., Hazewinkel, H.A. (2005) Prognostic factors in treating antebrachial growth deformities with a lengthening procedure using a circular external skeletal fixation system in dogs. *Veterinary Surgery* 34, 424-435.

VanDeWater, A.L., Olmstead, M.L. (1983) Premature closure of the distal radial physis in the dog: A review of 11 cases. *Veterinary Surgery* 12, 7-12.

Van Vechten, B.J., Vasseur, P.B. (1993) Complications of middiaphyseal radial ostectomy performed for treatment of premature closure of the distal radial physis in two dogs. *Journal of the American Veterinary Medical Association* 202, 97-100.

von Pfeil, D.J., DeCamp, C.E. (2009) The epiphyseal plate: physiology, anatomy, and trauma. *Compendium on Continuing Education for the Practicing Veterinarian* 31, E1-11.

Wagner, S.D., Desch, J.P. 2nd, Ferguson, H.R., et al. (1987) Effect of distal femoral growth plate fusion on femoral-tibial length. *Veterinary Surgery* 16 (6), 435-439.

Wendelburg, K.M., Lewis, D.D., Sereda, C.W., et al. (2011) Use of an interlocking nail-hybrid fixator construct for distal femoral deformity correction in three dogs. *Veterinary and Comparative Orthopaedics and Traumatology* 24, 236-245.

96 Avascular Necrosis

Dominique Griffon

College of Veterinary Medicine, Western University of Health Sciences, Pomona, CA, USA

Avascular necrosis of the femoral head occurs spontaneously in small breed dogs and is often referred to as Legg-Calvé-Perthes disease. However, this chapter focuses on avascular necrosis as a complication of fracture repair.

Definition

Avascular necrosis is defined as bone lysis caused by an interruption of the blood supply secondary to fracture, fracture fixation, or both. This complication has traditionally been described after repair of femoral epiphyseal separation ("slipped capital femoral epiphysis"), most commonly caused by Salter-Harris type I fractures (Figure 96.1). Avascular necrosis may also occur after femoral neck fractures and spontaneous slipped femoral capital epiphysis.

Risk factors

- Age of the patient: immature patients
- Physeal epiphyseal separation secondary to trauma
- Open reduction and fixation

Diagnosis

The diagnosis is usually made during the first postoperative radiographic evaluation (Figure 96.2). Bone lysis is noted along the femoral neck and may extend into the femoral head. The lysis may progress and jeopardize fracture immobilization via implant loosening or migration. Lameness is present along with pain on manipulation of the hip. On histopathology, areas of necrosis are present within the femoral head and neck (Figure 96.3).

Treatment

The decision-making process takes into consideration clinical signs of pain and lameness, radiographic signs of disease of the articular surface, and implant stability. Figure 96.4 includes a general algorithm for the management of postoperative avascular necrosis.

Outcome

The outcome of dogs with avascular necrosis secondary to femoral capital physeal fracture is fair. Partial restoration of femoral neck width is noted at 8 weeks in dogs that respond to conservative management. Degenerative joint disease should be expected in all cases, and salvage procedures may be required in severe cases. Femoral head and neck ostectomy has been reported in 20% of femoral capital physeal fractures in dogs (Gibson *et al.* 1991).

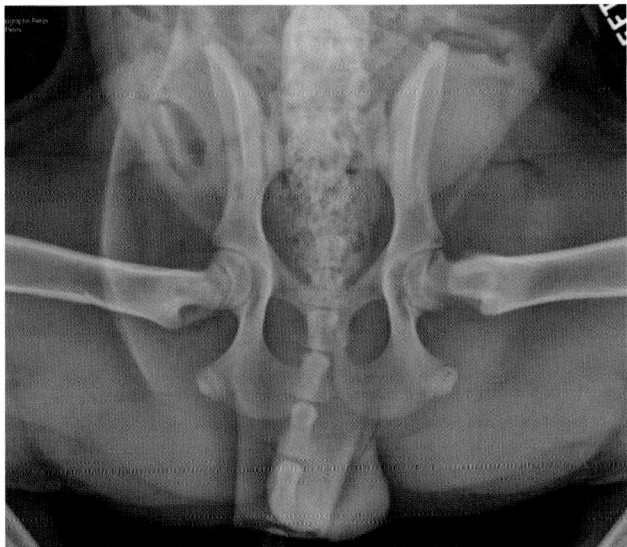

Figure 96.1 Femoral capital physeal fracture in an immature Labrador retriever. Notice the mild fracture displacement of the fracture on the left femoral head.

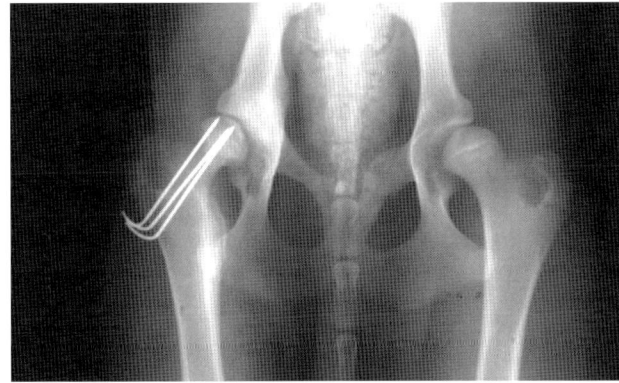

Figure 96.2 Avascular necrosis of the femoral neck 6 weeks after surgery in a 5-month-old medium mixed breed dog. The dog sustained a Salter I femoral epiphyseal fracture as a result of a motor vehicle accident. The fracture was repaired with three parallel Kirschner wires (0.54 inch) placed through a craniolateral approach to the hip. Note the lysis of the femoral neck.

Complications in Small Animal Surgery, First Edition. Edited by Dominique Griffon and Annick Hamaide.
© 2016 John Wiley & Sons, Inc. Published 2016 by John Wiley & Sons, Inc.
Companion website: www.wiley.com/go/griffon/complications

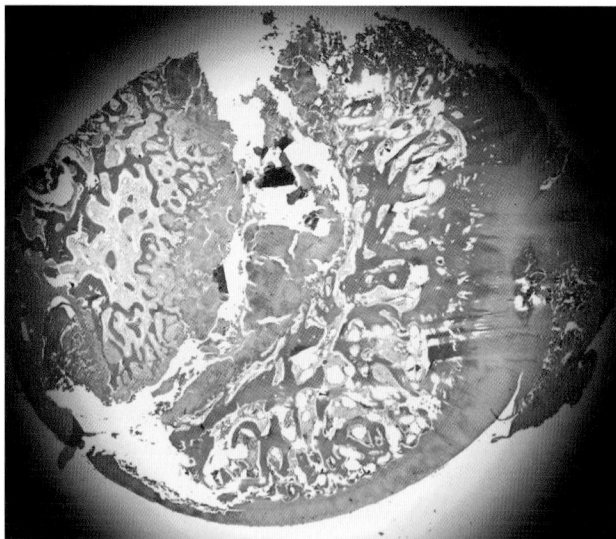

Figure 96.3 Histopathology of a femoral head with a Salter I fracture. Note the areas of necrosis around the physis and femoral neck.

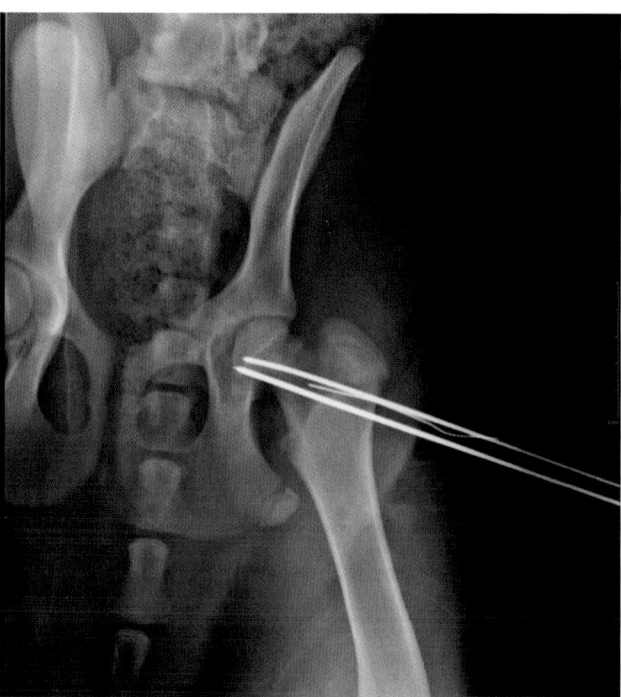

Figure 96.5 Femoral epiphyseal fracture repair under fluoroscopic guidance. Intraoperative view during closed reduction and pin fixation under fluoroscopic guidance in dog imaged in Figure 96.1. Placement of Kirschner wires is assessed until each pin engages the physis but does not penetrate the articular surface.

Prevention

Although further evidence is needed to establish this approach, closed reduction and fixation of femoral capital physeal fractures is the most promising approach to prevent postoperative avascular necrosis (Figures 96.5 and 96.6). The procedure is carried out under fluoroscopic guidance and include the following step:

• Reduction
• Placement of two or three Kirschner wires
• Passive range of motion is initiated after surgery. Exercise is limited to short walks on good surfaces for 6 weeks.

Relevant literature

Avascular necrosis is most commonly reported in dogs as a spontaneous disease of the femoral head in young small breed dogs. Several case reports document avascular necrosis of the femoral neck after spontaneous separation of the femoral capital epiphysis,

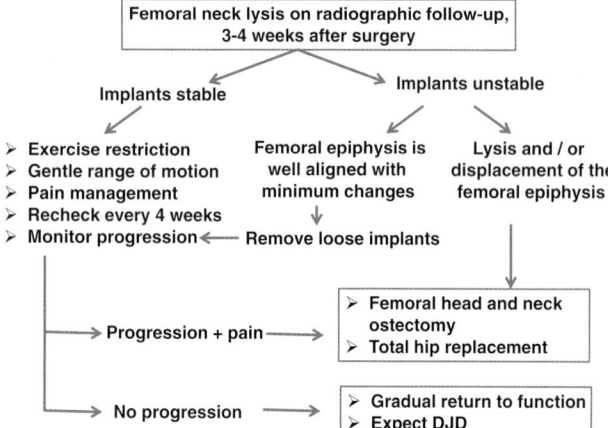

Figure 96.4 Algorithm for the management of avascular necrosis after femoral capital physeal fracture repair. DJD, degenerative joint disease.

with presentations resembling those of "slipped capital femoral epiphysis" in children (Moores *et al.* 2004). This condition has been reported in adult cats, most commonly affecting heavier neutered males with delayed physeal closure (McNicholas *et al.* 2002). In these cases, fracture of the femoral capital physis occurred without trauma and preceded metaphyseal resorption and sclerosis. The severity of osteolysis correlated with the duration of clinical signs and progressed on serial radiographic evaluation. The authors attributed these changes to the formation of a pseudoarthrosis, also observed after conservative management of traumatic femoral capital fractures.

As a surgical complication, avascular necrosis is most commonly reported after repair of traumatic femoral capital physeal fractures. Femoral neck narrowing, or "apple coring," has been reported in 38% to 100% of dogs after surgical repair of a proximal femoral epiphyseal fracture (Hulse *et al.* 1981; DeCamp *et al.* 1989; Tillson *et al.* 1996). Radiographic signs of femoral neck narrowing after femoral capital physeal fracture fixation are typically worse at 4 weeks after surgery. Partial restoration of the width of the femoral neck at 8 weeks has prompted authors to speculate that femoral thinning may be part of the normal reparative process (Tillson *et al.* 1994, 1996).

This complication has most commonly been attributed to compromised blood supply to the femoral neck and neck caused by initial trauma or fracture repair (or both). Approximately 70% of the extraosseous blood supply to the proximal femur and coxofemoral joint comes from the medial and lateral circumflex femoral arteries (Kaderly *et al.* 1982a, 1982b; Tillson *et al.* 1996).

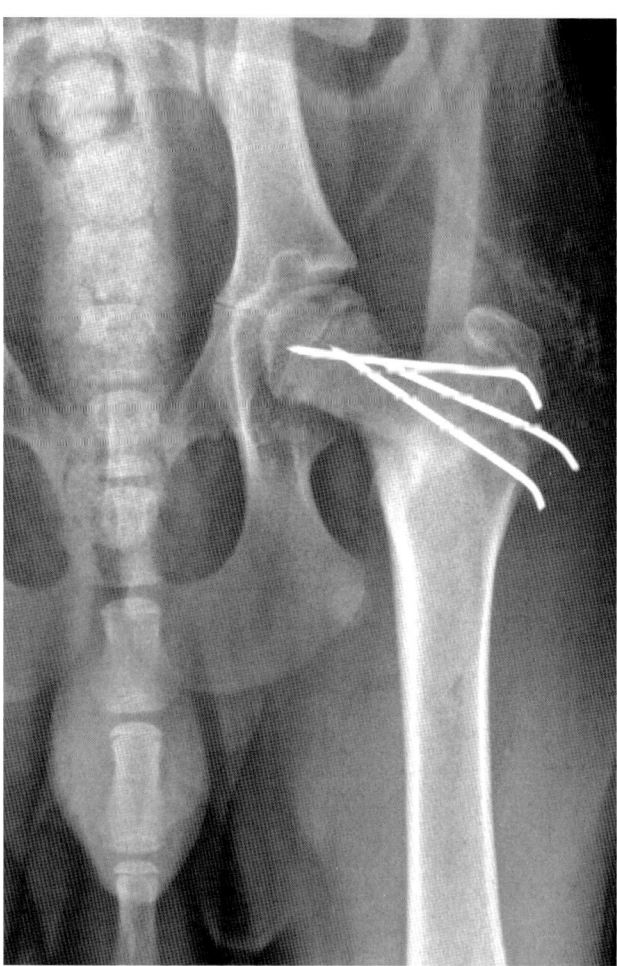

Figure 96.6 Radiographs obtained 3 weeks after pin fixation of a femoral epiphyseal fracture under fluoroscopic guidance (represented on Figure 96.5). One pin (central) has migrated out, but fracture reduction is satisfactory, with no evidence of bone lysis.

Continuation of these vessels within the coxofemoral joint capsule gives rise to an extraosseous vascular retinaculum at the base of the femoral neck. These vessels course along the femoral neck, forming an extraosseous, intracapsular network crossing the physis into the epiphysis. The dorsal retinacular artery supplies the majority of the proximal femoral epiphysis as a single vessel as well as through anastomoses with the vascular arcade formed by the retinacular artery.

A similar pathogenesis has been proposed in children, in whom avascular necrosis develops in 17% to 47% of femoral head or neck fractures (Hughes and Beaty 1994). In addition to compromised blood supply, the amount of initial fracture displacement correlates directly with the risk of avascular necrosis. Three types of avascular necrosis have been described in children: type I involves the entire femoral head, type II partially involves the femoral head, and type III includes an area of necrosis extending from the fracture line to the physis. Type I avascular necrosis is the most common and carries the poorest prognosis.

No treatment has been established for avascular necrosis, regardless of the species. In dogs, failure to respond to conservative management leads to salvage procedures. Consequently, femoral head and neck ostectomy has been reported in 20% of dogs in a retrospective study of 34 dogs with femoral capital fractures (Gibson et al. 1991). Recent strategies to manage these fractures focus on closed reduction and fixation early after diagnosis. This approach follows the general trend toward minimally invasive surgery and appears anecdotally promising. However, further clinical evidence is warranted to confirm its ability to prevent postoperative avascular necrosis in femoral capital fractures.

References

DeCamp, C.E., Probst, C.W., Thomas, M.W. (1989) Internal fixation of femoral capital physeal injuries in dogs: 40 cases (1979-1987). *Journal of the American Veterinary Medical Association* 194, 1750-1754.

Gibson, K.L., Vane, R.T., Pechman, R.D. (1991) Femoral capital physeal fractures in dogs: 34 cases (1979-1989). *Journal of the American Veterinary Medical Association* 198, 886-890.

Hughes, L.O., Beaty, J.H., (1994) Fractures of the head and neck of the femur in children. *Journal of Bone and Joint Surgery* 76 (Suppl. A), 283-292.

Hulse, D.H., Wilson, J.W., Abdelbaki, Y.Z. (1981) Revascularization of femoral capital physeal fractures following surgical fixation. *Journal of Veterinary Orthopedics* 2, 50-57.

Kaderly, R.E., Anderson, W.D., Anderson, B.G. (1982a) Extraosseous vascular supply to the mature dog's coxofemoral joint. *American Journal of Veterinary Research* 43, 1208-1214.

Kaderly, R.E., Anderson, B.G., Anderson, W.D. (1982b) Intracapsular and intraosseous vascular supply to the mature dog's coxofemoral joint. *American Journal of Veterinary Research* 44, 1805-1812.

McNicholas, W.T., Wilkens, B.E., Blevins, W.E., et al. (2002) Spontaneous femoral capital physeal fractures in adult cats: 26 cases (1996-2001). *Journal of the American Veterinary Medical Association* 221, 1731-1736.

Moores, A.P., Owen, M.R., Fews, D., et al. (2004) Slipped capital femoral epiphysis in dogs. *The Journal of Small Animal Practice* 45 (12), 602-8.

Tillson, D.M., McLaughlin, R.M., Roush, J.K. (1994) Evaluation of experimental proximal femoral physeal fractures repaired with two cortical screws placed from the articular surfaces. *Veterinary and Comparative Orthopaedics and Traumatology* 7, 136-139.

Tillson, D.M., McLaughlin, R.M., Roush, J.K. (1996) Fractures of the proximal femoral physis in dogs. *Compendium on Continuing Education for the Practicing Veterinarian* 18, 1164-1182.

97 Bone Resorption

Dominique Griffon

College of Veterinary Medicine, Western University of Health Sciences, Pomona, CA, USA

Definitions

Bone resorption results from an imbalance in bone homeostasis leading to predominant osteoclastic activity.

Risk factors

Causes of bone resorption in the early postoperative phase (within 3 months of fracture repair) include:

- Infection, osteomyelitis (see Chapter 5)
- Stress shielding: fixation of a fracture with an implant that is too rigid and compromises biomechanical loading of the bone
  - Current hybrid and linear external fixators (IMEX Veterinary, Inc., Longview, TX) are generally more rigid than similar traditional Kirschner-Ehmer construct (Figure 97.1).
  - Carbon fiber rods are stiffer than aluminium rods of the same diameter.
  - Stainless steel plates are stiffer and more likely to induce bone atrophy than titanium implants (Figure 97.2).
- Disuse: insufficient biomechanical stimulation of fracture healing caused by external coaptation, immobilization and/or loss of function of the limb (Figure 97.3)
- Loose implants and excessive interfragmentary motion: Bone resorption is a physiologic response that increases the surface area of the fracture site and decreases interfragmentary strain (Figures 97.4 and 97.5).

Long-term bone resorption after fracture repair may occur because of stress shielding, fracture-associated sarcoma (Figure 97.6), or development of an unrelated pathology on the limb leading to disuse.

Diagnosis

Clinical signs associated with bone resorption may not be immediately apparent, especially in the early postoperative phase, when some degree of lameness is expected. As bone loss progresses, function of the limb is affected and may eventually lead to non–weight-bearing lameness, especially if secondary complications such as fractures or implant failure develop. The presence of soft tissue swelling and draining tracts is consistent with bone neoplasia infection. Severe pain on palpation of the bone years after fracture fixation may be indicative of resorption secondary to neoplasia.

The diagnosis of bone resorption is made based on radiographic evidence of radiolucency within the fracture site. Early detection of bone resorption as a cause of delayed fracture healing is established

based on serial radiographs: callus formation may not appear to progress as expected, the fracture gap seems to widen and/or adjacent cortices become thinner (see Figures 97.1 to 97.4). The goal of the diagnostic workup is to establish the presence of bone resorption and identify its underlying cause. The apparatus should be critically evaluated for loosening and/or interference with the fracture site (see Figures 97.2 and 97.5). Culture and sensitivity are indicated in cases suspect of infection. Biopsy should be considered if neoplasia seems likely (see Figure 97.6).

Treatment

Bone resorption warrants treatment because it is unlikely to stop its progression or resolve spontaneously. Treatment options vary with the underlying cause, and an algorithm outlining general principles of management in the early postoperative phase is proposed in Figure 97.7. Surgical management of osteomyelitis and delayed fracture healing are described elsewhere is this book. Bone resorption caused by implant failure and/or excessive interfragmentary strain warrant revision of the fixation, combined with biologic stimulation of bone healing such as autogenous cancellous graft (see Figures 97.4 and 97.5). Bone resorption secondary to stress shielding and disuse is generally addressed by gradually increasing biomechanical loading of the limb. External fixators may undergo staged disassembly, while plates require removal (see Figure 97.2 and Figure 97.8). In these cases, external coaptation is generally indicated to protect the weakened bone. Bone resorption long term after fracture repair is unusual but may follow the same principles of management if stress shielding or implant-related complications are diagnosed. These cases warrant thorough evaluation because concurrent neurologic and/or orthopedic diseases may be the cause of disuse, such as fracture-induced sarcoma (see Chapter 104). Treatment should be targeted toward the underlying cause for loss of function.

Outcome

The prognosis for treatment of bone resorption varies with the extent and cause of bone destruction. Cases with early diagnosis of stress shielding and a healed fracture carry a very good prognosis, although implant removal may lead to fracture of the weakened bone. Fractures with delayed healing or nonunion caused by bone resorption carry a poorer prognosis, especially if disuse of the limb has decreased the quality of the remaining bone stock. In unstable

Complications in Small Animal Surgery, First Edition. Edited by Dominique Griffon and Annick Hamaide.

© 2016 John Wiley & Sons, Inc. Published 2016 by John Wiley & Sons, Inc.

Companion website: www.wiley.com/go/griffon/complications

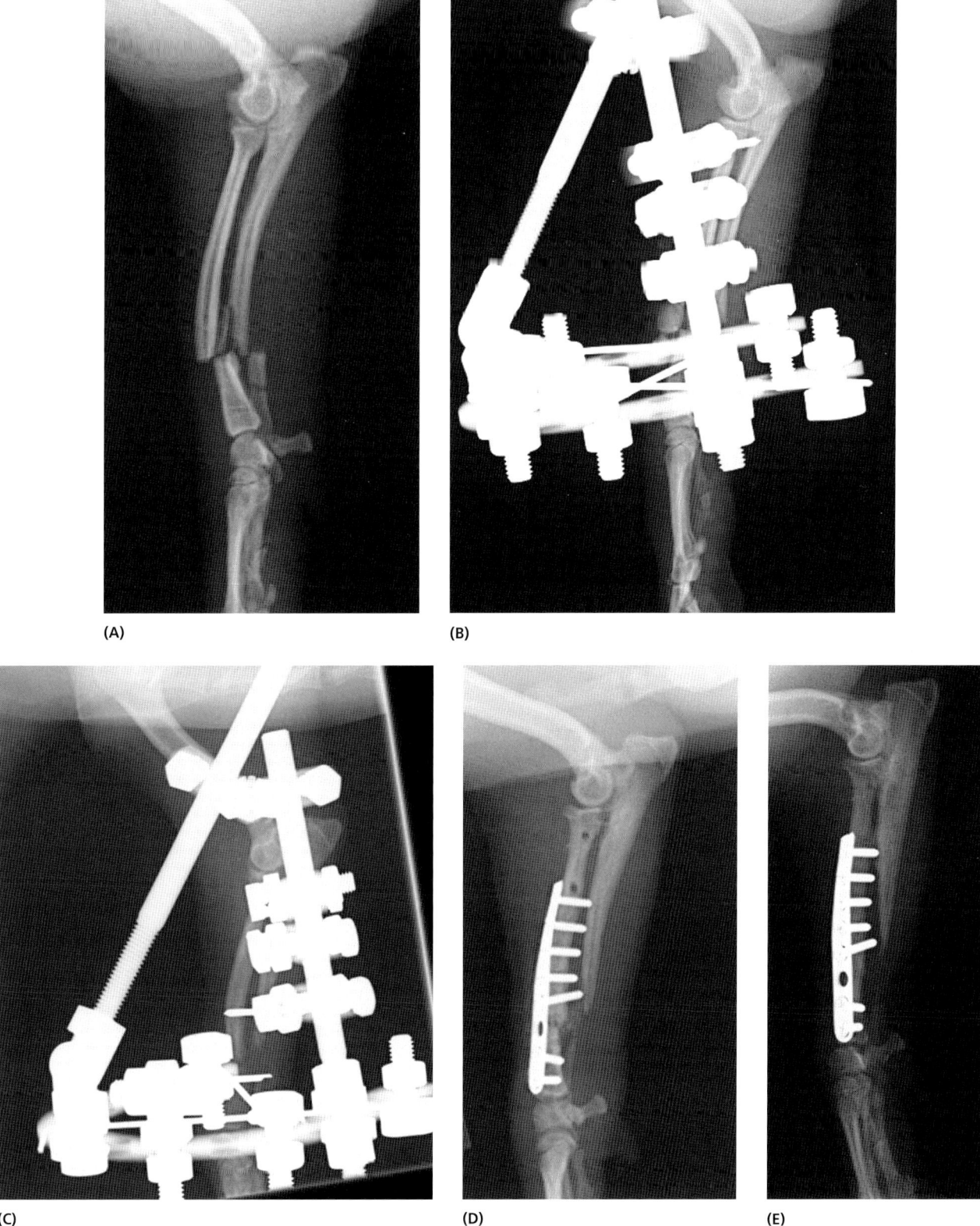

(A)

(B)

(C)   (D)   (E)

Figure 97.1 Bone resorption caused by stress shielding after hybrid fracture fixation. **A,** Preoperative mediolateral radiograph of a 3-year-old Maltese with grade II open comminuted fractures of the right radius and ulna secondary to dog bites. The limb had been bandaged for 5 days, and *Staphylococcus aureus* was isolated from the wound. **B,** Radiograph obtained immediately after fixation of a hybrid fixator and implantation of antibiotic-impregnated calcium sulfate beads within the fracture site. **C,** Radiograph obtained 6 weeks after surgery. The soft tissue injuries are healed, but bone resorption is present at the fracture site and in the distal ulna, presumably attributed to the stiffness of the implant. **D,** Radiograph obtained after revision with a plate and autogenous bone graft. A synostosis is noted between the proximal radius and ulna, and disuse osteopenia is present within the distal radius and metacarpal bones. **E,** Radiograph obtained 6 weeks after plate fixation. Callus formation around the fracture site is consistent with bone healing.

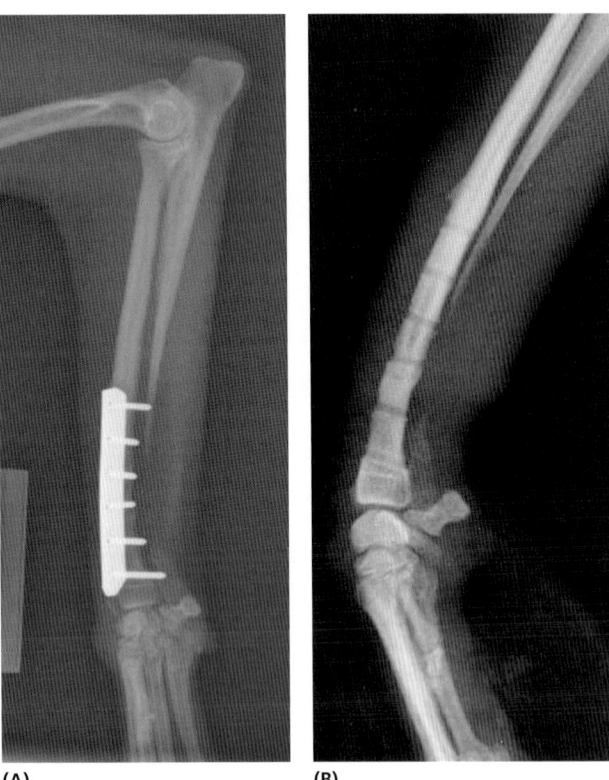

(A)   (B)

Figure 97.2 Bone resorption caused by stress shielding after plate fixation.
A, Radiograph obtained 9 weeks after repair of a transverse distal radial
plate with a 2-mm dynamic compression plate in a young Yorkshire terrier.
The dog had good function of the limb, but resorption of the ulna is
visible. **B,** Radiograph after plate removal. The radial fracture was healed;
autologous conditioned plasma was injected into the ulnar defect through
the screw holes. The dog was placed in a light splint (made from a syringe
case) for 3 weeks before a gradual increase in exercise.

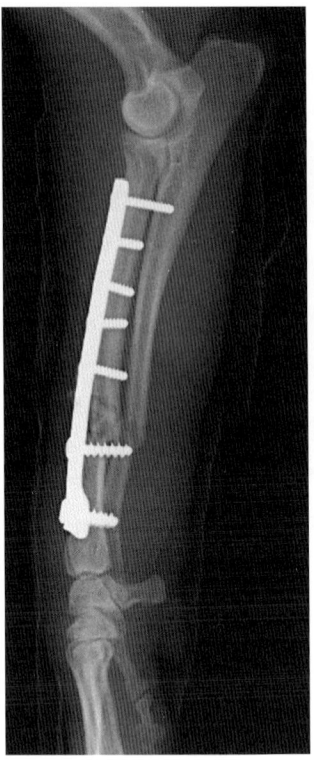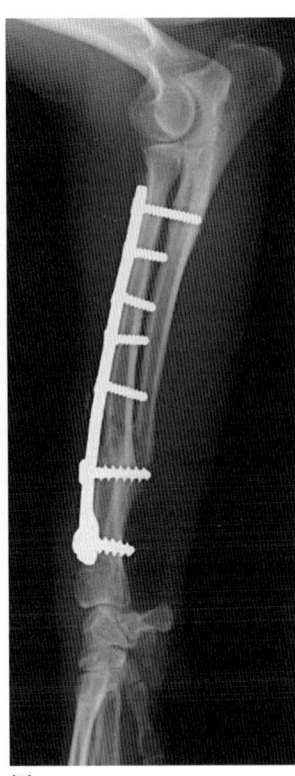

(A)   (B)

Figure 97.3 Bone resorption caused by loss of function after plate fixation.
A, Radiograph obtained immediately after plate fixation of a comminuted
fracture of the distal radius and ulna in a small mixed breed dog. The
proximal screw is too long and engaging the ulna. One screw in the distal
segment seems too close to the fracture site. **B,** Radiographs obtained at 12
weeks after surgery. The dog presented with lameness, presumably caused
by periosteal irritation associated with the most proximal screw (too
long). The loss of radiopacity of the radius and resorption of the ulna were
attributed to disuse and stress shielding from the plate. The proximal screw
was removed and use of the limb encouraged with analgesia and physical
therapy. The plate was removed 4 weeks later, and after 2 weeks of external
coaptation, the dog was allowed a gradual increase in exercise.

conditions, biologic factors such as age and size of the patient, location of the fracture, presence of infection, and amount and quality
of bone available for surgical revision of the implant greatly influence the prognosis. Disuse caused by immobilization is reversible,
although a remobilization period of at least twice the duration of
immobilization should be expected for full reversal of bone loss
(Kaneps *et al.* 1997).

Prevention

Prevention of bone resorption focuses primarily on providing a biomechanical environment favorable to bone healing by:
- Proper selection of fixation technique and size of implants based
  on consideration of biologic and mechanical characteristics of the
  fracture
- Consider biologic fixation techniques for comminuted nonar-
  ticular fractures, emphasizing preservation of soft tissues and restoration of limb alignment with less-than-rigid fixation.
- Early return to function via surgical fixation of fractures, postoperative pain management and physical therapy
- Whenever possible, external coaptation should be limited to
  compression bandages applied for a few days after fracture repair

to control postoperative swelling. Alternatives should be considered (see Chapter 16) if external coaptation is considered for a
longer duration.
- Monitor fracture healing via serial radiographs until bony union
  to allow early diagnosis and treatment of postoperative bone
  resorption.

Prevention of infections and fracture-associated sarcoma are
addressed in Chapters 104.

Relevant literature

This section focuses primarily on the mechanical conditions that
favor bone resorption. Literature related to clinical entities responsible for bone loss, such as osteomyelitis (see Chapter 5) and
fracture-associated sarcoma (see Chapter 104), are reviewed elsewhere in the book. If adequate vascularity is a prerequisite for bone
healing, the biomechanical environment surrounding a fracture
determines the pattern of repair (Griffon 2005). Bone resorption

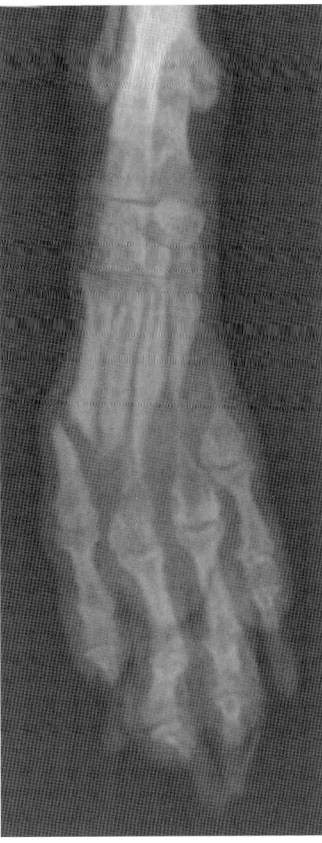

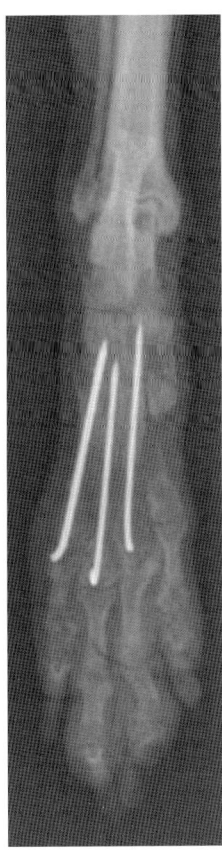

(A)   **(B)**

Figure 97.4 Bone resorption caused by excessive interfragmentary strain and disuse. This small breed dog was presented 6 weeks after conservative management of open fractures of all metacarpal bones secondary to bite wounds inflicted by an opossum. The dog had been treated with antibiotics based on culture and sensitivity results of wound swabs. Soft tissues were healed at the time of presentation, but the dog was not bearing weight on the limb. **A,** Initial radiograph. Decreased radiopacity of the metacarpal and carpal bones, combined with severe bone resorption at all fracture sites. Fractures were treated via intramedullary pins and autogenous graft. Cancellous bone was placed in bone defects, and corticocancellous bone from the iliac crest was placed served as onlay graft between fragments. A splint was applied after surgery. **B,** Radiographs 12 weeks after surgery. The dog had regained some function of the limb, but healing appears delayed on radiographs. Autogenous stem cells were injected percutaneously into the fracture site.

is a normal process of fracture healing and correlates in magnitude with the motion and gap present at the site. Whereas primary bone formation occurs without bone resorption under extreme conditions of reduction and immobilization, spontaneous healing represents the opposite end of the spectrum and best illustrates the mechanisms involved in secondary bone healing. Spontaneous healing of complete fractures typically occurs in the **presence of highly unstable fragment ends**. Bone repair must develop despite high interfragmentary strain, defined as the deformation occurring at the fracture site relative to the size of the gap. However, bone formation can only occur in a stable biomechanical environment with an interfragmentary strain lower than 2% (Perren and Cordey 1980). Under unstable conditions, healing proceeds

via initial contraction of adjacent muscles, resorption of fragment ends, orderly repair with tissues suitable for the mechanical environment, and formation of a prominent external callus. Bone resorption at the fracture site allows distribution of motion over a larger surface area and can be recognized radiographically as a local loss of radiopacity and widening of the gap. If the fracture gap is well vascularized, interfragmentary motion will stimulate callus formation, further increasing the surface area; the fracture will progress to a cartilaginous callus, but if this callus is unable to stabilize the fragments, a hypertrophic nonunion and pseudoarthrosis will develop. However, compromised vascularization and excessive instability will only allow formation of fibrous tissue and development of an atrophic nonunion.

Similarly, large gaps do not heal spontaneously and have been used as experimental models of nonunions (Claes et al. 1998). In mixed breed dogs, a 2.5-cm diameter defect in the diaphysis of the radius is an established model for nonunions (Sciadini et al. 1997). Removal of a 21-mm-long section of femoral diaphysis produced critically sized defects in dogs (Kraus et al. 1999). One of the first and most common nonunion models in dogs was developed for the evaluation of bone morphogenetic proteins on bone healing (Nilsson et al. 1986). Resection of a length of ulna equal to twice the diameter of the midshaft created a defect that consistently failed to heal. This model does not require fixation and is therefore less invasive.

On the other end of the spectrum, bone resorption is induced by **disuse** and lack of biomechanical stimulation. These conditions occur after prolonged immobilization in a cast or splint, stress shielding secondary to plate fixation of fractures, absence of gravitational forces (space flights), or loss of limb function (Waters et al. 1991). Disuse may result from pain, musculoskeletal disease, or neurologic disorders. Immobilization osteoporosis results from an imbalance in bone homeostasis (resorption vs. formation) caused by insufficient dynamic biomechanical stimulation. The response of bone to mechanical usage was initially proposed in Julius Wolff's 1892 treatise and has since been expanded (Frost 1988). According to this mechanostat theory, if bone loading generates strains that drop below a minimum threshold, bone mass and architecture are adjusted until the bone strains are within the minimum effective strain range (Frost 1987). In addition to direct forces placed on bone, muscle contraction against gravity is believed to play a crucial role in the biomechanical loading of bones (Giangregorio and Blimkie 2002). Therefore, muscle atrophy secondary to immobilization would be expected to contribute to bone loss. However, the exact mechanisms responsible for immobilization osteoporosis remain unclear. Reduced calcium and phosphorus concentrations, resistance to cytokines such as insulin-like growth factor-1, reduction in transforming growth factor-β, and increases in prostaglandin E2 have all been implicated in the bone response to biomechanical unloading (Giangregorio and Blimkie 2002). In small animals, disuse osteoporosis is most commonly associated with other complications of fracture management (e.g., implant failure) that compromise limb function and bone healing. The veterinary literature focuses mainly on the clinical aspects of these conditions and is summarized in corresponding chapters in this book. Prolonged immobilization caused by external coaptation is well accepted as a clinically relevant cause of bone resorption in small animals, although most of the evidence published on this complication stems from experimental studies. Immobilization of a limb in a cast or non–weight-bearing bandage is well established as a canine model of immobilization disuse in studies focusing

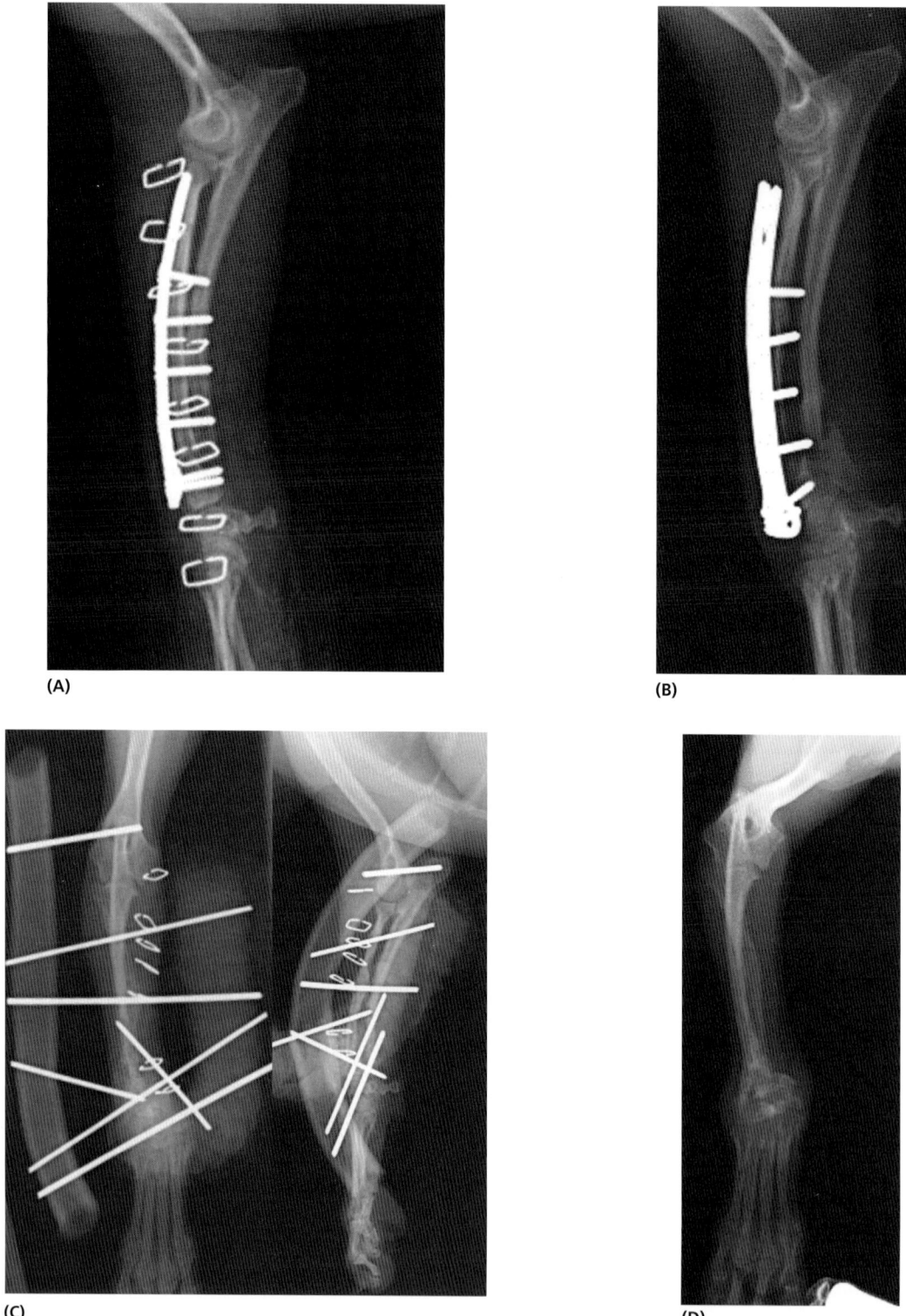

(A)

(B)

(C)

(D)

Figure 97.5 Bone resorption and implant failure after plate fixation of a distal radial fracture in an 11-month-old, 4-kg miniature Yorkshire terrier. **A,** Postoperative radiograph. The fracture was repaired with a 1.5-mm-diameter canine distal radial plate and six cortical screws, two in the distal fragment. **B,** Radiographic appearance 6 weeks after surgery. Catastrophic implant failure of the two distal screws and atrophic nonunion of the radius. Note the decreased radiopacity and bone resorption affecting the radius and ulna. **C,** Craniocaudal and mediolateral radiographs after revision with an acrylic external fixator. Because of the limited bone stock, Kirschner wires have been placed in multiple planes in the radius and ulna, bridging the radiocarpal joint. The repair was augmented with autogenous cancellous bone and demineralized bone matrix. **D,** Final radiographic follow-up 5 months after initial fracture repair. The limb was placed in a splint (made of a syringe case) after removal of the external fixator. The dog regained some function of the limb despite the pseudoarthrosis formed at the fracture site and ankylosis of the carpus. This case was managed before the development of mini-circular external fixators.

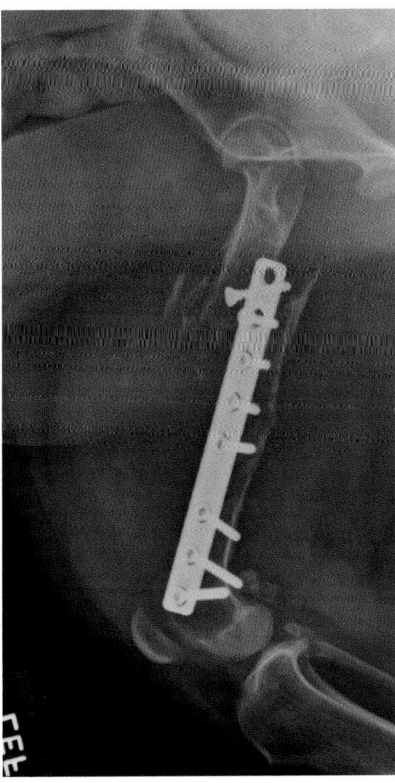

Figure 97.6 Bone resorption caused by fracture-associated sarcoma. This radiograph was obtained on a 7-year-old large mixed breed dog that sustained a femoral fracture at 1 year of age.

on the pathophysiology, treatment, and prevention of this condition. In healthy immature dogs (12- to 16-week-old mixed breed dogs), immobilization of the hindlimb in a fiberglass cast extending from the midfemur to the digits for 28 days decreased the bone mass of the distal tibial metaphysis by 30.6% (Waters *et al.* 1991). In another study, bandaging the forelimb of adult mixed breed dogs in a non–weight-bearing position for 16 weeks reduced the bone mineral density of immobilized humeri by about 30% and significantly affected the biomechanical properties of affected bones (Kaneps *et al.* 1997). Similar to the case in other species, changes were more significant in cancellous bone, where biomechanical properties ranged between 28% and 74% of control values, than in cortical bone, where similar parameters varied between 71% and 96% of control values. Loss of biomechanical strength and stiffness are accompanied by histologic changes, including trabecular thinning and increased trabecular spacing (Lane *et al.* 1996). The ability of remobilization to reverse changes induced by disuse varies among studies, most likely because of differences in experimental design such as duration of immobilization and remobilization. The minimum duration of immobilization required to induce bone loss is unclear in dogs, but in rats, number of osteoclasts and active resorption surfaces doubled after 7 days of hindlimb suspension (Vico *et al.* 1991). Decreases in bone mineral content and bone formation rate have also been reported as early as 14 days after limb immobilization in rats (Sessions *et al.* 1989). Bone response to disuse varies with species and mechanism of immobilization, preventing straight extrapolation of these results to dogs placed in a splint or cast after surgery. Nonetheless, they provide a rationale for minimizing the extent and duration of postoperative immobilization.

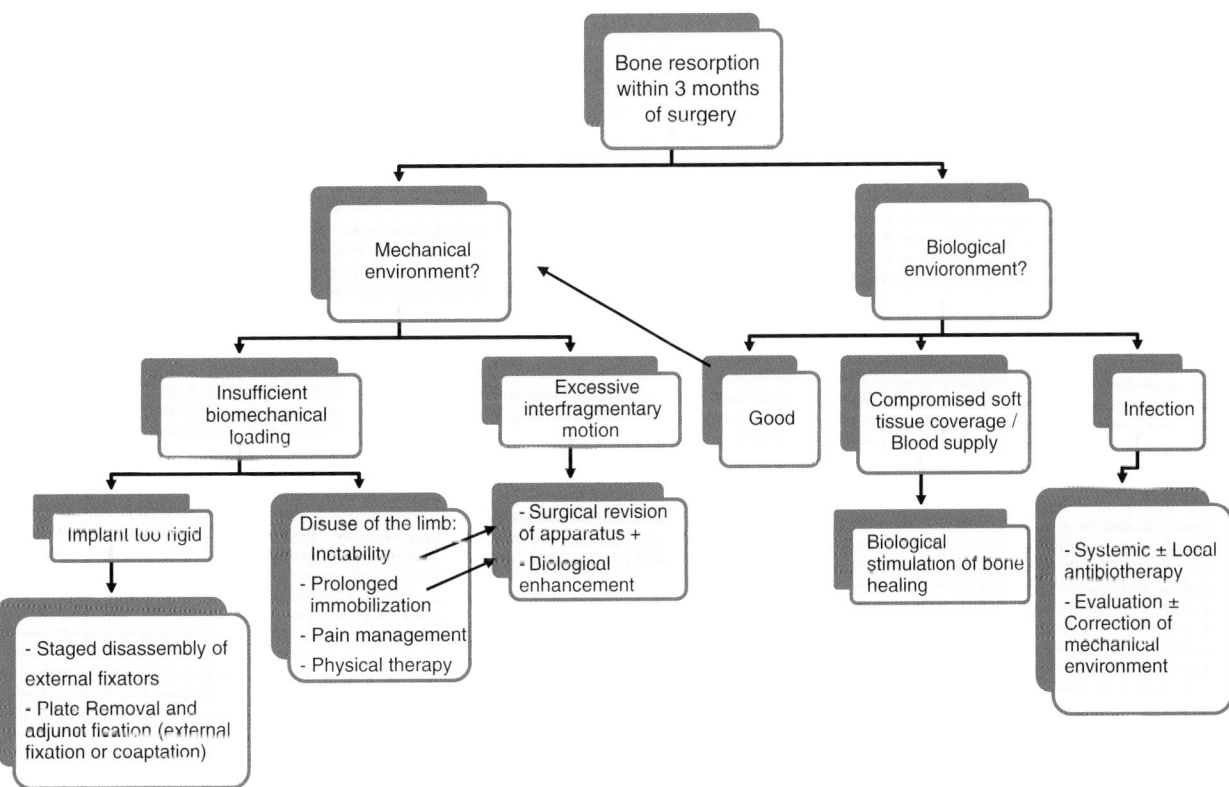

Figure 97.7 Algorithm for management of bone resorption in the early postoperative phase of fracture fixation.

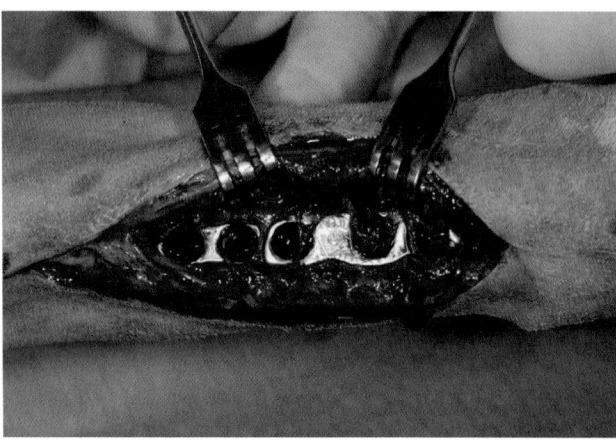

(A)

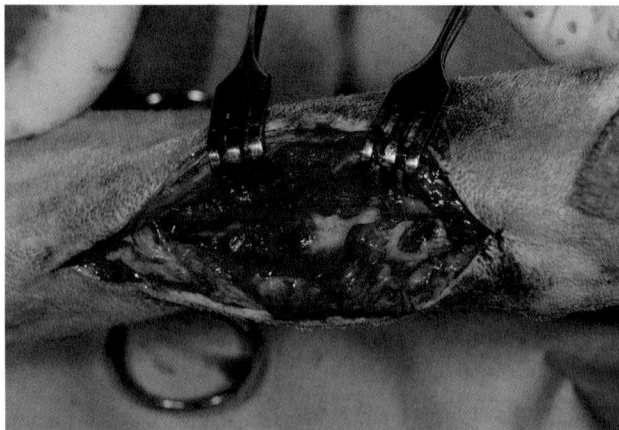

(B)

Figure 97.8 Plate removal. **A,** The plate remains attached to the bone after screw removal because bone has formed around it. **B,** Appearance of the bone after plate removal. Bony ridges that formed in contact with the plate should be preserved to provide support.

References

Claes, L.E., Heigele, C.A., Neidlinger-Wilke, C., et al. (1998) Effects of mechanical factors on the fracture healing process. *Clinical Orthopaedics and Related Research* 355 (Suppl.), S132-S147.

Frost, H.M. (1987) Bone "mass" and the "mechanostat": a proposal. *The Anatomical Record* 219 (1), 1-9.

Frost, H.M. (1988) Structural adaptations to mechanical usage. A proposed "three-way rule" for bone modeling. *Veterinary and Comparative Orthopaedics and Traumatology* 1, 7-17.

Giangregorio, L., Blimkie, C.J. (2002) Skeletal adaptations to alterations in weight-bearing activity: a comparison of models of disuse osteoporosis. *Sports Medicine* 32 (7), 459-476.

Griffon, D. (2005) Fracture healing. In Johnson, A., Houlton, J. (eds.) *AO Principles of Fracture Management in the Dog and Cat.* Thieme, New York, pp. 73-97.

Kaneps, A.J., Stover, S.M., and Lane, N.E. (1997) Changes in canine cortical and cancellous bone mechanical properties following immobilization and remobilization with exercise. *Bone* 21 (5), 419-423.

Kraus, K.H., Kadiyala, S., Wotton, H., et al. (1999) Critically sized osteo-periosteal femoral defects: a dog model. *Journal of Investigative Surgery* 12 (2), 115-124.

Lane, N.E., Kaneps, A.J., Stover, S.M., et al. (1996) Bone mineral density and turnover following forelimb immobilization and recovery in young adult dogs. *Calcified Tissue International* 59, 401-406.

Nilsson, O.S., Urist, M.R., Dawson, E.G., et al. (1986) Bone repair induced by bone morphogenetic protein in ulnar defects in dogs. *Journal of Bone and Joint Surgery* 68 (4), 635-642.

Perren, S.M., Cordey, J. (1980) The concept of interfragmentary strain. In Uhthoff, H.K. (ed.) *Current Concepts of Internal Fixation of Fractures.* Springer, Berlin, p. 63.

Sciadini, M.F., Dawson, J.M., Johnson, K.D. (1997) Bovine-derived bone protein as a bone graft substitute in a canine segmental defect model. *Journal of Orthopaedic Trauma* 11 (7), 496-508.

Sessions, N.D., Halloran, B.P., Bikle, D.D., et al. (1989) Bone response to normal weight bearing after a period of skeletal unloading. *American Journal of Physiology* 257 (4), E606-E610.

Vico, L., Novikov, V.E., Very, J.M., et al. (1991) Bone histomorphometric comparison of rat tibial metaphysis after 7-day tail suspension vs. 7-day spaceflight. *Aviation, Space, and Environmental Medicine* 62 (1), 26-31.

Waters, D.J., Caywood, D.D., Turner, R.T. (1991) Effect of tamoxifen citrate on canine immobilization (disuse) osteoporosis. *Veterinary Surgery* 20 (6), 392-396.

98 Delayed Union

Ann Johnson
College of Veterinary Medicine, University of Illinois, Champaign, IL, USA

Definition

Fractures that are not healing as quickly as anticipated based on biologic, mechanical, and clinical factors and the method of fracture fixation are considered delayed unions. Adult dogs and cats with long bone fractures generally have radiographic evidence of bone bridging all fracture lines by 12 weeks. Immature dogs and cats generally have radiographic evidence of fracture healing by 6 weeks. Bone healing may take months to occur in elderly animals, particularly old cats. The anticipated rate of fracture healing should take into account the nature of the traumatic injury, the location of the fracture, the systemic state of the animal, the fixation of the fracture, and the postoperative management (Hayda *et al.* 1998).

Risk factors

- Systemic illness
- Compromised vascular supply
- Unstable implants
- Extremely rigid fixation
- Infection
- Poor postoperative management
- Radiation therapy
- Pharmacologic factors, including corticosteroids and nonsteroidal antiinflammatory drugs (NSAIDs)

Diagnosis

Determination of fracture delayed union is generally based on serial clinical and radiographic evaluations. Although weight bearing and pain response to palpation at the fracture site are two important clinical measures to assess fracture healing, radiography is the standard method for evaluating bone healing. Radiographic observations used to assess fracture healing include presence of cortical continuity, loss of fracture line(s) on serial radiographs, and presence of bridging callus. Delayed union is a subjective diagnosis based on observation of serial orthogonal radiographs of the fracture made over time and the clinician's experience with similar fractures (Figure 98.1). In general, fractures that are not healed by 12 to

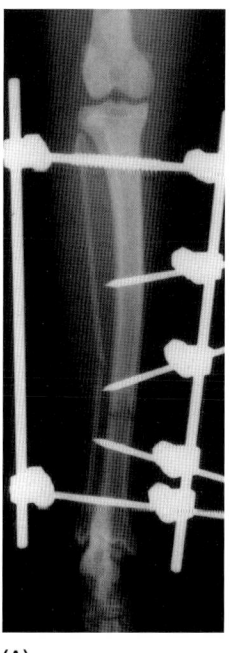

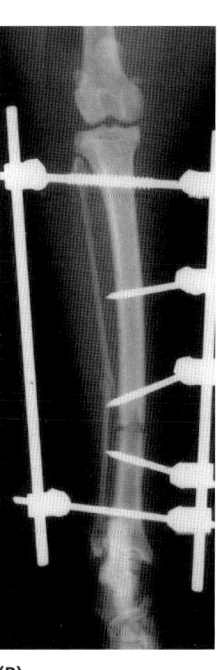

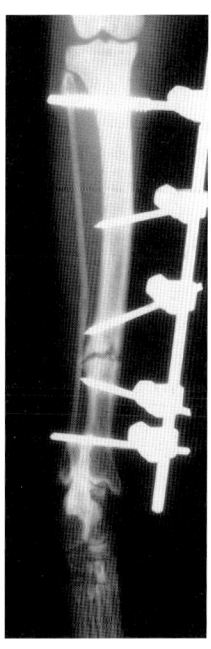

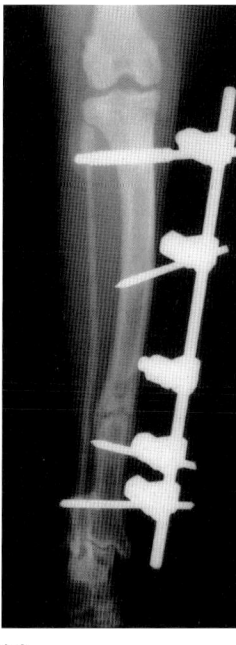

(A) (B) (C) (D)

Figure 98.1 **A,** Postoperative radiograph of a 3-year old cat with a transverse tibial fracture stabilized with a type II external fixator. **B,** Six weeks later, the fracture line had widened, and there was minimal evidence of bridging callus. The fixator was destabilized. **C** and **D,** The 12- and 18-week follow-up radiographs show slowly progressive healing.

Complications in Small Animal Surgery, First Edition. Edited by Dominique Griffon and Annick Hamaide.
© 2016 John Wiley & Sons, Inc. Published 2016 by John Wiley & Sons, Inc.
Companion website: www.wiley.com/go/griffon/complications

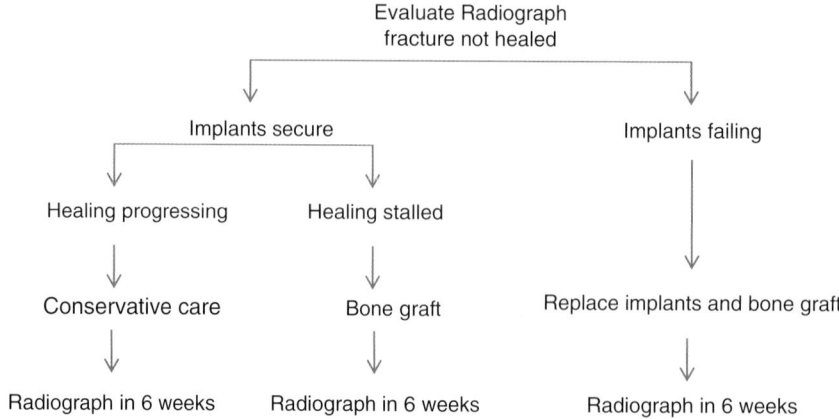

Figure 98.2 Algorithm for management of delayed union.

16 weeks and have evidence of progressive healing activity but with some doubt about the outcome are diagnosed as delayed unions.

Treatment

Treatment of a delayed union depends on the stability and potential longevity of the fixation. If the fixation is appropriate with no evidence of impending failure and there is evidence of bone healing, then continued confinement and serial evaluations are in order (see Figure 98.2). A cancellous bone autograft or allograft with demineralized bone matrix may be inserted surgically to address concerns over the minimal progression of healing relative to the longevity of implants.

If the fixation is unstable, it must be modified or replaced. External fixators may be modified to increase stability if needed or alternatively to destabilize to modulate bone healing (see Chapter 109). Other methods of fixation are not as amenable to modification without surgical intervention. If surgical intervention is needed to replace implants, a bone graft should be added (Figures 98.3 and Figure 98.4).

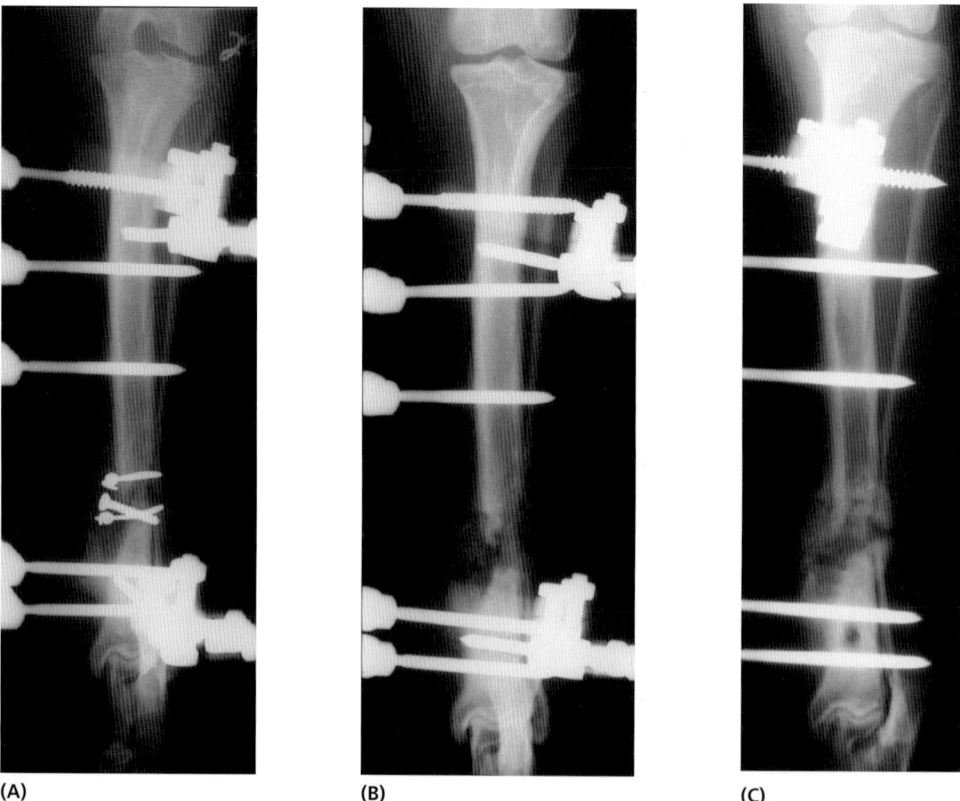

(A) (B) (C)

Figure 98.3 **A,** Six-week postoperative radiograph of a tibial fracture with evidence of loose implants and a sequestered piece of bone. **B,** The implants and bone were removed and a bone graft placed. **C,** Two months later, healing is progressing slowly.

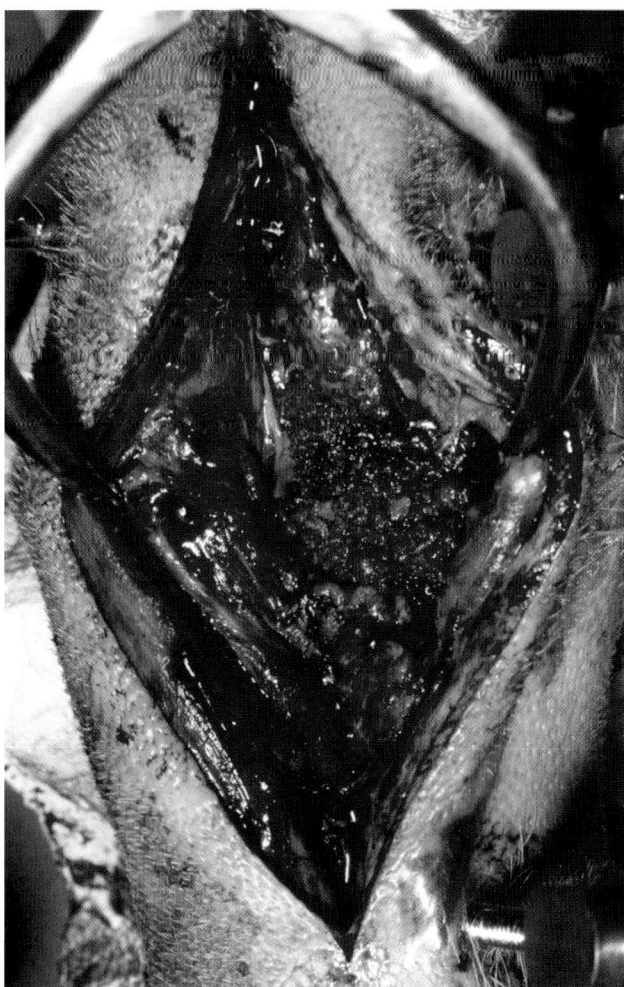

Figure 98.4 Cancellous bone autograft placed in the bone defect after implant and sequestrum removal.

Similarly, if there is an unstable or sequestered piece of bone, it should be removed. The site should be cultured and appropriate antimicrobials administered.

Owners must be counseled regarding confinement, implant care (external fixators), and uncertain prognosis. The fracture should be evaluated radiographically in 6-week intervals. As long as healing progresses, union generally will occur. If there is no evidence of progressive healing or if implant failure occurs, the fracture is reclassified as a nonunion and requires surgery for optimal outcome.

Outcome

If there is radiographic evidence of healing activity and the implants maintain the stability of the fracture, most delayed unions will heal. Implant instability or failure may lead to a nonunion.

Prevention

Appropriate fracture and patient assessment will help the clinician either avoid delayed unions or plan for them by incorporating bone graft materials and using implants that maintain the bone implant interface integrity for an extended time.

Relevant literature

Causes of delayed bone healing are varied but include poor vascularization at the fracture, systemic illness, implant issues, and pharmacologic influences. Excessive trauma to surrounding soft tissue at the fracture destroys vasculature and delays healing. A lack of arterial blood supply to the distal radius of toy breed dogs has been credited with a high incidence of delayed union and nonunion (Welch *et al.* 1997). Although the feline tibia shows a similar predisposition to delayed and nonunion (Nolte *et al* 2005), a decrease in intramedullary arterial supply could not be documented (Dugat *et al.* 2011). Excessively rigid implants protect the bone from mechanical forces that stimulate bone production. Conversely, unstable implants impair new vascularization at the fracture and delay healing. NSAIDs have been shown to inhibit bone healing in experimental animal models using mice, rats, and rabbits (Barry 2010). Long-term administration of carprofen appeared to inhibit bone healing in tibial osteotomies in dogs (Ochi *et al.* 2011). However, extrapolation of these experimental data to clinical cases warrants is affected by species differences, as well as dose and duration of treatment used in these studies. Overall, the benefits of short-term postoperative administration of NSAIDs outweigh their potential and transient effect on fracture healing (Griffon 2010).

The criterion for diagnosis of a delayed union is elusive. The assessment is generally made from orthogonal radiographs, which is the standard of practice (Axelrad and Einhorn 2011). However, there is wide variation not only in individual surgeons' interpretation of bone healing based on radiographs but also in their definition of a delayed union, nonunion, and malunion (Bhandari *et al.* 2002; Axelrad and Einhorn 2011). In one study, orthopedic surgeons' interpretation of a delayed union ranged from 1 to 8 months (Bhandari *et al.* 2002). Alternative imaging has been used to differentiate delayed union from nonunion and guide treatment. Computed tomography is valuable to detect bone bridging throughout the fracture (Axelrad and Einhorn 2011). Ultrasonography has been used to identify the amount of vascularization at a fracture and guide treatment of delayed union. Fractures with moderate to large amount of vascularization present on power Doppler examination were managed conservatively, and one fracture with minimal vascularization was treated with bone graft and a plate (Risselada *et al.* 2008).

Because assessment and diagnosis vary, appropriate treatment can also vary. Most delayed unions are simply slow bone healing and will eventually unite with conservative management. The limiting factor is the longevity of implants. Speeding healing with bone graft or bone graft substitutes may prevent problems. Autologous bone graft is the gold standard, but allograft with demineralized bone matrix is effective clinically (Hoffer *et al* 2008). Bone marrow injections have been used, but the osteogenic capacity of this treatment has been variable with some investigators very positive and others cautious about the outcome (Tshamala and van Bree 2006; Fayaz 2011).

References

Axelrad, T.W., Einhorn, T.A. (2011) Use of clinical assessment tools in the evaluation of fracture healing. *Injury* 42, 301-305.

Barry, S. (2010) Non-steroidal anti-inflammatory drugs inhibit bone healing: a review. *Veterinary and Comparative Orthopaedics and Traumatology* 23 (6), 385-392.

Bhandari, M., Guyatt, G.H., Swiontkowski, M.F., et al. (2002) A lack of consensus in the assessment of fracture healing among orthopaedic surgeons. *Journal of Orthopaedic Trauma* 16, 562-566.

Dugat, D., Rochat, M., Ritchey, J., et al. (2011) Quantitative analysis of the intramedullary arterial supply of the feline tibia. *Veterinary and Comparative Orthopaedics and Traumatology* 24 (5), 313-319.

Fayaz, H.C., Giannoudis, P.V., Vrahas, M.S., *et al.* (2011) The role of stem cells in fracture healing and nonunion. *International Orthopaedics* 35 (11), 1587-1597.

Griffon, D.J. (2010) Secondary bone healing. In Bojrab, M.J. (ed.) *Disease Mechanisms in Small Animal Surgery* 3rd ed. Teton NewMedia, Jackson, WY.

Hayda, R.A., Brighton, C.T., Esterhai, J.L. (1998) Pathophysiology of delayed healing. *Clinical Orthopaedics and Related Research* 355 (Suppl.), S32.

Hoffer, M., Griffon, D.J., Schaeffer, D., et al. (2008) Clinical applications of demineralized bone matrix: a retrospective and case-matched study of 75 dogs. *Veterinary Surgery* 37 (7), 639-647.

Nolte, D.M., Fusco, J.V., Peterson, M.E. (2005) Incidence of and predisposing factors for nonunion of fractures involving the appendicular skeleton in cats: 18 cases (1998-2002). *Journal of the American Veterinary Medical Association* 226 (1), 77-82.

Ochi, H., Hara, Y., Asou, Y, Harada, et al. (2011) Effects of long-term administration of carprofen on healing of a tibial osteotomy in dogs. *American Journal of Veterinary Research* 72 (5), 634-641.

Risselada, M., van Bree, H., Kramer, M., et al. (2008) Use of ultrasonography to guide the management of delayed unions in three dogs. *Veterinary Record* 162 (22), 725-727.

Tshamala, M., van Bree, H. (2006) Osteoinductive properties of the bone marrow Myth or reality. *Veterinary and Comparative Orthopaedics and Traumatology* 19, 133-141.

Welch, J.A., Boudrieau, R.J., DeJardin, L.M., et al. (1997) The intraosseous blood supply of the canine radius: implications for healing of distal fractures in small dogs. *Veterinary Surgery* 26 (1), 57-61.

99 Nonunion

Ann Johnson

College of Veterinary Medicine, University of Illinois, Champaign, IL, USA

Definitions

A nonunion is a fracture in which the healing process has apparently stopped progressing and surgical intervention is necessary to create an environment conducive to bone healing. Nonunions are classified biologically as viable and nonviable. Viable nonunion is a fracture with good biology at the fracture site but failing to heal because of mechanical instability hampering the tissue responses. Variable amounts of callus are evident on radiographs. Hypertrophic nonunions produce callus, but the cartilage at the fracture is unable to vascularize and bridge the fracture cortices with bone (Figure 99.1). A nonviable nonunion is a fracture that fails to heal because the biologic responses leading to bony union are inadequate. There is an absence of callus, with rounding or resorption of the bone ends. Sclerosis of the medullary canal may occur (Figure 99.2).

Risk factors

- Dogs with femoral fractures treated with single intramedullary pins
- Distal radial diaphyseal fractures in toy breed dogs stabilized with external coaptation
- Fractures treated with plates of inadequate size or length
- Comminuted fractures inadequately stabilized with cerclage wires
- Fractures treated with external fixators of inadequate frame and pin size (see Chapter 109)
- Fractures with poor biology (i.e., vascularization) caused by fracture location, high-energy injury with extensive soft tissue destruction, or excessive surgical intervention.
- Fractures of the proximal ulna and of the tibia in cats (Nolte *et al.* 2005)

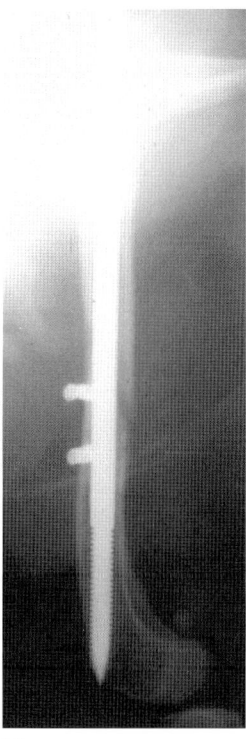
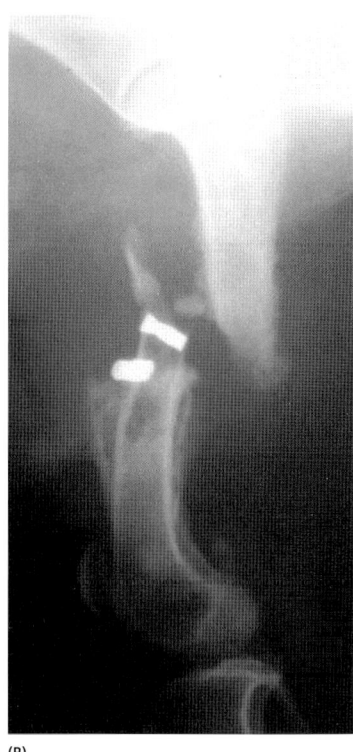
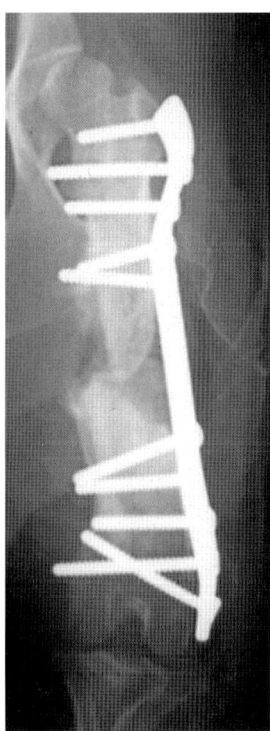
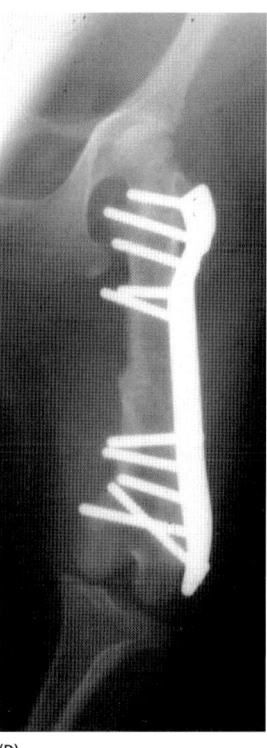

(A)   (B)   (C)   (D)

Figure 99.1 **A,** Inadequate stabilization of a femur with an intramedullary pin, suture, and crimp clamps. **B,** Development of a hypertrophic nonunion with a sequestered bone piece and loose implants. **C,** Stabilization of the nonunion with a bone plate. **D,** Healed nonunion 12 weeks after surgery.

Complications in Small Animal Surgery, First Edition. Edited by Dominique Griffon and Annick Hamaide.

© 2016 John Wiley & Sons, Inc. Published 2016 by John Wiley & Sons, Inc.

Companion website: www.wiley.com/go/griffon/complications

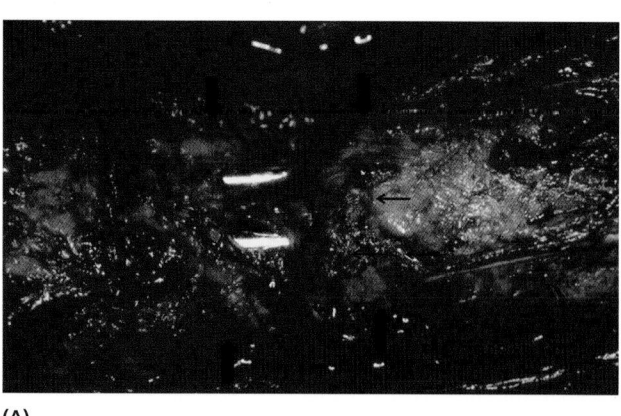
(A)

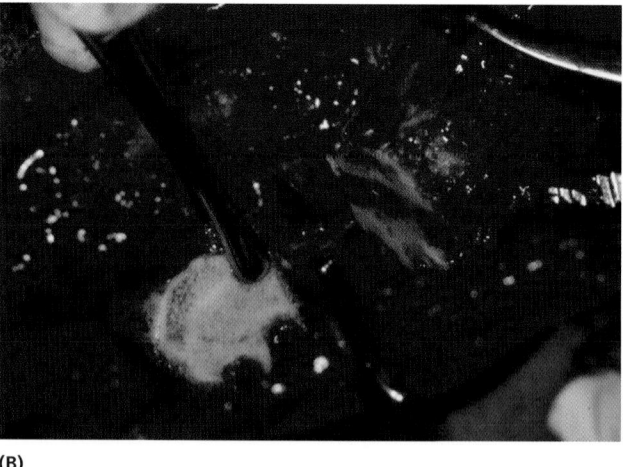
(B)

Figure 99.2 Intraoperative appearance of a femoral nonunion. **A,** Two intramedullary pins failed to stabilize a transverse femoral fracture. Note the atrophy of the bone at the fracture site with closure of medullary canal around the pins. **B,** Appearance of the fracture site after ostectomy of the atrophied ends of the proximal and distal bone fragments. *Source:* D. Griffon, Western University of Health Sciences, Pomona, CA, 2014. Reproduced with permission from D. Griffon.

Diagnosis

The diagnosis of nonunion is usually based on observation of orthogonal radiographs of the fractured bone. Nonunions are often diagnosed from one set of radiographs because there is evidence of unstable implants or bone pieces (sequestra), loss of fracture reduction, bone resorption, or sclerosis of the medullary canal. However, in fractures with adequate stabilization, serial radiographs may be necessary to confirm that healing is not progressing based on the presence of a persistent lucent line at the fracture, ineffective callus formation, and absence of bone bridging the cortical pieces. Computed tomography is a valuable option for detecting bone bridging throughout the fracture when the diagnosis of nonunion is questionable (Axelrad and Einhorn 2011).

The presumptuous diagnosis of viable or nonviable nonunion is made based on the amount of callus present around the fracture. Fractures with abundant periosteal callus are considered viable. However, it may be difficult to distinguish a viable nonunion with minimal callus from a nonviable nonunion. Ultrasonography or scintigraphy may be useful in determining the presence of vascularity at the nonunion (Risselada *et al.* 2006).

Osteomyelitis often occurs concurrently with nonunion. See Chapter 5 for information.

Treatment

Treatment is determined by the assessment of the stability of the fracture and fixation and the biologic viability of the site (Figure 99.3). Bone healing in stable fractures with functional implants may be stimulated with cancellous bone graft, autologous bone marrow, or growth factors. Unstable fractures with obvious loose implants or sequestered bone fragments require removal of the offending items (see Figure 99.1). Biologic viability also affects treatment. Fractures with adequate vascularity usually respond to stabilization alone. Fractures with limited vascularity benefit from stimulation of the biologic healing process using cancellous bone graft, autologous bone marrow, or growth factors.

Stable nonunions may be treated with:
- Limited approach to the fracture site to place a cancellous bone autograft, cancellous bone allograft with demineralized bone matrix (DBM), autologous bone marrow, or bone morphogenic protein (rhBMP-2).
- Percutaneous injection of autologous bone marrow under fluoroscopic guidance
- Percutaneous injection of growth factors such as rhBMP-2 under fluoroscopic guidance.

Unstable viable nonunions with hypertrophic callus are treated by:
- Removing any loose implants and necrotic cortical bone pieces
- Opening the medullary canal (see Figure 99.2): Although this is often unnecessary, removing callus in the area will allow easier visualization of the cortex for plate contouring and provide cancellous bone for grafting.
- Carefully aligning the joints and stabilizing the fracture with a bone plate contoured to approximate the normal shape of the bone and used as a compression plate (see Figure 99.1) or external fixation (Figure 99.4)
- Stabilization via external fixation is especially relevant to nonunions of the distal long bones or suspected infections
- Cancellous bone grafts may be used, although often the hypertrophic callus provides adequate cancellous bone for healing.

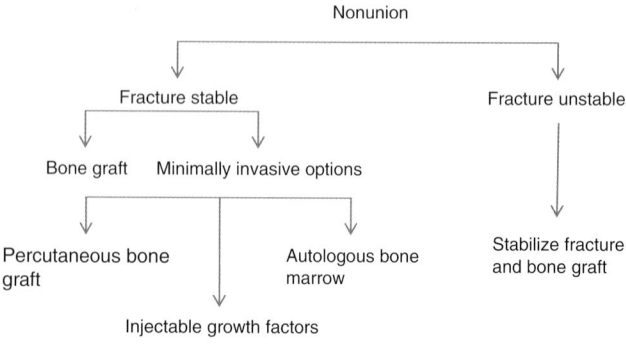

Figure 99.3 Algorithm for treatment of nonunion.

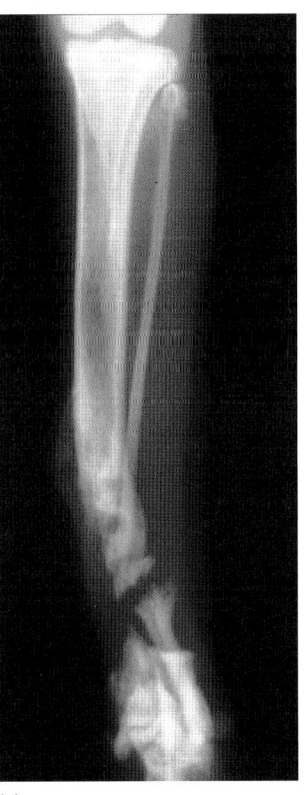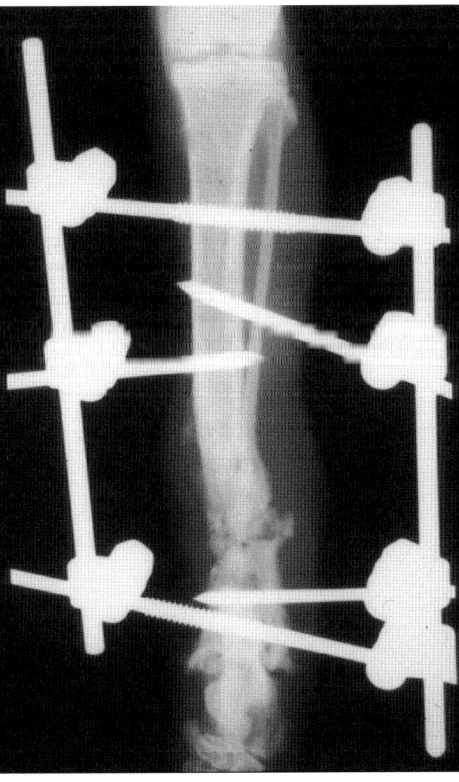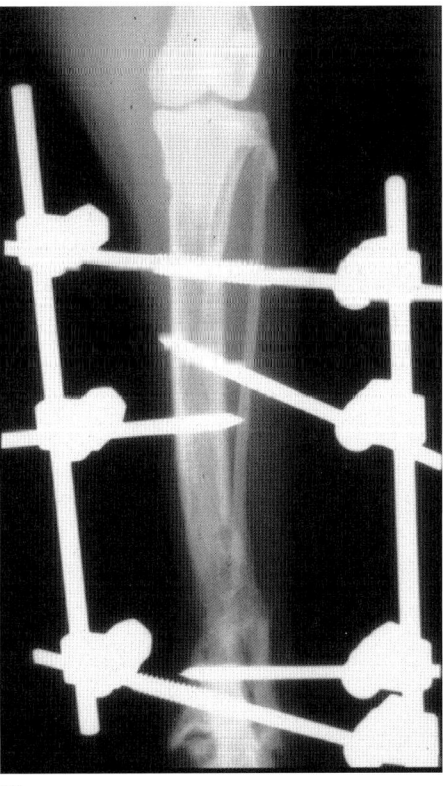

(A)   (B)   (C)

Figure 99.4 A, Atrophic nonunion of the distal tibial diaphysis in a cat. The fibula exhibits callus. **B,** Resection of the fibrous tissue, addition of cancellous bone from the fibular callus site, and stabilization of the tibia with an external fixator. **C,** Healed nonunion 12 weeks later.

- Obtaining swabs for bacterial culture and sensitivity because concurrent osteomyelitis is common
- If a radiographic or clinical diagnosis of osteomyelitis is made, treatment must include appropriate antimicrobial therapy.
- Plate removal is recommended after healing of infected nonunions because plates may serve as a nidus for continued infection.

Nonviable unstable nonunions are treated by:
- Surgically removing fibrous tissues and sclerotic bone occluding the medullary canal (see Figure 99.2) or en-bloc resection of the inactive bone and fracture site
- Stabilizing the fracture with a durable implant: bone plate and screws or external fixation
- Packing the area with cancellous bone autograft or allograft with DBM
- Obtaining swabs for bacterial culture and sensitivity and, if necessary, appropriate antimicrobial therapy.

Outcome

Unstable hypertrophic nonunions generally heal rapidly after being adequately stabilized (see Figure 99.1). Nonviable nonunions may be more problematic unless the healing process can be reinitiated.

Prevention

Nonunions may be prevented by accurate fracture and patient assessment to choose the appropriate implants and with fracture planning that respects the surrounding soft tissues and incorporates bone graft materials during fracture stabilization. Good client communication regarding postoperative fracture management is also essential.

Relevant literature

Despite the best efforts of surgeons, nonunion occurs in around 5% of fractures in reported case series. The incidence of nonunion appears consistent over the years when past literature is examined and compared with current outcomes (Nolte *et al.* 2005). Dogs and cats have a similar incidence of nonunions (Nolte *et al.* 2005). The most common sites for nonunion in dogs are the radius and ulna, femur, and humerus, and the most common sites for nonunion in cats are the tibia and proximal portion of the ulna (Nolte *et al.* 2005). Most nonunions result from instability, but a lack of vascularity is considered a contributing factor in the distal radius of toy breed dogs (Welch *et al.* 1997). There is similar speculation about the feline tibia, but intramedullary arterial supply appears similar in cats and dogs (Dugat *et al.* 2011).

The treatment of nonunion relies primarily on stabilization for vascular nonunions and resection and stabilization for atrophic nonunions (Blaeser *et al.* 2003). In all cases, the implant selected should remain rigid for an extended period of time, whether it relies on plate or external fixation. Assessing the vascularity of a nonunion may be difficult from radiographs, although abundant callus infers adequate vascularity. Doppler evaluation is more sensitive than radiographic evaluation in detecting vascularity (Risselada *et al.* 2006). Scintigraphy is also useful to evaluate vascularity (Averill *et al.* 1999).

Augmenting treatment with bone graft or bone graft substitutes is very important in stable nonunions and nonviable nonunions. Autologous bone graft is the gold standard, but several studies in the human and veterinary literature support the use of osteoinductive agents as substitutes for autogenous cancellous graft in noninfected nonunions. The type of osteoinductive agents most commonly used in small animals consist of a naturally occurring mixture of growth factors such as DBM. This type of allograft has been found equally effective to autogenous cancellous bone in comminuted fractures and arthrodesis in dogs (Hoffer *et al.* 2008). Several reports have documented the efficiency of BMP2 in the treatment of nonunions in dogs, but the application of recombinant agents remains limited by cost (Schmökel *et al.* 2004; Milovancev *et al.* 2007). Some experimental evidence supports the effectiveness of omentum in achieving healing in a confirmed nonunion model (Saifzadeh *et al.* 2009). A plethora of osteoconductive agents have become commercially available to veterinarians, largely for use in corrective osteotomies or treatment of cruciate ligament deficiency via tibial osteotomies. However, the efficiency of these agents has not been well established, especially in cases with compromised bone healing. Some authors see the future of bone grafting in combining stem cells and scaffolds (Fayaz *et al.* 2011).

References

Axelrad, T.W., Einhorn, T.A. (2011) Use of clinical assessment tools in the evaluation of fracture healing. *Injury* 42 (3), 301-305.

Averill, S.M., Johnson, A.L., Chambers, M., et al. (1999) Qualitative and quantitative scintigraphic imaging to predict fracture healing. *Veterinary and Comparative Orthopaedics and Traumatology* 12, 142-158.

Blaeser, L.L., Gallagher, J.G., Boudrieau, R.J. (2003) Treatment of biologically inactive nonunions by a limited en bloc ostectomy and compression plate fixation: a review of 17 cases. *Veterinary Surgery* 2 (1), 91-100.

Dugat, D., Rochat, M., Ritchey, J., et al. (2011), Quantitative analysis of the intramedullary arterial supply of the feline tibia. *Veterinary and Comparative Orthopaedics and Traumatology* 24 (5), 313-319.

Fayaz, H.C., Giannoudis, P.V., Vrahas, M.S., *et al.* (2011) The role of stem cells in fracture healing and nonunion. *International Orthopaedics* 35 (11), 1587-1597.

Hoffer, M., Griffon, D.J., Schaeffer, D., et al. (2008) Clinical applications of demineralized bone matrix: a retrospective and case-matched study of 75 dogs. *Veterinary Surgery* 37 (7), 639-647.

Milovancev, M., Muir, P., Manley, P.A., et al. (2007) Clinical application of recombinant human bone morphogenetic protein-2 in 4 dogs. *Veterinary Surgery* 36 (2), 132-140.

Nolte, D.M., Fusco, J.V., Peterson, M.E. (2005) Incidence of and predisposing factors for nonunion of fractures involving the appendicular skeleton in cats: 18 cases (1998-2002). *Journal of the American Veterinary Medical Association* 226 (1), 77-82.

Risselada, M., van Bree, H., Kramer, M., et al. (2006) Evaluation of nonunion fractures in dogs by use of B-mode ultrasonography, power Doppler ultrasonography, radiography, and histologic examination. *American Journal of Veterinary Research* 67 (8), 1354-1361.

Saifzadeh, S., Pourreza, B., Hobbenaghi, R., et al. (2009) Autogenous greater omentum, as a free nonvascularized graft, enhances bone healing: an experimental nonunion model. *Journal of Investigative Surgery* 22 (2), 129-137.

Schmokel, H.G., Weber, F.E., Seiler, G., et al. (2004) Treatment of nonunions with non-glycosylated recombinant human bone morphogenetic protein-2 delivered from a fibrin matrix. *Veterinary Surgery* 33 (2), 112-118.

Welch, J.A., Boudrieau, R.J., DeJardin, L.M., et al. (1997) The intraosseous blood supply of the canine radius: implications for healing of distal fractures in small dogs. *Veterinary Surgery* 26 (1), 57-61.

100 Malunion

Andrew Worth

Massey University Veterinary Teaching Hospital, Palmerston North, New Zealand

Definition

Malunion is faulty union of the fragments of a fractured bone (O'Toole 2003). The term is derived from the Latin *male,* meaning "badly," and "union," the action of joining together.

Malunions are the result of successful fracture healing in the presence of a nonanatomic fracture alignment (Boudrieau *et al.* 1999). Malunions are common in fractures that heal naturally without veterinary intervention (Figure 100.1). Malunions can also result from suboptimal alignment during fracture repair or postoperative loss of immobilization and alignment before fracture healing. The resultant anatomic abnormalities may be in one or more planes:

- Rotational deformities: The limb heals with internal or external rotation around its long axis.
- Angular deformities: The limb heals with a deviation away from the median axis.
- Combinations of angular and rotational deformities

Additionally, a malunion of a long bone may be associated with shortening of the limb as a consequence of severe angulation, overriding of fracture fragments, collapse of a highly comminuted section of a bone shaft, or premature physeal closure in a growing animal.

The clinical relevance of a malunion varies with the severity of the deviation or limb shortening. In a functional malunion, the abnormality in alignment does not affect the use of the limb, and subsequent degeneration of adjacent joints is not clinically apparent. A malunion is considered nonfunctional when the change in alignment or limb length limits limb use, causes degeneration of adjacent joints, or impedes the animal's gait in an unacceptable way.

Angulations oriented in the major plane of motion of the limb (craniocaudal) are better tolerated than mediolateral deformities, which are more likely to affect limb function. However, extreme craniocaudal malunions can severely shorten a limb, thereby affecting the gait (Figure 100.2).

Quadripeds with a digitigrade stance are far less affected by limb shortening than plantigrade bipeds because of their ability to adjust proximal joint angles to effectively lengthen the limb. However, a length disparity exceeding 20% is likely to cause functional impairment.

The clinical relevance of a malunion may also relate to the presence of a callus inherent to secondary bone healing. Callus formation is especially relevant to pelvic fractures and osteotomies because of the potential for secondary obstipation and megacolon (Figure 100.3).

Risk factors

Risk factors for the development of a malunion include:
- A fracture that is untreated (undiagnosed or neglected)
- Conservative management of a fracture
- Closed reduction of a fracture
- Biologic strategies for fracture fixation
- Postoperative implant failure
- Premature removal of fracture fixation
- Revision of a previous fracture complication
- Osteomyelitis leading to abnormal bone healing

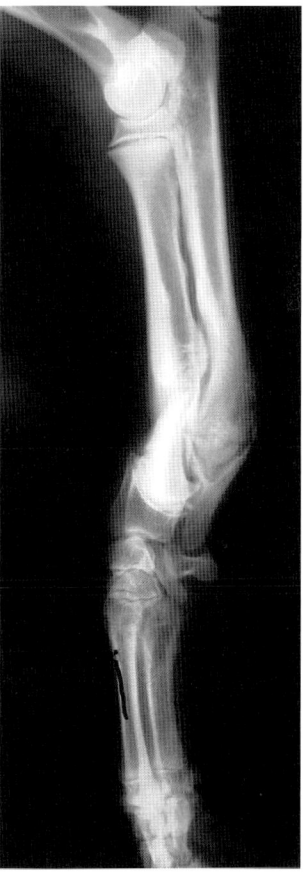

Figure 100.1 Mediolateral radiograph of an antebrachial malunion in a Doberman puppy after a neglected fracture that underwent natural healing. In addition to the angular deformity, there was significant limb shortening.

Complications in Small Animal Surgery, First Edition. Edited by Dominique Griffon and Annick Hamaide.
© 2016 John Wiley & Sons, Inc. Published 2016 by John Wiley & Sons, Inc.
Companion website: www.wiley.com/go/griffon/complications

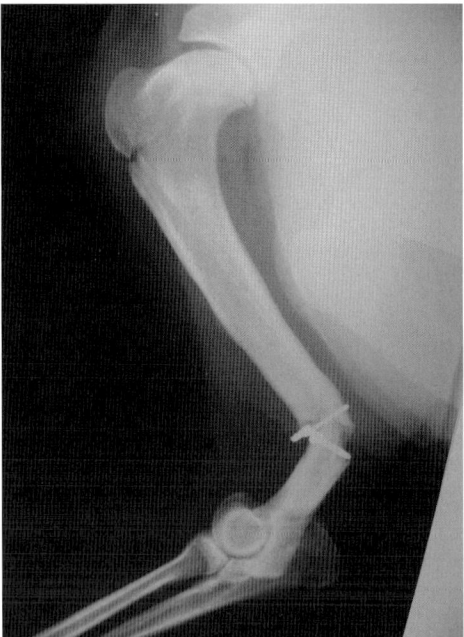

Figure 100.2 Mediolateral radiograph of a malunion with severe angulation in the craniocaudal plane resulting in significant shortening of the limb. An intramedullary pin and cerclage had been used for fracture fixation, but the pin had migrated and was removed before expected healing. The dog was caged, and the fracture went on to heal as a malunion.

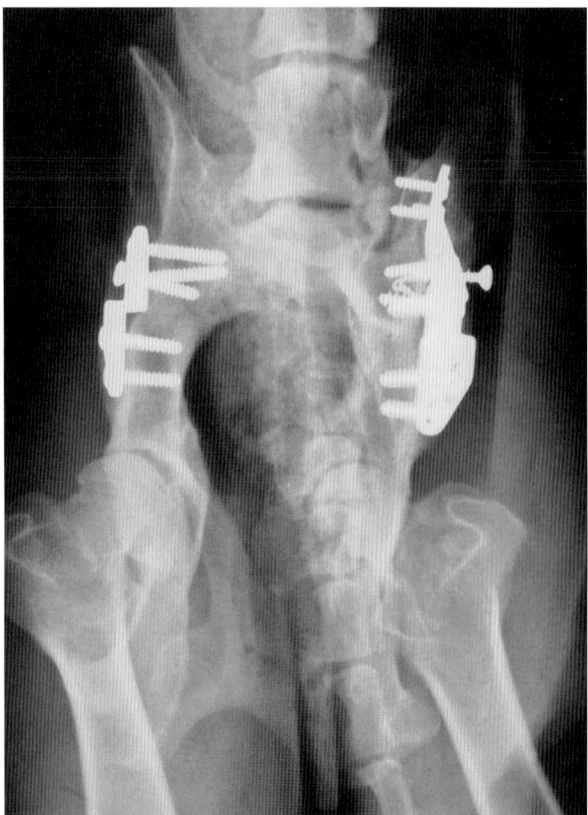

Figure 100.3 Narrowing of the pelvic canal after triple pelvic osteotomy. Secondary bone healing and malunion has resulted from loss of fixation stability.

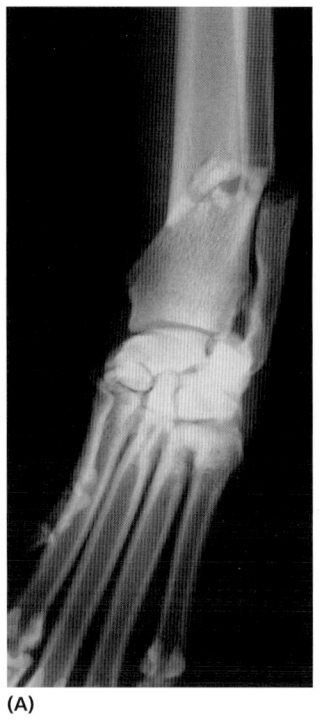 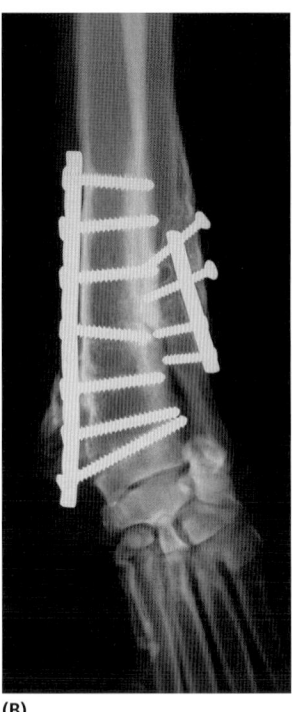

(A) **(B)**

Figure 100.4 Cranio-caudal radiograph of comminuted radial, and transverse ulnar, distal diaphyseal fractures in a large breed dog (**A**). Open reduction and internal fixation with plates resulted in a malunion with a valgus deviation of the carpus (**B**) as the result of suboptimal anatomic alignment permitted by the comminution, and inadequate contouring of the medially applied radial plate.

Based on the author's clinical impression, the following procedures seem prone to malunions in small animals:

- Long bone fractures treated by intramedullary pinning without adequate rotational stability
- Bone plating of metaphyseal fractures resulting in suboptimal plate contouring (Figure 100.4)
- Bone plating of transverse radial fractures in toy breeds where there is difficulty restoring and maintaining rotational alignment during plate application
- Biologic osteosynthesis of long bone fractures caused by the difficulty of restoring and maintaining correct alignment of the bone simultaneously in all planes (Figure 100.5)
- Pelvic osteotomies in immature dogs affected by postoperative screw loosening, loss of reduction, and early callus formation
- Revision of a previous fracture complication (e.g., implant failure or delayed healing) carries a greater risk of postoperative malunion because early callus formation may cause loss of anatomic landmarks. The surgeon cannot visualize the correct bone alignment and has to rely on limb alignment or intraoperative radiography (Figure 100.6).

Diagnosis

Many malunions are functional and do not warrant intervention for purely cosmetic reasons. The clinician should evaluate the animal's gait and comparative alignment of the contralateral limb, rotational deformity, and limb length. Assessment of the animal's gait and verification of the functional or nonfunctional status of a malunion

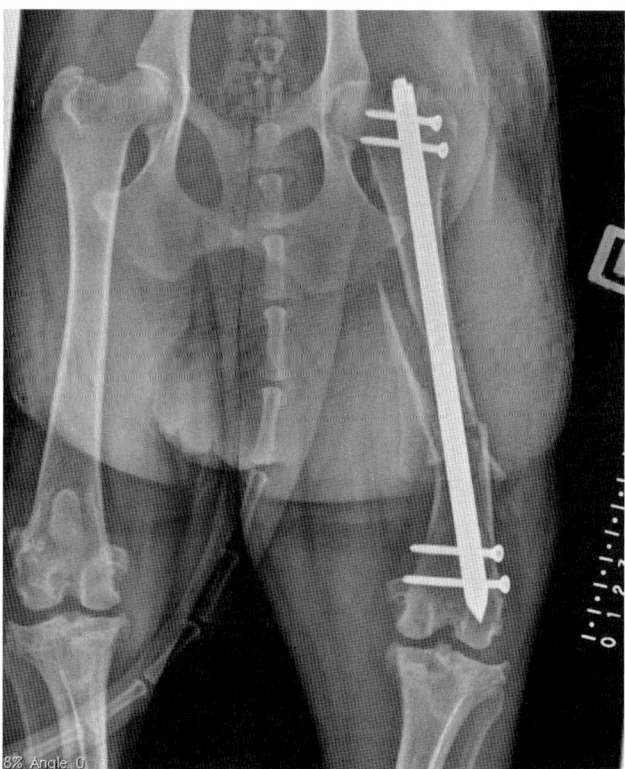

Figure 100.5 A comminuted femoral fracture was stabilized using an interlocking nail according to biologic fracture repair principles. Limited open reduction was used to insert the nail into the distal fragment, but anatomic alignment was not attempted. The limb was aligned by reference to adjacent joint angles. The fracture healed with angulation in the mediolateral plane. Although the dog walked with a bow-legged gait, the malunion was functional, and no intervention was required.

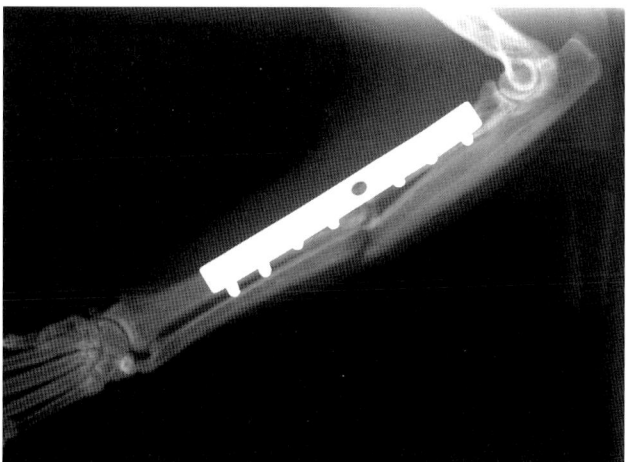

Figure 100.6 A domestic cat presented for fractures of the radius and ulna. Stabilization with an intramedullary pin in the ulna and a dowel pin in the radius failed because of rotational instability and bending of the implants. During revision surgery, a more appropriate repair was attempted with a plate applied to the dorsal surface of the radius. However, because of early fibrous callous formation, the correct orientation of the fracture fragments was not achieved, and the result was a 90-degree rotational malalignment. Note the craniocaudal radiographic appearance of the carpus and the mediolateral view of the elbow. Postoperatively, the cat had difficulty ambulating with a severely supinated paw (nonfunctional malunion), and the fracture had to be revised again to return alignment to normal.

is paramount. Nonfunctional malunions cause lameness through abnormal joint loading (sprains), ambulatory impediment, or abnormal joint mechanics (Halpers von Lande and Worth 2010). Joint manipulation should be performed to determine presence of pain, ligamentous sprain, or evidence of osteoarthrosis. A complete diagnostic approach is aimed at characterizing the severity and location of the angulation and assessing its functional impact before establishing a therapeutic plan for the patient. Radiographs are crucial to the preoperative planning of patients undergoing corrective osteotomies.

Radiographs of the malunion should include orthogonal projections, including the joints proximal and distal to the fracture site. The contralateral limb should be radiographed as a reference. Pelvic radiographs should be performed to assess pelvic diameter in animals presenting with constipation after traumatic pelvic fracture. Pelvic fractures involving the ilium or iliosacral joint can lead to displacement of the bone fragments and subsequent pelvic canal narrowing.

Radiographic assessment of malunions

Whereas single-plane malunions are easily corrected from standard radiographs complex deformities are best assessed via segmental radiography or computed tomography (CT) evaluation. Limb alignment quantified by way of joint angulation has been reported for a selected population of dogs, but breed-specific data are unavailable (Fox *et al.* 2006; Dismukes *et al.* 2008a). However, unlike developmental angular limb deformities in which both limbs may be affected, radiographs of the contralateral limb serve as a reliable reference in a malunion. Complex deformities with rotational components prevent imaging of the joints proximal and distal to the malunion in true orthogonal planes. A segmental radiographic technique should be considered in these cases; orthogonal views of the joints proximal and distal to the malunion are obtained independently and then composited, as described by Dismukes *et al.* (2008b). CT provides a superior assessment of complex deformities and is considered as the gold standard for three-dimensional surgical planning of osteotomies. Rapid prototype printing technology creates life-size models, which, along with saw guides, allow realistic rehearsal (using models) of the corrective surgery. This technology also enables preoperative plate contouring as well as accurate intraoperative osteotomy (using the saw guide) (Crosse and Worth 2010).

Several methods have been described for the assessment of malunions and preoperative planning of corrective osteotomies:

Radiographic tracing method

Orthogonal radiographs of the affected limb include the joints proximal and distal to the malunion (Figure 100.7). In cases with monoplanar, single malalignments, the radiographic outline of the

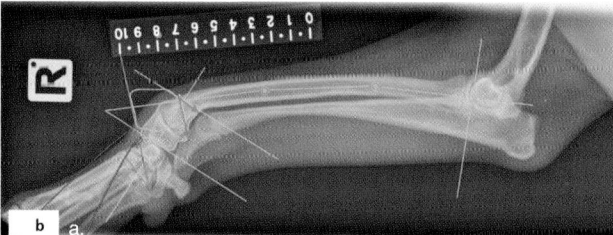

Figure 100.7 Mediolateral radiograph of the antebrachium of a dog with a distal angular limb deformity. The radiographic outline can be traced on a transparency sheet or tracing paper then reoriented to calculate the correction required (see text below).

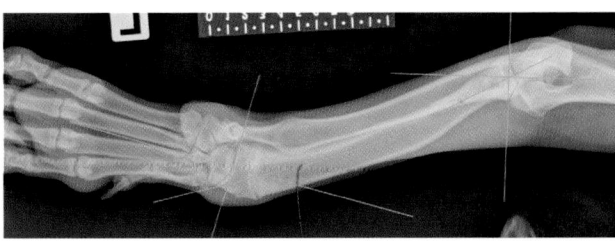

Figure 100.8 Cranio-caudal radiograph of a young dog with a developmental angular limb deformity showing the centre of rotational angulation (CORA) methodology (Fox et al. 2006). Asymmetrical distal physeal development has led to compensatory bone changes proximally. Using the CORA method the joint planes and anatomic bone axes are determined and the intersections of these lines demarcate one or more CORA.

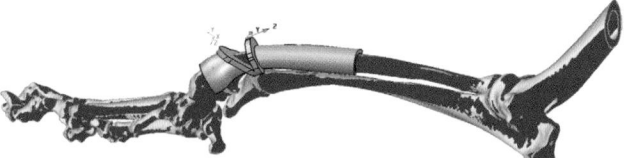

Figure 100.10 Three dimensional reconstruction based on CT data showing the antebrachum of a dog with angular deformity for which a closing wedge osteotomy is being planned. A saw guide (jig) has been created that can be printed in plastic using rapid prototyping technology, then used intra-operatively to guide an osteotomy ensuring a more accurate correction of the patients limb.

bone is traced on a transparency or tracing paper. A line is drawn parallel to the joint surfaces at either end of the bone to be corrected. The mid-diaphyseal line is traced to the point of maximum curvature, and a line is drawn across the diaphysis parallel to the closest of the two joint lines (green lines). A second transparent sheet is placed over the first, and the other fragment is traced (a in Figure 100.8) and then rotated (b in Figure 100.8) around the cortical intersection of the osteotomy line. The osteotomy is defined (orange arrows in Figure 100.8) so that the axes of the proximal and distal articular surfaces are parallel with each other (Johnson 2005).

The center of rotational angulation method

Malunions in immature animals may induce compensatory growth that lead to conformational changes at a second site (Figure 100.8). These cases tend to display more complex malunion or growth deformities that complicates the surgical planning. The center of rotational angulation method (CORA) can be used to plan correction (Fox *et al.* 2006). The surgeon determines the plane of the articular surface at either end of the bone and the central diaphyseal line in mediolateral and craniocaudal radiographs. The intersection of the diaphyseal vectors is the CORA (arrow in Figure 100.8) and determines the site of the radial osteotomy. In compensated deformities, a second CORA will be identified, and a double dome osteotomy may be required to prevent residual translational deformity after correction of the major CORA (Fox *et al.* 2006).

Advanced imaging techniques

Computed tomography data can be reformatted into three-dimensional images and manipulated to allow quantification of the deformity (Figure 100.9). The CT data are exported as a file compatible with

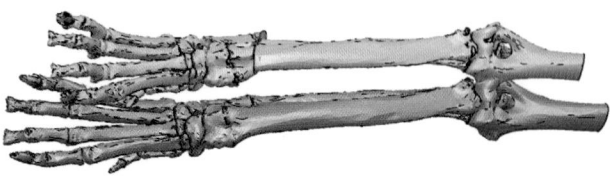

Figure 100.9 Three dimensional images generated from CT scan data of a dogs antebrachiae (radiographs of the same dog are featured in Figure 100.8). The green image (top) shows the affected limb with the deformity resolved by a simulated closing wedge osteotomy. A a mirror image of the unaffected contralateral limb is shown below (purple) and is used to generate the landmarks on which to base the correction.

engineering software designed for three-dimensional manipulation. The affected limb can be overlaid on a mirror image of the normal contralateral limb for direct comparison. The data can be manipulated to rehearse a corrective osteotomy and assess the end result. Rapid prototyping (RP) technology is used to create models of the limb in acryl-nitrile butadiene styrene plastic. The surgery can be rehearsed on the plastic model, and appropriate implants can be contoured and sterilized before surgery. Jigs can also be printed to use as saw guides to ensure accurate orientation of the osteotomy (Figure 100.10).

Treatment

Functional malunions, by definition, do not require treatment. Nonfunctional angular malunions can be treated by refracture or osteotomy followed by fixation in a more functional alignment (Anson 1991; Rovesti 2005).

Several types of osteotomy have been described to manage malunions. Osteotomy techniques are selected based on consideration for limb length discrepancy, available equipment, postoperative compliance, and the desirability of plating over external skeletal fixation (ESF) or circular ring fixation (CRF).

- Oblique osteotomy (Figure 100.11): The bone is transected at the center of angulation so that the tip of the proximal fragment can be seated within the medullary cavity of the distal fragment to provide load sharing and accelerate healing caused by contact between fragments.
- Transverse osteotomy with an opening or closing wedge: In an opening wedge osteotomy, the diaphysis is transected at the point of maximal angulation, and the concave cortex is displaced to open a wedge-shaped defect sufficiently wide to correct the malalignment (Figure 100.12). The gap is left open or packed with a graft. The opening side of the wedge must be beneath the fixation plate. A gap in the far cortex of the bone relative to the plate would increase strain and affect bone healing. In a closing osteotomy (Figure 100.13), a wedge is defined with the apex on the concave cortex at the point of maximum angulation and the base of the wedge along the convex cortex. The wedge is removed and the fragment reduced to oppose the osteotomy, thus straightening the limb. This technique usually preserves cortical apposition between the proximal and distal segments but creates some loss in length. Torsional deformities may be corrected acutely during wedge osteotomy. The degree of correction may be estimated by direct visualization of the range of motion of the foot (the foot should only move in the craniodorsal plane during flexion) or via reference to Kirschner wires placed before the osteotomy parallel to the adjacent joint surfaces of each fragment but in the true mediolateral plane of the bone.

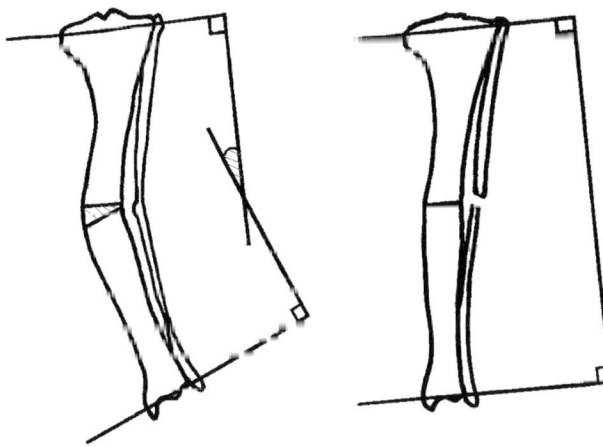

Figure 100.13 Diagram of a tibial malunion corrected by an closing wedge osteotomy. A medial plate or external skeletal fixator is used to stabilise the new alignment.

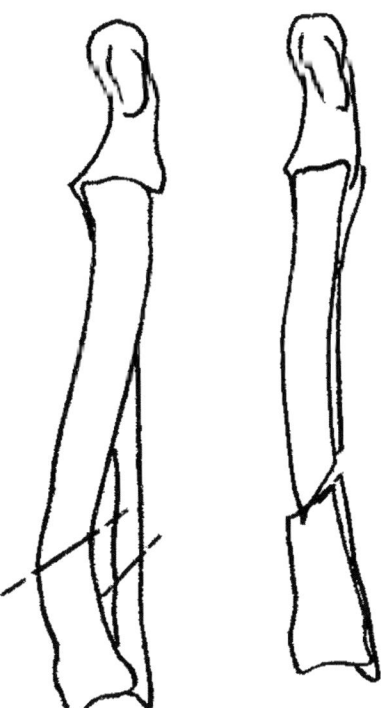

Figure 100.11 Diagram of an oblique osteotomy of a malunion of the antebrachium. The radius is cut on an angle to allow the proximal fragment to be placed inside the distal fragment and the correction is stabilised by an external skeletal fixator.

After osteotomy and realignment of the limb, the bone may be maintained in position via:

• ESF: Oblique and open wedge osteotomies are traditionally immobilized with external fixation for complex malunions in more than one plane (Fox *et al.* 1995). The osteotomy is performed at the area of greatest deformity, and the end of the proximal fragment is reduced to lie within the medullary cavity of

• Dome (crescentric) osteotomy (Figure 100.14): A concentric saw is required to perform a radial cut. Incomplete reduction allows reorientation of the bone in a second plane. Dome osteotomy preserves limb length over closing wedge osteotomy and, compared with an opening wedge osteotomy, does not create a gap at the osteotomy site. In this technique, the saw blade is offset from the CORA location by the radius of the saw blade arc, such that the center of the osteotomy is positioned concentrically over the CORA (Fox *et al.* 2006).

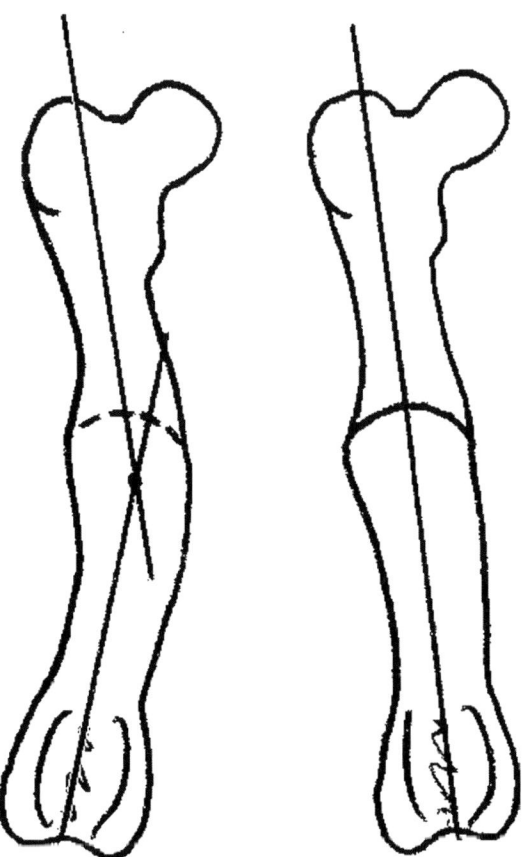

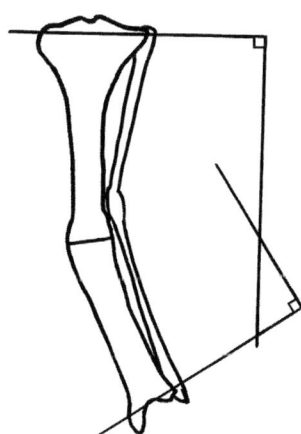 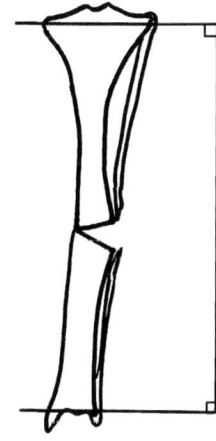

Figure 100.12 Diagram of a tibial malunion corrected by an opening osteotomy using the CORA or tracing paper methods. A lateral plate or external skeletal fixator is used to stabilise the new alignment.

Figure 100.14 A dome osteotomy is performed using a radial saw blade centered on the CORA. The fragments are rotated into alignment then fixed in position with internal or external fracture fixation.

the distal fragment. The rotational deformity is corrected around the newly established bone axis, and an ESF is used to maintain optimal limb alignment by reference to the adjacent joints and radiographs. Continuous adjustment can be made with the use of hinges and angular motors. Transverse osteotomies may also be stabilized with ESF as well as internal fixation with plates.

- CRF: The small size of the tensioned wires is an advantage in areas with limited bone stock for implant placement (e.g., small distal fragments). CRF is highly compatible with both linear and angular motors. CRF with angular motors allows gradual angular correction, thereby mitigating soft tissue tightness significant enough to prevent acute correction. Limb shortening significant enough to affect function can be treated by distraction osteogenesis using linear motors (Figure 100.15). Distraction rates of 1.0 to 1.5 mm per day in two to four adjustments are commonly used, but lengthening may be limited by the soft tissue tension and patient compliance (Lewis *et al.* 1999).
- Plate fixation: Plate fixation requires accurate preoperative planning using radiography or CT. Because the fixation is

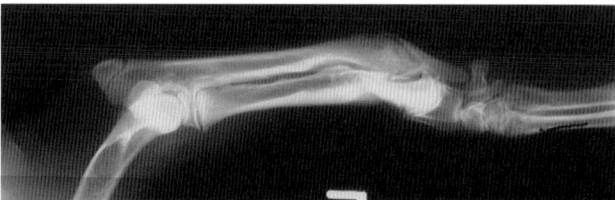

(A)

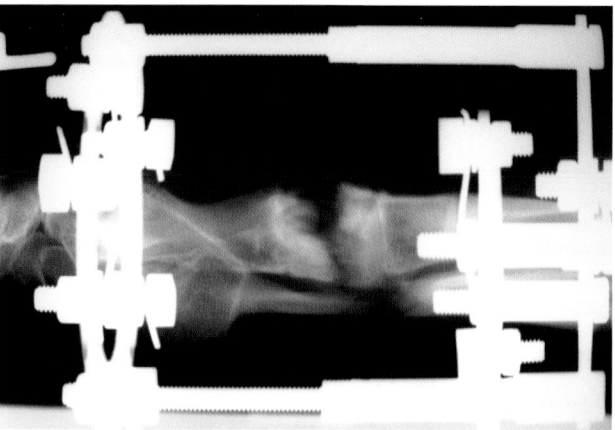

(B)

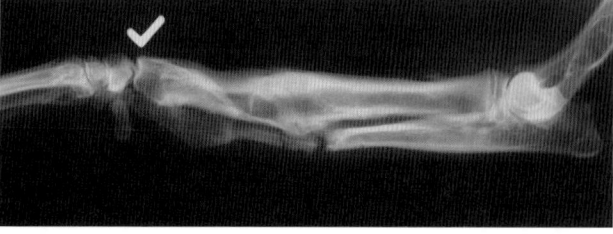

(C)

Figure 100.15 A circular ring fixator has been applied to the antebrachial malunion shown in Figure 100.1 (**A**) An acute correction of the angular deformity was performed, and two linear motors were used to produce distraction osteogenesis and gain length (**B**). The end result was significant limb lengthening as well as angular correction.

finalized intraoperatively, there is no opportunity for postoperative adjustment. Precontouring the plate from radiographs of the contralateral limb or based on RP models is advantageous.
- Pelvic malunions with pelvic narrowing sufficient enough to cause obstipation refractory to medical management warrant surgical intervention. The pubis can be separated with an oscillating saw via a midline approach. A bone graft fashioned from a section of rib or ilium (typically an allograft) is wired into place to act as a spacer. Alternatively a Kirschner wire can be fashioned into a spring-like spacer. An ilial osteotomy or a triple pelvic osteotomy may be required in cases in which additional pelvic widening is needed.

Prevention

- When anatomic alignment is adopted as a fracture repair strategy, accuracy and stability are paramount, such that alignment is optimal and maintained.
- When a biologic strategy is used, careful planning and a good understanding of limb alignment and relevant bony landmarks are paramount.
- Postoperative radiographs should be assessed for errors in alignment and revision performed if a nonfunctional malunion in likely.
- Fracture healing should be investigated with radiographs at 4 to 6 weeks and then every 3 to 4 weeks until healing is verified.
- Implants should not be removed before radiographic and clinically apparent union; otherwise, additional fixation is required.
- Femoral fractures present a particular problem when treated with closed or limited open reduction. Spasm or contracture of the iliopsoas or gluteal muscles can lead to external or internal rotation of the proximal femur, respectively. If rotation of the proximal femur in relation to the distal fragment is not completely corrected, a malunion can develop and affect the version angle of the coxofemoral joint (Newton and Nunamaker 1985).
- Pelvic malunions following triple pelvic osteotomy can be prevented by the use of cancellous screws, ensuring screw penetration into the sacrum where possible, adding a ventral plate, eight-hole triple pelvic osteotomy plates (versus traditional six-hole plates), and the use of locking plates (versus standard plates).

Relevant literature

The degree of angulation or shortening of a limb requiring correction is largely unknown. Mild angulations (up to 10–15 degrees) are tolerated well in most animals, and loss of bone length up to 20% can be compensated for by joint extension or compensatory growth of a long bone in the same limb (in animals with remaining growth potential). Surgical decision making should be based on clinical signs (i.e., functional use of the limb vs. a nonfunctional impediment). The most common cause of a malunion is failure of fracture fixation. Failure of fracture fixation generally results in a nonunion, but occasionally there is still sufficient stability to allow healing to occur, albeit in an abnormal position.

Premature removal of fracture fixation may occur when implants migrate or radiographic fracture healing was inappropriately assessed as sufficient to allow fixation removal. Catastrophic refracture may occur but some cases may display a loss of limb alignment but eventual healing, resulting in a malunion.

Open reduction and internal fixation with bone plates is a standard method of repair for anatomically reconstructable fractures. Accurate anatomic reconstruction prevents malunion. However, metaphyseal fractures represent a greater risk of malunion because of the flared and irregular profile of the bone fragments involved in the fixation. Metaphyseal fractures managed with standard (non-locking) plates require a more significant and accurate plate contouring than diaphyseal fractures. If the plate is not well contoured, the fragments will be displaced during screw tightening, leading to a malalignment.

Biologic strategies of fracture fixation rely on the surgeon aligning the limb in the absence of anatomic bone reconstruction. Biologic strategies are most suited to comminuted fractures of the diaphysis of long bones. A fully closed or an "open-but-do-not-touch" reduction is used, and limb alignment has to be optimized in the absence of anatomic bone reconstruction. Reference to the hinge angle of the adjacent joints is used to maintain the limb in a functional position during fixation. Limb alignment can be optimized with intraoperative fluoroscopy, and interfragmentary Kirschner wires or stopper (olive) wires can be used to drag fragments into better alignment.

When plating techniques are used as a biologic strategy (biologic osteosynthesis is traditional bridging or plate-rod constructs), limb alignment can be improved by precontouring the plate to a radiograph of the nonfractured limb before surgery. Dimensionally accurate orthogonal projections are required, and aluminium templates are used to guide the contouring of an appropriately sized plate with hand irons or a bending press or pliers.

External skeletal fixation is a common biologic fracture strategy, offering opportunities for postoperative adjustment, thereby minimizing the risk of malalignment. The surgeon can loosen clamps and make adjustments guided by direct visualization of the limb and by reference to radiographs. However, external skeletal fixation is associated with greater patient morbidity than internal fixation because of soft tissue irritation and stress transfer through the frame to the bone. ESF constructs that use acrylic or methyl meth acrylate bars or clamps increase the versatility in the location and angle of fixation pin placement. This type of apparatus facilitates the placement of the connecting bar compared with conventional systems (Ross and Matthiesen 1993).

References

Anson, L.W. (1991) Malunions. *Veterinary Clinics of North America: Small Animal Practice* 21 (40), 761-780.

Boudrieau, R.J., Birchard, S.J., Sherding, R.G. (1999) Delayed unions, nonunions, and malunions. *Saunders Manual of Small Animal Practice* 2, 1218-1223.

Crosse, K.R., Worth, A.J. (2010) Computer-assisted surgical correction of an antebrachial deformity in a dog. *Veterinary and Comparative Orthopaedics and Traumatology* 23 (5), 354-361.

Dismukes, D.I., Fox, D.B., Tomlinson, J.L., et al. (2008a) A determination of pelvic limb alignment in the large-breed dog: a cadaveric radiographic study in the frontal plane. *Veterinary Surgery* 37, 674-682.

Dismukes, D.I., Fox, D.B., Tomlinson, J.L., et al. (2008b) Use of radiographic measures and three-dimensional computed tomographic imaging in surgical correction of an antebrachial deformity in a dog. *Journal of the American Veterinary Medical Association* 232, 68-73.

Fox, S.M., Bray, J.C., Guerin, S.R., et al. (1995) Antebrachial deformities in the dog: treatment with external fixation. *Journal of Small Animal Practice* 36 (7), 315-320.

Fox, D.B., Tomlinson, J.L., Cook, J.L., et al. (2006) Principles of uniapical and biapical radial deformity correction using dome osteotomies and the center of rotation of angulation methodology in dogs. *Veterinary Surgery* 35, 67-77.

Johnson, A.L. (2005) Corrective osteotomies. In Johnson, A.L. Houlton, J.E.F., Vannini, R. (eds.) *AO Principles of Fracture Management in the Dog and Cat.* Thieme, New York.

Kuipers von Lande, R.G., Worth, A.J. (2010) Femoral fracture malunion corrected with a closing wedge osteotomy and distal femoral osteotomy plate. *Australian Veterinary Practitioner* 40 (4), 154-160.

Lewis, D.D., Radasch, R.M., Beale, B.S., *et al.* (1999) Initial clinical experience with the IMEX™ circular external skeletal fixation system. *Veterinary Comparative Orthopedics and Traumatology* 12, 118-127.

Newton, C.D., Nunamaker, D.M. (1985) *Textbook of Small Animal Orthopaedics.* JB Lippincott, Philadelphia.

O'Toole, M.T. (2003) Miller-*Keane Encyclopedia and Dictionary of Medicine, Nursing, and Allied Health*, 7th edn. Saunders, St. Louis.

Ross, J.T., Matthiesen, D.T. (1993) The use of multiple pin and methylmethacrylate external skeletal fixation for the treatment of orthopaedic injuries in the dog and cat. *Veterinary and Comparative Orthopaedics and Traumatology* 6, 115-121.

Rovesti, G.L. (2005) Malunions. In Johnson, A.L. Houlton, J.E.F., Vannini, R. (eds.) *AO Principles of Fracture Management in the Dog and Cat.* Thieme, New York.

101 Loss of Function in Performance Dogs

Lauren Pugliese[1] and Jon Dee[2]

[1]The Ohio State University College of Veterinary Medicine, Columbus, OH, USA
[2]Hollywood Animal Hospital, Hollywood, FL, USA

Racing greyhounds are the most established elite canine athletes. Other canine athletes have gained recognition in field trials, agility, sled pulling, herding, hunting, and search and rescue. All of these dogs are subjected to demanding physical functions and are therefore often presented for mild lameness or a decrease in performance. This chapter focuses on complications associated with the management of injuries in racing greyhounds, leading to a loss of function in these athletes.

Injuries frequently affect the racing careers of greyhound dogs and may potentially end their careers. Valuable dogs will be maintained as breeding stock; the remaining dogs are relinquished to become pets or euthanized. Conceptually, the ideal treatment of complications lies in prevention and early recognition before failure of the structure. Postoperative recovery and return to function are affected by the management of the injury; postinjury outcomes tend to spiral and compound upon themselves as the number of errors, either management related or technical in nature, increase in a given patient. Identification of these errors, surgical skills, and correct instrumentation may aid in decreasing these complications.

Definition

Loss of function in a canine athlete may be broadly defined as an inability to maintain athletic performance as a result of injury or an inability to return to racing after treatment of an injury. It may also include a decrease in expected performance or refusal to perform previously accomplished tasks.

Racing greyhounds are affected by an array of musculoskeletal injuries that are not commonly seen in other working or performance dogs (Hickman 1975; Prole 1976, Sicard *et al.* 1999). These injuries often involve the carpus and tarsus, complex joints with injuries often involving multiple components. Greyhounds racing on a circular track in a counterclockwise manner develop site-specific bone adaptation with compaction of trabecular bone and an increase in bone mineral density in the right central tarsal bone; this is the most common site for a fatigue fracture. While galloping around the bend, the left forelimb acts as a pivot, and the right hind limb provides propulsion (Hickman 1975). As the running dog negotiates a turn, the stresses applied to these two limbs are important contributing factors to the unique injuries that racing greyhounds sustain (Hickman 1975).

A study evaluating joint kinematics comparing greyhounds with Labrador retrievers found that although moment and power patterns were similar for the tarsal joints, the greyhounds had larger amplitude to the wave form (Colborne *et al.* 2005; Bergh 2008). These variations in kinematics may explain predisposition to certain injury types, such as central tarsal bone fractures, in greyhounds (Bergh 2008). Fractures commonly associated with tarsal bone lesions conform to three patterns: the triads of the tarsus and the tetrad of the tarsus.

Triad of the tarsus (two combinations):
- Central tarsal fracture
- Fourth tarsal fracture
- Lateral aspect of base of metatarsal V

or
- Central tarsal fracture
- Fourth tarsal fracture
- Medial sagittal slab fracture of the base of the calcaneus
  Tetrad of the tarsus:
- Type IV central tarsal fracture
- Fourth tarsal compression
- Avulsion of the base of metatarsal V
- Tarsal bone II fracture

Risk factors

Loss of function in performance dogs may result from injuries associated with exercise, such as fatigue failure, or from complications associated with the management of these injuries.

Risk factors for injuries include:
- Intense, repetitive exercise
- Age and duration of training
- Location: bones of distal extremities
- Failure to recognize early deterioration in performance
- Inadequate recovery time
- Track design and quality

Risk factors for postoperative loss of function include:
- Chronicity of the injury
- Preoperative degenerative joint disease
- Presence of undiagnosed lesion (misdiagnosis)
- Presence of intraarticular lesions and postoperative reduction of these lesions
- Presence of concurrent injuries

Complications in Small Animal Surgery, First Edition. Edited by Dominique Griffon and Annick Hamaide.
© 2016 John Wiley & Sons, Inc. Published 2016 by John Wiley & Sons, Inc.
Companion website: www.wiley.com/go/griffon/complications

- Conservative treatment
- Skin closure under tension over implants
- Inadequate padding and external coaptation
- Inadequate postoperative rehabilitation
- Delay in presentation for definitive correction between injury and surgery

Diagnosis

The history and clinical signs in racing greyhounds vary from subtle loss of performance to non–weight-bearing lameness, depending on the injury. Often, catastrophic career-ending fractures occur during a race or intense training. Loss of function in canine athletes should prompt clinicians to recommend early diagnostic evaluation, including complete orthopedic examination and imaging of the affected area. There is no substitute for thorough and repetitive orthopedic examination of the affected and contralateral extremity. Patients should be assessed for pain, instability, crepitation, and swelling.

During the orthopedic examination, careful palpation of the soft tissue structures, the palpable bony landmarks appropriate to each joint, and each joint and long bone are assessed in a routine, consistent manner. Each joint should be isolated and manipulated in isolation from other joints. Comparison between the right and left sides can be made, although this can be complicated by the presence of bilateral disease. The following should be routinely evaluated during the orthopedic examination:

- Extension
- Flexion
- Range of motion (ROM) to the end points
- Internal rotation
- External rotation
- Varus
- Valgus
- Stressed and evaluated through ROM

Physical examination may be complicated by swelling and soft tissue injuries in acute cases. These cases may warrant stabilization or soft padded bandages to aid in reduction of associated swelling and inflammation before evaluation under sedation. Careful examination for defects in the skin surface should be made as well as monitoring of extension of bruising and changes from day to day.

Excellent radiographic technique is a prerequisite to identification of small, nondisplaced fractures; exposure and positioning must be well adjusted, and additional views are frequently indicated. A complete radiographic evaluation of the tarsus requires four projections (Figure 101.1) to visualize all tarsal bones:

- Dorsomedial to plantarolateral (DMPL-O) view
- Dorsolateral plantaromedial (DLPM-O) view
- Craniocaudal view
- Mediolateral view

Additional radiographs such as oblique, flexed, extended, and stressed views may be indicated to assess the extent of the damage. Radiographs of the contralateral limb may be obtained for comparison.

Computed tomography (CT) is indicated in elite athletes and when a definitive diagnosis cannot be established on radiographs (Figure 101.2). Advanced imaging may be particularly useful when decreased performance is noted before catastrophic failure or definitive fracture. CT may help diagnose the cause of a loss of performance in dogs without radiographic abnormalities and can improve the assessment of the extent of injuries in cases with uncertain diagnostic abnormalities.

Treatment

The decision to pursue surgical management has to result in a better outcome than nonsurgical conservative medical therapy. Financial

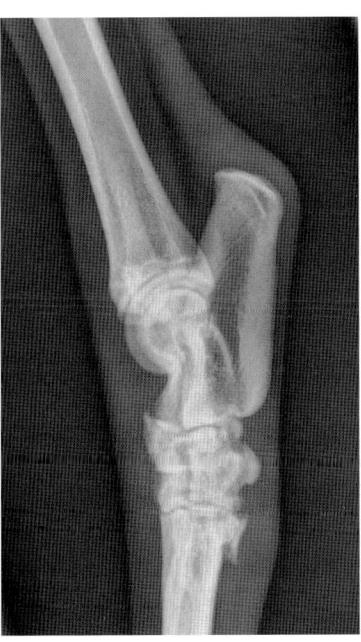 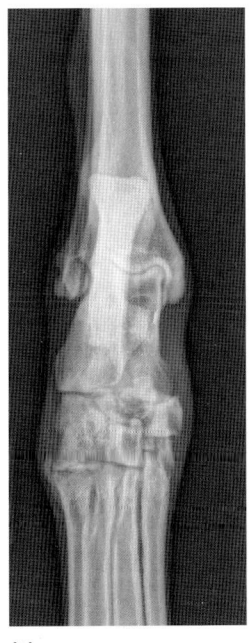 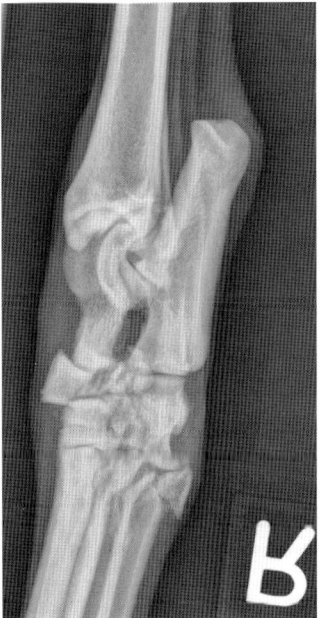 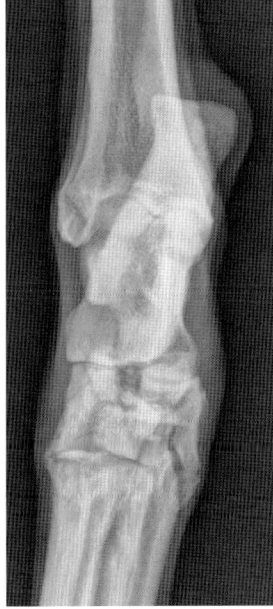

(A) (B) (C) (D)

Figure 101.1 Radiographic evaluation of tarsal injuries using an example of a central tarsal fracture. Oblique projections improve the evaluation of injuries. **A,** Lateral view of the right tarsus. The dorsal margin of the central tarsal bone and the proximal aspect of metatarsal V are mildly but visibly displaced. **B,** Craniocaudal projection of the right tarsus. A medial displacement of the central tarsal bone can be detected. **C** and **D,** Oblique projections separate the tarsal bones and highlight the level of the displacement of the central tarsal bone, metatarsal V, and the fourth tarsal bone. *Source:* J. Dyce, OSU Veterinary Medical Center, Colombus, OH. Reproduced with permission from J. Dyce.

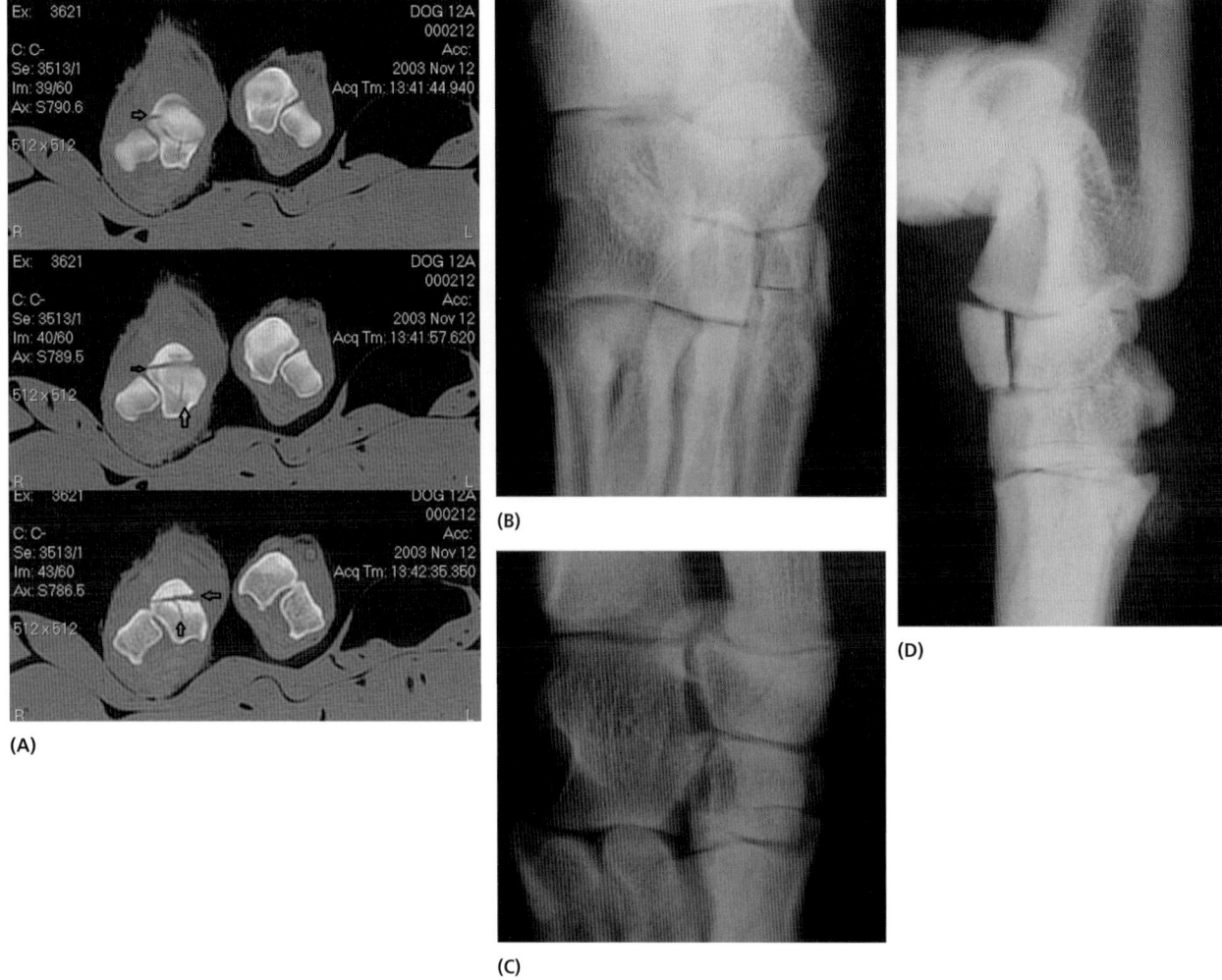

Figure 101.2 Radiographs and computed tomography (CT) scan of a tarsus with a type IV central tarsal fracture. **A,** CT allows detection of a second fracture line (arrow) that is not clearly visible in the radiographic projections (**B, C,** and **D**). On radiographic projections, only the dorsal slab is visible and would result in a type II classification. *Source:* Reproduced with permission from A. Piras.

considerations such as the quality of the dog, the genetic breeding potential, and the future anticipated usage of the dog often influence the choice of treatment. An algorithm for treatment of injuries in racing greyhounds is provided in Figure 101.3.

Current recommendations for acute management include:
- Minimize swelling and discomfort via a modified Robert Jones bandage with splint support for 24 to 48 hours.
- Reassess under analgesia or anesthesia after the swelling has subsided.
- Perform physical and radiographic examination before and after any closed joint stabilization (reduction).
- Address avulsions, fragments, and fractures via anatomic reduction and internal fixation.
- Address soft tissue components via "capture techniques," soft tissue anchors, or anatomically based transosseous tunnels.

Prognosis

The prognosis varies with the type of injury, duration of signs, and treatment modality. Return to racing has been reported in more than 80% of central tarsal bone fractures treated via open reduction

and lag screw fixation (Boudrieau *et al.* 1984a). Fractures treated conservatively carry a guarded to poor prognosis for return to function. Calcaneal fractures are associated with central tarsal bone injuries have a guarded to poor return to racing function; reducible fractures of the calcaneus with surgical repair have a good prognosis. When reconstruction of articular surfaces is compromised, ankylosis of affected joints may eventually decrease pain. Alternatively, arthrodesis may be considered to provide a pain-free outcome in retired racing dogs.

Prevention

Strategies to prevent injuries in racing greyhounds include:
- Appropriate track design and management of racing conditions
- Proper fitness training before racing
- Early identification of stress or fatigue fracture changes in endosteal bone, cortical thickening, or subchondral sclerosis
- Identification of mild soft tissue changes such as mild swelling, weight-bearing lameness, and loss of performance capability

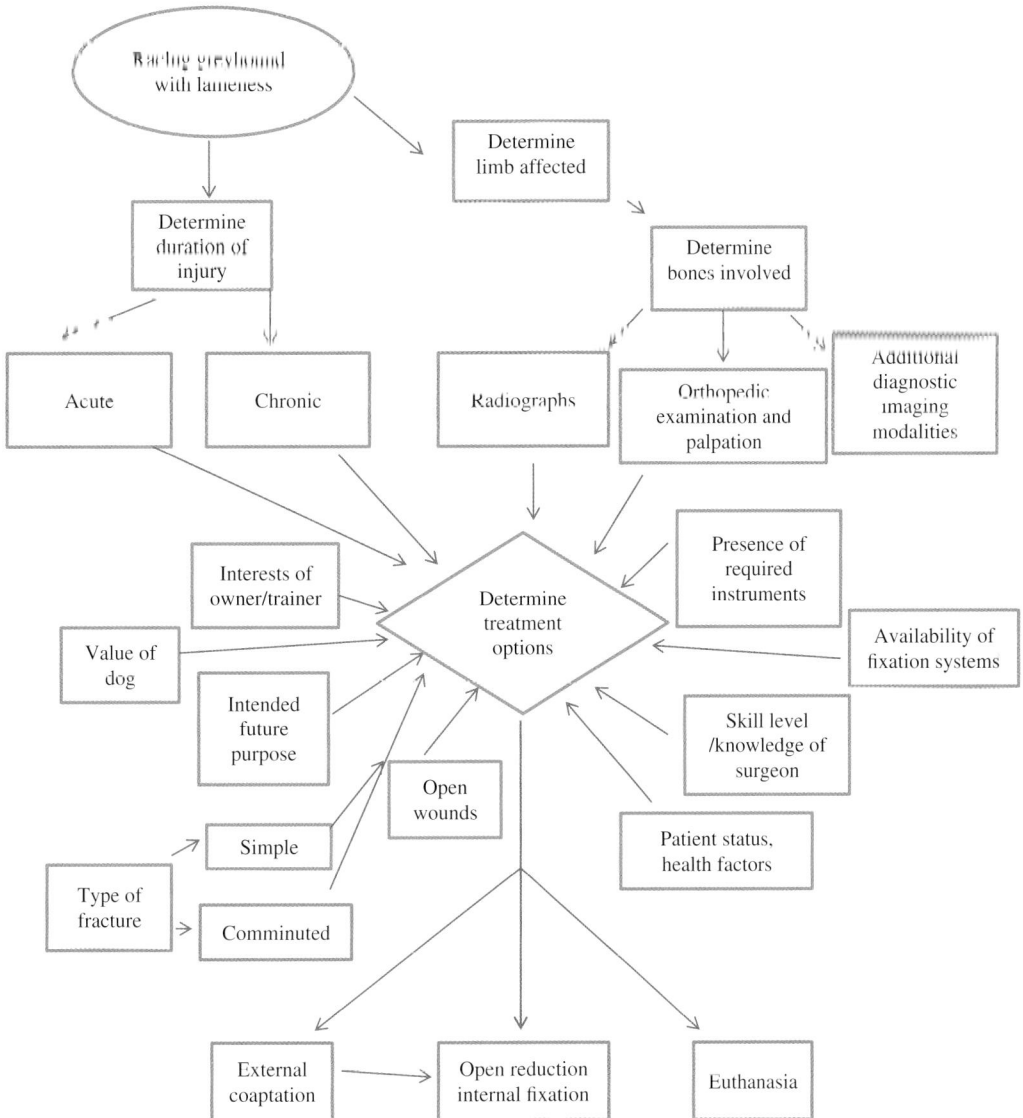

Figure 101.3 Flow chart illustrating the decision-making process for managing orthopedic injuries in racing greyhounds.

Strategies to optimize the return to racing after surgical treatment of tarsal and carpal fractures in greyhounds generally include:
- Complete and accurate diagnosis of all injuries
- Stable positioning in dorsal recumbency (or sternal recumbency for calcaneal fractures), with the distal limb off the table to allow manipulation of the joint
- Avoid fragment removal (to serve as bone graft).
- Accurate reduction and temporary compression with the use of forceps (Figure 101.4)
- Avoid closing skin under tension over implants, such as thick plates; locking plates have a lower profile, which may allow for easier closure. Consider pins, a tension band, and screws combined with external coaptation as an alternative whenever possible.
- Apply well-padded external coaptation, especially over bony prominences.
- Regular bandage changes with evaluation of bony prominences for soft tissue injuries

Relevant literature

In racing greyhounds, the tarsus is affected in 3% to 6% of all injuries seen in dogs running on turf and from 43% to 56% in surveys of injuries from dogs running on dirt (Prole 1976). The carpus is injured in 21% of cases in one review (Prole 1976). Carpal and tarsal fractures in greyhounds have been described and classified (Boudrieau *et al.* 1984a; Johnson 1987).

Racing greyhounds remain the model for stress or fatigue fractures in dogs. Research in racing greyhound injuries has also been used as a model for stress fractures in human athletes and equine competitors. These fractures have a different etiology than those resulting from acute trauma (Tomlin *et al.* 2000). Fractographic, histologic, and scanning electron microscopy studies of central tarsal bone fractures support the concept that fatigue fractures occur because of an imbalance between remodeling and microdamage, leading to fatigue fracture of the central tarsal bone with potential concomitant injuries (Tomlin *et al.* 2000). These fractures occur

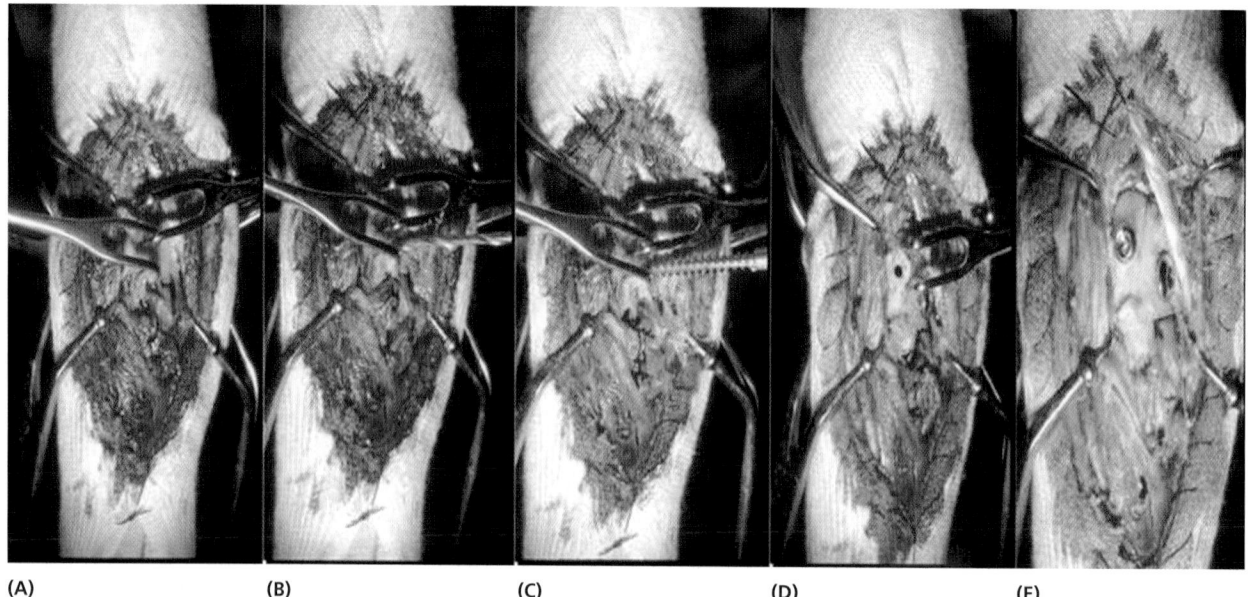

(A)   (B)   (C)   (D)   (E)

Figure 101.4 A to E, Open reduction and fixation of a tarsal fracture. Note the use of Vulsellum forceps to attain reduction. The use of special instruments and fine-tipped point-to-point reduction forceps can aid in accurate anatomic reduction.

with a reproducible pattern in a specific site as a result of asymmetric cyclic loading during racing and training (Muir *et al.* 1999; Johnson *et al.* 2000; Tomlin *et al.* 2000).

Injuries concurrently diagnosed in dogs with central tarsal bone fractures include fractures of other bones within the same tarsus, reported in 64% of cases in one study (Boudrieau *et al.* 1984b). Consequently, the types of injuries seen, the surgical repair options available, and the outcomes of the repair will vary markedly in racing greyhounds versus other dogs.

Return to function in greyhounds is influenced by the duration of injuries before presentation (acute vs. chronic), the mode of treatment (surgical vs. conservative), the type or combinations of lesions present, the ability of the clinician to identify all injuries present, the ability to achieve adequate reduction, and the postoperative considerations and management.

Similar to many orthopedic injuries, patients with acute presentation and management often carry a better prognosis than those with chronic injuries, in which remodeling and malunion have occurred. However, acute management often has significant soft tissue injury that can limit palpation and manipulation and cause increased pain compared with a chronic injury. Valuable dogs should preferably be evaluated early with this examination including radiographs and possibly CT.

Often, a delay to surgery may exist as the dog is managed for an injury conservatively with rest and bandaging before more definitive surgical management. This delay may complicate the repair and reduce the ability to return to normal function with ongoing cartilage damage leading to degenerative joint changes, the accumulation of muscle atrophy secondary to disuse, and the natural healing process interfere with accurate reduction and reconstruction.

Identification of all of the injuries present is essential to adequately plan and surgically address these injuries (Boudrieau *et al.* 1984b). The diagnosis is generally based on physical examination and a complete set of high-quality radiographs. Closed reductions of tarsocrural and antebrachiocarpal luxations should always be radiographed again before surgical intervention. Pathology that

was not apparent on the images obtained before reduction often becomes apparent. This is key to planning and achieving adequate repair of all elements of the injury.

The growing availability of CT may also enhance recognition of fractures and concurrent injuries within the complex joints of the tarsus and carpus. To date, there has only been one recent publication evaluating the accuracy of radiographs compared with CT (Hercock *et al.* 2011). This study found that CT improved the observer's ability to identify fractures of the central tarsal bone and related injuries compared with radiographic evaluation (Hercock *et al.* 2011). CT has proven valuable in other joints as well. To support this, a recent study identified a dorsal slab fracture in the fourth carpal bone that was not visible on radiographs but noted on CT scan (Rutherford and Ness 2012). The role of advanced imaging may aid in diagnosing minimally displaced fractures, subtle injuries, or early fractures.

Surgical technique and decision making play roles in reducing the incidence of complications and promoting return to function. Patient positioning for surgery of the extremities should focus on providing stable alignment of the long axis of the limb parallel to the ground. For a distal hindlimb, the patient should be placed in dorsal recumbency with the limb over the end of the table. This positioning allows manipulation of the pes to assess ROM throughout the procedure. Maintaining a straight alignment and avoiding rotation help to prevent iatrogenic creation of a varus or valgus deformity.

Achieving and maintaining adequate reduction during fracture fixation are crucial to restoring articular surface and improving outcome. Achieving adequate reduction may require specific instrumentation such as Vulsellum forceps, small fragment forceps, and human patella forceps. (see Figure 101.4) Fragment removal is generally discouraged because it deprives the fracture site from bone graft and seems to negatively impact return to racing (Boudrieau *et al.* 1984b; Guilliard 2000).

Surgeons generally tend to select robust implants, particularly for the fixation of complex fractures subjected to significant tension or compression. The string of pearls locking plate is the strongest implant and would conceptually seem an ideal candidate for repair of comminuted fractures of the calcaneus, for example (DeTora and Kraus 2000, Miller et al. 2011). However, the high profile of this plate system leads to tension of the skin over the implant. The thin skin of greyhounds is unable to tolerate this tension during skin closure. Locking plates may have a lower plate profile with an increased strength provided by the larger internal screw diameter, which makes them a suitable alternative. Wound dehiscence associated with exposure of implants may lead to secondary infection and necessitate future implant removal.

If there is no comminution and anatomic reconstruction can be achieved a simple fixation with a pin and tension band may be used to stabilize calcaneal fractures. Occasionally, a lag screw may provide additional support and reconstruction. This "less is more" approach to fracture reduction may require adjunct external coaptation for a short duration after surgery. The support provided via external coaptation can be gradually decreased over several weeks, substituting an initial splint with a modified Robert Jones bandage.

When applying bandages and splints on the distal extremities in greyhounds, special consideration must be given to the vulnerability of the skin over bony prominences, predisposing these areas to pressure points and sores. Adequate padding must be placed over bony prominences and around the first digit to prevent open wounds. Padding over the plate can be minimized by cutting the padding away from this area in a doughnut configuration. Padding over areas of the metatarsophalangeal joint prominence medially and laterally, the medial and lateral sides of the digit where the neighboring toenail is compressed into the digit, evaluation of the calcaneus, and the area over the lateral plate at the level of the tarsometatarsal joint should be modified to protect these areas. Frequent bandage changes are also recommended to identify early complications.

The outcome varies depending on several factors, including the degree of injury, type of injury, concurrent injury, accurate diagnosis, and whether surgical repair was performed. In a study of central tarsal bone fractures managed either by external coaptation or surgery, return to racing was achieved in 88% of dogs treated via internal reduction with screw fixation compared with only 58% of those treated by coaptation (Boudrieau et al. 1984b). The progression of osteoarthritis is also minimized in cases repaired with open reduction and internal fixation (Boudrieau et al. 1984b).

Reconstruction of comminuted interarticular fractures of the tarsus may be impossible. The bone fragments will help to promote intertarsal ankylosis, which may provide a more stable and pain-free joint after tarsal injury (Guilliard 2000). This allows for fusion between the mostly immobile tarsal bones and aids in formation of an arthrodesis.

Conservative management of tarsal injuries generally carries a poor prognosis for return to racing (Guilliard 2010). Surgical repair results in a shorter and more predictable recovery than conservative management, allowing any dog that may potentially return to racing to do so sooner (Guilliard 2010). Subsequently, surgical repair should be pursued whenever possible for tarsal injuries. Fractures of the metatarsal bones may be managed conservatively with success (Guilliard 2013). This was supported in a study in which 14 of 18 dogs evaluated returned to racing after metatarsal III fractures that were allowed to heal with rest, a supportive dressing, or both (Guilliard 2013).

Precise surgical correction with anatomic reduction, complete identification of all injuries present, and careful management of the soft tissue components can result in a successful return to function. Tolerance for less than an anatomic reconstruction is often inadequate for a return to high-performance function. Careful planning, improved surgical execution, and conscientious postoperative management can lead to a return to high-level performance.

References

Bergh, M. (2008). Radiographic, computed tomographic, and histologic study of central tarsal bone fractures in racing greyhounds. (Electronic thesis or dissertation). Retrieved from https://etd.ohiolink.edu/.

Boudrieau, R.J., Dee, J.F., Dee, L.G. (1984a) Central tarsal bone fractures in the racing Greyhound: a review of 114 cases. *Journal of the American Veterinary Medical Association* 184 (12), 1486-1491.

Boudrieau, R.J., Dee, J.F., Dee, L.G. (1984b) Treatment of central tarsal bone fractures in the racing Greyhound. *Journal of the American Veterinary Medical Association* 184 (12) 1482-1500.

Colborne, G.R., Innes, J.F., Comerford, E.J., et al. (2005). Distribution of power across the hind limb joints in Labrador retrievers and greyhounds. *American Journal of Veterinary Research* 66 (9), 1563-1571.

DeTora, M., Kraus, K. (2008) Mechanical testing of 3.5 mm locking and non-locking bone plates. *Veterinary and Comparative Orthopaedics and Traumatology* 21 (4), 318-322.

Guilliard, M.J. (2000) Fractures of the central tarsal bone in eight racing greyhounds. *Veterinary Record* 147, 512-515.

Guilliard, M.J. (2010) Third tarsal bone fractures in the greyhound. *Journal of Small Animal Practice* 51 (12), 635-641.

Guilliard, M.J. (2013) Conservative management of fractures of the third metatarsal bone in the racing Greyhound. *Journal of Small Animal Practice* 54 (10), 507-511.

Hercock, C.A., Innes, J.F., McConnell, et al. (2011) Observer variation in the evaluation and classification of severe central tarsal bone fractures in racing Greyhounds. *Veterinary and Comparative Orthopaedics and Traumatology* 24, 215-222.

Hickman, J. (1975) Greyhound injuries. *Journal of Small Animal Practice* 16 (1-12), 455-460.

Johnson, K.A. (1987) Accessory carpal bone fractures in the racing greyhound: classification and pathology. *Veterinary Surgery* 16 (1), 60-64.

Johnson, K.A., Muir, P., Nicoll, R.G., Roush, J. K. (2000). Asymmetric adaptive modeling of central tarsal bones in racing greyhounds. *Bone* 27 (2), 257-263.

Miller, E.I., Acquaviva, A.E., Eisenmann, D.J., et al. (2011) Perpendicular pull-out force of locking versus non-locking plates in thin cortical bone using a canine mandibular ramus model. *Veterinary Surgery* 40, 870-874.

Muir, P., Johnson, K.A., Ruaux-Mason, C.P. (1999). In vivo matrix microdamage in a naturally occurring canine fatigue fracture. *Bone* 25 (5), 571-576.

Prole, J.H.B. (1976) A survey of racing injuries in the Greyhound. *Journal of Small Animal Practice* 17 (4), 207-218.

Rutherford, S., Ness, M.G. (2012) Dorsal slab fracture of the fourth carpal bone in a racing Greyhound. *Veterinary Surgery* 41 (8), 944-947.

Sicard, G.K., Short, K., Manley, P.A. (1999) A survey of injuries at five greyhound racing tracks. *Journal of Small Animal Practice* 40 (9), 428-432.

Tomlin, J.L., Lawes, T.J., Blunn, G.W., et al. (2000) Fractographic examination of racing greyhound central (navicular) tarsal bone failure surfaces using scanning electron microscopy. *Calcified Tissue International* 67, 260-266.

102 Carpal Contracture

Alessandro Piras[2] and Tomas Guerrero[1]
[1]St. George's University, School of Veterinary Medicine, True Blue, Grenada, West Indies
[2]Surgical Referral Services and Canine Sport Medicine Centre, Russi Vet Hospital; College of Veterinary Medicine University of Dublin, University College Dublin, Dublin, Ireland

Carpal contracture or flexural contracture of the carpus is defined as the inability to extend the carpal joint in a physiological range of motion (ROM). This condition may be a complication of secondary wound healing, when skin loss exceeds one third of the circumference of the distal limb. In these cases, the normal repair processes may not suffice to restore skin coverage, leading to an abnormal contraction of soft tissues and restricted ROM. This chapter focuses on carpal contracture secondary to orthopedic procedures such as limb lengthening procedures and prolonged external coaptation of the joint in flexion.

Flexural contracture of the carpus associated with limb lengthening procedures

Definition
This is loss of carpal extension secondary to distraction osteogenesis of the radius and ulna.

Risk factors
- Limb lengthening procedures
- Fast rate of lengthening
- Patients requiring large amounts of lengthening
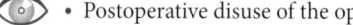
- Postoperative disuse of the operated limb (**Video 102.1**)
- Postoperative pain (leading to disuse)

Diagnosis
- Diagnosis is based on clinical examination of the carpal joint. The normal ROM of the carpus in Labrador Retrievers varies from 31 to 34 degrees in flexion to 194 to 197 degrees in extension (Jaegger *et al.* 2002). Carpal contracture usually affects a single limb, allowing use of the contralateral limb as reference. A loss of extension combined with abnormal weight bearing is consistent with carpal contracture.
- Radiographic examinations of the affected joint and radius (Figure 102.1) are indicated to evaluate the bone regeneration at the distraction site and the presence of joint pathology, such as degenerative joint disease (DJD).

Treatment
- Aggressive physiotherapy based on forced extension of the joint. In the first sessions, the physiotherapy is carried out having the dog deeply sedated or anesthetized. The carpal joint is manually extended along its maximum ROM. Later during the treatment, with the patient's increased tolerance to the manipulations, it is possible to avoid anesthesia and sedation.
- Place a bandage to maintain the carpus in extension.
- Pain management (see Chapter 14), including nonsteroidal anti-inflammatory drugs (NSAIDs) and opioids.
- Decrease the distraction rate.
- Encourage the use of the affected limb through low-impact exercise.

Outcome
The prognosis depends on early measurements to prevent this complication. Patients detected early enough and aggressively treated have a good prognosis to recover full ROM.

Chronic contractures rarely resolve with physical therapy because solo treatment and surgical intervention is usually required. Severe cases of carpal flexural contracture have a guarded prognosis, and full ROM recovery is not expected to occur.

Prevention
Prevention of carpal contracture associated with distraction osteogenesis relies mainly on encouraging postoperative use of the limb via physiotherapy and analgesia. Early implementation of these measures is essential in dogs that require significant lengthening.

Preventive measures include:
- It is generally agreed that some period of latency subsequent to the osteotomy enhances the formation of bone. The duration of the latency in most clinical reports ranges from 3 days (in young patients) to 10 days (in older patients). The recommended rate of distraction ranges from 0.5 mm/day to 1.0 mm/day with a rhythm of two or four times a day. In general, exceeding 1-mm distraction rate a day can decrease or stop the formation of bone regenerate and have a negative impact on soft tissues (tendons, muscles). The physician must choice a balanced rate that avoids early consolidation of the regenerate but does not exceed the lengthening and adapting potential of the soft tissues. A rate of 1 mm/day seems to be a rational choice, but individual patients must be evaluated, particularly when the lengthening procedure is associated with simultaneous correction of a deformity (Aronson 1997).
- Provide detailed postoperative instructions and demonstrations to owners regarding the lengthening device to avoid technical errors during distraction.
- Prescribe postoperative analgesia (see Chapter 14).

Complications in Small Animal Surgery, First Edition. Edited by Dominique Griffon and Annick Hamaide.
© 2016 John Wiley & Sons, Inc. Published 2016 by John Wiley & Sons, Inc.
Companion website: www.wiley.com/go/griffon/complications

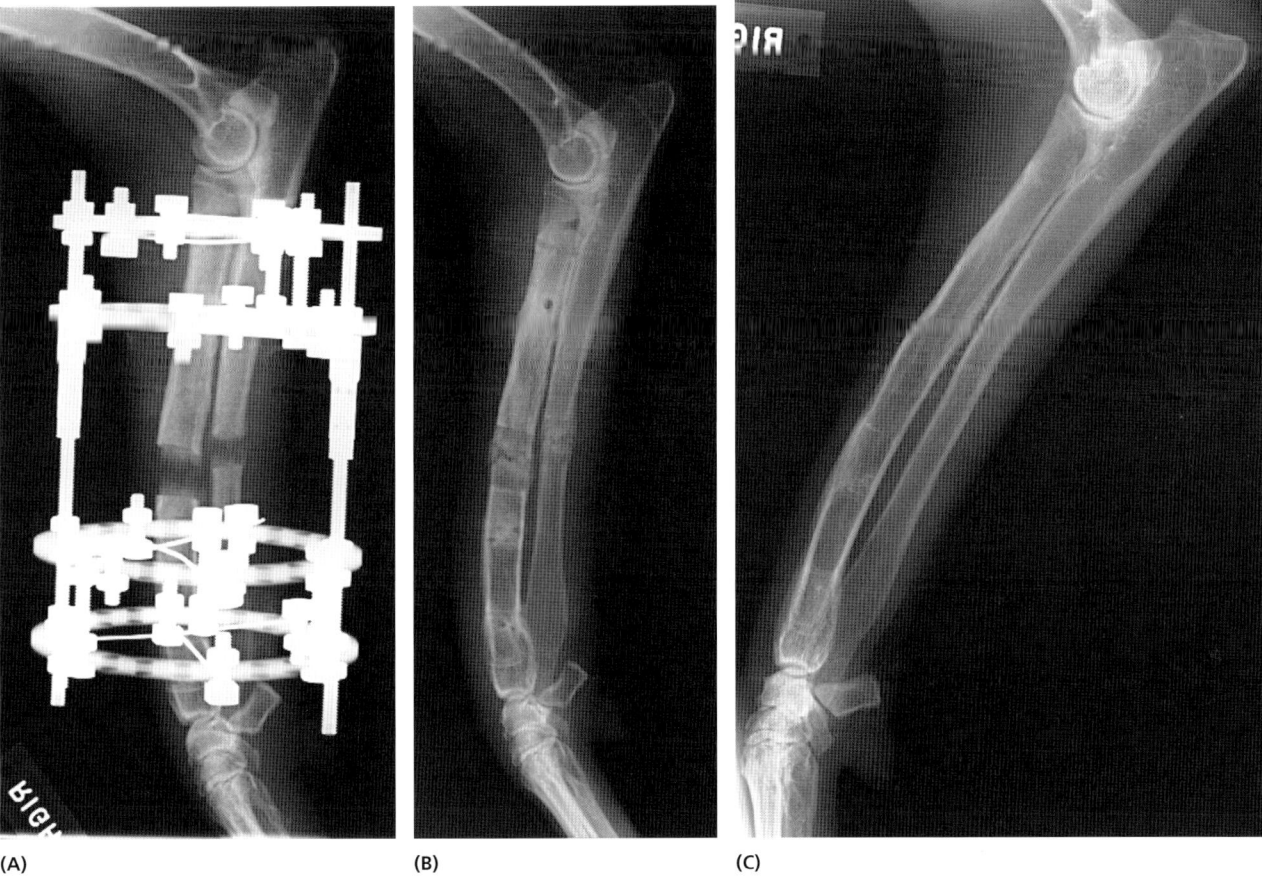

Figure 102.1 Radiographic evaluation of dogs with carpal contracture during limb lengthening. These radiographs were obtained on the dog shown in Video 102.1. **A,** Three weeks after surgery. Note the bone regeneration at the distraction site and flexed position of the carpus. **B,** Radiograph obtained immediately after removal of the apparatus. The dog was managed with placed in an extended splint for 2 weeks followed by physical therapy and gradual return to exercise. **C,** Three months after removal of the apparatus. The bone is healed, and the dog has regained normal function, although carpal extension remained slightly decreased on palpation. *Source:* D. Griffon, Western University of Health Sciences, Pomona, CA, 2014. Reproduced with permission from D Griffon.

- Daily home physical therapy, including passive ROM of the carpus, and cold compresses until inflammation has subsided
- Postoperative analgesia: NSAID, opioid analgesic drugs, or both
- Use of elastic devices or bandages connected to the limb lengthening apparatus to maintain the foot in extension during lengthening, especially if significant lengthening is planned (Figure 102.2)
- Weekly postoperative evaluation of the patient allows early detection of complications and adjustment of distraction rate.

Flexural contracture of the carpus associated with bandages

Definition

This is loss of carpal extension secondary to prolonged external coaptation.

Risk factors

Postoperative immobilization of the distal forelimb is routinely performed with the carpus in slight varus and flexion to prevent carpal valgus and hyperextension. This complication is commonly seen as a result of ligament laxity induced by prolonged external coaptation, especially in immature dogs. However, flexural contracture of the

carpal joint has been reported as a complication of bandages applied to prevent weight bearing of the forelimb. The Velpeau sling (Figure 102.3) is used to immobilize the shoulder region, and the carpal flexion bandage (Figures 102.4 Figure 102.5) is intended solely to prevent weight bearing while maintaining passive motion of the shoulder and elbow joints. The carpal flexion bandage has also been used to protect internal fixation of fractures of the accessory carpal bones (ACB) and surgical repair of the flexor carpi ulnaris (Piermattei *et al.* 2006). Other indications have included comminuted fractures of the ACB (type V) that are not amenable to open reduction and internal fixation and minimally displaced epiphyseal fractures in young dogs. After internal fixation of the ACB, the carpus is protected with a fiberglass molded palmar splint or a padded bandage for 4 to 6 weeks. In these cases, the carpus should initially be immobilized at about 40 degrees of flexion but should subsequently be adjusted in incremental degrees of extension with every splint or bandage change to gradually restore the weight-bearing position (Johnson 1998; Johnson and Piras 2005). Risk factors for carpal contracture subsequent to external coaptation therefore include:

- Prolonged immobilization of the carpus in a moderate to severe flexion, such as a Velpeau sling (more than 2 weeks).
- Failing in gradually extending the carpus at every bandage change in case of a carpal flexion bandage (Figure 102.6).

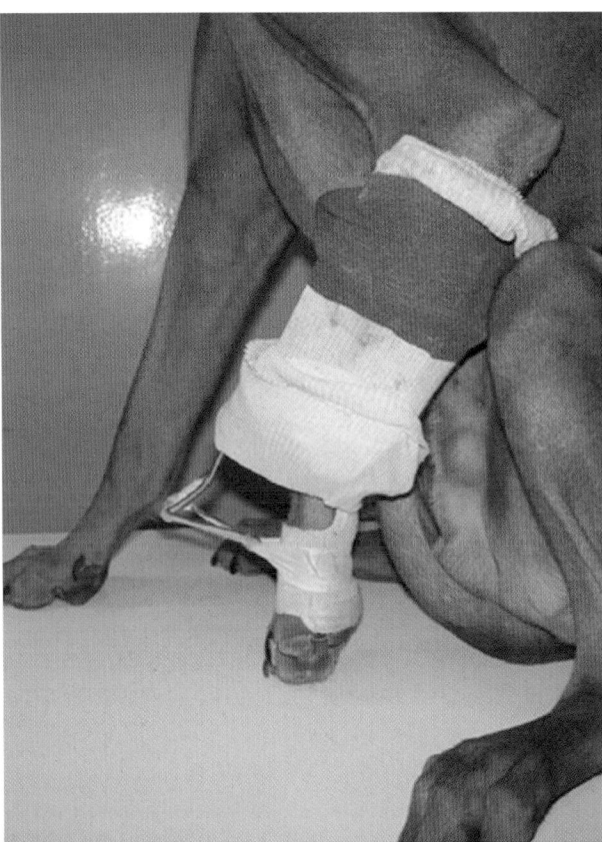

Figure 102.2 Treatment of carpal contracture during limb lengthening. A bar attached to the most distal ring of the circular fixator was used as a support for a stirrup. The paw was bandaged and connected to the bar by elastic bands, tensioned as needed to keep the carpus in extension. *Source:* G. L. Rovesti, Clinica Veterinaria Miller, Reggio nell'Emilia, Italy. Reproduced with permission from G. L. Rovesti.

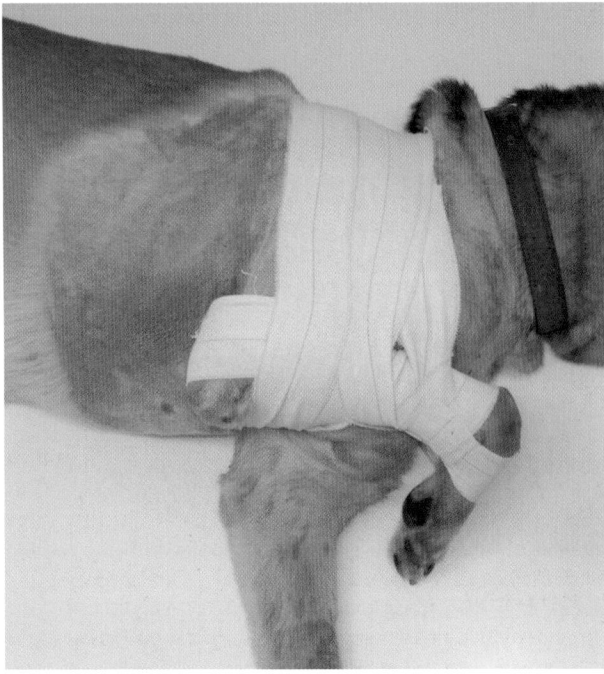

Figure 102.3 Velpeau sling. The sling was applied to protect fixation of a proximal humeral fracture. To prevent for flexural contracture of the carpus, the carpal joint was not completely flexed.

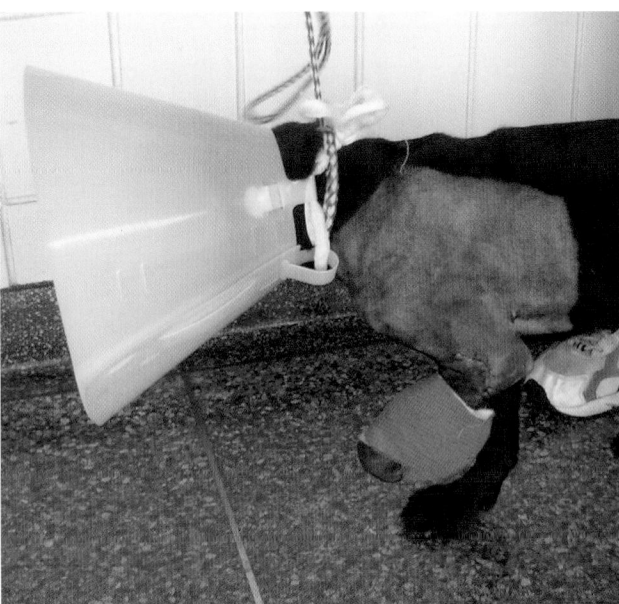

Figure 102.4 Carpal flexion bandage. Note the degree of flexion of the carpus. *Source:* D. Griffon, Western University of Health Sciences, Pomona, CA, 2014. Reproduced with permission from D. Griffon.

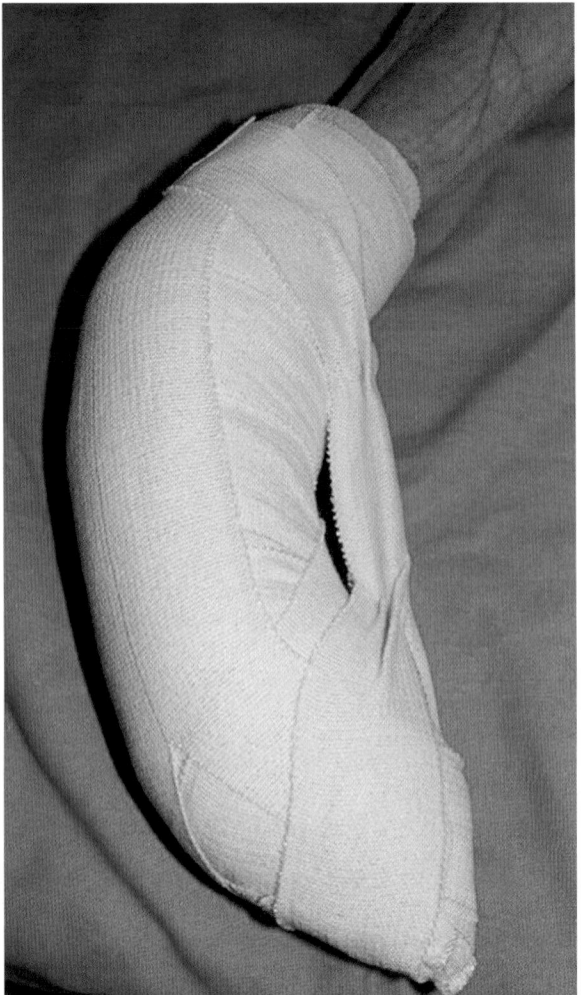

Figure 102.5 Carpal flexion bandage applied after the repair of a fracture of the accessory carpal bone. The stirrup of Elastoplast regulate the amount of flexion applied.

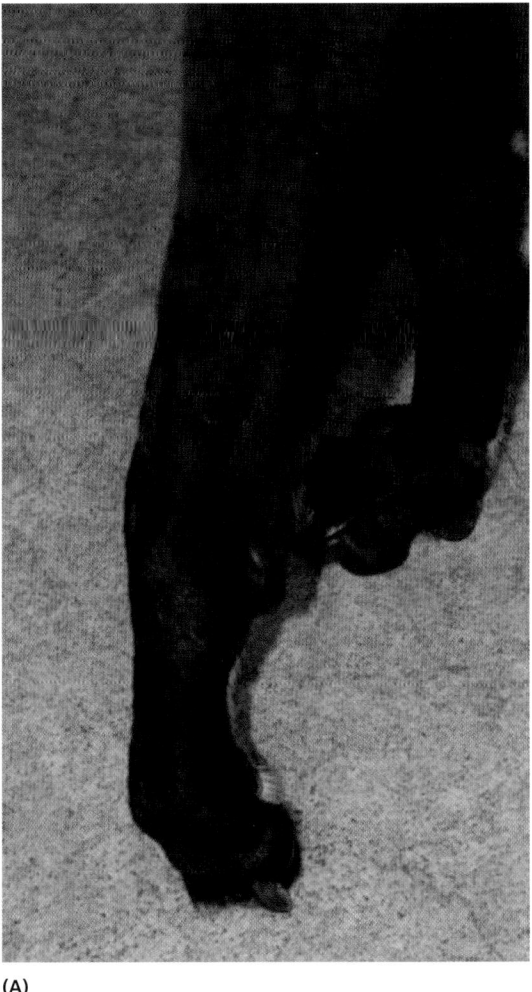

(A)

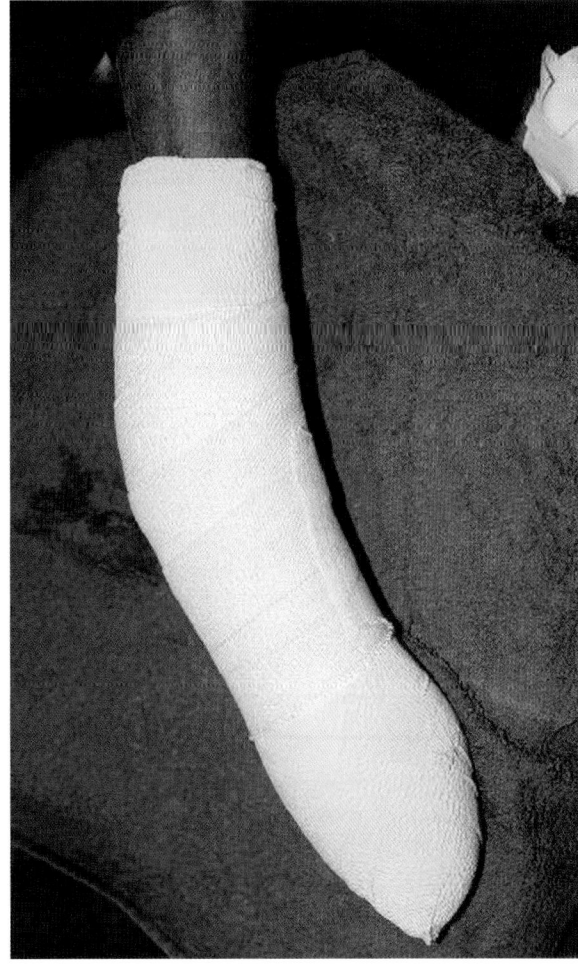

(B)

Figure 102.6 Flexural contracture in a greyhound. **A,** The bandage was kept for 8 weeks in 30 degrees of flexion without gradual extension. **B,** Three weeks later, a bandage in extension has been applied to allow gradual extension and weight bearing.

Diagnosis

In case of a Velpeau sling, the contracture appears evident at the time of bandage removal: the patient cannot fully extend the shoulder, elbow, and carpal joints. Muscle atrophy can be present along with pain when carpal extension is attempted.

The clinical presentation of carpal contracture resulting from a carpal flexion bandage is different because the contracture affects only the carpal joint. The patient presents with a decreased extension of the carpus with decreased weight bearing (tendency to tip toe) (**Video 102.1**) during the stance phase.

In both cases, radiographs of the affected joint may be warranted to evaluate the presence of pathology (fracture healing, DJD).

Treatment

This bandage-related complication is usually treated with physiotherapy aiming to eliminate pain and inflammation and to return the contracted carpus to normal ROM and function.

Different protocols have been anecdotally reported, including:
- Magneto-therapy: once a day for 15 to 20 minutes. The recommended frequency is 7 Hz of 10 Hz with an intensity ranging between 25% and 60%.
- Laser therapy: once or twice a day; frequency of 18 Hz; intensity, 100%, 4 Joules/cm². The duration varies according to the extension of the area to be treated.

- Cryotherapy: once or twice a day; suggested maximum application time is 10 minutes.
- Tecar therapy (device for resistive-capacitive energy transmission and integrated transdermal transport): applied once a day (in selected cases can be applied twice a day) in capacitive modality with maximum intensity 9% to increase microcirculation without production of heat (Figure 102.7).
- Ultrasonography: 1 to 3 MHz according to deep of the lesion; intensity, 0.5/2 W/cm²; duty cycle of maximum 20%. The duration of every treatment varies according to the extension of the area to be treated (This modality has been mostly substituted by Tecar therapy, which grants better results in shorter time.).
- In chronic cases, it is possible to add electrostimulation and continue with Tecar therapy associated with mobilization and stretching exercises. The Tecar treatment starts with capacitive modality of 23% maximum intensity followed by the use of the probe for resistive modality with 1% to 3% maximum intensity. Within 20 to 30 minutes from the treatment starts the mobilization and stretching of the carpal joint for another 15 to 20 minutes. The treatment ends with the Tecar in capacitive modality to facilitate the venous drainage of the area.
- Standing exercises to stimulate weight bearing and proprioception for 15 to 20 minutes two or three times a day.

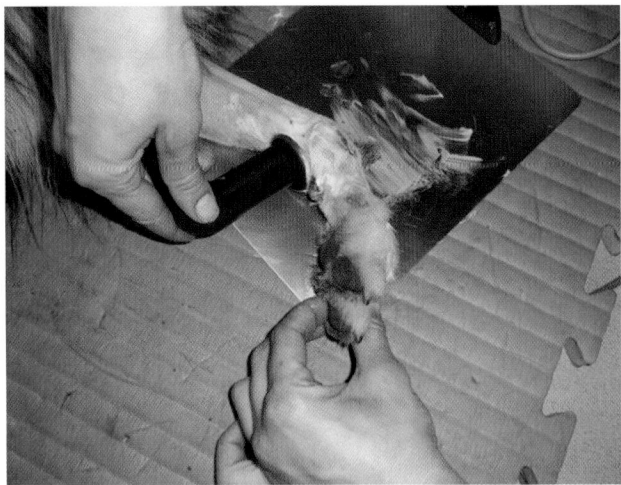

Figure 102.7 The capacitive probe of the Tecar is run along the flexor ulnaris carpi. A conductive paste is applied to facilitate the energy transmission. *Source:* E. R. Nutini, Mathi, Italy. Reproduced with permission from E. R. Nutini.

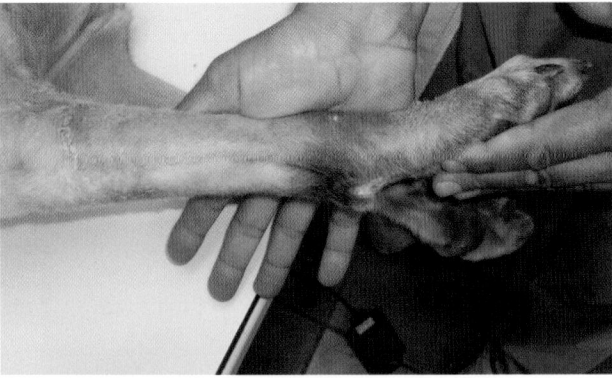

Figure 102.8 Passive range of motion is done at bandage changes to prevent flexural contracture of the carpus. *Source:* E. R. Nutini, Mathi, Italy. Reproduced with permission from E. R. Nutini.

- Underwater treadmill starting with water level to the chest and slow speed for 15 minutes and continuing along the treatment with water level at elbow level slow speed for 15 minutes. Once or twice a day of water treadmill exercise is generally sufficient.
- Aggressive physiotherapy based on forced extension of the joint, as previously described for the treatment of limb lengthening–associated contractures (Figure 102.8).
- Surgical release of the superficial and deep digital flexor tendons has been anecdotally reported as a successful option for patients that are not responsive to physiotherapy (A. Ferretti and P.M. Piga, personal communication).

Outcome
Physiotherapy is usually the treatment of choice and in the majority of the cases results in complete return to function in within 8 weeks.

Prevention
- The use of the Velpeau sling and carpal flexion bandage should generally be avoided and always limited to specific indications.
- Regular bandage changes: once daily for a few days after surgery and at least once weekly thereafter.
- Passive ROM every time the bandage is changed (see Figure 102.7)
- Avoid immobilization for more than 2 weeks.
- Incremental extension of the carpus during use of a carpal flexion bandage: starting from fully flexed position and gradually extending the carpus weekly at time of bandage change.

Relevant literature
Flexural contracture of the carpus is a common complication associated with limb lengthening procedures of the antebrachium (Langley-Hobbs *et al.* 1996; Lewis *et al.* 1999; Theyse *et al.* 2005; Rovesti *et al.* 2009); it is reported in 13.3% of cases (Rovesti *et al.* 2009). The flexor muscles of the antebrachium are larger than the extensor group, and the inability of flexor tendons and muscles to keep up with distraction rates combined with limb disuse causes its

relative shortening traction and the subsequent loss of carpal motion in flexion (Lewis *et al.* 1999; Theyse *et al.* 2005; Rovesti *et al.* 2009).

The management of carpal flexural contractures is challenging and often results in frustrating results (Theyse *et al.* 2005). Prevention of this complication is therefore preferable and may include strategies such as decreasing the distraction rate (Marcellin-Little *et al.* 1998) or even stopping lengthening procedures at first signs of carpal flexure contracture (Theyse *et al.* 2005; Rovesti *et al.* 2009). Other preventive measures such as physiotherapy and supportive bandaging during lengthening should be instituted before onset of clinical signs (Theyse *et al.* 2005). An early case report described prevention and treatment by bandaging the foot in extension (Langley-Hobbs *et al.* 1996).

Other reports on prevention and treatment of carpal contracture propose an approach based on physiotherapy combined with NSAIDs or opioid analgesic drugs (or both) along with placement of elastic bands to counteract flexion forces (Rovesti *et al.* 2009). Rovesti *et al.* (2009) described the placement of a bar on the cranial aspect of the limb connected by nuts to the most distal ring of the frame to function as a stirrup. In this report, the paw was bandaged and connected to the bar by elastic bands tensioned as needed to keep the carpus in extension. Physiotherapy was performed at least twice a day. The authors also recommended stopping limb lengthening if flexural contracture did not resolve, even if a discrepancy in length would be expected. Early implementation of these preventive measures was recommended in cases that required significant lengthening (Rovesti *et al.* 2009).

Bandaging of the carpus in flexion by means of a splint or a cast is indicated to manage comminuted fractures of the accessory carpal bone that are not amenable to open reduction. The carpal flexion bandage is also commonly used to provide postoperative protection after internal fixation of reducible fractures of the accessory carpal bone or other carpal bones. The carpus is initially immobilized at 40 degrees of flexion and gradually extended to normal standing position through a period of 4 to 6 weeks (Johnson 1988). Prolonged immobilization of the carpus in flexion should be avoided to prevent the development of carpal flexural contracture (Johnson and Piras 2005).

All videos cited in this chapter can be found on the book companion website at www.wiley.com/go/griffon/complications.

References

Aronson, J. (1997) Current concepts review: limb-lengthening, skeletal reconstruction, and bone transport with the Ilizarov method. *Journal of Bone and Joint Surgery* 79 (8) 1243-1258.

Jaegger, G., Marcellin-Little, D.J., Levine, D. (2002) Reliability of goniometry in Labrador Retrievers. *American Journal of Veterinary Research* 63 (7), 979-986.

Johnson, K.A. (1988) In Bloomberg, M.S., Dee, J.F., Taylor, R.A. (eds.) *Canine Sport Medicine and Surgery*. Saunders, Philadelphia, pp. 115-117.

Johnson, K.A, Piras, A. (2005) Fractures of the carpus. In Johnson, A.L., Houlton, J.E.F., Vannini, R. (eds.) *AO Principles of Fracture Management in the Dog and Cat*. Thieme, Stuttgart, p. 347.

Langley-Hobbs, S.J., Carmichael, S, Pead, M.J., et al. (1996) Management of antebrachial deformity and shortening secondary to a synostosis in a dog. *Journal of Small Animal Practice* 37 (8), 359-363.

Lewis, D.D., Radasch, R.M., Beale, B.S., et al. (1999) Initial clinical experience with the IMEX circular external skeletal fixation System. *Veterinary and Comparative Orthopaedics and Traumatology* 12, 118-127.

Marcellin-Little, D.J., Ferretti, A., Roe, S.C., et al. (1998) Hinged Ilizarov external fixation for correction of antebrachial deformities. *Veterinary Surgery* 27 (3), 231-245.

Piermattei, D.L., Flo, G.L, Decamp, C.E. (2006) Fractures and other orthopedic conditions of the carpus, metacarpus, and phalanges. In *Brinker, Piermattei, and Flo's Handbook of Small Animal Orthopedics and Fracture Repair*, 4th edn. Saunders Elsevier, St Louis, pp. 387-399.

Rovesti, G.L., Scwarz, G., Bogoni, P. (2009) Treatment of 30 angular limb deformities of the antebrachium and the crus in the dog using circular external fixators. *The Open Veterinary Science Journal* 3, 41-54.

Theyse, L.F., Voorhout, G., Hazewinkel, H.A.(2005) Prognostic factors in treating antebrachial growth deformities with a lengthening procedure using a circular external skeletal fixation system in dogs. *Veterinary Surgery* 34 (5), 424-435.

103 Quadriceps Contracture

Darryl Millis

CARES Center for Veterinary Sports Medicine, Department of Small Animal Clinical Sciences, University of Tennessee College of Veterinary Medicine, Knoxville, TN, USA

Definition

Quadriceps contracture results from fibrous adhesions between the quadriceps muscles (most commonly the vastus intermedius) and the distal femur, usually involving a fracture callus. It may develop as a complication of distal femoral fracture management. Contracture of the quadriceps muscles can occur because of trauma, poor stabilization of a femoral fracture, or prolonged stifle extension caused by either external coaptation or disuse because of pain (Bardet 1987). Other reported causes of quadriceps contracture include toxoplasmosis, *Neospora* spp. infection, and *Clostridium tetani* infection (Knowler and Wheeler 1995; Barber and Trees 1996; Goldhammer *et al.* 2008).

Risk factors

- Immature dogs (age 3–5 months) with distal to mid-diaphyseal femoral fractures
- Failure of fracture stabilization
- Delayed return to function
- Prolonged stifle extension due to pain or external coaptation
- Protozoal infections at a young age, including toxoplasma or *Neospora* spp.

Many biomechanical, biochemical, and structural changes are affected by long-term joint immobilization. These changes affect the bone, joint capsule, skeletal muscle, articular cartilage and other connective tissue (Figure 103.1).

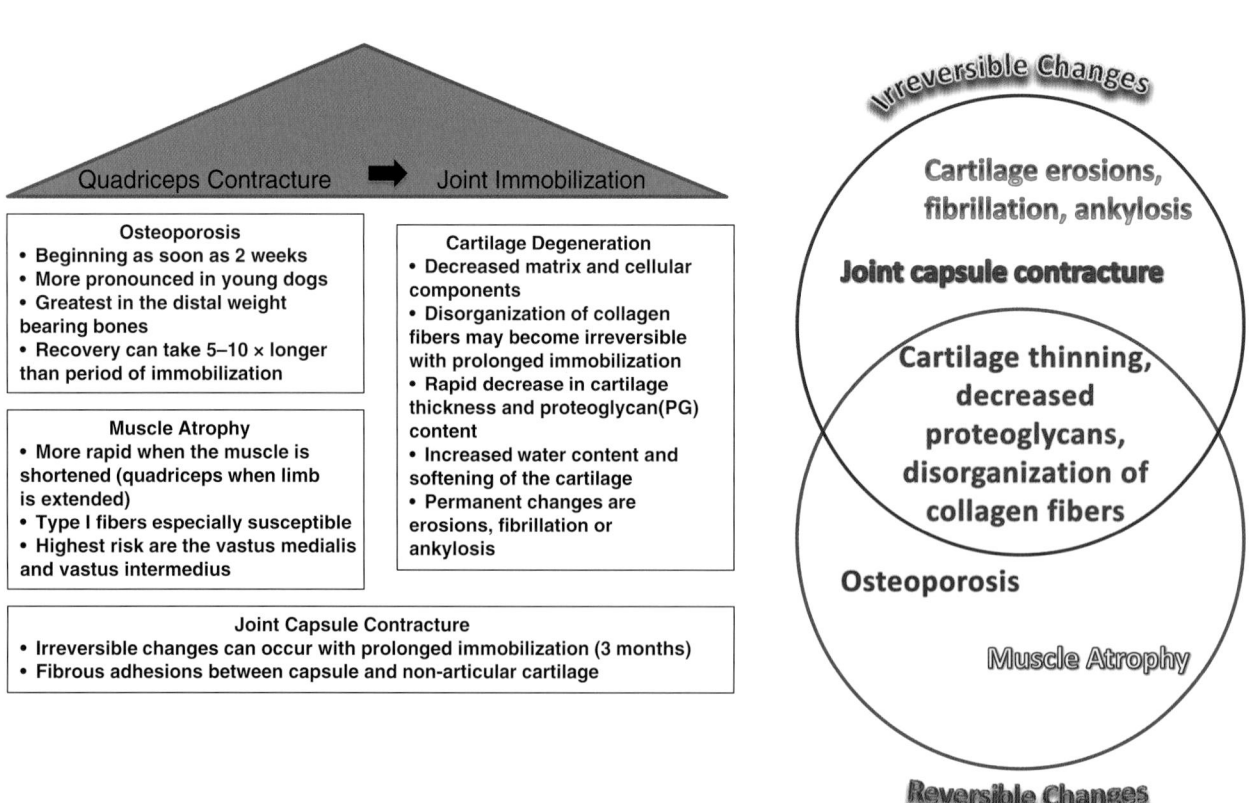

Figure 103.1 Pathophysiology of quadriceps contracture. PG, proteoglycan; ROM, range of motion.

Complications in Small Animal Surgery, First Edition. Edited by Dominique Griffon and Annick Hamaide.
© 2016 John Wiley & Sons, Inc. Published 2016 by John Wiley & Sons, Inc.
Companion website: www.wiley.com/go/griffon/complications

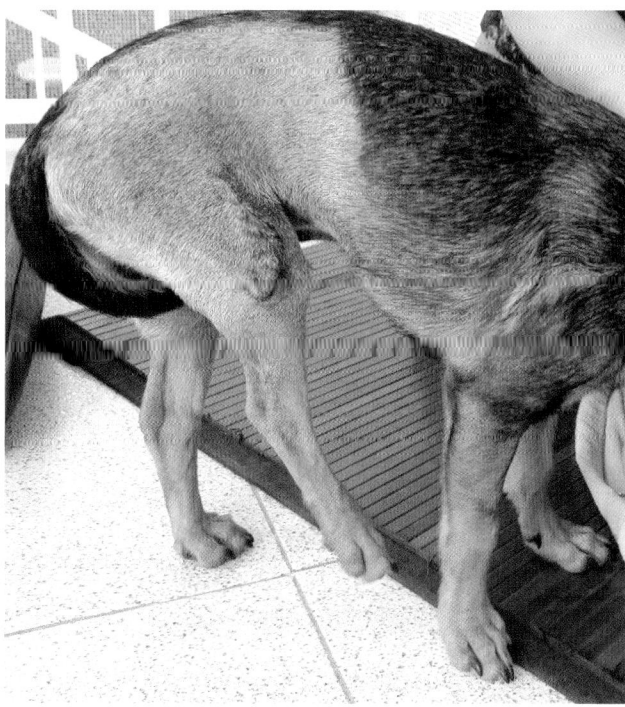

Figure 103.2 Clinical signs of quadriceps contracture. Note the extension of the stifle and muscle atrophy.

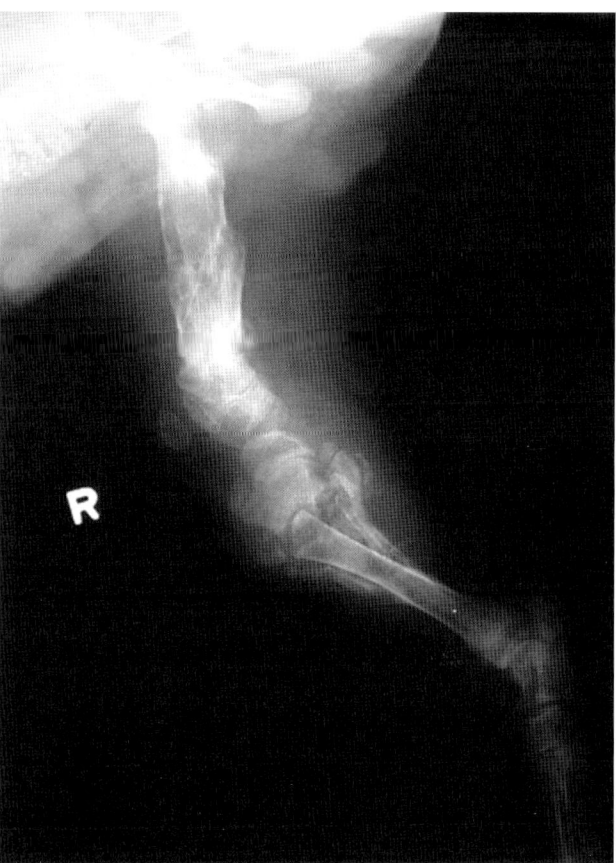

Figure 103.3 Radiographic abnormalities in a dog with quadriceps contracture secondary to femoral fracture.

Diagnosis

The diagnosis can be concluded based on history and physical examination. Clinical signs include:

- Severe hindlimb lameness
- Extensor rigidity of the hindlimb (Figure 103.2)
- Inability or greatly reduced ability to flex the hock and stifle
- Firm and atrophied quadriceps muscles, with concurrent atrophy of the thigh muscles

Additional signs may include:

- Patella alta or medial patella luxation
- Coxofemoral subluxation
- Genu recurvatum in extreme cases

Radiographic changes associated with this condition may include disuse osteopenia, stifle osteoarthritis, severe muscle atrophy, patella alta or luxation, and genu recurvatum in extreme cases (Figure 103.3).

Treatment

Algorithm

The treatment of a patient with quadriceps contracture depends on the length of time since injury and surgery and the maturity of the contracture (Figure 103.4).

Dogs with quadriceps contracture lasting longer than 3 to 4 weeks are candidates for surgical release of adhered tissue followed by intense rehabilitation. The progression of quadriceps contracture is faster in younger animals, and surgical treatment may be indicated earlier than in older dogs. Surgical intervention may include elevation of muscle tissue from the fracture callus, especially on the cranial aspect of the femur; dissection of adherent tissue from the joint capsule; and possibly release of restrictive joint capsule. Mild forced flexion of the stifle may result in release of remaining restrictive tissues, but caution must be exercised to prevent unwanted tissue damage and refracture. Postoperatively, the limb is maintained in a 90-90 flexion splint for several days until swelling and pain resolve and the dog begins active weight bearing. It is critical to follow surgical intervention with proper rehabilitation, or the condition will likely recur. Hospitalization and rehabilitation by trained personnel is recommended because owners often perform the therapy incorrectly or infrequently.

In dogs with early quadriceps contracture or in dogs after surgery for contracture, the main goals of physical rehabilitation include immediate passive range of motion (ROM) and stretching exercises to encourage joint motion and decrease the likelihood of fibrous tissue reformation and exercises that encourage active contraction and relaxation of the quadriceps muscle.

Surgical treatment

A variety of surgical procedures have been recommended, most of which focus on breaking down fibrous adhesions and increasing the ROM of the stifle. Options differ depending on the severity and duration of the condition and the probability of returning the limb to function. If the prospect of some joint function remains, surgical options include:

- Separation of quadriceps muscle from fracture callus and fibrous tissue
- Lengthening Z-plasty of the quadriceps muscle or patella ligament
- Release of rectus femoris from pubis

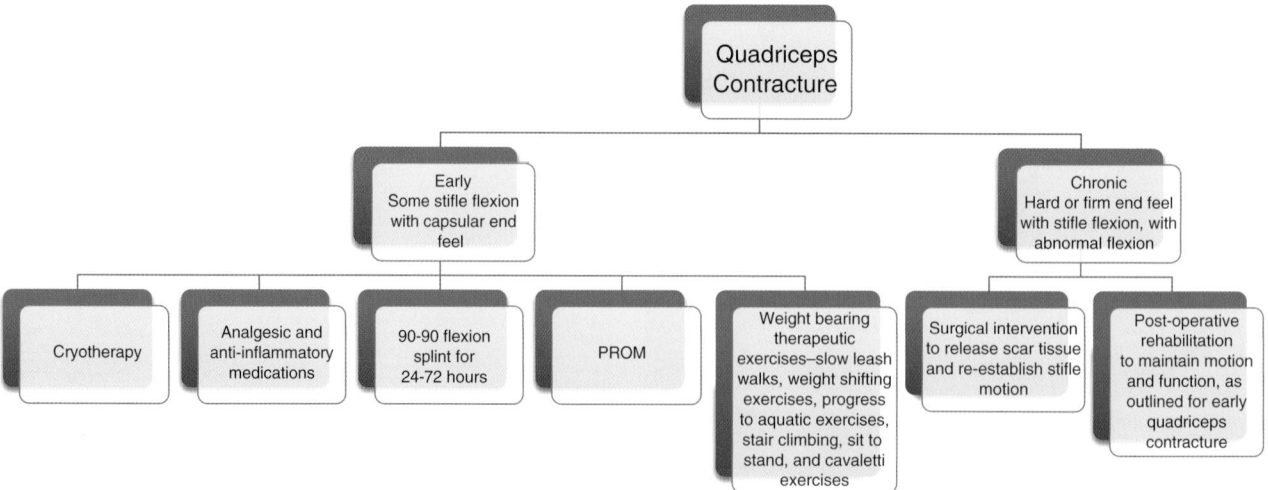

Figure 103.4 Algorithm for treatment of quadriceps contracture. ROM, range of motion.

- Excision of fibrous muscle fibers, especially vastus intermedius
- Sliding myoplasty
- Arthrotomy with separation or transection of joint capsule components limiting motion
- Cuneiform osteotomy of the femur
- Excision arthroplasty for coxofemoral luxation

Contraindications to the above surgeries include severe limb shortening (>25% difference in the length of the femur), replacement of quadriceps muscle with fibrous tissue (nonfunctional muscle), or severe disuse osteopenia in young dogs because of the risk of pathologic fracture.

If the joint is unlikely to return to function because of severe degenerative changes, other salvage procedures include:
- Stifle arthrodesis
- Limb amputation

Static and dynamic stifle flexion

Dynamic flexion devices have been successfully used in several cases to return the stifle to a more acceptable ROM. Devices that are most relevant allow for earlier return to function and aggressive physical rehabilitation, encouraging active ROM of the stifle. These techniques include:
- Loops of monofilament line attached to the ischial tuberosity and the calcaneus (Moores and Sutton 2009)
- External fixator components attached to the pelvis and lower limb connected by rubber bands (Wilkens *et al.* 1993)
- 90-90 flexion splints to prevent stifle stiffness after femoral fracture repairs (Aron and Crowe 1986) (Figure 103.5)

The detrimental effects of joint immobilization are minimized when the stifle is held in flexion rather than extension because extreme shortening and subsequent rapid atrophy of the quadriceps muscles are eliminated. Disuse muscle atrophy should still be expected but to a milder degree. Cartilage is more likely to atrophy with short-term immobilization in a flexed rather than extended position. Conversely, immobilization with the stifle in extension may result in degenerative changes. Atrophic changes are reversible with low-impact loading after several weeks, but degenerative changes result in permanent alteration of cartilage structure (Setton *et al.* 1997).

Physical rehabilitation

Treatment

A program for postoperative distal femoral fracture and quadriceps contracture repair may begin with massage and passive ROM several times a day followed by cryotherapy to alleviate inflammation and pain. After postoperative inflammation has subsided, heat may be applied to the area to facilitate stretching and ROM. Neuromuscular electrical stimulation of the quadriceps and hamstrings can be applied before weight bearing to prevent the progression of muscle atrophy. After several days, weight-shifting exercises can be added to encourage use of the limb and build muscle strength. As the patient progresses, hydrotherapy such as underwater treadmill walking can be added to increase active ROM in the stifle while relying on the buoyancy of the water to limit loading of the limb. Beyond 4 weeks, therapy may shift toward jogging and swimming to build muscle strength and improve the amplitude of motion of

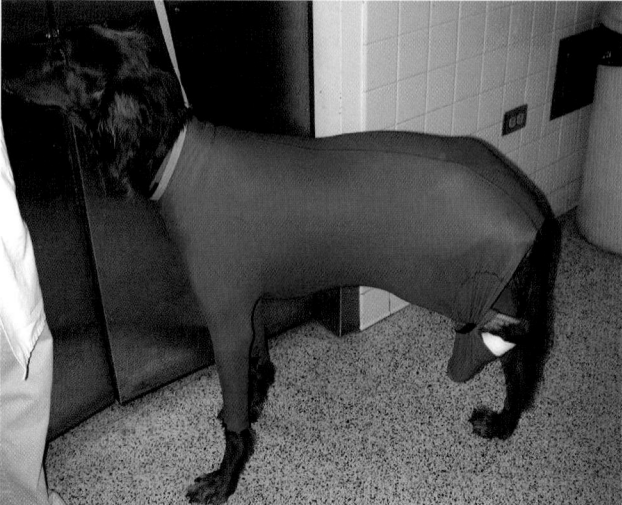

Figure 103.5 Dynamic flexion of the stifle: a device using a body suit maintains flexion of the stifle.

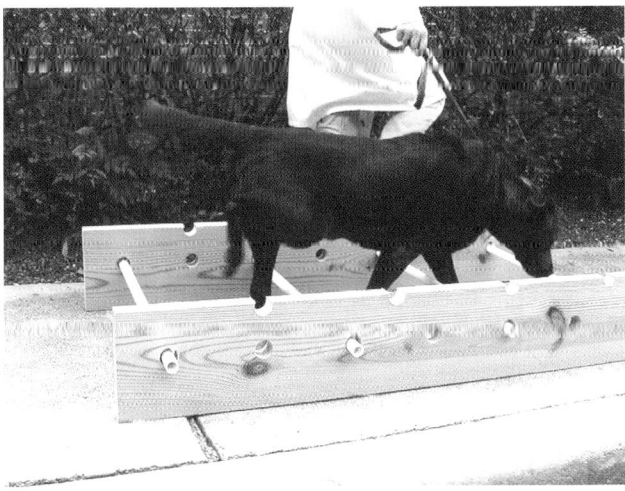

Figure 103.6 Cavaletti rail walking, an exercise used in the management of quadriceps contracture.

the stifle, especially in flexion. Other exercises to promote active stifle flexion include sit-to-stand exercises, cavaletti rail walking (Figure 103.6), and stair walking. Each patient should be assessed regularly to adjust the level of physical rehabilitation accordingly.

Prognosis

Unfortunately, the majority of quadriceps contracture cases have a poor prognosis for return to normal function if the condition has persisted for some time after injury. Some degree of lameness will persist in most dogs, even those that regain some ROM in the stifle and hock. The prognosis depends somewhat on the chronicity of the contracture and is worse if degenerative changes have already occurred in the stifle.

Prevention

The main strategies to prevent quadriceps contracture include (Figure 103.7):
- Early, rigid fracture stabilization with an emphasis on early return to function
- Never apply external coaptation as a means of repair for a femoral fracture, especially in an immature patient.
- Appropriate pain management to encourage weight bearing and use of the limb. The following approaches may be considered:
  ◦ Opioid medication, nonsteroidal antiinflammatory drugs (NSAIDs), epidural analgesia, α_2 blockers, and other analgesic agents (e.g., gabapentin).

Prevention of Quadriceps Contracture

- Early surgical fixation with adequate stability
- Cryotherapy to reduce inflammation, swelling, and pain
- Analgesic and anti-inflammatory medications
- 90-90 flexion splint for 24–72 hours
- Gentle, passive range of motion exercises
- Weight bearing exercises – slow leash walks, weight shifting exercises
- Progress to aquatic exercises, stair climbing, sit to stand, and cavaletti exercises to improve active range of motion

Figure 103.7 Strategies to prevent post-operative quadriceps contracture

◦ Cryotherapy can reduce the pain and swelling associated with surgery.
- Transcutaneous electrical stimulation may also be beneficial for pain control. Physical rehabilitation with an individualized program should be combined with appropriate and regular monitoring.

In general, weight bearing may not occur for 1 to 3 days after surgery. During this period of limited weight bearing, the limb may be maintained in a 90-90 flexion bandage to maintain the quadriceps muscles in an elongated position. At least twice daily, the bandage is removed to perform passive ROM exercises, an opportunity to weight bear, and cryotherapy. Passive ROM exercises are continued for at least 3 weeks after surgery. After the dog is toe touching on the limb at a stance or walk, weight-shifting exercises and slow leash walks may be initiated. A gradually increasing therapeutic exercise program, within the realm of safety to avoid fixation complications, is instituted after the patient is weight bearing, generally within 1 week (Figure 103.6).

Relevant literature

Quadriceps contracture is a detrimental complication of distal femur fractures. The quadriceps muscles, especially the vastus intermedius, form fibrous adhesions that are incorporated into the fracture callus, resulting in poor muscle function and permanent stifle extension. In addition to lameness and decreased weight bearing, this complication may lead to coxofemoral subluxation, patella alta, and patella luxation. The lack of joint motion associated with quadriceps contracture can lead to permanent changes in the soft and bony tissues of the affected limb, including disuse osteoporosis, muscle atrophy, muscle fibrosis, joint contracture, and changes to the articular cartilage. Some changes, such as muscle atrophy and changes in synovial fluid composition, may start as early as 1 to 2 weeks but usually improve with proper management. Synovial fluid is essential to maintaining the health of the articular cartilage, and the loading and unloading of the joint produced by weight bearing is needed to transport nutrients and water into the articular cartilage (Millis *et al.* 2004). Articular cartilage changes secondary to immobilization include fibrillation, deep erosions, fibrous ankylosis, and cartilaginous or even bony ankylosis (Bardet 1987). These changes become permanent after months of immobilization.

Return to normal function has been reported in rare cases. Most attempts at quadriceps contracture repair fail at restoring the ROM of the stifle and eliminating lameness. Regaining flexion even beyond 90 degrees is often impossible. Failed attempts at forceful flexing of the stifle under general anesthesia may result in proximal tibial epiphysiolysis (Ulusan *et al.* 2011) or fracture. The few successful cases that have been reported generally involve some form of static or dynamic flexion of the stifle during the immediate postoperative recovery period (Aron and Crowe 1986; Wilkens *et al.* 1993; Moores and Sutton 2009; Ulusan *et al.* 2011). Concurrent physical rehabilitation seems to result in the greatest recovery of flexion and the least amount of subjective lameness (Moores and Sutton 2009).

The principles of prevention include good surgical technique with minimal tissue trauma and adequate biomechanical stabilization of the fracture site; pain control; reduction of swelling and edema; and early, active use of the limb. Good surgical technique and minimal soft tissue disruption result in less swelling and pain postoperatively. Adequate fracture fixation allows early limb use and increasingly active ROM exercises along with muscle strengthening exercises. Perioperatively, efforts are directed to administration of analgesics, including opioid medications, NSAIDs, epidural analgesia, α_2 blockers, and other analgesic agents (e.g., gabapentin). In addition to pharmaceuticals, cryotherapy can reduce the pain and swelling associated with surgery. Transcutaneous electrical stimulation may also be beneficial for pain control. Physical rehabilitation is likely to prevent quadriceps contracture after surgical repair, eliminating the need for treatment of this devastating condition. A flexion bandage may be placed and changed twice daily for a few days after surgery. Passive ROM and massage are initiated immediately after surgery. A rehabilitation plan tailored to the patient is indicated until fracture healing and return to normal function.

References

Aron, D., Crowe, D. (1986) The 90-90 flexion splint for prevention of stifle joint stiffness with femoral fracture repairs. *Journal of the American Animal Hospital Association* 23, 447-454.

Barber, J., Trees, A. (1996) Clinical aspects of 27 cases of neosporosis in dogs. *Veterinary Record* 139, 439-443.

Bardet, J. (1987). Quadriceps contracture and fracture disease. *Veterinary Clinics of North America: Small Animal Practice* 17 (4), 957-973.

Goldhammer, M., Chapman, P., Grierson, J. (2008) Coxofemoral luxation in a border collie as a complication of a Clostridium tetani infection. *Journal of Small Animal Practice* 49, 159-162.

Knowler, C., Wheeler, S. (1995) Neospora caninum infection in three dogs. *Journal of Small Animal Practice* 36, 172-177.

Millis, D., Levine, D., Taylor M. (2004) *Canine Rehabilitation and Physical Therapy*, 1st edn. WB Saunders, St. Louis.

Moores, A.P., Sutton, A. (2009) Management of quadriceps contracture in a dog using static flexion apparatus and physiotherapy. *Journal of Small Animal Practice* 50, 251-254.

Setton, L.A., Mow, V.C., Muller, F.J., et al. (1997) Mechanical behavior and biochemical composition of canine knee cartilage following periods of joint disuse and disuse with remobilization. *Osteoarthritis and Cartilage* 5, 1-16.

Ulusan, S., Captug-Ozdemir, O., Gul-Sancak, I., et al. (2011) Treatment techniques of femoral quadriceps muscle contracture in ten dogs and two cats. *Kafkas Üniversitesi Veteriner Fakültesi Dergisi* 17 (3), 401-408.

Wilkens, B., McDonald, D., Hulse, D. (1993) Utilization of a dynamic stifle flexion apparatus in preventing recurrence of quadriceps contracture: a clinical report. *Veterinary and Comparative Orthopaedics and Traumatology* 6, 219-223.

104 Fracture-Associated Sarcoma

G. Elizabeth Pluhar

Department of Veterinary Clinical Sciences, College of Veterinary Medicine, University of Minnesota, St. Paul, MN, USA

Definition

A fracture-associated sarcoma is a primary tumor of bone that arises at a previous fracture site, presumably secondary to the original trauma or placement of implants to stabilize a fracture. Plate fixation seems most commonly associated with this condition, although tumors have also been reported after intramedullary nailing. Histologically, these tumors most commonly consist of osteogenic sarcomas or osteosarcomas, but undifferentiated sarcomas, fibrosarcomas, and other tumor types have also been reported. Independent of traumatic fractures, implant-associated sarcomas have been reported after total joint replacement or tibial plateau leveling osteotomy (TPLO).

Risk factors

Similar to spontaneous primary bone tumors, these tumors are more frequent in large and giant breed dogs. The median time from the initial trauma to diagnosis is 5.5 years, so most dogs are middle to older age. Approximately 50% of these tumors occur in the femur. There may be an increased risk of developing TPLO-associated sarcoma after bilateral procedures (Figure 104.1). Unlike spontaneous osteosarcoma, tumors associated with fracture are more common in the diaphysis at the previous fracture site rather than in the metaphysis of long bones. Proposed pathogenic factors are summarized in Figure 104.2.

Diagnosis

The most common clinical signs consist of lameness, pain, and soft tissue swelling over a previous fracture or surgical site. Non–weight-bearing lameness, instability, and crepitus are present if a pathologic fracture exists.

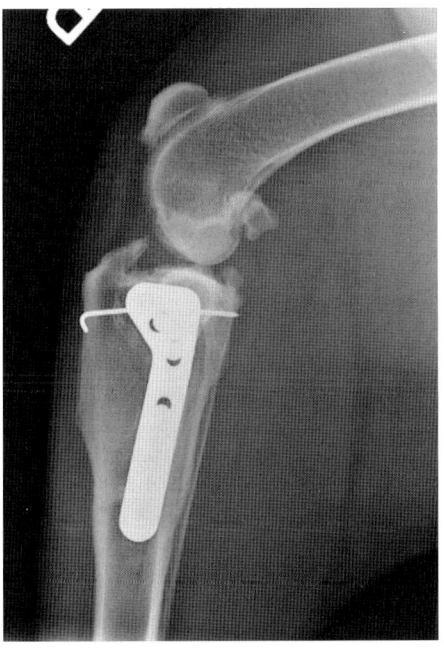
(A)

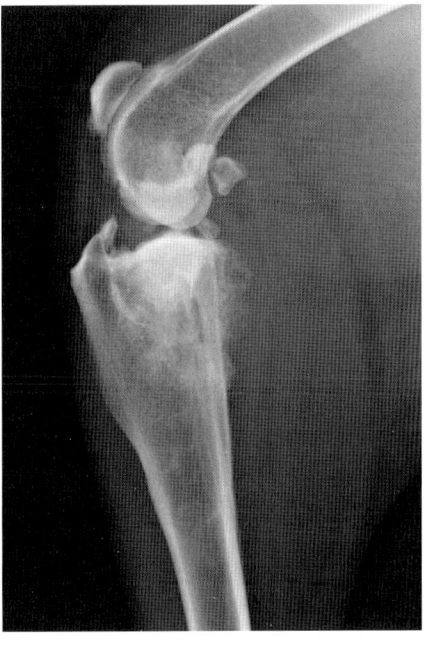
(B)

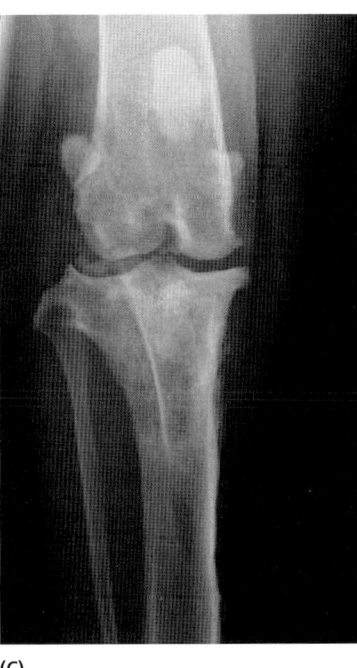
(C)

Figure 104.1 Tibia with radiolucency around the plate 2 years after tibial plateau leveling osteotomy (A). Tibia with fracture (implant) associated sarcoma 3 years after plate removal lateral (B) and craniocaudal (C) projections.

Complications in Small Animal Surgery, First Edition. Edited by Dominique Griffon and Annick Hamaide.

© 2016 John Wiley & Sons, Inc. Published 2016 by John Wiley & Sons, Inc.

Companion website: www.wiley.com/go/griffon/complications

Intrinsic Factors	Extrinsic Factors
• Initial trauma • Surgical trauma • Medullary infarct • Altered cellular activity	• Alloy toxicity • Corrosion secondary to electrolysis from dissimilar metals • Chronic instability

NEOPLASTIC TRANSFORMATION

Figure 104.2 Pathogenesis of fracture-associated sarcomas.

The diagnosis is confirmed with radiography of the affected bone. Radiographic signs include:
• Periosteal proliferation in a spiculated (sunburst pattern) or a lamellar pattern

• Bone lysis may be severe enough to create a "moth–eaten" appearance (Figure 104.3).

Radiographs of the thorax, including right and left lateral and ventrodorsal projections, are indicated to evaluate the presence of metastases.

A definitive diagnosis of neoplasia requires histologic examination of a tumor biopsy, confirming the presence of neoplastic cells, often multinucleate, and surrounded by osteoid. No diagnostic tool can definitely differentiate fracture-associated sarcomas from spontaneous tumors. A presumptive diagnosis is made based on history of trauma or placement of implants, and, in some cases, the unusual location of the tumor (Figure 104.4).

Treatment

The treatment for fracture-associated sarcomas is similar to spontaneously occurring primary bone sarcomas. Surgical options include amputation of the affected limb, or more rarely, limb-sparing procedures. Interlocking nail fixation of pathologic fractures has recently been reported in three dogs with fracture-associated sarcoma (Bhandal and Boston 2011). Adjunctive chemotherapy with a platinum or doxorubicin-based protocol is currently recommended (Chun and de Lorimier 2003).

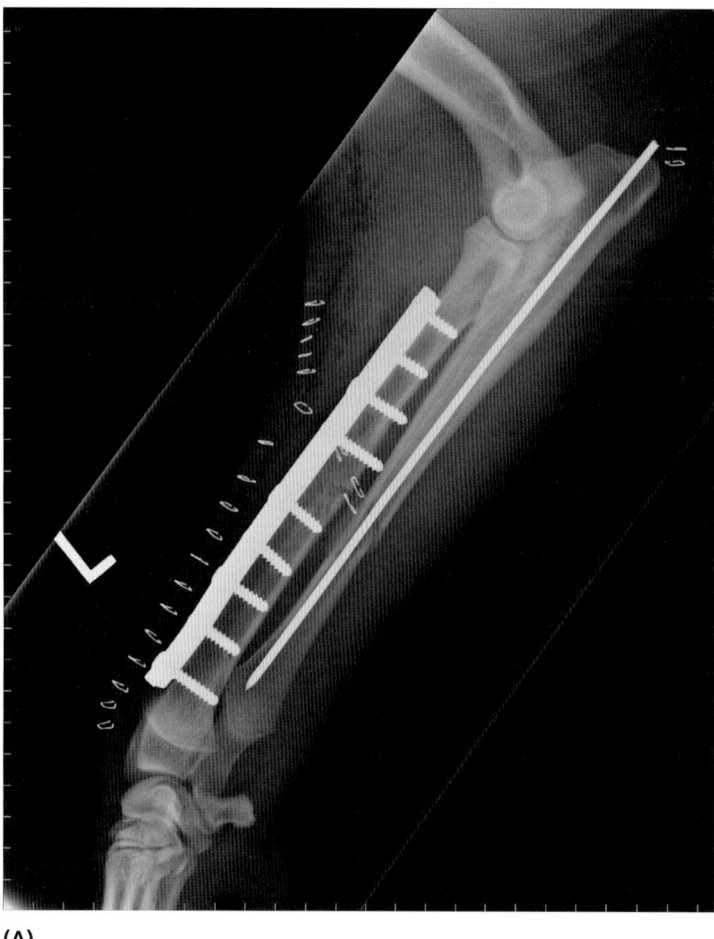

(A)

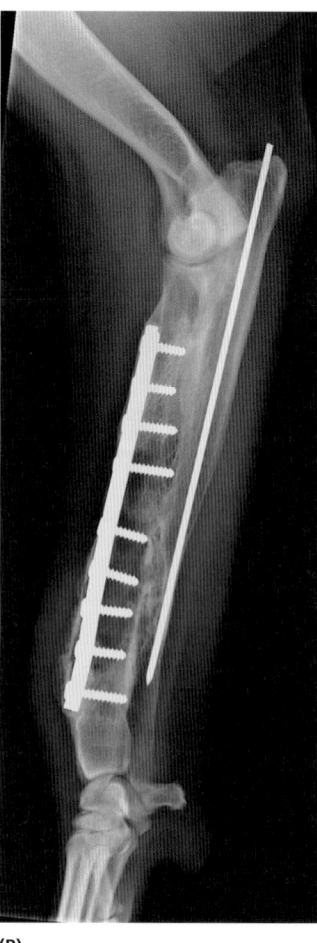

(B)

Figure 104.3 Radiograph of a radius and ulna fracture in a 9-month-old Bernese mountain dog stabilized with a plate immediately after surgery (**A**) and 4 years later after development of a fracture-associated sarcoma (**B**). Note the combination of bone lysis and periosteal proliferation in the radial diaphysis.

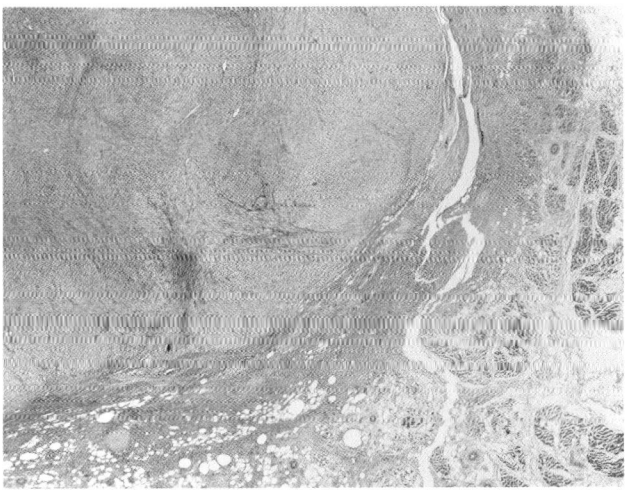

(A)

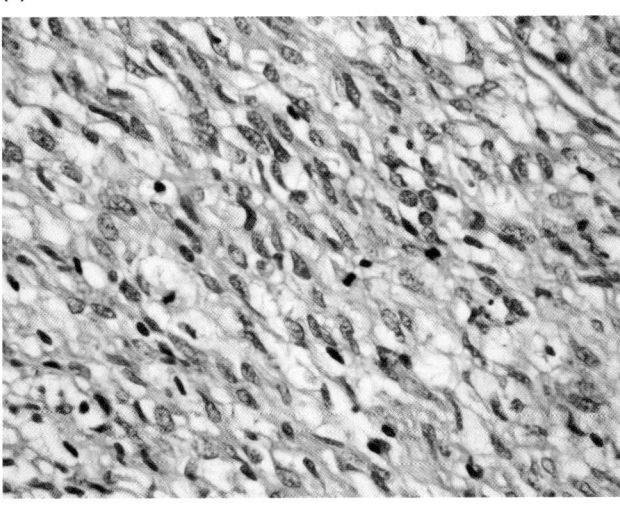

(B)

(C)

Figure 104.4 Photomicrograph of tibial plateau leveling osteotomy–associated sarcoma of the proximal tibia. **A**, Well-demarcated lobule composed of neoplastic spindle-shaped cells (left) with adipose tissue and skeletal muscle (right) (2×; hematoxylin and eosin [H&E] stain). **B**, Neoplastic spindle cells are arranged in streams and intersecting bundles (herringbone pattern) (20×; H&E stain). **C**, A moderate number of mitotic figures are present (60×; H&E stain).

Outcome

Similar to spontaneous osteosarcoma, the prognosis for fracture-associated sarcomas is poor. The median survival time with treatment is approximately 1 year.

Prevention

As logic would dictate, the only way to avoid this fracture complication is to avoid the fracture. It may be possible to decrease the probability of tumor development by avoiding the use of implants made of alloys that contain high levels of cobalt, chromium, and nickel or dissimilar metals or that are manufactured by casting rather than forging. Contact between these metals leads to electrolysis, thereby accelerating corrosion (Figure 104.5).

The degree of corrosion may be further increased in scratches and crevices caused by plate contouring, so minimizing iatrogenic damage to the plate may result in decrease this risk. Sarcomas have not been reported after fracture fixation with external skeletal fixators or titanium implants. Because of its rare occurrence, prevention of fracture-associated sarcoma is generally not considered in the decision-making process for fracture management.

Relevant literature

Several reports have documented the presence of osteosarcoma after fractures or fracture fixation in small animals (Harrison *et al.* 1976; Sinibaldi *et al.* 1976; Knecht and Priester 1978; Bennett *et al.* 1979; van Bree *et al.* 1980; Sinibaldi *et al.* 1982; Stevenson *et al.* 1982; Ward *et al.* 1990; Sonnenschein *et al.* 2012). More recently, this complication has been reported after total hip replacement (see Chapter 113) (Roe *et al.* 1996; Marcellin-Little *et al.* 1999). However, an actual causal relationship between fractures and the development of osteosarcoma has yet to be shown. A large case-controlled study found no significant positive association between metal materials and the development of soft tissue or bone tumors in dogs (Li *et al.* 1993).

The epidemiology of fracture-associated sarcomas shares common features with that of spontaneous bone tumors in that both occur most commonly in large to giant breed dogs of middle or older age, but they can affect any breed of dog or cat. The incidence of fracture-associated sarcomas in cats is low (Fry and Jukes 1995). The median time between fracture and fracture-associated sarcoma development is 5.5 years in dogs (Stevenson *et al.* 1982; Vasseur and Stevenson 1987) and 6 to 15 months in cats (Fry and Jukes 1995).

The location and distribution of appendicular osteosarcoma in large breed dogs seem to differ between spontaneously occurring and fracture-associated tumors. The vast majority (95.3%) of spontaneously occurring osteosarcomas arise in metaphyseal bone, but most (86.2%) tumors that develop after fractures involve the diaphysis (Ling *et al.* 1976). The femur is the most common site for fracture-associated sarcomas (~50%), but only 20% to 25% of spontaneously occurring osteosarcomas arise in the femur (Ling *et al.* 1976; Stevenson *et al.* 1982; Vasseur and Stevenson 1987). A study focusing on the correlation between osteosarcomas and previous trauma noted the absence of trauma in all cases of ulnar, tarsal, or metacarpal osteosarcoma, but 25% of femoral osteosarcomas included a history of previous trauma of the affected femur (Fry and Jukes 1995).

Fracture-associated sarcomas are found in sites of previous trauma, but the role of trauma in neoplastic development is unclear. Controversy remains regarding the respective roles of trauma and

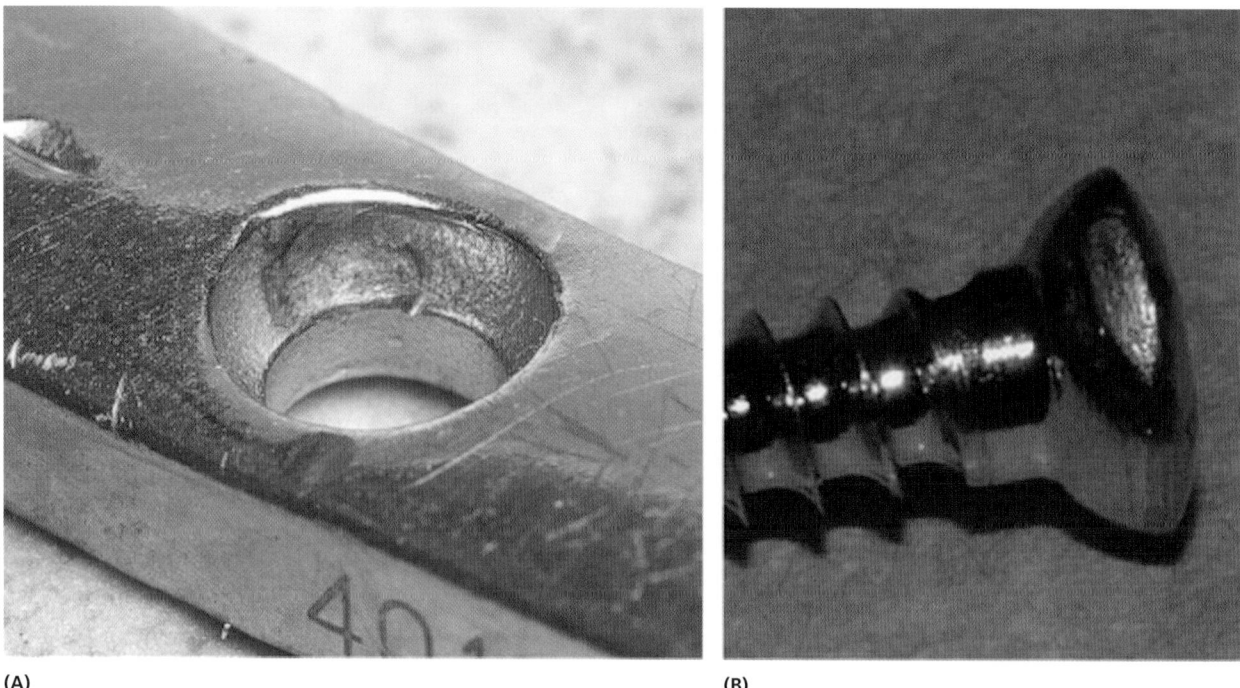

(A)   (B)

Figure 104.5 Corrosion damage in the screw hole of a tibial plateau leveling osteotomy plate at the site of contact between the screw head and plate (**A**). Corrosion damage on the corresponding screw head that was in tight contact with the corroded site in the hole of the plate (**B**).

implants in the pathogenesis of this complication. Increased bone turnover may play a role along with tissue damage from the initial trauma, altered cellular activity associated with healing of the fracture, infection, corrosion of the implants, and electrolysis between dissimilar metals (Harrison *et al.* 1976) (see Figure 104.5).

Some authors have proposed that tumor development most likely results from the fracture trauma and cellular changes during the healing process rather than the implant itself (Bennett *et al.* 1979). In support of this theory, the development of fracture-associated sarcomas has been documented with postoperative complications that include infection, delayed union, implant loosening, and draining tracts. Other factors implicated in the development of fracture-associated sarcomas include pathologic conditions associated with increased bone turnover, such as bone infarcts, irradiation, nutritional osteodystrophy, chronic subclinical bacterial proliferation, and use of cortical allografts (Sinibaldi *et al.* 1982; Vasseur and Stevenson 1987; Ward *et al.* 1990; Stevenson 1991).

Other reports discredit the predominant role of traumatic injuries, documenting the development of sarcomas after placement of surgical implants on the bone. For example, three reports of osteosarcoma have been reported after total hip arthroplasty in dogs; one was attributed to a chronically unstable femoral prosthesis (Roe *et al.* 1996), another to bone infarction (Marcellin-Little *et al.* 1999), and a third was thought to have no association with the surgery (Murphy *et al.* 1997). When carcinogenic effects of metallic particles and corrosion products from implants were tested in mice, cobalt, cadmium, nickel, and cobalt–chromium–molybdenum alloys produced malignant tumors (Heath and Freeman 1971). A small increase in malignancies in a rat population was associated with orthopedic implants containing alloys with a high content of cobalt, chromium, and nickel (Memoli *et al.* 1986). These experimental studies support the concept that the mere presence of implants, based on their composition, may trigger tumor

formation. Secondary changes, such as wear particles and corrosion, may further compound the predisposition to tumor formation after placement of implants. Indeed, wear products from metal-on-metal prostheses caused malignant tumors when injected in the muscle of rats (McKenna *et al.* 1966; Swanson *et al.* 1973). Several reports document sarcomas of the proximal tibia in dogs after TPLO (Boudrieau *et al.* 2005; Straw 2005; Harasen and Simko 2008; Atherton and Arthurs 2012; Selmic 2011; Selmic *et al.* 2013). The reported incidence of osteosarcoma after TPLO is 1 in 100 dogs over 12 years, but dogs undergoing bilateral procedures are 8.4 times more likely to develop a tumor (Sartor *et al.* 2013). Establishing a causative relationship between TPLO and sarcoma is complicated by the fact that osteosarcomas spontaneously develop in the proximal tibia. Nonetheless, corrosion of the stainless steel implants was proposed as a cause of increased osteolytic activity in adjacent bone and chronic synovitis, both potentially contributing to the neoplastic transformation. These concerns prompted the explantation of TPLO plates after clinical union of the osteotomy, as well as investigations of commercially available plates.

The plates in the early reports of TPLO associated sarcoma were made of cast 316L stainless steel and met the general requirements for chemical composition for a cast 316L alloy (Boudrieau *et al.* 2006; Charles and Ness 2006; Lackowski *et al.* 2007). Two studies reported that the surface irregularities and porosity of the cast plates led to corrosion products that could cause local soft tissue damage (Boudrieau *et al.* 2006; Charles and Ness 2006). A conflicting study found no evidence of chemical or topographic changes consistent with corrosion in explanted TPLO plates (Lackowski *et al.* 2007). Plates containing more ferrite had higher chromium and lower nickel contents and were more strongly magnetic compared with those composed of pure austenite (Boudrieau *et al.* 2006; Lackowski *et al.* 2007). Although cast plates were suspected to play a role in the development of TPLO-associated sarcoma, reports of sarcoma developing after TPLO have been persisted after introduction of wrought plates that meet higher material standards (Atherton and Arthurs 2012; Selmic *et al.* 2013).

Dogs diagnosed with fracture or implant-associated sarcoma are not usually treated because of their poor prognosis. Treatment options for these tumors are the same as for primary bone tumors and include amputation with or without chemotherapy, limb-sparing procedures, or primary stabilization of the fracture in the diseased bone. Ten of 29 dogs diagnosed with proximal tibial osteosarcoma at least 1 year after TPLO had a median survival time of 313 days after limb amputation and adjuvant chemotherapy (Selmic *et al.* 2013). Dogs with pathologic fractures secondary to osteosarcoma survived 379 and 434 days after amputation alone and 623 days with adjuvant carboplatin (Bhandal and Boston 2011). These pathologic fractures have also been stabilized by either external or internal fixation using a variety of implants to reduce pain, improve limb use, and extend median survival time to 161 days (Boston *et al.* 2011). Bone healing does occur but may be delayed, so internal stabilization may be a better option than external fixation.

References

Atherton, M.J., Arthurs, G. (2012) Osteosarcoma of the tibia 6 years after tibial plateau leveling osteotomy. *Journal of the American Animal Hospital Association* 48, 188-193.

Bennett, D., Campbell, J.R., Brown, P. (1979) Osteosarcoma associated with healed fractures. *Journal of Small Animal Practice* 20, 13-18.

Bhandal, J., Boston, S.E. (2011) Pathologic fracture in dogs with suspected or confirmed osteosarcoma. *Veterinary Surgery* 40 (4), 423-430.

Boston, S.E., Bacon, N.J., Culp, W.T., et al. (2011) Outcome after repair of a sarcoma-related pathologic fracture in dogs: a Veterinary Society of Surgical Oncology Retrospective Study. *Veterinary Surgery* 40 (4), 431-437.

Boudrieau, R.J., McCarthy, R.J., Sisson, Jr. R.D. (2005) Sarcoma of the proximal portion of the tibia in a dog 5.5 years after tibial plateau leveling osteotomy. *Journal of the American Veterinary Medical Association* 227 (10), 1613-1617.

Boudrieau, R.J., McCarthy, R.J., Specher, C.M., et al. (2006) Material properties of and tissue reaction to the Slocum TPLO plate. *American Journal of Veterinary Research* 67 (7), 1258-1265.

Charles, A.E., Ness, M.G. (2006) Crevice corrosion of implants recovered after tibial plateau leveling osteotomy in dogs. *Veterinary Surgery* 35, 438-444.

Chun, R., de Lorimier, L.P. (2003) Update on the biology and management of canine osteosarcoma. *Veterinary Clinics of North America: Small Animal Practice* 33, 491-516.

Fry, P.D., Jukes, H.F. (1995) Fracture associated sarcoma in the cat. *Journal of Small Animal Practice* 36, 124-126.

Harasen, G.L., Simko, E. (2008) Histiocytic sarcoma of the stifle in a dog with cranial cruciate ligament failure and TPLO treatment. *Veterinary and Comparative Orthopaedics and Traumatology* 21 (4), 375-377.

Harrison, J.W., McLain, D.L., Hohn, R.B., et al. (1976) Osteosarcoma associated with metallic implants. *Clinical Orthopedics* 116, 253-257.

Heath, J.C., Freeman, M.A. (1971) Carcinogenic properties of wear particles from prosthesis made in cobalt-chromium alloy. *Lancet* 1, 564-566.

Knecht, C.D., Priester, W.A. (1978) Osteosarcoma in dogs: a study of previous trauma, fracture and fracture fixation. *Journal of the American Animal Hospital Association* 14, 82-84.

Lackowski, W.M., Vasilyeva, Y.B., Crooks, R.M., et al. (2007) Microchemical and surface evaluation of canine tibial plateau leveling osteotomy plates. *American Journal of Veterinary Research* 44, 1040-1048.

Li, X.Q., Hom, D.L., Black, J., et al. (1993) Relationship between metallic implants and cancer: A case-control study in a canine population. *Veterinary and Comparative Orthopaedics and Traumatology* 6, 70-74.

Ling, G.V., Morgan, J.P., Pool, R.R. (1976) Primary bone tumors in the dog: a combined clinical, radiographic and histologic approach to early diagnosis. *Journal of the American Veterinary Medical Association* 165, 55-67.

Marcellin-Little, D.J., DeYoung, D.J., Thrall, D.E., et al. (1999) Osteosarcoma at the site of bone infarction associated with total hip arthroplasty in a dog. *Veterinary Surgery* 28, 54-60.

McKenna, R.J., Schwinn, C.P., Soong, K.Y. (1966) Sarcomata of the osteogenic series (osteosarcoma, fibrosarcoma, chondrosarcoma, periosteal osteogenic sarcoma, and sarcomata arising in abnormal bone). *Journal of Bone and Joint Surgery* 48 (Suppl. A), 1-26.

Memoli, V.A., Urban, R.M., Alroy, J., et al. (1986) Malignant neoplasms associated with orthopedic implant materials in rats. *Journal of Orthopaedic Research* 4, 346-355.

Murphy, S.T., Parker, R.B., Woodard, J.C. (1997) Osteosarcoma following total hip arthroplasty in a dog. *Journal of Small Animal Practice* 38, 263-267.

Roe, S.C., DeYoung, D.D., Weinstock, D., et al. (1996) Osteosarcoma eight years after total hip arthroplasty. *Veterinary Surgery* 25, 70-74.

Sartor, A., Selmic, L.E., Withrow, S.J., et al. (2103) Retrospective case series evaluating the incidence and risk factors affecting development of osteosarcoma following consecutive tibial plateau leveling osteotomies performed at a single institution between 1999-2009 [abstract 6]. In *The 40th Annual Conference of the Veterinary Orthopedic Society* Park City, UT.

Selmic, L. (2011) TPLOs and osteosarcoma. In *The Proceedings of the Veterinary Symposium of the American College of Veterinary Surgeons* Chicago, IL. pp. 277-279.

Selmic, L.E., Ryan, S.D., Boston, S., et al. (2013) Proximal tibial osteosarcoma following tibial plateau leveling osteotomy in 29 dogs: a Veterinary Society of Surgical Oncology Retrospective Case Series [abstract 38]. In *The 40th Annual Conference of the Veterinary Orthopedic Society* Park City, UT.

Sinibaldi, K., Rosen, H., Liu, S.K. (1976) Tumors associated with metallic implants in animals. *Clinical Orthopedics* 118, 257-266.

Sinibaldi, K.R., Pugh, J., Rosen, H., et al. (1982) Osteomyelitis and neoplasia associated with the use of the Jonas intramedullary splint in small animals. *Journal of the American Veterinary Medical Association* 181, 885-890.

Sonnenschein, B., Dickomeit, M.J., Ball, M.S. (2012) Late-onset fracture-associated sarcoma in a cat. *Veterinary Comparative Orthopaedics and Traumatology* 25 (5), 418-420.

Stevenson, S. (1991) Fracture-associated sarcomas. *Veterinary Clinics of North America: Small Animal Practice* 21, 859-872.

Stevenson, S., Hohn, R.B., Pohler, O.E.M., et al. (1982) Fracture-associated sarcoma in the dog. *Journal of the American Veterinary Medical Association* 180, 1189-1196.

Straw, M. (2005) What's your diagnosis? Fracture/implant-associated osteosarcoma following TPLO procedures. *Journal of Small Animal Practice* 46 (9), 457-459.

Swanson, S.A., Freeman, M.A.R., Heath, J.C. (1973) Laboratory tests on total joint replacement prosthesis. *Journal of Bone and Joint Surgery* 55 (Suppl. B), 759-773.

van Bree, H., Verschooten, F., Hoorens, J., et al. (1980) Internal fixation of a fractured humerus in a dog and late osteosarcoma development. *Veterinary Record* 107, 501-502.

Vasseur, P.B., Stevenson, S. (1987) Osteosarcoma at the site of a cortical bone allograft in a dog. *Veterinary Surgery* 16, 70-74.

Ward, J.J., Thornbury, D.D, Lemons, J.E., et al. (1990) Metal-induced sarcoma: a case report and literature review. *Clinical Orthopaedics and Related Research* 252, 299-306.

105 Thermal Pain

G. Elizabeth Pluhar

Department of Veterinary Clinical Sciences, College of Veterinary Medicine, University of Minnesota, St. Paul, MN, USA

Definition

Thermal pain is caused by the conduction of external cold temperatures to the bone through a bone plate with minimal soft tissue coverage. Thermal pain is also commonly called *thermal* or *cold conduction* and *temperature* or *cold sensitivity*. Thermal conduction has been anecdotally reported as a problem with the use of internal fixation with bone plates and is listed as an indication to remove the plate. However, no reference supports this phenomenon in the veterinary literature. Stainless steel plates are made of alloys or mixtures of different metals, which generally have lower thermal conductivity relative to pure elements. For example, the thermal conductivity of pure iron is 529 BTU-in/hr-ft²-°F and 300 series stainless steel used to make medical implants, an iron alloy, is 173 BTU-in/hr-ft²-°F (http://www.matweb.com/index.aspx).

Risk factors

- Fractures of the bones with little soft tissue coverage, such as the radius and tibia (Figure 105.1)
- Animals living in regions with extremely low temperatures with deep snow

Diagnosis

The most common history in affected dogs consists of lameness occurring during exposure to outdoor cold weather and resolving upon returning indoors. No test allows definitive diagnosis of thermal pain. However, it may be possible to reproduce clinical signs by soaking the limb with the plate in ice water to induce lameness. The lameness should resolve after the limb is dried and returns to room temperature.

Treatment

Implant removal usually alleviates pain and lameness if the underlying bone has healed sufficiently. This problem is rarely, if ever, severe enough to warrant plate removal before fracture healing.

Outcome

The prognosis is excellent with implant removal as long as measures are taken to prevent bone fracture in the early postoperative

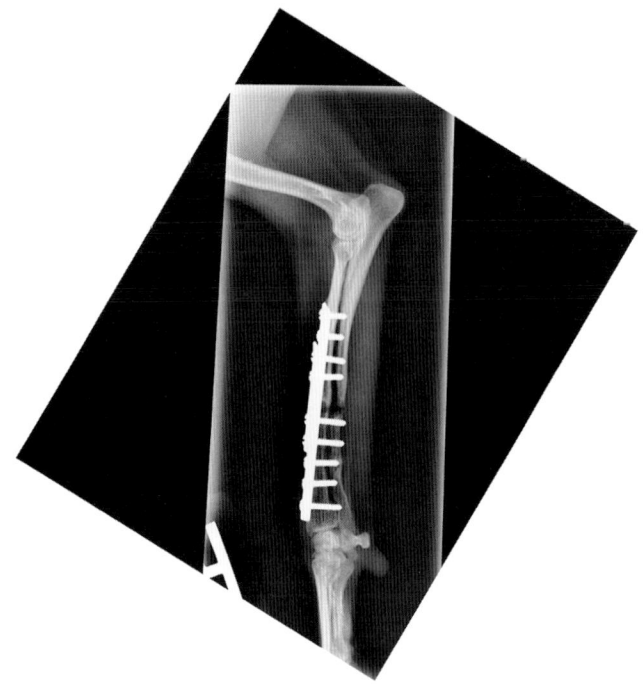

Figure 105.1 Fixation of a radial fracture with a large plate on a fractured radius. The plate has been applied over the anterior surface of the radius, an area with little soft tissue coverage.

phase. (See Chapter 97 for more information regarding implant removal.)

Prevention

Because this phenomenon rarely, if ever, occurs, it is difficult to address prevention. However, thermal pain would be avoided by using some other methods of fracture fixation such as external skeletal fixation, interlocking nailing, and so on. This should only be a consideration if the animal lives in an area that experiences extremely cold temperatures. Another consideration is to use titanium alloy implants because they have a lower thermal conductivity (46.5 BTU-in/hr-ft²-°F) than 316L stainless steel (http://www.matweb.com/index.aspx).

---

prove cold conduction even if cold associated lameness resolves after plate removal. It has been theorized that thermal conduction pain is caused by differential expansion of the plate and bone when exposed to temperature extremes (Brinker *et al.* 1975). No objective data have been published in the veterinary literature about thermal pain and plate removal.

Similar to the veterinary literature, few articles report temperature sensitivity in human patients after internal fixation of fractures with bone plates (Alpert and Seligson 1996). Among them, two patients underwent removal of eight craniofacial plates used to stabilize LeFort I osteotomies, procedures aimed at repositioning the maxilla (Schmidt *et al.* 1998). These patients complained of both cold sensitivity and pain, but the article did not discuss whether symptoms resolved after plate removal. Another report describes two patients with traumatic defects of the skull repaired with a titanium mesh (Figure 105.2). Both developed thermal sensitivity that improved after hair grew and covered the surgery site (Sahoo *et al.* 2010). This apparent protective effect of hair may explain the rare incidence of thermal pain in veterinary patients in which hair covers most of the body. In a recent review of plate removal after facial fractures in Finland, plates were removed in only 20% of patients (Thorén *et al.* 2010). The most common subjective reason for removal was cold sensitivity, thereby supporting the concept that cold climate may influence the need for plate removal.

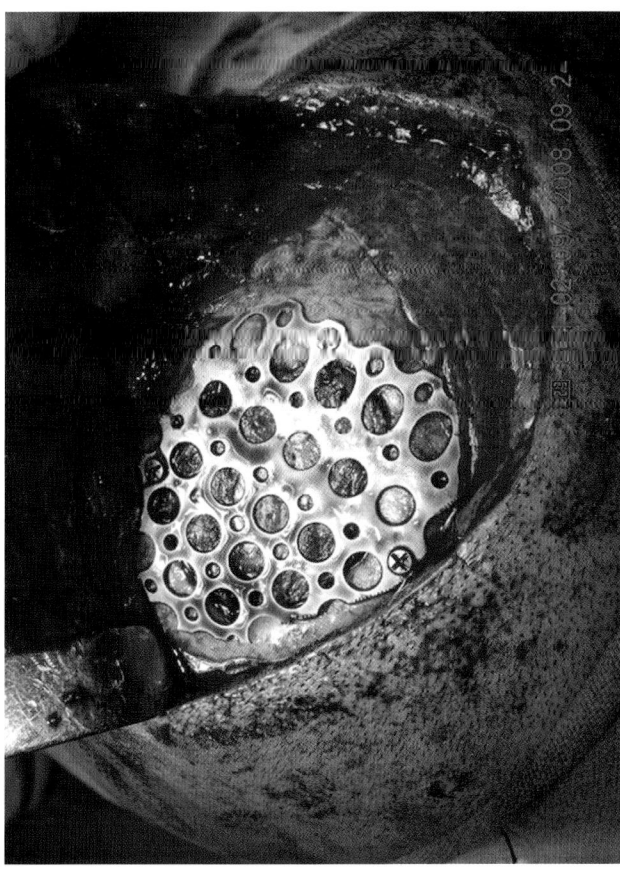

Figure 105.2 Fixation of a cranial defect with a titanium mesh in a human patient. The mesh caused cold sensitivity that resolved with hair growth. *Source:* Sahoo *et al.* (2010). Reproduced with permission from Lippincott, Wilkins and Williams.

Relevant literature

Thermal pain or cold conduction is an anecdotally reported complication of open reduction and internal fixation with bone plates. It is mentioned as a justification for plate removal in veterinary orthopedic textbooks (Brinker *et al.* 1998; Johnson *et al.* 2005; Piermattei *et al.* 2006). It may be impossible to definitively

References

Alpert, B., Seligson, D. (1996) Removal of asymptomatic bone plates used for orthognathic surgery and facial fractures. *Journal of Oral and Maxillofacial Surgery* 54, 618.

Brinker, W.O., Flo, G. L., Braden, T., et al. (1975) Removal of bone plates in small animals. *Journal of the American Animal Hospital Association* 11, 577-586.

Brinker, W.O., Olmstead, M.L., Sumner-Smith, G., et al. (1998) *Manual of Internal Fixation in Small Animals*, 2nd edn. Springer-Verlag, New York.

Johnson, A., Houlton, E.F., Vannini, R. (2005) *AO Principles of Fracture Management in the Dog and Cat*. AO Publishing, Davos Platz, Switzerland.

Piermattei, D., Flo G.L., DeCamp C.E. (2006) *Brinker, Piermattei, and Flo's Handbook of Small Animal Orthopedics and Fracture Repair*, 4th edn. Saunders/Elsevier, St. Louis.

Sahoo, N., Del Roy, I., Desai, A.J., et al. (2010) Comparative evaluation of autogenous calvarial bone graft and alloplastic materials for secondary reconstruction of cranial defects. *Journal of Craniofacial Surgery* 21, 79-82.

Schmidt, B.L., Perrott, D.H., Mahan, D., et al. (1998) The removal of plates and screws after Le Fort I osteotomy. *Journal of Oral and Maxillofacial Surgery* 56, 184-188.

Thorén, H., Snall, J., Kormi, E., et al. (2010) Symptomatic plate removal after treatment of facial fractures. *Journal of Craniomaxillofacial Surgery* 38 (7), 505-510.

106 Complications in External Skeletal Fixation

Gian Luca Rovesti

Clinica veterinaria M. E. Miller Via della Costituzione 10 Cavriago, Italy

Postoperative edema

Definition

Postoperative edema is fluid accumulation in the extravascular space of soft tissues. Postoperative edema may lead to more severe complications if the swelling is severe enough to force the skin to contact the fixator frame, causing skin necrosis and pain.

Risk factors

- Aggressive manipulation of tissues
- Soft tissue damage secondary to traumatic fractures
- Acute correction of severe angular deformities

Diagnosis

The diagnosis is established through clinical examination of the affected limb. Pitting edema is diagnosed by applying pressure to the swollen area and depressing the skin with a finger. If an indentation persists after the release of pressure, the edema is referred to as pitting edema and is caused by water retention (Figure 106.1).

Treatment

Some degree of edema should be expected in the immediate postoperative phase, especially after fracture repair. The intensity varies

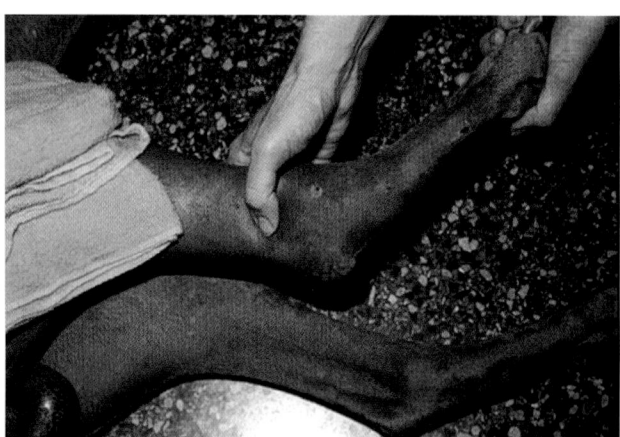

Figure 106.1 Clinical appearance of pitting edema in a dog with traumatic fractures. The limb was treated with twice-daily massages and cold compresses combined with application of compressive bandage. The swelling resolved in a few days after fracture fixation. *Source:* D. Griffon, Western University of Health Sciences, Pomona, CA, 2014. Reproduced with permission from D. Griffon.

greatly, and mild to moderate edema represents a minor complication. In most cases, it resolves in a few days and responds to postoperative care, including massage, limb elevation, hydrotherapy, and compressive bandages (Figure 106.2). If the edema does not resolve within a few days of surgery, underlying complications such as infection should be investigated.

Prevention

- When possible, fractures should be immediately immobilized via external coaptation to limit fracture-associated trauma in the preoperative phase.
- Delicate manipulation of soft tissues during surgery
- Create a stab incision (~1 cm) through the skin and tunnel to the bone that are large enough to accommodate external fixator pins and remain aligned directly with the axis of the pin.
- Placement of compression bandage such as a Robert Jones bandage immediately after external fixation of a closed fracture (see Figure 106.2B): foam sponges (e.g., recycled and sterilized scrub sponges) may be placed between the connecting bars and the skin to improve the distribution of pressure around the limb (see Figure 106.2A). The bandage should be changed 12 to 24 hours later and replaced as needed for a few days until the edema has resolved.
- A sterile wet bandage (see Figure 106.2C) should be applied on open fractures to avoid further soft tissue damage.
- Limit acute correction of angular deformities to avoid tension of the soft tissues.
- Leave at least 1 cm (width of a finger) between the skin and the inner part of the fixator to accommodate for postoperative swelling.

Pin and wire tract drainage

Definition

This is discharge from the pin or wire tract. Depending on the underlying cause, the discharge can be serous, mucous, purulent, or any combination of the above. Pin tract drainage represents the most frequent complication in external skeletal fixation (ESF).

Risk factors

- Poor postoperative care: lack of owner or patient compliance
- Superficial sepsis (see also Chapter 1)
- Osteomyelitis or deep sepsis (see later)
- Pin or wire breakage (see section on implant failure)

Complications in Small Animal Surgery, First Edition. Edited by Dominique Griffon and Annick Hamaide.
© 2016 John Wiley & Sons, Inc. Published 2016 by John Wiley & Sons, Inc.
Companion website: www.wiley.com/go/griffon/complications

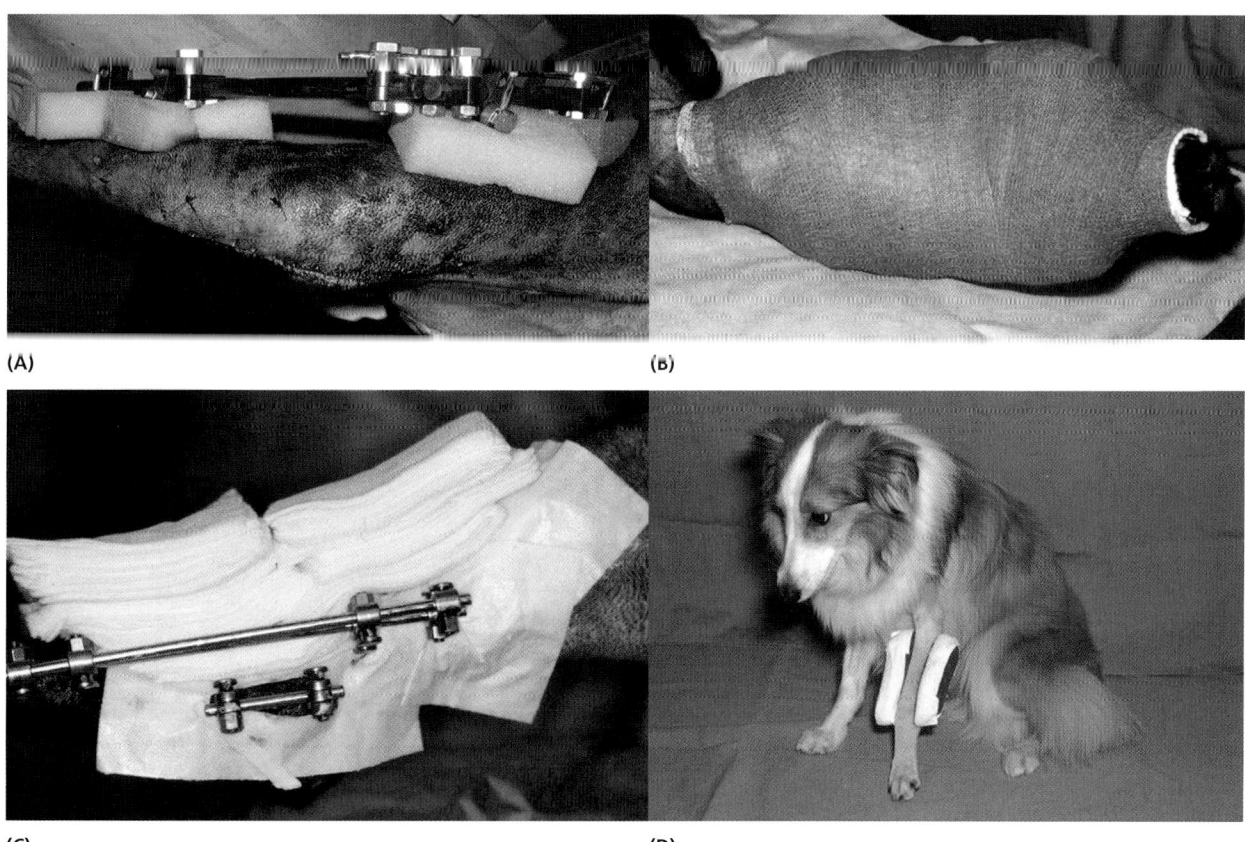

(A)   (в)

(C)   (D)

Figure 106.2 Bandages used in the postoperative management of external fixators. **A,** Recycled, sterilized scrub sponges may be placed between the connecting bars and the skin to provide compression over pin tracts in the immediate postoperative phase. **B,** The external fixator can then be incorporated in a soft padded compressive bandage changed every day until resolution of postoperative edema. **C,** Open wounds are managed with a wet-to-dry bandage until formation of a granulation bed. **D,** After postoperative edema has resolved, patients can be discharged from the hospital with a bandage that protects the apparatus but leaves the skin and pin tracts exposed to air. *Source:* D. Griffon, Western University of Health Sciences, Pomona, CA, 2014. Reproduced with permission from D. Griffon.

- Loosening of the pin (see section on implant failure)
- Periarticular areas are predisposed to this complication because of the friction between the pin and soft tissues during movement of the limb is greater than along the diaphysis, thereby increasing the risk of peri-implant tissue damage and secondary infection

Diagnosis

The initial diagnosis is based on observation of the amount and nature of the drainage around the pin. A clear and mild amount of drainage is expected for a few days after placement of an external fixator. Mucopurulent drainage surrounding one or several pins warrants further evaluation. The goal of this evaluation is to identify biomechanical or biologic factors causing the discharge. Radiographic evaluation of the limb is indicated to evaluate the stability of the implant (see section on implant failure) and look for evidence of infection (see osteomyelitis). In the absence of osteomyelitis and implant failure, excessive drainage may be attributed to poor postoperative care or wound infection. The first signs of superficial infection usually consist of swelling, redness, and serous discharge. No severe pain is elicited upon palpation of the area.

Treatment

The treatment is based on identification of the underlying cause for the excessive drainage. In the absence of signs consistent with

implant loosening or osteomyelitis, the treatment will be similar to that of superficial wound infection. Increasing the quality and frequency of postoperative care (see section on prevention) is usually enough to control the problem. Antibiotherapy may be considered to avoid systemic distribution and deep sepsis, especially if pin removal is not an option. Usually, the removal of the involved pin as soon as possible during the treatment course resolves this complication.

Prevention

External fixation requires a high level of owner's compliance because daily postoperative care is required until removal of the fixator. Strategies to prevent pin tract drainage and superficial infection after the animal has been discharged from the hospital include:
- Strong communication with the owners before and after surgery to ensure compliance.
- Daily cleaning of the skin and pin interface with an antiseptic along with application of antiseptic ointment.
- Placement of a bandage around the connecting bars and clamps, leaving the skin exposed to air (see Figure 106.2D). A plastic bag or a sock may be placed around the limb before exposure to outdoors on rainy days. If the bag is non-breathable, it should be removed once the dog comes back to the house environment. The bandage may be changed once weekly or as needed to stay clean and dry.

Clear communication of discharge instructions is a prerequisite to good postoperative care of the fixator. The surgical team should take the time to discuss home instructions individually with the owners before releasing the dog. Written discharge instructions should be provided for future reference along with detailed instances when the owner should contact the clinic. It is also good practice to call the owners a few days after releasing the patient to obtain a progress report and answer any questions they may have. Incorrect communication with the owner may shorten the life span of the fixator because sepsis along the pins or wires shortens their holding capacity, thus posing a significant problem if the scheduled treatment is not completed. The capability of the owner to manage the postoperative care required should therefore be evaluated before surgery and becomes a factor in the selection of fracture repair technique.

Postoperative care is slightly more complex in cases undergoing progressive correction. This approach is typically selected for progressive corrections of angular deformities. It may also be used to create compression between fracture segments by modifying the spatial conformation of the frame. In these cases, specific instructions along with a precise scheme of the procedure should be provided to the owner, and frequent rechecks should be scheduled to monitor the progression of the correction. Inadvertent displacement of a fracture in the direction opposite to that intended to provide interfragmentary compression led to the discovery of distraction osteogenesis by Ilizarov. However, mismanagement of external fixators generally leads to unfavorable outcome in terms of bone healing and is best prevented via clear communication and demonstration of postoperative care before discharge.

Osteomyelitis and deep sepsis

Definition
This is an infection that involves deep tissues and bone. It can spread in surrounding tissues. Osteomyelitis is covered in Chapter 5. This section focuses on aspects that are specific to external fixation.

Risk factors
Deep sepsis usually develops as a complication of superficial wound infection and pin tract drainage. The duration of signs therefore tends to be more prolonged (weeks) than in dogs with superficial wound infections. Superficial sepsis tends to prompt dogs to lick the surgical site, thus exacerbating the contamination. Infection spreads through superficial tissues and eventually spread to deeper structures, including bone.

Diagnosis
Compared with superficial wound infection, deep sepsis tends to induce more diffuse and severe swelling and redness. Lameness and pain on palpation of the surgical site are noticed on orthopedic examination. The discharge present around pins is mucopurulent and sticky (Figure 106.3). The patient can be depressed, and a leukocytosis may be found on a cell blood count. Radiographic signs of osteomyelitis (see section on osteomyelitis) may be noted.

Treatment
The treatment includes systemic antibiotics, local antiseptic lavages, and cool compresses to reduce edema. Loose pins are removed. Revision of the fixator may be required if the apparatus does not provide enough stability and fracture healing is not complete. In

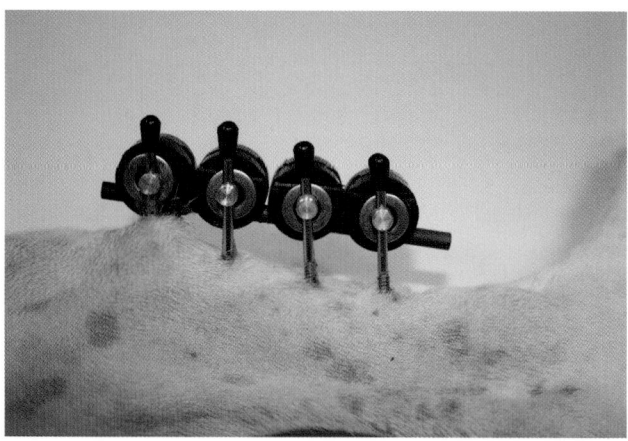

Figure 106.3 Clinical appearance of a pin with a deep infection. Swelling and redness are evident, and a sticky exudate is present around the pin.

these cases, new pins or wires are added in different locations, away from the infected pins. When infection occurs in the late repair phase, with callus bridging the fracture gap, infected pins may not need to be replaced. A splint should be placed to allow gradual loading of the limb.

Prevention
- Aggressively treat any sign of swelling and redness.
- Instruct correctly the owner about the postoperative management.
- Keep the dog in a clean environment.
- Avoid interference (e.g., licking) of other dogs living in the same house as the dog with the external fixator.
- Protect the fixator with a sleeve of fabric to avoid external contamination.

Implant failure

Definition
General principles of implant failure are presented in Chapter 94. The most common types of external fixator failures involve loosening or breakage of pins or wires. When a pin or wire loosens or breaks, its instability can cause discharge (Figure 106.4). Left untreated, this loss of fixation may lead to catastrophic failure of the apparatus, bone healing complications, or both.

Risk factors
- Weakness of the fixator frame (Figure 106.5): configuration of the frame or pins and wires number and distribution. The configuration of the external fixator should take into consideration the orientation of forces acting on the fracture. The number and size of pins and wires placed per segment should be selected based on the support required, including the load-sharing capability of the bone, the dimensions of each segment, and the weight of the patient.
- Transfixation of large muscle groups
- Placement of pins in a periarticular area
- Insufficient length of the fixator frame, causing a disadvantageous lever arm and a stress riser point at the level of the most distal or proximal pin or wire
- Implant design: Smooth pins are prone to loosening.

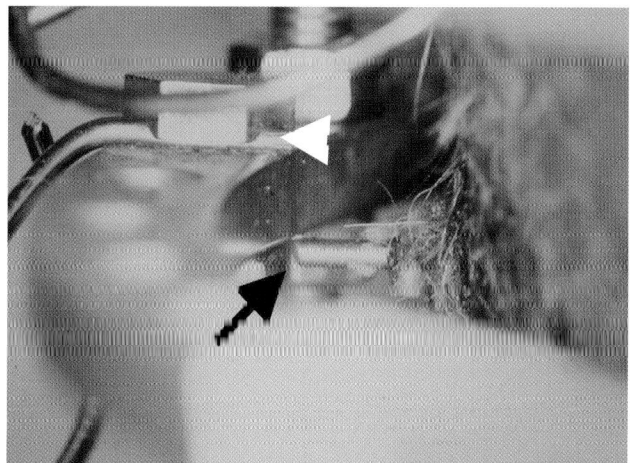

Figure 106.4 Clinical appearance of a broken wire (black arrow). Note the gap between the wire and the clamp (white arrowhead) to which the wire was connected. The discharge present at the pin and skin interface is a sign of instability.

- Technique used to insert pins, such as high-speed drilling (see section on prevention)
- Hyperactive patient

Diagnosis

Implant breakage can be easily noticed on physical examination (see Figure 106.4). However, when a pin or wire breaks close to or inside the bone cortex, surrounding soft tissues do not allow direct visualization and complicate the diagnosis of failure. To easily check the soundness of pins and wires, pull with the index finger on the pin or wire while stabilizing the frame with the hand. If the implant is intact, the dog should not resent the maneuver. If the pin or wire is broken, instability can usually be appreciated, and a painful reaction is typically induced. Radiographic evaluation is indicated to confirm a clinical suspicion of breakage. Oblique views may be needed to visualize the loss of continuity of the wire or pin. Pin or wire breakage is usually accompanied by periosteal reaction.

Treatment

Removal of the broken implant is required in all cases. Leaving a loose implant in place causes discomfort and increases the risk of infection.

Implant failure in the late stages of fracture healing may be a sign of increased activity. If bone healing has progressed to a bridging callus, loose pins may not need to be replaced.

Any sign of early pin or wire breakage should be regarded as a sign of overall frame weakness and treated consequently. Replacement of the pin or wire is indicated if needed to maintain the stability of the implant, considering the stage of healing of the fracture. In addition, the surgeon should consider revising the apparatus to increase the overall stiffness of the fixation. The first step consists in a critical review of the apparatus and correction of technical mistakes.

In the absence of technical errors, external fixation now offers a great deal of versatility in terms of strategies to adjust the stiffness of a frame:
- Increasing the number of pins or wires per segment, within existing plane(s) of fixation: A minimum of two pins should be placed in each segment, and little benefit is obtained by exceeding three points of fixation per segment. With hybrid or circular fixators, dropped wires may be added to rings.
- Changing the structure of the frame: Adding a plane of fixation significantly increases the stiffness of the frame and the ability to counteract bending forces in the plane of fixation. For example, adding half pins connected to a bar modifies a type I fixator into a type Ib or a type II fixator into a type III, the stiffest configuration available in linear fixators.
- Increasing the diameter of connecting bars: The connecting bar tends to be the weakest link in an external fixator, especially in type I configurations. Several systems of external fixation offer the possibility of adjusting the diameter of connecting bars without changing pins because clamps allow placement of overlapping ranges of pin and bar diameters.
- Changing the composition of connecting bars: The traditional Kirschner-Ehmer apparatus relied on stainless steel bars, which are weaker than the bars made of more recently developed materials. Among these, 6.3-mm-diameter titanium bars have a greater resistance to bending forces than carbon bars of similar size, and 9.5-mm-diameter carbon bars are more resistant than aluminium rods of similar size.

Prevention

- Apply proper principles of external fixation in terms of selection and placement of fixators.
- Use a fixator of correct size, structure, and length based on consideration of biologic and biomechanical factors affecting the fracture.
- Use pins and wire of correct size for the patient's weight and bone diameter.
- Use positive threaded pins or negative threaded pins with blended transition between the thread and the shaft of the pin rather than smooth pins. A sharp transition between the thread and the shaft of the pin is a stress riser area in both positive and negative threaded pins, and this shape should be avoided. Smooth pins should never be placed perpendicular to the bone and even when angled do not reach the same holding power as threaded pins.

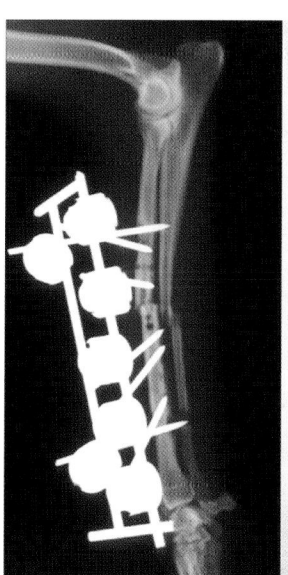
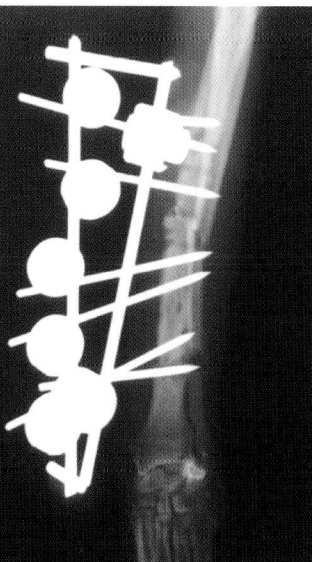

Figure 106.5 Radiographs of a linear external fixator illustrating several elements of weakness: the fixator frame was not well distributed along the bone segment; the use of smooth pins reduced the bone holding power; fracture segments were not fully in contact, thereby reducing the load sharing with the bone; multiple attempts at pin insertion predisposed the bone to secondary fractures and reduced the holding power of adjacent pins.

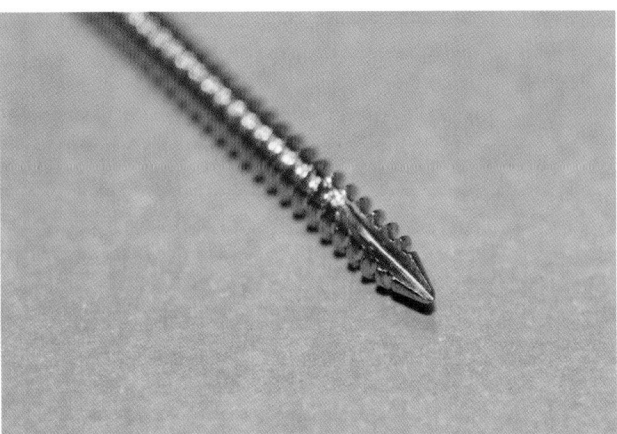

Figure 106.6 Self-tapping threaded pin. A self-tapping tip and interference of the thread are the most important parameters influencing radial holding power.

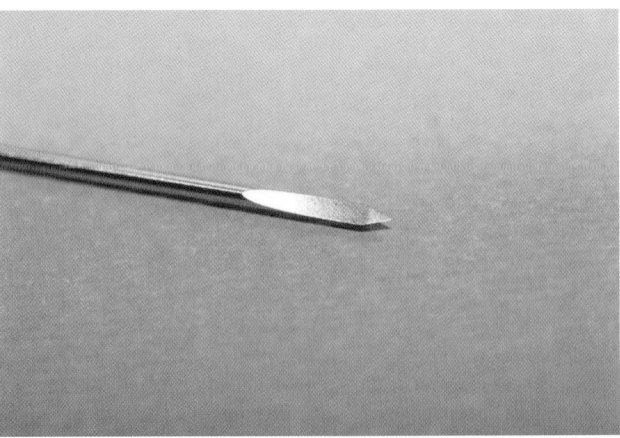

Figure 106.7 Half-tip Kirschner wire. This tip facilitates the penetration of the wire through hard cortical bone, reducing the likelihood of thermal bone necrosis and subsequent wire instability.

- Insertion technique: predrilling a hole before slow insertion of threaded pins (Figure 106.6).
- Use half-tip Kirschner wires in cortical bone to facilitate penetration and avoid thermal necrosis (Figure 106.7).
- Use hybrid or circular fixation to manage periarticular fractures. These fractures are characterized by a short bone segment, thereby reducing the lever arm of the fixator. In addition, the available bone stock and adjacent joint limit the number of points of fixation in the segment. Transarticular fixators have been used to manage these cases but require prolonged postoperative immobilization of the joint, thereby compromising articular cartilage. Hybrid or circular fixation circumvents this limitation through placement of fine wires connected to a ring in the short bone segment.

- Restrict postoperative exercise to leash walks until radiographic evidence of callus formation.

Iatrogenic and iterative bone fractures

Definition

Bone fractures associated with the placement of external fixators may develop under two circumstances. The first type occurs during or shortly after placement of pins in the bone (Figure 106.8). Late occurrence of a fracture occurs around the time of removal of the fixator and may be located at the original fracture site or through a pin tract (Figure 106.9).

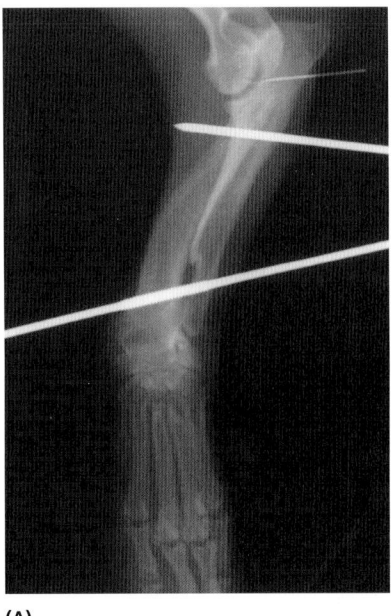

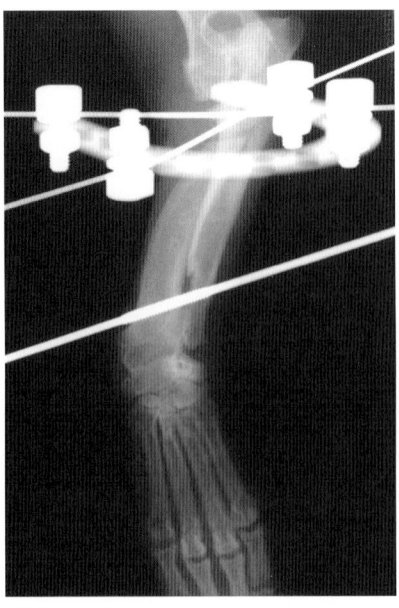

(A)   (B)

Figure 106.8 Iatrogenic fracture of the proximal radius during closed placement of a pin in the proximal radius during corrective osteotomy (**A**). The pin did not penetrate the center of the bone and instead compromised the cranial cortex of the bone, leading to an intraoperative fracture. A circular ring was consequently placed proximal to the fracture (**B**). *Source:* D. Griffon, Western University of Health Sciences, Pomona, CA, 2014. Reproduced with permission from D. Griffon.

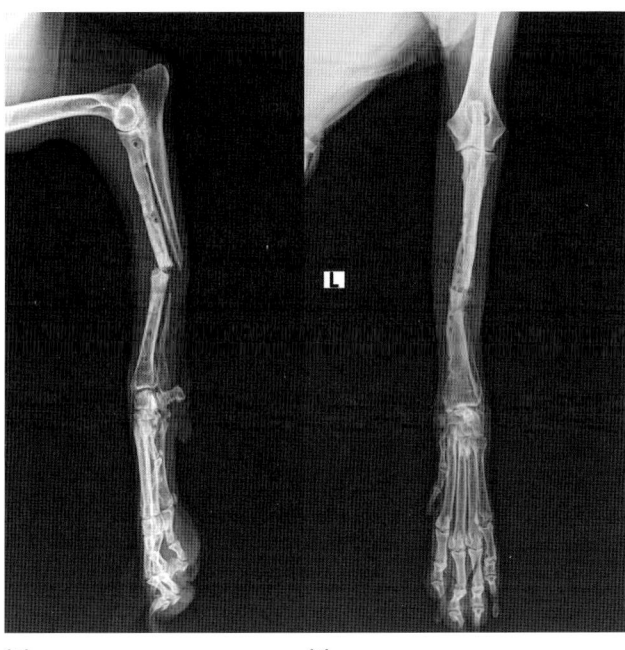

(A)   **(B)**

Figure 106.9 Lateral (**A**) and sagittal (**B**) projections of a secondary fracture 10 days after fixator removal. The original fracture healed, and the secondary fracture is located at the level of the proximal pin closest to the original fracture.

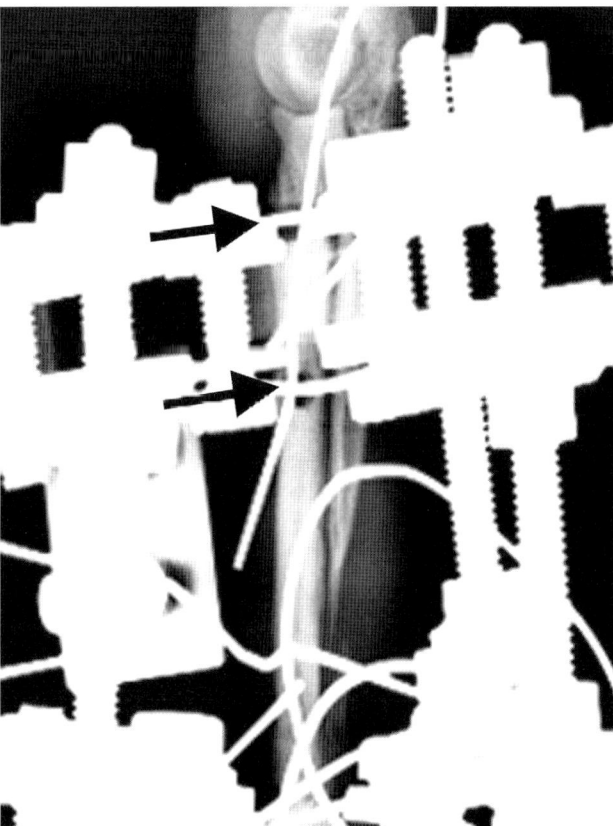

Figure 106.10 Radiographic appearance of bone erosion around two wires (black arrows). This situation is potentially dangerous, increasing the risk of instability, discharge, infection, and secondary fracture.

Risk factors

- Excessive diameter of the pin relative to the bone: As a general guideline, pins should approximate 25% of the bone diameter. This factor is especially relevant when the bone (e.g., the radius) varies in dimension along its axis and the pin diameter is not adjusted accordingly (see Figure 106.8).
- Small bones such as metacarpal and metatarsal bones are predisposed to this complication along with radial fractures in toy breeds and cats.
- Incorrect placement of pins, failing to engage the medullary cavity of a long bone and compromising a cortex: This complication is more likely during closed placement of pins because of a lack of visualization (see Figure 106.8).
- Too short fixator, which causes a stress rising effect at the most proximal and most distal pin or wire.
- Incorrect evaluation or interpretation of fracture healing, leading to premature removal of the fixator.
- Excessive stiffness of the frame and stress shielding predispose to fractures after removal of the fixator (see Figure 106.9).
- Pin loosening and secondary osteolysis predispose the bone to fracture through the affected pin tract after removal of the fixator (Figure 106.10).

Diagnosis

Clinical signs are consistent with those of fractures. The diagnosis is confirmed via radiographs. Iatrogenic fractures occurring during or shortly after placement of the fixator usually involve one or several pin tracts (see Figure 106.8). Fractures caused by premature removal of the fixator tend to develop at the original fracture site. Alternatively, secondary fractures may occur through a pin tract, especially if pin loosening led to osteolysis (see Figures 106.9 and 106.10).

Treatment

Iatrogenic fractures require fixation. Depending on its location and configuration, the fracture may be treated by extending the previously existing frame (see Figure 106.8) or changing the overall structure of the fixator.

Prevention

The following factors contribute to the prevention of iatrogenic fractures during or shortly after placement of an external fixator:

- Use an external fixator in which connecting bars and clamps accommodate a range of pin diameters. This allows the surgeon to tailor pin selection to the local dimensions of the bone.
- The external fixator should span the entire length of the bone with threaded pins.
- Opt for circular fixation in areas with limited bone stock.
- Maintain visualization of the bone during pin placement. Placing a Hohmann retractor on each side of the bone facilitates closed placement of pin through the medullary canal (i.e., in the center) of the bone. Alternatively, a fluoroscopic-guided insertion may be helpful in critical areas, when dealing with small-sized bones.

Several strategies may be considered to avoid iterative fractures after removal of the external fixator:

- Avoid stress shielding via simple frames with adequate pin number and size. External fixators using carbon, titanium and aluminum connective bars are stronger and stiffer than those using stainless steel bars. Transitioning from traditional Kirschner-Ehmer fixation to newer systems has been associated with a simplification of frames.

- Staged destabilization or dynamization allows gradual biome-chanical loading of the bone and stimulate bone formation. These techniques are most effective if initiated around 6 weeks after fixation.
- A correct radiographic evaluation is mandatory to decide when the frame removal is appropriate. At least two orthogonal projections should be obtained. Oblique projections are indicated if interference with the frame affects visualization of the fracture site.
- Placement of a splint for 2 weeks followed by a gradual return to exercise allows gradual loading of the fracture after removal of the fixator.

Neurovascular damage

Definition
This is iatrogenic damage to a vessel or nerve of clinical significance. The damage may be acute (intraoperative) or delayed (caused by movements or adjustments of the fixator).

Risk factors
- Positioning of pins and wires too close to a high-risk area for neu-rovascular (NV) bundles.
- Intraoperative swelling secondary to the original trauma can preclude a clear appreciation of the anatomic relationships and landmarks.
- Bone transport or lengthening procedures that do not take cor-rectly into account the position of a NV bundle potentially inter-fering with pin or wire translation.

Diagnosis
- Pain progressively worsening
- Neurapraxia
- Pulsating arterial hemorrhage

Treatment
- When the problem ensues during bone transport, distraction should be stopped and the position of the offending pin or wire reevaluated.
- When the problem shows immediately after the surgery, the offending pin or wire should be identified and removed. If the painful area is not easily identified, the pins or wires can be care-fully hammered. Usually, a pin or wire placed in a safe area does not induce any response, but a pin placed too close to a nerve will induce acute pain upon manipulation.
- Treatment of arterial hemorrhage requires removal of the pin or wire.

Prevention
Neurovascular damage is most frequently caused by inadvertent intraoperative lesions during insertion of pins or wires insertion. For close insertion of pins and wires, safe corridors should be fol-lowed. As a general rule, NV bundles tend to shift away from the pin or wire during insertion through soft tissues. Instead, wrapping of tissues around the pin or wire should be avoided because this does not allow the NV bundle to shift away, damaging it.

A very specific case of NV damage is caused by the wire used for bone transport, usually with circular fixators. The wire connected to the transport ring cuts through soft tissues during the transport of the bone cylinder. Soft tissues heal immediately after the wire cut, so that the wound is always in a healing phase, until the transport

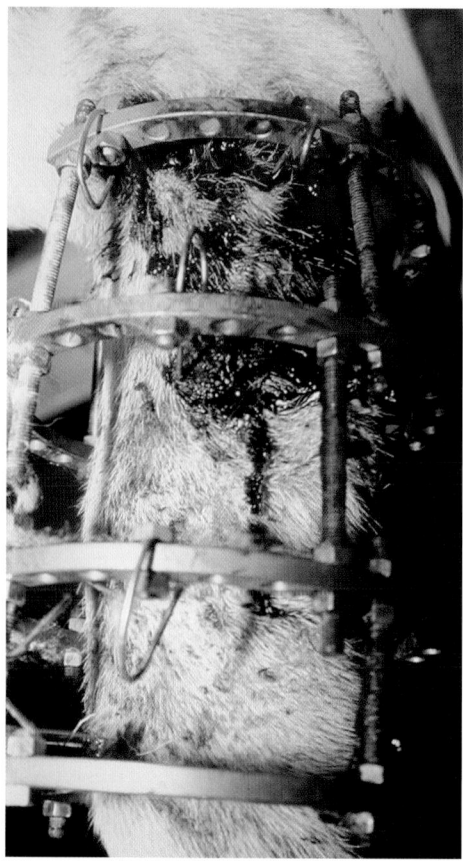

Figure 106.11 Hemorrhage 35 days after placement of a periarticular external fixator. Removal of the involved wire and placement of a compression bandage usually resolve this complication.

is performed. The path of the wire should be scheduled to avoid it to cross a NV bundle because it can cut it during its progression.

Sometimes a postoperative adjustment of the fixator frame is required, mostly to correct residual angular deformities. When the correction is performed acutely, caution should be used to avoid too a big change in the frame configuration because of the distortion of soft tissues that may cause. If this is the case, a damage to the NV bundle may ensue, causing neurapraxia or vascular disturbances.

A late vascular damage can occur days or weeks after the surgery. It is usually caused by a pin or wire inserted close to a vessel in a periarticular area. Because of the shifting of soft tissues during limb movement, the vessel wall is progressively eroded by the contact with the pin or wire and eventually ruptures, causing focal hemor-rhage (Figure 106.11).

Residual deformities

Definition
Residual deformities can be defined as abnormal limb alignment after fracture fixation or correction of an angular limb deformity. This complication is addressed in Chapter 100, and aspects specific to external fixation are discussed here.

Risk factors
- In transverse fractures of bones with a fairly cylindrical shape, reduction may be difficult to evaluate, increasing the risk of

torsion. Flexing the distal joint helps verify the alignment of the limb.
- In comminuted fractures, the alignment should be evaluated based on the alignment of adjacent joints.
- Closed fracture reduction: Interference with soft tissues and lack of visualization complicate the realignment of the limb.

Diagnosis
- Clinical examination. abnormal posture of the limb in an awake patient, with displacement of the distal end of the limb. Gait may be affected, depending of the severity of the residual deformity.
- Radiographic signs: The relative position of adjacent joints is abnormal. The severity of the deformity and the point of maximum deformation should be measured.

Treatment
Although residual deformities represent a challenging complication, ESF offers the potential for managing those complications without the need to revise the surgical procedure. In most cases, the correction is performed immediately after the evaluation of postoperative radiographs while the patient is still under anesthesia. Minor adjustments may be made subsequently under sedation. The most common residual deformities are in the plane perpendicular to the plane of fixation of type Ia or type II fixators. In general, correction should be considered when it has a significant clinical impact. Although 15 to 20 degrees of deformity has been anecdotally considered worthy of correction, the kind of deformity, its location, and the fact that is simple (on a single plane) or complex (on multiple planes) greatly influence its clinical impact. Varus and internal rotation are less tolerated than valgus and external rotation, prompting correction in the majority of cases.

Correction of deformities tends to be more difficult in the plane of the fixator. When the deformity is perpendicular to the plane of the fixator, bending the connecting bar may be technically less challenging than releasing the clamps and adjusting the angulation of the pins. Indeed, releasing the clamps to adjust the alignment of the bone carries the risk of losing the reduction of the bone segments. If the connecting bar is made of rigid material such as carbon bars, it can be temporarily replaced by a malleable bar (i.e., stainless steel), which is bent as required to realign the bone axis. After the realignment is achieved, the rigid bar is again connected to the pins, and the malleable bar is removed. Although this is not always possible, it is a useful technique to take advantage of both types of connecting bars. The sequence of changing should be carefully scheduled because some external fixator clamps cannot be connected to the pin if a bar is already connected, and this may require clamp prepositioning along the pins to allow for bar changing.

Correction of residual deformities is easier with circular and hybrid fixation: the connection between the rings, or between the ring and the linear component, is released, allowing correction. The connection is tightened again after alignment has been restored (Figure 106.12).

Prevention
- Position the patient on the surgical table so that it is possible to evaluate the limb in its full range of motion.
- Flex and extend the joints during the surgery to check if adjacent joints move on the correct plane.

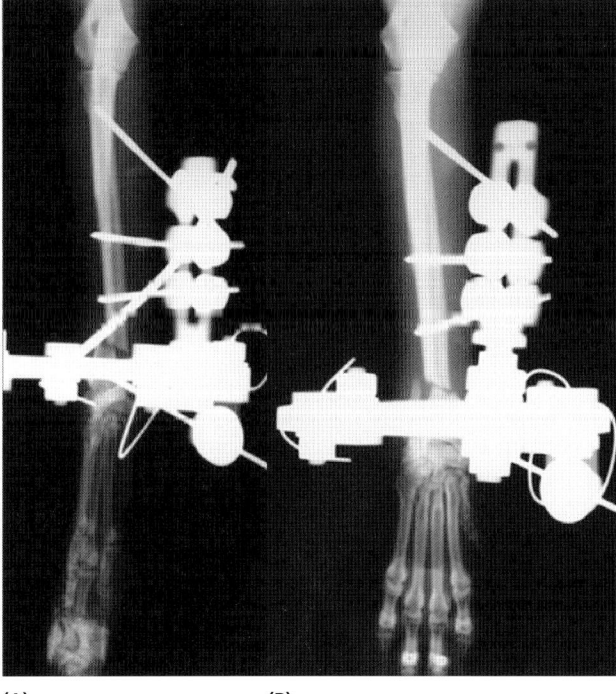

(A)   **(B)**

Figure 106.12 Immediate postoperative radiograph of a hybrid fixator. Residual torsional deformity of the forelimb is present (**A**). The clamp connecting the linear bar to the circular ring was released and moved to a different location on the ring to correct the alignment of the bone (**B**).

- Draping the normal contralateral limb in the surgical field, if possible, offers a reference for aligning the affected limb. This strategy is especially relevant in chondrodystrophic breeds.
- Intraoperative fluoroscopy allows evaluation of fracture reduction.
- Perform a reduced approach to the fracture area to verify proper reduction if fluoroscopy is not available.

Relevant literature
The pin–bone interface is the least stable component of the external fixator (Keeley et al. 2008). For this reason, the purchase of pins and wires in the bone should be given careful consideration, especially if prolonged immobilization of the fracture is expected. Interference, defined as the difference between the major and minor diameter of the pin, is one of the main factors influencing the holding power, regardless of the thread's shape and pitch (Halsey et al. 1992). Ideally, pins should be inserted by hand or at low speed after predrilling (Aron and Dewey 1992). This is very important because pins inserted with a torque resistance less than 68 Ncm loosen in 69% of cases, but those inserted with a torque resistance higher than 68 Ncm loosen in only 9% of cases (Pettine et al. 1993). Self-perforating, self-tapping, trocar-tipped pins have become very popular because of the possibility of inserting them in a single procedure, thereby decreasing the duration of surgery. Although they do not require predrilling, their holding power in the bone is often affected by two factors. The first is the thermal necrosis induced as the trocar tip advances into the bone. The trocar tip is not suited for cutting the bone while it advances, and the high friction generates heat. The second source of loosening comes from the fact that

they perforate and tap the near cortex and then advance to contact the far cortex. The resistance met against the far cortex delays their progression and causes biomechanical stress of each cortex of the bone. Two complications may develop: the pin may be forced to rotate within the previously tapped near cortex, thus destroying the bone thread. As a consequence, only the far cortex will be threaded after placement of the pin, decreasing its stability and increasing the risk of loosening. Alternatively, the progression caused by the thread in the near cortex while the pin contacts the far cortex generates pressure against the far cortex. This pressure may fracture the far cortex, especially if fracture lines are already present adjacent to this site. Postoperative radiographs should be carefully evaluated for the presence of fractures at the pin–bone interface. In human orthopedics, cylindrical pins with hydroxyapatite coating offer the best duration in terms of torque at removal. If the holding power of pins decreases too rapidly in the postoperative period, secondary instability causes drainage from the pin tract and potentially jeopardizes the overall stiffness of the frame. The diameter of pins should be carefully selected and should be about 25% of the bone diameter. Defects exceeding 20% of the bone diameter reduces the torsional strength of the bone by 34%, and a hole exceeding 50% of the bone diameter reduces it by 62%, thus predisposing to secondary fractures (Giotakis and Narayan 2007).

Similarly, the selection of Kirschner wires influences the stability of circular and hybrid fixators. Trocar-tipped wires may be safely inserted in cancellous bone. Kirschner wires with lance or double-lance tips should be avoided because their perforation is slightly larger than the shaft diameter of the wire, rapidly affecting their holding capability. For hard cortical bone, half-tip Kirschner wires are preferred because they penetrate easily in cortical bone, avoiding the thermal necrosis that tends to occur with trocar-tipped wires. If thermal necrosis develops, the radial holding capability of the wire is lost, and instability ensues.

Pins and wires should be inserted following **safe corridors** (Marti and Miller 1994a, 1994b). When muscle bellies are transfixed, postoperative pain and potential neurovascular damages are more likely to occur. Small-sized Kirschner wires can be inserted through muscle bellies as long as tendons are not locked and muscles can move. This can be achieved by inserting Kirschner wires through extensor muscles while keeping the adjacent joints flexed and through flexor muscles keeping the adjacent joint extended (Ilizarov 1992).

Discharge from the pin or wire tract is the most common complication in ESF in both fracture treatment and angular deformity correction (Rovesti *et al.* 2007, 2009). This complication can usually be managed as long as irritation and sepsis remain superficial, but it becomes a more serious complication if deep infection and osteomyelitis develop. An aggressive treatment is required when redness, swelling, and pain on palpation are present around a pin or wire. Systemic antibiotics, local cleaning, and removal of the involved pin or wire are to be considered.

The type and frame of external fixator should be selected based on biomechanical consideration with regards to the fracture configuration and the ability to share loads and forces that need to be counteracted. In general, external fixators are especially effective at counteracting forces that are aligned with the plane of the pins (Fragomen and Rozbruch 2007). Specific frame designs, such as hybrid fixators, should be considered to manage fractures with limited bone stock, such as peri- and juxtaarticular fractures (Marcellin-Little 2002; Kirkby *et al.* 2008; Phelps *et al.* 2010).

External fixators distinguish themselves form other means of fracture fixation by their versatility (Aro and Chao 2008). Indeed,

they provide multiple strategies to adjust the stiffness of the apparatus by modifying different components such as size, composition and number of pins and connecting bars, distance between the bars and the bone, the structure of the frame, the size and thickness of the rings, and the strut constructs used for frame stabilization (Cross *et al.* 2001; Lewis *et al.* 2001; Fragomen and Rozbruch 2007; Socie *et al.* 2012).

The stiffness of the frame can therefore be set to match the specific requirements of callus development, thereby preventing **instability or stress protection**. Both situations can delay or hinder callus formation because of opposite mechanisms. Adjustment of fixators requires an accurate evaluation and good understanding of bone healing, mainly based on radiographic examination. The introduction of radiolucent materials for external fixation has greatly enhanced this capability, reducing the interference of the frame.

Residual angular or torsional deformities can result from incorrect appreciation of the axis of the limb or intraoperative difficulties manipulating the bone fragments. When deformities warrant correction in the postoperative period, external fixators allow adjustments under heavy sedation or general anesthesia. As a general rule, residual deformities are more difficult to correct with linear rather than circular fixators, especially in the plane of the pins. Hybrid or circular fixators are more favorable to postoperative adjustments, allowing correction of fracture reduction between the immediate postoperative phase to final outcome (Rovesti *et al.* 2007).

Secondary fractures usually result from technical errors in the structure or distribution of the frame or inappropriate pin selection and placement. Iterative fractures are usually caused by incorrect evaluation of healing progression or premature removal of the fixator. The apparatus may interfere with postoperative radiographic evaluation caused by the superimposition of the frame with the bone to be examined. This may hinder the evaluation of bone healing and should prompt the clinician to obtain oblique projections. This is particularly true for circular fixation, in which interference may occur 360 degrees around the limb. The recent introduction of radiolucent materials greatly addressed this problem, facilitating the evaluation of callus formation.

References

Aro, H.T., Chao, E.Y. (1993) Biomechanics and biology of fracture repair under external fixation. *Hand Clinics* 9 (4), 531-542.

Aron, D.N., Dewey, C.W. (1992) Application and postoperative management of external skeletal fixators. *Veterinary Clinics of North America Small Animal Practice* 22 (1), 69-97.

Cross, R.A., Lewis, D.D., Murphy, S.T., et al. (2001) Effects of ring diameter and wire tension on the axial biomechanics of four-ring circular external skeletal fixator constructs. *American Journal of Veterinary Research* 62, 1025-1030.

Fragomen, A.T., Rozbruch, S.R. (2007) The mechanics of external fixation. *Hospital for Special Surgery Journal* 3 (1), 13-29.

Giotakis, N., Narayan, B. (2007) Stability with unilateral external fixation in the tibia. *Strategies in Trauma and Limb Reconstruction* 2 (1), 13-20.

Halsey, D., Fleming, B., Pope, M.H., et al. (1992) External fixator pin design. *Clinical Orthopaedics and Related Research* 278, 305-312.

Keeley, B.J., Heidari, B., Mahony, N.J., et al. (2008) Biomechanical comparison of the pullout properties of external skeletal fixation pins in the tibiae of intact and ovariectomised ewes. *Veterinary and Comparative Orthopaedics and Traumatology* 21 (5), 418-426.

Kirkby, K.A., Lewis, D.D., Lafuente, M.P., et al. (2008) Management of humeral and femoral fractures in dogs and cats with linear-circular hybrid external skeletal fixators. *Journal of the American Animal Hospital Association* 44, 180-197.

Ilizarov, G.A. (1992) *Transosseous Osteosynthesis: Theoretical and Clinical Aspects of the Regeneration and Growth of Tissue.* Springer-Verlag, New York.

Lewis, D.D., Bronson, D.G., Cross, A.R., et al. (2001) Axial characteristics of circular external skeletal fixator single ring constructs. *Veterinary Surgery* 30, 386-394.

Marcellin-Little, D.J. (2002) External skeletal fixation. In Slatter, D. (ed.) *Textbook of Small Animal Surgery*, 3rd edn. WB Saunders, Philadelphia, pp. 1818-1834.

Marti, J.M., Miller, A. (1994a) Delimitation of safe corridors for the insertion of external fixator pins in the dog 1: hindlimb. *Journal of Small Animal Practice* 35, 16-23.

Marti, J.M., Miller A. (1994b) Delimitation of safe corridors for the insertion of external fixator pins in the dog 2: forelimb. *Journal of Small Animal Practice* 35, 78-85.

Pettine, K.A., Chao, E.Y., Kelly, P.J. (1993) Analysis of the external fixator pin-bone interface. *Clinical Orthopaedics and Related Research* 293, 18-27.

Phelps, H.A., Lewis, D.D., Aiken-Palmer, C., et al. (2010) Use of a linear-circular hybrid external fixator for stabilization of a juxta-physeal proximal radial fractures in a deer (Odocoileus virginianus). *Journal of Zoo and Wildlife Medicine* 41, 688-696.

Rovesti, G.L., Bosio, A., Marcellin-Little, D.J. (2007) Management of 49 antebrachial and crural fractures in dogs using circular external fixators. *Journal of Small Animal Practice* 48, 194-200.

Rovesti, G.L., Schwarz, G., Bogoni, P. (2009) Treatment of 30 angular limb deformities of the antebrachium and the crus in the dog using circular external fixators. *The Open Veterinary Science Journal* 3, 41-54.

Socic, M.J., Rovesti, G.L., Griffon, D.J., et al. (2012) Biomechanical comparison of strategies to adjust axial stiffness of a hybrid fixator. *Veterinary and Comparative Orthopaedics and Traumatology* 25, 224-230.

107 Complications Specific to Locking Plates

Randy Boudrieau

Cummings School of Veterinary Medicine at Tufts University, North Grafton, MA, USA

Application of locking plates requires an understanding not only of the technique of applying locking plate fixation but also of its philosophy. Furthermore, not all locked plating systems are created equal, and the nuances and differences of the various systems must also be understood, including the limitations of each. Locking plate systems currently available for use in small animals (and discussed in this chapter) are listed in Table 107.1. The primary rationale for applying locking plates is preservation of the biology (vascular supply) to the bone, not an improvement in the mechanics, although there are situations in which the latter also is obtained. The complications that ensue usually are a result of technical failures (surgeon error), improper application related to these tenets of locking plate fixation, and limitations of the different systems when applying them to specific situations in veterinary surgery. Readers are encouraged to read the section at the end of this chapter for an in-depth review of the literature relevant to this topic.

Implant failure

Definition

Implant failure is loosening or breakage of the implant occurring before fracture healing has reached a stage where the bone can resume its function and sustain physiological loads.

Risk factors

Factors leading to failure of locking plate fixation can be listed under three categories, technical failures, improper application related to the tenets of locking plate fixation, and risk factors inherent to specific systems.

Technical failures

Some complications are due to the orthogonal position (in most fixed-angle construct designs) of the screws, which is required to allow the locking mechanism:

- Insufficient screw purchase in the bone (Figure 107.1) when the plate is not centered over the bone or if the plate should rotate away from the axis of the bone during tightening of the first screw, known as the "helicopter effect" (Figure 107.2)
- Intraarticular placement of a screw (Figure 107.3) as a result of plate contouring when locking plates are placed in periarticular regions

Other complications result from compromised screw purchase in the plate:

- Deformation of the screw hole associated with plate contouring
- Misalignment of the screw with the locking mechanism in the plate hole during its insertion, resulting in a cross-threaded or poorly seated screw head at the locking interface, predisposing it to loosening

Table 107.1 Locking plate systems

Plate System	Acronym	Manufacturer	Advantages	Disadvantages
Advanced Locking Plate System	ALPS	Kyon Pharma, Inc. (Boston, MA)	Standard or locking fixation Absolute or relative stability Infection resistance Wide size range Cut to length Custom bending instrumentation In-plane plate bending	Short locking screw length Low plate stiffness (Ti) Manually aligned locking drill guide Poor screw-holding (screwdriver)
FIXIN		TraumaVet S.r.l (Rivolito, Italy)	Relative stability Locking screw mechanism (conical coupling system)	No absolute stability Limited size, length, and hole pattern Insert Screw size and thread Combination stainless steel support/Ti screws and inserts
Locking Compression Plate	LCP®	DePuy Synthes® Vet (West Chester, PA)	Standard or locking fixation Absolute or relative stability Specialty plate pre-contour Wide size range Custom bending instrumentation Screw holding (screwdriver)	Preservation of blood supply at bone/plate interface technique dependent
String of Pearls	SOP™	Orthomed (Vero Beach, FL)	Relative stability In-plane plate bending with torsion (6 degrees freedom)	No absolute stability High plate stiffness Screw locking mechanism No dedicated locking screw

Complications in Small Animal Surgery, First Edition. Edited by Dominique Griffon and Annick Hamaide.

© 2016 John Wiley & Sons, Inc. Published 2016 by John Wiley & Sons, Inc.

Companion website: www.wiley.com/go/griffon/complications

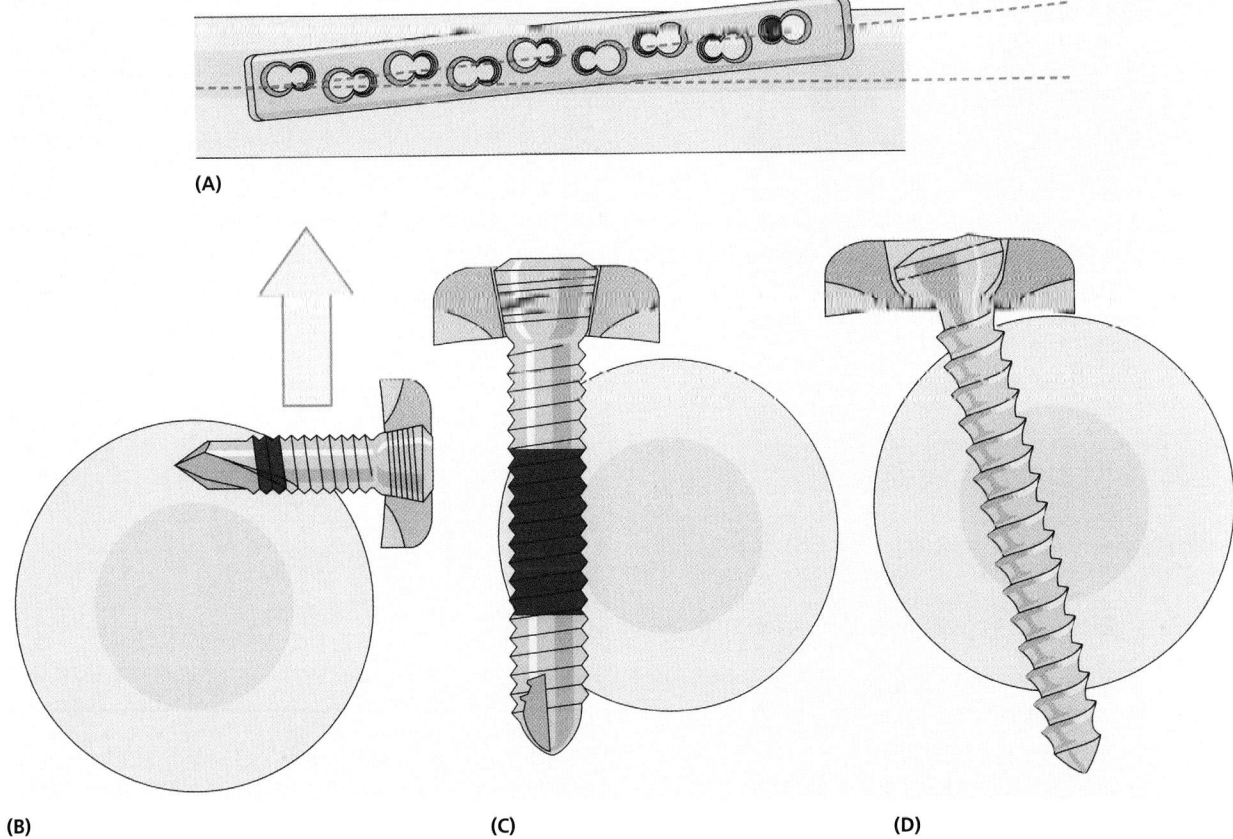

Figure 107.1 Inadequate placement of a locking screw in a long bone. Improper alignment of the plate with the bone axis will result in the screw hole not directly over the bone isthmus (**A**). Orthogonal insertion of locking screw places the screw eccentrically, compromising anchorage of a monocortical (**B**) or bicortical screw (**C**). Alternatively, a standard cortex screw may be angled under this circumstance and placed appropriately within the bone (**D**). *Source:* Wagner and Frigg, 2009. Reproduced with permission from Elsevier.

- Insufficient application of screw torque during insertion, which again predisposes to loosening
- Locking screws placed in the nonlocking portion of combination holes designed for standard screws

Improper application related to the tenets of locking plate fixation

Locking plates were primarily designed to provide noncontact with the underlying bone at the bone–plate interface, thereby preserving the blood supply. Additionally, monocortical screw fixation was the principle to also preserve the endosteal circulation. Better preservation of vascularity stimulates bone healing and reduces infection. There is some evidence to suggest a mechanical advantage under certain circumstances. Although locking plates may be biomechanically advantageous in areas with limited bone stock (periarticular and periprosthetic fractures) or compromised bone (osteoporotic), these systems are not designed for applications in high-strain environments. The following factors may therefore increase the risk of failure of a locking construct:
- Simple two-piece fractures
- Plates that do not span a long portion of bone
- A limited number of screws (three or fewer) placed in each bone segment
- Monocortical fixation of short bone segments
- Inherent limitations of minimally invasive plate osteosynthesis (MIPO): Limited visualization and manipulation of the bone and adjacent soft tissues complicate fracture reduction and accurate screw positioning and insertion, along with a potential for plate impingement on soft tissues. These factors may increase the biomechanical loads placed on the construct and ultimately affect its strength.
- Fractures subjected to overloading or high torsional loads (full weight bearing) (Figure 107.4)
- Thin cortices that affect the stability of monocortical screws (Figure 107.5)
- Delayed healing caused by compromised fracture biology (e.g., multiple plate fixation with plate–bone contact) (Figure 107.6)

Risk factors inherent to specific systems

Advanced Locking Plate System (ALPS; Kyon Pharma, Inc., Boston, MA)
- Monocortical fixation as sole fixation in cases when bicortical screw fixation is indicated
- Insufficient plate size with a titanium construct (low stiffness)

Locking Compression Plate (LCP; DePuy Synthes Vet, West Chester, PA)
- Combination of standard and locking screws in the same construct (see Figure 107.6) warrants careful consideration: The biologic principle of noncontact is compromised because standard screws are applied first in a well-contoured plate (ensuring bone plate contact and compromise of the vascularity directly under the plate).

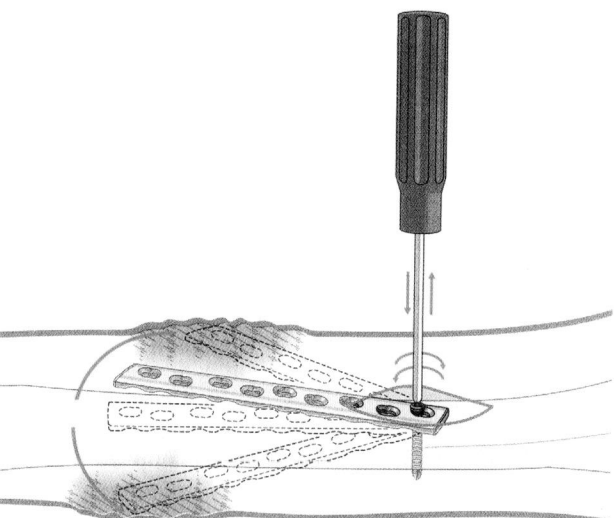

Figure 107.2 Rotation of a locking plate along the axis of the bone. After the first screw is engaged in the screw hole of the plate, the entire plate can rotate around this screw unless it is secured on the opposite end. *Source:* Wagner and Frigg, 2006. Copyright by AO Foundation, Switzerland.

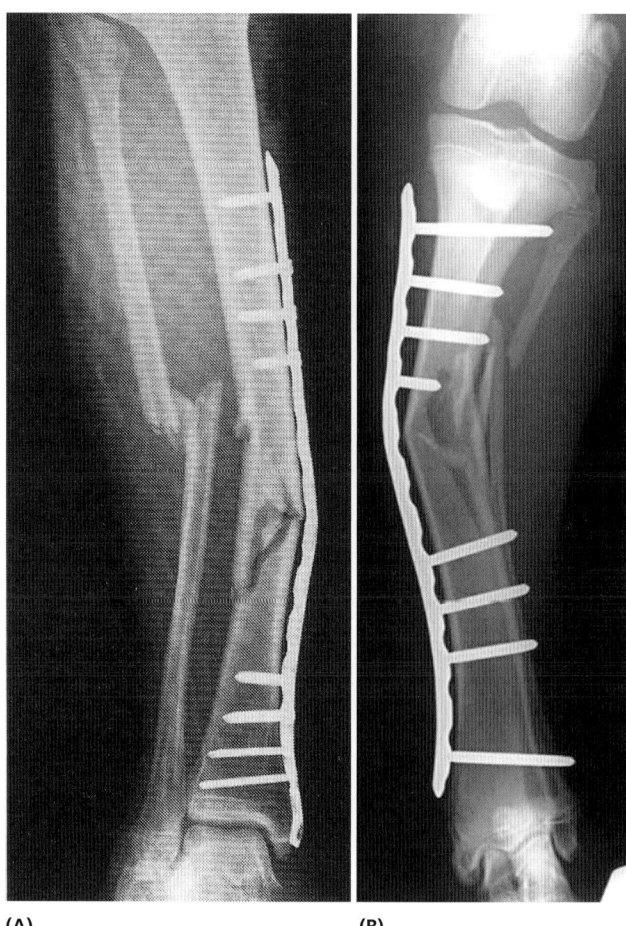

(A)   **(B)**

Figure 107.4 Single overload of an implant with plastic deformation of the plate. **A,** Radiograph of a tibial fracture in a human patient bearing full weight on the repair 1 day after surgery. *Source:* Wagner and Frigg, 2006. Copyright by AO Foundation, Switzerland. **B,** Radiograph of a tibial fracture in a 6-month-old male Bernese mountain dog 2 days after surgery. *Source:* Schwandt and Montavon, 2005.

Note that the identical mechanism of acute overload occurs in all long bones postoperatively in small animals (vs. the weight-bearing bones of the lower extremities in humans, which should be protected in the early postoperative period); therefore, the recommendations made for locking plates in humans needs to be adjusted appropriately when applied to animals.

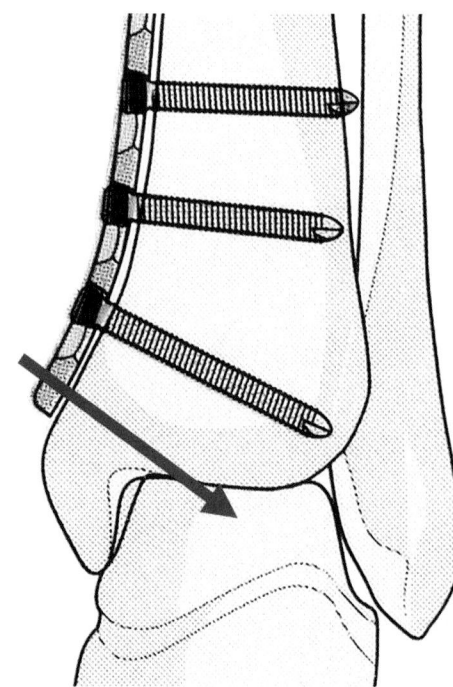

Figure 107.3 Locking plate placed on the distal tibia. All locked screws are orthogonal to the plate, which is contoured to the bone surface. The arrow illustrates the path of a screw placed in a distal and orthogonal position on the plate, resulting in intraarticular placement. Options to prevent this complication include (1) limiting the length of the screw to the bone stock in tibia or (2) angling a standard screw away from the joint (see Figure 107.1).

Fixin (TraumaVet S.r.l, Rivolito, Italy)
- Placement of a short plate to repair a simple fracture with a small gap is especially prone to failure because of the lower strength of this implant compared with other locking systems.
- Empty screw holes in the "support" (The terminology used for this implant include the concepts of "support" and "insert," the latter of which secures the screw in place. The system is termed a "plate" only when the support and inserts are combined. Lack of an "insert" creates a stress riser, especially if located over the fracture site.) (Figure 107.7)

String-of-Pearls (SOP; Orthomed, Vero Beach, FL)
- Constructs are more prone to screw breakage than other systems because standard screws (generally with smaller core diameters than comparable locking screws) are used in a plate that has comparatively high stiffness.

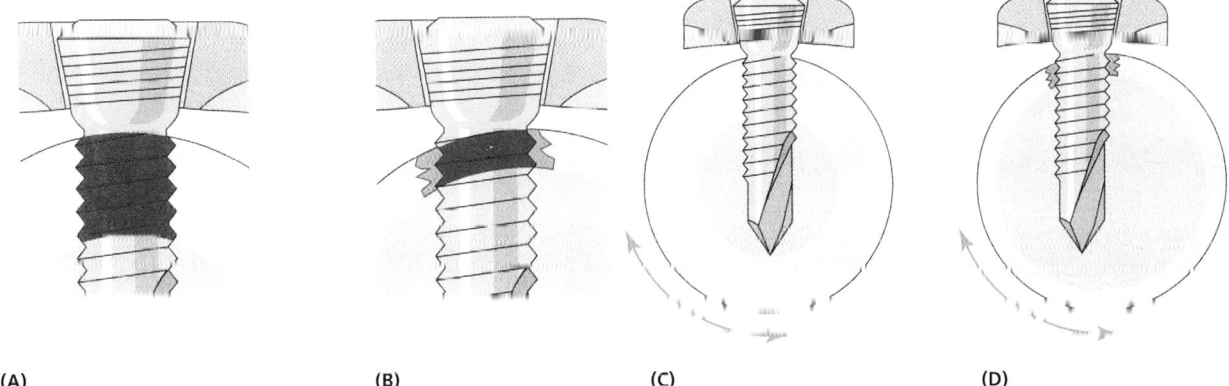

(A)   **(B)**   **(C)**   **(D)**

Figure 107.5 Influence of cortical thickness of the bone on the working length of monocortical screws. In normal bone, the working length may be sufficient (**A**); however, thinner cortices decrease the working length of a monocortical screw (**B**). With a long working length, the anchorage can sufficiently withstand applied torque loads (**C**); with a short working length, the same torque load is concentrated over a smaller area of anchorage, thereby prompting rotational displacement (**D**). *Source:* Wagner and Frigg, 2009. Reproduced with permission from Elsevier.

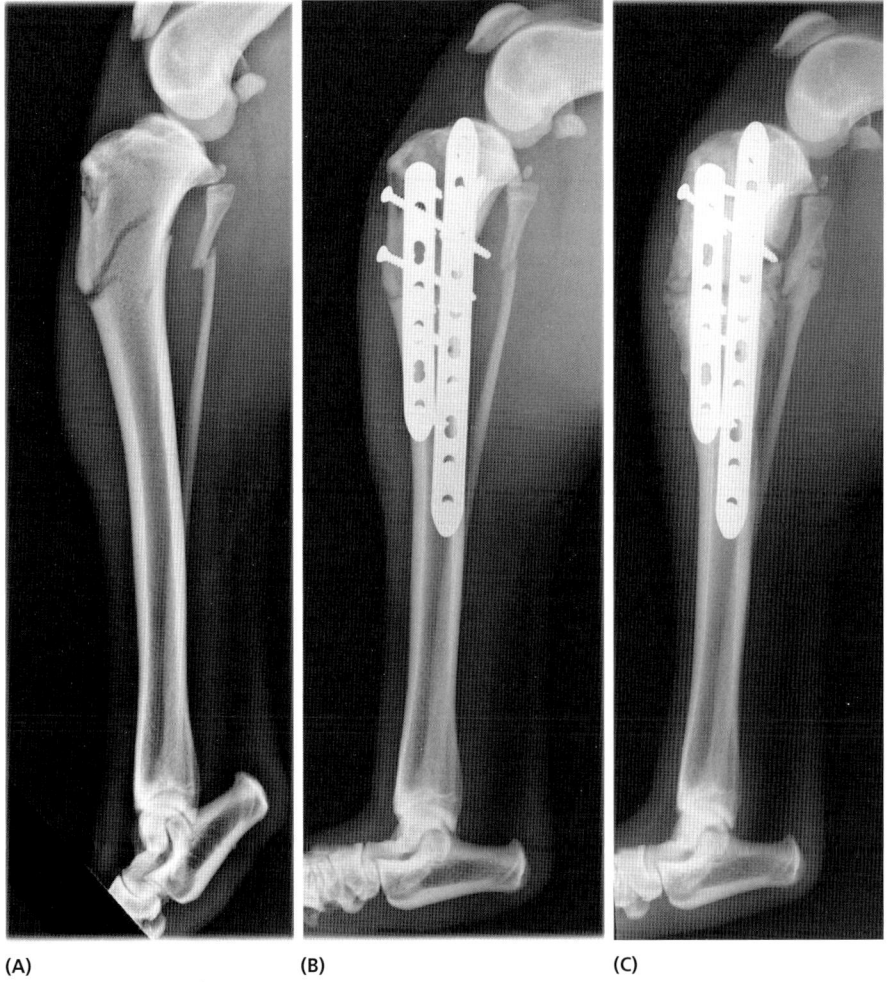

(A)   **(B)**   **(C)**

Figure 107.6 Delayed bone healing and infection after combined locking and standard plate fixation. Preoperative (**A**) and immediate (**B**) and 8-week (**C**) postoperative lateral radiographs of the tibia in a 1.5-year-old, MC, Bernese mountain dog. A, Incomplete fracture of the proximal tibial metaphysis. B, Craniocaudal interfragmentary compression was obtained with two lag screws; two medial plates (7- and 10-hole 3.5-mm Locking Compression Plate) were applied medially (total of two standard cortex and four locking 3.5-mm) screws were placed in the proximal bone fragment, and seven standard cortex 3.5-mm screws were placed in the distal bone fragment (one screw in each plate was eccentrically plated to achieve further dynamic compression across the fracture site). C, Despite the rigid fixation, delayed union and infection are diagnosed at 8 weeks. The two plates were contoured to the bone surface because combination fixation was used. The extent of tibia covered by the plates may have compromised the vascular supply, compounding the inherently limited soft tissue coverage in this region. Combined, these factors may have compromised the biologic environment of the fracture, affecting healing and resistance to infection.

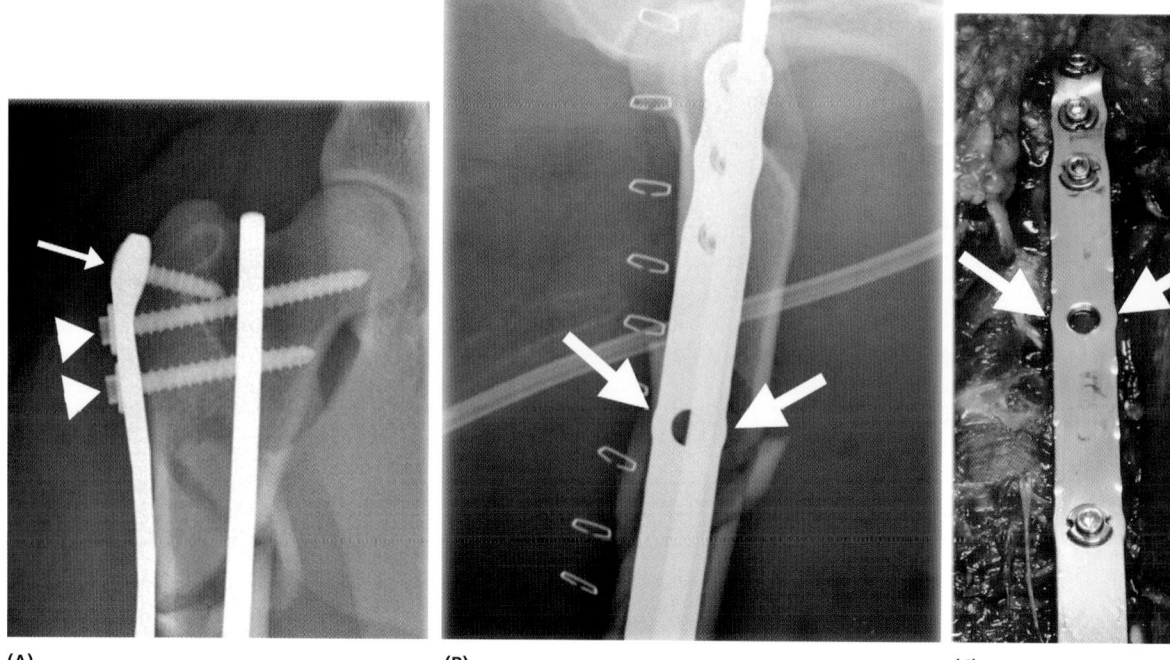

(A) **(B)** **(C)**

Figure 107.7 Inadequate screw fixation in a Fixin system. Immediate postoperative craniocaudal (**A**) and lateral (**B**) radiographs of the comminuted femoral fracture immobilized with a 3.5-mm Fixin plate (and intramedullary [IM] pin). A, The first proximal screw is seated appropriately (small arrow), but the second and third screws are insufficiently seated (arrowheads); notice the slight angulation of these latter because as they are not orthogonal to the plate surface. **B**, The insert of this plate hole has been removed, which will weaken the plate at this location (large arrows); the position directly over the comminution further compromises the plate strength (although this effect is somewhat mitigated by the presence of the IM pin). **C**, Intraoperative photograph showing the open screw hole without insert (large arrows), creating a potential stress riser at this location. The comparison between the seating of the proximal three screws can be appreciated because the first screw is appropriately seated with minimal protrusion of the screw head from the insert (small arrow) compared with inadequate seating of the other two screws, where some protrusion of the screw head above the insert (arrowheads).

Diagnosis

Factors predisposing locking plates to failure, such as inaccurate placement of a screw or misalignment of the plate over the bone, may be noticed during surgery by direct inspection. Insufficient bone purchase may go undiagnosed during screw placement because the feedback obtained by the surgeon during screw insertion reflects solely the interface between the screw and the plate.

Implant failure becomes clinically significant when fracture immobilization is compromised before healing, and clinical signs will be similar to those observed in other cases of implant failure (see Chapter 94). A definitive diagnosis of implant failure is made on orthogonal radiographic projections of the affected bone. The most common radiographic signs of locking plate failure include:

- Screw breakage, usually directly under the screw head (near the screw–plate interface) (Figures 107.8 and 107.9)
- Screw pullout, especially with monocortical screws in a fully loaded bone (Figure 107.10)
- Screw loosening or migration caused by a poorly seated or aligned screw (see Figure 107.7)
- Plastic deformation of the plate and loss of limb alignment caused by acute overload (see Figure 107.4)
- Breakage of the plate (fatigue failure) caused by low stiffness or strength (Figure 107.11)

Treatment

The management of locking implant failure follows the same general principles outlined in Chapter 94.

Outcome

Implant failure occurring after the bone has regained enough biomechanical function to sustain physiological loads carries an excellent prognosis. Most fractures warranting revision of a locking system carry a good prognosis for healing; however, any revision procedure can further compromise the tissues, adversely affecting healing and simultaneously potentiating infection.

Prevention

- Locking plates are especially relevant to biologic fracture management of comminuted fractures. Standard plate fixation, with accurate reduction, compression and rigid fixation (absolute stability) is recommended for simple (two-piece) diaphyseal fractures
- Locking plates must span a long segment of bone to provide effective bridging fixation. Recommendations have been proposed for the LCP; these include plate length greater than three times the length of the fracture segment, with a screw-to-hole ratio of less than 0.5, at least three or four screws per segment, and at least two or three holes open at the fracture or defect area (Figure 107.12)

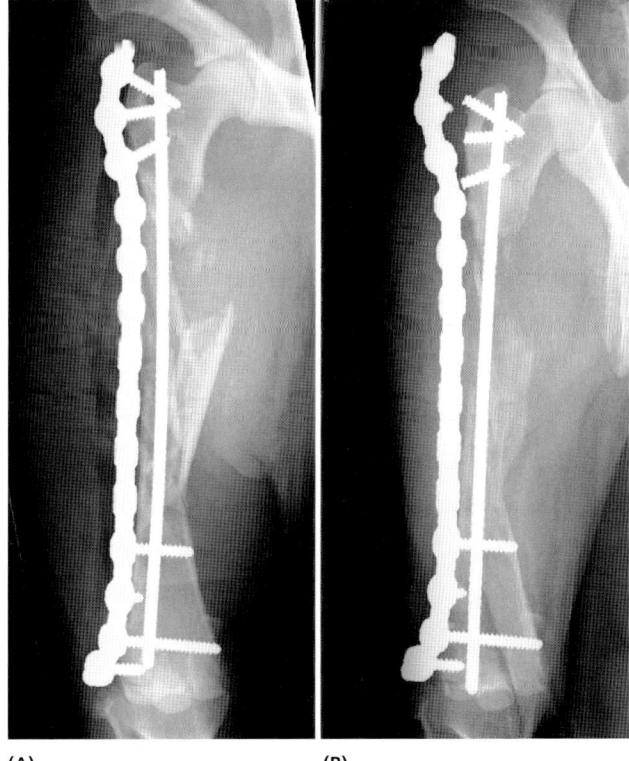

(A)   **(B)**

Figure 107.8 Breakage of screws in a String-of-Pearls (SOP) construct. Immediate (**A**) and 8-month (**B**) postoperative craniocaudal radiographs of the femur in a 5.8-year-old female mixed breed dog. A 14-hole, 3.5-mm SOP bridges the fracture along with an intramedullary (IM) pin (~40% of the medullary diameter) in a plate-rod configuration (**A**). Bridging is incomplete in the proximal third of the diaphysis, and the bridging further distally is not robust; the three proximal cortex screws have sheared just below their heads in the plate. This construct may not have had sufficient elasticity because of the combination of a very stiff plate and IM pin combination; a smaller diameter IM pin may be indicated in this situation with this plate. Fatigue failure of the screws is a result of nonhealing; however, the smaller screw diameter (compared with similarly sized plates) makes this mode of failure more common. *Source:* Reproduced with permission from T. Gemmill.

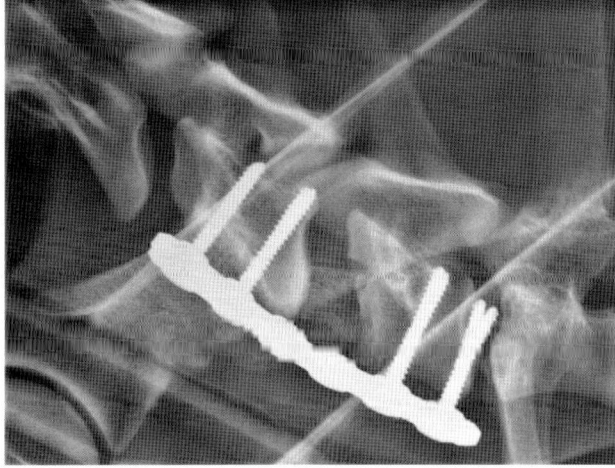

(A)

(B)

Figure 107.9 Implant failure after vertebral fracture repair with a String-of-Pearls (SOP) construct. Immediate (**A**) and 4-week (**B**) postoperative lateral radiographs of the lower cervical spine in a 1.5-year-old, MC, Great Dane dog. **A**, A distraction-stabilization has been performed with two ventral six-hole SOPs of C6 and C7; a cancellous bone block has been used at the C6 to C7 interspace (a cancellous graft also was placed ventrally between these plates). **B**, All four screws in C6 have sheared just below their heads in the plate, and C6 to C7 has collapsed.

- Use of larger diameter screws so as to better resist shear and bending forces (as opposed to pullout with standard screws)
- The concept of low versus high strain for both the bone and the plate (Figures 107.13 and 107.14); locking fixation is more conducive to bridging or low strain
- Hand tightening of screws to ensure accurate and complete seating within their corresponding holes (a torque limiter is recommended when power-driving screws for safety; its use will not ensure satisfactory screw seating)
- Bicortical screw fixation or supplemental fixation (e.g., intramedullary [IM] pin, second plate, ESF) in bones with thin cortices (most dogs and cats), which is subject to high loads (full weight bearing or short fracture segments) (see Figure 107.5).
- Bicortical screw fixation or adjunct fixation with monocortical fixation.
- Larger or longer implants with titanium (ALPS) or more elastic constructs (Fixin) (see Figures 107.13 and 107.14).

- Preserving vascularity directly under the plate to maintain the biologic benefits (improved bone healing and infection resistance), such as ensuring noncontact at the bone–plate interface (e.g., "wave" in the plate under the portion intended for locking [LCP] (Figure 107.15), or point contact [ALPS] or using a fully bridging plate [Fixin or SOP])
- Recognizing the different stiffness of the various plates; the variations between plate and construct stiffness also must be recognized. Constructs with low stiffness are best suited for biologic management (relative stability) of low-strain (comminuted) fractures. Adjunct fixation should be considered in cases that require maximal stability (absolute stability) of high strain (two-piece) fractures.

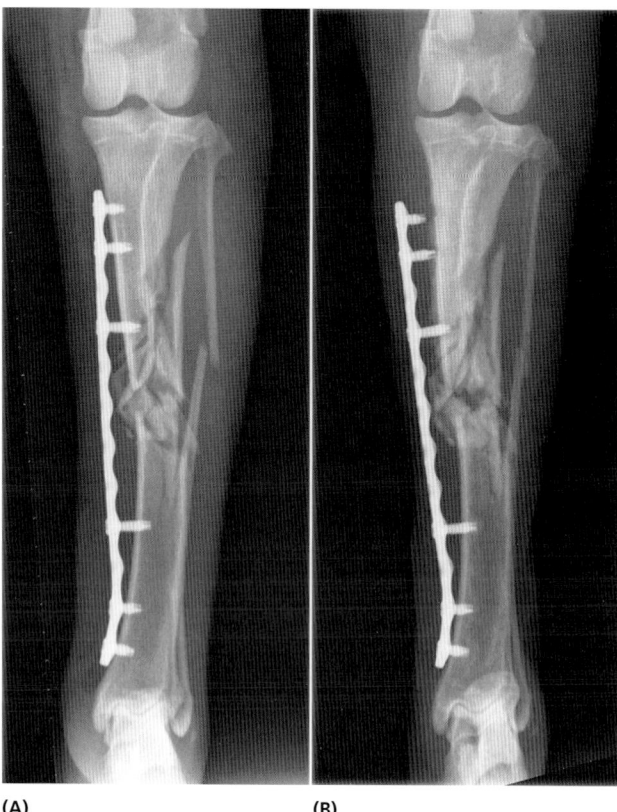

(A)   **(B)**

Figure 107.10 Screw failure in a locking Advanced Locking Plate System (ALPS) construct. Immediate (**A**) and 3-week (**B**) postoperative craniocaudal radiographs of the tibia in a 4-year-old female German shepherd dog. **A**, A single ALPS 10 plate (12-hole with three monocortical screws in each bone fragment; note the absence of plate contouring) spans a comminuted tibial fracture. **B**, Fixation failure (overload) has occurred because all screws in the proximal fragment have pulled out of the bone. *Source:* Reproduced with permission from I. Pfeil.

Relevant literature

Technical failures

All of the systems have some form of locking mechanism of the screw to the plate in order to obtain a fixed-angle construct of the plate to the bone, and in most cases, this fixed angle is orthogonal to the surface of the plate (exceptions include anatomically contoured plates, e.g., the DePuy Synthes Vet tibial plateau leveling osteotomy [TPLO] plate). Herein is the first potential for problems when the plate is not directly centered over the bone. The screw cannot be angled to ensure bone purchase; therefore, **insufficient screw purchase** is obtained (see Figure 107.1). Similarly, if a plate is contoured near a joint, the locking screw cannot be redirected and as such can then result in intraarticular placement (see Figure 107.3). This is an occasional issue in the anatomically contoured plate if it also is contoured beyond the preplanned screw positioning designed to avoid the joint. {Using the same example of the TPLO plate, the proximal locking screws will be directed intraarticularly if the plates are contoured to match a large medial buttress as a result of the greater concavity present to this area of the bone surface.

If **contouring a locked plate**, care also must be taken not to alter or deform the screw hole because the locking mechanism

may then be compromised, and the plate can no longer secure or hold the head of the screw sufficiently. Some systems have "blanks" (i.e., screw heads only that are secured into the holes during the bending process), and others have instrumentation that is designed to preserve the screw-hole integrity during plate bending.

Screw purchase with the plate or bone can be adversely affected when using locking plates. Screws can "jam" when they are not appropriately aligned with the screw hole and thus become cross-threaded in screw holes with threads or incorrectly seated within the screw hole in plates with some form of a conical taper. Insufficient purchase of the screw may lead to screw loosening from these issues. Screw loosening also may occur simply because of insufficient application of torque during screw insertion. The latter may occur, for example, when using a torque limiter device because this limiter may prevent full seating of the screw, especially in cases in which some malalignment is present between the screw and screw hole. A torque limiter is recommended in instances when torque is poorly controlled, such as during power driving of screws, because it prevents injury to the bone or the implants; however, the concept of "cold welding" to prevent overtightening (and the original rationale provided to use the torque limiter) is not an issue with stainless steel (SS) implants; therefore, hand tightening should be performed to ensure that the screw is fully seated within the plate hole. In plates with combination holes (e.g., Combi hole of the LCP), a locking screw should not be placed in the wrong side of the hole because this will preclude any locking mechanism and not result in the same plate–bone interface compression as obtained with a standard screw). Whenever contact with the plate is incomplete, screw-plate purchase is decreased, diminishing the overall construct strength. There is complete loss of feedback ("feel") of screw–bone purchase when tightening a locking screw because the feedback obtained is with the screw to the plate and not with the screw to the bone. Therefore, screw purchase into bone may be compromised without any knowledge of the surgeon.

Soft tissue injury may occur during tightening (or loosening with implant removal) if the plate spins or rotates along the axis of the screw, known as the "helicopter effect." This effect may be more problematic when placing or removing locked implants using minimally invasive operative techniques (see Figure 107.2).

Improper application related to the tenets of locking plate fixation

As noted, the primary aspect in development of locking plates was with regard to the biology and preservation of the blood supply, both cortical and endosteal. This concept led to the idea of noncontact of the plates to the bone surface (or point contact) and further avoidance of any disturbance to the medullary circulation (via monocortical fixation) (Perren *et al.* 1988; Perren 2002). Secondarily, several mechanical advantages were proposed such as preservation of both primary and secondary reduction and improved purchase in osteoporotic bone (Sommer *et al.* 2007). Although a multitude of publications compare the mechanical properties between standard and locking plate fixation, the mechanical advantages of the locking plate are not clearly established. Most studies report comparable fixation strength, but others have shown biomechanical superiority of the locking system over conventional plating (Korner *et al.* 2004; Florin *et al.* 2005; Liporace *et al.* 2005; Redfern *et al.* 2006; Richter *et al.* 2005; Trease *et al.* 2005; Chiodo *et al.* 2006; Boswell *et al.* 2007; Leitner

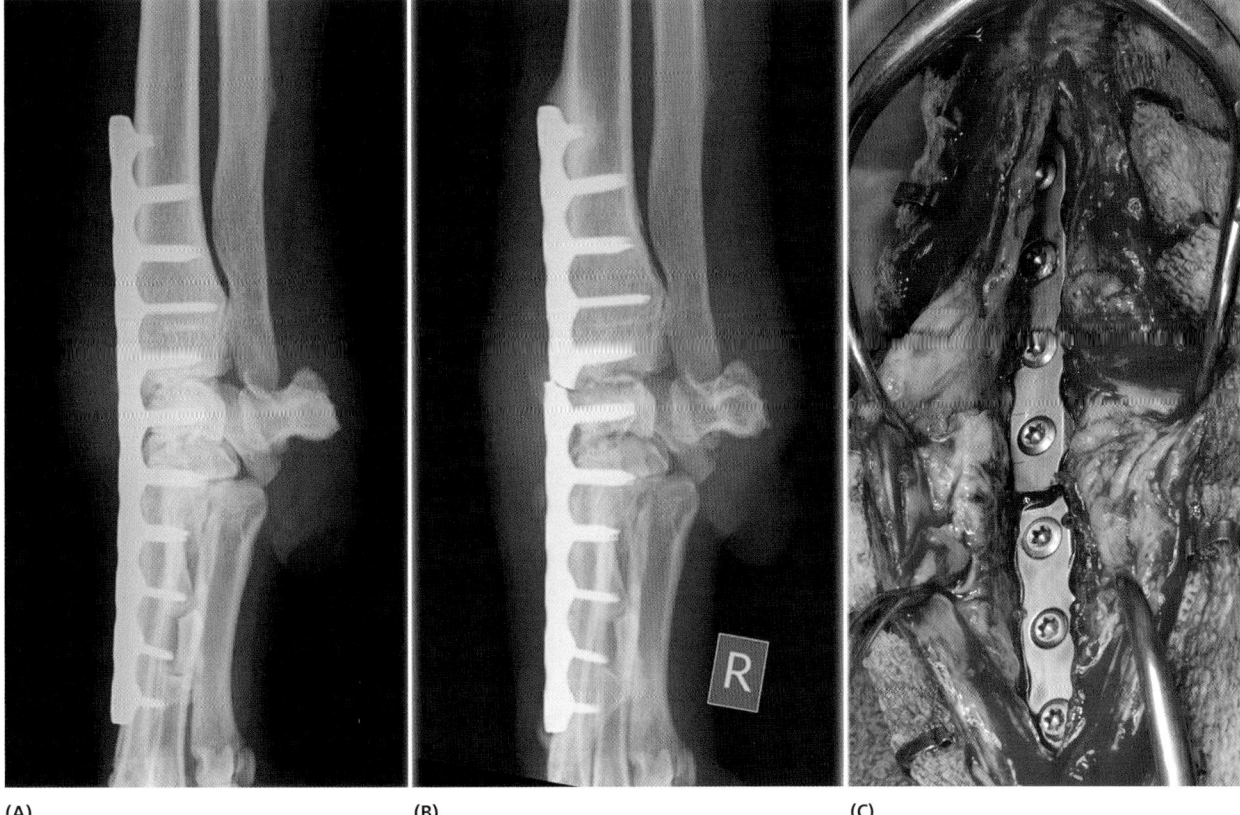

(A)   (B)   (C)

Figure 107.11 Fatigue failure of an Advanced Locking Plate System (ALPS) locking plate. Immediate (**A**) and 10-week (**B**) postoperative lateral radiographs of the antebrachiocarpal joint in an 8-year-old female German shepherd dog; intraoperative photograph of the plate (10 wk). **A**, An 11-hole ALPS 10 has been placed to span the distal radius to the third metacarpal bone (the articular cartilages all joint surfaces was removed, and cancellous autograft was placed intraarticularly). **B** and **C**, Fatigue failure of the plate is observed just above the radiocarpal bone. *Source:* A. Vezzoni, Clinica Veterinaria Vezzoni srl, Cremona, Italy. Reproduced with permission from A. Vezzoni.

et al. 2007; Schupp *et al.* 2007). As such, the current recommendations established for use of locked plating in humans include osteoporotic bone and periarticular and periprosthetic fractures (Zura and Browne 2006; Haidukewych and Ricci 2008; Strauss *et al.* 2008).

The concept of using locking plate fixation is founded on the premise that bridging fixation with an internal fixator provides relative (rather than absolute) stability and is adequate for early functional treatment so as to stimulate healing via callus formation (Wagner and Frigg 2006). These locking systems are not designed to be applied to high-strain situations because the concept of preservation of the biology foregoes precise anatomic reconstruction with its inherent surgical dissection. Locking plates must therefore span a fracture such that excessive loads are not placed on the screws or the plate.

The area that has received the most attention for locking plate fixation deals with minimally invasive surgical techniques (**minimally invasive plate osteosynthesis [MIPO]**). Locked plating is especially appealing to MIPO because these plates do not require accurate contouring to the bone to achieve adequate fixation. This advantage has prompted the development of a plethora of anatomically contoured plates for almost every bone in the human body. Within this area of application, the concept of relative stability strain was developed (Perren 2002). A number of guidelines have consequently been proposed for locking plate application

under these conditions, all involving bridge plating of fractures via MIPO. As noted, the first concept limiting bridging fixation to low-strain situations eliminates simple (two-piece) fractures. In these cases, standard plating techniques are still preferred so as to provide absolute stability (Gardner *et al.* 2004; Wagner and Frigg 2009). With **bridging fixation**, long segments of the bone must be spanned to ensure low strain on the bone and the plates (>three times the length of the fracture segment); in addition, a screw-to-hole ratio of less than 0.5 is recommended along with a recommendation to leave at least two or three holes open at the fracture or defect (see Figure 107.12) (Wagner *et al.* 2007). The locked construct, along with its screw-only mode of transfer, creates a stress riser at the screw-plate junction, thus, forces must be dispersed throughout the length of the plate (and bone) over at least three or four screws in each major bone fragment spanning the fracture (Wagner and Frigg 2006). The greater stresses on the screw itself also calls for a different screw design where the screws are subject to additional shear and bending stresses, as opposed to pullout with standard plating techniques (Wagner and Frigg 2006). The LCP **screw design** is such that it has an increased projection area of 40%, thereby distributing forces to a larger bone area (see Figures 107.13 and 107.14) (Wagner and Frigg 2006). Furthermore, the larger screw core diameter allows for 100% increase in shear stress and 200% more bending stress, thus reducing the incidence of screw failure under such application techniques (Wagner and

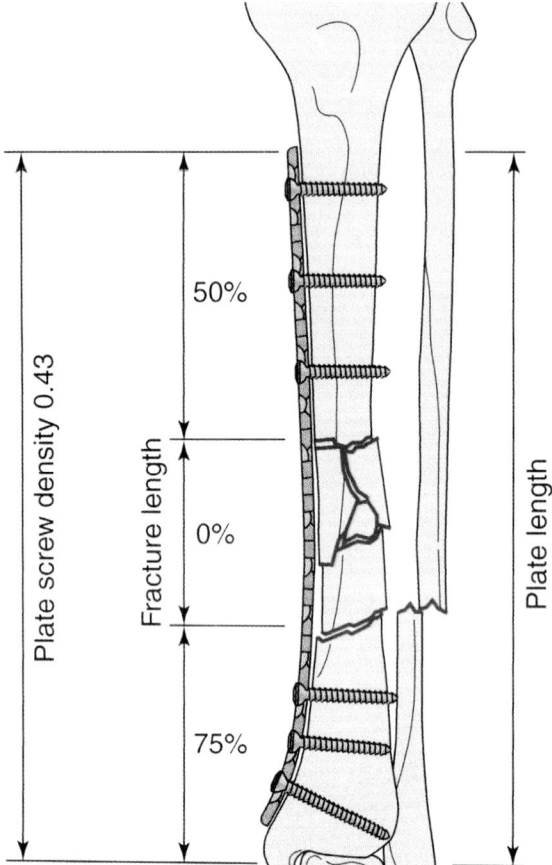

Figure 107.12 Importance of the plate-span ratio and plate-screw density in the bridge plating technique. The plate-span ratio should be greater than 2:1 or 3:1; the plate-screw density values below 0.5 to 0.4 are recommended. In this example, the plate span ratio is ~3:1 (ratio between the length of the plate to the length of the fracture); the plate-screw ratio is 0.43 (6 of 14 holes filled)[proximal fragment 0.5 (3 of 6 holes filled), fracture segment 0 (0 of 4 holes filled), distal fragment 0.75 (3 of 4 holes filled)]. *Source:* Wagner and Frigg, 2009. Reproduced with permission from Elsevier.

Frigg 2006). Most manufacturers abide by this principle in which locking screws are larger (core diameter) than their standard counterparts.

The advantages of locking plate fixation in humans were noted in the treatment of fractures of osteoporotic bone and in the improved stability obtained with application of monocortical screws in the diaphysis, whereby both the periosteal (under the plate) and the medullary blood supply also were preserved, and maintained structural integrity with no loss of bone in the opposite cortex. These advantages led to the application techniques described with the MIPO techniques where screws lend themselves to more optimal use as monocortical fixation (no necessity to select screw length precisely and no soft tissue damage or irritation with a screw tip protruding from the bone surface). It must also be recognized, however, that overall reduction or fixation can more easily be compromised using MIPO techniques. Although this may occur with any fixation system applied using MIPO methods, the locking plate systems are specifically recommended to be applied in this manner because of their very design, where location-specific plates are used

and plate contouring is not required. MIPO technique has a number of inherent issues that the surgeon must be aware of in addition to screw positioning, such as the potential for greater difficulty in reduction and fixation, soft tissue injury (inadvertent damage to unseen vessels and nerves), or plate impingement of other soft tissues (tendons or muscles). The **disadvantages to this closed technique** also must recognize that stability of the fracture depends on the rigidity of the construct (because no load sharing with bone is present in such bridging techniques). The latter can place excessive demands on the system, in addition to the aforementioned factors that acknowledge closed reduction and intraoperative control of alignment, and minimally invasive plate application and fixation are not easy to perform.

There is, moreover, the recognition that **bicortical screw anchorage** is still needed for sufficient mechanical stability in situations where thin cortices exist (or in osteoporotic bone) or in bones subjected to high torsional loads (e.g., humerus in humans) (see Figure 107.5). In a thin cortex, there is an insufficient working length for the screw to retain sufficient mechanical stability (Wagner and Frigg 2006). In addition, in short bone fragments, where screws are placed closer to each other, bicortical anchorage continues to be recommended (Wagner and Frigg 2006).

Bridging plate application results in relative stability and no contribution of the bone to the overall construct stability. This environment creates a potential for **irreversible plastic deformation** of the plate within the fracture zone if there is unacceptable loading or overloading; this risk is recognized in lower limb fractures in humans, prompting recommendations for additional support. For example, locking plate fixation of tibial fractures may be complemented by addition of a plate on the fibula or placement of an additional (temporary) external fixator (ESF) on the opposite side of the bone (see Figure 107.4) (Wagner and Frigg 2006).

The primary advantage of the fixed-angle internal fixation consists of the preservation of the biology, minimizing postoperative bone necrosis as a result of plate contact at the plate–bone interface that compromises the vascularity in these areas and in turn also lowering infection rates. The pursuit of these particular advantages also led to the introduction of titanium with these implants. The prototype locking implant was the PC-Fix, a point contact titanium construct, which was (Arens *et al.* 1999) found to not only preserve the vascularity at the bone–plate interface but also significantly decrease the formation of a foreign body membrane around the implant as compared with SS (Arens *et al.* 1999). Additionally, titanium was found to be more inert, allowing revascularization to occur up to the edges of the plate, as opposed to SS, where vascularity was reduced adjacent to the plate (Arens *et al.* 1999). The larger foreign body membrane and avascular area observed with SS plates creates dead space where bacteria can grow and spread without defense. Combined, limited plate–bone contact and titanium implants were shown experimentally to drastically improve the local resistance to infection (factor of 750×) compared with SS plates placed in rabbits (Arens *et al.* 1999). In addition, the PC-Fix was thought to improve axial stability because of its minimal point contact to the bone, the latter aspect increasing overall stability compared with no contact (Wagner and Frigg 2009).

The LCP was developed in lieu of the PC-Fix, partly because of its enhanced ability to be applied as either a standard implant or a locking implant, depending on the needs of the surgeon. This plate allows standard plate fixation, with the application of

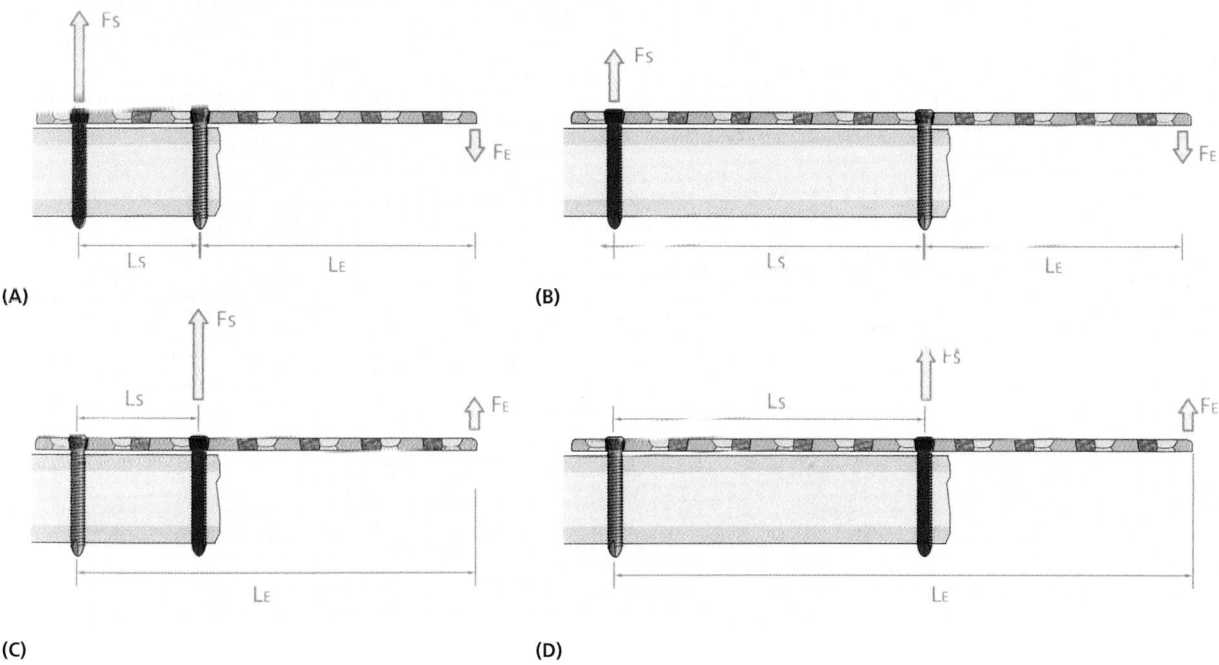

Figure 107.13 Pull-out force on screws and its relationship to the working leverage of the plate. With a short plate, screw loading is high because of the short working leverage on the screws with an applied bending moment (**A** and **C**). With a longer plate, the screw loading is decreased because of the longer working leverage with an applied bending moment (**B** and **D**). F_E, external force creating a bending moment on the plate; F_S, pull-out force of the screw; L_E, lever arm of the external force; L_S, lever arm of the screw. *Source:* Wagner and Frigg, 2006. Copyright by AO Foundation, Switzerland.

interfragmentary compression for absolute stability in simple (two-piece) fractures or locking plate fixation in cases with application of bridging fixation with relative stability in comminuted fractures. Mixing techniques, or hybrid fixation (using both locking and standard screws in the same bone fragment) was originally discouraged so as to adhere to the underlying philosophy behind the development of locking plates; however, this philosophy was not always followed in clinical use. These philosophical concepts remain unchanged but perhaps are overlooked. Keeping in mind the principles of biologic fixation and preservation of the blood supply, locking fixation meets these goals only by maintaining some space between the plate and bone (point contact

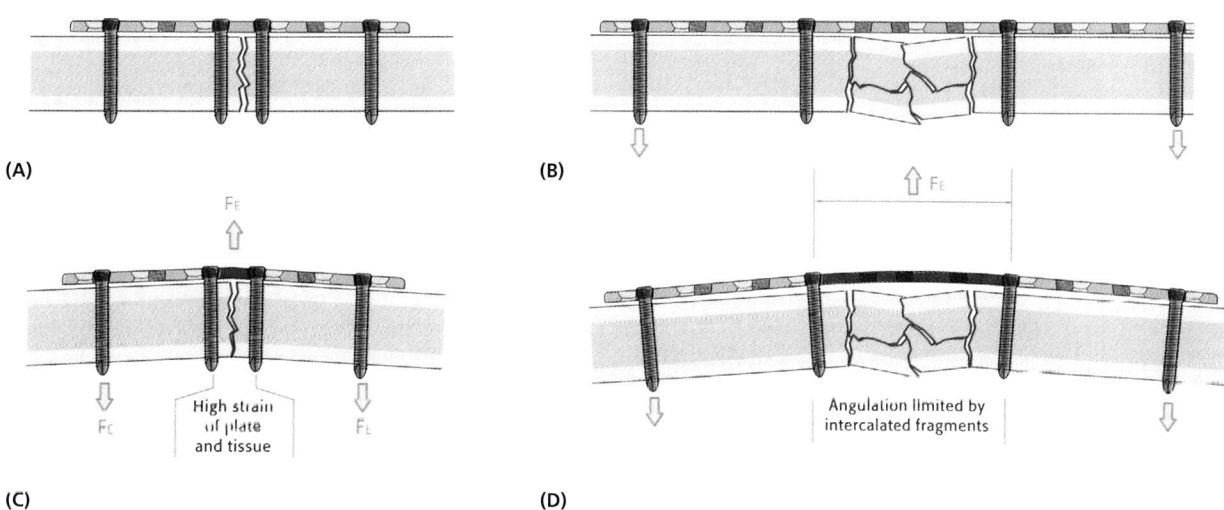

Figure 107.14 Plate strain in three-point bending. When the bent segment is short (**A** and **C**), the relative deformation (strain) is high, increasing the risk of fatigue failure of the implant. In areas where the plate spans a longer distance (e.g., across a comminuted segment of a fracture; **B** and **D**), the same bending moment leads to less stress concentration of the plate because the deformation is distributed over a longer distance. The latter leads to low implant strain and a higher resistance against fatigue failure. FE, external force creating a bending moment on the plate. *Source:* Wagner and Frigg, 2006. Copyright by AO Foundation, Switzerland.

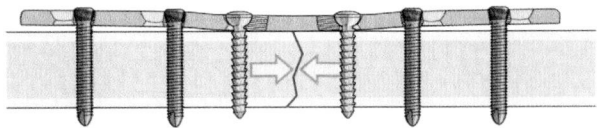

Figure 107.15 Combination of locking and standard plate fixation. Standard cortex screws must be placed first and the plate adapted to the bone surface to ensure interface contact at this level (in this example, interfragmentary compression is being used with the dynamic compression plate holes, arrows). Note that the plate contacts the cortex only in the area immobilized with conventional screws. *Source:* Wagner and Frigg, 2006. Copyright by AO Foundation, Switzerland.

only, or ensuring a gap remains present at the plate–bone interface); therefore, combining standard and locking screws can violate this principle because standard screws must be placed first to press the plate to the bone—the mechanism required for stability. Subsequent application of locking screws does not increase the strength of the fixation unless there is a potential for compromised bone purchase (e.g., short fragment, thin cortex, osteoporosis). An apparently forgotten technique when applying both methods in the same bone fragment is to ensure that areas of locking screws maintain a space between the plate and bone (thus preserving the biology, and the philosophy of application); this is done by bending the plate to create a "wave" in areas immobilized with locking screws (e.g., LCP) (see Figure 107.15). Whether failure to preserve the vasculature in this manner leads to complications of delayed healing or greater infection rates remains to be determined.

Limitations of the different locking plate systems

Several locking systems have become commercially available in veterinary surgery, and some have recently been evaluated experimentally (LCP, SOP, Fixin, ALPS) (Blake *et al.* 2011; Cabassu *et al.* 2011). These systems vary in their ability to follow the philosophy of locking plate application so as to best preserve the biology while simultaneously providing sufficient mechanical support in animals. The importance of preserving the vascularity at the bone–plate interface may also be overstated because of the variation of bone contours, especially in small animals. Some evidence has been published to suggest that, even with standard plate application, the "best" plate–bone contact is limited to about 30% of the plate surface (Field *et al.* 1997). In this scenario, combination techniques may not have adverse effects on the biology or healing. Nevertheless, recognition of the differences in the specific implants and their application methods (and better or less preservation of the biology) may dictate their use and the complications observed.

Not all locking systems share similar **biomechanical properties**, and they differ not only when comparing plates themselves but also as constructs encompassing screw–bone and screw–plate interfaces (Blake *et al.* 2011; Cabassu *et al.* 2011). Furthermore, their ability to preserve the biology while providing adequate mechanical support is influenced by their design. Finally, locking systems vary in their methods of placement. A lack of familiarity with a specific system can lead to a variety of technical issues and subsequent problems.

By virtue of their design, the ALPS, SOP, and Fixin implants all meet the goal of preservation of the vascularity at the bone–plate interface, but only the ALPS is designed to preserve endosteal

vascularity with application of monocortical screw fixation. Bicortical or monocortical screws can be placed regardless of the manufacturer; however, there is limited ability to place bicortical screw with the ALPS because longer screws are not available. Bone cortices are much thinner in small animals than in humans, thereby preferentially supporting bicortical screw placement. In lieu of bicortical screw fixation, supplemental fixation, such as dual (orthogonal or opposite) plate application, may be necessary to counteract the forces of weight bearing; this tenet has been alluded to in humans, in whom overload can easily occur (lower limb fractures, high torsion, or osteoporotic bone) (see Figure 107.10). Recognizing the limitations of fracture fixation in small animals, where both fracture overload is a constant issue and torsional loads are not unusual, **bicortical screws are indicated unless additional support is combined to monocortical screw fixation,** as was alluded to in humans.

The **LCP** can be applied either as a conventional or locking construct, but combined fixation with standard and locking screws requires contouring of the plate to the bone surface to generate the frictional contact at the plate–bone interface necessary with standard screws. This strategy comes at a cost to the biology of fracture healing because of the impact of standard fixation on the blood supply. This is especially true when multiple plates are applied. In these instances, the mechanical environment may also be suboptimal because the stiffness of these plates amplifies the stress-shielding effect associated with multiple plate fixation (see Figure 107.6). The LCP can be applied as an internal fixator that does not disturb the bone–plate interface vascularity but only by actively seeking to do so. Methods to minimize contact between locking plates and underlying bones include (1) a lack of plate contouring, whereby the curve of the bone does not conform to the straight plate; (2) contouring the plate to form "waves" and maintain gaps at the plate–bone surface (see Figure 107.15); and (3) temporary placement of a "spacer" (e.g., Kirschner wire) during initial placement of the plate. Neither of these latter two techniques, however, appears to be used clinically in veterinary surgery. With minimal plate contouring, long plates (e.g., applying an LCP over the full length of the bone) can suffice to preserve a gap at the bone–plate interface. Surgeons must, however, be aware that gaps exceeding 2 mm between an LCP and the bone surface will reduce the axial stiffness and torsional rigidity of the construct, thereby increasing the risk of plastic deformation of the implant during cyclic loading (Ahmad *et al.* 2007). The application of shorter plates enhances plate–bone contact, thereby affecting the biology of the fracture and violating the principle of creating the low-strain environment with relative stability by spanning the bone with an internal fixator (Perren 2002).

Application of **Fixin plates** induces compression of the plates against the bone surface; however, lack of plate contouring, combined with the use of longer plates, decreases plate–bone contact. The Fixin plates thus are better suited in fractures managed via relative stability, where they serve as bridging internal fixators with low stiffness (greater elasticity) (Blake *et al.* 2011; Cabassu *et al.* 2011). Surgeons must be cognizant of the lower strength of these implants compared with other locking systems such as the LCP and consider adjunct fixation in situations prone to excessive loading (e.g., weight-bearing loads). Strategies to supplement this fixation include the addition of an IM pin or second plate, as has been previously noted. Use of short plates with small gaps is thus contraindicated with these implants.

Alternatively, the **SOP** is a plate that allows three-dimensional contouring and uses standard screws but can only be applied as a fixed-angle locking construct. It does, however, have some limitations that surgeons must keep in mind when applying this system. The implant is very stiff (DeTora and Kraus 2008; Blake *et al.* 2011) and is applied to the bone using standard screws, which weakens the overall strength of the construct (Blake *et al.* 2011). As a result, the screws become the weak link of the construct, increasing the risk of screw failure, either as a loss of contact between the screw head and plate, or more often, as shearing or failure of the screws just below the heads (see Figures 107.8 and 107.9).

The specific details of the respective systems are, indeed, different. It is reasonable to consider the LCP system as a reference for comparison because it was the first locking plate available, and its design derives from the limited contact dynamic compression plate (LC-DCP), an implant that surgeons are most familiar with because it has been available for the longest time. In addition, the biomechanical properties of this implant have been evaluated in several studies (Blake *et al.* 2011; Cabassu *et al.* 2011).

The **ALPS** are composed of all titanium implants, which may allow them to better match the modulus of elasticity of bone (Blake *et al.* 2011; Cabassu *et al.* 2011). The lower stiffness associated with the use of titanium, combined with monocortical fixation may, however, result in insufficient construct stiffness or strength, depending on the relative size of implants used (see Figure 107.11). Furthermore, the implant design requires plate–bone contact, and using this plate without contact may result in screw or plate failure; this issue may, however, be circumvented with newly manufactured screws (as of 2011).

The **SOP system**, as noted earlier, is the stiffest plate, which could create a mismatch between the modulus of elasticity of the bone and the implant; however, despite the greater stiffness of the plate, SOP constructs display similar stiffness to other locking systems, such as LCP constructs (Blake *et al.* 2011; Cabassu *et al.* 2011). These results reflect the influence of screw–plate and bone–screw interactions in the constructs and the relative weakness of standard screws in the SOP construct. In addition, the conventional screw is not specifically designed to match a comparable surface within the node of the SOP, thereby potentially affecting the quality of the screw–plate interface.

In the **Fixin system**, complete seating of the screw within the insert of the plate at the plate hole is crucial to the construct. A slight malalignment of the screw within the insert may result in difficult or inadequate seating in the conical coupling system with failure to advance the screw under these conditions. Furthermore, all inserts must be retained within the support. Empty screw holes without this spacer create an additional stress riser, predisposing the implant to failure at this level (see Figure 107.7).

Locking plate fixation is a relatively new and quickly evolving technology in veterinary medicine, warranting further investigation to determine the specific indications for the plethora of new but different implants currently manufactured. In the meantime, surgeons must be well informed of the variability in mechanical properties and limitations of each design. This information will aid the decision-making process and individualize selection of a locking implant for a specific fracture and patient. **These systems should not be approached with identical philosophies** but instead take into consideration their differences, even if subtle, because they may affect the outcome of a fracture, influencing both the mechanical stability and biology of the environment (Blake *et al.* 2011; Cabassu *et al.* 2011).

Conclusion

Although fixed-angle constructs have gained popularity in small animal surgery and have led to the development of many variations of this form of fixation, surgeons should be reminded that indications for standard plating techniques also continue to remain valid (Wagner 2003). Conventional versus locked plating techniques result in different biomechanics and subsequent healing response; being cognizant of the appropriate indications for each strategy will help minimize complications (Gardner *et al.* 2004).

References

Ahmad, M., Nanda, R., Bajwa, A.S., et al. (2007) Biomechanical testing of the locking compression plate: when does the distance between bone and implant significantly reduce construct stability? *Injury* 38, 358-364.

Arens, S., Eijer, H., Schlegel, U., et al. (1999) Influence of the design for fixation implants on local infection: experimental study of dynamic compression plates versus point contact fixators in rabbits. *Journal of Orthopaedic Trauma* 13, 470-476.

Blake, C.A., Boudrieau, R.J., Torrance, B.S., et al. (2011) Single cycle to failure in bending of 3 standard and 5 locking plates and plate constructs. *Veterinary and Comparative Orthopaedics and Traumatology* 24, 408-417.

Boswell, S., McIff, T., Trease, C.A., et al. (2007) Mechanical characteristics of locking and compression plate-constructs applied dorsally to distal radius fractures. *Journal of Hand Surgery* 32, 623-629.

Cabassu, J.B., Kowaleski, M.P., Shorinko, J.K., et al. (2011) Single cycle to failure in torsion of 3 standard and 5 locking plate constructs. *Veterinary and Comparative Orthopaedics and Traumatology* 24, 418-425.

Chiodo, T.A., Ziccardi, V.B., Janal, M., et al. (2006) Failure strength of 2.0 locking versus 2.0 conventional Synthes mandibular plates: a laboratory model. *Journal of Oral and Maxillofacial Surgery* 64, 1475-1479.

DeTora, M., Kraus, K. (2008) Mechanical testing of 3.5 mm locking and non-locking bone plates. *Veterinary and Comparative Orthopaedics and Traumatology* 21, 318-322.

Field, J.R., Hearn, T.C., Caldwell, C. (1997) Bone plate fixation: an evaluation of interface contact area and force of the dynamic compression plate (DCP) and the limited contact-dynamic compression plate (LC-DCP) applied to cadaveric bone. *Journal of Orthopaedic Trauma* 11, 368-373.

Florin, M., Arzdorf, M., Linke, B., et al. (2005) Assessment of stiffness and strength of 4 different implants available for equine fracture treatment: a study on a 20 degree oblique long bone fracture model using a bone substitute. *Veterinary Surgery Journal* 34, 231-238.

Gardner, M.J., Helfet, D.L., Lorich, D.G. (2004) Has locked plating completely replaced conventional plating [review]? *The American Journal of Orthopedics* 33, 439-446.

Haidukewych, G.J., Ricci, W. (2008) Locked plating in orthopaedic trauma: a clinical update [review]. *Journal of the American Academy of Orthopaedic Surgeons* 16, 347-355.

Korner, J., Diederichs, G., Arzdorf, M., et al. (2004) A biomechanical evaluation of methods of distal humerus fracture fixation using locking compression plates versus conventional reconstruction plates. *Journal of Orthopaedic Trauma* 18, 286-293.

Leitner, M., Pearce, S., Windolf, M., et al. (2007) Evaluation of tibia plateau positioning and biomechanical stability of TPLO plate fixation using either locking or conventional screws. *Veterinary Surgery Journal* 36, E15.

Liporace, F.A., Gupta, S., Jeong, G.K., et al. (2005) A biomechanical comparison of a dorsal 3.5-mm T-plate and a volar fixed angle plate in a model of dorsally unstable distal radius fractures. *Journal of Orthopaedic Trauma* 19, 187-191.

Perren, S.M. (2002) Evolution of the internal fixation of long bone fractures: the scientific basis of biological internal fixation: choosing a new balance between stability and biology. *The Journal of Bone & Joint Surgery* 84 (Suppl. B), 1093-1110.

Perren, S.M., Cordley, J., Rahn, B.A., et al. (1988) Early temporary porosis of bone induced by internal fixation implants: a reaction to necrosis, not stress protection? *Clinical Orthopaedics and Related Research* 232, 139-255.

Redfern, D.J., Oliveira, M.L., Campbell, J.T., et al. (2006) A biomechanical comparison of locking and nonlocking plates for the fixation of calcaneal fractures. *Foot & Ankle International* 27, 196-201.

Richter, M., Gosling, T., Zech, S., et al. (2005) A comparison of plates with and without locking screws in a calcaneal fracture model. *Foot & Ankle International* 26, 309-319.

Schupp, W., Arzdorf, M., Linke, B., et al. (2007) Biomechanical testing of different osteosynthesis systems for segmental resection of the mandible. *Journal of Oral and Maxillofacial Surgery* 65, 924-930.

Sommer, C., Schütz, M., Wagner, M. (2007) Internal fixator. In Rüedi, T.P., Buckley, R.E., Moran, C.G. (eds.) *AO Principles of Fracture Management*, 2nd edn. AO Publishing, Davos Platz, Switzerland, pp. 321-335.

Strauss, E.J., Schwarzkopf, R., Egol, K.A. (2008) The current status of locked plating: the good, the bad, and the ugly. *Journal of Orthopaedic Trauma* 22, 479-486.

Trease, C.A., McIff, T., Toby, E.B. (2005) Locking versus nonlocking T-plates for dorsal and volar fixation of dorsally comminuted distal radius fractures: a biomechanical study. *Journal of Hand Surgery* 30,756-763.

Wagner, M. (2003) General principles for the clinical use of the LCP. *Injury* 34 (Suppl. 2), SB31-SB42.

Wagner, M., Frigg, R. (2006) Techniques and procedures in LCP and LISS. In Buckley, R., Gautier, E., Schütz, M., Sommer, C. (eds.) *AO Manual of Fracture Management: Internal Fixators, Concepts and Cases Using LCP and LISS*. AO Publishing, Davos Platz, Switzerland, pp. 87-161.

Wagner, M., Frenk, A., Frigg, R. (2007) Locked plating: biomechanics and biology and locked plating: clinical indications. *Techniques in Orthopaedics* 22, 209-218.

Wagner, M.A., Frigg, R. (2009) Locking plates: development, biomechanics, and clinical application. In Browner, B.D., Jupiter, J.B., Levine, A.M., et al. (eds.) *Skeletal Trauma: Basic Science, Management, and Reconstruction*. Saunders, Philadelphia, pp. 143-176.

Zura, R.D., Browne, J.A. (2006) Current concepts in locked plating. *Journal of Surgical Orthopaedic Advances* 15, 173-176.

Salvage Orthopedic Procedures

108 Arthrodesis

Dominique Griffon

College of Veterinary Medicine, Western University of Health Sciences, Pomona, CA, USA

Arthrodeses are most commonly performed on the carpus and tarsus to manage severe traumatic injuries such as intraarticular fractures, luxations, ligament injuries, and shearing injuries. Other indications include chronic instability and end-stage diseases such as degenerative joint disease (DJD), septic arthritis, immune-mediated arthritis, shearing injuries, and some peripheral nerve deficits.

The complication rate after dorsal carpal arthrodesis ranges from 7% to 50% of pancarpal arthrodesis (PCA) achieved via dorsal plating (Johnson 1980; Whitelock *et al.* 1999; Denny and Barr 1991; Worth and Bruce 2008). In a retrospective study of 22 carpal arthrodesis in 20 cats, nine complications were encountered in seven joints (~33% complication rate) (Calvo *et al.* 2009). Complication rates associated with tarsal arthrodeses range from 25% to 80% of dogs immobilized via plate fixation (Allen *et al.* 1993; Muir and Norris 1999; McKee *et al.* 2004). In a recent study of tarsal arthrodesis using plate fixation, major complications occurred in 32.5%, and minor complications developed in 42.5% of cases (Roch *et al.* 2008). Complications were more common with pantarsal rather than partial tarsal arthrodeses and more severe when the plate was applied on the medial rather than the lateral aspect of the joint.

Based on a review of the literature covering all types of arthrodeses, the most common complications seem to consist of soft tissue lesions caused by external coaptation (see Chapter 16) followed by implant failure. The incidence of other complications, such as bone fractures or loss of function, appears to vary with the joint and method of fixation used for the arthrodesis.

Complications associated with bandages and splints
Chapter 16.

Delayed healing
Chapter 98,

Infection
See Chapters 5, 7 and 8.

Implant failure

Definition
Implant failure is loss of fixation of an orthopedic implant. The most common type of implant failure after arthrodesis consists of screw loosening. Pin loosening is the second most common complication after arthrodesis by external fixation. Pin or plate breakage is less common but often leads to major complications, requiring revision surgery. Implant failure after arthrodesis usually results from fatigue failure secondary to cyclic loading of the implant and is more common after dorsal pantarsal arthrodesis.

Risk factors
Factors that predispose arthrodeses to implant failure are summarized in Figure 108.1.

Diagnosis
The most common clinical sign consists of lameness and pain on palpation of the area surrounding the failed implant. Depending on the implant and extent of the failure, additional signs may include:
- Soft tissue swelling
- Draining tract (over an isolated loose screw or around a loose pin)

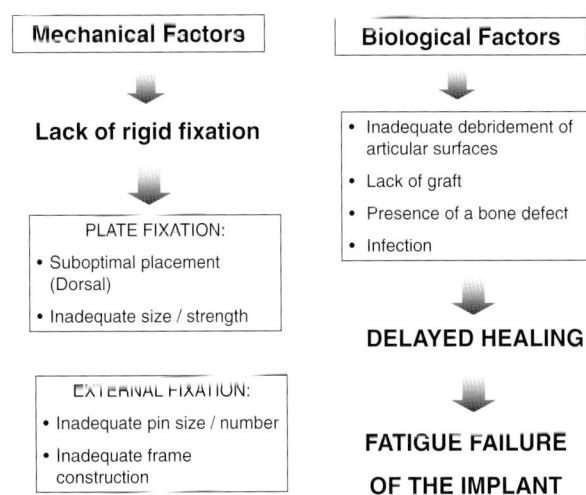

Figure 108.1 Risk factors for complications after arthrodesis.

Complications in Small Animal Surgery, First Edition. Edited by Dominique Griffon and Annick Hamaide.

© 2016 John Wiley & Sons, Inc. Published 2016 by John Wiley & Sons, Inc.

Companion website: www.wiley.com/go/griffon/complications

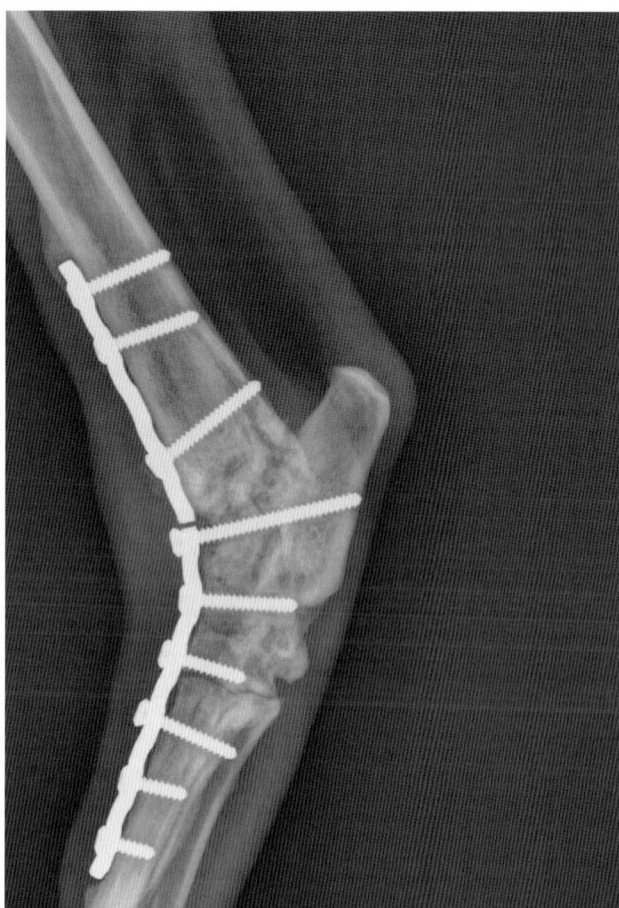

Figure 108.2 Implant failure after arthrodesis. A dorsally applied plate failed 6 months after pantarsal arthrodesis as a result of delayed healing.

- Broken pin or connective bar
- Unstable arthrodesis (motion of the joint)

The diagnosis is confirmed via radiography (Figure 108.2). Signs include a broken implant, implant migration, radiolucency around the implant, and/or periosteal reaction.

Treatment

Implant removal alleviates signs if the arthrodesis is complete at the time of failure.

Revision is indicated if the joint is unstable. The principles of a revision in these cases include:

- Revise joint surfaces (may consider en-bloc distal ostectomy of the tibia and fibula).
- Ensure good apposition of the joint at a standing angle, based on preoperative measurement of the contralateral side. This angle is typically between 135 and 145 degrees for pantarsal arthrodesis in dogs and between 115 and 125 degrees in cats. PCAs are maintained at 10 degrees of hyperextension.
- Restore rigid fixation.
- Apply a bone graft.
- Obtain intraoperative sample for culture (aerobic and anaerobic) and sensitivity.

Regardless of the method used to restore rigid immobilization, the implant should extend proximal and distal to the previous implant. Revision may be achieved with a longer plate, placing screws

between previous screw holes. Alternatively, a locking plate may be selected to prevent screw loosening. External fixation is preferred if infection is suspected. A type II linear fixator may be placed with angled acrylic bars on each side of the joint or triangulation of rigid (carbon) connective bars (Figure 108.3). Circular or hybrid fixation is especially relevant to the management of cats and toy breeds.

Outcome

Although the outcome of revision arthrodeses has not been specifically addressed in the literature, the prognosis and healing times are similar to those of an initial arthrodesis if the underlying cause of implant failure has been addressed.

Prevention

Biologic strategies to enhance bone union:

- Strive for removing articular cartilage while avoiding excessive bone removal (creation of bone defects).
- Pack defects with a grafting agent (autogenous cancellous graft or demineralized bone matrix).
- Percutaneous plate arthrodesis has been proposed to preserve extraosseous bone supply and accelerate healing in pancarpal and pantarsal arthrodeses (Pozzi et al. 2012).

Mechanical strategies to provide long-term rigid fixation:

- Appropriate implant selection
- Consider the use of locking plates, such as String-of-Pearl (SOP) plates for shoulder arthrodesis (Fitzpatrick et al. 2012).

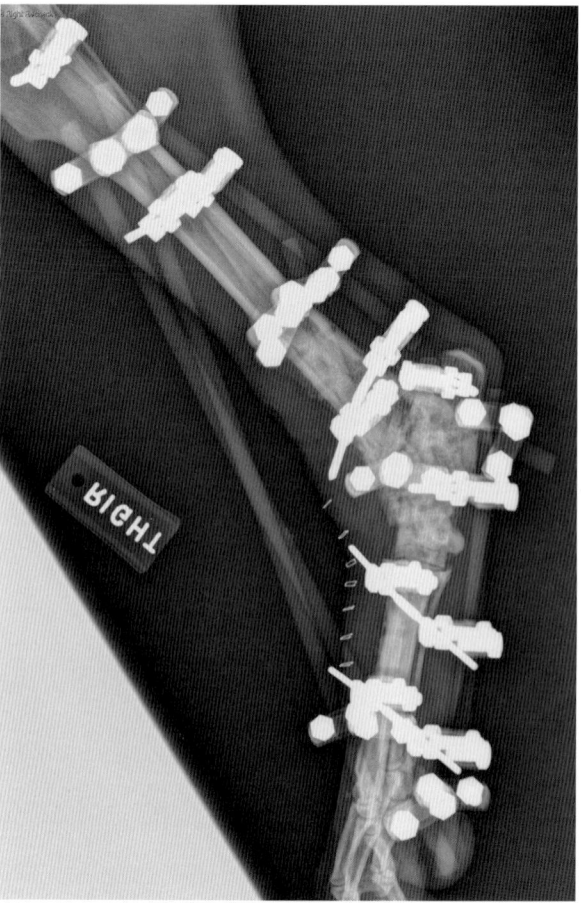

Figure 108.3 Revision of a failed plate with external fixation. Postoperative radiograph of the failed arthrodesis in Figure 108.2.

- Placement of a screw into the calcaneus during dorsal pantarsal arthrodesis (calcaneoquartal screw)
- Addition of a calcaneotibial screw as an adjunct to plating.
- Consider medially applied plates for pantarsal arthrodeses.
- Lateral plate fixation is associated with a lower rate of complications than pin and tension–band–wire fixation for arthrodesis of the calcaneoquartal joint (Barnes *et al.* 2013).

Bone fractures

Definition

Fracture of a bone secondary to arthrodesis. This complication involves most commonly the metacarpal (MTC) and metatarsal (MTT) bones but may also affect larger bones.

Risk factors

- Stress-rising effect caused by implant size (diameter of the screw >45% of the bone diameter)
- Eccentric placement of screws through MTC and MTT
Insufficient coverage of the bone by the implant (implant too short)

Diagnosis

Clinical signs include soft tissue swelling and lameness. Weight-bearing lameness may accompany a fracture of an MTC or MTT bone, but tibial or radial fractures will completely compromise the use of the limb. Pain, crepitus, and abnormal motion of the fracture site can be noted on palpation. The diagnosis is confirmed via radiographs (Figure 108.4).

Treatment

- Isolated MTC or MTT fractures occurring through a screw hole may be treated by removal of the screw without additional fixation. Undisplaced MTC and MTT fractures occurring distal to the bone plate have been treated conservatively with external coaptation.
- Fractures occurring through the tibia or radius warrant revision and fixation (Figure 108.5).
- Fixation may consist of a plate or external fixation extending beyond the level of the fracture.

Outcome

Conservative management of isolated MTC or MTT bone fractures usually results in a functional nonunion with intermittent lameness. The prognosis after fixation of a radial or tibial fracture is identical to that of an uncomplicated arthrodesis.

Prevention

- Select implants with a diameter equal to a maximum of 30% of the diameter of the bone.
- Select plates that accommodate different screw diameters for carpal arthrodesis. Options include:
  ○ Stacked veterinary cuttable plates in smaller patients,
  ○ Hybrid dynamic compression plates
  ○ Castless plate for PCA (Figure 108.6)

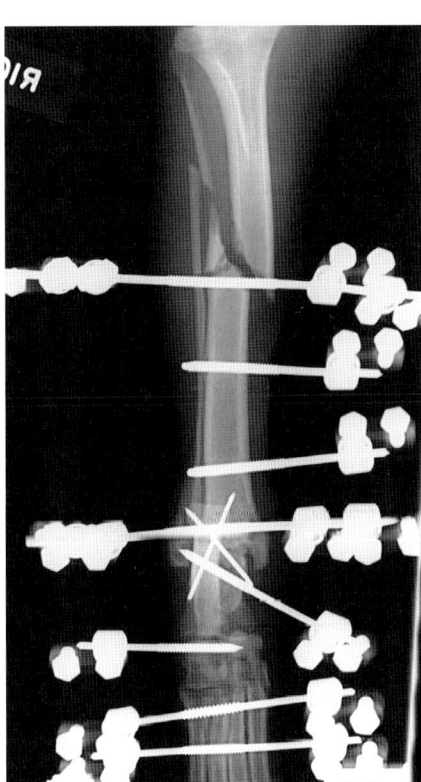

Figure 108.4 Fracture of the tibia secondary to pantarsal arthrodesis via external fixation. The bone fractured at the level of the most proximal pin, most likely because the apparatus did not extend into the proximal tibia.

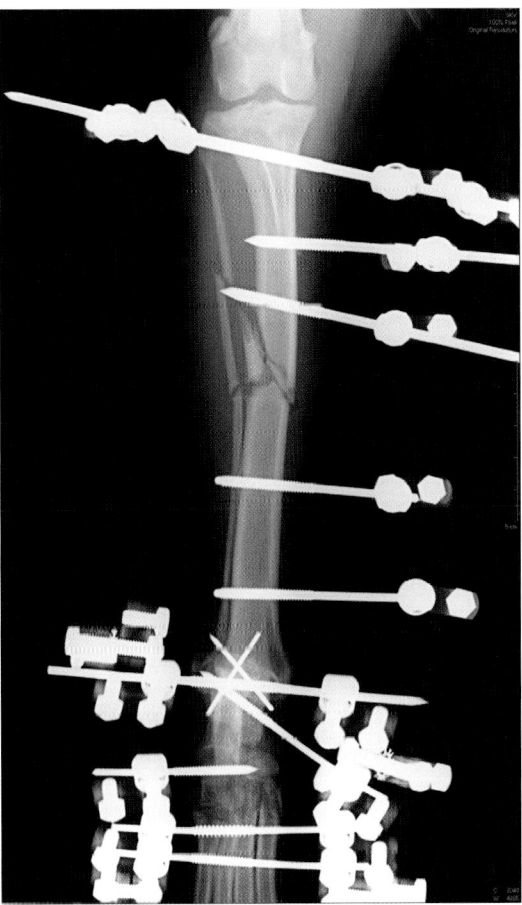

Figure 108.5 Revision of a tibial fracture secondary to pantarsal arthrodesis. The pin interfering with the fracture site has been removed and the external fixation extended proximally.

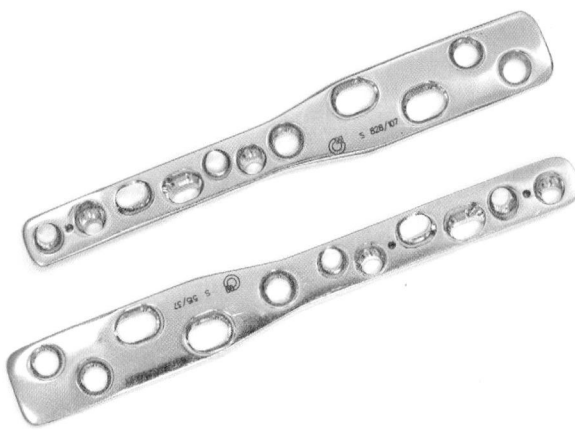

Figure 108.6 Prevention of metacarpal bone fractures with plates specifically designed for carpal arthrodesis. The CastLess plate for pancarpal arthrodesis (CLP; Orthomed Ltd., Halifax, UK) features smaller holes on its distal portion, offset so screws can engage metacarpal bones 3 and 4.

- Select a type of external fixator that allows placement of pins of several diameters.
- Select implants that cover at least 50% of the MTC or MTT bones.
- Avoid eccentric placement of implants (aim for penetration of the medullary canal).
- Extend external fixation for pantarsal arthrodesis into the proximal metaphysis of the tibia.

Loss of function

Definition
The definition varies among studies and clinicians. Loss of function is generally defined as a failure to return to normal activity, especially in working dogs. Loss of function is occasionally considered a deterioration or lack of improvement of the preoperative function. Poor function can occur despite a successful arthrodesis.

Risk factors
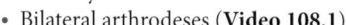
- Arthrodesis of highly mobile joints such as the stifle and elbow
- Limited ability of adjacent joints to compensate for the lack of mobility
- Bilateral arthrodeses (**Video 108.1**)
- Complete arthrodesis compared to partial arthrodesis of the tarsus
- Partial arthrodesis compared to complete arthrodesis of the carpus
- Presence of concurrent orthopedic disease
- Fusion in malposition of the joint
- Tendon contraction (digital flexor tendon, gastrocnemius tendon)

Diagnosis
The diagnosis is generally based on the owner's assessment of the dog's function. Clinical signs may include varying degrees of lameness, pain on palpation of the joint, abnormal angle of the operated joint, decreased range of motion of adjacent joints, or presence of a draining tract or soft tissue swelling. Abnormal wear of the toes

may be noted if the joint is fused in a position that is too extended. Orthopedic examination may be normal if lameness is intermittent.

Radiographic evaluation of the joint is indicated to verify implant integrity, appropriate length of positioning of implant, bone healing, and functional angle of fusion. The angle for pantarsal arthrodesis is typically between 135 and 145 degrees in dogs and between 115 and 125 degrees in cats. Pancarpal arthrodeses maintain the joint at 10 degrees of extension. The clinician should also look for signs of infection (Figure 108.7) and/or degenerative changes in adjacent joints.

Treatment
Treatment options are limited to cases in which an underlying cause of the poor limb function can be established. Conservative treatment is considered if the dog can function as a pet or is able to fulfill most functions of a working dog.

Degenerative joint disease of the radiocarpal after partial arthrodesis can be treated via PCA. Fusion in poor position of the joint may be corrected by revision of the arthrodesis in a functional angle. Interference of a screw with soft tissues can be corrected by replacement or removal of the screw. Low-grade osteomyelitis responds to implant removal, lavage, and

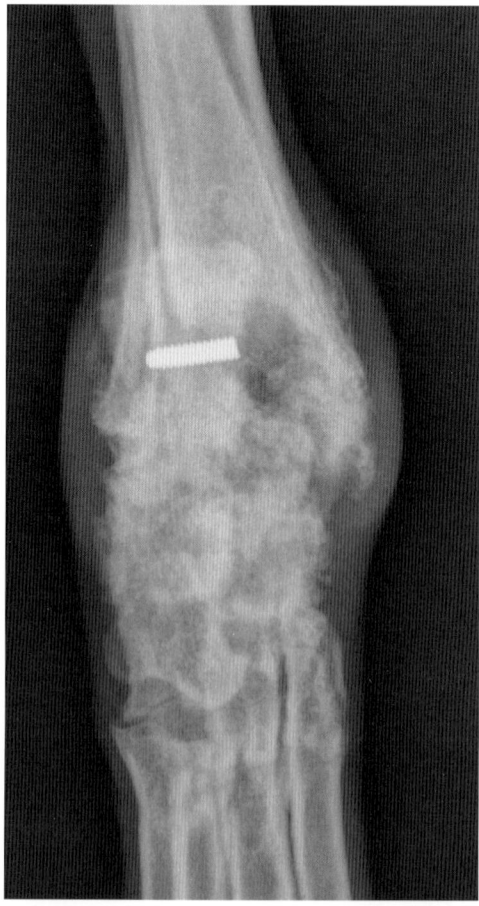

Figure 108.7 Low-grade infection resulting in poor limb function 7 months after arthrodesis. Weight-bearing lameness persisted after removal of the external fixator (shown in Figure 108.3) applied to revise the failed arthrodesis shown in Figure 108.2. The presence of a radiolucent area adjacent to a broken screw was suggestive of a low-grade infection confirmed via guided fine-needle aspiration and culture.

implantation of antibiotic beads. Systemic antibiotherapy is prescribed postoperatively based on culture and sensitivity results. The first line of treatment for postoperative tendon contraction consists of physical therapy. Tenotomy may be considered in unresponsive cases.

Outcome

The prognosis in dogs with poor postoperative limb function is overall guarded. The chances of improving function are greater in cases where an underlying cause, such as interference of a screw with soft tissues or DJD secondary to partial arthrodesis, can be identified. Tendon contraction, low-grade osteomyelitis, or malunion of an arthrodesis carry a poorer prognosis.

Prevention

- Setting owner's expectations regarding postoperative function and complications
- Placement of screws in the distal aspect of the radiocarpal bone prevents interference with the radiocarpal joint during extension of the carpus after partial carpal arthrodesis.
- Recommend a pancarpal rather than a partial arthrodesis of the carpus if any sign of pathology is found in the radiocarpal joint preoperatively.
- Partial arthrodesis of the tibiotarsal joint is contraindicated because it will lead to DJD of the tarsal and tarsometatarsal joints; a panarthrodesis of the tarsus is indicated if there is pathology of the tibiotarsal joint.
- Splint the limb with the digits in extension to limit the risk of digital tendon contraction.
- Consider castless means of fixation (castless plates or external fixation) to avoid long-term immobilization of adjacent joints and encourage early return to function.
- Consider joint replacement rather than arthrodesis of highly mobile joints (elbow).

Relevant literature

The most common major postoperative complication associated with carpal and tarsal arthrodeses consists of **implant failure**, specifically screw loosening, reported in 2% to 23% of cases (Johnson 1980; Denny and Barr 1991; DeCamp *et al.* 1993; Clarke *et al.* 2009). Failure of a dorsally applied plate (see Figure 108.1) is infrequent but may occur because the tension side of the bone is plantar. The highest plate stress was located at the level of the radiocarpal bone in a biomechanical and computational evaluation of PCAs fixed with a hybrid dynamic compression plate (HDCP) or CastLess plate (CLP) (Rothstock *et al.* 2012). The same study identified the most distal and proximal screws as exposed to the highest stress. Implant failure is more likely to occur in cases of delayed healing, resulting from lack of bone apposition, inadequate debridement of the articular cartilage, absence of bone graft, poor regenerative properties, or infection. Filling the debrided joints with fresh autogenous cancellous bone has been found to improve the healing of carpal arthrodesis in dogs (Johnson and Bellenger 1980). More recently, grafting tarsal and carpal arthrodeses with a commercially available frozen mixture of allogenic cancellous chips and demineralized bone matrix resulted in similar complication rates and healing times in a case-matched clinical study of dogs (Hoffer *et al.* 2008). Because of the mechanical disadvantage associated with a dorsal positioning of the plate, external coaptation is routinely used as an adjunct to carpal and tarsal arthrodesis. Splints are commonly associated

with complications such as pressure sores and require frequent rechecks, increasing the cost of the surgery. In a clinical review of 219 dogs with PCAs, external coaptation related complications occurred in 32% of dogs treated with HDCP (Bristow *et al.* 2015). This rate increased to 45% when a cast was applied. Readers are invited to review Chapter 16 further information on complications related to bandages and splints. Implant failure and complications caused by external coaptation have prompted the search for alternative techniques. Among these, a the CLP for PCA (Orthomed Ltd Halifax, UK) has been designed to (1) provide compression across the joints, (2) allow placement of smaller screws in the MTC bones, and (3) engage MTC 3 and 4. The proposed advantages of this plate are to minimize the risk of fractures of the MTCs and eliminate the need for external coaptation. However, the CLP was found to offer similar bending resistance to HDCP when each implant (not construct) was tested in vitro (Meeson *et al.* 2012). From a clinical standpoint, no difference in postoperative complication rates was found in a review of 105 PCAs with CLP compared with 125 PCAs with HDCP (Bristow *et al.* 2015). However, the duration of external coaptation was shorted in dogs with CLP (median, 7 days) than HDCP (median, 42 days). This difference in management explained the lower incidence of complications related to external coaptation in dogs with CLP (18%) compared with those with HDCP (32%). In the same study, implant loosening or breakage was reported infrequently, in 11% and 7.6% of PCAs immobilized with HDCP or CLP, respectively.

Alternative strategies to limit the risk of implant failure consist of applying plates to the lateral and medial aspect of the tarsus (McKee *et al.* 2004; Guerrero and Montavon 2005; Guillou *et al.* 2008). In these cases, plantar necrosis has been reported as the most common complication, occurring in 15% of cases (Roch *et al.* 2008). The skin of the plantar metatarsus and the deep tissues of the MTT pad become devitalized over the second and fifth digits. Management varied from open wound management to amputation of the affected digit. Percutaneous placement of a lateral plate has recently been described (Pozzi *et al.* 2012). Although evidence is currently lacking to substantiate these benefits, minimally invasive plate fixation would be expected to preserve adjacent soft tissues, thereby preventing skin tension and ischemia. This approach would be expected to enhance bone healing and minimize soft tissue complications while offering mechanical advantages in term of plate location.

Bone fractures after arthrodesis occur as a result of a stress-rising effect created by the implant. This complication is most likely to occur in the MTT and MTC bones because of the small diameters of these bones compared with the tibia and radius. Ensuring proper coverage of the bone and using smaller diameter screws in this area decrease the risk of fractures (Whitelock *et al.* 1999). Plates specifically designed for PCAs such as HDCP and CLP are now routinely used. Biomechanical testing of hybrid plates (3.5- and 2.7-mm screws) with 3.5-mm limited contact dynamic compression plates (LC-DCPs) concluded that the slight superiority in compliance and angular deformation of LC-DCP constructs may have limited clinical significance but that the lower plate strain detected in hybrid constructs should improve resistance to acute and fatigue failure (Guillou *et al.* 2012).

Although not as common, fracture of the tibia may occur after arthrodesis of the tarsus via external fixation (see Figure 108.4). Extending the fixation proximally into the metaphysic of the bone improves the distribution of loads on the bone and seems to prevent this complication. External fixators require more postoperative patient care to prevent complications associated with pin tracts. This type of fixation remains relevant to the management of open wounds, such as shearing injuries. Indeed, their application minimizes elevation of soft tissues around the joint, maintains implants away from infected joints, and allows removal under sedation after the arthrodesis is complete.

Owners' expectations should be set before surgery in terms of **limb function** after arthrodesis. Function is overall very good with arthrodeses of the carpus and tarsus as long as limb alignment is preserved and the joint immobilized at a normal standing angle. Return to full function has been reported in 74% of pets undergoing PCA (Denny and Barr 1991). The long-term function of working dogs with PCA is also good, with 50% of dogs returning to preoperative levels of function and another 33% being able to perform most of their duties (Worth and Bruce 2008). Despite these good clinical outcomes, a recent kinetic study reported kinetic parameters lower than normal, especially in propulsion, 2 years after carpal arthrodesis in dogs (Andreoni *et al.* 2010). In a study of 25 carpi with third-degree carpal sprains, all owners reported improvements in function after partial carpal arthrodesis, and none of the dogs required a PCA (Willer *et al.* 1990). However, the outcome of partial arthrodesis is generally described as less favorable, with 50% to 70% of cases considered successful (Denny and Barr 1991; Andreoni *et al.* 2010). Poor limb function is often attributed to DJD of the radiocarpal joint, reported in 11.5% to 89% of dogs (Willer *et al.* 1990; Andreoni *et al.* 2010). These changes may be due to interference of the screws placed in the radiocarpal bone during extension of the radiocarpal joint or to the presence of preexisting disease. After carpal arthrodesis, cats have been found to be more reluctant to jump and climb and to jump lower heights than normal (Calvo *et al.* 2009). Complications were diagnosed in 35% of cats reviewed in this study, the most common type being related to the use of pins. The long-term outcome after tarsal arthrodesis is poorly documented in the literature. Partial tarsal arthrodesis of the tarsus is generally believed to result in a better outcome than pantarsal arthrodesis because the talocrural joint accounts for about 90% of the mobility of the tarsus (Gorse *et al.* 1991; Muir and Norris 1999). Isolated arthrodesis of the talocrural joint is contraindicated as the procedure will inevitably lead to degenerative disease of the tarsal and tarsometatarsal joints. A recent multicenter case series documented the outcome of 14 dogs with shoulder arthrodesis (Fitzpatrick *et al.* 2012). Complications occurred in 9 dogs, with minor complications in 5 dogs (e.g., incidental implant migration) and major complications in 2 dogs (infection and implant failure). The last two complications consisted of poor function leading to amputation in 1 case and infection leading to euthanasia in another case. In dogs in which morbidity was successfully managed, long-term function was overall evaluated positively by veterinarians and owners. Limb circumduction was the most common sign in dogs with persistent lameness.

All videos cited in this chapter can be found on the book companion website at www.wiley.com/go/griffon/complications.

References

Allen, M., Dyce, J., Houlton, J.E.F. (1993) Calcaneoquartal arthrodesis in the dog. *Journal of Small Animal Practice* 34, 205-210.

Andreoni, A.A., Rytz, U., Vannini, R., et al. (2010) Ground reaction force profiles after partial and pancarpal arthrodesis in dogs. *Veterinary and Comparative Orthopaedics and Traumatology* 24 (1), 1-6.

Barnes, D.C., Knudsen, C.S., Gosling, M., et al. (2013) Complications of lateral plate fixation compared with tension band wiring and pin or lag screw fixation for calcaneoquartal arthrodesis: treatment of proximal intertarsal subluxation occurring secondary to non-traumatic plantar tarsal ligament disruption in dogs. *Veterinary and Comparative Orthopaedics and Traumatology* 26 (6), 445-452.

Bristow, P.C., Meeson, R.L., Thorne, R.M., et al. (2015) Clinical comparison of the hybrid dynamic compression plate and the castless plate for pancarpal arthrodesis in 219 dogs. *Veterinary Surgery* .44 (1), 70-77.

Calvo, I., Farrell, M., Chase, D., et al. (2009) Carpal arthrodesis in cats. *Veterinary and Comparative Orthopaedics and Traumatology* 23 (6), 1-7.

Clarke, S.P., Ferguson, J.F., Miller, A. (2009) Clinical evaluation of pancarpal arthrodesis using a castless plate in 11 dogs. *Veterinary Surgery* 38, 852-860.

DeCamp, C.E., Martinez, S.A., Johnston, S.A. (1993) Pantarsal arthrodesis in dogs and a cat: 11 cases (1983-1991). *Journal of the American Veterinary Medical Association* 203, 1705-1707.

Denny, H.R., Barr, A.R.S. (1991) Partial arthrodesis in the dog: a review of forty-five cases. *Veterinary Surgery* 10, 35-43.

Fitzpatrick, N., Yeadon, R., Smith, T.J., et al. (2012) Shoulder arthrodesis in 14 dogs. *Veterinary Surgery* 41 (6), 745-754.

Gorse, M.J., Earley, T.D., Aron, D.N. (1991) Tarsocrural arthrodesis: long term functional results. *Journal of the American Animal Hospital Association* 27, 231-234.

Guerrero, T.G., Montavon, P.M. (2005) Medial plating for carpal arthrodesis. *Veterinary Surgery* 34, 153-158.

Guillou, R.P., Frank, J.P., Sinnott, M.S., et al. (2008) In vitro mechanical valuation of medial plating for pantarsal arthrodesis in dogs. *American Journal of Veterinary Research* 69 (11), 1406-1412.

Guillou, R.P., Demianiuk, R.M., Sinnott, M.T., et al. (2012) In vitro mechanical evaluation of a limited contact dynamic compression plate and hybrid carpal arthrodesis plate for canine pancarpal arthrodesis. *Veterinary and Comparative Orthopaedics and Traumatology* 25 (2), 83-88.

Hoffer, M. Griffon, D.J., Schaeffer, D., et al. (2008) Clinical applications of demineralized bone matrix: a retrospective and case-matched study of 75 dogs. *Veterinary Surgery* 37 (7), 639-647.

Johnson, K.A. (1980) Carpal arthrodesis in the dog. *Australian Veterinary Journal* 56, 565-573.

Johnson, K.A., Bellenger C.R. (1980) The effects of autologous bone grafting after carpal arthrodesis in the dog. *Veterinary Record* 107 (6), 126-132.

McKee, W.M., May, C., Macias, C., et al. (2004) Pantarsal arthrodesis with a customized medial or lateral bone plate in 13 dogs. *Veterinary Record* 154, 165-170.

Meeson, R.L., Goodship, A.E., Arthurs, G.I. (2012) A biomechanical evaluation of a hybrid dynamic compression plate and a castless arthrodesis plate for pancarpal arthrodesis in dogs. *Veterinary Surgery* 41 (6), 738-744.

Muir, P., Norris, J.L. (1999) Tarsometatarsal subluxation in dogs: partial arthrodesis by plate fixation. *Journal of the American Animal Hospital Association* 35, 155-162.

Pozzi, A., Lewis, D.D., Hudson, C.C., et al. (2012) Percutaneous plate arthrodesis in small animals. *Veterinary Clinics of North America: Small Animal Practice* 42 (5), 1079-1096.

Roch, S.P., Clements, D.N., Mitchell, R.A.S., et al. (2008) Complications following tarsal arthrodesis using bone plate fixation in dogs. *Journal of Small Animal Practice* 49, 117-126.

Rothstock, S., Kowaleski, M.P., Boudrieau, R.J., et al. (2012) Biomechanical and computational evaluation of two loading transfer concepts for pancarpal arthrodesis in dogs. *American Journal of Veterinary Research* 73 (11), 1687-1695.

Whitelock, R.G., Dyce, J., Houlton, J.E. (1999) Metacarpal fractures associated with pancarpal arthrodesis in dogs. *Veterinary Surgery* 28, 25-30.

Willer, R.L., Johnson, K.A., Turner, T.M., et al. (1990) Partial carpal arthrodesis for third degree carpal sprains. A review of 45 carpi. *Veterinary Surgery* 19, 334-340.

Worth, A.J., Bruce, W.J. (2008) Long-term assessment of pancarpal arthrodesis performed on working dogs in New Zealand. *New Zealand Veterinary Journal* 56, 78-84.

109 Amputation

Maria Fahie

Western University of Health Sciences, College of Veterinary Medicine, Pomona, CA, USA

Limb amputation is performed relatively commonly in small animal veterinary practice. Indications for surgically planned amputation include bone or soft tissue neoplasia of an extremity, complicated fracture healing (malunion or nonunion), debilitating peripheral nerve damage, congenital deformity, severe arthritis, ischemic necrosis, and revision of a traumatic injury. Contraindications to limb amputation include any patient with a debilitating condition in its remaining limbs or with an obese body condition score that would impair a three-legged gait. Thorough orthopedic and neurologic examination of patients is highly recommended preoperatively. This chapter focuses on specific aspects of complications associated with limb amputation and onychectomy.

Tissue swelling

Definition

Swelling of an amputation site should be distinguished as hemorrhage, seroma, or cellulitis. Swelling caused by hemorrhage would be expected within hours of surgery and would result in a fluid pocket at the surgical site and possibly frank blood drainage from the incision. Swelling caused by seroma could occur at any point within the first 2 to 3 weeks after surgery. Fluid content should be serous or serohemorrhagic but not purulent. Swelling caused by cellulitis (Figure 109.1) could occur within the first 24 hours postoperatively or at any time in the healing process if infection developed. Cellulitis is a palpable firm swelling that may be edematous and does not have fluid pockets. General information about seroma and cellulitis can be found in Chapters 1 and 10.

Risk Factors

- Poor adherence to Halsted's principles of surgery, especially with regards to tissue trauma and hemostasis
- Trauma predisposing the proximal portion of the limb, near the planned amputation site, to ischemia
- Neoplastic or infectious process in the limb causing preoperative inflammation
- Extensive dissection of subcutaneous tissues
- Inappropriate hemostasis during muscle incisions and incorporation of muscle tissue rather than fascia in sutures
- Use of electrocautery or laser without appropriate control of thermal damage via lavage
- Inadequate protection and hydration of tissues exposed during surgery

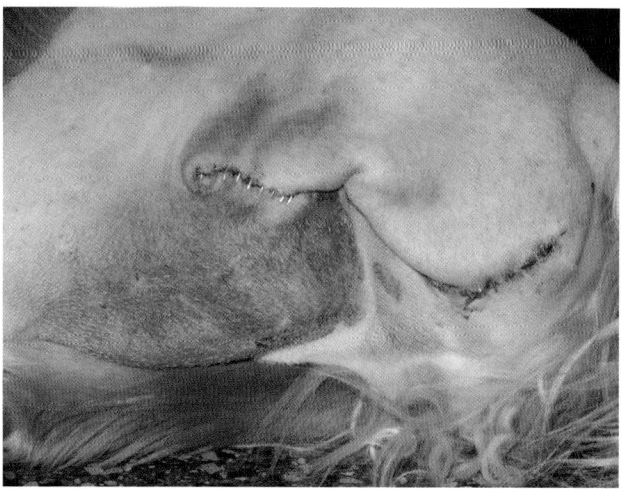

Figure 109.1 Postoperative swelling and erythema consistent with cellulitis. Appearance of the surgical area 2 days after amputation of a hindlimb in a golden retriever. *Source:* D. Griffon, Western University of Health Sciences, Pomona, CA, 2014. Reproduced with permission from D. Griffon.

- Distal location of the ostectomy, leading to excessive motion of the remaining bone within soft tissues
- Bone marrow hemorrhage, especially humerus or femur, when the medullary cavity is not occluded with Gelfoam or bone wax
- Skin tension during wound closure, usually caused by inappropriate location of initial skin incisions
- Compromised vascular supply to skin edges caused by overzealous suture placement, especially in patients already at risk for ischemia
- Inadequate elimination of dead space during closure
- Preoperative hypoalbuminemia or negative nutritional energy balance contributing to delayed wound healing
- Predisposition to intraoperative hypotension, electrolyte imbalance, or anemia in compromised patients (because the limb to be amputated contains a portion of total body fluids)
- Patients in which disease invades into pelvic bones and requires hemipelvectomy may be predisposed to incisional healing problems, postoperative pain, and slower return to function (Kramer et al. 2008). These complications have been attributed to the degree of tissue dissection and manipulation required for these procedures.

Complications in Small Animal Surgery, First Edition. Edited by Dominique Griffon and Annick Hamaide.

© 2016 John Wiley & Sons, Inc. Published 2016 by John Wiley & Sons, Inc.

Companion website: www.wiley.com/go/griffon/complications

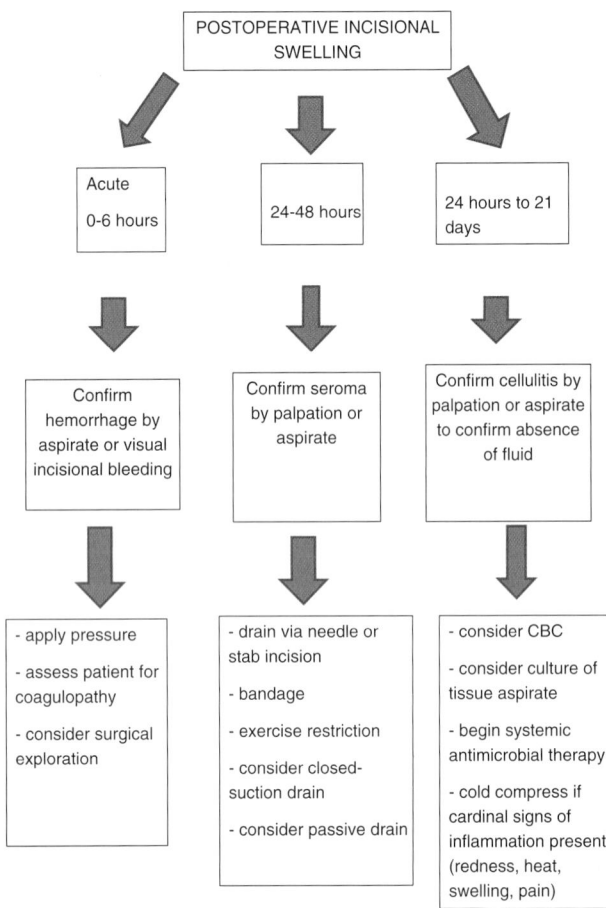

Figure 109.2 Algorithm for the diagnosis and management of swelling after limb amputation. CBC, complete blood count.

Diagnosis

The cardinal signs of inflammation include redness, heat, swelling, pain and loss of function (see Figure 109.1). Fine-needle aspiration (FNA) of the swelling allows samples for cytology and culture. An algorithm for diagnosis and management of postoperative cellulitis is proposed in Figure 109.2.

Treatment

- Appropriate medical management with antiinflammatory agents and antibiotics based on cytology and culture
- Cryotherapy (cold packing): Vascular constriction and reduced muscle spasm help control inflammation, edema, and pain in the acute postoperative phase (Clark and McLaughlin 2001; Davidson et al. 2005).
- Early postoperative recognition and management (see Figure 109.2)
- Placement of surgical drains should be considered in cases with seroma formation. Closed suction drains are preferred over passive drainage (Penrose drain); both types of drains should be covered by a bandage (tie-over [Figure 109.3] or body wrap) and managed appropriately to prevent ascending infection
- Consider emerging modalities in physical rehabilitation such as low-energy laser or extracorporeal shockwave therapy. Specific evidence on mechanisms and the ability to reduce pain may be published in the future as popularity increases in human medicine. These modalities may reduce pain, promote tissue repair, and stimulate cell metabolism and growth (Millis et al. 2005).

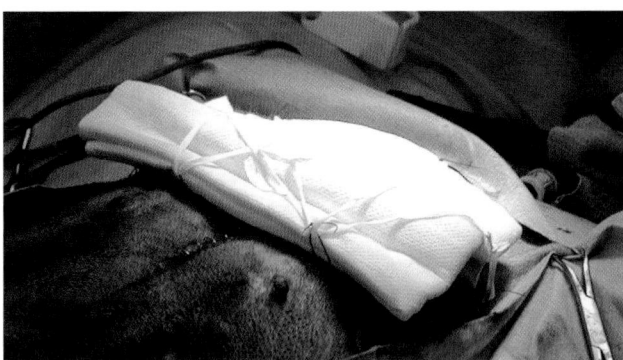

Figure 109.3 Tie-over bandage. This bandage is designed to protect surgical wounds located in areas prone to bandage slipping.

Outcome

The outcome is generally favorable, although surgical intervention (revision of the osteotomy, placement of drains) is occasionally warranted. Within discussion forums, there are reports of reexploration of amputation sites in order to identify and appropriately ligate bleeding vessels. Patient monitoring is important to determine whether hemorrhage warrants transfusion or other volume-expanding medical management.

Prevention

- Postpone surgery when possible for compromised patients and those with traumatized limbs (allow a minimum of 3–5 days posttrauma for the degree of devitalized tissue to be obvious).
- Meticulous intraoperative hemostasis, tissue handling, and wound closure should be ensured.

Strategies to improve hemostasis include:

- Minimize the amount of perivascular tissues incorporated to improve ligature security.
- Maintain a few millimeters between ligatures and a hemostatic forceps because the clamp keeps the vessel flat and may affect the tightness of the ligature.
- Avoid clamping thin-walled vessels to prevent iatrogenic tearing.
- Gentle perivascular tissue dissection helps expose enough vessel for placement of at least two appropriately spaced ligatures.
- During double ligation of vessels, the first ligature should be placed proximally on an artery and distally on a vein. This chronology facilitates the placement of the second ligature over a vessel that is not enlarged because of vascular occlusion.
- Consider the use of stapling devices, vessel-sealing devices, or a Harmonic scalpel if available.

Inappropriate level of amputation

Definition

Amputation of the thoracic limb has been described with scapulectomy or disarticulation of the scapulohumeral joint. The second option is less popular because of increased intraoperative difficulty, unnecessary weight carried by the patient, and prominent bony prominences secondary to muscle atrophy (Seguin and Weigel 2012). In the author's experience, scapulohumeral disarticulation is preferable in many patients because the incision is smaller and the amount of intraoperative tissue manipulation is reduced. **Videos 109.1 and 109.2** illustrate the motion of the scapula in both a small

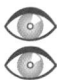

and large dog, which may be physically displeasing to owners. These videos also illustrate the level of postoperative muscle atrophy after 6 months in the large dog and 4½ years in the small dog.

Traumatic amputation of an extremity can occur in any level of the limb and does not necessarily require revision to the level described in textbooks. **Video 109.3** illustrates a cat with thoracic limb amputation performed with mid-diaphyseal humeral osteotomy when she was about 10 weeks old. Partial amputations can be in the best interest of patients presented on emergency basis or with a risk of sepsis. Revision can always be performed after the patient is stable if it is necessary based on the patient's gait and quality of life.

Amputation of the pelvic limb is usually performed either via coxofemoral disarticulation or femoral osteotomy midway on the diaphysis. The stance and gait of a cat after pelvic limb amputation by coxofemoral disarticulation are illustrated in **Video 109.4**.

A femoral osteotomy located too distal during amputation of a hindlimb can result in healing complications or disease recurrence. Limited soft tissue coverage of the bone generates tension on the skin and pressure on the remaining muscle. With the exception of coxofemoral and scapulohumeral disarticulations, complications are more likely to occur if the articular surface is left intact at the amputation site, particularly for digit amputation (Piermattei *et al.* 2006).

Risk factors
- Pediatric patient with traumatized limb
- Traumatic amputation necessitating emergent surgical exploration to stop the hemorrhage
- Disarticulation at joints distal to the hip or shoulder
- Excessive intraoperative periosteal stripping may contribute to ectopic bone formation.
- Significant preoperative muscle atrophy

Diagnosis
- Obvious protrusion of bone through an amputation site associated with skin irritation or signs of pain
- Diagnosis of recurrent or residual disease may require FNA for cytology and culture or biopsy for histopathology in patients in which neoplasia or infection were the cause for amputation.

Treatment
- Surgical revision of the amputation is preferred. An osteotomy is performed proximally, preserving all soft tissues to improve bone coverage. A file may be used if necessary to smooth edges.
- Myodesis (stabilization of distal muscles and fascia to the bone) and myoplasty (stabilization of dissected muscles to other muscles over the end of the bone) are used for human patients with distal limb or tibial amputation (Pasquina *et al.* 2006).
- Residual or recurrent disease requires appropriate medical or oncologic management.

Outcome
In surgical textbooks and within a discussion forum, revision surgery is reported to successfully resolve an inappropriate level of amputation.

Prevention
- Preoperative in-depth anatomic knowledge of limb vascular supply, bone, and musculature
- Preoperative planning of initial incision and type and location (Weigel 2002; Piermattei and Johnson 2004; Johnson *and* Dunning 2005; Piermattei *et al.* 2006; Fossum 2007).

Loss of function

Definition
Loss of function is delayed recovery or permanent loss of presurgical function and mobility.

Patients are generally expected to have adapted to their three-legged state within 4 weeks after amputation. Thoracic limb amputees generally adduct their remaining thoracic limb toward midline to compensate (**Video 109.5**). When moving more quickly and turning, they sometimes lose their balance and use their jaws to help regain control ("face plant") (**Video 109.6**).

Risk factors
- Concurrent neurologic disease or severe osteoarthritis in remaining limbs
- Lack of preexisting lameness (dogs or cats that are lame before amputation have already adapted to three-legged mobility; if the patient was not lame before, the adaptation period may be prolonged)
- Obesity
- Concurrent orthopedic or neurologic diseases affecting multiple limbs
- Owners' expectations for postoperative performance
- Postoperative pain or neuropathic pain
- Persistent lameness should be expected after amputation of digits 3 and 4 specifically because those are the primary weight-bearing digits.
- Lameness should be expected if more than two digits are removed.
- Recommendations regarding the level at which phalangeal (P) amputation of P1 or P2 should be performed varies; some sources recommend amputation via osteotomy, but others prefer disarticulation (Weigel 2002; Piermattei *et al.* 2006). In the author's opinion, removing the articular surface facilitates soft tissue closure over the bone.
- The size of the dog is not considered a risk factor based on surveys of dog owners regarding their impression of quality of life and speed of recovery

Diagnosis
Loss of function is generally diagnosed based on history (owners' observations) and orthopedic examination by the veterinarian. If available, serial gait analysis provides objective monitoring of the gait. Response to appropriate pain management can be diagnostic for the cause of immobility. Chewing at the surgical site of an amputated digit, tail, or limb can be an indication of pain.

Long-term loss of function in pets that made a full postoperative recovery should prompt a thorough orthopedic and neurologic examination of the remaining limbs. Further diagnostic work-up should be based on findings and may lead to consideration of treatment options if concurrent disease is confirmed (Figure 109.4).

Treatment
- Prosthetic devices are not considered standard of practice in small animals, as they are in human amputees; however, they are becoming available (Figure 109.5). Some of these consist of a socket (contacting the residual limb), pylon or shank (for structural support), and ground contact device (artificial paw) that are attached by a harness or suspension system with air or skin contact with silicone or urethane (Adamson *et al.* 2005).
- Postoperative rehabilitation: learning to stand and walk on three legs, then adapting to new center of gravity with walking on

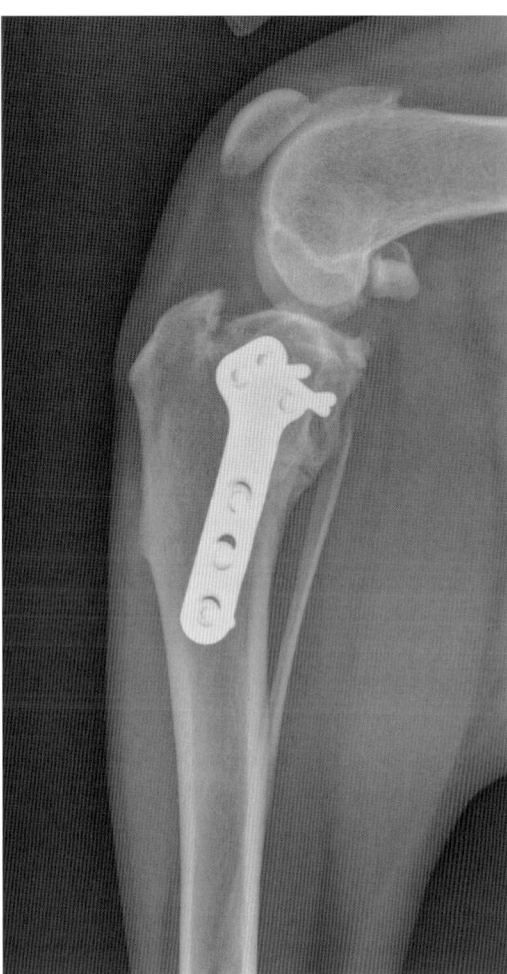

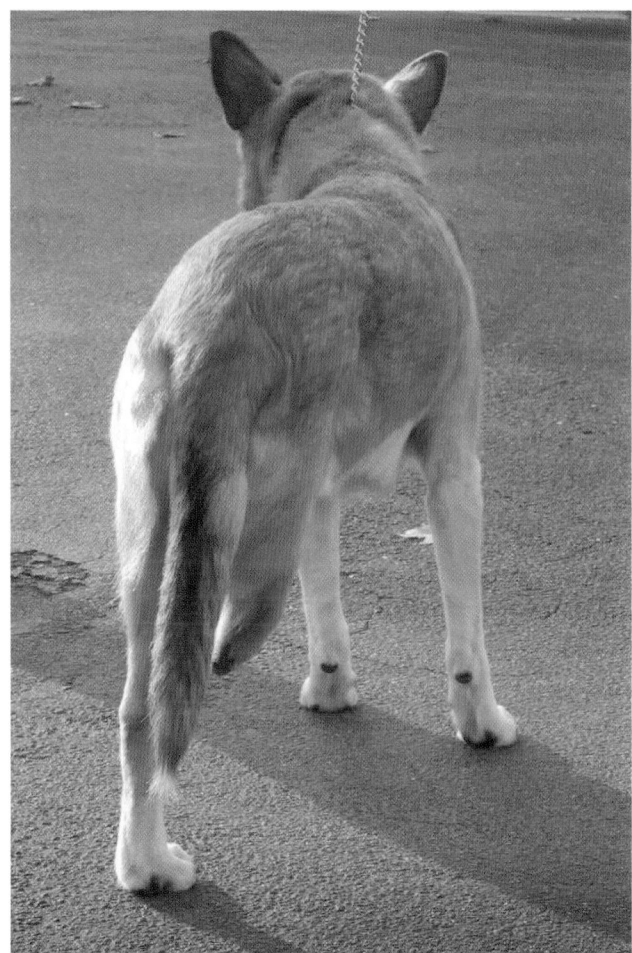

(A)

Figure 109.4 Radiograph obtained 12 weeks after tibial plateau leveling osteotomy (TPLO) in an amputee with cranial cruciate ligament disease. The large breed dog shown in Video 109.7 was referred 2 years after amputation of the right hindlimb for a sudden onset of an inability to walk. The dog was diagnosed with cranial cruciate ligament disease (CCLD) in the contralateral limb. A TPLO was selected for this patient to promote early return to a walk, and a locking plate was placed to improve fixation of the bone. *Source:* D. Griffon, Western University of Health Sciences, Pomona, CA, 2014. Reproduced with permission from D. Griffon.

uneven terrain, including sand or balance boards. Encourage full range of motion of joints proximal to the amputation site to prevent contracture (Davidson *et al.* 2005).

- Behavioral therapy, including owner's awareness, training, and potentially use of medications to appease the patient (Simpson and Papich 2003)
- Neuropathic pain management: massage, analgesics, dog-appeasing pheromone (DAP) diffuser, morphine–lidocaine–ketamine (MLK) administered as a constant-rate infusion (CRI), amantadine, acupuncture, ketamine CRI, topical capsaicin, gabapentin, fluoxetine (Mathews 2008)
- For conditions affecting the digits, follow surgical recommendations (Piermattei *et al.* 2006) and consider reconstructive procedures, such as fusion podoplasty (Pavletic 2010).
- Loss of function caused by disease in the remaining limbs may warrant surgical treatment. Examples include degenerative joint disease, elbow dysplasia, hip dysplasia, and cranial cruciate disease (see Figure 109.4 and **Video 109.7**).

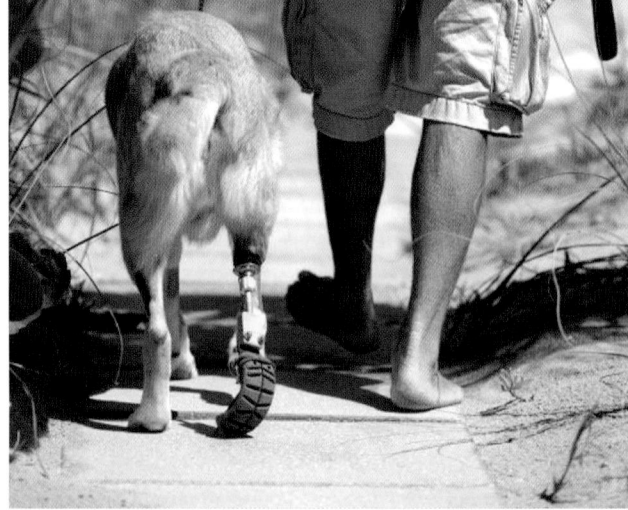

(B)

Figure 109.5 Preoperative (**A**) and postoperative (**B**) appearance of a canine amputee with a prosthetic limb. (Courtesy of Dennis Marcellin-Little, North Carolina State University College of Veterinary Medicine.)

Outcome

Appropriate identification of the cause for loss of function is a prerequisite to proper management. Owners of dogs with risk factors for poor function on three legs should be thoroughly informed of alternative options such as physical rehabilitation or limb-sparing procedures before amputation.

The prognosis after surgical treatment of diseases or injuries in the remaining limbs varies with the nature of the disease but can be excellent. However, these dogs may be predisposed to complications (reported for total hip replacements in amputees), and surgeons should tailor their management to anticipate earlier and higher mechanical loading of the implant (see Figure 109.4 and **Video 109.7**).

Prevention

Educating owners regarding patient's postoperative behavior and functional deficits combined with rehabilitation and pain management, is likely to improve the recovery phase and accelerate return to function in dogs when proper surgical technique has been applied.

- Consider palliative therapy rather than amputation if postoperative function is likely to be compromised and outweighs benefits (Liptak *et al.* 2004b)
- Consider limb-sparing or osseointegrating transcutaneous tibial implants for qualified patients at risk for poor postoperative mobility (Straw and Withrow 1996; Liptak *et al.* 2004a; Drygas *et al.* 2008; Fitzpatrick 2011).
- Advanced pre-, intra-, and postoperative pain management (see Chapter 14)
- Avoid neuroma formation.
  - Apply local anesthetic around or near but not directly into the nerve 5 minutes before incising if possible.
  - Plan the level of nerve incision proximal to that of the muscle and bone to avoid entrapment and excessive pressure.
  - Incise the nerve with minimal tissue crushing and trauma; use a tongue depressor to stabilize it before transection with a sharp scalpel blade.
  - Avoid including a nerve and a vessel in the same ligature; whenever possible, dissect the two structures apart.

Complications associated with onychectomy

Definition

Onychectomy refers to amputation of the claw of a digit. Because the claw develops from germinal tissue at the ungual crest of the third phalanx (P3), removal of P3 along with the claw is required to prevent regrowth of the claw after surgery. Therefore, the "declaw" procedure would more appropriately be termed a phalangectomy. Surgical techniques for declaw include scalpel blade dissection, carbon dioxide laser, and radiofrequency (RF). Deep digital tendonectomy is not currently recommended by the American Association of Feline Practitioners (2008). The procedure has not been shown to decrease postoperative complications compared with declaw (Swiderski 2002).

Early postoperative complications of declaw include pain, hemorrhage, lameness, swelling, and non–weight bearing. The complication most commonly mentioned on discussion forums is related to placement of postoperative bandages that are too tight. This can result in vascular compromise that can be severe enough to necessitate amputation of the limb.

Longer term postoperative complications include infection, regrowth of the claw, protrusion of P2, palmigrade stance (Figure 109.6), and prolonged intermittent lameness (Tobias 1994). Flexor tendon contracture has also been reported (Soiderer 2005).

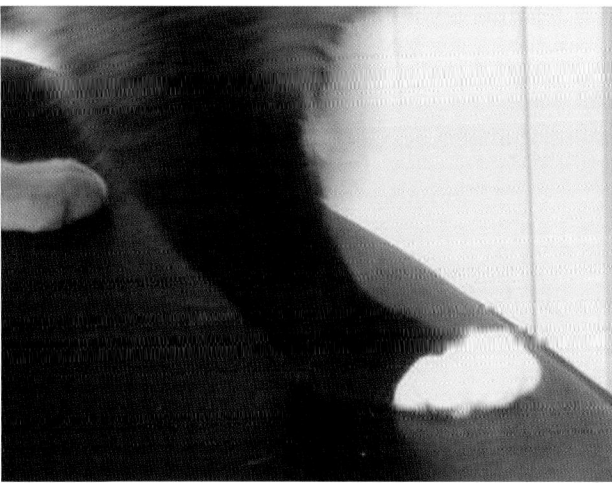

Figure 109.6 Palmigrade stance after onychectomy.

Risk factors

- Failure to remove the entire P3: presence of a bone fragment increases the risk of postoperative lameness, and remnants of ungual crest lead to regrowth of the claw
- Inappropriate wound apposition
- Presence of tissue glue within the subcutaneous tissues is a risk factor for foreign body reaction and infection.
- Inadequate postoperative pain assessment and analgesia
- Age: Older cats tend to exhibit more signs of postoperative pain than kittens.
- Surgical technique: Amputation with nail clippers is more likely to result in incomplete excision is the blade is not accurately placed through the palmar aspect of the interphalangeal joint.
- Ischemia of the limb caused by intraoperative application of the tourniquet
- Ischemia of the limb caused by inappropriate bandaging

Diagnosis

Wound dehiscence and infection can be observed grossly. Regrowth of P3 or protrusion of P2 can occur months after declaw surgery and result in lameness. Ischemic limb injury is usually evident within the first 24 hours postoperatively when limb swelling or pain is evident grossly. Postoperative pain assessment is challenging in cats; general principles are discussed in Chapter 14, but signs associated specifically with declaw include cats lying on their sides, rather than sternal, and absence of grooming.

Radiographs can be used to confirm the presence of remaining or protruding bone.

Treatment

- Regrowth of P3 requires revision surgery to remove the fragment.
- Protrusion of P2 may require revision surgery with amputation of additional phalanges in that digit to provide adequate tissue for appropriate wound apposition to prevent dehiscence.
- Infection and wound dehiscence should be treated as described in Chapters 1 and 9, and with digital lesions, wound soaking is easier to perform.
- Appropriate multimodal analgesia and pain assessment should be used.
- Reliable methods to manage limb ischemia are not reported in the veterinary literature; however, use of massage and warm therapy

may enhance vasodilation and circulation, and Epsom salt soaks may reduce limb swelling.

Outcome

With appropriate choice of technique and application of multimodal analgesia, declaw can be performed without complication. Revision surgery can successfully resolve regrowth and protrusion.

Prevention

- Use of a carbon dioxide laser may prevent complications, alleviating the need for a tourniquet (thereby reducing risks of neuropraxia and limb swelling from the pressure of the tourniquet compromising nerves and blood vessels) and reducing the need for postoperative bandages (which eliminates the chance of bandage related complications).
- Use scalpel blade dissection if carbon dioxide laser not available or the technique not mastered.
- Avoid tissue adhesive within the wound.
- Avoid tourniquet and bandage application.
- Administer multimodal analgesic therapy for appropriate duration (at least 2 weeks).

Relevant literature

Complication rates associated with amputation are not well documented in the veterinary literature. Most complications of limb amputation are reported anecdotally in forums such as the Veterinary Information Network (VIN; http://www.vin.com) and most commonly report **physical complications**. These include hemorrhage, wound dehiscence, infection, seroma, recurrence of disease at the stump, and loss of function.

Some of these complications may result from **inadequate soft tissue coverage** of the bone or inappropriate level of amputation (Weigel 2002; Fossum 2007; Seguin and Weigel 2012). These patients have poor wound healing or chronic incisional pain as a result. Recommendations for management of surgical site infection and seroma are described in Chapter 1. Surgical options for distal extremity reconstruction for amputated or traumatized digits, and use of tie-over bandages and drains, which are all relevant to amputation wounds are also described in textbooks (Campbell 2006; Pavletic 2010). Specific complications of digit amputation are mostly associated with wound healing, exposed bone, and persistent postoperative lameness depending on which digits are amputated. The increased load of weight-bearing nature on digits 3 and 4 may exacerbate healing complications (Muir and Pead 1998; Liptak et al. 2005; Pavletic 2010). In a subjective comparison of declaw techniques, carbon dioxide laser (0.25-mm tip, 1–2 mm away from tissue, 3–6 W continuous) and RF (cutting setting for skin; blended setting for remainder) resulted in similar healing based on histology. However, postoperative hemorrhage necessitating placement of a bandage was more common in the RF group (Burns 2010). Apposition of the wound after removal of P3 can be performed using tissue adhesive or suture material. No evidence clearly establishes the superiority of one method over the other. Closure with tissue adhesives seems to predispose cats to postoperative inflammation and infection, especially if the adhesive penetrates subcutaneous tissues. These complications are less likely when suture material is used to apposed skin edges but is more time consuming. Based on her clinical experience, the author recommends closure with 4-0 polyglactin 910 (Vicryl).

Return to function as a pet after amputation is generally excellent in patients with normal function of the three remaining limbs and proper level of amputation. However, the primary literature emphasizes the benefit of detailed preoperative communication with the owner regarding surgical goals, anticipated prognosis, short- and long-term postoperative care, and outcome expectations (Kirpensteijn et al. 1999; Forster et al. 2010). Owners' perception of the value of amputation for their pets, factors that influenced their decision, and the effects of amputation on their pets' quality of life and adaptation abilities were evaluated in a phone survey of 44 owners of canine amputees (Kirpensteijn et al. 1999). Nineteen of 22 owners stated that their initial reluctance to amputation for cosmetic reasons was unfounded. Thirty-three of 44 owners said that the recovery period was shorter than anticipated. In another study, 89% of 204 cat owners believed their pets regained a normal quality of life, and 94% reported they would make the same decision for amputation if recommended for another pet. Most of the cats were young males with pelvic limb amputation due to trauma (Forster et al. 2010). Ground reaction forces measured after amputation indicate that dogs adapt by reducing the amount of time they load their remaining limbs without increasing their gait velocity, thereby increasing the rhythm of their leg movement (cadence) (Kirpensteijn et al. 2000). After forelimb amputation, dogs have reduced braking ability, making it more difficult for them to keep their balance. Use of a harness when walking may therefore be helpful. Dogs with hindlimb amputation may have difficulties propelling themselves to gain speed. Prosthetics may be considered in dogs with unsatisfactory postoperative function or amputees with concurrent diseases of remaining limbs. Internet access provides a wealth of video resources (e.g., YouTube at http://www.youtube.com) for tibial implants and prosthetic limbs in dogs and cats. Several companies offer prostheses (My Pet's Brace at http://www.mypetsbrace.com or Animal Ortho Care at http://www.animalorthocare.com), and some clinical research has focused on the development of osseointegrating limb implants (Fitzpatrick 2011).

Loss of function in amputees may be associated with disease affecting the remaining limb(s). Treatment of injury or disease in the contralateral remaining limb has been reported in small animals, including total hip replacement, femoral head ostectomy (FHO), and shoulder luxation repair (Preston et al. 1999; Carpenter et al. 1996; Burton and Owen 2007). Total hip arthroplasty has been evaluated in nine dogs with pelvic limb amputations; seven of them ultimately had good or excellent results. However, five dogs required revision surgeries because of implant luxation, and the complication rate was high at 56% (Preston et al. 1999). FHO has also been performed on the contralateral limb of a 6-month-old shepherd dog treated with left pelvic limb amputation by disarticulation at 6 weeks of age because of quadriceps contracture and left coxofemoral luxation. The right coxofemoral joint developed arthritis, which caused significant pain before the FHO. The dog's quality of life after surgery was reported acceptable because he was able to walk up to 3 miles daily and run without apparent pain for 4 more years (Carpenter et al. 1996). Discussion boards on VIN mention cases of contralateral hind limb cruciate ligament injuries treated with tibial plateau leveling osteotomy and traditional extracapsular stabilization. With regards to the forelimbs, a case report describes an 8-year-old Whippet with right thoracic limb amputation and a subsequent lateral luxation of the contralateral shoulder. Surgical management included bicipital tendon transposition, modified Campbell scapulohumeral encircling prosthesis, and a novel body cast spica splint, eventually leading to a successful outcome (Burton and Owen 2007).

Postoperative neuropathic pain or altered behavior can contribute to loss of function. Owners perceiving postoperative pain in their pets tend to find their recovery to a good quality of life prolonged. Neuropathic pain may present as sporadic episodes of aggression or excitability (Mathews 2008). Neuropathic pain after amputation is initiated or caused by a primary lesion to the nerve. Phantom limb pain (PLP) is a form of neuropathic pain. PLP is not definitively documented in dogs and cats, but some evidence supports the potential for amputated rats to experience pain memory (Forster et al. 2010). PLP is believed to result from injury to peripheral nerves with central sensitization and changes in the cortical recognition of pain and sensation. Patients with severe preoperative pain could be predisposed to postoperative neuropathic or PLP.

The ability to identify and quantify pain in veterinary patients remains a challenge in diagnosing and monitoring pain after amputation. For example, altered grooming habits are considered a potential pain indicator in cats. However, overgrooming and lack of grooming are both known to occur because of stress without surgery in cats (Mathews 2008; Forster et al. 2010). A case report describes neuropathic pain and sciatic neuroma in a 2-year-old cat after midfemoral amputation because of sciatic nerve entrapment during a femoral fracture repair. This cat exhibited two episodes of inappropriate urination and pain at the amputation surgical site 1 and 2 months after surgery (O'Hagan 2006). Resolution was eventually obtained of intensive treatment, including hospitalization for administration of MLK at a CRI for 37 hours followed by sublingual administration of buprenorphine and oral administration of amitriptyline for 21 days.

General management of **postoperative pain** is discussed in Chapter 14. Two randomized controlled studies specifically reported on pain management protocols for routine intra- and postoperative use during amputation (Wagner et al. 2002, 2010). The earlier study included 27 dogs undergoing thoracic limb amputation and found a significant improvement in postoperative pain scores at 12 and 18 hours and improved mobility at 3 days after surgery when fentanyl was administered as a 5–mg/kg bolus preoperatively and then as a CRI of 10 µg/kg/min intraoperatively and 2 µg/kg/min for 18 hours after surgery. The second study compared administration of gabapentin preoperatively (10 mg/kg orally [PO] once) and postoperatively (5 mg/kg PO twice a day) for 3 days but did not detect a significant improvement in pain scores compared with a placebo group. In addition to systemic analgesia, wound soaker catheters have become commercially available to allow local administration of analgesics in amputation wounds. Local analgesia provided via these diffusion catheters versus 5-Fr red rubber catheter modified with 20-gauge needle holes was assessed in 52 dogs and 2 cats (Abelson et al. 2009). Dogs received CRIs of 2% lidocaine at 3.5 to 6 mL/hr (~2 mg/kg/hr), and cats received a 0.5% bupivacaine bolus (1–1.5 mg/kg) every 6 hours. Complications included one case of suspected lidocaine neurotoxicity as exhibited by ataxia and tremors. Signs resolved after the infusion was discontinued. Catheter disconnection occurred in four cases, three of which occurred with the modified red rubber catheters.

Postoperative pain resulting from the declaw procedure in cats has been described with subjective and objective methods when comparing surgical techniques and pain management protocols. A study comparing declaw methods with subjective assessment found that cats lying on their sides, rather than sternal, and absence of grooming were consistent signs of postoperative pain (Cloutier 2005). The use of a visual analog scale and response to palpation of the paw are recommended as the optimal subjective methods

to assess postoperative pain for declaw. Measures of plasma cortisol and β-endorphin levels were not accurate (Cambridge 2000). Pain after the declaw procedure is best managed with multimodal analgesia. A study found no difference in subjective indicators of pain in cats receiving a four-point bupivacaine block in addition to systemic buprenorphine (Curcio 2006). Another subjectively assessed study reported a significant improvement in postoperative pain scores when meloxicam was administered preoperatively subcutaneously in addition to systemic butorphanol administration (Carroll 2005).

Postoperative lameness after declaw is generally assessed based on orthopedic examination. However, gait analysis via force plate and pressure walkway systems has been used to provide objective comparisons between techniques and analgesics (Romans et al. 2004, 2005; Robinson 2007). In a pressure walkway analysis, gait characteristics did not differ between 26 cats declawed at least 6 months before the study and cats without declaw (Romans et al. 2004). Improvement of peak vertical force within the first 12 days after declaw was greater when the procedure was performed with carbon dioxide laser compared with scalpel dissection (Robinson 2007). Serial monitoring of peak vertical force after declaw was also used to demonstrate that the administration of transdermal fentanyl or intramuscular butorphanol was superior than sole topical bupivacaine. However, when the peak vertical force of all operated cats in that study was considered, the gait remained abnormal at 12 days after surgery, emphasizing the recommendation for long-term analgesics after declaw (Romans et al. 2005).

Nonphysical complications include behaviors such as anxiety and depression. They may be more prominent in human amputees than in animals. The only published evidence that veterinary patients may experience nonphysical consequences of amputation consists of two studies documenting altered behavior that could be attributed to anxiety in canine amputees (Kirpensteijn 1999; Shepherd 1999). The behaviors included increased aggression (6 of 44 dogs), increased anxiety (5 of 44 dogs), increased submissiveness or reduced dominance (2 of 44 dogs), and lack of interest in other dogs (1 of 44). As a surgical procedure, amputation is generally associated with anxiety and negative connotations by owners, who assume that impairment of function is inevitable. In many situations, the recommendation to perform amputation is based on the diagnosis of a condition that is associated with a very poor prognosis, such as appendicular osteosarcoma. The potential for compromised long-term survival contributes to the negative feelings associated with amputation. Owners contemplating or having experienced amputation of their pets' limb can easily communicate online (e.g., Tripawds at http://www.tripawds.com). This can greatly enhance owners' confidence in their decision-making process and during the postoperative recovery period. It is important to remember that amputation can provide ideal palliative relief of pain. An advantage of amputation in animals compared with humans consists in animals' natural capability to adapt in order to survive. Animals are not concerned about their cosmetic appearance, although they may behave differently after amputation if their stature in their environment is altered. Positive consequences of amputation may include pain relief, enhanced human–animal bond, improved mobility if the limb was dysfunctional before surgery, and increased life span in cases with non- or low metastatic neoplasia or osteomyelitis.

All videos cited in this chapter can be found on the book companion website at www.wiley.com/go/griffon/complications.

References

Abelson, A.L., McCabe, E.C., Shaw, S., et al. (2009) Use of wound soaker catheters for the administration of local anesthetic for post-operative analgesia: 56 cases. *Vet Anaesth Analg* 36 (6), 597-602.

Adamson, C., Kaufmann, M., Levine, D., et al. (2005) Assistive devices, orthotics and prosthetics. *Vet Clin North Am Small Anim Pract* 35 (6), 1441-1451.

American Association of Feline Practitioners. (2008) Position statement: feline declawing. *J Feline Med Surg* 10, XIV-XVI.

Burns, S.M., Howerth, E.W., Rawlings, C.A., et al. (2010) Comparison of the carbon dioxide laser and the radiofrequency unit for feline onychectomies. *J Am Anim Hosp Assoc* 46, 375-384.

Burton, N.J., Owen, M.R. (2007) Treatment of a shoulder luxation in a forelimb amputee dog. *Vet Comp Orthop Traumatol* 20 (2), 146-149.

Cambridge, A.J., Tobias, K.M., Newberry, R.C., et al. (2000) Subjective and objective measurement of postoperative pain in cats. *J Am Vet Med Assoc* 217, 685-690.

Campbell, B.G. (2006) Dressings, bandages, and splints for wound management in dogs and cats. *Vet Clin North Am Small Anim Pract* 36 (4), 759-791.

Carpenter, L.G., Oulton, S.A., Piermattei, D.L. (1996) Femoral head and neck excision in a dog that had previously undergone contralateral hind limb amputation. *J Am Vet Med Assoc* 208 (5), 695-696.

Carroll, G.L., Howe, L.B., Peterson, K.D. (2005) Analgesic efficacy of preoperative administration of meloxicam or butorphanol in onychectomized cats. *J Am Vet Med Assoc* 226, 913-919.

Clark, B., McLaughlin, R.M. (2001) Physical rehabilitation in the small animal orthopedic patient. *Vet Med* 96 (3), 234-246.

Cloutier, S., Newberry, R.C., Cambridge, A.J., (2005) Behavioral signs of postoperative pain in cats following onychectomy or tenectomy surgery. *Appl Anim Behav Sci* 92, 325-335.

Curcio, K., Bidwell, L.A., Bohart, G.V., et al. (2006) Evaluation of signs of postoperative pain and complications after forelimb onychectomy in cats receiving buprenorphine alone or with bupivicaine administered as a 4 point regional block. *J Am Vet Med Assoc* 228, 65-68.

Davidson, J.R., Kerwin, S.C., Millis, D.L. (2005) Rehabilitation for the orthopedic patient. *Vet Clin North Am Small Anim Pract* 35 (6), 1357-1388.

Drygas, K.A., Taylor, R., Sidebotham, C.G., et al. (2008) Transcutaneous tibial implants: a surgical procedure for restoring ambulation after amputation of the distal aspect of the tibia in a dog. *Vet Surg* 37, 322-327.

Forster, L.M., Bessant, C.M.C., Corr, S.A. (2010) Owner's observations of domestic cats after limb amputation. *Vet Rec* 167 (19), 734-739.

Fitzpatrick, N., Smith, T.J., Pendegrass, C.J., et al. (2011) Intraosseous transcutaneous amputation prosthesis (ITAP) for limb salvage in 4 dogs. *Vet Surg* 40, 909-925.

Fossum, T.W. (2007) Small Animal Surgery, 3rd edn. Mosby/Elsevier, St. Louis.

Fitzpatrick, N., Smith, T.J., Pendegrass, C.J., et al. (2011) Intraosseous transcutaneous amputation prosthesis (ITAP) for limb salvage in 4 dogs. *Vet Surg* 40, 909-925.

Johnson, A.L., Dunning D. (2005) Atlas of Orthopedic Surgical Procedures of the Dog and Cat. W.B. Saunders, St. Louis.

Kirpensteijn, J., van den Bos, R., Endenburg, N. (1999) Adaptation of dog to the amputation of a limb and their owners' satisfaction with the procedure. *Vet Rec* 144 (5), 115-118.

Kirpensteijn, J., van den Bos, R., van den Brom, W.E., Hazewinkel, H.A.(2000) Ground reaction force analysis of large breed dogs when walking after the amputation of a limb. *Vet Rec* 146 (6), 155-159.

Kramer, A., Walsh, P.J., Seguin, B. (2008) Hemipelvectomy in dogs and cats: technique overview, variations and description. *Vet Surg* 37, 413-419.

Liptak, J.M., Dernell, W.S., Ehrhart N., et al. (2004a) Canine appendicular osteosarcoma: curative-intent treatment. *Compend Contin Educ Pract Vet* 26 (3), 186-196.

Liptak, J.M., Dernell, W.S., Ehrhart N., et al. (2004b) Canine appendicular osteosarcoma: diagnosis and palliative treatment. *Compend Contin Educ Pract Vet* 26 (3), 172-182.

Liptak, J.M., Dernell, W.S., Rizzo, S.A., et al. (2005) Partial foot amputation in 11 dogs. *J Am Anim Hosp Assoc* 41 (1), 47-55.

Mathews, K.A. (2008) Neuropathic pain in dogs and cats: if only they could tell us if they hurt. *Vet Clin North Am Small Anim Pract* 38, 1365-1414.

Millis, D.L., Francis, D., Adamson, C. (2005) Emerging modalities in veterinary rehabilitation. *Vet Clin North Am Small Anim Pract* 35 (6), 1335-1355.

Muir, P., Pead, M.J. (1998) Chronic lameness after digit amputation in three dogs. *Vet Rec* 143 (16), 449-450.

O'Hagan, B.J. (2006) Neuropathic pain in a cat post-amputation. *Aust Vet J* 84 (3), 83-86.

Pasquina P.F., Bryant P.R., Huang M.E., et al. (2006) Advances in amputee care. *Arch Phys Med Rehabil* 87 (3), 34-43.

Pavletic, M.M. (2010) Atlas of Small Animal Reconstructive Surgery, 3rd edn. Wiley Blackwell, Somerset, NJ

Piermattei, D.L., Johnson, K.A. (2004) An Atlas of Surgical Approaches to the Bones and Joints of the Dog and Cat, 4th edn. W.B. Saunders, St. Louis.

Piermattei, D.L., Flo, G.L., DeCamp, C.E. (2006) Brinker, Piermattei and Flo's Handbook of Small Animal Orthopedics and Fracture Repair, 4th edn. Saunders/Elsevier, St. Louis.

Preston, C.A., Schulz, K.S., Vasseur, P.B. (1999) Total hip arthroplasty in nine canine hind limb amputees: a retrospective study. *Vet Surg* 28 (5), 341-347.

Robinson, D.A., Romans, C.W., Gordon-Evans, W.J., et al. (2007) Evaluation of short term limb function following unilateral carbon dioxide laser or scalpel onychectomy in cats. *J Am Anim Hosp Assoc* 230, 353-358.

Romans, C.W., Conzemius, M.G., Horstman, C.L., et al. (2004) Use of pressure platform gait analysis in cats with and without bilateral onychectomy. *Am J Vet Res* 65, 1276-1278.

Romans, C.W., Gordon, W.J., Robinson, D.A., et al. (2005) Effect of postoperative analgesic protocol on limb function. *J Am Vet Med Assoc* 227, 89-93.

Seguin, B., Weigel, J.P. (2012) Amputations. In: Johnston, K.M., Tobias, S.J. (eds.) Veterinary Surgery Small Animal. Elsevier Saunders, St. Louis, pp. 1029-1036.

Shepherd, K. (1999) Behavioral changes following hind limb amputation in dogs. *Vet Rec* 144 (7), 185-186.

Simpson, B.S., Papich, M.G. (2003) Pharmacologic management in veterinary behavior medicine. *Vet Clin North Am Small Anim Pract* 33, 365-404.

Straw, R.C., Withrow, S.J. (1996) Limb-sparing surgery versus amputation for dogs with bone tumors. *Vet Clin North Am Small Anim Pract* 26 (1), 135-143.

Soiderer, E.E. (2005) Bilateral flexor tendon contracture post declaw in 2 cats. *Can Vet J* 46, 244-246.

Swiderski, J. (2002) Onychectomy and its alternatives in the feline patient. *Clin Tech Small Anim Pract* 17, 158-161.

Tobias, K.S. (1994) Feline onychectomy at a teaching institution: a retrospective study of 163 cases. *Vet Surg* 23, 274-280.

Wagner, A.E., Walton, J.A., Hellyer, P.W., et al. (2002) Use of low doses of ketamine administered by constant rate infusion as an adjunct for postoperative analgesia in dogs. *J Am Vet Med Assoc* 221 (1), 72-75.

Wagner, A.E., Mich, P.M., Uhrig, S.R., et al. (2010) Clinical evaluation of perioperative administration of gabapentin as an adjunct for postoperative analgesia in dogs undergoing amputation of the forelimb. *J Am Vet Med Assoc* 236 (7), 751-756.

Weigel, J.P. (2002) Amputations. In: Slatter, D (ed.) Textbook of Small Animal Surgery, vol. 2, 3rd edn. W.B. Saunders, Philadelphia, pp. 2180-2185.

110 Limb-Spare Procedures

Jennifer Covey[1] and Nicholas Bacon[2]

[1]Pittsburgh Veterinary Specialty and Emergency Center, Pittsburgh, PA, USA
[2]Surgical Oncology, University of Surrey School of Veterinary Medicine, Fitzpatrick Referrals Oncology and Soft Tissue, Guildford, Surrey, UK

Osteosarcoma (OSA) is the most common canine primary bone tumor. Approximately 75% of cases occur in the appendicular skeleton, with the distal radius being the most common site. Therapy for dogs with OSA involves treatment of the primary tumor and adjuvant chemotherapy to control metastatic disease. Limb amputation is considered the standard of care for local tumor control and analgesia. However, dogs may be poor candidates for amputation if they have preexisting neurologic conditions or concurrent severe joint disease, and some owners are opposed to amputation. In these cases, limb-sparing procedures should be considered and may include radiation, surgery, or a combination of both.

Stereotactic radiosurgery (SRS) (Farese *et al.* 2004) and stereotactic body radiotherapy (SBRT) are promising and evolving limb-sparing techniques that can be considered for bone tumors in almost any appendicular location. Current limitations to these approaches include tumor size, extent of soft tissue involvement, and amount of cortical bone destruction at the time of treatment, as well as limited access to specialized equipment and facilities.

Surgical limb sparing is a more widely available option. Because appendicular OSA most commonly involves the metaphyseal region of the bone, surgical limb-sparing procedures typically entail arthrodesis of the adjacent joint. Tumors involving the distal radius have been considered the most amenable to limb salvage because function after limb-sparing and carpal arthrodesis has produced the most positive results. Limb-sparing techniques for mid-diaphyseal tumors of the radius, ulna, humerus, and tibia have also been described with favorable results (Liptak *et al.* 2004a). Current methods of limb salvage surgeries involving the scapulohumeral, coxofemoral, stifle, and tarsal joints are only recommended in exceptional cases when no other options exist because limb function after arthrodesis of these joints is often considered poor (LaRue *et al.* 1989; Kuntz *et al.* 1998; Morello *et al.* 2001).

This chapter focuses on complications after surgical limb sparing of the distal radius because this is the most commonly performed procedure.

Implant failure

Definition

Implants for limb-sparing surgery include any device used within the procedure to provide support to the limb, including the bone plate(s), screws, endoprosthesis, and allograft. Implant failure is defined as loss of fixation of the implant, which can be caused by loosening or breakage of the screws or bone plate or fracture of the endoprosthesis, allograft, or host bone.

Risk factors

The underlying etiology of implant failure for limb-sparing surgeries most commonly involves a combination of biologic and mechanical factors that lead to implant loosening or breakage over time.

Mechanical causes of failure include:
- Inappropriate implant size
- Insufficient implant fixation
- Cyclic loading at the host bone–endoprosthesis or bone–allograft interface

Biologic factors leading to failure include:
- Infection
- Compromised immune function secondary to neoplasia and concurrent use of chemotherapy
- Preoperative radiation therapy
- Patient comorbidities (obesity, preexisting sites of infection, concurrent endocrinopathies, severe neuropathy or arthropathy)

Diagnosis

History and clinical signs vary from the patient being relatively asymptomatic to an acute onset of non–weight-bearing lameness. Limb swelling varies with the magnitude of the implant failure and the implants involved.

Plain radiographs are most commonly used to diagnose implant failure (Figure 110.1). Advanced imaging (e.g., nuclear scintigraphy or whole-body computed tomography [CT]) may be considered to evaluate distant metastatic disease before repair.

Treatment

Implant failure does not necessarily require surgical intervention. Revision is not warranted in patients with minimal to no clinical signs and a stable implant. This is especially true for broken or loosening screws (Figure 110.2).

Surgery is only indicated if pain or lameness can clearly be attributed to implant instability.

Complications in Small Animal Surgery, First Edition. Edited by Dominique Griffon and Annick Hamaide.
© 2016 John Wiley & Sons, Inc. Published 2016 by John Wiley & Sons, Inc.
Companion website: www.wiley.com/go/griffon/complications

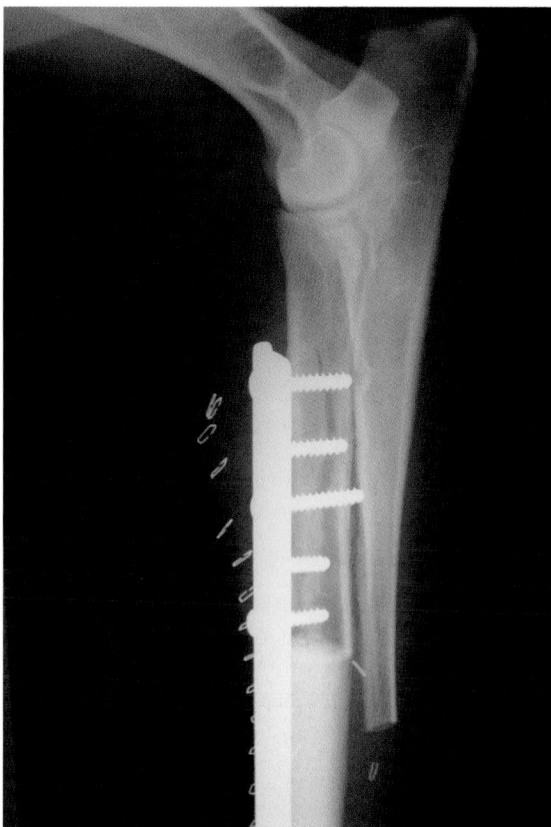

Figure 110.1 Implant failure after cortical allograft limb spare. Note the longitudinal fracture of the radius compromising screw fixation in the proximal segment of the radius.

Surgical repair can include a combination of the following options (Figure 110.3):

• Replace loose or broken screws with screws of a larger diameter.
• Place screws into adjacent bone (e.g., ulna) to improve placement in cortical bone.
• Replace the bone plate with one of a larger size.
• Move the bone plate to improve contact between screws and bone (e.g., placement over the fourth rather than the third metacarpal bone).
• Remove the implant(s) and replace with an external fixator.
• Supplemental fixation (e.g., external fixator or additional orthogonal bone plate) if the host bone has fractured.
• Amputation should be considered for catastrophic failure or for financial reasons.

Outcome

The prognosis for function of the limb after limb-spare revision should be good provided that the underlying cause of failure is suitably addressed. Owners should, however, be forewarned that infection should be expected after surgical revision of a canine limb spare.

Prevention

• Apply the plate as far proximally along the cranial aspect of the radius as possible.
• Limit surgical candidates to those with tumors involving less than 50% of radius.
• If considering endoprosthesis, use a 98-mm-long spacer (rather than the longer 122-mm version) whenever possible based on tumor size (a distance of 10–30 mm of grossly visible normal bone is recommended as the surgical margin).
• Aim for an ideal 80% coverage of the metacarpal bone and obtain a minimum of 50% coverage.

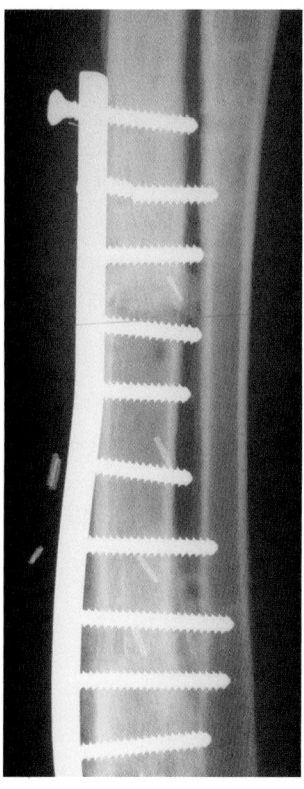

Figure 110.2 Stable implant with one broken and one loose screw.

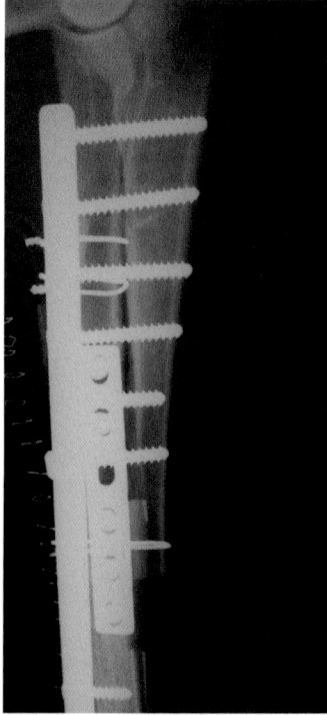

Figure 110.3 Radiograph after revision of the failed implant shown in Figure 110.1. Revision entailed replacement of proximal screws with screws engaging the ulna along with addition of cerclage wires and a mediolateral plate.

- Place the screws centrally in the metacarpal bone (either the third or fourth metacarpal can be used).
- If using an allograft, inject antibiotic impregnated polymethyl methacrylate (PMMA) into the medullary canal to reduce the incidence of screw loosening and allograft failure.
- Consider a locking plate or screws to improve torsional stiffness and increase resistance to pullout. (As a minimum, place a locking screw adjacent to the osteotomy and in the most proximal and distal holes.)
- Avoid empty screws holes at the bone–allograft or bone–endo-prosthesis interface.
- For large breed patients with radiographically thin cortices, a short proximal radial segment, and simultaneous excision of the ulna, consider adding a plate on the lateral surface between the radius and ulna.

Infection

See Chapter 8.

Definition

Although implant associated infection is described elsewhere in this book, it is appropriate to discuss limb spare–associated infection because it is the commonest postoperative complication. The infection rate for radial limb-sparing surgeries in veterinary medicine ranges from 30% to 70%, which is significantly higher than the rates reported for routine fracture repair, even those affecting the distal antebrachium.

Risk factors

The causative factors for the higher infection rate associated with limb salvage surgery are not fully understood. Infection has been attributed to:

- Extensive surgical resection, soft tissue dissection, and damage to the vascular and lymphatic supply

- Creation of dead space and reluctance to use indwelling active suction drains
- Long duration of procedure and anesthesia
- Implantation of large metallic endoprosthesis
- Implantation of large avascular cortical allograft
- Limited soft tissue coverage over the distal antebrachium
- Immunocompromise from neoplasia and chemotherapy
- Potential undiagnosed sources of infection from the skin, intestine, or urogenital system
- Concomitant use of radiation therapy

Diagnosis

Signs of infection can occur from a few days to a few months after surgery. It is more likely, however, that signs are seen 3 to 6 months after surgery.

Clinical symptoms commonly manifest as localized signs (Figure 110.4):
- Heat
- Pain or discomfort on manipulation
- Swelling
- Draining sinus tracts, commonly along the incision site. These can progress to exposed implants, typically at the level of the allograft or endoprosthesis.
- Lameness

Radiographic changes are variable:
- Bone resorption
- Periosteal bone proliferation
- Widening of the allograft–bone or endoprosthesis–bone interface
- Increased medullary density
- Soft tissue swelling
- Lucencies around implants, particularly screws (Figure 110.5)

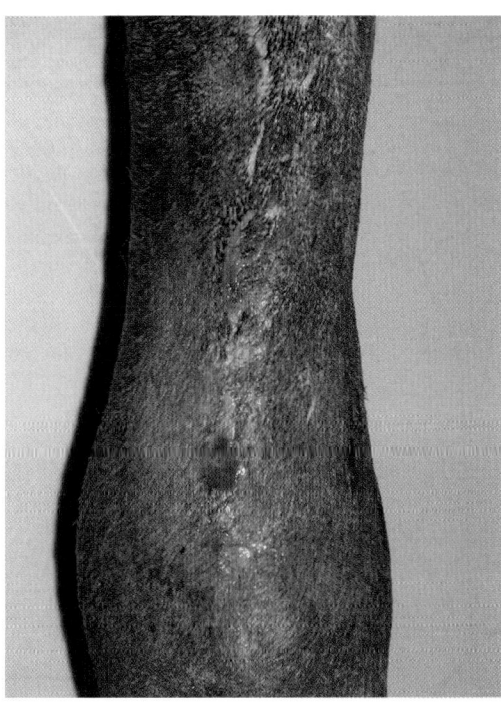
(A)

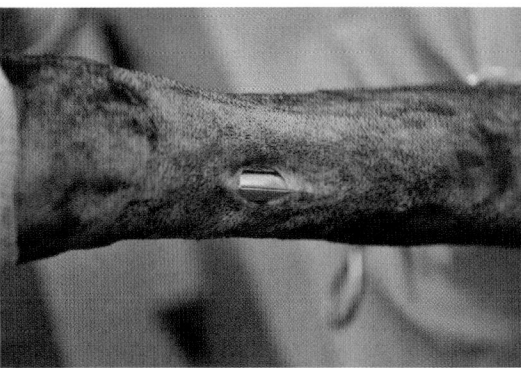
(B)

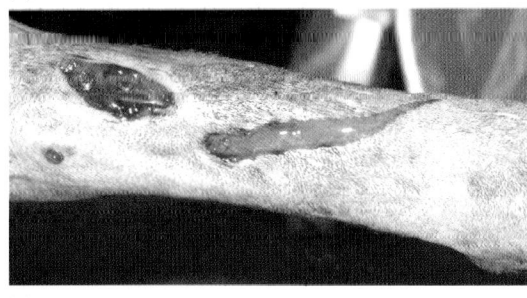
(C)

Figure 110.4 A, Common manifestations of infection can include a small draining sinus. **B**, Plate exposure with minimal drainage. **C**, Plate exposure with a copious volumes of purulent exudate.

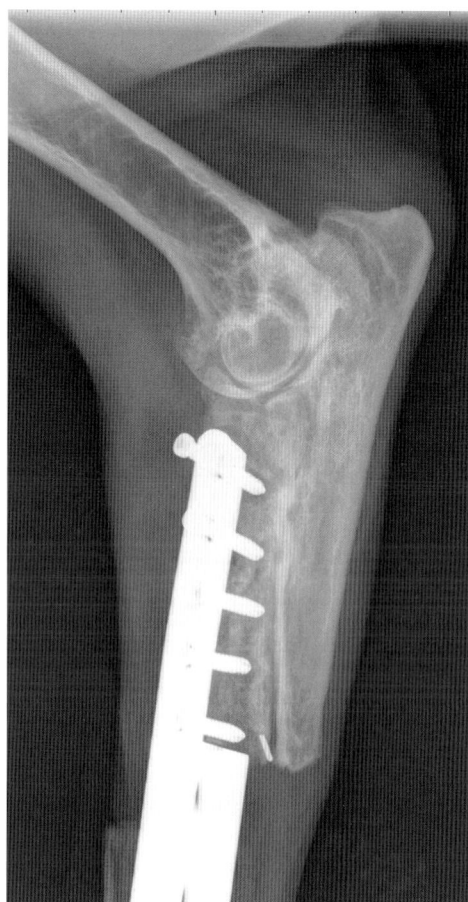

Figure 110.5 Radiograph of a dog with osteomyelitis along the proximal radius.

Treatment

The majority of patients respond, at least in the beginning, to systemic antibiotics. Initial treatment should consist of culture and sensitivity followed by appropriate antibiotic therapy. Any culture should be collected in a sterile fashion with anesthesia or heavy sedation, clip, sterile skin preparation, and surgical gloves. Infections are most often monomicrobial. The duration of treatment varies and is based on response to therapy. Patients with recurrent draining tracts or wound drainage may need either chronic or pulsatile antibiotic therapy.

Local therapy should be considered for infections refractory to systemic antibiotics. This can be achieved by use of antibiotic-impregnated PMMA beads, as well as isolated regional limb perfusion (Figure 110.6). Other novel carriers have been proposed as well, including calcium sulfate beads, absorbable gelatin sponges, plaster of paris, and R-gel. Use of negative-pressure wound therapy in conjunction with local delivery of antibiotics has also been helpful to decrease bacterial load in a handful of cases.

Judicious surgical debridement is indicated when draining tracts develop and implants become exposed because it is unlikely that these wounds will heal by second intention. Because of the lack of available skin, it is important to minimize the amount of skin removed so that primary closure is achievable. It is often necessary to use a releasing incision along the caudal antebrachium to close the primary wound (Figure 110.7). In extreme cases (cases refractory to more conservative debridement, large area of bone plate

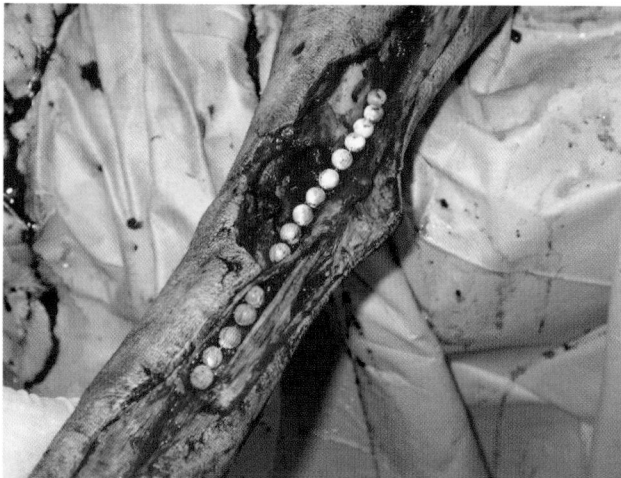

Figure 110.6 Placement of antibiotic-impregnated polymethylmethacrylate beads at the time of surgical debridement.

exposure, etc), wound closure may warrant use of a skin flap (e.g., distant direct, axial pattern flap, myocutaneous, microvascular free tissue transfer).

In the majority of cases, it is not possible to fully eliminate the biofilm-producing bacteria from the implant surface, and explantation of the infected implant(s) is required to remove the source of infection. However, doing so would require replacement with another implant, temporary implantation of a cement spacer with antibiotics, or amputation.

Outcome

Because of the challenge in eradicating biofilm-producing bacteria, infection is likely to persist in some capacity for as long as the limb is preserved. In some cases, the battle against infection will be daily,

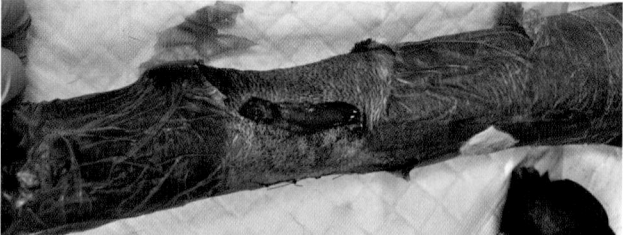

(A)

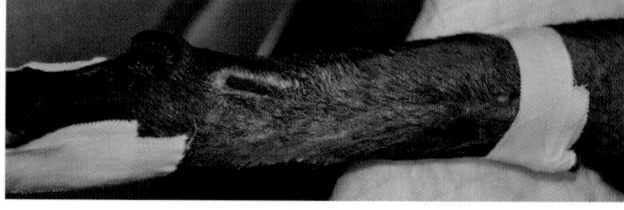

(B)

Figure 110.7 Skin closure during surgical management of an infected limb spare. **A**, A releasing incision allows closure of the primary wound. **B**, Two weeks later, the releasing incision has almost healed. (Photos are from the same dog shown in Figure 110.4B.)

requiring multiple bandage changes, additional surgeries, extended hospital stays, and long-term administration of antibiotics. Management of these patients can become extremely costly, sometimes more than the cost of the original surgery. It is important to counsel owners extensively on these risks before surgery.

Infection associated with limb-spare surgery for OSA has been documented to improve overall survival time in canine patients. Dogs with infection have been documented to live a median of 250 to 396 days longer than dogs without infection (Lascelles *et al.* 2005; Liptak *et al.* 2006; Thrall *et al.* 1990). The mechanism of action remains unclear; however, upregulation in cell-mediated or humoral antitumor activity has been proposed.

Prevention

A multitude of surgical techniques have been performed in an attempt to lower the infection rate seen with limb-sparing surgery, but thus far the answer remains elusive.

The use of a metal endoprosthesis instead of allografts was hoped to reduce the infection rate but without success to date (Liptak *et al.* 2006).

Lameness and limb function

Definition

The definition of limb function generally implies a return to normal activity, albeit after arthrodesis of the carpus. Subjective assessment of limb function after limb-sparing surgery of the distal radius has been good to excellent in up to 92% of cases. However, at this time, objective gait analysis is lacking to quantify the return to normal function after a surgical limb spare.

Risk factors

Loss of function after limb-sparing surgery and carpal arthrodesis is generally attributable to the other complications described in this chapter (implant failure, infection, local tumor recurrence); however, other causative factors can include temporary lymphedema and transient nerve palsy.

Diagnosis

The diagnosis is typically based on the owner's subjective assessment of function. Clinical signs may include:
- Lameness
- Soft tissue swelling
- Draining sinus tracts
- Pain on direct palpation
- Radial nerve deficits (walk on dorsal surface of paw caused by an inability to extend digits; hypoalgesia can be present if sensory branches involved)

Radiographic changes are often indicative of the underlying cause (implant failure, infection, local recurrence).

Treatment

Treatment involves delineating the causative factors and addressing them as needed. Lymphedema and radial nerve palsy are typically temporary and should resolve.

A multitude of pharmacologic agents are available to aid medical management of chronic pain in cancer patients (Gaynor 2008). A brief summary of options include a combination of any of the following:
- Opioids (dose depending on the drug selected)
- Tramadol: 2 ot 10 mg/kg every 6 to 12 hours as needed

- Nonsteroidal antiinflammatory drugs (dose depending on the formulation used)
- Bisphosphonates
  - Pamidronate 1 to 2 mg/kg diluted in 500 mL of saline, given over 2 hours
  - Can be given every 3 to 5 weeks
- Gabapentin
  - 2 to 10 mg/kg every 8 to 12 hours (Doses are extrapolated from human medicine; no evidence-based studies have been performed in dogs.)
  - Increases up to 50 mg/kg every 8 hours have been reported.
- Amantadine: 3 to 5 mg/kg once daily

Outcome

The outcome depends on the ability to successfully treat the underlying cause.

Prevention

- Appropriate case selection
- Careful soft tissue dissection to minimize trauma to lymphatics and nerves.

Local recurrence

Definition

Local recurrence is defined as regrowth of the neoplasm at the surgical site and is commonly the result of incomplete tumor excision or residual tumor cells remaining in the soft tissues after marginal excision. With limb-sparing procedures, the goal of surgery is to achieve a wide margin of resection. Wide margins may be achievable within the bone; however, within the soft tissue compartment surrounding the tumor, the surgeon is often working just outside of the tumor pseudocapsule, thus increasing the likelihood of leaving microscopic satellite disease behind. Local recurrence has been reported in 14% to 46% of distal radial surgical limb-spare procedures (Kent *et al.* 2004; Withrow *et al.* 1993). Time to recurrence in this location has ranged from 80 to 582 days after surgery (LaRue *et al.* 1989; Withrow *et al.* 1993; Morello *et al.* 2001; Morello *et al.* 2003; Liptak *et al.* 2004b; Ehrhart 2005; Liptak *et al.* 2006; Hodge *et al.* 2011).

Risk factors

- Invasion of tumor into surrounding soft tissues
- Incomplete surgical margins
- Skip metastasis: not reported in animals but documented in approximately 2% of human patients (Kager *et al.* 2006)

Diagnosis

Clinical signs
- Pain
- Lameness
- Soft tissue swelling
- Firm bony swelling

Radiographic signs
- Soft tissue swelling in the limb-spare site (early change)
- Proliferative or destructive bone change in the remaining section of radius
- Mineralized mass within the adjacent soft tissues at the ostectomy site

It can be difficult to differentiate infection from local recurrence; therefore, fine-needle aspirate or biopsy is recommended to confirm the diagnosis (Figure 110.8).

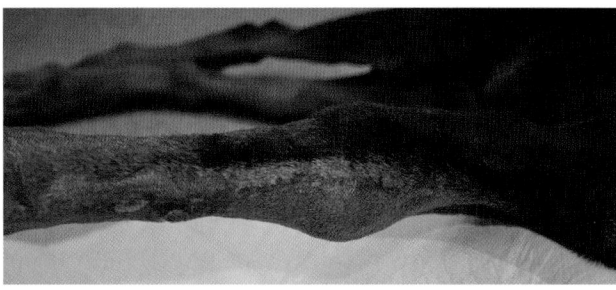

(A)

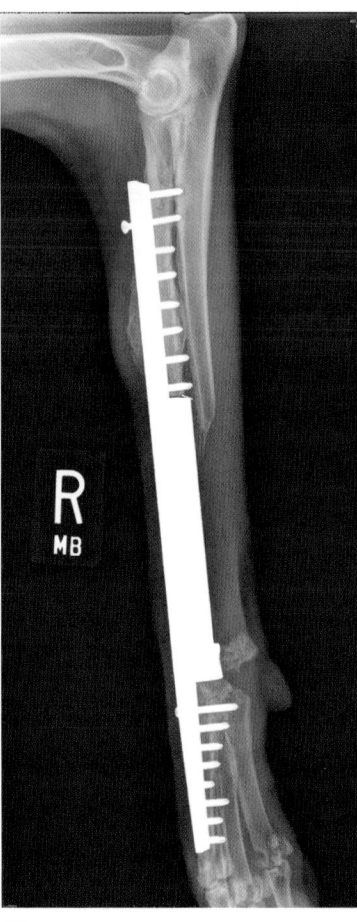

(B)

Figure 110.8 Local recurrence. **A**, Findings on physical examination. **B**, Radiographic appearance. Note the presence of draining sinuses along the incision site in **A**.

Treatment

Recurrence can be treated similar to the primary bone tumor, with amputation; limb spare; or palliative therapy, including radiation, bisphosphonates, and analgesics.

Outcome

Veterinary studies have shown conflicting evidence regarding local recurrence and outcome. However, based on extrapolations from human medicine, it is assumed that local recurrence has a negative effect on overall survival.

Prevention

- Use advanced imaging preoperatively to determine what surgical margins are achievable.
- Consider either neoadjuvant chemotherapy or local cisplatin delivery.
- Careful patient selection (caution owners of surgical technique, especially in dogs with large soft tissue component)
- Submit a marrow sample from the medullary canal of the remaining radius for histopathology to rule out sarcoma extension in the canal.
- Ink the osteotomized radial segment to help pathology determine the presence or absence of tumor cells at the specimen margin.
- Consider excising adjacent ulna to increase the excisable margin

Relevant literature (and comparative aspects)

Implant failure after surgical limb-sparing surgery of the distal radius occurs in up to 40% of cases with a median time to failure of 72 to 237 days after surgery (Liptak *et al.* 2004b, 2006). Limb-sparing surgery is unique compared with typical internal fixation fracture repair. With routine fracture repair, there are a finite number of cycles before the plate fails, and the objective of the repair is to achieve union before failure occurs (Gardner *et al.* 2009). Although studies have shown that allografts and irradiated autografts may incorporate into the host bone, this process typically takes years before providing sufficient stability to the repair and is therefore not relevant for most canine limb-spare patients, with a median survival time after curative intent treatment of 8 to 12 months. Unless a vascularized graft is used, it is generally accepted that the implant, whether allograft or endoprosthesis, essentially acts a spacer that provides stability to the repair.

Aseptic loosening is a common cause of implant failure after tumor resection and limb-sparing surgery in human medicine and may also contribute to implant failure in veterinary medicine. In humans, newer prostheses have been introduced, with a porous coating encouraging extracortical bone bridging and bone ingrowth. This process is enhanced by use of autogenous bone graft placed along the cortical bone–implant junction (Tanzer *et al.* 2003; Chao *et al.* 2004). Other methods to promote osseointegration, including use of bisphosphonates, hydroxyapatite, and growth factors (e.g., bone morphogenetic protein 7) have also been investigated with encouraging results (Fukuroku *et al.* 2007; Jakobsen *et al.* 2009).

Implant failure has not been identified as having an impact on survival in most studies. Interestingly, however, one study found a positive correlation of construct failure and survival. Dogs without construct failure were 17 times more likely to die of tumor-related causes. In this study, construct failure significantly increased the median survival time from 322 to 685 days (Liptak *et al.* 2006).

The infection rate of up to 70% after limb-sparing procedures is significantly higher than the rates reported for other implant-related surgeries. Infection after internal fixation of routine distal radial fractures is rare, reported in fewer than 1% of cases, even after multiple revision surgeries (Larsen *et al.* 1999). In humans, the rate of infection after limb salvage surgery ranges from 5% to 18%, increasing to 43% with revision surgery (Choong *et al.* 1996; Capanna *et al.* 2007; Myers *et al.* 2007). In both veterinary and human medicine, higher infection rates are seen in areas with limited soft tissue coverage. Use of vascularized muscle flaps has helped decrease the rate of infection in humans and has also been proposed as a strategy to decrease infection in dogs (Liptak *et al.* 2006). The use of silver-coated megaprostheses is also showing promise in reducing the infection rates associated with limb-sparing surgery in humans (Hardes et al. 2010).

Limb-sparing surgery in dogs has primarily been recommended for tumors involving the distal radius because function following carpal arthrodesis is good to excellent in the majority of cases. The outcome after allograft-arthrodesis in humans is considered less successful, with high complication rates and good functional results reported in only approximately 50% of cases (Muscolo et al. 2006). As a result, there has been an increasing trend for use of composite allograft–prosthetic composites, modular tumor endoprosthesis, and rotating hinge megaprostheses for reconstruction and joint replacement after limb salvage surgeries, with good to excellent function reported in most studies. The veterinary literature includes a case report describing excellent function after a custom allograft prosthetic had been used for treatment of a proximal femoral OSA (Liptak et al. 2005).

Local recurrence has been reported in 15% to 46% of dogs undergoing surgical limb salvage surgery. This is in contrast to human medicine, in which the local recurrence rate is less than 10%. The difference may be explained by the common use of intensive chemotherapy protocols before limb-sparing in humans to consolidate the tumor capsule and kill tumor cells in and around the pseudocapsule. Patients with greater than 90% necrosis after neoadjuvant chemotherapy are significantly less likely to develop local recurrence than those with less than 90% necrosis. The local recurrence rate has also been found to be lower in dogs in which a higher percent necrosis was attained preoperatively with neoadjuvant chemotherapy and radiation (Powers et al. 1991; Withrow et al. 1993). However, these protocols lead to increased costs, longer hospital stays, and more complications (Dernell 2003) and thus have been largely abandoned.

The completeness of the surgical margins has been shown to be prognostic for the development of local recurrence. Several studies have been performed to evaluate different diagnostic modalities and their reliability in identifying tumor margin. In human medicine, magnetic resonance imaging (MRI) is considered the gold standard for identifying intramedullary tumor extension, with an accuracy of 96% to 99%. In veterinary medicine, radiography, nuclear scintigraphy, CT, and MRI have all been evaluated. MRI appears to have less of a tendency to overestimate tumor length compared with the other imaging modalities (Wallack et al. 2002), although CT has also shown good correlation in predicting the extent of endosteal or intramedullary involvement (Karnik 2011). In addition to plain radiographs, it is currently recommended that either CT or MRI be used for margin evaluation before limb-sparing surgery.

Pathologic fracture associated with a primary malignant bone tumor has previously been considered a contraindication to human limb-spare surgery because it was postulated that fracture results in local hematoma formation, dissemination of tumor cells into adjacent tissue and between fascial planes; and damage to the microcirculation, facilitating metastasis, thus leading to reduced survival times (Scully et al. 2002; Ebeid et al. 2005). Recent evidence, however, suggests that limb salvage surgery for pathologic fractures provides similar long-term prognosis to amputation, and pathologic fracture is no longer considered a contraindication to limb salvage surgery in humans (Jeon et al. 2009). Two recent veterinary studies evaluated internal fixation of sarcoma-related pathologic fractures with evidence to suggest that treatment was technically feasible, alleviated pain, and led to a prolonged survival time in some dogs (Bhandal and Boston 2011; Boston et al. 2011).

Treatment for local recurrence has not been thoroughly evaluated in veterinary medicine. In humans, complete surgical excision of the recurrent disease is the only treatment modality with proven efficacy, and the benefit of adjuvant chemotherapy remains controversial (Ferrari et al. 2003; Bielack et al. 2009). The development of local recurrence has been reported to have a negative effect on overall survival in human patients, with a 5-year survival rate of 16%. In veterinary patients, local recurrence or incomplete margins at surgery has a negative to negligible effect on survival. A study by Kuntz et al. (1998) showed that completeness of surgical margins for limb-spare surgery of the proximal humerus was prognostic for the development of metastatic lesions and for overall survival, with patients 7.7 times more likely to develop metastatic lesions and 4.16 times more likely to die of tumor-related causes with incomplete margins. Liptak et al. (2006) found no significant difference in survival times with local recurrence (351 vs. 562 days); however, the ability to detect a statistical difference was only 14%. Withrow et al. (2004) found that survival time was significantly decreased with incomplete resection on univariate analysis but not on multivariate analysis.

Local slow-release chemotherapy, an open-cell lactic acid polymer containing 8% cisplatin (OPLA-Pt), has been shown to decrease the overall local recurrence rate. A randomized, prospective study of 80 dogs showed a reduction in the overall local recurrence from 30% to 16% for dogs that received OPLA-Pt (Withrow et al. 2004). At this time, however, OPLA-Pt is not commercially available. In 2009, a compounded cisplatin bead was released for treatment of equine skin tumors (Wedgewood Pharmacy, Swedesboro, NJ), but information regarding its efficacy for canine patients with OSA has not been performed. A recent study evaluated a novel localized delivery system for carboplatin. The system involves the subcutaneous administration of 300 mg/m^2 of aqueous carboplatin over a single hospital stay. Of the 17 cases evaluated, three had limb salvage surgery performed, with no local recurrence seen (Simcock et al. 2012).

References

Bhandal, J., Boston, S.E. (2011) Pathologic fracture in dogs with suspected or confirmed osteosarcoma. *Veterinary Surgery* 40 (4), 423-430.

Bielack, S., Jurgens, H., Jundt, G., et al. (2009) Osteosarcoma: the COSS experience. *Cancer Treatment and Research* 152, 289-308.

Boston, S.E., Bacon, N.J., Culp W.T.N., et al. (2011) Outcome after repair of a sarcoma-related pathologic fracture in dogs: a veterinary society of surgical oncology retrospective study. *Veterinary Surgery* 40 (4), 431-437.

Capanna, R., Campanacci, D.A., Belot, N., et al. (2007) A new reconstructive technique for intercalary defects of long bones: the association of massive allograft with vascularized fibular autograft. Long-term results and comparison with alternative techniques. *Orthopedic Clinics of North America* 38 (1), 51-60.

Chao, E.Y.S., Fuchs, B., Rowland, C.M., et al. (2004) Long-term results of segmental prosthesis by extracortical bone-bridging and ingrowth. *The Journal of Bone & Joint Surgery* 86-A(5), 948-955.

Choong, P.F.M., Sim, F.H., Pritchard, D.J., et al. (1996) Megaprostheses after resection of distal femoral tumors. *Acta Orthopaedica Scandinavica* 67 (4), 345-351.

Dernell, W.S. (2003) Limb-spring surgery for dogs with bone neoplasia. In Slatter, D. (ed.) *Textbook of Small Animal Surgery*, 3rd edn. Saunders, Philadelphia, p. 2275.

Ebeid, W., Amin, S., Abdelmegid, A. (2005) Limb salvage management of pathologic fractures of primary malignant bone tumors. *Cancer Control* 12 (1), 57-61.

Ehrhart, N. (2005). Longitudinal bone transport for treatment of primary bone tumors in dogs: techniques and outcome in 9 dogs. *Veterinary Surgery* 34, 24-34.

Farese, J.P., Milner, R., Thompson, M.S., et al. (2004) Stereotactic radiosurgery for treatment of osteosarcomas involving the distal portions of the limbs in dogs. *Journal of the American Veterinary Medical Association* 225 (10) 1567-1572.

Ferrari, S., Briccoli, A., Mercuri, M., et al. (2003) Postrelapse survival in osteosarcoma of the extremities: prognostic factors for long-term survival. *Journal of Clinical Oncology* 21 (4), 710-715.

Fukuroku, J., Inoue, N., Rafiee, B., et al. (2007) Extracortical bone-bridging fixation with use of cortical allograft and recombinant human osteogenic protein-1. *The Journal of Bone & Joint Surgery* 89 (7), 1486-1496.

Gardner, M.J., Evans, J.M., Dunbar, R.P. (2009) Failure of fracture plate fixation. *Journal of the American Academy of Orthopaedic Surgeons* 17 (10), 647-657.

Gaynor, J.S. (2008) Control of cancer pain in veterinary patients. *Veterinary Clinics of North America: Small Animal Practice* 38 (6), 1429-1448.

Hardes, J., Von Eiff, C., Streitbuerger, A., et al. (2010) Reduction in periprosthetic infection with silver-coated megaprostheses in patients with bone sarcoma. *Journal of Surgical Oncology* 101, 389-395.

Hodge, S.C., Degner D., Walshaw, R., et al. (2011) Vascularized ulnar bone grafts for limb-sparing surgery for the treatment of distal radial osteosarcoma. *Journal of the American Animal Hospital Association* 47 (2), 98-111.

Jakobsen, T., Baas, J., Kold, S., et al. (2009) Local biphosphonate treatment increases fixation of hydroxyapatite-coated implants inserted with bone compaction. *Journal of Orthopaedic Research* 27 (2), 189-194.

Jeon, D.G. (2009) Prognostic effect of pathologic fracture in localized osteosarcoma. *Asia-Pacific Journal of Oncology & Hematology.* 2 (1), 131-135.

Kager, L., Zoubek, A. Kempf-Bialek B., et al. (2006) Skip metastases in osteosarcoma: experience of the cooperative osteosarcoma study group. *Journal of Clinical Oncology* 24 (10), 1535-1541.

Karnik, K.S. (2011) Accuracy of computed tomography in determining lesion size in canine osteosarcoma of the appendicular skeleton. Masters thesis, The Ohio State University.

Kent, M.S., Strom, A., London C.A., et al. (2004) Alternating carboplatin and doxorubicin as adjunctive chemotherapy to amputation or limb-sparing surgery in the treatment of appendicular osteosarcoma in dogs. *Journal of Veterinary Internal Medicine* 18 (4), 540-544.

Kuntz, C.A., Asselin, T.L., Dernell, W.S., et al. (1998) Limb salvage surgery for osteosarcoma of the proximal humerus: outcome in 17 dogs. *Veterinary Surgery* 27 (5), 417-422.

Larsen, L.J., Roush, J.K., McLaughlin R.M. (1999) Bone plate fixation of distal radius and ulna fractures in small- and miniature-breed dogs. *Journal of the American Animal Hospital Association* 35 (3), 243-250.

LaRue, S.M., Withrow, S.J., Powers, B.E., et al. (1989) Limb-sparing treatment for osteosarcoma in dogs. *Journal of the American Veterinary Medical Association* 195 (12), 1734-1744.

Lascelles, B.D.X., Dernell, W.S., Correa, M.T., et al. (2005) Improved survival associated with postoperative wound infection in dogs treated with limb-salvage surgery for osteosarcoma. *Annals of Surgical Oncology* 12 (12), 1073-1083.

Liptak, J.M., Dernell, W.S., Lascelles, B.D.X., et al. (2004a) Intraoperative extracorporeal irradiation for limb sparing in 13 dogs. *Veterinary Surgery* 33 (5), 446-456.

Liptak, J.M., Dernell, W.S., Straw, R.C., et al. (2004b) Intercalary bone grafts for joint and limb preservation in 17 dogs with high-grade malignant tumors of the diaphysis. *Veterinary Surgery* 33 (5), 457-467.

Liptak, J.M., Pluhar, G.E., Dernell, W.S., et al. (2005) Limb-sparing surgery in a dog with osteosarcoma of the proximal femur. *Veterinary Surgery* 34 (1), 71-77.

Liptak, J.M., Dernell, W.S., Ehrhart N., et al. (2006) Cortical allograft and endoprosthesis for limb-sparing surgery in dogs with distal radial osteosarcoma: a prospective clinical comparison of two different limb-sparing techniques. *Veterinary Surgery* 35 (6), 518-533.

Morello, E., Buracco, P., Martano, M., et al. (2001) Bone allografts and adjuvant cisplatin for the treatment of canine appendicular osteosarcoma in 18 dogs. *Journal of Small Animal Practice* 42 (2), 61-66.

Morello, E., Vasconi, E., Martano, M., et al. (2003) Pasteurized tumoral autograft and adjuvant chemotherapy for the treatment of canine distal radial osteosarcoma: 13 cases. *Veterinary Surgery* 32 (6), 539-544.

Muscolo, D.L., Ayerza, M.A., Aponte-Tinao, L.A. (2006) Massive allograft use in orthopedic oncology. *The Orthopedic Clinics of North America* 37 (1), 65-74.

Myers, G.J.C., Abudu, A.T., Carter, S.R., et al. (2007) The long-term results of endoprosthetic replacement of the proximal tibia for bone tumours. *The Journal of Bone & Joint Surgery* 89 (12), 1632-1637.

Powers, B.E., Withrow, S.J., Thrall, D.E., et al. (1991) Percent tumor necrosis as a predictor of treatment response in canine osteosarcoma. *Cancer* 67 (1), 126-134.

Scully, S.P., Ghert M.A., Zurakowski D., et al. (2002) Pathologic fracture in osteosarcoma; Prognsotic importance and treatment implications. *TheJjournal of Bone and Joint Surgery* 84-A (1), 49-57.

Simcock, J.O., Withers, S.S., Prpich, C.Y., et al. (2012) Evaluation of a single subcutaneous infusion of carboplatin as adjuvant chemotherapy for dogs with osteosarcoma: 17 cases (2006-2010). *Journal of the American Veterinary Medical Association* 241 (5), 608-614.

Tanzer, M., Turcotte, R., Harvey, E., et al. (2003) Extracortical bone bridging in tumor endoprostheses. *The Journal of Bone & Joint Surgery* 85 (12), 2365-2370.

Thrall, D.E., Withrow, S.J., Powers, B.E., et al. (1990) Radiotherapy prior to cortical allograft limb sparing in dogs with osteosarcoma: a dose response assay. *International Journal of Radiation Oncology*Biology*Physics* 18 (6), 135-1357.

Wallack, S.T., Wisner, E.R., Werner, J.A., et al. (2002) Accuracy of magnetic resonance imaging for estimating intramedullary osteosarcoma extent in pre-operative planning of canine limb-salvage procedures. *Veterinary Radiology & Ultrasound* 43 (5), 432-441.

Withrow, S.J., Thrall, D.E., Straw, R.C., et al (1993) Intra-arterial cisplatin with or without radiation in limb-sparing for canine osteosarcoma. *Cancer* 71 (8), 2484-2490.

Withrow, S.J., Liptak, J.M., Straw, R.C., et al. (2004) Biodegradable cisplatin polymer in limb-sparing surgery for canine osteosarcoma. *Annals of Surgical Oncology* 11 (7), 705-713.

Surgery of the Coxofemoral Joint

111 Femoral Head and Neck Excision

Wing Tip Wong
WTW Veterinary Surgical Service, Melbourne, Australia

Femoral head and neck excision (FHNE) is a common surgical procedure performed to relieve pain and salvage limb function in a variety of conditions, including hip dysplasia, avascular necrosis of the femoral head, osteoarthritis of the coxofemoral joint from any cause, comminuted acetabular or femoral neck fractures, fractures of the femoral head, and chronic hip luxation (Piermattei *et al.* 2006).

Reports of complications associated with FHNE have mainly focused on poor use of the limb (Gendreau and Cawley 1977; Off and Matis 2010). The most common cause proposed for this complication involves bone-to-bone contact between the femur and the acetabulum (Berzon *et al.* 1980; Lewis *et al.* 1988; Lippincott 1992) resulting from inadequate removal of the femoral neck. Other proposed reasons for this loss of function include biomechanical restriction from a poor pseudoarthrosis, body weight, and preexisting muscle atrophy. The other occasionally reported complication after FHNE consists of sciatic nerve entrapment (Walker 1981; Jeffery 1993; Liska *et al.* 2010). Fracture of the proximal femur involving the greater trochanter or down the femoral shaft was described as a possible complication from the use of an osteotome and mallet in osteoporotic bone and in traumatic fractures with unrecognized fissures (Berzon *et al.* 1980).

Fracture of the proximal femur

Definition
Fractures of the proximal femur generated during osteotomy of the femoral neck may involve the greater trochanter and proximal metaphysis or diaphysis of the femur.

Risk factors
- Poor exposure
- Existing pathology such as osteoporosis, unrecognized fissures, and severe end-stage osteoarthritis obscuring anatomy
- Poor plane of osteotomy
- Failure to disarticulate the hip
- Inappropriate equipment to perform osteotomy

Diagnosis
Clinical findings of pain and lameness may resemble the postoperative morbidity seen with the procedure. Crepitus is usually indicative of a problem.

Radiography provides the definitive diagnosis (Figure 111.1).

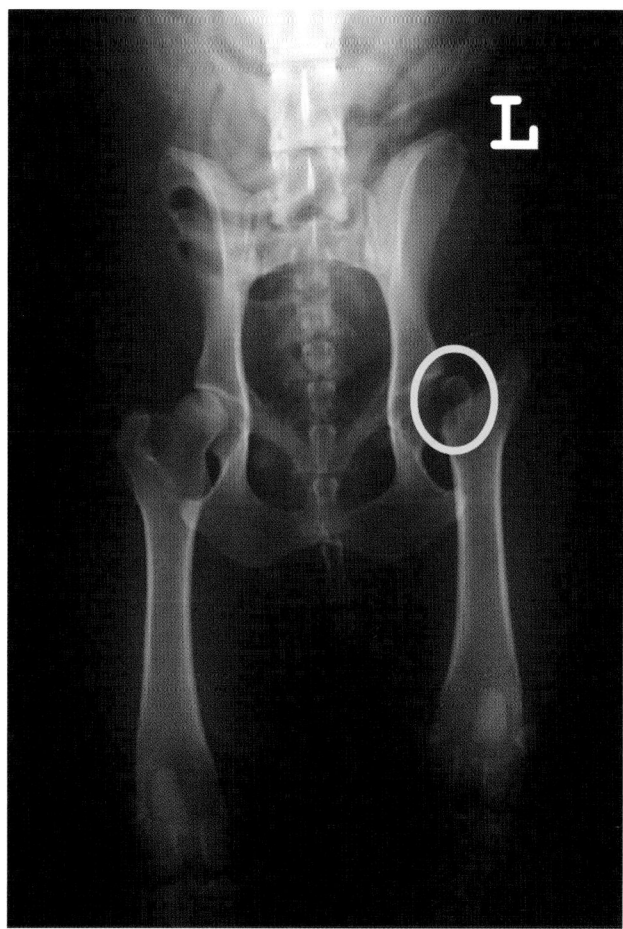

Figure 111.1 Fracture of the greater trochanter (circled) noted in a postoperative radiograph after a femoral head and neck excision.

Treatment
Fractures in the greater trochanter where the fragment is of a sufficient size and includes attachment of tendons should be reduced and repaired with pins and tension band wire. Smaller fragments that are not associated with tendon attachment may be removed.

Fractures in the proximal metaphysis or diaphysis running parallel to the long axis of the femur can be repaired with cerclage wires. Fractures running in a transverse plane can be repaired with a plate.

Complications in Small Animal Surgery, First Edition. Edited by Dominique Griffon and Annick Hamaide.
© 2016 John Wiley & Sons, Inc. Published 2016 by John Wiley & Sons, Inc.
Companion website: www.wiley.com/go/griffon/complications

Outcome

The outcome is generally favorable because the fractures are associated with low-energy and mild soft tissue trauma and are usually repaired immediately. Fractures at the greater trochanter or those occurring in osteoporotic bone may result in delayed healing or develop into a nonunion.

Prevention

- Obtain current preoperative radiographs to appreciate existing bone changes.
- Use an approach that provides good visualization and access.
- Review the chosen approach using available resources such as instructional DVDs and practice the approach on a cadaver.
- Disarticulate the femoral head before the osteotomy.
- Rotate the femur laterally until the stifle is pointing perpendicular to the sagittal plane of the pelvis.
- Extend the osteotomy from adjacent to the greater trochanter to the proximal aspect of the trochanter minor, proximal to the insertion of the iliopsoas muscle.
- Do not orient the osteotomy (osteotome or saw) in a proximo-distal direction. In small patients, the osteotomy can be performed in a strictly cranial to caudal direction. In larger dogs, the osteotomy is initiated at its most distal point and progresses proximally.
- Use a sharp osteotome or an oscillating saw.

Inadequate removal of the femoral neck

Definition

This refers to insufficient bone removal at the femoral neck resulting in bone contact with the pelvis. This is the most common complication leading to residual lameness.

Risk factors

- Poor exposure
- Existing pathology obscuring anatomy
- Poor plane of osteotomy, usually resulting from poor positioning of the limb during osteotomy. If the stifle is internally rotated rather than perpendicular to the sagittal plane of the pelvis (the patella should be pointing toward the ceiling), excess bone is left along the caudal aspect of the femoral neck.
- Failure to disarticulate the hip
- Inappropriate equipment to perform osteotomy

Diagnosis

The most common clinical signs are lameness and pain. Lameness can range from weight-bearing lameness exacerbated by activity to non–weight-bearing lameness at all times. Pain is elicited by manipulation of the joint. This is usually accompanied with crepitus. Radiography confirms residual bone at the femoral neck (Figure 111.2).

Treatment

Revision surgery is done to remove more bone along the femoral neck (Figures 111.3 and 111.4). Excess bone is usually located along the caudal and distal aspect of the osteotomy. Exposure will be more difficult because of fibrosis from the previous surgery. Consider using an oscillating saw to produce a smoother osteotomy surface. Soft tissue interposition with a biceps femoris or deep gluteal muscle sling can be incorporated. Early physical therapy together with nonsteroidal anti-

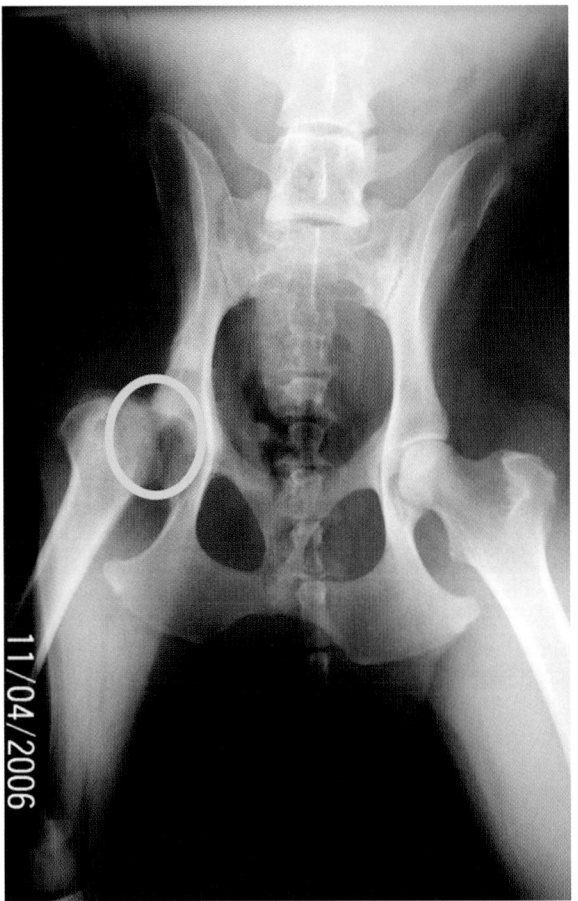

Figure 111.2 Inadequate removal of femoral head and neck (circled) noted in postoperative radiograph.

inflammatory drugs to encourage range of motion (ROM) in the joint and usage of the leg are important (Figures 111.3 and 111.4).

Outcome

The prognosis for return in function is usually good if treated early before severe muscle atrophy sets in. The prognosis is guarded if muscle contracture is present.

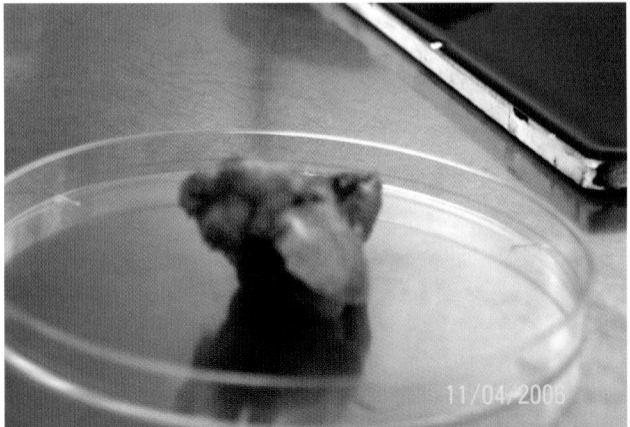

Figure 111.3 Fragment containing the remainder of the femoral head and neck removed during revision of the femoral head and neck excision in Figure 111.2.

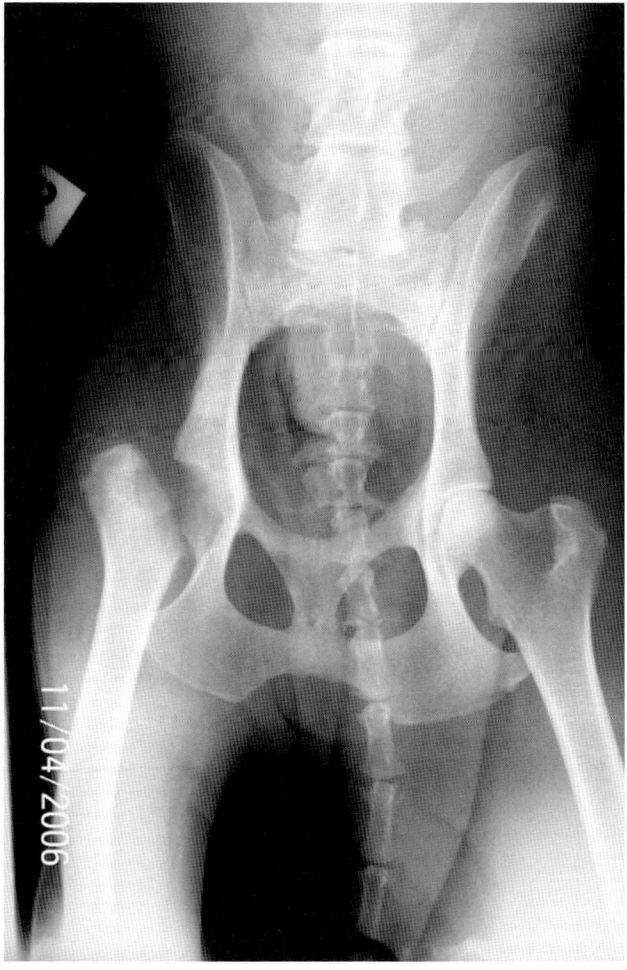

Figure 111.4 Postoperative radiograph after revision surgery in Figure 111.2 showing adequate removal of the femoral neck.

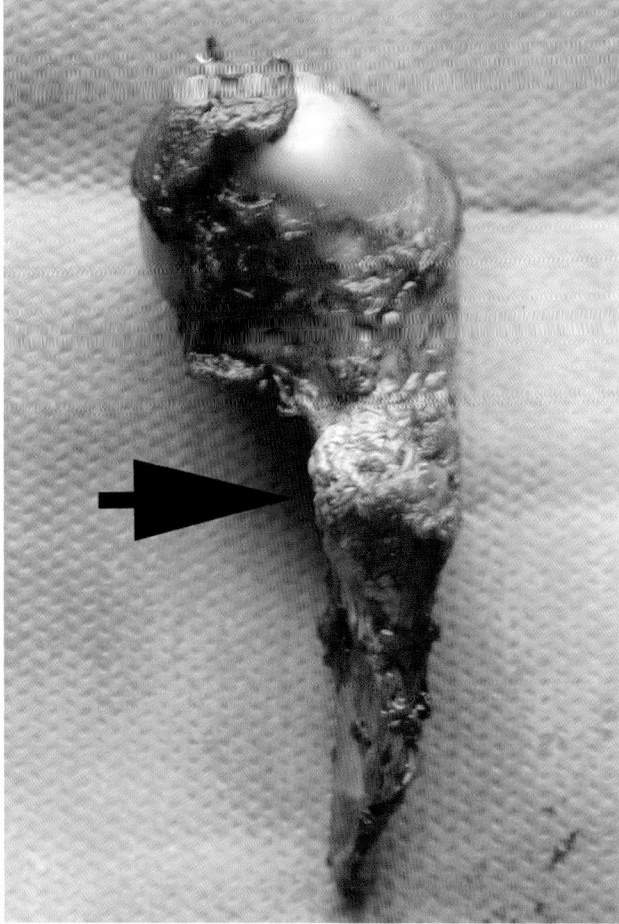

Figure 111.5 Plane of osteotomy to include the trochanter minor (arrow) preferred by this author. This is best performed using an oscillating saw.

Prevention

- Obtain current preoperative radiographs to appreciate existing bone changes in relation to the plane of osteotomy.
- Use an approach that provides good visualization and access.
- Review the chosen approach using available resources such as instructional DVDs and practice the approach on a cadaver.
- Disarticulate the femoral head before the osteotomy.
- Rotate the femur laterally until the stifle is pointing perpendicular to the sagittal plane of the pelvis, the patella being oriented toward the ceiling.
- Extend the osteotomy from adjacent to the greater trochanter and to the proximal aspect of the trochanter minor proximal to the insertion of the iliopsoas muscle.
- Use a sharp osteotome or an oscillating saw.
- This author aims to include the trochanter minor in the osteotomy whenever possible (Figures 111.5 and 111.6).

Injury to the sciatic nerve

Definition

Injury to the sciatic nerve may occur during or after surgery. The severity of injury can range from transient neuropraxia caused by stretching or constriction to permanent neurotmesis or axonotmesis caused by crushing or transection.

Risk factors

- Iatrogenic surgical trauma from careless retraction, incorrect positioning of the osteotome, and overzealous use of the oscillating saw
- Excessive soft tissue trauma leading to fibrotic entrapment
- Full-thickness biceps femoris muscle sling

Diagnosis

- Clinical signs relating to neurologic dysfunction specific to sciatic nerve noted.
- Radiography is unrewarding.
- Electromyographic examination will reveal abnormal nerve conduction velocity.

Treatment

- External neurolysis and repositioning of the sciatic nerve to an area with minimal inflammatory reaction
- Resection of caudolateral portion of ischium
- Immobilizing the limb in a cast with stifle and hock in slight flexion and digits in full extension to allow weight bearing and stop trauma to dorsum of foot

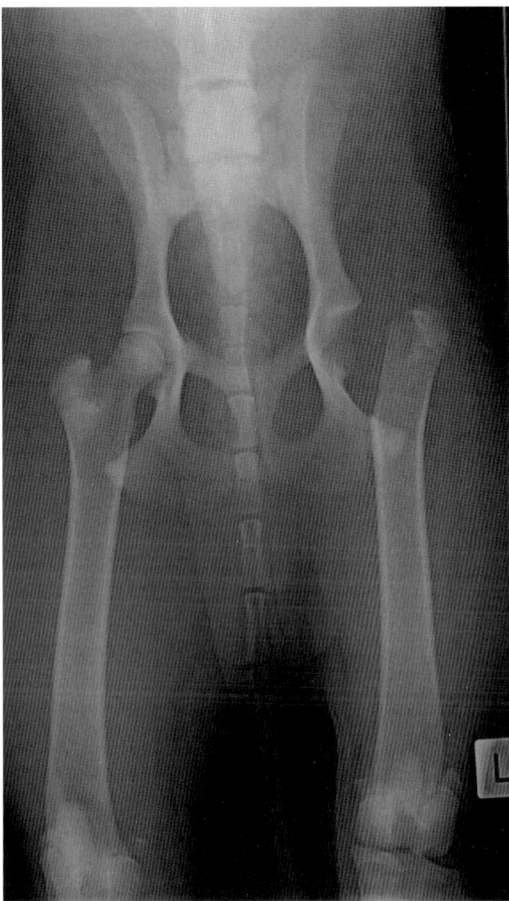

Figure 111.6 Postoperative radiograph after femoral head and neck excision where the trochanter minor has been removed together with the femoral neck.

- Long digital extensor tendon transfer to vastus lateralis
- Arthrodesis of hock
- Amputation

Outcome

The prognosis depends on the severity of the injury. Neuropraxia usually allows complete return of neurologic function, although recovery can take up to 6 months.

The prognosis for neurotmesis or axonotmesis is guarded.

Prevention

- Careful placement of a retractor to protect the sciatic nerve. Retraction should be released every 20 minutes.
- Minimize soft tissue trauma in the vicinity of the sciatic nerve.
- Attain good surgical exposure.
- Use a partial-thickness biceps femoris muscle sling in preference to the full-thickness sling.

Loss of function

Definition

Loss of function can range from lameness incompatible with normal activity to lack of improvement from preoperative function. Some dogs, particularly small breed dogs, will continue to use the leg poorly despite a good surgical outcome. A biomechanically abnormal gait should be expected after FHNE because the procedure does not preserve the joint and normal alignment of the limb. A proximal displacement of the greater trochanter can be noted as the dog bears weight. However, biomechanical lameness can be differentiated from loss of function because it is not associated with pain.

Risk factors

- Undiagnosed concurrent orthopaedic or neurologic problem
- Poor technique
- Poor physical therapy program
- Iatrogenic neurologic trauma

Diagnosis

Loss of function of a significant magnitude is easily appreciated from lameness, pain, and neurologic deficits. More subtle changes, especially as noted by the owner when the patient is more relaxed, can be difficult to assess. In these cases, the following steps may be considered to further assess function:

- Compare the amount of wear of the nails between the hindlimbs.
- Walk the patient on soft sand and assess the depth of the footprints.
- Assess gait objectively with a pressure mat or force plate.
- View video footages of the patient's movements away from the clinic setting.

Treatment

Definitive treatment options are easier to formulate when an underlying cause of the loss of function can be identified. Many concurrent orthopedic and neurologic problems such as cruciate disease, medial patellar luxation, and intervertebral disc disease can be resolved with additional surgery.

Failure to remove sufficient bone or leaving an uneven edge or shelf at the osteotomy can be rectified with revision surgery. Incorporating adjunctive soft tissue interposition to improve limb function can be considered.

Qualified animal physical therapists can be engaged to formulate and supervise an appropriate program to encourage better use of the leg.

Minor iatrogenic sciatic nerve trauma can improve with time. More severe deficits can be treated with arthrodesis of the hock.

Revision to total hip replacement is questionable because the difference in conformation of the osteotomy may lead to implant instability and previous surgery increases the risk of infection. A thorough discussion of treatment options should occur before FHNE.

Outcome

Improvement in function is generally achievable if intervention is instigated early. Many dogs regain normal function.

Prevention

Ideal candidates for FHNE include small dogs with unilateral coxofemoral disease and good muscle mass. Increased body weight, concurrent orthopedic disease, and poor muscle mass increase the risk of poor postoperative function. Owners should be informed of the postoperative biomechanical lameness observed after FHNE, and their expectations should be set accordingly.

- Thorough clinical examination to avoid missing a concurrent problem or recognizing a postoperative problem

- Use an oscillating saw for the osteotomy.
- Consider a muscle sling for large dogs.
- Start passive ROM exercise immediately after surgery and active exercise such as walking and swimming after 1 week.
- Beware of the proximity of the sciatic nerve.

Relevant literature

The most frequently cited early reports on the use of FHNE (Ormrod 1961; Spreull 1961; Piermattei 1965) recorded encouraging results. Reports on larger number of cases have emerged since that time (Duff and Campbell 1977; Lippincott 1987; Off and Matis 2010), and outcomes from these have not been consistently favorable, largely because of differences in the methods of evaluation. The less than ideal outcome in function was most evident in studies that did not rely solely on owner satisfaction. Based on follow-up examination of 66 dogs and 15 cats ranging from 7 months to 10 years after surgery, lameness and pain were detected in 56% and 32%, respectively, of the animals (Off and Matis 2010). Slow return to function in the early postoperative period has been attributed to bone-to-bone contact (Lippincott 1992).

Inadequate removal of the femoral neck is the most common immediate postoperative complication leading to bone contact between the femur and the acetabulum and early postoperative lameness. The contact area is usually located along the distal aspect of the osteotomy as the gluteal muscles displace the limb proximally during weight bearing. This complication usually results from poor surgical exposure or limb positioning, leading to incorrect plane of osteotomy. The recommended plane of osteotomy for dogs weighing less than 20 kg spared the trochanter minor, and an additional step to remove this structure was recommended for dogs weighing over 20 kg (Lippincott 1992). A wedge resection technique has been described to remove the femoral head and neck and an adjacent wedge of metaphyseal bone (Montgomery et al. 1987). This technique required fixation of the greater trochanter to the metaphysis with cross pins. Various methods have been used to perform FHNE. Although the skill of the individual surgeon has a major impact on the effectiveness, each method has its inherent features that should be appreciated. A powered oscillating saw provides the greatest accuracy and smoothness of the osteotomy (Lippincott 1992). Inadvertent maldirection of the osteotomy when using an osteotome can be prevented by using a sharp osteotome and drilling a series of holes along the proposed plane of osteotomy. After the osteotomy and removal of the femoral head and neck, the femur should be returned to the neutral position and moved through its normal ROM to check for crepitus. If present, the osteotomy surface will require further debridement until crepitus is no longer palpable.

Injury to the sciatic nerve can occur during or after surgery because of its proximity to the femoral head. Forterre et al. (2007) reviewed 18 dogs and 9 cats with iatrogenic sciatic nerve injury, but none was caused by FHNE. Although acute injury to the sciatic nerve during FHNE has rarely been reported (Liska et al. 2010), the inherent risk of sciatic nerve impingement during external rotation of the femur without coxofemoral disarticulation was clearly demonstrated in a cadaver study (Andrews et al. 2008). Delayed development of sciatic nerve neuropraxia after FHNE has been reported in a total of four dogs (Walker 1981; Jeffery 1993). All four animals regained normal neurologic function after release of the sciatic nerve entrapment by removal of part of the ischium or by external neurolysis to free the nerve from fibrous tissue. Recovery times varied from at least 3 weeks to 6 months.

Sciatic nerve paralysis can occur with a full-thickness biceps femoris muscle sling (Stanton et al. 1988). This condition has been attributed to stretching of the nerve from tension exerted by the full-thickness sling. A partial-thickness sling can avoid this complication (Prostredny et al. 1991).

When recovery has not been sufficient to provide acceptable function, such as hock extension and dorsiflexion of the digits for weight bearing, hock arthrodesis and transfer of the long digital extensor tendon have been reported to improve plantar contact of the foot on the ground (Lesser 1978).

Persistent lameness after FHNE is a form of **loss of function.** Various tissues have been used as interposition between the osteotomy site and acetabulum to improve limb function. These include the joint capsule (Off and Matis 2010), the deep gluteal muscle (Berzon et al. 1980), the biceps femoris muscle (Lippincott 1987; Prostredny et al. 1991), and the rectus femoris muscle (Remedios et al. 1994). The benefits of muscle slings remain controversial. Although there has been strong advocacy for its use (Berzon et al. 1980; Lippincott 1987), several studies failed to demonstrate an advantage (Mann et al. 1987; Montgomery et al. 1987). A more recent investigation in dogs with normal coxofemoral conformation indicated that a partial-thickness biceps femoris muscle flap was superior to the deep gluteal muscle flap (Prostredny et al. 1991). Monitored for 3 weeks after surgery, dogs with a partial-thickness biceps flap showed better improvement in limb function and ROM than dogs with a deep gluteal flap. This was attributed to more complete coverage of the osteotomy site by the partial-thickness biceps flap. Both flaps ultimately underwent fibrous replacement, which provided the long-term benefit of limiting contact between the femur and the acetabulum. It is fair to say that the controversy over the use of muscle slings in FHNE is not resolved. Soft tissue interposition, particularly with a partial-thickness biceps femoris muscle flap, may be beneficial in cases of irreparable acetabular fractures in which bone contact after FHNE is common, chronic coxofemoral disorders in which extensive periarticular fibrosis and muscle atrophy exist, and revision surgery to remove more femoral neck (Lewis 1992).

Revision of unsuccessful FHNE to a total hip replacement can yield excellent and pain-free function (Gofton and Sumner-Smith 1982; Liska et al. 2010). However, the presence of fibrous tissue and altered anatomy at the surgery site will complicate the surgery, and manipulation of a previous surgical site increases the risk of infection. Complications are therefore more likely after revision of FHNE with total hip replacement than after primary total hip replacement. Therefore, in dogs that are initially better candidates for a hip replacement, FHNE should not be offered as a primary option. Revision to a hip replacement should only be attempted by a surgeon with considerable experience in this procedure.

Although fracture of the proximal femur during FHNE has been listed as a potential complication of FHNE (Berzon et al. 1980), no report has been published regarding its occurrence and management.

References

Andrews, C.M., Liska, W.D., Roberts, D.J. (2008) Sciatic neuropraxia as a complication in 1000 consecutive canine total hip replacements. *Veterinary Surgery* 37, 254–262.

Berzon, J.L., Howard, P.E., Covell, S.J., et al. (1980) A retrospective study of the efficacy of femoral head and neck excisions in 94 dogs and cats. *Veterinary Surgery* 9, 88–92.

Duff, R., Campbell, J.R. (1977) Long term results of excision arthroplasty of the canine hip. *Veterinary Record* 101, 181–184.

Forterre, F., Tomek, A., Rytz, U., et al. (2007) Iatrogenic sciatic nerve injury in eighteen dogs and nine cats (1997–2006). *Veterinary Surgery* 36, 464–471.

Gendreau, C., Cawley, A.J. (1977) Excision of the femoral head and neck: the long-term results of 35 operations. *Journal of the American Animal Hospital Association* 13, 605-608.

Gofton, N., Sumner-Smith, G. (1982) Total hip prosthesis for revision of unsuccessful excision arthroplasty. *Veterinary Surgery* 11, 134-139.

Jeffery, N.D. (1993) Femoral head and neck excision complicated by ischiatic nerve entrapment in two dogs. *Veterinary and Comparative Orthopaedics and Traumatology* 6, 215-218.

Lesser, A.S. (1978) The use of a tendon transfer for the treatment of a traumatic sciatic nerve paralysis in the dog. *Veterinary Surgery* 7, 85-89.

Lewis, D.D. (1992) Femoral head and neck excision and the controversy concerning adjunctive soft tissue interposition. *Compendium on Continuing Education for the Practicing Veterinarian* 14, 1463-1471.

Lewis, D.D., Bellah, J.R., McGavin, M.D., et al. (1988) Postoperative examination of the biceps femoris muscle sling used in excision of the femoral head and neck in dogs. *Veterinary Surgery* 17, 269-277.

Lippincott, C.L. (1987) A summary of 300 surgical cases performed over an 8 year period: excision arthroplasty of the femoral head and neck with a caudal pass of the biceps femoris muscle sling. *Veterinary Surgery* 16, 96.

Lippincott, C.L. (1992) Femoral head and neck excision in the management of canine hip dysplasia. *Veterinary Clinics of North America* 22, 721-737.

Liska, W.D., Doyle, N.D., Schwartz, Z. (2010) Successful revision of a femoral head ostectomy (complicated by postoperative sciatic neurapraxia) to a total hip replacement in a cat. *Veterinary and Comparative Orthopaedics and Traumatology* 23, 119-123.

Mann, F.A., Tangner, C.H., Wagner-Mann, C., et al. (1987) A comparison of standard femoral head and neck excision and femoral head and neck excision using a biceps femoris muscle flap in the dog. *Veterinary Surgery* 16, 223-230.

Montgomery, R.D., Milton, J.L., Horne, R.D., et al. (1987) A retrospective comparison of three techniques for femoral head and neck excision in dogs. *Veterinary Surgery* 16, 423-426.

Off, W., Matis, U. (2010) Excision arthroplasty of the hip joint in dogs and cats. *Veterinary and Comparative Orthopaedics and Traumatology* 5, 297-305.

Ormrod, A.N. (1961) Treatment of hip lamenesses in the dog by excision of the femoral head. *Veterinary Record* 73, 576-577.

Piermattei, D.L. (1965) Femoral head ostectomy in the dog: indications, techniques and results in ten cases. *Journal of the American Animal Hospital Association* 1, 180-188.

Piermattei, D.L., Flo, G.L., DeCamp, C.E. (2006) Femoral head and neck excision. In Piermattei, D.L., Flo, G.L., DeCamp, C.E. (eds.) *Brinker, Piermattei, and Flo's Handbook of Small Animal Orthopaedics and Fracture Repair,* 4th edn. Saunders, St. Louis, pp. 501-504.

Prostredny, J.M., Toombs, J.P., VanSickle, D.C. (1991) Effect of two muscle sling techniques on early morbidity after femoral head and neck excision in dogs. *Veterinary Surgery* 20, 298-305.

Remedios, A.M., Clayton, H.M., Skuba, E. (1994) Femoral head excision arthroplasty using the vascularised rectus femoris muscle sling. *Veterinary and Comparative Orthopaedics and Traumatology* 7, 82-87.

Spreull, J.S.A. (1961) Excision arthroplasty as a method of treatment of hip joint diseases in the dog. *Veterinary Record* 73, 573-576.

Stanton, M.E., Weigel, J.P., Henry, R.E. (1988) Ischiatic nerve paralysis associated with the biceps femoris muscle sling: case report and anatomic study. *Journal of the American Animal Hospital Association* 24, 429-432.

Walker, T.L. (1981) Ischiadic nerve entrapment. *Journal of the American Veterinary Association* 178, 1284-1288.

112 Complications of Double and Triple Pelvic Osteotomies

Aldo Vezzoni

Clinica Veterinaria Vezzoni srl via Massarotti 60/A, Cremona CR, Italy

In young dogs with early diagnosis of hip dysplasia (HD), correct ive pelvic osteotomies, such as double pelvic osteotomy (DPO) or triple pelvic osteotomy (TPO), are carried out to halt or minimize hip joint subluxation and subsequent development of degenerative joint disease (DJD). TPO, and recently DPO, have been used to improve coverage of the femoral head through ventroversion of the dorsal acetabular rim (DAR) (Slocum and Devine 1986, 1987, 1992, 1998). DPO differs from TPO in that it does not involve ischial osteotomy; this modification was proposed in 2006 by Haudiquet and Guillon and has since been evaluated in clinical studies (Haudiquet 2008; Vezzoni *et al.* 2010). In this procedure, the rotation of the ilium caudal to the osteotomy relies on the deformation of the ischial table and on the flexibility of the cartilaginous pubic symphysis in growing dogs (Punke *et al.* 2011). The acetabular rotation effectively produced after DPO appeared to be about 5 degrees less than the amount of rotation obtained at the level of the iliac osteotomy (Haudiquet and Guillon 2006; Punke *et al.* 2011).

Implant failure

Definition

Implant failure is defined as loosening of bone fixation because of implant breakage, screw loosening, or plate pullout. Implant failure is the most common complication reported after TPO and was seen when TPO plates were first used for DPO. Implant failures have different modalities in TPO versus DPO: they most commonly involve the cranial fixation in TPO and the caudal fixation in DPO.

Risk factors

Risk factors for implant failure after both TPO and DPO include:
- Insufficient postoperative exercise restriction
- Excessive body weight
- Simultaneous bilateral procedures (Figure 112.1)

With the TPO technique, insufficient purchase of the screws in the sacrum has been reported to increase the risk of screw loosening (Simmons *et al.* 2001; Whelan *et al.* 2004). In addition, screws placed in the cranial segment of the ilium are more likely to fail than those placed in the caudal segment (Figures 112.2 and 112.3).

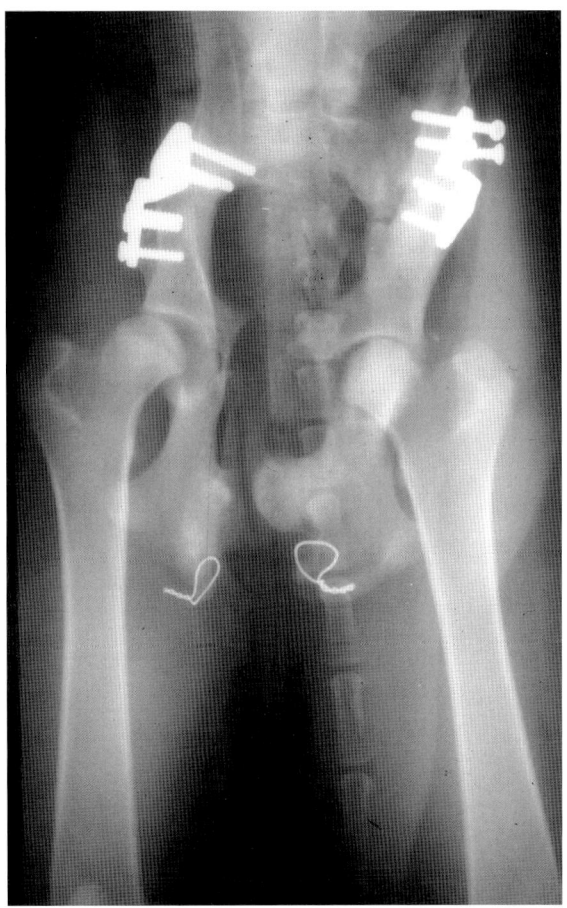

Figure 112.1 Bilateral malunion after simultaneous bilateral triple pelvic osteotomy (TPO) in a young golden retriever. The TPOs were fixed with cortical screws that did not penetrate the sacroiliac joint. Although cerclage wires were placed on both ischial osteotomies, insufficient exercise restriction led to the loosening of multiple screws on the left side and caudal screws on the right side. Loss of fixation resulted in migration of both iliac segments, loss of acetabular coverage, and pelvic narrowing. The owners did not return the dog until 8 weeks after the initial surgery, at which point malunions were diagnosed. Source: A. Johnson, University of Illinois at Urbana-Champaign, Urbana, IL. Reproduced with permission from A. Johnson

Complications in Small Animal Surgery, First Edition. Edited by Dominique Griffon and Annick Hamaide.
© 2016 John Wiley & Sons, Inc. Published 2016 by John Wiley & Sons, Inc.
Companion website: www.wiley.com/go/griffon/complications

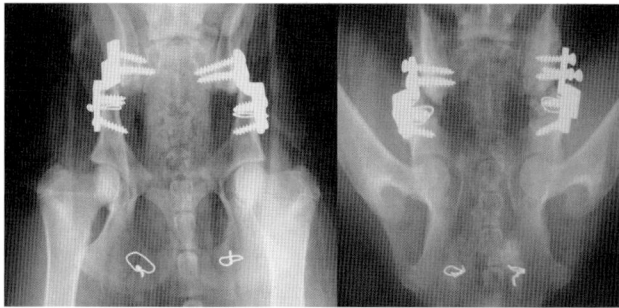

Figure 112.2 Extended (**A**) and frog-leg (**B**) ventrodorsal pelvic radiographic view of an 8-month-old German shepherd dog 1 month after single-session bilateral triple pelvic osteotomy. Several cortical screws have loosened, and there is pelvic narrowing.

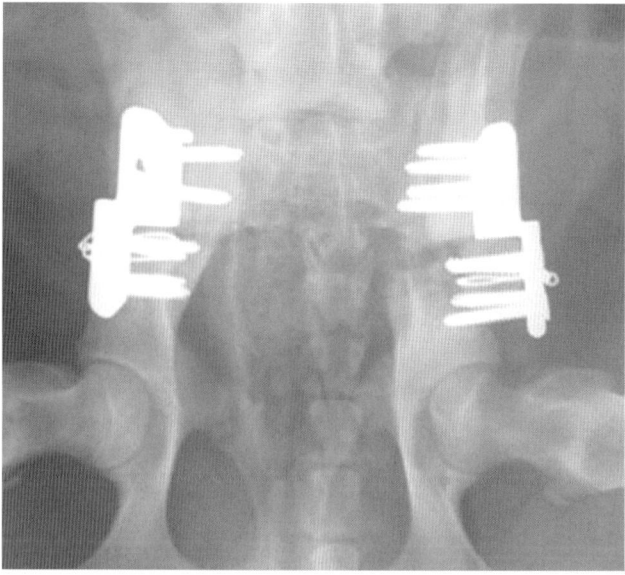

Figure 112.4 Frog-leg ventrodorsal pelvic radiographic view of a 7-month-old Labrador retriever. Follow-up 1 month after single-session bilateral double pelvic osteotomy. There is complete pullout of the distal (caudal) part of the plate despite the use of a cerclage wire. The parallel locking screws pulled out a segment of bone, thus creating an "avulsion" fracture.

With the DPO technique, the use of parallel screws in the caudal segment of the ilium increased the risk of screw and plate pullout (Figure 112.4) (Vezzoni *et al.* 2010).

Diagnosis

Most cases of isolated screw loosening (Figure 112.5) consist of incidental findings detected at the first postoperative radiographic reevaluation of the patient, typically 4 to 6 weeks after surgery. Callus formation may appear more prominent than usual, and migration of a screw is noted without failure of the fixation.

Severe implant failure occasionally occurs when multiple screws become loose, compromising the fixation and leading to loss of alignment of the iliac shaft (see Figures 112.1 and 112.6). Implant failure rarely occurs as a result of plate breakage. Loss of fixation is commonly associated with acute lameness and sudden onset of patient discomfort. If the animal is not reevaluated at that time,

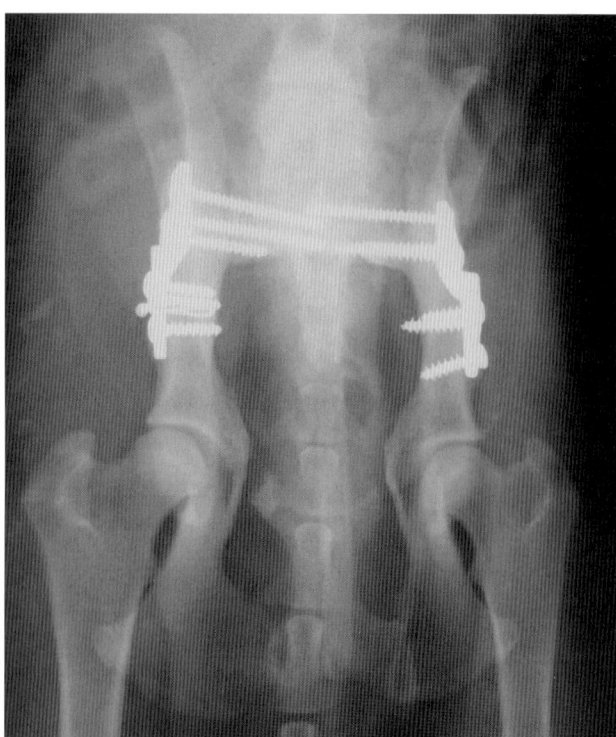

Figure 112.3 Follow-up 1 year after single-session bilateral triple pelvic osteotomy in a Labrador retriever. Screws placed in the cranial ilial segment engaged the sacroiliac joint to prevent implant loosening.

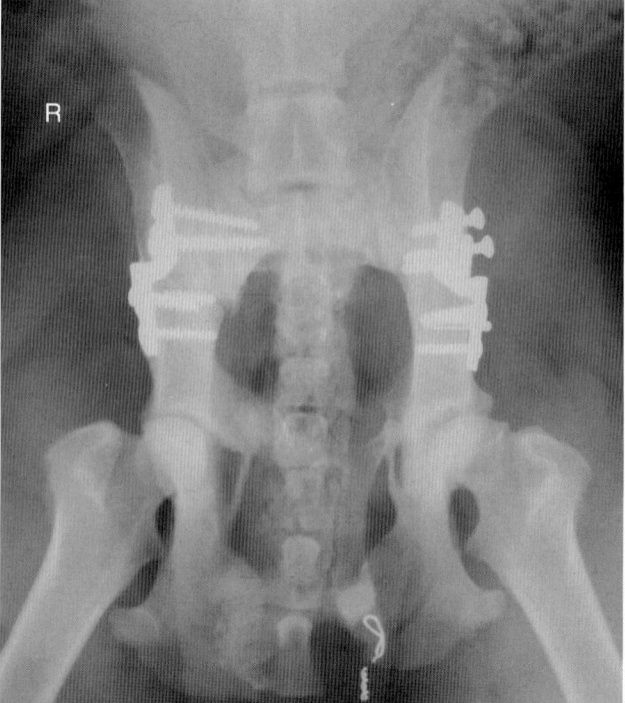

Figure 112.5 Follow-up 3 years of bilateral triple pelvic osteotomy in a Labrador, retriever with cancellous screws on the right side and cortical screws and cerclage wire on the left side. Two cortical screws became loose, and one cancellous screw fractured. The ischial cerclage wire on the left side also ruptured.

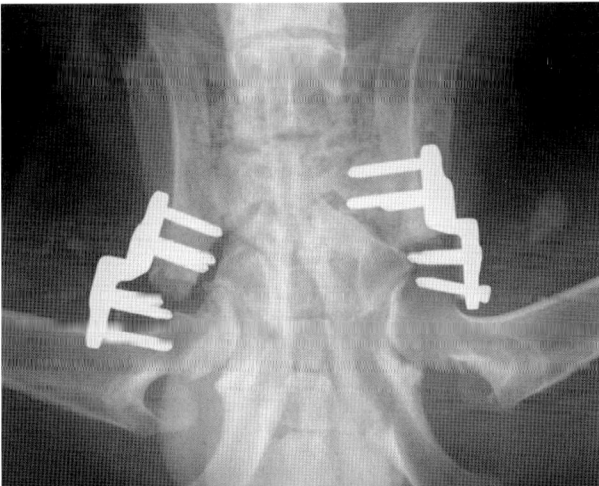

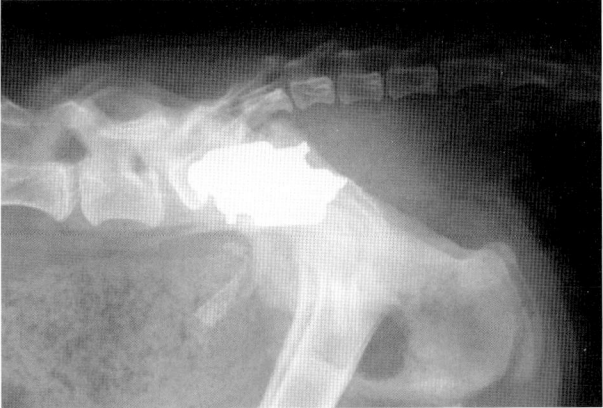

Figure 112.6 Bilateral simultaneous double pelvic osteotomy in an 8-month-old Rottweiler with complete implant failure 1 week after surgery, including avulsion of the plates fixed with parallel locking screws. Note the ventral deviation of the ischium on the lateral projection.

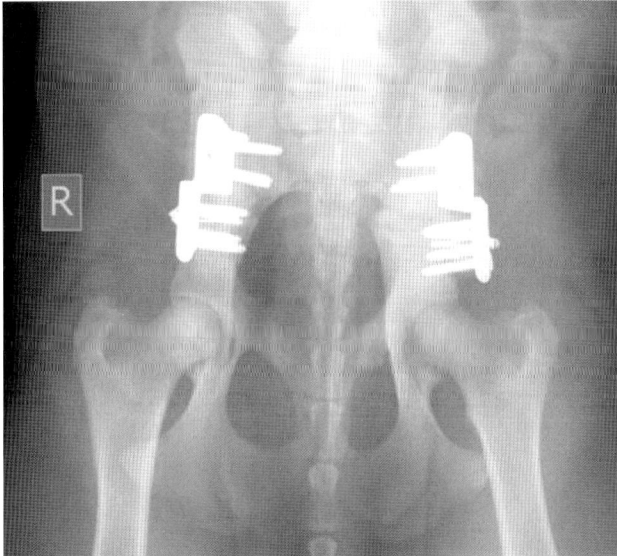

Figure 112.7 Radiographs obtained 2 months after surgery of the case illustrated in Figure 112.4. Conservative treatment resulted in complete fracture healing without significantly affecting joint congruity.

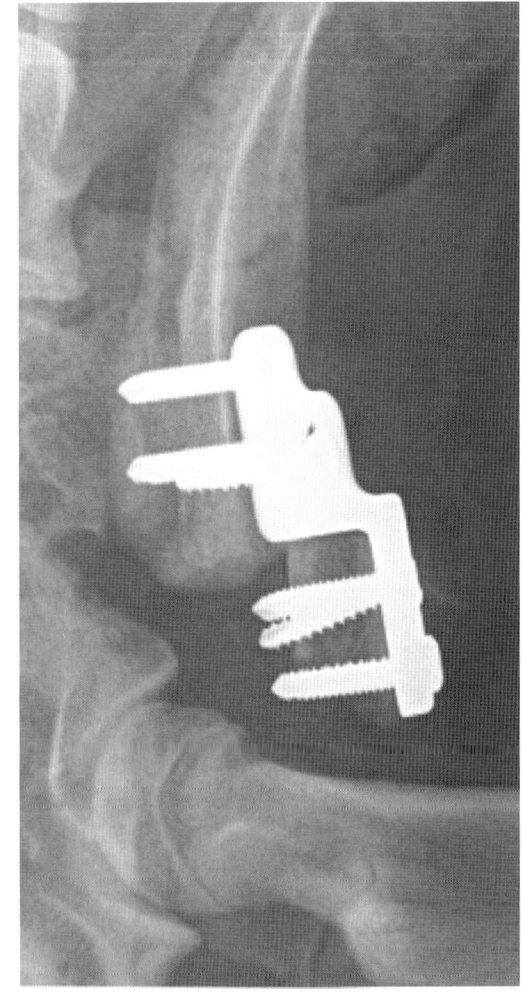

clinical signs tend to improve spontaneously, leading to a malunion noted at the next recheck (Figure 112.7).

Radiographic signs of implant failure after both TPO and DPO include:

- Migration of one or several screws: loss of contact between the screw head and the plate, presence of a radiolucent bone tunnel extending beyond the tip of the screw
- Loss of contact between the plate and the underlying bone
- Migration of the caudal segment of the plate with or without avulsion fracture of the underlying cortex after locking plate fixation (Figures 112.8 and 112.9)
- Loss of apposition between the cranial and caudal segments of the ilium
- Change in acetabular version (increased or decreased)
- Loss of alignment of the axis of the ilium
- Narrowing of the pelvic canal, most common after bilateral TPO (Figure 112.10); after DPO, narrowing occurs only with implant failure (Figure 112.11)
- Excessive callus formation

Treatment

The management of implant failure after pelvic osteotomy depends on the type of failure, its clinical significance, and the stage of bone

Figure 112.8 Avulsion fracture 5 days after double pelvic osteotomy in a 6-month-old golden retriever. A locking plate was applied without orienting the most caudal screw in a caudal direction. This orientation would have allowed the plate to span bone caudal to the plate and prevent iliac fracture at that location.

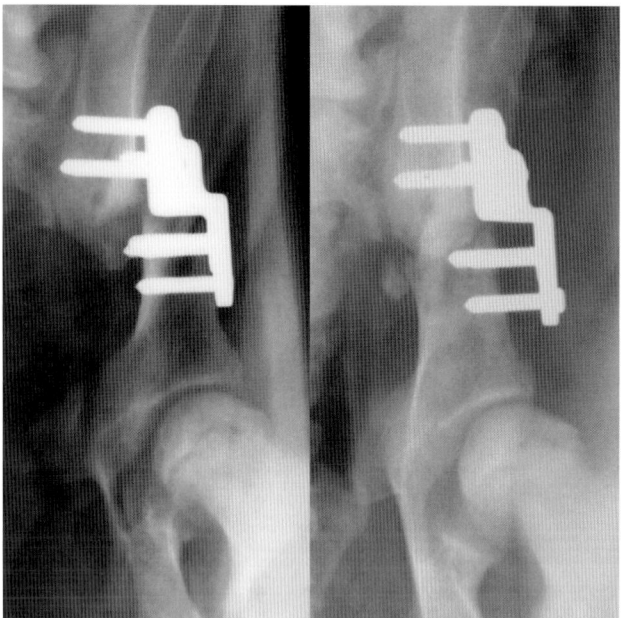

Figure 112.9 Double pelvic osteotomy fixed with parallel locking screws and plate in a 6-month-old Labrador retriever. Radiographs obtained immediately after surgery (**A**) and a week later (**B**). Note the full avulsion of the plate from the caudal iliac segment.

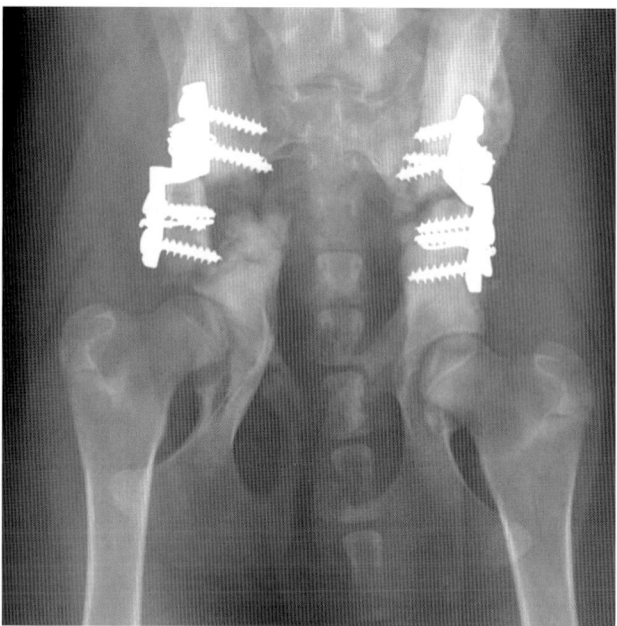

Figure 112.11 Ventrodorsal radiograph of the pelvis in a 5.5-month-old Rottweiler 1 month after single-session bilateral double pelvic osteotomy. On the right side, there are a complete iliac fracture caudal to the plate, callus formation, pelvic narrowing, and loss of dorsal coverage of the femoral head.

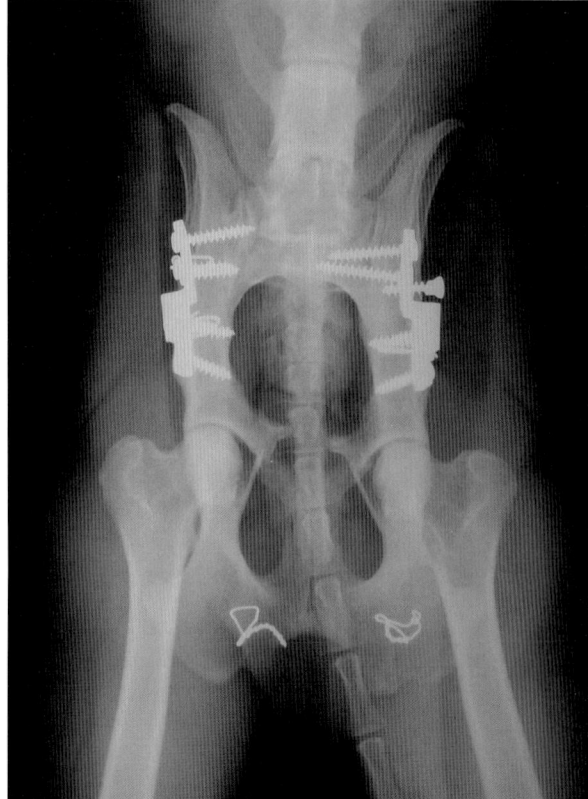

Figure 112.10 Ventrodorsal radiograph of the pelvis in a 2-year-old border collie 17 months after single-session bilateral triple pelvic osteotomy. There is some narrowing of the pelvic canal along with excessive coverage of the femoral heads and loosening of a screw but no apparent progression of degenerative joint disease.

repair at the time of diagnosis. Screw loosening without clinical signs or failure of the fixation is treated by strict exercise restriction and serial evaluation of bone healing until union. Surgical revision of one or a few loose or broken screws is usually not required because the remaining fixed screws, musculature, and callus, which forms quickly in young immature dogs, stabilize the osteotomy adequately (see Figure 112.7). Some degree of pelvic collapse should be expected after minor implant loosening after TPO but does not require surgical revision.

Surgical revision should be considered when implant failure leads to loss of bone alignment and acetabular ventroversion. Examples include loosening of multiple screws and plate pull-out, especially if the complication is bilateral. Revision should be undertaken as soon as possible and before a callus has formed. Ideally, the osteotomy should be stabilized with a new plate and diverging screws, possibly one or two directed caudally toward the acetabulum. In addition, a second straight plate may be applied to the ventral iliac border. In severely unstable conditions, a long dorsal plate that extends over the acetabulum and ischial body should be applied.

Treatment of pelvic malunions (see Figure 112.1) resulting from failed TPOs is very complex. In cases with loss of dorsal acetabular coverage, a total hip replacement may be considered to manage the HD. However, collapse of the pelvic canal and hypertrophic callus formation may lead to obstipation. (See the section on treatment of pelvic collapse.)

Outcome

Delayed healing of the iliac osteotomy is an outcome common to all cases of implant failure, but healing is usually not prevented by implant failure. The consequences of implant failure after TPO are pelvic collapse and pelvic canal narrowing along with excessive coverage of the femoral head by the acetabular labium (Slocum and Devine 1986, 1987; Hunt and Litsky 1988). Excessive coverage

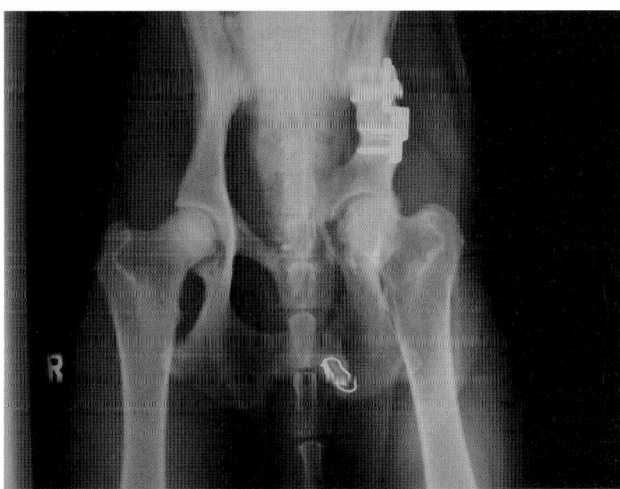

Figure 112.12 One year follow-up of a left triple pelvic osteotomy with a 30-degree plate in a golden retriever. Coverage of the femoral head appears excessive, and impingement between the dorsal acetabular rim and the femoral neck limits hip abduction and extension. Excessive rotation combined with partial screw loosening of the cranial fixation caused pelvic narrowing.

of the femoral head results in impingement of the femoral neck by the DAR (Figure 112.12); femoral abduction is limited, causing an abnormal gait with internal rotation of the limb (Schrader 1986; Slocum and Devine 1986; Tomlinson and Johnson 2000). The main consequence of implant failure after DPO consists of loss of acetabular coverage, which reduces the effect of DPO (Figure 112.13) and enhances the progression of osteoarthritis (OA). In contrast to TPO, pelvic canal narrowing is a minor problem after DPO because the ischium is not cut, except in cases with subsequent iliac fracture.

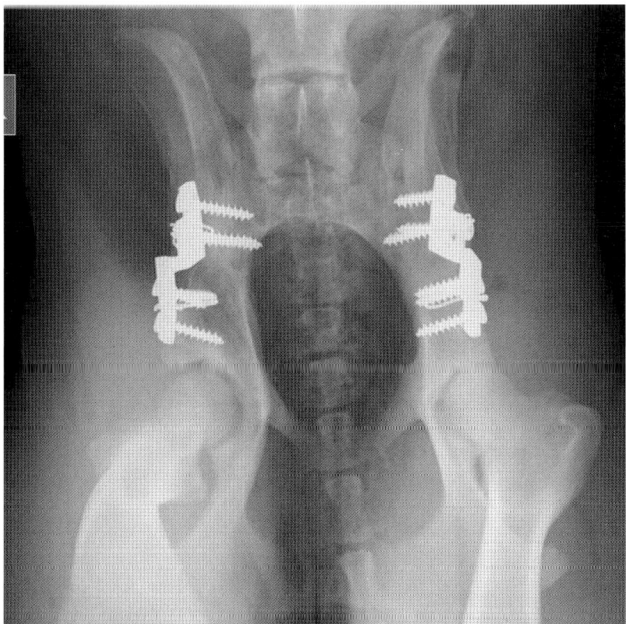

Figure 112.13 Six-month follow-up of the case illustrated in Figure 112.11. Spontaneous healing of the iliac fracture resulted in loss of dorsal coverage of the femoral head and early signs of degenerative joint disease.

Table 112.1 Strategies proposed to prevent implant loosening after triple pelvic osteotomies

Strategy	Potential limitation(s)
Use of cancellous screws	Increase risk of screw breakage
Engage >50% of the sacral body	Penetration into the vertebral canal
Ischial wiring	Draining tract
Placement of a small screw in standard TPO plate cerclage hole	Limited effect
PMMA augmentation	Thermal damage to the bone, foreign body
Calcium phosphate augmentation	Not available on the veterinary market
Adjunct ventral plate	Cost, surgical time, soft tissue retraction
Eight-hole rectangular plate	Bone size may not be sufficient in smaller dogs
Locking TPO plate	None

PMMA, polymethylmethacrylate; TPO, triple pelvic osteotomy.

Prevention

After TPO, the fixation cranial to the iliac osteotomy is subjected to higher loads and is therefore predisposed to implant failure. Strategies proposed to prevent implant loosening after TPO (Table 112.1) include:

- The use of cancellous screws, especially if they do not engage the sacrum, decrease the risk of screw loosening (Doornink *et al.* 2006). However, these screws may be predisposed to breakage compared with cortical screws, especially if there is a gap between the plate and underlying bone.
- Insertion of at least one cranial screw into the sacrum, engaging at least 50% of the sacral body (see Figure 112.3; Whelan *et al.* 2004)
- Placement of cerclage wires over the plate and fixation of the ischial osteotomy with a hemicerclage (Simmons *et al.* 2001). This adjunct fixation decreases the risk of screw loosening, but wires placed in the ischium may lead to draining tracts.
- Placement of a 2.0-mm cortical screw in the additional hole located in the caudodorsal aspect of a standard TPO plate (Figure 112.14)
- Cement augmentation of screws (Hutchinson *et al.* 2005): Injection of polymethylmethacrylate or calcium phosphate cement into the screw hole before inserting the screw increases the pull out strength of screws placed in the sacrum and ilium of dogs by about 30 and 20%, respectively.
- Placing the screw in divergent directions and not parallel (Vezzoni *et al.* 2000). (Figure 112.15)
- Placement of a straight plate on the ventral aspect of the ilium (Fitch *et al.* 2002a) (Figure 112.16). This strategy requires significant contouring of the plate and additional surgical time.
- Placement of an eight-hole rectangular plate (Figure 112.17).
- Use of locking screws (Rose *et al.* 2012).

The last two options listed above are the most effective and simplest to prevent screw loosening, especially in large to giant dogs (Figure 112.18). Staging bilateral TPOs by at least 6 weeks has been recommended to palliate complications associated with simultaneous procedures. This approach carries the risk of DJD progressing in the contralateral, unoperated hip while the operated side heals.

After DPO, the fixation of the caudal iliac segment is the most subject to stress, and implant failure more commonly affects the caudal part of the fixation. The implants appear subject to higher

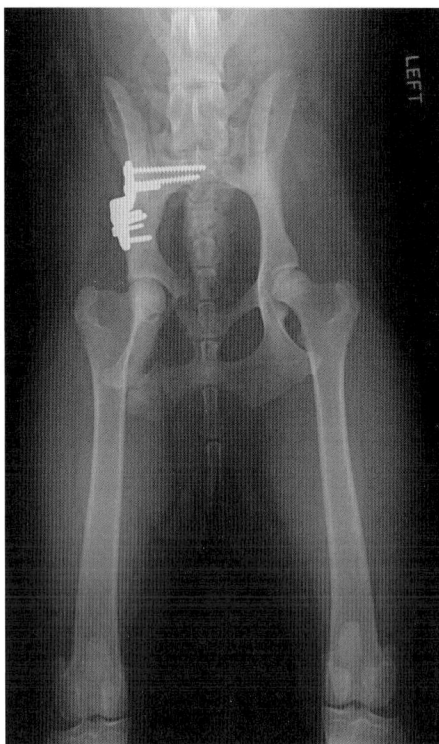

Figure 112.14 Ventrodorsal radiograph of the pelvis 1 year after triple pelvic osteotomy (TPO) with a standard 20-degree, six- hole plate. Two 4-mm-diameter cancellous screws (40 and 36 mm long) were placed across the sacroiliac joint as a strategy to prevent screw migration in a young active dog. In addition, a 2-mm cortical screw was placed in the additional hole for cerclage wire located in the caudodorsal aspect of the TPO plate. *Source:* D. Griffon, Western University of Health Sciences, Pomona, CA, 2014. Reproduced with permission from D. Griffon.

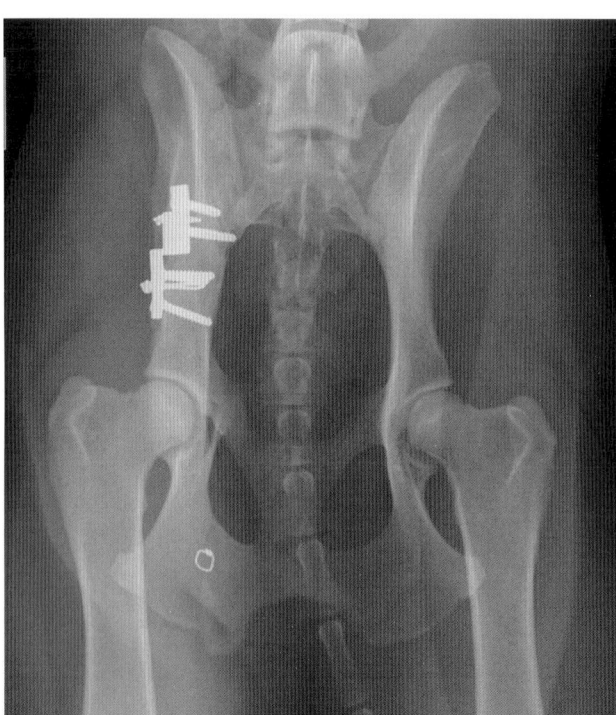

Figure 112.15 One-year follow-up after right triple pelvic osteotomy without implant loosening or pelvic collapse. All of the screws were oriented in a divergent way.

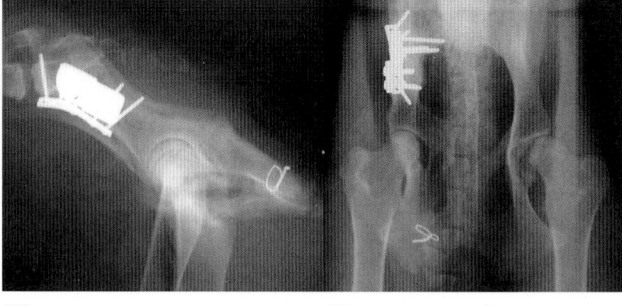

(A)　　　　　　　　　　　　　　　　(B)

Figure 112.16 Ventrodorsal (**A**) and lateral (**B**) radiographs of the pelvis obtained three months after triple pelvic osteotomy (TPO) in a Saint Bernard. A 2.7-mm DCP plate and screws were placed on the ventral aspect of the ilium as an adjunct to the standard TPO plate. In addition, two cortical screws are placed through the cranial iliac segment and into the body of the sacrum.

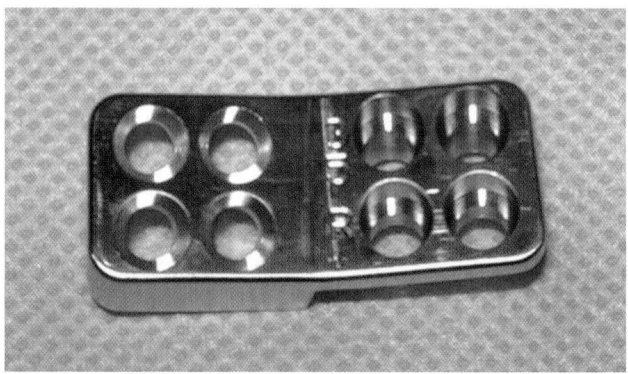

Figure 112.17 Eight-hole plate for triple pelvic osteotomy (Rooks plate). *Source:* D. Griffon, Western University of Health Sciences, Pomona, CA, 2014. Reproduced with permission from D. Griffon.

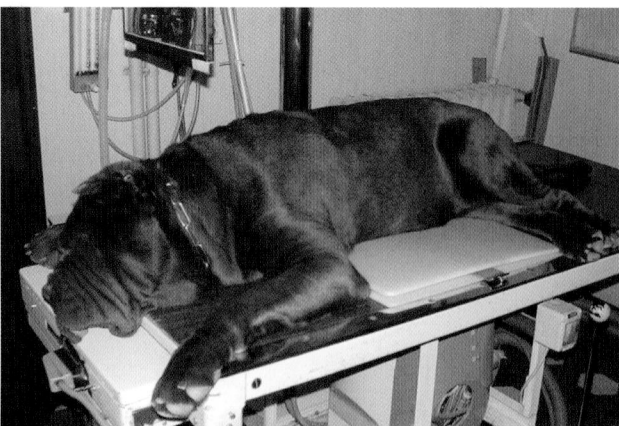

Figure 112.18 An eight-month-old Neapolitan mastiff, a candidate for triple pelvic osteotomy and double pelvic osteotomy and weighing 50 kg. In giant dogs, bilateral simultaneous surgical procedures are contraindicated, and additional fixation of the iliac osteotomy is recommended.

stress caudally, with a tendency for the ilium to return to its original anatomic position in the first days postoperatively. This phenomenon has been attributed to the elastic memory of the rotated bone. However, the stability achieved 1 week after surgery is greater with DPO than TPO because of the intact ischium.

Table 112.2 Strategies proposed to prevent implant loosening after double pelvic osteotomies

Strategy	Potential limitation (s)
Use of DPO-dedicated plates	None
Minimum of two distal screws locking	None
Most distal dorsal screw oriented distally	Joint invasion when plate is too caudal
Divergent locking screws to increase bone purchase	None
Adjunct ventral plate in older and heavier dogs	Cost, surgical time, soft tissue retraction
Sedation for 2–3 weeks	None

DPO, double pelvic osteotomy.

Strategies proposed to prevent implant loosening after DPO (Table 112.2) include:

- Use of plates and screws designed specifically for DPO, preferably with locking screws (Figure 112.19). Four of the screws are used to fix the distal segment; at least two of them are inserted as locking screws in diverging or converging directions. This improves stability of the fixation and greatly reduces the risk of plate pull-out.(Figure 112.20) Cerclage wires failed to prevent plate pullout after DPO in one case (Vezzoni *et al.* 2010) (see Figure 112.4).
- The most distal dorsal screw should be oriented caudally, toward the acetabulum, to span the bone caudal to the plate and prevent iliac fracture at that location (Figure 112.21).
- Fixation of the cranial part of the plate is not as critical as with TPO. Engaging a screw in the sacrum is therefore not required, and is in fact not recommended, to preserve the function of the sacroiliac joint.

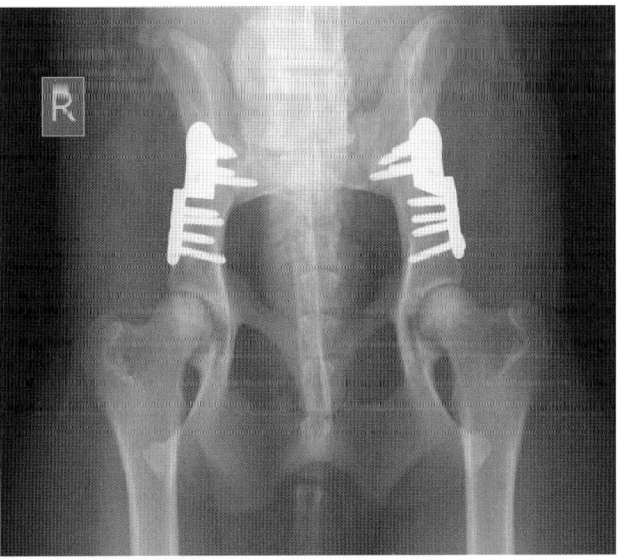

Figure 112.20 Six-month follow-up of a bilateral simultaneous double pelvic osteotomy in a Bernese mountain dog. Normal healing and stable apparatus were obtained after fixation with New Generation Devices (NGD, Glen Rock, NJ) plates and orientation of the most caudal screw toward the acetabulum.

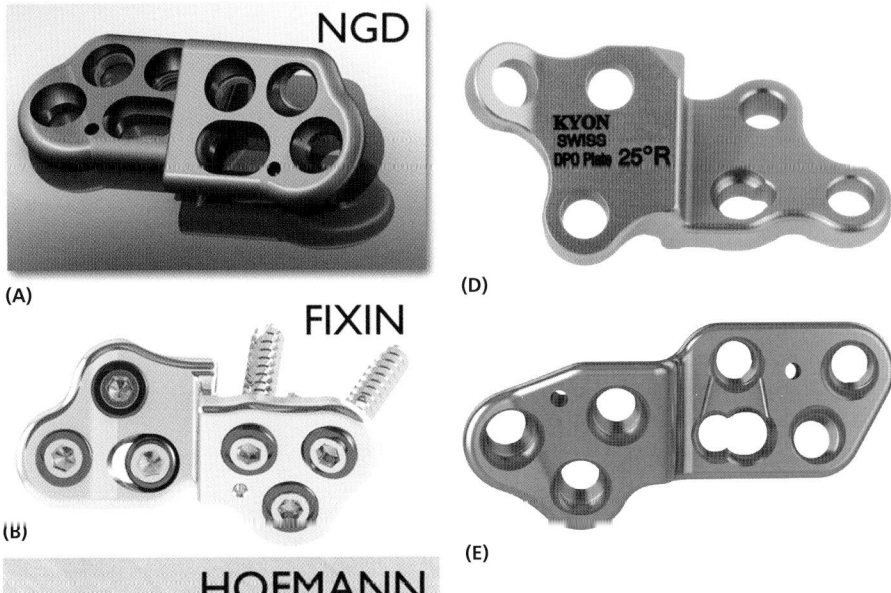

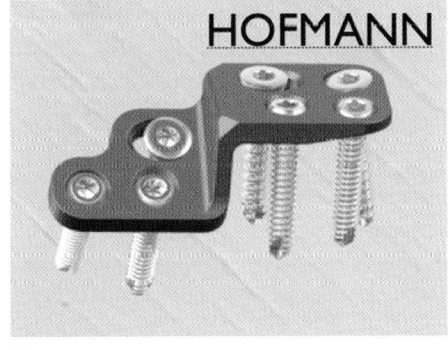

Figure 112.19 Plates specifically designed for double pelvic osteotomy, with locking screws. **A**, New Generation Devices (NGD), Glen Rock, NJ. *Source:* Reproduced with permission from New Generation Devices, USA. **B**, Fixin, TraumaVet S.r.l, Rivoli, TO, Italy. *Source:* Reproduced with permission from INTRAUMA SRL, Italy. **C**, Hoffman, Italy. *Source:* Reproduced with permission from Hofmann® s.r.l., Italy. **D**, Kyon AG, Zurich (CH) and Kyon Veterinary Products, Boston (MA), **E**, DePuy Synthes Vet, West Chester, PA.

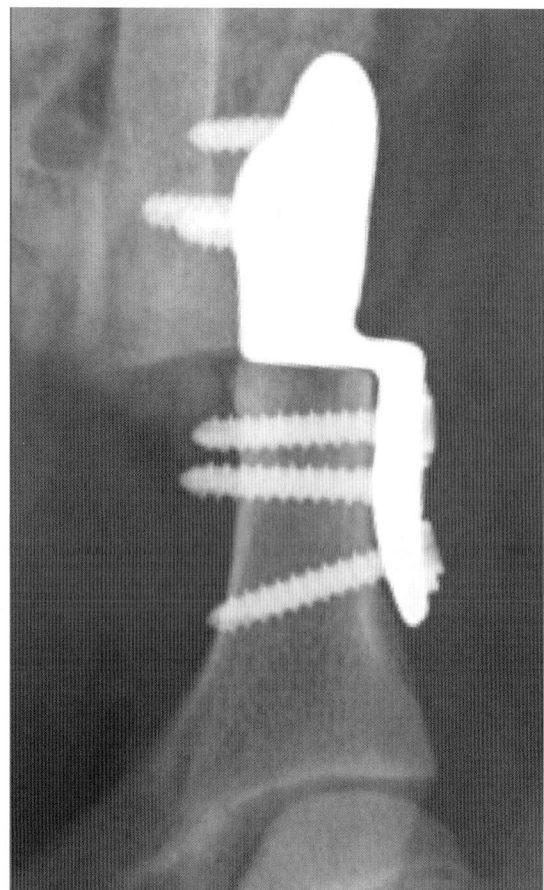

Figure 112.21 Fixin (TraumaVet S.r.l, Rivoli, TO, Italy) double pelvic osteotomy plate with locking screws. The most caudal screw is oriented toward the acetabulum to span the bone caudal to the plate and prevent iliac fracture at that location.

- At least two locking screws should be placed in the cranial portion of the plate.
- Placement of a straight plate on the ventral aspect of the ilium (Vezzoni *et al.* 2010) (Figure 112.22) is recommended in more mature and heavier patients. Sedation of the dog for 2 to 3 weeks after surgery may be considered to relieve the tension caused by the elastic memory of the twisted bone.
- Bilateral DPOs are best staged at least 6 weeks apart in more mature and heavier patients to avoid complications associated with simultaneous procedures. This approach, as with TPO, carries the risk of DJ progressing in the contralateral, unoperated hip while the operated side heals.

Intraoperative hemorrhage

Definition

Intraoperative physical injury of large vessels can result in severe and potentially fatal hemorrhage. Blood vessels located near the ilium and susceptible to injury during TPO and DPO include the cranial gluteal artery and vein dorsolateral to the ilium and the internal iliac artery and vein medial to the ilium (Figure 112.23). The femoral artery and vein, as well as the medial circumflex femoral artery and vein, are in the area of the pubic osteotomies. The caudal gluteal artery and vein become exposed near the osteotomy of the ischium, close to the insertion of the sacrotuberous ligament.

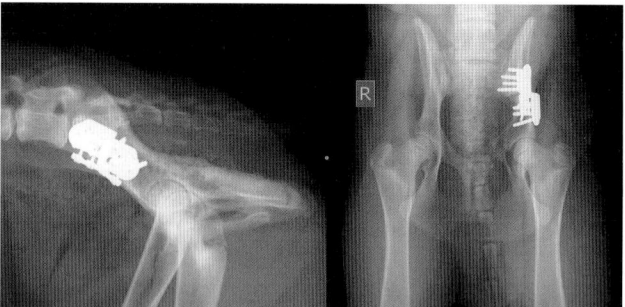

(A)

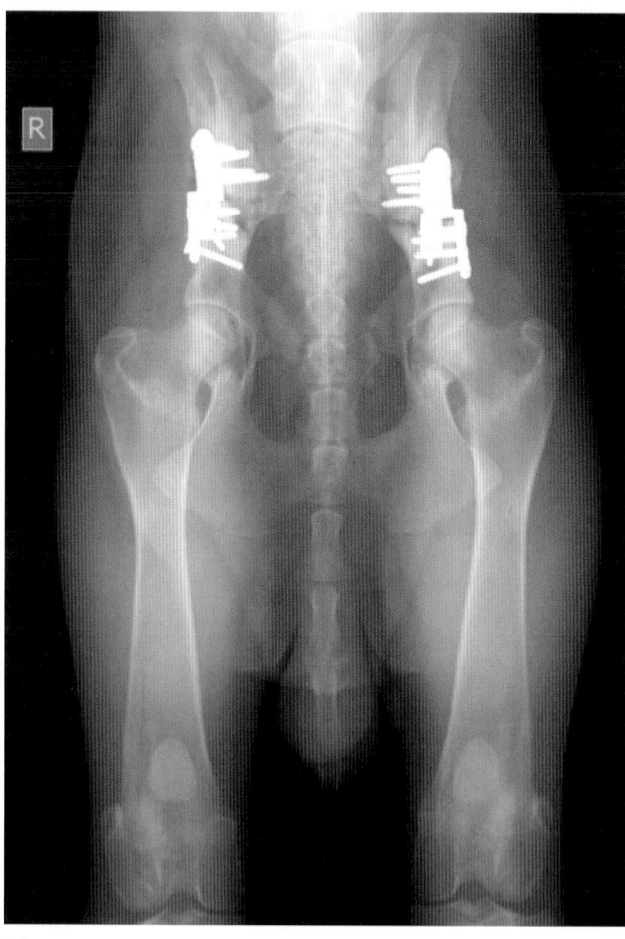

(B)

Figure 112.22 Placement of a ventral iliac plate for adjunct fixation. **A**, Ventrodorsal and lateral radiographs of the pelvis 1 month after double pelvic osteotomy (DPO) in a 7-month-old German shepherd dog. A 2.7-mm Koenigsee plate with locked screws were placed on the ventral aspect of the ilium as an adjunct to the DPO plate (Next Generation Device, Glen Rock, NJ). In the cranial iliac segment, the screws are not inserted into the body of the sacrum to preserve the function of the sacroiliac joint. **B**, Ventrodorsal and lateral radiographs of the pelvis obtained 1 month after bilateral DPO in an 8-month-old German shepherd dog. A 2.7-mm cuttable plate and screws were placed on the ventral aspect of the ilium as an adjunct to the DPO plates. In the cranial iliac segment, the screws are designed not to engage the body of the sacrum.

Risk factors

General risk factors for iatrogenic vascular damage during TPO and DPO include poor knowledge of the surgical anatomy, lack of visualization, and technical errors:

- During osteotomy of the ilium, pubis, and ischium during the drilling of the screw holes
- While passing periosteal elevators, retractors, and cerclage wire around the ilium

Specific risk factors for iatrogenic laceration relate to the location of blood vessels relative to the surgical site (see Figure 112.23):

- Cranial gluteal artery and vein dorsal to the ilium
- Internal iliac artery and vein medial to the ilium
- Iliolumbar artery and vein near the ventral border of the ilium
- Femoral artery and vein near the osteotomy site of the pubis
- Medial circumflex femoral artery near the osteotomy site of the pubis
- Caudal gluteal artery and vein near the obturator foramen close to the insertion of the sacrotuberous ligament

Diagnosis

The diagnosis of hemorrhage is straightforward because injury of large vessels causes sudden, severe bleeding. Bleeding from smaller vessels may result in a postoperative hematoma if ligation or cauterization was inadequate.

Treatment

Hemorrhage from smaller vessels, such as the cranial gluteal and the iliolumbar arteries and veins, is controlled by routine hemostasis, including occlusion, ligation, and cauterization. Periosteal elevation of soft tissues may result in retraction of the severed iliolumbar vessels into the soft tissues, requiring additional dissection. Control of bleeding from large vessels such as the femoral or internal iliac arteries and veins can be very difficult or impossible. An injury to the femoral artery and vein is unlikely, but the internal iliac artery and vein may be perforated while drilling holes in the ilium and constitutes a very severe complication. Bleeding from an injured internal iliac vein can be stopped by packing the area medial

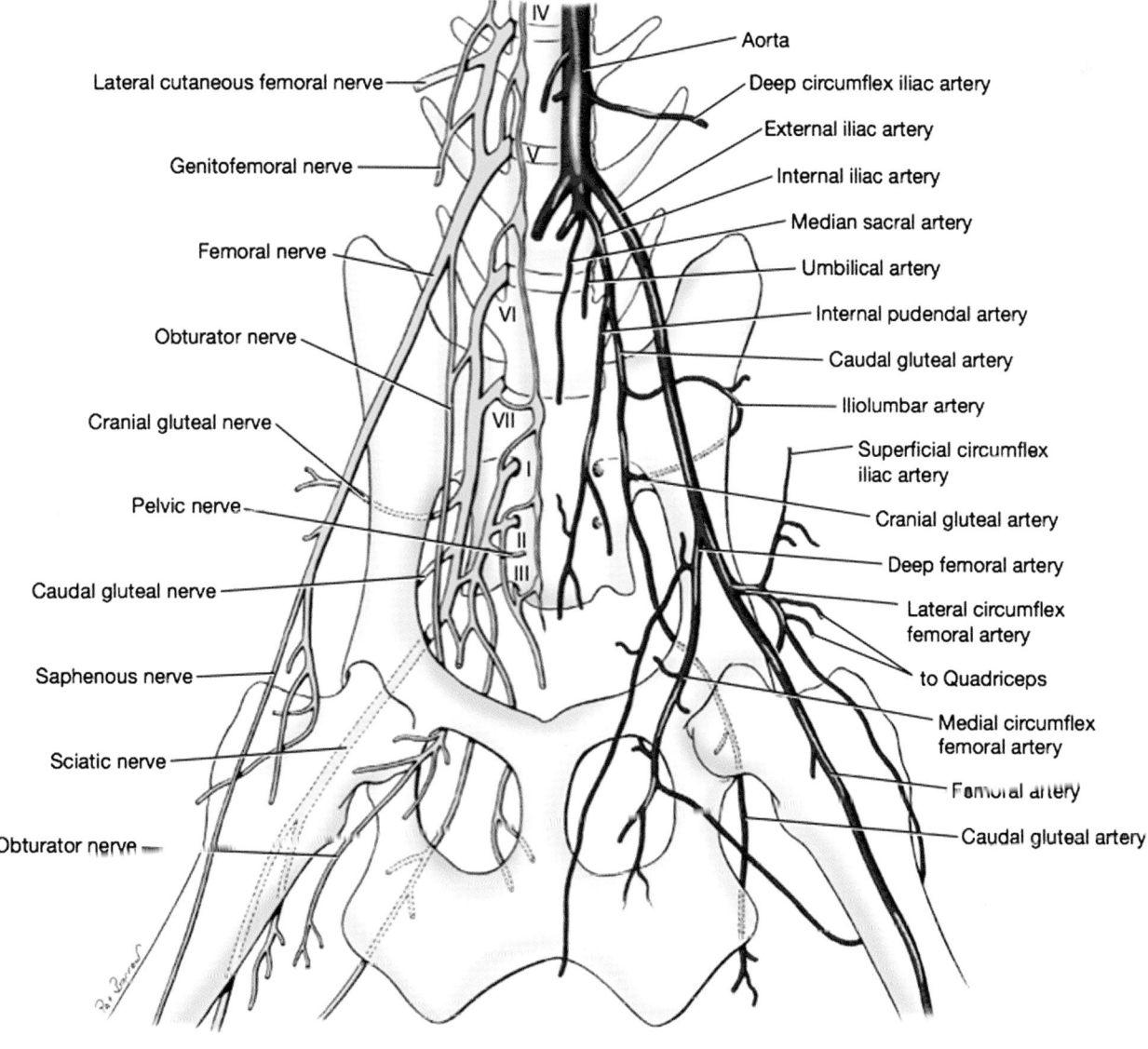

(A)

Figure 112.23 Surgical anatomy of the vasculature relevant to pelvic osteotomies. **A,** Ventrodorsal representation of pelvic arteries.   *(Continued)*

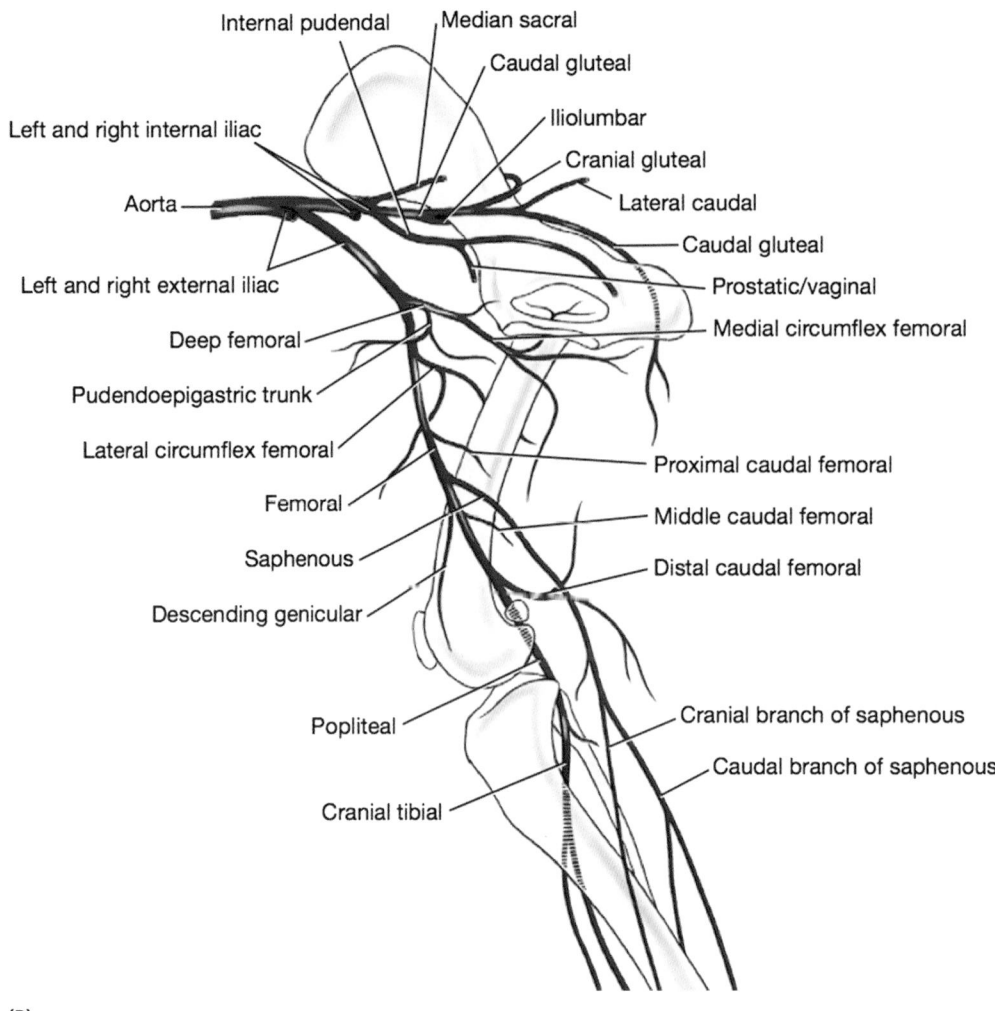

(B)

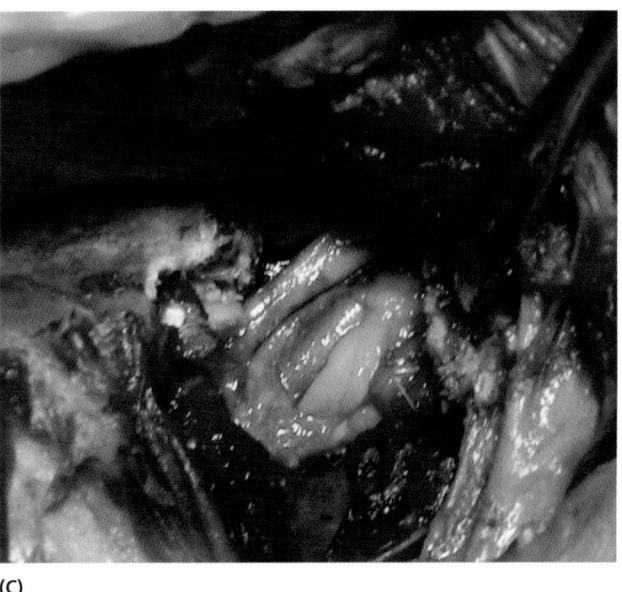

(C)

Figure 112.23 *(Continued)* **B**, Medial view of pelvic arteries. **C**, Postmortem specimen after creation of a window in the ilium in the same location as the iliac osteotomy in double pelvic osteotomy and triple pelvic osteotomy. Note the position of the iliac vein ventral to the sciatic nerve. *Source:* Evans and de Lahunta, 2010. Reproduced with permission from Elsevier.

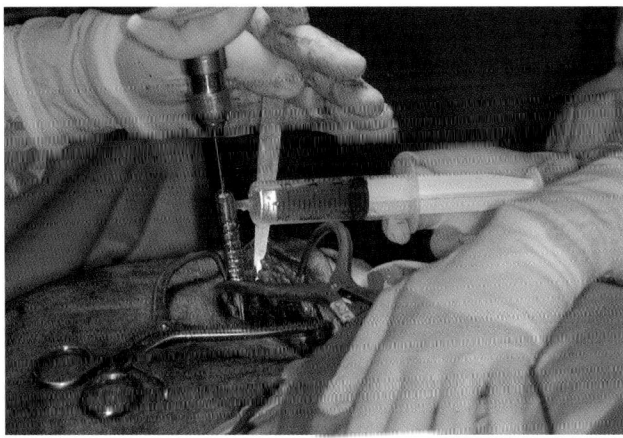

Table 112.3 Iatrogenic damage to peripheral nerves during pelvic osteotomies

Nerve	Risk factors	Clinical signs
Sciatic nerve	Iliac osteotomy, nerve root impingement, elevation and nerve compression	Decreased or absence conscious proprioception; neurologic deficit of tibial and fibular nerves with impairment of hock extension
Obturator nerve	Iliac, pubic, and ischium osteotomies	Lateral sliding of the limb on slippery surfaces
Cranial gluteal nerve	Surgical approach and muscle retraction	Not observed
Pudendal nerve	Iliac osteotomy too caudal	Urinary and fecal incontinence

Figure 112.24 Prevention of injury to the deep iliac vessels during drilling. The power drill should be held with both hands, with one hand resting on a periosteal elevator placed against the ilium. This technique improves control of the drill as well as the ability to stop drilling immediately after the bone has been perforated.

to the iliac body with collagen haemostatic sponges. Bleeding from an injured internal iliac artery can be dramatic, extremely fast, and potentially fatal; a finger can be inserted under the iliac body to compress the artery while another member of the surgical team creates a window in the ilium to gain access to the injured vessel to repair it. Smaller blood vessels that have been damaged are simply clamped and ligated.

Outcome

Hemorrhage that is not addressed may result in a hematoma, and injury to a major blood vessel can easily cause death.

Prevention

A sound knowledge of the vascular anatomy of the pelvic region is critical for preventing injury to blood vessels during TPO and DPO. Hemorrhage of the iliolumbar vessels is prevented via careful elevation of the soft tissues in a caudocranial direction ventral to the ilium. At the level of the iliac crest, the dissection is moved slightly off the bone to allow identification of the vessels and hemostasis. To avoid accidental injury to the deep iliac vessels under the iliac body while drilling, the power drill should be held with both hands (Figure 112.24), with one hand resting on a periosteal elevator placed against the ilium. This technique improves the ability of the surgeon to control the drill and stop drilling immediately after the bone has been perforated. Passing a cerclage wire around the ilium should be done using a gouge to protect nerves and blood vessels.

Nerve damage

Definition

Nerve damage is defined as a physical injury to peripheral nerves caused by compression, contusion, traction, or laceration. Sciatic nerve damage is of major concern in relation to TPO and DPO, but other nerves may also be affected. Compression, contusion, and traction of a nerve may cause neurapraxia (paralysis in the absence of structural changes), which may take weeks to months to resolve. Laceration of the axons with preservation of the perineurium causes axonotmesis (disruption of the axon and myelin

sheath but with preservation of connective tissue fragments), which is followed by possible return of nerve function after several months. Neurotmesis is defined as a complete laceration of the nerve, including the perineurium, thereby causing permanent loss of function.

Risk factors

See Table 112.3.

Iatrogenic damage to the sciatic nerve typically occurs during osteotomy of the ilium, especially as the blade of the oscillating saw penetrates the dorsal third of the far cortex of the Ilium. Placing a Hohmann retractor behind the greater ischiatic notch has been recommended to protect the sciatic nerve and retract soft tissues during iliac osteotomy. However, iatrogenic damage may result because the tip of the retractor may pinch the nerve. The risk of injury during osteotomy is increased if the sciatic nerve has inadvertently been trapped between the retractor and the medial surface of the bone. To prevent this complication, soft tissues may be elevated from the ventral and medial aspect of the ilium to allow insertion of a finger medial to the bone. This finger allows palpation of the nerve as the tip of the Hohmann retractor is maneuvered to make sure that the nerve is effectively placed behind the tip of the Hohman. Alternatively, a Hohman retractor with a very short tip could also be used and anchored only on the cranial edge of the greater ischiatic notch. Nerve damage may occur during periosteal elevation medial to the iliac body if the elevator pinches the ventral nerve branch (Figures 112.25 and 112.26). The most common neurologic complication consists of sciatic neurapraxia caused by excessive retraction of the nerve by the Hohmann retractor during the osteotomy of the ilium or by ventral compression of the nerve with a periosteal elevator.

The obturator nerve (Figures 112.27 and 112.28) may be damaged during the osteotomy of the ischium, especially if an osteotome is used to cut the bone blindly. The obturator nerve travels through the cranial portion of the obturator foramen and can be damaged if the osteotome inadvertently penetrates this area. The obturator nerve may also be damaged during pubic osteotomy because the nerve runs medial to the pubic ramus, as well as during iliac osteotomy because it runs ventral to the ilium. During surgical procedures, the obturator nerve should be protected by a blunt periosteal elevator.

The cranial gluteal nerve may be damaged during the surgical approach to the ilium, iliac osteotomy, or placement of the plate. The branch innervating the tensor fascia lata muscle crosses the surgical field and is therefore predisposed to surgical trauma; however, injury to this nerve does not appear to have clinical consequences.

Injury to the pudendal nerve may occur when the iliac osteotomy site is placed too far caudally and involves the roots of the sacral

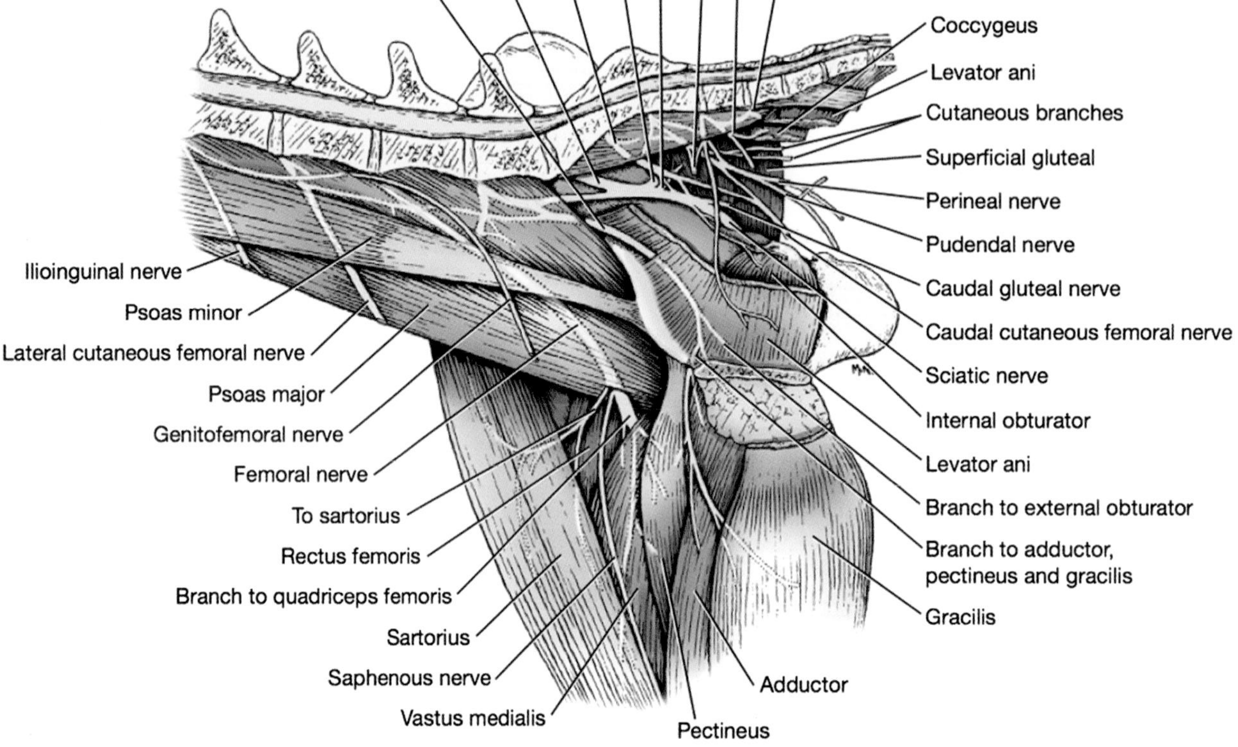

Nerve to piriformis

Cranial gluteal nerve

Pelvic nerve

Ventral branch of 1st sacral nerve

Nerve to levator ani

Ventral branch of 7th lumbar nerve

1st caudal nerve

Obturator nerve

Coccygeus

Levator ani

Cutaneous branches

Superficial gluteal

Perineal nerve

Pudendal nerve

Ilioinguinal nerve

Caudal gluteal nerve

Psoas minor

Caudal cutaneous femoral nerve

Lateral cutaneous femoral nerve

Sciatic nerve

Psoas major

Internal obturator

Genitofemoral nerve

Levator ani

Femoral nerve

Branch to external obturator

To sartorius

Branch to adductor, pectineus and gracilis

Rectus femoris

Branch to quadriceps femoris

Gracilis

Sartorius

Saphenous nerve

Adductor

Vastus medialis

Pectineus

Figure 112.25 Surgical anatomy of the innervation relevant to pelvic osteotomies. Medial view of pelvic nerves. *Source:* Evans and de Lahunta, 2010. Reproduced with permission from Elsevier.

nerves or through carelessness when drilling screw holes into the sacrum. The errors that result in pudendal nerve damage may also cause pelvic nerve injury.

Diagnosis

A diagnosis of nerve damage is made based on postoperative clinical signs and electromyography. These vary with the degree of damage and may range from mild, temporary monoparesis to permanent monoplegia of the affected limb (see Table 112.3).

Sciatic nerve damage causes combined deficiencies of the tibial and fibular nerves, including monoparesis or paralysis, with dysfunction of the cranial tibial and gastrocnemius muscles. This causes the foot to rest on its dorsal aspect; extension of the stifle and hock is also present (Figure 112.29). The tone of the quadriceps muscle is maintained by the femoral nerve but is not offset by the hamstring muscles because of sciatic nerve damage. Abnormalities noted on neurologic examination of the operated limb will include a decrease or loss of conscious proprioception, decreased sciatic nerve reflex, and increased patellar reflex.

Injury of the obturator nerve may cause lateral sliding of the limb in dogs standing on a slippery surface because of weakness of the adductor muscles.

Pudendal nerve injury causes urinary and fecal incontinence because of loss of sphincter tone and paresis or paralysis of the perineal muscles. There is also sensory impairment of the corresponding

dermatomes. Damage to the pelvic nerves causes disorders of micturition such as urine retention associated with bladder paresis or paralysis.

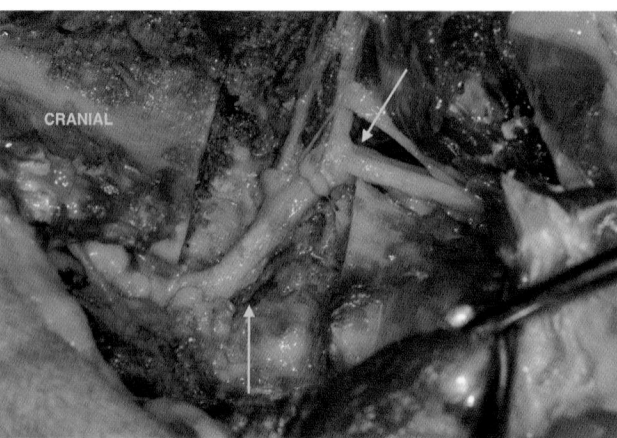

Figure 112.26 Postmortem specimen of the iliac region of a dog. A window has been created through the bone at the level of the iliac osteotomy. Note how the sciatic nerve can easily be damaged by the tip of a Hohmann retractor (upper arrow), a periosteal elevator (lower arrow), the oscillating saw blade, the osteotome, the drill bit, or a cerclage wire.

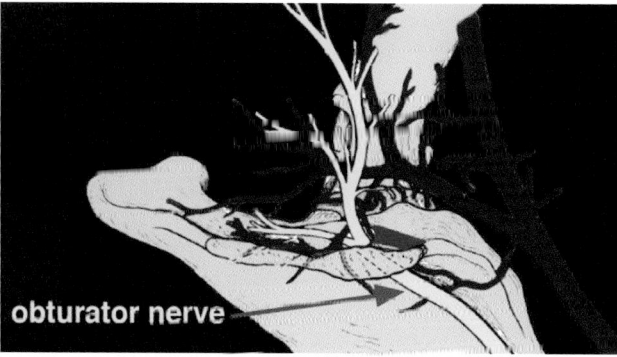

Figure 112.27 Surgical anatomy relevant to the pubic osteotomy. The obturator nerve travels under the pubis and medial circumflex femoral artery *Source:* Miller et al., 1964. Reproduced with permission from Elsevier.

Treatment

The most common neurologic deficit noted after pelvic osteotomies consists of mild sciatic neurapraxia. These cases are treated conservatively: a sling may be placed under the abdomen to assist ambulation, and a bandage (or socks) may be placed over the foot to protect the skin and maintain plantar footing until conscious proprioception has returned. In selected cases of severe sciatic deficit, treatment may be attempted by providing temporary support of the hock with transarticular external fixation to maintain the foot in a weight-bearing position and the hock in flexion. This approach is suggested in cases of severe but incomplete sciatic nerve damage; the goal is to avoid further damage to the limb during the recovery time.

Outcome

The outcome of nerve damage depends on the type of damage and degree of dysfunction. Most cases of postoperative neurologic deficits consist of sciatic neurapraxia and fully return to function within a few weeks after surgery. The prognosis is usually poor when complete loss of motor and sensory function has occurred. If the nerve sheath is intact, the prognosis is better, provided that reinnervation occurs within no more than 1 year of the damage. Electromyograms, nerve conduction studies, and evoked potential findings have great value when making a prognosis and assessing the progression of recovery.

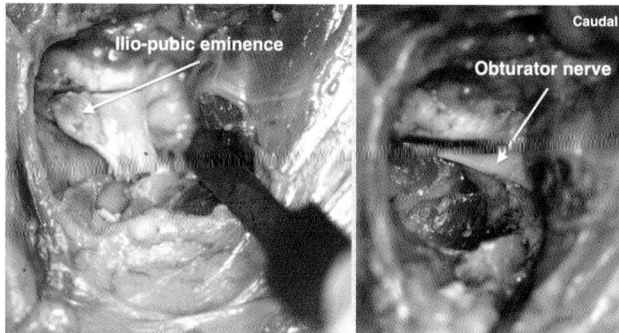

Figure 112.28 Postmortem specimen of the pubic region of a dog. A window has been created in the bone over the location of the pubic osteotomy. The picture illustrates how the obturator nerve can be damaged by instruments during periosteal elevation of tissues and ostectomy.

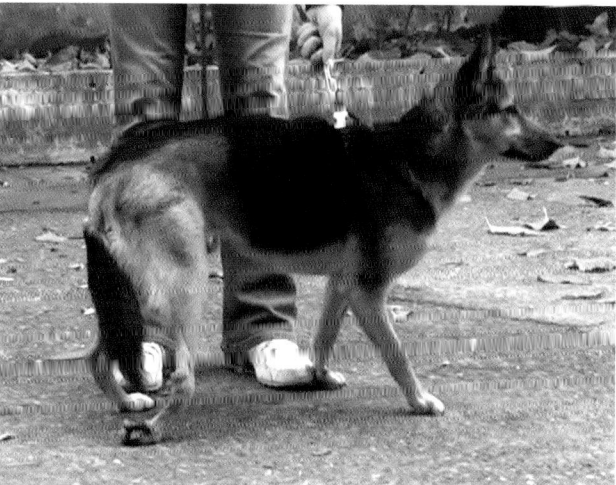

Figure 112.29 Physical examination of an 8-month-old mixed breed dog with severe sciatic nerve deficit 1 month after right double pelvic osteotomy.

Prevention

Prevention of sciatic nerve damage should focus on avoiding the use of regular Hohmann retractors on the greater ischiatic notch when exposing the surgical field. The Langenbeck periosteal elevator or a modified Hohmann retractor with a very short tip, positioned flat to the ilium just caudal to the sacrum, should be used instead, taking care not to pinch the nerve. Another suggestion is to use delicate oscillating saw blades and to stop the osteotomy when the inner iliac cortex is reached in the dorsal third of the ilium; the final piece of cortex is then cut with a sharp, thin, and uniform (not wedged) osteotome (Hardt Delima osteotome) directed in a ventral to dorsal direction. Oscillating saw blades or osteotomes with a predetermined stop can also be useful. The precautions described for the prevention of vascular injury must be used when drilling the screws holes and passing a cerclage wire under the ilium

Pelvic canal narrowing

Definition

Pelvic canal narrowing is defined as the loss of pelvic geometry secondary to iatrogenic reduction of the horizontal diameter of the pelvic canal. Severe pelvic canal narrowing is more likely after bilateral TPO and is very uncommon after bilateral DPO, except when plate pullout or fracture of the ilium. After DPO, fracture of the ischium (Figure 112.30) could occur because of the tension exerted by the rotation and favored by poor postoperative care, such as lack of compliance with strict rest. A partial dorsal osteotomy of the ischial table has been proposed to facilitate pelvic rotation (Petazzoni et al. 2012) but could predispose the bone to subsequent fracture. Severe pelvic canal narrowing may cause constipation, urethral impingement and dysuria, and dystocia in cases of mismating.

Risk factors

Factors associated with pelvic canal narrowing during or after TPO include:
- Implant failure, which is the most common cause of pelvic narrowing (see Figure 112.2)
- Excessive acetabular rotation (see Figure 112.12)

- Bilateral TPOs
- Pubic osteotomy, especially if placed on the medial aspect of the ramus. A long pubic remnant is then rotated toward the pelvic canal.
- Immobilization of the iliac osteotomy with a conventional dynamic compression plate (Figure 112.31) torqued to the desired angle of acetabular version. This technique is contraindicated because the implant aligns the axis of pelvic rotation with the ventrodorsal midsection of the iliac shaft, resulting in an internal rotation of the ventral portion of the ilium and pubic remnant.

Factors associated with pelvic canal narrowing during or after DPO include:
- Implant failure with caudal pull-out of the plate (see Figures 112.6 and 112.11)
- Iliac fracture
- Fracture of the ischium after DPO

Diagnosis

A diagnosis of subclinical pelvic canal narrowing is possible with ventrodorsal radiographs of the pelvis. When narrowing is clinically apparent, signs related to urethral compression may occur immediately postoperatively or later if they are caused by the callus, and constipation and obstipation may appear weeks to months later. Obstipation may lead to secondary megacolon.

Treatment

Treatment of pelvic narrowing is not required in the absence of clinical signs. Severe and acute pelvic collapse can cause urethral compression and dysuria (Dudley and Wilknes 2004; Papadopoulos and Tommasini Degna 2006), which may constitute a medical emergency requiring immediate surgical correction. Urethral impingement between long pubic remnants after bilateral TPO and pubic osteotomies is treated by bilateral pubic ostectomy. Acute pelvic narrowing caused by implant failure should be treated by revision as early as possible to prevent malunion. The use of an external fixator device has been described to pull the acetabular fragments apart (Papadopoulos and Tommasini Degna 2006). Severe, chronic narrowing resulting in megacolon is rare and usually associated with complete or almost complete pelvic collapse. Corrective iliac osteotomies and removal of callus may be attempted, but adhesions with

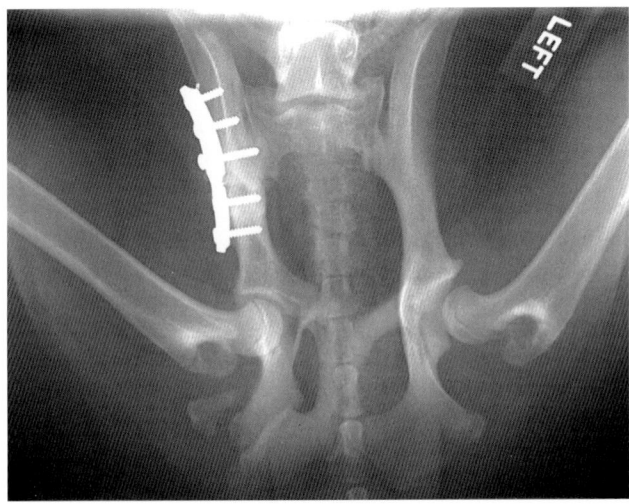

Figure 112.31 Frog-leg radiograph of the pelvis of a dog presented 1 month after a right triple pelvic osteotomy. The osteotomy had been immobilized with a straight, twisted plate, resulting in moderate pelvic canal narrowing. Note the displaced ischial tuberosity, resulting from a malpositioned osteotomy of the ischium. *Source:* D. Griffon, Western University of Health Sciences, Pomona, CA, 2014. Reproduced with permission from D. Griffon.

intrapelvic structures and soft tissue contracture complicate the surgery. An iliac fracture caudal to the plate after DPO should be repaired with a dorsal plate that extends over the acetabulum and ischial body (Figure 112.32). Complete and incomplete fractures of the ischial table after DPO heal spontaneously (see Figure 112.30).

Outcome

The outcome depends on the degree of pelvic canal narrowing. The prognosis is good if the narrowing represents an incidental radiographic finding. In contrast, the prognosis is poor when the pelvic collapse is severe, mainly because of obstipation and gait abnormalities secondary to excessive femoral head coverage. Although owners of dogs with HD are cautioned against breeding the animal, pelvic canal narrowing prohibits natural birth, and a cesarean section is necessary.

Prevention

The following strategies should be considered to prevent pelvic narrowing:
- Pubic ostectomies should be preferred over pubic osteotomies to minimize the length of pubic remnants rotated toward the pelvic canal.
- Limit the degree of acetabular ventroversion through proper case selection. An acetabular rotation of 20 degrees with TPO is sufficient to restore acetabular coverage in good candidates.
- Iliac osteotomies should not be stabilized with dynamic compression plates because these locate the axis of rotation of the iliac shaft midway between the dorsal and ventral aspects of the bone, thereby inducing a medial displacement of the bone ventral to the plate. Plates designed for TPO and DPO locate the axis of rotation along the ventral border of the ilium, thereby inducing a lateral displacement of the dorsal aspect of the bone.
- The DPO technique preserves the integrity of the ischium, thereby limiting pelvic narrowing compared with the TPO.

In addition, strategies to prevent implant failure should be considered, especially during bilateral TPO or DPO in a heavy dog. In these cases, a ventral plate may be placed as an adjunct fixation

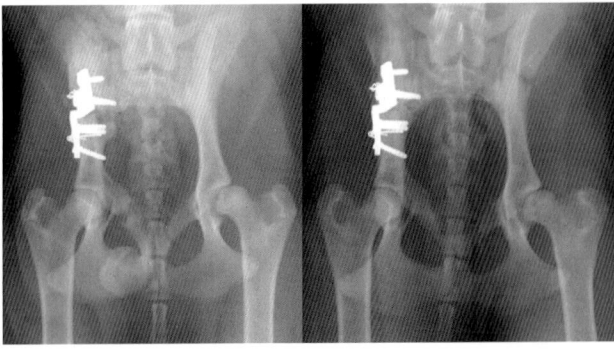

(A)   **(B)**

Figure 112.30 Ventrodorsal pelvic radiograph of a 7-month-old Labrador retriever 1 month (**A**) and 3 months (**B**) after right double pelvic osteotomy. The incomplete fracture of the right ischial table, which has healed, is an incidental finding.

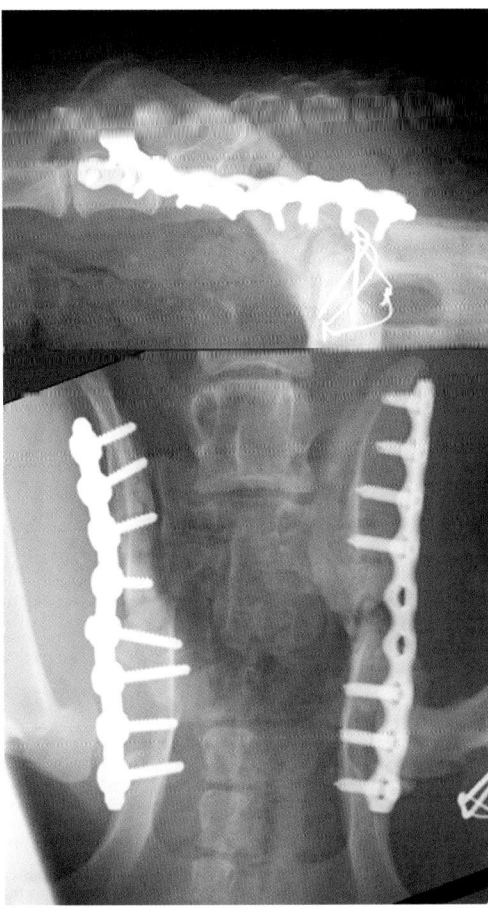

Figure 112.32 Lateral and ventrodorsal radiographs after repair of the implant failure illustrated in Figure 112.6. A String-Of-Pearl locking plate was placed on the right ilium, and an Advanced Locking Plate System (ALPS) Kyon AG, Zurich (CH) and Kyon Veterinary Products, Boston (MA). plate was placed on the left ilium.

on the ilium on each operated side to protect the iliac osteotomies (Fitch *et al.* 2002; Vezzoni *et al.* 2010) (see Figures 112.16 and 112.22). To reduce the risk of an iliac fracture caudal to the plate, the most caudal screw should be inserted in a caudal direction to span the line where the fracture is most likely to occur (see Figure 112.21). Finally, to reduce the risk of ischial fracture after DPO, postoperative restriction of exercise is critical and may be combined with sedation (Vezzoni *et al.* 2010).

Progression of degenerative joint disease

Definition
This complication is characterized by an inability of TPO or DPO to prevent or halt the development of joint degeneration secondary to HD. Progression of radiographic signs of DJD should be expected in most cases but may not be associated with clinical signs.

Risk factors
The majority of risk factors associated with postoperative DJD involve case selection, and the majority of them remain controversial and surgeon dependent. These risk factors include:
- Dogs older than 1 year of age
- Preoperative signs of DJD

- "Soft" or subtle Ortolani sign (consistent with the presence of fibrous tissue filling the acetabulum)
- Angle of subluxation greater than 20 degrees
- Minimum hip DAR based on arthroscopy DAR radiographic projection
- Low Norberg angle and severe loss of femoral head coverage (Rasmussen *et al.* 1998)
- Less than 50% head coverage in the frog view

Degenerative joint disease may also progress as a result of surgical complications such as insufficient acetabular ventroversion and persistence of a postoperative Ortolani sign (Figures 112.33 and 112.34). Acetabular coverage increases in the weeks after pelvic osteotomy as a result of soft tissue healing and muscle contraction. Persistence of an Ortolani sign beyond 2 months after surgery is consistent with incomplete correction of the laxity and increases the risk of secondary DJD. Implant failure and loss of fixation may also predispose a joint to postoperative DJD by altering its conformation.

Diagnosis
A diagnosis of progression of DJD is based on serial orthopedic examinations and evaluations of pelvic radiographs. Progression of radiographic signs can usually be detected at the follow-up examination 6 months to 1 year after surgery. In these cases, joint laxity (distraction index [DI] and Ortolani's sign) has persisted, the angle of reduction (AR) and subluxation (AS) and the DI are similar to preoperative values. Adequate restoration of acetabular coverage by TPO or DPO should lead to an Ortolani's sign that is negative or at least significantly less than before surgery. When joint laxity persists after a corrective procedure, progression of DJD will be become obvious on long-term follow-up examinations.

Treatment
Treatment is indicated when function is affected by DJD (see Chapter 18). Multimodal medical management is often the first line of treatment, especially if the owners do not wish to pursue further surgery. This approach combines nutritional management (weight control and supplementation), low-impact exercise, and antiinflammatory agents. Total hip prosthesis is the treatment of choice in cases when the progression of DJD cannot be managed by conservative treatment (see Figure 112.33).

Outcome
The outcome and prognosis of a dog with DJD depends on the severity of the condition but is overall similar to the prognosis of dogs with HD and secondary DJD.

Prevention
Most efforts at preventing DJD after corrective pelvic osteotomy have focused on strict case selection and careful planning of the surgical procedure. Criteria considered as ideal for pelvic osteotomies include:
- Dogs between 4.5 to 8 months of age, with still fertile growth plates, to optimize postoperative remodeling of the hip
- Absence of preoperative signs of DJD on physical and radiographic examinations
- Palpation of a "crisp," clear Ortolani's sign, consistent with a reduction of the femoral head into an intact acetabulum with a preserved dorsal rim
- Angle of subluxation equal or inferior to 25 degrees for a TPO and 20 degrees for a DPO; difference between AR and AS = or > 15 degrees

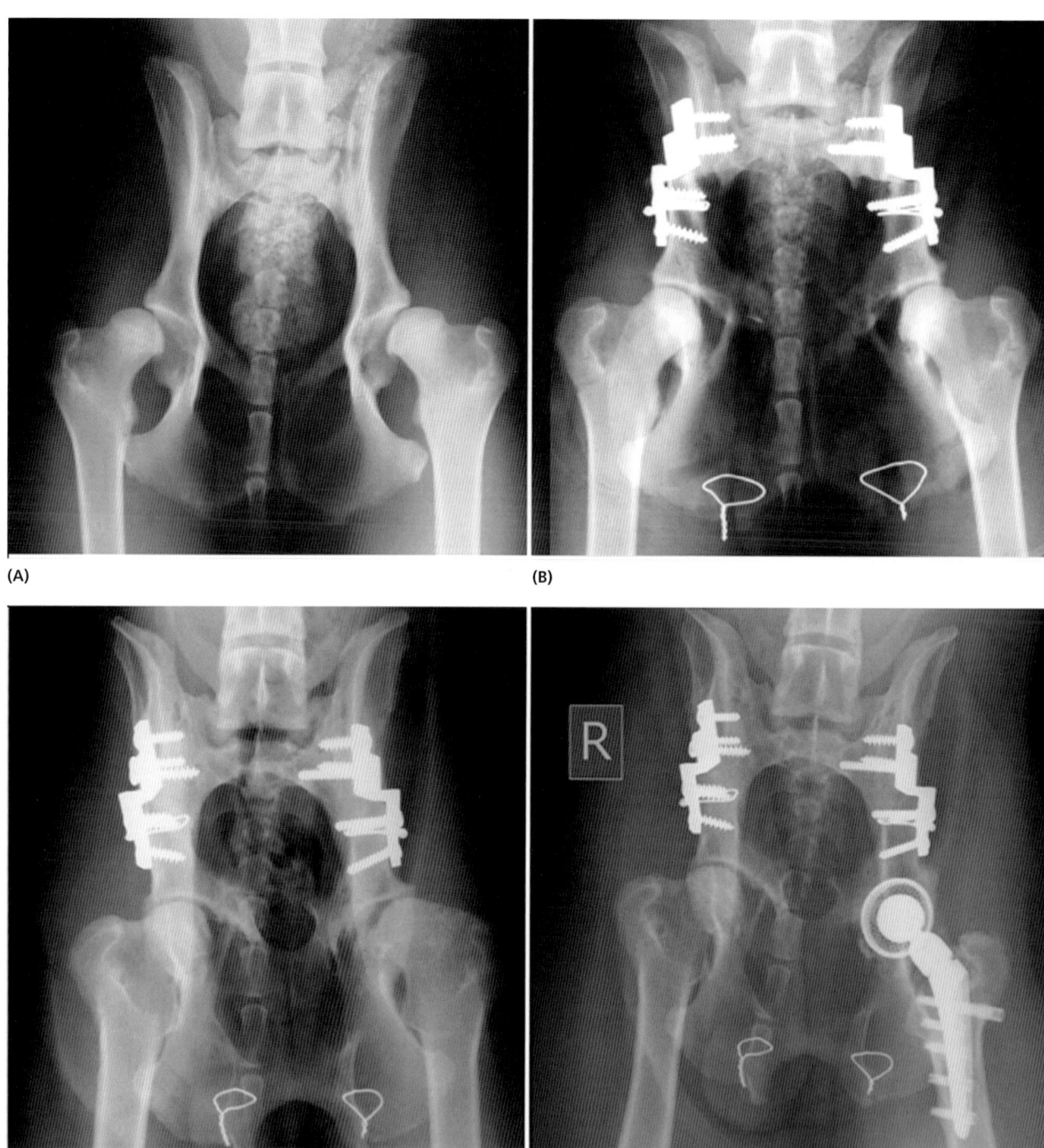

(A)

(B)

(C)

(D)

Figure 112.33 Progression of degenerative joint disease (DJD) after bilateral triple pelvic osteotomy in an 8-month-old boxer. **A**, Preoperative radiograph of the pelvis. DJD and erosion of the dorsal acetabular rim are visible on the left hip. Findings on orthopedic examination included for the right hip, angle of reduction (AR), 40 degrees; angle of subluxation (AS), 15 degrees; and distraction index (DI), 0.7 and for the left hip, AR, 40 degrees; AS, 30 degrees; and DI, 0.9. **B**, Immediate postoperative radiograph after placement of a 25-degree plate on the right ilium and a 30-degree plate on the left ilium. **C**, Two-year follow-up. Severe progression of DJD warranted a left total hip replacement (THR). **D**, Three-year follow-up after left THR and 5 years after right triple pelvic osteotomy (TPO). The right femoral head remains well covered without progression of DJD. The left prosthetic cup appears quite closed because of the TPO-induced acetabular ventroversion.

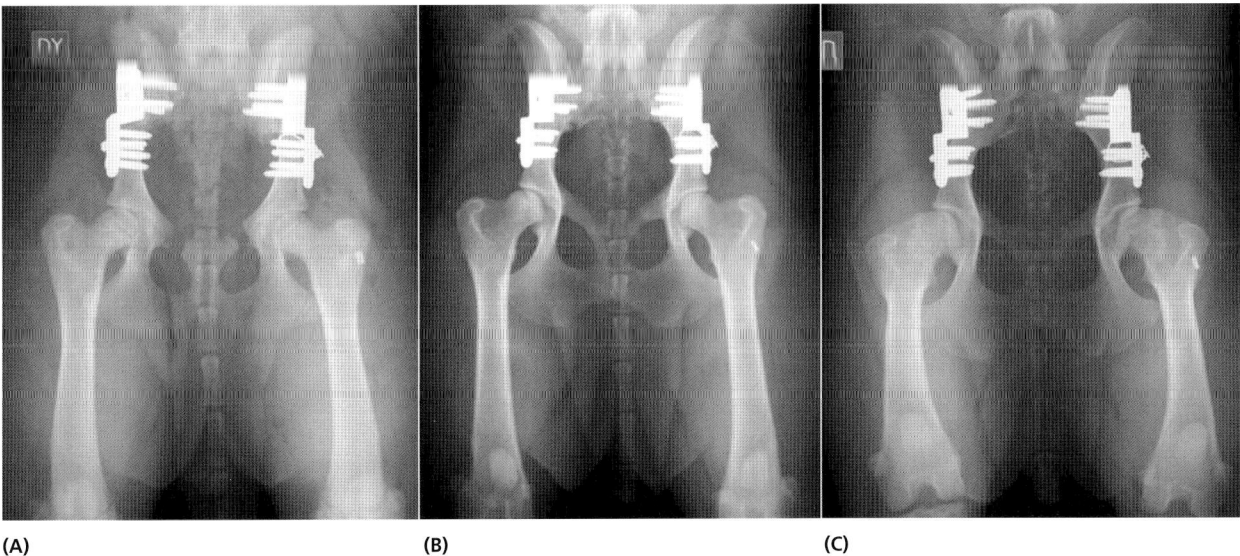

(A)   (B)   (C)

Figure 112.34 Bilateral hip dysplasia in a 6-month-old Labrador retriever. Preoperative orthopedic findings included on the right hip, angle of reduction (AR), 37 degrees; angle of subluxation (AS), 20 degrees; distraction index (DI), 0.83; and dorsal acetabular rim (DAR), 12.5 and for the left hip joint, AR, 40 degrees; AS, 22 degrees; DI, 0.91; and DAR, 16.5. **A**, Extended ventrodorsal radiograph of the pelvis immediately after single-session bilateral double pelvic osteotomy with 25-degree plates. A figure-of-eight nylon suture was added on the left side to counteract joint laxity. **B**, Follow-up 6 months after surgery. Coverage of the right femoral head is incomplete, and sclerosis is visible on the cranial acetabular border (AR, 34 degrees; AS, 15 degrees). **C**, Radiograph 3.5 years after surgery. Severe bilateral progression of DJD with deformation of the femoral heads. Multiple osteophytes are present on the acetabular rim, femoral head, and neck of hips.
This was not an ideal candidate for double pelvic osteotomy. In addition, placement of 30-degree plates may have produced better results.

- Intact and DAR on arthroscopy or DAR projection, with only minimal rounding
- No or minimal acetabular filling in the frog Ventro-Dorsal (VD) view with head compression inside the acetabula
- DI over normal values for each breed, but not over 1.0

Although a 30-degree plate for TPO should not be used to avoid excessive acetabular coverage of the femoral head, the same plate effectively rotates the pelvis by a maximum of 25 degrees in DPO and does therefore not result in excessive coverage of the femoral head. Therefore, when carrying out a DPO, a 30-degree plate can be used safely when subluxation is more severe, and a 25-degree plate is reserved for less severe subluxation.

After surgery, general preventive measures against DJD are often recommended, including weight control and nutritional management.

Relevant literature

Complication rates associated with TPO range in the literature from 35% to 70% of cases. Screw loosening is the most common complication and has been reported in 10% to 62% of cases, with clinical consequences affecting the management in up to 25% of dogs. Screw loosening may result in pain, lameness, narrowing of the pelvic canal, delayed healing of the osteotomy, catastrophic implant failure, and surgical revision. Pelvic canal collapse and narrowing, excessive head coverage with subsequent impingement of the femoral head, delayed healing of iliac and ischial, nerve damage, and overall high morbidity have also been frequently reported (Hoo good and Lewis 1993; Koch et al. 1993; Remedios and Fries 1993; Plante et al. 1997; Whelan et al. 2004; Doornink et al. 2006). The TPO technique was consequently modified to reduce the compli-

cation and morbidity rates, particularly after simultaneous bilateral operations (Koch et al. 1993; Sukhiani et al. 1994a, b; Graehler et al. 1994; Borostyankoi et al. 2003). Because of the limited number of clinical studies on DPO published to date, the complication rate associated with DPO remains unclear. However, excessive femoral head coverage, delayed union of the osteotomies, or patient discomfort after bilateral procedures were not reported in a recent study of 53 DPOs (Vezzoni et al. 2010). Implant failure was the most frequently encountered complication after DPO performed with standard TPO plates, but this complication decreased greatly when plates specially designed for DPO were used (Vezzoni et al. 2010). The use of a locking seven-hole plate with 3.5-mm-diameter locking screws has recently been found to lower the rate of minor and major complications reported with the use of conventional six-hole plates. In particular, the rate of screw loosening was decreased to 0.4% of screws and 2.6% of hips operated on (Rose et al. 2012). However, en-bloc pull-out of the caudal portion of the plate appears to be an occasional complication of the TPO locking plate.

Implant failure is the most common complication reported after TPO and was seen when TPO plates were first used for DPO. In TPO, whereas screw loosening seems to be more frequently associated with the use of cortical screws, screw breakage is more common with cancellous screws (see Figure 112.1). Loosening and breakage of screws after TPO occurred mainly in the cranial segment of the ilium, but loosening decreased when screw purchase into the sacrum was achieved (Simmons et al. 2001, Whelan et al. 2004). Application of an adjunct plate to the ventral portion of the ilium has been found to double the stiffness of a standard six-hole TPO plate in axial bending and decreases the rate of screw loosening by a factor of 9 (Fitch et al. 2002a, b). The ventral plate may consist of a 2.0-mm dynamic compression plate or a

2.0- to 2.7-mm veterinary cuttable plate. Placement of the screws is complicated by the presence of soft tissues ventral to the ilium, requiring significant retraction. This strategy is especially relevant in giant active breeds but has not gained much popularity because of the increased cost and surgical time. Instead, eight-hole and locking plates are generally preferred in these cases because of the ease and speed of application.

In the only published clinical report on DPO to date, the rate of screw loosening was very low, at 3.5 % (13 of 371 screws) (Vezzoni *et al.* 2010). This finding was attributed to an improved stability of the pelvic fixation in DPO because preservation of the ischium reduces stress on the implants. There were 3 cases of plate pull-out from the caudal segment of the ilium after DPO, all associated with the use of TPO locking plates and parallel screws (see Figures 112.4 and 112.11). Even locking parallel screws were not strong enough to withstand the pull-out forces created by the elastic memory of the ilium rotated along its long axis. For this reason, the risk of implant failure after DPO depends mainly on the stability of the caudal segment of the fixation; thus, a strong caudal fixation is crucial to a successful outcome. Indeed, plate pull-out did not occur when plates designed for DPO were used when two locking and two nonlocking screws, all diverging, were inserted in the caudal segment (Vezzoni *et al.* 2010).

The most common risk factor for **pelvic canal narrowing** in dogs after TPO is screw loosening. Narrowing of the pelvic canal may occur after simultaneous bilateral operations, mainly because of excessive acetabular rotation, implant failure, and excessive length of the pubic remnants (Sukhiani *et al.* 1994a, b; Fitch *et al.* 2002a, b). Severe pelvic narrowing secondary to complete pelvic collapse represents a critical complication of catastrophic, early implant failure. Slocum and Devine (1987) described postoperative dysuria in three cases caused by urethral impingement by the inwardly rotated acetabular branch of the pubic bone. The occurrence of this complication gave rise to a modification of the original TPO technique, which entailed a pubic ostectomy instead of an osteotomy to shorten the pubic remnants. In contrast to TPO, pelvic narrowing has not been described after bilateral uncomplicated DPO, and the preservation of pelvic geometry is one of the advantages of DPO. Nevertheless, some degree of pelvic collapse is possible after DPO when plate pull-out or fracture of the ilium or ischium occurs. Plate pull-out was described earlier in the chapter. Fracture of the ilium caudal to the plate may occur after DPO when the osteotomy site is too far cranial (Vezzoni *et al.* 2010). Fracture of the ischium after DPO usually occurs at the site of the ischial osteotomy and may be complete or incomplete (green-stick fracture) (Vezzoni *et al.* 2010) (see Figures 112.5 and 112.6). The main cause of this type of fracture is the tension exerted by the ilial rotation during the first 2 to 3 weeks after surgery when bone is undergoing remodelling.

Progression of DJD has been considered as an expected outcome after TPO. Indeed, TPO has been found to slow, but not stop, the progression of DJD in dogs with bilateral HD and unilateral surgery (Johnson *et al.* 1998). In a subsequent prospective study of 34 dogs, DJD progressed in 40% of dogs at long-term follow-up (Rasmussen *et al.* 1998). Eighty-seven percent of dogs received excellent or good physical examination scores, and 76% received excellent or good at-home activity scores. The progression of radiographic signs of OA should therefore be expected after surgery, but these may not translate into clinical signs. An important risk factor for progression of DJD is inadequate case selection. Criteria for selection of candidates to TPO have become more stringent with time in response to the high rate of postoperative progressive DJD initially noted. Ideal candidates for DPO or TPO include dogs between 4.5 and 8 months

of age (the younger, the better) with coxofemoral joint subluxation and laxity that predispose them to future development of severe HD. Younger dogs are much more likely to benefit from corrective pelvic osteotomy because of their residual growth potential and associated improvement of joint congruity. In more mature dogs, on the other hand, the adaptive ability of bone is decreased, which leads to mismatching of joint surfaces, incongruity, and subsequent DJD. Clinical and radiographic evidence of DJD should be minimal or absent. On palpation, the angle of subluxation should not exceed 25 degrees for TPO and 20 degrees for DPO. On radiographic evaluation of the hip, there should be no or minimal acetabular filling on the ventrodorsal frog view, and the lateral border of the DAR should appear sharp and intact, with minimal rounding. The DI should not exceed a value of 1 (Vezzoni *et al.* 2008, 2010). Older dogs and dogs with more severe clinical signs and a diagnosis of DJD are more likely to develop progressive DJD. Persistent joint laxity after corrective pelvic osteotomy is usually caused by inappropriate case selection, a plate with insufficient angulation, or an excessive DI and represents another risk factor for the development of DJD.

References

Borostyankoi, F., Rooks, R.L., Kobluk, C.N., et al. (2003) Result of single-session bilateral triple pelvic osteotomy with an eight-hole iliac bone plate in dogs: 95 cases (1996-1999). *Journal of the American Veterinary Medical Association* 222, 54-59.

Doornink, M.T., Nieves, M.A., Evans, R. (2006) Evaluation of ilial screw loosening after triple pelvic osteotomy in dogs: 227 cases (1991-1999). *Journal of the American Veterinary Medical Association* 229, 535-541.

Dudley, R.M., Wilknes, B.E. (2004) Urethral obstruction as a complication of staged bilateral triple pelvic osteotomy. *Journal of the American Animal Hospital Association* 40, 162-164.

Fitch, R.B., Hosgood, G., Staatz, A. (2002a) Biomechanical evaluation of triple pelvic osteotomy with and without additional ventral plate stabilization. *Veterinary and Comparative Orthopaedics and Traumatology* 145-149.

Fitch, R.B., Kerwin, S., Hosgood, G., et al. (2002b) Radiographic evaluation and comparison of triple pelvic osteotomy with and without additional ventral plate stabilization in forty dogs—part 1. *Veterinary and Comparative Orthopaedics and Traumatology* 15, 164-171.

Fitch, R.B., Kerwin, S., Hosgood, G., et al. (2002c) Treatment of mechanically failed triple pelvic osteotomies in four dogs—part 2. *Veterinary and Comparative Orthopaedics and Traumatology* 3, 172-176.

Graehlerr, R.A., Weigel, J.P., Pardo, A.D. (1994) The effects of plate type, angle of ilial osteotomy, and degree of axial rotation on the structural anatomy of the pelvis. *Veterinary Surgery Journal* 23, 13-20.

Haudiquet, P.H. (2008) Other strategies for HD—DPO vs TPO. *Proceedings of 14th ESVOT Congress*, September 10-14. Munich, Germany, pp. 85-86.

Haudiquet, P.H., Guillon, J.F. (2006) Radiographic evaluation of double pelvic osteotomy versus triple pelvic osteotomy in the dog: an in vitro experimental study. *Proceedings of 13th ESVOT Congress*, September 7-10. Munich, Germany, pp. 239-240.

Hosgood, G., Lewis, D.D. (1993) Retrospective evaluation of fixation complications of 49 pelvic osteotomies in 36 dogs. *Journal of Small Animal Practice* 34, 123-130.

Hunt, C.A., Litsky, A.S. (1988) Stabilization of canine pelvic osteotomies with AO/ASIF plates and screws. *Veterinary and Comparative Orthopaedics and Traumatology* 1, 52-57.

Hutchinson, G.S., Griffon, D.J., Siegel, A.M., et al. (2005) Evaluation of an osteoconductive resorbable calcium phosphate cement and polymethylmethacrylate for augmentation of orthopedic screws in the pelvis of canine cadavers. *American Journal of Veterinary Research* 66 (11), 1954-1960.

Johnson, A.L., Smith, C.W., Pijanowski, G.J., et al. (1998) Triple pelvic osteotomy: effect on limb function and progression of degenerative joint disease. *Journal of the American Animal Hospital Association* 34, 260-264.

Koch, D., Hazewinkel, H., Nap, R., et al. (1993) Radiographic evaluation and comparison of plate fixation after triple pelvic osteotomy in 32 dogs with hip dysplasia. *Veterinary and Comparative Orthopaedics and* Traumatology 6, 9-15.

Papadopoulos, G., Tommasini Degna, M, (2006) Two cases of dysuria as a complication of single-session bilateral triple pelvic osteotomy. *Journal of Small Animal Practice* 47, 741-743.

Petazzoni, M., Tamburro, R., Nicetto, T., et al. (2012) Evaluation of the dorsal acetabular coverage obtained by a modified triple pelvic osteotomy (2.5 pelvic osteotomy). *Veterinary and Comparative Orthopaedics and Traumatology* 25, 385-389.

Plante, J., Dupuis, J., Beauregard, G., et al. (1997) Long term results of conservative treatment, excision arthroplasty, and triple pelvic osteotomy for the treatment of hip dysplasia in the immature dog. *Veterinary and Comparative Orthopaedics and Traumatology* 10, 101-110.

Punke, J.P., Fox, D.B., Tomlinson, J.L., et al. (2011) Acetabular ventroversion with double pelvic osteotomy versus triple pelvic osteotomy: a cadaveric study in dogs. *Veterinary Surgery Journal* 40, 555-562.

Rasmussen, L.M., Kramek, B.A., Lipowitz, A.J. (1998) Preoperative variables affecting long-term outcome of triple pelvic osteotomy for treatment of naturally developing hip dysplasia in dogs. *Journal of the American Veterinary Medical Association* 213 (1), 80-85.

Remedios, A.M., Fries, C.L. (1993) Implants complications in 20 triple pelvic osteotomies. *Veterinary and Comparative Orthopaedics and Traumatology* 6, 202-207.

Rose, S.A., Peck, J.N., Tano, C.A., et al. (2012) Effect of a locking triple pelvic osteotomy plate on screw loosening in 26 dogs. *Veterinary Surgery Journal* 41 (1), 156-162.

Schrader, S.C. (1986) Triple pelvic osteotomy of the pelvis and trochanteric osteotomy as a treatment for hip dysplasia in the immature dog: the surgical technique and results of 77 consecutive operations. *Journal of the American Veterinary Medical Association* 189, 659-665.

Simmons, S., Johnson, A.L., Schaeffer, D.J. (2001) Risk factors for screw migration after triple pelvic osteotomy. *Journal of the American Veterinary Medical Association* 37, 269-273.

Slocum, B., Devine, T. (1986) Pelvic osteotomy technique for axial rotation of the acetabular segment in dogs. *Journal of the American Animal Hospital Association* 22, 331-338.

Slocum, B., Devine, T. (1987) Pelvic osteotomy in the dog as treatment for hip dysplasia. *Seminars in Veterinary Medicine & Surgery (Small Animal)* 2, 107-116.

Slocum, B., Devine, T. (1992) Pelvic osteotomy for axial rotation of the acetabular segment in dogs with hip dysplasia. *Veterinary Clinics of North America: Small Animal Practice* 22, 645-683.

Slocum, B., Devine, T. (1998) Triple pelvic osteotomy. In: Bojrab, M.J., Ellison, G.W., Slocum, B. (eds.) *Current Techniques in Small Animal Surgery*, 4th edn. Lippincott Williams & Wilkins, Baltimore, pp. 1159-1165.

Sukhiani, H.R., Holmberg, D.L., Binnington A.G., et al. (1994a) Pelvic canal narrowing caused by triple pelvic osteotomy in the dog. Part II: a comparison of three pubic osteotomy techniques. *Veterinary and Comparative Orthopaedics and Traumatology* 7, 114-117.

Sukhiani, H.R., Holmberg, D.L., Hurtig, M.B. (1994b) Pelvic canal narrowing caused by triple pelvic osteotomy in the dog. Part I: the effect of pubic remnant length and angle of acetabular rotation. *Veterinary and Comparative Orthopaedics and Traumatology* 7, 110-113.

Tomlinson, J.L., Johnson, J.C. (2000) Quantification of measurement of femoral head coverage and Norberg angle within and among four breeds of dogs. *American Journal of Veterinary Research* 61, 1492-1500.

Vezzoni, A., Baroni, E., Petazzoni, M. (2000) Triple pelvic osteotomy: multicentric retrospective study on implant failure in 218 cases. *Proceedings of the 40th SCIVAC Congress*, Montecatini, Italy.

Vezzoni, A., Dravelli, G., Vezzoni, L., et al. (2008) Comparison of conservative management and juvenile pubic symphysiodesis in the early treatment of canine hip dysplasia. *Veterinary and Comparative Orthopaedics and Traumatology* 21, 267-279.

Vezzoni, A., Boiocchi, S., Vezzoni, L., et al. (2010) Double pelvic osteotomy for the treatment of hip dysplasia in young dogs. *Veterinary and Comparative Orthopaedics and Traumatology* 23, 444-452.

Whelan, M.F., McCarthy, R.J., Boudrieau, R.J., et al. (2004) Increased sacral screw purchase minimizes screw loosening in canine triple pelvic osteotomy. *Veterinary Surgery Journal* 33, 609-614.

113 Total Hip Replacement

William Liska[1] and Jonathan Dyce[2]
[1] Global Veterinary Specialists, Sugar Land, TX, USA
[2] Ohio State University, Columbus, OH, USA

Introduction

A wealth of knowledge has accumulated since the early pioneers of hip replacement in dogs reported their experiments (McElfresh 1991). The importance of durable materials, especially polyethylene, was immediately recognized and led to generations of implants with improved composition and design (Judet and Judet 1950; Newman and Scales 1951; Markowitz *et al.* 1964). Efforts focused on improving function of the hip through the development of a hemiarthroplasty with an acrylic, stainless steel, or vitallium femoral head on a short stem combined with acetabular reaming. Many generations of implants later, the search for perfection still continues, fueled by high expectations for postoperative function.

The expectations for hip replacement in humans in essence consist of reduced pain and improved mobility. Much higher expectations are placed on veterinary hip replacement surgeons by pets' owners. Dogs and cats undergoing hip replacement are expected to be pain free and functioning normally every day for their remaining life span. Mild dysfunction is critiqued as an intolerable failure to restore function regardless of the preoperative severity and chronicity of the disease. Similarly, whereas ambulation after reconstructive knee surgery and clinical union after fracture repair with fair function are viewed as milestones for abdication of clinical oversight, a lifetime of ongoing responsibility is placed on the hip replacement surgeon.

Total hip replacement (THR) is a technically challenging procedure and as such can result in complications. Fortunately, almost all can be resolved successfully. The level of technical difficulty of the procedure requires that surgeons go through a learning curve (Hayes *et al.* 2011) to develop the skill set required to ensure reproducible success, case after case. This learning curve may be multiphasic. The surgeon's confidence can be buoyed after performing 50 to 100 procedures in medium-sized dogs with mild or moderate osteoarthritis (OA). Then humbling moments begin, when the procedure is complicated by factors such as old age, atypical anatomy, end-stage OA, severe preoperative chronic subluxation, undiagnosed concomitant diseases of the knee or spine, exceptionally small or large patients, animals that elude necessary postoperative behavioral modification, owners that do not perceive the importance of compliance with aftercare instructions, and other unpredictable adverse events. Variable duration of signs and degree of severity of the arthropathy at the time of presentation contribute to the learning curve associated with THR (Lockwood and Liska 2011). The complication rate may reach levels deemed unacceptably high by the surgeon, prompting discontinuation of the procedure as an in-house service. This attitude is acceptable but should lead to referring hip replacement candidates to other surgeons rather than femoral head and neck ostectomy (Off and Matis *et al.* 2010).

Hip replacement surgery requires a commitment to become a high-volume surgeon to attain and maintain proficiency. Likewise, there must be a commitment by the instrumentation and prosthesis supplier to provide superbly designed and durable products along with a willingness to upgrade technology as indicated. Surgeons should maintain a registry of every patient receiving a THR, and patients should be examined at regular intervals (preferably annually) throughout their life span. The recheck examinations should be conducted with the understanding that clinical signs may not be observed by owners or even overtly evident to trained eyes. Multiple follow-up parameters should be recorded, especially with regards to complications (incidence and types), as a personal audit of the surgeon's performance. Surgeons should be aware of the clinical relevance of their observations because some findings considered as complications in humans may not be detectable in animals or, if detected, may not be clinically significant. Inclusion of gait analysis during follow-up examinations adds objective evidence of function when subjective evaluation is inadequate (Dogan *et al.* 1991; Budsberg *et al.* 1996; Braden *et al.* 2004; Lascelles *et al.* 2010; Kalis *et al.* 2012; Jankovits *et al.* 2012).

Complications of cemented hip replacement have been described in several publications (Massat *et al.* 1994; Olmstead 1995; Conzemius and Vandervoort 2005; Bergh *et al.* 2006; Iwata *et al.* 2008). Survival analysis of an uncemented prosthesis has also been reported (DeYoung *et al.* 1992; Marcellin-Little *et al.* 1999a). When examining these reports, readers should be aware that the reported complication rate for THR is accurate only to the moment of the last examination of each and every animal in a particular study group. At that point, the complication rate in the study is at its lowest and can only rise subsequently because the prosthesis is expected to last the entire life span of the patient (Dyce 2010). Identifying the true complication rate of the procedure precludes loss of animals to follow-up and requires examining complications over the animals' entire life span. Quite candidly, the prostheses and instrumentation are superior and not at fault for the complications. Owners are

Complications in Small Animal Surgery, First Edition. Edited by Dominique Griffon and Annick Hamaide.
© 2016 John Wiley & Sons, Inc. Published 2016 by John Wiley & Sons, Inc.
Companion website: www.wiley.com/go/griffon/complications

ultimately responsible for their decision to have their pets undergo THR or not. The surgeon's responsibility is to engineer success and minimize the risk of complications through adequate preparation of the entire surgical team, patient and client (communication), surgical expertise, and competence in addressing complications. Noncompliance with aftercare instructions can jeopardize success, along with unfortunate and unpredictable events. However, complications are overall rare, and it is extremely rare for a technically perfectly executed hip replacement to encounter complications. Nonetheless, guaranteeing absence of complications would require eliminating THR in pets. This would unjustifiably deprive many dogs and cats of a good quality of life.

By default, the complications are presented in alphabetical order throughout the chapter, except for less recognized miscellaneous complications at the end of the chapter. Complications discussed in this chapter focus exclusively on prostheses manufactured by BioMedtrix (Boonton, NJ). No attempt was made to compare complications related to other implant and instrumentation vendors. Sparse reports have been published regarding other cementless hip replacement systems (Vezzoni *et al.* 2004; Vezzoni 2010; Hummel *et al.* 2010). Complications inevitably occur with other systems and will eventually be reported in detail.

Aseptic loosening

Definition
Aseptic loosening is defined as a loosening of a hip prosthesis in the absence of clinical or microbiologic evidence of infection. Aseptic loosening may result from a biologic process associated with wear of contact surfaces, or from biomechanical failure. Both mechanisms result in unacceptable motion at the bone–implant or bone–cement interface.

The biologic process resulting in aseptic loosening originates from the migration of submicron particles of ultra-high-molecular-weight polyethylene (UHMWPE) causing a macrophage-mediated osteoclastic activity. Bone resorption, combined with the formation of a fibrovascular membrane between the host and implant, leads to unacceptable motion, more commonly located at the bone–cement interface (Figure 113.1). Tribology confirms that every articular surface normally undergoes wear. However, this process is exacerbated when synthetic surfaces, such as metal on polyethylene are in contact, implanted in vivo, and must function beyond a decade. This biologic process is affected by a combination of parameters, including prosthesis design, composition, surgical technique, loading forces, thermal and chemical factors, and host response.

In addition to the biologic process associated with wear, mechanical failure can also lead to aseptic loosening, more commonly located between the implant and cement. Examples include cement–implant debonding, cementless stem **subsidence**, implant malpositioning, implant displacement, third body wear, early excessive repetitive interface micromotion, and traumatic events. Polyethylene failure is primarily a result of in vivo oxidation (Birman *et al.* 2005), but oxidation can be present in implants with an expired shelf life (see Figure 113.1). Implants with an expired shelf life date should not be used. Mechanical failures can lead to excessive production of particulate UHMWPE, metal, and cement debris and contribute to the common final pathway of biologic aseptic loosening. If left untreated, the foreign body reaction can eventually lead to **granuloma** formation.

Aseptic loosening has traditionally been described as a long-term complication of cemented total hip arthoplasty, prompting the development of cementless technology. Nonetheless, both cemented and cementless implants are subject to loosening, although less frequently with the latter.

Incidence goal
Although the incidence varies between reports, it is reasonable to expect an incidence of asymptomatic aseptic loosening below 2% after 10 years or at the end of life, whichever is less (Edwards *et al.* 1997; El-Warrak *et al.* 2001; Skurla *et al.* 2005).

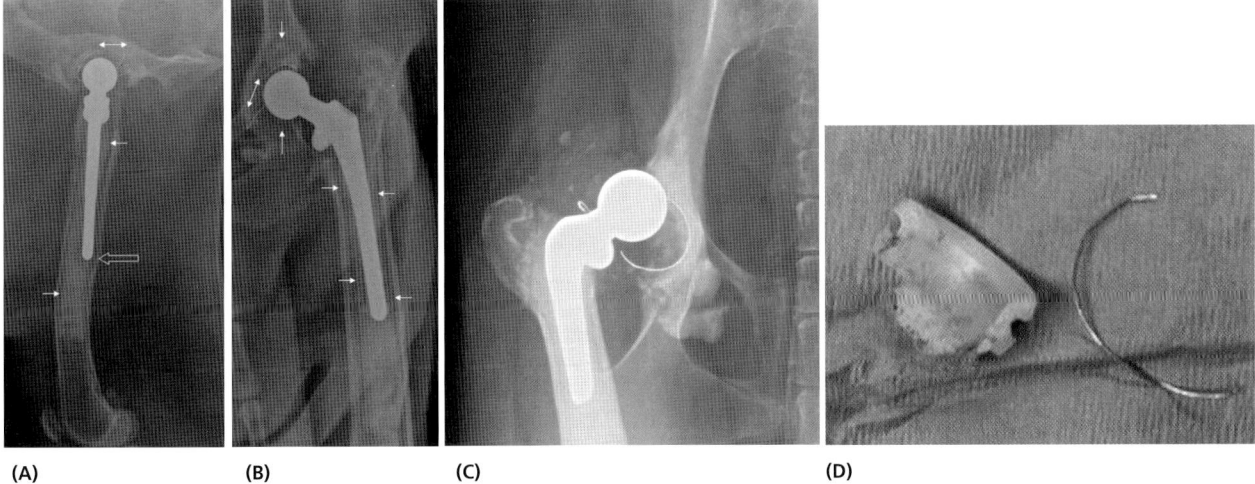

(A)   (B)   (C)   (D)

Figure 113.1 Aseptic loosening of the acetabular and femoral implants in a 10-year-old female golden retriever 9 years after hip replacement. **A** and **B**, A wide lucent space is present at the bone–cement interface (arrows) on both the lateral and ventral-dorsal view. The identification wire encircling the acetabular component is broken (double arrow), indicating either deformation of the cup or cup displacement with the wire restrained by the cement mantle. Remodeling of the femoral cortex is noted (open arrow) in close proximity to the tip of the femoral stem. **C**, The wire in the acetabular component is broken, and femoral head subluxation is present similar to the wire in Figure 113.1 A with aseptic loosening. In this instance, cup aseptic loosening is not present. **D**, Wire failure and head subluxation resulted secondary to polyethylene failure. The acetabular component had an expired shelf life when it was implanted.

Risk factors

- Cobalt chrome and titanium metal, UHMWPE, and polymethylmethacrylate (PMMA) used in hip arthroplasty are proven relatively inert materials in a bulk stable environment. In a particulate form, they all elicit a granulomatous response when pro-inflammatory cytokines recruit macrophages (<2-μm particles) and giant cells (larger particles) that attempt to carry away debris (Palmisano *et al.* 2003). This process directs osteoclast-mediated osteolysis.
- Poor cementing technique is the greatest factor predisposing to aseptic loosening of cemented implants. The cement mantle should distribute loads equally through a consistently adequate mantle thickness that has no pores, defects, or other flaws.
- Malpositioned implants increase the formation of wear debris.
- Placement of reduction instruments on the ventral aspect of the cup during trial and implant head rearticulation can lever the cup out of the acetabular bed.
- Femoral stems composed of titanium are softer and less resistant to wear particles than implants made of cobalt chromium (Edwards *et al.* 1997). This abrasion of titanium on cement can result in metallosis (Figure 113.2), cement granuloma, and loosening. Cobalt chromium is less susceptible to wear, but the debris, when present, produces a more pronounced inflammatory reaction than those derived from titanium (Kim *et al.* 1994).
- UHMWPE is subject to wear, but several factors can affect this process. UHMWPE wear rates are lower in dogs than in humans (Skurla and James 2001). The process used for manufacturing implants affects wear rates along with the sterilization technique. The degradation rate of the UHMWPE is reduced by gamma sterilization in a nitrogen atmosphere and sealed packaging.

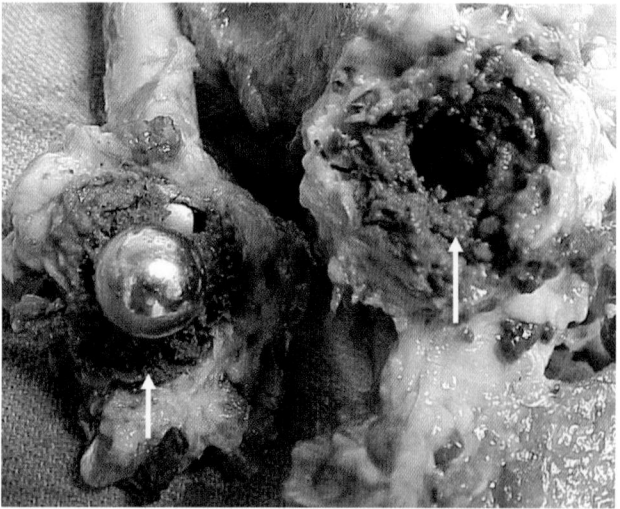

Figure 113.2 Metallosis after cemented total hip replacement. An ultra-high-molecular-weight polyethylene (UHMWPE) acetabular cup and a titanium femoral stem were implanted in this 13-year-old chow chow. Note the discoloration of the soft tissue surrounding the femoral neck (left arrow) and the rim of the acetabulum (right arrow). Metallosis is caused by embedded titanium particulate debris generated by abrasion of bone cement at the debonded implant–cement interfaces. The implant was retrieved 12 years after surgery when the dog died of an unrelated cause.

- The path of least resistance facilitates the dispersion of UHMWPE wear debris in the tissues and resulting inflammation. These inflammatory mediators recruit macrophages and activate osteolysis. Holes in the UHMWPE-lined cup provide an open port of exit as they are pumped out by cyclical loading. Holes present in the metal shell allow passage directly to the tissues where the osteolytic response can begin.
- Third-body wear accelerates wear debris accumulation in the tissues. Metal, cement, bone, or any other debris trapped or pumped into the articular surface between the head and cup accelerates wear. Third-body wear at the articulation of the metal head on the UHMWPE cup increases friction at the interface. This in turn transfers greater loads to the bone–implant interfaces and accelerates loosening.
- Femoral stem implant–cement debonding results in regional metal circular and longitudinal polished wear lines as the stem rotates and pistons in the mantle. This abrasive action generates both metal and cement wear debris that leads to aseptic loosening and potentially granuloma formation (Figure 113.3) (see Cement granuloma).
- Owner compliance restricting vigorous and strenuous activity during the first 1 or 2 months after surgery is important. Excessive cyclical mechanical strain at the bone–cement interface disrupts angiogenesis, cell differentiation, early bone on growth production or osteointegration, and eventually stability. The excessive activity (micromotion) may be responsible for bone loss instead of bone production and destabilization of the prosthesis.
- Radiation of 1000 centigrays has been shown to decrease fixation strength of porous-coated implants at 2 weeks but not at 4 or 8 weeks. Thus, the prosthesis should be shielded from radiation (Sumner *et al.* 1990b). THR cementless fixation subsequent to radiation therapy has compromised osteointegration ability (Wise *et al.* 1990).
- A perpetual pathophysiological "race" exists between particulate wear debris production and removal by macrophages. The winner determines loosening or maintained stable fixation.
- Poor surgical technique resulting in an initially unstable cementless fixation: This situation is characterized by the presence of a loose implant without evidence of sepsis but should be differentiated from the traditional description of aseptic loosening because of the difference in pathogenesis. Several factors can cause inadequate fixation of cementless implants, including errant acetabular reaming with a cranial-caudal wobble will wallow out the bone bed and preclude press-fit implantation. Excessive reaming of the dorsal acetabular rim may compromise bone coverage of the cup. The same complication may occur if the acetabular rim is reamed to a thin layer of bone, increasing the risk of fracture during impaction of the cup. In joints with severe wear of the dorsal acetabular rim, the lateral aspect of the saucerized neoacetabulum may be displaced dorsally and toward the midline. In this instance, reaming should extend to the lateralmost aspect of the rim to improve bone coverage of the cup with the hard sclerotic bone present in that area. Caudal deflection of the reamer away from hard sclerotic bone at the cranial pole can lead to excessive bone removal at the caudal acetabular wall, thereby precluding a tight press fit. Large osteophytes are sometimes present along the ventral acetabulum over the transacetabular ligament. These osteophytes should be removed before cup implantation. If they are not removed, they can deflect the direction of cup impaction. Also, they can obstruct impaction, resulting in incomplete

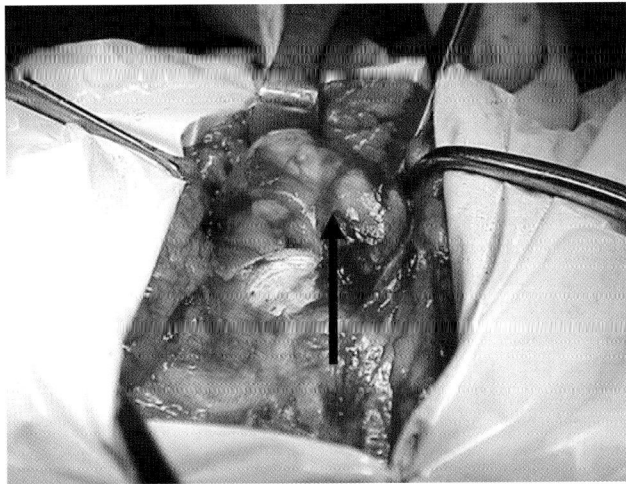

(A)

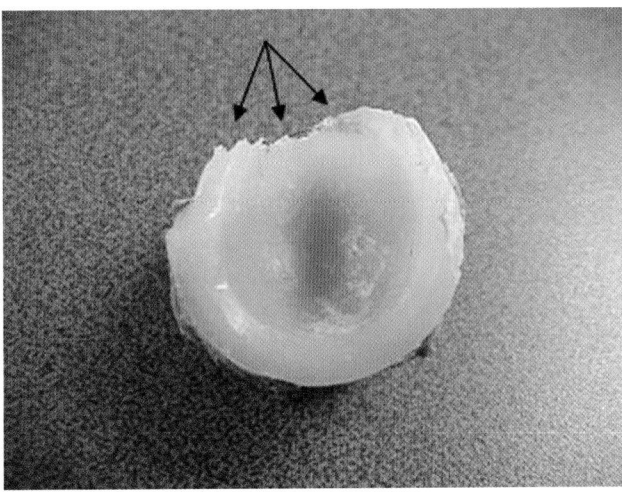

(B)

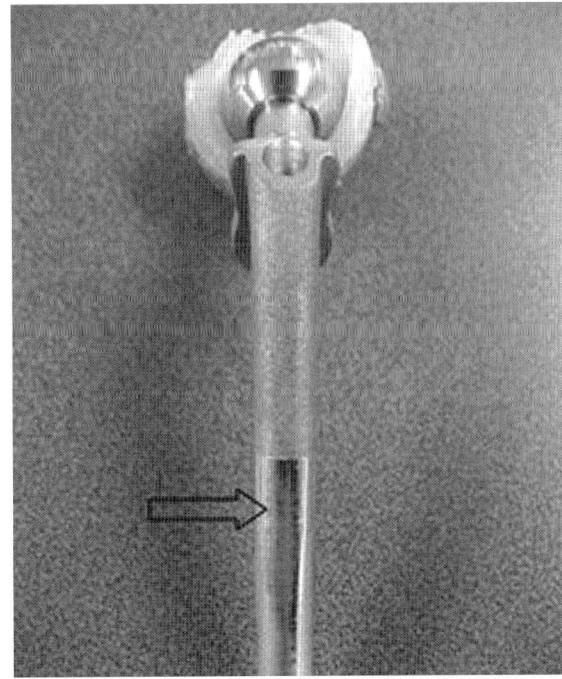

(C)

Figure 113.3 Granuloma formation following chronic aseptic loosening of a cemented hip replacement. On the intraoperative image (**A**), a multilobulated cement granuloma (arrow) extends lateral to the hip. Prolonged aseptic loosening led to dorsiversion of the cup, with particulate cement third body wear of its dorsal rim (three arrows; **B**). Cement debris appeared embedded in the surface of the cup, creating a rough surface. Loosening at the cement–femoral stem junction led to rotational instability, as evidenced by the presence of wear on the polished metal (open arrow; **C**).

cup seating. Peripheral synovium and other soft tissue should be debrided to prevent its interposition between the bone and the cup. Before the first cup impaction blow, a crescent-shaped space should be present between the reamed dorsal acetabular rim and the dorsal margin of the cup shell. This space allows for cup impaction at a 45-degree angle dorsal-medially into the bed preparation. If the crescent-shaped space is not present, incomplete seating or a malpositioned cup may be the result.

Diagnosis

Clinical signs of aseptic loosening include pain with intermittent, subtle lameness during range of motion (ROM) exercises, especially in extension if the cup is loose; if the femoral stem is loose, deep digital pressure of the proximal femoral diaphysis or internal rotation will elicit pain and exaggerate the lameness; progressive pelvic and crural muscle atrophy; and manipulation of the prosthesis can sometimes cause palpable or audible crepitus.

Radiographically, a nonfocal, radiolucent zone 1 mm or thicker is present over most or all of the bone–cement (cemented) or bone–implant (cementless) interface. A variable degree of asymmetrical periosteal change may be present. Implant position may be altered compared with postoperative positioning (see Figures 113.1 and 113.4).

A thin, faint, radiolucent line involving a small portion of the entire interface does not establish the definitive diagnosis of aseptic loosening (Konde *et al.* 1982). Although a thin or partial lucent line can be seen radiographically and histologically, the prosthesis is usually clinically stable. Only a progressively widening and more extensive lucent line around the cement or prosthesis seen on serial radiographic examinations indicates loosening, infection, or both.

- Exostosis of the medial acetabular cortex into the pelvic canal in the presence of a radiolucent zone indicates loosening but does not discriminate aseptic loosening from loosening secondary to infection (see Figure 113.4).
- Migration of the femoral stem tip or the entire femoral stem with adjacent cortical remodeling and thickening is sometimes but not always present despite endosteal osteolysis. Stem version angle changes may accompany stem loosening.
- Cement mantle transverse fissures or fractures are often present near the stem tip with cement fixation loosening.
- Chronic rotational instability of a loose cemented femoral stem collar contacting the calcar area results in cortical sclerosis in the contact area. Attrition of the calcar leads to cemented implant subsidence evidenced by relationship changes of the collar to landmarks, such as the lesser trochanter, compared with

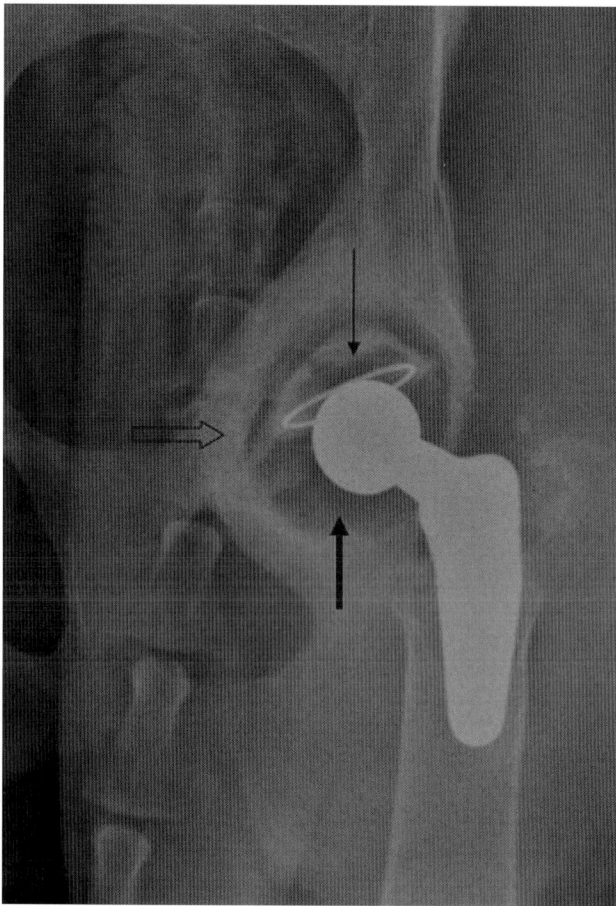

(A)

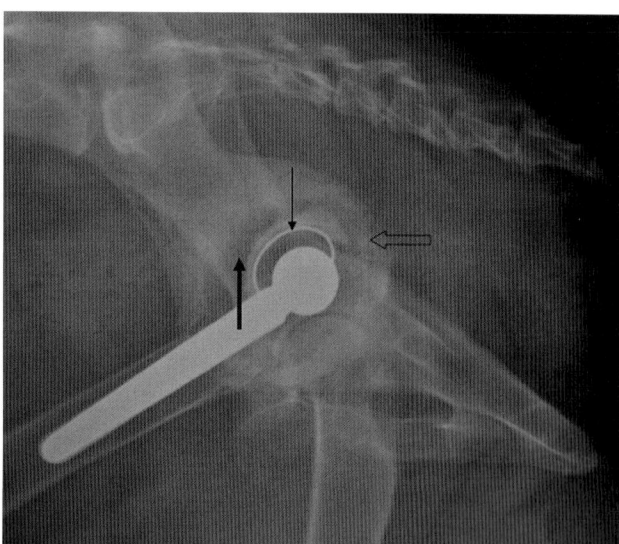

(B)

Figure 113.4 Ventral-dorsal (**A**) and medial-lateral (**B**) radiographs of the pelvis of a dog with aseptic loosening of the acetabular prosthesis (thin arrows). This dog became lame 6 years after total hip replacement, prompting the owners to seek a first follow-up evaluation since the surgery. The acetabular cup is retroverted and remained bonded to the cement mantle. This mantle is surrounded by a wide wallowed out bone bed (wide arrows). The prosthesis is displaced medially toward the pelvic canal. Bone (open arrows) is present around the medial aspect of the loose component (open arrows).

postoperative images. Prolonged osteoclastic activity can weaken the cortical bone and lead to femur fracture (Figure 113.5).

- The use of plain radiography does not always provide enough information to reliably assess if a cemented femoral implant is stable or unstable; however, the following indicators of rotational instability or stem pistoning can be indicative of loosening: implant position change, cement cracks, stem–cement interface lucency distal to the tip, and bone–cement interface lucency.
- A cement mantle less than 2.0 mm thick is not necessarily indicative of imminent loosening either, but an incomplete or inferior mantle with metal touching bone (endosteum) trends toward loosening (Frankel *et al.* 2004; Skurla *et al.* 2005).

Scintigraphy can assist in localizing increased vascularity and osteoblastic activity associated with bone pathology but does not definitively discriminate between aseptic and septic loosening.

A fluoroscopic examination is inherently insensitive because of the difficulty manipulating the prosthesis while avoiding the x-ray beam and therefore does not significantly add to information gained from clinical signs, orthopedic examination, and radiographs.

Aseptic loosening of a well-osteointegrated biologic fixation prosthesis is extremely rare. If loosening is suspected of a previously well-osteointegrated implant, septic loosening should be ruled out (see Infection).

Incidence goal

The incidence of aseptic loosening in cemented implants is less than 1% in the animal's lifetime. The incidence of loosening in cementless osteointegrated implants is anecdotally known to be exceptionally low but has not been reported in a large study with long-term follow-up.

Treatment

When osteoclastic activity is present, single-stage revision of the cup or stem is more successful if performed before extensive remodeling. Fibrovascular membrane and bone specimens should be cultured to rule out occult infections.

Cemented THR can be revised with cementless components (Massat *et al.* 1998; Torres and Budsberg 2009).

- Loose implants are not difficult to remove because bone beds are usually devoid of cancellous bone; however, cemented implants can be vulnerable to loosening again because of the absence of cancellous bone and stable fixation. Thus, replacement implants should be cementless whenever possible with bone stock voids and defects packed with an impacted autogenous cancellous bone graft.
- Preventive placement of cerclage wires may be indicated to avoid intraoperative or postoperative femoral fissures or fractures on account of thin or weak femoral cortical bone resulting from endosteal osteolysis. Optionally, the stem can be cemented and stability augmented by a lateral neutralization plate with screws extending from the greater trochanter to the distal femur.
- Explantation of the prosthesis is sometimes the best option in cases with advanced osteolysis and extensive bone changes. The acetabular component can be grasped and removed intact with the cement mantle if the changes are advanced. If necessary, an osteotome can be used to mobilize or cut cemented implants into pieces. Loose cementless cups are impacted on the metal shell along their dorsal rim until they "rotate" ventrally on the cranial-caudal axis out of the bed.

Cemented femoral stems can be easily extracted by impacting the stem collar. Well-bonded cement at the implant–cement interface will come out still attached to the stem, but the cement mantle

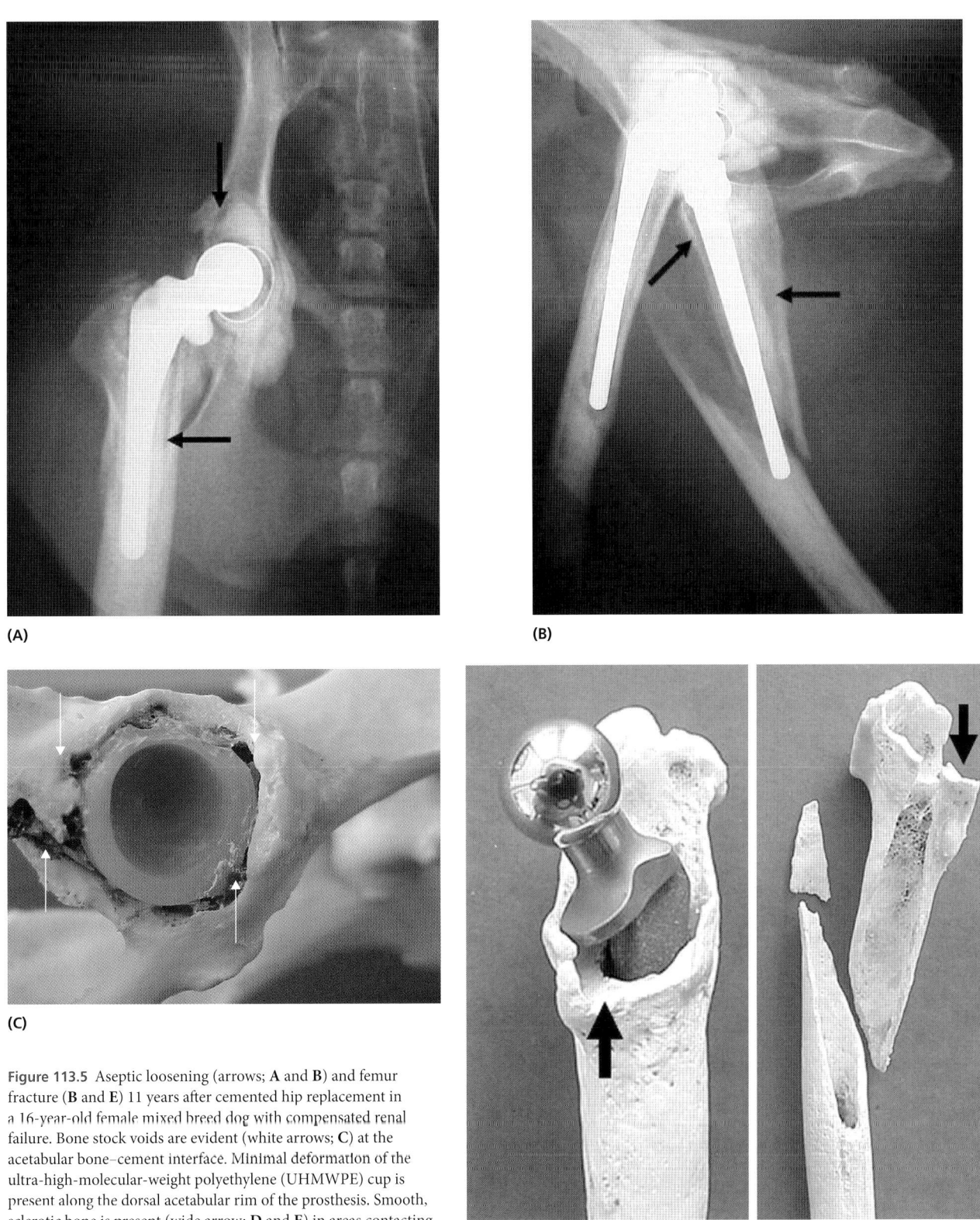

(A)

(B)

(C)

(D)

(E)

Figure 113.5 Aseptic loosening (arrows; **A** and **B**) and femur fracture (**B** and **E**) 11 years after cemented hip replacement in a 16-year-old female mixed breed dog with compensated renal failure. Bone stock voids are evident (white arrows; **C**) at the acetabular bone–cement interface. Minimal deformation of the ultra-high-molecular-weight polyethylene (UHMWPE) cup is present along the dorsal acetabular rim of the prosthesis. Smooth, sclerotic bone is present (wide arrow; **D** and **E**) in areas contacting the unstable femoral stem collar.

will remain in the medullary canal if it has debonded. Removal of the cement from the canal is accomplished through a diaphyseal cortical or extended trochanteric osteotomy window. Osteotomies split the femur cranially and caudally and extend beyond the end of the cement mantle inside the canal. The osteotomies are beveled to

prevent creation of a stress riser that could lead to a postoperative fracture. After cement removal, the osteotomy window is replaced and stabilized with full cerclage wires (Figure 113.6). Bone along the proximal femoral prosthesis osteotomy opening is removed to resemble a femoral head ostectomy.

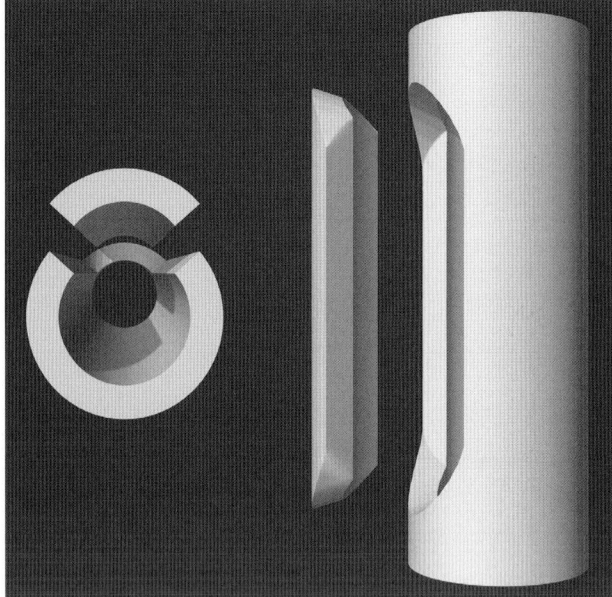

(A)

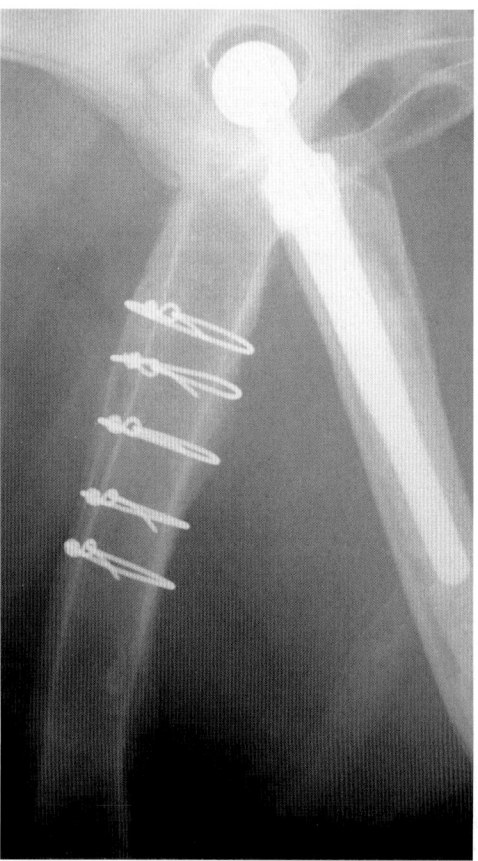

(B)

Figure 113.6 Removal of cement from the medullary canal through a beveled femoral window. The diagram (**A**) illustrates the orientation of all femoral osteotomy lines used to gain access to the medullary canal. After removal of cement from the medullary canal, the diaphyseal femoral segment is reduced and stabilized with cerclage wires spaced 1 cm apart (**B**). On this radiograph obtained 6 weeks after explantation, the periosteal bone formation is unchanged from preoperative images that were consistent with osteomyelitis. The osteotomy lines are no longer visible. Wire removal is rarely necessary.

Although ultrasonic cement removal instruments can be used in humans, these instruments must be used with caution in animals with thin cortical bone because improper use can overheat causing thermal necrosis of or even dissolve bone.

Very little information is available about the consequences of residual cement in the medullary canal if loosening is positively aseptic and not septic. It is not always necessary to remove aseptic cement from the femoral canal.

Outcome

Revision of an aseptic loose hip replacement prosthesis may recreate a pain-free joint with return to objectively normal function. Explantation will result in function similar to a femoral head ostectomy. The minimum expectation should be subjectively normal function during normal daily activity.

Expectations after explantation should include leg length discrepancy; an unpredictable degree of pain relief; likely persistent thigh muscle atrophy; discomfort during hip extension or abduction; and a prolonged, but necessary, period of rehabilitation therapy.

Prevention
Implant selection

The design and composition should be optimized for osteointegration through selection of porosity and pore size:
- Prosthesis design influences fixation and distribution of forces along host–implant interfaces. An implant will loosen if its design concentrates excessive force along an interface. For example, prostheses with pointed or sharp corners can create a stress riser effect; conversely, cylindrical implants do not adequately resist rotation.
- Prosthesis materials must be durable enough to last 10 to 15 years, or the life span of dogs and cats, and must meet standards that minimize particulate wear debris, known to promote osteolysis. Metal bearing on UHMWPE inevitably results in wear debris over time. Future research in the development of prostheses should be aimed at preventing wear debris–mediated osteolysis (Shanbhag *et al.* 1997).
- The prosthesis size must be carefully tailored to the patient so as to not affect implant stability. In active animals, an undersized implant will generate excessive load over an area too small to withstand the stresses.

Implantation technique

- Prosthesis fixation materials and design have varying effects on implant stability. Micromotion at the bone–cement or implant–cement interface can eventually lead to cement and metal particulate wear debris, which, similar to polyethylene, can lead to osteolysis. The optimal thickness of the cement mantle has not been reported, most likely because of the wide variation of animal breeds, body weights, and body condition scores.
- New-generation cementing techniques rely on vacuum cement mixing, bed preparation pulsatile lavage with suction, intramedullary cement restrictor plugs, stem centralizers, cement injection, stem preheating, and pressurized implantation (Schultz *et al.* 2000). These techniques are recommended to reduce the risk of aseptic loosening.
- The technique for implantation of a THR must result in stable fixation at the time of surgery. Ideally, the cement mantle should be uniform at the time of fixation (Edwards *et al.* 1997; Schultz *et al.* 2000).

- Version, inclination, and axial alignment of the components must be appropriately positioned to maximize load dispersion and minimize wear (Dyce et al. 2000b).
- Cancellous bone structure should be meticulously preserved and debris carefully removed from trabecular spaces in the implant bed to allow cement intrusion. Inadequate cement intrusion will result in less overall bone–cement contact surface area; suboptimal implant fixation; and, ultimately, implant loosening.
- To avoid dislodging the cup, reduction instruments should not be placed on the ventral aspect of the cup. A Hohmann retractor serves as a good lever to achieve trial and implant head rearticulation as long as its tip is placed on the shaft of the ischium, caudal to the acetabular implant.
- Protect the lining of the acetabular cup from postmanufacture scratches. Pack the cup with gauze during femoral bed preparation and copiously lavage before rearticulation to remove debris that could cause third body wear (Dyce et al. 2000b). The suction tip should be used carefully when removing lavage fluid to avoid damage to the cup lining.
- Metal skids and metal-on-metal contact of the head with the metal shell of the cementless acetabular component should be avoided because scratches on the femoral head accelerate polyethylene wear (Wood et al. 2003).
- Cementless implants must be stable immediately after surgery because animals will load the prosthesis within days of surgery. Excessive micromotion caused by poor surgical technique can result in inadequate fixation during the first 6 to 8 weeks of osteointegration. Severely disrupted osteointegration leads to fibrous ingrowth instead of bone ingrowth. Fibrous ingrowth will not ossify and jeopardizes long-term fixation.

Relevant literature

Excellent osteointegration is expected with initially stable proximally porous surfaced tapered femoral stems. The failure rate due to aseptic loosening varies around 0.6% in humans, and a similar expectation seems a reasonable goal in animals (Casper et al. 2011). In humans, risk factors for failure of osteointegration are reported to include male sex, a smaller canal flare index, larger stem size, and greater canal fill at the mid and distal thirds of the stem. In the latter, a proximal-distal mismatch with the stems wedged distally can produce a mechanical environment unfavorable for proximal osteointegration (Cooper et al. 2011). Awareness of variability in proximal femoral morphology helps minimize the risk of femoral aseptic loosening in animals. The wide anatomic variability also justifies the need for options in terms of implant design, size, and fixation techniques. Based on measurements in a canine model, changes in femoral neck length do not significantly affect cement strains. A shortened femoral stem length improved implant positioning to a magnitude of questionable clinical relevance. At this point, the properties of the shortened stem do not justify alteration of the implant design (Dassler et al. 2003; Dearmin and Schulz 2004).

Coating prosthetic implants with hydroxyapatite (HA) can improve osteoconductivity and accelerate osteointegration. These properties are attractive even though the volume of bone ingrowth in porous versus HA-coated surfaces seem similar at about 12 weeks. HA-coated surfaces may also limit particulate debris migration to sites where osteoclastic activity could eventually cause aseptic loosening. Even though HA contributes to overall particulate load and increased synovitis, it is unlikely to be a major contributor to overall periprosthetic inflammatory processes in dogs (Anderson et al. 2001).

Tribology has been the everlasting focus of many long-term human studies since inception of joint replacement surgery. Novel materials are developed and clinically applied, largely because of their perceived superiority in reducing wear debris and incidence of aseptic loosening (Greenwald 2011). Among those, ceramics display improved friction, wear, purity, durability, and lubrication properties. However, the advantages and disadvantages of novel biomaterials remain under investigation and will not necessarily be practical or even applicable for animal use. As an additional incentive to prevent wear debris, osteosarcoma has been reported as a possible late complication of THR secondary to chronic bone irritation associated with chronic aseptic loosening (Roe et al. 1996).

Some intraoperative techniques have been proposed to improve the mechanical stability of the implant. Among these, prewarming polyethylene acetabular components before implantation was found to have no benefit (Shields et al. 2002). New-generation cementing techniques rely on vacuum cement mixing, bed preparation pulsatile lavage with suction, intramedullary cement restrictor plugs, stem centralizers, cement injection, stem preheating, and pressurized implantation (Schultz et al. 2000). No deleterious effects were identified after short-term pressurization of the cement during implantation (Shields et al. 2002). These cementing techniques are therefore recommended to reduce the risk of aseptic loosening.

Cement granuloma

Definition

A cement granuloma is a late complication of THR caused by a foreign body reaction to excessive cement particulate debris. The wear debris is generated at the bone–cement or the implant–cement interface secondary to severe chronic femoral implant loosening (see Aseptic loosening) and less frequently acetabular loosening (Palmisano et al. 2003). Migration of this wear debris into periarticular soft tissues induces the formation of a granuloma.

Risk factors

- Chronic aseptic loosening untreated by revision arthroplasty generates particulate wear debris that leads to granuloma formation.

Diagnosis

- Progressive lameness can develop years (usually >4 years) after cemented arthroplasty. A chronic lameness with acute deterioration can be a premonitory sign of a pathological fracture.
- Muscle atrophy and pain from decreased passive ROM of the hip accompany aseptic prosthesis loosening.
- A firm, palpable, soft tissue mass will be found near the acetabulum or proximal femur (see Figure 113.3). If the mass extends into the pelvic canal, signs associated with pelvic canal obstruction, such as obstipation, may be present. The mass will be palpable during a rectal examination.
- A variably sized and shaped soft tissue opacity containing radiodensities can be seen radiographically. Aseptic loosening of the prosthesis cement fixation will be evident (Figure 113.7).
- A thin-walled, cavitary, extraosseous mass filled with echogenic fluid surrounding irregular, homogeneous, granular debris is usually noted on ultrasonographic examination.
- Fluid aspirated from the cavity is slightly cloudy with sterile, flocculent to caseous debris. Dark discoloration is consistent with a large amount of metal debris (see Figure 113.2).

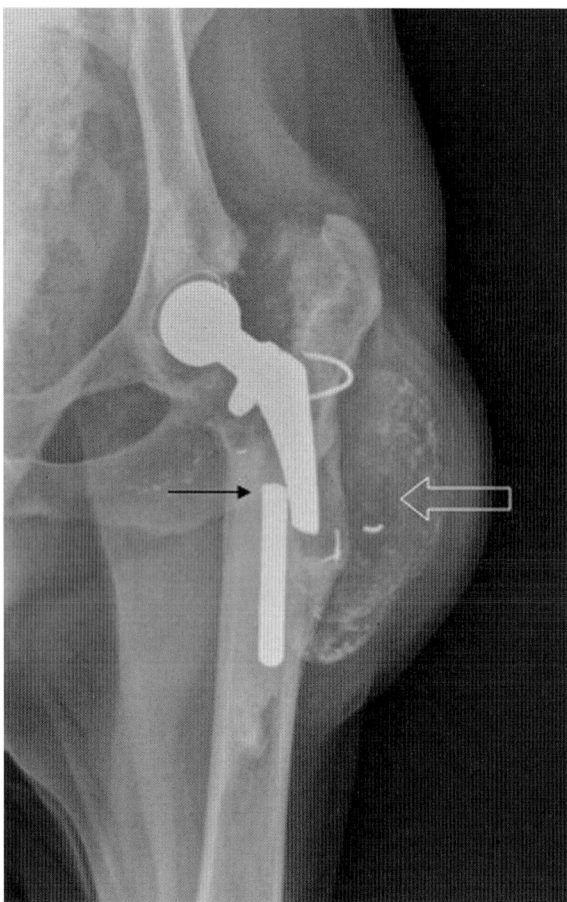

(A)

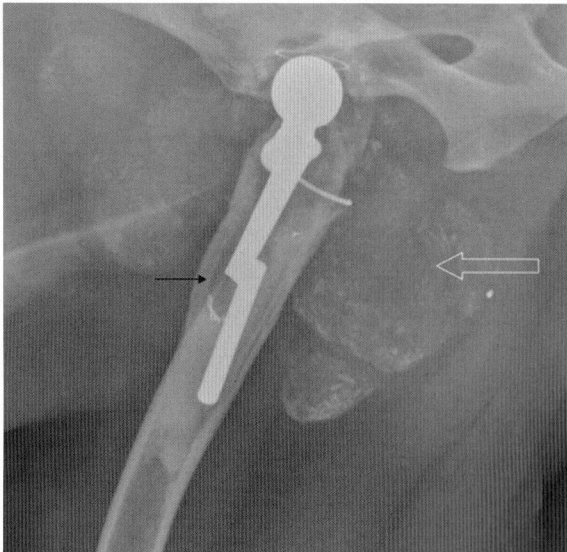

(B)

Figure 113.7 Granuloma formation and femoral stem failure (small arrows) 7 years after total hip replacement in a mixed breed dog. **A** and **B**, These images were acquired 2 years later (9 years after surgery). The femoral stem was chronically aseptically loose, causing metal fatigue and failure. The tip of the proximal segment migrated through the lateral cortex. The large cement granuloma (open arrows) is especially evident on the lateral view (**B**).

- Findings on histologic examination include a dense fibrous capsule; a heavy burden of birefringent; UHMWPE; refractile, crystalline, bone cement debris; and other amorphous debris.
- Periosteal reaction is absent, which would be expected with septic loosening.

Incidence goal

Cement granuloma formation is a very rare complication (<0.2%).

Treatment

- Intrapelvic masses are removed via a ventral celiotomy.
- If the prognosis after revision surgery is expected to be poor, implant removal with conversion to a femoral head and neck ostectomy is indicated for a chronically, aseptically loose prosthesis.

Outcome

Explantation of an aseptically loose prosthesis combined with granuloma excision results in limb function similar to a femoral head and neck ostectomy.

Prevention

- Avoid or minimize the risks of anything that could lead to aseptic loosening.
- Avoid perforation of the acetabular medial cortical wall when using acetabular component cement fixation.
- Recommend annual radiographic monitoring of THR recipients. If aseptic loosening is present, early revision has a greater chance to be successful if performed before extensive changes are present secondary to a large granuloma.

Relevant literature

An intrapelvic, cement granuloma has been reported in a dog 6 years after implantation of a cemented, titanium femoral stem. The medial acetabular cortical wall was perforated during the original surgery, and the granuloma extended from the cement through the wall. The dog in this report had no evidence of aseptic loosening, so this case is a variant of the typical cement granuloma (Freeman *et al.* 2003). Polyethylene (Korkala and Syrjanen 1998) or titanium wear debris can contribute to granuloma formation in similar scenarios.

Cortical perforation (acetabulum and femur)

Definition

This is inadvertent or iatrogenic creation of a bone defect through the cortex of the acetabulum or femur during bed preparation for prosthesis implantation.

Risk factors

Risk factors for perforation of the medial acetabulum include (Figure 113.8):
- Juvenile dogs with developmental subluxation have medial cortical wall hypoplasia. The thin cortex can be easily penetrated during inattentive reaming.
- The acetabular wall in middle-aged and older dogs with chronic end-stage OA is composed of a thick layer of soft cancellous bone separating the sclerotic articular surface from the atrophic medial cortical wall. The blades of the reamer can plunge through the cancellous layer, and inattention can quickly result in medial cortex perforations varying in size (see Figures 113.8 and 113.10).

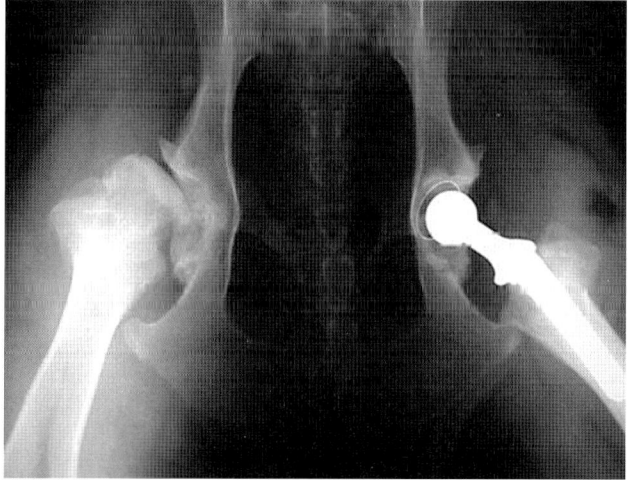

(A)

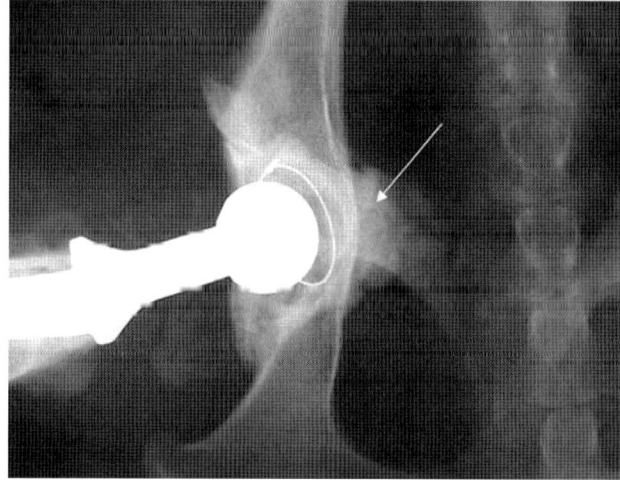

(B)

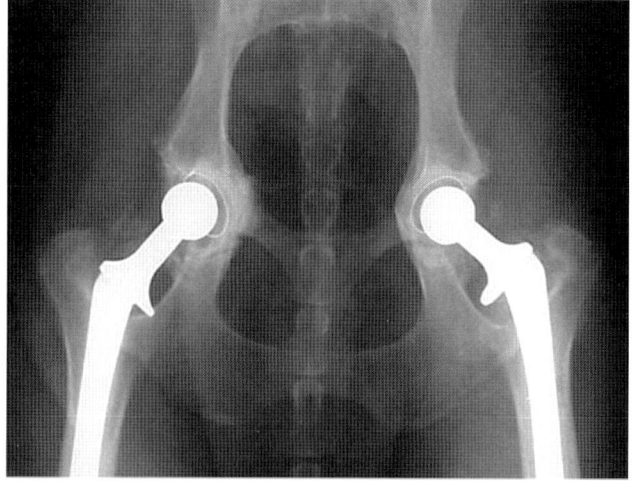

(C)

Figure 113.8 Cortical perforation of the acetabulum. The medial cortical wall of the acetabulum was inadvertently perforated during bed preparation in this 7-year-old, 43-kg female Weimaraner. **A**, The preoperative ventrodorsal radiograph of the pelvis is consistent with advanced osteoarthritis of the right coxofemoral joint, with a thick layer of cancellous bone between the articular surface and cortical bone. A total hip replacement had been performed on the left hip 4 months earlier. **B**, Postoperative radiograph. Perforation of the acetabular cortex was recognized during surgery and treated with an autogenous cancellous bone graft (arrow), harvested from reamings to prevent cement extrusion into the pelvic canal. **C**, Three-year radiographic follow-up. The acetabular component appears stable, and the graft is remodeled.

- Extensive bone sclerosis between the articular surface and the medial cortical wall can obscure the acetabular reaming depth. In most instances, the medial cortical wall can be found at the depth of the thin cleft of soft tissue in the original acetabular fovea.

Risk factors for perforation of the femur include (Figure 113.9):
- Perforation of the femoral cortex generally results from a misalignment of the femoral reaming pilot hole with regards to the long axis of the femoral diaphysis. Visualization of the proximal axis of the femur is limited by surrounding soft tissues, thereby jeopardizing the alignment of the pilot hole.
- Patient size: Centering the pilot hole over the femoral diaphysis is more challenging in small dogs.
- Proximal femoral medullary canal sclerosis precludes the identification of cancellous bone as an anatomic reference to position the pilot hole. This sclerosis occurs secondary to chronic OA, spontaneous and chronic capital physeal fractures, and avascular necrosis of the femoral head.
- Malunion of a proximal femur fracture complicates axial alignment of the stem with a deviated femoral canal. The femoral canal may be decreased in diameter, sclerotic, or difficult to identify. Additional exposure of the proximal femur may be warranted to improve visualization (see Figure 113.9).

- Revision of a femoral head ostectomy to a THR creates challenges identical to those encountered in limbs with malunion of the proximal femur (Fitzpatrick *et al.* 2012c).

Diagnosis
- Perforation of the medial cortical wall of the acetabulum is easily identified via direct inspection during surgery. Partial loss of the cortical wall can be suspected before full perforation by palpation with a pointed tipped instrument. Cortical perforation can occur while preserving an intact medial periosteum.
- Femoral perforation most commonly involves the caudal cortex and can go unrecognized because of the covering of surrounding soft tissues. The diagnosis is suspected when there is misalignment of a small-diameter (blunt-tipped) rod placed in the femoral canal, with respect to the axis of the femoral diaphysis. Perforation can be confirmed by direct palpation of the hole through which the rod exits the femoral canal and penetrates soft tissues. The blunt-tipped rod can also be used to gently palpate the internal walls of the femoral canal to identify a "soft spot" consistent with the site of perforation.
- A perforation of the femur can be confirmed by extending the exposure of the femur using the surgical approach used to manage proximal femoral fractures.

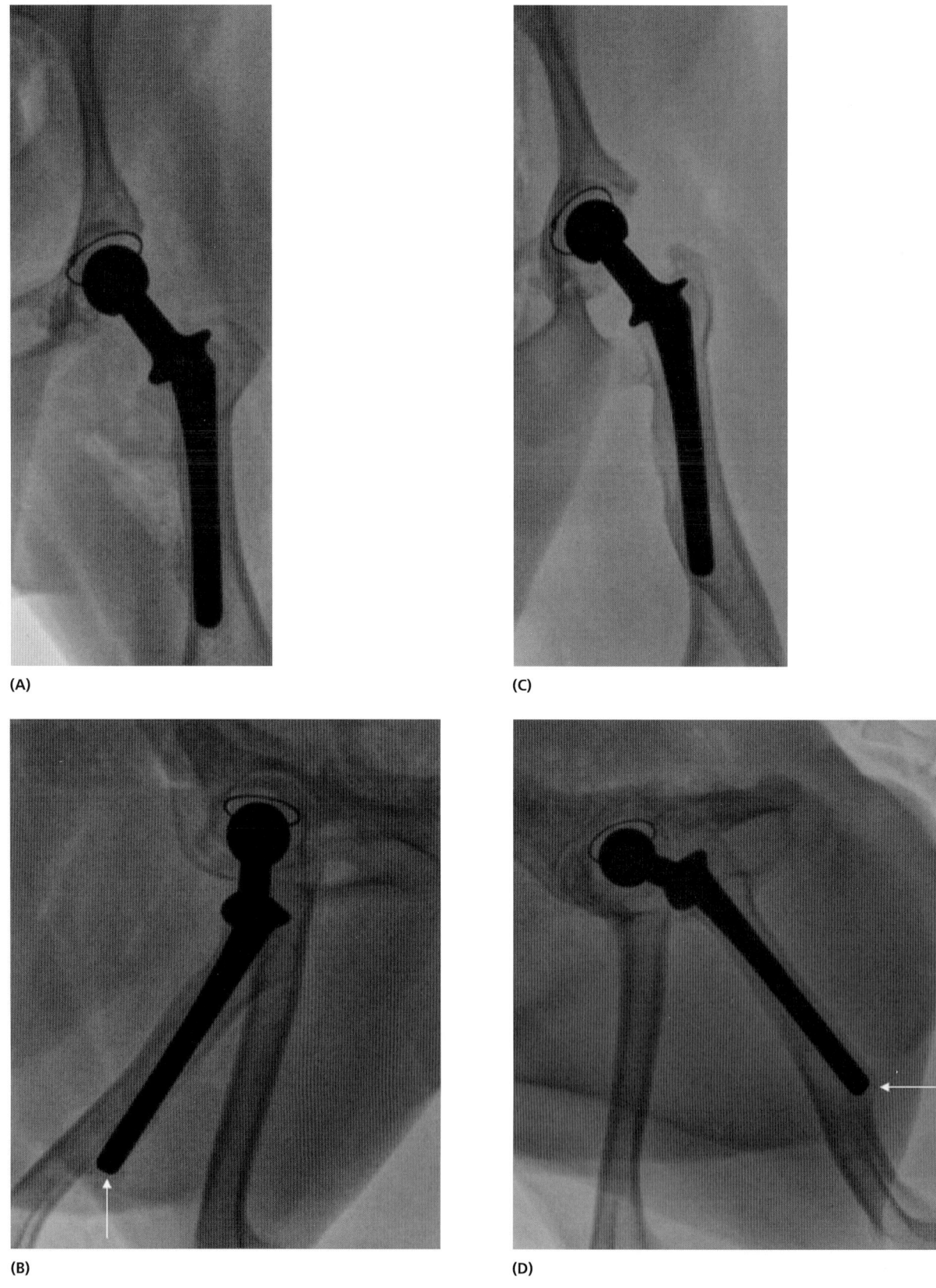

(A)

(B)

(C)

(D)

Figure 113.9 Perforation of the femoral cortex. An 8-month-old, 2.5-kg female Maltese with avascular necrosis of the femoral head was treated with a micro total hip replacement. **A**, A slight coxa valga and a medial tilt of femoral stem's tip are noted on the postoperative ventral-dorsal projection. **B**, On the medial-lateral view, the stem tip (arrow) is clearly extending outside of the medullary canal. Note the proximal deformation of the femur. **C** and **D**, Radiographic follow-up 6 years after surgery. Medial femoral cortical remodeling is evident on the ventral-dorsal view. The femoral stem tip is encased in bone (arrow). The dog's peak vertical force and impulse on the z-axis force plate data were similar to those of the normal contralateral limb. This case provides an example of good functional outcome despite the technical errors made during the original surgery.

Incidence goal

The risk is surgeon dependent. A 5% incidence is a realistic goal

Treatment

- Acetabular defects in a bed preparation for a cemented cup should be filled with an autogenous cancellous or corticocancellous graft typically obtained from the femoral head. Cancellous bone obtained from reamed bone or from the femoral head is adequate for a small (<3 mm) perforation. A corticocancellous

graft can be fashioned from the femoral head to cover a large perforation of the medial acetabular cortex. This type of graft is more occlusive to restrain flow of cement into the pelvic canal. This corticocancellous grafting technique can also be used to treat unintentionally large perforations created during cementless cup implantation (Figure 113.10).
- Intentional acetabular perforation to gain additional cup seating depth may be inconsequential in a large dog receiving a cementless cup with an outer metal shell (Figure 113.11). However,

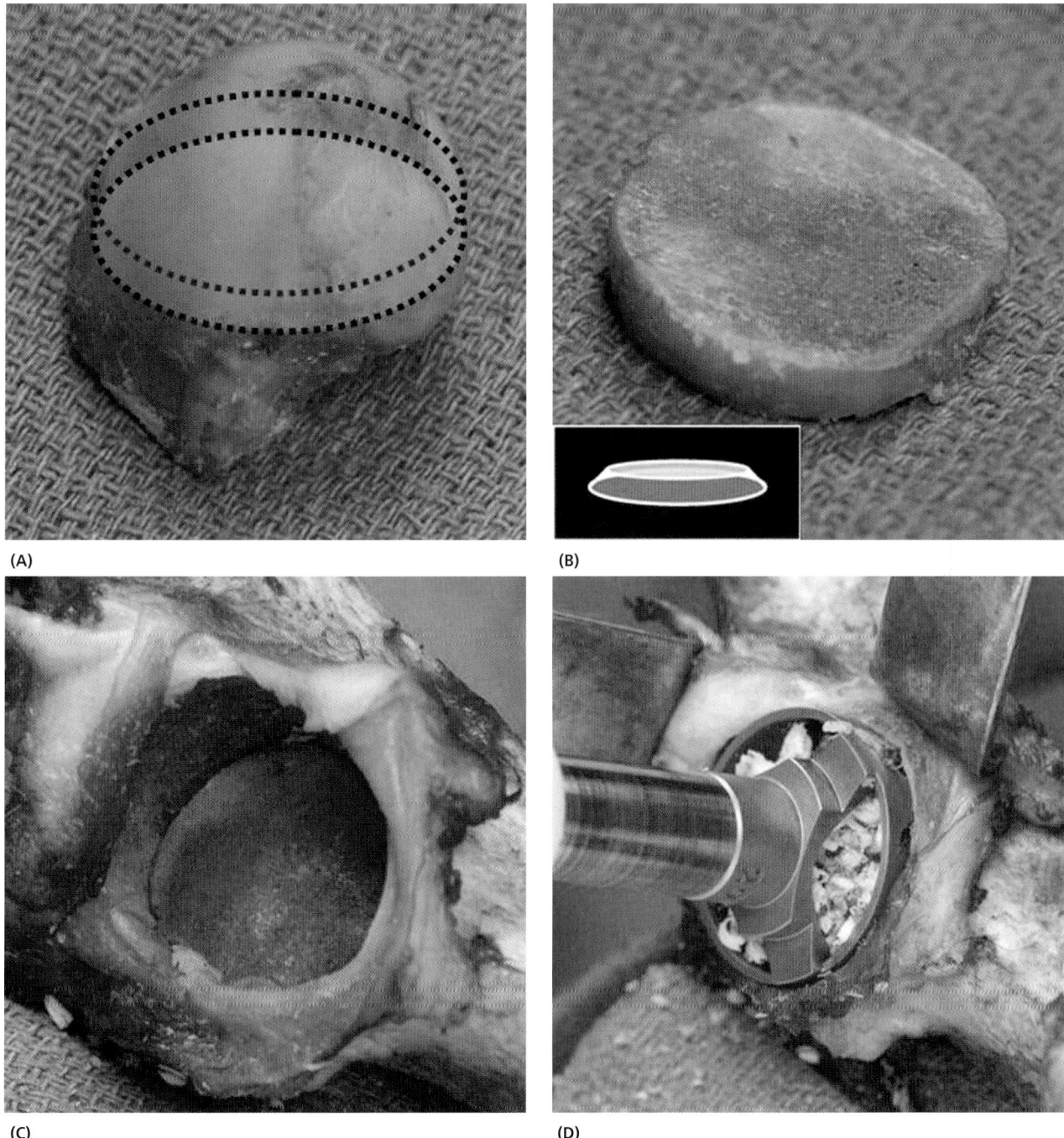

(A)

(B)

(C)

(D)

Figure 113.10 Treatment of an acetabular defect with a corticocancellous graft obtained from the femoral head during total hip replacement. **A**, The lines indicate the intended saw cuts to create the graft. **B**, The circumference of the disc is beveled to create a plug (see shape on insert) slightly larger than the defect. **C**, The graft is tamped into the acetabular cortical defect. **D**, Additional reaming may be considered to adjust the shape of the bed or allow implantation of a larger cup, if necessary. **E**, The bed preparation for either cemented or cementless cup implantation is complete. **F**, On this cadaveric specimen, the view from within the pelvic canal confirms complete occlusion of the acetabular perforation. Note the extent of the defect that can be successfully treated with this technique. *(Continued)*

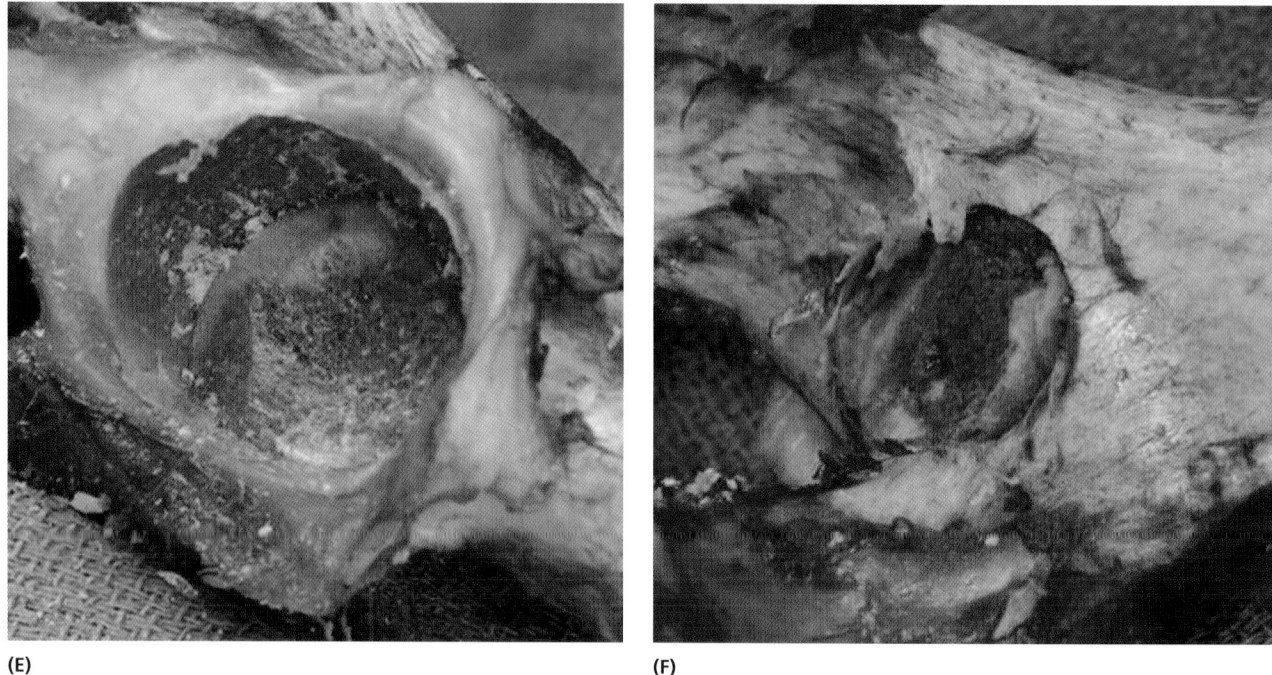

(E)   (F)

Figure 113.10 *(Continued).*

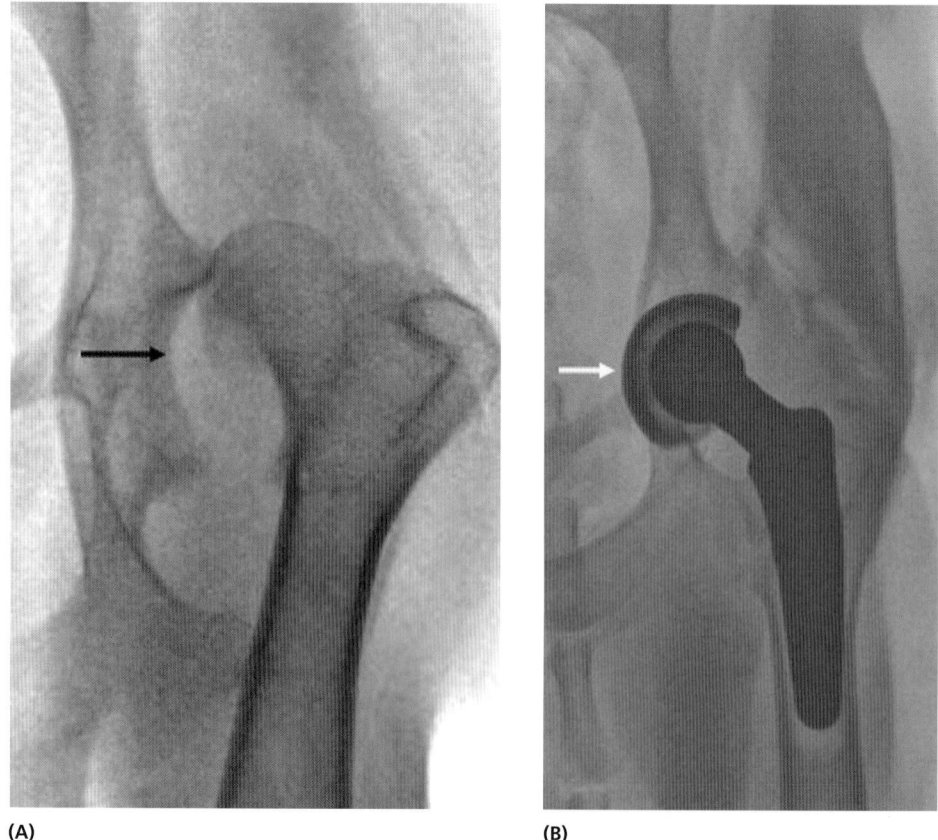

(A)   (B)

Figure 113.11 Conservative management of an intentional acetabular perforation. **A**, Chronic coxofemoral subluxation and luxation associated with advanced osteoarthritis and extensive wear of the dorsal acetabular rim (arrow) were noted on this preoperative radiograph. **B**, Postoperative radiograph. The medial wall of the acetabulum was intentionally perforated with the finishing reamer during bed preparation. As a result, the metal shell of the acetabular cup could be implanted several millimeters farther medially. This maneuver is designed to improve dorsal acetabular rim coverage and may be considered as a strategy to improve stability of the acetabular cup in dogs with a severe bone stock void.

additional femoral neck length may be necessary to assure correct transarticular tension with a cup deeply seated through a perforation. A short neck length leaves the prosthesis at risk of luxation.

- Cerclage wires should be placed around the femur before implantation of a cementless stem if the cortical bone has been weakened. A large perforation of the femoral cortex may preclude cementless stem implantation, depending on the location.
- Before implantation of a cemented femoral stem, any perforation of the femur must be occluded during cement introduction and pressurization.
- Arthroplasty may need to be aborted if a perforation is large enough to jeopardize permanent fixation.

Outcome
Perforations can be successfully managed in most cases.

- Iatrogenic, small-diameter acetabular perforations can be made at the surgeons' preference to gain depth and dorsal coverage of a cementless cup (see Figure 113.11). If the cortical perforation is not disproportionately large, a press-fit, cementless cup impacted partially through the medial cortical wall is adequately stable to withstand normal physiological loads (Margalit *et al.* 2010).
- A disproportionately large acetabulum perforation increases the risk of cup protrusio (see Protrusio).
- Femoral perforation is of little consequence if the integrity of the cortical strength is uncompromised and the remainder of the implantation is acceptable (Figure 113.12).

Prevention
- Critical review of the preoperative radiographs is essential to identify anatomic variants, such as femoral procurvatum. These variations warrant thorough intraoperative adjustments of the angle and position of the pilot hole relative to the femoral canal.
- The acetabulum should be reamed with care with intermittent pausing to determine the depth and alignment of the preparation bed. An instrument should be used to palpate the medial wall of the acetabulum if the depth cannot be ascertained by visual inspection alone.
- Femoral positioning is critical to minimize the risk of caudal cortical perforation. The proximal femur must be elevated and the distal femur must be depressed so the diaphysis is parallel (or the distal femur is lower than proximal) to the table. An assistant should push down (toward the floor) on the stifle while maintaining 90 degrees of limb external rotation with the patella toward the ceiling and the crus in a slight varus position. This is especially relevant in obese dogs, in which proper positioning is complicated by the presence of a thick layer of subcutaneous adipose tissues over the gluteal muscles.
- A bone forceps on the proximal third of the diaphysis can serve as an "aiming device" to center the pilot hole. This is particularly helpful if the proximal medullary canal is sclerotic.
- An instrument or blunt-tipped rod can gently be placed against the internal walls of the femoral canal to palpate the endosteal cortex and identify any perforation.

Femoral fractures (fissures and displaced)

Definition
Femoral fractures associated with both cemented and cementless hip replacement range from nondisplaced fissures to catastrophic failure with full displacement of fragments. Fissures and fractures can occur intraoperatively, but most occur within the first week after surgery. Fissures can propagate to catastrophic failure whether they were created during surgery or occurred during early weight bearing. Fracture classification helps understand the mechanism of injury, anticipate the level of difficulty associated with fracture stabilization, and determine the prognosis (Box 113.1).

Pelvic fractures involving the cranial pole, caudal pole, or dorsal rim of the acetabulum have not been reported. These fractures occur primarily intraoperatively.

Risk factors
- Periprosthetic femoral fracture is a risk inherent to THR caused by differences in the modulus of elasticity of bone, bone cement, and the metal femoral component. These differences result in a concentration of forces around the tip of the stem.

Surgical technique
- Femoral fractures tend to be more common during the learning curve for cementless THR than during placement of a cemented stem because of the impaction required to establish a press fit fixation. Overzealous impaction, especially with misalignment relative to the femoral axis, can lead to iatrogenic fissures or fractures.
- Overzealous reaming of the femoral canal during bed preparation for cemented implants weakens the bone and therefore must be avoided to decrease the risk of fracture.
- Overzealous broaching of the femoral canal during bed preparation for cementless implants removes all cancellous bone. Preservation of a cancellous bone envelop along the osteotomy line reduces contact between the endosteal surface and the stem, thereby preventing excessive loading of the cortical bone.
- Varus malalignment of the stem may overload the proximal medial femoral cortex.
- Excessive femoral neck length increases the cantilever load on the proximal medial cortex.
- Subsidence of the femoral stem may lead to an overload of the medial femoral cortex and secondary fracture. Note: A femoral fissure or fracture can result in secondary subsidence (see Subsidence).
- Excessive impaction of a cementless cup can lead to an acetabular fracture.
- Fracture of the cranial or caudal acetabulum can occur as a result of excessive force applied during removal of osteophytes.
- Overzealous force applied to the distal femur during challenging rearticulation, such as with a chronic developmental luxation or concomitant severe transarticular muscle fibrotic contracture, can apply excessive torque or angular loads to the femur; both can predispose to fracture.

Anatomic factors
- Preexisting femoral cortical atrophy often accompanies severe thigh muscle atrophy secondary to chronic OA.
- Concurrent osteopathy affecting cortical bone strength (see Figure 113.5)
- Previous surgery of the hip (Liska 2004; Ganz *et al.* 2010)
- Postoperative trauma, even sometimes minor, resulting in excessive local loading or torque on the bone
- Anatomic conformation of the femur with a low canal flare index ("stovepipe femur") of the proximal femoral morphology increases the risk of fracture during cementless implantation (Ganz *et al.* 2010).

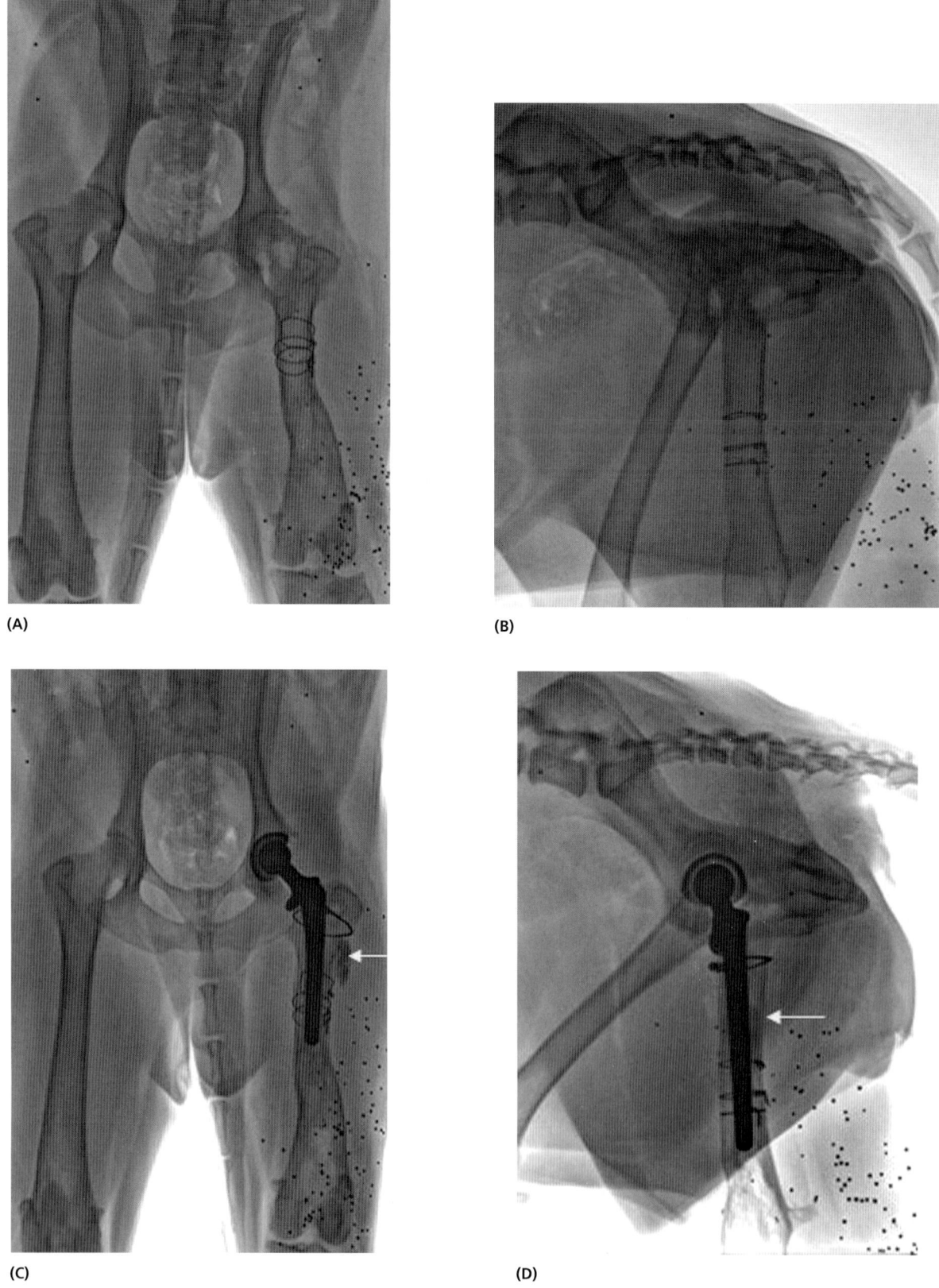

(A)

(B)

(C)

(D)

Figure 113.12 Successful outcome of a hybrid hip replacement after femoral perforation, cement extrusion, and wire placement. The preoperative ventral-dorsal (**A**) and medial-lateral (**B**) radiographs illustrate a valgus malunion of the left femoral neck and a mid-diaphyseal malunion secondary to gunshot injury. The implants used to stabilize the original fractures had been removed several years earlier except for three full cerclage wires. Buckshot remains from the time of the original injuries. Postoperative ventral-dorsal (**C**) and medial-lateral (**D**) radiographs after hybrid hip replacement with a cementless acetabular cup and a cemented femoral stem. A globule of bone cement (arrows) extruded through a cortical perforation accidentally created during preparation of the femoral canal. The proximal femoral cortex was thin and brittle. A full cerclage wire was placed around the proximal femur to minimize the risk of fissure or fracture. The extruded cement was not removed and resided harmlessly in the soft tissues.

Classification of femoral fractures associated with canine total hip replacement*

Type A1: greater trochanter

Type A2: lesser trochanter or calcar

Type B1: stable stem; proximal to stem tip

Type B2: stable stem; within 1 cm of tip

Type B3: stable stem; distal to tip

Type C1: unstable stem; proximal to stem tip

Type C2: unstable stem; within 1 cm of tip

Type C3: unstable stem; distal to tip

Type D: comminuted

Type E1: fissure; proximal to tip

Type E2: fissure; within 1 cm of tip

*Types A, B, and C are noncomminuted with transverse, oblique, or spiral orientation. Types A to D have some degree of fracture displacement.

Calcar = limited to proximal medial cortex of the femur, with or without fissure; Distal = >1 cm distal to the tip of the stem; Proximal = >1 cm proximal to the tip of the stem; Stable = well-fixed femoral prosthesis; Stem = femoral prosthesis; Unstable = aseptic or septic loosening.

- Conversely, a femur with a high canal flare may be predisposed to fracture if excessive reaming or impaction is required to accommodate the femoral stem through a relatively narrow isthmus.
- Proximal femoral remodeling can occur in some dogs with chronic subluxation or luxation secondary to severe hip dysplasia.

A lateral drift of the proximal medial cortex of the femur can excessively increase the direct contact of the broach or stem against the medial endosteal surface. Medialization of the greater trochanter results in overhang to the central axis of the medullary canal and demands incremental trochanter reaming to prevent stem medialization or coxa vara implantation. Both scenarios can result in femoral fissure and should be identified during preoperative planning.

- Medullary canal sclerosis secondary to chronic osteopathy such as spontaneous capital physeal fracture and avascular necrosis of the femoral head
- Older dogs with brittle bones (Liska 2004; Ganz *et al.* 2010)
- Younger dogs with an open physeal plate at the base of the greater trochanter can sustain a slipped physeal plate during reduction or a fracture postoperatively (Figure 113.13).
- Greater trochanter fractures may occur if a narrow isthmus of bone is created at the base during biplanar femoral osteotomy.

Diagnosis

- Femoral fissures located along the medial or cranial osteotomy line can be seen during surgery. Fissures that originate caudally in the vicinity of the trochanteric fossa may be obstructed from the surgeon's view and go undetected. The proximal femoral diaphysis distal to the osteotomy line should be inspected visually before closure if a fissure is suspected based on intraoperative findings and technical difficulties. An example of such a scenario would include arduous stem implantation caused by a narrow femoral

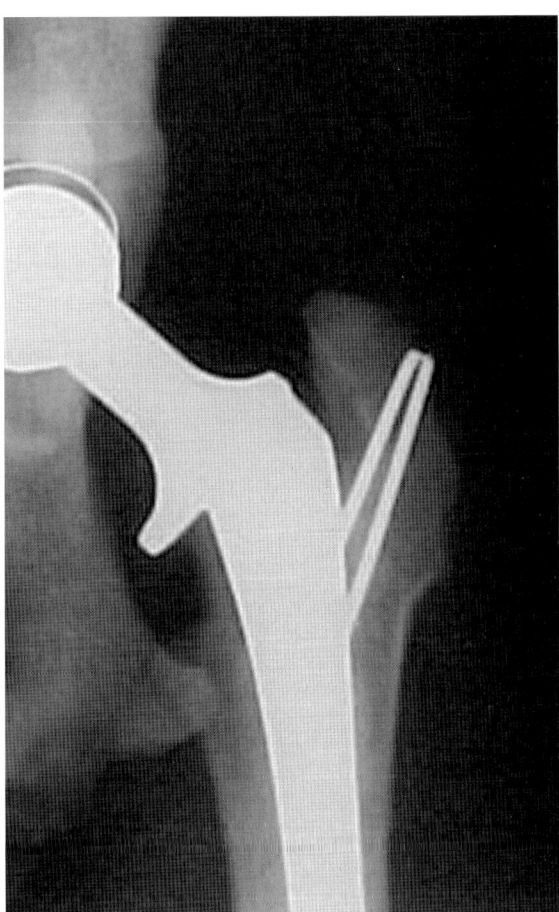

(A)

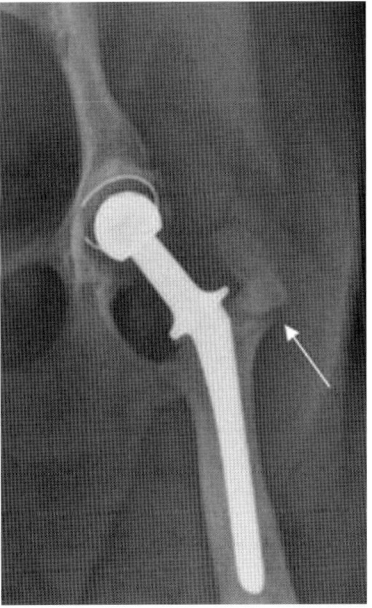

(B)

Figure 113.13 Salter-Harris fracture of the greater trochanter during total hip replacement (THR) in immature dogs. **A**, A cemented THR was performed in a 7-month-ld female chow with chronic and severe coxofemoral subluxation. A physeal fracture of the greater trochanter occurred during the difficult rearticulation of the prosthesis. After reduction, the fracture was stabilized with two pins anchored in polymethylmethacrylate. Recovery and healing were uneventful. **B**, A cemented micro THR was performed in a 7-month-old female Havanese dog with avascular necrosis of the femoral head. This highly active dog became acutely lame 4 weeks after surgery. Pain was elicited by palpation of the greater trochanter and a minimally displaced fracture at the base of the greater trochanter (arrow) was diagnosed. The fracture healed with 4 weeks of conservative management and strict exercise restriction.

isthmus. Another example would arise when the larger of two stems selected based on preoperative templates is placed because the smaller stem was judged as being too small during surgery.

- The femur can be inspected for fissures through elevation and cranial retraction of the vastus lateralis.
- Early postoperative fractures may be underlain by unidentified or unprotected intraoperative fissures. These fractures may occur when physiological loads are applied during early mobility.
- Catastrophic fractures occur most frequently within a few days after surgery but can occasionally occur later in the healing phase as a result of trauma (Figure 113.14). An acute non–weight-bearing lameness will be present. Rotation of the limb at the knee may occur without a corresponding rotation of the greater trochanter. Crepitation at the fracture may or may not be palpable.
- An acetabular fissure, or worse a fracture, can occur during impaction of a cementless acetabular implant. A minimally displaced fissure can go undetected until a gap can be seen on follow-up radiographs caused by revascularization osteolysis during healing. Callus formation will appear later, confirming the previous presence of a fissure (Figure 113.15).
- Fracture location, orientation, and displacement are confirmed on radiographs. Displaced fractures are obvious and typically display a long oblique or spiral orientation passing in the vicinity of the femoral stem tip.
- Orthogonal radiographic projections are required to confirm the presence of a minimally displaced fracture. Sedation or anesthesia is recommended if painful positioning causes movement that could convert a fissure or minimally displaced fracture into a catastrophic failure.
- Fissures can occur days or weeks after surgery as loading increases and result in an acute onset of lameness. Palpation of the diaphysis, usually near the tip of the femoral stem, elicits pain and briefly aggravates the lameness. A fissure may not be evident on the initial set of radiographs. Multiple radiographic projections may be required to visualize the fissure. Fissures that remain undiagnosed become apparent on serial radiographs taken 2 to 4 weeks after the onset of lameness as bone healing and callus formation progress (see Figure 113.15).

Incidence goal
The incidence goal is less than 3% (Liska 2004).

Treatment
- Intraoperative fissures that develop during terminal broaching or cementless stem implantation can be stabilized (Roe 1997; McCulloch *et al.* 2012) with multiple single- or double-loop cerclage wires placed 1 cm apart at least 1 cm beyond the fissure and the tip of the stem. The surgeon may also opt to remove the cementless stem, secure the fissures, and place a cemented stem.
- Postoperative fissures can be managed by strict cage confinement for 4 to 5 weeks or until there is radiographic evidence of bone union. Owners should be strongly advised that noncompliance could lead to fracture. The alternative approach involves a proactive application of internal fixation via plate, screw, and cerclage wires.
- Displaced fractures should have immediate open anatomic reduction and internal fixation using plate and screw fixation augmented by full cerclage wires if the fracture configuration is long oblique or spiral (Figure 113.16) (Liska 1985; Liska 2004; Fitzpatrick *et al.* 2012b).

- Acetabular fractures may preclude cup implantation if the preparation of the bed is extensively compromised and the fracture cannot be immediately stabilized. Periprosthetic acetabular fractures require immediate reconstruction to reestablish a stable functional acetabular prosthesis. Corticocancellous grafting should be considered to augment the reconstruction (Torres *et al.* 2009).

Outcome
Stabilized operative and postoperative fissures will heal if propagating forces are neutralized. Anatomically reduced and stabilized fractures have an excellent prognosis for healing and maintenance of the prosthesis integrity and function within about 60 days (Figure 113.17) (Liska 2004). The clinical signs of femoral fracture are not always severe enough to prompt owners to return for radiographic evaluation. It is therefore possible for a displaced femoral fracture to go unrecognized and present as a healed fracture in the long term (Figures 113.18 and 113.19 and **Video 113.1**).

Prevention
- Thorough preoperative planning is crucial to identify the presence of risk factors.
- Owners of at-risk patients should be counseled before surgery about the importance of restricting postoperative activity for about 6 weeks.
- Preparation of the femoral bed should be initiated in the trochanteric fossa and follow the diaphyseal axis of the femur to prevent excessive force on the cortex at the tip of the broach. A desirable neutral implant position can be achieved via a cranial lateral approach to the hip without a trochanteric osteotomy (Wylie *et al.* 1997). The latter only adds to the risk of creating another complication, such as a delayed or nonunion of the osteotomy.
- Adherence to surgical principles during implantation helps prevent iatrogenic fissure or fracture.
- Implant design or materials change may eventually improve the mismatch in modulus of elasticity between implant and bone at the tip of the femoral stem.
- The osteotomy of the femoral neck should be located proximally to preserve bone stock and limit the length of the femoral neck required to ensure stability.
- The end of the osteotomy window should be beveled during cement removal from the canal to prevent stress riser formation (see Figures 113.6 and 113.20).
- Full cerclage wires can be used as a precautionary measure if there is a perceived risk of fissure or fracture (Figure 113.21).

Relevant literature
Femoral fractures have been reported in 2.3% of 2551 uncemented (25% of the total) and cemented (75% of the total) total hip arthroplasties in humans. Uncemented femoral fixation has been identified as a risk factor for fractures compared with cemented fixation. Femoral component survivorship was 95.8% for uncemented stems and 91.7% for cemented stems at a mean of 6.8 years (Berend *et al.* 2006).

The degree of variability of the cross-sectional geometry is greater in dogs than in humans. Dogs have a relatively large ratio of medullary canal to total area and hence relatively thin cortexes (Sumner *et al.* 1990a). Other interspecies anatomic differences include: anteversion angles, femoral offset, age-related changes, and gait pattern (Jaecques *et al.* 1998; Kuo *et al.* 1998). The morphologic and functional differences combined with dogs' early return to

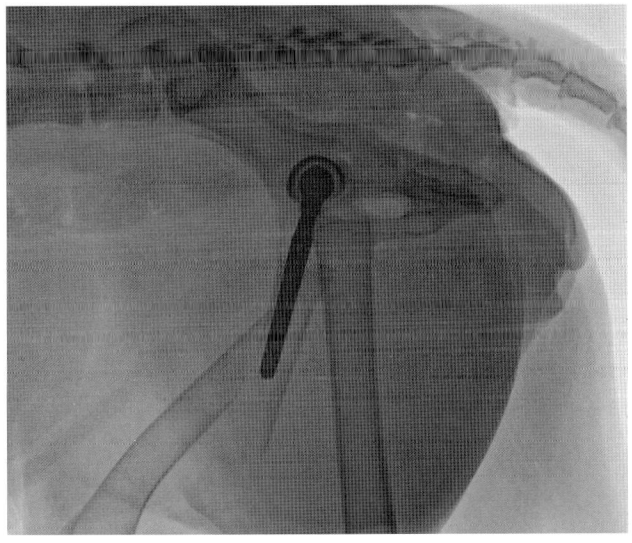

(A)

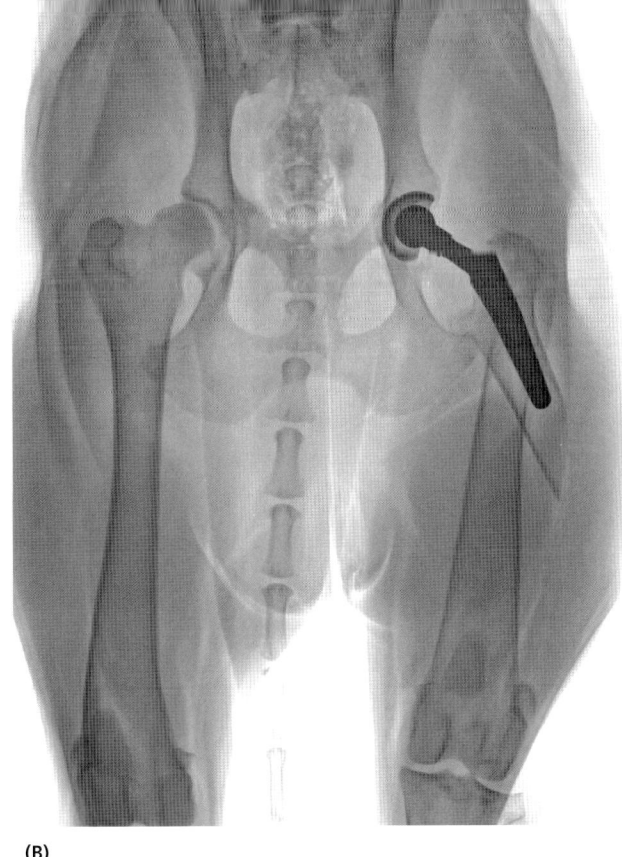

(B)

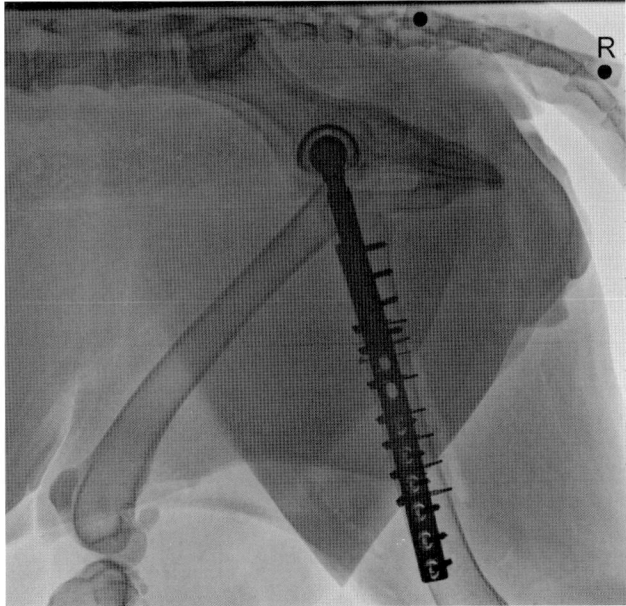

(C)

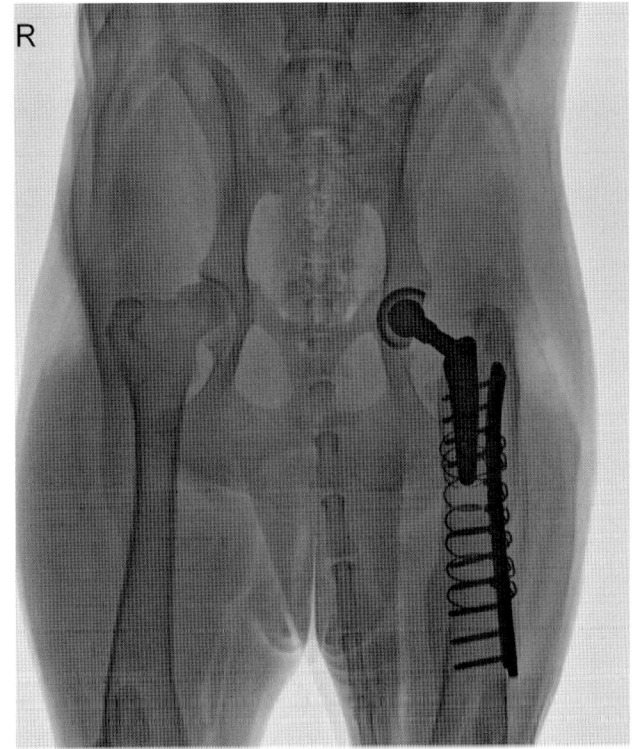

(D)

Figure 113.14 Femoral fracture after trauma 4 years after total hip replacement. **A** and **B**, Preoperative radiographs of a 40-kg female mastiff that fell on a slippery wet floor and sustained a short oblique femoral fracture distal to a cementless femoral stem. **C** and **D**, Postoperative radiographs. The fracture was stabilized with seven full cerclage wires and a neutralization plate. The fracture was healed 6 weeks later.

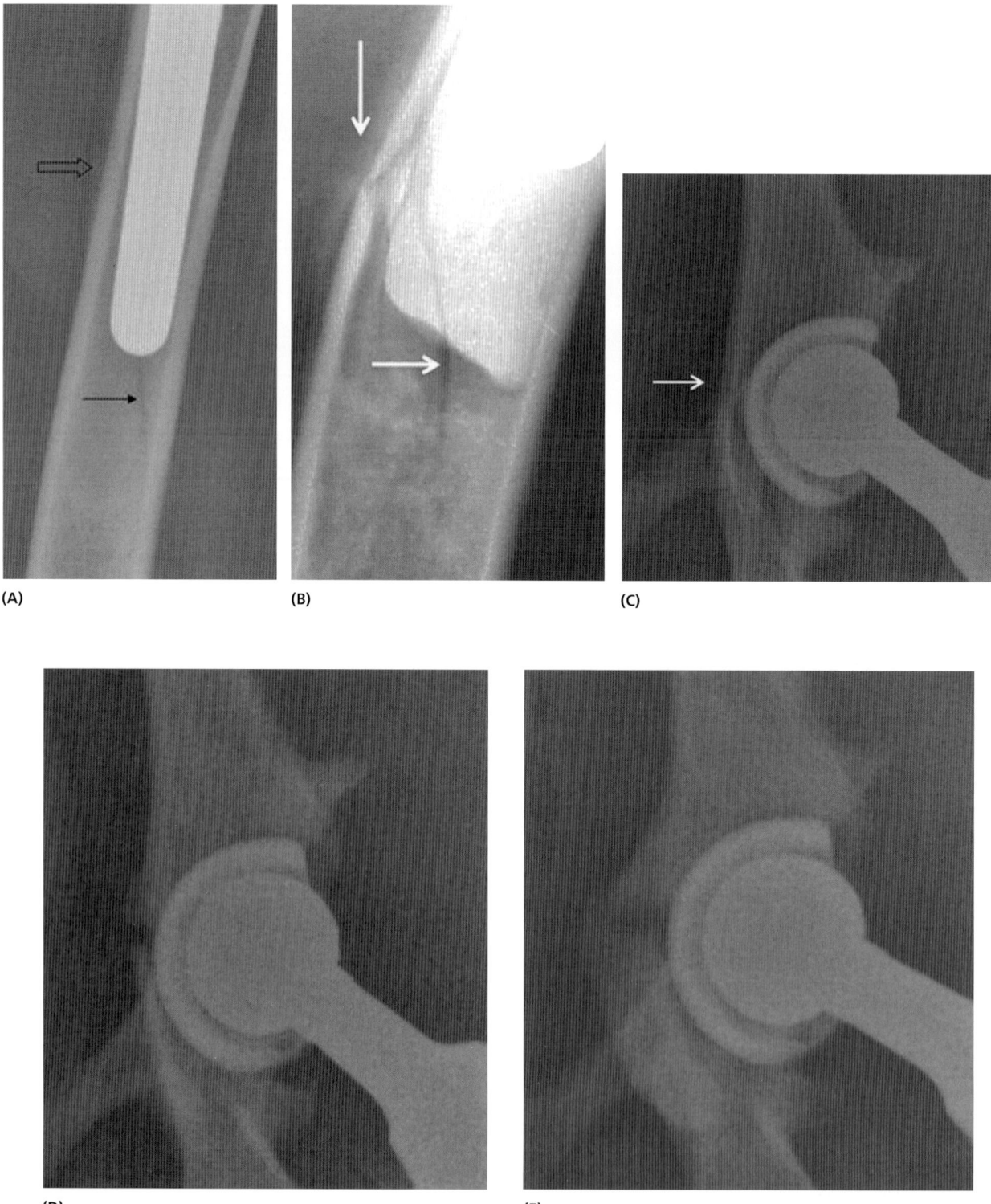

(A)   (B)   (C)

(D)   (E)

Figure 113.15 Examples of femoral and acetabular fissures detected after implantation of a cementless femoral stem. **A**, This radiograph obtained 6 weeks after surgery is consistent with a femoral fissure at the tip of the femoral stem. Note the presence of periosteal bone formation (open arrow) indicative of healing. The patient, an active 9-year-old male Belgian shepherd, had become acutely lame and painful on palpation of the femur 3 weeks after surgery. The fissure was not visible on radiographs obtained at the time of original presentation. The fissure healed without surgery, and the prosthesis was maintained. Fissures at the end of the cement mantle (arrows; **B**) did not require internal fixation. The dog's activity was severely restricted for 6 weeks to allow the fissures to heal and to prevent a catastrophic fracture. In another case, the dog's rehabilitation and weight bearing were slower than expected, prompting an early follow-up radiograph at 3 weeks. A fissure present in the medial cortical wall of the acetabulum (**C**) was retrospectively visualized on the postoperative radiographs (**C**), becoming more evident at 3 weeks (**D**). Callus formation (**E**) is present 10 weeks after surgery, at which point the dog was fully weight bearing and showed no discomfort on hip extension.

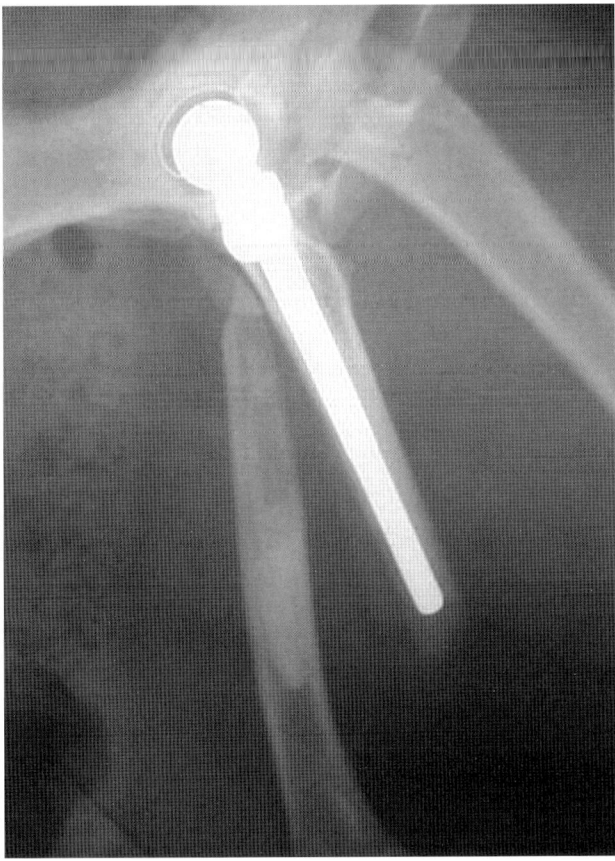

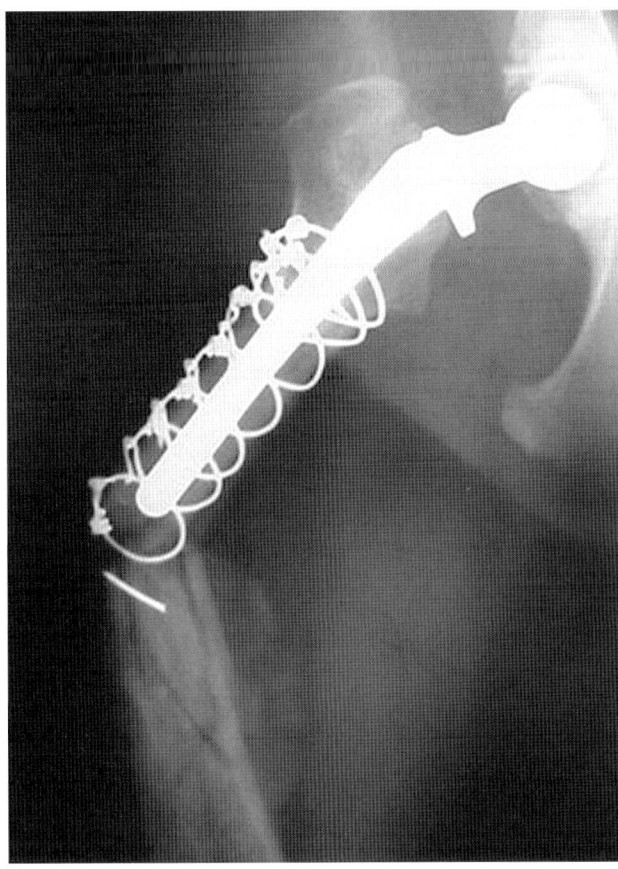

(A)   **(B)**

Figure 113.16 Long oblique fracture originating near the tip of the femoral stem. This configuration is the most common encountered after total hip replacement, in this case, secondary to trauma 90 days after surgery (**A**). Radiograph obtained after repair with seven full cerclage wires and a small pin. This repair does not neutralize bending forces adequately, and predictably, a second fracture occurred 27 days later (**B**). Other circumferential devices used to stabilize long oblique or spiral fractures, such as double-loop cerclage wires (Roe *et al.* 1997) or cables (Blaeser *et al.* 1999), provide a more secure construct but would not have improved the neutralization of bending forces along the fracture line in this dog.

function may, at least in part, explain differences in the incidence of periprosthetic femur fractures between humans and dogs.

The influence of distal femoral fracture repair technique on healing complications is documented for locking plates in humans: a delayed union rate as high as *et al.* 20% was reported in 86 fractures treated with locking plates. In this study, empty holes in the plate adjacent to the fractures healed, and comminuted fractures failed to heal more frequently than less comminuted fractures. Callus formation was lower in nonunion fractures and in patients treated with stainless steel plates compared with those treated with titanium plates. From this study, we can surmise that the primary problem causing late presentation of a nonunion-without-hardware failure results from limited callus formation rather than hardware failure (Henderson *et al.* 2011). In the future, the outcomes of dogs with femoral fractures secondary to THRs treated with (Fitzpatrick *et al.* 2012b) or without locking plates (Liska 2004) should be compared. Intuitively, the incidence of nonunion should be lower with locking plates, but this is not the clinical impression of the author based on experience with a limited number of cases.

A cause and effect relationship between femoral stem stiffness, stress shielding, and bone adaptation (Sumner *et al.* 1992; Bergh *et al.* 2004; Mostafa *et al.* 2012) leading to femoral fractures has

not been established in dogs; therefore, their respective roles in the pathogenesis of THR-related fractures remain unclear.

Incision granuloma

Definition

An incision granuloma is a marked, diffuse, chronic, and proliferative dermatitis and folliculitis developing along a portion of the surgical skin incision. This condition is often associated with a superficial discharge and fibrosis.

Risk factors
- German shepherd breed
- Uncontrolled licking of the surgical incision and postoperative self mutilation

Diagnosis
- On physical examination, there is a moist, ulcerated, hairless lesion of variable size contiguous to the surgical incision. This lesion is typically associated with a history of recurrent self-mutilation and failure to heal (Figure 113.22).

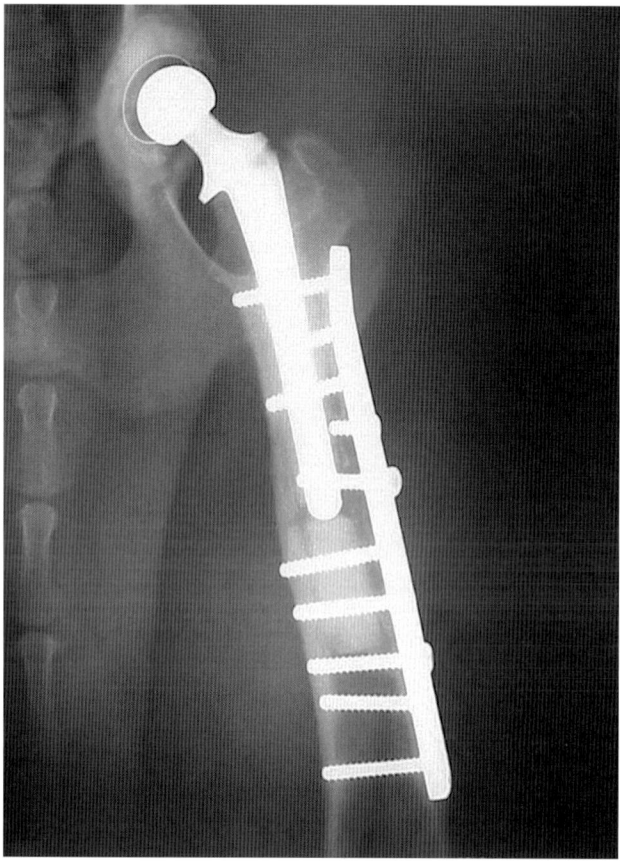

Figure 113.17 Radiograph obtained 698 days after repair of a short oblique fracture near the tip of the femoral stem and concurrent fracture of the cement mantle. The fracture, repaired with a neutralization plate, healed without further complication. The cemented implants remain stable at long-term follow-up.

- Histopathologic findings include marked, diffuse, epidermal and follicular hyperkeratosis and acanthosis. Hair follicles may be dilated and obstructed with keratin. If the follicles rupture, they may provoke pyogranulomatous inflammation. Multifocal, diffuse infiltration of neutrophils and lesser numbers of lymphocytes, plasma cells, and macrophages is noted in the superficial dermis and around hair follicles. Neutrophils may even infiltrate the overlying epidermis. Bacteria will be present in variable numbers.

Incidence goal
The incidence goal is less than 0.5%.

Treatment
- Prevent self-mutilation through restraint devices and coverage of the incision.
- Antibiotherapy is indicated to prevent expansion of the lesion, extension to deep structures, and systemic distribution that could lead to infection of the prosthesis.
- Local excision and primary closure of the lesion may be warranted if restraint and medical therapy fail.

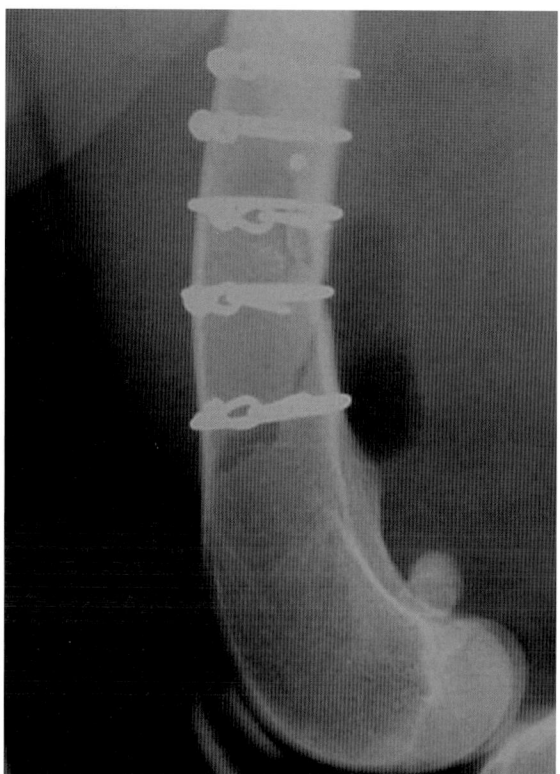

(A)

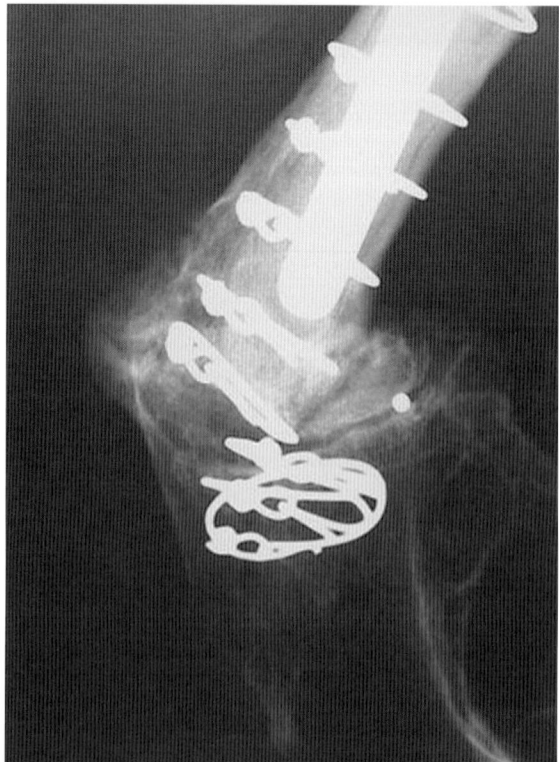

(B)

Figure 113.18 Failed repair of a long spiral distal femoral fracture after total hip replacement. The fracture (**A**) was anatomically reconstructed but inadequately repaired with full cerclage wires alone. The absence of a neutralization plate compromised the stability of the repair, and predictably, led to a second fracture. Surprisingly, this fracture healed. However, radiographs obtained 585 days after the original reduction are consistent with a malunion (**B**). A gait abnormality was present during weight-bearing ambulation.

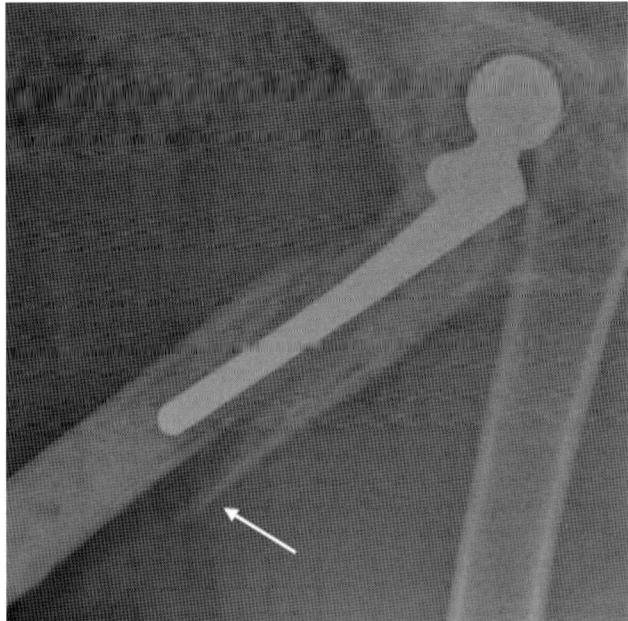

(A)

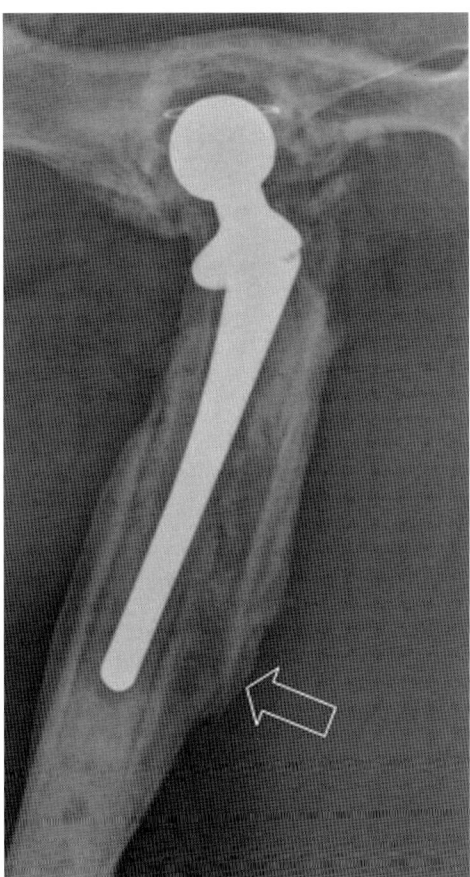

(B)

Figure 113.19 Conservative management of a spiral femoral fracture 8 years after cemented hip replacement. This 11-year-old female golden retriever was referred for evaluation of a lameness secondary to a right femoral fracture (arrow; **A**) and aseptic loosening of the femoral stem. Financial constraints limited treatment to restricted activity for 3 months. Eight months later, the fracture had healed (open arrow; **B**) as a malunion, and a mild lameness was noted on orthopedic examination of the dog (see **Video 113.1**).

Outcome

When treated promptly with restraint devices, coverage of the incision and associated inflammation should resolve without complication. Inflammation of the skin and subcutaneous tissue may occur and should be addressed if present. Excision will be successful as long as proper postoperative care is taken to prevent self-mutilation during healing.

Prevention

- Animal owners should be strongly advised to monitor their dogs and prevent licking of the surgical site. If this behavior cannot be controlled, the surgeon should take immediate precautionary action.
- Meticulous subcutaneous and intradermal skin suture closure. Staples are not used because they create a deeper and larger tract for bacteria to migrate to subcutaneous tissue, they are more likely to retain debris on the skin surface, and there is more microtrauma to the hypodermis during removal compared with fine skin suture material.
- Suture material selection may influence the outcome: Irritating material that must be phagocytized is more likely to draw attention to the incision than monofilament material that is hydrolyzed.

Infarction of the femoral medullary canal

Definition

Femoral medullary infarction is a benign finding, presumably attributed to the vascular disruption caused during preparation of the femoral bed before stem implantation during THR. Factors contributing to ischemia most likely include trauma to the nutrient artery, intraoperative thromboembolic events, or a combination of both events in the absence of other metabolic or vascular diseases. Femoral infarction can be experimentally induced by occlusion, ligation, or transection of the femoral artery (Foster *et al.* 1951). Radiographic signs appear months after surgery as radiodensities in the distal femoral medullary canal.

Risk factors

- Young dogs with predominantly intramedullary and centrifugal cortical bone blood supply (Sebestyen *et al.* 2000; Marsolais *et al.* 2009)
- Greater than average distance between the greater trochanter and the nutrient foramen (Sebestyen *et al.* 2000)
- Excessively deep reaming and rasping of the medullary canal (Haney and Peck 2009)
- Interference with healing of the nutrient artery, possibly by placement of the femoral stem adjacent to the nutrient foramen (Sebestyen *et al.* 2000)
- Massive bone infarction detected shortly after surgery may be an early indicator of future neoplasia (Marcellin-Little *et al.* 1999b).
- Body weight, gender, breed and femoral morphology do not seem to influence the risk of femoral infarction (Marsolais *et al.* 2009; Sebestyen *et al.* 2000).
- Medullary infarction is reported with the same frequency after either cemented or cementless hip arthroplasty (Sebestyen *et al.* 2000). This may suggest that additional research is warranted to elucidate the pathogenesis because the nutrient artery should likely be more disrupted during the aggressive reaming of a cemented implantation. Similarly, the presence of a cement mantle would intuitively be expected to obliterate the microvasculature and therefore increase the risk of ischemia compared with cementless implantation. Therefore, use of other THR systems may have similar risk factors as noted in the Incidence goal.

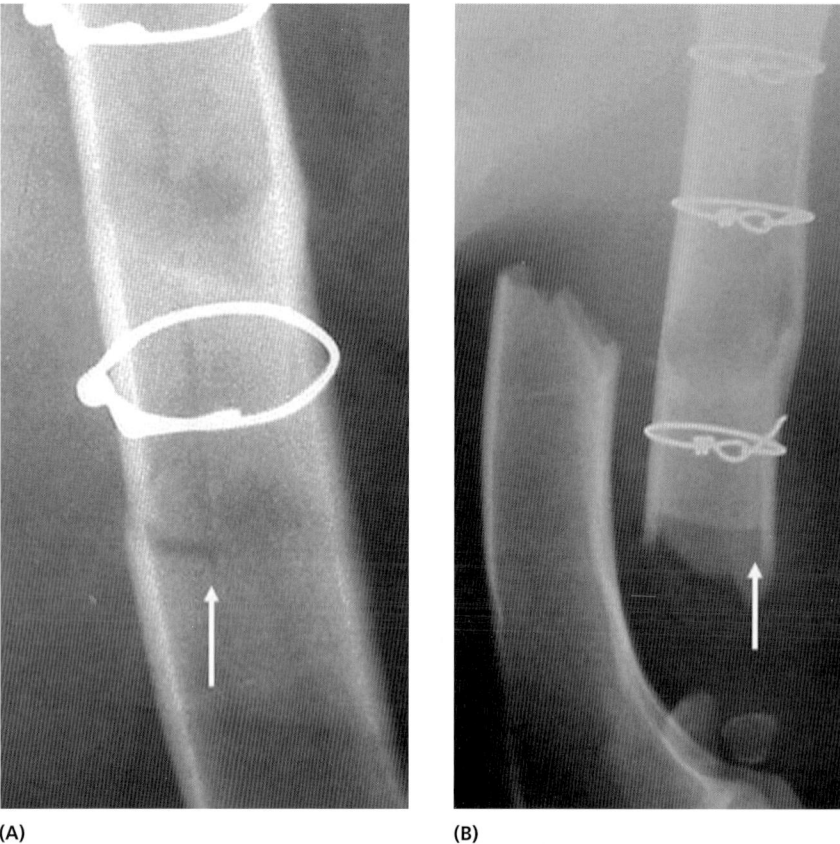

(A)   (B)

Figure 113.20 Fracture secondary to explantation of a cemented hip replacement: a 90-degree corner (arrow; **A**) was created at the distal end of the osteotomy window made to allow explantation of the cemented stem and polymethylmethacrylate. Instead of creating a beveled osteotomy (see Figure 113.6), the surgeon made a distal transverse cut, thereby creating a stress riser. A fracture subsequently originated at this location (arrow, **B**). The fracture healed after plate and screw fixation.

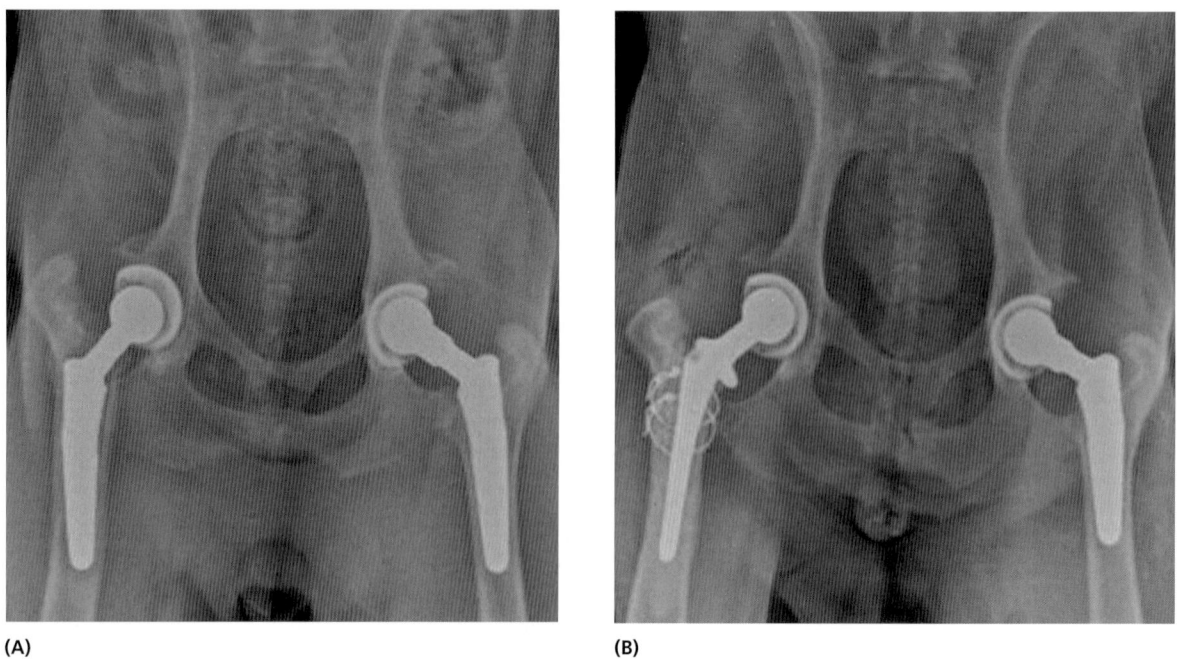

(A)   (B)

Figure 113.21 Femoral stem subsidence after cementless total hip replacement. This subsidence (**A**) was diagnosed 3.5 months after surgery in a 9-year-old female Old English sheepdog. A revision (**B**) was performed with a cemented stem. Although no fissures could be seen during the surgery, cerclage wires were applied to minimize the risk of a postoperative fracture.

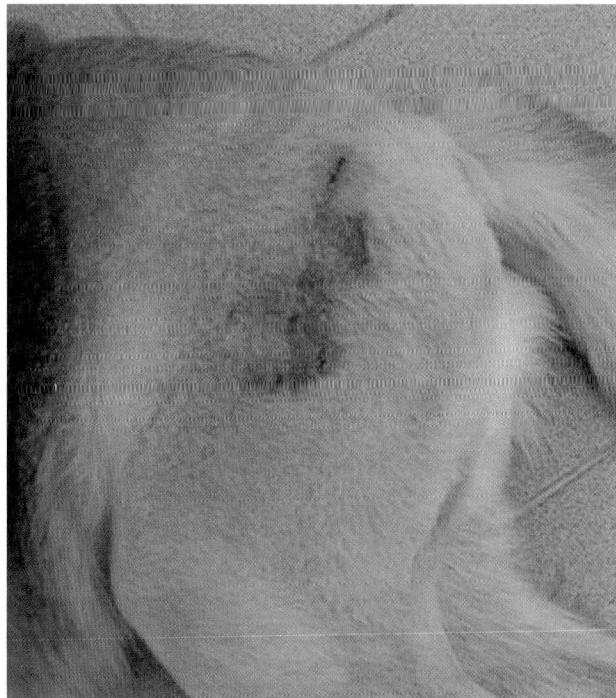

(A)

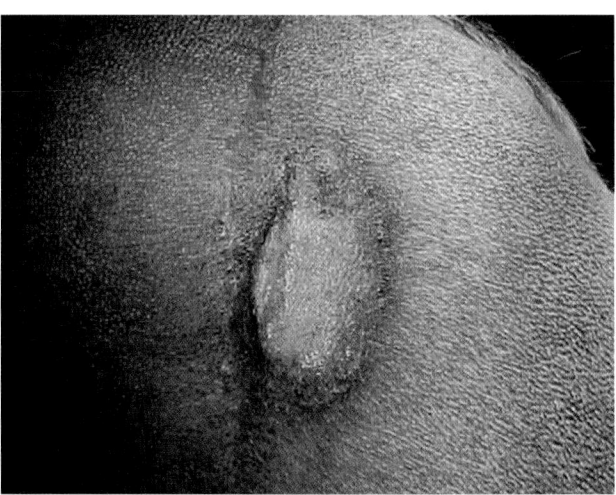

(B)

Figure 113.22 Incision granulomas after total hip replacement in two German shepherd dogs. A diffuse (**A**) and a smaller, moist (**B**) incision granuloma was present caudal to the incision 3 weeks after surgery in each dog. The diffuse granuloma was treated with antibiotics and restraint against self-mutilation. The moist granuloma was treated with antibiotics for 10 days before excision and primary closure.

Incidence goal

The overall risk of infarction appears to be about 14% (Sebestyen *et al.* 2000) to *et al.* 19.5% (Marsolais *et al.* 2009) in dogs undergoing surgery before 1 year of age when using different THR systems.

Diagnosis

- Radiopaque, irregular, serpiginous, noninvasive lesions in the medullary canal that are asymptomatic and do not seem to progress more than 1 year after surgery are pathognomonic for

medullary infarction. The nonspecific opacities generally do not appear to contact the endosteal cortex (Figure 113.23).

- The length of infarction varies from 17 to 110 mm long, comprising 7% to 45% of the femoral length. Infarction may also involve, to a lesser extent, the adjacent cortical bone (Sebestyen *et al.* 2000).
- Infarction can be tentatively diagnosed early postoperatively via perfusion scintigraphy and magnetic resonance imaging (MRI) (Munk *et al.* 1989).
- On histologic examination, the infarcts are typical of ischemic osteonecrosis, with dead marrow elements intermixed with osteocytes; a reactive zone of dystrophic mineralization surrounds the ischemic necrotic core; osteoclastic activity is low, and new bone formation extends from the endosteum into the canal (Sebestyen *et al.* 2000).

Treatment

- No specific treatment is indicated for asymptomatic dogs.
- It is prudent to differentiate between infarction and other postoperative complications by correlating clinical signs, radiographic appearance, and serial radiographic evaluations.
- Femoral infarction has been associated with an increased incidence of stem loosening in dogs (Marsolais *et al.* 2009) and neoplasia in humans (Visuri *et al.* 2006). Although further research is warranted to confirm the clinical relevance of femoral infarction in small animals, periodic radiographic monitoring of affected dogs is warranted.

Outcome

Most lesions remain unchanged on serial radiographic examinations, but they have the potential to change in size. Infarction does not lead to pathological fracture. The incidence of aseptic loosening seemed unchanged in one report (Sebestyen *et al.* 2000) and increased in another (Marsolais *et al.* 2009). An osteosarcoma at the site of a bone infarction associated with total hip arthroplasty has been reported (Marcellin-Little *et al.* 1999b). Annual radiographic evaluation is warranted because of the remote possibility of conversion to neoplasia (Figure 113.24). The long-term outcome in dogs has not been reported.

Prevention

- Limiting rasping and reaming depths of the medullary canal, thus minimizing potential damage to the nutrient artery significantly decreased the incidence of femoral medullary infarction in one report (Haney and Peck 2009).
- Delaying surgery beyond 18 months of age has been proposed to prevent femoral infarction, but this option may not be practical for pain relief (Marsolais *et al.* 2009). Further evaluation of this scenario is indicated.

Relevant literature

In humans, bone infarction from radiation necrosis may be clinically relevant because of its association with the development of tumors, such as fibrosarcoma, malignant fibrous histiocytoma, osteogenic sarcoma, and angiosarcoma (Visuri *et al.* 2006). The topic of arthroplasty-related sarcoma raises concerns but is likely unwarranted in dogs. It is not rare for dogs to be presented for hip replacement surgery and have a periarticular neoplasm identified during the diagnostic workup. The incidence of periprosthetic sarcomas reported in humans is very low considering the total number of arthroplasty procedures performed. Chronic particle-induced inflammation around the prosthesis does not seem to increase the risk of carcinogenesis. The mean latency period is 6

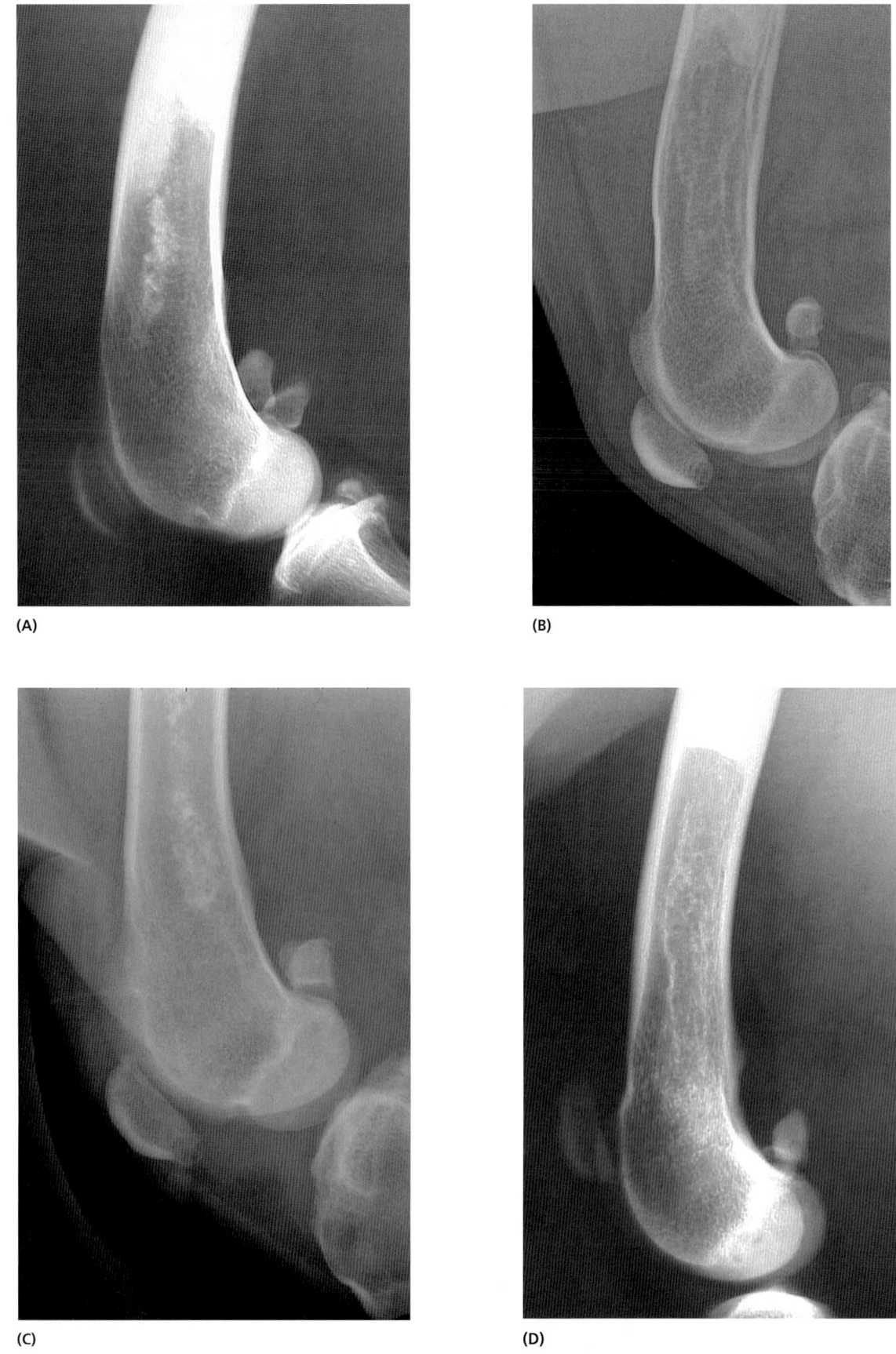

(A)

(B)

(C)

(D)

Figure 113.23 Femoral medullary infarction after total hip replacement. Note the variable radiographic appearance: small, discrete radiopaque densities (**A**), "rising smoke" (**B**), "clouds" (**C**), and extensive long serpiginous "trails" (**D**).

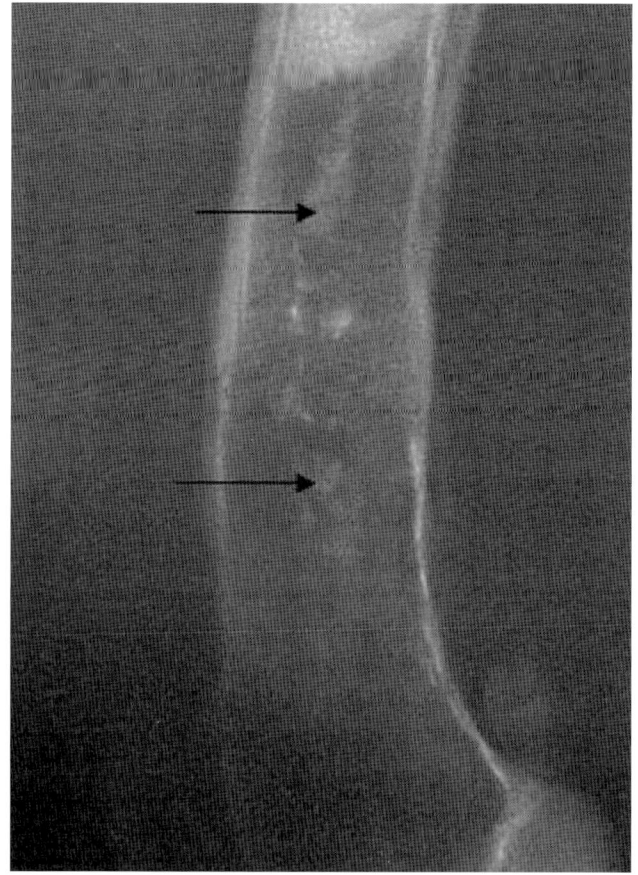

(A)

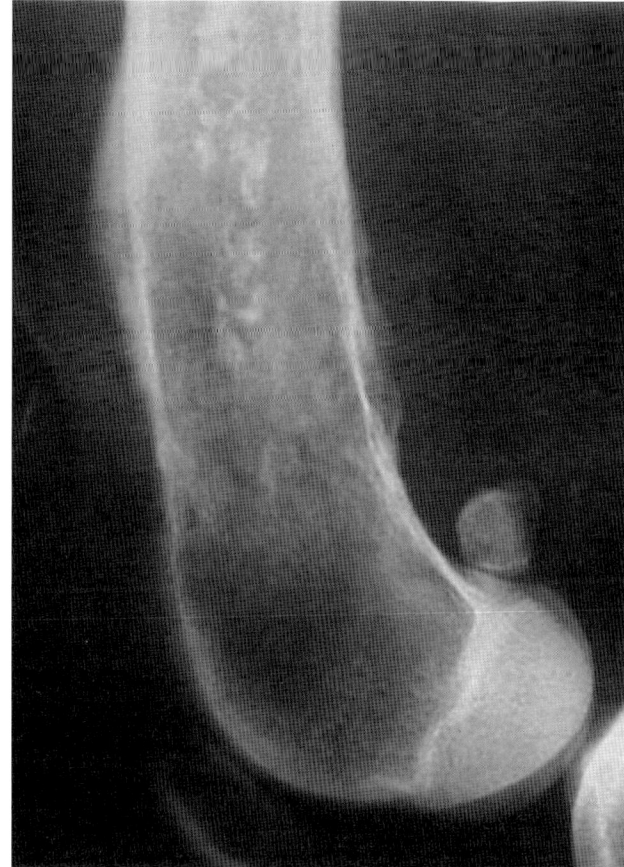

(B)

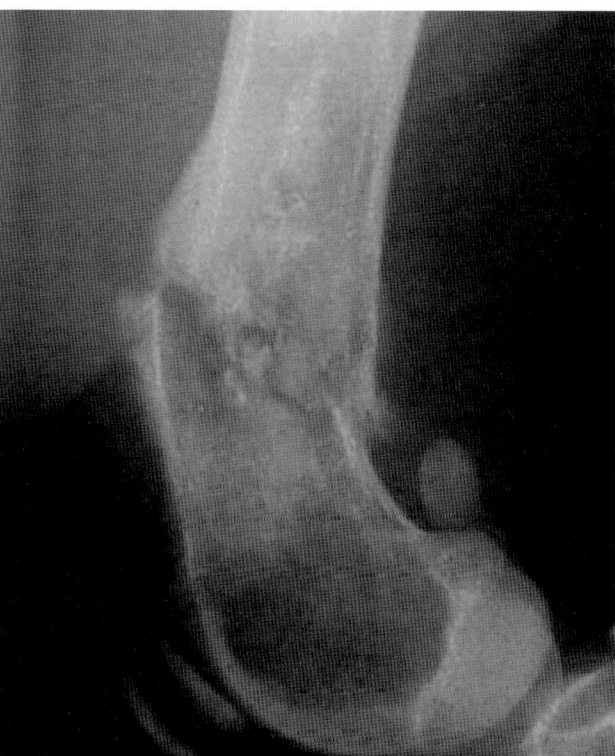

(C)

Figure 113.24 Femoral medullary infarction and pathological fracture after cemented hip replacement at 11 months of age, in a female mixed breed dog. Femoral medullary infraction was noted within 6 months after surgery on radiographic follow-up (arrows, **A**). The dog became painful over the distal femur 7.8 years after surgery. Radiographs (**B**) were consistent with increased medullary radiopacity and periosteal new bone formation. Histopathology confirmed the presence of an osteoblastic osteosarcoma. A pathological fracture (**C**) occurred 2 weeks after the biopsy. The limb was amputated. The dog died shortly thereafter of unrelated causes with no evidence of metastatic disease.

years after surgery, and prolonged latency does not correlate with an increased risk of cancer (Visuri *et al.* 2006).

Infection

Definition

Bacterial infection around a hip replacement is present when an organism resides and proliferates on the surface of the prosthesis or in the periarticular tissues as a result of operative or hematogenous contamination or as an extension of wound infection.

Postoperative infection is classified as early, late, hematogenous, or incidentally positive, if diagnosed at the time of revision arthroplasty for "aseptic" loosening of the implant (Tsukayama *et al.* 1996). Early signs of infection include delayed wound healing and purulent discharge. Late infections originate during surgery but can have a delayed (>6 months in some instances) presentation. Late infection is the most common presentation in dogs (Dyce and Olmstead 2002). Dysfunction caused by pain is progressive, and the response to pain management is poor.

Hematogenous infection is rare, and its origin may be suspected but is rarely established. This type of infection can appear at any time during the life span of the animal, but it is usually not considered as hematogenous in origin unless signs develop at least 6 months after surgery. Culture of the same organism, with the same sensitivity pattern, from the surgical wound and the remote suspected origin is nearly conformational of hematogenous infection.

Risk factors

- Preexisting infection in a patient considered for THR regardless of the location, severity, or duration of the condition.
- Bacterial dermatitis within the draped field is a strict contraindication for surgery.
- Occult septic arthritis present at the time of surgery will result in periprosthetic infection (Figure 113.25) (Benzioni *et al.* 2008).
- Failure to follow meticulous aseptic technique: Strict maintenance and cleaning of the operating theater, poor air quality, intraoperative contamination, traumatic technique, pathogen carriers (e.g., methicillin-resistant *Staphylococcus* organism dermatitis, subclinical rhinitis, or harbored elsewhere in the body), poor hospital hygiene, and poor animal husbandry all increase the infection rate.
- Patients with a suppressed immune system
- Preexisting *Brucella canis* infection (Smeak and Olmstead 1987)
- Prolonged surgery duration from skin incision to skin closure
- Previous surgical exposure of the joint. For example, revision surgery is predisposed to infection compared with primary THR.
- Formation of a glycocalyx biofilm on the surface of the implant shields local bacteria from contemporary opsonizing antibiotic delivery systems and may be responsible for harboring infection many months after surgery.

Diagnosis

- No single test can accurately predict early or late infection of a canine THR.
- A tentative diagnosis of periprosthetic infection is based on clinical findings such as swelling, erythema, pain, lameness, therapeutic responsiveness to antibiotics, and radiographic appearance.
- Radiographic signs include a gap of variable width (≥1 mm) at the bone–cement interface, cortical osteolysis, and periosteal new bone formation (Figure 113.26) (Konde *et al.* 1982; Dyce

and Olmstead 2002). Radiographic changes may or may not be initially present on both the acetabular and femoral components of the joint replacement (Figure 113.27).
- Three-phase scintigraphy with high isotope uptake during the vascular phase is supportive, but not pathognomonic, of a diagnosis of infection. Increased uptake during the bone phase may help differentiate early infection from inflammation. Specific isotope labeling is helpful in humans (Peremans *et al.* 2002) as is erythrocyte sedimentation rate, C-reactive protein, and polymerase chain reaction.
- Cytologic examination of the fluid obtained via prosthetic synoviocentesis is indicative of infection if a severe neutrophilic infiltration with intracellular bacteria is present. However, the sensitivity of this test is low, and false-negative results are common.
- A diagnosis of infection is confirmed via positive cultures. However, both false-positive and false-negative results affect the accuracy of this test. Failure to achieve growth from synovial fluid does not rule out infection.
- The sensitivity and specificity of bacterial cultures are improved when multiple, robust, representative samples of periprosthetic tissues are obtained rather than aspirates.

Tissues from patients undergoing revision surgery for aseptic loosening should always be processed for cultures to detect the potential presence of low-grade infection as an underlying cause for loosening.

Incidence goal

The incidence goal is less than 0.5%.

Treatment

Periprosthetic infection is very difficult to cure as long as the prosthesis remains in situ. Eradication of infection usually requires explantation of the prosthesis (and surrounding cement mantle if present), debridement of surrounding infected and necrotic soft tissue, and prolonged administration of antibiotics selected based on the sensitivity of the causative organism.

A femoral window has been adapted from techniques described in humans to allow explantation of the femoral prosthesis and all cement while preserving the remaining bone stock. In this technique, a segment of cortical bone is removed to access the medullary canal. Beveled osteotomy lines facilitate accurate reduction, and full cerclage wires stabilize the segment (see Figure 113.6) (Dyce and Olmstead 2002). Osteotomy lines should not be created perpendicular to the cortex to avoid collapse of the segment into the medullary canal after fixation and to avoid sharp corners acting as stress risers predisposing the bone to fracture (see Figure 113.20).

The approach may be an extended trochanteric osteotomy to improve exposure of the proximal femur. Hand instruments and ultrasonography can be used to remove cement via the femoral neck osteotomy opening. A chronically infected loose cement mantle can occasionally be extracted as a block if it is still intact and bonded to the femoral stem (Figure 113.28).

One-stage revision of a cemented prosthesis with another cemented prosthesis is not advisable because of the high probability of unresolved infection and recurrence. One-stage revision of cementless components is more feasible if antibiotherapy has been initiated before surgery based on the sensitivity of the organisms cultured from the site and is continued for weeks to months after surgery. The two-stage revision approach often preferred in humans

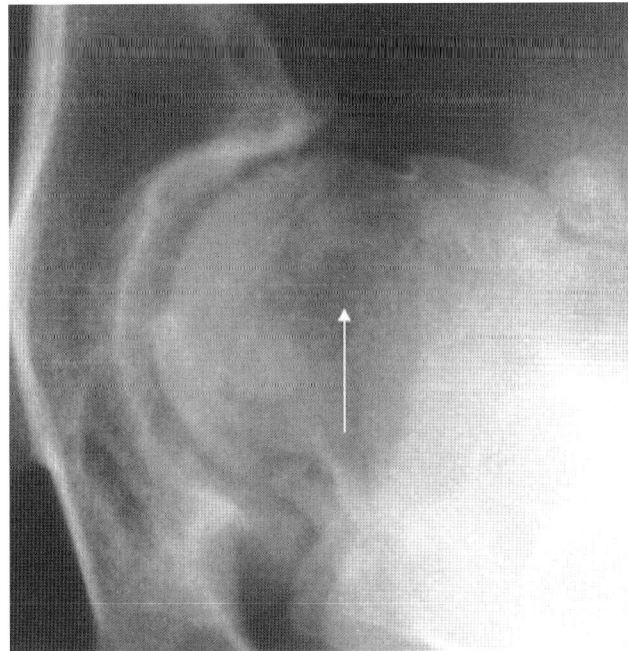

(A)

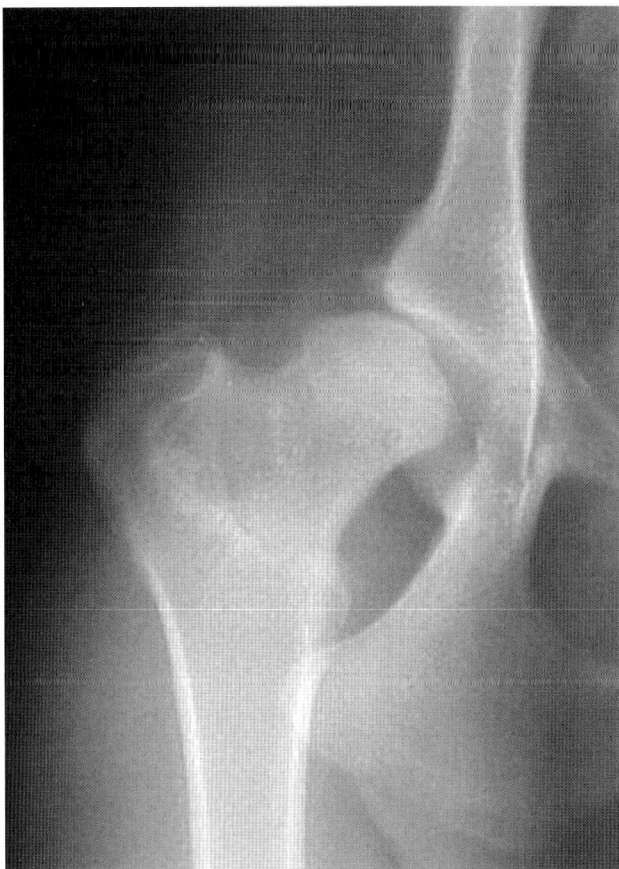

(B)

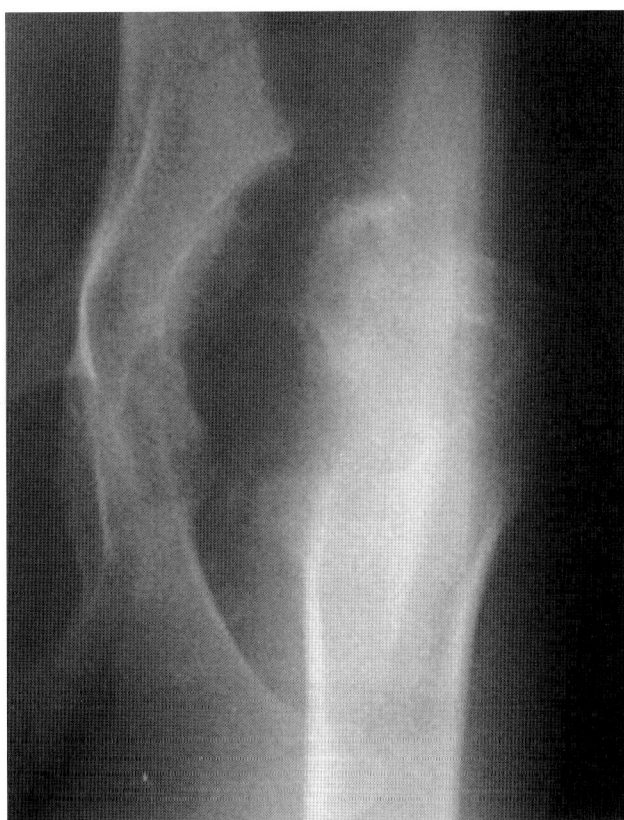

(C)

Figure 113.25 Variable radiographic appearance of coxofemoral septic arthritis. Infection can develop secondary to chronic osteoarthritis (OA), complicating the preoperative screening of candidates for total hip replacement. Septic arthritis may be associated with radiolucent lesions (arrow, A) or mild OA (**B**). Advanced OA with femoral head osteolysis (**C**) was present in a 5-year-old male English pointer hunting dog. Infection was suspected in each of these three joints because manipulation of the joints was more painful than anticipated based on the radiographic appearance.

is often not feasible in animals because of the need for prolonged and strict immobilization, failure to eliminate organisms harbored in infected bone, the severity of bone resorption, the risk of creating other complications, and financial constraints.

Revision of an infected cemented prosthesis to a cementless prosthesis is promising, but long-term results have not been reported.

Outcome

Invariably, periprosthetic joint infection has deleterious effects that limit function, require additional surgery, and increase cost. Infected implants are often treated by removal and conversion into a femoral head and neck ostectomy. Explantation and eradication of the infection can result in limb function similar to that of a

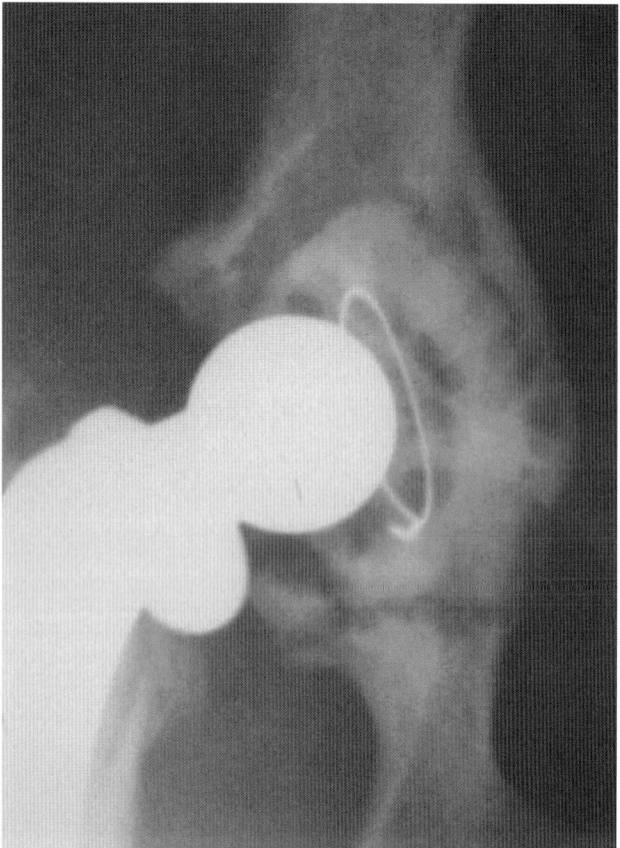

Figure 113.26 Radiographic signs of septic loosening of an acetabular cup. A wide lucent bone–cement interface, new bone formation, implant malpositioning, and medial migration are consistent with infection of this cemented prosthesis. This radiograph was obtained 6 months after an onset of lameness in a 9-year-old female English setter. The lameness started about 2 months after a large right anal sac abscess developed. The prosthesis had remained stable and functional for 5 years before the anal sac abscess event. The infected prosthesis was subsequently explanted.

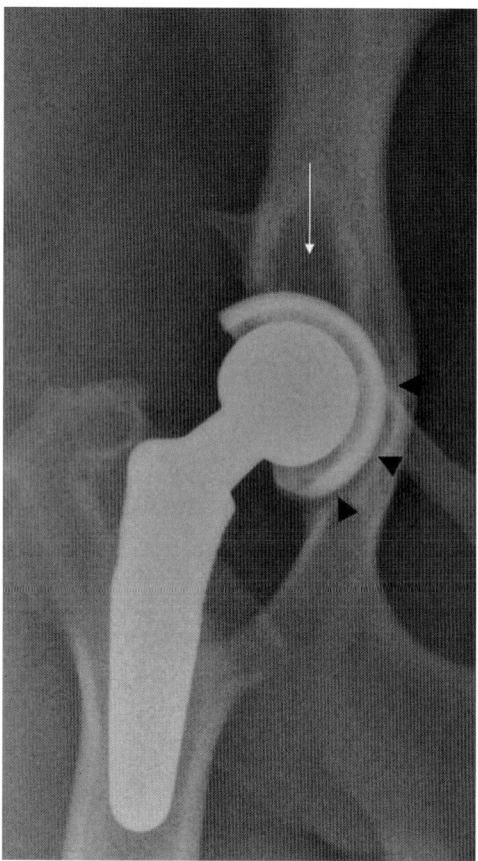

Figure 113.27 Radiographic evidence of osteolysis secondary to infection in the cancellous bone of the ilium cranial to the cup (long arrow) as well as around the bone–implant interface (three short arrows). A cementless hip replacement had been performed 2 years before a sudden onset of lameness in this 3-year-old female Labrador retriever. *Pseudomonas* organisms were isolated from tissue specimens harvested from the iliac lesion. A diffuse infiltrate of neutrophils, lymphocytes, plasma cells, and macrophages in areas of osteonecrosis and fibrosis were found on histological examination.

primary femoral head and neck excision but inferior to an uncomplicated THR.

Prevention

- Meticulous adherence to the principles of aseptic technique, including the operating room environment, is essential (Howard and Hanssen 2007).
- Before surgery, eradicate any dental pathology responsible for harboring bacteria associated with chronic oral infection.
- Defer surgery until resolution of any bacterial dermatitis (Figure 113.29).
- Potential sources of hematogenous infection should be resolved preoperatively and treated promptly if they arise after surgery. Examples of potential sources include wound abscesses, urinary tract infection, otitis, chronic sinusitis, discospondylitis, and chronic enteritis (Figure 113.30).
- Use iodophor-impregnated waterproof barriers on the skin and sew in a waterproof barrier under the skin surface to completely isolate the skin from the surgical wound.
- Follow proper prophylactic antibiotherapy: Cefazolin should be administered at 22 mg/kg body weight every 2 hours to maintain

serum concentrations above 20 µg/mL during surgery and up to 2 hours after the last administration of antibiotic (Marcellin-Little *et al.* 1996).
- Prolonged surgery increases the likelihood of infection.
- The suction tip can be the most contaminated surface at the end of the procedure (Medl *et al.* 2012). Suction should be clamped off when not in use. Using a new suction tip to aspirate debris and fluid from the femoral canal before cement injection may limit intramedullary contamination and infection.
- The relative risk of infection between cemented and cementless fixation is not reported but is generally considered to be lower with cementless fixation.
- PMMA decreases the bacterial load required to induce osteomyelitis in experimental studies. To mitigate this effect, cement is routinely impregnated with antibiotics before injection in cemented hip replacements (Weisman *et al.* 2000).

Relevant literature

Infection is a significant source of morbidity, mortality, and expense in hip replacement surgery. Defining periprosthetic joint infection is a complex and constantly evolving concept, compounded by the

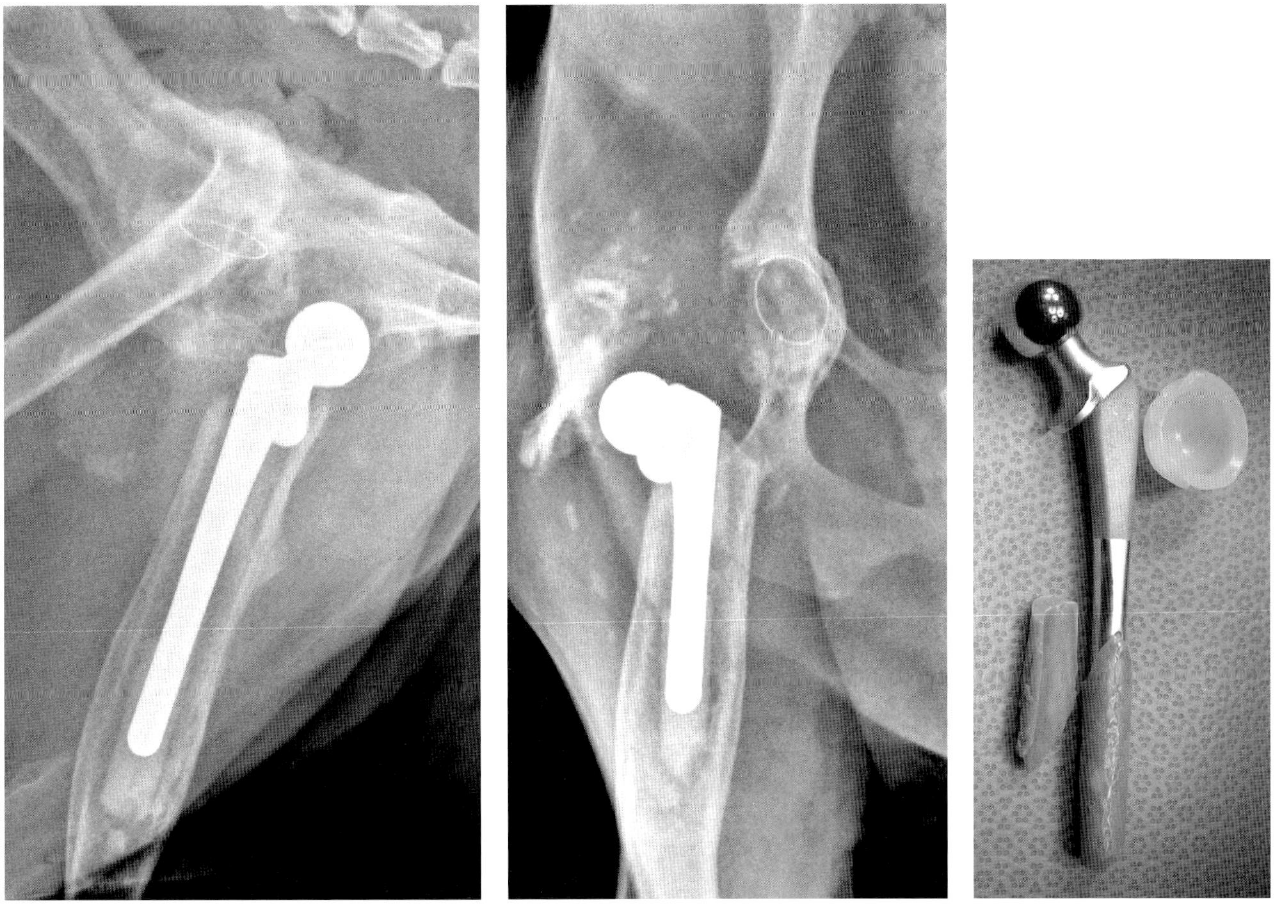

(A)   (B)   (C)

Figure 113.28 Catastrophic failure secondary to septic loosening. A 37-kg male 9-year-old mixed breed dog was referred for a non–weight-bearing lameness 8 years after total hip replacement (THR) with no follow-up examinations since surgery. **A** and **B**. Radiographs are consistent with a subtrochanteric femoral fracture (a trochanteric osteotomy was not performed at the time of THR), prosthesis luxation, a loose rotated malpositioned femoral implant, and soft tissue densities compatible with a cement granuloma. **B**. Prosthesis explantation was performed. The cement was still bonded to the tip of the stem. The medullary canal of the proximal femur was opened to remove the remainder of the cement. Methicillin-resistant *Staphylococcus* organisms were cultured from the periprosthetic tissues.

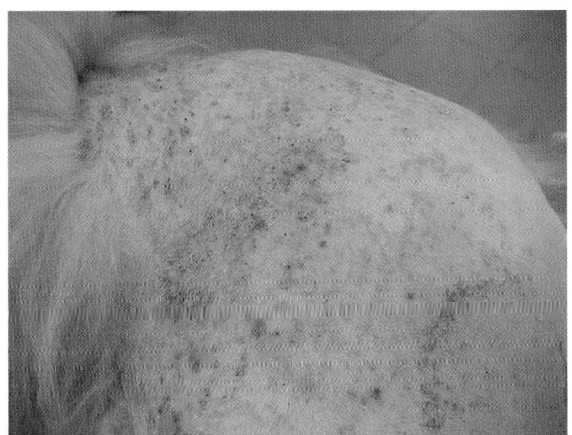

Figure 113.29 Bacterial dermatitis in a candidate for total hip replacement. Surgery should be delayed until resolution of the dermatitis. Seborrhea, folliculitis, and patches of *Staphylococcus* pyoderma were more obvious after the hair was clipped on this 2-year-old female golden retriever (left hindlimb with the head to the left). The dermatopathy was treated for 2 weeks with antibiotics and regular baths with chlorhexidine shampoo before reexamination for surgery.

difficulty in establishing a definitive diagnosis (Spanghel *et al.* 1997; Parvizi *et al.* 2011). Treatment relies on culture-based antibiotherapy and remains challenged by the difficult removal of all implants and debris, along with the development of resistant pathogens (Nelson 2011). Surgeons are therefore encouraged to develop surveillance strategies to reduce the incidence of infection.

The incidence of preoperative dental pathology in animals has not been reported in the veterinary literature. In humans, the incidence of dental disease was 23% in a group of consecutive patients (Barrington *et al.* 2011). Dental disease was treated in all patients in that group before arthroplasty, and no postoperative infection was diagnosed (Barrington *et al.* 2011). These data support the concept of clearing dental pathology in animals before joint replacement surgery. The protocol of the American Dental Association (ADA) concerning antibiotic prophylaxis in patients with total joint replacements undergoing dental procedures provide useful guidelines for the management of small animals. Patients at increased risk of hematogenous total joint infection include those with joint replacement surgery during the prior 2 years and those that are immunocompromised, malnourished, have diabetes, have malignancy, have inflammatory arthropathies, or have had previous prosthetic joint infections (Ching *et al.* 1989). The risk in animals is increased if there are extractions, endodontic

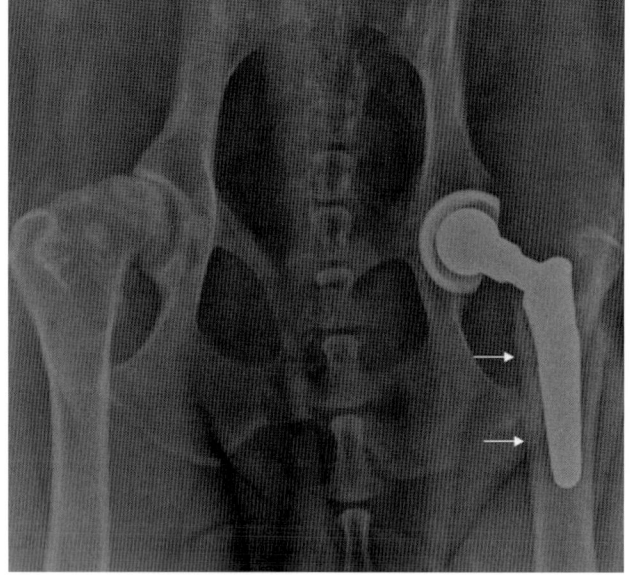

(A)

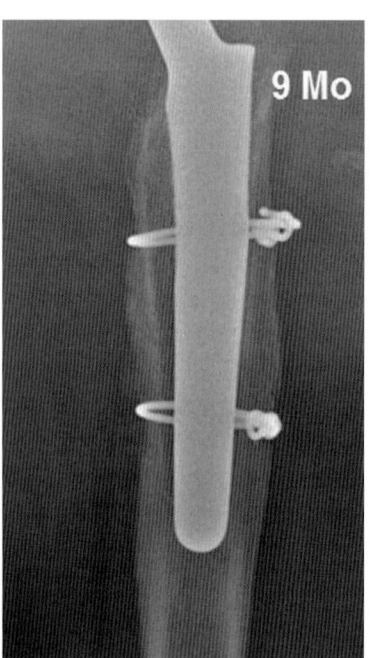

(C)

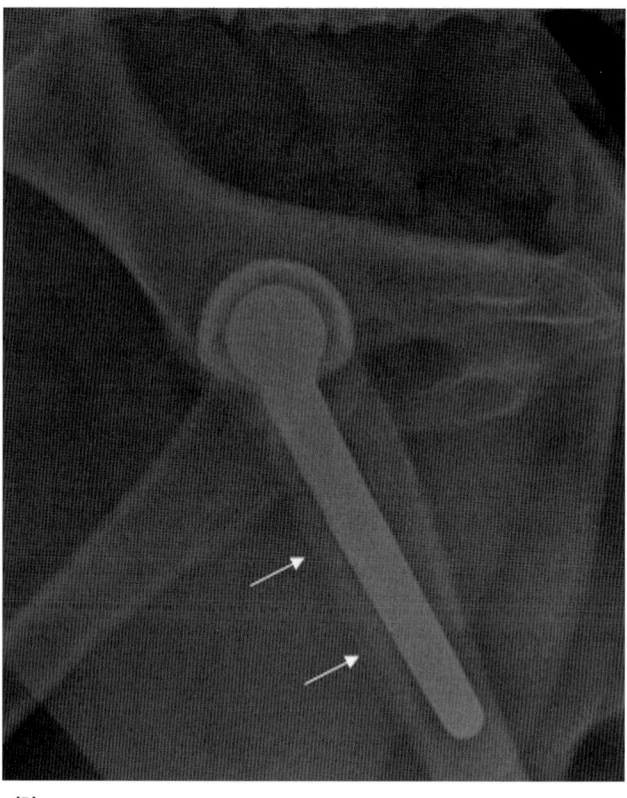

(B)

Figure 113.30 One-stage revision of a septic cementless total hip replacement. A subtle, slowly progressive lameness began in a 7-year-old male golden retriever 3.3 years after hip replacement. Pain was elicited on deep palpation of the femoral diaphysis. On radiographs (**A** and **B**), lucency was present around the retroverted femoral stem, and periostitis (arrows) was visible along the medial and cranial proximal femoral cortices. No change was present around the acetabular component. *Enterococcus* spp. was isolated during one-stage revision, which included removal of all biofilm and implantation of a size larger femoral stem. Antibiotics (doxycycline and marbofloxin) were administered for 6 weeks after surgery. No lameness was present, and the prosthesis was stable 9 months after revision surgery at the last follow-up examination (**C**). The origin of infection was presumed to be hematogenous.

procedures, periodontal disease, and bleeding during prophylactic cleaning. Dental procedures should not be performed during the same anesthesia episode as joint replacement surgery.

The American Academy of Orthopedic Surgeons (AAOS) regularly reviews and updates recommendations on antibiotic prophylaxis for bacteremia in patients with joint replacements (AAOS 2010). This information is posted on their website. The information from the ADA and AAOS is helpful, but veterinary surgeons are encouraged to consider human recommendations as such and to consider their own specific patient needs as well as to seek consultation with appropriate clinical and scientific sources before making antibiotic prophylaxis decisions.

The value of systematic intraoperative bacterial cultures during primary THR is questionable. Indeed, positive cultures have not been found to correlate with postoperative infection in several studies (Lee and Kapatkin 2002; Bergh *et al.* 2006; Frank *et al.* 2011; Ireifej *et al.* 2012). The ability to investigate this correlation is complicated by the fact that antibiotics are typically prescribed in dogs with positive intraoperative cultures as a preventive measure against postoperative infection. This practice is ethically acceptable, and it is difficult to justify withholding antibiotics given the consequences of infection on a joint replacement.

The organism responsible for periprosthetic infection should ideally be identified from cultures of retrieved periprosthetic tissues or synovial fluid aspirates before revision surgery. The timing of antibiotic administration with regards to revision surgery is debatable when no organism has been identified. A prominent concern is that preoperative administration of antibiotics could result in a false-negative intraoperative culture, affecting diagnosis and treatment. As a consequence, antibiotherapy is often withheld until intraoperative samples have been collected for cultures. However, when this concept was questioned in a prospective study of 25 patients with 26 infected total knee replacements, preoperative prophylactic antibiotics did not affect the results of intraoperative cultures (Burnett *et al.* 2010). The authors concluded that antibiotherapy should be initiated at the time of induction before surgery on an infected knee replacement if an organism has been identified on preoperative aspirates and no antimicrobial has been administered in the 4 weeks before surgery. Further investigations would be warranted to verify that these results can be extrapolated to small animals.

Luxation

Definition
Dislocation of the prosthetic femoral head from the cup of the acetabular component following THR is a disappointing complication that invariably requires additional surgery.

Risk factors
- High (>60-degree) or low (<30-degree) angle of lateral opening (ALO) for dorsal or ventral luxation, respectively. Extreme angles eliminate passive capture of the head (Dyce *et al.* 2001).
- Cup anteversion can create soft tissue impingement between the femoral neck and the caudal rim of the cup during external rotation and thus "lever" the head out of the acetabulum.
- If the femoral neck contacts an osteophyte on the caudal pole of the acetabulum during external rotation, the lever effect can lift the head out of the acetabulum.
- Cemented cups are suspected to have a higher incidence of luxation than cementless cups with a metal shell. Although the underlying cause of this difference has not been clearly established, the additional several millimeters of cup lateralization of the cementless cup are speculated to protect the implant from luxation. The lower luxation rate with cementless cups may be related to the lower risk of deformation of UHMWPE along the dorsal acetabular rim, where it is reinforced by the metal backing. Cemented cups may also have a tendency to be placed in high ALOs by surgeons who strive for complete bone coverage at the acetabular rim, thereby inducing a dorsiversion of the cup.
- Dogs with chronic or severe preoperative, cranial, dorsal subluxation (or luxation) carry a higher risk of postoperative luxation (Hayes *et al.* 2009). Chronic muscle contracture and muscle memory initially tend to direct the rearticulated prosthetic femoral head to the preoperative positioning of the femoral head. If the prosthesis remains in place, muscle contracture may be replaced by muscle relaxation and elongation, potentially leading to laxity and subsequent luxation.
- Giant breed dogs with rounded torsos such as St. Bernards and mastiffs, are predisposed to ventral luxation. The underlying mechanism for this predisposition is not clear, and no risk factors have been clearly identified. A short prosthetic femoral neck, undersized implants, high body weight, inept coordination during rising and lying down, a tendency to lay in sternal recumbency with the hindlimbs fully abducted, and the leverage created by long hindlimbs may all be underlying causes.
- Ventroversion of the acetabular cup increases the risk of ventral luxation, but the optimum version and inclination angles for each breed have not been established (Nelson *et al.* 2007).
- Small breed dogs and cats have an incidence of luxation similar to that of large dogs (Warnock *et al.* 2003; Liska *et al.* 2010; Witte *et al.* 2010; Marino *et al.* 2012).
- Subsidence tends to lead to luxation because of the associated "shortening" of the femoral neck. The shorter distance between the femoral head and the proximal femur allows impingement of bone on the face of the cup and levers the head out of the cup.
- Retroversion or anteversion of the femoral stem, especially with concomitant stem subsidence (Figure 113.31), can lead to neck impingement on the acetabular rim and luxation, whether or not it is associated with a fracture of the medial femoral cortex fracture (Figure 113.32).
- Excessive ventroversion of the cup may result from the surgeon's concerns to avoid dorsal luxation.

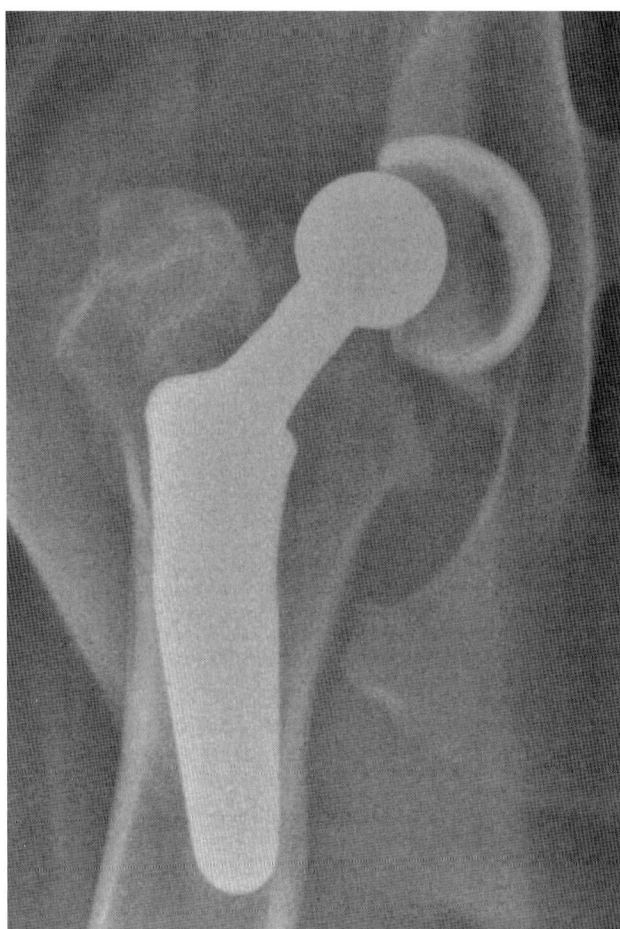

Figure 113.31 Luxation secondary to subsidence of a cementless femoral stem. Subsidence of this undersized cementless femoral stem is present 2 weeks after surgery in this 11-month-old female German shepherd. As a result of this subsidence, bone along the femoral neck osteotomy contacts the acetabular rim, causing subluxation of the femoral head. Revision involved implantation of a larger femoral stem. The larger stem underwent postoperative osteointegration and remains stable 4 years after surgery.

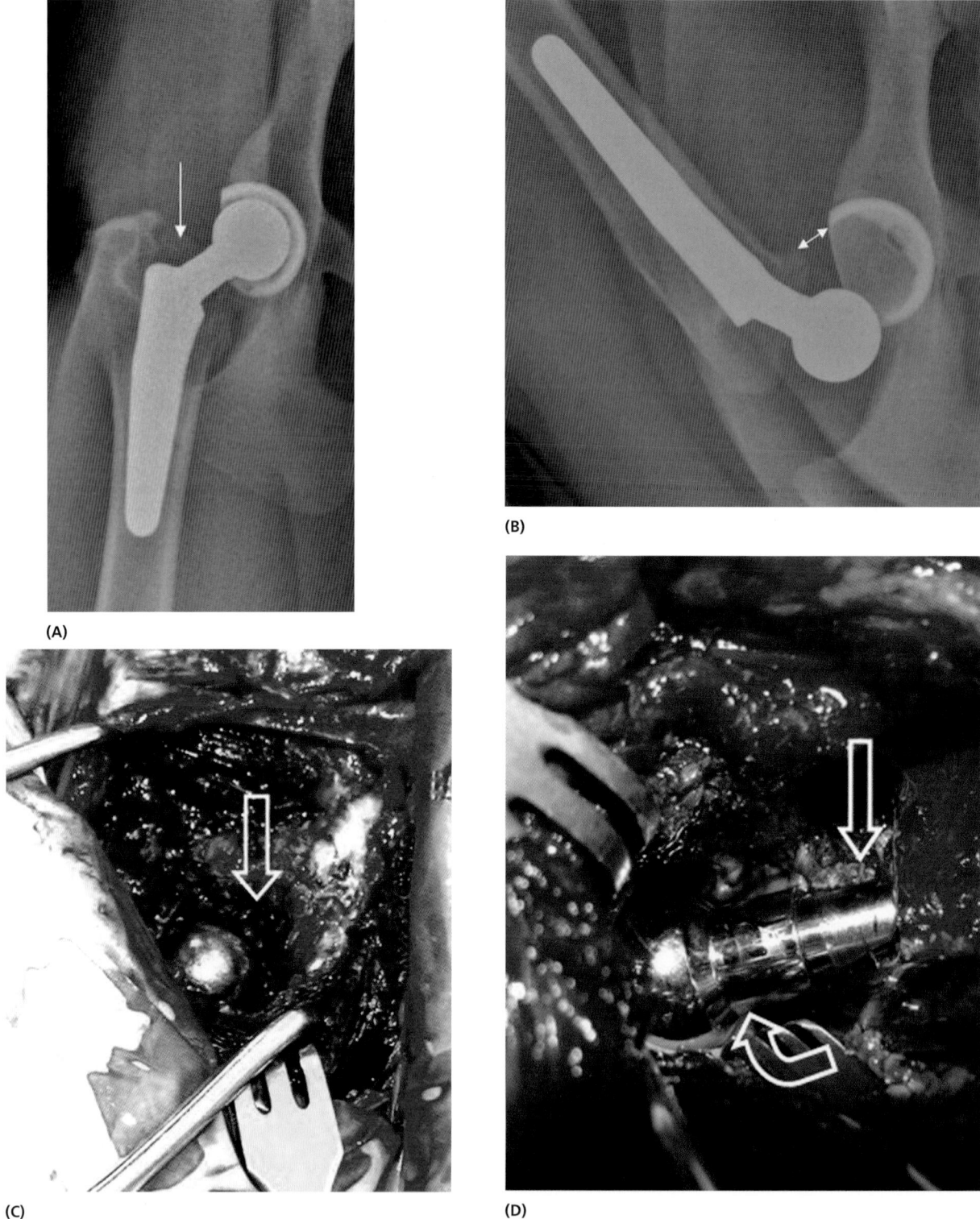

Figure 113.32 Neck lengthening in a dog with subsidence of the femoral stem and subsequent impingement with the acetabular rim. Femoral stem subsidence (>5 mm) and osteoproliferation along the osteotomy line (arrow; **A**) were diagnosed in this 2-year-old female golden retriever 1 year after cementless hip replacement. The subsidence likely occurred within 6 weeks after surgery but was not detected until the annual recheck. The shortened neck length caused bone impingement on the rim of the acetabulum (double arrow; **B**), leading to subluxation of the femoral head, which would spontaneously rearticulate. The decreased length of the femoral neck (open arrow; **C**) was evident intraoperatively because the portion of implant extending from the proximal femur was limited to the femoral head. Bone was removed along the femoral neck osteotomy (open arrow; **D**), and the femoral head was replaced with a femoral neck whose length was 6 mm longer than the original implant (open curved arrow; **D**). The revised femoral neck osteotomy (arrow; **E**) and the elongated neck (open curved arrow; **E**) are evident on the postoperative radiographs. No subluxation has recurred after 3 years of follow-up. A collared cementless femoral stem (**F**) will prevent subsidence when the collar is in contact with calcar cortical bone. *(Continued)*

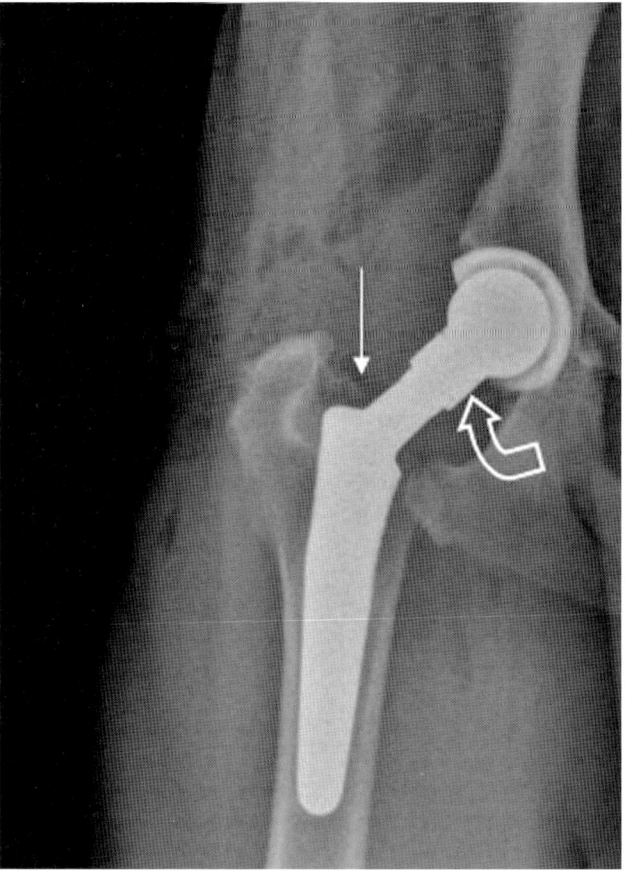

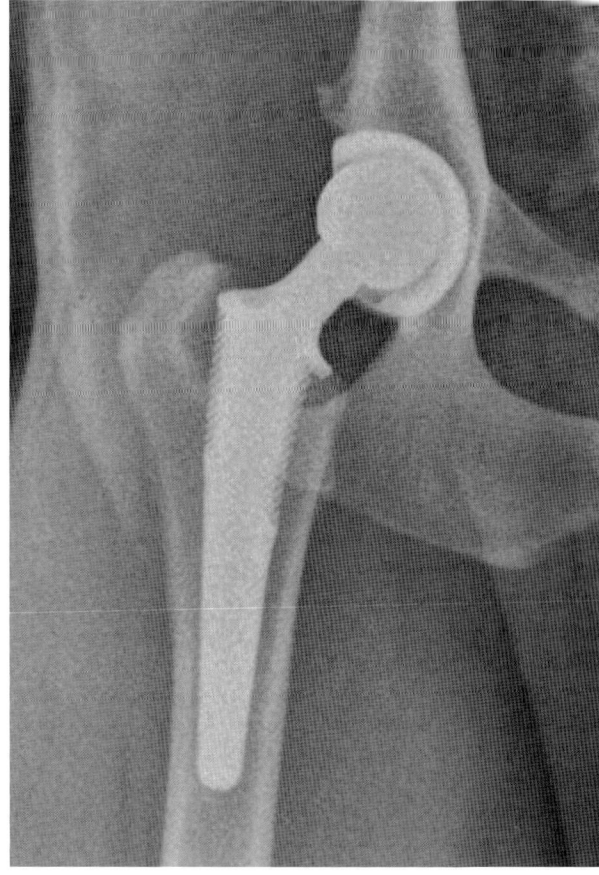

(E)   (F)

Figure 113.32 *(Continued).*

- Deficient strength of the transarticular muscle caused by muscle atrophy may compromise passive muscles stabilization of the head in the acetabular implant. This deficiency can lead to postoperative luxation alternating dorsally and ventrally.
- Luxation that occurs more than 1 year after surgery is generally related to trauma, implant malpositioning that survived short-term usage, or instability resulting from implant wear.
- Contralateral amputation (Figure 113.33), either before (Preston *et al.* 1999) or subsequent to hip replacement, increases the risk of luxation.
- Dogs that have a tendency to sit or lie in abdominal recumbency with the hindlimb in extreme abduction (Figure 113.34) are at risk for postoperative ventral luxation. Hobbles should be considered postoperatively when this posture is observed preoperatively.

Diagnosis

- Lameness with minimal weight bearing: Luxation almost always occurs within the first 5 weeks, frequently within the first 2 weeks, but usually within the first few days after surgery.
- Dogs with craniodorsal luxation carry the affected limb in a variable degree of external rotation and exhibit pain on abduction (Figure 113.35). The craniodorsal displacement of the greater trochanter can be noted on palpation and compared

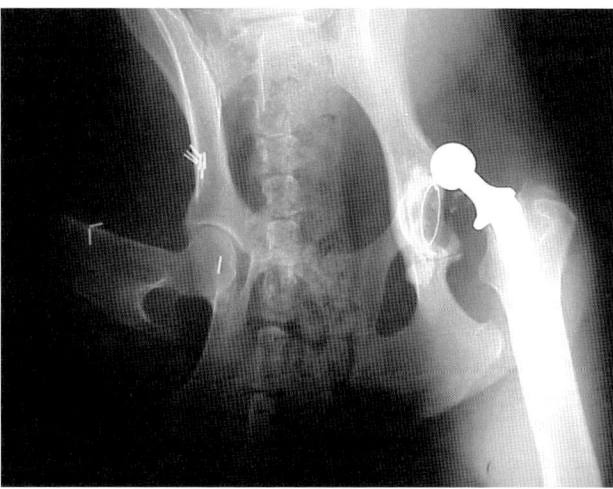

Figure 113.33 Luxation of a cemented total hip replacement (THR) after contralateral amputation. A left THR performed on this 3-year-old female, 57-kg Kuvasz had remained stable and fully functional until an osteosarcoma was diagnosed in the contralateral proximal tibia 2 years after the hip replacement. The previously stable hip prosthesis luxated 3 months after the amputation of the right hindlimb.

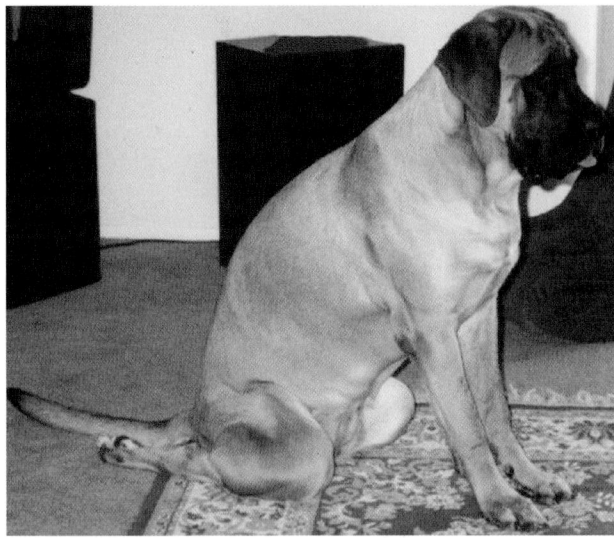

Figure 113.34 Ventral luxation of a total hip replacement in a dog with postoperative abduction of the limbs. This 1-year old female mastiff is sitting with both hindlimbs in full abduction while watching television and slept with the hindlimbs in the same position. Ventral hip luxation occurred within 24 hours of total hip replacement. The dog was successfully managed with rearticulation of the implant and placement of hobbles for 4 weeks.

with the contralateral side. A thumb placed between the greater trochanter and the ischial tuberosity is not pushed out of its location by the greater trochanter upon external rotation of the limb. The respective triangular alignment of the ischial tuberosity, greater trochanter, and wing of the ilium is modified.
- Dogs with ventral luxation carry the affected limb in internal rotation and exhibit pain on adduction. Abnormalities identified on palpation of landmarks are opposite in direction to those described above for dorsal luxation.
- The diagnosis is confirmed based on radiographic evidence of luxation (dorsal or ventral) of the femoral head prosthesis out of the acetabular cup (Figures 113.36 and 113.37).

Incidence goal

The incidence goal is less than 3% for an experienced surgeon with more than 100 procedures performed (Nelson *et al.* 2007).

Treatment
- Treatment of luxation begins with a critical review of radiographs, specifically evaluating the possibility of implant malpositioning that would predispose to impingement. With impingement of the neck on the acetabular rim, the head is "lifted" out of the cup by the fulcrum effect. The acetabular and femoral implants should be evaluated in their relative orientation (which determines passive ROM), not in isolation to each other.

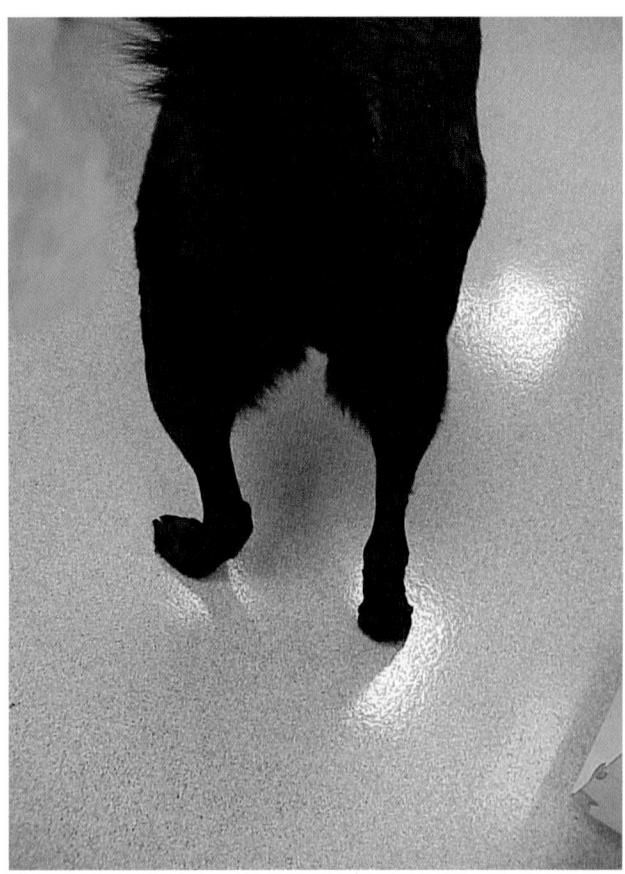

(A)

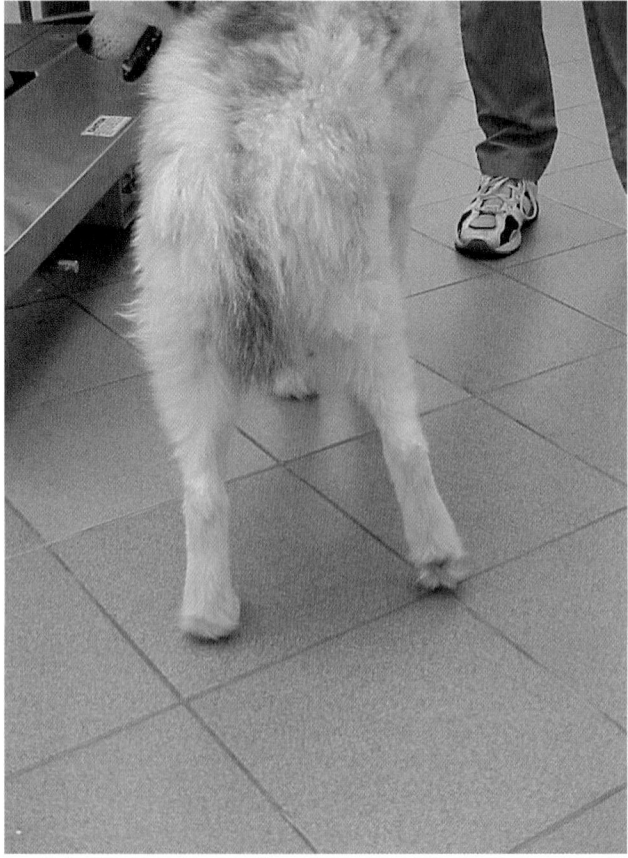

(B)

Figure 113.35 Positioning of the limb in dogs with coxofemoral luxation after total hip replacement. The limb is often placed in variable degrees of external (left hind; **A**) or internal (right hind; **B**) rotation if a cranial dorsal or ventral prosthesis luxation is present, respectively.

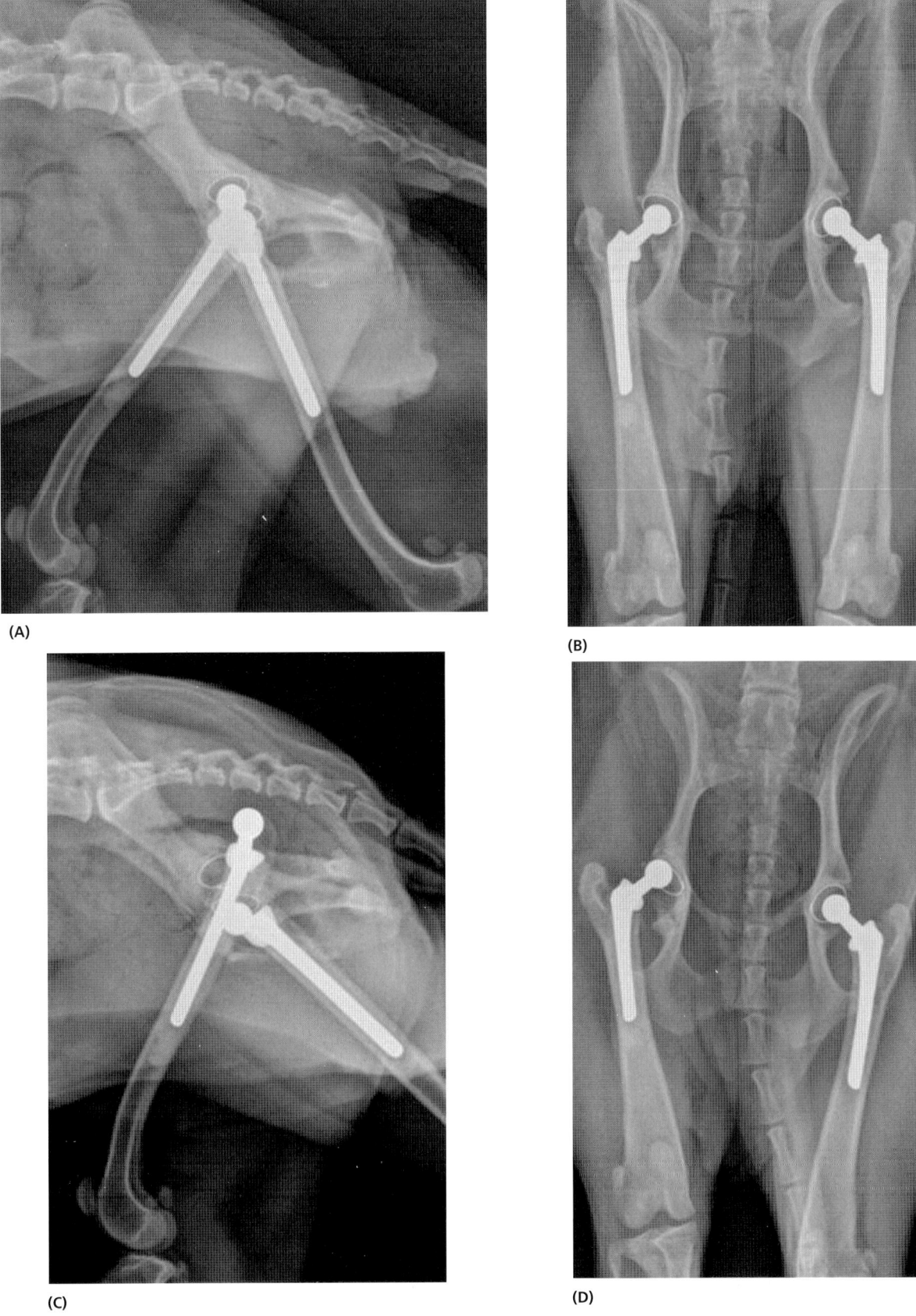

(A)

(B)

(C)

(D)

Figure 113.36 Dorsal luxation secondary to malpositioning of an acetabular prosthesis. Postoperative radiographs of a 10-year-old female King Cavalier spaniel with staged bilateral hip replacements (**A** and **B**): The left acetabular cup is well positioned, but the right cup is poorly positioned in dorsiversion and retroversion. Eight weeks after surgery, a dorsal luxation of the right hip is diagnosed (**C** and **D**). Revision of the cup position was required to maintain reduction.

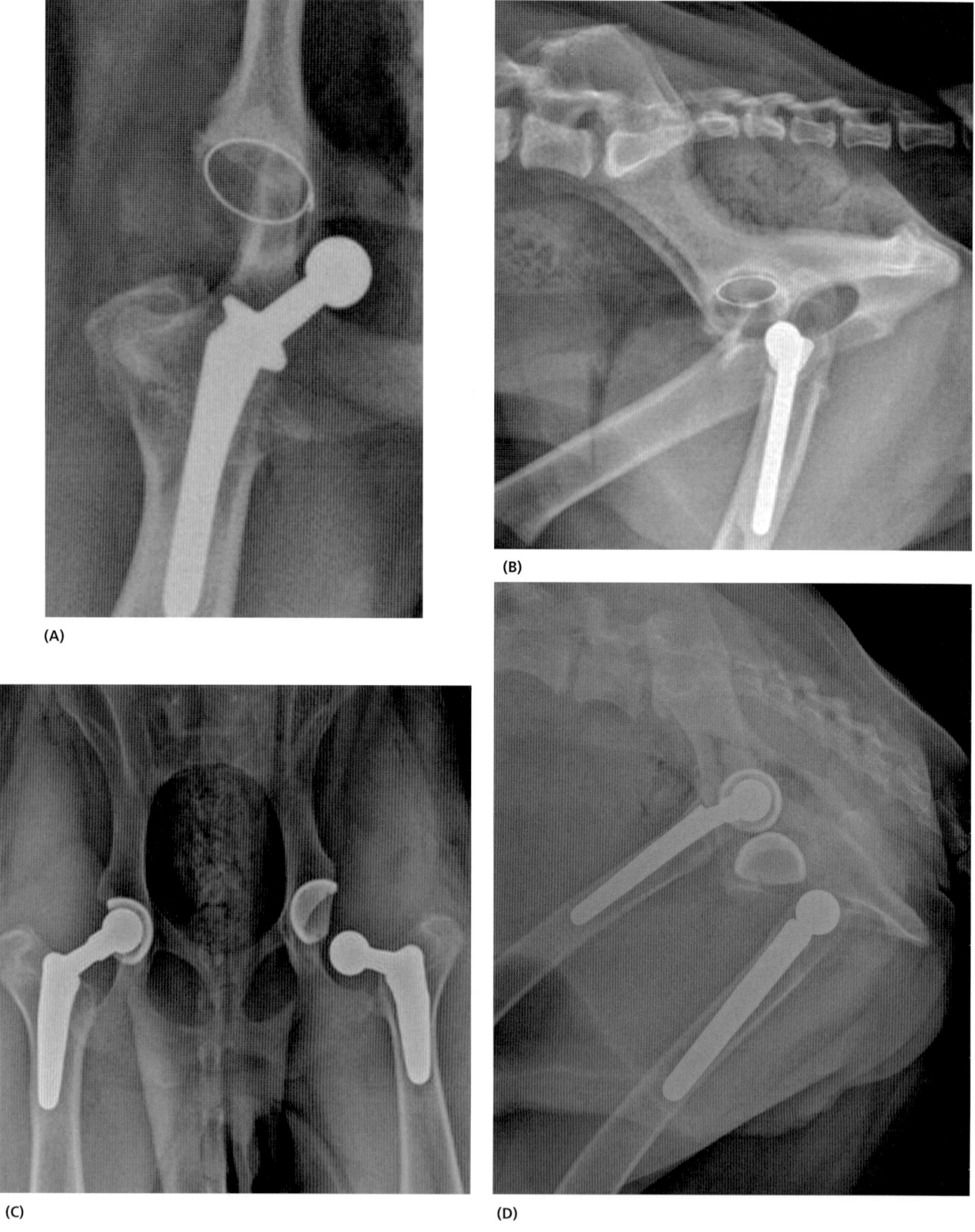

(A)

(B)

(C)

(D)

Figure 113.37 Radiographic appearance of a caudal-ventral luxation of a cemented (**A** and **B**) and cementless (**C** and **D**) prosthesis.

- Dorsal luxation invariably requires a revision of the cup position.
- Luxation of well-positioned implants caused by preoperative luxation and subsequent laxity can be revised by extending the length of the femoral neck.
- Dorsal dislocation of the cup and cement mantle (Figure 113.38) on a cemented fixation requires revision surgery to securely implant another cup. Cementless cup dislocation (Figure 113.39) can be revised with a larger sized, cementless cup or with a cemented cup. Revision using a cementless cup is preferable, but is not always feasible.
- The postoperative management of ventral luxation treated via reduction and femoral neck lengthening should include the placement of hobbles (Figure 113.40) to prevent limb abduction for 3 to 6 weeks.
- Explantation may be considered in dogs with uncontrollable luxation, particularly in cases that luxate both dorsally and ventrally.
- Pelvic osteotomy is rarely successful in the long term as a method to manage prosthesis luxation.
- Closed reduction for dorsal luxation is difficult and nearly uniformly unsuccessful in the long term. Closed reduction of ventral luxation is rarely possible. If so, maintaining limb adduction for 4 to 6 weeks in hobbles may be a successful treatment provided the implant positioning is within acceptable limits.

Outcome

Although revisions are technically challenging, the stability of the joint can usually be restored permanently, and a satisfactory outcome can be expected. Uncontrollable, multidirectional luxation may require explantation with revision into a femoral head and neck ostectomy. Limb function after explantation is similar to that of a femoral head and neck ostectomy.

Prevention

Intraoperative assessment of the cup positioning should be done before closure. The following steps lower this risk of luxation:

- Use a positioning device to maintain the dog in position relative to the surgery table with the hemipelvii superimposed. This device is designed to prevent the pelvis from shifting during the surgery.
- Giant dogs require the largest size implants that the anatomy will permit.
- Verifying the alignment of both ischial tuberosities, in a plane perpendicular to the surgery table, before insertion of the cup
- Removal of osteophytes ventral to the acetabulum to prevent dorsal rotation of the cup during insertion
- Inserting the cup in alignment with the normal cranial and caudal poles of the acetabulum
- Inserting the cup so the truncation is parallel to the orientation of the transacetabular ligament
- Using guides to facilitate positioning of the cups
- The relative positions of the femoral head and acetabular cup should be evaluated before closure. The circle formed by the face of the cup should be concentric to the ring formed where the neck enters the channel of the femoral head (Figure 113.41).
- It is crucial to check the stability of the prosthesis after rearticulation. The limb should be placed through full ROM before closure to be sure the head is stable in the cup.

The positioning of the acetabular and femoral components should always be evaluated on postoperative radiographs

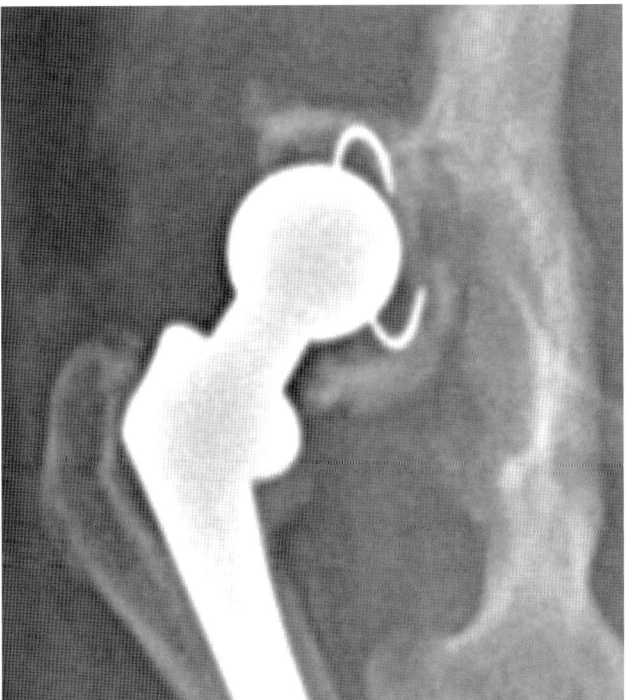

(A)

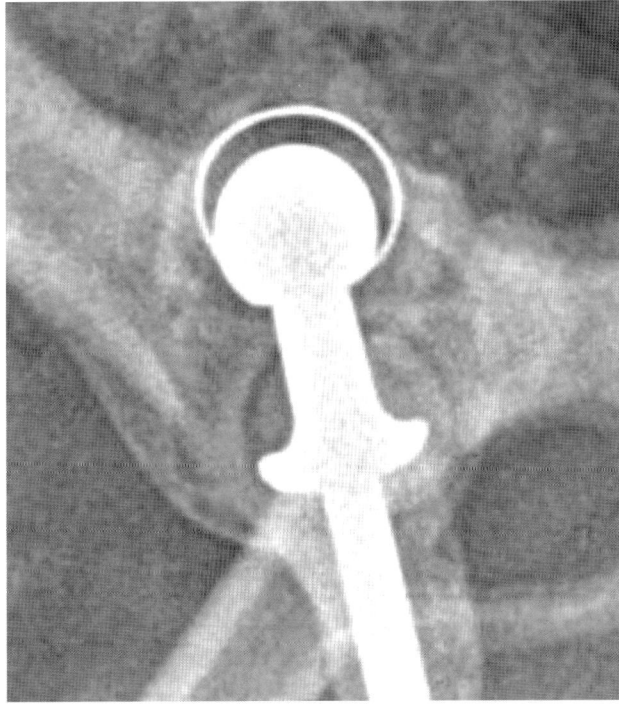

(B)

Figure 113.38 Dorsal dislocation of an inadequately fixed acetabular cup still bonded to the cement mantle 7 months after cemented hip replacement in a 1-year old female miniature poodle. The head remains articulated with the dislocated cup. Loss of bone stock along the dorsal acetabular rim and caudal pole of the acetabulum precluded satisfactory revision of the cup, thereby requiring explantation of the prosthesis.

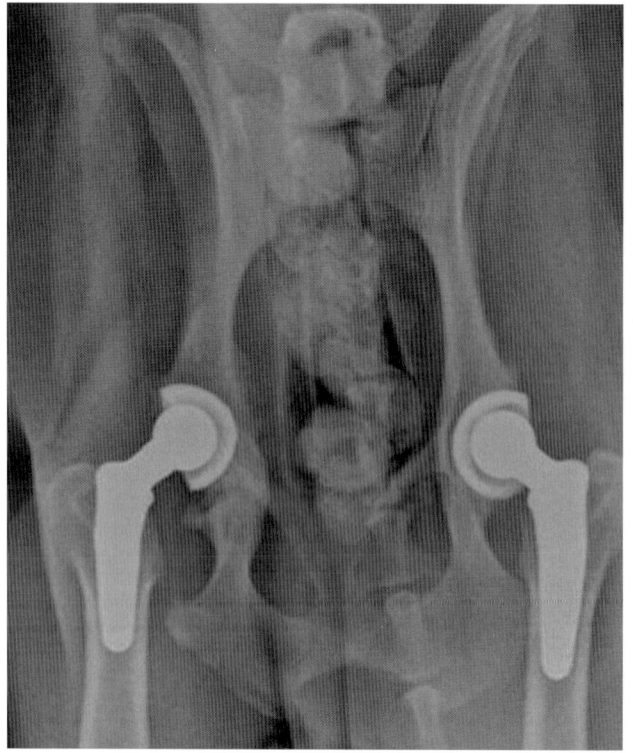

(A)

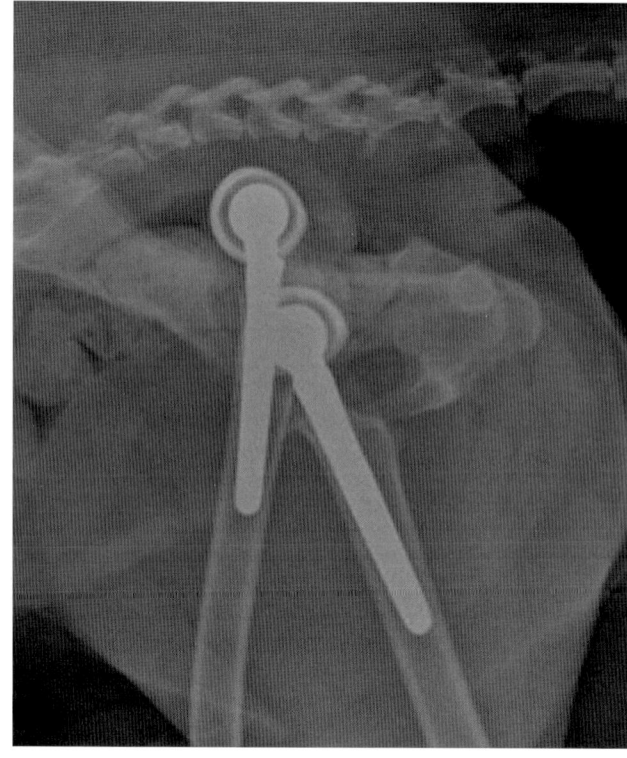

(B)

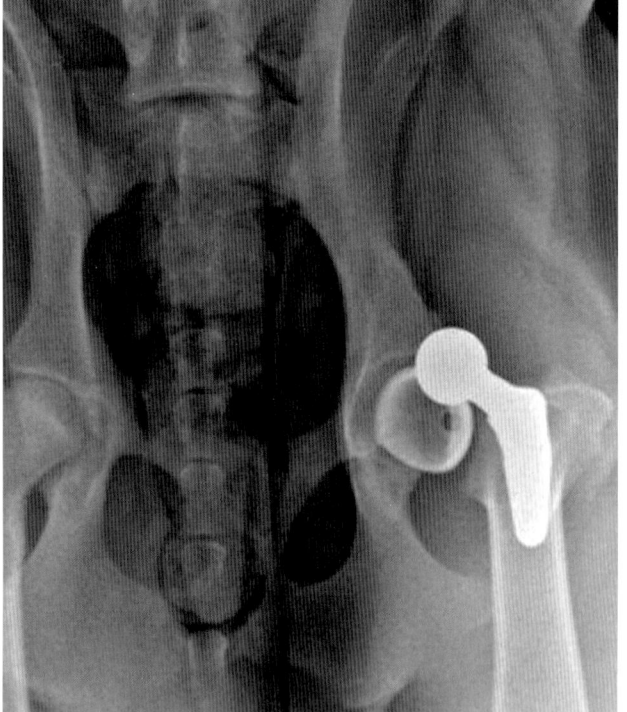

(C)

Figure 113.39 Dorsal dislocation of a cementless acetabular cup with the head still articulated in a 4-year-old, 24-kg mixed breed dog 5 weeks after surgery. Cup placement is acceptable postoperatively (**A**). Simultaneous dislocation of the cup and luxation of the head can occur if the cup has not been implanted correctly (**B** and **C**) as shown in this 10-month-old female Labrador retriever.

using criteria described in the literature (DeYoung *et al.* 1993; Marcellin-Little *et al.* 1999a; Cross and Newell 2000; Dyce *et al.* 2001; Jehn and Manley 2002; Jehn *et al.* 2003; Renwick *et al.* 2011; Aman and Wendelburg 2011, 2013; Bausman and Wendelburg 2012). The ALO of the femoral cup should ideally approximate 45 degrees and should always be within 30 to 60 degrees. The

ALO will be within the acceptable range if the patient was positioned correctly during surgery and the intraoperative assessment before closure was confirmed to be acceptable prosthesis positioning.
- Dorsal acetabular rim augmentation techniques have been proposed to improve dorsal coverage of all-UHMWPE cups in joints

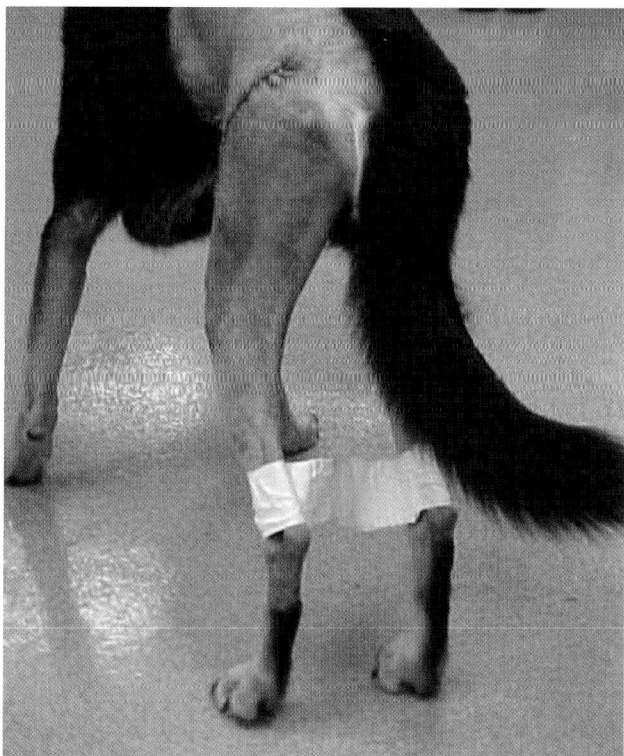

Figure 113.40 Postoperative use of hobbles to prevent ventral luxation of a total hip prosthesis. These hobbles interconnect the hind legs, allowing ambulation while preventing abduction of the limbs.

with acetabular rim wear. Mixed results have been reported in the short term (Pooya *et al.* 2003; Fitzpatrick *et al.* 2012a). Long term follow-up is needed to draw any conclusion regarding the efficacy of these procedures.

- Femoral stem subsidence (see Subsidence) must be avoided because it increases luxation risk.
- Timing the surgical intervention before excessive disuse muscle atrophy may decrease the probability of luxation.

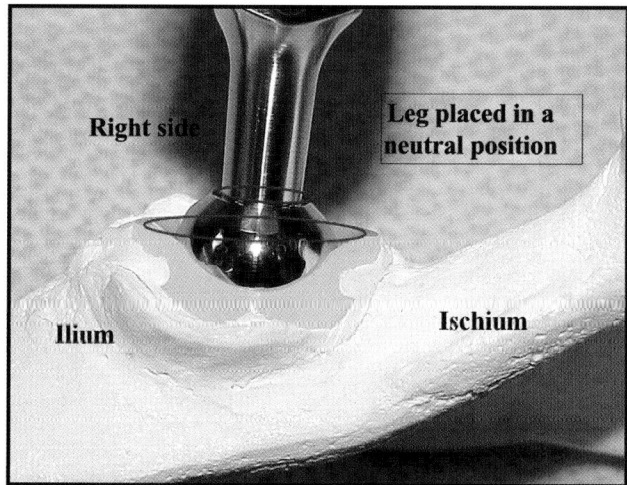

Figure 113.41 Intraoperative evaluation of the prosthesis positioning. Before closure, the limb is placed in a neutral position as if the dog is standing. Implant positioning is optimal if the circles (red rings) formed by the face of the cup, excluding the truncation, and the junction of the neck entering the head channel are concentric.

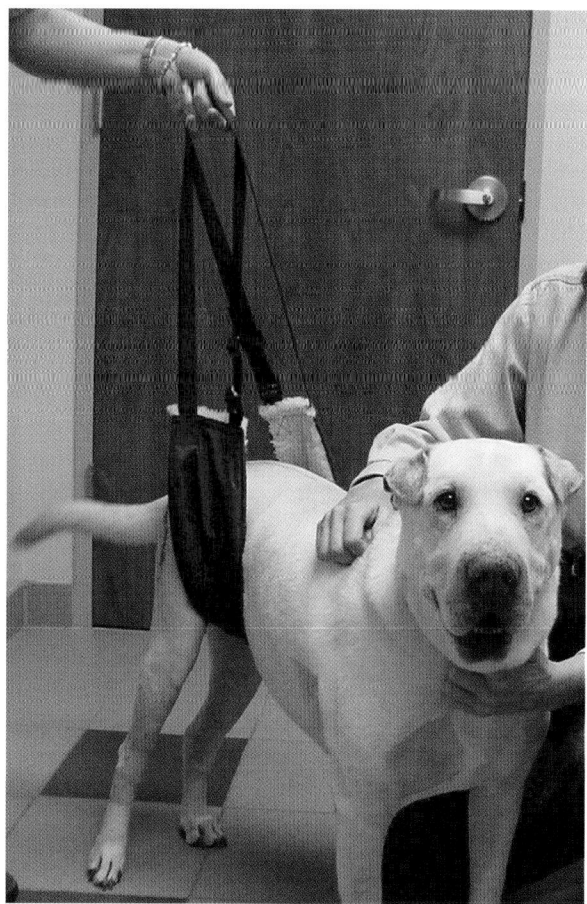

Figure 113.42 Use a sling to assist early postoperative ambulation. This type of device is advisable during the first 1 to 2 weeks after surgery if the dog must walk on slippery surfaces, such as smooth tile or hard wood floors, and when going up or down stairs.

- Precautionary measures to prevent excessive activity and falls during the early (4–5 weeks) postoperative period: A walking assist device (Figure 113.42), such as a sling, is advisable during transit across smooth surfaces; activity should be limited to good traction surfaces indoors and to a leash outdoors.

Relevant literature

Total hip replacement is a successful treatment of traumatic coxofemoral luxation, irrespective of the dysplastic status of the joint before injury (Pozzi *et al.* 2004).

Several novel treatment methods to maintain reduction of hip prosthesis luxation have been reported, including the use of a DeVita pin (Marti *et al.* 1999) and iliofemoral external fixator for ventral luxation (Ben Amotz *et al.* 2009). Pin migration and sciatic injury must be prevented if a DeVita pin is used. The risk of infection would intuitively increase with external fixator pins placed near the prosthesis, but evidence is not available to document this risk. Therefore, these devices and methods should be used only with good presurgical planning and with caution.

The acetabular inclination and version angles are generally considered to have a wide acceptable range in which there is a negative predictive value for luxation and a positive predictive value when the angles are extremely out of range. However, luxation can occur when the angles are optimum and does not always occur even though the angles are outside accepted norms.

Neurapraxia

Definition

Neurapraxia is defined as a temporary interruption of peripheral nerve conduction. This condition results from ischemia or compression damaging the myelin sheath. Loss of motor function is the most obvious clinical sign even though sensory dysfunction is also present. Neurapraxia is the mildest form of peripheral nerve injury because the axon remains intact, as opposed to axonotmesis or neurotmesis, in which there is loss of axon continuity. Wallerian degeneration does not occur with neurapraxia, and full recovery is expected, typically within 6 to 8 weeks of the injury. Sciatic neurapraxia is a potential complication of THR.

Risk factors

The following factors have been proposed to increase the probability of sciatic neurapraxia after hip replacement surgery.

- Age at the time of surgery: Tissues in older dogs may be less resilient and less able to respond to the surgical trauma.
- Duration of the surgical procedure: This parameter reflects the presence of factors increasing the difficulty of the surgical procedure itself such as the presence of severe, advanced OA or a joint previously operated on (Figure 113.43).
- Improper and nonchalant retraction of the gluteal muscles with stretching the sciatic nerve located dorsal and medial to the acetabulum can cause nerve injury.
- Retraction of the proximal femur in a caudomedial rather than caudolateral direction during preparation of the acetabular bone bed (Andrews *et al.* 2008): Caudomedial retraction can stretch and compress the nerve between the femur, thickened joint capsule, and ischium. Dogs with a short ischiatic shaft, a prominent tuber ischium, and a greatly thickened joint capsule from chronic OA may be more vulnerable to this kind of impingement (Figure 113.44). Sciatic nerve compression between the tuber ischium and the gluteal tendons has been documented via MRI in humans (Hurd *et al.* 2006).
- Surgeon inexperience has been speculated to correlate with neurapraxia, but such a relationship could not be established in a series of 1000 consecutive cases performed by one surgeon (Andrews *et al.* 2008).
- Other factors that may marginally increase the risk of neurapraxia include body weight and revision surgery.
- Preoperative coxofemoral luxation has been suggested as a predisposing factor, but this role was not confirmed in a recent retrospective study of THRs (Andrews *et al.* 2008).
- The exothermic reaction of bone cement could cause neurologic injury if a large amount of cement is resting directly on the nerve. Extruding large amounts of PMMA through a dorsal medial acetabular cortical perforation or over the dorsal medial aspect of the acetabulum directly onto the nerve could theoretically result in a neurapraxia from the exothermic reaction. This is also true if PMMA came to rest directly on the nerve caudal to the acetabulum. Technical errors this obvious must be avoided.

Diagnosis

- Proprioception deficits such as knuckling (Figure 113.45), dragging the foot with decreased ability, or inability to extend the digits is present immediately when the animal first stands or ambulates after surgery
- Flexor withdrawal reflexes of the hock are diminished.
- In severe cases, there will be decreased sensory perception over the dermatome supplied by the sciatic nerve.

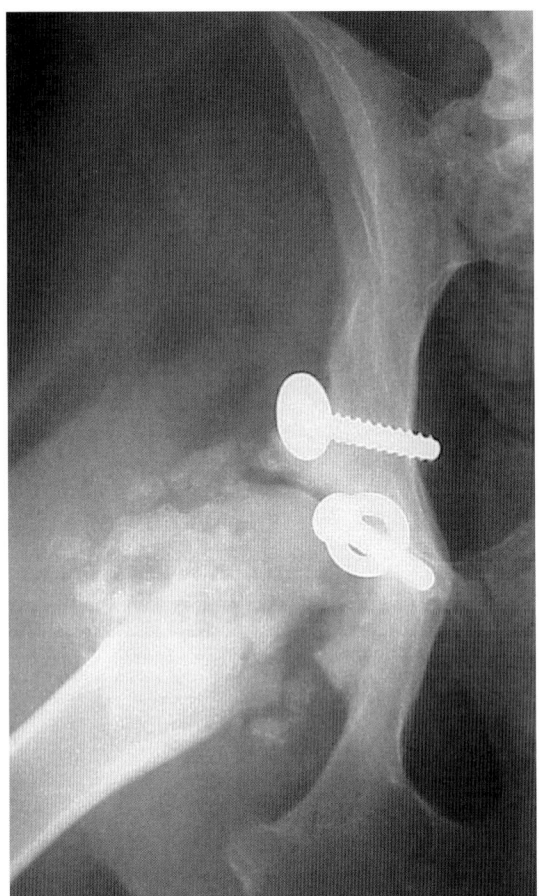

Figure 113.43 Example of a case in which the risk of neurapraxia is increased because of the technical challenges and prolonged duration of surgery. Advanced osteoarthritis and extensive periarticular fibrosis are present after an open reduction and internal fixation of an acetabular fracture 8 years earlier. The approach to the hip, screw removal, exposure of the acetabulum, an excessively thick caudal joint capsule, caudal retraction of the proximal femur, and limb in 90 degrees of external rotation all contribute to an increased risk of intraoperative sciatic nerve compression and postoperative neurapraxia.

- Nerve conduction and electromyography studies can provide additional information about the extent of nerve dysfunction.

Incidence goal

The incidence goal is less than 1.9% (Olmstead *et al.* 1983; Massat *et al.* 1994; Andrews *et al.* 2008).

Treatment

- The sciatic nerve should be explored if there is any perceived risk of nerve entrapment. Persistent stretching or impingement must be relieved.
- Rehabilitation therapy should be used to provide orthotic support and prevent flexion contracture or self-mutilation.
- Spontaneous nerve recovery must occur for full functional recovery.

Outcome

Sciatic neurapraxia is a transient problem, but the time to full recovery (placing the foot appropriately during every step with

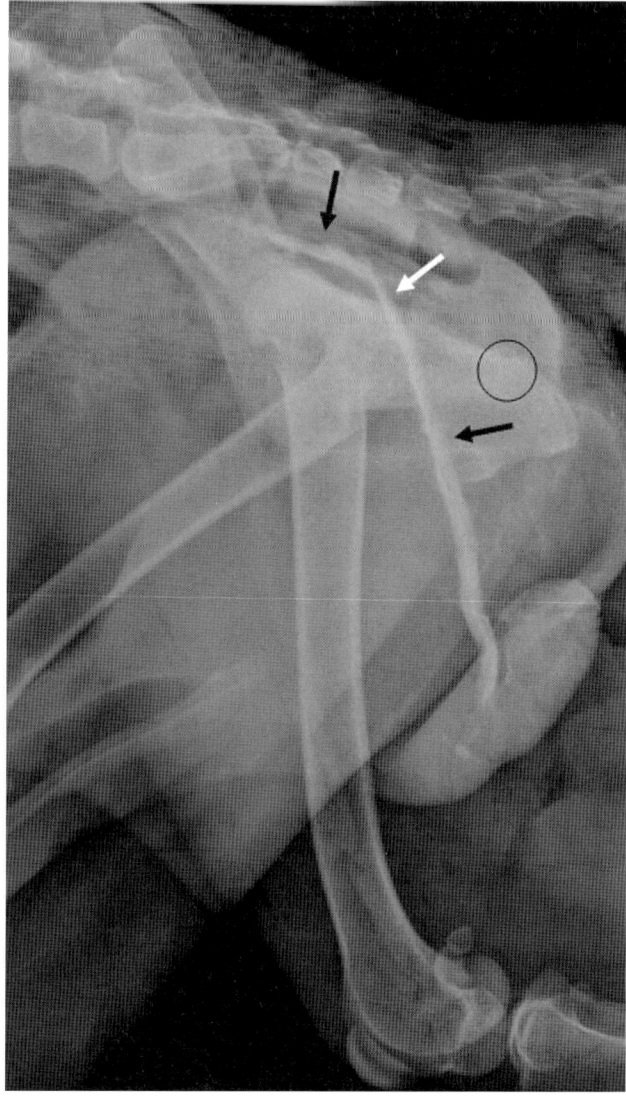

(A)

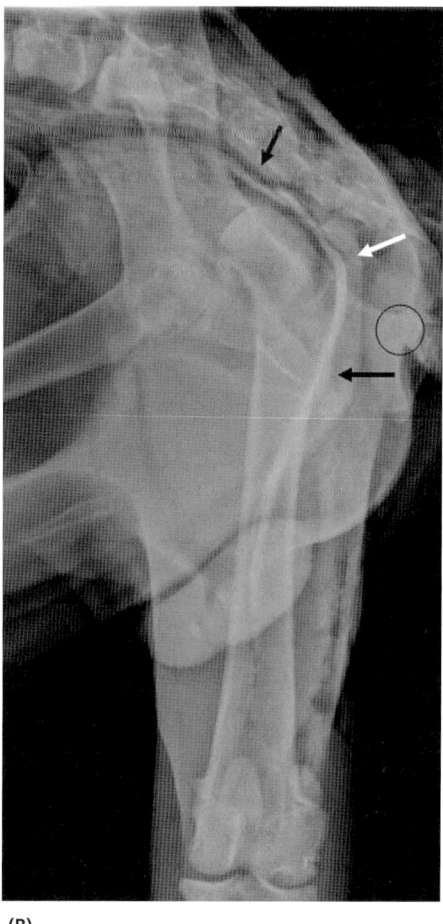

(B)

Figure 113.44 Sciatic neurogram (arrows) illustrating the normal course of the sciatic nerve (**A**). The course of the nerve is caudally displaced (compare white arrow location with the normal course white arrow) during 90-degree external rotation of the limb during surgery (**B**). Caudal retraction, especially in a medial rather than lateral direction, decreases the space between the greater trochanter and the tuber ischium (circled). Caudal medial retraction of the proximal femur should be avoided during acetabulum access because it increases the risk of nerve compression and is particularly relevant in dogs with short ischial shafts, severe osteoarthritis, and thickened joint capsules.

normal ability to flex the tibial-tarsal joint) is variable and proportional to the degree of severity. The mean recovery time is about 35 days with a range of about 10 to 120 days. Recovery can take as long as 5 months (Andrews et al, 2008).

Prevention
- Early intervention of OA treated with hip replacement will counter risk factors related to age and the duration of the procedure.
- Careful use of retractors to prevent nerve compression or stretching is indicated when accessing the acetabulum and during bed preparation.
- Proper cementing technique and removal of excess cement before curing: Extrusion of PMMA directly medial to the acetabular fossa or ventral to the transacetabular ligament is unlikely to be

problematic. The adverse effect of cement extrusion medial to the acetabulum has not been reported in dogs.
- Although not a complication of hip replacement surgery, surgeons should consider the possibility of preexisting subclinical or early neurologic deficits. Degenerative myelopathy is known to occur in some breeds that also develop chronic, bilateral, coxofemoral OA secondary to hip dysplasia. Peripheral neuropathy can also develop secondary to advanced coxofemoral OA (Sorjonen et al. 1990).

Relevant literature
Peripheral nerve injury has also been reported as a complication of pelvic fractures or fracture-dislocation. Despite these traumatic events, the probability to return to good or excellent limb function is overall high, reaching 81% in one report (Jacobson and Schrader

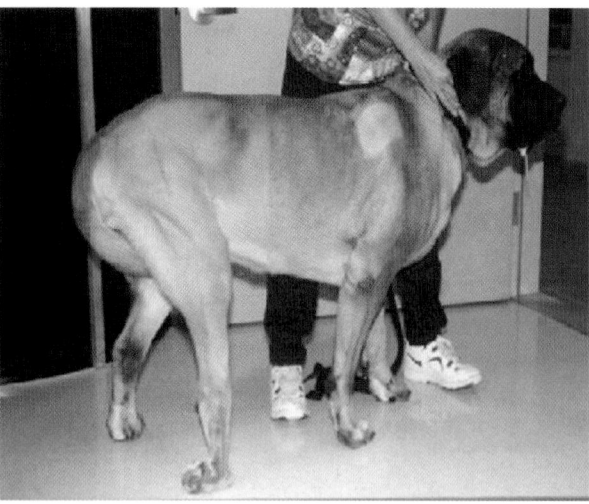

Figure 113.45 Postoperative sciatic neurapraxia. Note the "knuckling" of the foot on the affected limb, resulting from a deficit in conscious proprioception. Sensory perception is usually present with neurapraxia. Recovery time from this transient complication varies from days to months.

1987). However, a good prognosis should not be offered unless the exact nature of the neuropathy is known and progressive improvement on serial examination is observed (Forterre *et al.* 2007).

Neurapraxia must be differentiated from other, more severe peripheral nerve injuries, such as neurotmesis, in which the neural tube is severed. Axonotmesis consists of axonal disruption while sparing the myelin sheath. Neurotmesis and axonotmesis are associated with permanent damage or prolonged recovery of neural function, respectively (Schmalzried *et al.* 1991; DeHart and Riley 1999).

The reported prevalence of neurapraxia in humans ranges from 1.09% to 1.9% after primary hip replacement and up to 7.6% after revision surgery. The cause of sciatic neurapraxia in humans is unknown in about 50% of the cases (Johanson *et al.* 1983; Schmalzried *et al.* 1991; Schmalzried *et al.* 1997; DeHart and Riley 1999). Antiprotrusio devices and acetabular revision can induce late lesions of the sciatic nerve (Vastamaki *et al.* 2008). Excessive femoral neck lengthening has not been reported to cause nerve stretching and subsequent nerve dysfunction in dogs but has been reported in humans (Sakai *et al.* 2002; May *et al.* 2008). Postoperative hematoma formation can also cause nerve palsy (Butt *et al.* 2005).

The incidence of sciatic neurapraxia after canine primary hip replacement has been reported as 2.3% (221 dogs) (Olmstead *et al.* 1983), 3.6% (96 dogs) (Massat *et al.* 1994), and 1.9% (1000 dogs) (Andrews *et al.* 2008). THR has been reported as a successful treatment of sciatic neurapraxia after femoral head ostectomy in a cat (Liska *et al.* 2010).

Protrusio acetabuli

Definition
Protrusio is defined as medial migration or abrupt displacement of the acetabular component through a central, medial acetabular, cortical wall defect into the pelvic canal (Figure 113.46).

Risk factors
- Excessive penetration of the medial acetabular cortical wall during reaming can subsequently lead to acute medial cup displacement

during weight bearing. Protrusio occurs as a displacement of the cup through the thin, weak bone.
- If the cup is unstable, its medial migration can slowly lead to protrusio. A correlation between excessive, unoccluded, cortical perforation and eventual protrusio is suspected but is not documented.
- Juvenile dogs with severe dysplasia, subluxation, and disuse atrophy are vulnerable because the reamer can easily penetrate the hypoplastic, medial acetabular cortical wall.
- Penetration can occur in adult dogs with full-thickness bone sclerosis between the articular surface subchondral bone and the medial wall. Perforation occurs because of the absence of a defined layer of cancellous bone. The absence of this landmark complicates the decision of when to stop reaming before perforation occurs.
- Penetration during reaming can occur in adult dogs with end-stage OA and a thick layer of cancellous bone between the subchondral bone and the medial wall. As in juvenile dogs, an inattentive surgeon can easily penetrate the atrophied medial cortical wall during reaming.
- Protrusio can also occur as chronic aseptic loosening progresses. Osteolysis of the medial cortical wall and concurrent new bone forming in the pelvic canal can expand the acetabular bone bed. Osteolysis extending in a circular manner from the central portion of the acetabular cortex can extend into the acetabular ventral bone to the transacetabular ligament. These changes allow the acetabular cup to migrate medially (see Figure 113.4).

Diagnosis
- Penetration of the medial cortical wall while reaming can be visualized during surgery.
- Postoperative protrusion is associated with an abnormal gait and external rotation of the limb (**Video 113.2**).
- Displacement of the cup through the medial cortical wall is confirmed on radiographs.

Incidence goal
Although the true incidence has not been reported, this complication is rare.

Treatment
- Acetabular protrusio subsequent to THR requires revision surgery to reconstruct the cavitary defect.
- The acetabular rim is generally intact. The dorsal, cranial, and caudal portions of the acetabular rim must be strong enough to provide peripheral support for a large, porous-coated, biologically fixed component.
- An autogenous cancellous bone graft or a corticocancellous allograft can be used to fill the cavitary defect in the medial wall. Defects in the bone bed are filled with impacted graft.
- Preoperative imaging of the ventral acetabular rim via computed tomography (CT) helps evaluate the extent of bone loss. Chronic aseptic loosening can erode the cortical bone in this area, leaving only weak callus bone. A cementless revision cup can migrate medially if the acetabular rim bone stock is inadequate for fixation.
- A custom porous metal shell is used if the acetabular bed is larger than the largest canine off-the-shelf acetabular component. After the shell is impacted and stable, a canine acetabular component is then cemented into place. If the acetabular rim support is inadequate for initial fixation, screws are placed through the porous metal shell or cage. An alternative to the use of a metal cementless shell consists of a metal mesh, cage, or other metal

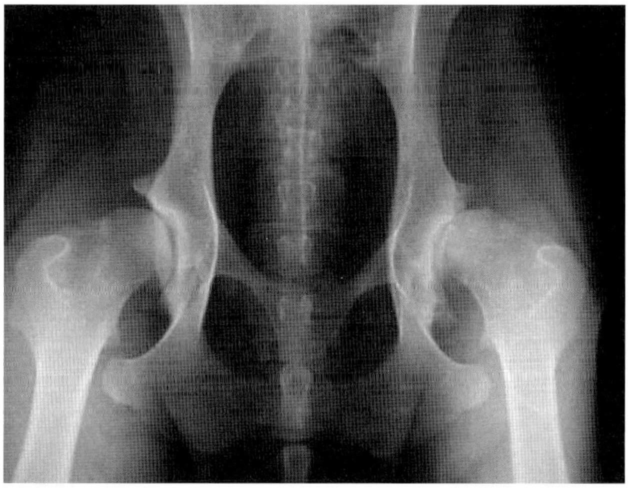

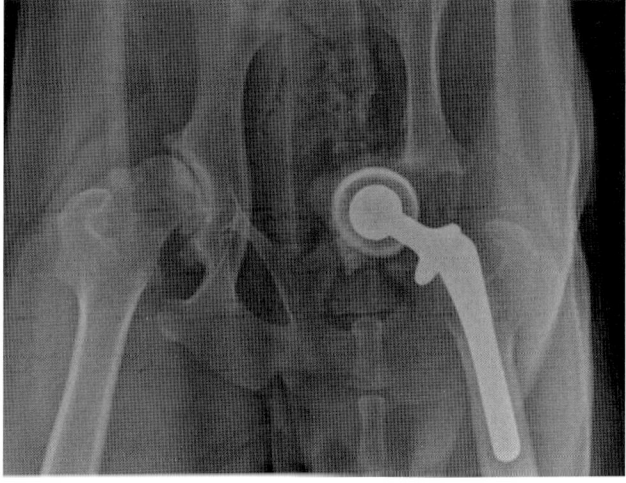

(A)

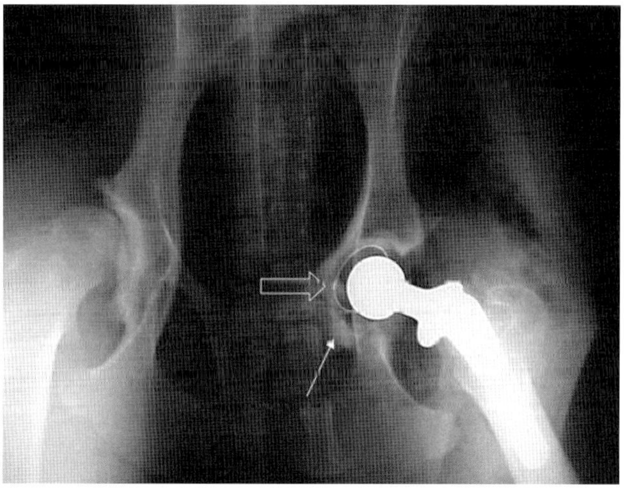

(B)

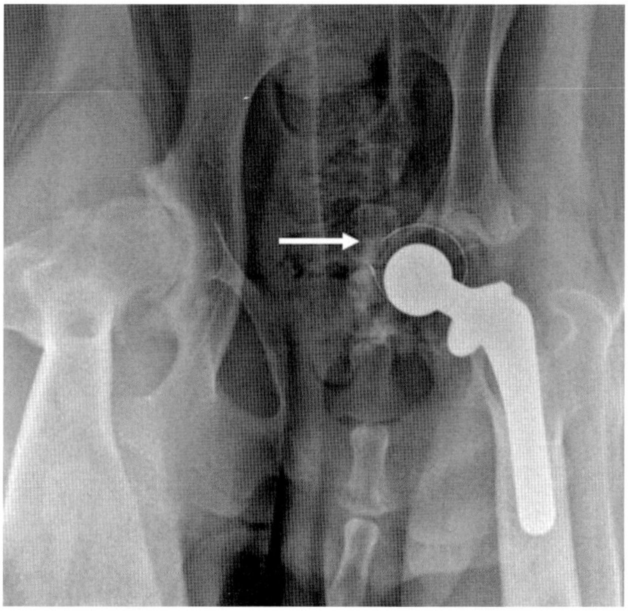

(C)

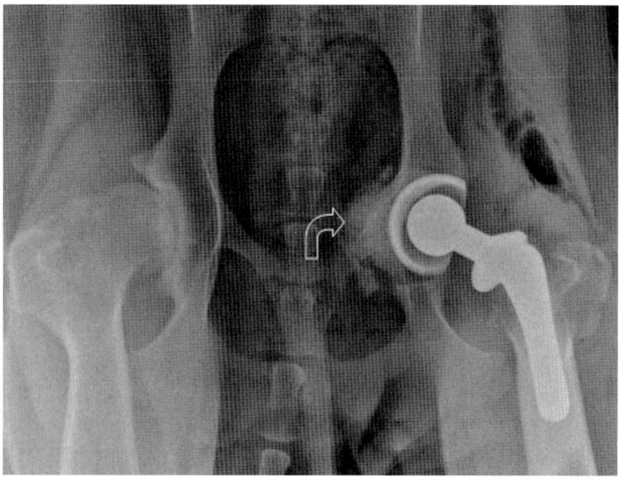

(D)

(E)

Figure 113.46 Acetabular protrusio after penetration of the medial acetabular cortex during total hip replacement (THR). Preoperative radiograph of a dog with bilateral coxofemoral osteoarthritis (**A**, evaluated as a good candidate for staged bilateral THR. The medial acetabular cortex was penetrated during surgery, and a large portion of the ventral acetabular wall was lost. On postoperative radiographs (**B**), the acetabular component is displaced too far medially (open arrow), and some bone cement extruded into the pelvic canal (small arrow). Protrusio was diagnosed on radiographs (**C**). Follow-up was 3.3 years after surgery. The cup is in ventroversion. The encircling wire (thin arrow) is broken, indicating motion of the ultra-high-molecular-weight polyethylene (UHMWPE) cup (see Video 113.2). Radiographs were obtained after revision of the cup (**D**) with a cementless component. An autogenous cancellous bone graft was placed medial to the component (curved open arrow). Protrusio recurred 6 months later (**E**). Implantation of a larger cementless cup may have prevented this complication either initially or during revision surgery. In addition, a more robust reconstruction with graft should have been performed during the initial surgery. The entire prosthesis was eventually explanted after two episodes of protrusio in the same dog. The cement was not removed from the femoral medullary canal.

device to augment the reconstruction of the medial wall. These devices are less favorable for long-term biologic fixation because they are not conducive to osteointegration.

• Explantation of the prosthesis is indicated if prosthesis revision is not possible.

Outcome

Preoperative planning is important to determine the extent of bone loss, the size of revision implants, and the optimal position of the revision prosthesis. Femoral inset should be corrected, and a minor leg length discrepancy may result. The results are favorable and similar to other types of revisions if leg length is maintained and remaining bone stock allows placement of an oversized cementless cup (Hansen and Ries 2006). Factors influencing the outcome include (1) restoring adequate support, (2) stabilization of implants, (3)biologic fixation of the new component in native and grafted bone, and (4) providing dorsal bone coverage at the cranial and caudal acetabular poles. The number of protrusio acetabular revisions properly reported with radiographic and clinical follow-ups is too low to document success rates in dogs.

Prevention

• Precautions should be taken to prevent medial cortical wall penetration in cases evaluated as predisposed based on preoperative radiographs. Reaming should be progressive, with frequent interruptions to probe the medial wall and evaluate landmarks relative to cup positioning.

• The stability of the acetabular component must be confirmed before closure.

• Annual radiographic evaluation of THR prostheses is recommended for early detection of complications such as aseptic loosening and medial migration of the acetabular component. Early detection can lead to early intervention and avoidance of an acute onset of pain and lameness caused by protrusio.

Relevant literature

Preoperative planning should take into consideration femoral offset and leg length (Hansen and Ries 2006). Femoral inset and leg length discrepancy are present with protrusio. An attempt should be made to return both to normal.

Pulmonary embolism

Definition

Pulmonary embolism (PE) consists of the migration of an embolus (particle or fragment) from a distant site via the systemic venous circulation to the pulmonary vasculature. A pulmonary thromboembolism results from the embolus acting as a nidus for formation of a thrombus that occludes a pulmonary artery. During THR surgery, globules of fat, small blood clots, fragments of bone marrow, and air can intravasate into the venous circulation of the cancellous bone and become emboli. Although rare, massive embolemia could potentially lead to fatal pulmonary vascular occlusion (Figures 113.47 and 113.48).

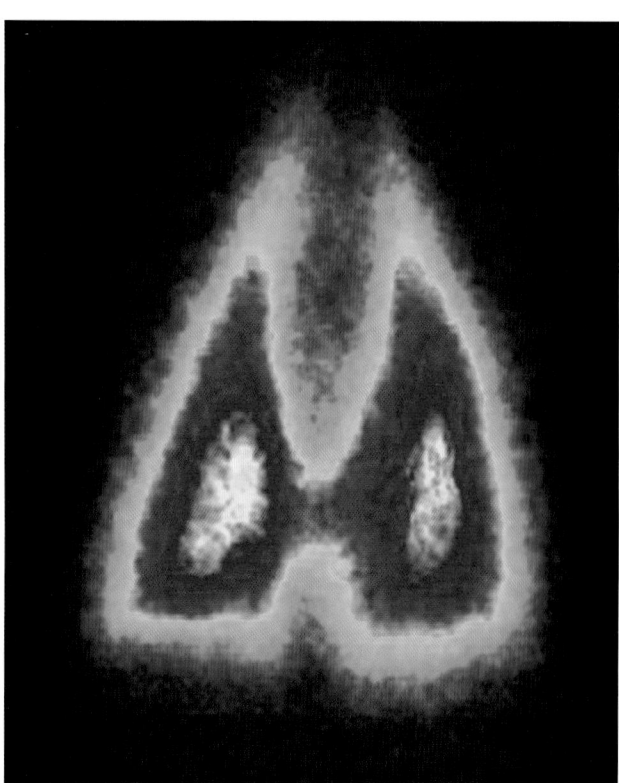
(A)

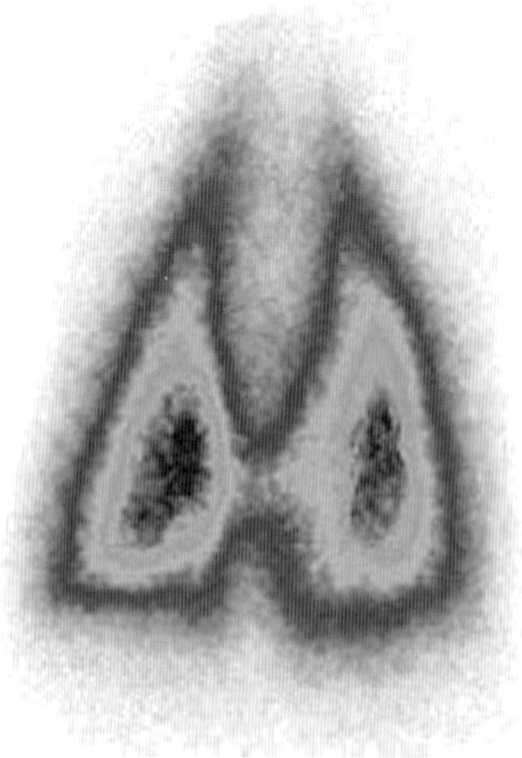
(B)

Figure 113.47 Normal ventrodorsal lung perfusion scintigraphy. Note the uptake homogeneously tapering in areas that contain higher lung volumes. Uptake gradually decreases toward the periphery of the lobes where there is less pulmonary volume, and therefore less perfusion. Color (**A**) and grey scale (**B**) images can be obtained.

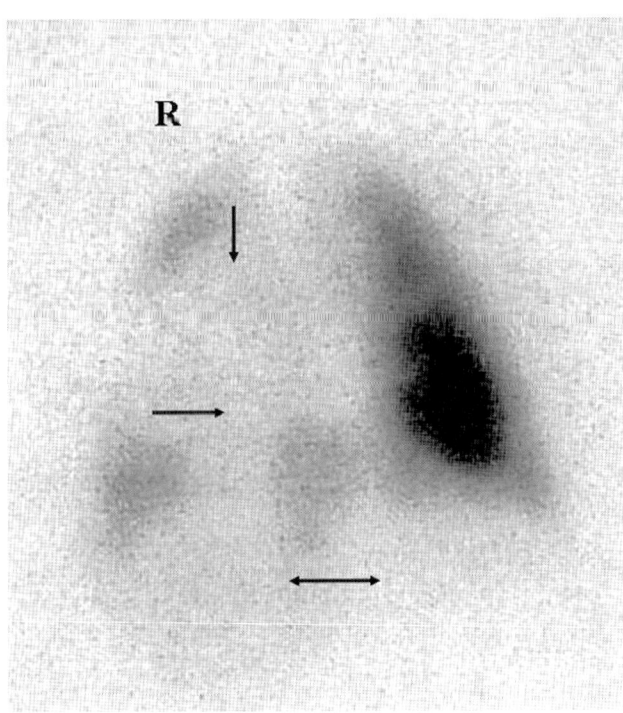

Figure 113.48 Nuclear scintigraphy of a dog with fatal pulmonary thromboembolism. Perfusion appears nearly absent in the right cranial, middle, and caudal as well as the left caudal lobes (arrows).

Risk factors

- Disruption of cancellous bone commonly occurs during orthopedic surgery procedures (Lozman *et al.* 1986; Hofmann *et al.* 1998; Shine *et al.* 2010). Embolemia can occur during sawing, drilling, or reaming of bone or during other peracute, traumatic, architectural changes to bone and its vasculature.
- The influence of cemented THR and pressurized cementing techniques remains controversial in dogs(see Literature review) Animals with systemic diseases, such as poor cardiopulmonary function, hyper-adrenolcorticism, immune mediated diseases, anemia, glomerular disease, sepsis, trauma, coagulation disorders, moribundancy, and neoplasia, may be predisposed to pulmonary thromboembolism (Laack and Goyal 2004).
- PE causes increased pulmonary ventilation dead space and a decrease in the platelet count (Otto and Matis 1994).

Diagnosis

- The majority of dogs with PE remain asymptomatic.
- Clinical signs of pulmonary thromboembolism include tachypnea, systemic hypoxia, cyanosis, respiratory distress, low oxygen saturation seen on pulse oximetry, and a decreased PO_2.
- Intraoperative ultrasonography (intercostal or transesophageal) of the right atrium and pulmonary outflow tract can be used to visualize embolemia (Figure 113.49 and **Video 113.3**; Figure 113.50 and **Video 113.4**; Figure 113.51; Figure 113.52 and **Video 113.5**). Embolemia will typically be present 5 to 8 seconds after stem insertion. Particle embolemia is about four times more common than pneumoembolism (Liska and Poteet 2003). In humans with transesophageal ultrasonography, the incidence of embolemia approaches 100% (Reindl and Matis 1998).

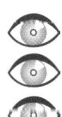

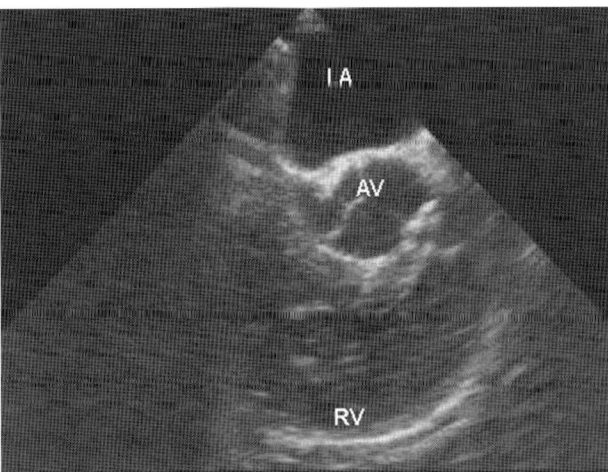

Figure 113.49 Ultrasonographic image of embolemia. A "snowstorm" of small particle embolemia is evident in the right ventricle (RV) in this still image captured from a video made during ultrasonographic imaging. For contrast, note the anechoic appearance within the left atrium (LA) and area of the aortic valve (AV) that lacks emboli (see **Video 113.3**).

- Pulmonary perfusion scintigraphy is used to detect segmental and subsegmental perfusion defects (Figure 113.53). A modified Prospective Investigation of Pulmonary Embolism Diagnosis (PIOPED) classification system can be used to evaluate lung scans. About 82% of dogs will have patchy defects with about 32% being severe (Liska and Poteet 2003).
- PE is not evident on plain radiographs (Liska and Poteet 2003).

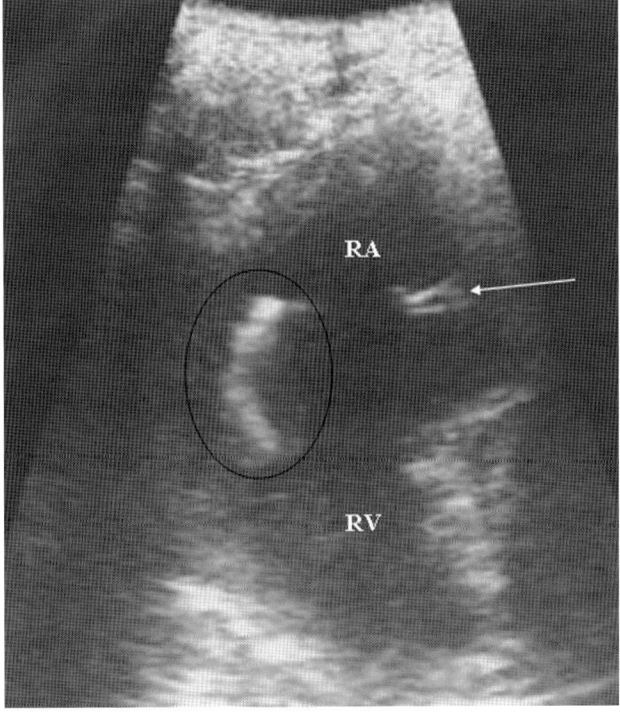

Figure 113.50 Ultrasonographic image of pulmonary embolism. A long cylindrical embolus (circled) enters the right ventricle 52 seconds after stem insertion in a 41-kg German shepherd. Another smaller embolus (small arrow) is trailing behind (see **Video 113.4**).

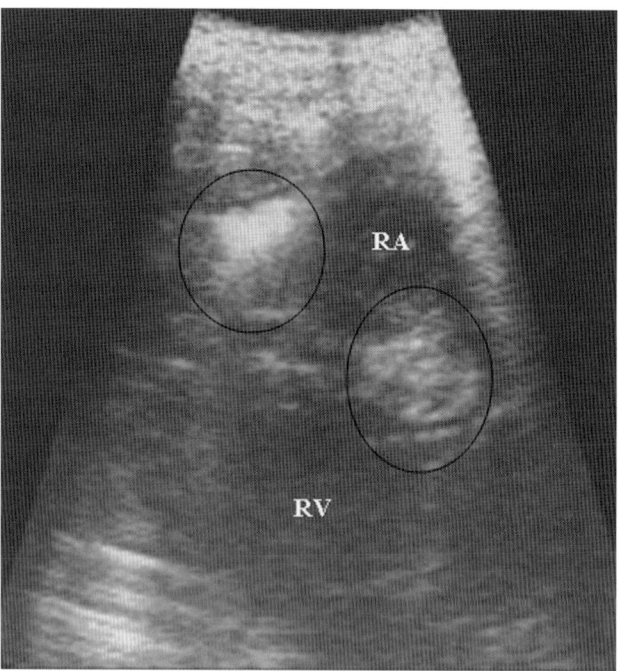

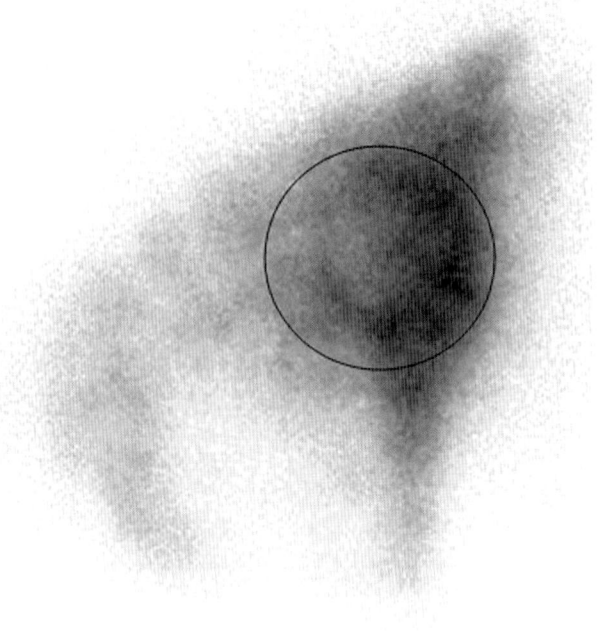

Figure 113.51 Ultrasonographic image of pulmonary thromboembolism. A 4-mm globular embolus (upper circle) is evident in the right atrium (RA) of a 90-lb German shepherd. The embolus was rapidly ejected into the pulmonary outflow tract. This embolus appeared 21 seconds after insertion of the femoral stem into the cement in the femoral medullary canal. Another large embolus (lower circle) is about to enter the right ventricle (RV).

Figure 113.53 Lateral projection of lung perfusion scintigraphy (nuclear scan) in a dog with asymptomatic pulmonary embolism. The patchy irregular mottled perfusion defect (circled) was presumably caused by a fat embolus–induced subsegmental occlusion.

- Spiral CT is the first-line gold standard for diagnosing pulmonary thromboembolism in humans. This tool allows direct visualization of the vasculature, differentiate this condition from others, is highly specific (few false negative diagnoses), and produces images quickly. Scoring the magnitude of involvement can

help determine the prognosis. The disadvantages of this technology revolve around its limited ability to see small, subsegmental arteries unless high-resolution technology is used. Other limitations include exposure to radiation and administration of intravenous contrast agent. CT data acquisition coupled with electrocardiography-gated recording can lead to a better assessment of cardiovascular function, thereby improving monitoring, accuracy of prognosis, and effectiveness of treatment (Ghaye *et al.* 2006; Kim *et al.* 2008).

Incidence goal

Segmental and subsegmental pulmonary perfusion defects have been detected on lung perfusion scans in 82% of dogs after insertion of a cemented stem, but none of these dogs displayed radiographic signs of pulmonary disease (Liska and Poteet 2003). Although the incidence of PE likely exceeds 80% (Liska and Poteet 2003), the incidence of pulmonary thromboembolism and mortality rate is so low that it is not known.

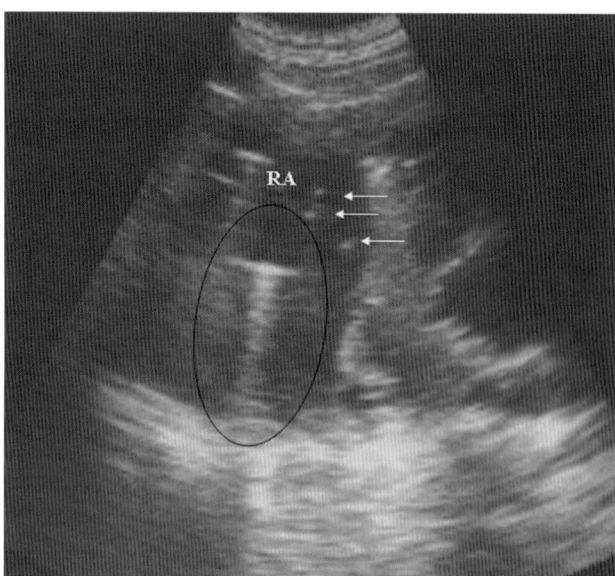

Figure 113.52 Ultrasonographic image of air bubble embolemia. The characteristic appearance of shadowing around the bubble embolus (circled) is evident along with three small particle emboli (small arrows) in the right atrium (RA) (see **Video 113.5**).

Treatment

- Most dogs recover spontaneously from PE. Despite the extremely low mortality rate, this complication must be taken seriously.
- If dogs are symptomatic, supportive care of ventilation–perfusion mismatch, including oxygen supplementation, should be provided.
- The impact of embolic events depends not only on the magnitude of the emboli but also on the release of vasoactive substances, platelet activity, extent of reflex pulmonary artery vasoconstriction, and cardiopulmonary status of the patient (Ghaye *et al.* 2006).

Outcome

The pulmonary changes that occur are almost always subclinical in healthy dogs with good cardiopulmonary function and reserve. Dogs generally spontaneously recover from embolemia, as evidenced by the low mortality rate. The extent of systemic effects is unknown, but potential risks exist if emboli travel to the heart, kidneys, nervous system, or other vital locations.

Prevention

The possibility of embolemia exists during any orthopedic surgery and cannot be fully prevented. Nonetheless, the following steps should be considered to avoid this complication:

- Use copious pulsatile lavage of the cancellous bone to remove embolic substrate.
- Fluid therapy helps maintain normovolemia, thereby minimizing the effects of embolemia on short-term cardiopulmonary depression (Reindl *et al.* 1998).

The use of anticoagulants to decrease thrombus formation in dogs is not indicated because the morbidity of bleeding is greater than the mortality risk from pulmonary thromboembolism.

Relevant literature

The incidence of postoperative PE resulting in human deaths varies from 0.19% in 42 days after surgery (Fender *et al.* 1997) to 0.067% after revision surgery with mobilization limited for 3 weeks (Wroblewski *et al.* 2000) and 0.67% within 1 year after surgery (Wroblewski *et al.* 1998). The exact mortality rate is unknown in dogs, with one death reported out of 678 procedures (Liska and Poteet 2003) and no deaths in the ensuing 1000 procedures. Fatal intraoperative fat embolism has been reported in a dog (Terrell *et al.* 2004). The filtration capacity of the lungs is affected by the composition of the emboli. For example, large (50 μ) fat globules can deform and move through the canine pulmonary vasculature of 15-μ diameter easier than other solid debris (Byrick *et al.* 1994). For this reason, fat may be less likely to act as a nidus for thrombus formation. However, for the same reason, fat can move on to other vital structures, where it can cause vascular occlusion. Fat emboli were found in the liver and kidney of a dog with fatal fat embolism (Terrell *et al.* 2004).

Changes in cardiopulmonary function and platelet count occur after implantation of a cemented femoral prosthesis. A decrease in end-tidal carbon dioxide tension, increase in arterial to end-tidal pCO_2 gradient, decreased platelet count, and physiological dead space develop between 2 and 5 minutes after insertion of the PMMA. The increased femoral medullary pressure and subsequent pulmonary microembolism of medullary contents is the most likely cause of changes in pulmonary function. However, hemoglobin oxygen saturation is not significantly altered (Otto *et al.* 1994). Despite these changes, one study in humans reported similar rates of embolemia during cemented and cementless stem insertion (Kim *et al.* 2002). Fatal marrow embolism has been reported after cementless implantation (Arroyo *et al.* 1994).

Second- and third-generation cementing techniques, relying on pressurization to improve the distribution of bone cement into cancellous bone, have been found to promote the intravasation of debris into the venous circulation (Kallos *et al.* 1974; Tronzo *et al.* 1974; Pitto *et al.* 1998). In dogs, emboli were identified in 82% of dogs undergoing cemented THR, but the embolism resolved spontaneously in all dogs in that study (Liska and Poteet 2003). By contrast, none of 11 dogs treated with a cementless hip replacement

had evidence of embolism on postoperative CT pulmonary angiography (Tidwell *et al.* 2007). Although the significance of this study is limited by sample size and the lack of intraoperative transesophageal ultrasonography, these findings would support a lower risk of PE after cementless rather than cemented hip replacement. Overall, the selection of cemented versus cementless THR in a given dog is influenced by factors other than concerns over pulmonary thromboembolism.

The risk of exposure of operating room personnel to PMMA fumes, and patients' risks from embolization of PMMA fumes is low considering decades of use in millions of procedures and patients (Becker *et al.* 2011). Nonetheless, vacuum mixing systems are strongly recommended to minimize the exposure of operating room personnel to PMMA fumes (Schlegel *et al.* 2004).

Subsidence

Definition

Subsidence is defined as a distal migration of the femoral stem implant into the femoral medullary canal before cementless fixation by osteointegration is complete (see Figure 113.31). Subsidence does not occur with well-fixed cemented stems or after osteointegration of cementless stems.

Risk factors

- Cementless collarless femoral stems
- Undersized femoral stem with inadequate femoral canal fill
- Incomplete canal bed preparation
- Low (distal) femoral neck osteotomy
- Catastrophic subsidence occurs if there is a proximal medial femoral fracture (see Fracture).
- An inadequately supported prosthesis by soft, spongy, cancellous bone in the proximal femur
- Cylindrical femoral medullary canals (low canal flare index) seen most commonly in German shepherd dogs
- Proximal femoral cortical and cancellous bone atrophy caused by age or chronicity of the lameness
- Timid or inadequate femoral stem impaction
- Excessive postoperative activity
- Proximal femoral fissure or fracture

Diagnosis

- Subsidence is radiographically evident on the anterior-posterior view of the proximal femur when follow-up images (see Figure 113.31) are compared with the immediate, postoperative radiographs.
- In the presence of subsidence, radiographs should also be critically evaluated for stem retroversion and for the presence of a proximal medial femoral fracture. Likewise, **luxation** of a cementless prosthesis should be evaluated for the presence of underlying problems, one of which is stem subsidence.

Incidence goal

The incidence goal is less than 2%.

Treatment

A few millimeters of subsidence or less than 10 degrees of retroversion may be inconsequential. However, excessive (>3–5 mm) distal migration or rotation requires revision. Moderate stem subsidence can result in impingement of the remaining femoral neck on the acetabular rim. This can cause intermittent lameness, subluxation, or luxation (see Luxation).

- A well-positioned, stable stem with subsidence that is causing luxation of the prosthesis can be revised by removing several millimeters of bone along the femoral neck osteotomy and extending the length of the prosthetic femoral neck (see Figure 113.32).
- Femoral stem revision is indicated if subsidence results in stem malpositioning, in the presence of a fracture, or if concomitant luxation is present with either of the above. Revision to stabilize the malpositioned stem should be undertaken immediately while stem extraction is still possible and before osteointegration is complete. Delays can result in progression of the osteointegration, thereby greatly complicating stem removal. Options for revision include implantation of a larger cementless stem, implantation of a collared cementless stem, or implantation of a collared cemented stem.

Outcome

Successful revision provides an excellent prognosis to maintain the prosthesis and return the limb to normal function.

Prevention

- Avoid a low femoral neck osteotomy when implanting a cementless collarless femoral stem.
- Implantation of a cementless collarless femoral stem requires careful consideration of all risk factors. If the risks are high, alternative options include:
  ○ Cementless collared femoral stem (see Figure 113.32)
  ○ Cemented femoral stem
  ○ Hybrid hip replacement using a cementless acetabular implant and a cemented stem (Gemmill *et al.* 2010)
  ○ Screw fixation of a cementless stem (Guerrero and Montavon 2009)
- Any indication of an intraoperative fissure should be fully explored and adequately stabilized. Cerclage wires applied to fissures resist subsidence (McCulloch *et al.* 2012) (see Fractures).
- Seating the stem to full depth may not be possible during initial impaction because of resistance to elastic and plastic deformation of bone, especially cancellous bone. Whereas elastic deformation correlates directly with the degree of bone mineralization, plastic deformation is more dependent on collagen maturity (Bala *et al.* 2011).
- After initial impaction, the surgeon selects the length of the femoral neck. Before reducing the selected prosthetic femoral head, the stem should be impacted again into its final position. This step is intended to nullify any remaining visco-elasto-plastic resistance to expansion and elastic deformation of the canal bed, thereby potentially decreasing the risk of subsidence.
- Subsidence has not been reported as a late (>6 weeks after surgery) complication, occurring after radiographic evidence of osteointegration and stable fixation. Sepsis should be suspected if subsidence of a previously stable implant develops several months after surgery.

Miscellaneous complications

Intraoperative instability of a cementless acetabular cup

The acetabular cup occasionally fails to achieve stability in its acetabular bone bed after impaction. Instability is usually noticed immediately after impaction of the cup. Despite its rare occurrence, this complication is significant because it can lead to cup dislocation and subsequent revision surgery.

The reaming process must be precise. The tolerance between the outside diameter of the slightly elliptical cup equator and the smaller cranial to caudal acetabular poles is 0.8 mm. Excessive "wobble" during reaming enlarges the bone bed beyond the acceptable dimensions required to achieve press-fit implantation.

Dorsal acetabular rim wear, secondary to chronic OA, can also leave inadequate bone coverage over the dorsal medial aspect of the cup. Excessive dorsal medial reaming will remove a portion of the dorsal bone coverage. Both can preclude a secure press-fit implantation and lead to cup dislocation. Cementless cups rely on craniocaudal press-fit fixation and are therefore more tolerant to lack of dorsal acetabular coverage than cemented implants. However, our clinical impression prompts us to suggest that dorsal exposure of a cementless cup approximating 3 mm is generally acceptable; exposure ranging between 3 and 5 mm dorsally increases the risk of cup dislocation; and exposure exceeding 5 mm is a high risk that can lead to cup dislocation. Excessive dorsal reaming can also result in excessively thin dorsal acetabular bone, which can fracture during cup impaction.

Caution is warranted when reaming a sclerotic acetabulum to prevent removal of the caudal acetabular pole. An initial, small directional reaming bed in the correct position, aiming at the acetabular fossa, helps to prevent caudal, ventral, or dorsal deflection of the reamer. Erroneous reaming of the caudal pole of the acetabulum can also leave a thin shelf of bone that can fracture during the final reaming process or during cup impaction. This complication is rare and is more likely to happen in small, young dogs.

Instability of a cup may also result from interposition of synovium or joint capsule between the cup and its bone bed. With interposition, the cup may appear to be stable intraoperatively, but soft tissue necrosis can later lead to instability and cup dislocation. If soft tissue is interposed, revision with excision of the interposing tissue should be performed immediately before closure.

The cementless cup must be impacted at the same 45-degree angle of attack along the reaming vector. When the cup is introduced, a crescent-shaped space should be present between the cup and the acetabular rim. If this space is not present at the initial impaction, seating of the medial aspect of the cup is impeded by the dorsal acetabular rim and will prevent full seating or will deflect the cup into ventroversion. Correct impaction at a 45-degree angle allows complete seating of the cup against the medial acetabular cortical wall and under the dorsal acetabular rim.

Incomplete cup seating

If the cup is not impacted at a 45-degree angle, incomplete seating (Figure 113.54) can result in inadequate press-fit support at the acetabular poles. This technical error can lead to a dislocation of the acetabular cup (Figure 113.55) from the bed preparation. Displacement of a cup and its cement mantle can occur with cemented fixation if the cup is not compressed deeply into the cement mantle or if the bone–cement fixation is inadequate. Failure of cementless or cemented acetabular implant fixation is rare and occurs primarily if initial fixation is inadequate. Cup-mantle displacement requires revision surgery (see Figure 113.38).

Cemented cup displacement

Acetabular cup displacement after debonding of the polyethylene–cement interface is a clinical entity that is distinct from aseptic

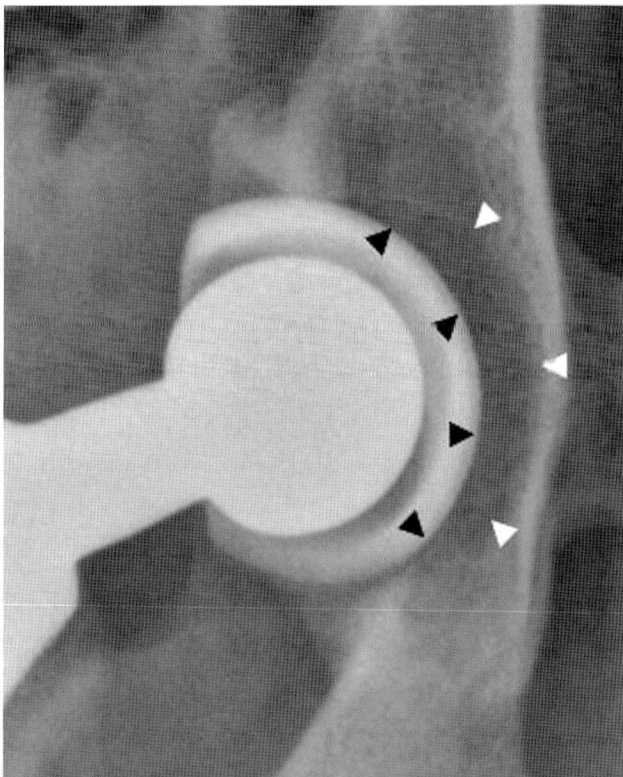

Figure 113.54 Incomplete seating of a cementless cup. Note the crescent-shaped radiolucent space between the medial aspect of the cup (black arrowheads) and the depth of the reaming bed preparation (white arrowheads) near the medial cortical wall. This technical error predisposes the cup to dislocation from its prepared bed.

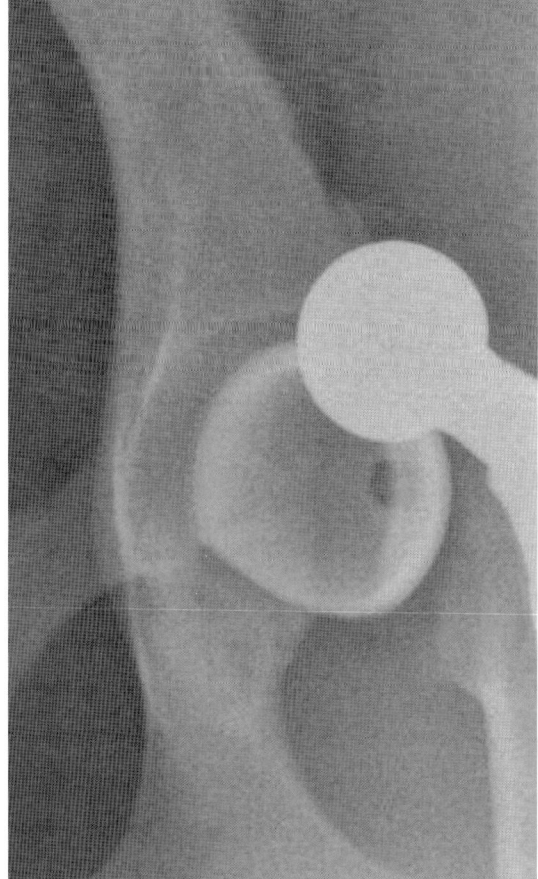

Figure 113.55 Dislocation of a cementless cup from its bed. Initial fixation was inadequate, which lead to cup dislocation and simultaneous head luxation.

loosening. This complication can be the result of a technical error and results in a lateral migration of the cup while still articulated with the femoral head. Acetabular cup displacement is significantly more likely to occur if the acetabular cup displacement ratio (ACDR) is less than 1.00. Measurements in the transverse plane are taken from the medial cortex of the acetabulum to the most medial portion of the acetabular rim (x) and from the medial cortex of the acetabulum to the center of the prosthetic head (y). The ACDR is x/y. A lower ratio results in decreased contact surface area between the cup and cement, and it indicates higher shear forces at the interface that can subsequently debond.

The complication is easily recognized on radiographs and requires revision of the cup. A preemptive revision can be performed if the ACDR is recognized to be low on postoperative radiographs. Revision surgery is successful provided other complications, such as infection, do not occur. Strategies to prevent cup displacement include reaming all the way to the acetabular medial cortical wall; medialization of the cup in an appropriately thin cement mantle against the medial cortical wall; and downsizing the cup, if necessary, in the presence of dorsal acetabular rim wear to achieve dorsal bone coverage of the implant (Hunter et al. 2003) (Figure 113.56).

Resorption of the proximal medial femoral cortex

Total hip replacement alters load transfer and stress to bone. A stable femoral stem shields the proximal medial femoral cortex

from its normal stresses, which can lead to disuse osteopenia. This phenomenon is evident primarily in dogs that are younger than 12 months old at the time of surgery (Figure 113.57). Whether resorption is more likely when the implant is in direct apposition to the endosteal surface or when the implant is encased in a trabecular bone envelop remains unclear. The diagnosis of bone resorption is based on radiographic evidence of thinning or disappearance of cortical bone around the femoral stem with the remainder of the cortical bone circumference intact. The process does not progress longer than about 6 months after surgery. No treatment is necessary, and long-term, adverse consequences have not been described or reported. Concern about cortical resorption does not warrant delaying surgery until dogs are more than 12 months old.

Femoral cortical hypertrophy

Cortical hypertrophy occurs at the tip of the femoral stem in response to stress concentration at the junction between bone and metal, where the modulus of elasticity changes dramatically. This finding is not a true complication but rather a physiological response to increased loading on bone, as described by Wolf's law (Figure 113.58). Cortical hypertrophy should not be confused with periosteal new bone formation (callus bone) that is evident on follow-up images of healed fissures or periostitis from sepsis.

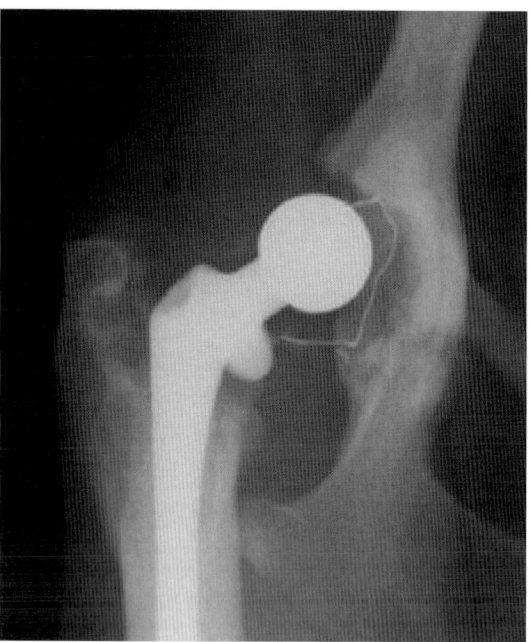

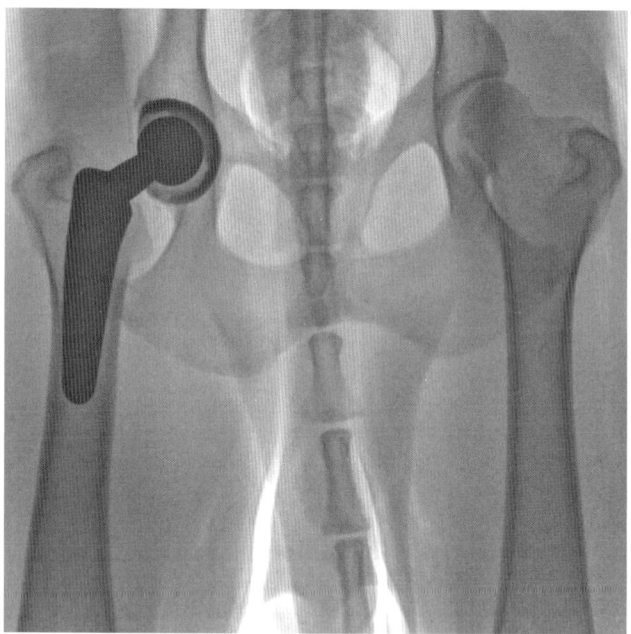

Figure 113.56 Displacement of a cemented acetabular cup 1 month after implantation in a 22-month-old female Rottweiler. The thickness of the cement mantle around the acetabulum is indicative of inadequate medialization of the cup combined with limited dorsal acetabular rim coverage resulted in an acetabular cup displacement ratio less than 1.00. This predisposed to mechanical failure (debonding) of the polyethylene–cement interface. The head remains articulated with the cup, but the positional wire is deformed and broken.

Figure 113.58 Femoral cortical hypertrophy 15 months after hip replacement in a 27-kg active 9-year-old male Belgian shepherd with osteoarthritis. Compared with the contralateral limb, the femoral cortex is hypertrophied near and distal tip of the femoral stem in response to the new load distribution.

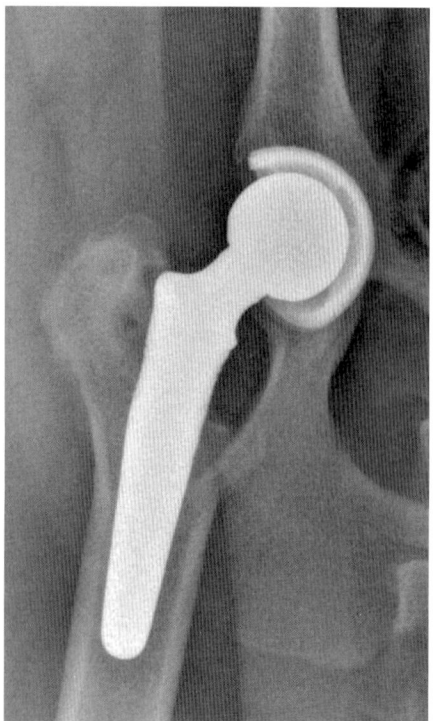

Figure 113.57 Resorption of the proximal medial femoral cortex 2 years after cementless hip replacement in a 9-month-old, 23-kg mixed breed dog with a capital physeal fracture. The resorption did not progress on serial radiographic evaluations and had no clinical relevance on the dog. Distal femoral medullary infarction (not shown) was also present.

Implant failure

Implant failure, or breakage of a prosthesis component, is extremely rare. Prosthesis engineering, implant design, metallurgical composition, in vitro testing, quality control, and improved surgical techniques have virtually eliminated the risk of implant failure after accurate implantation and adequate fixation. For example, concerns over potentially inadequate implant strength have been addressed by changing the manufacturing process from cast cobalt chrome (ASTM F-75) to wrought cobalt chrome (ASTM F-799. The resistance of implants to fatigue more than doubled as a result (BioMedtrix 2011). Although failure could still occur under prolonged and excessive loading, the onset would be delayed. Another upgrade is the use of titanium femoral stems that have a modulus of elasticity that is closer to that of bone compared with cobalt chrome.

Nonetheless, two cases of femoral stem breakage have been reported. In both cases, failure occurred at least 4 years after surgery in the presence of proximal aseptic loosening (Yates *et al.* 2010). The authors are also aware of a case of implant failure related to aseptic loosening and further complicated by formation of a **cement granuloma** (see Figure 113.7). The cases of femoral stem failure occurred more than 4 years after surgery, in medium-sized, overweight, active dogs. These dogs received undersized implants that became aseptically loose at the bone–cement interface. In some cases, the surgery was performed when the dogs were immature and sustained significant weight gain over the years leading up to stem failure. Aseptic loosening of the femoral stem increases cyclic loading from cantilever bending forces during ambulation, eventually leading to fatigue failure, most commonly located over the middle third of the stem.

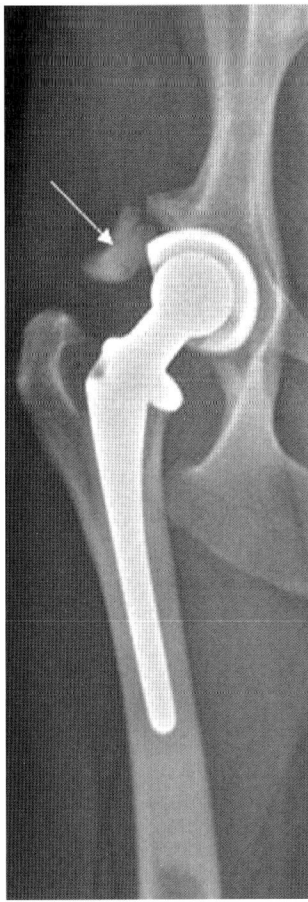

(A)

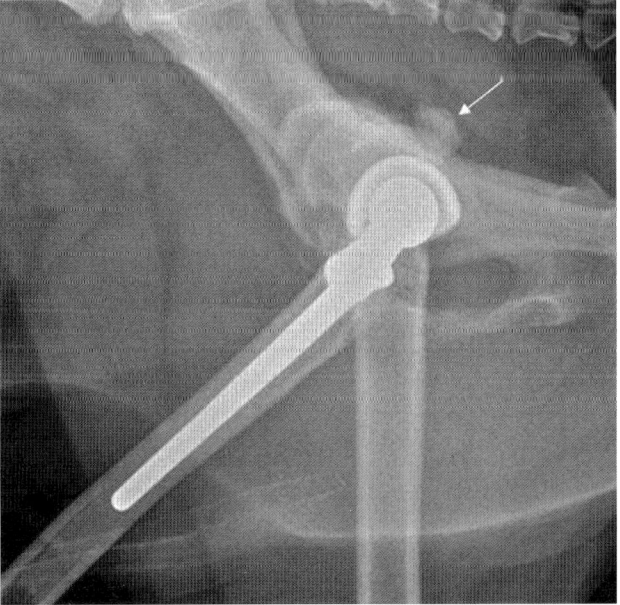

(B)

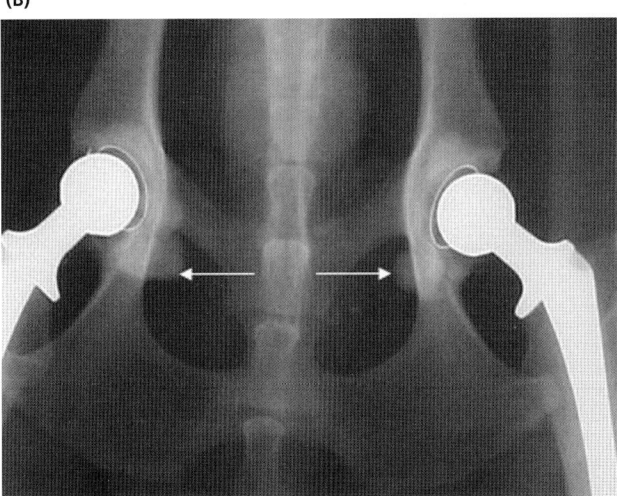

(D)

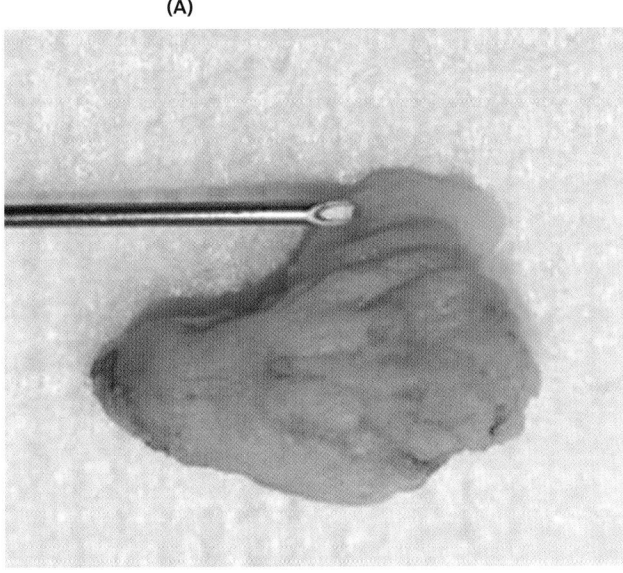

(C)

Figure 113.59 Presence of a cement fugitive (arrows) on the immediate ventrodorsal (**A**) and mediolateral (**B**) radiographs of a hybrid cementless acetabular cup and cemented femoral stem placed in a 3-year-old male border collie. The cement globule (**C**) was removed. Bilateral cement fugitives (arrows; **D**) are present ventral-medial to the ventral border of the acetabulum 2 years after staged bilateral hip replacements in a 7-year-old male Labrador retriever. The globules were not removed and remained quiescent for the dog's life span.

Failure of the UHMWPE acetabular component is almost always secondary to technical errors or a chronic complication such as malpositioning, either operative or subsequent to loosening or displacement. The wire embedded in the UHMWPE cup bends or breaks when the cup deforms. Therefore, radiographic evidence of wire deformation is consistent with failure of the acetabular component (see Figures 113.1 and 113.56).

Resolution of implant failure usually requires explantation of the prosthesis.

Cement fugitive

Variable amounts of bone cement periodically escape from view during cementing or go unnoticed before closure. The most common location for these cement fugitives is ventral to the transacetabular ligament, just inside the pelvic canal. Occasionally, a globule of cement will lodge between the gluteal muscles medial to the greater trochanter (Figure 113.59). These obvious oversights are evident on postoperative radiographs.

Cement fugitives are more likely if an excessive amount of liquid cement is placed in the prepared bed. During implantation, the excess cement will extrude in the path of least resistance and end up in an undesirable location. If cement is seen extruding into an undesirable location, it is easier to remove as one large piece by waiting until it is firm. Attempting to remove cement when it is still soft tends to tear the globule, leaving an undetected portion buried in the surgical site or between muscle planes. This complication is rare after the surgeon's first experience of inattention to this detail.

Removal of a cement fugitive can be difficult, especially if it is located within the pelvic canal (see Figure 113.59D). Small globules are generally of no consequence and are left in place. Large globules should be removed because they may impinge on the prosthesis or generate harmful debris. Globules embedded in the periarticular soft tissues lateral to the acetabulum should be removed immediately when seen on the postoperative radiographs while the animal is still under anesthesia.

All videos cited in this chapter can be found on the book companion website at www.wiley.com/go/griffon/complications.

References

Aman, A.M., Wendelburg, K.L. (2011) Assessment of acetabular cup positioning following total hip replacement from a lateral radiographic projection. *ACVS Scientific Presentation Ab*, Chicago, 11/3-5, E18.

Aman, A.M., Wendelburg, K.L. (2013) Assessment of acetabular cup positioning from a lateral radiographic projection after total hip replacement. *Veterinary Surgery* 42 (4), 406-417.

American Academy of Orthopedic Surgeons. (2010) Antibiotic prophylaxis for bacteremia in patients with joint replacements. *Information Statement 1033*, revised. Rosemont, IL.

Anderson, G.I., Orlando, K., Waddell, J.P. (2001) Synovitis subsequent to total-hip arthroplasty with and without hydroxyapatite coatings: a study in dogs. *Veterinary Surgery* 30, 311-318.

Andrews, C.M., Liska, W.D., Roberts, D.J. (2008) Sciatic neurapraxia as a complication in 1000 consecutive canine total hip replacements. *Veterinary Surgery* 37, 254-262.

Arroyo, J.S., Garvin, K.L., McGuire, M.H. (1994) Fatal marrow embolization following a porous-coated bipolar hip endoprosthesis. *The Journal of Arthroplasty* 9, 449-452.

Bala, Y., Depalle, B., Douillard, T., et al. (2011) Respective roles of organic and mineral components of human cortical bone matrix in micromechanical behavior: an instrumented indentation study. *Journal of the Mechanical Behavior of Biomedical Materials* 4 (7), 1473-1482.

Barrington, J.W., Barrington, T.A. (2011) What is the true incidence of dental pathology in the total joint arthroplasty population? *The Journal of Arthroplasty* 26 (6), 88-91.

Bausman, J.A., Wendelburg, K.L. (2012) Femoral prosthesis version angle calculation from a sagittal plane radiographic projection of the femur. *Veterinary Surgery* 42 (4), 398-405.

Becker, L.C., Bergfeld, W.F., Belsito, D.V., et al. (2011) Final report of the Cosmetic Ingredient Review Expert Panel safety assessment of polymethyl methacrylate (PMMA), methyl methacrylate crosspolymer, and methyl methacrylate/glycol dimethacrylate crosspolymer. *International Journal of Toxicology* 30 (13), 54-65.

Ben-Amotz, R., Liska, W.D., Beale, B.S., et al. (2009) Ilio-femoral external fixator application for temporary stabilization of recurring caudal ventral hip joint luxation after total hip replacement. *Veterinary and Comparative Orthopaedics and Traumatology* 22, 159-162.

Benzioni, H., Shahar, R., Yudelevitch, S., et al. (2008) Bacterial infective arthritis of a coxofemoral joint in dogs with hip dysplasia *Veterinary and Comparative Orthopaedics and Traumatology* 21, 262-266.

Berend, M.E., Smith, A., Meding, J.B., et al. (2006) Long-term outcome and risk factors of proximal femoral fracture in uncemented and cemented total hip arthroplasty in 2551 hips. *The Journal of Arthroplasty* 21 (6), 53-59.

Bergh, M.S., Muir, P., Markel, M.D, et al. (2004) Femoral bone adaptation to unstable long-term cemented total hip arthroplasty in dogs. *Veterinary Surgery* 33, 238-245.

Bergh, M.S., Gilley, R.S., Shofer, F.S., et al. (2006) Complications and radiographic findings following cemented total hip replacement: A retrospective evaluation of 97 dogs. *Veterinary and Comparative Orthopaedics and Traumatology* 19, 172-179.

BioMedtrix. (December 2011) Personal communication, Boonton, NJ.

Birman, M.V., Noble, P.C., Conditt, M.A., et al. (2005) Cracking and impingement in ultra-high-molecular-weight polyethylene acetabular liners. *The Journal of Arthroplasty* 20, 87-92.

Blaeser, L.L., Cross, A.R., Lanz, O.I. (1999) Revision of aseptic loosening of the femoral implant in a dog using cable cerclage. *Veterinary and Comparative Orthopaedics and Traumatology* 12, 97-101.

Braden, T.D., Olivier, N.B., Blaiset, M.A., et al. (2004) Objective evaluation of total hip replacement in 127 dogs utilizing force plate analysis. *Veterinary and Comparative Orthopaedics and Traumatology* 17, 78-81.

Budsberg, S.C., Chambers, J.N., Van Lue, S.L., et al. (1996) Prospective evaluation of ground reaction forces in dogs undergoing unilateral total hip replacement. *American Journal of Veterinary Research* 57, 1781-1785.

Burnett, R.J., Aggarwal, A., Givens, S.A., et al. (2010) Prophylactic antibiotics do not affect cultures in the treatment of an infected TKA. *Clinical Orthopaedics and Related Research* 468, 127-134.

Butt, A.J., McCarthy, T., Kelly, I.P., et al. (2005) Sciatic nerve palsy secondary to postoperative haematoma in primary total hip replacement. *Journal of Bone and Joint Surgery* 87 (Suppl. B), 1465-1467.

Byrick, R.F., Mullen, J.B., Mazer, C.D., et al. (1994) Transpulmonary systemic fat embolism. Studies in mongrel dogs after cemented arthroplasty. *American Journal of Respiratory and Critical Care Medicine* 150, 1416-1422.

Casper, D.S., Kim, G.K., Restrepo, C., et al. (2011) Primary total hip arthroplasty with an uncemented femoral component. Five-to nine-year results. *The Journal of Arthroplasty* 26, 638-641.

Ching, D.W., Gould, I.M., Rennie, J.A., et al. (1989) Prevention of late haematogenous infection in major prosthetic joints. *Journal of Antimicrobial Chemotherapy* 23, 676-680.

Conzemius, M.G., Vandervoort, J. (2005) Total joint replacement in the Dog. In Renberg, W.C. (ed.) *Veterinary Clinics of North America*, vol. 35. Saunders, Philadelphia, pp. 1213-1231.

Cooper, J.H., Jacob, P.C., Rodriquez, J.A. (2011) Distal fixation of proximally coated tapered stems may predispose to a failure of osteointegration. *The Journal of Arthroplasty* 26 (6 Suppl.), 78-83.

Cross, A.R., Newell, S.M. (2000) Definition and determination of acetabular component orientation in cemented total hip arthroplasty. *Veterinary Surgery* 29, 507-516.

Dassler, C.L., Schulz, K.S., Kass, P., et al. (2003) The effects of femoral stem and neck length on cement strains in a canine total hip replacement model. *Veterinary Surgery* 32, 37-45.

Dearmin, M.G., Schulz, K.S. (2004) The effect of stem length on femoral component positioning in canine total hip arthroplasty. *Veterinary Surgery* 33, 272-278.

DeHart, M.M., Riley, L.H. (1999) Nerve injuries in total hip arthroplasty. *Journal of the American Academy of Orthopaedic Surgeons* 7, 101-111.

DeYoung, D.J., DeYoung, B.A., Aberman, H.A., et al. (1992) Implantation of an uncemented total hip prosthesis technique and initial results of 100 arthroplasties. *Veterinary Surgery* 21, 168-177.

DeYoung, D.J., Schiller, R.A., DeYoung, B.A. (1993) Radiographic assessment of a canine uncemented porous-coated anatomic total hip prosthesis. *Veterinary Surgery* 22, 473-481.

Dogan, S., Manley, P.A., Vanderby, R., et al. (1991) Canine intersegmental hip joint forces and moments before and after cemented total hip replacement. *Journal of Biomechanics* 24 (6), 397-407.

Dyce, J. (2010) Emerging complications of BioMedtrix cementless (BFX) total hip replacement. *Proceedings ACVS Surgical Forum*, 459-461.

Dyce, J., Olmstead, M.L. (2002) Removal of infected canine cemented total hip prostheses using a femoral window technique. *Veterinary Surgery* 31, 552-560.

Dyce, J., Wisner, E.R., Wang, Q., et al. (2000a) Evaluation of risk factors for luxation after total hip replacement in dogs. *Veterinary Surgery* 29, 524-532.

Dyce, J., Tompkins, D., Bhushan, B., et al. (2000b) Polyethylene wear in retrieved canine acetabular components. *Veterinary and Comparative Orthopaedics and Traumatology* 13, 78-86.

Dyce, J., Wisner, E.R., Schrader, S.C., et al. (2001) Radiographic evaluation of acetabular component position in dogs. *Veterinary Surgery* 30, 28-39.

Edwards, M.R., Egger, E.L., Schwarz, P.D. (1997) Aseptic loosening of the femoral implant after cemented total hip arthroplasty in dogs: 11 cases in 10 dogs (1991-1995) *American Journal of Veterinary Research* 211, 580-586.

El-Warrak, A.O., Olmstead, M.L., Rechenberg, B., et al. (2001) A Review of aseptic loosening in total hip arthroplasty. *Veterinary and Comparative Orthopaedics and Traumatology* 14, 115-124.

Fender, D., Harper, W.M., Thompson, J.R., et al. (1997) Mortality and fatal pulmonary embolism after primary total hip replacement. Results from a regional hip register. *Journal of Bone and Joint Surgery* 6, 896-899.

Fitzpatrick, N., Bielecki, M., Yeadon, R., et al. (2012a) Total hip replacement with dorsal acetabular rim augmentation using the SOP implant and polymethylmethcrylate cement in seven dogs with dorsal acetabular rim deficiency. *Veterinary Surgery* 41, 168-179.

Fitzpatrick, N., Nikolaou, C., Yeadon, R., et al. (2012b) String-of-pearls locking plate and cerclage wire stabilization of periprosthetic femoral fractures after total hip replacement in six dogs. *Veterinary Surgery* 41, 180-188.

Fitzpatrick, N., Pratola, L., Yeadon, R., et al. (2012c) Total hip replacement after failed femoral head and neck excision in two dogs and two cats. *Veterinary Surgery* 41, 136-142.

Forterre, F., Tomek, A., Rytz, U., et al. (2007) Iatrogenic sciatic nerve injury in eighteen dogs and nine cats (1997-2006). *Veterinary Surgery* 36, 464-471.

Foster, L.N., Kelly, R.P., Watts, W.M. (1951) Experimental infarction of bone and bone marrow; sequelae of severance of the nutrient artery and stripping of periosteum. *Journal of Bone and Joint Surgery* 33, 396-406.

Frank, C.B., Adams, M., Kroeber, M., et al. (2011) Intraoperative subcutaneous wound closing culture sample: a predicting factor for periprosthetic infection after hip- and knee replacement? *Archives of Orthopaedic and Trauma Surgery* 131 (10), 1389-1396.

Frankel, D.J., Pluhar, E., Skurla, C.P., et al. (2004) Radiographic evaluation of mechanically tested cemented total hip arthroplasty femoral components retrieved post-mortem. *Veterinary and Comparative Orthopaedics and Traumatology* 17, 216-224.

Freeman, C.B., Adin, C.A., Lewis, D.D., et al. (2003) Intrapelvic granuloma formation six years after total hip arthroplasty in a dog. *Journal of the American Veterinary Medical Association* 223, 1446-1449.

Ganz, S.M., Jackson, J., VanEnkevort, B. (2010) Risk factors for femoral fracture after canine press-fit cementless total hip arthroplasty. *Veterinary Surgery* 39, 688-695.

Gemmill, T.J., Pink, J., Renwick, A., et al. (2010) Hybrid cemented/cementless total hip replacement in dogs: seventy-eight consecutive joint replacements. *Veterinary Surgery* 40, 621-630.

Ghaye, B., Ghuysen, A., Bruyere, P.J., et al. (2006) Can CT pulmonary angiography allow assessment of severity of prognosis in patients presenting with pulmonary embolism? What the radiologist needs to know. *RadioGraphics* 26, 23-40.

Greenwald, A.S. (ed) (2011) Seminars in arthroplasty ceramics. In *Orthopedic Surgery: The Contemporary Landscape*, vol 22. Elsevier, Philadelphia.

Guerrero, T.G., Montavon, P.M. (2009) Zurich cementless total hip replacement: retrospective evaluation of 2nd generation implants in 60 dogs. *Veterinary Surgery* 38, 70-80.

Haney, D.R., Peck, J.N. (2009) Influence of canal preparation depth on the incidence of femoral medullary infarction with Zurich cementless canine total hip arthroplasty. *Veterinary Surgery* 38, 673-676.

Hansen, E., Ries, M.D. (2006) Revision total hip arthroplasty for large medial (protrusio) defects with a rim-fit cementless acetabular component. *The Journal of Arthroplasty* 21, 72-79.

Hayes, G.M., Ramirez, J., Langley-Hobbs, S.J. (2009) Does the degree of preoperative subluxation or soft tissue tension affect the incidence of postoperative luxation in dogs after total hip replacement? *Veterinary Surgery* 40, 6-13.

Hayes, G.M., Ramirez, J., Langley-Hobbs, M.A. (2011) Use of the cumulative summation technique to quantitatively assess a surgical learning curve: canine total hip replacement. *Veterinary Surgery* 40, 1-5.

Henderson, C.E., Lujan, T.J., Kuhl, L.L., et al. (2011) 2010 Mid-America Orthopedic Association Physician in Training Award: healing complications are common after locked plating for distal femur fractures. *Clinical Orthopaedics and Related Research* 469, 757-765.

Hofmann, S., Huemer, G., Salzer, M. (1998) Pathophysiology and management of the fat embolism syndrome. *Anaesthesia* 53 (2), 35-37.

Howard, J.L., Hanssen, A.D. (2007) Principles of a clean operating room environment. *The Journal of Arthroplasty* 22(13), 6-11.

Hummel, D.W., Lanz, O.I., Were, S.R. (2010) Complications of cementless total hip replacement. A retrospective study of 163 cases. *Veterinary and Comparative Orthopaedics and Traumatology* 23, 424-432.

Hunter, S., Dyce, J., Butkus, L., et al. (2003) Acetabular cup displacement after polyethylene-cement interface failure: a complication of total hip replacement in seven dogs. *Veterinary and Comparative Orthopaedics and Traumatology* 16, 99-104.

Hurd, J.L., Potter, H.G., Dua, V., et al. (2006) Sciatic nerve palsy after primary total hip arthroplasty. A new perspective. *The Journal of Arthroplasty* 21, 796-802.

Ireifej, S., Marino, D., Loughin, C.A., et al. (2012) Risk factors and clinical relevance of positive intraoperative bacterial cultures in dogs with total hip replacement. *Veterinary Surgery* 41, 63-68.

Iwata, D., Broun, H.C., Black, A.P., et al. (2008) Total hip arthroplasty outcomes assessment using functional and radiographic scores to compare canine systems. *Veterinary and Comparative Orthopaedics and Traumatology* 21, 221-230.

Jacobson, A., Schrader, S.C. (1987) Peripheral nerve injury associated with fracture or fracture-dislocation of the pelvis in dogs and cats: 34 cases (1978-1982). *Journal of the American Veterinary Medical Association* 190, 569-572.

Jaecques, S.N., Helsen, J.A., Mulier, M., et al. (1998) Geometric analysis of the proximal medullary cavity of the femur in the German Shepherd dog. *Veterinary and Comparative Orthopaedics and Traumatology* 11, 29-36.

Jankovits, D.A., Liska, W.D., Kalis, R.H. (2012) Treatment of avascular necrosis of the femoral head in small dogs with micro total hip replacement. *Veterinary Surgery* 41, 143-147.

Jehn, C.T., Manley, P.A. (2002) The effects of femur and implant position on the radiographic assessment of total hip femoral implants in dogs. *Veterinary Surgery* 31, 349-357.

Jehn, C.T., Bergh, M.S., Manley, P.A. (2003) Orthogonal view analysis for evaluating the femoral component position of total hip implants in dogs using postoperative radiographs. *Veterinary Surgery* 32, 134-141.

Johanson, N.A., Pellicci, P.M., Tsairis, P., et al. (1983) Nerve injury in total hip arthroplasty. *Clinical Orthopaedics and Related Research* 214-222.

Judet, J., Judet, R. (1950) The use of an artificial head for arthroplasty of the hip joint. *The Journal of Bone & Joint Surgery* 32B, 166-173.

Kalis, R.H., Liska, W.D., Jankovits, D.A. (2012) Total hip replacement as a treatment option for capital physeal fractures in dogs and cats. *Veterinary Surgery* 41, 148-155.

Kallos, T., Enis, J.E., Gollan, F., et al. (1974) Intramedullary pressure and pulmonary embolism of femoral medullary contents in dogs during insertion of bone cement and a prosthesis. *Journal of Bone and Joint Surgery* 56A, 1363-1367.

Kim, K.F., Chiba, J., Rubash, H.E. (1994) In vivo and in vitro analysis of membranes from hip prosthesis inserted without cement. *The Journal of Bone & Joint Surgery* 76, 172-180.

Kim, Y.H., Oh, S.W., Kim, J.S. (2002) Prevalence of fat embolism following bilateral simultaneous and unilateral total hip arthroplasty performed with or without cement: a prospective, randomized clinical study. *Journal of Bone and Joint Surgery Am* 84A, 1372-1379.

Kim, H.J., Walcott-Sapp, S., Leggett, K., et al. (2008) The use of spiral computed tomography scans for the detection of pulmonary embolism. *The Journal of Arthroplasty* 23 (1), 31-35.

Konde, L.J., Olmstead, M.L., Hohn, B.R. (1982) Radiographic evaluation of total hip replacement in the dog. *Veterinary Radiology* 23, 98-106.

Korkala, O., Syrjanen, K.J. (1998) Intrapelvic cyst formation after hip arthroplasty with a carbone fiber-reinforced polyethylene socket. *Archives of Orthopaedic and Trauma Surgery* 118, 113-115.

Kuo, T.Y., Skedros, J.G., Bloebaum, R.D. (1998) Comparison of human, primate, and canine femora: implications for biomaterials testing in total hip replacement. *Journal of Biomedical Materials Research* 40, 475-489.

Laack, T.A., Goyal, D.G. (2004) Pulmonary embolism: an unsuspected killer. *Emergency Medicine Clinics of North America* 22 (4), 961-983.

Lascelles, B.X., Freire, M., Roe, S.C., et al. (2010) Evaluation of functional outcome after BFX total hip replacement using a pressure sensitive walkway. *Veterinary Surgery* 39, 71-77.

Lee, K.C., Kapatkin, A.S. (2002) Positive intraoperative cultures and canine total hip replacement: risk factors, periprosthetic infection, and surgical success. *Journal of the American Animal Hospital Association* 38, 271-278.

Liska, W.D. (1985) Wires in long bone fracture repair. In Slatter, D.H. (ed.) *Textbook of Small Animal Surgery*, vol. II, 1st edn. WB Saunders, Philadelphia, pp. 2003-2013.

Liska, W.D. (2004) Femur fractures associated with canine total hip replacement. *Veterinary Surgery* 33, 164-172.

Liska, W.D. (2010) Micro total hip replacement for dogs and cats: surgical technique and outcomes. *Veterinary Surgery* 39, 797-810.

Liska, W.D., Poteet, B.A. (2003) Pulmonary embolism associated with canine total hip replacement. *Veterinary Surgery* 32, 178-186.

Liska, W.D., Doyle, N.D., Schwartz, Z. (2010) Successful revision of a femoral head ostectomy (complicated by postoperative sciatic neurapraxia) to a total hip replacement in a cat. *Veterinary and Comparative Orthopaedics and Traumatology* 23, 119-123.

Lockwood, A.A., Liska, W.D. (2011) Duration of clinical signs before total hip replacement in dogs. *Journal of the American Veterinary Medical Association* 238, 1-4.

Lozman, J., Deno, D.C., Feustel, P.J., et al. (1986) Pulmonary and cardiovascular consequences of immediate fixation or conservative management of long bone fractures. *Archives of Surgery* 121, 992-999.

Marcellin-Little, D.J., Papich, M.J., Richardson, D.C., et al. (1996) Pharmacokinetic model for cefazolin distribution during total hip arthroplasty in dogs. *American Journal of Veterinary Research* 57, 720-726.

Marcellin-Little, D.J., DeYoung, B.A., Doyens, D.H., et al. (1999a) Canine uncemented porous-coated anatomic total hip arthroplasty: results of a long-term prospective evaluation of 50 consecutive cases. *Veterinary Surgery* 28, 10-20.

Marcellin-Little, D.J., DeYoung, D.J., Thrall, D.E., et al. (1999b) Osteosarcoma at the site of bone infarction associated with total hip arthroplasty in a dog. *Veterinary Surgery* 28, 54-60.

Margalit, K.A., Hayashi, K., Jackson, J., et al. (2010) Biomechanical evaluation of acetabular cup implantation in cementless total hip arthroplasty. *Veterinary Surgery* 39, 818-823.

Markowitz, J., Archibald, J., Downie, H.G. (1964) Surgery of bone and joints. In Markowitz, J., Archibald, J., Downie H.G. (eds.) *Experimental Surgery*, 5th edn. Williams & Wilkins, Baltimore, pp. 297-331.

Marsolais, G.S., Peck, J.N., Berry, C., et al. (2009) Femoral medullary infarction prevalence with the Zurich cementless canine total hip arthroplasty. *Veterinary Surgery* 38, 667-680.

Marti, J.M., Marcellin-Little, D.J., Roe, S.C. (1999) Use of a DeVita pin to maintain reduction of a dislocated total hip prosthesis in a dog. *Veterinary and Comparative Orthopaedics and Traumatology* 12, 85-87.

Massat, B.J., Vasseur, P.B. (1994) Clinical and radiographic results of total hip arthroplasty in dogs: 96 cases (1986-1992) *Journal of the American Veterinary Medical Association* 205, 448-454.

Massat, B.J., Miller, R.T., DeYoung, B.A., et al. (1998) Single-stage revision using an uncemented, porous-coated anatomic endoprosthesis in two dogs: case report. *Veterinary Surgery* 27, 268-277.

May, O., Girard, J., Hurtevent, J.F., et al. (2008) Delayed, transient sciatic nerve palsy after primary cementless hip arthroplasty. *Journal of Bone and Joint Surgery* 90B, 674-676.

Marino, D.J., Ireifej, S.J., Loughin, C.A. (2012) Micro total hip replacement in dogs and cats. *Veterinary Surgery* 41, 121-129.

McCulloch, R.S., Roe, M.S., Marcellin-Little, D.J., et al. (2012) Resistance to subsidence of an uncemented femoral stem after cerclage wiring of a fissure. *Veterinary Surgery* 41, 163-167.

McElfresh, E. (1991) History of arthroplasty. In Petty, W. (ed.) *Total Joint Replacement.* Saunders, Philadelphia, pp. 3-18.

Medl, N., Guerrero, T.G., Holzle, L., et al. (2012) Intraoperative contamination of the suction tip in clean orthopedic surgeries in dogs and cats. *Veterinary Surgery* 41, 254-260.

Mostafa, A.A., Druen, S., Nolte, I., et al. (2012) Radiographic evaluation of early periprosthetic femoral bone contrast and prosthetic stem alignment after uncemented and cemented total hip replacement in dogs. *Veterinary Surgery* 11, 69-77.

Munk, P.L., Helms, C.A., Holt, R.G. (1989) Immature bone infarcts: findings on plain radiographs and MR scans. *American Journal of Roentgenology* 152, 547-549.

Nelson, L.L. (2011) Surgical site infections in small animal surgery. *Veterinary Clinics of North America* 41, 1041-1056.

Nelson, L.L., Dyce, J., Shott, S. (2007) Risk factors for ventral luxation in canine total hip replacement. *Veterinary Surgery* 36, 644-653.

Newman, P.E., Scales, J.T. (1951) Unsuitability of polyethylene for moveable weight bearing prosthesis. *The Journal of Bone & Joint Surgery* 33B, 392-398.

Off, W., Matis, U. (2010) Excision arthroplasty of the hip joint in dogs and cats. Clinical, radiographic, and gait analysis findings from the Department of Surgery, Veterinary Faculty of the Ludwig-Maximilians-University of Munich, Germany. *Veterinary and Comparative Orthopaedics and Traumatology* 23, 297-305.

Olmstead, M.L. (1995) Canine cemented total hip replacements: state of the art. *Journal of Small Animal Practice* 36, 395-399.

Olmstead, M.L., Hohn, R.B., Turner, T.M. (1983) A five-year study of 221 total hip replacements in the dog. *Journal of the American Veterinary Medical Association* 183, 191-194.

Otto, K., Matis, U. (1994) Changes in cardiopulmonary variables in platelet count during anesthesia for total hip replacement in dogs. *Veterinary Surgery* 23, 266-273.

Palmisano, M.P., Dyce, J., Olmstead, M.L. (2003) Extraosseus cement granuloma associated with total hip replacement in 6 dogs. *Veterinary Surgery* 32, 80-90.

Parvizi, J., Zmistowski, B., Berbari, E.F., et. al. (2011) New definition for periprosthetic joint infection. *The Journal of Arthroplasty* 26, 1136-1138.

Peremans, K., DeWinter, F., Janssens, L., et al. (2002) An infected hip prosthesis in a dog diagnosed with a 99mTC-ciprofloxacin (infection) scan. *Veterinary Radiology & Ultrasound* 43, 178-182.

Pitto, R.P., Koessler, M., Draenert, K. (1998) The John Charnley Award. Prophylaxis of fat and bone marrow embolism in cemented total hip arthroplasty. *Clinical Orthopaedics and Related Research* 355, 23-34.

Pooya, H.A., Schulz, K.S., Wisner, E.R., (2003) Short-term evaluation of dorsal acetabular augmentation in 10 canine total hip replacements. *Veterinary Surgery* 32, 142-152.

Pozzi, A., Kowaleski, M.P., Dyce, J., et al. (2004) Treatment of traumatic coxo-femoral luxation by cemented total hip arthroplasty. *Veterinary and Comparative Orthopaedics and Traumatology* 17, 198-203.

Preston, C.A., Schultz, K.S., Vasseur, P.B. (1999) Total hip arthroplasty in nine canine hind limb amputees: a retrospective study. *Veterinary Surgery* 28, 341-347.

Reindl, S., Matis, U. (1998) Detection of embolic events by capnography and transeosophageal echocardiography during total hip replacement. *Veterinary and Comparative Orthopaedics and Traumatology* 11, 67-75.

Renwick, A., Gemmill, T., Pink, J., et al. (2011) Radiographic evaluation of BFX acetabular component position in dogs. *Veterinary Surgery* 40, 610-620.

Roe, S.C. (1997) Mechanical characteristics and comparisons of cerclage wires: introduction of the double-wrap and loop/twist tying methods. *Veterinary Surgery* 26, 310-316.

Roe, S.C., DeYoung, D., Weinstock, D., et al. (1996) Osteosarcoma eight years after total hip replacement. *Veterinary Surgery* 25, 70-74.

Sakai, T., Sugano, N., Fujii, M., et al. (2002) Sciatic nerve palsy after cementless total hip arthroplasty. Treatment by modular neck and calcar shortening: a case report. *Journal of Orthopaedic Science* 7, 400-4002.

Schlegel, U.J., Sturm, M., Ewerbeck, V., et al. (2004) Efficacy of vacuum bone cement mixing systems in reducing methylmethacrylate fume exposure: comparison of 7 different mixing devices and handmixing. *Acta Orthopaedica Scandinavica* 75, 559-566.

Schmalzried, T.P., Noordin, S., Amstutz, H.C. (1991) Nerve palsy associated with total hip replacement. Risk factors and prognosis. *The Journal of Bone & Joint Surgery* 73, 1074-1080.

Schmalzried, T.P., Noordin, S., Amstutz, H.C. (1997) Update on nerve palsy associated with total hip replacement. *Clinical Orthopaedics and Related Research* 188-206.

Schultz, K.S. (2000) Application of arthroplasty principles to canine cemented total hip replacement. *Veterinary Surgery* 29, 578-593.

Sebestyen, P., Marcellin-Little, D.J., DeYoung, B.A. (2000) Femoral medullary infarction secondary to canine total hip arthroplasty. *Veterinary Surgery* 29, 227-236.

Shanbhag, A.S., Hasselman, C.T., Rubash, H.E. (1997) Inhibition of wear debris medicated osteolysis in a canine total hip arthroplasty model. *Clinical Orthopaedics and Related Research* 344, 33-43.

Shields, S.L., Schulz, K.S., Hagan, C.E., et al. (2002) The effects of acetabular cup temperature and duration of cement pressurization on cement porosity in a canine total hip replacement model. *Veterinary Surgery* 31, 167-173.

Shine, T.J., Feinglass, N.G., Leone, B.J., et al. (2012) Transesophageal echocardiography for detection of propagating, massive emboli during prosthetic hip fracture surgery. *Iowa Orthopaedic Journal* 30, 211-214.

Skurla, C.T., James, S.P. (2001) A comparison of canine and human UHMWPE acetabular component wear. *Biomedical Sciences Instrumentation,* 37, 245-250.

Skurla, C.P., Pluhar, G.E., Frankel, J.F., et al. (2005) Assessing the dog as a model for human total hip replacement. *Journal of Bone and Joint Surgery* 87B, 120-127.

Smeak, D.D., Olmstead, M.L. (1987) Brucella canis osteomyelitis in two dogs with total hip replacements. *Journal of the American Veterinary Medical Association* 191, 986-990.

Sorjonen, D.C., Milton, J.L., Steiss, J.E., et al. (1990) Hip dysplasia with bilateral ischiatic nerve entrapment in a dog. *Journal of the American Veterinary Medical Association* 197, 495-497.

Spanghel, M.J., Younger, A.E., Masri, B.A., et al. (1997) Diagnosis of infection following total hip arthroplasty. *The Journal of Bone & Joint Surgery* 79A, 1578-1588.

Sumner, D.R., Devlin, T.C., Winkelman, D., et al. (1990a) The geometry of the adult canine proximal femur. *Journal of Orthopaedic Research* 8, 671-677.

Sumner, D.R., Turner, T.M., Pierson, R.H., et al. (1990b) Effects of radiation on fixation of non-cemented porous-coated implants in a canine model. *The Journal of Bone & Joint Surgery* 72A, 1527-1533.

Sumner, D.R., Turner, T.M., Urban, R.M., et al. (1992) Experimental studies of bone remodeling in total hip arthroplasty. *Clinical Orthopaedics and Related Research* 276, 83-89.

Terrell, S.P., Chandra, A.M., Pablo, L.S., et al. (2004) Fatal intraoperative pulmonary fat embolism during cemented total hip arthroplasty in a dog. *Journal of the American Animal Hospital Association* 40, 345-348.

Tidwell, S.A., Graham, J.P., Peck, J.N., et al. (2007) Incidence of pulmonary embolism after non-cemented total hip arthroplasty in eleven dogs: computed tomographic pulmonary angiography and pulmonary perfusion scintigraphy. *Veterinary Surgery* 36, 37-42.

Torres, B.T., Budsberg, S.C. (2009) Revision of cemented total hip arthroplasty with cementless components in three dogs. *Veterinary Surgery* 38, 81-86.

Torres, B.T., Chambers, J.N., Budsberg, S.C. (2009) Successful cementless cup reimplantation using cortical bone graft augmentation after an acetabular fracture and cup displacement. *Veterinary Surgery* 38, 87-91.

Tronzo, R.G., Kallos, T., Wyche, M.Q. (1974) Elevation of intramedullary pressure when methylmethacrylate is inserted in total hip arthroplasty. *Journal of Bone and Joint Surgery* 56, 714-718.

Tsukayama, D.T., Estrada, R., Gustilo, R.B. (1996) Infection after total hip arthroplasty. A study of a treatment of one hundred and six infections. *Journal of Bone and Joint Surgery* Am 78, 512-523.

Vastamaki, M., Ylinen, P., Puusa, A., et al. (2008) Late hardware-induced sciatic nerve lesions after acetabular revision. *Clinical Orthopaedics and Related Research* 466, 1193-1197.

Vezzoni, A. (2004) Total hip replacement seminar. *European Society of Veterinary Orthopaedics and Traumatology.* Munich, Germany, September 9.

Vezzoni, A. (2010) Surgical revisions in THR in-depth seminar. *World Veterinary Orthopedic Congress.* Bologna, Italy, September 15-18.

Visuri, T., Pulkkinen, P., Paavolainen, P. (2006) Malignant tumors at the site of total hip prosthesis. Analytic review of 46 cases. *The Journal of Arthroplasty* 21, 311-323.

Warnock, J.J., Dyce, J., Pooya, H., et al. (2003) Retrospective analysis of canine miniature total hip prostheses. *Veterinary Surgery* 32, 285-291.

Weisman, D.L., Olmstead, M.L., Kowalski, J.J. (2000) In vitro evaluation of antibiotic elution from Polymethylmethacrylate (PMMA) and mechanical assessment of antibiotic-PMMA composites. *Veterinary Surgery* 29, 245-251.

Weh, M.M., Hoer Leng, J.D., Guilermann, M.B., et al. (1990) The effect of radiation therapy on the fixation strength of an experimental porous coated implant in dogs. *Clinical Orthopaedics and Related Research* 261, 276-280.

Witte, P.G., Scott, H.W., Tonzing, M.A. (2010) Preliminary results of five feline total hip replacements. *Journal of Small Animal Practice* 51, 397-402.

Wood, I., Powell, H., Khom, A., et al. (2003) Evaluation of femoral head damage during canine total hip replacement. A comparison of reduction techniques. *Veterinary and Comparative Orthopaedics and Traumatology* 16, 184-190.

Wroblewski, B.M., Siney, P.D., Fleming, P.A. (1998) Fatal pulmonary embolism after total hip arthroplasty: diurnal variations. *Orthopedics* 21, 1271-1279.

Wróblewski, B.M., Siney, P.D., Fleming, P.A. (2000) Fatal pulmonary embolism and mortality after revision of failed total hip arthroplasties. *The Journal of Arthroplasty* 1, 137-139.

Wylie, K.R., DeYoung, D.J., Frost, W.T., et al. (1997) The effect of surgical approach on femoral stem position in canine cemented total hip replacement. *Veterinary Surgery* 26, 62-66.

Yates, G.D., Wasik, S.M., Edwards, G.A. (2010) Femoral component failure in canine cemented total hip replacement: a report of two cases. *Australian Veterinary Journal* 88 (6), 225-230.

114 Complications of Total Hip Replacement with the Zurich Cementless System

Aldo Vezzoni

Clinica Veterinaria Vezzoni srl, Via Angelo Massarotti 60/A, Cremona CR, Italy

The Kyon Hip Prosthesis (Kyon AG, Zurich (CH) and Kyon Veterinary Products, Boston MA), also known as the Zurich cementless total hip replacement (Z-THR), was the first cementless total hip replacement (THR) prosthesis introduced to the veterinary market in 2000. In this system, the cup is immediately fixed by press-fit insertion, and long-term stability is achieved by bone ingrowth through holes in the surface of the cup. Locking screws are used for immediate fixation of the stem, and osteointegration along the rough titanium surface of the implant provides long-term stability. The Kyon cup is made of pure titanium and the Kyon stem, head and neck unit, and screws are composed of titanium alloy (Tepic and Montavon 2004).

The type and incidence of complications associated with THR are time related; luxation, fracture, and early cup loosening usually occur within 6 months of surgery (short term); other complications, including stem loosening, late cup loosening, and implant breakage, occur later (long term). The likelihood of long-term complications increases with time. Thus, long-term complications are more likely to be seen in patients that are followed for extended periods of time and in dogs treated at an early age.

Luxation

Definition

Luxation is dislocation of the femoral head from the acetabular cup in a craniodorsal or in a caudoventral direction. Luxations are more common in the first weeks after surgery before healing of the joint capsule and periarticular tissues. Luxations occurring beyond 2 months after surgery are usually associated with major trauma or cup avulsion or implant breakage.

Risk factors

Risk factors for luxation of the prosthesis include:
- Insufficient postoperative exercise restriction
- Excessive body weight
- Poor musculature in young dogs with severe hip subluxation
- Preoperative hip dislocation
- Tall dogs with long limbs: The longer lever arm may increase the risk of luxation.
- Inadequate cup orientation (insufficient or excessive angle of lateral opening, with 45 degrees as a reference, and inadequate retroversion, with 15 degrees serving as a reference)

- Excessive or insufficient neck anteversion, with 25 degrees as a reference
- Too short neck and loose reduction
- Impingement of the neck with osteophytes or thickened joint capsule around the acetabulum
- Combination of multiple fore mentioned factors.

Diagnosis

A tentative diagnosis should be prompted by the presence of sudden lameness with non–weight-bearing stance, along with:
- Partial weight bearing
- Abnormal limb posture
- External rotation of the limb
- Appearance of a swelling at the level of the surgical wound
- Crepitus detected upon manipulation of the limb

The diagnosis is confirmed via radiography. The luxation is most obvious on a lateral projection (Figure 114.1), with the head usually located dorsally to the acetabulum in the most common dorsal and caudal dislocation. The femoral head is usually located in the obturator foramen after ventral dislocation (Figure 114.2).

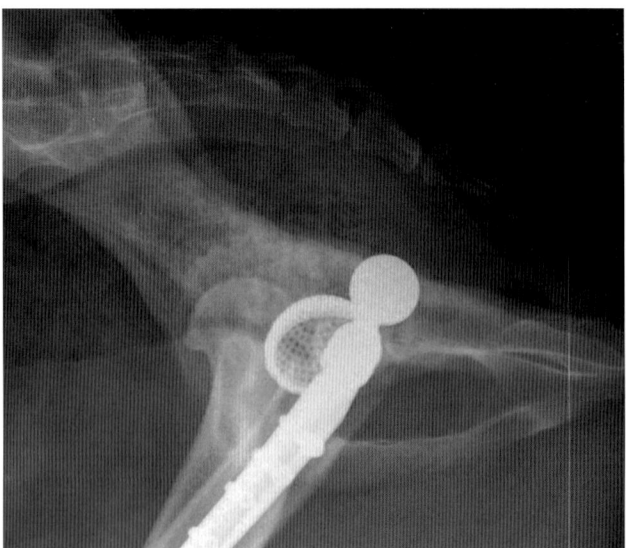

Figure 114.1 Lateral radiograph of the pelvis of a 9-month-old male German shepherd dog, with a dorsal luxation of the prosthesis, 10 days after total hip replacement.

Complications in Small Animal Surgery, First Edition. Edited by Dominique Griffon and Annick Hamaide.

© 2016 John Wiley & Sons, Inc. Published 2016 by John Wiley & Sons, Inc.

Companion website: www.wiley.com/go/griffon/complications

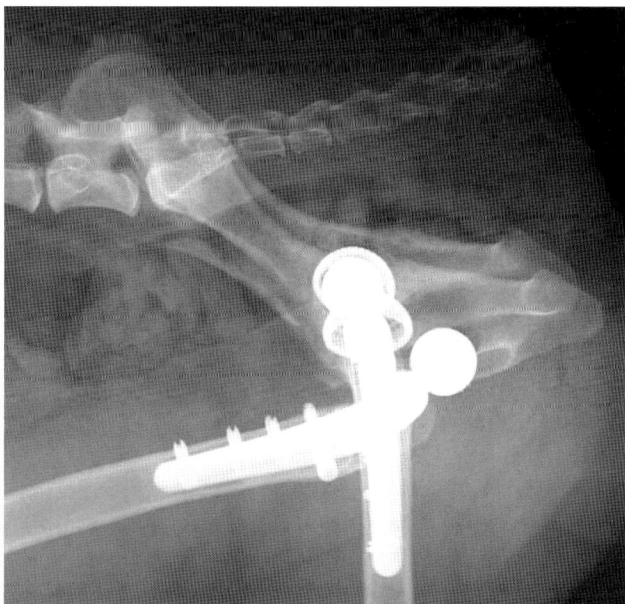

Figure 114.2 Lateral radiograph of the pelvis of a 2-year-old female Samoyed, with a ventral luxation of the prosthesis, 40 days after total hip replacement.

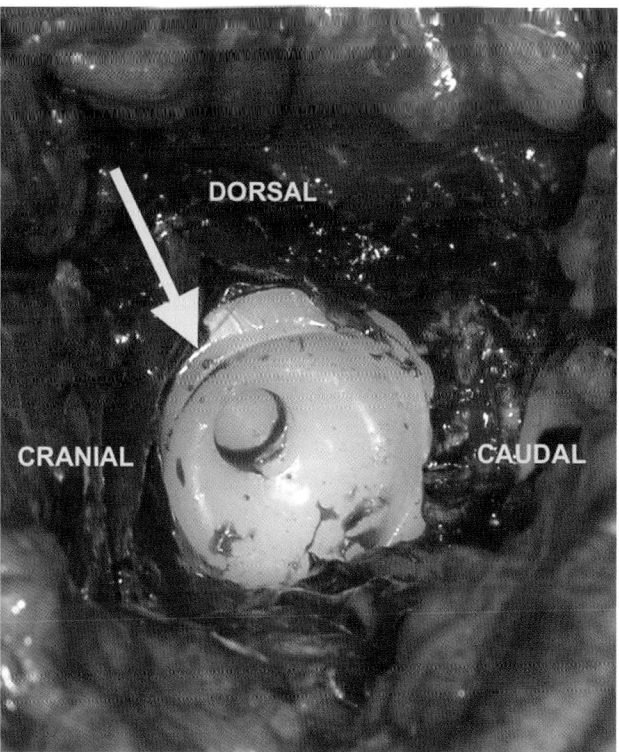

Figure 114.3 Intraoperative inspection of a cup during revision of a luxated implant. Note the depression in the border of the polyethylene insert (arrow), identifying the site of luxation.

Treatment

Prompt closed reduction may be attempted within a few hours of onset, maintaining the reduction with an Ehmer sling for 2 weeks.

Luxations of longer durations always require open reduction to change the head damaged by its rubbing against the metal of the cup. The principles of a revision in these cases include:

- Thorough preoperative assessment of the patient and review of previous records to evaluate the presence of risk factors
- General principles of revisions are listed in Box 114.1.
- Inspection of the acetabular cup: A depression is usually found along the border of the polyethylene insert, coinciding with the direction of the luxation: craniodorsal, caudal, or ventral. This assessment assists in the selection of revision procedures (Figure 114.3).
- If implants are correctly oriented, the first strategy consists of increasing neck length by one size, which is usually enough to provide sufficient stability of reduction.

Box 114.1 General principles for revisions of Zurich total hip replacements

Femoral Neck Length

Each revision may require a longer femoral neck to achieve a stable reduction, but longer necks apply more stress on the stem. Therefore, the use of long necks in primary surgeries should be avoided.

Protection of the Femoral Stem

Protection of the weakened femur after stem revision is required to avoid the risk of post-revision femoral fracture. High-speed burrs and tools for removing broken screws should be available when undertaking Z-THR revision surgeries.

ZHR, Zurich cementless total hip replacement; Kyon Veterinary Products, Zurich (CH) and Boston, MA.

- When the cause of luxation is identified as a poor cup orientation, the cup should be removed and reimplanted in the correct position.
- In cases with poor press-fit, a bigger cup should be considered. If increasing the size of the cup is not possible, a special revision cup can be selected instead.
- When luxation is due to an inappropriate orientation of the femoral neck, repositioning the stem is quite complex. Cases with moderate neck deviations may be revised via reorientation of the cup to match the neck anteversion, which is technically simpler than revising the positioning of the femoral stem.

Outcome

- When luxation is caused by poor stability, a longer neck is usually effective in preventing further luxation.
- The prognosis after revision of the acetabular cup is good if press-fit is achieved.
- If press-fit appears questionable after repositioning a cup the special revision cup armed with diverging screws should be used.
- If the origin of a recurrent luxation is not properly addressed, implant loosening and secondary infections are likely due to multiple revisions.

Prevention

The prevention of luxation is based on:

- Proper cup orientation with and angle of lateral opening (ALO) of approximately 45 degrees and a cup retroversion that matches the cranial and caudal acetabular borders
- Femoral neck anteversion approximating 25 degrees

- Intraoperative evaluation of the level of difficulty to luxate the implant prior to closing the wound: The pull test (pulling the neck up and distally) result should be negative.
- Evaluation of the stability of the hip throughout full range of motion (ROM), with external rotation up to 80 degrees, extension up to 120 degrees, and flexion up to 30 degrees to confirm the absence of instability or impingement against osteophytes or thickened joint capsule
- In case of loose reduction, a longer neck should be used to improve stability.
- Longer heads or necks increase the lever arm and stress applied on the stem, thereby increasing the risk of long-term failure of the neck (breakage or loosening). Proper planning of the neck osteotomy should therefore aim to use the short head–neck combination in medium to large size dogs and the medium head–neck combination in giant dogs.
- In large and giant dogs, the 29- or 32-mm cups should be used to accommodates the larger (19-mm-diameter head) because this implant will offer more resistance to luxation than the 16 mm-diameter head.
- The extra-short head–neck combination should be used with caution and be limited to small dogs, up to 20 kg. This combination has a more limited ROM compared with other head–neck sizes and consequently carries a higher risk of impingement and luxation.
- Whenever the extra-short head–neck combination is used, the cup orientation should be very accurate, and surgeons should verify the absence of friction between the polyethylene liner and the base of the neck before closure.
- Prevention of luxation is also based on proper post operative care, keeping the dog for 2 months in a limited space, avoiding slippery surfaces, and using a leash when walking outside and on the stairs.
- Tranquillization may be considered in the first 4 to 5 weeks to control young and active dogs.

Femoral fractures

Definition

A femoral fracture is loss of continuity of the femur caused by hip replacement with the Kyon system may occur during or after surgery.

Risk factors

Intraoperative femoral fractures or fissures may result from:

- Technical mistakes during overzealous femoral reaming while turning the rectangular shaped files or applying angular forces during reaming.
- During insertion of the femoral stem, with the aid of the jig: only axial movement is safe, and any torsion could lead to femoral fissure or fracture.
- Fracture of the trochanter may occur during reduction of the head inside the cup if excessive tension is required.
- While testing for luxation before closing the wound: External rotation of the limb may be limited by periarticular fibrosis in chronic coxarthrosis, and high torsional stress on the femur may lead to fracture.

Postoperative fracture can occur in the first 2 weeks after surgery and is more likely if the following conditions are present:

- Older patients, with chronic degenerative joint disease and osteopenia

- Excessive body weight
- Excessive quadriceps tension after forced reduction of the hip
- Uncontrolled postoperative activity, including jumping, slipping, or falling

Diagnosis

Intraoperative fissures and fractures are diagnosed by during inspection of the femur:

- A distinctive sudden and sharp noise coming from the surgical field should prompt suspicion.
- Elevation of the vastus lateralis from the proximal femur will expose a fissure extending distally from the femoral neck osteotomy site (Figure 114.4).

Postoperative fractures are diagnosed based on:

- A history of sudden lameness and cry after a jump, while rising from a sitting position, or after bumping against an obstacle
- The diagnosis is confirmed via radiographic examination (Figure 114.5). Fractures usually start from the femoral holes created for screw fixation of the stem.

Treatment

- Fissures of the proximal metaphysis that are diagnosed during surgery, and do not extend into the diaphysis can be fixed with two or three cerclage wires, well tightened and secured with the eyelet knot (see Figure 114.4).
- Fissures that extend into the diaphysis and complete femoral fractures require application combination of cerclage wires and a neutralization plate applied on the lateral-caudal aspect of the proximal femur and extending distally on the lateral aspect of the diaphysis with at least three or four bicortical screws distal to the fracture.

Postoperative fractures are treated as an emergency:

- Anatomic reconstruction is required to keep the stem locked inside the femur, using several strong cerclage wires (1.25 mm), secured with the eyelet knot (see Figure 114.5)
- Fracture stabilization is achieved with a long neutralization plate. Monocortical screws are used in the area of the stem, and bicortical screws are used away from the stem
- Since postoperative fracture usually occurs within 2 to 3 weeks after surgery, a surgical revision at a site closely located to the initial surgical site requires extra care to prevent infection. Local slow release antibiotic substances should be inserted in the surgical field (see Chapter 5). Among these, the author has used a collagen sponge (Septocoll; BIOMET DEUTSCHLAND, Berlin, Germany) impregnated with sulphate gentamicin (released within 24 hours) and crobefate gentamicin (released in 7 days). An injectable polymer hydrogel (VetriGel; Royer Biomedical, Frederick, ML) is currently undergoing clinical trials as a delivery system for amikacin in septic arthritis.

Outcome

- Femoral fissures and fractures diagnosed during surgery and immediately addressed will heal without consequences on implant stability and fixation.
- Undiagnosed intraoperative fissures usually evolve in postoperative fractures.
- Postoperative fractures have a good prognosis for restoring the stability of the stem fixation as long as anatomic reduction and stable fixation are achieved with cerclage wires and neutralization plate fixation.
- Unstable fixation generally leads to stem loosening.

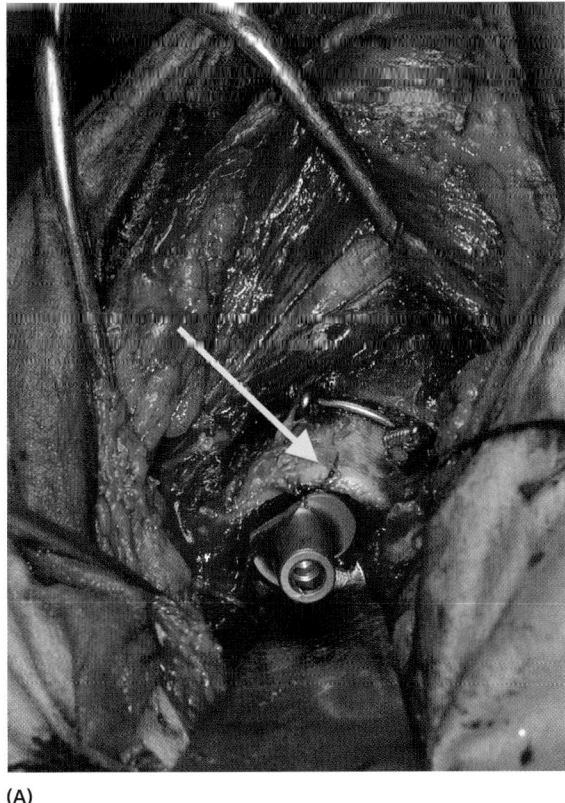

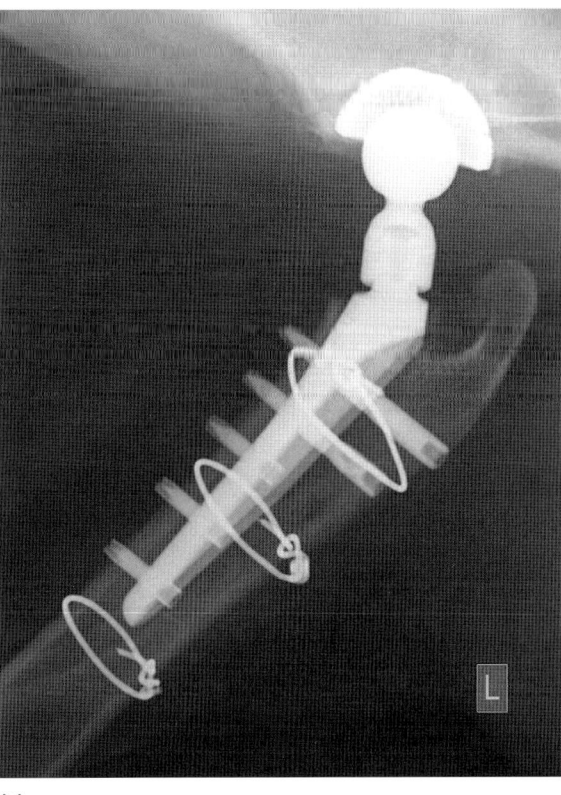

(A)   **(B)**

Figure 114.4 Femoral fissure during insertion of the femoral stem in an 8-year-old male Labrador retriever. **A**, Intraoperative appearance of the femoral fissure (arrow). The fissure does not extend distally and is treated with cerclage wires. **B**, Follow-up radiograph 2 months after surgery. Cerclage wires are unchanged and were effective in treating the femoral fissure.

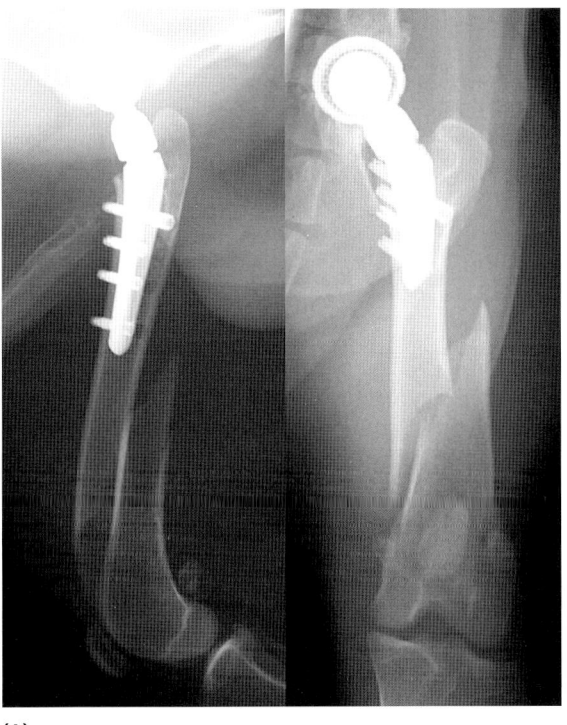

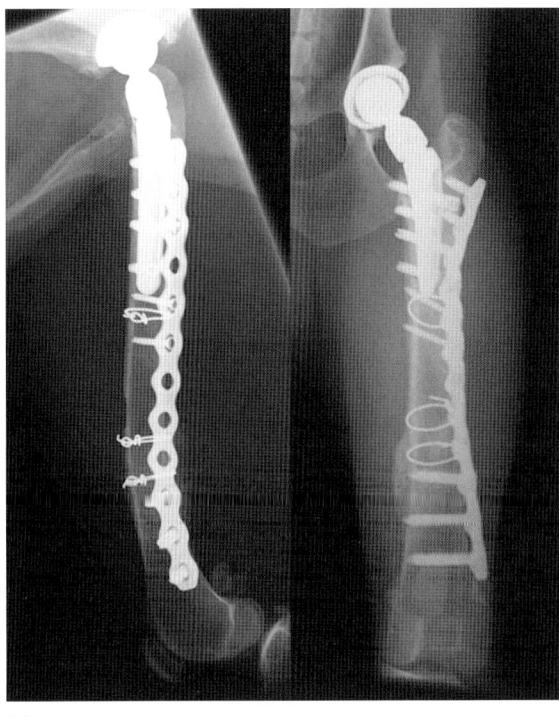

(A)   **(B)**

Figure 114.5 Postoperative femoral fracture in a 7-year-old male mixed breed dog 16 days after total hip replacement. **A**, Mediolateral (left) and anteroposterior (right) radiographs allow the diagnosis of a complete oblique fracture of the distal third of the femoral diaphysis distal to the femoral stem. **B**, Radiographs obtained 2 months after fracture repair with cerclage wires and neutralization plate (ALPS 10 [Advanced Locking Plate System], Kyon AG, Zurich (CH) and Kyon Veterinary Products, Boston MA). The apparatus is intact and the bone is undergoing callus formation.

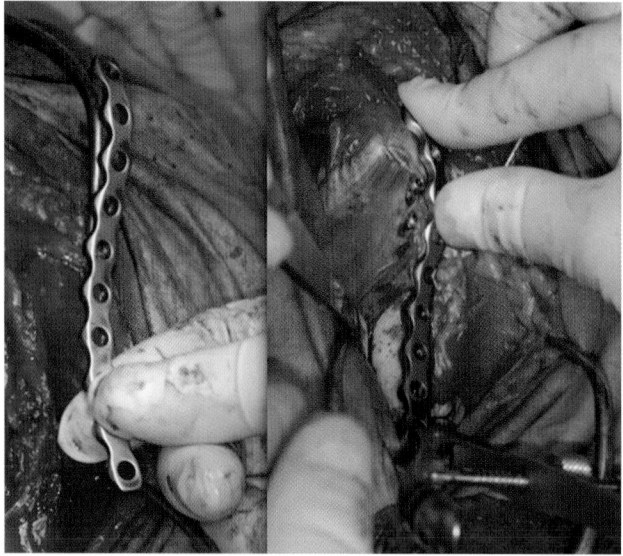

(A)

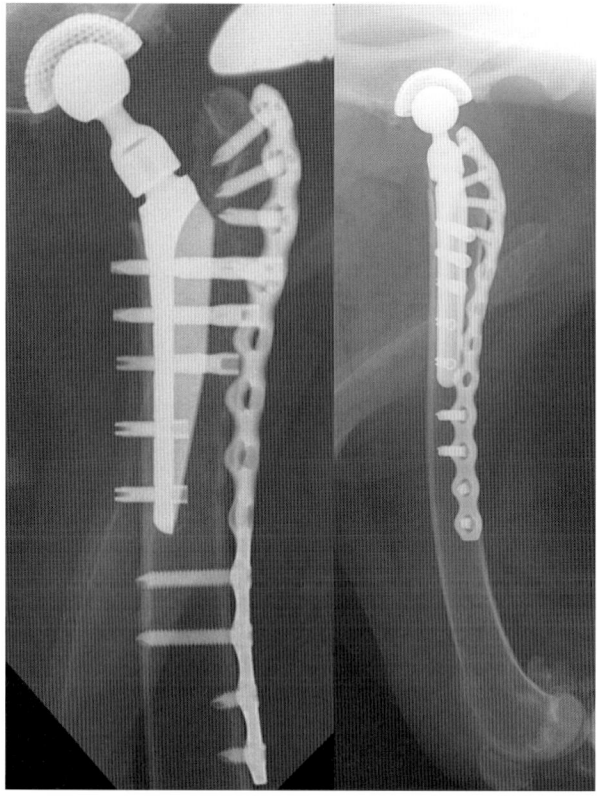

(B)

Figure 114.6 Prophylactic placement of a plate during hip replacement with a Kyon (Kyon AG,Zurich (CH) and Kyon Veterinary Products, Boston MA) implant. **A,** Intraoperative appearance of the femoral buttress plate. **B,** Radiographs obtained immediately after surgery (right) and 2 months later (left) in a 12-year-old male giant schnauzer. The 12-hole-long ALPS 10 (Advanced Locking Plate System, Kyon AG, Zurich (CH) and Kyon Veterinary Products, Boston MA) was applied to prevent postoperative femoral fracture in this older patient.

Prevention

Intraoperative fissures and fractures can be prevented via:

- Good surgical technique and sound understanding of maneuvers that increase the risk of fractures
- Thorough evaluation of the proximal femur throughout critical steps of the procedure

The following measures should be considered to prevent postoperative fractures:

- Preoperative identification of patients at risk for fractures (see Risk factors)
- Two bicortical screws can be inserted proximally (Vezzoni 2009) to improve rotational stability of the stem and reduce bone stress in cases deemed at risk for fractures.
- Placement of three single-loop 1-mm-diameter cerclage wires have been recommended to prevent fractures in an ex vivo study (Pozzi et al. 2013): One wire was placed between the fourth and the fifth screw and two were placed distally to the fifth screw.
- In the same study, protection was improved when a buttress plate fixed in the trochanteric area and in the distal femur bridged the area distal to the stem.
- Application of an S-shaped buttress plate extending over the entire length of the femur and fixed with monocortical screws (Vezzoni 2009, 2010) (Figure 114.6)

Cup loosening or breakage

Definition

Loosening of a cementless acetabular component is commonly the result of infection (septic loosening), lack of initial stability with subsequent failure of osteointegration (early aseptic

loosening), or osteolysis induced by polyethylene wear debris (late aseptic loosening).

Risk factors

Risk factors for early aseptic cup loosening, up to 6 month after surgery, include:

- Surgical site infection
- Systemic infection such as leishmaniasis or rickettsia
- Incomplete acetabular reaming leading to superficial (lateral) seating of the cup
- Partial insertion of the cup caused by incomplete reaming of the peripheral acetabulum
- Poor press-fit because of excessive acetabular reaming
- Premature weight bearing in young active dogs.

Risk factors for late aseptic loosening, at least 6 months after surgery, include:

- Excessive polyethylene wear
- THR performed in young dogs: A long life expectancy combined with implantation of small cups (21 and 23 mm) with a thinner polyethylene liner predispose these patients to aseptic loosening.
- Implantation of small cups in adult large dogs could lead to the same consequences, with severe polyethylene wear and eventual cup breakage a few years later.

Diagnosis

- Partial aseptic cup loosening is usually asymptomatic but may be diagnosed based on radiographic studies, including a tangent view of the cup, to evaluate the interface the cup and surrounding bone (Figure 114.9A).
- Septic cup loosening and advanced aseptic cup loosening cause persistent lameness and muscle atrophy.

- Arthrocentesis with cytology and culture is required to rule out infection; although false negative results are possible, positive results are always indicative of septic cup loosening
- Samples of synovial membrane must be collected during surgery and processed for cytology and culture to address postoperative antibiotic treatment and for prognostic purposes.

Treatment

Treatment options for loosening of the acetabular component include.

- Explantation is indicated when infection caused by multidrug-resistant bacteria is diagnosed. Second stage reimplantation may be considered after several months of selected antibiotic treatment.
- One-stage implant revision is indicated in cases with septic cup loosening caused by sensitive bacteria, after antibiotherapy based on culture and sensitivity, and with intraarticular placement of slow-release antibiotics before closure.
- Revision of aseptic cup loosening caused by polyethylene wear of cup breakage can be performed as one-stage revision.
- Revision of a loose cementless cup can be performed with a new cementless implant, usually of one to two sizes bigger, to achieve adequate press-fit in the presence of acetabular bone loss.
- Implantation of a new cementless cup can be particularly challenging when bone defects or poor bone quality jeopardize press-fit placement.
- Acetabular revision with a cementless cup must provide intimate contact between the acetabular implant and the host bone to be successful. The mechanical construct must also be stable and minimize micromotion to allow bone ingrowth into the cementless acetabular component.
- A cup specifically designed for revision surgeries (Figure 114.7) is now available (Kyon Veterinary ProductsZurich (CH) and Boston (MA)). The first component of the implant is a perforated titanium outer shell with holes for 2.4-mm titanium screws. The second component is an inner plain titanium cup with an ultra-high-molecular-weight polyethylene (UHMWPE) insert. The revision procedure starts with removal of the loose cup, and reaming of the acetabulum. The outer shell is fixed with a variable number of screws. The inner component is impacted into the outer shell to obtain press-fit stability (Figures 114.7 to Figure 114.9).

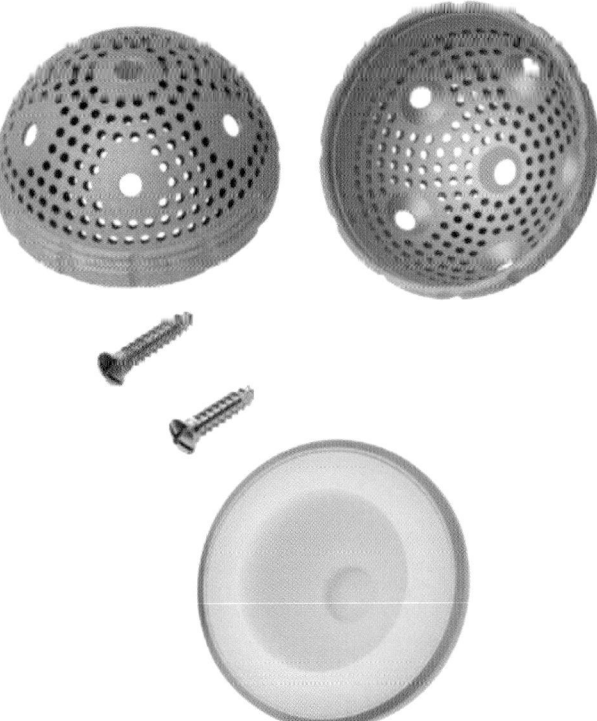

Figure 114.7 Zurich cementless total hip replacement Revision Cup (Kyon AG, Zurich (CH) and Kyon Veterinary Products, Boston MA). The outer shell is perforated for 2.4-screw fixation, and the inner shell contains a polyethylene liner.

- Prevention of infection is mandatory because any surgical revision of a THR is associated with a higher risk of infection. Strict asepsis is required, and slow-release antibiotic substances should be inserted inside the joint space before closure for that purpose. Among these, the author has used a collagen sponge (Septocoll) impregnated with sulphate gentamicin (released within 24 hours) and crobefate gentamicin (released in 7 days). An injectable polymer hydrogel (VetriGel) is currently undergoing clinical trials as a delivery system for amikacin in septic arthritis.

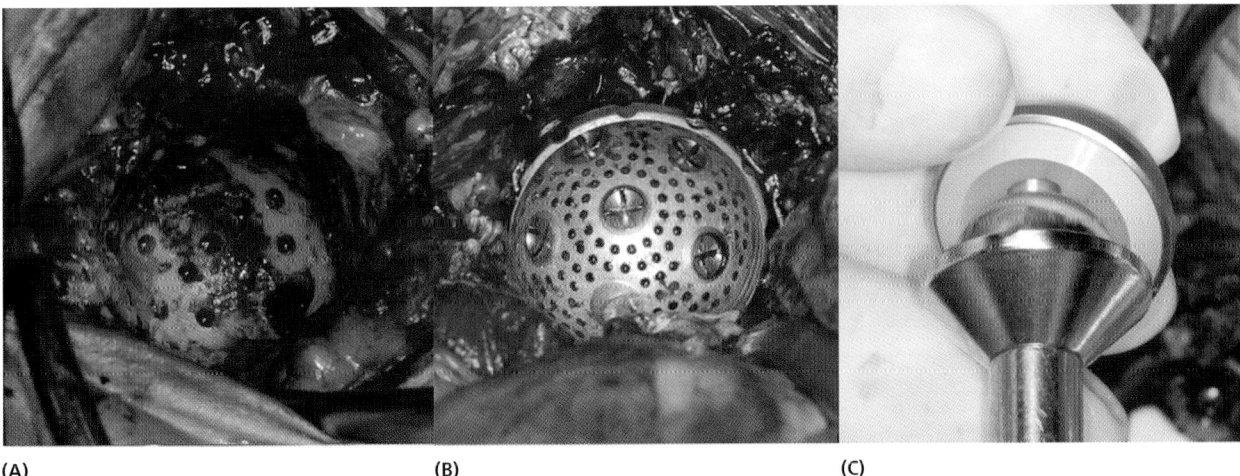

(A) (B) (C)

Figure 114.8 Revision of a cup after aseptic loosening. **A**, Curettage of the acetabulum and osteostixis. **B**, Fixation of the outer shell with cruciform-head screws. **C**, Close-up view of the inner shell and the cup impactor. **D**, The inner shell is mounted on the impactor. **E**, The inner shell is inserted coaxially in the outer shell and impacted in position. **F**, Final view of the inner shell well impacted inside the outer shell *(Continued)*.

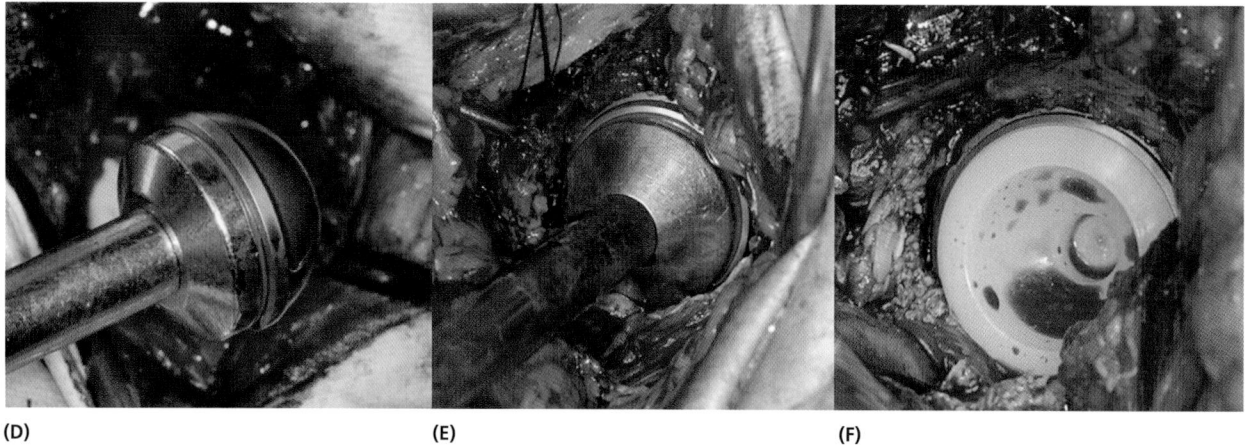

(D)   (E)   (F)

Figure 114.8 *(Continued).*

Outcome

- Revision of aseptic cup loosening is followed by osteointegration and normal joint function when adequate press-fit and stability of the new cup are achieved.
- The outcome of revision for septic cup loosening depends on the type of involved bacteria and on the ability to administer an effective antibiotic agent.

- The use of the revision cup can increase implant stability when the quality of the acetabular bone is poor.

Prevention

Early cup loosening can be prevented by:
- Proper reaming of the acetabulum and ability to achieve solid press-fit

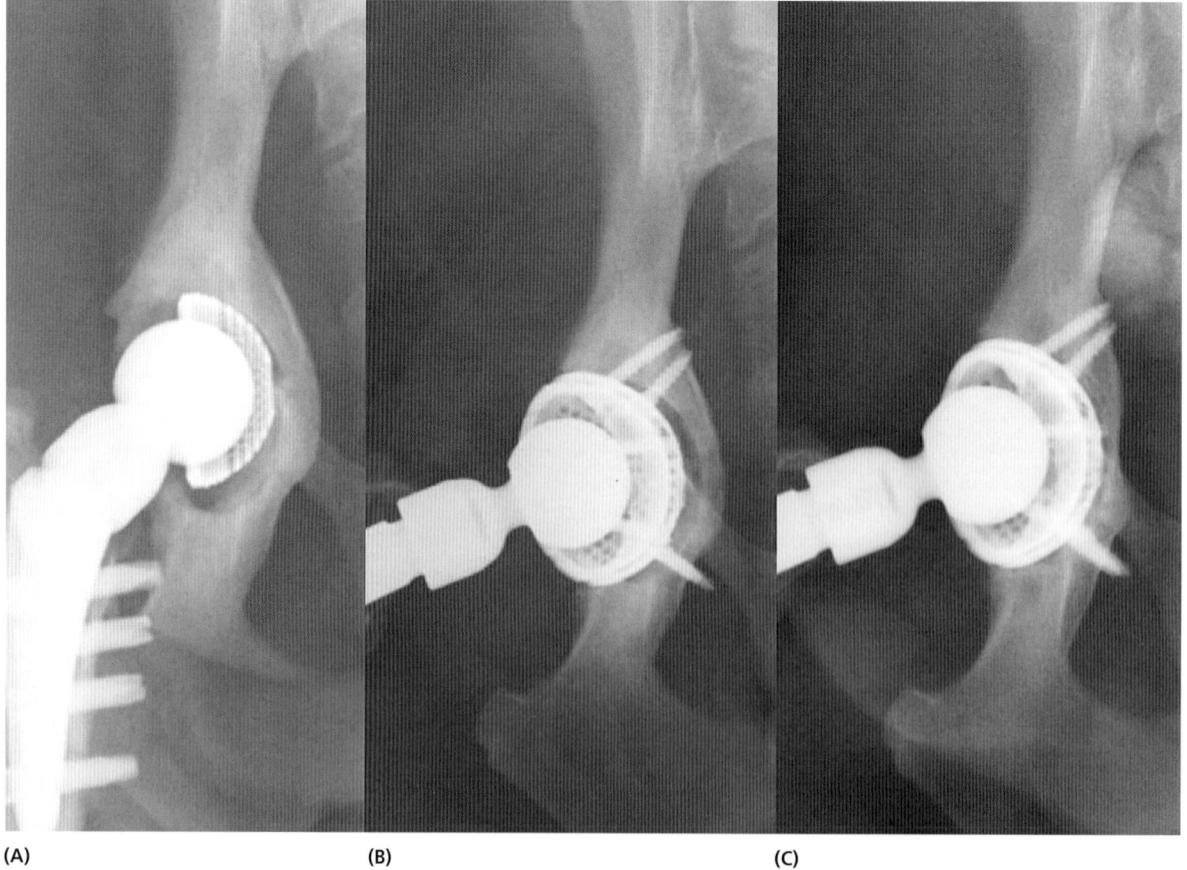

(A)   (B)   (C)

Figure 114.9 Aseptic loosening of the acetabular cup in an 8-year-old Epagneul Breton 5 years after THR. **A,** Preoperative radiographs. Note the radiolucency surrounding the cup. **B,** Radiographs after placement of a Revision Cup reinforced with 2.4-mm-diameter screws after revision. **C,** Radiographic appearance 1 year after revision.

- In case of acetabular saucerization, occasionally encountered with chronic luxation, and in immature dogs with luxated hips, initial implantation with a revision cup armed with diverging screws may be considered to prevent cup loosening

Late cup loosening can be prevented by:

- Using larger cups in young dogs; limiting the 21-mm-diameter cup to dogs weighing less than 20 kg and the 23-mm-diameter cup to dogs weighing up to 30 kg
- Whenever possible, the cup implanted during THR in growing dogs should be of the same size as the cup that would be selected in an adult dog of the same breed.
- Body condition score should be monitored and managed to remain within normal range for the entire life span of the dog.
- Physical activity should be controlled to avoid excessive exercising, and sports activity should be avoided or limited.
- Yearly radiographic follow-ups are recommended to intercept early signs of polyethylene wear, such as eccentricity of the head inside the cup and early signs of cup loosening.
- When performing THR in young and potentially active dogs, the possibility of a cup revision later in life should be discussed with to the owner.

Stem loosening or breakage

Definition

Early loss of stability of the femoral stem can result from infection and be combined with cup loosening. This complication may also occur in case of poor exercise restriction after surgery.

Late stem loosening may result from poor osteointegration, with cyclic failure of the screw fixation, screw breakage, or bone resorption. The femoral stem may undergo fatigue failure, usually because the stem is too small relative to the body weight.

Risk factors

- Early excessive physical activity may affect osteointegration and promote stem loosening.
- Poor selection of the femoral stem size relative to the body size and weight can cause fatigue failure of the screws or the stem.
- Bone loss in the proximal medial cortex from stress shielding can cause cyclic motion of the stem, eventually leading to its breakage.
- Excessive polyethylene wear activates osteoclasts, inducing bone resorption around both the cup and the stem.

Diagnosis

- Early aseptic loosening of the femoral stem may be overlooked clinically but can be diagnosed with radiographs oriented tangentially to the stem to evaluate the interface between stem, screws, and surrounding bone.
- Septic stem loosening and advanced aseptic stem loosening cause progressive lameness and reduction in muscle mass.
- Stem breakage usually causes sudden lameness that may resolve spontaneously when the broken stem locks itself in the bone.

Treatment

Surgical revision is indicated in all cases of femoral stem loosening or failure:

- General strategies are included in Box 114.1
- To remove the loose stem, access holes are created in the lateral femoral cortex using a high speed burr. A trial stem serves as a template to locate the screws (Figures 114.10 to 114.12)
- The screws are loosened with a sharp screwdriver, which must be well seated inside the hexagonal recess of the screw. Each screw

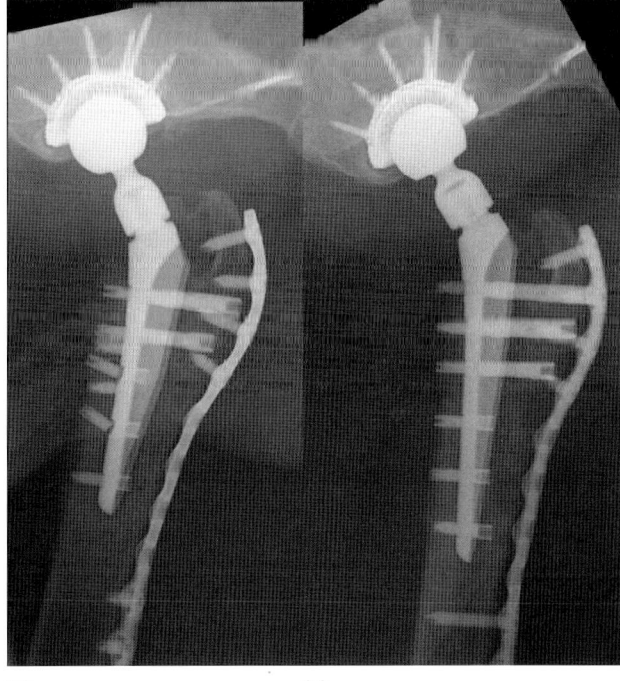

(A)   (B)

Figure 114.10 Femoral stem loosening. **A**, Recurrence of stem loosening with screws breakage in a 6-year-old, 65-kg male Rottweiler. **B**, Radiographic appearance 3 months after revision with an extra-long, custom stem.

head should first be cleaned from bone or fibrous tissue with a pointed tartar scaler.

- Screws that cannot be removed because the head has been stripped because of cold metal welding should be destroyed by overdrilling with a high-speed steel drill bit.
- Trying to remove stripped screws by hammering from a medial approach after cutting the bone all around the tip of the screw may result in femoral fracture.
- Tools specifically designed for this application should be used to remove bicortical screws with stripped hexagonal recesses.
- The new stem is inserted after preparation of the femoral canal. The revision stem must be fixed slightly proximal to the previous implant (to avoid the need for a longer head–neck unit) and with a slightly different anteversion to avoid existing screw holes.

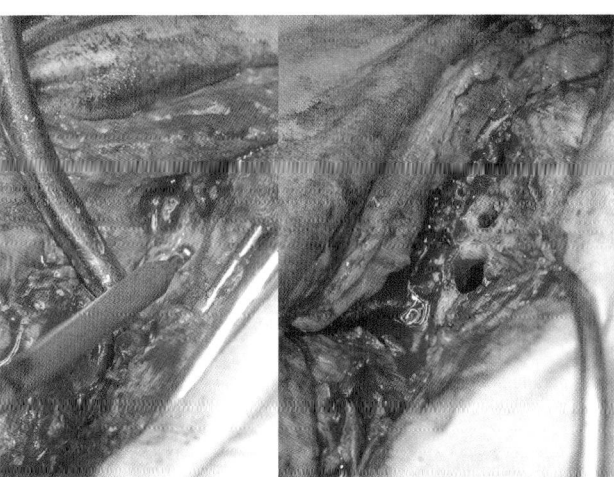

Figure 114.11 A high-speed burr is used to perforate the lateral cortex of the femur and identified embedded screws.

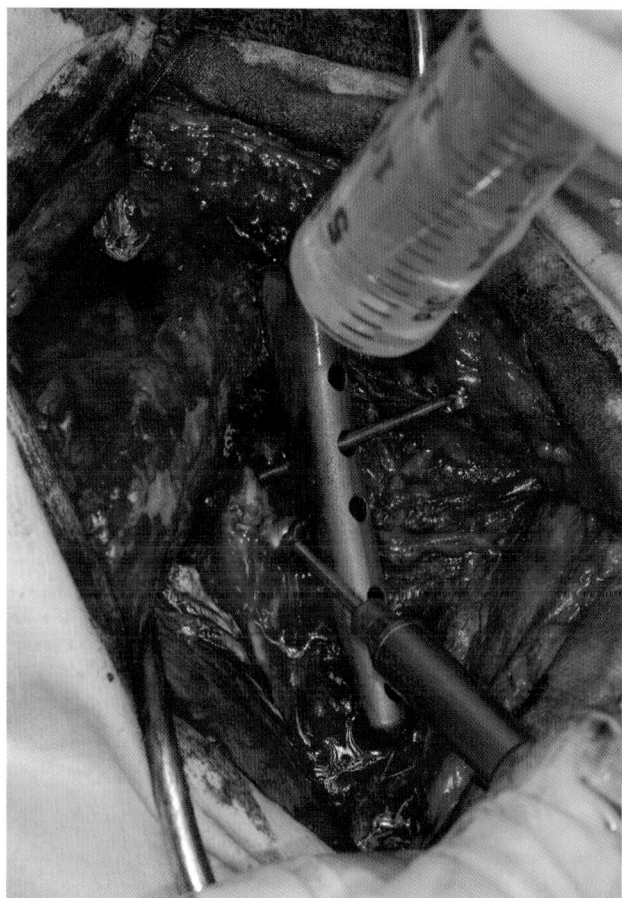

Figure 114.12 Use of a trial stem as a template to guide the placement of holes in the lateral femoral cortex.

- In case of a broken stem, the proximal part can be removed easily as well as the head–neck unit. The distal portion of the stem is usually well osteointegrated and requires creation of a lateral femoral window for its removal. The window is returned in position and the area protected by a buttress plate (Figures 114.13 to 114.15).

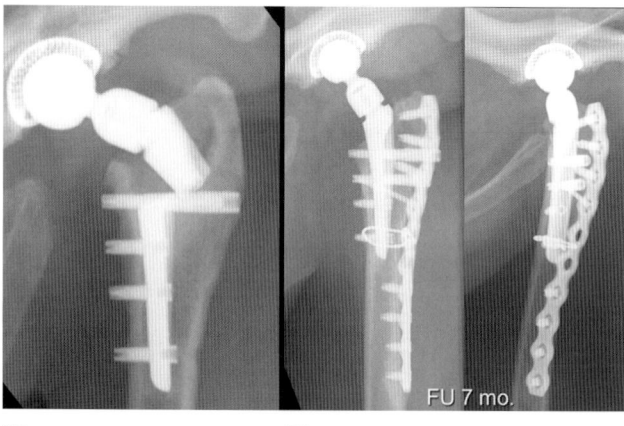

(A)   (B)

Figure 114.13 Revision of a broken femoral stem. **A,** Broken X-Small Stem in a 6-year-old border collie 4 years after Zurich cementless total hip replacement (Kyon AG, Zurich (CH) and Kyon Veterinary Products, Boston MA). **B,** Radiographs obtained 7 months after removal of the failed implant through a lateral femoral window, revision with a Small Stem, and protective femoral plating.

- Prevention of infection is mandatory because any THR surgical revision is associated with an increased risk of infection. Strict aseptic surgery is required, and slow-release antibiotic substances should be inserted inside the joint space before closure.

Outcome
- Septic stem loosening requires explantation and conversion of THR in a temporary or permanent femoral head and neck ostectomy (FHNO). After antibiotherapy based on culture and sensitivity, implantation of a new prosthesis can be considered several months after explantation in case of unsatisfactory function with the FHNO.
- Stem revision for aseptic stem loosening has a good prognosis if strong fixation of the screws is achieved via engagement in quality bone and avoidance of previous holes.

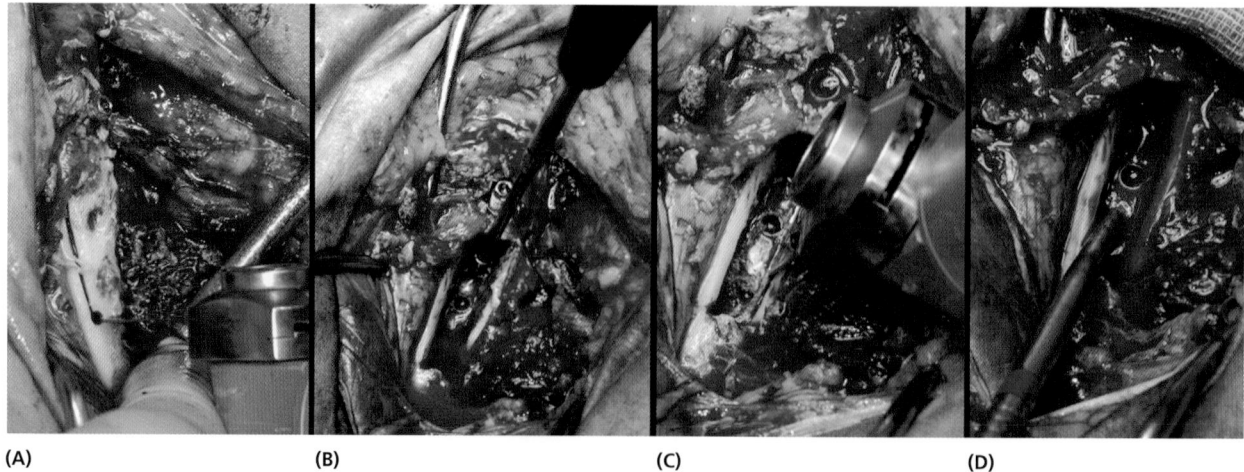

(A)   (B)   (C)   (D)

Figure 114.14 Lateral femoral window for implant revision in the case in Figure 114.13. **A,** Four holes are drilled at each corner of the intended window. The window is created in the lateral femoral cortex with an oscillating saw. **B,** Screws are loosened and removed. **C,** The interface between the integrated stem and surrounding bone is disrupted with a fine-blade oscillating saw. **D,** The stem is removed by hammering the impactor.

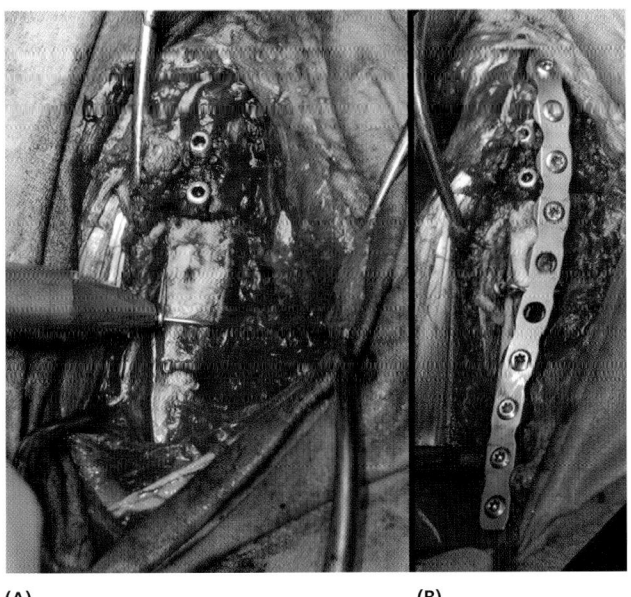

(A)   **(B)**

Figure 114.15 Fixation of the femoral window with a cerclage wire (**A**) and protection with an ALPS 10 (Advanced Locking Plate System, KYON AG, Switzerland) plate (**B**) in the case illustrated in Figure 114.13.

Prevention

Early stem loosening can be prevented by:
- Proper surgical technique
- Strict postoperative care and activity restriction.

Late stem loosening, breakage of the screws, and stem breakage can be prevented by:
- Proper sizing of the stem to the body weight
- Lifelong maintenance of body condition score within normal range to avoid imbalance with the implant size
- Extra-small stems should only be placed in dogs weighing less than 20 kg.
- Small stems should only be placed in dogs weighing up to 30 kg.
- Medium stem should only be placed in dogs weighing up to 40 kg.
- Large stems are indicated in dogs weighing more than 40 kg.
- As a general principle, the largest possible stem that can be inserted in the femoral canal should be selected to provide maximal strength.

Relevant literature

The literature concerning specifically the Z-THR is still quite limited. The risk of **infection** increases with each revision because of vascular impairment. Strict adherence to the principles of aseptic surgery is therefore critical in any revision. Gentamicin-impregnated equine collagen sponges are useful for providing a slow release of local antibiotics over several days (Owen *et al.* 2004; Vezzoni 2010). The sponge is left inside the joint capsule before closure in every revision.

The incidence of **luxation** after Z-THR has been reported from 3.7% to 11% in three different studies (Guerrero and Montavon 2009; Vezzoni 2009; Hummel *et al.* 2010). In Newfoundlands, the incidence of luxation reaches up to 20% (Vezzoni 2009).

Assessment of proper cup and neck orientation is critical for a stable hip reduction (Aman and Wendelburg 2013).

Intraoperative **fractures** of the femur and greater trochanter seem to occur frequently and have been reported in 9.2% of cases (Hummel *et al.* 2010) as a consequence of technical errors. Postoperative fractures seem less common because their incidence ranged from 1.1% to 1.2% in three different studies (Guerrero and Montavon 2009; Vezzoni 2009; Hummel *et al.* 2010). Several strategies have been proposed to prevent these complications. The insertion of two bicortical screws in the proximal femur is recommended to improve the rotational stability of the stem and reduce bone stress in weak bone (immature dogs; Vezzoni 2009). In an ex vivo study, placing three single-loop, 1-mm-diameter cerclage wires, one between the fourth and the fifth screw and two distally to the fifth screw, provided some protection against postoperative fractures (Pozzi *et al.* 2013). In the same study, more protection was provided by fixing a buttress plate from the trochanter to the distal femur. This buttress plate bridges the area distal to the stem, which is predisposed to postoperative fractures. In a clinical study, femoral fractures were prevented by applying a buttress plate to the femur. Monocortical screws were used to distribute loading forces over a wider area. The S-shaped plate was twisted proximally behind the stem and distally, lateral to the femur (Vezzoni 2009, 2010).

Cup loosening after Z-THR has been reported with an incidence of 3%, 3.7%, and 2.5% in three different studies; the latter study also reported cup breakage with subsequent loosening in 1.6% of cases (Guerrero and Montavon 2009; Hummel *et al.* 2010; Vezzoni 2011). Septic cup loosening and advanced aseptic cup loosening caused persistent lameness and muscle atrophy (Hanson *et al.* 2006; Guerrero and Montavon 2009; Vezzoni 2009). In human patients, adjunct fixation is advised in all cases of cup revision, including multiple screws to minimize micromotion and to promote bone ingrowth (Deirmengian *et al.* 2011). The Z-THR revision cup was used in 31 dogs with cup loosening and a minimum follow-up period of 6 months (Vezzoni *et al.* 2013). This study reported four intraoperative and two postoperative complications. The main intraoperative complication consisted of difficulties inserting the inner cup into its outer shell. Postoperative complications included craniodorsal hip luxation in one dog, which was successfully managed, and cup loosening in another dog, which required explantation of the prosthesis. Recent technical improvements in Z-THR have addressed several issues of the previous implants and are aimed at reducing the risk of luxation in giant dogs and the incidence of long-term implant failure (Tepic 2012). Implantation of a larger femoral head (measuring 19 mm in diameter) coupled with 29- and 32-mm-diameter cups in large and giant dogs has been shown to greatly reduce the risk of luxation in those predisposed dogs (Vezzoni 2009, 2011). In humans, increasing the diameter of the head has also been shown to generate resistance to luxation after THR (Howie *et al.* 2012).

The previous generation of Z-THR cups included 1 mm of space between the polyethylene inlay and the titanium shell, which was seen to cause some deformation of the liner over time and an increase in polyethylene wear. The current-generation Z-THR cups are composed of two shells: The inner shell supports the polyethylene inlay, thereby avoiding its deformation during loading, particularly in small cups. This shell also isolates the back side of the polyethylene inlay from the bone, possibly improving the osteointegration of the outer, perforated titanium shell. Moreover, the UHMWPE inlay has a special geometry, designed to reduce wear by modifying contact between the polyethylene and the metal head. These newly designed heads are coated with amorphous diamond to reduce the coefficient of friction and further minimize the polyethylene wear. The current generation of femoral stems benefit from micropinning metal treatment during manufacturing, making them 10% larger and 25% stronger than the previous generation.

References

Aman, A.M., Wendelburg, K.L. (2013) Assessment of acetabular cup positioning from a lateral radiographic projection after total hip replacement. *Veterinary Surgery* 42, 406-412.

Deirmengian, G.K., Zmistowski, B., O'Neil, J.T., et al. (2011) Management of acetabular bone loss in revision total hip arthroplasty. *Journal of Bone and Joint Surgery* 93, 1842-1852.

Guerrero, T.G., Montavon, P.M. (2009) Zurich cementless total hip replacement: retrospective evaluation of 2nd generation implants in 60 dogs. *Veterinary Surgery* 38 (1), 70-80.

Hanson, S.P., Peck, J.N., Berry, C.R., et al. (2006) Radiographic evaluation of the Zurich cementless total hip acetabular component. *Veterinary Surgery* 35 (6), 550-558.

Howie, D.W., Holubowycz, O.T., Middleton, R. (2012) Large femoral heads decrease the incidence of dislocation after total hip arthroplasty: a randomized controlled trial. *Journal of Bone and Joint Surgery* 94 (12), 1095-1102.

Hummel, D.W., Lanz, O.I., Were, S.R. (2010) Complications of cementless total hip replacement: a retrospective study of 163 cases. *Veterinary and Comparative Orthopaedics and Traumatology* 6, 424-432.

Owen, M.R., Moores, A.P., Coe, R.J. (2004) Management of MRSA septic arthritis in a dog using a gentamicin-impregnated collagen sponge. *Journal of Small Animal Practice* 45, 609-612.

Pozzi, A., Peck, J.N., Chao, P., et al. (2013) Mechanical evaluation of adjunctive fixation fro prevention of periprosthetic fracture with Zurich cementless total hip prosthesis. *Veterinary Surgery* 42, 529-534.

Tepic, S., Montavon, P.M. (2004) Concepts of Zurich cementless prosthesis. *European Society of Veterinary Orthopaedics and Traumatology Proceedings*, Munich, September.

Tepic S. (2012) Z-THR Development. http://www.kyon.ch. Accessed 2012.

Vezzoni A. (2009) Risk factors for complications in the Zurich cementless THR. *Proceedings ECVS Meeting*, Nantes.

Vezzoni, A. (2011) My last 1000 cases of Z-THR, what I have learned. *Proceedings of the 2011 ACVS Symposium*, Chicago, pp. 227-229.

Vezzoni A. (2012) Revision of Kyon THR. *Proceedings of 3rd World Veterinary Orthopaedic Congress ESVOT-VOS*, Bologna, September 15-18, pp. 464-467.

Vezzoni, L., Montinaro, V., Vezzoni, A. (2013) Use of a revision cup for treatment of Zurich cementless acetabular cup loosening. Surgical technique and clinical application in 31 cases. *Veterinary and Comparative Orthopaedics and Traumatology* 26, 408-415.

115 Open Reduction of Coxofemoral Luxations

Mark Rochat

Department of Veterinary Clinical Sciences, College of Veterinary Medicine, Purdue University, IN, USA

The coxofemoral (hip) joint is the most commonly affected by luxations in dogs (Basher *et al.* 1986; Ablin and Gambardella 1991). Craniodorsal luxation is by far most common, but ventral luxations occur on occasion. Closed reduction is often attempted initially in the absence of contraindications, such as hip dysplasia, Legg-Perthes disease, and concurrent articular or periarticular fractures. Closed reduction is generally followed by application of an Ehmer sling. Reluxation rates of 40% to 70% have been reported after closed reduction, and complications secondary to sling application are common.

Open reduction is pursued when closed reduction fails or preexisting factors advise against closed reduction. These factors include chronic luxation, concurrent preexisting disease processes, or the presence of a large avulsion fracture of the round ligament (Figure 115.1).

Success rates for open reduction techniques vary among studies and method of repair but generally range from 66% to 100%, with an average of approximately 85% (Fox 1991; McLaughlin 1995). Stabilization techniques after reduction of a coxofemoral luxation include toggle rod or other technique designed to mimic the round ligament of the femoral head, capsulorrhaphy, dorsal augmentation, antirotational suture, transacetabular pinning, and greater trochanteric transposition. Complications include recurrence of the luxation; implant failure; and, less commonly, sciatic neuropraxia.

Infection (see Chapters 1 and 6)

Recurrence

Definition

Recurrence is reluxation of the hip after reduction with or without stabilization.

Reluxation can occur for a number of reasons, including poor case selection, poor or intraoperative decision making, technical error, implant failure (see Chapter 94), and inadequate postoperative care.

Risk factors

Risk factors relevant to all cases of coxofemoral luxation include:
- Duration of the luxation: Maintaining reduction in chronic luxations is more difficult.
- Previous failed attempts at reduction: Attempting reduction may damage the joint capsule and other soft tissues.

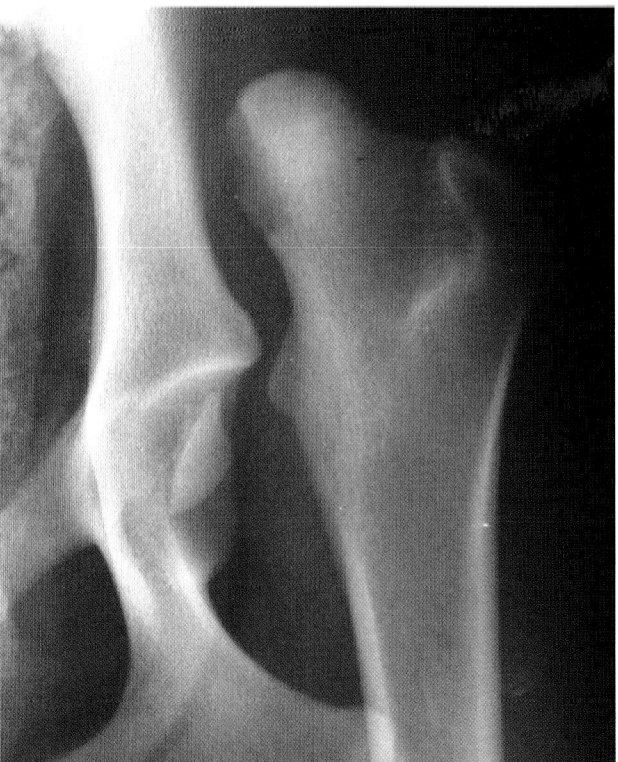

Figure 115.1 Dorsoventral radiograph of the pelvis of a dog with craniodorsal coxofemoral luxation and an avulsion fracture of the femoral head. Failure to identify concurrent injuries can complicate hip reduction and stabilization.

Both chronicity (often with some degree of weight bearing) and previous reduction attempts can aggravate damage to the joint capsule and surrounding soft tissues, leading to edema, inflammation, and destruction of supporting soft tissues. Failed reductions may be an indication of poor case selection.
- Poor case selection (Figure 115.2), and poor intraoperative decision making, or technical errors: Recurrence of the luxation can occur if poor decisions are made during surgery. These decisions are often technique dependent and require the surgeon to properly evaluate the situation at hand when selecting the surgical technique(s).

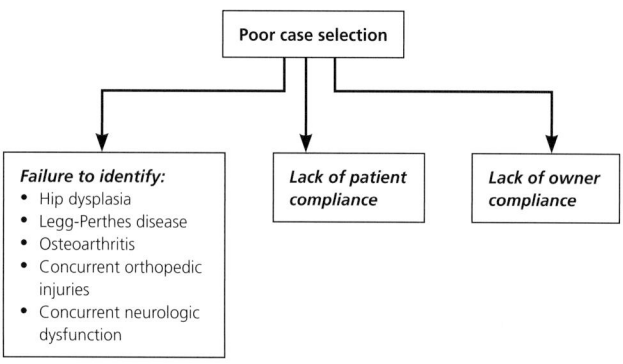

Figure 115.2 Contraindications to closed reduction of coxofemoral luxations.

Other risk factors, such as technical errors, vary with the surgical procedure.

Capsulorrhaphy

The technique stabilizes the hip by directly repairing the joint capsule (a primary stabilizer of the hip). Potential technical errors include:

- Inadequate integrity of joint capsule remnants
- Improper suturing of the joint capsule

Placement of a toggle rod (Çetinkaya and Olcay 2010)

The principle of this technique is to mimic the function of the ligament of the head of the femur with a suture secured medial to the acetabular medial cortex, entering the femoral head through the fovea capitis femoris, and exiting at the base of the greater trochanter.

Several technical errors can jeopardize the postoperative stability of the joint:

- Inadequate size, shape, or orientation of the toggle rod (mainly when using hand-made rods) (Demko *et al.* 2006)
- Failure to properly seat the rod against the medial acetabular wall
- Insufficient or inappropriate size or type of suture
- Failure of the suture knot or metal crimp
- Improper or inadequate reduction of the femoral head
- Excessive laxity of the prosthesis (suture, nylon line, or tape)
- Excessive tightness of the prosthesis

Fascia lata loop

The principle of this technique is the same as that for the toggle rod because it is designed to simulate the function of the ligament of the head of the femur.

Potential technical errors include:

- Inadequate width of fascial strip
- Improper or inadequate reduction of the femoral head: This may partially result from a failure to adequately debride the of the ligament of the head of the femur remnants from the acetabulum.
- Excessive laxity of the fascial strip
- Inadequate suturing of the loop to the third trochanter

Sacrotuberous ligament transposition

The principle of this technique is also aimed at simulating the function of the ligament of the head of the femur.

Potential technical errors include:

- Improper or inadequate reduction of the femoral head: This may partially result from a failure to adequately debride the ligament of the head of the femur remnants from the acetabulum.

- Excessive laxity of the sacrotuberous ligament
- Inadequate stabilization of the ligament or bone to the femur

Combined intra- and extraarticular stabilization (Venturini *et al.* 2010)

This technique uses a length of nylon (Bühner) tape to create a prosthetic round ligament as well as create a dorsal augmentation band secured to the femoral neck.

Potential technical errors include:

- Improper or inadequate reduction of the femoral head: This may partially result from a failure to adequately debride the round ligament remnants from the acetabulum
- Excessive laxity of the tape
- Failure of the knot
- Excessive tightness of the tape

Transacetabular pinning

This technique prevents luxation by rigidly securing the femoral head in the acetabulum by means of a metallic pin.

Potential technical errors include:

- Pin breakage (Figure 115.3) (Sissener *et al.* 2009)
- Femoral or acetabular fracture
- Pin migration
- Femoral head resorption (cats and dogs)

Tenodesis of the deep gluteal muscle (Rochereau and Bernardé 2012)

The technique is designed to prevent external rotational and adduction of the limb by compressing the deep gluteal tendon against the cranial edge of the acetabulum with a bone screw and spiked washer.

Potential technical errors include:

- Improper or inadequate seating of the screw and washer in the rectus femoris tuberosity
- Failure to abduct and internally rotate the femur during screw placement
- Inadequate or unhealthy deep gluteal muscle
- Inadequate or unhealthy joint capsule or failure to perform adjunct capsulorrhaphy

Dorsal augmentation (Johnson and Braden 1987)

The technique stabilizes the hip by applying tensioned sutures over the dorsal aspect of the joint capsule (Figure 115.4). The tight sutures prevent the lateral translocation and luxation of the femoral head.

Potential technical errors include:

- Pull out of screw(s) or anchor(s) placed in the dorsal acetabular rim
- Slipping of the suture off the screw head
- Suture breakage
- Failure of the anchor site on the femur

Antirotational suture

In this technique, suture is placed such that the hip is maintained in a neutral position, preventing external rotation.

Potential technical errors include:

- Improper screw or anchor placement cranial to the acetabulum
- Slipping of the suture off of the screw head
- Suture breakage
- Femoral or pelvic suture anchor site failure
- Improper positioning of the limb or joint when tightening the suture (neutral rotation and sagittal plane positioning is desired; excessive internal or external rotation will result in failure.)

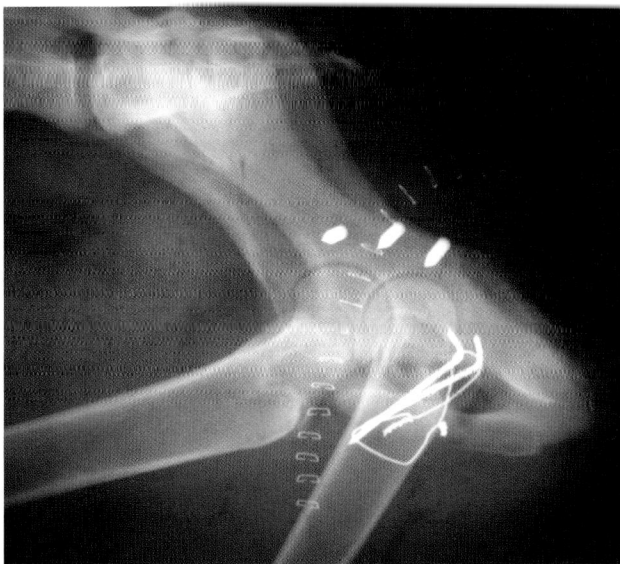

Figure 115.3 Lateral radiograph illustrating a combination of techniques to stabilize a craniodorsal luxation of the hip: 1, dorsal acetabular rim augmentation and antirotational sutures using suture anchors; 2, capsulorrhaphy; and 3, caudodistal transposition of the greater trochanter. Combining techniques tends to decrease the risk of recurrence.

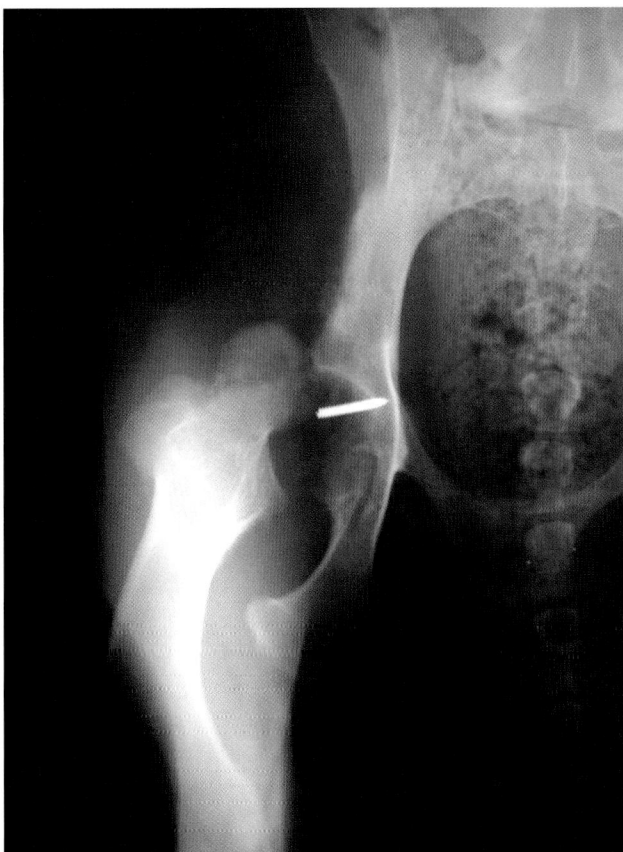

Figure 115.4 Dorsoventral radiograph of the pelvis of a dog with recurrent craniodorsal hip luxation after breakage of a transacetabular pin. The threaded portion of an end-threaded Steinman pin remains in the acetabulum. Osteolysis and irregular periosteal reaction were confirmed to result from concurrent joint sepsis.

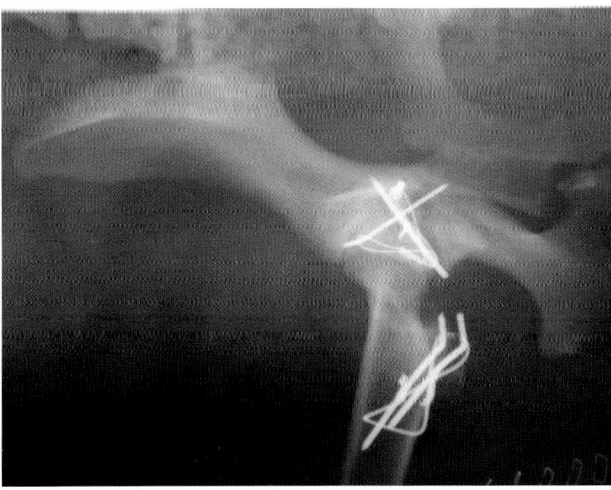

Figure 115.5 Lateral radiograph of a dog with a hip luxation and central acetabular fracture (repaired with Kirschner wires, interfragmentary wire, and polymethylmethacrylate cement). An osteotomy of the greater trochanter allowed repair of the fracture and reduction of the hip luxation. The trochanter has been reattached with pins and wire tension band to the femur distolateral to its normal location to increase gluteal muscle tension across the hip to support the primary repair.

Caudodistal transposition of the greater trochanter

This technique stabilizes the hip by stretching the dorsal gluteal muscles over the joint, imparting a short-term support.

Potential technical errors include:
- Insufficient bone stock due to inadequate osteotomy
- Improper implant placement
- Improper implant size
- Implant failure

See Figure 115.5.

Diagnosis

Recurrence of luxation after surgery is diagnosed based on a recurrence of clinical signs consistent with coxofemoral luxation (Table 115.1):
- Change in gait: The animal has become more cautious about bearing weight or non–weight bearing if allowed to bear weight. The limb is held in external rotation if the hip is luxated in a craniodorsal luxation

Table 115.1 Clinical Findings for Differentiating Craniodorsal Hip Luxation from Ventral Hip Luxation

Craniodorsal Hip Luxation
• Affected leg shorter
• Thigh adducted
• Stifle externally rotated
• Increased distance between greater trochanter and ischiatic tuberosity
• "V" formed by greater trochanter, dorsal iliac crest, and ischiatic tuberosity is shallow or nonexistent

Ventral Hip Luxation
• Affected leg longer
• Thigh abducted
• Stifle internally rotated
• Greater trochanter hard to palpate
• "V" formed by greater trochanter, dorsal iliac crest, and ischiatic tuberosity is deeper

Clinical Findings Common to Both Types of Luxations
• Variable degrees of lameness and pain
• Failed "thumb test"
• Crepitus

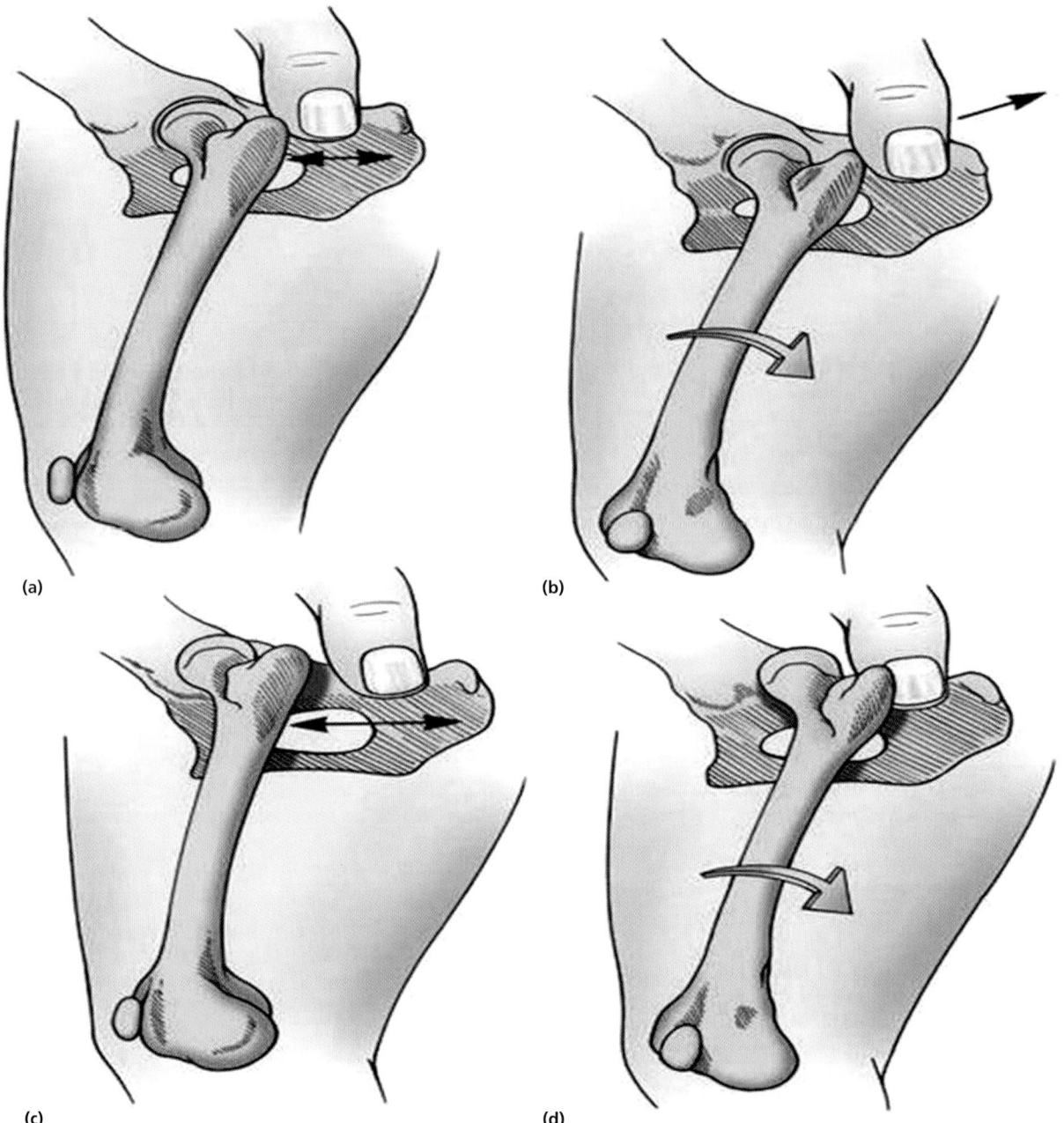

(a)

(b)

(c)

(d)

Figure 115.6 Line drawing illustrating the "thumb test" for diagnosis of cranidorsal coxofemoral luxation. The examiner's thumb is placed in the lesser ischiatic notch, and the pelvic limb is externally rotated. Failure of the greater trochanter to push the examiner's thumb from the notch, combined with a wider notch, is consistent with craniodorsal hip luxation. (Parts **A** and **B** demonstrate expulsion of the thumb from the lesser ischiatic notch with external rotation of the femur while Parts **C** and **D** demonstrate how external rotation of the femur fails to push the thumb from the notch). *Source:* Johnson 2013. Reproduced with permission from Elsevier.

- Increased pain beyond levels expected after surgery
- Excessive swelling around the hip
- Failure of the "thumb test" (Figure 115.6)
- Shortened limb length is consistent with craniodorsal luxation
- Loss of normal spatial alignment of the greater trochanter, ischiatic tuberosity, and dorsal iliac crest (Figure 115.7)

Any or all of these signs can suggest failure of the stabilization and recurrence of the luxation. The diagnosis is confirmed via radio-graphic examination. Specific aspects of failure are determined by the repair method used for stabilization.

Treatment

Correction of the recurrence begins by reassessing the patient for risk factors such as hip dysplasia, concurrent injuries, and preexisting conditions that created an imbalance between the demands placed on the hip and the biomechanical properties of

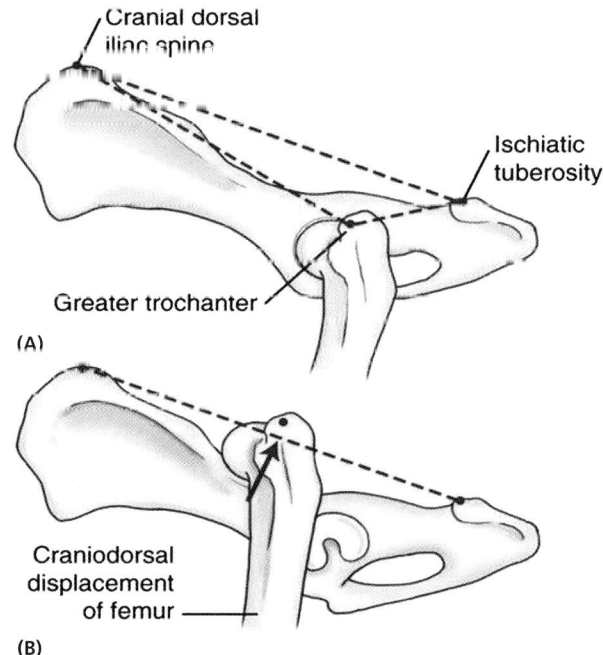

Figure 115.7 Line drawing illustrating the normal positional relationship of the ischiatic tuberosity, greater trochanter, and dorsal iliac crest. Craniodorsal hip luxation results in the three structures assuming a more linear alignment, as opposed to a shallow "V" conformation when the hip is not luxated. Additionally, the greater trochanter is closer to the iliac crest when the hip is dislocated. **A**, normal spatial relationship of the greater trochanter to the iliac crest and ischiatic tuberosity; **B**, change in spatial relationship of the above palpable structures when dislocation occurs). *Source:* Wardlaw and McLaughlin, 2012. Reproduced with permission from Elsevier.

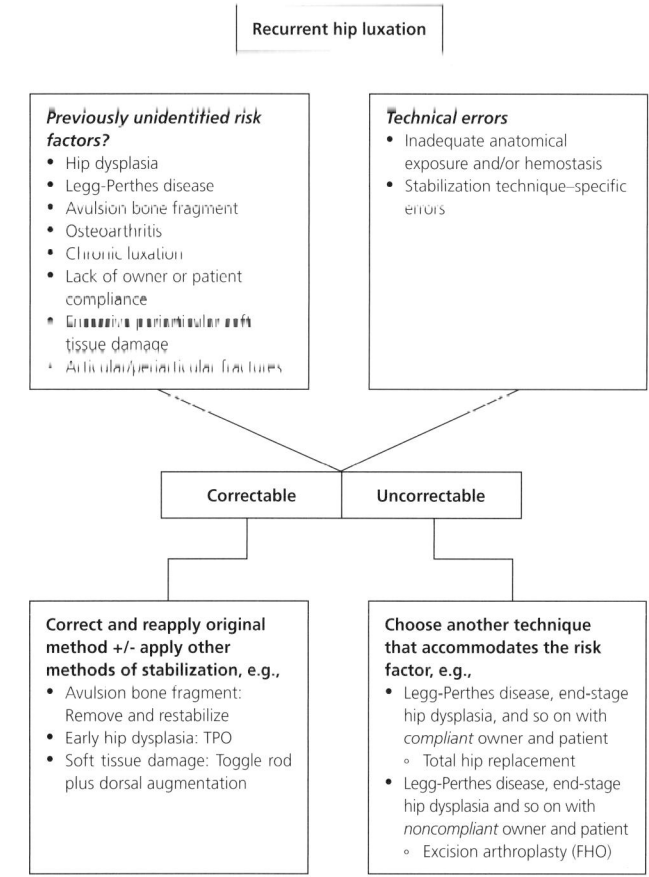

Figure 115.8 Algorithm for treatment of recurrent hip luxation.

the repair (Figure 115.8). Radiographs and surgical report should be reviewed to identify potential technical errors. Assuming open reduction is still appropriate and technical errors can be corrected, the original technique can be reapplied. More often than not, additional techniques must be combined or adjustments in post-operative care must be made to achieve success (Figure 115.9). Correction of poor intraoperative decision making varies largely with the technique that is used; steps taken to revise a failed repair are designed to prevent reluxation and are listed in this chapter under Prevention.

Outcome

The outcome after revision of failed hip luxation stabilization has not been described in detail in the veterinary literature. It is reasonable to assume that revision is appropriate if the patient was initially a good candidate for open reduction, infection is not present, and the articular surfaces of the femoral head and acetabulum do not appear severely damaged as a result of the failed repair. Unless technical errors were obvious in the original stabilization procedure, the use of other techniques or a combination of techniques is strongly advised to avoid repeated failure. Success rates with revision surgery can be considered high, assuming the factors above are addressed.

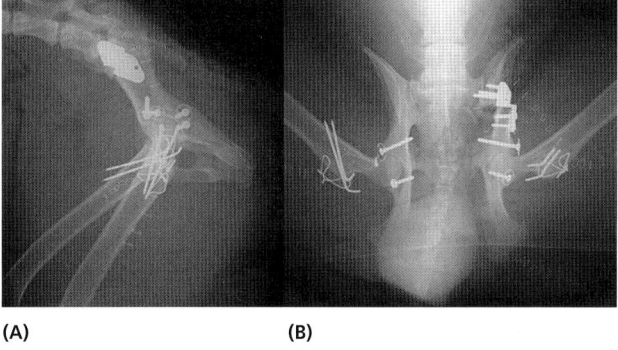

Figure 115.9 Bilateral coxofemoral luxations initially treated via capsulorrhaphy, dorsal augmentation, and transposition of the greater trochanter in a 7-year-old German shepherd that was hit by a car. Mild hip dysplasia and degenerative joint disease were observed after recurrence of the left coxofemoral luxation. The dog was successfully treated via revision of the left dorsal augmentation and triple pelvic osteotomy. **A**, lateral pelvic radiograph demonstrating placement of a triple pelvic osteotomy plate to rotate the acetabulum ventrally to improve stability of the joint. Screws and spiked washers have been placed as anchors for dorsal suture augmentation of the hip. The Kirschner wires and figure of eight tension bands have been placed to secure trochanteric osteotomies used to approach the hip for screw and washer placement. **B**, Ventro dorsal radiograph demonstrating the same features as in A. *Source:* H. Griffin, IMEX Veterinary, Longview, TX. Reproduced with permission from H. Griffin.

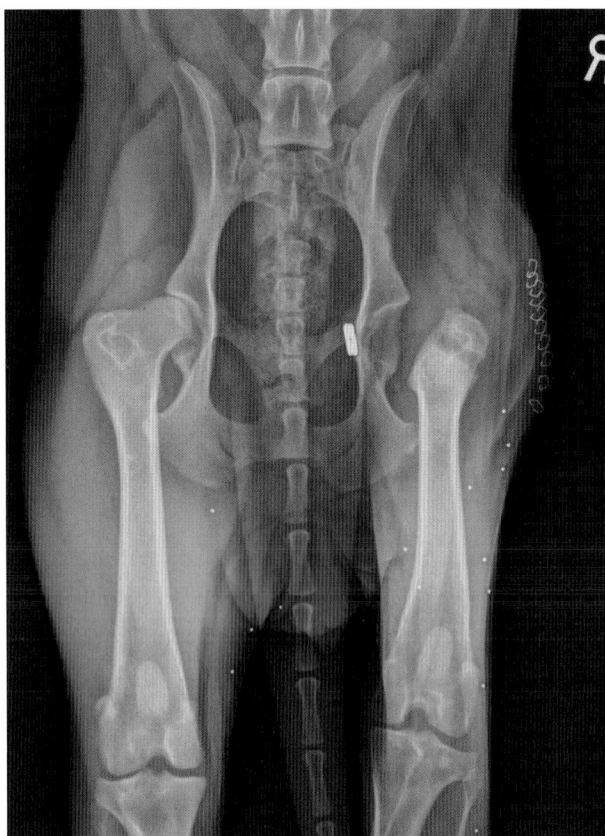

Figure 115.10 Ventrodorsal radiograph of an approximately 20-kg dog presented for a craniodorsal hip luxation. Mild hip dysplasia and lack of owner compliance resulted in recurrence of luxation 1 week after surgery following a dog fight. Revision by hip excision arthroplasty was performed.

Salvage procedures should be considered if factors predisposing the repair to failure are identified during evaluation. These factors may have been previously unidentified or may have developed after initial reduction. Such factors may include excessive damage of articular surfaces, infection, or lack of owner compliance. In these cases, excision arthroplasty or total hip arthroplasty may be preferable (Figure 115.10).

Prevention

Steps may be taken to avoid recurrence before, during, and after surgical treatment of a coxofemoral luxation.

Pre-operative phase:

- Good case selection: Dogs with preexisting coxofemoral disease may be better candidates for total hip replacement or excision arthroplasty.
- Accurate preoperative assessment of risk factors is a prerequisite to appropriate case selection. The assessment should focus on the radiographic detection of risk factors as well as evaluating the ability of the dog and its owner to follow postoperative instructions
- Patients should also be evaluated for their likelihood to comply with postoperative recommendations. A combination of procedures may be considered to immobilize the hip in combination with placement of a postoperative sling.

Excision arthroplasty may be considered as a last resort in patients that cannot be controlled, especially if owners are not willing to accept the risk of recurrence.

Intraoperative phase

General preventive measures include:

- Good knowledge of the relevant surgical anatomy to identify landmarks for placement of implants
- Good understanding of the principle behind each surgical procedure proposed for the treatment of coxofemoral luxation
- Maintain good visualization of the surgical site through:
  ○ Proper hemostasis and electrosurgery
  ○ Retraction of tissues: plan on surgical assistance being available during surgery
  ○ Lighting: Consider the use of a headlight.
  ○ Be prepared to perform a trochanteric osteotomy if needed.
- Careful removal of all soft tissues (usually edematous round ligament) present in the acetabulum to ensure good reduction of the femoral head
- Selection of the appropriate size and type of suture

Other preventive measures are specific to the repair technique and target a variety of complications:

Toggle rod repair (modified Knowles technique)

A commercial toggle rod of appropriate size and length should be considered to prevent pull-out (migration) of the toggle rod. General guidelines to select implant size include:

- 2.7-mm-diameter toggle system (IMEX Veterinary, Longview, TX) or mini TightRope fibertape (Arthrex Vet Systems, Naples, FL) for dogs weighing less than 5 kg and cats
- 3.2-mm-diameter toggle system or standard TightRope fibertape for dogs weighing 6 to 30 kg
- 4-mm-diameter toggle system or standard TightRope fibertape for dogs weighing more than 30 kg

The size of the anchor varies somewhat with the suture or tape used to create the neoligament. For example, fibertape and braided suture are not as big and bulky as monofilament nylon and therefore most likely to fit through the eyelet of a smaller anchor. Two smaller anchors can be placed to provide the needed strength and avoid complete failure if one suture breaks. Preference should be given to newer, two-hole toggle rods.

Although excessive tightness can lead to suture breakage, laxity predisposes to reluxation. Laxity of the toggle repair may be decreased by the following steps:

- Verifying that the rod is well seated against the acetabular wall: The rod should be fully pushed through the acetabular drill hole and turned sideways.
- Thoroughly checking stability and placement of the toggle completely through the acetabular hole and turned sideways
- Pulling the suture tight and cycling gently several times before tying to eliminate creep from the suture and resulting laxity
- Tightening each knot appropriately, with a surgeon's knot including at least six to eight throws depending on size and type of material

In cats and small dogs, a toggle technique with braided polyblend material (TightRope fibertape) may decrease the risk of suture breakage and prevent inadequate placement of the femoral tunnel with the use of a guidewire and cannulated drill bit (Ash *et al.* 2012).

Fascia lata loop

The fascial strip should measure at least 1 cm and should be adequately fixed to the third trochanter. Suture should be placed in dense fascia and engage enough tissue to prevent it from pulling through tissue.

Sacrotuberous ligament transposition

To ensure adequate stabilization of the ligament and bone to the femur, the osteotomy of the ischiatic tuberosity should be positioned to create a bony attachment of at least 1 cm in length and 0.7 mm in width and depth, thereby allowing placement of a screw of at least 2 mm in diameter (Kiliç *et al.* 2002)

Deep gluteal tenodesis (Rochereau and Bernardé 2012)

To ensure adequate placement of the screw and washer in the rectus femoris tuberosity:
- Review anatomic landmarks to locate the origin of the rectus femoris.
- Identify the bone margins and cranial acetabular rim with a needle, probe, or similar pointed instrument.

The limb should be maintained in abduction and internal rotation during screw placement:
- To release tension during screw placement
- To ensure adequate tensioning of the muscle posttransposition

Good surgical technique is essential to preserve the viability of the deep gluteal muscle and joint capsule.

Capsulorrhaphy

- Verify the viability and integrity of the joint capsule available for closure.
- Maintain the limb in abduction during closure.
- Careful reconstruction of the capsule
  - Proper retraction, hemostasis, and lighting (headlamp) to visualize the joint capsule
  - Consider using a special (smaller) needle on larger suture (polydioxanone [PDS] II, 2-0, UCL needle, Ethicon, Somerville, NJ)
  - Consider trochanteric osteotomy for a more precise placement of suture.
  - Use a tension-sparing suture pattern such as a horizontal mattress.

Dorsal augmentation

Proper placement of the screw and anchor in the acetabular rim is crucial:
- Review anatomy to position the screws in the dorsal and craniodorsal acetabular rim in a dorsolateral to ventromedial direction that allows sufficient bone purchase while avoiding the articular surface.

Placing a screw of appropriate size under a flat washer is essential to prevent suture migration. The following recommendations are based on the author's experience:
- Dogs weighing less than 5 kg and cats: 1.5-to 2.0-mm screws
- Dogs weighing 6 to 15 kg: 2.0- to 2.4-mm screws
- Dogs weighing more than 16 kg: 2.7-mm screws

Several measures may be considered to prevent or revise suture breakage:
- Use subcortical anchors: Traditional "prong" anchors, such as the Bone Biter anchor (Veterinary Instrumentation Limited, Broadfield Road, Sheffield, United Kingdom), are very hard to place properly in the dense bone and narrow acetabular rim. Recent anchors incorporate a screw type of design (e.g., FASTak anchors, Arthrex) that facilitates proper insertion.
- Use anchors with chamfered eyelet (e.g., 2.7-mm-diameter SECUROS bone anchors, DogLeggs, Reston, VA, and IMEX anchors) if using islet-style anchors: depending on the design of the anchor eyelet, the edges of the eyelet may not be chamfered or rounded.
- Use a larger or stronger type of suture, such as FiberWire (Arthrex).
- Use more than one anchor

To prevent failure of the suture anchor site on the femur:
- Review the local anatomy to make sure that the hole is located in the craniomedial aspect of the junction between the femoral neck and the greater trochanter, several millimeters from the edge of the bone (ensure sufficient bone stock surrounds the hole to avoid fracture)

Placement of an antirotational suture

To ensure proper placement of the screw or anchor cranial to the acetabular rim:
- Review anatomic landmarks to identify the origin of the rectus femoris
- Identify the bone margins of the cranial acetabular rim with a needle, probe, or similar pointed instrument

To prevent the suture from migrating off the screw:
- Use a flat washer with a screw.
- Substitute a suture anchor (islet or subsurface type) for the screw-washer combination.

To prevent suture breakage:
- Use a larger or stronger type of suture, such as FiberWire.
- After placement of the suture, check its tension with the limb in neutral position to make sure the suture is not too tight.

To prevent failure of femoral or acetabular suture anchor sites:
- Drill bone tunnels away from the edge of bone with several millimeters of surrounding bone.
- Use longer bone screws and washers or longer or larger suture anchors (islet or subsurface (Kunkel *et al.* 2013).

Transacetabular pinning

To avoid pin breakage:
- Limit this technique to small dogs.
- Maintain the limb in a non–weight-bearing sling until pin removal.
- Select a large-diameter, nonthreaded pin (Hunt and Henry 1985):
  - Dogs weighing less than 7 kg: 1.6-mm Kirschner wire
  - Dogs weighing 8 to 29 kg: 2.4-mm (3/32-in) Steinman pin
  - Dogs weighing more than 30 kg: 3.2-mm (1/8-in) Steinman pin

The pin should enter the acetabulum at the origin of the ligament of the head of the femur ventral to the lunate surface of acetabulum.

To ensure proper placement:
- A guide (Figure 115.11) should be used to facilitate accurate placement of the pin through the femoral neck into the fovea capitis.
- Fully reduce the hip before seating the pin in the acetabulum.

To prevent femoral or acetabular fracture:
- Apply the technique in small dogs only.
- Maintain the limb in a non–weight-bearing sling until pin removal.
- Use a small-diameter pin (see guidelines for size selection earlier).
- Accurate placement of the pin (see earlier).

Greater trochanteric transposition

To prevent implant failure:
- Select Kirschner wires and roll wire of appropriate size:
  - Dogs weighing less than 2 kg: 0.9-mm Kirschner wire
  - Dogs weighing 2 to 7.5 kg: 1.1-mm Kirschner wire
  - Dogs weighing more than 7.5 kg: 1.6-mm Kirschner wire

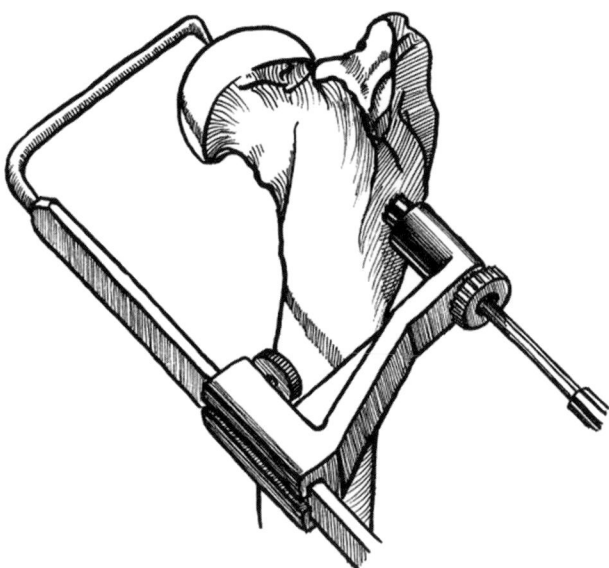

Figure 115.11 Line drawing of an aiming device used to drill a hole from the fovea capitis femoris to the base of the greater trochanter. The use of this device allows more accurate drilling of the tunnel through the femoral neck while protecting surrounding structures such as the sciatic nerve and articular cartilage. *Source:* Canapp *et al.*, 2012. Reproduced with permission from Elsevier.

- Kirschner wires should fully engage the femur from the center of the greater trochanter to the lesser trochanter.
- Drill the femoral bone tunnel distally at a distance from the osteotomy at least equal to the distance between the osteotomy and the proximal edge of the greater trochanter. This amount of bone stock should prevent the wire from tearing through the bone.
- Tighten the figure-of-eight wire evenly on both sides with proper twist technique.

Postoperative phase

Analgesia, including preemptive analgesics and multimodal therapies (see Chapter 14), is crucial to avoid undesirable activity and uncontrolled motion from the dog. These therapies should include nonsteroidal antiinflammatory drugs (see Chapter 15), opioids and tramadol, NMDA receptor antagonists, cold therapy, proper nursing care, and so on.

The use of an Ehmer sling has been advocated to maintain the limb in internal rotation and abduction, especially after closed reduction of a coxofemoral luxation. This sling has generally lost popularity because of its lack of proven efficiency and common soft tissue complication (Figure 115.12). Alternatively, commercial Ehmer slings can potentially be easier to use with less risk of soft tissue complications (DogLeggs VEST with Ehmer Sling, Reston, VA) (Figure 115.13).

Non–weight-bearing slings such as the Robinson sling may be applied for 3 to 4 weeks to avoid recurrence after capsulorrhaphy, dorsal augmentation, trochanteric transposition, and transacetabular pin.

Using a sling or placing a towel under the abdomen is the approach most commonly taken to assist walking in the early postoperative phase of patients treated with a combination of techniques and no predisposing risks to recurrence.

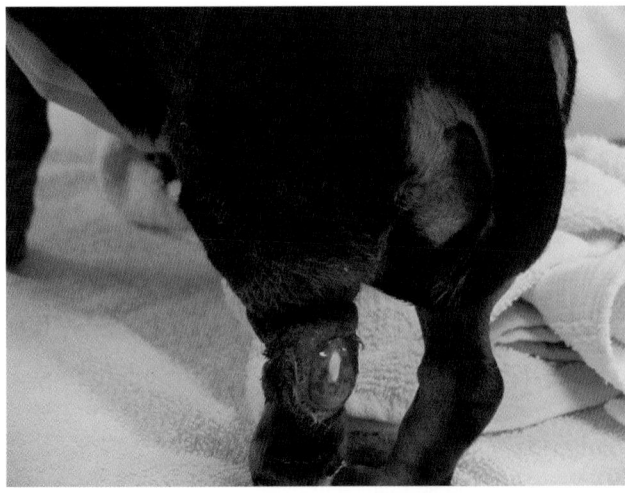

(a)

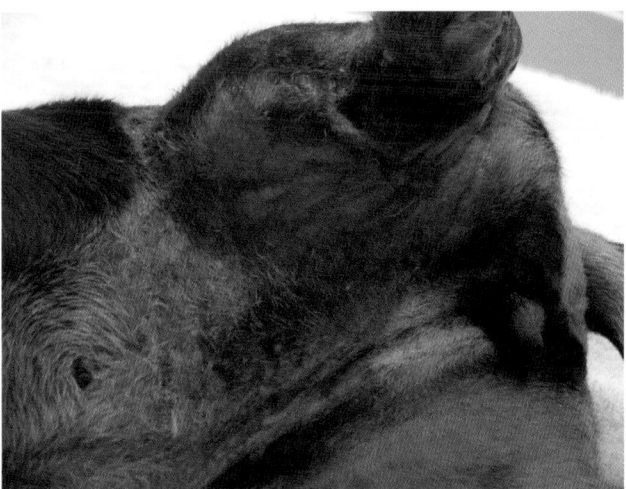

(b)

Figure 115.12 Cutaneous lesions on the tarsus (**A**) and around the proximal thigh (**B**) 1 week after application of an Ehmer sling on a dog with a coxofemoral luxation treated via closed reduction.

Applying a non–weight-bearing sling or mild sedation (trazodone or acepromazine) should be considered in patients that fail to comply with recommendations for exercise restriction. Providing written, very detailed discharge instructions with an accompanying verbal explanation at the time of discharge is crucial to ensure the owner's compliance.

Implant failure

Definition

Implant failure occurs when the surgical implant used to secure the reduced hip joint fails in some mechanical manner. Implants used for stabilizing luxated hips can include screws, washers, suture anchors, metallic toggle rods of varying designs, Kirschner wires, surgical roll wire, and a variety of types of suture. Implant failure can occur as a result of preoperative, intraoperative, and postoperative factors.

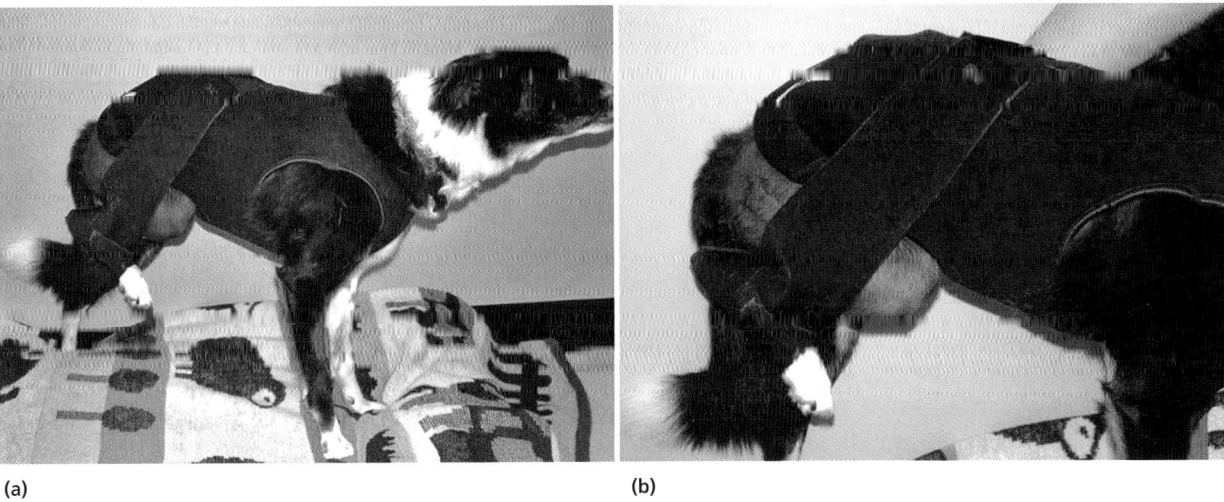

(a)   (b)

Figure 115.13 Photograph of the DogLeggs VEST with Ehmer Sling (DogLeggs, Reston, VA) on a dog after reduction of a hip luxation. The sling maintains internal rotation and abduction of the hip. (Reproduced with permission from Canapp, S.O., Campana, D.M., Fair, L.M. (2012) Orthopedic coaptation devices and small-animal prosthetics. In Tobias, K.M., Johnston, S. (eds.) *Veterinary Surgery: Small Animal*, 1st edn. St. Louis, Saunders, p. 636.)

Risk factors

Poor case selection
See Figure 115.2.

- Poor intraoperative decision making or technical error
Recurrence of hip luxation can result from implant failure. Factors associated specifically with implant failure are often technique dependent. Risk factors unique to implant failure are included in those listed for recurrence of luxation (see earlier discussion).
- Inadequate postoperative care
The most common causes of poor postoperative care are summarized in Figure 115.14.

Diagnosis

Implant failure after surgery is usually diagnosed if it becomes clinically relevant and leads to recurrence of coxofemoral luxation. In these cases, clinical signs of coxofemoral luxation are observed (see earlier discussion). Implant breakage or migration is observed on radiographic examination (see Figure 115.4).

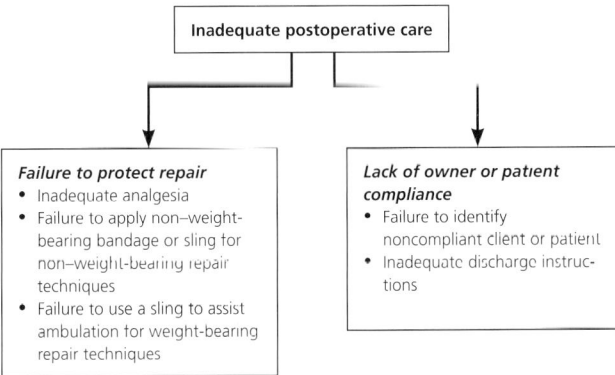

Figure 115.14 Cause of recurrent coxofemoral luxation associated with postoperative care.

Treatment

Correction of the implant failure follows the same guidelines as for those addressing recurrence of luxation (see earlier discussion).

Inadequate postoperative care is addressed by following the same principles as outlined earlier for recurrence.

Outcome

See the Outcome section for recurrence.

Prevention

Prevention of implant failure is accomplished by adhering to the same guidelines as for recurrence.

Sciatic neuropraxia

See also Chapter 82.

Definition

Sciatic neuropraxia results from damage to the sciatic nerve as it runs along the medial side of the acetabulum and then crosses dorsally over the lesser ischiatic notch immediately caudal to the acetabulum. Nerve injury is rare with hip luxation and usually occurs during surgical stabilization of the luxated hip (Fox 1991). Neuropraxia is defined as damage of the myelin sheath that surrounds the nerve axon. Although this complication is almost always temporary in small animals, efforts should focus on its prevention because abnormal weight bearing may predispose to recurrence of the luxation. Neuropraxia should be differentiated from more severe injuries such as axonotmesis and neurotmesis, both of which can occur if stabilization hardware or surgical instruments cause direct damage to the nerve.

Risk factors

- Improper surgical approach: An improper surgical approach can result in inadvertent damage to the sciatic nerve either by direct damage to the nerve or indirectly, by requiring excessive retraction of the soft tissues surrounding the hip, thereby stretching the nerve.

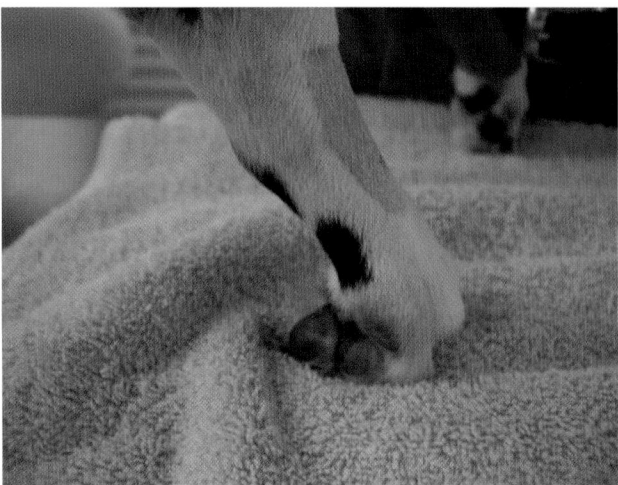

Figure 115.15 Photograph of a dog with conscious proprioceptive deficits of the rear limb, consistent with postoperative neuropraxia.

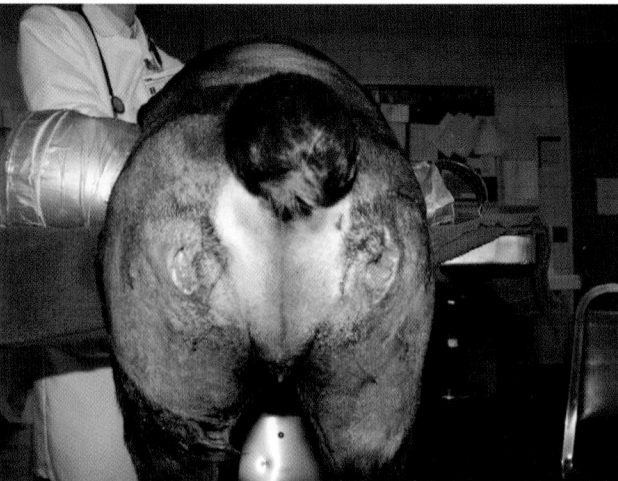

Figure 115.16 Neuropraxia and draining tracts in a dog presented with a history of bilateral coxofemoral luxations treated by ilioischial (DeVita) pinning.

- Chronic luxation: Muscle contracture and scar tissue associated with chronic luxation can increase the amount of force required to retract the contracted muscles or scar tissue, thereby stretching the nerve.
- Muscle spasm resulting from the luxation or concurrent injuries a can lead to overzealous retraction and nerve damage.
- Improper surgical technique, including poor hemostasis, poor lighting of the surgical field, and technical errors with implant or instrument placement, can result in nerve injury.

Diagnosis

Neuropraxia does not result in permanent loss of motor or sensory functions but does result in some degree of proprioceptive and motor dysfunction for a short period of time (Figure 115.15). This deficit may not be noticed in patients placed in a postoperative non–weight-bearing sling, thereby delaying the diagnosis until the limb is allowed to bear weight. Other techniques, such as the toggle rod technique, that allow cautious, limited weight bearing immediately after surgery may allow early detection of the proprioceptive loss. In these cases, radiographs should be considered to evaluate the potential for surgical implants impinging on the sciatic nerve. In dogs with a delayed postoperative onset of neurologic dysfunction, radiographs should be obtained to determine if implants have migrated and are now causing neurologic signs.

Treatment

Conservative management is indicated if the only abnormality found on the patient consists of a proprioceptive loss or diminution that cannot be attributed to the placement of surgical implants. Surgical exploration is indicated if implants are judged to be near or in the path of the nerve on radiographic examination. In these cases, revision of the implants or stabilization technique should occur as soon as possible.

Outcome

Neuropraxia generally resolves in a few days to several weeks as long as the cause of the neurologic damage has been eliminated. Implant placement should therefore be assessed as appropriate or adequately corrected.

Prevention

Preventive measures include:
- Use proper, anatomically based surgical approaches.
- Maintain adequate visualization of the surgical field via lighting (a headlight may be considered) and proper hemostasis.
- Epidural analgesia is generally helpful in dogs with coxofemoral luxation because of its effects on muscle relaxation.
- Avoid overzealous retraction. If required to reduce the hip, forceful retraction should be limited to a few minutes interspersed with periods of rest for the retracted tissues.
- Avoid stabilization techniques that require blind placement of implants in proximity of the nerve, such as transacetabular and ischioilial pinning (Hunt and Henry 1985) (Figure 115.16).
- Avoid technical maneuvers that increase the risk of nerve injury. For example, the tunnel extending from the fovea capitis to the base of the femoral neck in the toggle rod technique should not be drilled with the femur externally rotated. Instead, a combined aiming device or similar drill guide may be used to safely and accurately drill the femoral neck tunnel (see Figure 115.11).

Relevant literature

Complications associated with surgical repair of coxofemoral luxation are infection; sciatic neuropraxia; and recurrence caused by a number of factors, including implant failure, poor decision making both preoperatively and intraoperatively, technical errors in surgery, and inadequate postoperative care (primarily poor owner or patient compliance). A summary of complications after open reduction of coxofemoral luxation is presented in Table 115.2.

Although a detailed discussion of techniques that are currently favored for stabilization of luxated hips is included in the practical section of this chapter, several specific procedures warrant additional discussion. Ischioilial (or DeVita) pinning was originally described as a method of percutaneous stabilization of a hip after closed or open reduction. The basic intent is to pass a pin ventral to the ischiatic tuberosity, dorsal to the femoral neck, and anchor the pin in the ilial wing. Although conceptually simple, the technique can be challenging, and failure to closely adhere to several specific technical points sets the stage for failure. Threaded pins have been

Table 115.2 Complications reported in the literature (1996–2013) after treatment of traumatic coxofemoral luxations in dogs

Reference	Technique(s)	Number of cases	Complication rate	Most common complication
Ash et al. 2012	Modified toggle rod using TightRope	9 (4 cats, 5 small dogs)	11% (1)	Incisional swelling
Rochereau and Bernardé 2012	Capsulorrhaphy and deep gluteal tenodesis	46 dogs and 19 cats (26 dogs and 8 cats followed long term)	12% (8)	Screw placement errors, seroma, dehiscence
McCartney et al. 2011	Transacetabular pin	70 dogs	6% major; 45% minor	Incisional swelling and discharge; insufficient reduction
Venturini et al. 2010	Combined intra- and extraarticular technique	2 dogs	None	N/A
Demko et al. 2006	Toggle rod	62 dogs	26%	Recurrence (11.2%)
Onyılır et al. 2002	Sacrotuberous ligament transposition	10 dogs (experimental study)	0% reported	All markedly lame initially with varying degrees of resolution
Martini et al. 2001	Antirotational suture	11 dogs	0%	N/A

N/A, not applicable.

recommended to improve purchase of the pin in the ilial wing; failure to do so can result in migration of the pin through the epaxial musculature. Furthermore, it is critical to pass the pin ventral to the ischiatic tuberosity to provide a solid anchor against dorsal displacement of the pin with weight bearing. Because of the lack of curvature of the ischium and ilial wing, DeVita pinning is not possible in cats. Despite the procedure's longevity, serious complications, such as pin migration and injury to the sciatic nerve during placement or with activity, when combined with improvements in other surgical techniques, have largely relegated DeVita pinning to historical archives.

Another implant concept that merits comment is the increased use of suture anchors that serve as an alternative to bone screws or anchor holes for sutures used for dorsal augmentation and antirotational techniques. Suture anchors can either be subsurface anchors (Arthrex FASTak being the currently best example for use in the hip) and eyelet anchors that protrude above the bone's surface (IMEX 2.7-mm-diameter anchor being the currently best example). Both require a pilot hole to be drilled in the very dense periacetabular bone and are screwed into the bone. Both anchors can be applied with suture already loaded into the anchor and are of comparable cost to bone screws and washers. The primary advantage of suture anchors is the ease and accuracy with which the anchoring device can be placed in the usually deep, narrow confines of the hip.

The use of the Ehmer sling as a postoperative adjunct to open reduction has also begun to come into question. The modified Ehmer sling, as originally described, purportedly holds the limb in internal rotation and abduction, thereby maximally stabilizing the hip while healing occurs. Nevertheless, the sling has been historically fraught with soft tissue complications ranging from moderately severe dermatitis to full-thickness skin erosions. Consequently, there has been an anecdotal clinical trend toward using the less problem-fraught Robinson sling, recently available commercial slings, or no sling at all if the reduction is judged to be stable.

Although no study has directly compared the mechanical stability of the variously reported methods of surgical stabilization of the luxated hip, those that recreate the round ligament or repair the joint capsule (normally, the two primary stabilizers of the hip) subjectively tend to provide the most stability the joint. Further stability is provided by combining these techniques with those that provide peripheral support and become more critical to use when risk factors for failure (more chronic luxations with associated muscle contracture, concomitant injuries or arthropathies in other limbs, questionable owner and patient compliance, obesity, mild hip dysplasia, and irreparable joint capsular damage).

Finally, some coxofemoral luxations cannot be repaired nor normal hip function restored. In this scenario, salvage procedures, such as excision arthroplasty (femoral head and neck ostectomy [FHO]) or total hip arthroplasty, are required. Hopefully, careful consideration of all factors is given before attempting reduction of a hip luxation but if failure of an open reduction occurs, a salvage procedure may be the best solution. Although there is no doubt that total hip arthroplasty, even in very small dogs and cats, affords better functional outcomes over excision arthroplasty, other factors that contribute to success or failure of a total hip arthroplasty (see Chapter 113), such as cost, availability, lack of postoperative compliance, and preexisting infection or neurologic disease, can lead the surgeon to perform a FHO, usually with improved function when compared with that associated with the luxation.

References

Ablin, L.W., Gambardella, P.C. (1991) Orthopedics of the feline hip. *Compendium on Continuing Education for the Practicing Veterinarian* 13, 1379-1383.

Ash, K., Rosselli, D., Danielski, A., et al. (2012) Correction of craniodorsal coxofemoral luxation in cats and small breed dogs using a modified Knowles technique with the braided polyblend TightRope systems. *Veterinary and Comparative Orthopaedics and Traumatology* 25, 54-60.

Basher, A.W.P., Walter, M.C., Newton, C.D. (1986) Traumatic coxofemoral luxation in the dog and cat. *Veterinary Surgery Journal* 15, 356-362.

Çetinkaya, M.A., Olcay, B. (2010) Modified Knowles toggle pin technique with nylon monofilament suture material for treatment of two caudoventral hip luxation cases, *Veterinary and Comparative Orthopaedics and Traumatology* 23, 114-118.

Demko, J.L., Sidaway, B.K., Thieman, K.M., et al. (2006) Toggle rod stabilization for treatment of hip joint luxation in dogs: 62 cases (2000–2005). *Journal of the American Veterinary Medical Association* 229, 984-989.

Fox, S.M. (1991) Coxofemoral luxations in dogs. *Compendium on Continuing Education for the Practicing Veterinarian* 13, 381-389.

Hunt, C.A., Henry, W.B. (1985) Transarticular pinning for repair of hip dislocation in the dog: a retrospective study of 40 cases. *Journal of the American Veterinary Medical Association* 187, 828-833.

Johnson, M.E., Braden, T.D. (1987) A retrospective study of prosthetic capsule technique for treatment of problem cases of dislocated hips. *Veterinary Surgery Journal* 16, 346-351.

Kiliç, E., Osaydin, I., Atalan, G., et al. (2002) Transposition of the sacrotuberous ligament for the treatment of coxofemoral luxation in dogs. *Journal of Small Animal Practice* 43, 341-344.

Kunkel, K.A.R., Rusly, R.J., Basinger, R.R., et al. (2013) In vitro acute load to failure and eyelet abrasion testing of a novel veterinary screw-type mini-anchor design. *Veterinary Surgery* 42, 217-222.

Martini F.M., Simonazzi B., Del Bue M. (2001) Extra-articular absorbable suture stabilization of coxofemoral luxation in dogs. *Veterinary Surgery* 30, 468-475.

McCartney, W., Kiss, K., McGovern, F. (2011) Treatment of 70 dogs with traumatic hip luxation using a modified transarticular pinning technique. *Veterinary Record* 168, 355-357.

McLaughlin, R.M. (1995) Traumatic joint luxations in small animals. *Veterinary Clinics of North America: Small Animal Practice* 25, 1175-1196.

Rochereau, P., Bernardé, A. (2012) Stabilization of coxo-femoral luxation using tenodesis of the deep gluteal muscle. Technique description and reluxation rate in 65 dogs and cats (1995-2008). *Veterinary and Comparative Orthopaedics and Traumatology* 25, 49-53.

Sissener, T.R., Whitelock, R.G., Langley-Hobbs, S.J. (2009) Long-term results of transarticular pinning for surgical stabilization of coxofemoral luxation in 20 cats. *Journal of Small Animal Practice* 50, 112-117.

Venturini, A., Pinna S., Tamburro, R. (2010) Combined intra-extra-articular technique for stabilization of coxofemoral luxation. Preliminary results in two dogs. *Veterinary and Comparative Orthopaedics and Traumatology* 23, 182-185.

Wardlaw, J.L., McLaughlin, R. (2012) Coxofemoral luxation. In Tobias, K.M., Johnston. S.A. (eds.) *Veterinary Surgery: Small Animal,* vol. 1, 1st edn. WB Saunders Company, St. Louis, pp. 816-823.

Surgery of the Stifle

116

Complications Associated with Open Versus Arthroscopic Examination of the Stifle

Antonio Pozzi[1] and Stanley Kim[2]

[1]Vetsuisse Faculty, University of Zurich, Zürich, Switzerland
[2]Department of Small Animal Clinical Sciences, University of Florida, Gainesville, FL, USA

Lack of visualization of intraarticular structures

Definition

The intraarticular structures are not sufficiently exposed for diagnostic and/or therapeutic purposes. This complication is most commonly encountered during evaluation of the medial meniscus, potentially leading to the misdiagnosis of meniscal injury. Additionally, poor exposure can increase the risk of iatrogenic damage of intraarticular structures because instruments are often inserted blindly.

Risk factors

During arthrotomy, insufficient exposure commonly results from poor positioning of the surgical approach through the skin and deeper tissue layers. If the incision is too caudal, a large flap of fascia may obstruct the view of the joint. Similarly, an incision that is too proximal or too distal requires significantly more tissue retraction or extending the incision.

Factors affecting the visualization of intraarticular structures during arthroscopy include:

- Positioning of the initial skin incisions: The location of each portal dictates the access to all relevant areas in the joint. Proximal positioning of the scope portal facilitates initial visualization of the joint but complicates the evaluation of the caudal compartment. Distal positioning complicates initial visualization caused by interference of the fat pad.
- Presence of hemorrhage or debris in the joint.
- Limited intraarticular space. Fibrosis of the joint capsule secondary to chronic cranial cruciate ligament (CCL) deficiency limits the ability to distend and manipulate the stifle.
- Defective arthroscopic equipment: insufficient light or perfusion of the joint.

Diagnosis

Poor visualization of intraarticular structures is noted by the surgeon during surgery. For example, an inability to perform a partial meniscectomy because of insufficient exposure may prompt surgeons to convert an arthroscopy into an arthrotomy. In other instances, the consequences of a limited exposure to intraarticular structures may be delayed; undiagnosed meniscal tears may lead to poor postoperative recovery, recurrent lameness, or both, requiring second look arthroscopy or arthrotomy. The timing of clinical signs and the level of function attained postoperatively may help differentiate undiagnosed meniscal tears from postoperative tears, although the two conditions cannot be definitively differentiated.

Treatment

When visualization is inadequate for diagnostic or therapeutic purposes, time should be taken to analyze possible problems that occurred in the previous steps. Strategies to improve visualization of intraarticular structures are described under Prevention.

Outcome

The outcome of poor visualization includes increased surgical time, misdiagnosis of intraarticular pathology, and technical errors during treatment.

Prevention

A good knowledge of anatomy and landmarks previously described for arthrotomies are prerequisite to proper technique (Piermattei and Johnson 2004a, 2004b, 2004c) The strategy to achieve good exposure during stifle arthrotomy is summarized in Figure 116.1. It should be noted that technique varies between dogs and that despite good technique, visualization of intraarticular structures after stifle arthrotomy is inherently limited by a lack of magnification and poorer illumination compared with arthroscopy (see Figure 116.1).

The optimum position of an arthroscopic portal site is determined by reference to the palpable anatomic structures and any specific conformation. In the case of stifle arthroscopy, these landmarks include the distal aspect of the patella, patellar ligament, and proximal aspect of the tibial tuberosity. The instrument portal should be positioned to give optimal access to the pathologic structures requiring treatment. The conformation of the tibial plateau should be considered when positioning the arthroscope portal. For example, in dogs with very steep angles, it is recommended to move the scope port more proximal than in normal dogs.

For both arthrotomy and arthroscopy, some basic principles should be applied:

- Skin incision and portal site placement should be precise and based on consistently palpable landmarks.
- Appropriate surgical instruments including retractors, distractors, meniscal blades, and punches, are recommended. During arthrotomy the combined use of a Volkmann retractor for the

Complications in Small Animal Surgery, First Edition. Edited by Dominique Griffon and Annick Hamaide.
© 2016 John Wiley & Sons, Inc. Published 2016 by John Wiley & Sons, Inc.
Companion website: www.wiley.com/go/griffon/complications

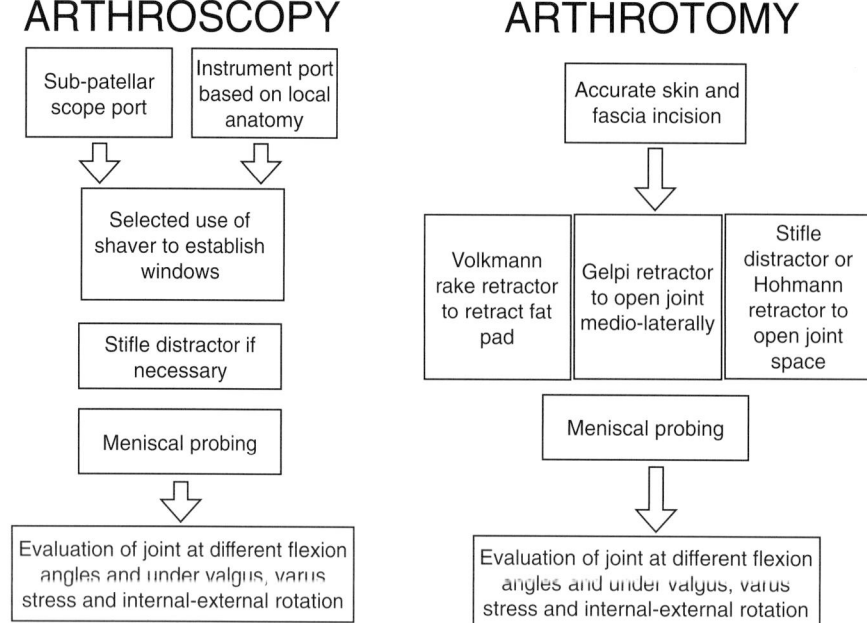

Figure 116.1 Strategies to improve visualization of intraarticular structures during arthrotomy and arthroscopy.

fat pad, a Gelpi retractor for the joint capsule, and a Hohmann retractor to subluxate the tibia or a stifle distractor allows optimal exposure (Figure 116.2). Stifle distractors can also be used during stifle arthroscopy (Figure 116.3).

• Illumination and magnification greatly facilitate evaluation of the stifle (especially the medial meniscus). Preoperative factors such as severe peri-articular fibrosis, partial CCL injury with stable joint, or previous surgery should be considered as they may complicate the exposure of intraarticular structures. The use of headlamps and surgical loupes should be considered.

• The stifle should be evaluated at multiple angles of flexion. In most dogs, exposure of the medial meniscus is improved when the stifle is extended. Cranial subluxation (see Figure 116.2B) of the tibia with a Hohmann retractor usually improves exposure of the menisci. The risk of misdiagnosis of meniscal tears and the risk of iatrogenic damage increase when distraction is not performed (Figure 116.4). The meniscus should be evaluated both on the femoral and tibial surfaces (see Figure 116.4B). With appropriate joint distraction, the peripheral edge of the meniscus can be evaluated for complete or partial peripheral tears (see Figure 116.4B).

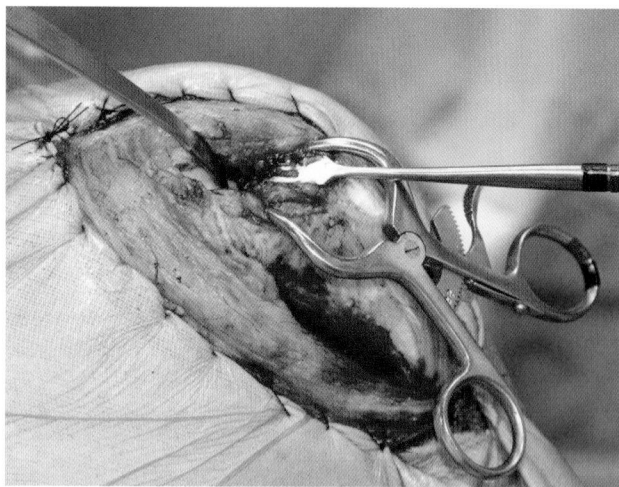

(A)

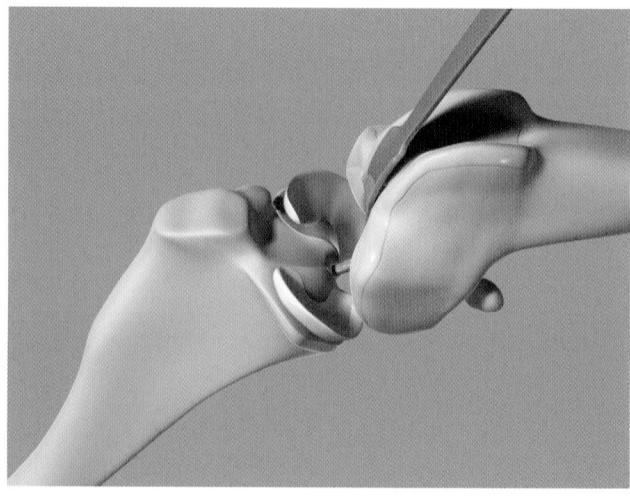

(B)

Figure 116.2 Retraction of intraarticular structures. **A**, Combined use of Volkmann retractor, a Gelpi retractor, and a Hohmann retractor to improve visualization of the medial meniscus. The Volkmann retractor allows retraction of the fat pad, the Gelpi retractor maintains the joint open mediolaterally, and the Hohmann retractor is placed caudal to the tibial plateau and used as a lever against the femoral condyle to induce a cranial subluxation of the tibia. **B**, The tip of Hohmann retractor can be placed on the tibial plateau between the caudal cruciate ligament and the caudal meniscotibial ligament of the medial meniscus to achieve both distraction and subluxation of the tibia.

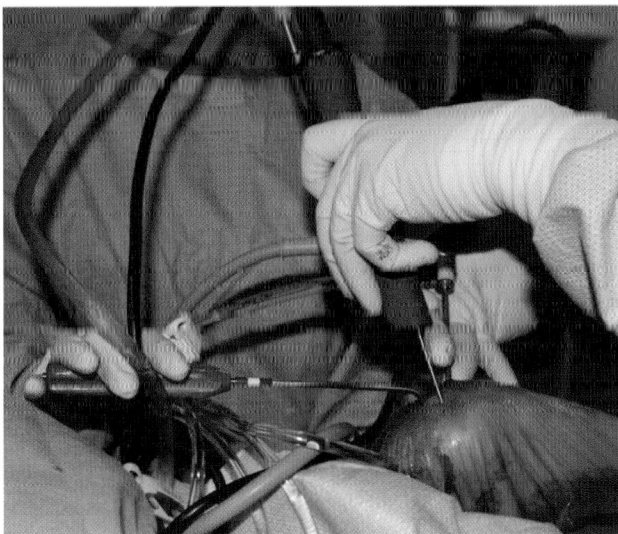

Figure 116.3 Use of a stifle distractor during arthroscopy. The stifle distractor can be inserted through a separate, proximal and lateral port or through the medial instrument port. Distraction during stifle arthroscopy minimizes the risk of iatrogenic cartilage damage during meniscectomy and improves the ability to diagnose meniscal tears.

• Varus and internal rotation of the crus should be used to expose the lateral femorotibial compartment. Conversely, valgus and external rotation facilitate exposure of the medial aspect of the stifle.

Iatrogenic damage

Definition

Iatrogenic damage is a new injury resulting from treatment by a surgeon during arthrotomy or arthroscopy.

Risk factors

Risk factors for specific iatrogenic lesions are listed in Table 116.1. Conditions that increase the overall risk of iatrogenic damage include:

• Poor adherence to surgical landmarks during surgical approach.
• Factors limiting intraarticular space such as fibrosis of the joint capsule, small dogs, or partial CCL rupture.
• Factors affecting the visualization of intraarticular structures.
• Proximity of intraarticular structures (i.e., caudal cruciate ligament and caudal meniscotibial ligament, CCL and intermeniscal ligament) (Figure 116.5).

Diagnosis

Most iatrogenic lesions are diagnosed immediately as the surgeon gains sufficient exposure to the joint. However, the structures at risk should be checked before closing the joint.

• Transection of long digital extensor: A complete transection of the tendon causes distal retraction of the tendon, which may not be visible in the joint.
• Transection of the patellar tendon causes proximal displacement of the patella because of the unrestricted tension of the quadriceps muscle.
• Injury to the medial or lateral collateral ligament is diagnosed as medial or lateral stifle instability.
• Injury to the caudal cruciate ligament is rarely complete. More commonly, a partial transection may occur during meniscal release or meniscectomy (see Figure 116.5) or during CCL debridement (see Figure 116.6A). A simple maneuver to evaluate the caudal cruciate ligament is to hyperflex the stifle, which allows exposing most of the caudal cruciate ligament. In addition, the caudal drawer test should be performed to evaluate the integrity of the caudal cruciate ligament.
• Injury to the cranial meniscal and intermeniscal ligaments can occur during CCL debridement (see Figure 116.6B). In most

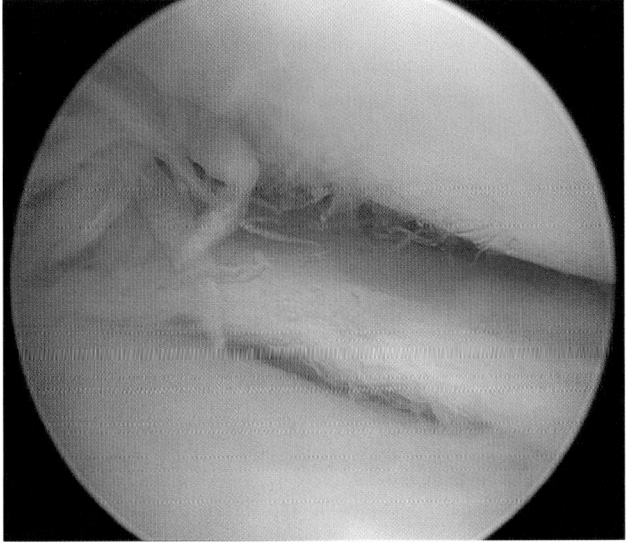

(A)

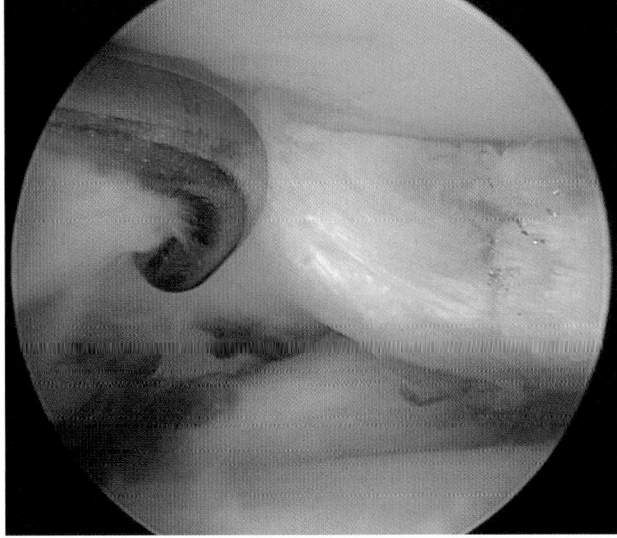

(B)

Figure 116.4 Effect of joint distraction on arthroscopic evaluation of the medial meniscus. **A**, Only the most axial part of the meniscus can be recognized. In addition to the limited joint space, the view of the meniscus is partially obstructed by fibers of the cranial cruciate ligament. **B**, After joint distraction, both the tibial and femoral surfaces of the meniscus can be evaluated. The most axial edge of the meniscus is probed for peripheral tears. Note that the tendon of the semimembranosus muscle can be visualized behind the medial meniscus.

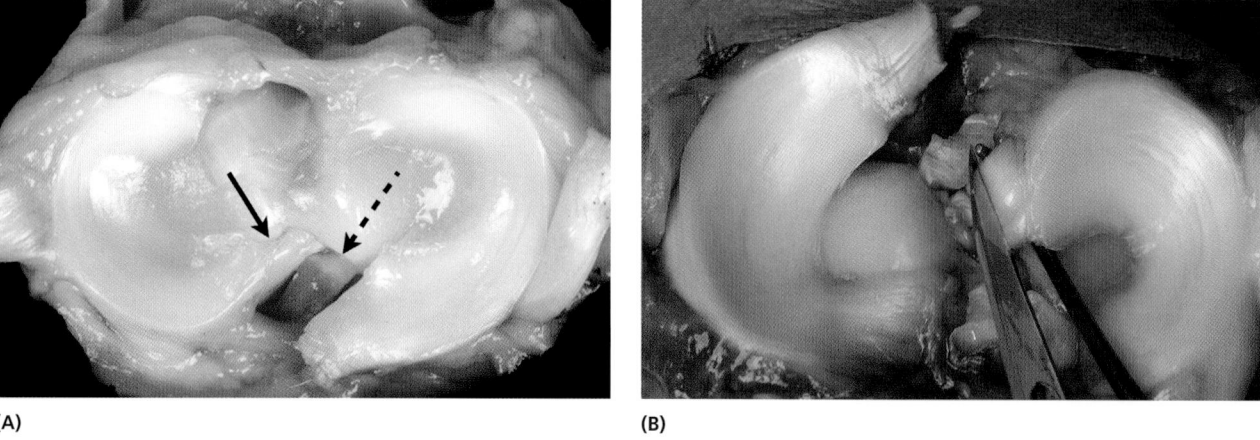

(A)   (B)

Figure 116.5 Proximity of anatomical structures in the stifle increases the risk of iatrogenic injuries. **A**, Damage to the caudal cruciate ligament (dashed arrow) can occur during meniscal release or meniscectomy (black arrow). **B**, A meniscal probe hooked around the meniscotibial ligament helps control the position of the blade during meniscal release or meniscectomy.

cases, it may be difficult to recognize these structures because they are covered by fat tissue (see Figure 116.6B, black arrow). To prevent this iatrogenic injury, the surgical blade should not be directed toward the tibial plateau; rather, it should be kept parallel to the plateau.

- Iatrogenic cartilage damage is common, and lesions may not be readily apparent during the exploratory surgery and can occasionally be difficult to distinguish from preexisting pathology. Linear or focal disruptions to the smooth articular surface may be iatrogenic injuries (Figure 116.7).

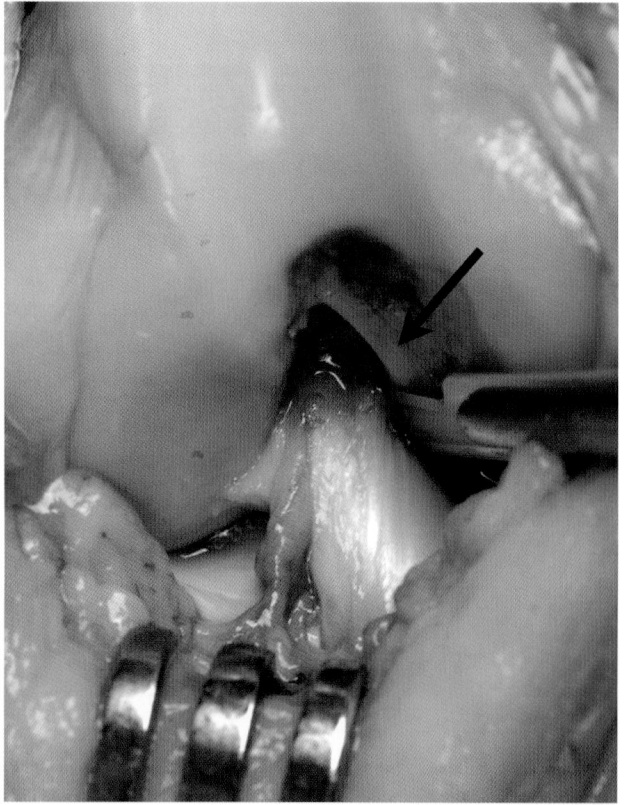
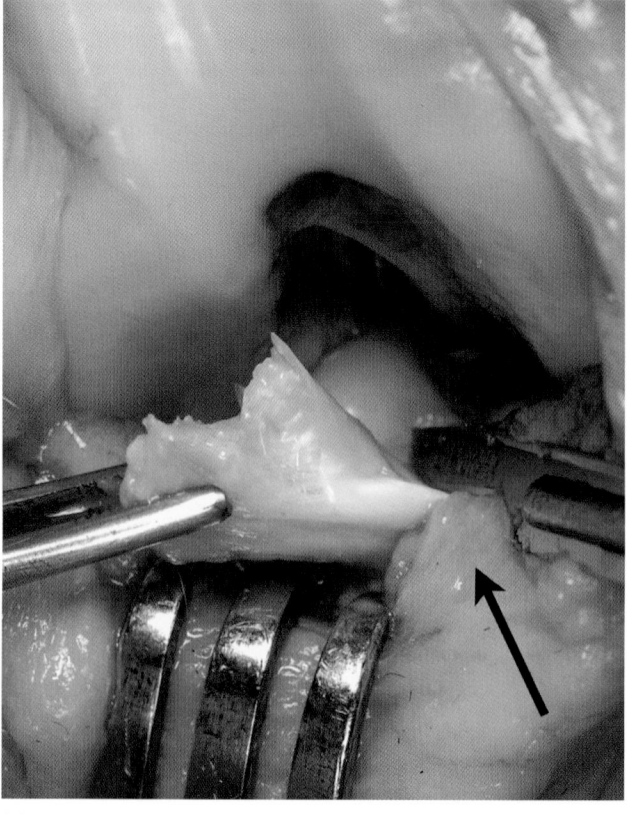

(A)   (B)

Figure 116.6 Risk of iatrogenic injuries during debridement of the cranial cruciate ligament (CCL). **A**, To avoid iatrogenic damage to the caudal cruciate ligament during debridement of the CCL, the blade should always be tangent to the caudal cruciate ligament. **B**, To prevent injuries to the cranial meniscal ligaments and the intermeniscal ligament, the blade should not be directed toward the tibial plateau.

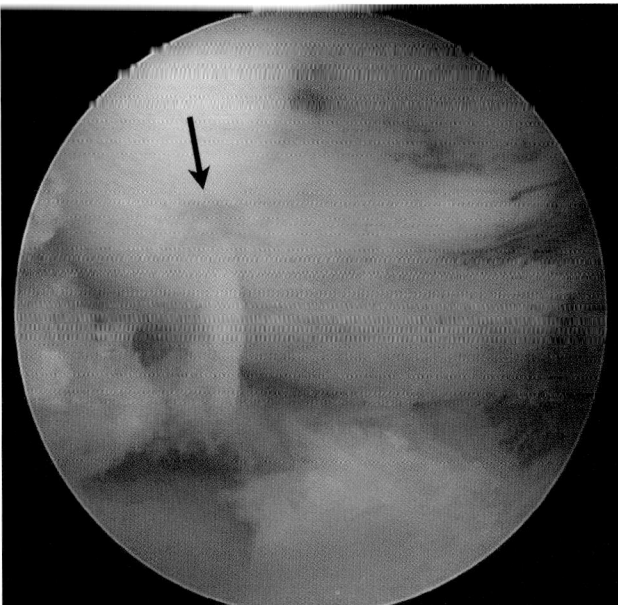

Figure 116.7 Iatrogenic cartilage damage. A partial-thickness lesion (arrow) has been created on the femoral condyle by surgical instruments during debridement of the cranial cruciate ligament and meniscectomy.

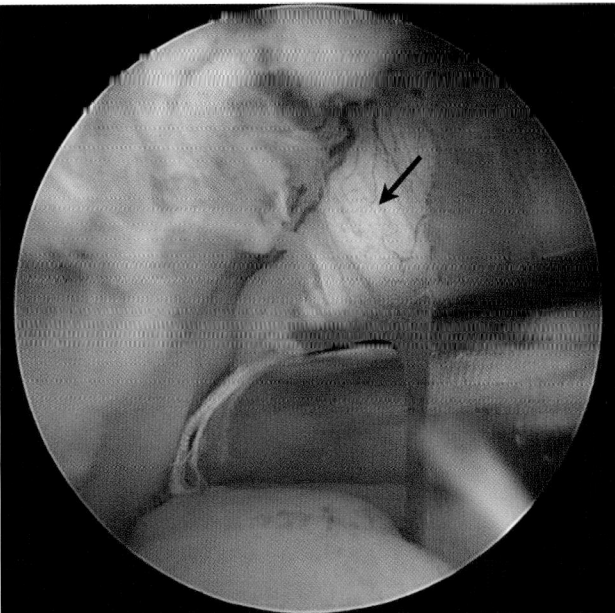

Figure 116.8 Arthroscopic debridement of the origin of the cranial cruciate ligament. The blade of the shaver is oriented medially so that the sleeve of the shaver protects the caudal cruciate ligament (arrow).

Treatment

The management of iatrogenic lesions varies from conservative treatment to surgical intervention:

- Transection of long digital extensor: This muscle–tendon unit is not required for normal ambulation and may not necessitate repair. Tenorrhaphy or tenodesis can be performed.
- Transection of the patellar tendon: This is a potentially catastrophic injury that always requires repair and joint immobilization until adequate healing has occurred.
- Injury to the medial or lateral collateral ligament: These ligaments play a vital role in ensuring stifle stability. Repair (primary repair, prosthetic repair, or both) and joint immobilization are required until adequate healing has occurred.
- Injury to the caudal cruciate ligament: Partial-thickness injury may not require repair. An extraarticular ligament prosthesis can be used for complete transection; primary repair may be difficult, and healing capacity is poor.
- Injury to the cranial meniscal and intermeniscal ligaments: If trauma is severe, then resection may be required. Repair with direct appositional sutures may be applied; however, the healing capacity of these structures is poor.
- Iatrogenic cartilage damage: Cartilage injury is often partial thickness and does not need treatment (see Figure 116.7). Large full-thickness lesions can be treated with microfracture or resurfacing techniques.

Outcome

The outcome varies with the type of lesion:

- Transection of the long digital extensor is typically of no appreciable consequence.
- Transection of the patellar tendon: Limb function will be markedly compromised by full-thickness loss of the patellar tendon.

The prognosis with repair depends on proper rehabilitation and the development of other complications.

- Injury to the medial or lateral collateral ligament: Without treatment, loss of either the lateral or medial collateral ligament will create marked chronic lameness. The prognosis associated with uncomplicated repair is good.
- Injury to the caudal cruciate ligament: Limb use may be adequate despite a damaged caudal cruciate ligament. However, this lesion will significantly affect the ability of restoring joint stability if there is concurrent CCL deficiency, which may be detrimental to long-term limb function.
- Injury to the cranial meniscal and intermeniscal ligaments: Full-thickness transection of the attachments compromise meniscal function and osteoarthritis will progress. Satisfactory limb use is still typically attainable.
- Iatrogenic cartilage damage: Small, partial thickness injuries may not be clinically significant. Lameness and osteoarthritis may occur with large or full-thickness injuries.

Prevention

General preventive measures include:

- Good knowledge of the anatomy and landmarks
- Maintain adequate visualization of the surgical field.
- Sharp instruments should be handled with care and under good visualization. The cutting edge of instruments should be directed away from adjacent, vital structures. For example, the blade of the shaver is oriented medially so that the sleeve of the shaver protects the caudal cruciate ligament (Figure 116.8).

Strategies to prevent specific iatrogenic injuries are listed in Table 116.1.

Table 116.1 Causes of iatrogenic damage during arthroscopy and arthrotomy and strategies to avoid them

Procedure	Iatrogenic damage	Preventive measures
Lateral arthrotomy	Partial or complete transection of long digital extensor	Incise the joint capsule more proximally than the long digit extensor tendon, such as between the patella and the trochlear ridge.
Medial or lateral arthrotomy	Partial or complete transection of the patellar ligament	Identify landmarks. Incise the fascia and joint capsule about 5 mm away from the tendon.
	Iatrogenic damage to the cartilage	Avoid the use of electrocautery to incise the joint capsule and control the depth of the scalpel blade.
Caudomedial arthrotomy	Injury to the medial collateral ligament	Place the joint in valgus to palpate the medial collateral ligament before incising the joint capsule.
Debridement at the origin of the CCL	Partial or complete transection of the caudal cruciate ligament	A #15 blade should be used to perform two incisions into the CCL converging in the notch. The blade is maintained parallel to the caudal cruciate ligament and to the medial aspect of the lateral femoral condyle and advanced at the level of the intercondylar notch. (see Figure 116.6A).
Debridement at the insertion of the CCL	Partial or complete transection of cruciate ligament or intermeniscal ligament	Keep the blade parallel to the tibial plateau when transecting the CCL from its tibial attachment (see Figure 116.6B).
Establishment of arthroscopy ports	Iatrogenic cartilage damage	Use blunt trocars to insert the cannulas. Insert the trocar distal to proximal on one side of the joint, with the limb extended. Avoid inserting cannulas or instruments in the patellofemoral joint in small dogs or tight joints.
Caudal pole hemi-meniscectomy	Partial or complete transection of the caudal cruciate ligament	Use the Hohmann retractor or a stifle distractor and a meniscal probe to protect the caudal cruciate ligament while transecting the caudal medial meniscotibial ligament (see Figure 116.5B).
Partial and caudal pole hemi-meniscectomy	Iatrogenic cartilage damage	Distract the joint using a stifle distractor. Use appropriate instruments for meniscal debridement such as meniscal punches or a meniscal knife (Figure 116.3).
Use a of shaver to debride the fat pad	Iatrogenic damage of the caudal cruciate ligament, the cranial meniscal ligament and poles, or intermeniscal ligament	Always shave in the "safe" zone and especially toward "safe directions." For example, it is important to direct the cutting side of the shaver in the opposite direction of the caudal cruciate ligament (see Figure 116.7).

CCL, cranial cruciate ligament.

Infection

See Chapter 6.

Postoperative pain

Definition

Postoperative pain is pain occurring after a medical operation. It is also defined as acute pain or pain temporarily related to injury and that resolves during the appropriate healing time.

Postoperative pain and its management are described in Chapter 14. Literature comparing pain after arthrotomy versus arthroscopy and aspects of pain management specific to stifle surgery is discussed next.

Relevant literature

Approaching the stifle with an arthrotomy or arthroscopy is widely accepted as a mandatory step during surgical management of stifle diseases (Kowaleski *et al.* 2012). The goal of these approaches is to provide **visualization of intraarticular lesions** to allow accurate diagnosis and treatment while minimizing morbidity. Open approaches to the stifle include lateral and medial arthrotomies, with or without patellar luxation, and caudomedial arthrotomy (Piermattei and Johnson 2004a, 2004b). Complications can occur during the surgical approach and while evaluating intraarticular structures. Recently, stifle arthroscopy has gained significant popularity among orthopedic surgeons (Whitney 2003). The magnification and illumination provided by arthroscopy allow evaluation of intraarticular structures that are otherwise difficult to observe via conventional arthrotomy. For example, the tibial surface of the meniscus can be directly inspected with arthroscopy but cannot be exposed with an arthrotomy. In addition, the joint can be evaluated in positions approaching the natural range of motion of the joint, which is not easily attainable with arthrotomy. Indications for

arthroscopic management of stifle diseases have expanded, and surgeons have consequently become aware of associated complications. Although the vast majority of stifle arthroscopic procedures occur without incident, complications such as poor exposure, iatrogenic damage, infection, and postoperative pain may occur.

The most important indication for surgical exposure during stifle arthrotomy and arthroscopy is accurate evaluation of the meniscus. Meniscal injury secondary to CCL insufficiency occurs in 40% to 70% of cases (Flo and DeYoung 1978; Bennett and May 1991; Flo 1993; Ralphs and Whitney 2002; Fitzpatrick and Solano 2010). Reports of meniscal tears in 10% to 20% of CCL insufficiency raise concerns over undiagnosed meniscal lesions. Most meniscal tears cause persistent lameness if left untreated (Thieman *et al.* 2006; Case *et al.* 2008). Improving surgical exposure should improve the detection of meniscal lesions and the accuracy of their treatment while minimizing the risk of iatrogenic damage to the cartilage. Techniques such as stifle distraction (Böttcher *et al.* 2009) and meniscal probing (Pozzi *et al.* 2008) can improve the accuracy of a surgical evaluation of the menisci. In a cadaveric study, meniscal probing increased the diagnostic accuracy for meniscal injury by 2.6- and 8-fold for arthrotomy and arthroscopy, respectively. Good exposure of the intraarticular structures and meniscal probing are of utmost importance for diagnosing meniscal injury because they potentially decrease the rate of surgical revision caused by meniscal pathology (Thieman *et al.* 2006; Case *et al.* 2008; Fitzpatrick and Solano 2010; Kalff *et al.* 2011).

Iatrogenic damage of intraarticular structures may occur during both arthrotomy and arthroscopy. Although its clinical relevance remains unclear, cartilage damage is the most common iatrogenic damage encountered during stifle surgery regardless of the approach. During stifle arthrotomy, damage to the cartilage or intra- and extraarticular ligamentous structures may occur when inserting the blade or other sharp instrument through the joint. During craniomedial and craniolateral arthrotomies, the patellar ligament may be damaged if the fascia is incised too medially. The long digital extensor tendon can be traumatized during a craniolateral approach to the stifle. During a caudomedial approach, the medial collateral ligament must be protected from inadvertent transection.

Care must be taken not to injure the underlying articular cartilage when the joint capsule is incised; this most commonly occurs when making the arthrotomy with an electrocautery or by inadvertently inserting the scalpel blade too deeply.

Iatrogenic injury to the caudal cruciate ligament can occur during careless or blind (1) debridement of a ruptured CCL, (2) placement of a stifle distractor or Hohmann retractor, or (3) medial meniscal debridement or meniscal release. Risk of iatrogenic damage of the caudal cruciate ligament exists while treating meniscal injury because the caudal pole of the medial meniscus is close to the tibial insertion of the caudal cruciate ligament. Iatrogenic damage to the caudal cruciate ligament, articular cartilage, and medial collateral ligament while performing meniscal release has been reported in a cadaveric model (Austin et al. 2007).

Iatrogenic injury to a normal CCL is uncommon. The intermeniscal ligament can be damaged during an aggressive incision into the infrapatellar fat pad or during debridement of the origin of a diseased CCL. Iatrogenic damage of the meniscus has been reported from the insertion of a needle intraarticularly to mark the joint during tibial plateau leveling osteotomy (O'Brien and Martinez 2009).

The narrow femorotibial joint space puts the articular cartilage at high risk of injury during meniscal surgery. Sharp instruments such as scalpel blades, meniscal knives, and punches should be maneuvered carefully because they can easily create cartilage defects on the weight-bearing aspects of the joint.

During arthroscopy, iatrogenic damage may occur during the creation of portals or during arthroscopic treatment of lesions caused by interference of instruments with adjacent structures. Cartilage damage is the most common type of iatrogenic lesion; sharp instruments or even sharp points of edges of cannulas can elevate a cartilage flap. Grasping forceps can cause cartilage damage when these instruments are opened in tight caudal joint areas. Electrosurgical instruments can be a source of iatrogenic damage because accidental contact of the noninsulated part of an electrocautery probe with cartilage will produce chondrocytes death and cartilage degeneration (Horstman and McLaughlin 2006; Horstman et al. 2009). Radiofrequency-treated cartilage has been shown to have reduced permeability and considerable histologic damage (Cook et al. 2004). In addition, radiofrequency causes greater chondrocyte death and more severe morphologic changes than mechanical debridement in experimental models. It should also be noted that joint space is always limited in small animals, potentially increasing the risk of damage from radiofrequency. Because of the risk of cartilage damage, radiofrequency has become less popular in small animal arthroscopy. Meniscal knives are particularly hazardous because after cutting completely through the meniscus, the blade will inevitably cut into the underlying soft cartilage.

Postoperative pain and subsequent lameness is expected to occur after arthrotomy or arthroscopy. Because the degree of discomfort is associated with the extent of nociceptive stimuli created from tissue trauma, it is reasonable to expect higher morbidity after arthrotomy than arthroscopy. In a prospective, experimental study performed in normal dogs, morbidity was greater after arthrotomy than arthroscopy (Hoelzler et al. 2004). The pain-free range of motion was wider in dogs that underwent arthroscopy, particularly on stifle flexion. The greater level of pain observed after arthrotomy may be attributed to the size of the incision into the joint capsule, stretching of the joint capsule during retraction, prolonged and

substantial subluxation during exploration and manipulation of intraarticular structures, and placement of sutures for closure of the arthrotomy.

Pain should be managed with a multimodal approach to analgesia. Systemic opioids should be routinely provided in the perioperative period. Nonsteroidal antiinflammatory drugs are reliable analgesics and can be used safely in conjunction with opioids. Regional anaesthesia such as epidurals and nerve blocks are also highly effective (Day et al. 1995; Muir 2008). Intraarticular morphine has been shown to provide a level of analgesia comparable to that of epidural morphine (Day et al. 1995). The use of intraarticular local anesthetics (e.g., bupivacaine) is controversial because some evidence supports their potential role in causing chondrocyte death in experimental studies (Hennig et al. 2010); thus, their use is not advocated at this time. Cold compression therapy has been successfully used to control postoperative swelling and pain after stifle surgery (Drygas et al. 2011). Use of cold compression therapy during the first 24 hours after tibial plateau leveling osteotomy has been found to decrease pain scale values and threshold scores (Drygas et al. 2011).

References

Austin, B., Montgomery, R.D., Wright, J., et al. (2007) Evaluation of Three approaches to meniscal release. *Veterinary Comparative Orthopaedics and Traumatology* 20, 92-97.

Bennett, D., May, C. (1991) Meniscal damage associated with cruciate disease in the dog. *Journal of Small Animal Practice*, 32, 111-117.

Böttcher, P., Winkels, P., Oechtering, G. (2009) A novel pin distraction device for arthroscopic assessment of the medial meniscus in dogs. *Veterinary Surgery* 38, 595-600.

Case, J.B., Hulse, D., Kerwin, S.C., et al. (2008) Meniscal injury following initial cranial cruciate ligament stabilization surgery in 26 dogs (29 stifles). *Veterinary Comparative Orthopaedics and Traumatology* 21, 365-367.

Cook, J.L., Marberry, K.M., Kuroki, K., Kenter, K. (2004) Assessment of cellular, biochemical, and histologic effects of bipolar radiofrequency treatment of canine articular cartilage. *American Journal of Veterinary Research* 65 (5), 604-609.

Day, T.K., Pepper, W.T., Tobias, T.A., et al. (1995) Comparison of intra-articular and epidural morphine for analgesia following stifle arthrotomy in dogs. *Veterinary Surgery* 24, 522-630.

Drygas, K.A., McClure, S.R., Goring, R.L., et al. (2011) Effect of cold compression therapy on postoperative pain, swelling, range of motion, and lameness after tibial plateau leveling osteotomy in dogs. *Journal of the American Veterinary Medical Association* 238, 1284-1291.

Fitzpatrick, N., Solano, M.A. (2010) Predictive variables for complications TPLO with stifle inspection by arthrotomy in 1000 consecutive dogs. *Veterinary Surgery* 39, 460-474.

Flo, G.L. (1993) Meniscal injuries. *Veterinary Clinics of North America Small Animal Practice* 23, 831-843.

Flo, G.L., DeYoung, D. (1978) Meniscal injuries and medial meniscectomy. *Journal of the American Animal Hospital Association* 14, 683-689.

Hennig, G.S., Hosgood, G., Bubenik-Angapen, L.J., et al. (2010) Evaluation of chondrocyte death in canine osteochondral explants exposed to a 0.5% solution of bupivacaine. *American Journal of Veterinary Research* 71, 875-883.

Hoelzler, M.G., Millis, D.L., Francis, D.A., et al. (2004) Results of arthroscopic versus open arthrotomy for surgical management of cranial cruciate ligament deficiency in dogs. *Veterinary Surgery* 33, 146-153.

Horstman, C.L., McLaughlin, R.M. (2006) The use of radiofrequency energy during arthroscopic surgery and its effects on intraarticular tissues. *Veterinary Comparative Orthopaedics and Traumatology* 19, 65-71.

Horstman, C.L., McLaughlin, R.M., Elder, S.H., et al. (2009) Changes to articular cartilage following remote application of radiofrequency energy and with or without Cosequin therapy. *Veterinary Comparative Orthopaedics and Traumatology* 22 (2), 103-112.

Kalff, S., Meachem, S., Preston, C. (2011) Incidence of medial meniscal tears after arthroscopic assisted tibial plateau leveling osteotomy. *Veterinary Surgery* 40 (8), 952-956.

Kowaleski, M.P., Boudrieau, R.J., Pozzi, A. (2011) Stifle joint. In Tobias, K.M., Johnston, S.A. (eds.) *Veterinary Surgery Small Animal*, 4th edn. Saunders, Philadelphia, pp. 906-998.

Muir, W.W. (2007) Local anesthesia in dogs and cats. In Muir, W.W. (ed.) *Handbook of Veterinary Anesthesia.* Mosby, St. Louis, pp. 1118-139.

O'Brien, C.S., Martinez, S.A. (2009) Potential iatrogenic medial meniscal damage during tibial plateau leveling osteotomy. *Veterinary Surgery* 38, 868-873.

Piermattei, D.L., Johnson, K.A. (2004a) Approach to the stifle joint through medial incision, In Piermattei, D.L., Johnson, K.A. (eds.) *An Atlas of Surgical Approaches to the Bones and Joints of the Dog and Cat,* 4th edn. Saunders, Philadelphia, pp. 347-349.

Piermattei, D.L., Johnson, K.A. (2004b) Approach to the stifle joint through a lateral incision, In Piermattei, D.L., Johnson, K.A. (eds.) *An Atlas of Surgical Approaches to the Bones and Joints of the Dog and Cat,* 4th edn. Saunders, Philadelphia, pp. 342-346.

Piermattei, D.L., Johnson, K.A. (2004c) Approach to the medial collateral ligament and caudo-medial part of the stifle joint. In Piermattei, D.L., Johnson, K.A. (eds.) *An Atlas of Surgical Approaches to the Bones and Joints of the Dog and Cat,* 4th edn. Saunders, Philadelphia, pp. 360-363.

Pozzi, A., Hildreth, B.E. 3rd, Rajala-Schultz, P.J. (2008) Comparison of arthroscopy and arthrotomy for diagnosis of medial meniscal pathology: an ex vivo study. *Veterinary Surgery* 37, 749-755.

Ralphs, S.C., Whitney, W.O. (2002) Arthroscopic evaluation of menisci in dogs with cranial cruciate ligament injuries: 100 cases (1999-2000). *Journal of the America Veterinary Medical Association* 221, 1601-1604.

Thieman, K.M., Tomlinson, J.L., Fox, D.B., et al. (2006) Effect of meniscal release on rate of subsequent meniscal tears and owner assessed outcome in dogs with cruciate disease treated with tibial plateau leveling osteotomy. *Veterinary Surgery* 35, 705-710.

Whitney, W.O. (2003) Arthroscopically assisted surgery of the stifle joint. In Beale, B.S., Hulse, D.A., Schulz, K.S. (eds.) *Small Animal Arthroscopy*. Saunders, Philadelphia, pp. 116-157.

117 Complications associated with cranial cruciate ligament repair

Dominique Griffon

College of Veterinary Medicine, Western University of Health Sciences, Pomona, CA, USA

Introduction

Cranial cruciate ligament disease (CCLD) is the leading cause of stifle-associated lameness in dogs and is the primary cause of degenerative joint disease (DJD) in that joint. As such, surgical management of CCL insufficiency represents one of the preponderant activities of small animal practices. Primary repair of cranial cruciate ligament (CCL) tears or avulsion are rarely attempted because of technical limitations inherent to preexisting CCL degeneration, poor regenerative capacities of damaged ligament, or small size of the avulsed bone fragment. Up until the 1990s, procedures recommended for surgical treatment of CCL insufficiency were designed to improve joint stability by replacing the damaged ligament (intracapsular techniques) or by creating a new restraint in a direction approaching that of the ligament but located out of the joint (transposition or existing structures or placement of a prosthesis). Among these, fibular head transposition (FHT) relies on the lateral collateral ligament of the stifle to prevent excessive internal rotation and cranial translation of the tibia (Smith and Torg 1985). This technique became popular in the early 1990s because it uses an autogenous graft, and was experimentally found more effective than intracapsular techniques in restoring the stability of the stifle. Although the technique provided good results in large dogs, force plate analysis of operated limbs failed to return to normal. Within 6 to 12 months after surgery, cranial drawer could be elicited, presumably because of stretching of the lateral collateral ligament (Dupuis et al. 1994). These findings along with complications associated with the procedure (fibular head fracture, implant migration, peroneal nerve damage) contributed to the subsequent decline in popularity of this technique.

Retinacular imbrication techniques rely on periarticular fibrosis to provide a long-term restraint to cranial translation of the tibia. Initial stability is achieved by tightening large nonabsorbable sutures between fabellae and the tibial crest. The original technique has been simplified with the use of heavy monofilament suture passed around the lateral fabella through a hole in the tibial crest (5 mm distal to the joint, 1 cm caudal to the cranial edge of the tibial crest) and under the patellar tendon. A crimp clamp system has gained popularity in clinical cases to facilitate the tightening of heavy nylon leader material and improve the biomechanical properties of the repair (Anderson et al. 1998). However, the location of the suture and periarticular fibrosis are not isometric and therefore do not restore the biomechanics of the stifle. In fact, overzealous tightening

of the suture in flexion may restrict postoperative range of motion (ROM). Recent advances in extracapsular repair have focused on (1) minimally invasive placement of a lateral fabellar suture (LFS) after arthroscopic evaluation of the knee and treatment of meniscal disease, (2) isometric placement of the suture, and (3) anchorage of the suture to bone rather than soft tissues. These goals prompted the development of suture anchors and the TightRope (TR) CCL system (Arthrex, Naples, FL). The TR technique involves the creation of a femoral tunnel (created with a 3.5- or 2.7-mm cannulated drill bit) originating just distal to the attachment of the lateral fabellar-femoral ligament and angled proximally through the distal femur (Cook et al. 2010). A tibial tunnel is created 3 to 4 mm distal to the knee, directed from the cranial aspect of the tubercle of Gurdey (caudal to the long digital extensor tendon) directed distally, cranially and medially. The tunnels are connected with FiberTape, a nonresorbable braided material that is stronger and stiffer than the leader line currently used with the crimp clamp system in large dogs.

Conversely, tibial osteotomies provide functional joint stability only during weight bearing but make no attempt at restoring anatomic stability. The tibial plateau leveling osteotomy (TPLO) does not restore the anatomic stability of the CCL-deficient stifle but modifies the joint geometry to neutralize cranial tibial thrust during weight bearing. The rationale behind the procedure relies on the magnitude of the cranial tibial thrust correlating with the slope of the tibial plateau. Accordingly, the slope of the medial tibial plateau is determined on a straight lateral radiograph of the stifle and tarsus. Intraobserver variability of this slope can reach up to ±3.4 degrees; while readings obtained from different readers may vary by up to ±4.8 degrees (Caylor et al. 2001). Limb alignment is evaluated on a posteroanterior radiograph of the leg. A radial osteotomy (of a predetermined radius) allows rotation of the tibial plateau before immobilization with a custom plate to create a postoperative tibial slope within 5 to 7 degrees of the long axis of the tibia. The TPLO procedure is more technically challenging than LFS repair but may improve function and owners' satisfaction (Gordon-Evans et al. 2013). The procedure also allows concurrent correction of tibial angulation or rotation. However, it does not restore the rotational stability lost as a result of CCLD.

Tibial tuberosity advancement (TTA) is based on the same principles as the TPLO in that it is aimed at eliminating the cranial tibial thrust generated during weight bearing. However, its premise is that the compression force generated during the stance phase is aligned

Complications in Small Animal Surgery, First Edition. Edited by Dominique Griffon and Annick Hamaide.
Companion website: www.wiley.com/go/griffon/complications

along the patellar tendon rather than the tibial axis. The procedure is therefore designed to eliminate the cranial component of the force by realigning the patellar tendon at 90 degrees with the tibial plateau. An osteotomy of the tibial crest allows its cranial transposition and immobilization with a specially designed plate. The amount of translation is based on preoperative measurement on a mediolateral projection of the tibia. In its original description, the osteotomy gap is implanted with a metallic cage filled with bone graft. The TTA is technically easier to perform than a TPLO and allows simultaneous mediolateral transposition of the tibial crest in dogs with patellar luxation. However, the cost is similar to that of a TPLO, and it does not allow correction of tibial torsion.

In a survey published in 1999, lateral suture stabilization was the technique most commonly used in small and large dogs (87% and 33%, respectively) (Leighton 1999). A more recent survey in the United Kingdom confirms that if surgical treatment was selected, extracapsular suture stabilization was performed in 63% of small dogs, but corrective osteotomies were only performed in 33% of cases (Comerford *et al.* 2013). Tibial osteotomies are currently commonly performed, especially in large breed dogs, although modifications of these techniques and new implants are constantly proposed. In a recent systematic review of surgical treatment for CCLD in dogs, English peer reviewed publications most commonly reported on TPLO, lateral extracapsular suture, and TTA (Bergh *et al.* 2014). This chapter focuses on complications associated with these three procedures.

Degenerative joint disease
See Chapter 18.

Infection
See Chapters 1 and 5.

Delayed bone healing
See Chapters 98

Postliminary meniscal disease

Definition
Postliminary meniscal disease involves meniscal lesions that were not diagnosed during initial treatment of CCLD but are detected in the postoperative phase. This condition is one of the most common major complications after CCL repair, with an overall incidence approximating 3% to 6% but varying greatly among reports (Tables 117.1 to 117.3). These lesions consist most commonly of bucket handle tears affecting the medial meniscus (~76% of cases reported by Case *et al.* 2008). Less common lesions include frayed caudal horn tears of the medial meniscus (~20% of cases) and longitudinal tears of the lateral meniscus (~3% of cases).

Risk factors
- Undiagnosed meniscal tears present at the time of CCLD treatment: evaluation of the joint via exploratory arthrotomy rather than arthroscopy
- Persistent cranial tibial thrust:
  - Undersized cage or insufficient advancement in TTAs
  - Insufficient rotation of the tibial plateau during TPLO

- Procedure: This complication seems more commonly reported after TTA (incidence varies between 2% and 27%; Wolf *et al.* 2012) and TPLO (incidence ranging between 1% and 5% of cases; Bergh and Peirone 2012) than extracapsular repairs (1.9% of cases reported by Casale and McCarthy 2009)

Diagnosis
Dogs with postoperative meniscal disease are typically presented for persistent lameness, failure to progress to expected levels of function, or acute onset of lameness. Presence of pain upon flexion of the stifle is four times more likely if meniscal disease is present (Dillon *et al.* 2014). An audible clicking is occasionally noticed during flexion and extension of the stifle (noticed in 28% of cases reported by Case *et al.* 2008). When present, a meniscal click increases the likelihood of medial meniscal disease by a factor of 11 (Dillon *et al.* 2014). A definitive diagnosis is made by direct inspection via arthrotomy or, preferably, by second-look arthroscopy (Figure 117.1 and **Video 117.1**).

Treatment
Meniscal tears are traditionally treated via partial meniscectomy (removal of a damaged portion involving less than half of the meniscus; see Figure 117.1), hemi-meniscectomy (removal of the caudal pole of the meniscus), or complete meniscectomy. Medical management for DJD should be prescribed after surgery (see Chapter 18).

Outcome
The prognosis for postoperative meniscal tears is fair. Lameness improves or resolves in about 95% of cases (Case *et al.* 2008), and function returns to levels adequate for pets. However, partial meniscectomy alters the biomechanics of the stifle, resulting in progression of DJD.

Prevention
Medial meniscal release has been proposed to prevent meniscal tears subsequent to TPLOs. Caudal meniscal release via transection of the caudal meniscotibial ligament is currently preferred over a radial (or abaxial) release. The efficacy of this procedure remains controversial (see Relevant literature).

The current recommendation to prevent postoperative meniscal disease is to improve the detection of preexisting lesions at the time of initial CCLD. This is best achieved via arthroscopy (Plesman *et al.* 2013; Ritzo *et al.* 2014) (see Chapter 116).

Detection of medial meniscal lesions may be improved during arthroscopy by:
- Using a stifle distractor (Böttcher *et al.* 2009)
- Probing the medial meniscus (Pozzi *et al.* 2008a)

Complications specific to extracapsular suture placement

Incorrect implant placement

Definition
Incorrect implant placement is defined as a positioning of the implant that differs from the standard description and affects the outcome. The placement of the implant may be incorrect in tension or location. Whereas loose implants lead to residual cranial drawer, excessive tension may restrict ROM and increase lateral compartment pressure

Table 117.1 Complications reported after tibial plateau leveling osteotomy in the literature*

Reference	Garnett and Daye 2014	Gordon-Evans et al. 2013	Nelson et al. 2013	Oxley et al. 2013	Gatineau et al. 2011	Fitzpatrick and Solano 2010	Conkling et al. 2010	Cook et al. 2010	Duerr et al. 2008	Corr and Brown 2007	Stauffer et al. 2006	Carey et al. 2005	Pacchiana et al. 2003	Priddy et al. 2003	Average
TPLOs performed (n)	98	40	15	100	476	1146	118	23	146	21	696	34	397	253	
Infection	2 2.0%			3 3.0%	14 2.9%	66 5.8%	1 0.8%	1 4.3%		3 14.3%			3 0.8%	9 3.6%	4.1%
Seroma	2 2.0%					8 0.7%	1 0.8%	3 13.0%					13 3.3%		4.0%
Meniscal tear		3.0%	1 6.7%	4 4.0%	10 2.1%	28 2.4%		1 4.3%	1 0.7%			2 5.9%	4 1.0%		2.9%
Patellar tendonitis	8 8.0%	0.0%				3 0.3%	1 0.8%	1 4.3%			19 2.7%	24 25.5%	2 0.5%		5.3%
Incisional edema, hematoma, bruising, or drainage	5 5.0%							1 4.3%	1 0.7%	1 4.8%	50 7.2%		7 4.3%		5.7%
Traumatic wound dehiscence	2 2.0%						3 2.5%		2 1.4%		13 1.9%		7 1.8%		1.9%
Draining tract													1 0.3%	1 0.4%	0.3%
Bandage complications									1 0.7%				14 3.5%		2.1%
Tibial fracture					1 0.2%			2 8.7%	1 0.7%	1 4.8%	3 0.4%				3.0%
Tibial tuberosity fracture	4 4.0%	0.0%	1 6.7%			5 0.4%	2 1.7%		7 4.8%	1 4.8%	28 4.0%	4 4.3%	14 3.5%	6 2.4%	3.2%
Fibular fracture		0.0%			2 0.4%	1 0.1%	1 0.8%		4 2.7%	1 4.8%	3 0.4%		1 0.3%	3 1.2%	1.2%
Patellar fracture					1 0.2%	1 0.1%						1 1.1%	1 0.3%		0.4%
Osteomyelitis									4 2.7%				7 1.8%	14 5.5%	3.3%
Medial patellar luxation				2 2.0%	5 1.1%	3 0.3%									1.1%
Internal tibial torsion												12 12.8%			12.8%
Delayed union	9 9.0%					3 0.3%	6 5.1%								4.3%
Ring sequestrum														1 0.4%	0.4%
Pivot shift					15 3.2%	3 0.3%	1 0.8%		4 2.7%						1.3%
Broken screw						1 0.1%	1 0.8%			2 9.5%			2 0.5%	4 1.6%	2.5%
Screw loosening											6 0.9%		4 1.0%	2 0.8%	0.9%
Kirschner wire loosening						2 0.2%									0.2%
Implant failure, other				1 1.0%					4 2.7%						1.3%
Intraoperative complications	2 2.0%										7 1.0%		6 1.5%		1.5%
Residual thrust	2 2.0%	3.0%													2.5%
Total number and percentage	36 36.0%	6.0%	4 26.7%	10 10.0%	48 10.1%	124 10.8%	17 14.4%	9 39.1%	29 19.9%	8 38.1%	129 18.5%	43 45.7%	96 24.2%	40 15.8%	22.5%

*For each reference, the total number of tibial plateau leveling osteotomies is listed along with the number and percentage of each complication reported. In each column, all complications are added to calculate the total number and overall percentage of complications in each study. These percentages are averaged in the bottom right cell. In each row, data collected from all studies are averaged in the last column to represent the average rate of each specific complication.

Table 117.2 Complications reported after lateral fabellar suture repair in the literature*

Reference	Gordon-Evans 2013		Nelson et al. 2013		Cassle McCarthy 2009		Average
LFS repairs (n)	40		23		363		
Postoperative meniscal tear	2	5.0%	1	4.3%	7	1.9%	3.8%
Incisional drainage or swelling			3	13.0%	22	6.1%	9.6%
Implant failure					10	2.8%	2.8%
Other					1	0.3%	0.3%
Infection					14	3.9%	3.9%
Bandage related					10	2.8%	2.8%
Total number and percentage	**2**	**5.0%**	**4**	**17.4%**	**64**	**17.6%**	**23.0%**

*For each reference, the total number of lateral fabellar sutures (LFSs) is listed along with the number and percentage of each complication reported. In each column, all complications are added to calculate the total number and overall percentage of complications in each study. These percentages are averaged in the bottom right cell. In each row, data collected from all studies are averaged in the last column to represent the average rate of each specific complication.

in the joint (Tonks et al. 2010). Incorrect location of the implant is somewhat specific to the technique:
- LFS technique:
  ◦ Failure to pass the suture around the fabellae (see Figure 117.2)
  ◦ Incorrect positioning of the hole in the tibial crest (see Figure 117.2)
- "TR CCL system:
  ◦ Incorrect placement of bone tunnels (Figures 117.3 and 117.4)

◦ Interposition of soft tissue between the toggle or button and bone (Figure 117.5)

Risk factors
- Surgical experience (Biskup and Griffon 2014)
- The TR technique is more likely to be associated with technical deviations than LFS (Biskup and Griffon 2014).
- "Reverse" TR: In this modification, the TR is placed in the opposite direction than in the standard technique. The toggle is therefore blindly placed against the femur, where it is more difficult to palpate (and therefore assess placement; see Figure 117.4).
- Minimally invasive placement of TR or LFS: Mini approaches are created over points of anchorage and the suture is tunneled under the skin.

Diagnosis
Persistence of a cranial drawer immediately after placement of the implant should trigger suspicion and warrant surgical exposure of the repair for direct inspection.

Incorrect implant placement undiagnosed immediately after surgery will usually result in slow and incomplete recovery of function after surgery. Persistent cranial drawer are noticed at follow-up examinations.

The sensitivity of radiographs for detection of technical deviations approximates 39% after TR and 50% after percutaneous LFS (Biskup and Griffon 2014). Technical errors most commonly identified on radiographs include inappropriate location of bone tunnels (see Figures 117.3 and 117.4) and implant (see Figure 117.4) along with interposition of soft tissues (see Figure 117.5).

Table 117.3 Complications reported after tibial tuberosity advancement in the literature*

Reference	Hirshenson et al. 2012		Wolf et al. 2012		Steinberg et al. 2011		Yeadon et al. 2010		Lafaver et al. 2007		Average
TTAs (n)	101		501		193		39		114		
Incisional inflammation	4	4.0%	33	6.6%	5	2.6%	2	5.1%	2	1.8%	4.0%
Tendonitis			2	0.4%							0.4%
Seroma			3	0.6%			2	5.1%			2.9%
Tibial tuberosity fracture	2	2.0%	18	3.6%	2	1.0%			4	3.5%	2.5%
Tibial fracture			3	0.6%					3	2.6%	1.6%
Breakage of fork			6	1.2%	1	0.5%			3	2.6%	1.4%
Failure of cage or screw	2	2.0%	4	0.8%	1	0.5%			1	0.9%	1.0%
Meniscal tear	5	5.0%	6 of 231 with MMR (2.6%) 10 of 36 without MMR (21.8%)		10	5.2%	1	2.6%	7	6.1%	4.7%
Medial patellar luxation	1	1.0%			1	0.5%	4	10.3%	1	0.9%	3.2%
Infection	1	1.0%			1	0.5%	2	5.1%	2	1.8%	2.1%
Lick granuloma		0.0%							2	1.8%	0.9%
Poor graft mineralization									3	2.6%	2.6%
Postoperative swelling of limb	2	2.0%							2	1.8%	1.9%
Wound dehiscence									1	0.9%	0.9%
Chronic poor performance									1	0.9%	0.9%
Patella baja	3	3.0%									3.0%
Total number and percentage	**20**	**19.8%**	**69**	**13.8%**	**21**	**10.9%**	**11**	**28.2%**	**32**	**28.1%**	**20.1%**

*For each reference, the total number of tibial tuberosity advancements (TTAs) is listed along with the number and percentage of each complication reported. In each column, all complications are added to calculate the total number and overall percentage of complications in each study. These percentages are averaged in the bottom right cell. In each row, data collected from all studies are averaged in the last column to represent the average rate of each specific complication. MMR: Medial meniscal release; † Dogs with CCLD and medial patellar luxation.

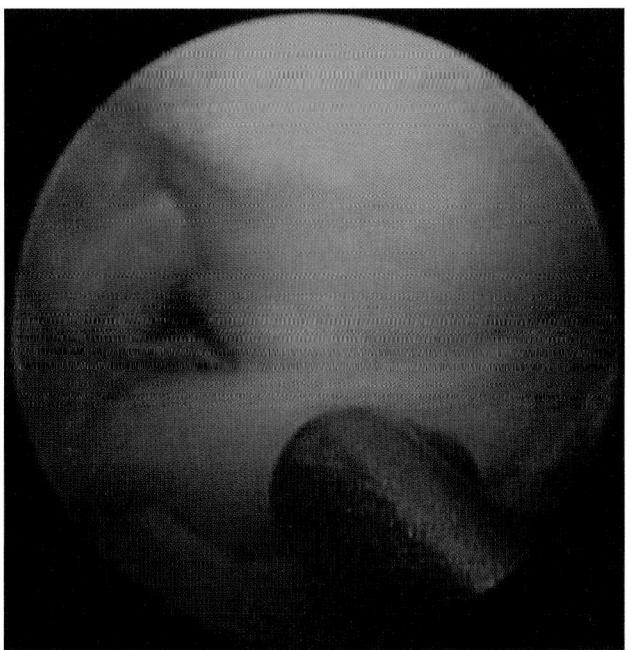

(A)

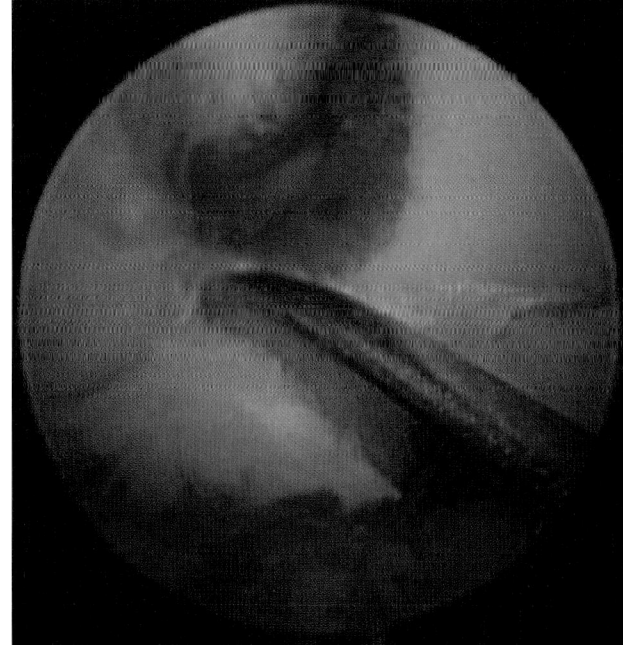

(B)

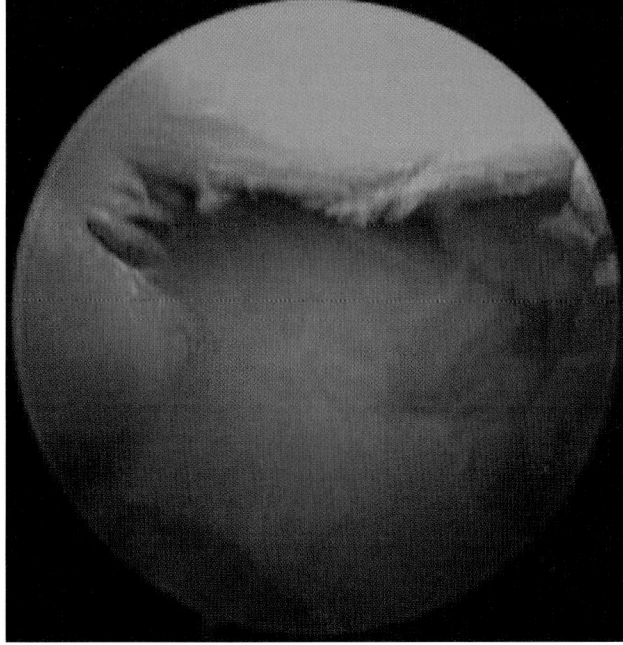

(C)

Figure 117.1 Medial meniscal tear in a dog 3 months after tibial plateau leveling osteotomy without meniscal release. **A,** A probe is used to confirm the type and extent of the lesion. **B,** The lesion is treated by partial meniscectomy using meniscal knives and a shaver. **C,** Postoperative appearance of the medial meniscus. Note the presence of iatrogenic trauma on the articular surface of the medial femoral condyle.

Treatment

Minor technical deviations, such as bone tunnels or holes placed a couple of millimeters off from the standard location, may not be clinically relevant. Technical deviations combined with lameness or laxity require surgical revision (see Figure 117.4). Loose suture or interposition of soft tissue can be treated by removing the suture and replacing it using the same landmarks and tunnels.

Revision strategies for LFS include:

- Suture that is loose or not placed around the fabella is removed and replaced appropriately. Alternatively, tibial osteotomy may be considered.

- Use of a crimp clamp kit and tensioner improves tightness of the suture compared with hand-tied knots in large dogs.
- If the hole in the tibial crest is malpositioned, options include creation of a second hole or tibial osteotomy.

Bone tunnels in the TR technique cannot be repositioned without increasing the risk of femoral or tibial fracture. In these cases, revision with an LFS is a safer option. Loose implants should be removed and may be replaced through the same bone tunnels if those are appropriately placed. Use of a tensioner and double-strand kit allow better control of the knot's tightness.

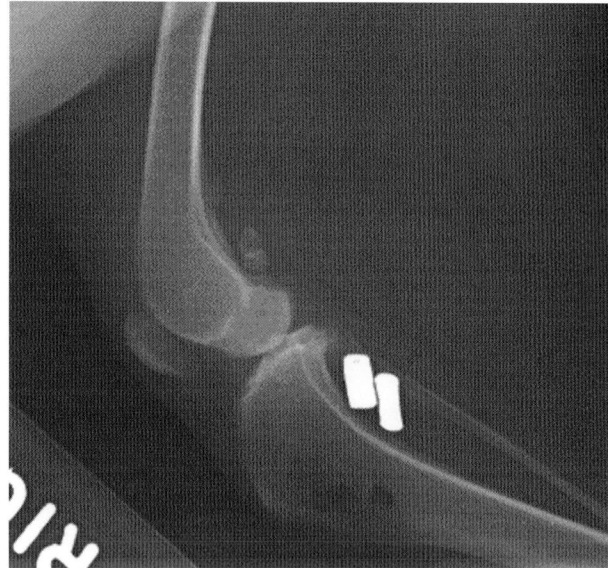

Figure 117.2 Radiograph of a small breed dog referred for persistent lameness and cranial drawer after cranial cruciate ligament disease treated via lateral fabellar suture (LFS). Abnormalities identified on radiographs included stifle effusion, presence of degenerative joint disease, and distal positioning of two holes in the tibial crest and of the two crimp clamps. During surgical exploration, the suture was found to pass around the fibular head rather than the lateral fabella. Implants were removed and replaced with an LFS.

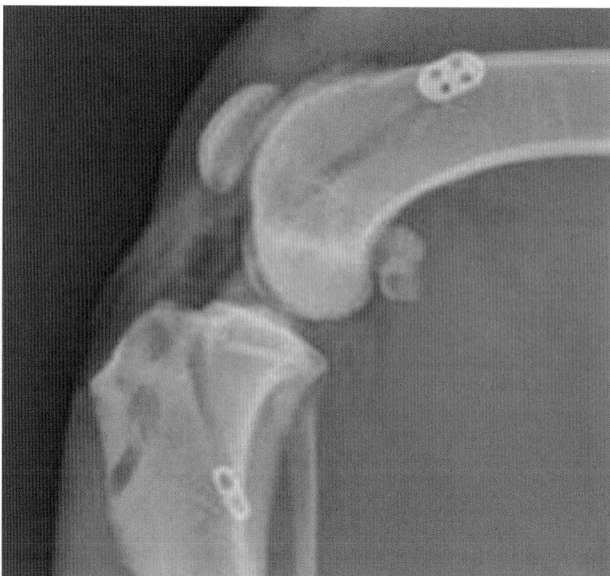

Figure 117.3 Incorrect positioning of tunnels during the TightRope (Arthrex, Naples, FL) technique. Note two failed attempts at positioning the tibial tunnel. The point of entry of the femoral tunnel is also misplaced. This specimen was created during a teaching laboratory on cadaver limbs. *Source:* Biskup and Griffon, 2014. Reproduced with permission from John Wiley & Sons.

Outcome

The prognosis after revision of a loose or misplaced implant is good overall, although the risk of postoperative complications may be greater than during initial surgery. Delayed revision of a defective implant and prolonged joint instability lead to secondary degenerative changes that are irreversible.

Prevention

Incorrect placement of implants results from technical errors, usually associated with lack of experience and knowledge of anatomic landmarks. This complication is therefore best prevented by obtaining training specifically focused on each technique before application in clinical cases.

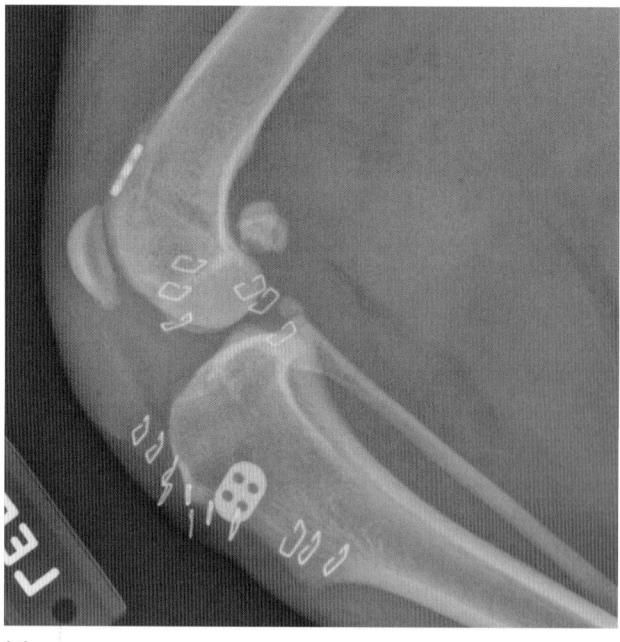

(A)

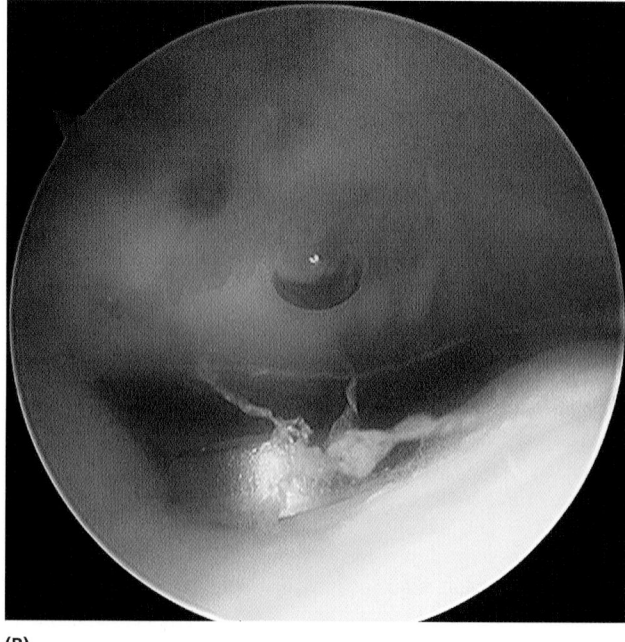

(B)

Figure 117.4 Incorrect positioning of the femoral tunnel during reverse TightRope (Arthrex, Naples, FL) repair in a mixed breed dog with cranial cruciate ligament disease. **A,** The exit point of the femoral tunnel is too cranial and distal, warranting revision. **B,** Arthroscopic view of the implant within the joint. The implant was removed and the repair revised with a lateral fabellar suture.

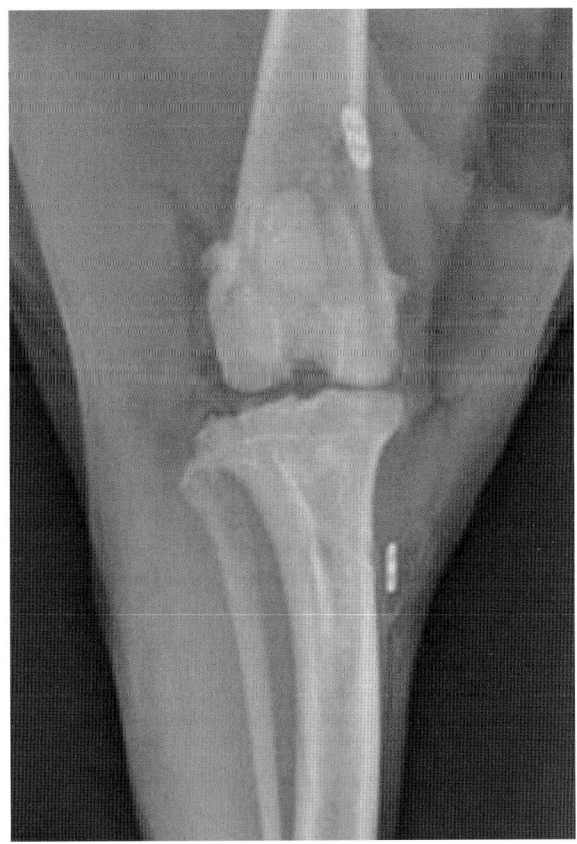

Figure 117.5 Interposition of the soft tissues between the tibial toggle and the bone in a traditional TightRope (Arthrex, Naples, FL) cranial cruciate ligament disease repair. This specimen was created during a teaching laboratory on cadaver limbs. *Source:* Biskup and Griffon, 2014. Reproduced with permission from John Wiley & Sons.

Proper placement of the suture LFS is facilitated by:
- Identification of the lateral fabella, which is facilitated by exposing the original of the gastrocnemius, and its fibers oriented in a caudocranial direction.
- Placement of the suture around the fabella can be checked by applying tension on each end of the suture; this tension should induce a displacement of the fabella.

Proper placement of tunnels and implant in TR is facilitated by:
- Using a traditional rather than reverse technique
- Using guide pins before drilling bone tunnels, as recommended by the manufacturer
- Using self-retaining retractors to expose the femoral button and verify appropriate location
- Using tensioner with a double-strand kit to control the tension of the knot

Postoperative implant loosening

Definition
Implant loosening leading to recurrence of joint instability and loss of function after CCLD repair. A slight loss of tension in suture commonly occurs after LFS as suture elongates because of cyclic

loading. A mild cranial drawer (1–2 mm) may be present without signs of pain or lameness. In a randomized, blinded, controlled clinical trial, a cranial drawer could be palpated in 15% of dogs 1 year after LFS (Gordon-Evans et al. 2013). This section focuses on joint instability affecting clinical outcome after placement of an extracapsular suture.

Risk factors
- Suture breakage
- Failure of a crimp clamp
- Loosening of a hand-tied knot
- Interposition of soft tissues between the implant and bone (see Figure 117.5)
- Bone necrosis and widening of bone tunnels after TR CCLD repair (Figure 117.6)
- Superficial placement of bone anchors

Diagnosis
Recurrence of joint laxity is diagnosed on orthopedic examination by palpation of a cranial drawer and positive tibia compression test result. The clinical significance of residual instability is not clearly established and is likely to vary with the degree of laxity. Clinically relevant instability is associated with secondary DJD and incomplete return to function. Dogs with persistent loss of function and joint instability should be evaluated for caudal cruciate ligament deficiency and meniscal lesions.

Treatment
Conservative treatment can be considered in small dogs with mild residual cranial laxity and mild or absent clinical signs. Conservative management includes neuromuscular rehabilitation targeted at strengthening active restraints to cranial tibial thrust (i.e., hamstring muscles). A multimodal approach to DJD should also be initiated (see Chapter 18). Surgical revision is indicated in patients with obvious cranial drawers (>5 mm) and unsatisfactory function of the limb. The management of these cases should include the following steps:
- Removal of loose or failed implants
- Assessment of the joint via arthrotomy or arthroscopy combined with probing of the menisci
- Submission of intraoperative samples for culture and sensitivity
- Restoration of joint stability based on the following options:
  - Consider tibial plateau osteotomy along with pin fixation of the tibial tuberosity to avoid stress fracture.
  - Replace a lateral suture using the same points of insertion if those were appropriate.
  - TR with widening of the femoral tunnel may be revised with an LFS or TPLO.
  - In cases with significant bone loss in the proximal tibia, bone anchors or pins (tension band) may be placed in the proximal tibia to anchor a suture.

If present, caudal cruciate ligament deficiency should be addressed with extracapsular repair (see Figure 117.6). Postliminary meniscal tears are generally managed via resection of the diseased portion of the medial meniscus (see section above). Postoperative antibiotherapy may be prescribed based on culture sensitivity.

Outcome
The prognosis for dogs with postoperative implant loosening is very good if stability can be restored. Secondary diseases such as caudal

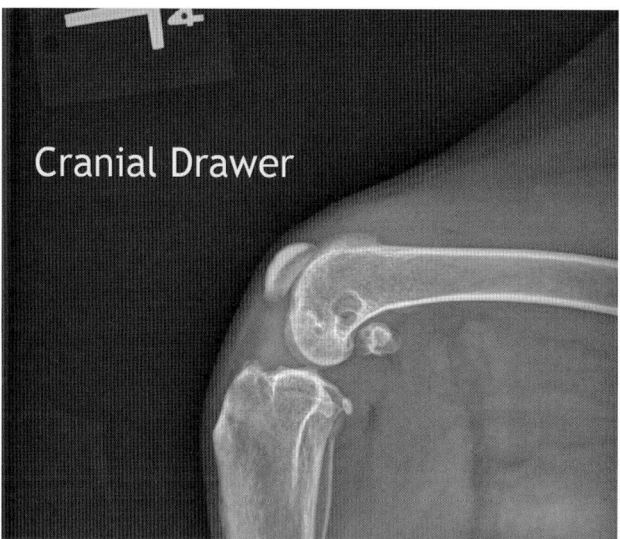

(A)

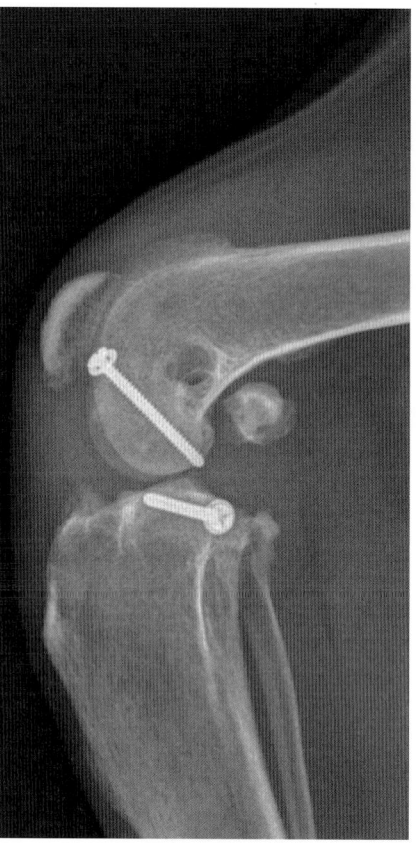

(B)

Figure 117.6 Bone necrosis and implant loosening after TightRope (TR; Arthrex, Naples, FL) repair. This dog was referred for potential knee replacement 1 year after initial TR cranial cruciate ligament disease repair. After surgery, the dog did not return to function, and bone necrosis of the femoral tunnel was noted (**A**). The dog underwent treatment caudal cruciate ligament deficiency (**B**) but failed to improve. Upon evaluation after referral, braided suture material was found along with septic arthritis. Amputation was recommended. *Source:* L. M. Déjardin, Michigan State University, East Lansing, MI. Reproduced with permission from L. M. Déjardin.

cruciate ligament deficiency, postliminary meniscal tear, infection, and DJD may affect the prognosis.

Prevention

Proper technique is a general strategy to avoid surgical complications in general. A good knowledge of relevant anatomy and landmarks recommended for each technique is a prerequisite to optimize suture location. Isometric placement is ideal to restore joint biomechanics and ensure constant suture tension throughout the ROM. Suture selection plays a controversial role: braided material is generally less prone than nylon to elongation with cyclic loading (Cabano *et al.* 2011; Rose *et al.* 2012). However, this factor can be subjectively anticipated and accounted for by setting the initial tension at which the suture is tied or crimped. The pathogenesis and prevalence of bone necrosis around bone tunnels in the TR technique remain undefined. In the absence of established preventive measures, aligning tunnels as much as possible with the long axis of the bone may limit friction of the suture around sharp bone edges. Alternatively, selecting bone anchors instead of femoral tunnels eliminates this risk of complication while achieving bone anchorage of a lateral suture.

Complications specific to tibial plateau leveling osteotomies

Osteosarcoma

See Chapter 104.

Patellar tendon thickening and tendonitis

Definition

Whereas postoperative patellar tendon thickening refers to an anatomic change in the dimensions of the patellar tendon after TPLO, patellar tendonitis is defined as a clinical condition resulting from postoperative inflammation of the tendon. Patellar tendon thickening may be an incidental radiographic finding, but patellar tendonitis is associated with clinical signs. The reported incidence of this condition varies among reports (see Table 117.1) and is higher (80%–100% of cases) in studies specifically focusing on the effect of TPLOs on patellar tendon, most likely because other reports may not consider patellar thickening as a complication of TPLO.

Risk factors

Potential risk factors include:

- Intraoperative retraction of the tendon during the tibial osteotomy
- Placement of an antirotational holding pin through the patellar tendon
- Iatrogenic trauma resulting from contact between the saw blade and tendon
- Cranially positioned tibial osteotomy (Carey *et al.* 2005)
- Body weight (Mattern *et al.* 2006)
- Postoperative tibial plateau angle (TPA) (Mattern *et al.* 2006)
- Excessive postoperative exercise, especially swimming during the first 6 weeks after TPLO
- Cranial closing wedge osteotomy combined with TPLO: Patellar thickening was reported in 61% of cases (Talaat *et al.* 2006).

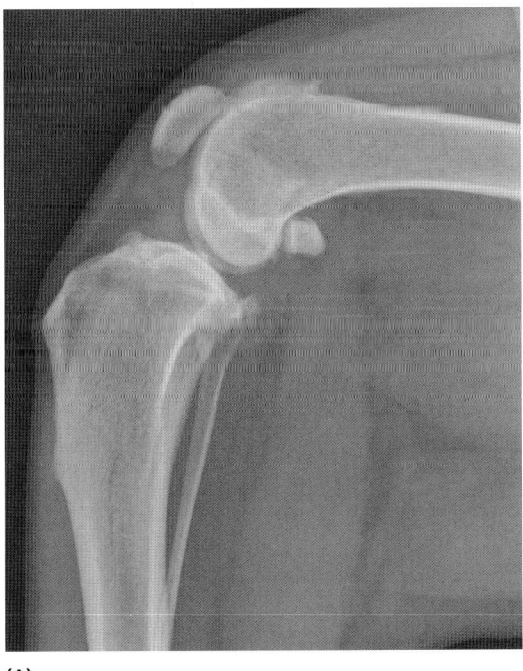

(A)

Figure 117.7 Patellar tendon thickening after tibial plateau leveling osteotomy (TPLO). Mediolateral radiographs obtained before (**A**) and 6 weeks (**B**) after TPLO. Thickening of the patellar tendon and unclear margins were incidental radiographic findings.

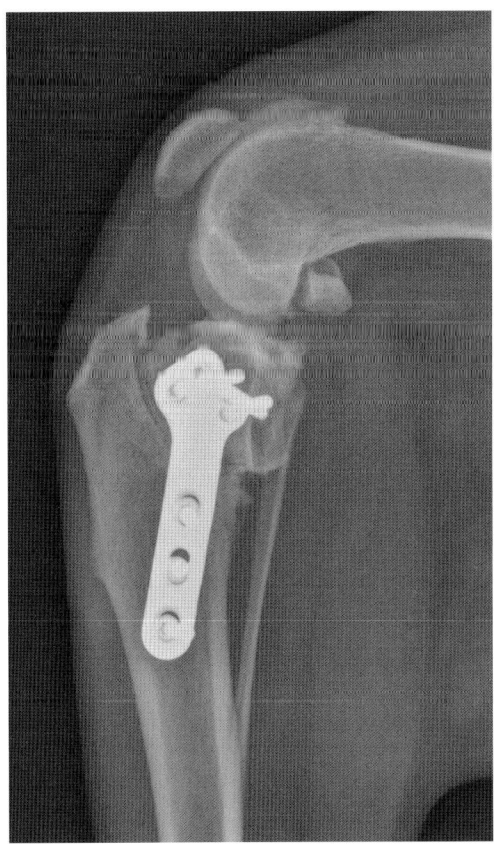

(B)

Diagnosis

Clinical signs associated with patellar tendonitis include pain on palpation of the tendon and delayed return to function (lameness). Patellar tendon thickening is diagnosed on mediolateral radiographs of the stifle, comparing pre- and postoperative dimensions (Figure 117.7). A radiographic grading system has been proposed by Carey *et al.* (2005), where grade 0 is assigned to tendons measuring a maximum of twice the preoperative thickness, grade 1 is assigned to tendons measuring 6 to 11 mm in thickness, and grade 2 is given to tendons exceeding 12 mm in thickness or displaying unidentifiable borders. Changes are usually more pronounced along the distal portion of the tendon (Mattern *et al.* 2006). Ultrasonographic changes include thickening and hypoechoic or anechoic central lesions with disruption of longitudinal ligamentous fibrils (Mattern *et al.* 2006).

Treatment

Patellar thickening may be an incidental finding on postoperative radiographs and may not warrant specific treatment. Patellar tendonitis resolves with rest and antiinflammatory drugs.

Outcome

The outcome is excellent. Clinical signs in dogs with patellar tendonitis generally resolve in 1 to 2 months.

Prevention

Retraction of the patellar tendon during the osteotomy is unlikely to play a significant role in the pathogenesis of this disease because retraction during procedures other than TPLO has not been found to produce postoperative changes. Protection of the tendon during the osteotomy therefore remains strongly indicated.

Positioning the tibial osteotomy caudal is recommended to optimize the rotation of the proximal tibia while avoiding complications such as patellar tendonitis and tibial tuberosity fractures.

Cranial closing wedge osteotomies were initially combined with TPLOs in stifles with TPAs exceeding 30 degrees. However, dogs with postoperative TPA exceeding the recommended 7 degrees have been found to regain function, questioning the indication for a cranial closing wedge osteotomy. In dogs with steep TPAs, incomplete correction limited to a TPLO may provide satisfactory outcome while decreasing morbidity.

Implant failure

Definition

Implant loosening or breakage compromising immobilization of the osteotomy and subsequent bone healing. Screw loosening is the most common type of implant failure associated with TPLO.

Risk factors

- Use of nonlocking screws or failure to obtain bicortical fixation (Figure 117.8)
- Cranial closing wedge osteotomy of the tibia combined with TPLO: Implant loosening or breakage has been reported in 28% of cases (Talaat *et al.* 2006; (Figure 117.9).

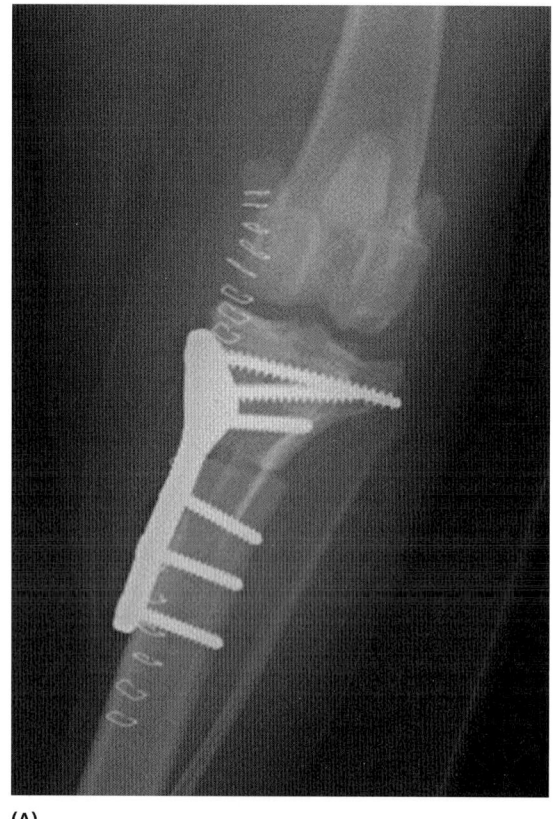
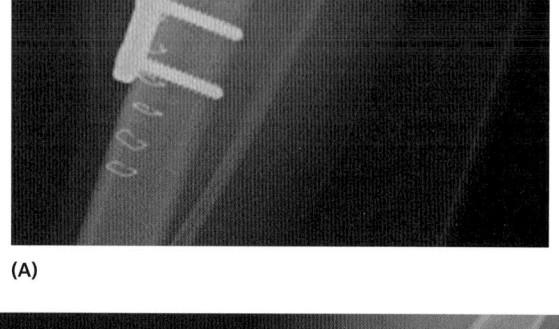

(A)

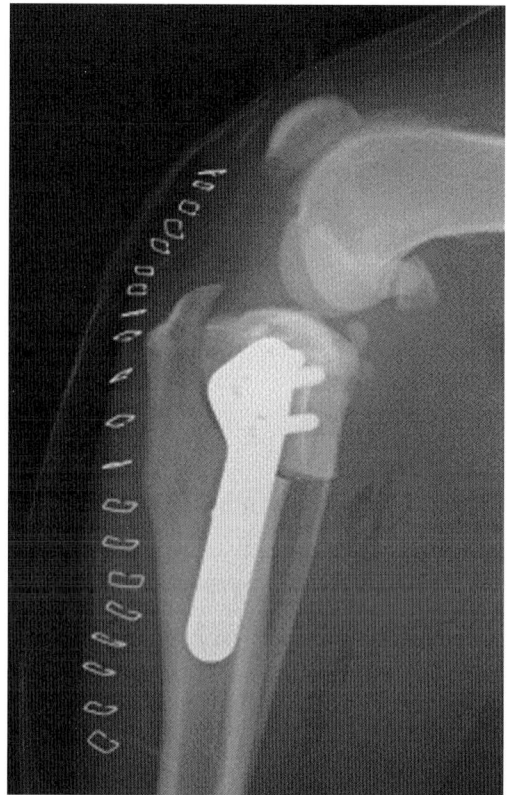

(B)

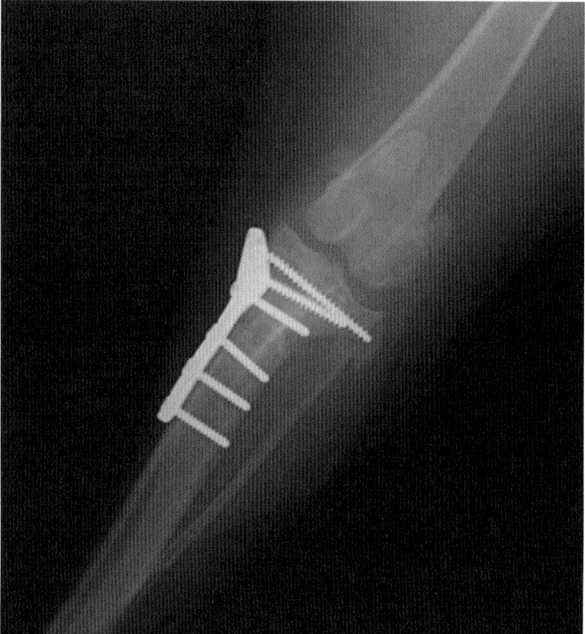

(C)

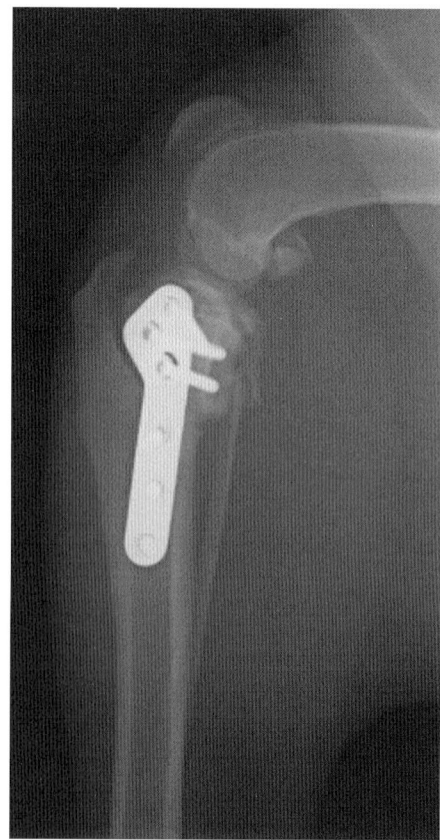

(D)

Figure 117.8 Screw loosening and fibular head fracture after tibial plateau leveling osteotomy (TPLO). Craniocaudal and mediolateral obtained immediately after TPLO with a nonlocking implant (**A** and **B**) and 3 weeks later (**C** and **D**). Engagement of the third proximal screw through the far cortex appeared questionable on postoperative radiographs (A and B). Radiolucency around this screw is consistent with loosening 3 weeks later (C and D). A fracture of the proximal fibula is also noticed but was not present on postoperative radiographs. Note the widening of the osteotomy gap consistent with micromotion. Management included replacement of the third proximal screw, tightening of the other screws, and strict exercise restriction.

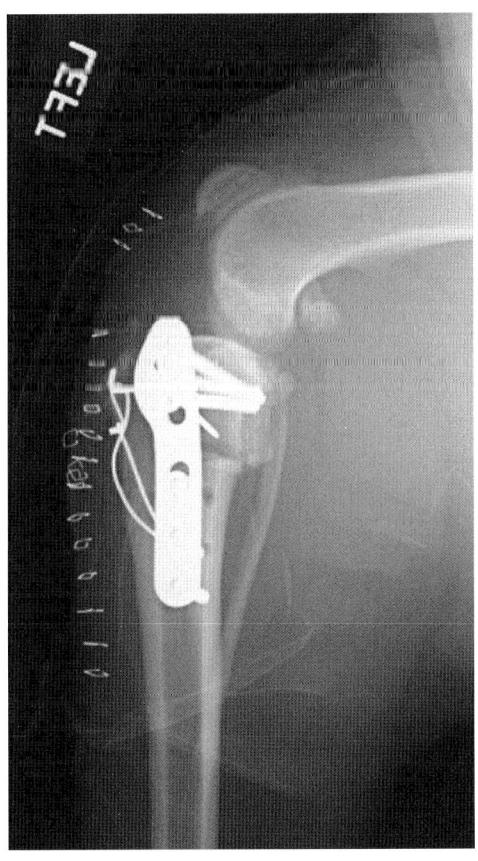

(A)

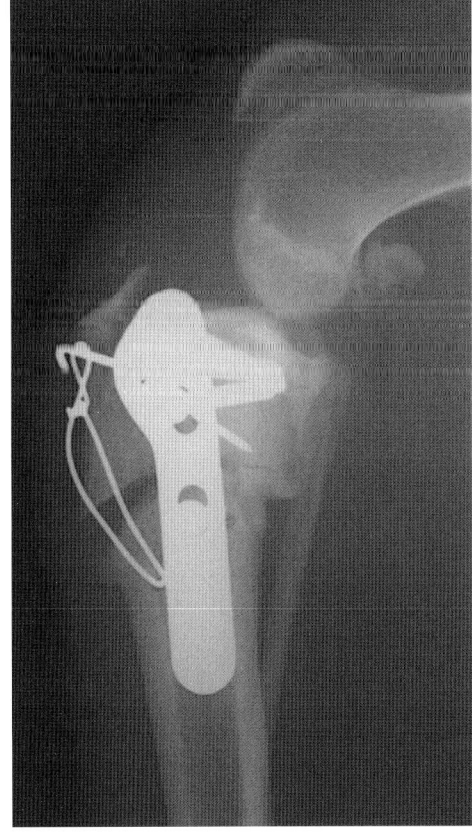

(B)

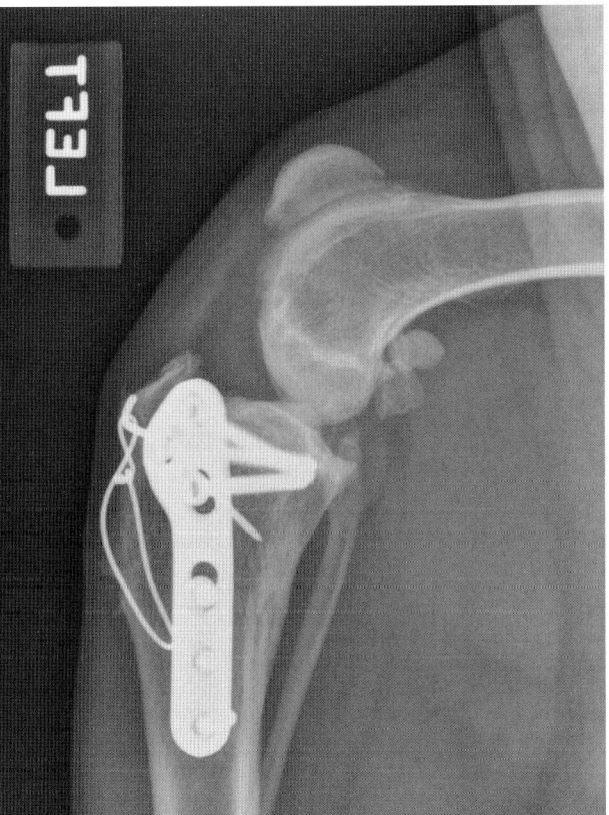

(C)

Figure 117.9 Pin migration and loss of reduction after tibial plateau leveling osteotomy (TPLO) and cranial closing wedge in an obese 3-year-old Labrador retriever female with a preoperative tibial plateau angle of 39 degrees and a medial meniscal tear. **A**, Postoperative radiograph. The dog was treated with a 30-degree TPLO correction and a 6-mm cranial closing wedge. A locking implant was used to immobilize the osteotomy, but locking screws of adequate length were not commercially available at the time of surgery. **B**, Radiograph obtained 6 weeks after surgery. Note the migration of the pin and loss of reduction of the cranial closing wedge. This complication most likely resulted from the poor placement of a single pin in the tibial tuberosity. Conservative management allowed bone union at 16 weeks. **C**, Radiograph 18 months after surgery. The implant remains unchanged, and degenerative joint disease has progressed.

- Excessive postoperative exercise
- Infection
- Excessive micromotion at the osteotomy site
- Concurrent tibial tuberosity or fibular head fractures
- Delayed bone healing

Diagnosis

Clinical signs vary with the type of implant failure and its consequence on the stability of the osteotomy. Loosening of single screw may be an incidental finding at follow-up. Catastrophic failure leads to sudden non–weight-bearing lameness and crepitus on palpation of the osteotomy site.

Implant failure is confirmed on radiographs (see Figures 117.8 and 117.9). Signs include:

- Radiolucency around the implant
- Implant migration
- Loss of reduction of the osteotomy
- Delayed healing
- Bone fracture (fibula or tibia)

Treatment

Conservative management and exercise restriction can be considered if implant loosening is an incidental finding on follow-up radiographs in dogs with normal progression of bone healing and stable fixation. Revision should be considered if stability of the osteotomy appears questionable or bone healing appears delayed. Catastrophic failure of implants warrants immediate surgical revision. Revision of the TPLO varies from replacing a loose screw to augmentation or replacement with an external fixator or another plate.

Outcome

The outcome with incidental screw loosening is similar to that of uncomplicated TPLOs. The prognosis after revision of a failed implant is generally good, although delayed bone healing should be expected. Complications secondary to implant failure, such as bone fractures, infection, or DJDs, can affect the prognosis.

Prevention

Implant failure is an infrequent complication reported in fewer than 2% of cases (see Table 117.1). Following proper technique for plate contouring and bicortical screw fixation is crucial to maintaining stability with traditional plate fixation. Alternatively, developments in implant design have led to the commercialization of locking TPLO plates. Among these, the TPLO locking plate (De Puy Synthes Vet, West Chester, PA) is a precontoured plate with plate head holes angled away from the articular surface and osteotomy, optimizing the placement of locking screws. Regardless of the implant selected for TPLO, postoperative exercise restriction until bony union is essential to prevent postoperative complications.

Bone fractures

Definition

Bone fractures secondary to TPLO include fractures of the fibula, tibia, and tibial tuberosity. The incidence of bone fractures varies among studies (see Table 117.1). Among these, tibial tuberosity avulsion fractures were reported in 4% of 213 TPLOs in a retrospective study specifically focusing on this complication (Bergh et al. 2008). The incidence of fibular fractures varied between 5.4% (of 168 TPLOs) and 15% (of 355) TPLOs in two retrospective studies

focusing specifically on this complication (Tuttle and Manley 2009; Taylor et al. 2011). Tibial fractures are uncommon but major complications after TPLO.

Risk factors

Tibial tuberosity fractures are believed to result from the tension applied by the quadriceps on the patella tendon. Proposed risk factures for these avulsion fractures include:

- Cranial tibial osteotomy (Figure 117.10)
- Simultaneous bilateral TPLOs
- Placement of an antirotational holding pin perpendicular to the long axis of the tibia
- Correction of steep TPAs (≥34 degrees)
- Previous extracapsular repair with a hole or a tunnel drilled in the proximal tibia (Figure 117.11)

Proposed risk factors for fibular fractures include:

- Body weight: The odds of a fibular fracture have been reported to increase by 1.5 times greater for every 4.5-kg increase in body weight (Taylor et al. 2011).
- Steep preoperative TPA and magnitude of the TPA correction
- Presence of a drill hole in the fibula
- TPLO performed without the use of a jig (Tuttle and Manley 2009; Flynn et al. 2014)

Tibial fractures occur most commonly as a result of implant failure or infection. Use of an oversized and eccentrically placed jig pin has been suggested as a predisposing factor (Bergh and Peirone 2012).

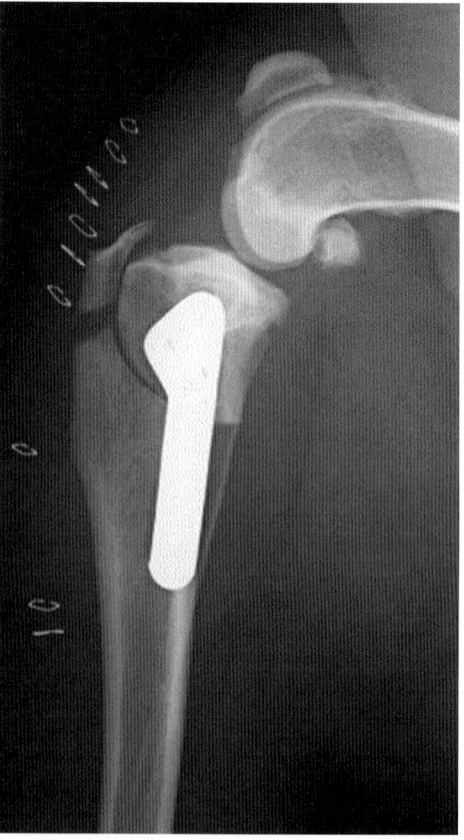

Figure 117.10 Tibial tuberosity fracture 10 days after tibial plateau leveling osteotomy. Note the cranial placement of the osteotomy, creating a narrow tibial tuberosity.

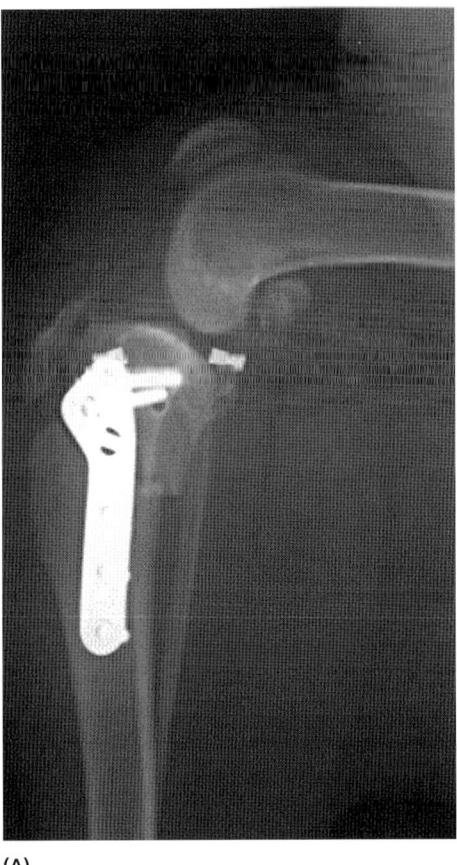
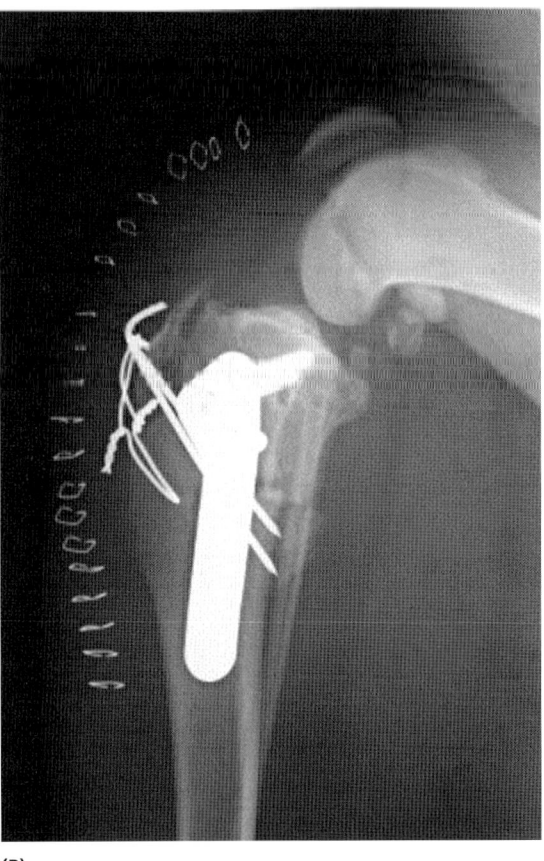

(A)   **(B)**

Figure 117.11 Tibial tuberosity fracture revision of a failed lateral fabellar suture (LFS) with a tibial plateau leveling osteotomy (TPLO).
A, Mediolateral radiograph obtained 2 weeks after the TPLO. An avulsion fracture of the tibial tuberosity probably resulted from the
stress rising effect of the hole drilled in the tibial tuberosity during the LFS. **B**, Radiograph obtained after revision with a tension band. The dog
recovered uneventfully. This complication may have been prevented by incorporating the antirotational holding pin placed during the TPLO
into a tension band.

Diagnosis

Tibial tuberosity fractures are occasionally diagnosed as incidental
findings on routine follow-up radiographs. Fractures that occur in
the early postoperative phase and are displaced (see Figure 117.10)
may be associated with delayed return to function (lameness) along
with swelling and pain over the tibial crest. The diagnosis is confirmed on radiographs, and most fractures appear as transverse or
short oblique avulsion fractures. The apparatus and bone healing
should be carefully evaluated for loss of stability and delayed callus
formation.

Fibular fractures may occur intraoperatively if a synostosis or
ankylosis between the fibula and lateral tibia prevents rotation of
the osteotomized tibial segment. In these cases, the fracture may be
heard during manipulation of the osteotomized tibial segment, suddenly free to rotate. However, fibular fractures are generally diagnosed on follow-up radiographs (see Figure 117.8). Most fractures
occur at the level of the fibular neck, some involve the body, and a
few affect the fibular head. The TPA of dogs with these fractures may
be higher at recheck than immediately postoperatively, suggesting
construct instability. The apparatus and osteotomy gap should be
carefully evaluated and monitored for concurrent implant failure
and delayed healing.

Tibial fractures are major complications inducing non–weight-
bearing lameness. The diagnosis is confirmed based on radiographs, and these fractures are commonly combined with implant
failure.

Treatment

Tibial tuberosity fractures may be treated conservatively if they
appear mildly displaced and do not appear to affect implant stability or bone healing. Unstable fractures diagnosed early in the
postoperative phase are best treated with a tension band to avoid
secondary implant failure (see Figure 117.11).

Fibular fractures are treated conservatively unless they are associated with implant failure and loss of stability.

Tibial fractures require surgical revision and treatment of any
concurrent disease, such as infection. Surgical revision is aimed
at restoring stability of the osteotomy site and ability of the tibia
to sustain biomechanical loads. Revision may be achieved via
plate fixation, external fixation, or a combination of both. Augmentation of bone repair with bone grafts or substitutes is recommended to accelerate healing. Antibiotherapy should be based on
analysis of intraoperative samples submitted for bacteriology and
sensitivity.

Outcome

The outcome of fibular and tibial tuberosity fractures is very good if stability is maintained until bony union. Complications may include delayed bone healing and implant failure. The prognosis after tibial fractures is more variable, depending on the type and location of the fracture(s), ability to restore stability and alignment of the osteotomy, and presence of infection. Complications after revision of TPLO with secondary tibial fractures may be severe enough to justify amputation.

Prevention

Careful planning of the tibial osteotomy appears to be the most effective strategy for preventing tibial tuberosity fractures; the osteotomy should be located caudally, preserving a craniocaudal width of at least 1 cm for the tibial tuberosity (Bergh et al. 2008). Angling the antirotational holding pin in a proximodistal direction rather than perpendicular to the long axis of the tibia may also limit the stress rising effect created by the pin. Incorporating this holding pin into a tension band may also help prevent postoperative tibial tuberosity fractures in dogs with preexisting bone defects in the proximal tibia.

Prevention of fibular fractures relies on the use of a TPLO jig and careful drilling of screw holes in the proximal tibia. No strategy has specifically been recommended to prevent tibial fractures.

Complications specific to tibial tuberosity advancement

Bone fracture

Definition

Bone fractures secondary to TTA include tibial fractures involving the tuberosity or less commonly the diaphysis. Overall, these are unusual complications, described in about 4% to 5% of TTAs (see Table 117.3) (Wolf et al. 2012; Calvo et al. 2014).

Risk factors

The following factors may increase the risk of tibial tuberosity fractures:
- Cranial placement of the tibial osteotomy
- Placement of the fork close to the osteotomy
- Surgeon's level of experience
- Large preoperative patellar tendon angle, large cage
- Iatrogenic damage

No risk factors have been specifically proposed for other tibial fractures, although poor apposition of the osteotomy, poor conformation of the osteotomy, and iatrogenic damage to the tibia adjacent to the osteotomy would be expected to create stress risers.

Diagnosis

Most tibial tuberosity fractures are diagnosed as incidental findings on radiographic follow-up 6 weeks after surgery and are not associated with obvious clinical signs. These fractures typically consist of avulsion fracture with a short oblique fracture line involving the most proximal portion of the fork hole while preserving the cranial cage screw (Calvo et al. 2014). A caudal and proximal displacement of the tibial tuberosity is usually present along with a mild loss of advancement of the tibial tuberosity.

Alternatively, tibial tuberosity fractures induce a sudden, non–weight-bearing lameness within the first weeks after surgery (Calvo et al. 2014). These fractures generally involve multiple fork holes and compromise the stability and advancement of the tibial

tuberosity (Figure 117.12). Tibial fractures will also induce a sudden onset of non–weight-bearing lameness and are confirmed on radiographs (Figure 117.13).

Treatment

Tibial tuberosity fractures that are not associated with clinical signs are generally managed conservatively. Fractures that induce clinical signs and jeopardize the advancement of the tibial tuberosity must be revised. If the cage screw fixation is intact, the revision may be limited to tension band fixation of the tibial tuberosity. If not, replacement of the cage can be attempted and combined with tension band (see Figure 117.12). If this is not possible, the tibial tuberosity is fixed against the tibia. The advancement of the crest is lost, and an LFS should be placed in these cases. Tibial fractures can be repaired via plate (see Figure 117.13) or external fixation.

Outcome

In a small case series, the outcome after tuberosity fractures was generally favorable. Fractures managed conservatively delayed the recovery by about 5 weeks, but those requiring surgical revision extended the convalescence by 8.5 weeks (Calvo et al. 2014). This complication appeared to create a partial loss of advancement and may therefore lead to residual joint instability.

Prevention

Overall, fractures may be prevented via sound technique, proper location and distal apposition of the osteotomy, and good implant selection and placement. Tibial tuberosity fractures may be prevented by placing the osteotomy slightly farther caudal and placing the fork as far cranial as possible on the tuberosity. This placement increases the distance between the fork and the osteotomy and would therefore engage a larger proportion of cortical bone.

Implant failure

Definition

Implant failure is loss of function or migration of the implant. It is a fairly uncommon complication, reported in about 2% of TTAs (see Table 117.3) (Wolf et al. 2012). The most common failures include breakage of the body of the fork, screw loosening on the cranial or caudal flange of the cage, and breakage of the cage flanges.

Risk factors

No factor has been reported to specifically increase the risk of implant failure after TTA. The risk factors for this complication are most likely similar to those reported to increase the overall risk of complication after TTA:
- Body weight greater than 40 kg
- Limited surgeon's experience (< 22 TTAs) (Proot and Corr 2013)
- Small cage size (6 mm)

Diagnosis

Implant failure may be an incidental finding on follow-up radiographs. In these cases, the stability of the implant is generally preserved, especially the cranial screw fixation of the cage, and the osteotomy may be at least partially healed. Alternatively, implant failure may delay the recovery (lameness) and jeopardize the advancement of the crest. Implant failure is confirmed on radiographs (Figure 117.14). The position of the tibial tuberosity and stability of the osteotomy should be evaluated because they will influence the management of the patient.

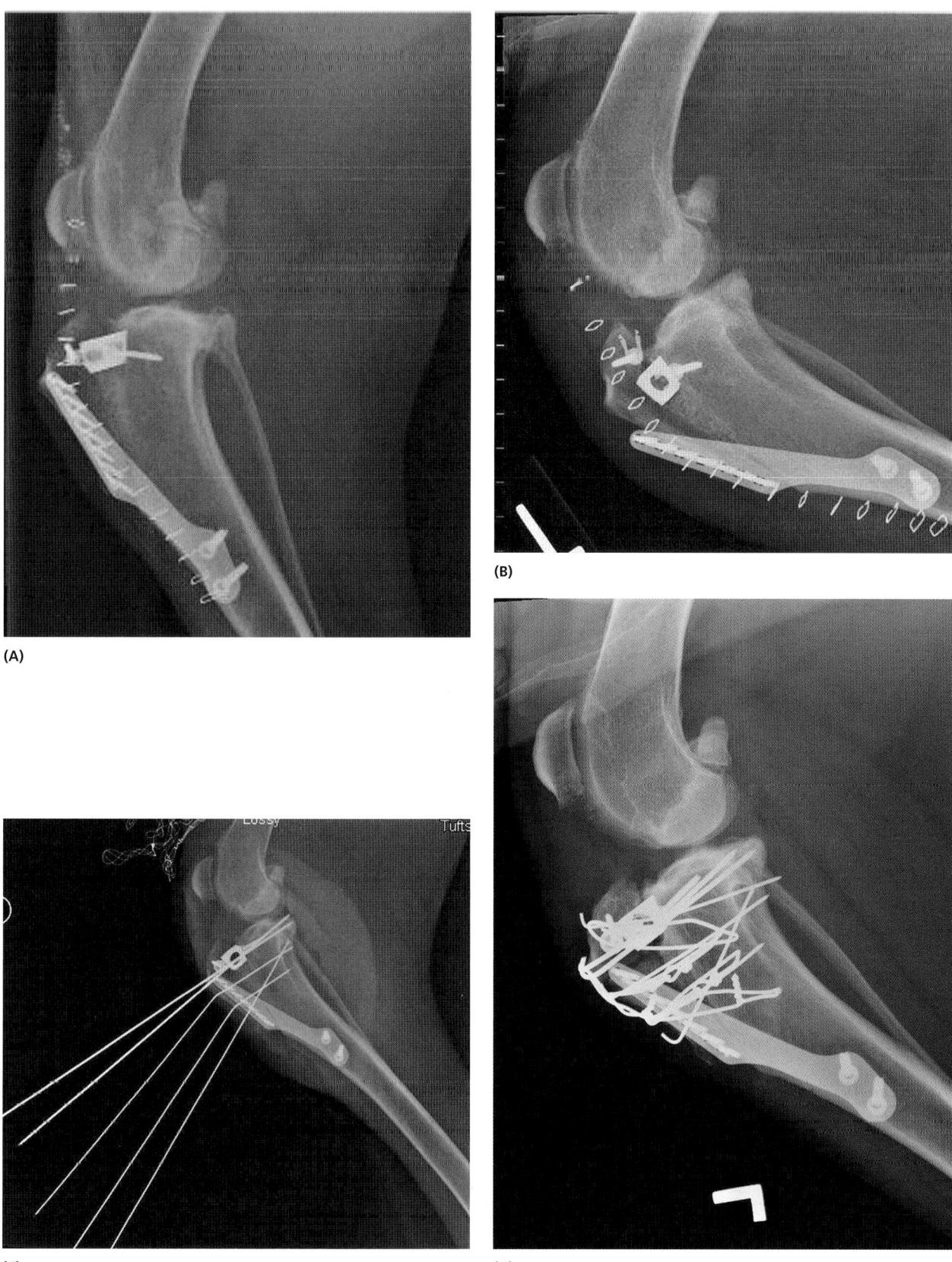

(A)

(B)

(C)

(D)

Figure 117.12 Tibial tuberosity fracture secondary to tibial tuberosity advancement (TTA). **A**, Radiograph obtained immediately after TTA. **B**, Radiograph obtained 1 week after TTA: the fracture of the tibial tuberosity is accompanied by failure of the cranial fixation of the cage and displacement of the tibial tuberosity. **C**, The cage has been replaced, and the placement of multiple Kirschner wires is verified intraoperatively before wires are placed in a tension band fashion. **D**, Radiographic appearance 12 weeks after revision. *Source:* R. Boudrieau, Tufts University, North Grafton, MA. Reproduced with permission from R. Boudrieau.

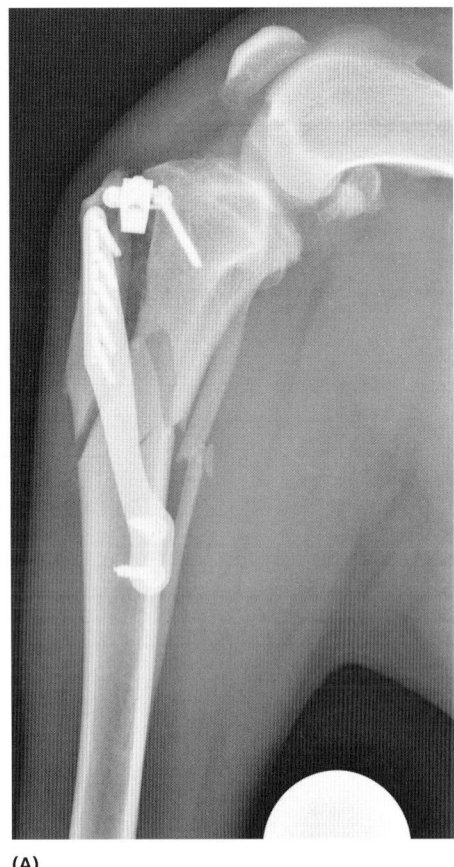

(A)

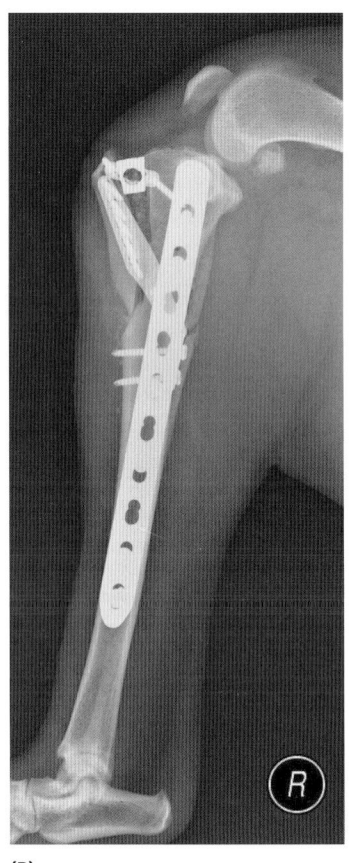

(B)

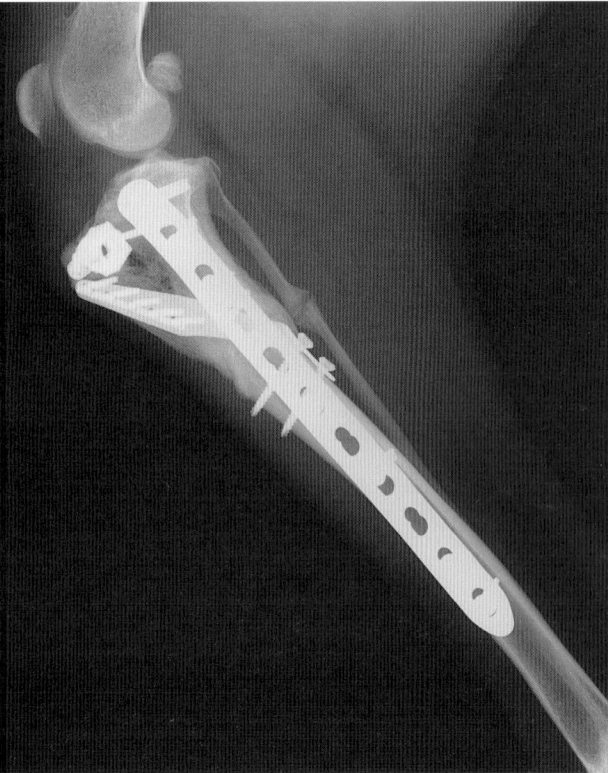

(C)

Figure 117.13 Tibial fracture secondary to tibial tuberosity advancement (TTA) in a 5-year-old golden retriever. **A**, Radiograph 2 weeks after TTA. The tibial fracture originates from the distal extent of the osteotomy and extends caudally with some comminution. The fibula is also fractured. **B**, Radiograph obtained after revision with a locking Synthes plate. **C**, Bony union is obtained 13 weeks later. The dog had a TTA on the contralateral side and eventually returned to full function. *Source:* R. Boudrieau, Tufts University, North Grafton, MA. Reproduced with permission from R. Boudrieau.

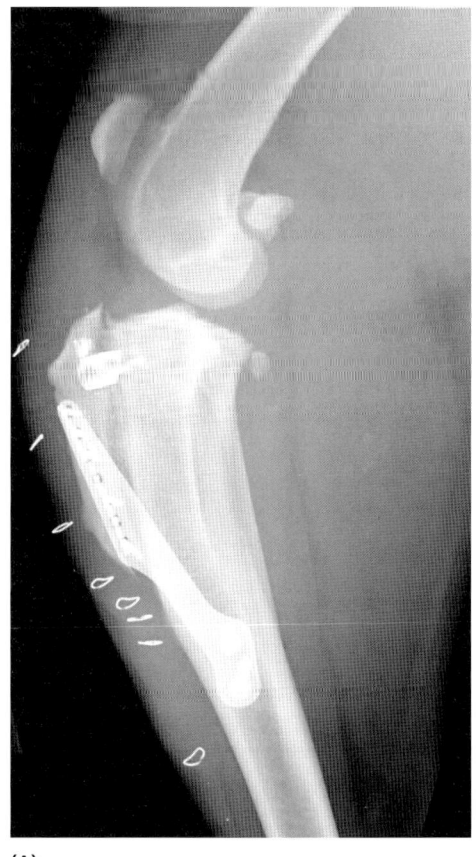

(A)

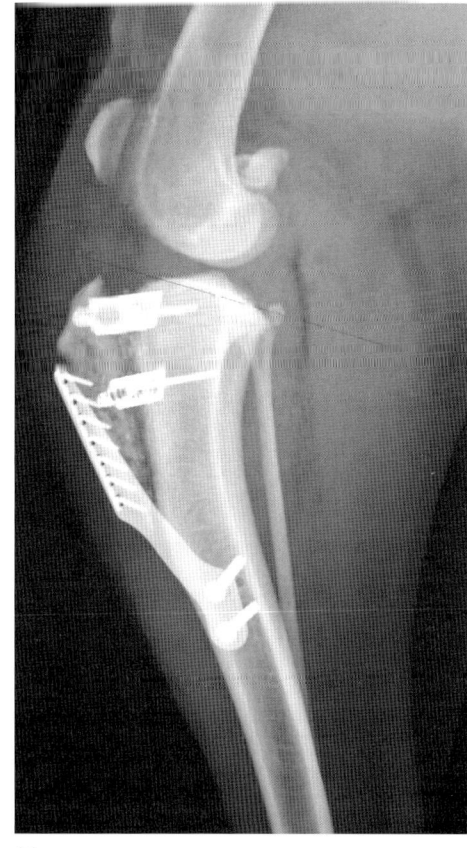

(B)

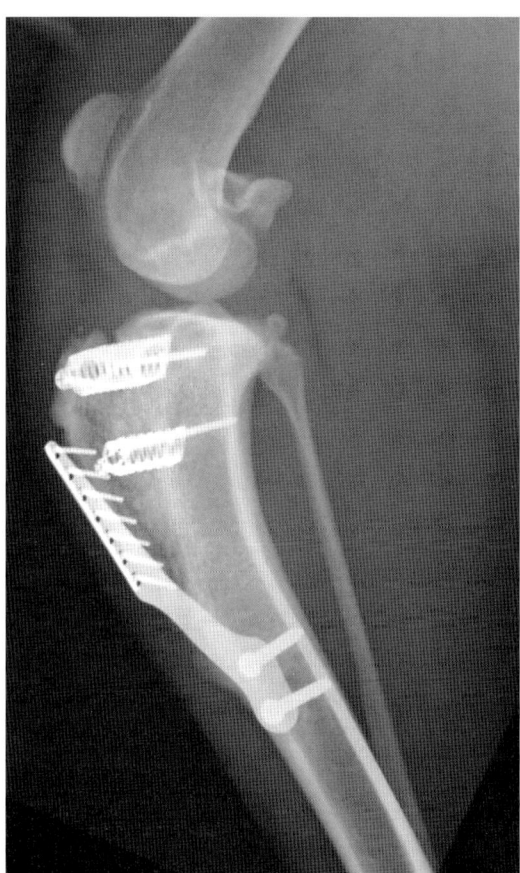

(C)

Figure 117.14 Implant failure after tibial tuberosity advancement (TTA).
A, Failure of the fork and collapse of a 6-mm cage, subsequently judged
as undersized. Note the caudal displacement of the tibial tuberosity.
B, Radiograph after revision. The proximal cage has been replaced with
a larger cage, and a smaller cage is positioned distally. **C**, Bone healing
6 weeks after revision. *Source:* R. Boudrieau, Tufts University, North
Grafton, MA. Reproduced with permission from R. Boudrieau.

Treatment

Conservative management can be considered if the implant failure does not interfere with the position of the tibial tuberosity and has a minor influence on bone healing. Caudal screw loosening or breakage of the caudal flange of the cage may fall into this category. Removal of loose implants may be indicated in patients with healed TTAs. Implant failure that alters the advancement of the tibial crest or is likely to affect bone healing warrants revision (see Figure 117.14). Revision generally involves replacement of failed implants, and adjunct fixation may be considered.

Outcome

Implant failure is relatively uncommon complication and has not been specifically studied. However, a positive outcome can be expected if advancement and stability of the tibial tuberosity are restored.

Prevention

Prevention of this complication relies on proper implant selection and application. General measures to prevent implant failure in TTAs include:
- Achieving good cortical purchase of the prongs in cortical bone to prevent failure of the fork
- Good apposition of the distal osteotomy against the caudal tibial cortex to prevent failure of the body of the fork
- Contouring the flanges of the cage to create good contact with the underlying bone while avoiding sharp bending may prevent breakage of the flanges.

Medial patellar luxation

Definition

Post-operative medial patellar luxation (MPL), or spontaneous dislocation of the patella medial to the trochlea groove, is reported in about 1% to 3% of TTAs (see Table 1173.3).

Risk factors

Proposed risk factors for MPL after TTA include:
- Loss of retropatellar contact: Advancing the tibial tuberosity may also lead to a cranial displacement of the patella, thereby affecting its contact with the trochlea.
- Patella baja: Advancing the tibial tuberosity creates tension along the patellar tendon, thereby displacing the patella distally.
- Oblique osteotomy: This factor plays a role if the osteotomy is angled cranially as the blade moves in a medial to lateral plane.
- Contouring of the plate: If the plate is not contoured adequately toward the lateral aspect of the limb, the tibial tuberosity will be displaced medially, especially in its proximal region.

Diagnosis

Patellar luxation is diagnosed based on orthopedic examination at follow-up. Most cases are mild and scored as 1 or 2. Clinical signs are generally present in patellar luxation grades 2 and above. Radiographs of the pelvis and stifle are indicated to evaluate limb conformation and the presence of underlying factors. The proximodistal location of the patellar should be evaluated and compared with pre-operative values; the distance between the proximal aspect of the patellar and the femoral condylar axis is measured on a craniocaudal projection and divided by the length of the patellar ligament. A ratio less than 1.9 has been found consistent with patella baja in dogs with patellar luxation (Mostafa *et al.* 2008).

Treatment

Surgical treatment should be considered in dogs with patellar luxations grades 2 and above. TTA-induced MPL most likely results from a misalignment of the extensor mechanism. The treatment therefore aims at correcting this alignment rather than deepening the trochlear groove (Figure 117.15). This correction is achieved by transposing the tibial tuberosity laterally, which can be achieved by contouring the TTA plate and placing washers under the cranial flange of the cage screw. This technique has been described for the treatment of concurrent CCLD and MPL (Yeadon *et al.* 2011). The proximodistal alignment of the patella can be corrected simultaneously by adjusting the position of the implant. Kirschner wires may be used for preliminary immobilization of the crest and as adjunct to plate fixation.

Outcome

This is an uncommon complication, and no study has specifically reported on the success rate of these revisions. However, a good outcome can be expected if the alignment of the extensor mechanism is achieved, other underlying factors are addressed, and stability of the tibial crest is achieved.

Prevention

The pathogenesis of this condition has not been fully established, and preventive measures are therefore unclear. However, the following recommendations seem reasonable:
- Thorough preoperative assessment of the patient to detect preexisting concurrent MPL and CCLD
- Evaluate the limb alignment of the patient before surgery.
- Proper alignment of the osteotomy
- Contour the plate to avoid medial deviation of the tibial crest.
- Intraoperative assessment of the stability of the patella

Relevant literature

Cranial cruciate ligament disease is the leading cause of stifle lameness in dogs, and as such, surgical management of this condition is one of the most active fields of investigations in small animal orthopedics. Surgical techniques are constantly evolving, along with rates and types of complications. A great deal of interest has focused on complications since tibial osteotomies were introduced in 1990s. However, comparing complication rates among procedures is challenging because of the variations between studies. These variations stem from factors such as duration of follow-up, measures of outcome (subjective vs. objective), types of complications included (minor vs. major), assessment of the joint (none, arthrotomies, arthroscopy), presence of concurrent lesions (e.g., meniscal disease), and modifications of the technique (type of implant, use of a jig, placement of graft). In addition, articles published early after introduction of a new procedure generally seem to report higher complication rates than those published later. These differences may reflect an initial learning curve combined with subsequent refinements aimed at decreasing morbidity. Tables 117.1 to 117.3 summarize the types and rates of complications reported with extracapsular repair, TPLO, and TTA in the veterinary literature.

Postliminary meniscal disease is one of the most common major complications after surgical repair of CCLD regardless of the repair technique. The pathogenesis for meniscal disease after CCLD repair can generally be attributed to residual joint instability and abnormal distribution of loads across the joint. The majority of research in this area has focused on TPLO. This procedure does not seem to

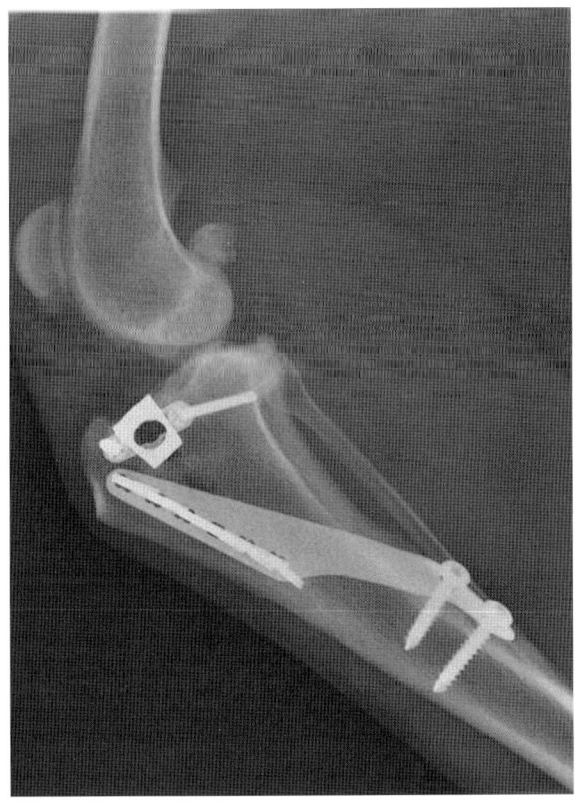

(A)

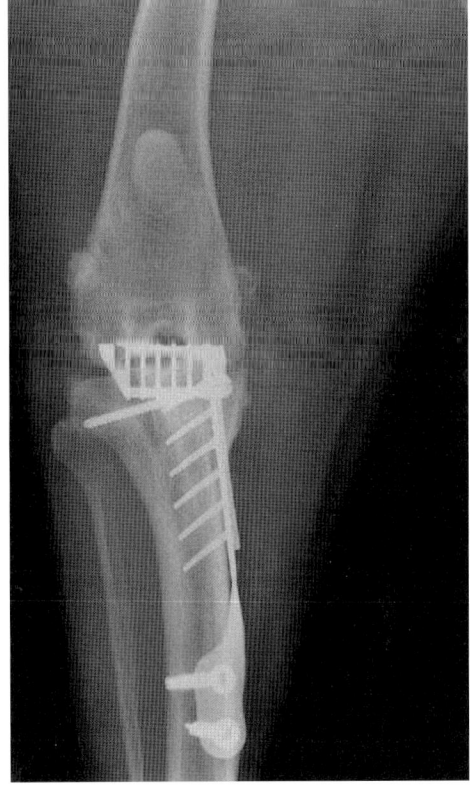

(B)

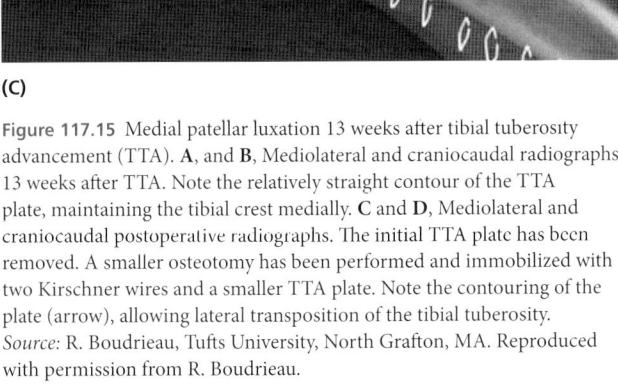

(C)

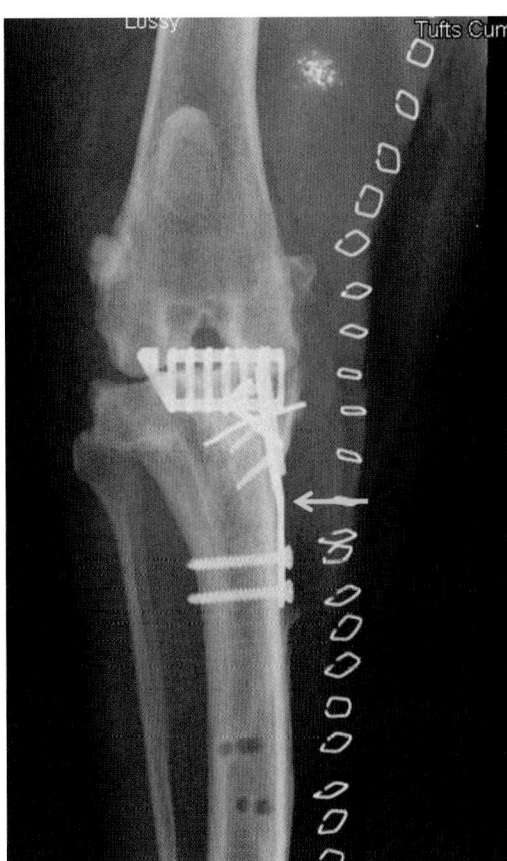

(D)

Figure 117.15 Medial patellar luxation 13 weeks after tibial tuberosity advancement (TTA). **A**, and **B**, Mediolateral and craniocaudal radiographs 13 weeks after TTA. Note the relatively straight contour of the TTA plate, maintaining the tibial crest medially. **C** and **D**, Mediolateral and craniocaudal postoperative radiographs. The initial TTA plate has been removed. A smaller osteotomy has been performed and immobilized with two Kirschner wires and a smaller TTA plate. Note the contouring of the plate (arrow), allowing lateral transposition of the tibial tuberosity. *Source:* R. Boudrieau, Tufts University, North Grafton, MA. Reproduced with permission from R. Boudrieau.

consistently eliminate femorotibial subluxation during standing in dogs (Kim *et al.* 2012) and does not address the rotational instability generated by CCLD. Conversely, the TTA preserves the anatomy of the tibial plateau and was found to maintain similar femorotibial contact patterns as normal stifles in two in vitro studies (Kim *et al.* 2009, 2010). However, the same research group later found that TTA did not normalize sagittal plane stability during standing despite a good return to function (Skinner *et al.* 2013). TTA was consequently found to be three times more likely to be associated with postliminary meniscal tears than TPLO (incidence of 27% in 18 TTAs vs. 12% in 65 TPLOs; Christopher *et al.* 2013). However, none of the dogs with TTA were assessed via arthroscopy at the time of surgery, whereas arthroscopy and probing were performed in most dogs with TPLO. Another study identified meniscal tear as the most common complication after TTA, diagnosed in 9.4% of 104 dogs with an initially intact meniscus (Steinberg *et al.* 2011).

Meniscal diseases can be broadly classified into five types based on their appearance: radial, vertical longitudinal (capsular detachment), bucket handle, flap, and complex meniscal tears (Thieman *et al.* 2009). In a recent clinical study of 223 stifles, the most common meniscal lesions diagnosed at the time of initial CCLD repair or in the postoperative phase were described as a single bucket handle tear in 28% of cases followed by complex tears (multiple full-thickness tears or maceration, 22%) and interstitial tears (partial-thickness tears, including horizontal or cleavage, 18%). Radial tears (8%) and capsular detachments (including caudal peripheral tears and folded caudal poles, 5%) were uncommon (Ritzo *et al.* 2014). Conservative management has been suggested for radial and vertical longitudinal tears based on their absence of influence on contact mechanics in an ex vivo study of canine stifles (Thieman *et al.* 2009). Meniscal repair of peripheral bucket handle tears has been described by placement of vertical, horizontal, or cruciate sutures. In an ex vivo study of normal stifles, all three suture techniques restored contact mechanics after experimental tears, prompting the authors to suggest meniscal repair for peripheral meniscal tears located in the vascular zone of normal meniscal parenchyma (Thieman *et al.* 2010). However, the tears most commonly diagnosed after CCLD repair involve the avascular portion of the meniscus and were found to increase by at least 45% the peak contact pressure in cadaveric stifles (Thieman *et al.* 2009). These lesions are therefore treated by resection of the affected area via partial, hemi-, or complete meniscectomy. These procedures have been found to induce osteoarthritis in normal dogs (Johnson *et al.* 2004), most likely secondary to alterations in pressure distribution (Pozzi *et al.* 2008b; Thieman *et al.* 2010) as well as loss of stabilization by the meniscus (Kim *et al.* 2012). Medial meniscectomy affected was also found to affect return to function and was identified as a risk factor for "pivot shift" in a retrospective study of 476 TPLOs (Gatineau *et al.* 2011). The morbidity associated with postliminary meniscal disease and its treatment justifies the development of preventive measures. Medial meniscal release was introduced shortly after TPLOs to allow motion of the caudal horn and avoid its impingement between the femur and tibia. A caudal release by transection of the medial meniscotibial ligament is preferred over a radial release and may be performed via arthroscopy or mini-arthrotomy. This procedure was found effective at decreasing the risk of postliminary meniscal disease in a recent clinical study of 163 dogs with CCLD (Ritzo *et al.* 2014). In this study, patients treated with meniscal release did not have subsequent meniscal lesions, whereas these were diagnosed in 11% of dogs that did not undergo initial meniscal release. This comparison may

have been influenced by inclusion of dogs with meniscal lesions diagnosed at the time of CCLD (concurrent lesions treated by partial meniscectomy), a factor found in itself to protect against subsequent tears. On the other end, medial meniscal release caused lameness and medial compartment cartilage pathology in dogs with normal stifles (Luther *et al.* 2009). These changes most likely result from alteration in the distribution of loads across the articular surface, thereby encouraging DJD (Pozzi *et al.* 2010). These undesirable effects, weighed against the relatively low incidence of postliminary meniscal tears have prompted some surgeons to restrict meniscal release to cases in which the status of the medial meniscus is uncertain (Thieman *et al.* 2006; Gatineau *et al.* 2011). Instead, clinicians should aim for accurate assessment of the medial meniscus during CCLD repair to eliminate undiagnosed concurrent tears. In that regard, arthroscopic assessment of the medial meniscus appears superior to open exploratory arthrotomy (see Chapter 116). The detection of concurrent meniscal diseases was 1.5 to 2 times more likely via arthroscopy than arthrotomy in two clinical studies of dogs with CCLD (Plesman *et al.* 2013; Ritzo *et al.* 2014). Probing with a meniscal probe (Small Joint Hook Tip Probe; Arthrex, Naples, FL) was found to improve the diagnostic ability of evaluations conducted via caudomedial or craniomedial arthrotomies as well as arthroscopy in an ex vivo study of experimental tears (Pozzi *et al.* 2008). In this study, the highest sensitivity (80%) and specificity (95%) were obtained when arthroscopy and probing were combined. This enhanced detection of concurrent meniscal lesions may explain the relatively low incidence of subsequent meniscal lesions (5.6%) reported in 357 stifles with CCLD managed via arthroscopy, probing, and TPLO (Kalff *et al.* 2011).

Relatively few articles report on **complications associated with extracapsular suture repairs** for CCLD. The largest and most recent study consists of a retrospective review of 363 LFS in 305 dogs (Casale and McCarthy 2009). More than 90% of limbs treated in this study received prophylactic antibiotics, were implanted with nylon leader line, and were bandaged after surgery for an unknown duration. Complications were recorded in about 17% of cases, about half of them consisting of self-resolving incisional complications. The second most common complications consisted of surgical site infection followed by implant-related issues and postliminary meniscal lesions. Overall, 7.2% of limbs treated with LFS required additional surgery to treat a complication. The only factors associated with a higher risk of complications included high body weight (>35 kg) and young age (younger than 5 years of age) at the time of surgery. Overall, LFS appears associated with a lower rate of complications than TPLO and TTA, especially with regards to major complications.

Complications after TR repair of CCLD remain poorly documented. A prospective clinical cohort study of 24 dogs treated with TR initially reported complications in about 30% of cases, nearly half of them (17% of cases) requiring further treatment (Cook *et al.* 2010). Complications included implant failure, infection, meniscal tear, and seroma. More recently, the same group reported minor complications in about 9% of 79 dogs with TR, major complications in 9% of cases, and postliminary meniscal tears in 6% of cases (Christopher *et al.* 2013). In an ex vivo study in which TR repairs were assessed via radiographs, biomechanical tests, and dissection, technical deviations were found in approximately half of the specimens prepared by surgery residents or diplomates (Biskup and Griffon 2014). Interestingly, only 39% of limbs with technical deviations were detected on radiographs.

Complications after TPLO have been well documented in the veterinary literature, although the rate and type of complications vary among studies (see Table 117.1). Infection has been reported as a serious complication after TPLO, with a prevalence exceeding that expected for clean elective orthopedic procedures. Readers are invited to review Chapter 5, which deals with osteomyelitis, for further information on this topic. Combined, incisional complications such as inflammation, drainage, swelling, seroma, and infection represent the majority of the morbidity associated with TPLO. Most are benign and do not require further surgical treatment. Among self-limiting soft tissue complications, patellar tendonitis is specific to TPLO and is reported in an average of 5% of cases. The most common complications requiring a second surgery (often defined as major complications) include postliminary meniscal tear, osteomyelitis, tibial fractures, and nonunion. Predisposing factors to complications vary among studies and include increased age and body weight, breed (Rottweiler), complete preoperative CCL tear, exposure via parapatellar arthrotomy, single-session bilateral TPLO, steep TPA, TPLO without jig, medial meniscectomy, thin craniocaudal crest, and surgeon's experience (Pacchiana *et al.* 2003; Bergh *et al.* 2008; Tuttle and Manley 2009; Fitzpatrick and Solano 2010; Gatineau *et al.* 2011; Taylor *et al.* 2011; Bergh and Peirone 2012). The identification of risk factors and wide clinical application of TPLOs have led to refinement in the technique, reduction in surgical time, and preventive measures against complications. Among those, locking implants specifically designed for TPLOs have likely contributed to reducing the technical difficulty of the procedure, limiting the risk of improper placement of implants and potentially accelerating bone healing. Adjustments in the postoperative management of patients are aimed at avoiding postoperative contamination and accelerating return to function without premature loading of the limb.

The largest and most recent publication focusing on **complications after TTAs** current consists of a retrospective study of 501 TTAs reported in 2012 (Wolf *et al.* 2012). In this study, the overall complication rate was 19%, which the authors deemed comparable to that reported for TPLOs and lower than rates initially reported for TTAs. Similarly to TPLOs, incisional issues such as infection and inflammation were the most common complications, identified in approximately 35% of cases (see Table 117.3). These complications were generally minor, resolving with medical treatment. Major complications occurred in 11% of cases, 37% of them consisting of fractures (overall incidence, 4%), followed by implant failures (17% of major complications; 2% of 501 cases). In that regard, issues most commonly encountered included fractures through the fork holes and breakage of the body of the fork. The majority of complications in this study were chronic, including fractures, implant failure, infection, and postliminary meniscal lesions diagnosed at follow-up. Revision surgery was required in half of the stifles with major complications. The most common complication requiring a second surgery consisted of postliminary meniscal tears. Complications were overall more common in dogs weighing more than 40 kg. Small cage size (6 mm) has also been identified as a predisposing factor to complications (Steinberg *et al.* 2011). The authors suggested that some dogs may have been undersized, which would lead to residual instability. This finding prompted the recommendation to select a 9-mm cage for cases with preoperative measurements between 6 and 9 mm. In a smaller retrospective study of 68 dogs with 101 TTAs, bilateral single-session TTA was not found to increase the risk of complications (Hirshenson *et al.* 2012).

The body of literature dealing with complications associated with surgical treatment of CCLD supports the concept that tibial osteotomies are generally more prone to complications, especially major complications, than extracapsular suture techniques. The same literature provides some evidence that TPLO results in a more favorable outcome, including functional outcome, than LFS (Gordon-Evans *et al.* 2013; Bergh *et al.* 2014). However, more evidence is needed to establish a clear comparison between the outcome of TTA and that of TPLO and LFS (Bergh *et al.* 2014). Despite the morbidity associated with tibial osteotomies, client satisfaction remains high. In a randomized, blinded, controlled clinical trial, owners unaware of the treatment received by their dogs ranked their satisfaction 1 year after surgery as a minimum score of 9 (out of 10) in 95% of TPLOs and only 75% of LFS (Gordon-Evans *et al.* 2013). Similarly for TTAs, 84% of owners retrospectively evaluated stated that they would be willing to repeat the procedure (Steinberg *et al.* 2011). Regardless of the technique selected, the most effective strategies to prevent complications include careful surgical planning, thorough application of the technique, and excellent client education before and after surgery.

The video cited in this chapter can be found on the book companion website at www.wiley.com/go/griffon/complications.

References

Anderson C.C., Tomlinson J.L., Daly W.R. et al. (1998) Biomechanical evaluation of a crimp clamp system for loop fixation of monofilament nylon leader material used for stabilization of the canine stifle joint. *Vet Surg* 27:533-539.

Bergh, M.S., Peirone, B. (2012) Complications of tibial plateau levelling osteotomy in dogs. *Veterinary and Comparative Orthopaedics and Traumatology* 25 (5):349-358.

Bergh, M.S., Rajala-Schultz, P., Johnson, K.A. (2008) Risk factors for tibial tuberosity fracture after tibial plateau leveling osteotomy in dogs. *Veterinary Surgery* 37 (4), 374-382.

Bergh, M.S., Sullivan, C., Ferrell, C.L. (2014) Systematic review of surgical treatments for cranial cruciate ligament disease in dogs. *Journal of the American Animal Hospital Association* 50 (5), 315-321.

Biskup, J.J., Griffon, D.J. (2014) Technical difficulties during the training phase for TightRope percutaneous lateral fabellar suture techniques for cranial cruciate ligament repair. *Veterinary Surgery* 43, 347-354.

Böttcher, P., Winkels, P., Oechtering, G. (2009) A novel pin distraction device for arthroscopic assessment of the medial meniscus in dogs. *Veterinary Surgery* 38, 595-600.

Cabano, N.R., Troyer, K.L., Palmer, R.H. (2011) Mechanical comparison of two suture constructs for extra-capsular stifle stabilization. *Veterinary Surgery* 40 (3), 334-339.

Calvo, I., Aisa, J., Chase, D., et al. (2014) Tibial tuberosity fracture as a complication of tibial tuberosity advancement. *Veterinary and Comparative Orthopaedics and Traumatology* 27 (2), 148-154.

Carey, K., Aiken, S.W., DiResta, G.R., et al. (2005) Radiographic and clinical changes of the patellar tendon after tibial plateau leveling osteotomy 94 cases (2000-2003). *Veterinary and Comparative Orthopaedics and Traumatology* 18 (4), 235-242.

Casale, S.A., McCarthy, R.J. (2009) Complications associated with lateral fabellotibial suture surgery for cranial cruciate ligament injury in dogs: 363 cases (1997-2005). *Journal of the American Veterinary Medical Association* 234 (2):229-235.

Case, J.B., Hulse, D., Kerwin, S.C., et al. (2008) Meniscal injury following initial cranial cruciate ligament stabilization surgery in 26 dogs (29 stifles). *Veterinary and Comparative Orthopaedics and Traumatology* 21 (4):365-367.

Caylor K.B., Zumpano C.A., Evans L.S. et al. (2001) Intra- and interobserver measurement variability of tibial plateau slope from lateral radiographs in dogs. *J Am Anim Hosp Assoc* 37:263-268.

Christopher, S.A., Beetem, J., Cook, J.L. (2013) Comparison of long-term outcomes associated with three surgical techniques for treatment of cranial cruciate ligament disease in dogs. *Veterinary Surgery* 42 (3), 329-334.

Comerford, E., Forster, K., Gorton, K., et al. (2013) Management of cranial cruciate ligament rupture in small dogs: a questionnaire study. *Veterinary and Comparative Orthopaedics and Traumatology* 26 (6), 493-497.

Conkling A.L., Fagin B., Daye R.M. (2010) Comparison of tibial plateau angle changes after tibial plateau levelling osteotomy fixation with conventional or locking screw technology. *Vet Surg* 39(4):475-481.

Cook, J.L., Luther, J.K., Beetem, J., et al. (2010). Clinical comparison of a novel extracapsular stabilization procedure and tibial plateau leveling osteotomy for treatment of cranial cruciate ligament deficiency in dogs. *Veterinary Surgery* 39 (3), 315-323.

Corr S.A., Brown C. (2007) A comparison of outcomes following tibial plateau levelling osteotomy and cranial tibial wedge osteotomy procedures. *Vet Comp Orthop Traumatol* 20(4):312-319.

Dillon, D.E., Gordon-Evans, W.J., Griffon, D.J., et al. (2014) Risk factors and diagnostic accuracy of clinical findings for meniscal disease in dogs with cranial cruciate ligament disease. *Veterinary Surgery* 43 (4):446-450.

Duerr F.M., Duncan C.G., Savicky R.S. et al. (2008) Comparison of surgical treatment options for cranial cruciate ligament disease in large-breed dogs with excessive tibial plateau angle. *Vet Surg* 37(1):49-62.

Dupuis J., Harari J., Papageorges M. et al. (1994) Evaluation of fibular head transposition for repair of experimental cranial cruciate ligament injury in dogs. *Vet Surg* 23:1-12.

Fitzpatrick, N., Solano, M.A. (2010) Predictive variables for complications after TPLO with stifle inspection by arthrotomy in 1000 consecutive dogs. *Veterinary Surgery* 39 (4), 460-474.

Flynn, P., Duncan, C.G., Palmer, R.H., et al. (2014) In vitro incidence of fibular penetration with and without the use of a jig during tibial plateau leveling osteotomy. *Veterinary Surgery* 43 (4), 495-499.

Garnett, S., Daye, R.M. (2014) Short-term complications associated with tibial plateau leveling osteotomy in dogs using 2.0 and 2.7mm plates. *Journal of the American Animal Hospital Association* in press.

Gatineau, M., Dupuis, J., Planté, J., et al. (2011) Retrospective study of 476 tibial plateau levelling osteotomy procedures. Rate of subsequent "pivot shift," meniscal tear and other complications. *Veterinary and Comparative Orthopaedics and Traumatology* 24 (5), 333-341.

Gordon-Evans, W.J., Griffon, D.J., Bubb, C., et al. (2013) Comparison of lateral fabellar suture and tibial plateau leveling osteotomy techniques for treatment of dogs with cranial cruciate ligament disease. *Journal of the American Veterinary Medical Association* 243 (5), 675-680.

Hirshenson, M.S., Krotscheck, U., Thompson, M.S., et al. (2012) Evaluation of complications and short-term outcome after unilateral or single-session bilateral tibial tuberosity advancement for cranial cruciate rupture in dogs. *Veterinary and Comparative Orthopaedics and Traumatology* 25 (5), 402-409.

Johnson, K.A., Francis, D.J., Manley, P.A., et al. (2004) Comparison of the effects of caudal pole hemi-meniscectomy and complete medial meniscectomy in the canine stifle joint. *American Journal of Veterinary Research* 65 (8), 1053-1060.

Kalff, S., Meachem, S., Preston, C. (2011) Incidence of medial meniscal tears after arthroscopic assisted tibial plateau leveling osteotomy. *Veterinary Surgery* 40 (8), 952-956.

Kim, S.E., Lewis, D.D., Pozzi, A. (2012) Effect of tibial plateau leveling osteotomy on femorotibial subluxation: in vivo analysis during standing. *Veterinary Surgery* 41 (4), 465-470.

Kim, S.E., Pozzi, A., Banks, S.A., et al. (2009) Effect of tibial tuberosity advancement on femorotibial contact mechanics and stifle kinematics. *Veterinary Surgery* 38 (1), 33-39.

Kim, S.E., Pozzi, A., Banks, S.A., et al. (2010) Effect of cranial cruciate ligament deficiency, tibial plateau leveling osteotomy, and tibial tuberosity advancement on contact mechanics and alignment of the stifle in flexion. *Veterinary Surgery* 39 (3), 363-370.

Lafaver, S., Miller, N.A., Stubbs, W.P., et al. (2007) Tibial tuberosity advancement for stabilization of the canine cranial cruciate ligament-deficient stifle joint: surgical technique, early results, and complications in 101 dogs. *Veterinary Surgery* 36 (6), 573-586.

Leighton, R.L. (1999) Preferred method of repair of cranial cruciate ligament rupture in dogs: a survey of ACVS diplomates specializing in canine orthopedics. American College of Veterinary Surgery. *Veterinary Surgery* 28 (3), 194.

Luther, J.K., Cook, C.R., Cook, J.L. (2009) Meniscal release in cruciate ligament intact stifles causes lameness and medial compartment cartilage pathology in dogs 12 weeks postoperatively. *Veterinary Surgery* 38 (4), 520-529.

Mattern, K.L., Berry, C.R., Peck, J.N., et al. (2006) Radiographic and ultrasonographic evaluation of the patellar ligament following tibial plateau leveling osteotomy. *Veterinary Radiology & Ultrasound* 47 (2), 185-191.

Mostafa, A.A., Griffon, D.J., Thomas, M.W., et al. (2008) Proximodistal alignment of the canine patella: radiographic evaluation and association with medial and lateral patellar luxation. *Veterinary Journal* 37 (3), 201-211.

Nelson, S.A., Krotscheck, U., Rawlinson, J., et al. (2013) Long-term functional outcome of tibial plateau leveling osteotomy versus extracapsular repair in a heterogeneous population of dogs. *Veterinary Surgery* 42 (1), 38-50.

Oxley, B., Gemmill, T.J., Renwick, A.R. (2013) Comparison of complication rates and clinical outcome between tibial plateau leveling osteotomy and a modified cranial closing wedge osteotomy for treatment of cranial cruciate ligament disease in dogs. *Veterinary Surgery* 42 (6), 739-750.

Pacchiana, P.D., Morris, E., Gillings, S.L., et al. (2003) Surgical and postoperative complications associated with tibial plateau leveling osteotomy in dogs with cranial cruciate ligament rupture: 397 cases (1998-2001). *Journal of the American Veterinary Medical Association* 222 (2), 184-193.

Plesman, R., Gilbert, P., Campbell, J. (2013) Detection of meniscal tears by arthroscopy and arthrotomy in dogs with cranial cruciate ligament rupture: a retrospective, cohort study. *Veterinary and Comparative Orthopaedics and Traumatology* 26 (1), 42-46.

Pozzi, A. Kim, S.E., Lewis, D.D. (2010) Effect of transection of the caudal meniscotibial ligament on medial femorotibial contact mechanics. *Veterinary Surgery* 39 (4), 489-495.

Pozzi, A., Hildreth, B.E. 3rd, Rajala-Schultz, P.J. (2008a) Comparison of arthroscopy and arthrotomy for diagnosis of medial meniscal pathology: an ex vivo study. *Veterinary Surgery* 37, 749-755.

Pozzi, A., Litsky, A.S., Field, J., et al. (2008b) Pressure distributions on the medial tibial plateau after medial meniscal surgery and tibial plateau levelling osteotomy in dogs. *Veterinary and Comparative Orthopaedics and Traumatology* 21 (1), 8-14.

Priddy, N.H., Tomlinson, J.L., Dodam, J.R., et al. (2003) Complications with and owner assessment of the outcome of tibial plateau leveling osteotomy for treatment of cranial cruciate ligament rupture in dogs: 193 cases (1997-2001). *Journal of the American Veterinary Medical Association* 222 (12), 1726-1732.

Proot, L.L., Corr, S.A. (2013) Clinical audit for the tibial tuberosity advancement procedure: establishing the learning curve and monitoring ongoing performance for the tibial tuberosity advancement procedure using the cumulative summation technique. *Veterinary and Comparative Orthopaedics and Traumatology* 26, 280-284.

Ritzo, M.E., Ritzo, B.A., Siddens, A.D., et al. (2014) Incidence and type of meniscal injury and associated long-term clinical outcomes in dogs treated surgically for cranial cruciate ligament disease. *Veterinary Surgery* 43 (8), 952-958.

Rose, N.D., Goerke, D., Evans, R.B. (2012) Mechanical testing of orthopedic suture material used for extra-articular stabilization of canine cruciate ligament-deficient stifles. *Veterinary Surgery* 41 (2), 266-272.

Skinner, O.T., Kim, S.E., Lewis, D.D., et al. (2013) In vivo femorotibial subluxation during weight-bearing and clinical outcome following tibial tuberosity advancement for cranial cruciate ligament insufficiency in dogs. *Veterinary Journal* 196 (1), 86-91.

Smith, G.K., Torg J.S. (1985) Fibular head transposition for repair of cruciate-deficient stifle in the dog. *J Am Anim Hos Assoc* 187(4);375-383.

Stauffer, K.D., Tuttle, T.A., Elkins, A.D., et al. (2006) Complications associated with 696 tibial plateau leveling osteotomies (2001-2003). *Journal of the American Animal Hospital Association* 42 (1), 44-50.

Steinberg, E.J., Prata, R.G., Palazzini, K., et al. (2011) Tibial tuberosity advancement for treatment of CrCL injury: complications and owner satisfaction. *Journal of the American Animal Hospital Association* 47 (4), 250-257.

Talaat, M.B., Kowaleski, M.P., Boudrieau, R.J. (2006) Combination tibial plateau leveling osteotomy and cranial closing wedge osteotomy of the tibia for the treatment of cranial cruciate ligament-deficient stifles with excessive tibial plateau angle. *Veterinary Surgery* 35 (8);729-739.

Taylor, J., Langenbach, A., Marcellin-Little, D.J. (2011) Risk factors for fibular fracture after TPLO. *Veterinary Surgery* 40 (6), 687-693.

Thieman, K.M., Pozzi, A., Ling, H.Y., et al. (2009) Contact mechanics of simulated meniscal tears in cadaveric canine stifles. *Veterinary Surgery* 38 (7), 803-810.

Thieman, K.M., Pozzi, A., Ling, H.Y., et al. (2010) Comparison of contact mechanics of three meniscal repair techniques and partial meniscectomy in cadaveric dog stifles. *Veterinary Surgery* 39 (3), 355-362.

Thieman, K.M., Tomlinson, J.L., Fox, D.B., et al. (2006) Effect of meniscal release on rate of subsequent meniscal tears and owner-assessed outcome in dogs with cruciate disease treated with tibial plateau leveling osteotomy. *Veterinary Surgery* 35 (8), 705-710.

Tonks, C.A., Pozzi, A., Ling, H.Y., et al. (2010) The effects of extra-articular suture tension on contact mechanics of the lateral compartment of cadaveric stifles treated with the TightRope CCL or lateral suture technique. *Veterinary Surgery* 39 (3), 343-349.

Tuttle, T.A., Manley, P.A. (2009) Risk factors associated with fibular fracture after tibial plateau leveling osteotomy. *Veterinary Surgery* 38 (3), 355-360.

Wolf, R.E., Scavelli, T.D., Hoelzler, M.G., et al. (2012) Surgical and postoperative complications associated with tibial tuberosity advancement for cranial cruciate ligament rupture in dogs: 458 cases (2007-2009). *Journal of the American Veterinary Medical Association* 240 (12), 1481-1487.

Yeadon, R., Fitzpatrick, N., Kowaleski, M.P. (2011) Tibial tuberosity transposition-advancement for treatment of medial patellar luxation and concomitant cranial cruciate ligament disease in the dog. Surgical technique, radiographic and clinical outcomes. *Veterinary and Comparative Orthopaedics and Traumatology* 24 (1), 18-26.

118 Complications Associated with the Treatment of Patellar Luxation

Abimbola Oshin
North Georgia Veterinary Specialists, Buford, GA, USA

Patellar luxation is the medial or lateral displacement of the patella from the femoral trochlear groove. It is primarily a developmental disease and is one of the most common orthopedic conditions encountered in dogs; it has been described in all breed categories (LaFond *et al.* 2002). Cats are also affected, but the incidence is lower than in dogs. Clinical diagnosis occurs at any time from the first few months of age into the geriatric years. Luxation is most commonly in the medial direction, although it can be lateral and, rarely, bidirectional (Remedios *et al.* 1992; Roush 1993; Hayes *et al.* 1994; Gibbons *et al.* 2006; Alam *et al.* 2007; Bound *et al.* 2009; Wangdee *et al.* 2015). A total of 25% to 65% of patellar luxations are observed bilaterally (Trotter 1980; Hayes *et al.* 1994; Arthurs and Langley-Hobbs 2006; Alam *et al.* 2007; Bound *et al.* 2009). Traumatic patella luxation is much less common and is unilateral. Patella luxation is graded in terms of severity from grade I through IV (Putnam 1968; Singleton 1969; Roush 1993). Surgery is usually indicated early in the course of the disease with grade III and IV luxations to prevent worsening skeletal deformities and osteoarthritis (OA) (Willauer and Vasseur 1987). Surgery for the other lesser grades usually depends on a variety of considerations, including clinical history, physical findings, frequency of luxation, and the patient's age (Schulz 2007).

Successful surgical treatment of patella luxation involves selecting the proper combination of surgical techniques to realign the structures participating in the extensor mechanism of the stifle. Surgical techniques described for the management of patella luxation includes one, or more commonly, a combination of the following: deepening the femoral trochlea groove (chondroplasty or trochleoplasty, which could be abrasion, wedge ridge elevation trochleoplasty, or block), parapatellar soft tissue release (desmotomy) and/or contralateral tightening (imbrication), antirotational sutures, release of musculatures (quadriceps and cranial portion of the sartorius), tibial tuberosity transposition, and femoral corrective osteotomy or ostectomy. Restoration of the anatomy and function in the treatment of patella luxation requires accurate detection and treatment of all skeletal and soft tissue pathology. Guidelines for selection of appropriate technique or combination of techniques, however, remain subjective.

Surgical management is generally successful, but up to 43.1% of cases are reportedly at least occasionally lame, and up to 13% require revision surgery; poor or unsatisfactory results are reported in 4.3% to 11% of cases (DeAngelis and Holm 1970; Denny and Minter 1973; Willauer and Vasseur 1987; Remedios *et al.* 1992; Alam *et al.* 2007; Linney *et al.* 2011; Kalff *et al.* 2014). Postoperative lameness and poor or unsatisfactory results may be due to a variety of factors. Conditions present preoperatively such as condition of the articular cartilage (Daems *et al.* 2009), OA, and limb deformities may play a role. The presence of concurrent disorders such as cruciate ligament rupture and meniscal injuries will lead to persistent lameness unless addressed. Finally, persistence of lameness beyond the normal 2- to 4-week postoperative period may be secondary to complications of the repair procedures. Some of the possible complications are outlined below.

Wound complications

Surgical wound complications, including inflammation of the surgical site, seroma formation, superficial and deep infection, wound dehiscence, suture reactions, and so on, are discussed elsewhere.

Degenerative joint disease

See Chapter 18

Septic arthritis

See Chapter 6

Reluxation

Definition

Reluxation is the recurrence of patella luxation in the postoperative period.

Risk factors

- Insufficient restoration of quadriceps alignment
- Failure to address other significant underlying deformities such as femoral varus and shallow trochlear groove
- Overcorrection
- Higher grade of patella luxation and pre or postoperative patella alta have not been significantly associated with the risk for reluxation

Diagnosis

Reluxation is usually diagnosed on physical examination. It may or may not be associated with clinical lameness. The diagnosis can be confirmed by radiography (Figure 118.1).

Treatment

Surgical management is indicated in cases with persistent clinical lameness. The management strategy uses the same criteria and

Complications in Small Animal Surgery, First Edition. Edited by Dominique Griffon and Annick Hamaide.
© 2016 John Wiley & Sons, Inc. Published 2016 by John Wiley & Sons, Inc.
Companion website: www.wiley.com/go/griffon/complications

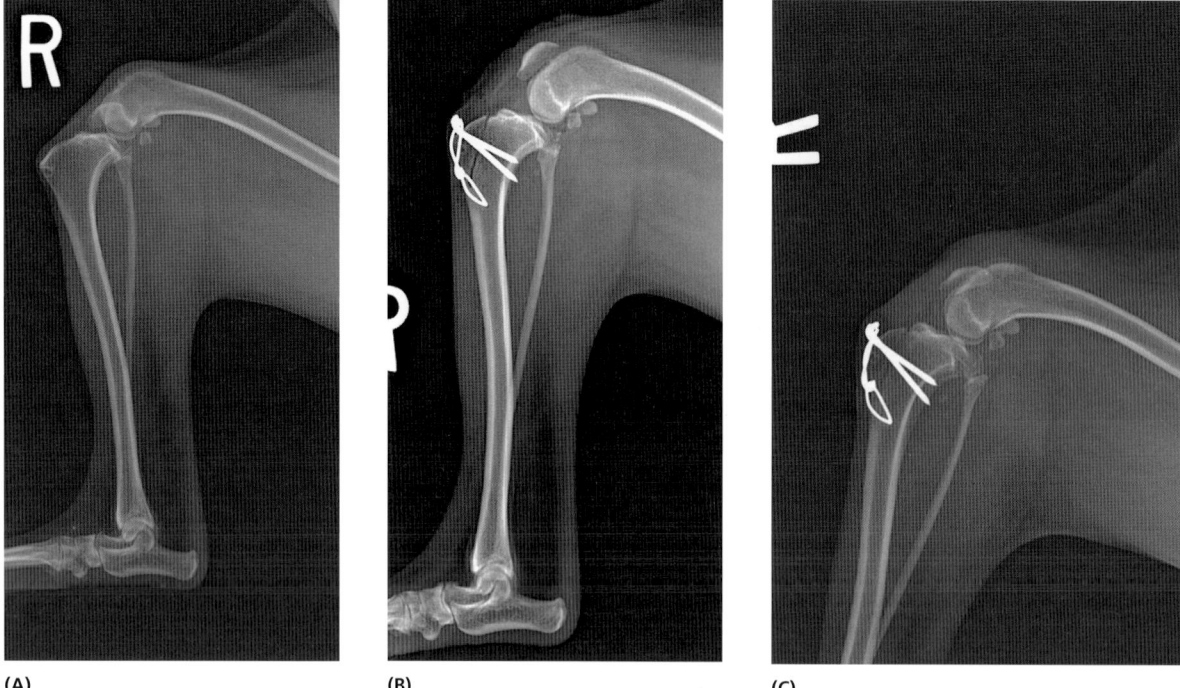

Figure 118.1 Preoperative (**A**) and immediate (**B**) and 3 weeks (**C**) postoperative lateral radiographs after repair of a grade II medial patella luxation demonstrating reluxation.

range of surgical techniques and procedures as with the original surgery.

- Deepen the femoral trochlea if the trochlea dimensions are inadequate.
- Address bony deformities with femoral corrective osteotomy or tibial tuberosity transposition to align the quadriceps mechanism.
- Parapatellar soft tissue release and contralateral tightening to maintain the patella within the trochlear groove
- Antirotational sutures to protect the soft tissue repair

Outcome

Unfortunately, reluxation is still possible after the second procedure. Therefore, as much care as was taken in the original surgery should be taken in the subsequent procedure. The risk of reluxation diminishes with subsequent surgery if additional techniques are added.

Prevention

To guard against reluxation, meticulous attention must be placed to the tendency for reluxation intraoperatively. Internal and external tibial rotation with the stifle in various degrees of flexion should be performed to assess the tendency for reluxation before completion of the procedure.

Complications of tibial crest transposition

Implant migration and implant failure

Definition

Implants used to secure the transposed tibial tuberosity might puncture the skin or migrate proximally or distally. Implant migration

may occur in association with implant failure in which parts of the implant breaks off before migration.

Risk factors

- Errors of technique where implants are not seated properly or deep enough or are not bent appropriately
- Repeated insertion and removal of the pins during the procedure
- Patient weight as a problem is more common in heavier patients.
- Omission of use of tension band wire when appropriate
- Use of inappropriately sized implants
- A patient that is allowed to be too active in the early postoperative period

Diagnosis

Diagnosis of implant problems is usually suspected when implants are seen poking through the skin at home or when a bump is seen in the cranial surface of the proximal tibia. The diagnosis is confirmed by physical examination and radiography.

Treatment

Treatment of migrating or failed implants depends on the time of occurrence. When these occur after the transposed tibial tuberosity is healed (usually >6 weeks postoperatively depending on age and size of patient), the implant can simply be removed. Implants migrating or failing before healing of the transposed tibial tuberosity may need to be replaced and any coexisting loss of transposition of the tibial tuberosity corrected.

Outcome

The outcome of treatment is usually good, especially if healing of the transposed tibial tuberosity is complete.

Prevention

The risk for implant migration or failure can be minimized by using appropriately sized implants, driving in the implants once, and avoiding repeated insertions and removal, and using tension band wire in all but the smallest dogs.

Fracture of tibial tuberosity

Definition

A fracture of the transposed tibial tuberosity allows distraction of the proximal fragment of the tibial tuberosity.

Risk factors

- Using inappropriately large Kirschner wires to fix the transposed tibial tuberosity
- Transposing a small segment of tibial tuberosity
- Tibial tuberosity transposition in immature animals where the growth plate is still wide open and the ossified portion of the tibial tuberosity is small
- Too much activity in the immediate postoperative periods

Diagnosis

Clinical signs may include exacerbation of lameness, patella alta, and loss of extension of the stifle. The diagnosis is ultimately confirmed radiographically (Figure 118.2).

Treatment

The decision to treat depends on the degree of clinical lameness seen. Conservative management with splinting is indicated when displacement of the proximal fragment and patella is minimal, especially when minimal lameness or advanced healing is already present. When lameness is associated, the patella tendon is usually attached to the distracted portion of the tibial tuberosity. Depending on the amount of bone distracted, fixation can be performed using appropriately sized pin and tension band wires, or screws with spiked washers may be used. The original implants may need to be removed to allow attachment of the distracted portion. The repair may need to be protected with a soft padded bandage for a couple of weeks. If only a small piece of tuberosity was avulsed, management is the same as for patella tendon rupture.

Outcome

The outcome after repair depends on the ability to fix the distracted portion and restore optimal patella length. If these can be achieved, the outcome is expected to be good.

Prevention

An adequate size of the tibial crest should be osteotomized for transposition. Also, implants should be appropriately sized to be no more than one third of the transposed tibial tuberosity. Tension band wire should be used whenever possible.

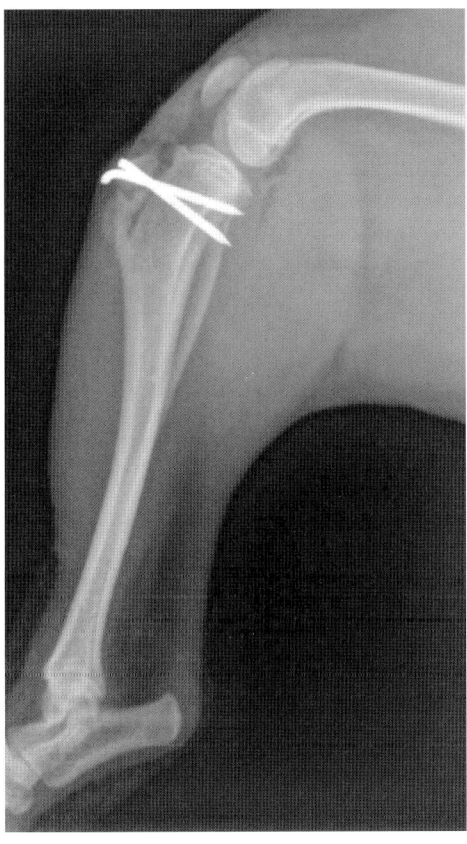
(A)

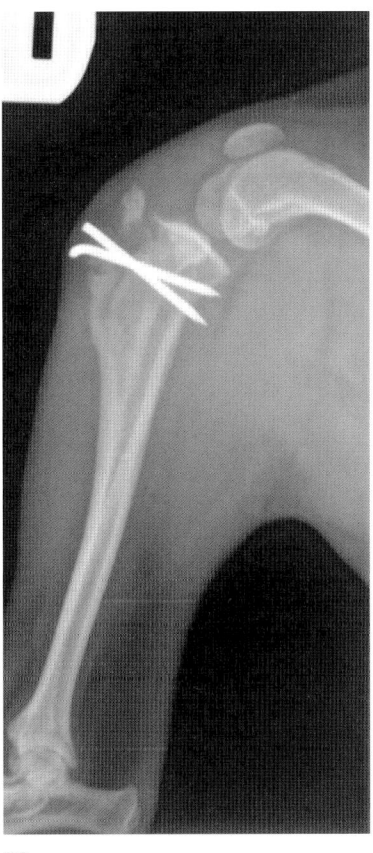
(B)

Figure 118.2 Immediate (**A**) and 8-week (**B**) postoperative radiographs demonstrating tibial tuberosity fracture.

Patella tendon rupture or severance

Definition
This is disruption of the patella tendon proximal to its attachment to the tibial tuberosity. This is usually recognized postoperatively, but it may also be an intraoperative or postoperative event.

Risk factors
Risk factors include lack of visualization of or protection of the patella tendon intraoperatively during tibial tuberosity transposition. This then leads to weakening or partial to complete severance of the tendon.

Diagnosis
Physical diagnosis is by palpation of patella riding higher than normal. The diagnosis can be confirmed by radiographs that demonstrated patella alta in the presence of intact and fixed tibial tuberosity.

Treatment
Repair is by primary suture of the ruptured tendons and protection of the repair by a mattress suture extending around and proximal to the patella or through a hole drilled into the patella and then through a holed drilled in the tibial tuberosity. The repair may need to be further protected with a soft padded bandage or a lateral splint.

Outcome
The outcome depends on the ability to restore optimal patella length. If these can be achieved, the outcome is expected to be good, although many patients have reduced stifle range of motion.

Prevention
Care should be taken to protect the patella ligament from iatrogenic damage during tibial tuberosity osteotomy. Also, patient activity should be restricted for an adequate period of time postoperatively.

Inadvertent severance of the long digital extensor tendon

Tibial fracture
Proximal tibial metaphyseal fracture is rare but has been seen secondary to tibial tuberosity transposition. The major risk factor is osteotomy of a large portion of the tibial tuberosity in a small dog, especially in patients with marked cranial bowing of the proximal tibia. The resulting fracture is characterized by an acute onset of severe lameness. Treatment is based on the degree of displacement seen and can be achieved with external coaptation if nondisplaced or by using internal fixation with bone plates.

Proximodistal patella malpositioning or malalignment

Definition
A malpositioned patella may be located too proximally or ride too high (patella alta). It may also be located too distally or too low (patella baja) in the femoral trochlear groove.

Risk factors
Patella malpositioning is usually an intraoperative complication associated with tibial tuberosity translocation, but it could also result postoperatively from tibial tuberosity avulsion, fracture, or patella ligament rupture.

Diagnosis
Diagnosis of proximodistal patella malposition can be made by palpating the patella during orthopedic evaluation. This subjective assessment is easy to make in cases of extreme patella malpositioning. The radiographic indices for establishing the presence of patella alta and patella baja have been well described (Mostafa *et al.* 2008). Briefly, it consists of measuring in lateral view the length of the patella tendon from the level of the tibial condyles to the distal pole of the patella and comparing it with the length of the patella from its proximal pole to its distal pole to obtain the PLL:PL index or measuring the distance from the proximal patella to the femoral transcondylar axis and comparing it with the patellar length in a craniocaudal or caudocranial view to obtain the A:PL index. The normal ratio was described as 1.97 to 2.06 and 1.92 to 2.03, respectively, for these indices but is most likely breed specific. Any ratio less than normal is patella baja and any ratio greater than normal is patella alta.

Treatment
Multiple surgical procedures have been reported. The most commonly reported procedure involves tibial tuberosity osteotomy if necessary, proximal, or distal translation of the tibial tuberosity as necessary and fixation using pin and tension band wires, lag screws with or without spiked washers, or a bone plate and screws (Paulos *et al.* 1994; Morshed and Ries 2002; Hockings 2004; Caton and Dejour 2010). When the length of the tibial tuberosity precludes adequate proximal translation of the tibial tuberosity for management of patella baja, management must incorporate patella lengthening procedures (Dejour *et al.* 1995; In *et al.* 2007). A proximal tibial tuberosity translation using tibial tuberosity advancement plate has been described (Edwards and Jackson 2012).

Outcome
The outcome after restoration of normal patella relationships in the stifle joint is good. Adequate protection of the repair in the immediate postoperative period combined with appropriate physical rehabilitation is indicated for the best possible outcome.

Prevention
Patella malpositioning can be prevented by taking care to prevent complications of tibial tuberosity fracture or avulsion and avoiding excessive distal translation during tibial tuberosity transposition.

Complications of trochlear recession
Abrasion trochleoplasty is reportedly successful as a component of surgical correction of patella luxation in small dogs. However, it is no longer recommended because loss of articular cartilage during the procedure means OA, and its associated deleterious effect on the joint is automatic. The most favored techniques are those that preserve the articular cartilage by itself, as in trochlear chondroplasty, or along with the underlying subchondral bone as with trochlear wedge and block recessions. Chondroplasty is only indicated in dogs younger than 6 months in which the articular cartilage can be gently separated from the underlying subchondral bone (Flo 1969). Chondroplasty in these young dogs should result in minimal complications because the cartilage is easily peeled of, and healing is quick after it is replaced.

Inadequate trochleoplasty dimensions

Definition

A trochlear groove that is not deep or wide enough to satisfy the requirement that approximately 50% or less of the patella protrudes above the trochlear ridges. The patella may therefore have the same tendency for reluxation as preoperatively.

Risk factors

The common predisposing factors for this complication include:
- Misshapen or eroded femoral trochlear from chronic grade II or III patellar luxations
- Operator inexperience
- Fear of condylar fracture

Diagnosis

Assessment of trochlear dimensions can be made visually during the surgical procedure. Other ways to assess the dimensions of the groove relative to that of the patella include the use of skyline views of the trochlear or computed tomography (Johnson *et al.* 2001; Towle *et al.* 2005).

Treatment

Treatment may not be necessary if reluxation does not occur. However with persistent and clinical reluxation, revision of the surgery is recommended and is aimed at creating adequate groove dimensions.

Outcome

The outcome after revision surgery is good. Care should be taken to make sure the dimension of the groove created is adequate. It is unlikely that groove dimension is the only reason for reluxation, so other procedures may be indicated during the revision surgery.

Prevention

When performing a procedure to deepen the femoral trochlear groove, make sure the width of the groove created is sufficient at its midpoint to accommodate the width of the patella but preserves the trochlear ridges.

Loss of osteochondral autograft

Definition

This is the accidental loss of the autograft tissue during the procedure. The tissue may be dropped or contaminated.

Risk factors

Loss of the osteochondral graft is associated with care not being taken during the trochleoplasty procedure, either during elevation of the graft or storing of the graft while the new femoral groove is being prepared.

Diagnosis

Loss of osteochondral autograft to contamination is an intraoperative complication that is immediately evident.

Treatment

After loss of the cartilage or osteochondral autograft, the procedure is converted into a trochlear sulcoplasty (abrasion trochleoplasty).

The resulting defect is smoothed with a high speed bur, an osteotome, a rongeur, or a bone rasp. Care should still be taken to ensure that at least 50% of the patella is positioned below the level of the trochlear ridges. A procedure to resurface the new groove with autogenous periosteal graft harvested from the medial surface of the proximal tibial metaphysis has been described (Hulse *et al.* 1986).

Outcome

Clinical reports suggest that trochlear sulcoplasty is very successful in small dogs and cats. Fibroplasia will result in a new groove lined with fibrocartilage, which is an acceptable substitute for hyaline cartilage in non–weight-bearing areas. The outcome can be improved, especially in larger patients, by resurfacing the defect with autogenous periosteal graft, which allows faster resurfacing of the groove and less patella cartilage damage (Hulse *et al.* 1986).

Prevention

For trochlear chondroplasty, maintaining either the proximal or distal attachment of the cartilage flap will prevent loss of the flap. With the other procedures, the osteochondral autograft should be removed carefully and the instrument used to make the cut should not be used to lever the final uncut segment of the autograft as it may be flicked off of the sterile field. Also, after the autograft is removed, it should be wrapped in a bloody sponge and stored on a flat surface within the sterile field where it can be protected.

Migration of the trochlear wedge

Definition

The wedge of bone created during recession trochleoplasty migrates into the joint.

Risk factors

Reluxation is a risk for migration of trochlear osteochondral fragment.

Diagnosis

The diagnosis is usually made radiographically and will demonstrate a joint mouse. The diagnosis has also been made during arthrotomy to manage persistent lameness from reluxation.

Treatment

Treatment is by reattachment or removal of the wedge depending on the duration of the migration and the state of the wedge and the trochlear groove.

Outcome

The outcome is good with either of the procedures described. If in doubt of which procedure to use, it is best to remove the wedge.

Prevention

Usually, there is no need to secure the wedge in place. It should be held in place from the quadriceps through the patella. If migration of the wedge is a concern intraoperatively, an appropriately sized Kirschner wire can be driven across the femoral condyles through the wedge to keep it in place (Figure 118.3).

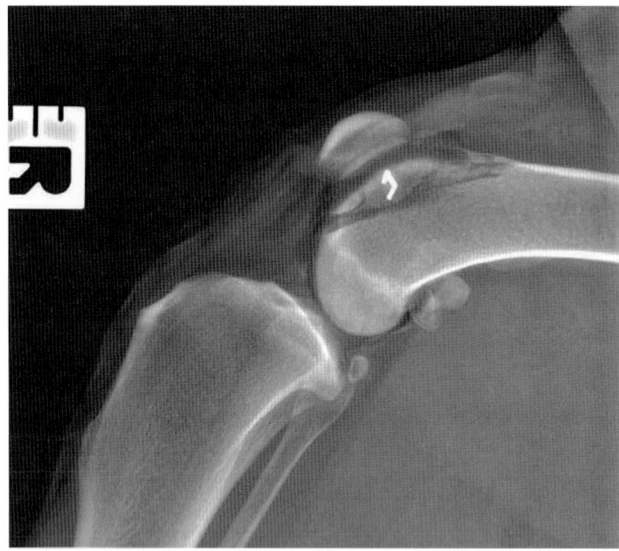

(A)

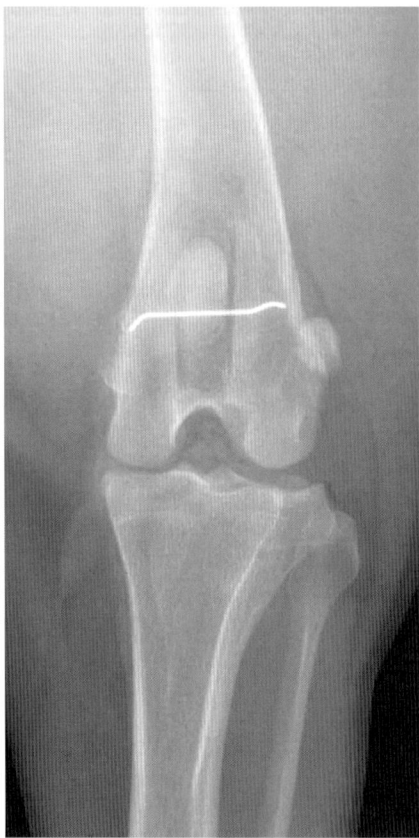

(B)

Figure 118.3 **A** and **B**, Postoperative lateral and caudocranial views of the right stifle showing trochleoplasty grooves with linear fissures and implant superimposed on the trochleoplasty. Incomplete fractures of the remaining bone of the trochleoplasty led to concerns about further fragmentation and migration. The wedge is held in place with a single Kirschner wire.

Fracture of the trochlear ridge

Definition
This is breaking off of the medial or lateral trochlear ridge.

Risk factors
Risk factors identified for trochlear ridge fracture include external trauma, inadequate thickness of residual trochlear ridge after trochleoplasty procedure, undermining of trochlear ridge by osteotomy, excessive abaxial force by the patella, and quadriceps mechanism from over or undercorrection.

Diagnosis
The diagnosis can be suspected based on physical examination findings of patella reluxation and stifle joint effusion. The diagnosis can be confirmed by orthogonal and skyline radiographic views of the stifle joint.

Treatment
Treatment is by open reduction internal fixation of the fracture with countersunk bone pins or screws. In a canine case report, a buttress plate using an acetabular plate was also used to reinforce the fractured trochlear ridge (Chase and Farrell 2010). Protection of the trochlear ridge from further abaxial force from the patella and quadriceps mechanism was achieved by biaxial patella antirotational sutures. A non-vascularized Ilial crest bone graft has also been reportedly used to treat trochlear ridge fracture (Ostberg et al. 2014).

Outcome
The outcome is excellent if the fracture ridge can be reduced and fixed successfully. Inadequate reduction or fixation is expected to result in varying degrees of OA that may affect the final outcome.

Prevention
This is a rare complication, but consideration and avoidance of the risk factors during the surgical procedure should help in preventing its occurrence.

Complications of femoral osteotomy
Complication of corrective osteotomy, including delayed union and fixation failure, are discussed in chapters 94 and 98 respectively.

Relevant literature
Complications occur in 18% to 29% of dogs undergoing patella luxation surgery. The complications are traditionally classified as major complications if they require revision surgery or minor complications if revision surgery is not required (Arthurs and Langley-Hobbs 2006; Gibbons et al. 2006; Cashmore et al. 2014). A greater risk for postoperative complications has been recognized in larger dogs. Single session bilateral surgery was not associated with increased complications in small dogs weighing less than 12 kg (Clerfond et al. 2014). The most commonly reported of the major complications of patella luxation surgery include patella reluxation and problems associated tibial tuberosity transposition such as loose or broken implants, tuberosity fracture or displacement, and fracture of the proximal tibia.

Reluxation is the most common postoperative complication of patella luxation repair. The incidence of patella reluxation from undercorrection ranges from 7.6% to 48% (Willauer and Vasseur 1987; Slocum and Slocum 1998; Arthurs and Langley-Hobbs 2006; Gibbons et al. 2006; Linney et al. 2011). It is usually in the same direction as the preoperative luxation, and reasons for this include insufficient restoration of quadriceps alignment, premature implant failure, and failure to address significant underlying limb deformities such as shallow trochlear groove and excessive femoral varus. Most studies have reported a relationship between high preoperative grades of patella luxation and high rates of reluxation (Singleton 1969; Remedios et al. 1992; Roush 1993; Arthurs and Langley-Hobbs 2006). However, this relationship is not statistically significant (Arthurs and Langley-Hobbs 2006; Linney et al. 2011; Cashmore et al. 2014). No significant relationships were also found between reluxation and age, sex, and weight (Linney et al. 2011). Reluxation in the opposite direction from overcorrection is less common but has been reported (Arthurs and Langley-Hobbs 2006; Linney et al. 2011). The time from surgery to reluxation has been evaluated and can range from 0.3 months to 31.1 months (Linney et al. 2011). Usually, when it occurs, reluxation is of a lower grade and frequently does not produce clinical signs (Willauer and Vasseur 1987; Roush 1993; L'Eplattenier and Montavon 2002; Piermattei et al. 2006). Historically, the proportion of cases of patella luxation repairs in which additional surgery was recommended for patellar reluxation ranges from 6.6% to 13.0% (Willauer and Vasseur 1987; Arthurs and Langley-Hobbs 2006; Linney et al. 2011). It is still, however, the most common reason for reoperation after surgery for patella luxation, accounting for 65% to 86% of revision surgeries (Arthurs and Langley-Hobbs 2006; Gibbons et al. 2006).

Tibial crest transposition is increasingly seen as a critical component of patella luxation repair. Translocation is in the direction opposite the patella luxation and is an attempt to realign the quadriceps mechanism. Complications of tibial crest transposition can be directly related to the procedure itself or to its effect on the proximodistal position of the patella. Common complications of tibial crest translocation procedure include implant migration or failure, fracture of the tibial tuberosity, and fracture for the proximal tibia and fibula (Arthurs and Langley-Hobbs 2006). Other less common complications are inadvertent severance of the patella tendon and inadvertent severance of the tendon of the long digital extensor.

In a normal stifle joint, patellofemoral contact facilitates extensor function of the stifle joint and provides a smooth gliding mechanism for the quadriceps apparatus while greatly increasing mechanical efficiency. A functioning patellofemoral joint also provides caudal compression and contributes to the overall stability of the stifle. Disruption of the patellofemoral joint is therefore likely to contribute to persistent postoperative lameness. Abnormal proximodistal positioning of the patella is referred to as patella alta or patella baja. In dogs, patella baja is associated with lateral patella luxation, and patella alta is associated with medial patella luxation. Abnormal patella positioning has, however, also been reported in dogs as a complication of patella luxation, either from direct injury and rupture of the patella or secondary to complications of tibial tuberosity transposition (Edwards and Jackson 2012).

A shallow trochlear groove is considered to be one of the major bony deformities associated with patellar luxation. Various trochleoplasty techniques have been described to deepen and widen the femoral trochlear groove to permit adequate sitting of the patella throughout the stifle range of motion. Whichever technique is used, the aim is to achieve a trochlear groove that is deep and wide enough that approximately 50% or less of the patella protrudes above the trochlear ridges (Slocum and Devine 1985). Performing trochlear recessions significantly reduces the frequency of patella reluxation (Arthurs and Langley-Hobbs 2006; Gibbons et al. 2006), but complications have been associated with these procedures. Complications of trochlear recession consist of those common to all procedures and those usually associated with the method of recession chosen. Common to all procedures are inadequate trochleoplasty dimensions (depth and width). A trochleoplasty that is too

deep may cause condylar fracture of the femur that will need to be repaired. With sulcoplasty and recession trochleoplasty, migration of elevated and recessed cartilage or osteochondral fragment, or fragmented portions of it, into the joint introduces an object that will exacerbate lameness and OA. After surgery, the compressive force of the articulating patella and the friction between the cancellous surfaces should keep a trochlear wedge in the deepened groove. If reduction is not maintained, the wedge can migrate. Migration of the trochlear wedge can be managed by removal or reattachment of the wedge (Remedios et al. 1992). Finally, trochleoplasty procedures, in an attempt to achieve adequate dimensions, may lead to prominent medial and lateral trochlear ridges that can subsequently fracture (Chase and Farrell 2010).

Secondary OA is a common sequela associated with patella luxation, and there is no evidence that its development and progression is influenced by the method of treatment (Willauer and Vasseur 1987; Roy et al. 1992).

Corrective distal femoral osteotomy has been advocated as a component of surgical correction of patella luxation when complicated by excessive femoral angular deformities (Peruski et al. 2006; Piermattei et al. 2006; Swiderski and Palmer 2007; Roch and Gemmill 2008). Use of appropriate implants and preservation of vascular supply via muscular attachments to the femur should result in predictable and relatively rapid healing. Complications associated with corrective osteotomies include healing problems, malalignment problems, and implant problems, which are discussed elsewhere.

Most of the other complications are minor and do not require revision surgery unless they lead to a major complication. Such minor complications include wound-related problems, swollen patella tendon, hock hyperextension, and proximal displacement of the tibial tuberosity.

References

Alam, M.R., Lee, J.I., Kang, H.S., et al. (2007) Frequency and distribution of patellar luxation in dogs. 134 cases (2000 to 2005). *Veterinary and Comparative Orthopaedics and Traumatology* 20, 59-64.

Arthurs, G.I., Langley-Hobbs, S.J. (2006) Complications associated with corrective surgery for patellar luxation in 109 dogs. *Veterinary Surgery* 35, 559-566.

Bound, N., Zakai, D., Butterworth, S.J., et al. (2009) The prevalence of canine patellar luxation in three centres. Clinical features and radiographic evidence of limb deviation. *Veterinary and Comparative Orthopaedics and Traumatology* 22, 32-37.

Cashmore, R.G., Havlicek, M., Perkins, N.R. et al. (2014) Major complications and risk factors associated with surgical correction of congenital medial patellar luxation in 124 dogs. *Veterinary and Comparative Orthopaedics and Traumatology* 27, 263-70.

Caton, J.H., Dejour, D. (2010) Tibial tubercle osteotomy in patello-femoral instability and in patellar height abnormality. *International Orthopaedics*, 34, 305-309.

Chase, D., Farrell, M. (2010) Fracture of the lateral trochlear ridge after surgical stabilisation of medial patellar luxation. *Veterinary and Comparative Orthopaedics and Traumatology* 23, 203-208.

Clerfond, P., Huneault, L., Dupuis, J. et al. (2014) Unilateral or single-session bilateral surgery for correction of medial patellar luxation in small dogs: short and long-term outcomes. *Veterinary and Comparative Orthopedics and Traumatology* 27, 484-90.

Daems, R., Janssens, L.A., Béosier, Y.M. (2009) Grossly apparent cartilage erosion of the patellar articular surface in dogs with congenital medial patellar luxation. *Veterinary and Comparative Orthopaedics and Traumatology* 22, 222-224.

DeAngelis, M., Hohn, R.B. (1970) Evaluation of surgical correction of canine patellar luxation in 142 cases. *Journal of the American Veterinary Medical Association* 156, 587-594.

Dejour, D., Levigne, C., Dejour, H. (1995) [Postoperative low patella. Treatment by lengthening of the patellar tendon]. *Revue de chirurgie orthopédique et réparatrice de l'appareil moteur* 81, 286-295.

Denny, H.R., Minter, H.M. (1973) The long term results of surgery of canine stifle disorders. *Journal of Small Animal Practice* 14, 695-714.

Edwards, G.A., Jackson, A.H. (2012) Use of a TTA plate for correction of severe patella baja in a Chihuahua. *Journal of the American Animal Hospital Association* 48 (2), 113-117.

Flo, G.L. (1969) Surgical correction of a deficient trochlear groove in dogs with severe congenital patellar luxations utilizing a cartilage flap and subchondral grooving. East Lansing, Michigan, Master of Science Thesis, Michigan State University.

Gibbons, S.E., Macias, C., Tonzing, M.A., et al. (2006) Patellar luxation in 70 large breed dogs. *Journal of Small Animal Practice* 47, 3-9.

Hayes, A.G., Boudrieau, R.J., Hungerford, L.L. (1994) Frequency and distribution of medial and lateral patellar luxation in dogs: 124 cases (1982-1992). *Journal of the American Veterinary Medical Association* 205, 716-720.

Hockings, M. (2004) Patella baja following chronic quadriceps tendon rupture. *The Knee*, 11, 95-97.

Hulse, D.A., Miller, D., Roberts, D., et al. (1986) Resurfacing canine femoral trochleoplasties with free autogenous periosteal grafts. *Veterinary Surgery* 15, 284-288.

In, Y., Kim, S.J., Kwon, Y.J. (2007) Patellar tendon lengthening for patella infera using the Ilizarov technique. *The Journal of Bone & Joint Surgery* 89, 398-400.

Johnson, A.L., Probst, C.W., Decamp, C.E., et al. (2001) Comparison of trochlear block recession and trochlear wedge recession for canine patellar luxation using a cadaver model. *Veterinary Surgery* 30, 140-150.

Kalff, S., Butterworth, S.J., Miller, A. et al. (2014) Lateral patellar luxation in dogs: a retrospective study of 65 dogs. *Veterinary and Comparative Orthopaedics and Traumatology.* 27, 130-4.

L'Eplattenier, H., Montavon, P. (2002) Patellar luxation in dogs and cats: management and prevention. *Compendium on Continuing Education for the Practicing Veterinarian* 24, 292-300.

LaFond, E., Breur, G.J., Austin, C.C. (2002) Breed susceptibility for developmental orthopedic diseases in dogs. *Journal of the American Animal Hospital Association* 38, 467-477.

Linney, W.R., Hammer, D.L., Shott, S. (2011) Surgical treatment of medial patellar luxation without femoral trochlear groove deepening procedures in dogs: 91 cases (1998-2009). *Journal of the American Veterinary Medical Association* 238, 1168-1172.

Morshed, S., Ries, M.D. (2002) Patella infera after nonoperative treatment of a patellar fracture a case report. *The Journal of Bone & Joint Surgery* 84, 1018-1021.

Mostafa, A.A., Griffon, D.J., Thomas, M.W., et al. (2008) Proximodistal alignment of the canine patella: radiographic evaluation and association with medial and lateral patellar luxation. *Veterinary Surgery* 37, 201-211.

Ostberg, S.E., Dimopoulou, M., Lee, M.H. (2014) Ilial crest bone graft transposition as treatment for fracture of the medial femoral trochlear ridge in a dog. *Veterinary and Comparative Orthopaedics and Traumatology* 27, 80-4.

Paulos, L.E., Wnorowski, D.C., Greenwald, A.E. (1994) Infrapatellar contracture syndrome. Diagnosis, treatment, and long-term followup. *The American Journal of Sports Medicine* 22, 440-449.

Peruski, A.M., Kowaleski, M.P., Pozzi, A., et al. (2006) Treatment of medial patellar luxation and distal femoral varus by femoral wedge osteotomy in dogs: 30 cases (2000-2005). In *2nd World Veterinary Orthopedic and 33rd Annual Veterinary Orthopedic Society Meeting*, February 25 to March 4, Keystone, CO, p. 240.

Piermattei, D.L., Flo, G.L., DeCamp, C.E. (2006) Patellar luxation. In Piermattei, D.L., Flo, G.L, DeCamp, C.E. (eds.) *Handbook of Small Animal Orthopedics and Fracture Repair*. Saunders Elsevier, St. Louis, pp. 562-582.

Putnam, R. (1968) Patellar luxation in the dog. Ontario, Canada, Master of Science Thesis, University of Guelph.

Remedios, A.M., Basher, A.W.P., Runyon, et al. (1992) Medial patellar luxation in 16 large dogs: a retrospective study. *Veterinary Surgery* 21, 5-9.

Roch, S.P., Gemmill, T.J. (2008) Treatment of medial patellar luxation by femoral closing wedge ostectomy using a distal femoral plate in four dogs. *Journal of Small Animal Practice* 49, 152-158.

Roush, J.K. (1993) Canine patellar luxation. *Veterinary Clinics of North America: Small Animal Practice* 23, 855-868.

Roy, R.G., Wallace, L.J., Johnston, G.R. (1992) A retrospective evaluation of stifle osteoarthritis in dogs with bilateral medial patellar luxation and unilateral surgical repair. *Veterinary Surgery* 21, 475-479.

Schulz, K. (2007) Medial patellar luxation. In Fossum, T.W. (ed.) *Small Animal Surgery*. Mosby Elsevier, St. Louis, pp. 1289-1297.

Singleton, W.B. (1969) The Surgical Correction of Stifle Deformities in the Dog. *Journal of Small Animal Practice* 10, 59-69.

Slocum, B., Devine, T. (1985) Trochlear recession for correction of luxating patella in the dog. *Journal of the American Veterinary Medical Association* 186, 365-369.

Slocum, B., Slocum, T.D. (1998) Patellar luxation algorithm. In Bojrab, M. (ed.) *Current Techniques in Small Animal Surgery*. Williams & Wilkins, Baltimore, pp. 1222-1231.

Swiderski, J.K., Palmer, R.H. (2007) Long-term outcome of distal femoral osteotomy for treatment of combined distal femoral varus and medial patellar luxation: 12 cases (1999-2004). *Journal of the American Veterinary Medical Association* 231, 1070-1075.

Towle, H.A., Griffon, D.J., Thomas, M.W., et al. (2005) Pre- and postoperative radiographic and computed tomographic evaluation of dogs with medial patellar luxation. *Veterinary Surgery* 34, 265-272.

Trotter, E. (1980) Medial patellar luxation in the dog. *Compendium on Continuing Education for the Practicing Veterinarian* 2, 58-67.

Wangdee, C., Hazewinkel, H.A., Temwichitr, J. et al. (2015) Extended proximal trochleoplasty for the correction of bidirectional patellar luxation in seven Pomeranian dogs. *Journal of Small Animal Practice* 56, 130-3.

Willauer, C.C., Vasseur, P.B. (1987) Clinical results of surgical correction of medial luxation of the patella in dogs. *Veterinary Surgery* 16, 31-36.

119 Complications Associated with Autogenous Osteochondral Repair

Noel Fitzpatrick

Fitzpatrick Referrals Orthopedics and Neurology, Godalming, Surrey, UK

Osteochondral plug fracture

Definition

Disruption of the graft core usually occurs transversely across the subchondral bone, leading to an inappropriately short sized graft; this causes the graft to sit below the articular surface. Fracture may occur during retrieval of the plug from the donor bed or during insertion of the plug into the recipient bed.

Risk factors

- Levering or toggling the graft removal device during plug retrieval
- Inappropriate graft handling
- Graft dehydration
- Incorrect graft alignment during insertion into the recipient bed
- Encroachment of donor core on an active growth plate

Diagnosis

The diagnosis is confirmed on obvious fracture of the plug during removal or during inspection of the graft core before insertion into the recipient bed. Careful attention should be paid to identify fissures in the graft that may proceed to overt fractures during implantation.

Treatment

The recipient bed depth must match the plug depth to ensure restoration of the topography of the articular surface. In the event of donor plug fracture, a second donor core could be retrieved to match the depth of the recipient bed. This may be taken from an adjacent site as outlined in Figures 119.1 and 119.2. Backfilling of the recipient bed to accommodate the fractured plug is possible with either packed autologous cancellous bone or allogenous packed corticocancellous bone chips, but it is essential to ensure packing and remeasurement of the recipient site and the donor core. It is also essential that at least 3 to 4 mm of original subchondral bone is still attached to the base of the cartilage donor core.

Prevention

- Ensure a smooth rotational motion of the graft retrieval device.
- Prevent levering or toggling movements during graft retrieval and graft insertion.
- Prevent graft dehydration by sparse application of flush solution if there is any delay in the insertion of the graft.

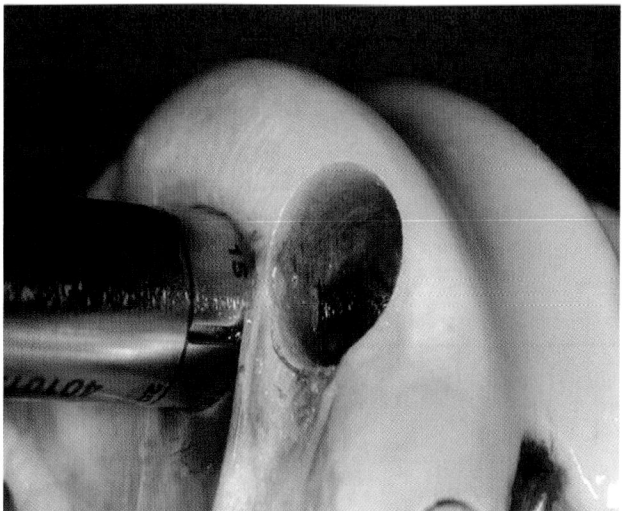

Figure 119.1 Collection of multiple donor grafts from the same condyle, one from the abaxial cartilaginous region of the medial trochlear ridge and one from the fibrous transition zone. An adequate amount of bone must be preserved between donor sites to avoid collapse.

- Remove the graft after preparation of the recipient bed, thus reducing the time between extraction and insertion and preventing dehydration of the graft material.
- Surgery should ideally be carried out on a joint when the associated growth plates have closed to prevent premature traumatic growth plate closure and the harvesting of mechanically unsound donor cores. In some juvenile larger breed dogs, graft acquisition is possible without encroaching the physes and can therefore be performed in such patients.

Donor site collapse

Definition

Donor site collapse is caused by subsidence of the subchondral bone surrounding the donor bed, leading to pain, swelling, lameness, and in some cases alteration of the topography of the joint surface above.

Complications in Small Animal Surgery, First Edition. Edited by Dominique Griffon and Annick Hamaide.
© 2016 John Wiley & Sons, Inc. Published 2016 by John Wiley & Sons, Inc.
Companion website: www.wiley.com/go/griffon/complications

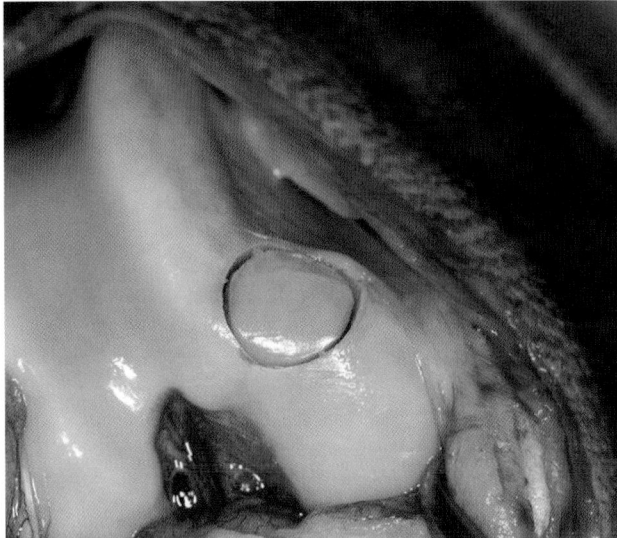

Figure 119.2 Donor site at the medial plateau of the intersect between the condyle and trochlea.

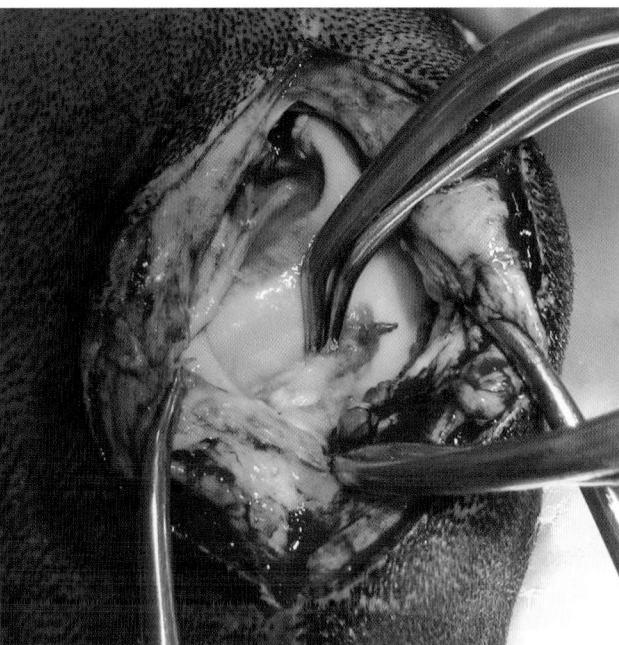

Figure 119.3 Examination of a recipient core site during tibial plateau leveling osteotomy surgery approximately 11 months after graft implantation. The surface appearance is consistent with hyaline cartilage. A donor site is also visible and is described in Figure 119.2.

Risk factors

- Multiple core retrieval; if the cores are orientated in a convergent pattern, there is an increased likelihood of donor site collapse
- Excessively deep core retrieval
- Juvenile patient
- Inappropriate anatomical position of donor site

Diagnosis

The diagnosis depends on the location of the donor site, within the contralateral joint or from the joint affected by the osteochondritis dissecans (OCD) lesion. Acute deterioration in limb function and pain over the donor site are indicative of donor site collapse if the graft has been harvested from the contralateral limb. Care must be taken when making this diagnosis if the graft was harvested from the same joint into which it is being placed; in these cases, it is essential to ascertain whether the lameness is caused by donor site collapse, failure of the graft, or a combination of both. Magnetic resonance imaging allows accurate evaluation of graft integration while also allowing evaluation of subchondral pathology. Diagnosis of donor site collapse may prove difficult without access to advanced imaging modalities. The typical appearance of appropriate donor and recipient sites are shown in Figures 119.3 and 119.4.

Treatment

Strict cage rest and appropriate analgesic management for 21 to 28 days should bring resolution of the issue, allowing the site to heal.

Outcome

Collapse of a donor site rarely requires revision surgery. The exception to this approach is in cases when collapse brings about a change in the topography of the articular surface. This can occur in graft sites situated close to the trochlear groove; subsidence of the trochlear ridges could cause pathology of the femoropatellar joint, which could require surgical intervention.

Prevention

- When multiple donor grafts are required, maintain 2 mm of bone stock between donor beds to allow adequate bone bridges to support loading (see Figure 119.1).

- Preoperative planning of multiple donor sites must be carried out to limit the degree of subchondral convergence at the donor sites.
- Backfilling the donor site with the bone stock removed from the recipient bed or using an allograft can prevent donor site collapse postoperatively.
- Donor cores should be harvested either from the abaxial aspect of the proximal medial trochlear ridge or from the plateau of the intersect of the condyle and trochlea (PICT); these areas

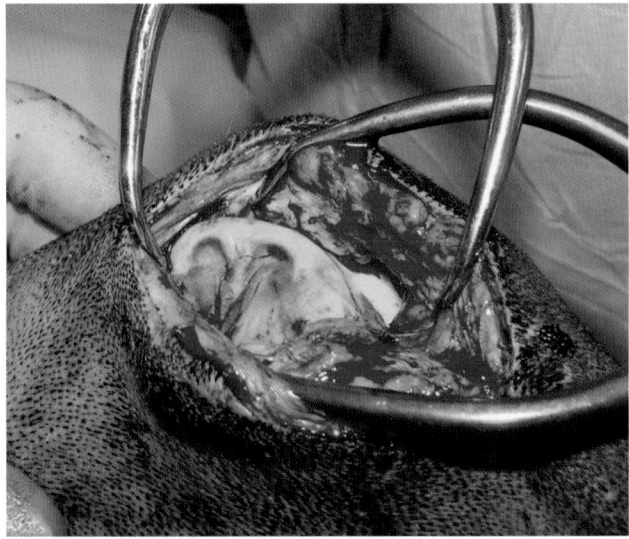

Figure 119.4 Examination of two donor sites during tibial plateau leveling osteotomy surgery approximately 11 months after harvest of grafts. The donor sites do not appear inflamed, and the defects are filled with fibrocartilage and fibrous tissue of the synovial reflection.

undergo little mechanical loading and thus should be resilient to collapse (see Figures 119.1 and 119.2). The abaxial aspect of the lateral trochlear ridge can also be used as a donor site for smaller grafts.

Donor plug recipient site mismatch

Definition
Integration of the graft and restoration of the articular surface require a perfect alignment between the surface of the graft and the surrounding cartilage. A mismatch between the core size and the recipient bed will cause the core to sit in an elevated position above the articular surface or subside beneath the level of the articular surface.

Risk factors
- Inaccurate recipient bed measurement
- Inaccurate donor core measurement
- Swarf contamination of the recipient bed
- If two or more contiguous overlapping grafts are required to resurface the lesion
- Excessive postoperative exercise reduces osteochondral integration and thus makes late postoperative core subsidence more likely

Diagnosis
The diagnosis is most frequently made during core placement and less frequently during second-look arthroscopy or a secondary surgical intervention. Subsidence of the donor plug produces a donor surface that is below the level of the articular cartilage. Proud donor cores fail to seat during insertion and remain proud compared with the patient's articular surface.

Treatment
Seating of the core 1 to 2 mm below the articular surface has been shown to have little negative effect on functional outcome. In contrast, donor plugs that sit proud have been found to generate abnormally high contact pressures on the opposing articular surface. This local overloading causes chondrocyte damage and may well perpetuate lameness caused by damage to the opposing articular cartilage or failure of the core caused by compression of chondrocytes (Koh *et al.* 2004). Plugs that are identified as proud during surgery should be removed immediately and replaced with a fresh plug from an alternate site. Explantation of the graft core can be carried out using a threaded Ellis pin introduced into the center of the graft, with care taken not to engage the base of the recipient bed, and pulling the plug out of the bed. If the recipient core edges are damaged, then a larger donor core must be implanted.

Prevention
- Ensure accurate measurement of the recipient bed before donor plug insertion.
- Double check the length of the donor core before placement.
- Check the recipient bed before plug insertion, removing all debris that may cause the plug to sit proud.
- If more than one graft is required to resurface the lesion, it is important that the first recipient site is filled first before the second graft site is drilled and filled, ensuring that the surface topography of each is satisfactory (Figure 119.5).
- Strict postoperative care facilitates osteochondral core integration, hence preventing late postoperative core subsidence.

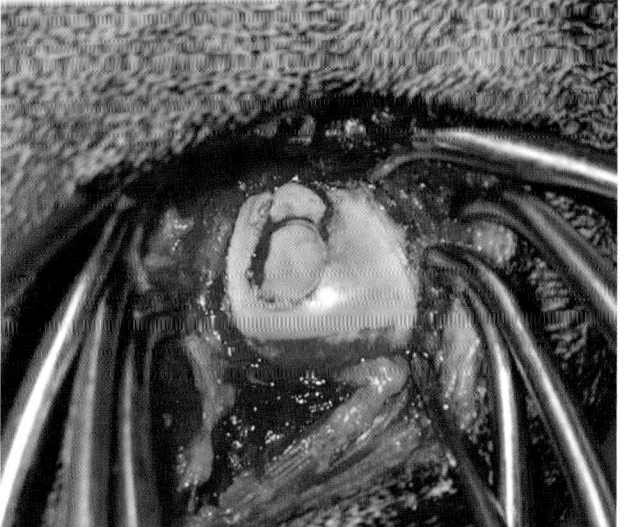

(A)

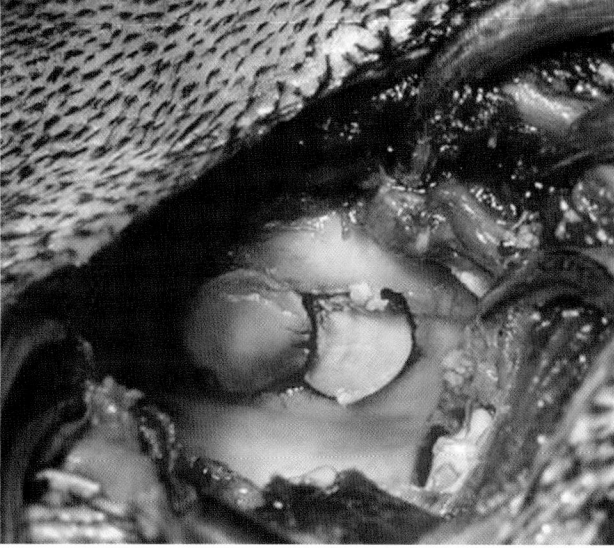

(B)

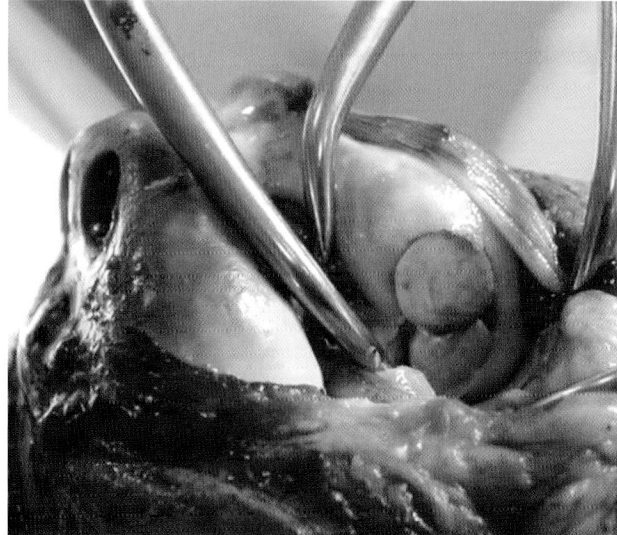

(C)

Figure 119.5 Double contiguous overlapping grafts for resurfacing of large osteochondral defects of the shoulder, elbow, and stifle.

Graft failure

Definition
This is loss of the functional integrity of the implanted graft. The most common causes of graft failure are chondrocyte death, failure of graft incorporation, and graft loosening.

Risk factors
- Excessive tamping during graft positioning; causing compression of the chondrocytes
- Poor correlation between the graft and recipient site size
- The subchondral changes seen with OCD may directly affect graft incorporation because trabecular disruption and subchondral bone edema may prevent adequate graft integration.
- An unstable press fit may cause overt graft loosening as will a poorly seated graft.
- Toggling during plug retrieval and implantation increases the likelihood of plug loosening.
- Postoperative joint sepsis is likely to cause graft failure.

Diagnosis
Clinically, patients with failed OATS™ (Osteochondral Autograft Transplantation Surgery) grafts exhibit ongoing pain, discomfort, and joint swelling. The diagnosis is confirmed via radiography or computed topography examination. Evidence of graft failure includes obvious intraarticular graft displacement, graft migration, and radiolucency around the graft. Arthrocentesis with subsequent culture and sensitivity will identify an infective cause of graft failure.

Treatment
Treatment ultimately involves surgical revision because conservative management of a failed osteochondral graft is not indicated. The principles of revision in these cases include:
- Explantation of the graft core as previously described.
- Current options for revision of a failed autogenous osteochondral graft usually involve overdrilling the original graft site with a larger reamer and then placing an autograft of a larger size harvested from a new donor site, a size-matched allograft, or synthetic graft resurfacing. It is especially important to ensure that the recipient bed is enlarged to expose viable bleeding cancellous bone edges.

Outcome
Unless revision surgery is carried out, the surgery is regarded as a failure with a high likelihood of ongoing pain and lameness.

Prevention
- Meticulous care must be taken during graft handling to prevent chondrocyte damage and death.
- Judicious tamping minimizes chondrocyte compression and subsequent cell death.
- Ensure proper seating of the graft into the recipient bed by carefully matching the recipient bed depth and graft length.
- Vigorous flushing of the recipient bed before measuring its depth will prevent unattached swarf from the reamer from causing erroneous measurements.
- Gentle tamping of the base of the recipient bed before measuring the depth will help seat any attached swarf and aid in producing an accurate measurement of recipient bed depth.
- When treating OCD lesions, make sure that the graft recipient bed extends deeply enough, beyond the zone of influence of the OCD lesion.

- Take great care during graft retrieval to guard against excessive torsional or toggling moments to maintain the architectural integrity of the graft.
- When more than one graft is placed, make sure that each is reamed and filled sequentially to best match the surface topography of the recipient site (see Figure 119.5).

Hemarthrosis

Definition
Hemarthrosis is postoperative intraarticular accumulation of blood causing lameness. It is usually associated with donor site hemorrhage, but in some cases, this complication may be caused by inherent clotting disorders.

Risk factors
- Excessive surgical trauma will cause postoperative hemarthrosis.
- Exposure of excessively deep subchondral bone
- Excessive postoperative exercise
- Clotting disorder

Diagnosis
Hemarthrosis may be suspected on the basis of a suggestive history, physical examination, or imaging studies, but definitive diagnosis usually requires arthrocentesis.

Treatment
Excessive joint distension may justify arthrocentesis to alleviate patient discomfort and prevent ischemic injury to the periarticular tissues. In cases of mild hemarthrosis, compression of the operated joint and strict rest may be sufficient to bring resolution.

Outcome
The outcome of postoperative hemarthrosis is usually favorable, and in the majority of cases resolution, will occur without the requirement for intervention.

Prevention
- Meticulous surgical technique and careful attention to hemostasis
- Backfilling the donor site with collagen hemostatic agents or bone graft obtained from the recipient bed may help prevent ongoing hemorrhage from the donor site.
- Strict postoperative exercise management
- Application of a light compressive bandage for the immediate 24 hours after surgery

Relevant literature
Osteochondritis dissecans affects, in decreasing order of frequency, the shoulder, elbow, tarsus, and stifle. The inherent difficulties in treating osteochondral defects arise from the poor intrinsic healing response of cartilage tissue (Bertrand et al. 1997). Without intervention, osteochondral defects fill with fibrocartilage, which has weaker biomechanical properties than hyaline cartilage (Sharpe et al. 2005). The goal in treating osteochondral defects is to reproduce normal hyaline cartilage within the defect and bring about restoration of the subchondral plate and articular surface topography. Up to 80% of patients will show an improved lameness score after autogenous osteochondral repair of an OCD lesion (Cook et al. 2008; Fitzpatrick et al. 2012). This is despite the difficulties documented with regard

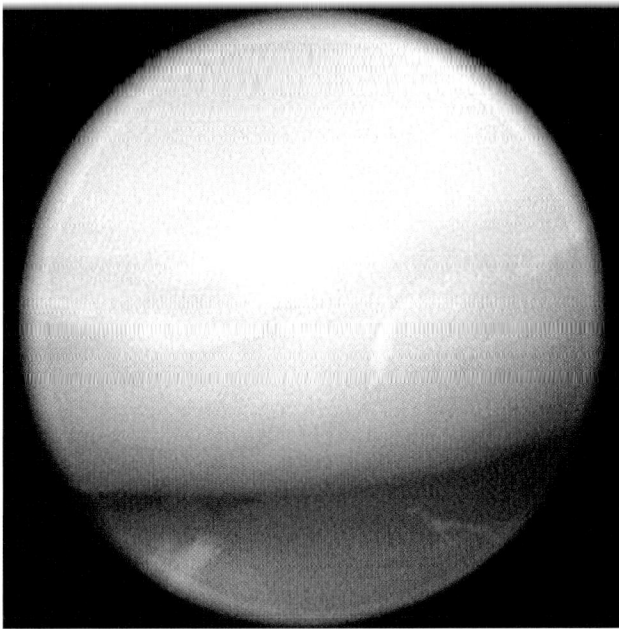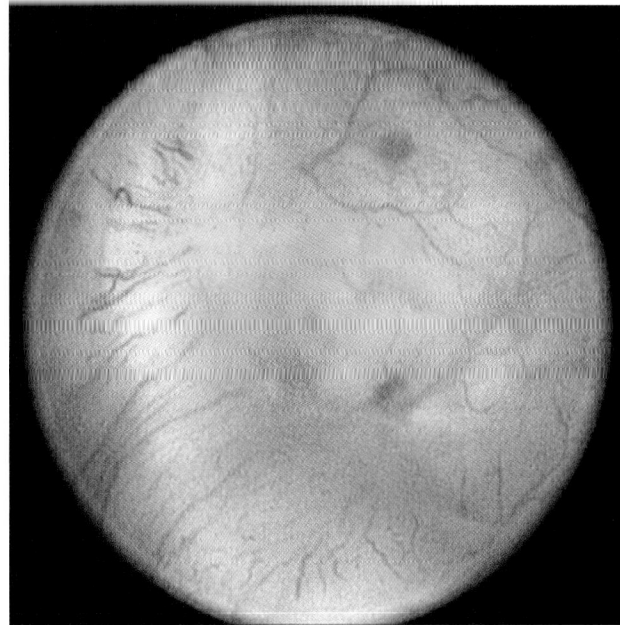

Figure 119.6 Second-look arthroscopy of recipient (Left) and (Right) donor sites after autograft repair of an osteochondritis dissecans defect of the medial femoral condyle. A hyaline cartilage–covered graft is evident in the recipient site and fibrous-tissue infill of the donor site.

to matching donor and recipient sites in respect of topography and morphologic characteristics of the cartilage surface (Böttcher *et al.* 2009, 2010). Second-look arthroscopy and arthrotomy (for unrelated surgical intervention) have confirmed robust graft integration and maintenance of hyaline cartilage on the graft over adjacent areas and on the opposing articular surface (see Figures 119.3, 119.4, and 119.6) (Fitzpatrick *et al.* 2009, 2010, 2012). There does, however, remain a paucity of long-term follow-up supporting the ongoing efficacy of this treatment modality, and there is no documentation in veterinary literature of the long-term fate of these grafts and the joints into which they are placed. Large-scale veterinary longitudinal studies examining complications at both donor and recipient sites are lacking. Long-term donor site complication rates in human surgery are reported at around 3% (Hangody and Fules 2003). Based on histologic examination, donor sites seem to fill with fibrocartilage, and long-term morbidity at the donor site has not been reported thus far in dogs (see Figures 119.4 and 119.6).

Meticulous attention to detail is the keystone to successful osteochondral transplant surgery. If the principles of graft retrieval, handling, and insertion are followed closely, the complication risk is low. As this technique evolves, it will likely move away from the use of autologous graft material and focus on the use of synthetic graft with biomechanical characteristics similar to those of hyaline cartilage (Fitzpatrick *et al.* 2013).

References

Bertrand, S.G., Lewis, D.D., Madison, J.B., et al. (1997) Arthroscopic examination and treatment of osteochondritis dissecans of the femoral condyle of six dogs. *Journal of the American Animal Hospital Association* 33, 451-455.

Böttcher, P., Zeissler, M., Maierl, J., et al. (2009) Mapping of split-line pattern and cartilage thickness of selected donor and recipient sites for autologous osteochondral transplantation in the canine stifle joint. *Veterinary Surgery* 38, 696-704.

Böttcher, P., Zeissler, M., Grevel, V., et al. (2010) Computer simulation of the distal aspect of the femur for assessment of donor core size and surface curvature for autologous osteochondral transplantation in the canine stifle joint. *Veterinary Surgery* 39, 371-379.

Cook, J.L., Hudson, C.C., Kuroki, K. (2008) Autogenous osteochondral grafting for treatment of stifle osteochondrosis in dogs. *Veterinary Surgery* 37, 311-321.

Fitzpatrick, N., Yeadon, R., Smith, T.J. (2009) Early clinical experience with osteochondral autograft transfer for treatment of osteochondritis dissecans of the medial humeral condyle in dogs. *Veterinary Surgery* 38, 246-260.

Fitzpatrick, N., Van Terheijden, C., Yeadon, R., Smith, T.J. (2010) Osteochondral autograft transfer for treatment of osteochondritis dissecans of the caudocentral humeral head in dogs. *Veterinary Surgery* 39, 925-935.

Fitzpatrick, N., Yeadon, Y., Van Terheijden, C., et al. (2012) Osteochondral autograft transfer for the treatment of osteochondritis dissecans of the medial femoral condyle in dogs. *Veterinary and Comparative Orthopaedics and Traumatology* 1, 135-143.

Fitzpatrick, N., Egan, P., Tucker, R., et al. (2013) Evaluation of an osteochondral implant for the treatment of OCD. Abstract presented at the ACVS Veterinary Symposium Surgical Summit, San Antonio, TX, October 25.

Hangody, L., Fules, P. (2003) Autologous osteochondral mosaicplasty for the treatment of full-thickness defects of weight-bearing joints: ten years of experimental and clinical experience. *The Journal of Bone & Joint Surgery* 85 (Suppl. A), 25-32.

Koh, J.L., Wirsing, K., Lautenschlager, E., et al. (2004) The effect of graft height mismatch on contact pressure following osteochondral grafting: a biomechanical study. *The American Journal of Sports Medicine* 32, 317-320.

Sharpe, J.R., Ahmed, S.U., Fleetcroft, J.P., et al. (2005) The treatment of osteochondral lesions using a combination of autologous chondrocyte implantation and autograft. *The Journal of Bone & Joint Surgery* 87, 730-735.

Surgery of the Scapulohumeral Joint

120 Shoulder Dislocation and Instability

Brian Beale

Gulf Coast Veterinary Specialists, Houston, TX, USA

Shoulder pain as a cause of lameness is becoming more frequently diagnosed in dogs. Instability of the shoulder is thought to be a common cause of shoulder pain and lameness (Bardet 1998). Shoulder instability allows abnormal translation of the humeral head relative to the glenoid cavity caused by disruption of the soft tissue supporting structures of the joint (Sidaway et al. 2004). Shoulder instability can range from mild to severe. Mild instability may be associated with mild pain and lameness with little evidence of instability on palpation. Moderate injury may result in palpable instability and subluxation. Severe instability is associated with injury to multiple soft tissue supporting structures of the shoulder, resulting in dislocation. Diagnosis of the condition can be difficult and controversial. It is important to carefully rule out elbow pathology as a cause of forelimb lameness as well because many dogs with shoulder pathology also have elbow disease. Conditions such as fragmented medial coronoid process of the elbow have been mistakenly diagnosed as lameness caused by shoulder pain in up to 20% of cases (Cook et al. 2005b).

Treatment of shoulder instability is equally controversial at the present time. Treatment options include conservative management with antiinflammatory therapy, controlled activity and physical rehabilitation exercises, simple debridement of damaged tissues, joint capsular shrinkage, joint capsular imbrication, ligament reconstruction, and arthrodesis. Surgical treatment can include a traditional arthrotomy or arthroscopy, depending on the surgical technique. Complications are common after treatment of shoulder instability and dislocation and include osteoarthritis (OA), recurrent instability and lameness, fracture, and infection.

Degenerative joint disease

See Chapter 18

Recurrent instability and lameness

Definition

Recurrent instability and dislocation of the shoulder can occur after conservative or surgical treatment. Instability is caused by tearing or stretching of the soft tissue supporting structures of the shoulder, including the:

- Biceps brachii tendon
- Subscapularis tendon

- Medial glenohumeral ligament (MGHL)
- Lateral glenohumeral ligament (LGHL)
- Supraspinatus tendon
- Infraspinatus tendon
- Joint capsule

Instability can occur cranially, medially, caudally, or laterally.

Risk factors

Predisposition factors include:

- Middle age, active, medium to large breed dogs
- Restriction of exercise and immobilization of the shoulder after injury

Diagnosis

Diagnosis of shoulder instability is based on:

- Physical examination:
  ○ Weight-bearing lameness of the forelimb
  ○ Pain localized to the shoulder during palpation
  ○ Measurement of abduction angles: The normal angle of abduction of the shoulder approximates 30 degrees when tested with the limb extended. Mild instability has been considered in dogs with abduction angles of 35 to 45 degrees, angles ranging between 45 and 65 degrees being consistent with moderate instability and angles exceeding 65 degrees suggesting severe instability (Marcellin-Little et al. 2007).
  ○ Assessment of the range of motion (ROM): Normal angles of passive flexion and extension approximate 45 to 60 degrees in dogs (30 degrees in cats) and 165 degrees, respectively (Marcellin-Little et al. 2007).
  ○ Cranial translation (cranial drawer)
- Radiographic examination: evidence of incongruity or luxation, or secondary changes such as degenerative joint disease
- Advanced imaging techniques (magnetic resonance imaging [MRI], computed tomography [CT]): evaluation of the biceps brachii, infraspinatus, supraspinatus, teres minor, and subscapularis muscles
- Arthroscopy is used for definitive diagnosis: synovitis, laxity or tears in the biceps brachii tendon, subscapularis tendon, and lesions of the articular surfaces of the glenoid and humeral head (Figure 120.1)

Although an excessive abduction angle is found with patients with medial shoulder instability, excessive abduction angles can also be seen with other causes of forelimb lameness (e.g., elbow dysplasia,

Complications in Small Animal Surgery, First Edition. Edited by Dominique Griffon and Annick Hamaide.
© 2016 John Wiley & Sons, Inc. Published 2016 by John Wiley & Sons, Inc.
Companion website: www.wiley.com/go/griffon/complications

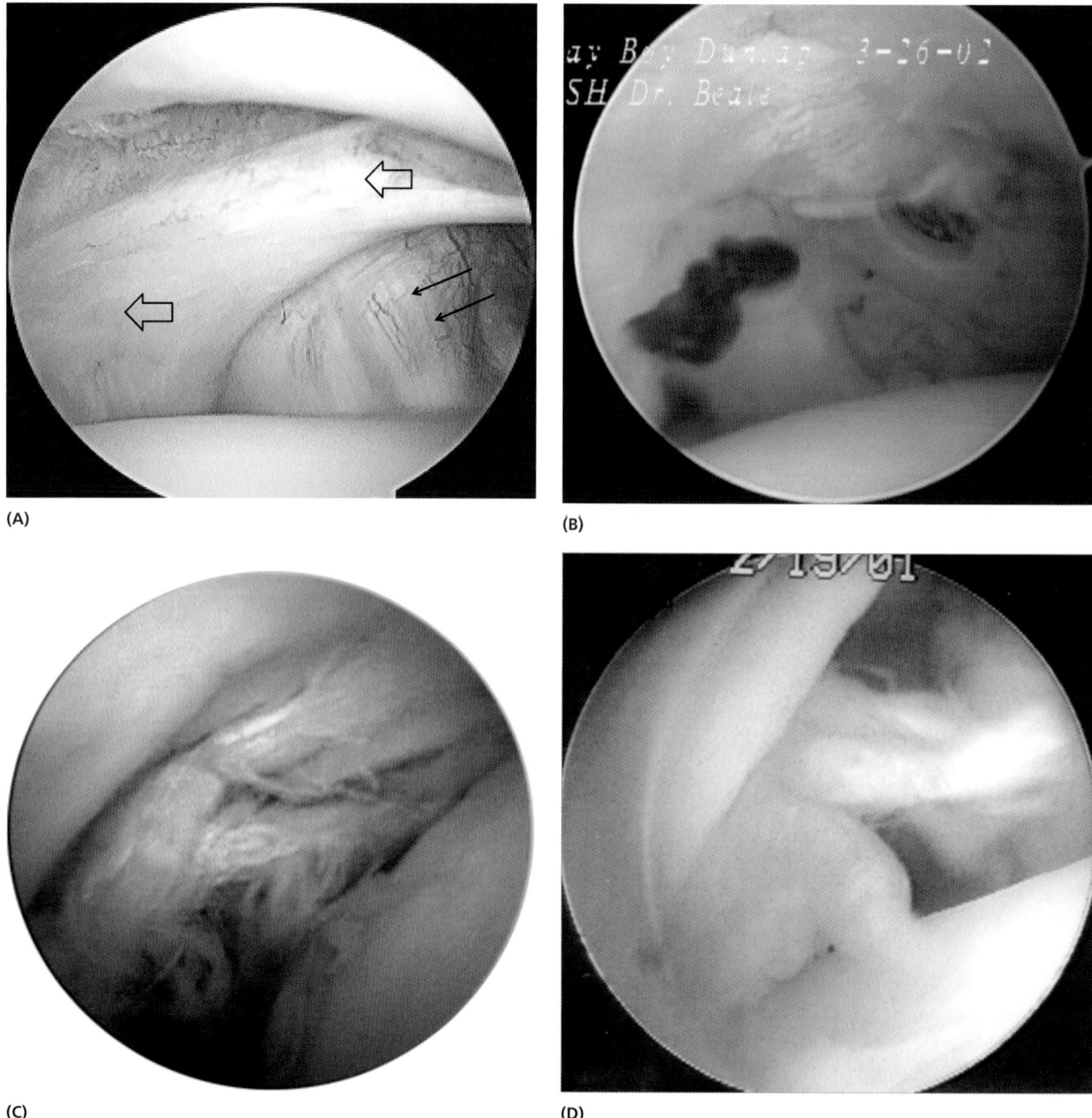

Figure 120.1 Arthroscopic diagnosis of shoulder instability. **A,** Normal appearance of the medial glenohumeral ligament (medial glenohumeral ligament [MGHL], block arrows) and subscapularis tendon (arrows). **B** and **C,** Variation in appearance of MGHL tears. **D,** Tear of the subscapularis tendon.

bone cancer, carpal injury) caused by muscle atrophy and loss of active (dynamic) restraints of the shoulder (Hulse and Beale 2006). It is particularly important to assess the entire forelimb of patients suspected of shoulder instability and to exclude the presence of elbow disease.

Treatment

The decision-making process is complicated because of the difficulty in assessing all of the potential anatomical structures of the shoulder and the lack of evidence-based evaluation of treatment modalities. The current management of shoulder instability remains largely based on the surgeon's opinion and preference.

If shoulder pain is present but minimal signs of translation or instability are evident, conservative treatment of shoulder instability can be considered initially:

- Activity restriction
- Anti-inflammatory and analgesic therapy (nonsteroidal anti-inflammatory drugs, corticosteroids)
- Intra-articular therapy: hyaluronic acid, autologous conditioned plasma, platelet rich plasma, or stem cells
- Shockwave therapy
- Physical therapy and use of a brace or sling that restricts abduction of the shoulder.

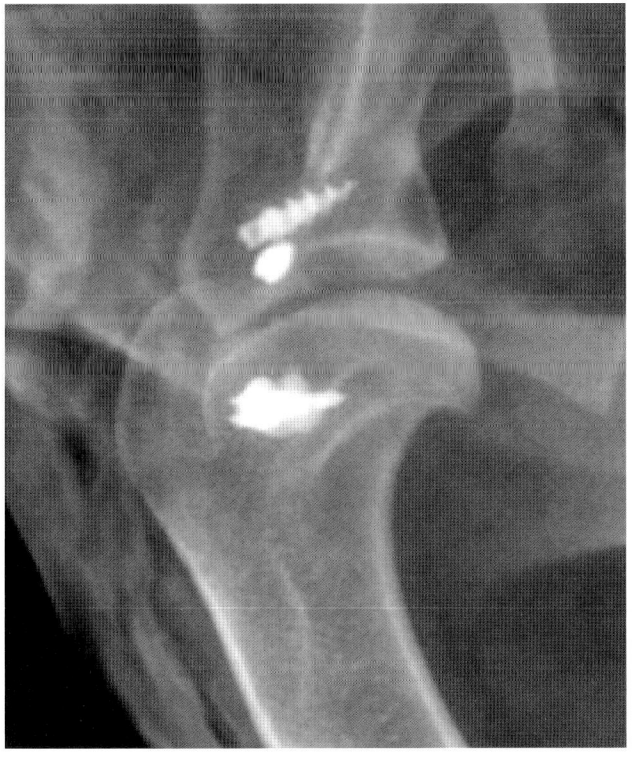 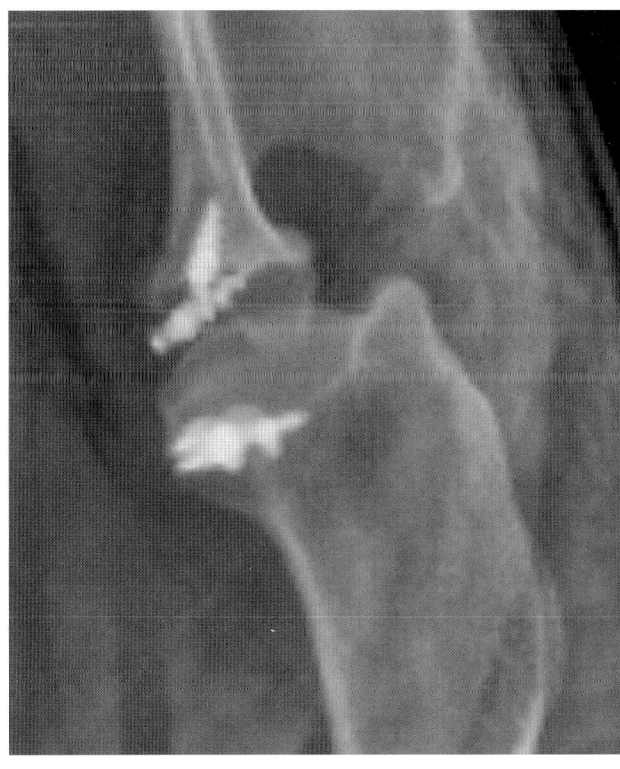

(A) **(B)**

Figure 120.2 Mediolateral (**A**) and craniocaudal (**B**) radiographs obtained after surgical repair of the cranial arm of the medial glenohumeral ligament (MGHL). Tearing of the cranial arm of the MGHL resulted in medial instability. Conservative therapy was unsuccessful. The cranial arm of the MGHL was reconstructed using two Fastak and one Corkscrew suture anchors and two strands of #2 FiberWire (Arthrex Vet Systems, Naples, FL).

Surgical treatment should be considered in:
- Dogs with obvious shoulder instability or dislocation, especially if combined with lesions of the articular cartilage
- Patients that fail to respond to conservative treatment after two to three months should be considered for surgical stabilization.

Surgical treatment may be accomplished via arthrotomy or arthroscopy, and techniques proposed to restore static shoulder stability include:
- Biceps tendon transposition
- Ligament reconstruction (MGHL or LGHL) (Figures 120.2 to 120.4).
- Imbrication of the subscapularis tendon
- Joint capsule imbrication
- Thermal shrinkage of the joint capsule

Reconstruction of the MGHL is typically performed through a craniomedial approach to the shoulder, followed by ligament reconstruction using bone tunnels, suture buttons or suture anchors and heavy braided suture (e.g., FiberWire or FiberTape, Arthrex Vet Systems, Naples, FL; Ethibond, Ethicon, Cincinnati, OH) (Fitch *et al*. 2001; Cook and Schulz 2008) (see Figures 120.2 to 120.4). It is important to reconstruct both arms of the ligament if they are both damaged (Figure 120.5). Most commonly, a small suture anchor or suture buttons are placed at the cranial and caudal aspects of the edge of the medial glenoid rim. The sutures are attached to the medial aspect of the proximal humerus using another suture anchor or suture button. When attaching to an anchor or suture button, the suture is tensioned and tied using four or five knots. A knotless suture anchor (SwiveLock, Arthrex Vet Systems) can also be used to eliminate the bulky knot as a source of infection or tissue irritation. When attaching to a Swivel Lock anchor, the suture is tensioned, but no knot is needed (see Figure 120.5).

After any type of surgical repair of surgical instability, the shoulder should be protected with restricted, controlled activity and a thoracic jacket or bandage. Immobilization of the shoulder has been recommended for six weeks followed by rehabilitation exercise for an additional six weeks (see Prevention) (Cook *et al*. 2005b; Pettitt *et al*. 2008).

Outcome

Good function of the affected shoulder can generally be expected by 12 to 16 weeks after surgery, but full return to function may require 5 to 6 months of rehabilitation. Surgical treatment of shoulder instability with prosthetic repair techniques was recently reported to lead to long-term successful outcome in about 85% of dogs compared with about 65% after nonsurgical management (Franklin *et al*. 2013). Major complications were encountered in 7% of cases.

Prevention

No strategy has been proposed to prevent the natural occurrence of shoulder instability in dogs. However, postoperative care of these patients is crucial to prevent residual or recurrent medial shoulder instability after surgical repair. During that phase, recommendations are designed to immobilize the shoulder until supporting tissues have healed while limiting the impact on muscle mass and

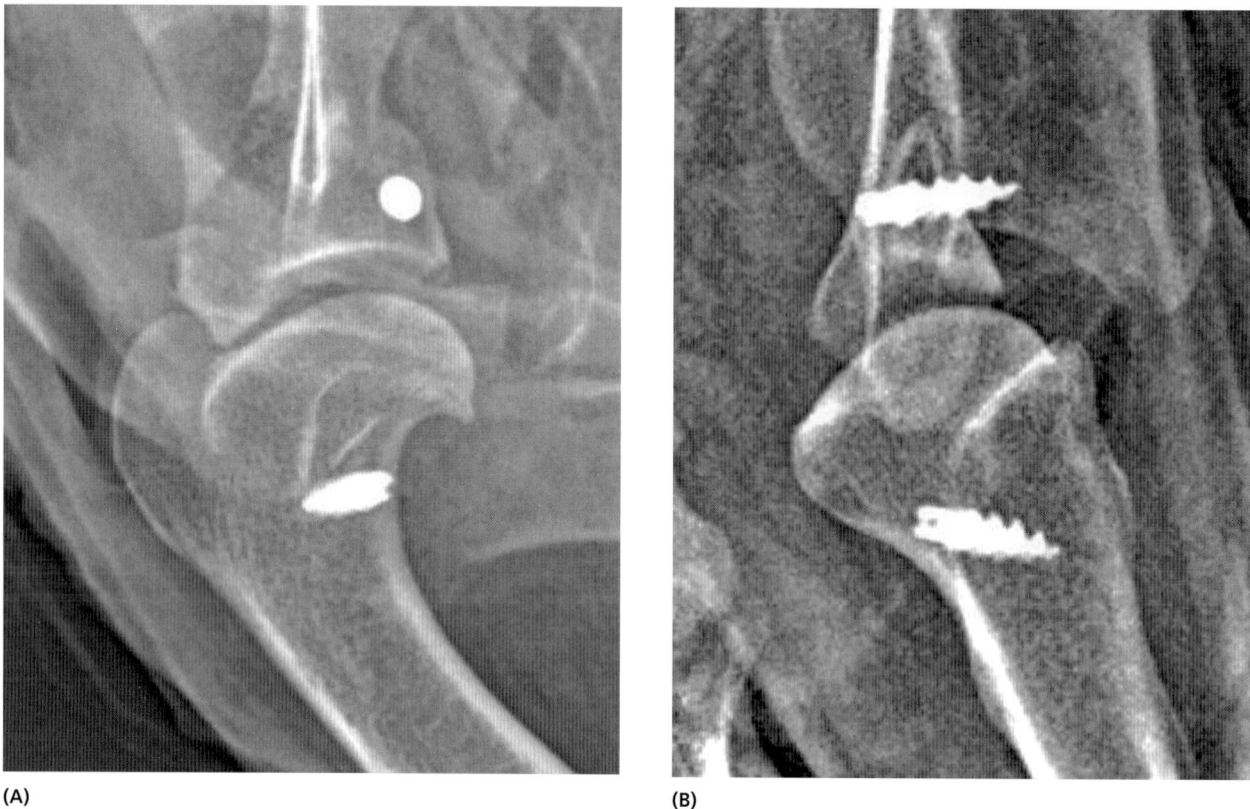

(A)   (B)

Figure 120.3 Mediolateral (**A**) and craniocaudal (**B**) radiographs obtained after surgical repair of the caudal arm of the medial glenohumeral ligament (MGHL). Tearing of the caudal arm of the MGHL resulted in medial instability. Conservative therapy was unsuccessful. The caudal arm of the MGHL was reconstructed using two Fastak suture anchors and one strands of #2 FiberWire (Arthrex Vet Systems, Naples, FL).

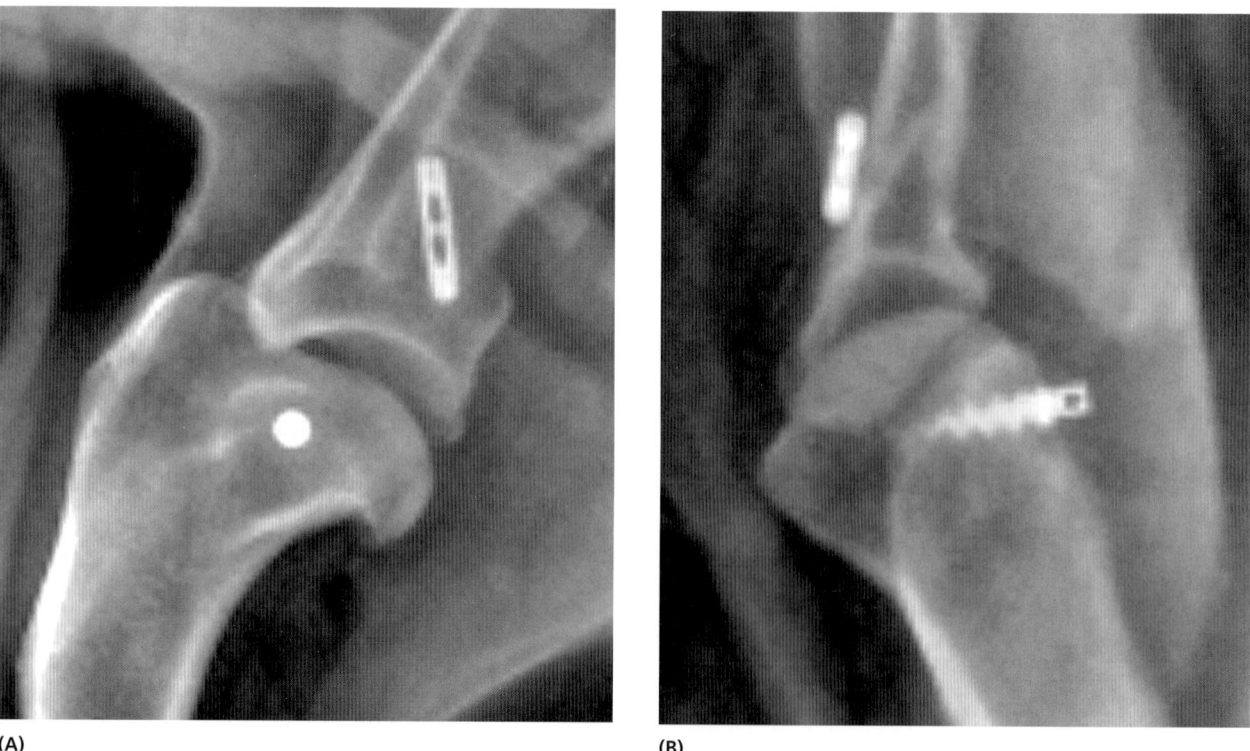

(A)   (B)

Figure 120.4 Mediolateral (**A**) and craniocaudal (**B**) radiographs obtained after surgical repair of the lateral glenohumeral ligament (LGHL). Tearing of the caudal portion of the LGHL resulted in lateral instability. Conservative therapy was unsuccessful. The caudal portion of the LGHL was reconstructed using a suture button and one Fastak suture anchors and one strand of #2 FiberWire using a toggle technique (Arthrex Vet Systems, Naples, FL).

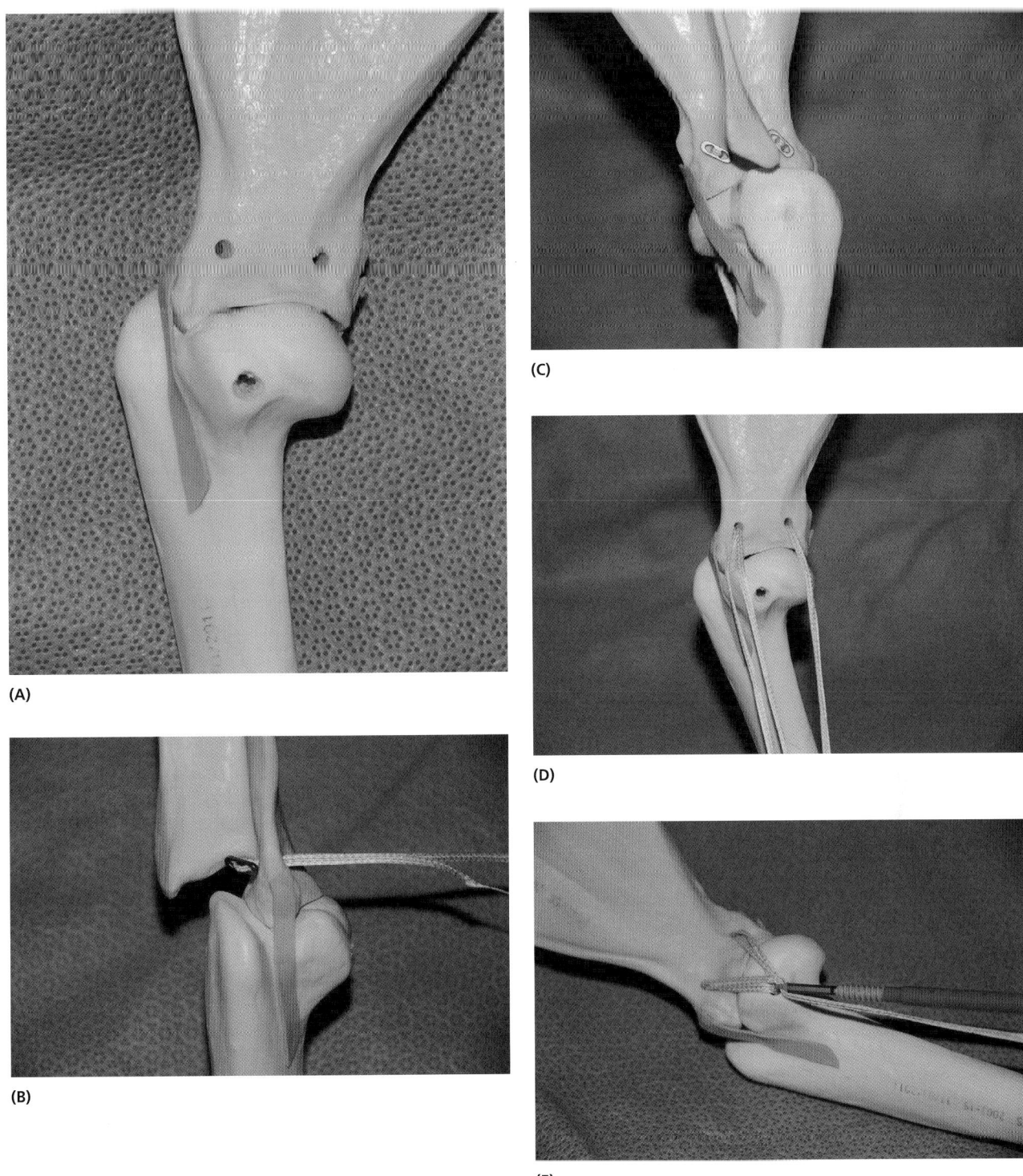

(A)

(B)

(C)

(D)

(E)

Figure 120.5 Reconstruction of the cranial and caudal arms of the medial glenohumeral ligament (MGHL) is recommended if the glenoid cavity and humeral head are normal and the entire MGHL is torn, resulting in substantial medial instability. The MGHL was reconstructed in this plastic bone model using two suture buttons and one knotless Swivel lock suture anchors and two strands of 2-mm FiberTape. (Arthrex Vet Systems, Naples, Florida). **A**, Bone tunnels. **B**, Suture button and FiberTape toggle. **C**, Cranial and caudal suture buttons (lateral scapular surface). **D**, Cranial and caudal arms of prosthetic MGHL (2-mm FiberTape). **E**, Prosthetic ligament attached to the eyelet of the Swivel Lock suture anchor, tensioned and introduced into bone tunnel.   *(Continued)*

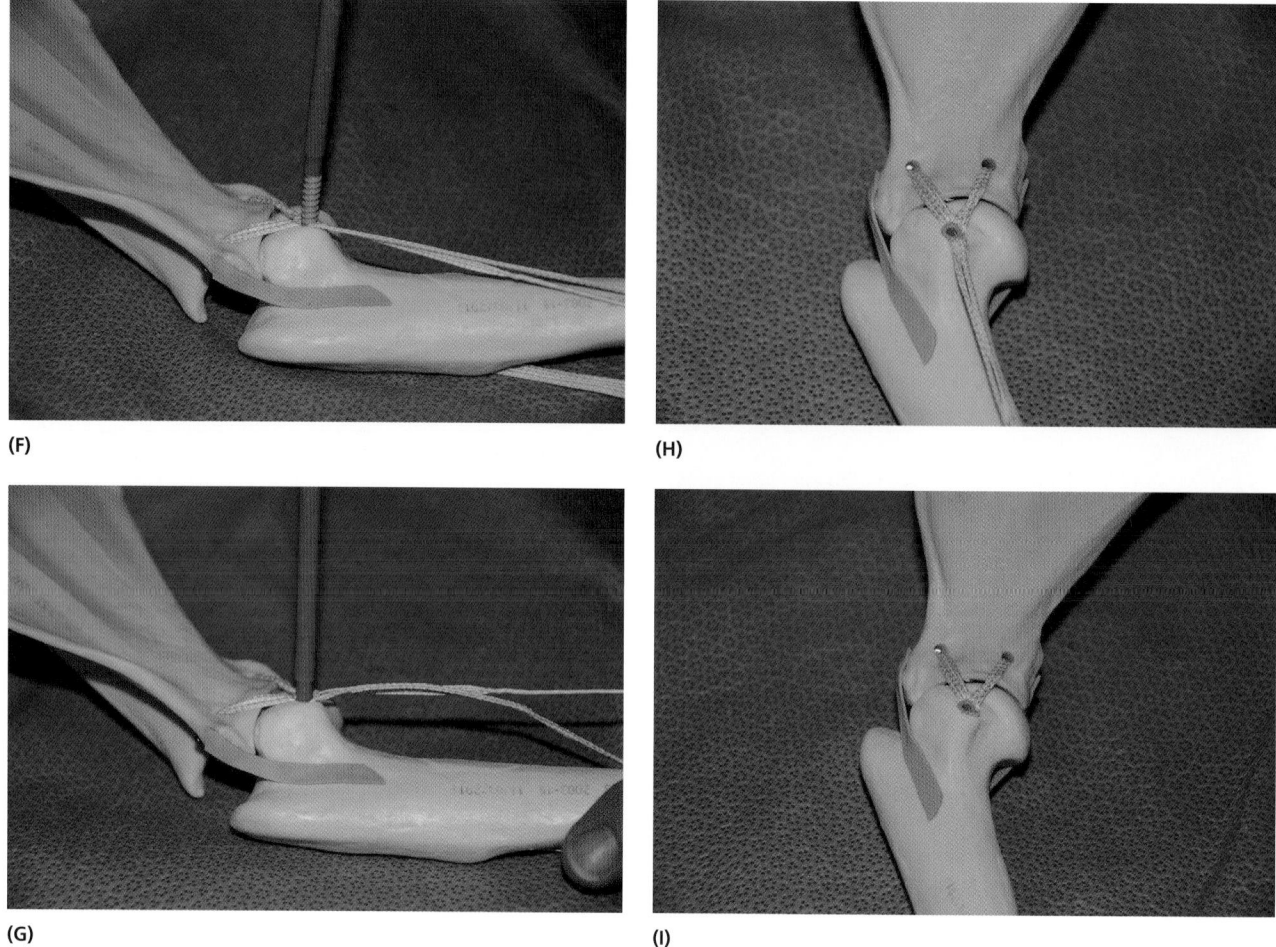

(F)   **(H)**

(G)   **(I)**

Figure 120.5 *(Continued)* **F**, Peek Swivel Lock anchor introduced into the bone tunnel to anchor the suture. **G**, Peek anchor screwed in place until flush with the surface of the humerus. **H**, Inserted tool removed, leaving the swivel lock anchor in place. **I**, The arms of the suture are cut flush, leaving a knotless prosthetic MGHL reconstruction.

ROM. The goals are to provide static stability with surgical correction and to increase dynamic stability during the postoperative period with appropriate limitations of abduction of the shoulder while performing rehabilitation exercises.

An example of rehabilitation program is proposed below:

- Weeks 0 to 2: A non–weight-bearing sling is used in dogs having marked instability. A Velpeau sling is often used, although a spica splint may be considered in more severe cases, with weak repairs. In these cases, manipulations to improve ROM are best delayed until hobbles or a weight-bearing sling is used. Dogs with mild instability treated via radiofrequency may not need a sling and instead may be immobilized directly with tape hobbles or a hobbles brace (e.g., Doggleggs, Reston, VA).
- Weeks 2 to 6: Shoulder hobbles and gradual return to weight bearing with physiotherapy. Although protocols for physiotherapy vary among clinicians, physioballs are often recommended to initiate non–weight-bearing exercises and gentle extension of the shoulder. Weight bearing is introduced by lifting one rear limb ("three-leg standing"), eventually progressing to para (two-leg) standing. Electrical stimulation can be applied to the shoulder muscles for pain management and treatment of atrophy. Around week 4, exercises are added to improve ROM and central core

strength. These exercises may include weave pole walking; handstands; hill walking; wobble board standing; Cavaletti poles; and eventually, the underwater treadmill.

- Weeks 6 to 18: Sport-specific exercises are gradually introduced, such as low-height, straight-line jumping; trotting through the weave poles; commando crawling through obstacles; and short leash runs. As strength, confidence, and evidence of body awareness improve, plyometric or "burst" activities can be initiated. A gradual return to full sport activities is done over the next 6 to 12 weeks. Burst activities should be limited to 3 to 5 minutes three times a day initially and then slowly increase duration and frequency over a 4-week period. A return to normal activity can be initiated after this period if clinical use of the affected limb is good.

Implant failure

Definition

Loss of stability associated with the orthopedic implant can result in recurrent pain and instability. The most common type of implant failure is suture breakage. Other modes of failure include suture anchor pullout.

Risk factors

Suture material used to reconstruct torn soft tissue structures of the shoulder must remain competent for a minimum of two to three months to provide long-lasting stability. The suture is expected to provide stability until healing occurs by fibrosis and repair of supporting soft tissues. The inherent instability of the shoulder poses a risk of implant failure because of the potential large loads placed on the implant.

Diagnosis

The diagnosis of a failed implant is made by orthopedic and radiographic examination. Failure of the implant by breakage is diagnosed by palpation of recurrent instability. Failure by suture anchor pull-out is diagnosed by palpation of recurrent instability and radiographic evidence of anchor migration.

Treatment

Treatment of implant failure can vary depending on the amount of instability and dysfunction present and the time after surgery.
- Mild instability or pain may be treated initially by conservative means as described earlier.
- Severe instability or obvious pain or lameness may require surgical revision. Surgical reconstruction of the damaged structures may be attempted again as described earlier. The surgeon should consider using a more robust implant or stabilization technique and use of postoperative immobilization of the shoulder (DogLeggs brace, sling or thoracic jacket) to protect the repair.

- Recurrent painful instability, concomitant damage to the glenoid, or extensive OA. Shoulder arthrodesis should be considered (Figures 120.6 and 120.7).

Outcome

Dogs and cats are expected to have a very good outcome after revision surgery if shoulder stability can be restored. Long-term stability is achieved only if the surgical repair remains intact for three months after surgery. Restricted activity and protection of the repair by limiting excessive motion of the joint (particularly abduction) during the rehabilitation period are paramount to success. Surgical revision using primary repair techniques may be difficult if excessive damage to the bone or regional soft tissues has occurred. Dogs and cats can have a favorable outcome with very good function after shoulder arthrodesis if primary repair is not practical (Beale 2012; Fitzpatrick *et al.* 2012).

Prevention

Strategies to prevent implant failure after prosthetic repair of shoulder instability include:
- Ensure proper positioning of anchors within bone. The most common cause of implant failure is suture breakage at the eyelet of the anchor or edge of the bone tunnel.
- Bone tunnels should be drilled in the direction of the pull of the suture.

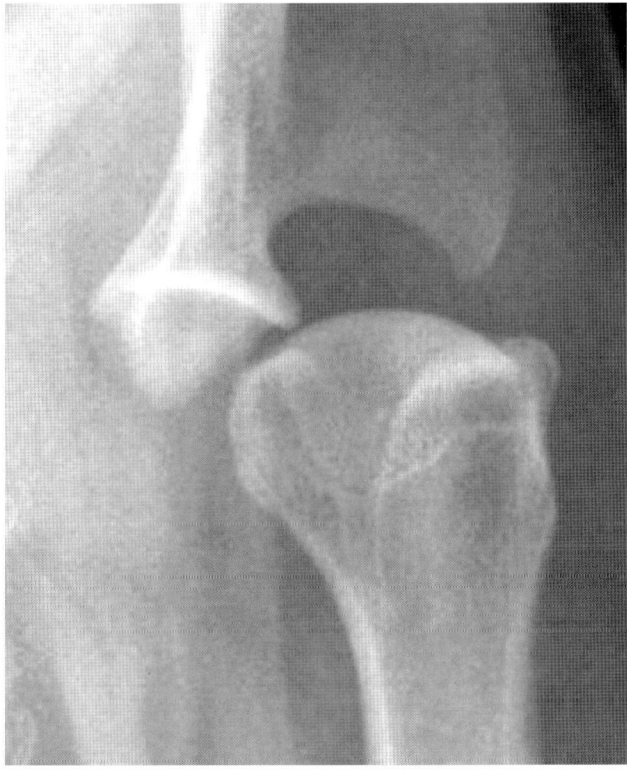

(A)

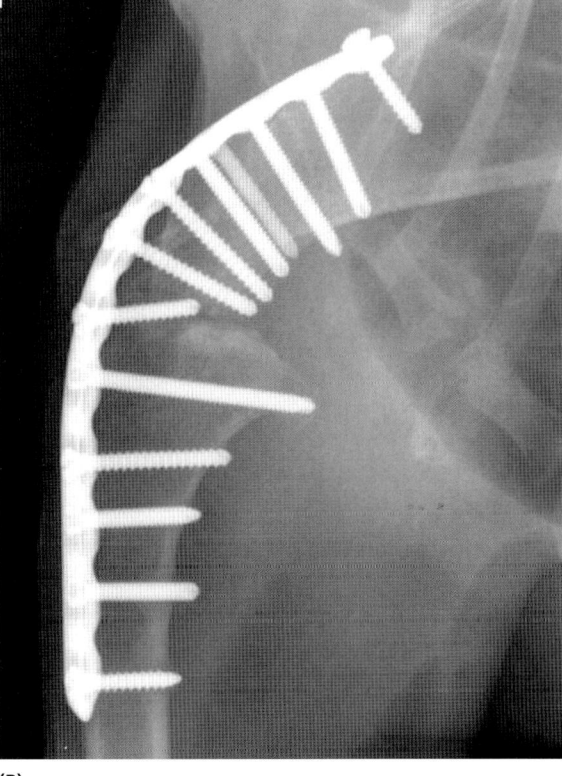

(B)

Figure 120.6 Preoperative (**A**) and postoperative (**B**) radiographs of a dog with a dislocation of the shoulder. This condition causes severe instability and substantial damage to the soft tissues supporting the shoulder. Ligament reconstruction has an increased chance of failure; therefore, shoulder arthrodesis can be used as a primary repair technique with a very good outcome.

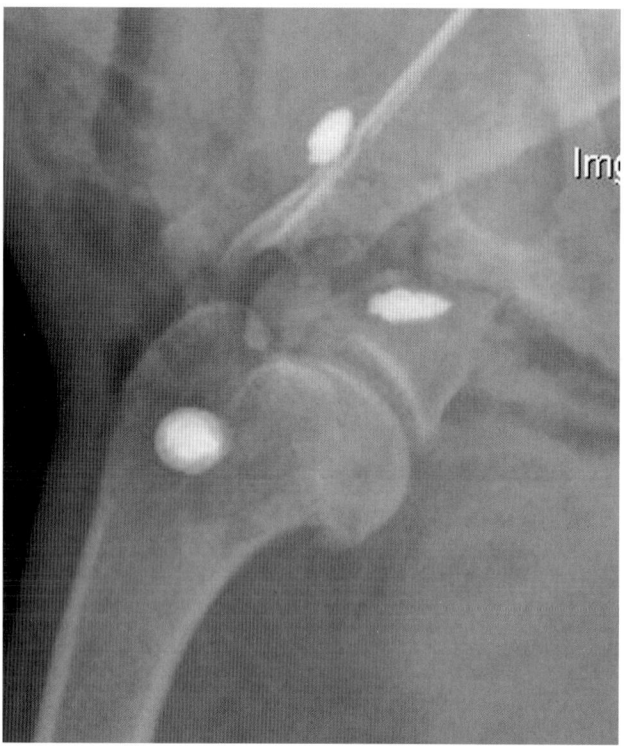

(A)

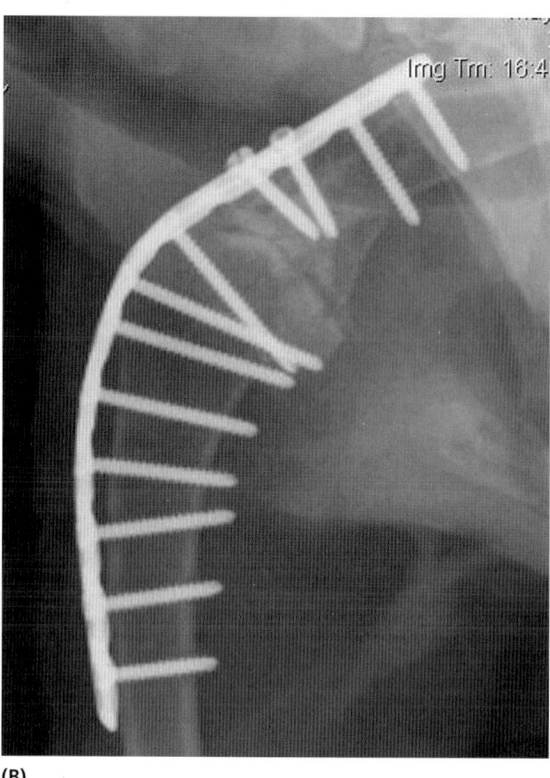

(B)

Figure 120.7 Failure of a surgical reconstruction of the medial glenohumeral ligament (MGHL). **A**, Fracture and suture anchor pull-out occurred in this patient after reconstruction of both arms of the MGHL ligament. **B**, The dog was treated with a shoulder arthrodesis, resulting in an excellent outcome.

- Any sharp edges of the bone tunnels should be smoothed using a countersink tool or curette.
- Suture anchors should be buried below the surface of the bone if possible to decrease stress on the suture material
- The largest practical diameter of suture material should be used when reconstructing the medial glenohumeral ligament because of the large forces placed on the shoulder. Adjust the suture size to the patient size. Toy breed dogs and cats are typically stabilized using #2 suture material, medium-sized dogs are stabilized using #5 suture, and large breed dogs are stabilized using multiple strands of #5 suture or heavier weaved materials (e.g., FiberTape, Arthrex Vet Systems).
- Postoperative immobilization and rehabilitation of the affected limb are crucial (see Prevention in the previous section).
- A locking plate and screw system should be used if performing shoulder arthrodesis because of the high chance of screw pull-out in the thin bone of the scapula when using traditional plating systems (Beale 2012) (see Figure 120.6).

Fracture

Definition

Fracture rarely occurs after reconstruction of the ligaments or tendons of the shoulder. Fractures typically occur through the holes drilled into the bone to anchor the prosthetic ligament (Figure 120.7). Fractures may involve the greater tubercle of the humerus or the scapular neck.

Risk factors

The drilling of holes in bone weakens the integrity of the bone until healing occurs. Several factors increase the risk of fracture after prosthetic treatment of shoulder instability in dogs:
- Fractures more commonly involve the scapula than the humerus.
- Holes positioned proximally, close to the neck of the scapula rather than along the glenoid.
- Multiple holes caused by failed attempts at creating bone tunnels or placement of multiple sutures (multidirectional instability, repair of both arms of the MGHL).
- The diameter of the hole drilled is proportional to the loss of strength of the bone; the hole diameter should be as small as possible to allow placement of the suture material, suture button, or anchor.
- The risk of fracture is greatest 4 to 6 weeks after surgery.

Diagnosis

The diagnosis of fractures of the shoulder is typically made with radiographic examination (see Figure 120.7). Occasionally, CT is used to evaluate the potential involvement of the fracture into the articular surface of the joint.

Treatment

Shoulder fractures are treated based on previously described methods, adhering to the (AO) principles of fracture repair (Cabassu 2005).
- Fractures of the greater tubercle: Consider use of lag screws and Kirschner wires.
- Fractures of the scapular neck: Consider the use of L-plates.

- Fractures of the glenoid: Consider use of lag screws and plates as needed.
- Revision of the prosthetic repair may partially rely on implants (screws and washers) used to treat the fracture.
- Postoperatively, these cases are placed in a spica splint for two to four weeks before rehabilitation depending on the severity of the fracture and stability of the repair. Activity should be restricted to leash walk until radiographic bone healing is achieved.
- Alternatively, scapular fractures involving the glenoid can also be treated using shoulder arthrodesis with an excellent outcome (Beale 2012). Shoulder arthrodesis may be the best option in a patient with concurrent shoulder instability and glenoid fracture (see Figure 120.7).

Outcome

The prognosis is very good after repair and healing of scapular neck fractures and greater tubercle fractures. One exception is if suprascapular nerve damage occurs as a result of the fracture or iatrogenic damage during surgical repair. Injury to this nerve can result in atrophy and weakening of the shoulder muscles and long-term lameness. Fractures of the glenoid are also expected to have a good prognosis as long as anatomic reduction and rigid stabilization are achieved. Comminuted or poorly reduced glenoid fractures have an increased likelihood of OA and chronic pain. The prognosis after shoulder arthrodesis is excellent if the surgical technique is good and proper postoperative care is given.

Prevention

Fractures after prosthetic repair of shoulder instability may be prevented if:
- The diameter of screw or suture anchor hole is selected appropriately based on the size of the bones: The hole diameter should be as small as possible to allow placement of the suture material, suture button, or anchor. In general, the hole diameter should be no greater than 25% of the width of the bone.
- Limit the number of holes. Consider the use of a small wire as a guide before creating tunnels.
- Position holes in the greater tubercle to allow enough bone stock, especially proximally and cranially.
- Position holes in the scapula close to the joint surface to optimize stabilization and avoid interfering with the neck of the scapula.
- Enforce exercise restriction (see Prevention in the first section of this chapter) to minimize the biomechanical loads applied on the repair.

Infection

This section focuses on aspects specific to shoulder luxation repair. Additional information about surgical infection is available in Chapters 5 and 6.

Definition

Infection can occur after any type of surgery of the shoulder. Infection is typically associated with pain, lameness, and occasionally draining tracts. Infection may be occult or latent.

Risk factors

The chance of infection increases as the surgical time increases and if implants are used in the repair. Surgical times should be minimized to lower the chance of infection. Surgery should be delayed if the skin appears infected. Typically, shoulder surgery is elective and can wait for 1 to 3 weeks until antibiotic therapy clears the skin infection. Surgical implants can act as a nidus for infection. Commonly used implants include suture material, prosthetic ligaments, suture anchors, suture buttons, bone plates, screws, and washers. Braided suture material has a higher risk of infection than monofilament suture. Metallic implants are most commonly made of stainless steel or titanium. Titanium is thought to be slightly more resistant to infection than stainless steel. Bacteria have the ability to survive in the body long term by formation of a biofilm on the surface of the implant (Donlan 2001). The biofilm protects the bacteria from attempts by the immune system and antibiotics to completely eliminate the bacteria. Surgeons should prevent contact of the implant with the skin during the surgical procedure using appropriate draping protocol.

Diagnosis

Infection is diagnosed by physical examination, radiographic examination, and appropriate laboratory tests. Palpation may reveal pain, swelling, or purulent drainage. Pyrexia may or may not be present. Radiographic evidence of increased radiolucency at the sites of attachment of the suture or suture anchor may indicate infection. Periosteal proliferation of bone, particularly of a rough character, is suggestive of infection. The complete blood count may reflect an increased neutrophil count in some patients. Culture of draining fluid and the implant should be performed to determine the type of bacteria and sensitivity to antibiotic therapy.

Treatment

Treatment can be attempted initially with antibiotic therapy based on culture and sensitivity. Chronic or recurrent infection is best treated by implant removal, debridement of damaged tissues, copious lavage, and appropriate antibiotic therapy (Budsberg 2005). If a revision surgery is needed to restore stability to the shoulder after implant removal, the surgery should be performed a minimum of one month following resolution of the infection. Delaying the revision for a longer period of time is advisable if possible to lessen the chance of recurrent infection. Shoulder arthrodesis is a very good surgical option if recurrent instability occurs after removal of infected implants. Shoulder arthrodesis should be performed using a locking plate and screw system after complete resolution of the infection (Beale 2012; Fitzpatrick et al. 2012).

Outcome

Most infections resolve with no long-term consequences if treated appropriately. The most common causes of chronic infection and pain are inappropriate antibiotic selection, lack of debridement of necrotic bone, and presence of foreign material (metallic or plastic implants or braided suture material). One study found that only 3% of infections resolved completely after antibiotic therapy if surgical implants were left at the surgical site (Savicky et al. 2013). Resolution of infection generally occurs within two weeks if necrotic bone and foreign material are removed and appropriate antibiotics are administered based on culture and sensitivity results.

Prevention

The infection rate is low if proper aseptic technique is used. Surgery should be delayed until pyoderma is resolved. The surgical site should be appropriately disinfected and draped. An adherent drape (e.g., Ioban drape; 3M, St. Paul, MN) and use of a scrub solution that has residual antiseptic activity (e.g., DuraRrep, 3M) are recommended. All implant material (metal, plastic, suture) should be prevented from contacting the skin to reduce the chance of accidental contamination. Exposure of the implant to bacteria can lead to colonization and biofilm production, increasing the likelihood of clinical infection. Prophylactic antibiotics are recommended intraoperatively and postoperatively for 7 to 14 days if surgical time exceeds 90 minutes or if braided suture material (e.g., FiberWire) is used.

Relevant literature

The joint capsule, tendons, and ligaments surrounding the shoulder provide the majority of support to the shoulder. Unlike the hip joint, the shoulder has a very shallow socket (glenoid fossa) that provides minimal resistance to instability and dislocation (Sidaway et al. 2004). Dogs place approximately 60% to 65% of their weight on the front limbs, resulting in weight-bearing loads that constantly challenge the integrity of the ligaments and tendons supporting the shoulder (Molsa et al. 2010). In addition, activity restriction and restraint of the shoulder after injury can be difficult to accomplish for extended periods of time because of the local anatomy as well as the morbidity associated with immobilization. Medial instability is the most commonly recognized form of shoulder instability in dogs (Cook et al. 2005a; Cook and Cook 2009). However, in a recent study of 130 dogs with shoulder instability, 23% of cases were diagnosed with lateral or multidirectional instability (Franklin et al. 2013).

The gait of a dog with shoulder instability is usually abnormal at the walk and the trot. Most patients have an obvious weight-bearing lameness with a prominent head bob on the affected limb. The first step in diagnosing shoulder instability consists of localizing pain to the shoulder joint. For that purpose, the shoulder should be isolated and evaluated independent of the elbow. The shoulder should be assessed for pain and instability in the conscious patient. The shoulder is assessed as it is manipulated in flexion, extension, abduction, adduction, internal rotation, and external rotation. It should be noted that ROM varies slightly among breeds. For example, German shepherds have less extension and more flexion of the shoulder than Labrador retrievers (Marcellin-Little et al. 2007). Cranial instability of the shoulder may be evident using a cranial drawer test similar to that used for the stifle. Abduction angles can be measured and used as a tool for diagnosis on medial shoulder instability (Cook et al. 2005a). Abduction angles greater than 50 degrees have been suggested as pathologic and indicative of medial shoulder instability (Cook et al. 2005a). Although an excessive abduction angle is found with patients with medial shoulder instability, excessive abduction angles can also be seen with other causes of forelimb lameness (e.g., elbow dysplasia, bone cancer, carpal injury) caused by muscle atrophy and loss of active (dynamic) restraints of the shoulder (Hulse and Beale 2006). Instability with dislocation is usually very noticeable and is associated with abnormal angulation of the limb. Diagnostic imaging is useful in assessment of the active restraints of the shoulder. MRI can be used to evaluate the biceps brachii, infraspinatus, supraspinatus, teres minor, and subscapularis muscles (Shaefer and Forrest 2006). Arthroscopy is used to evaluate the static stabilizers of the shoulder, including the medial glenohumeral ligament, lateral glenohumeral ligament, and joint capsule (Beale et al. 2003). Arthroscopy is also useful in assessing the biceps brachii tendon, subscapularis tendon, and articular surfaces of the glenoid and humeral head (Beale et al. 2003). Pathologic changes include mineralization, tendonitis, fibrosis and contracture, partial or complete tears of ligament or tendons, joint capsular stretching, cartilage erosion,

or fragmentation. Many patients have multiple pathologic changes, complicating the decision-making process.

In the absence of objective evidence, treatment remains largely based on individual experience and preference. Some surgeons elect to treat dogs diagnosed with shoulder instability surgically, but others prefer a more conservative approach (Butterworth et al. 2003). Both groups report anecdotal success, and at the present time, there are no criteria to unequivocally differentiate between the need for surgical and nonsurgical management. At the current time, it would be reasonable to use a surgical stabilization technique in dogs having obvious shoulder instability, especially if articular cartilage wear is seen, supporting the theory that abnormal translation of the humeral head is occurring. If shoulder pain is present but minimal signs of translation or instability are evident, conservative treatment of shoulder instability can be considered initially. Thermal shrinkage of the joint capsule was previously recommended as a means of stabilizing the shoulder (O'Neill and Innes 2004; Cook et al. 2005b), but this technique may be useful in patients with very mild instability only.

In a recent multicenter cohort study of dogs with medial shoulder instability treated via prosthetic repairs (no tendon transposition), minor complications were reported in 6% of cases, and major complications occurred in 7% (Franklin et al. 2013). Minor complications included transient pain, incisional complications, and sling-associated dermatitis. Major complications included loss of stability, infection, and sling-associated flexion contracture. Dogs with medial shoulder instability are three times more likely to have a successful outcome with surgical reconstruction compared with conservative therapy (Franklin et al. 2013). In the same study, dogs with multidirectional instability were five times more likely to have a good outcome if they were treated surgically rather than medically. Good results have been reported after stabilization of the MGHL via ligament reconstruction (Fitch et al. 2001), imbrication of the subscapularis tendon (Pettitt et al. 2007), or imbrication of the MGHL and medial joint capsule (Devitt 2006). Good results were recently reported in two dogs with tears of the lateral glenohumeral ligament treated by joint capsule imbrication using a suture anchor technique (Pettitt and Innes 2008).

References

Bardet, J.F. (1998) Diagnosis of shoulder instability in dogs and cats; a retrospective study. *Journal of the American Animal Hospital Association* 34, 42–54.

Beale, B.S. (2012) Shoulder arthrodesis using locking plates. *Proceedings of the 16th ESVOT Congress*, Bologna, Italy, pp. 51–53.

Beale, B.S., Hulse, D.A., Schulz, K.S., et al. (2003) Arthroscopically assisted surgery of the shoulder joint. In Beale, B.S., Hulse, D.A., Schulz, K.S., Whitney, W.O. (eds.) *Small Animal Arthroscopy*. Saunders, St. Louis, pp. 23–49.

Budsberg, S. (2005) Osteomyelitis. In Johnson, A.L., Houlton, J.E.F., Vannini, R. (eds.) *AO Principles of Fracture Management in the Dog and Cat*. AO Publishing, Davos, Switzerland, pp. 416–423.

Buttersworth, S.J. (2003) The use of intra-articular methylprednisolone in the management of shoulder lameness in the dog. *Proceedings of the 46th Annual BSAVA Congress*, Birmingham, UK, April 3 to 6, p. 598.

Cabassu, J.P. (2005) Fractures of the scapula. In Johnson, A.L., Houlton, J.E.F., Vannini, R. (eds.) *AO Principles of Fracture Management in the Dog and Cat*. AO Publishing, Davos, Switzerland, pp. 151–158.

Cook, J.L., Cook, C.R. (2009) Bilateral shoulder and elbow arthroscopy in dogs with forelimb lameness: diagnostic findings and treatment outcomes. *Veterinary Surgery* 38, 224–232.

Cook, J.L., Renfro, D.C., Tomlinson, J.L., et al. (2005a) Measurement of angles of abduction for diagnosis of shoulder instability in dogs using goniometry and digital image analysis. *Veterinary Surgery* 34, 463–468.

Cook, C.L., Schulz, K.S. (2008) TightRope canine shoulder stabilization technique guide, in Arthrex Systems, Naples, FL.

Cook, J.L., Tomlinson, J.L., Fox, D.B., et al. (2005b) Treatment of dogs diagnosed with medial shoulder instability using radiofrequency-induced thermal capsulorrhaphy. *Veterinary Surgery* 34, 469-475.

Devitt, C.M. (2006) Suture anchor techniques for medial shoulder imbrication. *Proceedings of the Advanced Arthroscopy Course, Naples, Italy, August 24 to 26.*

Donlan, R.M. (2001) Biofilm formation. A clinically relevant microbiological process. *Clinical Infectious Diseases* 33, 1387-1392.

Fitch, R.B., Breshears, L., Staats, A., et al. (2001) Clinical evaluation of a prosthetic medial glenohumeral ligament repair in the dog (ten cases). *Veterinary and Comparative Orthopaedics and Traumatology* 14, 222-228.

Fitzpatrick, N., Yeadon, R., Smith, T., et al. (2012) Shoulder arthrodesis in 14 dogs. *Veterinary Surgery* 41, 745-754.

Franklin, S.P., Devitt, C.M., Ogawa, J., et al. (2013) Outcomes associated with treatments for medial, lateral and multidirectional shoulder instability in dogs. *Veterinary Surgery* 42, 361-364.

Hulse, D.A., Beale, B.S. (2006) Shoulder laxity associated with chronic forelimb lameness in the dog. *Proceedings of the Advanced Arthroscopy Course, Naples, Italy, August 24 to 26.*

Marcellin-Little, D.J., Levine, D., Canapp, S.O. (2007) The canine shoulder: selected disorders and their management with physical therapy. *Clinical Techniques in Small Animal Practice* 22, 171-182.

Molsa, S.H., Hielm Bjorkman, A.K., Laitinen-Vapaavuori, O.M. (2010) Force platform analysis in clinically healthy Rottweilers; comparison with Labrador retrievers. *Veterinary Surgery* 39, 701-707.

O'Neill, T., Innes, J.F. (2004) Treatment of shoulder instability caused by medial glenohumeral ligament rupture with thermal capsulorrhaphy. *Journal of Small Animal Practice* 45, 25-28.

Pettitt, R.A., Innes, J.F. (2008) Arthroscopic management of a lateral glenohumeral ligament rupture in two dogs. *Veterinary and Comparative Orthopaedics and Traumatology* 21 (3), 302-306.

Pettitt, R.A., Clements, D.N., Guilliard, M.J. (2007) Stabilisation of medial shoulder instability by imbrication of the subscapularis muscle tendon of insertion. *Journal of Small Animal Practice* 48 (11), 626-31.

Savicky, R., Beale, B., Murtaugh, R., et al. (2013) Outcome following removal of TPLO implants with surgical site infection. *Veterinary and Comparative Orthopaedics and Traumatology* 26 (4), 260-265.

Shaefer, S.L., Forrest, L.J. (2006) Magnetic resonance imaging of the canine shoulder: an anatomic study. *Veterinary Surgery* 35 (8), 721-728.

Sidaway, K., McLaughlin, R.M., Elder, S.H., et al. (2004) Role of the tendons of the biceps brachii and infraspinatus muscles and the medial glenohumeral ligament in the maintenance of passive shoulder joint stability in dogs. *American Journal of Veterinary Research* 65, 1216-1222.

Surgery of the Elbow

121 Reduction of Elbow Luxations

Peter Böttcher

Diplomate ECVS, European Veterinary Specialist in Surgery, Department of Small Animal Medicine, University of Leipzig, Leipzig, Germany

Elbow luxation

Luxation of the cubital joint in dogs and cats is a relatively rare condition and occurs most often after a traumatic event, such as a car accident (Mitchell 2011; Meyer-Lindenberg *et al.* 1991; O'Brien *et al.* 1992). In dogs and cats, the antebrachium luxates almost exclusively laterally (Meyer-Lindenberg *et al.* 1991; O'Brien *et al.* 1992; Savoldelli *et al.* 1996; Mitchell 2011). Caudal luxations predominate in rabbits because of the very deep central ridge between the humeral trochlea and the humeral capitulum (Ertelt *et al.* 2010). Depending on the direction of the luxation and the degree of dislocation, rupture or avulsion (or both) of one or both collateral ligaments is present. In case of severe instability, the origins of the flexor or extensor muscles may also be ruptured or avulsed from the humeral condyle (Griffon 2012). Joint stability must be evaluated when the joint has been reduced to decide whether surgical repair is indicated. The integrity of collateral ligaments should be tested with the Campbell's test (Campbell 1971), which evaluates the degree of supination and pronation while the elbow is flexed to 90 degrees (Figure 121.1) (Farrell *et al.* 2007).

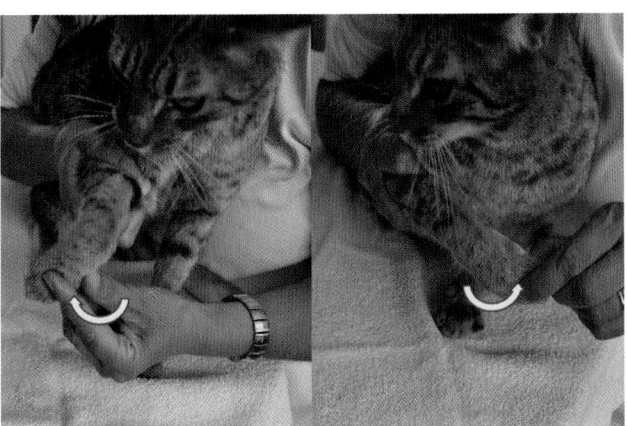

(A)   **(B)**

Figure 121.1 Campbell's test. When the elbow and carpus are held at 90 degrees of flexion, the medial and lateral collateral ligaments are responsible for the rotational stability of the elbow. Their integrity is therefore tested in that position. When these ligaments are intact, the paw can be rotated anywhere from 17 to 50 degrees laterally (**A**, supination) and 31 to 70 degrees medially (**B**, pronation). *Source:* D. Griffon, Western University of Health Sciences, Pomona, CA, 2014. Reproduced with permission from D. Griffon.

A luxated elbow may be reduced by closed reduction, which bears a more favorable prognosis than after an open reduction (Meyer-Lindenberg *et al.* 1991; Schaefer *et al.* 1999; Mitchell 2011). Chronic luxations and joints with instability severe enough to require surgical stabilization warrant open reduction.

Congenital elbow luxation is an uncommon anomaly and typically presents as a non–weight-bearing lameness when a puppy is a few weeks old. Three types of congenital luxation are recognized: humeroradial (type I), humeroulnar (type II), and combined humeroradial and humeroulnar (type III). Reduction is performed either in an open or closed fashion. Because of the inherent character of misalignment in the congenitally luxated elbow, additional procedures, such as transarticular pinning (Withrow 1977; Rahal *et al.* 2000) or external fixator (Milton *et al.* 1979), are generally indicated to maintain reduction. Reduction should be attempted as early as possible because animals older than 4 to 5 months of age require more invasive open reduction and stabilization techniques (Griffon 2012). The goal of surgical repair of congenital elbow luxation is to allow normal function of the affected limb but not full joint reconstruction (Rahal *et al.* 2000). When managed early in the course of the disease, acceptable limb function can be achieved (Rahal *et al.* 2000; Clark *et al.* 2010).

Degenerative joint disease

See Chapter 18.

Septic arthritis

See Chapter 6.

Recurrence

Definition

This is reluxation of the joint after either closed or open reduction. The incidence is relatively low (2%–12%) for traumatic luxations (Meyer-Lindenberg *et al.* 1991; O'Brien *et al.* 1992; Schaefer *et al.* 1999; Mitchell 2011) and high (38%) for congenital humeroulnar luxation (Rahal *et al.* 2000).

Complications in Small Animal Surgery, First Edition. Edited by Dominique Griffon and Annick Hamaide.
© 2016 John Wiley & Sons, Inc. Published 2016 by John Wiley & Sons, Inc.
Companion website: www.wiley.com/go/griffon/complications

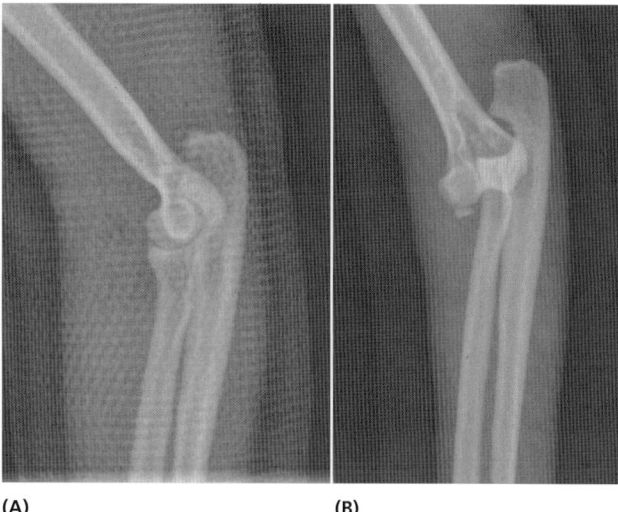

(A)   (B)

Figure 121.2 A, Closed reduction of an elbow luxation and external coaptation with the limb in full extension. **B**, Reluxation caused by an untreated collateral ligament or flexor/extensor muscle avulsion. Notice the bony fragment indicating substantial avulsion fracture. *Source:* D. Griffon, Western University of Health Sciences, Pomona, CA, 2014. Reproduced with permission from D. Griffon.

Risk factors
Traumatic luxations
- Elbow luxations carry a higher risk of recurrence in dogs than cats.
- Instability after reduction (abnormal Campbell's test result) (see Figure 121.1).
- Untreated avulsion of the extensor or flexor muscles (Figure 121.2)
- Duration of the luxation and previous failed attempts at maintaining reduction

Congenital luxations
- Placement of a transarticular pin into the condyle or the humeral metaphysis instead of the humeral body in humeroulnar luxation (Rahal *et al.* 2000)
- Excessive soft tissue tension at the time of initial reduction

Risk factors common to both types of luxations
- Insufficient owner or patient compliance; uncontrolled exercise after reduction
- Inability to apply slings, splints, or bandages to maintain immobilization of the joint

Diagnosis
Reluxation results in the same clinical signs as primary luxation and has to be expected in any case with recurrent lameness or worsening of limb function after previous reduction. On physical examination, the limb is held in a typical posture, with the elbow in slight flexion and the antebrachium in abduction and external rotation (Figure 121.3). The animal does not bear weight on the limb, and pain is elicited on palpation of the swollen joint. Range of motion (ROM) is reduced, and crepitus may be present, depending on the degree of degenerative joint disease (DJD) and cartilage damage. Orthogonal radiographs confirm the tentative diagnosis of reluxation and help characterize the direction and degree of luxation, as well as the presence of secondary osteoarthritis or concomitant fractures (Figure 121.4). Radiographs are also indicated in case of previous stabilization of the joint with implants to verify their actual position and integrity.

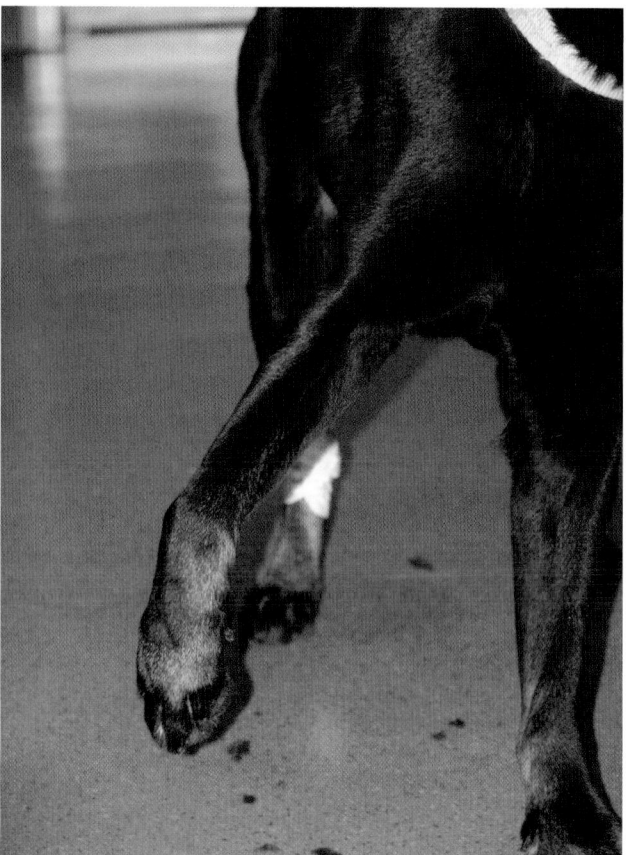

Figure 121.3 Typical posture with lateral elbow luxation, characterized by an elbow held in slight flexion and the antebrachium in abduction and external rotation.

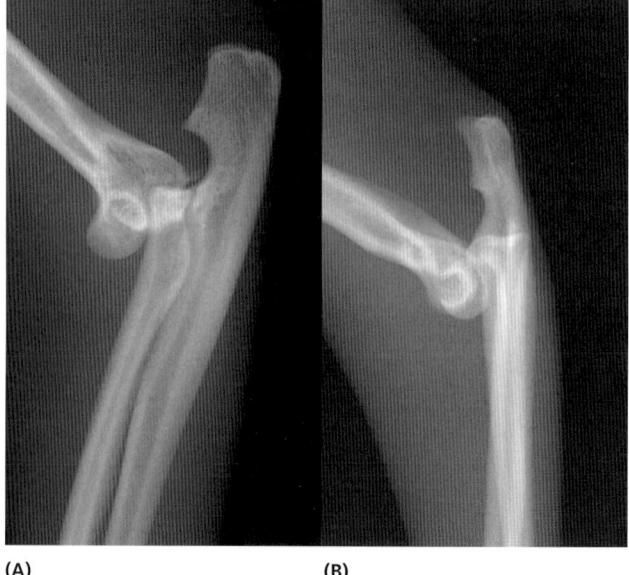

(A)   (B)

Figure 121.4 Orthogonal radiographs (**A** and **B**) are indicated to confirm the tentative diagnosis of luxation or reluxation and characterize the direction and degree of luxation, as well as the presence of secondary osteoarthritis or concomitant fractures.

Treatment

Traumatic luxation

- Open reduction is indicated in every case of malunion.
- Surgical repair of ruptured or avulsed ligaments as well as flexor and extensor muscles must be attempted.
- The lateral collateral ligament is approached via a caudolateral approach to the elbow; a medial approach is required to expose the medial collateral ligament.
- Repair techniques are aimed at restoring the function of the cranial (inserting on the radius) and caudal (inserting on the ulna) crura of each damaged collateral ligament
- Repair techniques vary with the location and severity of lesions (Table 121.1 and Figure 121.5).
- In case of significant soft tissue disruption, prosthetic repair and augmentation of collateral ligaments, as proposed by Farell *et al.* (2007) (Figure 121.6), should be performed.
- If stability cannot be restored, arthrodesis or amputation has to be considered. However, even in cats, limb function after elbow arthrodesis is severely compromised (Moak *et al.* 2000).

Congenital luxation

- Repeated transarticular pinning of humeroulnar luxation with two parallel pins aiming for the humeral body for another 10 days with splinting for 20 days (Rahal *et al.* 2000)

Postoperative care after treatment of any recurrent elbow luxation should include immobilization of the joint and limited exercise for 3 to 4 weeks. Immobilization may be achieved with a splint, a modified external fixator, or a flexible fixator (see Figure 121.5) (Schwartz and Griffon 2008). A modified external fixator relies on pins placed in the olecranon and the distal humerus to maintain the elbow in extension. To achieve flexible fixation, pins are connected with rubber bands rather than rigid connective bars on each side of the limb. Regardless of the technique, care must be taken to preserve enough bone (≥5 mm) around the pins to prevent a fracture of the olecranon (Figure 121.7). Physical therapy is indicated after immobilization to improve ROM and return to function.

Outcome

Reluxation of traumatic cases is generally caused by residual joint instability after closed reduction and can successfully be treated using an open approach and prosthetic ligament repair. However, joint function is often suboptimal in cases with severe soft tissue instability (see Loss of function).

Repeated fixation of congenital elbow luxation may provide good function overall.

Table 121.1 Repair of collateral ligaments in elbows with recurrent luxations

Type of lesion	Repair technique	Indication
Midsubstance tear	Primary suturing with nonabsorbable suture in a locking look pattern	Rare
Avulsion fractures of the origin (proximal) or insertion (distal) of a ligament	Tension band, screw, or spiked washer	Uncommon
Tear with severe disruption of the fibers	Prosthetic replacement with figure-of-eight placement of no absorbable suture around screws and washers or through bone anchors	Common
Bilateral ligament rupture with severe disruption of fibers	Biaxial suture repair through transcondylar tunnels	One report

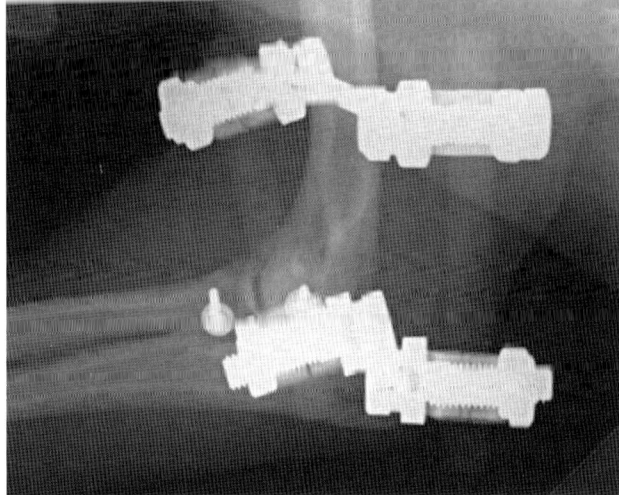

(A)

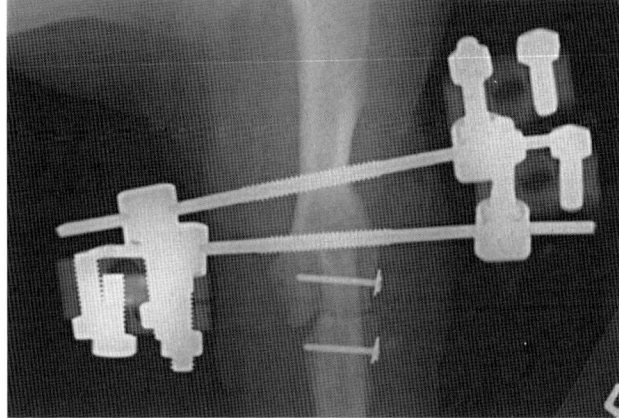

(B)

Figure 121.5 Recurrence of a traumatic luxation treated via prosthetic repair and immobilized with external fixation. Repair techniques vary with the location and severity of lesions. *Source:* D. Griffon, Western University of Health Sciences, Pomona, CA, 2014. Reproduced with permission from D. Griffon.

Prevention

Traumatic luxation

- Surgical treatment of severe joint instability after closed reduction
- Immobilization of the joint in extension for at least 7 days followed by leash walks and controlled exercise for about 4 to 6 weeks

Congenital luxation

- Rigid immobilization of the reduced humeroulnar luxation for a period of 10 to 14 days using one or two transarticular pins from the olecranon to the humeral body

Loss of function

Definition

Loss of function is generally defined as a failure to regain pain-free limb function without any sign of lameness. Poor function often occurs despite successful reduction.

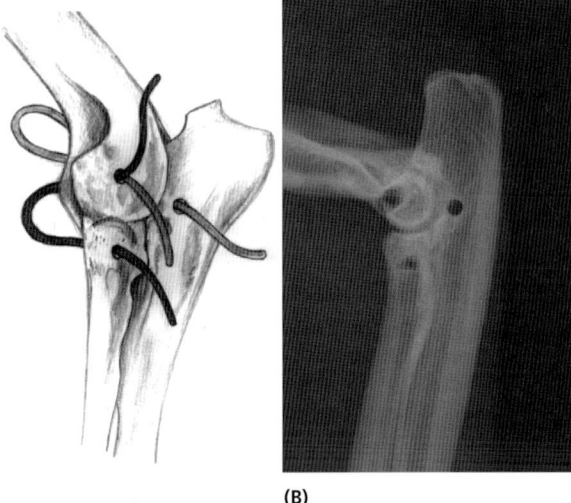

(A)   **(B)**

Figure 121.6 A, Prosthetic reconstruction of lateral and medial collateral ligaments proposed by Farell et al. (2007). *Source:* Farrell *et al.*, 2007. Reproduced with permission from John Wiley & Sons. **B**, Application in a cat. Notice the unintended anisometric configuration caused by eccentric positioning of the transcondylar bone tunnel.

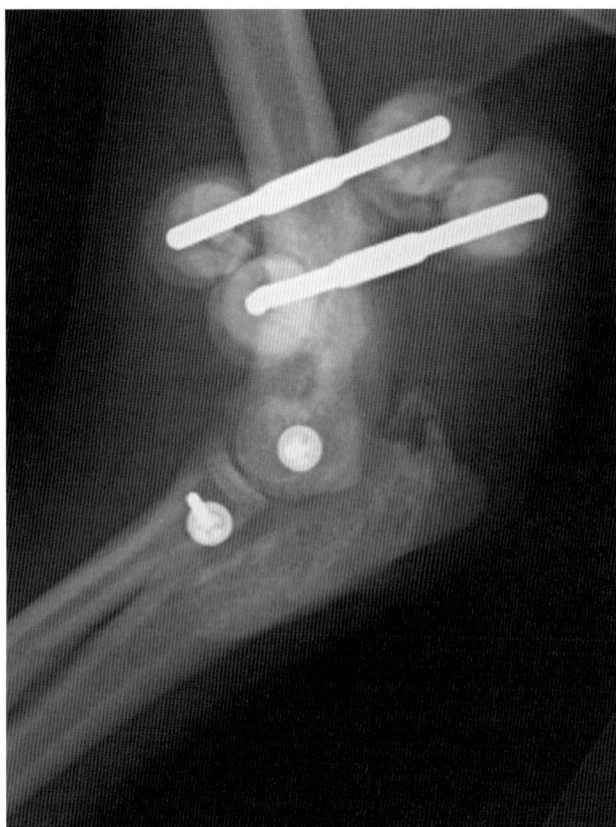

Figure 121.7 Fracture of the olecranon after application of a flexible fixator to maintain the elbow in extension. Care must be taken to preserve enough bone (≥5 mm) around the pins to prevent a fracture of the olecranon. *Source:* D. Griffon, Western University of Health Sciences, Pomona, CA, 2014. Reproduced with permission from D. Griffon.

Risk factors
Traumatic luxation
- Concomitant joint pathologies, such as cartilage damage, fragmentation of the medial coronoid process, or fracture of the anconeal process
- Any lesion requiring an open approach (instability after closed reduction, avulsion fractures, reluxation)
- Chronic luxation
- Extended immobilization of the joint (over 3 weeks; duration), inducing arthrofibrosis

Diagnosis
Clinical signs vary in the degree of lameness, in terms of severity and frequency. Lameness may be chronic or induced by exercise. Signs may be limited to stiffness after rest in mildly affected cases. Lameness may not be apparent in cats. Instead, jumping activity may be reduced and may go unnoticed by the owners. On orthopedic examination of the affected limb, pain is usually elicited on palpation, and ROM may be reduced. Overall, these clinical signs are similar to those associated with DJD (see Chapter 18).

Treatment
- Surgical reconstruction is considered in cases with persistent instability.
- Chronic lameness without obvious cause (instability, fragments) is treated conservatively (see Chapter 18).
- Function limited by arthrofibrosis can be improved with physiotherapy.
- Joint replacement, arthrodesis, or amputation may be considered in severe cases that do not respond to conservative management.

Outcome
The prognosis in dogs with poor postoperative limb function is overall guarded. Total or partial elbow replacement might provide significant improvement.

Prevention
Traumatic luxation
- Early reduction (<24 hours)
- Address instability after closed reduction (ligament repair).
- Removal of fragments
- Limit the duration of rigid immobilization (7–10 days; <3 weeks in all cases) and consider external flexible fixation.
- Postoperative physiotherapy: Maintain weight at the low end of the normal range and consider administration of nutraceuticals.

Relevant literature
The most common postoperative complication associated with elbow luxation is **loss of function**. Every dog with traumatic luxation requiring open reduction because of significant joint instability after closed reduction is at high risk for chronic lameness and DJD (Meyer-Lindenberg *et al.* 1991; O'Brien *et al.* 1992; Savoldelli *et al.* 1996; Mitchell 2011). According to previous reports, 67% to 77.1% of animals treated via closed reduction and good stabilization of the joint (Meyer-Lindenberg *et al.* 1991; O'Brien *et al.* 1992; Schaefer *et al.* 1999; Mitchell 2011) regain good to excellent function, but a similar outcome is obtained in only 0% to 56% of dogs requiring open intervention (Lindenberg *et al.* 1991; O'Brien *et al.* 1992; Schaefer *et al.* 1999; Meyer-Mitchell 2011). Removal of any fragment in combination with primary repair of avulsed collateral ligaments

of flexor or extensor muscles has been reported to improve joint function significantly (Schaefer *et al.* 1999). Because of its crucial impact on return to full function, joint stability should be meticulously assessed after closed reduction using Campbell's method (Campbell 1971) or stress radiographs (Montavon and Savoldelli 1995; Savoldelli *et al.* 1996). The variety of treatment algorithms proposed for traumatic elbow luxation reflects the lack of uniformly accepted method for addressing instability. The prosthetic repair proposed by Farell *et al.* (2007) has been successfully used in a cat with chronic luxation (Heitmann and Meyer-Lindenberg 2009) but has not been reported in dogs. Because chronic luxation bears a guarded prognosis, traumatic luxations should be considered as emergencies warranting immediate reduction (Meyer-Lindenberg *et al.* 1991). Depending on the type of luxation, a favorable prognosis for successful reduction of congenital luxations can be expected. However, the goal of the treatment in these cases differs from that of traumatic luxations in that full joint reconstruction and prevention of DJD are usually not achieved. Data on long-term outcome after reduction of congenital luxations are not available.

Reluxation is a rare complication, at least in traumatic cases. Because recurrence most commonly results from untreated joint instability, the prognosis for return to full function after open reduction, and management of joint stability is guarded.

The risk for postoperative **infection** is generally insignificant, with the exception of cases in which braided, unresorbable suture material is used for prosthetic repair of torn collateral ligaments. The placement of external fixators, as indicated in complicated reconstruction of either congenital elbow luxation or very instable traumatic luxations, may lead to draining tract infection and pin loosening (see Figure 121.7 and Chapter 106).

References

Campbell, J.R. (1971) Luxation and ligamentous injuries of the elbow of the dog. *The Veterinary clinics of North America* 1, 429-440.

Clark, K.J., Jerram, R.M., Walker, A.M. (2010) Surgical management of suspected congenital luxation of the radial head in three dogs. *New Zealand Veterinary Journal* 58, 103-109.

Ertelt, J., Maierl, J., Kaiser, A., et al. (2010) [Anatomical and pathophysiological features and treatment of elbow luxation in rabbits] *Tierarztliche Praxis. Ausgabe K, Klein Heim ?????*, ??? ? ??

Farell, M., ?????, Ph., Zimm.... Th. et al. (????) In vitro validation of a technique for assessment of canine and feline elbow joint collateral ligament integrity and description of a new method for collateral ligament prosthetic replacement. *Veterinary Surgery* 36, 548-556.

Griffon, D. (2012) Surgical diseases of the elbow. In Tobias, K.M., Johnston, S.A. (eds.) *Veterinary Surgery: Small Animal.* Elsevier, St. Louis.

Heitmann, W.H., Meyer-Lindenberg, A. (2009) Klinische Anwendung einer neuen Technik zur chirurgischen Stabilisierung der chronischen Luxatio antebrachii mittels transossärem Seitenbandersatz bei einer Katze. *Kleintierpraxis* 54, 25-32.

Meyer-Lindenberg, A., Fehr, M., N..., L. (1991) Die Luxatio antebrachii traumatica des Hundes—Häufigkeit, Symptome, Therapie und Ergebnisse. *Kleintierpraxis* 36, 307-616.

Milton, J.L., Horne, R.D., Bartels, J.E., et al. (1979) Congenital elbow luxation in the dog. *Journal of the American Veterinary Medical Association* 175, 572-582.

Mitchell, K.E. (2011) Traumatic elbow luxation in 14 dogs and 11 cats. *Australian Veterinary Journal* 89, 213-216.

Moak, P.C., Lewis, D.D., Roe, S.C., et al. (2000) Arthrodesis of the elbow in three cats. *Veterinary and Comparative Orthopaedics and Traumatology* 13, 149-153.

Montavon, P.M., Savoldelli, D. (1995) [Clinical and radiologic evaluation of the integrity of medial and lateral collateral ligaments of the elbow in dogs]. *Schweizer Archiv fur Tierheilkunde* 137, 475-479.

O'Brien, M.G., Boudrieau, R.J., Clark, G.N. (1992) Traumatic luxation of the cubital joint (elbow) in dogs: 44 cases (1978-1988). *Journal of the American Veterinary Medical Association* 201, 1760-1765.

Rahal, S.C., De Biasi, F., Vulcano, L.C., et al. (2000). Reduction of humeroulnar congenital elbow luxation in 8 dogs by using the transarticular pin. *Canadian Veterinary Journal* 41, 849-853.

Savoldelli, D., Montavon, P.M., Suter, P.F. (1996) [Traumatic elbow joint luxation in the dog and cat: perioperative findings]. *Schweizer Archiv fur Tierheilkunde* 138, 387-391.

Schaefer, I.G., Vwolvekamp, P., Mej, B.P., et al. (1999) Traumatic luxation of the elbow in 31 dogs. *Veterinary and Comparative Orthopaedics and Traumatology* 12, 33-39.

Schwartz Z, Griffon, D.J. (2008) Nonrigid external fixation of the elbow, coxofemoral and tarsal joints in dogs. *Compendium on Continuing Education for the Practicing Veterinarian* 30, 648-653.

Withrow, S.J. (1977) Management of a congenital elbow luxation by temporary transarticular pinning. *Veterinary Medicine, Small Animal Clinician* 72, 1597-1602.

122 Ulnar Osteotomy and Ostectomy

Dominique Griffon

College of Veterinary Medicine, Western University of Health Sciences, Pomona, CA, USA

Ulnar osteotomies and ostectomies are indicated in the management of elbow incongruity and premature closure of the distal ulnar growth plate. The location and configuration of the osteotomies vary with the indication. Dynamic proximal ulna osteotomies (DPUOs) are performed in dogs with radioulnar incongruity, generally associated with other components of elbow dysplasia. In these cases, the DPUO is designed to allow biomechanical loading during weight bearing, which, coupled with the action of the triceps, will modify the position of the proximal ulna and naturally restore the alignment of articular surfaces. An osteotomy is indicated in limbs with a relatively short ulna (negative radioulnar incongruence) because proximal migration of the bone is expected after surgery. Positive radioulnar incongruence (short radius) seems more common in dogs with elbow dysplasia, increasing biomechanical loading of the medial coronoid process. A proximal ostectomy is technically required in these cases to allow distal migration of the ulna. The most common complication after DPUO consists of a caudal tipping and varus deformation of the proximal ulna.

A distal ulnar osteotomy is indicated in immature dogs with premature closure of distal ulnar growth plate and secondary radius valgus. The purpose of this technique is to release the constraint created by the ulna on the remaining growth of the radius in immature dogs. A postoperative increase in radial length and correction of the angular deformity correlate with the growth potential in the radial physes. Owners should be warned that any rotational deformity will most likely persist and that additional surgical correction may be warranted at skeletal maturity. Premature healing of the distal ulna is the most common complication associated with ulnar osteotomy in immature dogs.

Infection

See Chapter 1.

Premature healing

Definition

Premature healing is defined as healing of a distal ulnar osteotomy before maturity and closure of the radial growth plates. This complication prevents the intended correction of a radius valgus. As bony union occurs across the ostectomy, remaining radial growth will aggravate the limb angulation.

Risk factors

- Age of the patient: This complication is more likely in patients undergoing surgery at a very young age because of their rapid rate of healing and growth potential in the radius (Figure 122.1).
- Ulnectomy less than 1 cm wide
- Incomplete resection of the periosteum

Diagnosis

The diagnosis is usually made during postoperative radiographic evaluation (see Figure 122.1). Callus formation and bony union across the ulnectomy are noted. Serial radiographs (every 6–8 weeks) are indicated until maturity to allow early diagnosis. Clinical signs, such as failure to improve or progression of the radius valgus, will develop in immature dogs that are not monitored radiographically.

Treatment

The principles of treatment are similar to those applied to manage radius valgus (See Chapter 95).

- If the ulnar ostectomy heals close to maturity and closure of the radial growth plates, treatment may not be warranted as long as the alignment of the limb is acceptable. Corrective osteotomies may be considered if the residual angulation is clinically relevant. As a general guideline, corrections are considered in limb angulations exceeding 10 degrees.
- If the ulnar ostectomy heals early after surgery and significant growth is expected from the radius (based on the age of patient and radiographic appearance of the growth plates), the ostectomy may be revised, making sure that preventive measures (see later) are taken.

Outcome

The outcome after premature healing of an ulnar ostectomy is good, although surgical correction is generally required.

Prevention

- Create two complete osteotomies of the distal ulna, at least 1 to 2 cm apart (minimum 1.5 times the diameter of the ulna) (Figure 122.2).

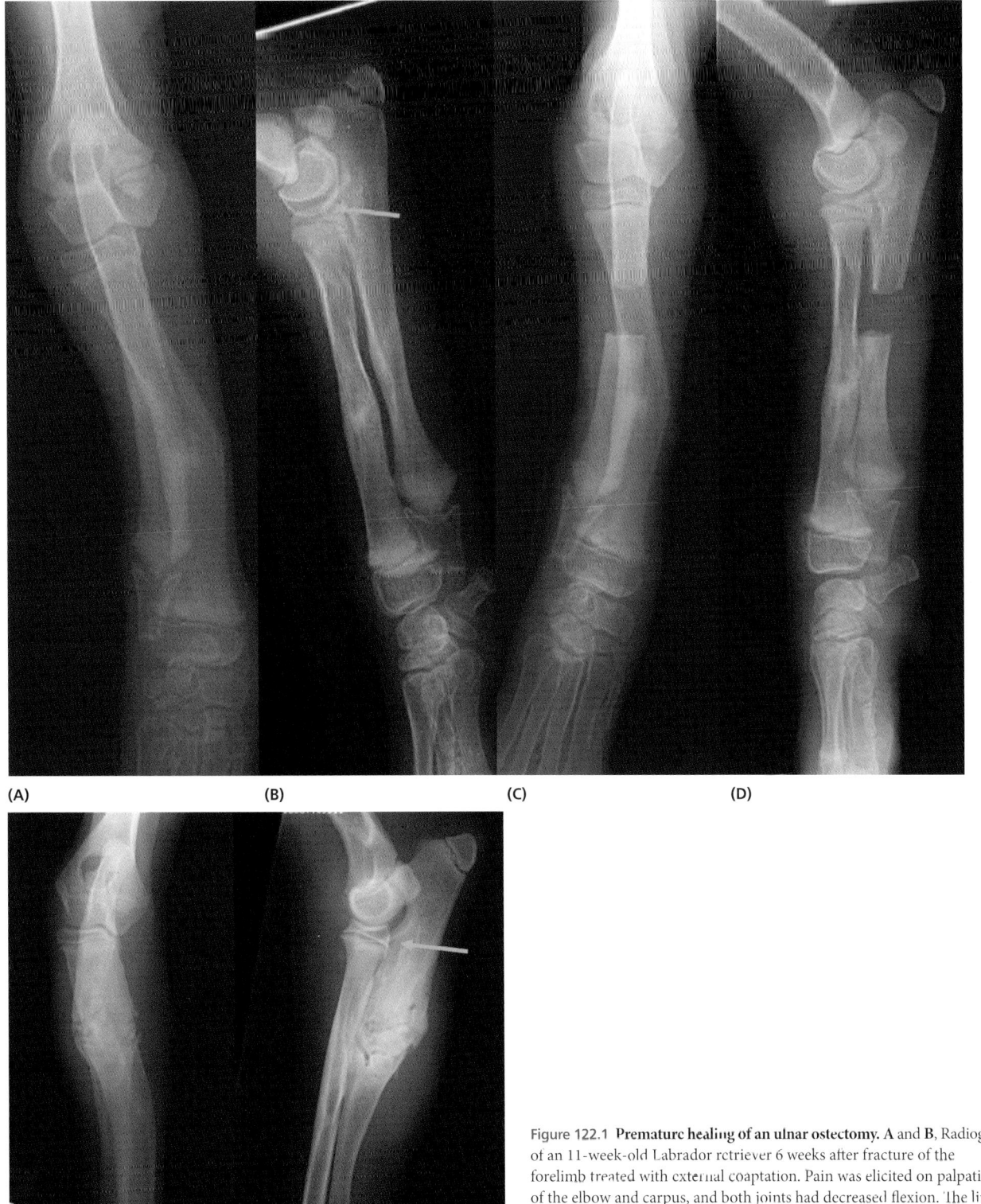

(A)   (B)   (C)   (D)

(E)   (F)

Figure 122.1 **Premature healing of an ulnar ostectomy. A** and **B**, Radiographs of an 11-week-old Labrador retriever 6 weeks after fracture of the forelimb treated with external coaptation. Pain was elicited on palpation of the elbow and carpus, and both joints had decreased flexion. The limb has a valgus deformity, and the affected radius is 0.5 cm shorter than the contralateral radius, resulting in radioulnar incongruency (arrow). **C** and **D**, Radiographs obtained immediately after ulnectomy and removal of the synostosis between the radius and ulna at the fracture site. **E** and **F**, Two months later, the dog was referred with a grade 4 lameness and pain on extension of the elbow. The limb angulation was improved, and both forelimbs were of similar length. Premature healing of the ulnectomy and synostosis between the radius and ulna led to a short ulna and associated radioulnar incongruence. The ulnectomy was surgically revised.

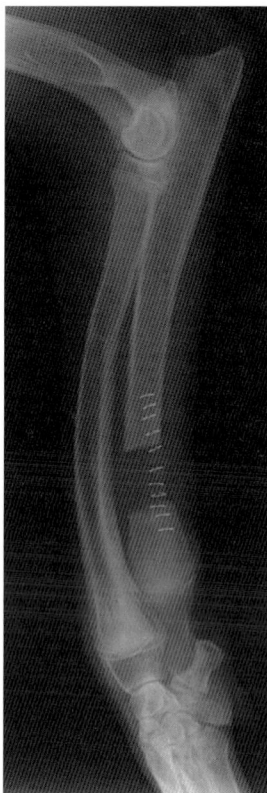

Figure 122.2 Distal ulnectomy. Osteotomies were created to ensure removal of a 2-cm-long segment of distal ulna along with its periosteum. A fat graft was placed in the defect to prevent bone healing.

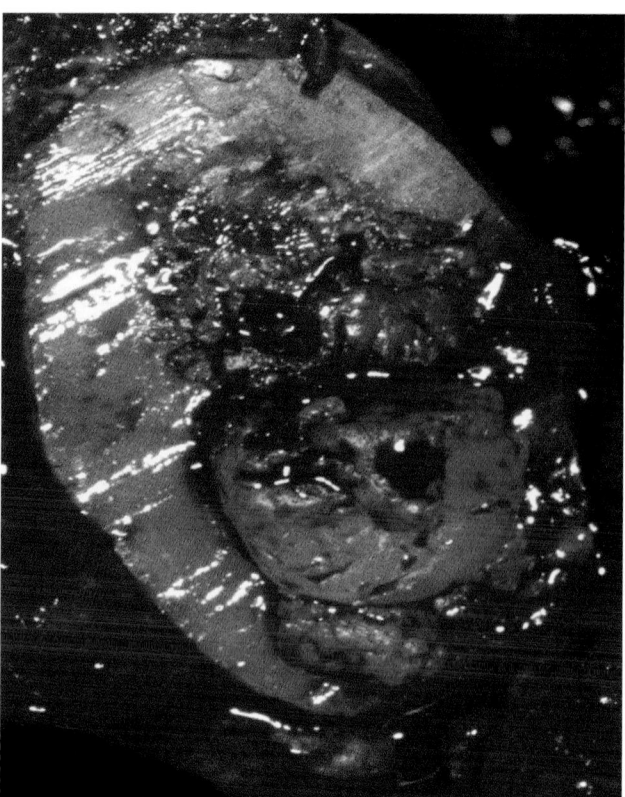

Figure 122.3 Bone wax may be placed over an osteotomy to prevent bone formation and provide hemostasis.

- Ensure complete removal the periosteum between the two bone segments. Alternatively, suturing the periosteum over the end of each bone fragment has been suggested to stop bone growth.
- Place a fat graft between the proximal and distal bone segments: A 2- to 3-cm-long skin incision is made in the ipsilateral flank, exposing subcutaneous fat. A large single piece of adipose tissue is sharply dissected free and placed in the ostectomy gap.
- Occlude the medullary cavity of the osteotomized bone segments with bone wax. This strategy is very efficient but may increase the risk of foreign body reaction (Figure 122.3).

Caudal tipping and varus deformation of the proximal ulna

Definition
This complication consists of a caudal tilting, medial angulation, and rotation of the proximal ulna after dynamic proximal ulnar osteotomy or ostectomy.

Risk factors
This postoperative finding is more common:
- After ulnar ostectomy: Contact between the proximal and distal ulnar segments is more likely to be maintained after osteotomy, thereby limiting the displacement of the proximal ulna.
- Radioulnar incongruity caused by a short ulna: Proximal displacement of the ulna is expected, thereby increasing the space between bone segments (Figure 122.4).

- Technical errors in the configuration of the osteotomy or ulnectomy: The bone is transected perpendicular to its long axis, for example.

Diagnosis
The diagnosis is based on radiographic evaluation; caudal tipping and varus deformation of the proximal ulna are typically apparent on the first follow-up radiographs obtained a few weeks after surgery (see Figure 122.4). A bony protuberance resulting from callus formation can be palpated over the caudal aspect of the surgical site (Figure 122.5). Lameness may be present but does not generally exceed what may be expected at this stage of the recovery.

Treatment
The clinical significance of this finding remains controversial (see Relevant literature). In fact, this migration of the proximal ulna has been suggested as a predominating effect of the DPUO rather than the axial shift. Treatment is generally not indicated. If return to function is less than expected or unsatisfactory, reevaluation of the elbow via computed tomography (CT) or arthroscopy should be considered to evaluate radioulnar incongruence and other lesions associated with elbow dysplasia.

Outcome
Callus formation may lead to the presence of a bony protuberance on the caudal aspect of the ulna. The functional outcome is generally similar to that expected after surgical management of elbow dysplasia.

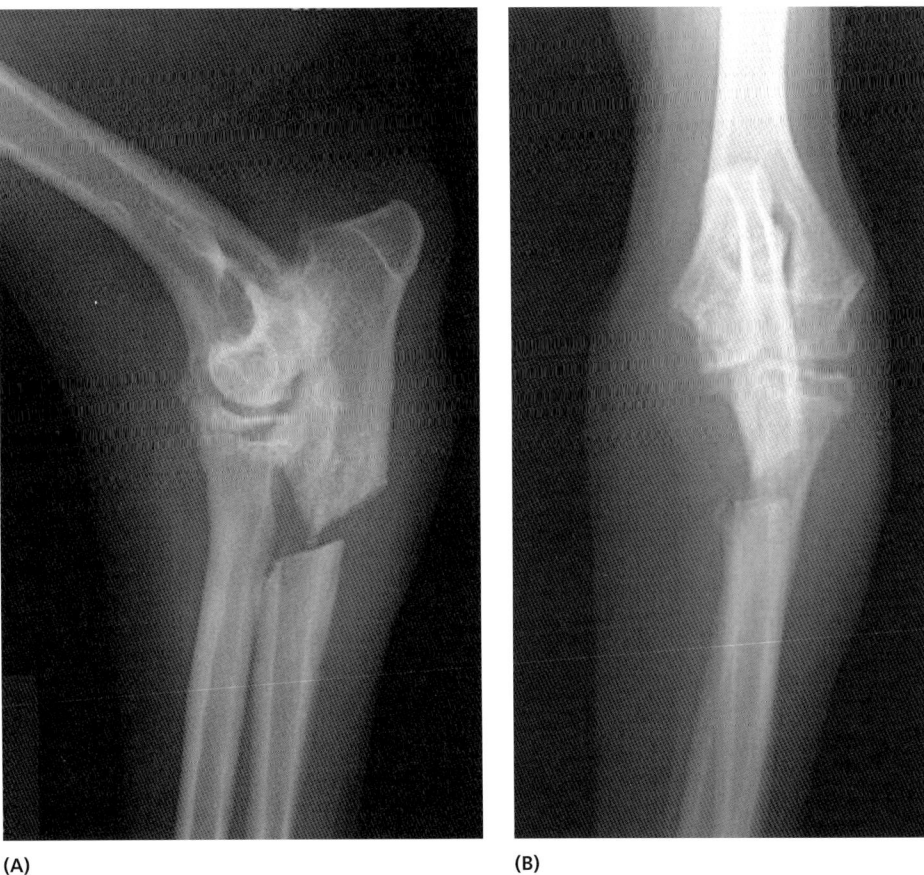

(A)   **(B)**

Figure 122.4 Caudal tipping and varus angulation after dynamic proximal ulna osteotomy. Mediolateral (**A**) and craniocaudal (**B**) projections obtained 3 weeks after surgery. The osteotomy was not angled sufficiently relative to the long axis of the ulna.

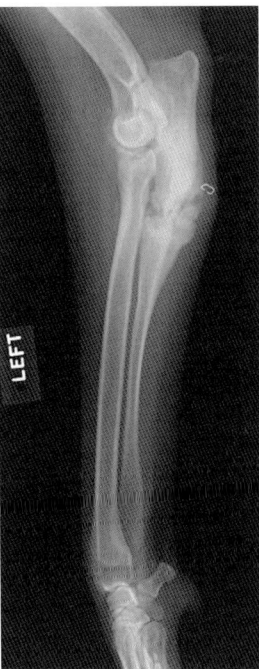

Figure 122.5 Callus formation 3 months after dynamic proximal ulnar osteotomy. A bony protuberance could be palpated in this dog because of the presence of callus and caudal tipping of the proximal ulna.

Prevention

Preventive measures include:

- Placement of an intramedullary pin in the ulna: The pin will guide the axial migration of the proximal ulna. This option is associated with complications such as pin migration, pin breakage, and draining tracts.
- Distal ulnar osteotomy or ostectomy, located 2 to 2.5 cm from the ulnar epiphysis, combined with a release of the interosseous ligament (Might *et al.* 2011)
- Oblique osteotomies are recommended to reduce postoperative mobility of the proximal ulna and limit callus formation. A bi-oblique DPUO (Fitzpatrick and Yeadon 2009; Fitzpatrick *et al.* 2013) is located at the level of proximal and midthird of the radius and directed caudoproximal to craniodistal (approximating 40 degrees to the long axis) and proximolateral to distomedial (approximating 30 degrees to the long axis) (Figure 122.6).

Relevant literature

Most of the literature related to ulnar osteotomies and ostectomies focus on dynamic proximal ulnar ostectomy because this procedure is commonly performed to treat length discrepancy between the radius and ulna, and restore radioulnar congruity. Despite its popularity, the efficacy of DPUO in restoring joint congruity, and its morbidity remained poorly defined (Griffon 2012). Initial descriptions of the procedure recommended an osteotomy performed 2 to 3 cm distal to the plane of the radial joint surface and perpendicular to

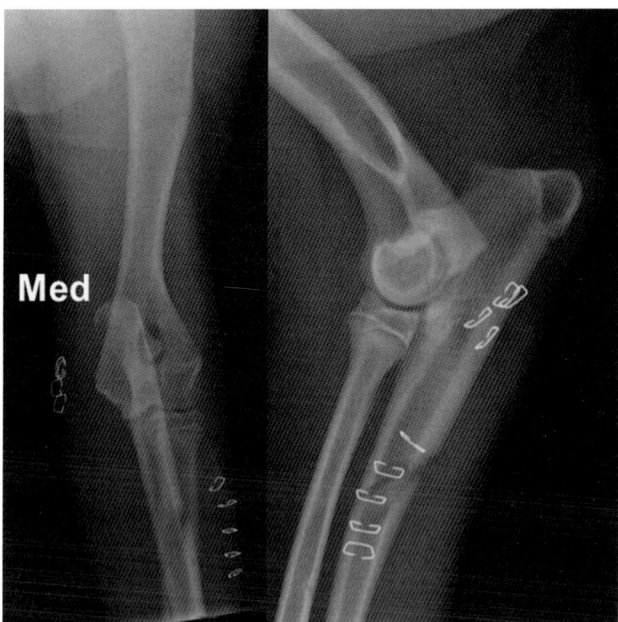

Figure 122.6 Oblique proximal ulnar osteotomies. Osteotomies are angled in the mediolateral and craniocaudal planes to improve bone contact during migration of the proximal ulnar segment.

the long axis of the ulna (Sjöström 1998). Removal of a slice of bone measuring 2 to 4 mm in thickness was also suggested to increase the diastasis and prevent premature healing. The postoperative deviation of the proximal ulna was recognized as consequence inherent to the procedure, with the only morbidity consisting in swelling and pain over the osteotomy site. The caudal tipping of the proximal ulna was reported by Bardet and Bureau (1996) in a series of 83 elbows with medial coronoid disease treated via arthroscopy and DPUO. The authors reported "good to excellent" clinical results in 93% cases despite the progression of radiographic signs of degenerative joint disease. In this study, the osteotomy was slightly angled in the craniocaudal plane, leading to bony union without noticeable side effects. Similar findings were reported Turner *et al.* in 1998, when DPUO was performed in a transverse plane to manage ununited anconeal process in 17 dogs (23 elbows). The authors consistently noticed a clinical sign of caudomedial rotation of the proximal ulna but encountered no complications. Osteotomies healed in approximately 21 weeks, with clinical improvement in 21 of 23 limbs. The same procedure was reported by Ness (1998) in 13 elbows with fragmented coronoid disease; the periosteum was sutured around the transverse osteotomy, performed 2.5 cm distal to the humeroradial joint. All osteotomies healed despite a consistent mild angulation of the proximal ulna, approximating 10 to 15 degrees caudally and 0 to 5 degrees medially.

Strategies have subsequently been developed to prevent excessive caudal and medial deviation of the proximal ulna after DPUO. Placement of small intramedullary pin (5/64 inch) in the osteotomized ulna was combined with lag screw placement to treat four immature dogs (6–8.5 months old) with ununited anconeal process (Krotscheck *et al.* 2000). Lameness and pain resolved in all dogs, and no complications were reported, although mild arthrosis was present in all treated joints. This approach has more recently been questioned because it limits the migration of the proximal ulna to a single plane, potentially affecting the ability of physiological loads

to correct the alignment of joint surfaces in all planes. Other strategies therefore focus on modifying the location and orientation of the osteotomy to avoid internal fixation of the segment. The proximal location of osteotomies was designed to maximize the ability of the proximal ulna to move under physiological loads and avoids interference with the interosseous ligament. This ligament measures about 2 cm in length and 0.5 cm in width and extends distally slightly beyond the middle of the ulna but not quite to the middle of the radius (Miller and Evans 1993). As a consequence, a distal osteotomy did not restore the radioulnar contact patterns in an experimental model of incongruity, presumably because the interosseous ligament prevented migration of the proximal ulna relative to the radius (Preston *et al.* 2001). Distal ulnar osteotomies and ostectomies are more commonly used to treat premature closure of the distal ulnar growth plates in immature dogs with or without elbow dysplasia. These procedures are usually not associated with a significant deviation of the proximal ulnar segment. In a recent cadaver study, similar displacements of the proximal ulnar segment were measured after DPUO and a distal osteotomy (2.0–2.5 cm proximal to the distal ulnar epiphysis) combined with release of the interosseous ligament (Might *et al.* 2011). Although not validated in clinical cases, the authors propose this approach as an equally effective and technically easier alternative to DPUO for the treatment of elbow incongruity in skeletally mature dogs. Another approach consists in a bi-oblique increasing the obliquity (>40 degrees relative the long axis of the ulna) and angling the osteotomy in both craniocaudal and mediolateral planes (Fitzpatrick and Yeadon 2009).

Recent studies have tried to elucidate the impact of DPUO on joint surfaces within the elbow in an attempt to determine the therapeutic value of this approach and its recent modifications. A recent prospective randomized clinical study included 32 elbows (16 elbows per group) with medial coronoid disease treated via fragment excision with or without DPUO (Krotscheck *et al.* 2014). DPUO had no effect on long-term outcome, including radiographic scores of osteoarthrosis and ground reaction forces. Böttcher *et al.* (2013) used three-dimensional CT to generate in silico models of the elbow in 10 dogs (12 elbows) with medial coronoid disease or osteochondritis dissecans (or both) of the elbow, combined with axial radioulnar incongruence exceeding 2 mm. Based on models generated before after subtotal coronoidectomy and oblique DPUO, DPUO reduced axial radioulnar incongruence and improved the focal contact area at the medial coronoid process. The authors concluded that these effects were due to a complex three-dimensional rotation of the proximal ulnar segment rather than axial migration alone. DPUO also appeared to improve humeroulnar subchondral joint space width primarily by caudal tipping of the proximal ulnar segment in the non–weight-bearing elbow. Rotational changes were also described in 26 dysplastic elbows treated via bi-oblique DPUO (Fitzpatrick *et al.* 2013). A CT method previously tested in experimental models of radioulnar incongruence (Holsworth *et al.* 2005; Wagner *et al.* 2007) was used to document a pos-operative increase of the radioulnar joint at the level of the base and midbody of the medial coronoid process and at the level of the lateral coronoid process. These changes are consistent with a cranial rotation of the medial coronoid process around the radial epiphysis. The medial coronoid process also had a tendency to tilt cranially, as the distal aspect of the proximal ulnar segment tipped caudally. Collectively, these two studies raise questions as to the value of limiting the migration of the proximal ulna to the axial plane. However, future studies are warranted to establish the clinical significance of the three-dimensional realignment observed in joints treated with DPUO.

References

Bardet, J.F., Bureau, S. (1996) La fragmentation du processus coronoide chez le chien. Etude rétrospective de 83 coudes traités par ostéotomie ulnaire de raccourcissement. Pratique Medicale et Chirurgicale De l'Animal De Compagnie 31, 451.

Böttcher, P., Brauer, S., Werner, H. (2013) Estimation of joint incongruence in dysplastic canine elbows before and after dynamic proximal ulnar osteotomy. Veterinary Surgery 42, 371-376.

Fitzpatrick, N., Yeadon, R. (2009) Working algorithm for treatment decision making for developmental disease of the medial compartment of the elbow in dogs. Veterinary Surgery 38, 285.

Fitzpatrick, N., Caron, A., Solano, M.A. (2013) Bi-oblique dynamic proximal ulnar osteotomy in dogs: reconstructed computed tomographic assessment of radioulnar congruence over 12 weeks. Veterinary Surgery 42, 727-738.

Griffon, D.J. (2012) Non-traumatic diseases of the elbow. In Tobias, K., Johnston, S. (eds.) Small Animal Surgical Practice. Elsevier, St. Louis, pp. 724-751.

Holsworth, I.G., Wisner, E.R., Scherrer, W.E. (2005) Accuracy of computerized tomographic evaluation of canine radio-ulnar incongruence in vitro. Veterinary Surgery 34, 108.

Krotscheck, U., Hulse, D.A., Bahr, A., et al (2000) Ununited anconeal process: Lag screw fixation with proximal ulnar osteotomy. Veterinary and Comparative Orthopaedics and Traumatology 13, 212.

Krotscheck, U., Böttcher, P.B., Thompson, M.S. et al (2014) Initial subchondral joint space width and radioabsorptiometry in dogs with and without fragmented medial coronoid process. Veterinary Surgery 43 (3), 330-338.

Might, K.R., Hanzlik, K.A., Case, J.B., et al. (2011) In vitro comparison of proximal ulnar osteotomy and distal ulnar ostectomy with release of the interosseous ligament in a canine model. Veterinary Surgery 40, 321-326.

Millan, M.L., Evans, H.E. (1993) Ligaments and joints of the thoracic limb. In Miller's Anatomy of the Dog, 3rd edn. Saunders, Philadelphia, pp. 219-257.

Ness, M. (1998) Treatment of FCP in young dogs by proximal ulnar osteotomy. Journal of Small Animal Practice 39, 15.

Preston, C., Schulz, K., Taylor, K.T., et al. (2001) In vitro experimental study of the effect of radial shortening and ulnar ostectomy on contact patterns in the elbow joint of dogs. American Journal of Veterinary Research 62, 1548.

Sjöström, L. (1998) Ununited anconeal process in the dog. Veterinary Clinics of North America 28, 75.

Turner, B.M., Abercromby, R.H., Innes J., et al. (1998) Dynamic proximal ulnar osteotomy for the treatment of ununited anconeal process in 17 dogs. Veterinary and Comparative Orthopaedics and Traumatology 11, 76-79.

Wagner, K., Griffon, D.J., Thomas, M.W., et al. (2007) Radiographic, computed tomographic, and arthroscopic evaluation of experimental radio-ulnar incongruence in the dog. Veterinary Surgery 36, 691.

123 Complications of Sliding Humeral Osteotomy

Noel Fitzpatrick

Fitzpatrick Referrals Orthopaedics and Neurology, Godalming, Surrey, UK

Implant or humeral failure

Definition

Loss of fixation of the orthopedic construct due to bone and/or implant failure after sliding humeral osteotomy (SHO). Biomechanical overload results either in a humeral fracture (more commonly proximal) or in implant failure. Both complications occur after SHO in disparate but repeated patterns and share similar risk factors.

Risk factors

Factors contributing to mechanical overload of the construct may be related to plate placement, core diameter of screws, or degree of cortical apposition between the proximal and distal segments (Figure 123.1).

Plate malpositioning

- Cranial placement of the plate within the proximal segment: Failure in centering the plate relative to the sagittal axis of the humerus places more stress on the proximal screws because of cranialization of the plate. Axial loading tends to displace the humeral head distally and may cause breakage of the exposed proximal screws (Figure 123.2).
- Caudal plate positioning: The humerus is shaped as an S when viewed from the lateral perspective, with a cranial

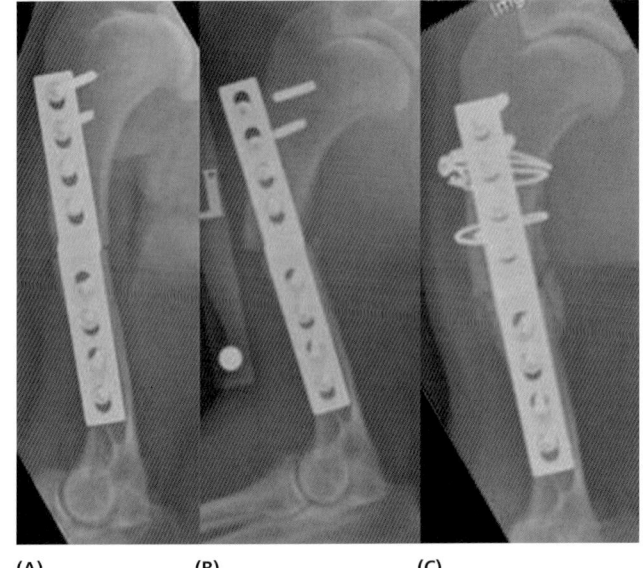

(A) (B) (C)

Figure 123.2 Postoperative radiograph illustrating the malpositioning of a sliding humeral osteotomy plate relative to the proximal humerus (**A**). The cranial placement of the plate contributed to the fracture of proximal screws (**B**) Surgical revision involved the placement of alternative screws (not locking) at divergent angles, as well as cerclage wires (**C**).

bow proximally and a caudal bow distally. Therefore, centering a straight diaphyseal plate on the mid-diaphysis creates a challenge. Failure to center the plate may result in a caudal placement of the distal screws within the proximal segment. Axial loading of the humeral head generates bending forces (compression caudal, tension cranial) that may lead to a sagittal fracture through the proximal screws, combined with a cranial tilting of the distal extent of the proximal segment (Figure 123.3).

- Torsion: Failure to place the plate at a neutral position with regards to the craniocaudal and lateromedial axes creates torsion within the plate–screw construct and between the bone segments during load bearing. Under these circumstances, chronic loading may result in a fracture, most likely involving the proximal segment (Figure 123.4).

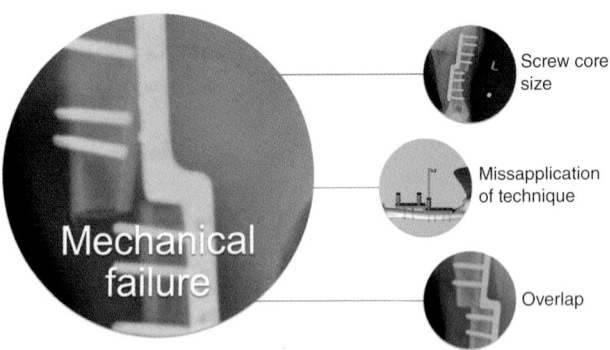

Screw core size

Missapplication of technique

Overlap

Mechanical failure

Figure 123.1 Factors contributing to the mechanical overload of a sliding humeral osteotomy construct.

Complications in Small Animal Surgery, First Edition. Edited by Dominique Griffon and Annick Hamaide.

© 2016 John Wiley & Sons, Inc. Published 2016 by John Wiley & Sons, Inc.

Companion website: www.wiley.com/go/griffon/complications

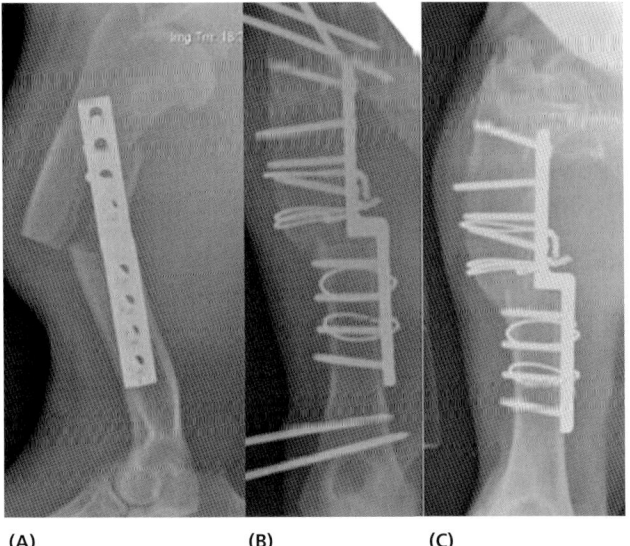

(A)   (B)   (C)

Figure 123.3 Radiographs obtained after sliding humeral osteotomy. The placement of the plate over the caudal aspect of the proximal humeral segment led to a fracture of the humerus proximal to the osteotomy site (**A**). The fracture is repaired with alternative screws (not locking) at divergent angles, cerclage wires and lateral external skeletal fixation (**B**). The revision leads to a favorable outcome with bony union and removal of the external fixator (**C**).

Lack of segmental bone overlap

- A minimum of 30% cortical bone overlap is recommended between the two osteotomy segments to avoid shear overload at the screw–plate junction and failure of the construct (Figure 123.5).

Screw diameter

- 3.5-mm screws were originally employed to secure the SHO plate in position and frequently failed (Figure 123.6).

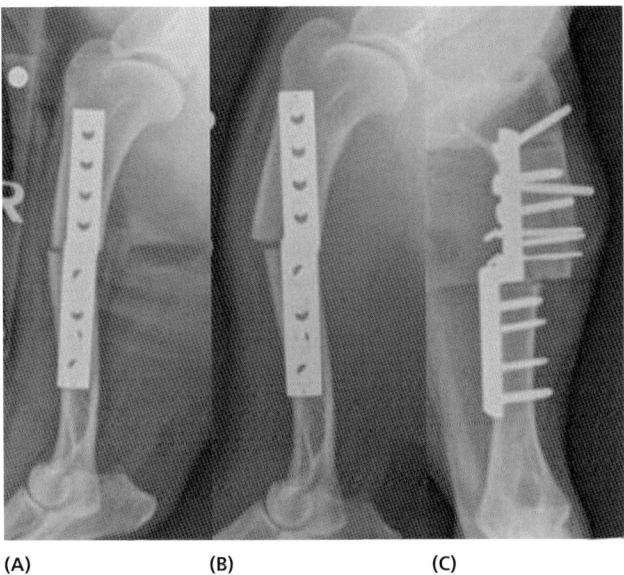

(A)   (B)   (C)

Figure 123.4 Radiographic view obtained immediately after sliding humeral osteotomy and placement of a plate creating torsion forces between bone segments (**A**). Fracture of the distal extent of the proximal humeral segment (**B**). Surgical revision relied on placement of alternative screws (not locking) at divergent angles, along with cerclage wires (**C**).

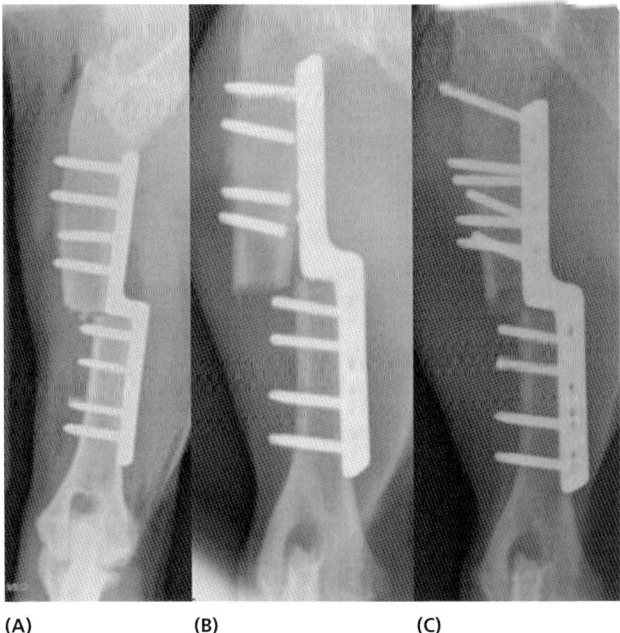

(A)   (B)   (C)

Figure 123.5 Postoperative radiograph of a sliding humeral osteotomy with insufficient apposition between the proximal and distal humeral segments (**A**). Screws placed within the proximal humeral segment consequently failed at the screw–plate interface (**B**). Implant failure was managed via reapposition of bone segments and placement of alternative screws (not locking) at divergent angles (**C**).

Lack of postoperative compliance

- Vigorous activity during the first 6 weeks should be strictly prohibited after the SHO procedure. Lack of compliance can result in catastrophic implant or bone failure, requiring surgical revision (Figure 123.7).

Diagnosis

A traumatic event may be noted during the history of these patients. Clinical signs are consistent with those of a long bone fracture:
- Lameness (weight bearing to non–weight bearing)
- Pain and crepitus on palpation over the implant area

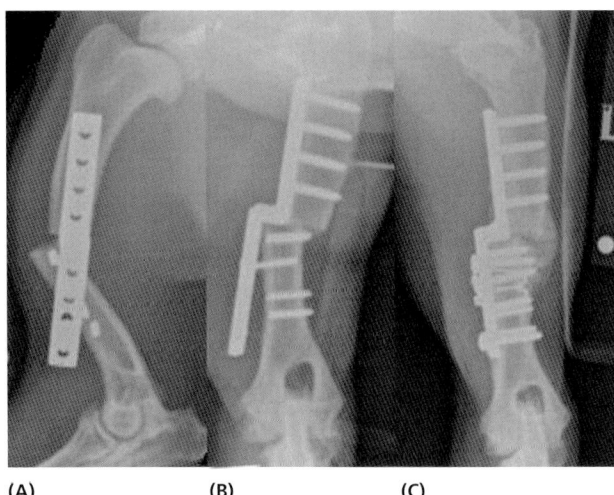

(A)   (B)   (C)

Figure 123.6 Mediolateral (**A**) and craniocaudal (**B**) radiographs of a failed sliding humeral osteotomy. Insufficient core diameter led to failure of screws at the screw–plate interface within the distal humeral segment. Repair involved the placement of alternative, larger screws and cerclage wires (**C**).

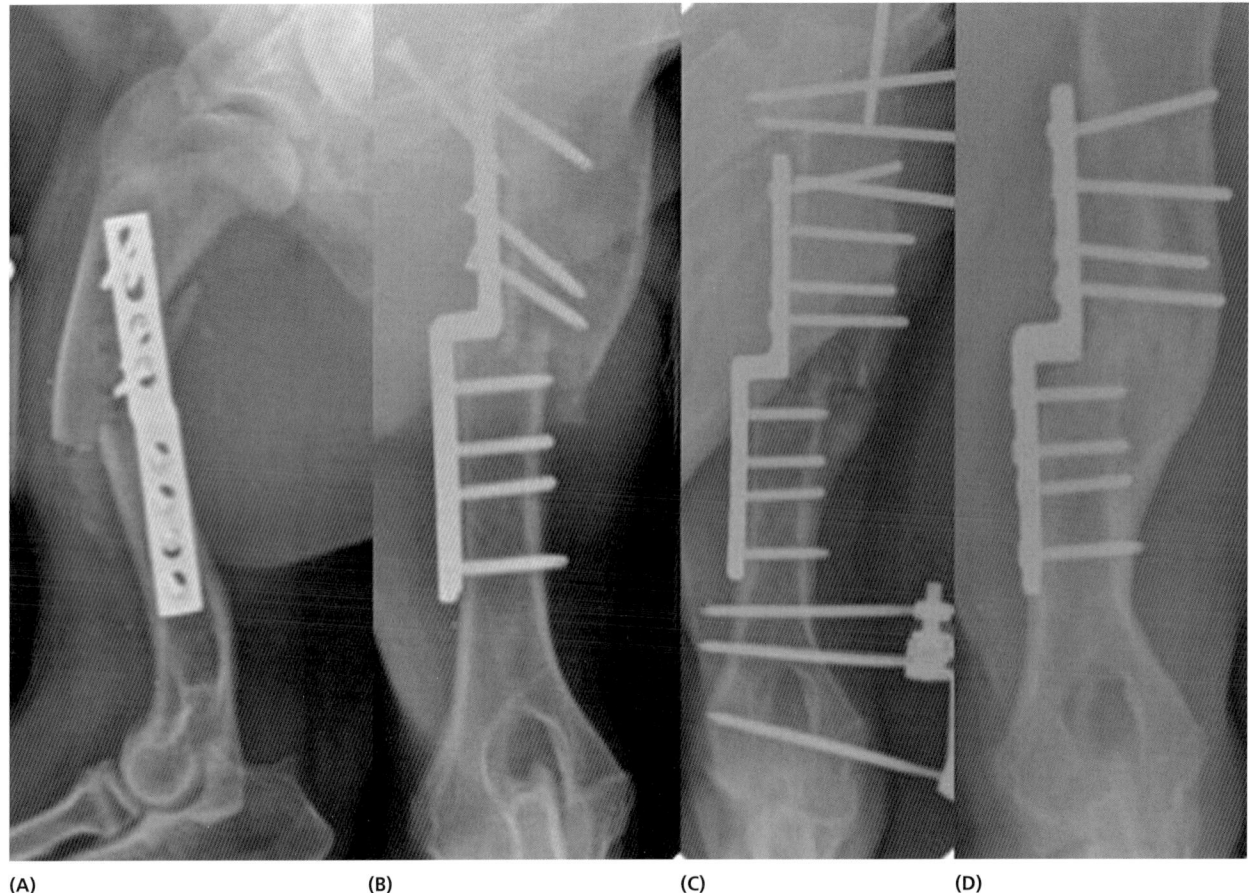

(A)   **(B)**   **(C)**   **(D)**

Figure 123.7 Implant failure secondary to lack of postoperative exercise restriction: Fracture of the caudal and distal aspect of the proximal humerus and screw loosening are visible on the mediolateral (**A**) and anteroposterior (**B**) postoperative radiographs. Revision included the placement of alternative screws (not locking) at divergent angles (**C**) and a lateral external skeletal fixator (**D**).

- Serosanguineous to viscous fluid discharge from the surgical wound
- Unstable osteotomy

Ultimately, the diagnosis is based on orthogonal plane radiographs (see Figures 123.2 to 123.7). Radiographic signs may include:

- Multiple or single screw breakage
- Bone fracture or fissure
- Soft tissue swelling
- Screw loosening

Treatment

Revision surgery and stabilization of the humerus are required to ensure a satisfactory outcome. Particular attention must be paid to preservation of neurovascular structures. The revision should be aimed at restoring rigid fixation, preserving limb alignment while maintaining appropriate translation of the humeral segments. External skeletal fixators types 1a or 1b or *tie-in* in combination with alternative screws and cerclage wire constructs have been successfully used (see Figures 123.2 to 123.7).

Prevention

Progressive improvement of the technique and implant resilience have decreased the major complication rate to 4.8% in the most recent publication (Fitzpatrick *et al.* 2009) and to 0% in the latest set of 60 elbows in 46 dogs cases presented (Fitzpatrick *et al.* 2015).

Refinement of the technique

- The plate should be centered over the craniocaudal surface of the humerus at the level of the fourth hole. Surgeons should be cognizant of the sigmoid shape of the humerus to ensure that the most proximal and distal extents of the plate are in contact with bone and screws engaging adequate bone stock.
- Screws should be parallel to the intercondylar humeral axis and perfectly perpendicular to the plate to achieve locking. It is imperative that all screws are locked completely. Because two screws, screws 6 and 7, are used to translate the distal segment after osteotomy, the screw holes are not perpendicular to the plate, and when replaced with locking screws, these are necessarily cold welded in the threaded hole.
- Preloading of the locking drill guides will optimize the working length of the plate-screw construct:
  - Drill guides in holes 1, 2, 7, and 8 are mounted on the end of the "combi-hole" farthest from the plate step (i.e., osteotomy site).
  - Drill guides in holes 3, 4, 6, and 7 are mounted on the end of the "combi-hole" closest to the osteotomy site (Figure 123.8).
- A monocortical screw placed in hole 4 improves the contact between the plate and underlying bone. The natural cranial sloping of the proximomedial humeral cortex induces a tendency for the drill bit to slide cranially. This shift is especially more likely to occur at the most proximal extent of the construct because the only portion of the plate in contact with the *cis*-cortex consists of its caudal edge. Ensuring that the plate is in close and contiguous

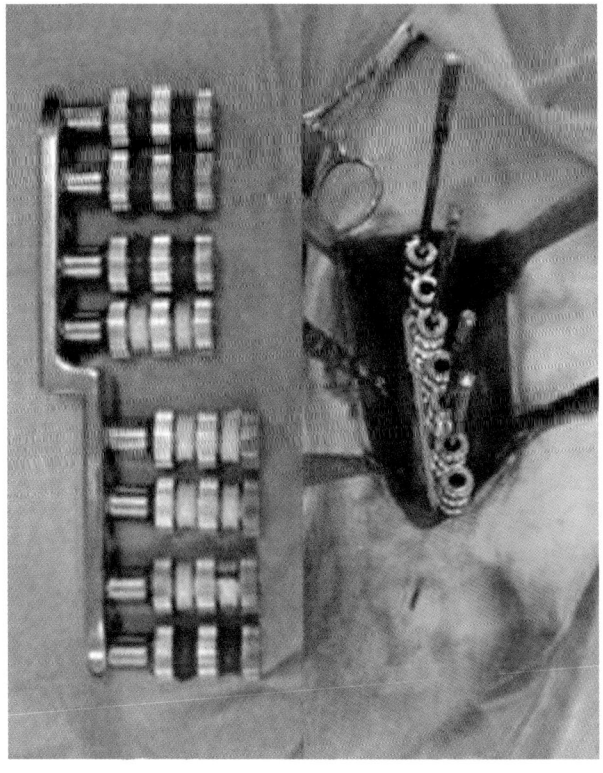

(A)   **(B)**

Figure 123.8 Image of preloaded drill guides on a stepped locking plate (**A**) and appropriate alignment of the implant on the medial cortex of the humerus (**B**).

contact with the bone and that the drill guides are appropriately locked avoids potential errors with regard to screw trajectory when drilling holes 1 and 2

Refinement of the implants

Third generation devices (narrower profile locking drill guides, 4.2-mm New Generation Devices (NGD) locking screws, 8 holes 3.5-mm NGD stepped plate) provide a stronger construct, allowing 7, 7.5 mm, or 10 mm of lateral translation at the level of the osteotomy. The stepped bone plate acts as a buttress with minimal to no load sharing at the osteotomy site. The use of locking screws (4.2 mm) with a larger core diameter maximizes construct stiffness and minimizes the risk of screw breakage. Drill guides have also been redesigned to ensure perpendicular placement of screws relative to the plate, thereby improving the contact between screw threads and plate and appropriate the locking of screw heads.

Early recognition of problems

Sliding humeral osteotomy is associated with a long and steep learning curve. The technique has undergone several refinements, focusing mainly on the importance of plate positioning, screw size, and order of screw placement. Strict adherence to the current recommendations is mandatory to avoid problems.

- Adjunct fixation: In most cases, the 7.5-mm stepped plate achieves adequate residual overlap and translation of forces to the lateral compartment of the elbow to ameliorate clinical signs. However, if the segmental overlap between the proximal and the distal humerus appears under 30% of the bone diameter, adjunct fixation should be considered in the form of a second plate (Figure 123.9).

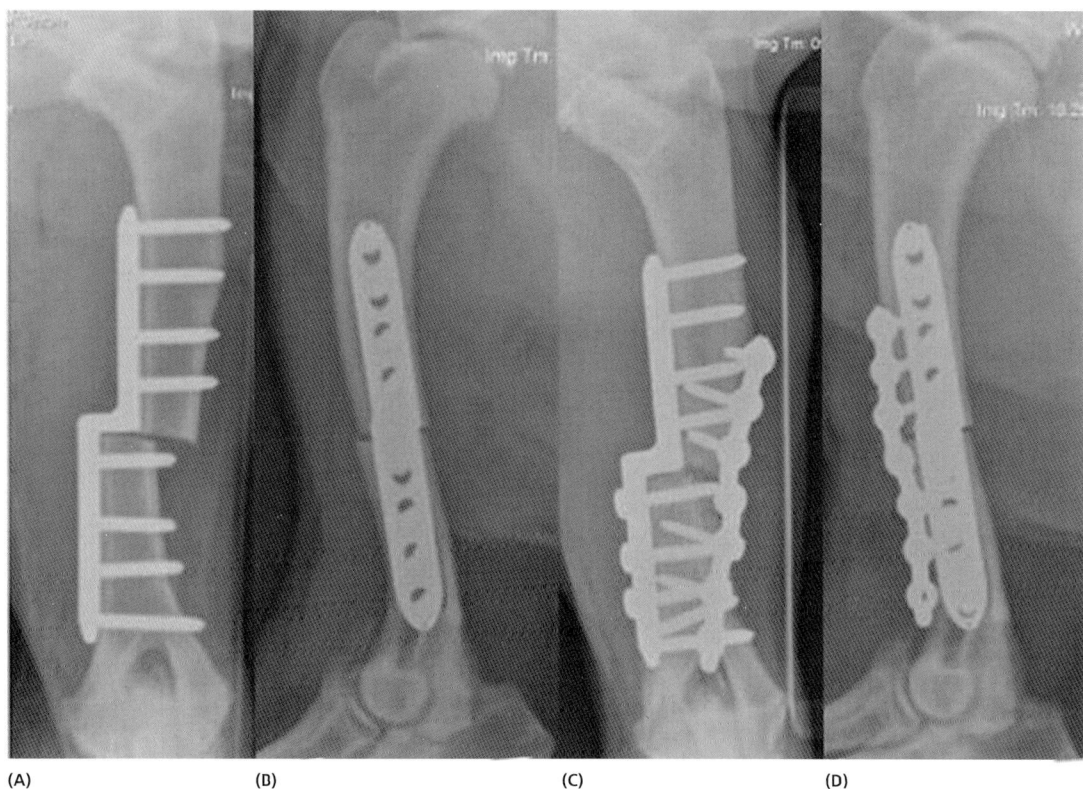

(A)   **(B)**   **(C)**   **(D)**

Figure 123.9 Early recognition of suboptimal segmental overlap (**A** and **B**). This allows application of a second plate (in this case, a 3.5-mm String of-Pearls plate) (**C**) to avoid complications (**D**).

• Exercise restriction is mandatory for all patients that undergo SHO until the 6-week postoperative clinical and radiographic reassessment. During that time, exercise should be limited to short, leashed walks on stable surfaces.

Delayed osteotomy union

Delayed bone healing is discussed as a complication of fracture management in Chapter 98. This section deals specifically with delayed healing of a SHO.

Definition

Bone healing progressing slower than expected, taking into account clinical observations collected over time on dogs undergoing SHO (bony union usually occurs by 6 weeks) along with mechanical and biological variables specific to the patient.

Risk factors

Delayed healing has been reported after SHO, but no specific causes or risk factors have been identified at this point. Based on our understanding of fracture healing, potential risk factors include:
• Contact between the proximal and the distal humeral segments: This factor does not seem to have a clinical influence on the healing of SHOs as long as the overlap is at least equal to 30% of the diameter of the bone.
• Incorrect plate positioning may cause fatigue of the implants and micromotion at the osteotomy, causing either implant failure (usual response) or delayed bone healing.
• Simultaneous bilateral procedures or contralateral surgery performed within 6 weeks of the first procedure increase the risk of overload of the construct, thereby affecting bone healing.

Diagnosis

Delayed union can appear as an incidental finding on radiographic reevaluation 6 to 12 weeks after SHO or may be accompanied by persistent moderate to severe thoracic limb lameness. An unexpected degree of pain and lameness is associated with the diagnosis of delayed union, but these signs are not pathognomonic for delayed bone healing.

Treatment

Delayed healing in the presence of stable implants and absence of clinical signs is typically managed conservatively. Exercise restriction should be enforced and radiographic evaluation rescheduled 6 weeks later. Cases with clinical signs of delayed union or lack of progression of bone-healing response on serial radiographs may benefit from autogenous cancellous or allogenous corticocancellous bone graft application. Cases with clinical signs and radiographic evidence of implant failure warrant immediate surgical revision.

Prevention

Despite the lack of data regarding the minimum overlap required for bone healing at the osteotomy site, a minimum of 30% is recommended. Cases that require bilateral SHOs should be staged by a minimum of 6 weeks, ensuring that acceptable osseous union at the osteotomy site is radiographically visible on one side before operating on the contralateral limb.

Surgical wound complications

These complications are addressed in Chapter 1. This section includes characteristics specific to sliding humeral osteotomies.

Definition

This is complications related to the surgical wound created through exposure of the bone during SHO. This broad definition may include:
• Wound infection: This complication was not seen in the published data, but it occurred in 2% of the latest presented data (Fitzpatrick *et al.* 2009).
• Wound dehiscence occurred in 2%.

Risk factors

Wound infection can occur because of pre- and intraoperative contamination, concurrent patient dermatitis, or skin abrasion.

Dehiscence after SHO may occur because of concomitant individual diseases interfering with wound healing (e.g., endocrinopathies), mechanical abrasion of the wound from self-trauma by the patient, tension across the surgical wound, or seroma formation secondary to poor tissue apposition.

Diagnosis

The most common clinical signs are:
• Bleeding from the wound
• Swelling around the wound or extensively around the surgical area
• Erythema
• Dermalgia or pain associated with the skin and underlying tissues on the medial aspect of the humerus

Treatment

The nature and the extent of the dehiscence determine the aggressiveness of the treatment required. Generally, surgical debridement of the wound is recommended when subcutaneous layers are disrupted and muscular layers are exposed or if infection produces deep discharging opening tracts. Antibiotherapy directed by culture and sensitivity should be implemented.

Prevention

Prevention of infection
• Strict adherence to the principles of aseptic surgery
• Prophylactic antibiotherapy
• Provision of an Elizabethan collar and close postoperative supervision of the patient are required to prevent self-trauma

Prevention of dehiscence
• Proper apposition of tissue planes to prevent seroma formation: Placement of a surgical drain is not necessary after SHO. Suture is preferred because the skin on the medial aspect of the humerus is generally hairless and thin. The author has experienced poor skin edge apposition with staples. A postoperative compressive bandage is not recommended.

Relevant literature

Sliding humeral osteotomy was developed in the Orthopedic Research Laboratory of the University of California Davis by Dr. Karl Schulz (Fujita *et al.* 2003; Schulz and Fitzpatrick 2009) and was refined for clinical application by the author. This procedure is derived from techniques developed in human patients, to manage advanced osteoarthritis (OA) of the knee. In these cases, progressive destruction of the cartilage covering articular surfaces has led to joint collapse over affected areas, accelerating OA damage and pain. A high tibial osteotomy has been developed in humans to decrease contact pressure in the diseased medial compartment of the knee, thereby attempting to retard progression of the cartilage damage and decrease pain. Following similar principles, SHO has been described as a modifying rather than corrective osteotomy. Indeed, the procedure has been designed to redirect axial forces placed on the limb during weight bearing away from the damaged cartilage covering areas of humeroulnar conflict toward the humeroradial joint. Translation of ground reaction forces toward the lateral compartment after SHO has been confirmed in ex vivo studies (Fujita et al. 2003, Mason et al. 2005). This redistribution of loads is believed to relieve the pain generated by bone-on-bone contact and promote the healing process of intraarticular lesions (Fitzpatrick et al. 2012).

Although SHO has become accepted as a valid modality for treatment of advanced medial compartment elbow disease, little clinical evidence has been published up to date. Fitzpatrick et al. published the first set of data reporting the evolution of the technique in 59 limbs of 49 dogs, including clinical outcomes and associated complication rates (Fitzpatrick et al. 2009). This study reported different complication rates, depending on the technique and generation of implants tested. The total complication rate improved in time, from 34.5% and 22.2% to 19%. Similarly, the rate of major complications, defined as those requiring surgical intervention, decreased from 17.2% and 22.2% to 4.8%, as the technique and implants improved.

The most consistent type of implant failure reported in the first retrospective review of 59 limbs (Fitzpatrick et al. 2009) consisted of the breakage of multiple screws. These screws failed in a sequential pattern from hole 4 through holes 3 and 2. The failure occurred at the junction of the screw with the *cis*-cortex of the proximal humeral segment. This phenomenon was likely attributable to a mismatch between the structural strength of the implant and the load applied in a non–load-sharing construct. Failure to center the

plate relative to the humeral caudocranial surface also contributed to this complication.

The author of this chapter has now performed more than 200 SHO procedures and recently, a new set of data has been presented for 60 elbows in 46 dogs (Fitzpatrick et al. 2015) showing a refined surgical technique and a reduction of total complication rate to 4.17%, with 0% major complications noted. Catastrophic postoperative fractures have not been seen after adoption of technique and implant modifications. There were three key elements to the avoidance of complications: (1) strict adherence to very specifically defined technique of plate application, osteotomy, and bone segment translation; (2) use of only 4.0-mm screws; and (3) insistence on locking all screws in holes 1, 2, 3, 4, 5, and 8. The locking screws in translational screw holes 6 and 7 are cold welded but still using 4.0 mm screws.

Finally, it is worth noting that the learning curve for this procedure is steep. The author would like to state for transparency that he has seen failures even with the refined technique when not personally performed by himself. As a result of this the author has further refined the technique and early results are encouraging. The objective is for any surgeon to perform the technique reproducibly well with minimal morbidity, early mobility and 0% major complications.

References

Fitzpatrick, N. (2012) Sliding humeral osteotomy: reduction of major complication rate to zero and clinical outcome equivalence with or without focal coronoid treatment. *Congress BSAVA*, Birmingham, UK.

Fitzpatrick, N., Bertran, J., Solano, M. (2015) Sliding humeral osteotomy: medium term objective outcome measures and reduction of complications with a modified technique. *Veterinary Surgery* 44 (2), 137-149.

Fitzpatrick, N., Yeadon, R., Smith, T., et al. (2009) Techniques of application and initial clinical experience with sliding humeral osteotomy for treatment of medial compartment disease of the canine elbow. *Veterinary Surgery* 38 (2), 261-278.

Fujita Y., Schulz K. S., Mason D. R., et al. (2003) Effect of humeral osteotomy on joint surface contact in canine elbow joints. *American Journal of Veterinary Research* 64 (4), 506-511.

Mason, D.R., Schulz, K.S., Fujita, Y., et al. (2005) In vitro force mapping of normal canine humeroradial and humeroulnar joints. *American Journal of Veterinary Research* 66 (1), 132-135.

Schulz K., Fitzpatrick, N. (2009) Sliding humeral osteotomy for treatment of elbow dysplasia in dogs. *Veterinary Surgery* 38 (2), 261-278.

Index